LIPPINCOTT Nursing Procedures

Seventh Edition

Wolters Kluwer

Philadelphia • Baltimore • New York • London
Buenos Aires • Hong Kong • Sydney • Tokyo

Publisher: Jay Abramovitz
Clinical Director: Joan M. Robinson, RN, MSN
Clinical Project Manager: Collette Bishop Hendler, RN, MS, CIC
Clinical Editor: Beverly Ann Tscheschlog, RN, MS
Product Director: David Moreau
Senior Product Manager: Diane Labus
Editor: Margaret Eckman
Editorial Assistant: Linda K. Ruhf
Art Director: Elaine Kasmer
Design: Joseph John Clark, Joseph DePinho (Cover)
Design Assistant: Karen Kappe Nugent
Senior Production Project Manager: Cynthia Rudy
Manufacturing Coordinator: Kathleen Brown
Production Services: Aptara, Inc.

9 8 7 6 5 4 3 2 1

Printed in China

Library of Congress Cataloging-in-Publication Data

Lippincott nursing procedures. – Seventh edition.
p. ; cm.
Nursing procedures
Preceded by Lippincott's nursing procedures. 6th ed. c2013.
Includes bibliographical references and index.
ISBN 978-1-4698-5303-1 (alk. paper)
I. Lippincott Williams & Wilkins, publisher. II. Title: Nursing procedures.
[DNLM: 1. Nursing Care. 2. Evidence-Based Nursing. WY 100.1]
RT41
610.73–dc23

2015019766

LWW.com

Contents

Contributors and consultants vi
How to use this book viii
ALPHABETICAL LISTING OF NURSING PROCEDURES ■ 1

A

Abdominal paracentesis, assisting 1
Admission 2
Admixture of drugs in a syringe 5
Advance directives 7
Airborne precautions 10
Air-fluidized therapy bed use 13
Alignment and pressure-reducing devices 15
Angioplasty care 17
Antiembolism stocking application 21
Aquapheresis 24
Arterial and venous sheath removal 29
Arterial pressure monitoring 31
Arterial puncture for blood gas analysis 37
Assessment techniques 40
Autologous blood collection, preoperative 43
Autologous blood transfusion, perioperative 45
Automated external defibrillation 47

B

Back care 50
Balloon valvuloplasty care 52
Bariatric bed use 56
Bed bath 57
Bed equipment, supplemental 59
Bedmaking, occupied 61
Bedmaking, unoccupied 64
Bedpan and urinal use 67
Bedside spirometry 69
Biliary drainage catheter care 71
Binder application 73
Bispectral index monitoring 76
Bladder ultrasonography 78
Blood culture sample collection 79
Blood glucose monitoring 81
Blood pressure assessment 84
Body jewelry removal 88
Body mechanics 90
Bone marrow aspiration and biopsy 92
Brain tissue oxygen monitoring and care 95
Brain tissue oxygen monitoring device, insertion, assisting 97
Bronchoscopy, assisting 99
Buccal and sublingual drug administration 103
Burn care 105
Burn dressing application, biological and synthetic 110

C

Canes 112
Capillary blood gas sampling 114
Carbon monoxide oximetry 115
Cardiac monitoring 117
Cardiac output measurement 121
Cardiopulmonary resuscitation, adult 124
Cardiopulmonary resuscitation, child 131
Cardiopulmonary resuscitation, infant 134
Cardioversion, synchronized 136
Care plan preparation 139
Cast application 140
Cast removal 144
Central venous access catheter 145
Central venous pressure monitoring 155
Cerebrospinal fluid drainage management 160
Cervical collar application 162
Chemotherapeutic drug administration 163
Chemotherapeutic drug preparation and handling 169
Chest physiotherapy 171
Chest tube drainage system monitoring and care 175
Chest tube drainage system setup 181
Chest tube insertion, assisting 184
Chest tube removal, assisting 187
Clavicle strap application 189
Closed-wound drain management 190
Code management 192
Cold application 198
Colostomy and ileostomy care 200
Colostomy irrigation 204
Contact lens care 206
Contact precautions 209
Continent ileostomy care 214
Continuous ambulatory peritoneal dialysis 218
Continuous bladder irrigation 221
Continuous passive motion device use 224
Continuous positive airway pressure use 226
Continuous renal replacement therapy 229
Credé maneuver 233
Cricothyrotomy, assisting 235
Crutch use 237

D

Defibrillation 240
Discharge 244
Documentation 246
Doppler use 248
Droplet precautions 249
Drug and alcohol specimen collection 252
Dying patient care 255

E

Eardrop instillation 257
Ear irrigation 259
Elastic bandage application 261
Electrical bone growth stimulation 263
Electrocardiogram, 12-lead 265
Electrocardiogram, right chest lead 267
Electrocardiogram, posterior chest lead 269
Electrocardiogram, signal-averaged 271
Endoscopic therapy, assisting 273
Endotracheal drug administration 276
Endotracheal intubation 278
Endotracheal tube care 283

End-tidal carbon dioxide monitoring 285
Enema administration 289
Epicardial pacing and care 291
Epidural analgesic administration 295
Esophagogastric tamponade tube care 298
Esophagogastric tamponade tube insertion and removal 301
External fixation management 303
Eye care 306
Eye compress application 307
Eye irrigation 308
Eye medication administration 311

F

Fall prevention and management 313
Fecal impaction removal, digital 317
Fecal occult blood tests 318
Feeding 320
Feeding tube insertion and removal 323
Femoral compression 325
Foot care 328
Foreign-body airway obstruction and management 329
Functional assessment 332

G

Gait belt use 333
Gastric lavage 336
Gastrostomy feeding button reinsertion 338

H

Hair care 339
Halo-vest traction management 340
Hand hygiene 343
Hearing aid care 346
Heat application 348
Height and weight measurement 350
Hemodialysis 353
Hemoglobin testing, bedside 359
Hip arthroplasty care 360
Hour-of-sleep care 362
Humidifier therapy 363
Hyperthermia-hypothermia blanket use 366

I

IM injection 368
Impaired swallowing and aspiration precautions 373
Implanted port use 376
Incentive spirometry 383
Incontinence device application, male 385
Incontinence management, fecal 387
Incontinence management, urinary 388
Indwelling urinary catheter care and removal 391
Indwelling urinary catheter insertion 394
Indwelling urinary catheter irrigation 398
Intermittent infusion device drug administration 400
Intermittent infusion device flushing and locking 402
Intermittent infusion device insertion 404
Intermittent positive-pressure breathing 407
Intermittent urinary catheterization 409
Internal fixation management 412
Intra-abdominal pressure monitoring 415
Intra-aortic balloon counterpulsation 417
Intracranial pressure monitoring 424
Intradermal injection 430
Intraosseous infusion 432
Intrapleural drug administration 435
Iontophoresis 440
Isolation garb use 441
IV bolus injection 444
IV catheter insertion and removal 446
IV catheter maintenance 456
IV infusion rates and manual control 461
IV pump use 462
IV secondary line drug infusion 466
IV therapy preparation 468

J

Jugular venous oxygen saturation monitoring 471

K

Knee arthroplasty postprocedure care 473

L

Laryngeal mask airway insertion 475
Laser therapy, assisting 479
Latex allergy protocol 481
Lipid emulsion administration 483
Low-air-loss therapy bed use 485
Lumbar puncture, assisting 487

M

Manual ventilation 489
Massive infusion device use 491
Mechanical traction management 494
Mechanical ventilation, positive pressure 497
Metered-dose inhaler use 501
Mixed venous oxygen saturation monitoring 503
Moderate sedation 505
Mucus clearance device 509

N

Nasal bridle insertion and removal 511
Nasal irrigation 514
Nasal medication administration 516
Nasal packing, assisting 518
Nasoenteric-decompression tube care 522
Nasoenteric-decompression tube insertion and removal 524
Nasogastric tube care 526
Nasogastric tube drug instillation 528
Nasogastric tube insertion and removal 531
Nasopharyngeal airway insertion and care 536
Nebulizer therapy 537
Negative-pressure wound therapy 541
Nephrostomy and cystostomy tube dressing changes 545
Neurologic assessment 547
Nutritional screening 552

O

Ommaya reservoir drug infusion 556
Oral care 560
Oral drug administration 564
Organ donor, identification 567
Oronasopharyngeal suction 569
Oropharyngeal airway insertion and care 571
Oxygen administration 573

P

Pain management 578
Parenteral nutrition administration 581

Parenteral nutrition monitoring 587
Passive range-of-motion exercises 589
Patient-controlled analgesia 592
Pericardiocentesis, assisting 595
Perineal care 598
Peripherally inserted central catheter use 600
Peripheral nerve stimulation 608
Peritoneal dialysis 610
Peritoneal lavage, assisting 614
Permanent pacemaker care 617
Personal protective equipment 621
Postmortem care 622
Postoperative care 624
Preoperative care 628
Preoperative skin preparation 631
Pressure dressing application 632
Pressure ulcer care 633
Progressive ambulation 639
Prone positioning 641
Protective environment guidelines 643
Pulmonary artery pressure and pulmonary artery wedge pressure monitoring 645
Pulse amplitude monitoring 648
Pulse assessment 649
Pulse oximetry 651

R

Radiation implant therapy 654
Radiation therapy, external 657
Radioactive iodine therapy 658
Rectal suppositories and ointments 660
Rectal tube insertion and removal 662
Residual limb care 664
Respiration assessment 667
Restraint application 669
Ring removal 673
Rotation beds 675

S

Safe medication administration practices, general 678
Seizure management 682
Self-catheterization 685
Sequential compression therapy 687
Sexual assault examination 690
Sharp debridement 692
Shaving 694
Sitz bath 695
Skin biopsy 697
Skin graft care 699
Skin staple and clip removal 701
Soaks 703
Spiritual care 705
Splint application 707
Sponge bath 709
Sputum collection 711
Standard precautions 713
Sterile technique, basic 715
Stool specimen collection 718
St-segment monitoring 719
Subcutaneous injection 721
Subdermal drug implants 725
Surgical drain removal 726
Surgical wound management 728
Suture removal 731
Swab specimen collection 734
Synchronized cardioversion 737

T

Temperature assessment 740
Therapeutic bath 742
Thoracentesis, assisting 744
Thoracic electrical bioimpedance monitoring 746
Tilt table 747
Topical skin drug application 748
Tracheal cuff–pressure measurement 750
Tracheal suctioning, intubated patient 752
Tracheostomy and ventilator speaking valve 756
Tracheostomy care 759
Tracheotomy, assisting 764
Transabdominal tube feeding and care 767
Transcranial Doppler monitoring 771
Transcutaneous electrical nerve stimulation 774
Transcutaneous pacing 776
Transdermal drug application 778
Transducer system setup 780
Transfer within a facility 782
Transfusion of blood and blood products 783
Transfusion reaction management 790
Transvenous pacing 793
Traumatic wound management 796
Tub baths and showers 799
Tube feedings 801

U

Ultraviolet light therapy 806
Unna boot application 808
Urinary diversion stoma care 810
Urine collection, 12- or 24-hour timed 813
Urine glucose and ketone tests 814
Urine pH 815
Urine specimen collection 817
Urine straining, for calculi 819

V

Vaginal medication administration 820
Venipuncture 821
Ventricular assist device care 825
Ventricular drain insertion, assisting 828
Volume-control set preparation 830

W

Walkers 832
Water intoxication assessment 834
Weaning a patient from a ventilator 836
Wound dehiscence and evisceration management 838
Wound irrigation 840

Z

Z-track injection 842

Index 845

Contributors and consultants

Tuesday Adams, RN-BC, MSN, WCC
Academics/Training Department Head
Navy Medicine Operation Training Center
Naval Expeditionary Medical Training Institute
Camp Pendleton, California

Erin Alden, RN-BC, MN, ACNS-BC, CMSRN
Acute Care Clinical Nurse Specialist
Harborview Medical Center
Seattle, Washington

Catherine Amero, RN, MSN/ED, CRNI
Infusion Specialist & Educator
Milford Regional Medical Center
Milford, Massachusetts

Katherine Balkema, RN-BC, BSN, BA, MM, CMSRN
Clinical Nurse Educator
Holland Hospital
Holland, Michigan

Donna Barto, RN, DNP, CCRN
Advanced Nurse Clinician
Virtua Health
Marlton, New Jersey

Lisa Ann Behrend, RN, MSN, AC-CNS, CCRN-CSC
Critical Care Nurse, Clinical Instructor
Fountain Valley Regional Medical Center
Fountain Valley, California

Debbie Berry, RN, MSN, CCN, CPHQ, CWCN, CPPS, LHRM
AVP of Quality and Clinical Operations
Hospital Corporation of America
West Florida Division
Tampa, Florida

Lorraine Bigony, RN, MSN, CNOR, ONC
Director of Perioperative Services
Nazareth Hospital
Philadelphia, Pennsylvania

Dorothy Borton, RN, BSN, CIC
Manager, Infection Prevention & Control
Albert Einstein Healthcare Network
Philadelphia, Pennsylvania

Cheyenne Brown, RN, BS, CEN
Charge Nurse
Intermountain Health Care
Salt Lake City, Utah

Sandra Burns, RN, MSN/ED, PHD[c]
Assistant Professor
Roseman University of Health Sciences
Henderson, Nevada

Janet Burton, RN, MSN, CMSRN
Administrative Coordinator
Aldersgate Distance Education Program
Cincinnati, Ohio

Marisa Bustillo, RN, BSES, MS, CCRN, C-NPT, CPEN, CPN
Staff Nurse, Pediatric & Neonatal Intensive Care Transport
Texas Children's Hospital
Houston, Texas

Shari A. Regina Cammon, RN-BC, MSN, PCCN
Clinical Education Specialist
St. Mary Medical Center
Langhorne, Pennsylvania

Melinda Anne Constantine, RN, MSN, CMSRN, ONC
Assistant Director Nursing Education & Operations
North-Shore Long Island Jewish Medical Center
New Hyde Park, New York

Jiajoyce Conway, DNP, AOCNP, CRNP, FNP-BC
Oncology Nurse Practitioner
Cancer Care Associates of York
York, Pennsylvania

Christopher Cox, RRT, BS
Clinical Education Specialist II
Mercy Hospital
Joplin, Missouri

Lisa DeSmidt, RN, MSN, APRN, CCNS, CCRN
Assistant Professor of Nursing
Roane State Community College
Harriman, Tennessee

Angela Dillahunty, RN, CA-CP SANE, CFN, CMI-V, SANE-A, SANE-P
Forensic Nurse Examiner, Program Coordinator
Christus St. Elizabeth Hospital
Beaumont, Texas

Yvonne Dobbenga-Rhodes, RNC-OB, MS, CNS, CNS-BC, CPN
Maternal-Child Health Clinical Nurse Specialist
Washington Hospital Healthcare System
Fremont, California

Laurie Donaghy, RN, BSN, CEN
Staff Nurse
Temple University Hospital
Philadelphia, Pennsylvania

Barbara Engram, RN, MSN, CPHM
Venous Access Nurse
Florida Hospital Celebration
Celebration, Florida

Ellie Z. Franges, RN, MSN, ANP-BC, CNRN, CRNP
Nurse Practitioner—Neurosurgery
Lehigh Valley Health Network
Bethlehem, Pennsylvania

Anthodith Garganera, RN, MSN/MHA, CMSRN
Patient Care Facilitator
Texas Health Presbyterian Hospital of Plano
Plano, Texas

Christine Hankerson, RN, MSN, MS/P, PHD
Director of Learning
Opis Management Resources, LLC
Tampa, Florida

Sharon Hansen, RN, MN, CCRN
Critical Care Educator, Lecturer
MultiCare Health System
Tacoma, Washington

Janice Hausauer, MS, FNP-BC, APRN
Assistant Clinical Professor
Montana State University
Bozeman, Montana

Kathleen Hill, RN, MSN, CCNS-CSC
Clinical Nurse Specialist
The Cleveland Clinic
Cleveland, Ohio

Christine Hoener, RN, BSN
Nursing Supervisor
Cape Fear Valley Healthcare
Fayetteville, North Carolina

Tammie Holcomb, RN, DNP/ACNP
Nurse Practitioner
Henry County Medical Center
Paris, Tennessee

Venecia Holmes, CMSRN, BSN, MHA, NE-BC
Nurse Manager
Bon Secours-Mary Immaculate Hospital
Newport News, Virginia

Abby Horton, RN, MSN
Adjunct Instructor
Shelton State Community College
Tuscaloosa, Alabama

Ron Hoyler, RN, MSN, MBA-HCM, CDE, CDTC
Diabetes Nurse Educator
Children's Mercy Hospital
Kansas City, Missouri

Lois Jackson, RN, MSN, CEN
Intensive Care Director
University Physicians Hospital
Tucson, Arizona

Fiona Johnson, RN, MSN, CCRN
Clinical Education Consultant
Memorial Health University Medical Center
Savannah, Georgia

Hope Johnson, RN, MSN, CNOR, NEA-BC
Director of Perioperative Services
Lehigh Valley Health Network
Allentown, Pennsylvania

Gary Rae Jones, MSN
Clinical Consultant
Pittsburg, Kansas

Tamara Kear, RN, MSN, PHD, CNN
Assistant Professor of Nursing/Nephrology Nurse
Villanova University
Villanova, Pennsylvania

Christine Kennedy, RN, MSN
Hospital Education Instructor
VA Connecticut Healthcare System
West Haven, Connecticut

Jennifer Lee, RN, MSN, FNP-C
Nurse Practitioner
Carolina Cardiology Consultants
Greenville Hospital System
Greenville, South Carolina

Phyllis Magaletto, RN, BC, MSN
Instructor (Medical-Surgical Nursing)
St. John's Riverside Hospital
Cochran School of Nursing
Yonkers, New York

Donna Martin, RN-BC, MSN, CDE, CMSRN
Assistant Professor, Nursing
Lewis University
Romeoville, Illinois

Patricia McBride, RN, MSN, CIC
Infection Preventionist
Bryn Mawr Hospital
Bryn Mawr, Pennsylvania

Rebecca McNeil, RN, BSN, CCRN
ICU Clinical Educator
Mount Carmel Health System
Columbus, Ohio

Pamela Moody, RN, DNP, PHD, FNP-BC
Nurse Administrator Public Health
Alabama Dept. of Public Health
Tuscaloosa, Alabama

Beth Norman, RN, MS, ACNS-BC, CNS
Medical Surgical Clinical Nurse Specialist
Legacy Health
Portland, Oregon

Timothy Orcutt, RN, MSN, CEN
Education and Training Specialist
North Valley Hospital
Whitefish, Montana

Karen Page, RN-BC, MSN, CMSRN
Clinical Educator
Lakeland Regional Medical Center
Lakeland, Florida

Pamela Pascarelli, RN-BC, MSN, APN, CCRN
Education Specialist, Critical Care
Hackensack University Medical Center
Hackensack, New Jersey

Cynthia Perry, RN, MS, AOCNP FNP, FNP-BC
Guthrie Cancer Center
Sayre, Pennsylvania

Rexann Pickering, RN, MS, MSN, PHD, CIM, CIP
Administrator, Human Protection, Director Continuing Education
Methodist Healthcare IRB
Memphis, Tennessee

Anabel Quintanar, RN-BC, MSN, CEN, PHN
Nurse Care Manager—PACT Team
Veterans Administration Greater Los Angeles Healthcare System
Santa Maria, California

Roseanne Hanlon Rafter, RN, MSN, GCNS, BC
Safety/Quality Specialist
Abington Memorial Hospital
Abington, Pennsylvania

Tara Rexroat, RN, MSN, CMSRN
Interim Director of Nursing
Concorde Career College
Kansas City, Missouri

Cynthia Rothenberger, RN, MSN, ACNS, BC
Assistant Professor, Nursing
Alvernia University
Reading, Pennsylvania

Amy Ruhf, MS, ATC, LAT, CES, CKTP
Athletic Trainer
Holy Redeemer Health System
Meadowbrook, Pennsylvania

Noraliza Salazar, RN-BC, MSN, CCNS
Assistant Clinical Professor
University of California
San Francisco, California

Cheryl Schmitz, RN, BC, MS, CEN, CNS-BC, CPEN
Clinical Specialist for Emergency Services
Inova Loudoun Hospital
Leesburg, Virginia

Angelia Sims, RN, CRNI, OCN
Nurse Manager Infusion Services & Hemodialysis
Portland Providence Medical Center
Portland, Oregon

Jennifer Smoltz, RN, MSN, ACNP-BC, CWOCN
Nurse Practitioner
Cleveland Clinic Health System
Fairview Regional Hospital
Cleveland, Ohio

Peggy Thweatt, RN, MSN
Nursing Faculty
Medical Careers Institute
Newport News, Virginia

Kathleen Ueland, RN, BSN, CCRN, CHFN
Cardiac Case Manager
Good Samaritan Hospital
Puyallup, Washington

Gail Viergutz, RN, MS, ANP-C
Nurse Practitioner—ED and Urgent Care
St. Michael's Hospital/Ministry Corporation
Stevens Point, Wisconsin

Deborah Walker, DNP, AOCN, CRNP
Assistant Professor/Nurse Practitioner
University of Alabama at Birmingham School of Nursing
Birmingham, Alabama

Marsha Walmsley, RN, MSN
Professor of Nursing
Sinclair Community College
Dayton, Ohio

Shelley Welch, RN, MSN, CCRN-CSC
Staff Development Educator, Cardiology
Trinity Mother Frances Hospitals and Clinics
Tyler, Texas

Julie Will, RN, MSN
Dean, School of Health Sciences
Ivy Tech Community College of Indiana
Terre Haute, Indiana

Joan Wilson, RN, BSN, CCRN alumnus
Critical Care Nurse Education, Clinical Education Specialist
Mercy Hospital
Joplin, Missouri

Wendy Woodall, MSN, CMSRN, CNE
Chief, Hospital Education Division
Martin Army Medical Center
Ft. Benning, Georgia

How to use this book

As a nurse, you're expected to know how to perform or assist with literally hundreds of procedures. From the most basic patient care, to complex treatments, to assisting with the most intricate surgical procedures, you need to be able to carry out nursing procedures with skill and confidence. But mastering so many procedures is a tall order.

Newly updated with the latest evidence-based research, this seventh edition of *Lippincott Nursing Procedures* provides step-by-step guidance on the most commonly performed nursing procedures you need to know, making it the ideal resource for providing the professional, hands-on care your patients deserve.

The A to Zs of organization

With over 400 procedures covered in detail, the current edition of *Lippincott Nursing Procedures* presents this wealth of information in the most efficient way possible. Many procedures books use such categories as fundamental procedures, body systems, and other types of procedures (such as psychiatric care) to organize the material. But with the proliferation in the number and types of procedures you need to understand, such an organization can become difficult to manage.

To address this, *Lippincott Nursing Procedures* organizes all procedures into an A-to-Z listing, making the book fast and easy to use. When you need to find a particular procedure quickly, you simply can look it up by name. No need to scan through the table of contents. No time lost turning to the index, looking for the name of the procedure you want, and then finding the right page in the book.

Once you've found the entry for a particular procedure in the alphabetical listing, you'll find that each entry uses the same clear, straightforward structure. An introductory section appears first. After that, most or all of the following sections appear, depending on the particular procedure:

- The *Equipment* section lists all the equipment you'll need, including all the variations in equipment that might be needed. For instance, in the "endotracheal intubation" entry, you'll see a general equipment list, which is followed by separate lists of the additional equipment you'll need for direct visualization intubation and blind nasotracheal intubation.
- As the name implies, the *Preparation of equipment* section guides you through preparing the equipment for the procedure.
- In the *Implementation* section—the heart of each entry—you'll find the step-by-step guide to performing the particular procedure.
- *Special considerations* alerts you to factors to keep in mind that can affect the procedure.
- *Patient teaching* covers procedure-related and home care information you need to teach to the patient and his family.
- *Complications* details procedure-related complications to watch for.
- The *Documentation* section helps you keep track of everything you need to document related to the procedure.
- The expanded *References* section includes numbered citations keyed to the main text of each entry. These numbered citations serve as the clinical evidence that underpins the information and step-by-step procedures presented in the entry. (There'll be more on this in the next section of this "how to" guide.)
- The *Additional references*—the final section in each entry—presents even more clinical background research for the reader who wants to delve deeper.

The continued use of the A-to-Z organization in the seventh edition and the clear structure of each entry make this book a powerful tool for finding and understanding the procedures you need to know.

Evidently speaking...

Lippincott Nursing Procedures strengthens its evidence-based approach to nursing care with an expanded numbered *References* section that appears in each entry. As mentioned earlier, the numbered citations are keyed to information that appears throughout each procedure.

As you read through an entry and come across a bullet describing a particular step in a procedure, you'll notice one or more red superscript numbers following the bullet. These numbers, in turn, refer to citations in the *References* section; the studies in these citations supply clinical evidence or detail best practices related to that bulleted step in the procedure. This is what is meant by *evidence-based practice*: A particular practice—say, performing hand hygiene—is supported by the clinical evidence. This evidence-based approach means the procedures you'll read about in *Lippincott Nursing Procedures* are best-practice procedures that rely on solid, authoritative evidence.

As you look at the numbered references in each entry, you may notice that many of them are followed by a level number. This level number appears in parentheses after the reference as the word "Level" followed by a Roman numeral that ranges from I to VII. These level numbers give you an indication of the strength of the particular reference, with Level I being the strongest and Level VII the weakest.

Here's how the rating system for this hierarchy of evidence works:

- *Level I:* Evidence comes from a systematic review or meta-analysis of all relevant randomized, controlled trials.
- *Level II:* Evidence comes from at least one well-designed randomized, controlled trial.
- *Level III:* Evidence comes from well-designed, controlled trials without randomization.
- *Level IV:* Evidence comes from well-designed case-control and cohort studies.
- *Level V:* Evidence comes from systematic reviews of descriptive and qualitative studies.
- *Level VI:* Evidence comes from a single descriptive or qualitative study.
- *Level VII:* Evidence comes from the opinion of authorities, reports of expert committees, or both.

In this book, the majority of cited references followed by a level are rated "Level I." These Level I references provide the strongest level of evidence to support a particular practice. You can use these levels to gauge the strength of supporting evidence for any particular practice or procedure.

Another important way *Lippincott Nursing Procedures* provides a more evidence-based approach is by offering rationales for many procedures' steps. These rationales are set off from the main text in italics. For instance, you may see a bullet like this: "Answer all the patient's questions *to decrease anxiety and improve cooperation.*" The second part of that bullet—the italicized portion—is the rationale, or reason, for performing the first part. The practice of answering the patient's questions is supported by the clinical evidence of the patient's decreased anxiety and increased cooperation.

Just the highlights, please

Lippincott Nursing Procedures, Seventh Edition, also benefits from other features that make it easy to use. Throughout, you'll find highlighting that greatly enhances the main text.

Some examples:

- As mentioned earlier, footnotes appear in red for easier spotting.
- Colored letter tabs at the top of each page make finding a particular entry quick and easy.
- Full-color photos and diagrams highlight the main text, illustrating many of the step-by-step procedures in the *Implementation* section of each entry.
- Special alerts—with colorful, eye-catching logos—appear in many entries:

NURSING ALERT lets you know about potentially dangerous actions or clinically significant findings related to a procedure

PEDIATRIC ALERT warns you of particular precautions to take concerning infants, young children, and adolescents

ELDER ALERT cautions you about the special needs of this growing population

HOSPITAL-ACQUIRED CONDITION ALERT, new to this edition, warns you about conditions that the Centers for Medicare and Medicaid Services has identified as conditions that can occur as the result of hospitalization. Following various best practices can reasonably help to prevent such conditions; when these conditions do occur, they have payment implications for health care facilities.

- Short, boxed-off articles appear throughout the book. These short pieces run the gamut, from explaining procedures in more detail, to highlighting equipment, to offering tips for clearer documentation, to name just a few. Several are set off with their own eye-catching icons and are enhanced with illustrations or full-color photos:

EQUIPMENT profiles an essential piece of equipment needed to help diagnose or treat the patient

TROUBLESHOOTING helps you to quickly identify problems and complications, isolate their probable cause, and guide you with step-by-step interventions

PATIENT TEACHING provides helpful tips, reminders, and follow-up instructions to share with patients being discharged following their procedure.

Your go-to guide

Now that you know what the seventh edition of *Lippincott Nursing Procedures* has to offer—and have learned how to use it quickly and adeptly—you're ready to take on the task of performing a variety of nursing procedures. Whether you're a nursing student, a recent graduate, or an experienced practitioner, you're ready to provide all your patients with expert nursing care, with your go-to guide at your fingertips.

A

ABDOMINAL PARACENTESIS, ASSISTING

As a bedside procedure, abdominal paracentesis involves the aspiration of fluid from the peritoneal space through a needle, trocar, or angiocatheter[1] inserted in the abdominal wall. Used to diagnose and treat massive ascites resistant to other therapies, the procedure helps to determine the cause of ascites while relieving the resulting pressure.

Abdominal paracentesis may also precede other procedures, including radiography, peritoneal dialysis, and surgery; detect intra-abdominal bleeding after a traumatic injury; and be used to obtain a peritoneal fluid specimen for laboratory analysis. The procedure must be performed cautiously in pregnant patients as well as in patients with bleeding tendencies, severely distended bowel, or infection at the intended insertion site.

Equipment

Stethoscope ■ blood pressure monitor ■ pulse oximeter ■ thermometer ■ scale ■ tape measure ■ sterile gloves ■ mask ■ gloves ■ gown ■ goggles ■ fluid-impermeable pads ■ four Vacutainer tubes ■ two large Vacutainer bottles (1,000 mL or larger) ■ laboratory biohazard transport bag ■ laboratory request forms ■ antiseptic cleaning solution (povidone-iodine, chlorhexidine) ■ local anesthetic (multidose vial of 1% or 2% lidocaine with epinephrine) ■ sterile 4″ × 4″ (10-cm × 10-cm) gauze pads ■ tape ■ sterile paracentesis tray ■ sterile drapes ■ marking pen ■ 5-mL syringe with 21G or 25G needle ■ Optional: alcohol sponge, 50-mL syringe, suture materials, IV albumin, IV insertion kit, indwelling urinary catheter insertion equipment, pain medication.

If a preassembled tray isn't available, gather the following sterile supplies: trocar with stylet, 16G to 20G needle, or angiocatheter; 25G or 27G 1½″ needle; 20G or 22G spinal needle; scalpel; #11 knife blade; three-way stopcock.

Implementation

- Perform hand hygiene and put on gloves.[2,3,4]
- Confirm the patient's identity using at least two patient identifiers.[5]
- Reinforce the practitioner's explanation of the procedure and answer questions. Reassure the patient that he should feel no pain but that he may feel a stinging sensation from the local anesthetic injection and pressure from the needle, trocar, or angiocatheter insertion. He may also sense pressure when the practitioner aspirates abdominal fluid.
- Check the patient's history for hypersensitivity to latex or to the local anesthetic.
- Confirm that written informed consent has been obtained and is in the patient's medical record.[6,7]
- Instruct the patient to void before the procedure. Alternatively, insert an indwelling urinary catheter, if ordered, *to minimize the risk of accidental bladder injury from insertion of the needle, trocar, or angiocatheter.*
- Conduct a preprocedure verification *to make sure that all relevant documentation, related information, and equipment are available and correctly identified to the patient's identifiers.*[8]
- Verify that the laboratory and imaging studies have been completed as ordered and that the results are in the patient's medical record. Notify the practitioner of any unexpected results.[8]
- Obtain the patient's vital signs, oxygen saturation level, weight, and abdominal girth *to serve as a baseline for comparison during and after the procedure.* Use the tape measure to measure the patient's abdominal girth at the umbilical level. Use a felt-tipped marker to indicate the abdominal area measured.
- Place the patient in the supine position or on his side *to allow the fluid to pool in dependent areas.*[1]
- Expose the patient's abdomen from diaphragm to pubis. Keep the rest of the patient covered *to avoid chilling him.*
- Make the patient as comfortable as possible and place a fluid-impermeable pad under him *for protection from drainage.*
- Remind the patient to stay as still as possible during the procedure *to prevent injury from the needle, trocar, or angiocatheter.*
- Perform hand hygiene.[2,3,4]
- Open the paracentesis tray using sterile technique *to ensure a sterile field.*
- Put on a gown, a mask, goggles, and gloves.[9]
- Label all medications, medication containers, and other solutions on and off the sterile field.[10]
- Conduct a time-out immediately before starting the procedure *to perform a final assessment that the correct patient, site, positioning, and procedure are identified and, as applicable, that all relevant information and necessary equipment are available during and after the procedure.*[11]
- Assist the practitioner as he prepares the patient's abdomen with antiseptic cleaning solution, drapes the insertion site with sterile drapes, and administers the local anesthetic.
- If the paracentesis tray doesn't contain a sterile ampule of anesthetic, wipe the top of a multidose vial of anesthetic solution with an alcohol sponge and allow it to dry, and then invert the vial at a 45-degree angle. *This step allows the practitioner to insert the sterile 5-mL syringe with the 21G or 25G needle and withdraw the anesthetic without touching the nonsterile vial.*
- Using the scalpel, the practitioner may make a small incision before inserting the needle, trocar, or angiocatheter (usually 1″ to 2″ [2.5 to 5 cm] below the umbilicus). Listen for a popping sound, *which signifies that the needle, trocar, or angiocatheter has pierced the peritoneum.*
- Assist the practitioner with collecting specimens in the proper containers. If the practitioner orders substantial drainage, aseptically connect the three-way stopcock and tubing to the needle, trocar, or angiocatheter. Run the other end of the tubing to a large, sterile Vacutainer. Alternatively, aspirate the fluid with a three-way stopcock and 50-mL syringe.
- Label the specimen tubes with the patient's name and identification number, as well as the date and time of the collection in the presence of the patient *to prevent mislabeling,*[10] and send them to the laboratory in a laboratory biohazard transport bag with the appropriate laboratory request forms. If the patient is receiving antibiotics, note this information on the request form for consideration during the fluid analysis.
- Gently turn the patient from side to side *to enhance drainage,* if necessary.
- As the fluid drains, monitor the patient's vital signs and oxygen saturation level frequently. Observe him closely for vertigo, faintness, diaphoresis, pallor, heightened anxiety, tachycardia, dyspnea, and hypotension, especially if more than 1,500 mL of peritoneal fluid was aspirated at one time. *This loss may induce a fluid shift and hypovolemic shock.*
- Immediately report signs of shock to the practitioner; he may prescribe IV albumin *to prevent hypovolemia and a decline in renal function.*
- When the procedure ends and the practitioner removes the needle, trocar, or angiocatheter, he may suture the incision.
- Remove and discard your gloves, perform hand hygiene, and put on sterile gloves.
- Tape sterile 4″ × 4″ (10-cm × 10-cm) gauze pads to the site *to serve as a pressure dressing.* When drainage becomes minimal, remove and discard the pressure dressing, apply dry sterile gauze pads, and tape them to the site.
- Help the patient assume a comfortable position.
- Monitor the patient's vital signs and oxygen saturation level, and check the dressing for drainage as determined by the patient's condition and at an interval determined by your facility *because no evidence-based research is*

available to indicate best practice for the frequency of vital sign assessment after a procedure.[12] Note the color, amount, and characteristics of the drainage.

- Perform a comprehensive pain assessment using techniques appropriate for the patient's age, condition, and ability to understand.[13] Administer pain medication as needed and ordered, following safe medication administration practice.
- Dispose of used supplies in the appropriate receptacles.
- Remove and discard your gloves and perform hand hygiene.[2,3,4]
- Document the procedure.[14]

Special considerations

- Throughout this procedure, help the patient remain still *to prevent accidental perforation of abdominal organs.*
- If the patient shows signs of hypovolemic shock, reduce the vertical distance between the needle, trocar, or angiocatheter and the drainage collection container *to slow the drainage rate.* If necessary, stop the drainage.
- *To prevent fluid shifts and hypovolemia,* limit aspirated fluid to between 1,500 and 2,000 mL. If peritoneal fluid doesn't flow easily, try repositioning the patient *to facilitate drainage.* Also, verify suction in the Vacutainer collection bottle when you connect it to the drainage tubing and be sure to use macrodrip tubing without a backflow device.
- After the procedure, observe for peritoneal fluid leakage. If this develops, notify the practitioner.
- Obtain the patient's weight (using the same scale) and abdominal girth daily. Compare these values with the baseline figures *to detect recurrent ascites.*
- Ultrasound may be used *to assist in locating the fluid and inserting the needle, trocar, or angiocatheter. Ultrasound-guided paracentesis has been shown to result in fewer adverse events than paracentesis performed without ultrasound guidance.*[15]
- Monitor the patient's respiratory changes during the procedure. *Ascites may place pressure on the diaphragm, leading to respiratory distress; removing ascitic fluid should help relieve this pressure and distress.*[1]

Complications

Removing large amounts of fluid may cause hypotension, oliguria, and hyponatremia. If an excessive amount of fluid (more than 2 L) is removed, ascitic fluid tends to form again, drawing fluid from extracellular tissue throughout the body. Other complications include perforation of abdominal organs, including of the bowel or bladder by the needle, trocar, or angiocatheter; wound infection; bleeding; and peritonitis.

Documentation

Record the date and time of the procedure, puncture site location, and whether the wound was sutured. Document the amount, color, viscosity, and odor of aspirated fluid in your notes as well as in the fluid intake and output record. Record the patient's vital signs, oxygen saturation, weight, and abdominal girth measurements before and after the procedure. Also note the patient's tolerance of the procedure, his vital signs, and any signs or symptoms of complications during the procedure. Note the number of specimens sent to the laboratory.

REFERENCES

1 Lynn-McHale Wiegand, D. (Ed.). (2011). *AACN procedure manual for critical care* (6th ed.). St. Louis, MO: Saunders.

2 The Joint Commission. (2015). Standard NPSG.07.01.01. *Comprehensive accreditation manual for hospitals: The official handbook.* Oakbrook Terrace, IL: The Joint Commission. (Level VII)

3 Centers for Disease Control and Prevention. (2002). Guideline for hand hygiene in health-care settings: Recommendations of the Healthcare Infection Control Practices Advisory Committee and the HICPAC/SHEA/APIC/IDSA Hand Hygiene Task Force. *MMWR Recommendations and Reports, 51* (RR-16), 1–45. Accessed March 2015 via the Web at http://www.cdc.gov/mmwr/pdf/rr/rr5116.pdf (Level II)

4 World Health Organization. (2009). "WHO guidelines on hand hygiene in health care: First global patient safety challenge, clean care is safer care" [Online]. Accessed March 2015 via the Web at http://whqlibdoc.who.int/publications/2009/9789241597906_eng.pdf (Level IV)

5 The Joint Commission. (2015). Standard NPSG.01.01.01. *Comprehensive accreditation manual for hospitals: The official handbook.* Oakbrook Terrace, IL: The Joint Commission. (Level VII)

6 The Joint Commission. (2015). Standard RI.01.03.01. *Comprehensive accreditation manual for hospitals: The official handbook.* Oakbrook Terrace, IL: The Joint Commission. (Level VII)

7 Centers for Medicare & Medicaid Services, Department of Health and Human Services. (2014). Condition of participation: Patient's rights. 42 C.F.R. § 482.13.

8 The Joint Commission. (2015). Standard UP.01.01.01. *Comprehensive accreditation manual for hospitals: The official handbook.* Oakbrook Terrace, IL: The Joint Commission. (Level VII)

9 Siegel, J. D., et al. (2007). "2007 guideline for isolation precautions: Preventing transmission of infectious agents in healthcare settings" [Online]. Accessed March 2015 via the Web at http://www.cdc.gov/hicpac/pdf/isolation/Isolation2007.pdf (Level II)

10 The Joint Commission. (2015). Standard NPSG.03.04.01. *Comprehensive accreditation manual for hospitals: The official handbook.* Oakbrook Terrace, IL: The Joint Commission. (Level VII)

11 The Joint Commission. (2015). Standard UP.01.03.01. *Comprehensive accreditation manual for hospitals: The official handbook.* Oakbrook Terrace, IL: The Joint Commission. (Level VII)

12 American Society of PeriAnesthesia Nurses. (2012). *2012-2014 Perianesthesia nursing standards, practice recommendations and interpretative statements.* Cherry Hill, NJ: American Society of PeriAnesthesia Nurses.

13 The Joint Commission. (2015). Standard PC.01.02.07. *Comprehensive accreditation manual for hospitals: The official handbook.* Oakbrook Terrace, IL: The Joint Commission. (Level VII)

14 The Joint Commission. (2015). Standard RC.01.03.01. *Comprehensive accreditation manual for hospitals: The official handbook.* Oakbrook Terrace, IL: The Joint Commission. (Level VII)

15 Patel, P. A., et al. (2012). Evaluation of hospital complications and costs associated with using guidance during abdominal paracentesis procedures. *Journal of Medical Economics, 15,* 1–7.

ADDITIONAL REFERENCES

Barsuk, J. H., et al., (2013). Clinical outcomes after bedside interventional radiology paracentesis procedures. *American Journal of Medicine, 126,* 349–356.

Sekiguchi, H., et al. (2013). Making paracentesis safer: A proposal for the use of bedside abdominal and vascular ultrasonography to prevent a fatal complication. *Chest, 143,* 1136–1139.

ADMISSION

Admission to a nursing unit prepares a patient for his stay in a health care facility. Whether the admission is scheduled or follows emergency treatment, effective admission procedures should include certain steps to accomplish important goals. These steps include verifying the patient's identity using at least two patient identifiers,[1] assessing his clinical status, making him as comfortable as possible, introducing him to roommates and staff members, orienting him to the environment and routines, and providing any supplies and special equipment needed for daily care.

The Joint Commission requires that each patient undergo an admission assessment by a registered nurse within 24 hours after inpatient admission.[2,3] The Healthcare Facilities Accreditation Program requires that an initial assessment be performed by a registered nurse within the timeframe established by the individual facility.[4] During this assessment, the nurse should prioritize the patient's needs, always remaining aware of the patient's levels of fatigue and comfort, and should maintain the patient's privacy while obtaining the health history. According to the

Patient Care Partnership, the patient has the right to expect that examinations, consultations, and treatment will be conducted in a manner that protects the patient's privacy.[5]

Efficient admission routines that show appropriate concern for the patient can ease the patient's anxiety and promote cooperation and receptivity to treatment. Conversely, admission routines that the patient perceives as careless or excessively impersonal can heighten anxiety, reduce cooperation, impair the patient's response to treatment, and possibly aggravate symptoms.

Equipment

Patient gown ■ personal property form ■ valuables envelope ■ admission form ■ nursing assessment form ■ sphygmomanometer ■ stethoscope ■ thermometer ■ hospital-grade disinfectant pad ■ patient scale ■ identification band ■ Optional: emesis basin, bedpan, urinal, bath basin, emergency equipment (crash cart with cardiac medications, defibrillator, handheld resuscitation bag with mask, intubation equipment), oxygen delivery system, suction, equipment for obtaining blood or urine specimens, patient care reminders, medical identification bracelet.

Preparation of equipment

Position the bed as the patient's condition requires. If the patient is ambulatory, place the bed in the low position; if he's arriving on a stretcher, place the bed in the high position. Fold down the top linens. Prepare emergency or special equipment, such as oxygen or suction, as needed.

Implementation

- Adjust the lights, temperature, and ventilation in the room.
- Quickly review the admission form and the practitioner's orders. Note the reason for admission, restrictions on activity and diet, and any orders for diagnostic tests requiring specimen collection.
- Gather and prepare the appropriate equipment.
- Perform hand hygiene.[6,7,8,9,10,11,12]
- Speaking slowly and clearly, greet the patient by his proper name and introduce yourself and any other staff members present.[13]
- Confirm the patient's identity using at least two patient identifiers.[1] Apply an identification band, verifying that the identifiers are correct, including the patient's name and its spelling. Notify the admission office of any corrections.
- Escort the patient to his room and, if he isn't in great distress, introduce him to his roommate. Alternatively, if the patient is being admitted from the emergency department and is on a stretcher, summon the help of coworkers to transfer the patient from the stretcher to the bed. Keep in mind that, depending on the patient's condition, he may require immediate treatment; treatment takes priority over routine admission procedures. (See *Managing emergency admissions*.)
- Help the patient change into a hospital gown or pajamas he has brought from home if appropriate; if the patient is sharing a room, provide privacy.[17]
- Itemize all valuables, clothing, and prostheses on the personal property form (or in your notes if your facility doesn't use such a form). Encourage the patient to store valuables or money in the safe or, preferably, to send them home along with any medications he may have brought.
- Orient the patient to the room. Show the patient how to use the equipment in his room; include the call system, bed controls, television controls, telephone, and lights. Show an ambulatory patient where the bathroom and closets are located.
- Explain the routine at your health care facility. Mention when to expect meals, vital signs assessments, and medications. Review visiting hours and any restrictions.
- Obtain and record the patient's vital signs.

Managing emergency admissions

After emergency department (ED) treatment, the patient arrives on the nursing unit with a temporary identification bracelet, a practitioner's orders, and a record of treatment. Read this record and receive hand-off communication from the nurse who cared for the patient in the ED *to ensure continuity of care and gain insight into the patient's condition and behavior.*

Perform hand hygiene and follow standard precautions.[6,7,8,9,10,11] Trace all catheters and tubing from the patient to their point of origin *to make sure that they're attached to the proper connection ports.* If the patient has more than one connection to a port of entry into the body (for example, if an IV catheter has more than one infusion infusing through it), label each tube near the insertion site. Label the infusion bag, ensuring that the label faces out so it can be easily read.[14] If the patient is receiving infusions by different administration routes, place the infusion pumps on opposite sides of the bed *to prevent administration errors.*[14] If the infusion pump or any other patient equipment has alarms, make sure the alarm limits are set according to the patient's current condition and that the alarms are turned on, functioning properly, and audible to staff members.[15,16]

Obtain and record the patient's vital signs, and follow the practitioner's orders for treatment. If the patient is conscious and not in great distress, explain any treatment orders. If family members accompany the patient, ask them to wait in the lounge while you assess the patient and begin treatment. Permit them to visit the patient after he's settled in his room. When the patient's condition allows, proceed with routine admission procedures.

- Measure the patient's height and weight if possible. If he can't stand, use a chair or bed scale and ask him his height. *Knowing the patient's height and weight is important for planning treatments and diet and for calculating medication and anesthetic dosages.* Record the patient's weight in kilograms and document it prominently in the chart *to help prevent medication errors.*[18]
- Collect blood and urine specimens, if ordered.
- Obtain a complete patient history. Include all previous hospitalizations, illnesses, surgeries, and food and drug allergies.
- Make sure that a complete list of the medications the patient was taking at home (including doses, routes, and frequency) has been obtained and documented in the patient's medical record. Compare this list with the patient's current medications and reconcile and document any discrepancies (omissions, duplications, adjustments, deletions, or additions) in the patient's medical record *to reduce the risk of transition-related adverse drug events.*[19]
- Determine whether the patient has an advance directive and, if so, place a copy in the medical record. If the patient doesn't have one, provide information about advance directives to the patient.[20,21] (See the "Advance directives" procedure, page 7.)
- Ask the patient to tell you why he came to the facility. Record the answers (in the patient's own words) as the chief complaint. Follow up with a physical assessment, emphasizing complaints. Record any marks, bruises, discolorations and wounds on the nursing assessment form.
- Perform a comprehensive pain assessment using techniques appropriate for the patient's age, condition, and ability to understand.[22]
- If required by your facility, attach a medical identification bracelet to the patient's arm if the patient has a drug allergy, is at risk for falls, or has another condition that requires a medical identification bracelet.
- Assess and address the patient's safety needs.

Using patient care reminders

When placed at the head of the patient's bed, care reminders call attention to the patient's special needs and help ensure consistent care by communicating these needs to the health care facility's staff members, the patient's family, and other visitors.

You can use a specially designed card or a plain piece of paper to post important information about the patient, such as:
- allergies
- dietary restrictions
- fluid restrictions
- needed specimen collection
- infection-control or isolation procedures
- hearing impairments, including whether the patient is deaf or hearing impaired and if so, in which ear
- whether a foreign language is spoken.

You can also use care reminders to post special instructions, such as:
- complete bed rest
- no blood pressure on right arm
- turn every hour
- nothing by mouth.

Don't violate the patient's privacy by posting his name, diagnosis, details about surgery, or other information he might find embarrassing.

- After assessing the patient, inform him of any tests that have been ordered and when they're scheduled. Describe what he should expect.
- Before leaving the patient's room, make sure he's comfortable. Adjust his bed, and place the call light and other personal items within easy reach.
- Post patient care reminders (concerning such topics as allergies and special needs) at the patient's bedside, as needed, *to notify coworkers.* (See *Using patient care reminders.*)
- Perform hand hygiene.[6,7,8,9,11]
- Clean and disinfect your stethoscope and other equipment, as needed, using a hospital-grade disinfectant pad.[23,24]
- Perform hand hygiene.[6,7,8,9,11]
- Document the procedure.[25,26,27]

Special considerations

- If the patient brings medications from home, take an inventory and record this information on the nursing assessment form. Instruct the patient not to take any medications unless authorized by the practitioner. Send authorized medications to the pharmacy for identification and relabeling.[28] Send other medication home with a responsible family member, or store them in the designated area outside the patient's room until he's discharged. *Use of unauthorized medications may interfere with treatment or cause an overdose.*
- Note that The Joint Commission issued a sentinel event alert concerning medical device alarm safety *because alarm-related events have been associated with permanent loss of function and death.* Among the major contributing factors were improper alarm settings, inappropriately turned off alarms, and alarm signals that were not audible to staff. Make sure alarm limits are appropriately set and that alarms are turned on, functioning properly, and audible to staff. Follow facility guidelines for preventing alarm fatigue.[29]
- Find out the patient's normal routine, and ask him if he would like to make adjustments to the facility regimen; for instance, he may prefer to shower at night instead of in the morning. *By accommodating the patient with such adjustments whenever possible, you can ease his anxiety and help him feel more in control of his potentially threatening situation.*
- Patients requiring isolation precautions should be placed in an isolation room *to reduce the risk of transmission.*[12,30]
- Teach the patient and his family about the importance of proper hand hygiene in preventing the spread of infection. Encourage them to speak up if a health care worker fails to perform hand hygiene before having contact with the patient or the patient's environment.

Documentation

After leaving the patient's room, document your assessment findings. Your documentation should include the patient's vital signs, height, weight, allergies, and drug and health history; a list of his belongings and those sent home with family members; the results of your physical assessment; and a record of specimens collected for laboratory tests.

REFERENCES

1 The Joint Commission. (2015). Standard NPSG.01.01.01. *Comprehensive accreditation manual for hospitals: The official handbook.* Oakbrook Terrace, IL: The Joint Commission. (Level VII)

2 The Joint Commission. (2015). Standard PC.01.02.03. *Comprehensive accreditation manual for hospitals: The official handbook.* Oakbrook Terrace, IL: The Joint Commission. (Level VII)

3 Centers for Medicare & Medicaid Services, Department of Health and Human Services. (2014). Condition of participation: Nursing services. 42 C.F.R. § 482.23.

4 American Osteopathic Association. (2014). Standard 10.01.24. *Healthcare Facilities Accreditation Program: Accreditation requirements for acute care hospitals.* Chicago, IL: American Osteopathic Association. (Level VII)

5 American Hospital Association. (2003). "The patient care partnership: Understanding expectation, rights, and responsibilities" [Online]. Accessed March 2015 via the Web at http://www.aha.org/aha/content/2003/pdf/pcp_english_030730.pdf

6 The Joint Commission. (2015). NPSG.07.01.01. *Comprehensive accreditation manual for hospitals: The official handbook.* Oakbrook Terrace, IL: The Joint Commission. (Level VII)

7 Centers for Disease Control and Prevention. (2002). Guideline for hand hygiene in health-care settings: Recommendations of the Healthcare Infection Control Practices Advisory Committee and the HICPAC/SHEA/APIC/IDSA Hand Hygiene Task Force. *MMWR Recommendations and Reports, 51*(RR-16), 1–45. Accessed March 2015 via the Web at http://www.cdc.gov/mmwr/pdf/rr/rr5116.pdf (Level II)

8 World Health Organization. (2009). "WHO guidelines on hand hygiene in health care: First global patient safety challenge, clean care is safer care" [Online]. Accessed March 2015 via the Web at http://whqlibdoc.who.int/publications/2009/9789241597906_eng.pdf (Level IV)

9 Centers for Medicare & Medicaid Services, Department of Health and Human Services. (2014). Condition of participation: Infection control. 42 C.F.R. § 482.42.

10 American Osteopathic Association. (2014). Standard 07.01.10. *Healthcare Facilities Accreditation Program: Accreditation requirements for acute care hospitals.* Chicago, IL: American Osteopathic Association. (Level VII)

11 American Osteopathic Association. (2014). Standard 07.01.21. *Healthcare Facilities Accreditation Program: Accreditation requirements for acute care hospitals.* Chicago, IL: American Osteopathic Association. (Level VII)

12 Siegel, J. D., et al. (2007). "2007 guideline for isolation precautions: Preventing transmission of infectious agents in healthcare settings" [Online]. Accessed March 2015 via the Web at http://www.cdc.gov/hicpac/pdf/isolation/Isolation2007.pdf (Level II)

13 The Joint Commission. (2015). Standard PC.02.01.21. *Comprehensive accreditation manual for hospitals: The official handbook.* Oakbrook Terrace, IL: The Joint Commission. (Level VII)

14 Institute for Safe Medication Practices. (2010). Preventing catheter/tubing misconnections: Much needed help is on the way. *Nurse Advise-ERR, 8,* 1–2. Accessed March 2015 via the Web at http://www.ismp.org/Newsletters/nursing/Issues/NurseAdviseERR201012.pdf

15 Graham, K. C., & Cvach, M. (2010). Monitor alarm fatigue: Standardizing use of physiological monitors and decreasing nuisance alarms. *American Journal of Critical Care, 19,* 28–37.
16 The Joint Commission. (2015). Standard NPSG.06.01.01. *Comprehensive accreditation manual for hospitals: The official handbook.* Oakbrook Terrace, IL: The Joint Commission. (Level VII)
17 The Joint Commission. (2015). Standard RI.01.06.05. *Comprehensive accreditation manual for hospitals: The official handbook.* Oakbrook Terrace, IL: The Joint Commission. (Level VII)
18 Emergency Nurses Association. (2012). "Position statement: Weighing patients in kilograms" [Online]. Accessed March 2015 via the Web at http://www.ena.org/SiteCollectionDocuments/Position%20Statements/WeighingPTsinKG.pdf
19 The Joint Commission. (2015). Standard NPSG.03.06.01. *Comprehensive accreditation manual for hospitals: The official handbook.* Oakbrook Terrace, IL: The Joint Commission. (Level VII)
20 Centers for Medicare & Medicaid Services, Department of Health and Human Services. (2014). Condition of participation: Patient's rights. 42 C.F.R. § 482.13(b).
21 The Joint Commission. (2015). Standard RI.01.05.01. *Comprehensive accreditation manual for hospitals: The official handbook.* Oakbrook Terrace, IL: The Joint Commission. (Level VII)
22 The Joint Commission. (2015). Standard PC.01.02.07. *Comprehensive accreditation manual for hospitals: The official handbook.* Oakbrook Terrace, IL: The Joint Commission. (Level VII)
23 Rutala, W. A., et al. (2008). "Guideline for disinfection and sterilization in healthcare facilities, 2008" [Online]. Accessed March 2015 via the Web at http://www.cdc.gov/hicpac/pdf/guidelines/Disinfection_Nov_2008.pdf (Level I)
24 American Osteopathic Association. (2014). Standard 07.02.03. *Healthcare Facilities Accreditation Program: Accreditation requirements for acute care hospitals.* Chicago, IL: American Osteopathic Association. (Level VII)
25 The Joint Commission. (2015). Standard RC.01.03.01. *Comprehensive accreditation manual for hospitals: The official handbook.* Oakbrook Terrace, IL: The Joint Commission. (Level VII)
26 Centers for Medicare & Medicaid Services, Department of Health and Human Services. (2014). Condition of participation: Medical record services. 42 C.F.R. § 482.24(b).
27 American Osteopathic Association. (2014). Standard 10.00.03. *Healthcare Facilities Accreditation Program: Accreditation requirements for acute care hospitals.* Chicago, IL: American Osteopathic Association. (Level VII)
28 The Joint Commission. (2015). Standard MM.03.01.05. *Comprehensive accreditation manual for hospitals: The official handbook.* Oakbrook Terrace, IL: The Joint Commission. (Level VII)
29 The Joint Commission. (2013). "Sentinel event alert: Medical device alarm safety in hospitals" [Online]. Accessed March 2015 via the Web at http://www.jointcommission.org/assets/1/18/SEA_50_alarms_4_5_13_FINAL1.PDF (Level VII)
30 Centers for Disease Control and Prevention. (2005). Guidelines for preventing the transmission of *Mycobacterium tuberculosis* in health-care settings, 2005. *MMWR Recommendations and Reports, 54*(RR-17), 1–140. Accessed March 2015 via the Web at http://www.cdc.gov/mmwr/PDF/rr/rr5417.pdf (Level II)

ADDITIONAL REFERENCES

American Association of Critical-Care Nurses (AACN). (2013). "AACN practice alert: Alarm management" [Online]. Accessed March 2015 via the Web at http://www.aacn.org/wd/practice/docs/practicealerts/alarm-management-practice-alert.pdf (Level VII)

Bickley, L. S., & Szilagyi, P. G. (2013). *Bates' guide to physical examination and history taking* (11th ed.). Philadelphia, PA: Lippincott Williams & Wilkins.

ADMIXTURE OF DRUGS IN A SYRINGE

Combining two drugs in one syringe avoids the discomfort of two injections. Usually, drugs can be mixed in a syringe in one of four ways: They may be combined from two multidose vials (for example, regular and long-acting insulin), from one multidose vial and one ampule, from two ampules, or from a cartridge-injection system combined with either a multidose vial or an ampule. Such combinations are contraindicated when the drugs aren't compatible and when combined doses exceed the amount of solution that can be absorbed from a single injection site.

The Association of Professionals in Infection Control and Epidemiology and the World Health Organization recommend using single-use or single-dose vials whenever possible. The risk of transmission posed by inappropriate handling of multidose vials has been clearly demonstrated and mandates a practice of one vial per one patient whenever possible.[1] Infection transmission risk is reduced when multidose vials are dedicated to a single patient.[2] The Infusion Nurses Society also recommends that nurses administer pharmacy-prepared or commercially available products whenever possible.[3]

Equipment

Prescribed medications ■ alcohol pads ■ sterile gauze pads ■ sterile syringe and needle ■ Optional: safety needle, 5-micron filter needle.[3]

The type and size of syringe and needle depend on the volume and viscosity of prescribed medications, the patient's body mass, and the injection site.

Implementation

- Before preparing the injection, make sure the preparation area is free from clutter, and clean the preparation surface with an alcohol pad.[1,4]
- Avoid distractions and interruptions when preparing medication *to prevent medication errors.*[5,6]
- Verify the order on the patient's medication record by checking it against the practitioner's order.[7,8,9]
- Gather the medications and equipment.
- Compare the medication labels with the order in the patient's medical record.[7,8,9]
- Verify the compatibility of the drugs to be combined.
- Check the patient's medical record for an allergy or a contraindication to the prescribed medications. If an allergy or contraindications exist, don't administer the medications; notify the practitioner.[6]
- Check the expiration date on each of the medications. If either of the medications is expired, return it to the pharmacy and obtain new medication.[7,8,9]
- Visually inspect each solution for particles or discoloration or other loss of integrity; don't administer the medications if either has compromised integrity.[7,8,9]
- Discuss any unresolved concerns about the medications with the patient's practitioner.[7,8,9]
- Calculate the doses to be administered.
- Have another nurse double-check your calculations if necessary.

NURSING ALERT If either of the prescribed medications is considered a high-alert medication, which can cause significant patient harm when used in error, before administering the medications have another nurse perform an independent double-check, if required by your facility, *to verify the patient's identity and make sure that the correct medications are drawn up in the prescribed concentrations, the indications for both medications correspond with the patient's diagnosis, the dosage calculations are correct and the dosing formula used to derive the final dose is correct, and the route of administration is safe and proper for the patient.*[10,11]

- Perform hand hygiene.[1,12,13,14,15,16]
- When preparing the medications, read the medication labels as you select the medications, as you draw each up, and after you have drawn each up *to verify the correct dose.*

Mixing drugs from two multidose vials

■ Remove the vial lid and disinfect the rubber stopper on the first drug vial and allow it to dry[1,3] *to decrease the risk of contaminating the medication as you insert the needle into the vial.*
■ Pull back the syringe plunger until the volume of air drawn into the syringe equals the volume to be withdrawn from the drug vial.
■ Without inverting the vial, insert the needle into the top of the vial, making sure that the needle's bevel tip doesn't touch the solution. Inject the air into the vial and withdraw the needle. *This step replaces air in the vial, which prevents the creation of a partial vacuum when you withdraw the drug.*
■ Repeat the steps above for the second vial. Then, after injecting the air into the second vial, invert the vial, withdraw the prescribed dose, and then withdraw the needle (as shown below).

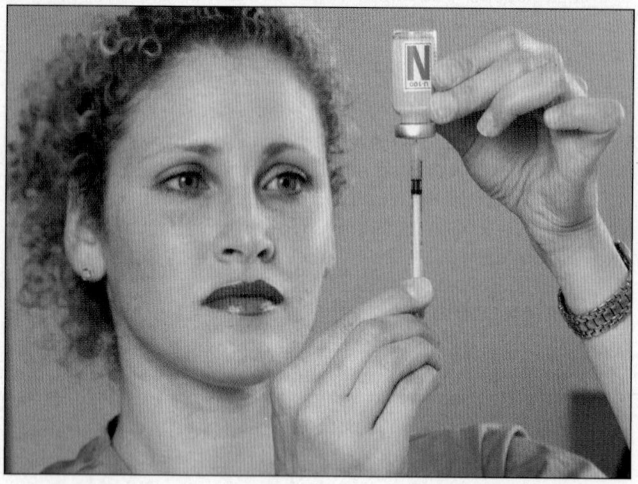

■ Wipe the rubber stopper of the first vial again, allow it to dry, and insert the needle, taking care not to depress the plunger. Invert the vial, withdraw the prescribed dose, and then withdraw the needle.
■ Change the needle on the syringe, if indicated, to a safety needle.
■ Discard any needle in a puncture-resistant sharps container and all additional equipment appropriately.[17]

Mixing drugs from a multidose vial and an ampule

■ Remove the medication vial's lid.
■ Disinfect the stopper with an alcohol pad using friction and allow it to dry.[1,3]
■ Pull back the syringe plunger until the volume of air drawn into the syringe equals the volume to be withdrawn from the drug vial.
■ Insert the needle into the top of the vial and inject the air. Then invert the vial and keep the needle's bevel tip below the level of the solution as you withdraw the prescribed dose.
■ Put the sterile needle cover over the needle.
■ Tap the stem of the ampule *to move any medication from the stem into the body of the ampule.*
■ Wrap a sterile gauze pad or an alcohol pad around the ampule's neck *to protect yourself from injury in case the glass splinters.*[2]
■ Quickly snap off the top of the ampule along the scored line at the neck.[1] Snap the neck in the direction away from your body.
■ Change to a 5-micron filter needle *to filter out any glass splinters.*[3,18,19,20]
■ Insert the needle into the ampule. Be careful not to touch the outside of the ampule with the needle.
■ Draw the correct dose into the syringe.
■ Change the 5-micron filter needle to a safety needle to administer the injection.
■ Discard the needles and the ampule in a puncture-resistant sharps container, and discard all additional equipment appropriately.[17]

Mixing drugs from two ampules

■ Tap the stems of the ampules *to move any medication from the stems into the body of the ampules.*
■ Open each ampule by wrapping a sterile gauze pad or an alcohol pad around the ampule's neck *to protect yourself from injury in case the glass splinters.*[2]
■ Quickly snap off the top of each ampule along the scored line at the neck.[1] Snap the neck in the direction away from your body.
■ Insert a syringe with a filter needle attached *to filter out any glass splinters* into the ampule without allowing the needle to come into contact with the rim of the ampule. Be sure the needle is in the solution.[3,18,19,20]
■ Withdraw the amount ordered from the first ampule and remove the needle from the solution.
■ Repeat the previous four steps with the second ampule, changing the needle before drawing up the medication from the ampule if possible.
■ When the syringe is prepared, change to a regular safety needle to administer the medication.

Completing the procedure

■ Discard all equipment in appropriate receptacles.[17]
■ Perform hand hygiene.[1,12,13,14,15,16]
■ Document the procedure.[21,22,23]

Special considerations

■ Insert a needle through the vial's rubber stopper at a slight angle, bevel up, and exert slight lateral pressure. *This way you won't cut a piece of rubber out of the stopper, which can then be pushed into the vial.*
■ When mixing drugs from multidose vials, be careful not to contaminate one drug with the other. Ideally, the needle should be changed after drawing the first medication into the syringe, although this isn't always possible *because many disposable syringes don't have removable needles.*
■ Never combine drugs if you're unsure of their compatibility, and never combine more than two drugs. *Although drug incompatibility usually causes a visible reaction, such as clouding, bubbling, or precipitation, some incompatible combinations produce no visible reaction, even though they alter the chemical nature and action of the drugs.* Check appropriate references and consult a pharmacist when you're unsure about specific compatibility. When in doubt, administer two separate injections.
■ Some medications are compatible for only a brief time after being combined and should be administered within 10 minutes after mixing. After this time, environmental factors, such as temperature, exposure to light, and humidity, may alter compatibility.
■ Always follow manufacturer's instructions for storage and use of medication vials, and label multidose vials with the date immediately upon opening.
■ Keep multidose vials away from the immediate patient environment.[2]
■ *To reduce the risk of contamination,* most facilities dispense parenteral medications in single-dose vials. Insulin is one of the few drugs still packaged in multidose vials. Be careful when mixing regular and long-acting insulin. Draw up the regular insulin first *to avoid contamination with the long-acting suspension.* (If a minute amount of the regular insulin is accidentally mixed with the long-acting insulin, it won't appreciably change the effect of the long-acting insulin.)
■ Use multidose vials only if there is no other alternative, and make sure the vials are dedicated for a single patient if possible. Label multidose vials with the date, the patient's name, and your signature immediately after piercing.[1,24]
■ Use vials labeled by the manufacturer as "single dose" or "single use" for only one patient. *These medications may lack antimicrobial preservatives and can become contaminated and serve as a source of infection if used inappropriately. Evidence shows that improper use of single-dose vials for more than one patient increases the risk of infection.*[25]
■ *To reduce the risk of contamination,* most facilities dispense parenteral medications in single-dose vials.

Complications

Infection may result from improper technique.

Documentation

Record the drugs administered, injection site, and time of administration. Document any adverse drug reactions and other pertinent information.

REFERENCES

1 World Health Organization. (2010). "WHO best practices for injections and related procedures toolkit" [Online]. Accessed March 2015 via the Web at http://whqlibdoc.who.int/publications/ 2010/9789241599252_eng.pdf (Level IV)

2 Dolan, S. A., et al. (2010). APIC position paper: Safe injection, infusion and medication vial practices in healthcare. *American Journal of Infection Control, 38,* 167–172. Accessed March 2015 via the Web at http://www.apic.org/Resource_/TinyMceFileManager/Position_Statements/AJIC_Safe_Injection0310.pdf (Level I)

3 Standard 20. Compounding of parenteral solutions and medications. Infusion nursing standards of practice. (2011). *Journal of Infusion Nursing, 34,* S27. (Level VII)

4 American Osteopathic Association. (2014). Standard 07.02.03. *Healthcare Facilities Accreditation Program: Accreditation requirements for acute care hospitals.* Chicago, IL: American Osteopathic Association. (Level VII)

5 Westbrook, J., et al. (2010). Association of interruptions with an increased risk and severity of medication administration errors. *Archives of Internal Medicine, 170,* 683–690. (Level IV)

6 Institute for Safe Medication Practices. (2013). Side tracks on the safety express: Interruptions lead to errors and unfinished... Wait, what was I doing? *Nurse Advise-ERR, 11*(2), 1–4. Accessed March 2015 via the Web at https://www.ismp.org/Newsletters/acutecare/showarticle.aspx?id=37 (Level VII)

7 The Joint Commission. (2015). Standard MM.06.01.01. *Comprehensive accreditation manual for hospitals: The official handbook.* Oakbrook Terrace, IL: The Joint Commission. (Level VII)

8 American Osteopathic Association. (2014). Standard 16.01.03. *Healthcare Facilities Accreditation Program: Accreditation requirements for acute care hospitals.* Chicago, IL: American Osteopathic Association. (Level VII)

9 Centers for Medicare & Medicaid Services, Department of Health and Human Services. (2014). Condition of participation: Nursing services. 42 C.F.R. § 482.23(c).

10 Institute for Safe Medication Practices. (2008). Conducting an independent double-check. *ISMP Medication Safety Alert! Nurse Advise-ERR, 6*(12), 1. Accessed March 2015 via the Web at http://www.ismp.org/Newsletters/nursing/Issues/NurseAdviseERR200812.pdf (Level VII)

11 Institute for Safe Medication Practices. (2012). "ISMP's list of high-alert medications" [Online]. Accessed March 2015 via the Web at http://www.ismp.org/tools/highalertmedications.pdf (Level VII)

12 The Joint Commission. (2015). Standard NPSG.07.01.01. *Comprehensive accreditation manual for hospitals: The official handbook.* Oakbrook Terrace, IL: The Joint Commission. (Level VII)

13 Centers for Disease Control and Prevention. (2002). Guideline for hand hygiene in health-care settings: Recommendations of the Healthcare Infection Control Practices Advisory Committee and the HICPAC/SHEA/APIC/IDSA Hand Hygiene Task Force. *MMWR Recommendations and Reports, 51*(RR-16), 1–45. Accessed March 2015 via the Web at http://www.cdc.gov/mmwr/pdf/rr/rr5116.pdf (Level II)

14 World Health Organization. (2009). "WHO guidelines on hand hygiene in health care: First global patient safety challenge, clean care is safer care" [Online]. Accessed March 2015 via the Web at http://whqlibdoc.who.int/publications/2009/9789241597906_eng.pdf (Level IV)

15 American Osteopathic Association. (2014). Standard 07.01.10. *Healthcare Facilities Accreditation Program: Accreditation requirements for acute care hospitals.* Chicago, IL: American Osteopathic Association. (Level VII)

16 Centers for Medicare & Medicaid Services, Department of Health and Human Services. (2014). Condition of participation: Infection control. 42 C.F.R. § 482.42.

17 Occupational Safety and Health Administration. (n.d.). "Bloodborne pathogens, standard number 1910.1030" [Online]. Accessed March 2015 via the Web at http://www.osha.gov/pls/oshaweb/owadisp.show_document?p_table=standards&p_id=10051 (Level VII)

18 Stein, H. G. (2006). Glass ampules and filter needles: An example of implementing the sixth 'R' in medication administration. *MedSurg Nursing, 15,* 290–294.

19 Hafez, M. A., & Al-Dars, A. M. (2012). Glass foreign bodies inside the knee joint following intra-articular injection. *The American Journal of Case Reports, 13,* 238–240. Accessed March 2015 via the Web at http://www.ncbi.nlm.nih.gov/pmc/articles/PMC3616057/

20 Standard 28. Filters. Infusion nursing standards of practice. (2011). *Journal of Infusion Nursing, 34,* S33–S34. (Level VII)

21 American Osteopathic Association. (2014). Standard 10.00.03. *Healthcare Facilities Accreditation Program: Accreditation requirements for acute care hospitals.* Chicago, IL: American Osteopathic Association. (Level VII)

22 Centers for Medicare & Medicaid Services, Department of Health and Human Services. (2014). Condition of participation: Medical record services. 42 C.F.R. § 482.24(b).

23 The Joint Commission. (2015). Standard RC.01.03.01. *Comprehensive accreditation manual for hospitals: The official handbook.* Oakbrook Terrace, IL: The Joint Commission. (Level VII)

24 American Osteopathic Association. (2014). Standard 25.01.18. *Healthcare Facilities Accreditation Program: Accreditation requirements for acute care hospitals.* Chicago, IL: American Osteopathic Association. (Level VII)

25 Centers for Disease Control and Prevention. (2012). "Single-dose/single-use vial position and messages" [Online]. Accessed March 2015 via the Web at http://www.cdc.gov/injectionsafety/PDF/CDC-SDV-Position05022012.pdf

ADDITIONAL REFERENCE

Nettina, S. M. (2014). *Lippincott manual of nursing practice* (10th ed.). Philadelphia, PA: Wolters Kluwer.

ADVANCE DIRECTIVES

The Patient Self-Determination Act of 1990[1] requires health care facilities to provide information about the patient's right to choose and refuse treatment. An advance directive is a legal document used as a guideline for providing life-sustaining medical care to a patient with an advanced disease or disability who is no longer able to indicate his own wishes.[2] Advance directives include living wills and health care proxies.

All patients should be encouraged to have an advance directive as part of an admission, before routine medical treatment, and during annual physical examinations at their primary practitioner's office. All adults, regardless of their current health status, should make their preferences about medical treatment known before a serious injury or unexpected illness occurs. The advance directive should be discussed with the patient's practitioner, family, and health care agent.

If a patient is terminally ill or in a persistent vegetative state or coma, a living will instructs health care providers about the patient's preferences for life-sustaining treatment. In making a living will, a legally competent patient states which procedures he does or doesn't want carried out, such as endotracheal intubation and mechanical ventilation, feeding tube insertion, parenteral or enteral nutrition and hydration, antibiotic therapy, dialysis, and cardiopulmonary resuscitation. The living will goes into effect when a patient can no longer communicate his choices regarding medical care. (See *The living will,* page 8.)

In the health care proxy (also called *durable power of attorney for health care*), the patient designates another person to make decisions; this person is commonly referred to as a health care agent. (See *Health care proxy,* page 9.)

The living will

The living will is an advance care document that specifies a patient's wishes with regard to medical care should he become terminally ill, incompetent, or unable to communicate. This will is commonly used in combination with the patient's health care proxy.

All states and the District of Columbia have laws that outline the documentation requirements for living wills. The sample document below is from Ohio.

Living Will

If my attending doctor and one other practitioner who examines me determine, to a reasonable degree of medical certainty and in accordance with reasonable medical standards, that I am in a terminal condition or in a permanently unconscious state, and if my attending doctor determines that at that time I no longer am able to make informed decisions regarding the administration of life-sustaining treatment, and that, to a reasonable degree of medical certainty and in accordance with reasonable medical standards, there is no reasonable possibility that I will regain the capacity to make informed decisions regarding the administration of life-sustaining treatment, then I direct my attending doctor to withhold or withdraw medical procedures, treatment, interventions, or other measures that serve principally to prolong the process of my dying, rather than diminish my pain or discomfort.

I have used the term "terminal condition" in this declaration to mean an irreversible, incurable, and untreatable condition caused by disease, illness, or injury from which, to a reasonable degree of medical certainty as determined in accordance with reasonable medical standards of my attending doctor and one other practitioner who has examined me, both of the following apply:

1. There can be no recovery.
2. Death is likely to occur within a relatively short time if life-sustaining treatment is not administered.

I have used the term "permanently unconscious state" in this declaration to mean a state of permanent unconsciousness that, to a reasonable degree of medical certainty, is determined in accordance with reasonable medical standards by my attending doctor and one other practitioner who has examined me, as characterized by both of the following:

1. I am irreversibly unaware of myself and my environment.
2. There is a total loss of cerebral cortical functioning, resulting in my having no capacity to experience pain or suffering.

Nutrition and hydration

I hereby authorize my attending doctor to withhold or withdraw nutrition and hydration from me when I am in a permanent unconscious state if my attending doctor and at least one other practitioner who has examined me determine, to a reasonable degree of medical certainty and in accordance with reasonable medical standards, that nutrition or hydration will not or no longer will serve to provide comfort to me or alleviate my pain.

[Sign here for withdrawal of nutrition or hydration] ____________________

I hereby designate [Print name of person to decide] as the person who I wish my attending doctor to notify at any time that life-sustaining treatment is to be withdrawn or withheld pursuant to this Declaration.

____________________ ____________________

[Sign your name here] [Today's date]

Witnessed by: ____________________

[Living will person's name] voluntarily signed or directed another individual to sign this Living Will in the presence of the following who each attests that the Declarant appears to be of sound mind and not under or subject to duress, fraud, or undue influence.

____________________ ____________________

[First witness signs here] [Second witness signs here]

Adapted from: Midwest Care Alliance. (2010). "State of Ohio living will declaration" [Online]. Accessed March 2015 via the Web at http://associationdatabase.com/aws/MCA/asset_manager/get_file/32895/choices_april_2011.pdf

Equipment

Advance directive forms or a copy of the previously established advance directive ■ Optional: written or audiovisual information on advance directives.

Implementation

- Perform hand hygiene.[3,4,5,6,7]
- Confirm the patient's identity using at least two patient identifiers.[8]
- Ask the patient whether he has an advance directive.[1]

If the patient has an advance directive

- Review the advance directive with the patient and confirm that it still reflects his wishes.
- Place the advance directive in the medical record *so that it's easily accessible to all health care providers.*[2,9,10]
- Notify the practitioner and the rest of the health care team that the patient has an advance directive *so that it can be used to guide care.*[2,11]
- Determine whether the health care agent has a copy of the advance directive.
- Encourage the patient to discuss his advance directive with his family and health care agent *so that they understand the patient's wishes and can ask questions while the patient is competent and can explain his decisions.*
- Perform hand hygiene.[3,4,5,6,7]
- Document the procedure and that the patient has an advance directive.[2,10,12,13,14]

A

Health care proxy

The sample document below is an example of a health care proxy, which allows a competent patient to delegate to another person the authority to consent to or refuse health care treatment for him. This document helps the patient ensure that his wishes will be carried out if he should become incompetent.

Each state with a health care proxy law has specific requirements for executing the document. The sample form below is from Nebraska.

Power of attorney for health care

I appoint ______________________________

whose address is ______________________________

and whose telephone number is ______________________________

as my attorney-in-fact for health care. ______________________________

I appoint ______________________________

whose address is ______________________________

and whose telephone number is ______________________________

as my successor attorney-in-fact for health care. ______________________________

I authorize my attorney-in-fact appointed by this document to make health care decisions for me when I am determined to be incapable of making my own health care decisions. I have read the warning that accompanies this document and understand the consequences of executing a power of attorney for health care.

I direct that my attorney-in-fact comply with the following instructions or limitations (optional):

I direct that my attorney-in-fact comply with the following instructions on life-sustaining treatment (optional):

I direct that my attorney-in-fact comply with the following instructions on artificially administered nutrition and hydration (optional):

I have read this power of attorney for health care. I understand that it allows another person to make life and death decisions for me if I am incapable of making such decisions. I also understand that I can revoke this power of attorney for health care at any time by notifying my attorney-in-fact, my physician, or the facility in which I am a patient or resident. I also understand that I can require in this power of attorney for health care that the fact of my incapacity in the future be confirmed by a second physician.

______________________________ ______________________________

[signature of person making designation] [date]

____

Adapted from: Nebraska Department of Health & Human Services, Division of Medicaid & Long-Term Care. (n.d.). "Nebraska Power of Attorney for Health Care" [Online]. Accessed March 2015 via the Web at http://dhhs.ne.gov/medicaid/Documents/Power-of-Attorney.pdf

If the patient doesn't have an advance directive

■ Provide the patient with verbal and written information about advance directives *so that he can make an informed decision about developing one.*[2,11]

■ Answer the patient's questions about advance directives or have a social worker or patient representative discuss advance directives with him *to provide accurate information.*[2,11]

■ Assist in the assessment of the patient's level of competency *to ensure that he can make decisions.* This process may include assessing his ability to understand information, consider the alternatives, evaluate the alternatives in relation to his own situation, make a decision, and communicate his choice. A doctor or advanced practice nurse may determine the patient's capacity for making decisions.

■ Perform hand hygiene.[3,4,5,6,7]

■ Document the procedure and note that the patient doesn't have an advance directive.[2,10,12,13,14]

Special considerations

■ If family members express opposition to the patient's advance directive, notify the patient's practitioner, the nursing supervisor, and the risk manager. Encourage family members to discuss their feelings with the patient and these individuals. A consult with the facility's ethics committee may be requested, as indicated.

■ The patient may revoke or change his advance directive at any time.[11] For example, the patient may revoke his directive if he changes his mind about his previous decision or if his condition mandates that he revise his directive. The patient can revoke an advance directive either orally or in writing.

Documentation

Document the presence of an advance directive[4] and that the practitioner was notified of its presence.[2,11] Include the name of the practitioner and the time of notification. Include the name, address, and telephone number of the health care agent. If the patient's wishes differ from those of his practitioner or family, note the discrepancies.

If the patient doesn't have an advance directive, document that he was given written information concerning his rights under state law to make decisions regarding health care. If the patient refuses information on an advance directive, document this refusal using the patient's own words, in quotes, if possible. Record any conversations with the patient regarding his decision making. Document that proof of competence was obtained.

References

1 Patient Self-Determination Act of 1990, 42 U.S.C. §§ 4206, 4751 (1990).

2 Centers for Medicare & Medicaid Services, Department of Health and Human Services. (2014). Condition of participation: Patient's rights. 42 C.F.R. § 482.13(b).

3 The Joint Commission. (2015). Standard NPSG.07.01.01. *Comprehensive accreditation manual for hospitals: The official handbook.* Oakbrook Terrace, IL: The Joint Commission. (Level VII)

4 Centers for Disease Control and Prevention. (2002). "Guideline for hand hygiene in health-care settings: Recommendations of the Healthcare Infection Control Practices Advisory Committee and the HICPAC/SHEA/APIC/IDSA Hand Hygiene Task Force" [Online]. *MMWR Recommendations and Reports, 51*(RR-16), 1–45. Accessed March 2015 via the Web at http://www.cdc.gov/mmwr/pdf/rr/rr5116.pdf (Level II)

5 World Health Organization. (2009). "WHO guidelines on hand hygiene in health care: First global patient safety challenge, clean care is safer care" [Online]. Accessed March 2015 via the Web at http://whqlibdoc.who.int/publications/2009/ 9789241597906_eng.pdf (Level IV)

6 Centers for Medicare & Medicaid Services, Department of Health and Human Services. (2014). Condition of participation: Infection control. 42 C.F.R. § 482.42.

7 American Osteopathic Association. (2014). Standard 07.01.21. *Healthcare Facilities Accreditation Program: Accreditation requirements for acute care hospitals.* Chicago, IL: American Osteopathic Association. (Level VII)

8 The Joint Commission. (2015). Standard NPSG.01.01.01. *Comprehensive accreditation manual for hospitals: The official handbook.* Oakbrook Terrace, IL: The Joint Commission. (Level VII)

9 The Joint Commission. (2015). Standard RC.02.01.01. *Comprehensive accreditation manual for hospitals: The official handbook.* Oakbrook Terrace, IL: The Joint Commission. (Level VII)

10 American Osteopathic Association. (2014). Standard 15.01.12. *Healthcare Facilities Accreditation Program: Accreditation requirements for acute care hospitals.* Chicago, IL: American Osteopathic Association. (Level VII)

11 The Joint Commission. (2015). Standard RI.01.05.01. *Comprehensive accreditation manual for hospitals: The official handbook.* Oakbrook Terrace, IL: The Joint Commission. (Level VII)

12 The Joint Commission. (2015). Standard RC.01.03.01. *Comprehensive accreditation manual for hospitals: The official handbook.* Oakbrook Terrace, IL: The Joint Commission. (Level VII)

13 Centers for Medicare & Medicaid Services, Department of Health and Human Services. (2014). Condition of participation: Medical record services. 42 C.F.R. § 482.24.

14 American Osteopathic Association. (2014). Standard 10.00.03. *Healthcare Facilities Accreditation Program: Accreditation requirements for acute care hospitals.* Chicago, IL: American Osteopathic Association. (Level VII)

Additional references

Bacon, D., et al. (2007). Position statement on laws and regulations concerning life-sustaining treatment, including artificial nutrition and hydration, for patients lacking decision-making capacity. *Neurology, 68,* 1097–1100.

Duke, G., et al. (2007). Factors influencing completion of advanced directives in hospitalized patients. *International Journal of Palliative Nursing, 13,* 39–43.

Nishimura, A., et al. (2007). Patients who complete advanced directives and what they prefer. *Mayo Clinic Proceedings, 82,* 1480–1486.

Watson, E. (2010). Advanced directives: Self-determination, legislation, and litigation issues. *Journal of Legal Nursing Consulting, 21*(1), 97–14.

Airborne precautions

Airborne precautions, used in addition to standard precautions, prevent the spread of infectious droplet nuclei (small particles that become suspended in the air and disperse over long distances by air currents). Because the infectious particles can become suspended in the air, they may be inhaled by susceptible individuals who haven't had face-to-face contact with their source (the infected individual).[1] (See *Conditions requiring airborne precautions.*)

Effective airborne precautions require an airborne infection isolation room—a single-patient room that's equipped with monitored negative pressure (in relation to the surrounding area). An airborne infection isolation room should have 12 air exchanges/hour if the room has been newly constructed or renovated, or 6 air exchanges/hour if it's an existing room. The air is either vented directly to the outside of the building or filtered through high-efficiency particulate air (HEPA) filtration before recirculation.[1,2,3] According to the Centers for Disease Control and Prevention (CDC), air pressure should be monitored daily, using visual indicators, while the room is in use.[3] The door to the room should be kept closed to maintain the proper air pressure balance between the isolation room and the adjoining hallway or corridor. An anteroom is preferred.

All people who enter an airborne infection isolation room must wear respiratory protection, provided by a disposable respirator (such as an N95 respirator or a HEPA respirator) or a reusable respirator (such as a HEPA respirator or a powered air-purifying respirator [PAPR]).[1,3] Regardless of the type you use, perform a user seal check each time you put on a respirator to make sure that it properly fits to your face.[1,3] When using a PAPR, also ensure proper functioning of the unit.

NURSING ALERT **When a patient comes to your facility complaining of respiratory signs and symptoms and an airborne infection is suspected, put a surgical mask on him (if tolerated) and immediately place him in a private room with the door closed until an airborne infection isolation room is available. If the patient is unable to tolerate a mask, place him in a private room with the door closed and wear a respirator to care for him.**

Equipment

Respirators (either disposable N95 or HEPA respirators or reusable HEPA respirators or PAPRs) ■ surgical masks ■ isolation sign ■ patient care reminders ■ tissues ■ no-touch receptacle.

Conditions requiring airborne precautions[1]

If a patient is known to have a condition requiring airborne precautions, the facility should follow the Centers for Disease Control and Prevention's (CDC's) isolation precautions *to prevent the spread of organisms spread by the airborne route.*[2] This table outlines some common conditions that require airborne precautions, including the required duration and any special considerations.

CONDITION	PRECAUTIONARY PERIOD	SPECIAL CONSIDERATIONS (AS APPLICABLE)
Avian influenza	■ For 14 days after onset of signs and symptoms or until an alternate diagnosis is confirmed	■ N/A
Chickenpox (varicella)	■ Until lesions are crusted and no new lesions appear	■ Susceptible health care workers shouldn't enter the room if immune caregivers are available. ■ Contact precautions should be instituted.
Herpes zoster (disseminated disease in any patient or localized disease in immunocompromised patient until disseminated disease is ruled out)	■ For duration of illness	■ Susceptible health care workers shouldn't enter the room if immune caregivers are available. ■ Contact precautions should be instituted.
Measles (rubeola)	■ For 4 days after onset of rash ■ For duration of illness in immunocompromised patients	■ Susceptible health care workers shouldn't enter the room if immune caregivers are available.
Monkeypox	■ Until disease is confirmed and smallpox is excluded	■ Contact precautions should be instituted until lesions have crusted.
Severe acute respiratory syndrome	■ For duration of illness plus 10 days after resolution of fever	■ Eye protection (goggles or face shield) should be worn. ■ Contact precautions should be instituted. ■ Vigilant environmental disinfection should be performed.
Smallpox	■ For duration of illness until all scabs have crusted and separated (typically 3 to 4 weeks)	■ Contact precautions should be instituted. ■ Unvaccinated health care workers shouldn't provide care when immune health care workers are available.
Tuberculosis, extrapulmonary, draining lesion	■ Until patient improves clinically and drainage has ceased or until three consecutive negative cultures of continued drainage are obtained	■ Contact precautions should be instituted.
Tuberculosis, pulmonary or laryngeal disease, confirmed	■ Until patient improves clinically while on effective therapy (decreased cough and fever, improved chest X-ray) and has three consecutive sputum smears negative for acid-fast bacillus, collected on separate days	■ N/A
Tuberculosis, pulmonary or laryngeal disease, suspected	■ Until active tuberculosis is deemed highly unlikely and either another diagnosis explains the clinical findings or the results of three consecutive sputum smears for acid-fast bacillus, collected 8 to 24 hours apart, are negative	■ At least one of the three sputum specimens should be collected in the morning.

Preparation of equipment

Keep all airborne precaution supplies outside the patient's room in a wall- or door-mounted cabinet, a cart, or an anteroom.

Implementation

■ Review the patient's medical record and verify the need for airborne precautions.

■ Gather the equipment.

■ Perform hand hygiene.[4,5,6,7,8]

■ Confirm the patient's identify using at least two patient identifiers.[9]

■ Situate the patient in a single-patient airborne infection isolation room with the door closed.[1] If possible, the room should have an anteroom. If a private bathroom is available, make sure the bathroom is also under negative air pressure. Monitor negative pressure according to regulations.

■ Explain isolation precautions to the patient and family *to ease patient anxiety and promote cooperation.*

EQUIPMENT

Respirator seal check

After you properly put on your respirator, perform a seal check. To do so, place your hands over the face piece, as shown below, and then exhale gently. The seal is considered satisfactory if a slight positive pressure builds up inside the face piece without air leaking from the seal. Evidence of air leaking from the seal includes fogging of your glasses, a feeling of air trickling down your uncovered face, and lack of pressure buildup under the face piece.

If the respirator has an exhalation valve, cover the filter surface with your hands as much as possible and then inhale. The seal is considered satisfactory if the face piece collapses on your face and you don't feel air passing between your face and the face piece.

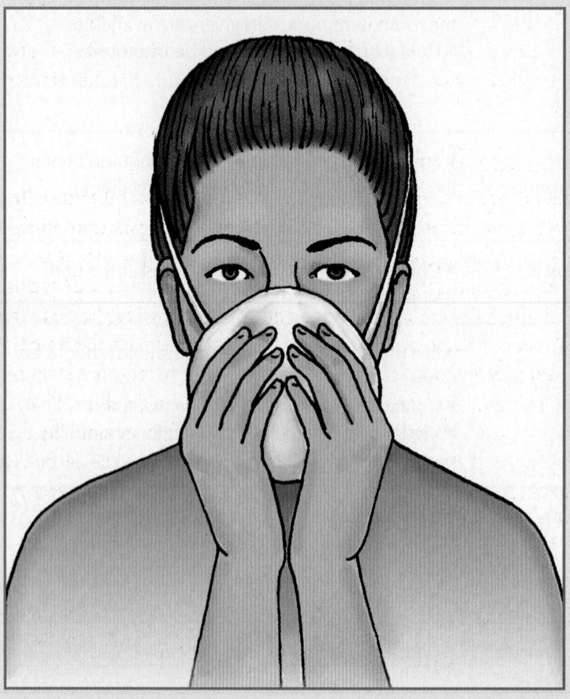

- Keep the patient's door (and the anteroom door) closed at all times *to maintain negative pressure and contain the airborne pathogens.*[1] Put an AIRBORNE PRECAUTIONS sign on the door *to notify anyone entering the room of the situation.*
- Put on a respirator according to the manufacturer's instructions. Adjust the straps for a firm but comfortable fit. Check the seal. (See *Respirator seal check.*)
- If you're using a PAPR, check for proper function, battery life, and air flow.
- Remove the patient's mask, if he's wearing one.
- Provide the patient with tissues, and instruct him to cover his nose and mouth with a tissue when coughing or sneezing. Place a sign in the patient's room as a reminder.[1]
- Provide the patient with a no-touch receptacle for used tissue disposal. Instruct him to dispose of tissues in the receptacle after use and to perform hand hygiene after contact with respiratory secretions and contaminated objects.[10]
- Perform hand hygiene.[4,5,6,7,8]
- Remove your respirator after leaving the patient's room and closing the door. To remove your respirator, grasp the bottom and then the top elastic; avoid touching the front of the respirator *because the front is considered contaminated.*
- Discard the respirator in the appropriate receptacle, or store it for reuse. You may reuse an N95 respirator according to the manufacturer's recommendations if it's not damaged or soiled.
- Perform hand hygiene.[4,5,6,7,8]
- Document the procedure.[11,12,13]

Special considerations

- Keep in mind that all health care workers should wear a respirator when entering an airborne infection isolation room *to minimize the transmission of airborne organisms such as* Mycobacterium tuberculosis.[3]
- Before entering the patient's room, check the seal on your respirator *to confirm that the respirator fits appropriately.* The seal should be checked both initially and then periodically at a frequency determined by federal, state, and local regulations.[3]
- Teach visitors the proper way to wear respiratory protection, and make sure that they wear respiratory protection while in the patient's room.[3]
- Limit the patient's movement from the room. If the patient must leave for essential procedures, make sure he wears a surgical mask, covering his nose and mouth.[1,3] Notify the receiving staff of the patient's isolation precautions *so that the precautions will be maintained and the patient will be promptly returned to his room.*
- Depending on the type of respirator and recommendations from the manufacturer, discard your respirator or store it until the next use.[1] If storing your respirator for reuse, store it in a dry, well-ventilated place (not a plastic bag) *to prevent microbial growth.* Clean nondisposable respirators according to the manufacturer's recommendations.
- If a patient on airborne precautions requires surgery, try to schedule the procedure when a minimal number of health care workers and other patients are present. If possible, schedule the procedure as the last case of the day *so that more time is available to clean and disinfect the operating room.* Use an operating room with an anteroom, if possible. Make sure that all staff members involved in the surgery wear respiratory protection.[3]
- After a patient with suspected or confirmed *M. tuberculosis* leaves an airborne infection isolation room, allow adequate time to elapse before allowing another patient to enter *to ensure that contaminated air is removed from the room.* The CDC recommends that a room with six air exchanges/hour be left empty for 69 minutes to effectively remove 99.9% of airborne contaminants.[3]

Complications

Social isolation is a complication of airborne precautions.

Documentation

Record the need for airborne precautions on the nursing care plan and as otherwise determined by your facility. Document initiation and maintenance of the precautions, the patient's tolerance of the procedure, and any patient or family teaching performed and their understanding of that teaching. Also document the date airborne precautions were discontinued.

REFERENCES

1 Siegel, J. D., et al. (2007). "2007 guideline for isolation precautions: Preventing transmission of infectious agents in healthcare settings" [Online]. Accessed March 2015 via the Web at http://www.cdc.gov/hicpac/pdf/isolation/Isolation2007.pdf (Level II)

2 The Joint Commission. (2015). Standard IC.01.05.01. *Comprehensive accreditation manual for hospitals: The official handbook.* Oakbrook Terrace, IL: The Joint Commission. (Level VII)

3 Centers for Disease Control and Prevention. (2005). Guidelines for preventing the transmission of *Mycobacterium tuberculosis* in health-care settings, 2005. *MMWR Recommendations and Reports, 54*(RR-17), 1–140. Accessed March 2015 via the Web at http://www.cdc.gov/mmwr/PDF/rr/rr5417.pdf (Level II)

4 Centers for Disease Control and Prevention. (2002). Guideline for hand hygiene in health-care settings: Recommendations of the Healthcare Infection Control Practices Advisory Committee and the HICPAC/SHEA/APIC/IDSA Hand Hygiene Task Force. *MMWR Recommendations and Reports, 51*(RR-16), 1–45. Accessed March 2015 via the Web at http://www.cdc.gov/mmwr/pdf/rr/rr5116.pdf (Level II)

5 The Joint Commission. (2015). Standard NPSG.07.01.01. *Comprehensive accreditation manual for hospitals: The official handbook.* Oakbrook Terrace, IL: The Joint Commission. (Level VII)

6 World Health Organization. (2009). "WHO guidelines on hand hygiene in health care: First global patient safety challenge, clean care is safer care" [Online]. Accessed March 2015 via the Web at http://whqlibdoc.who.int/publications/2009/9789241597906_eng.pdf (Level IV)

7 Centers for Medicare & Medicaid Services, Department of Health and Human Services. (2014). Condition of participation: Infection control. 42 C.F.R. § 482.42.

8 American Osteopathic Association. (2014). Standard 07.01.21. *Healthcare Facilities Accreditation Program: Accreditation requirements for acute care hospitals.* Chicago, IL: American Osteopathic Association. (Level VII)

9 The Joint Commission. (2015). Standard NPSG.01.01.01. *Comprehensive accreditation manual for hospitals: The official handbook.* Oakbrook Terrace, IL: The Joint Commission. (Level VII)

10 Centers for Disease Control and Prevention. (2012). "Respiratory hygiene/cough etiquette in healthcare settings" [Online]. Accessed March 2015 via the Web at http://www.cdc.gov/flu/professionals/infectioncontrol/resphygiene.htm

11 The Joint Commission. (2015). Standard RC.01.03.01. *Comprehensive accreditation manual for hospitals: The official handbook.* Oakbrook Terrace, IL: The Joint Commission. (Level VII)

12 Centers for Medicare & Medicaid Services, Department of Health and Human Services. (2014). Condition of participation: Medical record services. 42 C.F.R. § 482.24.

13 American Osteopathic Association. (2014). Standard 10.00.03. *Healthcare Facilities Accreditation Program: Accreditation requirements for acute care hospitals.* Chicago, IL: American Osteopathic Association. (Level VII)

ADDITIONAL REFERENCES

American Osteopathic Association. (2012). Standard 07.01.10. *Healthcare Facilities Accreditation Program: Accreditation requirements for acute care hospitals.* Chicago, IL: American Osteopathic Association. (Level VII)

Centers for Disease Control and Prevention (CDC). (2003). Guidelines for environmental infection control in health-care facilities: Recommendations of CDC and the Healthcare Infection Control Practices Advisory Committee (HICPAC). *MMWR Recommendations and Reports, 52*(RR-10), 1–42. Accessed March 2015 via the Web at http://www.cdc.gov/mmwr/preview/mmwrhtml/rr5210a1.htm (Level II)

Hughes, N. L. (2006). Respiratory protection, part 1: When and how to protect yourself. *American Journal of Nursing, 106*(1), 96.

Hughes, N. L. (2006). Respiratory protection, part 2: When and how to protect yourself. *American Journal of Nursing, 106*(2), 88.

AIR-FLUIDIZED THERAPY BED USE

Originally designed for managing burns, the air-fluidized therapy bed is now used for patients with various debilities. The surface of the bed conforms to the patient's bony surfaces. The patient's body is immersed into the bed's surface, which lowers the interface pressure by increasing the surface pressure distribution area.[1] By allowing harmless contact between the bed's surface and grafted sites, the bed promotes comfort and healing.

The traditional air-fluidized therapy bed is actually a large tub that supports the patient on a thick layer of silicone-coated microspheres of lime glass. Another version combines the air-fluidized section with a low-air-loss or cushioned section. (See *The air-fluidized therapy bed,* page 14.) A monofilament polyester filter sheet covers the microsphere-filled tub. Warmed air, propelled by a blower beneath the bed, passes through it. The resulting fluid-like surface reduces pressure on the skin to avoid obstructing capillary blood flow, which helps to prevent pressure ulcers and to promote wound healing.[2,3] The bed's air temperature can be adjusted to help control hypothermia and hyperthermia. The microprocessor technology also allows manipulation of various sections of the unit for optimum adjustment. Some models come with adjustable back and leg supports to promote positioning.

The air-fluidized therapy bed may be contraindicated for a patient with an unstable spine. It may also be contraindicated for a patient who can't mobilize and expel pulmonary secretions because the lack of back support impairs productive coughing. Operation of the air-fluidized therapy bed is complex and requires special training.

Equipment

Air-fluidized therapy bed with microspheres (about 1,650 lb [750 kg]) ■ filter sheet ■ flat sheet ■ elastic cord ■ patient transfer device ■ Optional: gloves, other personal protective equipment, foam wedge, humidifier and mask.

Preparation of equipment

A manufacturer's representative or a trained staff member usually prepares the bed for use. If you must help with the preparation, make sure the microspheres reach to within ½″ (1.3 cm) of the top of the tank. Then position the filter sheet on the bed with its printed side facing up. Match the holes in the sheet to the holes in the edge of the bed's frame. If the bed has detachable aluminum rails, place them on the frame, with the studs in the proper holes. Depress the rails firmly, and then secure them by tightening the knurled knobs to seal the filter sheet. Place a flat sheet over the filter sheet or use the specialized sheet provided by the bed company, and secure it with the elastic cord. Turn on the air current *to activate the microspheres and to ensure that the bed is working properly;* then turn it off.

Implementation

- Consult with a wound, ostomy, and continence nurse or an educated skin care team member before using an air-fluidized bed *to make sure it's the best choice of support surface for the patient.*
- Gather the equipment and help prepare the bed, if necessary.
- Perform hand hygiene and put on gloves and other personal protective equipment, if needed, *to comply with standard precautions.*[4,5,6,7,8,9,10,11]
- Confirm the patient's identity using at least two patient identifiers.[12]
- Explain and, if possible, demonstrate the operation of the air-fluidized therapy bed. Tell the patient the reason for its use and explain that he'll feel as though he's floating.
- With the help of three or more coworkers, transfer the patient to the bed using an appropriate transfer device.
- If the patient has a feeding tube, use a foam wedge to elevate the head of the bed *to prevent aspiration.*
- Turn on the air pressure *to activate the bed.*
- Remove the lift sheet.
- Adjust the air temperature as necessary. *Because the bed usually operates within 10° to 12°F (5.6° to 6.7°C) of ambient air temperature,* set the room temperature to 75°F (23.9°C). If the microsphere temperature reaches 105°F (40.6°C), the bed automatically shuts off; it restarts automatically after 30 minutes.
- Remove and discard your gloves and any other personal protective equipment worn.
- Perform hand hygiene.[4,5,6,8,10]
- Document the procedure.[13,14,15]

EQUIPMENT

The air-fluidized therapy bed

The air-fluidized therapy bed is a large tub filled with microspheres that are suspended by air pressure and give the patient fluidlike support. The bed provides the advantages of flotation without the disadvantages of instability, patient positioning difficulties, and immobility.

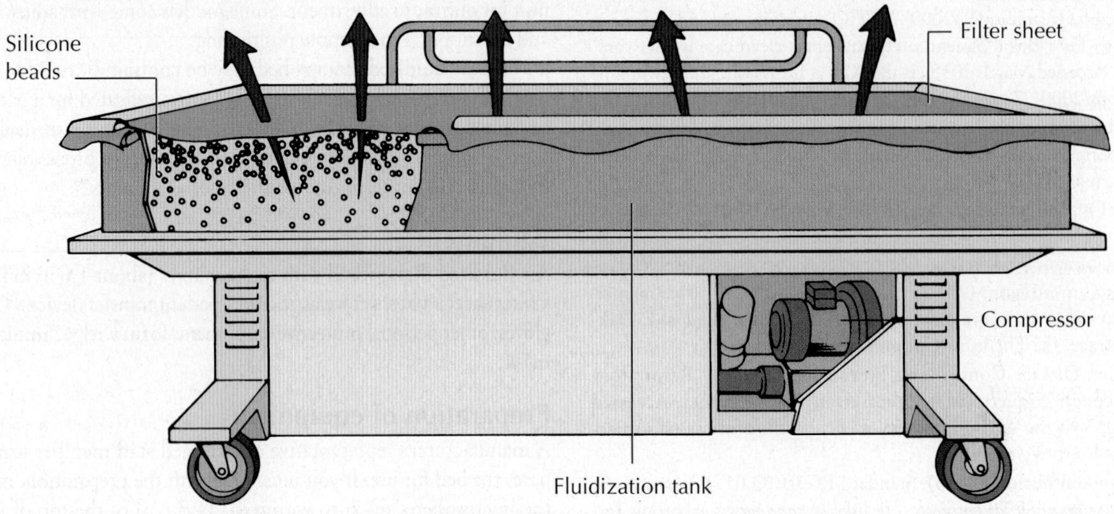

Special considerations

■ Monitor the patient's fluid and electrolyte status *because an air-fluidized therapy bed increases evaporative water loss.* Also, because of this drying effect, always cover a mesh graft for the first 2 to 8 days, as ordered. If the patient has excessive upper respiratory tract dryness, use a humidifier and mask, as ordered. Encourage coughing and deep breathing. After prolonged use of an air-fluidized bed, watch for hypocalcemia and hypophosphoremia.

■ To position a bedpan, roll the patient away from you, place the bedpan on the flat sheet, and push it into the microspheres. Then reposition the patient. To remove the bedpan, hold it steady and roll the patient away from you. Turn off the air pressure and remove the bedpan. Then turn the air on and reposition the patient.

■ Don't secure the filter sheet with pins or clamps *because they can puncture the sheet and release the microspheres.* Also take care to avoid puncturing the bed when giving injections. Repair holes or tears that occur with iron-on patching tape. Sieve the microspheres monthly or between patients *to remove any clumped microspheres.* Handle them carefully to avoid spills; *spilled microspheres can cause falls.* Treat a soiled filter sheet and clumped microspheres as contaminated items. Change the filter sheet and operate the unit unoccupied for 24 hours between patients.

■ Assess the patient's skin and reposition the patient every 2 hours. *Specialty beds don't eliminate the need for frequent assessment and position changes.*

■ For cardiopulmonary resuscitation, an emergency STOP/DEFLATE button immediately stops the action of the bed.

Documentation

Record the duration of therapy and the patient's response to it. Document the condition of the patient's skin, pressure ulcers, and other wounds.

References

1 Baranoski, S., & Ayello, E. A. (2012). *Wound care essentials: Practice principles* (3rd ed.). Philadelphia, PA: Lippincott Williams & Williams.

2 Ochs, R. F., et al. (2005). Comparison of air-fluidized therapy with other support surfaces used to treat pressure ulcers in nursing home residents. *Ostomy/Wound Management, 51,* 38–68.

3 Hickerson, W. L., et al. (2004). Comparison of total body tissue interface pressure of specialized pressure-relieving mattresses. *Journal of Long-Term Effects of Medical Implants, 14,* 81–94.

4 The Joint Commission. (2015). Standard NPSG.07.01.01. *Comprehensive accreditation manual for hospitals: The official handbook.* Oakbrook Terrace, IL: The Joint Commission. (Level VII)

5 Centers for Disease Control and Prevention. (2002). Guideline for hand hygiene in health-care settings: Recommendations of the Healthcare Infection Control Practices Advisory Committee and the HICPAC/SHEA/APIC/IDSA Hand Hygiene Task Force. *MMWR Recommendations and Reports, 51* (RR-16), 1–45. Accessed March 2015 via the Web at http://www.cdc.gov/mmwr/pdf/rr/rr5116.pdf (Level II)

6 World Health Organization. (2009). "WHO guidelines on hand hygiene in health care: First global patient safety challenge, clean care is safer care" [Online]. Accessed March 2015 via the Web at http://whqlibdoc.who.int/publications/2009/9789241597906_eng.pdf (Level IV)

7 Siegel, J. D., et al. (2007). "2007 guideline for isolation precautions: Preventing transmission of infectious agents in healthcare settings" [Online]. Accessed March 2015 via the Web at http://www.cdc.gov/hicpac/pdf/isolation/Isolation2007.pdf (Level II)

8 Centers for Medicare & Medicaid Services, Department of Health and Human Services. (2014). Condition of participation: Infection control. 42 C.F.R. § 482.42.

9 Perry, D., et al. (2012). "Institute for Clinical Systems Improvement: Pressure ulcer prevention and treatment protocol (3rd ed.)" [Online]. Accessed March 2015 via the Web at https://www.icsi.org/_asset/6t7kxy/PressureUlcer.pdf

10 American Osteopathic Association. (2014). Standard 07.01.21. *Healthcare Facilities Accreditation Program: Accreditation requirements for acute care hospitals.* Chicago, IL: American Osteopathic Association. (Level VII)
11 American Osteopathic Association. (2014). Standard 07.01.10. *Healthcare Facilities Accreditation Program: Accreditation requirements for acute care hospitals.* Chicago, IL: American Osteopathic Association. (Level VII)
12 The Joint Commission. (2015). Standard NPSG.01.01.01. *Comprehensive accreditation manual for hospitals: The official handbook.* Oakbrook Terrace, IL: The Joint Commission. (Level VII)
13 The Joint Commission. (2015). Standard RC.01.03.01. *Comprehensive accreditation manual for hospitals: The official handbook.* Oakbrook Terrace, IL: The Joint Commission. (Level VII)
14 Centers for Medicare & Medicaid Services, Department of Health and Human Services. (2014). Condition of participation: Medical record services. 42 C.F.R. § 482.24.
15 American Osteopathic Association. (2014). Standard 10.00.03. *Healthcare Facilities Accreditation Program: Accreditation requirements for acute care hospitals.* Chicago, IL: American Osteopathic Association. (Level VII)

ADDITIONAL REFERENCES

Hill-Rom. (2008). "Clinitron bed eLearning" [Online]. Accessed March 2015 via the Web at http://www.hill-rom.com/eLearningCourses/Clinitron/index.html?offline=true
VanGilder, C., & Lachenbruch, C. A. (2010). Air-fluidized therapy: Physical properties and clinical uses. *Annals of Plastic Surgery, 65,* 364–370.

ALIGNMENT AND PRESSURE-REDUCING DEVICES

Various assistive devices can be used to maintain correct body positioning and to help prevent complications that commonly arise when a patient must be on prolonged bed rest. Alignment and pressure-reducing devices, or pressure-redistribution devices, include boots to protect the heels and help prevent skin breakdown and footdrop; abduction pillows to help prevent internal hip rotation after femoral fracture, hip fracture, or surgery; trochanter rolls to help prevent external hip rotation; and hand rolls to help prevent hand contractures. Several of these devices—cradle boots, trochanter rolls, and hand rolls—are especially useful when caring for patients who have a loss of sensation, mobility, or consciousness.

Cradle boots, made of sponge rubber with heel cutouts, cushion the ankle and foot without completely enclosing it. Other commercial boots are available, but not all help to prevent external hip rotation. Footboards with antirotation blocks help prevent footdrop and external hip rotation, but they don't prevent heel pressure. High-topped sneakers may be used to help prevent footdrop, but they don't prevent external hip rotation or heel pressure. The abduction pillow is a wedge-shaped piece of sponge rubber with lateral indentations for the patient's thighs. Its straps wrap around the thighs to maintain correct positioning. Although a properly shaped bed pillow may temporarily substitute for the commercial abduction pillow, it's difficult to apply and fails to maintain the correct lateral alignment. The commercial trochanter roll is made of sponge rubber, but it can also be improvised from a rolled blanket or towel. The hand roll, available in hard and soft materials, is held in place by fixed or adjustable straps. It can be improvised from a rolled washcloth secured with roller gauze and adhesive tape. (See *Common preventive devices,* page 16.)

Equipment

Cradle boots ▪ abduction pillow ▪ trochanter rolls ▪ hand rolls ▪ Optional: washcloth, blanket or towel, roller gauze, hypoallergenic or adhesive tape.

Preparation of equipment

If you're using a device that's available in different sizes, select the appropriate size for the patient.

Implementation

- Gather the appropriate equipment.
- Perform hand hygiene.[1,2,3,4,5]
- Confirm the patient's identity using at least two patient identifiers.[6]
- Explain the purpose of the alignment and pressure-reducing device.
- Assess the patient's skin and perform a pressure ulcer risk assessment, paying special attention to where the device will be applied.

Applying a cradle boot

- Open the slit on the superior surface of the boot. Then place the patient's heel in the circular cutout area.
- Insert the other foot in the second boot and position the patient's legs properly *to prevent strain on hip ligaments and pressure on bony prominences.*

Applying an abduction pillow

- Place the patient in the supine position and slide the pillow between the patient's legs.
- Place the upper part of both of the patient's legs in the pillow's lateral indentations and secure the straps *to prevent the pillow from slipping.*

Applying a trochanter roll

- Position one trochanter roll, rolled towel, or blanket along the outside of the patient's thigh and place another roll along the other thigh. Make sure neither roll extends as far as the knee *to avoid peroneal nerve compression and palsy, which can lead to footdrop.*

Applying a hand roll

- Place one roll or rolled washcloth in each of the patient's hands *to maintain the neutral position.*
- Secure the strap, if present, or apply roller gauze and secure with hypoallergenic or adhesive tape.

Completing the procedure

- Reposition the patient at periodic *intervals to reduce the duration and magnitude of pressure over affected body surfaces.*[7,8,9,10]
- If the patient is able to reposition himself, teach him how to make small, frequent position changes.[9]
- Perform hand hygiene.[1,2,3,4,5]
- Document the procedure.[11,12,13]

Special considerations

- Remember that the use of assistive devices doesn't preclude regularly scheduled patient positioning, range-of-motion exercises, and skin care. Turn the patient a minimum of every 2 hours.[9]
- Assess the patient's pressure ulcer risk at regular intervals.[14]
- Monitor the skin integrity of skin that's located under a strap.
- Consult with a wound, ostomy, and continence nurse, as needed.

Patient teaching

Explain the proper use of each device, emphasizing proper alignment of extremities, and have the patient or caregiver give a return demonstration

EQUIPMENT

Common preventive devices

Equipment is available to reduce pressure or help maintain positioning, depending upon the patient's needs.

Cradle boot

Prevents footdrop, skin breakdown, and external hip rotation

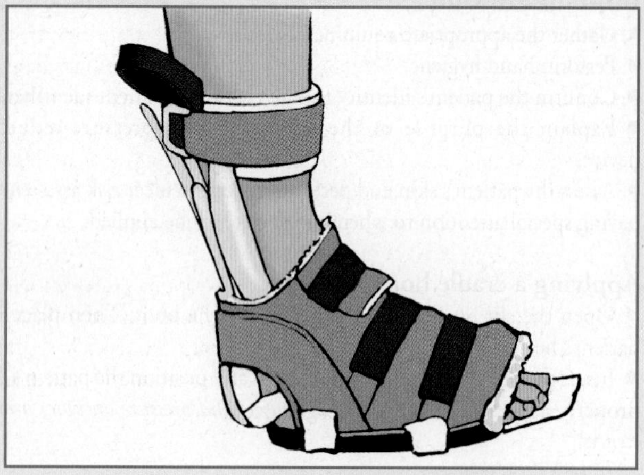

Trochanter roll

Prevents external hip rotation

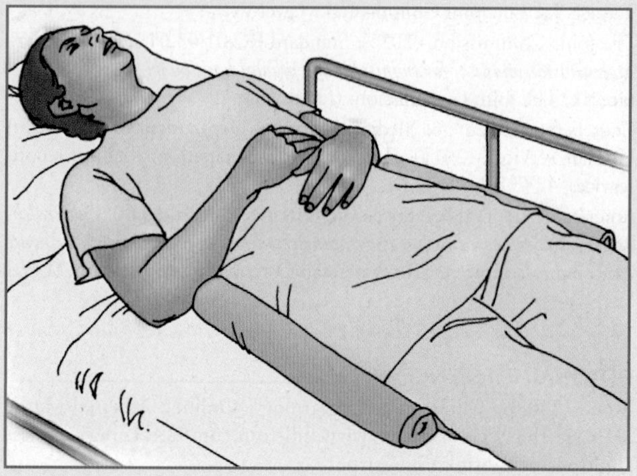

Abduction pillow

Prevents internal hip rotation and hip abduction

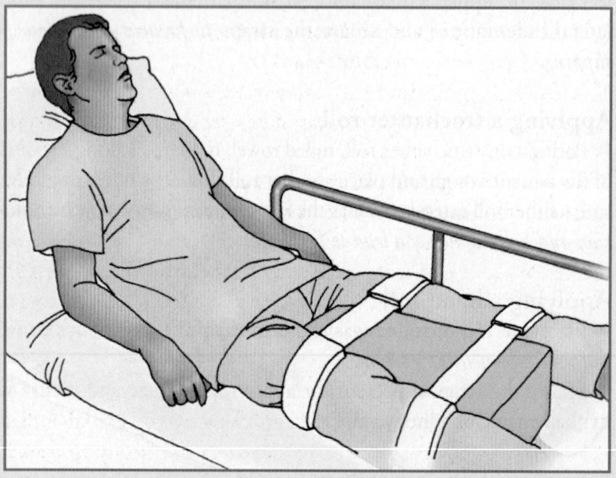

Hand roll

Prevents hand contractures

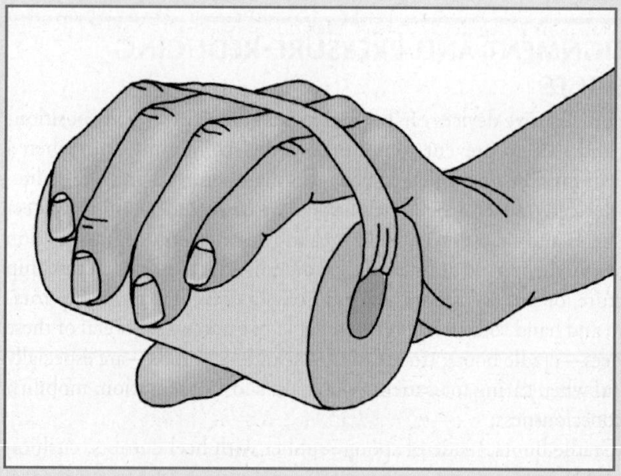

so you can check for proper technique. Emphasize measures needed to prevent pressure ulcers.

Complications

Contractures and pressure ulcers may occur with the use of a hand roll and possibly with other assistive devices. To avoid these problems, remove hand rolls every 2 hours.

Documentation

Record the use of these devices in the patient's chart and the nursing care plan, including the reason for the device. Document your assessment for complications as well as your pressure ulcer risk assessment. Also record any patient teaching performed and the patient's understanding. Reevaluate the patient care goals as needed.

References

1 The Joint Commission. (2015). Standard NPSG.07.01.01. *Comprehensive accreditation manual for hospitals: The official handbook.* Oakbrook Terrace, IL: The Joint Commission. (Level VII)

2 Centers for Disease Control and Prevention. (2002). Guideline for hand hygiene in health-care settings: Recommendations of the Healthcare Infection Control Practices Advisory Committee and the HICPAC/SHEA/APIC/IDSA Hand Hygiene Task Force. *MMWR Recommendations and Reports, 51* (RR-16), 1–45. Accessed March 2015 via the Web at http://www.cdc.gov/mmwr/pdf/rr/rr5116.pdf

3 World Health Organization. (2009). "WHO guidelines on hand hygiene in health care: First global patient safety challenge, clean care is safer care" [Online]. Accessed March 2015 via the Web at http://whqlibdoc.who.int/publications/2009/9789241597906_eng.pdf (Level IV)

4 Centers for Medicare & Medicaid Services, Department of Health and Human Services. (2014). Condition of participation: Infection control. 42 C.F.R. § 482.42.

5 American Osteopathic Association. (2014). Standard 07.01.21. *Healthcare Facilities Accreditation Program: Accreditation requirements for acute care hospitals.* Chicago, IL: American Osteopathic Association.
6 The Joint Commission. (2015). Standard NPSG.01.01.01. *Comprehensive accreditation manual for hospitals: The official handbook.* Oakbrook Terrace, IL: The Joint Commission.
7 Baranoski, S., & Ayello, E. A. (2012). *Wound care essentials: Practice principles* (3rd ed.). Philadelphia, PA: Lippincott Williams & Williams.
8 European Pressure Ulcer Advisory Panel & National Pressure Ulcer Advisory Panel. (2009). Treatment of pressure ulcers: Quick reference guide. Washington, DC: National Pressure Ulcer Advisory Panel. Accessed March 2015 via the Web at http://www.epuap.org/guidelines/Final_Quick_Treatment.pdf
9 Perry, D., et al. (2012). "Institute for Clinical Systems Improvement: Pressure ulcer prevention and treatment protocol (3rd ed.)" [Online]. Accessed March 2015 via the Web at https://www.icsi.org/_asset/6t7kxy/PressureUlcer.pdf (Level VII)
10 Black, J. (2012). Preventing pressure ulcers occurring on the heel. *Wounds International, 3*(3), 1–4. Accessed March 2015 via the Web at http://www.woundsinternational.com/pdf/content_10517.pdf
11 The Joint Commission. (2015). Standard RC.01.03.01. *Comprehensive accreditation manual for hospitals: The official handbook.* Oakbrook Terrace, IL: The Joint Commission.
12 Centers for Medicare & Medicaid Services, Department of Health and Human Services. (2014). Condition of participation: Medical record services. 42 C.F.R. § 482.24.
13 American Osteopathic Association. (2014). Standard 10.00.03. *Healthcare Facilities Accreditation Program: Accreditation requirements for acute care hospitals.* Chicago, IL: American Osteopathic Association. (Level VII)
14 National Pressure Ulcer Advisory Panel. (2007). "Pressure ulcer prevention points" [Online]. Accessed March 2015 via the Web at http://www.npuap.org/PU_Prev_Points.pdf

ADDITIONAL REFERENCE

Agency for Healthcare Research and Quality. (2011). "Preventing pressure ulcers in hospitals: A toolkit for improving quality of care" [Online]. Accessed March 2015 via the Web at http://www.ahrq.gov/research/ltc/pressureulcertoolkit/

ANGIOPLASTY CARE

A nonsurgical approach to opening coronary vessels narrowed by arteriosclerosis, percutaneous transluminal coronary angioplasty (PTCA) uses a balloon-tipped catheter that's inserted into a narrowed coronary artery. This procedure, performed in the cardiac catheterization laboratory under local anesthesia, helps restore circulation to the heart, relieving pain caused by angina and myocardial ischemia.

Angioplasty is a percutaneous coronary intervention. When it can be performed within 90 minutes of the patient's arrival at the emergency department, the American Heart Association recommends it as the treatment of choice for managing ST-elevation myocardial infarction (STEMI). The period of time from arrival at the emergency department until angioplasty is performed is commonly referred to as door-to-balloon time. When door-to-balloon time is less than 90 minutes, mortality rates are lower.[1,2]

When angioplasty is used to treat STEMI, it may be performed with or without stent placement. However, when a stent is placed, it decreases the risk of target vessel revascularization and may reduce the risk of myocardial reinfarction (MI). Because of this, stent placement has become routine during angioplasty in patients with STEMI.[3,4]

Cardiac catheterization usually accompanies PTCA to assess the stenosis and the efficacy of the angioplasty. Catheterization is used as a visual tool to direct the balloon-tipped catheter through the vessel's area of stenosis. After the balloon is in place, it's inflated, compressing the plaque against the vessel wall and allowing coronary blood to flow more freely. (See *Performing PTCA,* page 18.)

PTCA provides an alternative for patients who are poor surgical candidates because of chronic medical problems. It's also useful for patients who have total coronary occlusion, unstable angina, and plaque buildup in several areas and for those with poor left ventricular function. After angioplasty, it's important to monitor the patient closely for signs and symptoms of coronary spasm, MI, and bleeding at the insertion site.

Equipment

Antiseptic solution (preferably chlorhexidine-based) ■ local anesthetic ■ prescribed IV solution ■ IV administration set ■ electrocardiogram (ECG) monitor and electrodes ■ oxygen and oxygen delivery system ■ clippers ■ prescribed antiplatelet medication ■ prescribed sedative ■ contrast medium ■ emergency medications ■ emergency equipment, including a defibrillator, a handheld resuscitation bag, and intubation equipment ■ heparin (or other prescribed anticoagulant) for injection ■ introducer kit for PTCA catheter ■ eye protection ■ gloves ■ sterile gloves ■ sterile gown ■ surgical cap ■ mask ■ Optional: Doppler ultrasound flow detector, nitroglycerin, pulmonary artery catheter insertion kit, prescribed statin medication, eye protection, compression or hemostatic device, topical hemostatic agent as prescribed, semipermeable transparent dressing, supplies for venous blood sampling.

Implementation

Preprocedure care

- Verify the practitioner's orders.
- Check the patient's history for allergies; if he has had allergic reactions to any of the prescribed medications, notify the practitioner.[5]
- Make sure that informed consent has been obtained and the signed form is in the patient's medical record.[6]
- Perform a preprocedure verification *to make sure that all relevant documentation, related information, and equipment are available and correctly identified to the patient's identifiers.*[7]
- Verify that laboratory and imaging studies have been completed, as ordered, and that the results are in the patient's medical record; notify the practitioner of any unexpected results. Make sure that the results of coagulation studies, a complete blood count, serum electrolyte studies, and blood typing and crossmatching are available.[8] Review baseline hemodynamic parameters and patient medications for contraindications to the procedure.[5]
- Perform hand hygiene.[9,10,11]
- Confirm the patient's identity using at least two patient identifiers.[12]
- Explain the procedure to the patient and his family *to reduce the patient's fear and promote cooperation.*
- Inform the patient that the procedure lasts from 1 to 4 hours and that he may feel some discomfort from lying on a hard table for that long.
- Tell him that a catheter will be inserted into an artery or a vein in his groin and that he may feel pressure as the catheter moves along the vessel.
- Reassure him that, although he'll be awake during the procedure, he'll be given a sedative. Explain that the practitioner or nurse will ask him how he's feeling and that he should tell them if he experiences any chest pain.
- Explain that the practitioner will inject a contrast medium *to outline the lesion's location.* Warn the patient that he may feel a hot, flushing sensation or transient nausea during the injection.
- Administer a statin medication, as prescribed, following safe medication administration practices, *to reduce the risk for periprocedural MI.*[5]
- If PTCA isn't an emergency procedure, restrict food and fluids for a sufficient time to allow for gastric emptying, at least 2 hours for clear liquids and 6 hours for meals that include fried or fatty food or meat.[13]
- Perform hand hygiene.[9,10,11]

Performing PTCA

Percutaneous transluminal coronary angioplasty (PTCA) is a minimally invasive procedure that's performed to open an occluded coronary artery. It's performed in the cardiac catheterization laboratory after coronary angiography confirms the presence and location of an occlusion. After the occlusion is located, the practitioner threads a guide catheter through the patient's femoral artery and into the coronary artery under fluoroscopic guidance. A radial artery approach may also be used; it's particularly useful in patients with coagulopathy, elevated international ratio, or morbid obesity because this approach reduces the risk of bleeding.[5]

When the guide catheter's position at the occlusion site is confirmed by angiography, the practitioner carefully introduces into the catheter a double-lumen balloon that's smaller than the catheter lumen. He then directs the balloon through the lesion, where a marked pressure gradient will be obvious. The practitioner alternately inflates and deflates the balloon until an angiogram verifies successful arterial dilation and the pressure gradient has decreased.

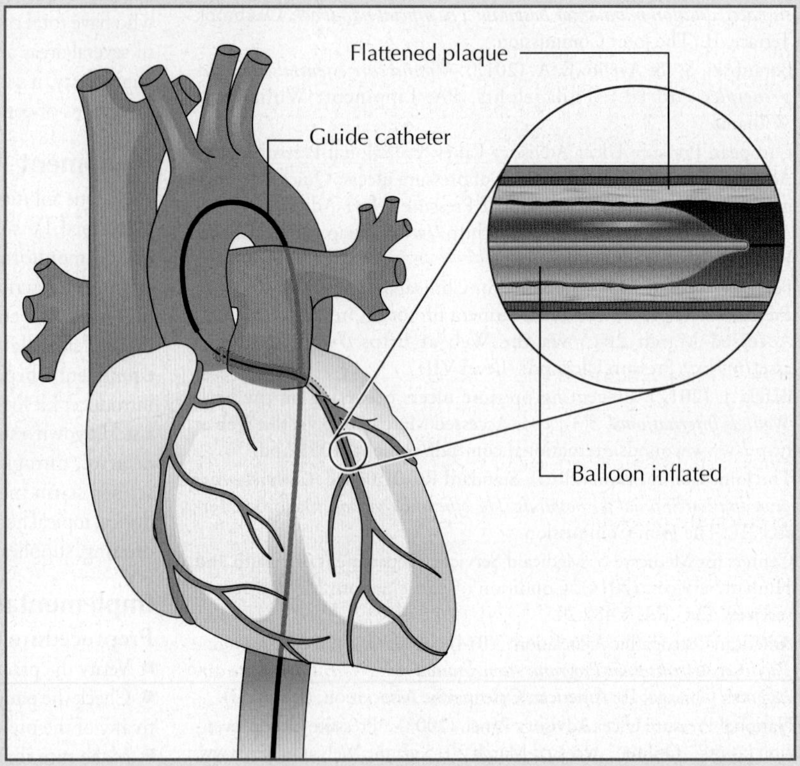

■ Insert an IV catheter, as needed, *in case emergency medications are required.* (See the "IV catheter insertion and removal" procedure, page 446.)

NURSING ALERT **Although the minimum effective aspirin dosage with percutaneous coronary intervention (PCI) hasn't been established, administer 325 mg of aspirin at least 2 hours, and preferably 24 hours, before a PCI (such as PTCA) as prescribed** ***because aspirin reduces the frequency of ischemic complications after PCI.***[5]

■ Clip hair from the insertion site.[14]

■ Clean the area of skin at the insertion site with antiseptic solution.

■ Administer a sedative as prescribed, following safe medication administration practices.

■ Obtain baseline vital signs.

■ Assess for the presence and quality of distal pulses *to evaluate the neuromuscular status of the patient's extremities.* If pulses are weak or nonpalpable, use a portable Doppler ultrasound flow detector *to help detect and assess pulses.* (See the "Doppler use" procedure, page 248.)

■ Perform hand hygiene.[9,10,11]

■ Communicate information about the patient's history, condition, and care to the nurse who will care for the patient during PTCA and then give her the opportunity to ask questions. *Handoff communication between caregivers promotes patient safety and prevents errors.*

■ Document the procedure.[15]

Intraprocedure care

■ Perform hand hygiene.[9,10,11]

■ When the patient arrives at the cardiac catheterization laboratory, confirm the patient's identity using at least two patient identifiers.[12]

■ Perform a preprocedure verification process *to make sure that all relevant documentation, related information, and equipment are available and correctly identified to the patient's identifiers.*[7]

■ Confirm that the correct procedure has been identified for the correct patient at the correct site.[7]

■ Apply ECG electrodes and ensure that the IV catheter is patent.

■ Administer oxygen through an appropriate oxygen delivery device.

■ The practitioner will put on a surgical cap, a mask, a sterile gown, sterile gloves, and eye protection, if needed. Put on the same personal protective equipment.[16]

■ Open the sterile supplies and label all medications, medication containers, and other solutions on and off the sterile field.[17]

■ The practitioner prepares the site, injects a local anesthetic, and then drapes the patient from head to toe, leaving the insertion site exposed. *Maximal barrier precautions prevent infection.*[18] If the patient doesn't have a pulmonary artery catheter in place, the practitioner may insert one now.

■ Conduct a time-out immediately before starting the procedure *to determine that the correct patient, site, positioning, and procedure are identified and confirm, as applicable, that relevant information and necessary equipment are available.*[19]

■ The practitioner inserts a large guide catheter into the artery and then threads an angioplasty catheter through the guide catheter. An angioplasty catheter is thinner and longer and has a balloon at its tip. Using a thin, flexible guide wire, he then threads the catheter retrograde through the aorta and into the coronary artery to the area of stenosis.

■ The practitioner injects a contrast medium through the angioplasty catheter and into the obstructed coronary artery *to outline the lesion's location and help assess the blockage.* He also injects heparin or another anticoagulant[5] *to prevent the catheter from clotting* and, if needed, intracoronary nitroglycerin *to dilate coronary vessels and prevent spasm.*

■ The practitioner alternatively inflates and deflates the catheter's balloon, gradually increasing the amount of time the balloon is inflated each time. *The expanding balloon compresses the atherosclerotic plaque against the arterial wall, expanding the arterial lumen.* Because balloon inflation blocks blood flow to the myocardium distal to the inflation area, the patient may experience angina at this time. If balloon inflation fails to decrease the stenosis, the practitioner may try a larger balloon; he may also insert a vascular stent *to prevent vessel closure.* (See *Vascular stents.*)
■ Monitor the insertion site for bleeding throughout the procedure. Monitor the patient's international normalized ratio, prothrombin time, partial thromboplastin time, activated clotting time, and platelet count, as ordered.[6,9]
■ Assist with obtaining serial angiograms *to help determine the effectiveness of treatment.*
■ The practitioner removes the angioplasty catheter, leaving the guide catheter in place *in case the procedure needs to be repeated because of vessel occlusion.* The guide catheter is usually sutured at this time and is generally removed 2 to 24 hours after the procedure; assist with suturing it in place, as appropriate.
■ Remove and dispose of personal protective equipment properly, and perform hand hygiene.[9,10,11]
■ Document the procedure.[15]

Postprocedure care

■ When the patient returns to the unit, perform hand hygiene.[9,10,11]
■ Confirm his identity using at least two patient identifiers.[12]
■ When the patient returns to the unit, he may be receiving anticoagulants. If he's bleeding at the catheter insertion site, he may also have a compression device on it *to prevent a hematoma.* Alternatively, manual pressure may be applied. If bleeding at the site occurs, apply pressure approximately 2 to 3 cm (¾" to 1") above the puncture site.[20]
■ Frequently monitor the patient's vital signs and peripheral pulses distal to the catheter insertion site as well as the color, temperature, and capillary refill of the affected extremity. *There's no evidence-based research available to indicate best practice for vital sign frequency.*[21] Watch for signs of neurovascular compromise and, if present, notify the practitioner. Immediate surgical consultation may be necessary if compartment syndrome develops.[22]
■ Monitor and record ECG rhythm and arterial pressures.

NURSING ALERT ***Because coronary spasm may occur during or after PTCA,* monitor the patient's ECG for ST- and T-wave changes, and obtain vital signs frequently. Be alert for signs and symptoms of ischemia, which requires emergency coronary revascularization.**

■ Instruct the patient to remain in bed for the amount of time specified by the practitioner and to keep the affected extremity straight and immobilized while he's on bed rest. Elevate the head of the bed 15 to 30 degrees, as ordered. Bed positioning and rest times vary depending on the arterial site selected, the technique used for closure during PTCA, the size of the sheath used, and whether the patient receives antiplatelet therapy after the procedure.
■ Assess the catheter site for hematoma, ecchymosis, and hemorrhage. If an area of expanding hematoma appears, mark the site and alert the practitioner. If bleeding occurs, locate the artery and apply manual pressure; then notify the practitioner.
■ Administer IV fluids, as ordered (usually 100 mL/hour) *to promote excretion of the contrast medium.* Be sure to assess for signs of fluid overload (distended jugular veins, atrial and ventricular gallops, dyspnea, pulmonary congestion, tachycardia, hypertension, and hypoxemia).
■ Perform hand hygiene[9,10,11] and then put on gloves.[18]
■ After the catheter is removed, apply direct pressure for at least 10 minutes; apply a compression or hemostatic device or a topical hemostatic agent, as ordered.[23]

EQUIPMENT

Vascular stents

Two serious complications of percutaneous transluminal coronary angioplasty (PTCA) are acute vessel closure and late restenosis. To prevent these complications, the practitioner may use a procedure called *stenting.*

The stent is typically made of metal, most commonly stainless steel. *Drug-eluting stents* are coated with a medication or polymer. The medication coating the stent is released at the implantation site to reduce the risk of restenosis. The polymer coating acts to decrease platelet aggregation; some polymers may also contain medication. The polymer allows the medication to be released gradually to help reduce inflammation at the site, which reduces the risk of restenosis. However, the medication's effect is localized.

A stent may be inserted in patients at risk for clotting after PTCA, after a failed PTCA to keep a patient stable until he can undergo coronary artery bypass surgery, or as an alternative to coronary artery bypass surgery.

To insert a stent, the practitioner places the stent on a standard balloon angioplasty catheter and positions it over a guide wire. Fluoroscopy verifies when the stent is correctly placed. The practitioner then inflates the balloon, which expands and presses against the plaque. The practitioner then removes the catheter, leaving the stent in place.

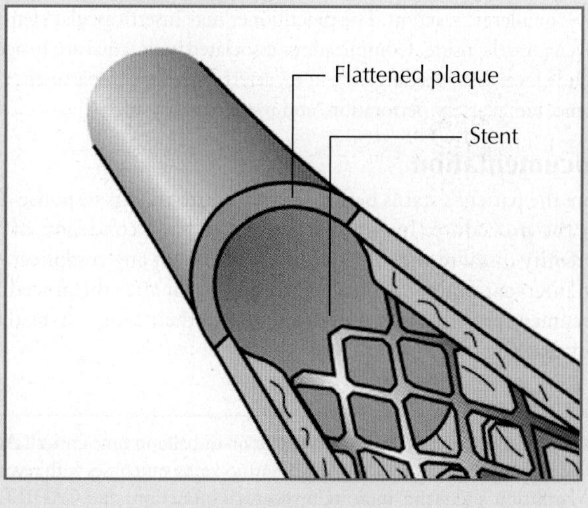

■ Monitor the site often and lace a dressing over the site, preferably a transparent semipermeable dressing.[24]
■ Remove and discard your gloves and perform hand hygiene.[9,10,11]
■ Document the procedure.[25]

Special considerations

■ Devices to prevent lower extremity embolism, such as a sequential compression device or an embolic capture device, are recommended for use during PTCA for a saphenous vein graft.[4,20]
■ The current recommendation is to administer 75 mg of clopidogrel (Plavix) daily or 10 mg of prasugrel (Effient) daily after the procedure for a period of 1 to 12 months, depending on the exact procedure completed. If the patient isn't already receiving long term aspirin therapy, 300 to 325 mg/day of aspirin may also be prescribed for 1 to 6 months, depending on the patient's condition and status. This is typically followed by a regimen of 75 to 162 mg/day.[4]

■ If the patient exhibits signs and symptoms of an MI after the procedure, expect the practitioner to order a 12-lead ECG and CK-MB and troponin levels.

■ Note that The Joint Commission issued a sentinel event alert concerning medical device alarm safety *because alarm-related events have been associated with permanent loss of function and death.* Among the major contributing factors were improper alarm settings, inappropriately turned off alarms, and alarm signals that were not audible to staff. Make sure alarm limits are appropriately set and that alarms are turned on, functioning properly, and audible to staff. Follow facility guidelines for preventing alarm fatigue.[26]

Patient teaching

Instruct the patient to avoid heavy lifting or strenuous activities after the procedure *because it could affect the puncture site.* Tell him to drink plenty of fluids during the first 24 hours following the procedure *to flush the contrast medium from his system.* Instruct the patient to report any signs of infection, such as fever or redness, drainage, or swelling at the puncture site.

Complications

The most common complication of PTCA is restenosis. Others include prolonged angina, coronary artery perforation, balloon rupture, reocclusion (necessitating a coronary artery bypass graft), MI, pericardial tamponade, hematoma, hemorrhage, reperfusion arrhythmias, vasospasm of the coronary artery, closure of the vessel, and contrast-induced nephropathy[27] or allergic reaction. The practitioner may insert vascular stents to prevent vessel closure. Complications associated with radial artery access include local area bleeding, infection, arterial spasm, compartment syndrome, radial artery perforation, and pseudoaneurysm.[28]

Documentation

Note the patient's status before the procedure and his response during the procedure. Include vital signs and the condition of the extremity distal to the insertion site. Document any complications and interventions performed before, during, or after the procedure. Document patient and family teaching and their comprehension of your teaching.

REFERENCES

1 Brodie, B. R., et al. (2010). When is door-to-balloon time critical? Analysis from the HORIZONS-AMI (Harmonizing outcomes with revascularization and stents in acute myocardial infarction) and CADILLAC (Controlled abciximab and device investigation to lower late angioplasty complications) trials. *Journal of the American College of Cardiology, 56,* 407–413. (Level II)

2 Kushner, F., et al. (2009). 2009 focused updates: ACC/AHA guidelines for the management of patients with ST-elevation myocardial infarction (updating the 2004 guideline and 2007 focused update) and ACC/AHA/SCAI guidelines on percutaneous coronary intervention (updating the 2005 guideline and 2007 focused update): A report of the American College of Cardiology Foundation/American Heart Association Task Force on Practice Guidelines. *Circulation, 120,* 2271–2306. (Level I)

3 American Heart Association. (2010). 2010 American Heart Association guidelines for cardiopulmonary resuscitation and emergency cardiovascular care. *Circulation, 122,* S787–S817. (Level II)

4 Levine, G. N., et al. (2011). 2011 ACCF/AHA/SCAI guideline percutaneous coronary intervention: A report of the American College of Cardiology Foundation/American Heart Association Task Force on Practice Guidelines and the Society for Cardiovascular Angiography and Interventions. *Circulation, 124,* e574–e651. Accessed March 2015 via the Web at http://circ.ahajournals.org/content/early/2011/11/07/CIR.0b013e31823ba622.full.pdf (Level II)

5 Merriweather, N., & Sulzbach-Hoke, L. M. (2012). Managing risk of complications at femoral vascular access sites in percutaneous coronary intervention. *Critical Care Nurse, 32*(5), 16–29. Accessed March 2015 via the Web at http://ccn.aacnjournals.org/content/32/5/16.full.pdf

6 The Joint Commission. (2015). Standard RI.01.03.01. *Comprehensive accreditation manual for hospitals: The official handbook.* Oakbrook Terrace, IL: The Joint Commission. (Level VII)

7 The Joint Commission. (2015). Standard UP.01.01.01. *Comprehensive accreditation manual for hospitals: The official handbook.* Oakbrook Terrace, IL: The Joint Commission. (Level VII)

8 Gulanick, M., & Myers, J. L. (2010). *Nursing care plans: Diagnosis, interventions, and outcomes* (7th ed.). St. Louis, MO: Mosby.

9 The Joint Commission. (2015). Standard NPSG.07.01.01. *Comprehensive accreditation manual for hospitals: The official handbook.* Oakbrook Terrace, IL: The Joint Commission. (Level VII)

10 World Health Organization. (2009). "WHO guidelines on hand hygiene in health care: First global patient safety challenge, clean care is safer care" [Online]. Accessed March 2015 via the Web at http://whqlibdoc.who.int/publications/2009/9789241597906_eng.pdf (Level IV)

11 Centers for Disease Control and Prevention. (2002). Guideline for hand hygiene in health-care settings: Recommendations of the Healthcare Infection Control Practices Advisory Committee and the HICPAC/SHEA/APIC/IDSA Hand Hygiene Task Force. *MMWR Recommendations and Reports, 51*(RR-16), 1–45. Accessed March 2015 via the Web at http://www.cdc.gov/mmwr/pdf/rr/rr5116.pdf (Level II)

12 The Joint Commission. (2015). Standard NPSG.01.01.01. *Comprehensive accreditation manual for hospitals: The official handbook.* Oakbrook Terrace, IL: The Joint Commission. (Level VII)

13 American Society of Anesthesiologists. (2011). Practice guidelines for preoperative fasting and use of pharmacologic agents to reduce the risk of pulmonary aspiration: Application to healthy patients undergoing elective procedures: An updated report by the American Society of Anesthesiologists Committee on Standards and Practice Parameters. *Anesthesiology, 11,* 495–511. (Level V)

14 The Joint Commission. (2015). Standard NPSG.07.05.01. *Comprehensive accreditation manual for hospitals: The official handbook.* Oakbrook Terrace, IL: The Joint Commission. (Level VII)

15 The Joint Commission. (2015). Standard RC.01.03.01. *Comprehensive accreditation manual for hospitals: The official handbook.* Oakbrook Terrace, IL: The Joint Commission. (Level VII)

16 Centers for Disease Control and Prevention. (2011). "Guidelines for the prevention of intravascular catheter-related infections" [Online]. Accessed March 2015 via the Web at http://www.cdc.gov/hicpac/pdf/guidelines/bsi-guidelines-2011.pdf (Level I)

17 The Joint Commission. (2015). Standard NPSG.03.04.01. *Comprehensive accreditation manual for hospitals: The official handbook.* Oakbrook Terrace, IL: The Joint Commission. (Level VII)

18 Occupational Safety and Health Administration. (n.d.). "Bloodborne pathogens, standard number 1910.1030" [Online]. Accessed March 2015 via the Web at http://www.osha.gov/pls/oshaweb/owadisp.show_document?p_table=STANDARDS&p_id=10051

19 The Joint Commission. (2015). Standard UP.01.03.01. *Comprehensive accreditation manual for hospitals: The official handbook.* Oakbrook Terrace, IL: The Joint Commission. (Level VII)

20 Zankar, A., et al. (2011). Embolic capture angioplasty of lower extremity lesion following distal embolization. *Cardiovascular, Revascularization Medicine, 12,* 337–340.

21 American Society of PeriAnesthesia Nurses. (2012). *2012–2014 Perianesthesia nursing standards, practice recommendations and interpretive statements.* Cherry Hill, NJ: American Society of PeriAnesthesia Nurses. (Level VII)

22 Balaji, N. R., & Shah, P. B. (2011). Cardiology patient page: Radial artery catheterization. *Circulation, 124,* e407–e408. Accessed March 2015 via the Web athttp://circ.ahajournals.org/content/124/16/e407.full

23 Kordestani, S. S., et al. (2012). A randomized controlled trial on the hemostasis of femoral artery using topical hemostatic agent. *Clinical and Applied Thrombosis/Hemostasis, 18,* 501–505. Accessed March 2015 via

the Web at http://chitotech.com/new/site/wp-content/uploads/2012/02/ChitoHem.pdf (Level II)

24 Mcle, S., et al. (2009). Transparent film dressing vs pressure dressing after percutaneous transluminal coronary angiography. *American Journal of Critical Care, 18,* 14–19. (Level IV)

25 American Osteopathic Association. (2014). Standard 10.00.03. *Healthcare Facilities Accreditation Program: Accreditation requirements for acute care hospitals.* Chicago, IL: American Osteopathic Association. (Level VII)

26 The Joint Commission. (2013). "Sentinel event alert: Medical device alarm safety in hospitals" [Online]. Accessed March 2015 via the Web athttp://www.jointcommission.org/assets/1/18/SEA_50_alarms_4_5_13_FINAL1.PDF (Level VII)

27 Caruso, M., et al. (2011). Contrast-induced nephropathy after percutaneous coronary interventions in simple lesions: Risk factors and incidence are affected by the definition utilized. *Internal Medicine, 50,* 983–989.

28 Altin, S. E., & Singh, V. P. (2012). Radial access complications. *Cardiac Interventions Today, 3,* 48–52. Accessed March 2015 via the Web at http://bmctoday.net/citoday/pdfs/cit0512_F5_Singh.pdf

ADDITIONAL REFERENCES

Barnason, S., et al. (2012). Patient recovery and transitions after hospitalization for acute cardiac events: An integrative review. *Journal of Cardiovascular Nursing, 27,* 175–191.

Carrillo, X., et al. (2012). Safety and efficacy of transradial access in coronary angiography: 8-year experience. *Journal of Invasive Cardiology, 24,* 346–351.

Laird, P. A., & Ruppert, S. D. (2012). Stent thrombosis in a clopidogrel nonresponder. *Critical Care Nursing Quarterly, 35,* 151–159.

Manoukian, S. V. (2009). Predictors and impact of bleeding complications in percutaneous coronary intervention, acute coronary syndromes, and ST-segment elevation myocardial infarction. *American Journal of Cardiology, 104*(Suppl. 5), 9C–15C.

McEnroe-Petitte, D. M. (2011). Preparing a patient for cardiac catheterization. *Nursing 2011, 41* (Suppl. 11), 14–15.

Mill, C., et al. (2012). Care of the post percutaneous coronary intervention patient. *Australian Nursing Journal, 19*(7), 26–27.

Rolley, J. X., et al. (2009). Review of nursing care for patients undergoing percutaneous coronary intervention: A patient journey approach. *Journal of Clinical Nursing, 18,* 2394–2405.

ANTIEMBOLISM STOCKING APPLICATION

Elastic antiembolism stockings help prevent venous thromboembolism (VTE), a disorder that includes deep vein thrombosis (DVT) and pulmonary embolism. They do so by compressing superficial leg veins. This compression increases venous return by forcing blood into the deep venous system rather than allowing it to pool in the legs and form clots.

HOSPITAL-ACQUIRED CONDITION ALERT **Keep in mind that VTE in patients who underwent total knee replacement or hip replacement is considered a hospital-acquired condition because it can be reasonably prevented using best practices.[1,2] Make sure to follow VTE prevention practices (such as using mechanical compression devices, including antiembolism stockings and an intermittent pneumatic compression device, early ambulation, and pharmacologic prophylaxis) to reduce the risk of VTE.[3]**

Antiembolism stockings should provide graduated compression and produce a calf pressure of 14 to 15 mm Hg.[2,3] They're usually indicated for postoperative, bedridden, and elderly patients as well as for those with varicose veins and other patients at risk for DVT. Because compression therapy has helped in the treatment of venous ulcers and chronic venous insufficiency, it's considered a standard of care.[4,5] For patients with chronic venous problems, intermittent pneumatic compression stockings may also be ordered during surgery and postoperatively. (See the "Sequential compression therapy" procedure, page 687.)

Elastic antiembolism stockings aren't recommended in patients with dermatoses or open skin lesions, gangrene, severe arteriosclerosis or other ischemic vascular diseases, pulmonary or any massive edema, recent vein ligation, or vascular or skin grafts, or severe leg deformity.[2] Studies have shown that graduated compression stockings don't reduce the risk of DVT in stroke patients and may even increase these patients' risk of skin complications.[6,7]

As of October 2008, the Centers for Medicare & Medicaid Services added DVT and pulmonary embolism in patients who underwent hip and total knee replacement surgery to their list of hospital-acquired conditions. These conditions are thought to be preventable with the use of evidence-based treatment guidelines and carry payment implications if a patient acquires them while recovering from hip or total knee replacement surgery.[8]

All types of antiembolism stockings—knee-length, thigh-length, and waist-length—provide thromboprophylaxis, with no evidence to support the use of one type over another. Because of this, choose which type of stocking to use based on patient compliance, ease of use, and cost.[9]

Equipment

Tape measure ▪ antiembolism stockings of correct size.

Preparation of equipment

Before applying a knee-length stocking

Measure the patient using a tape measure *to ensure a proper fit.* (See *Measuring for antiembolism stockings,* page 23.) Measure the circumference of the calf at its widest point[4] and the leg length from the popliteal fold (bend of the knee) to the base of the heel.

Before applying a thigh-length stocking

Measure the upper thigh circumference at the gluteal fold, then the calf circumference at the greatest dimension, and lastly the leg length from the gluteal fold to the base of the heel.

Before applying a waist-length stocking

To measure for a waist-length stocking, first measure the upper thigh circumference at the gluteal fold.[4] Next, measure the calf circumference at the greatest dimension.[5] Last, measure the leg length by measuring from the gluteal fold to the base of the heel.[4]

If the patient's thigh measurements are outside of the specified recommended range, knee-length stockings may be another option.[5]

Implementation

- Verify the practitioner's order.
- Review the patient's medical record for contraindications to antiembolism stocking use.
- Perform hand hygiene.[10,11,12,13,14]
- Confirm the patient's identity using at least two patient identifiers.[15]
- Provide privacy[16] and explain the procedure to the patient.
- Help the patient lie down if he isn't already doing so.
- Assess the condition of the patient's legs. If you suspect arterial disease, notify the practitioner before applying the stockings.[5]

Applying a knee-length stocking

- Insert your hand into the stocking from the top and grasp the heel pocket from the inside. Holding the heel, turn the stocking inside out. *This method allows easier application than gathering the entire stocking and working it up over the foot and ankle.*[5]
- Position the stocking over the foot and heel, making sure the heel is centered in the heel pocket.[5]

■ Pull a few inches of the stocking up around the patient's ankle and calf[5] (as shown below).

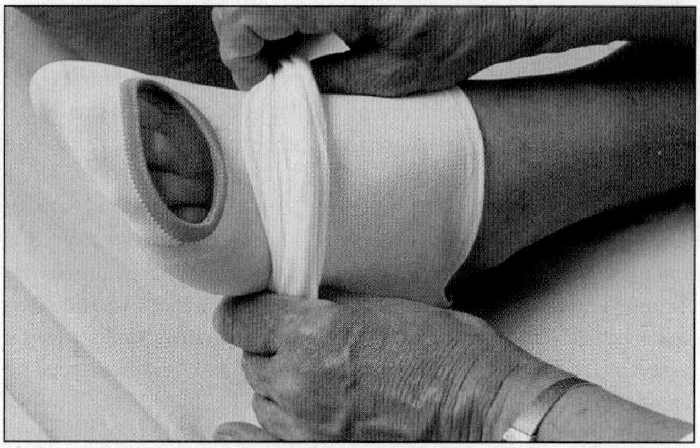

■ Continue pulling stocking up the patient's leg using short, alternating front and back pulls (as shown below). The bottom of the band (or change in the stocking's stitching) should fall 1″ to 2″ (2.5 to 5 cm) below the popliteal fold.

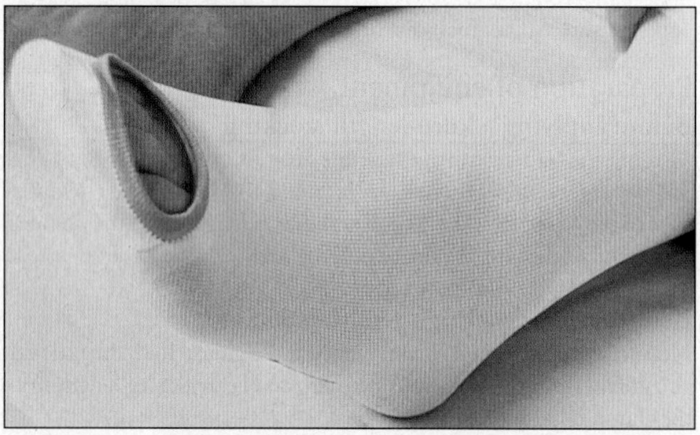

■ Continue easing the stocking upward. As you apply the thigh portion of the stocking, start rotating the stocking inward so the panel (if present) is slightly toward the inside of the patient's leg (as shown below). When the stocking is fully applied, the top band of the stocking should rest at the patient's gluteal fold.[5]

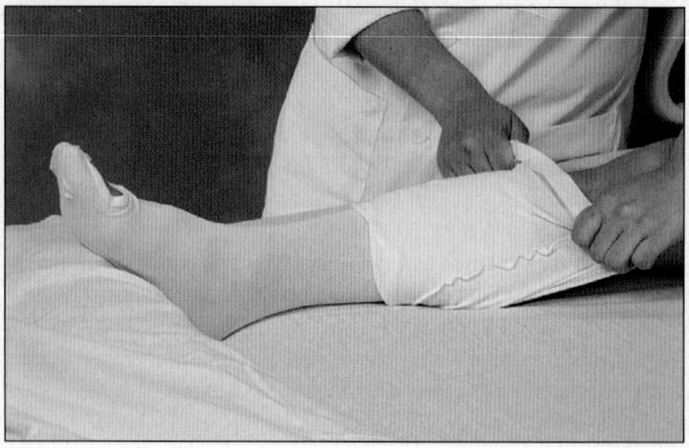

■ Smooth out wrinkles in the stocking fabric *to prevent skin breakdown.*[4]
■ Make sure the patient's toes are visible through the toe inspection area if present; the patient's toes shouldn't stick out of the inspection area opening.[4]
■ Repeat the procedure for the second stocking if ordered.
■ Perform hand hygiene.[10,11,12,13,14]
■ Document the procedure.[17,18]

Applying a thigh-length stocking

■ Follow the procedure for applying a knee-length stocking, taking care to distribute the fabric evenly below the knee before continuing the procedure.
■ With the patient's leg extended, stretch the rest of the stocking over the knee.
■ Flex the patient's knee, and pull the stocking over the thigh until the top is 1″ to 3″ (2.5 to 7.5 cm) below the gluteal fold.
■ Stretch the stocking from the top, front and back, *to distribute the fabric evenly over the thigh.*
■ Repeat the procedure for the second stocking if ordered.
■ Document the procedure.[17,18]

Applying a waist-length stocking

■ When the stocking reaches the patient's knee, begin turning the stocking to position the side panel. The stocking should be positioned so that the upper thigh hem rests in the groin and at the gluteal fold. Make sure the seam is flat against the body and the side panel is at the hip bone.[4]
■ Repeat the procedure for the second stocking.[4]
■ Unfold the waist belt and bring it around the patient's waist. The smooth side of the belt should rest against the patient's skin. Fasten the waist belt snaps to the stockings.[4]
■ Connect the waste belt buckle and adjust the waist belt *so that it's tight enough to secure the stockings in place.*[4]
■ Smooth out wrinkles in the stocking fabric *to prevent skin breakdown.*[4]
■ Pull the toe area forward to smooth the ankle and instep area to promote toe comfort.[4] Make sure the patient's toes are visible through the toe inspection area, if present; the toes shouldn't stick out of the inspection area opening.[4]
■ Perform hand hygiene.[10,11,12,13,14]
■ Document the procedure.[17,18]

Special considerations

■ If the patient has a fluctuation in weight or develops edema or postoperative swelling, remeasure the patient and obtain stockings of the appropriate size.[4,5]
■ Encourage the patient to wear the stockings day and night until they no longer have significantly reduced mobility.[4]
■ Remove the stockings at least once daily. Inspect the skin, provide skin care, and then reapply the stockings.[4,5] For patients with significant reduction in mobility, poor skin integrity, or sensory loss, inspect the skin two to three times per day, particularly over the heels and bony prominences.[4,19]
■ Discontinue the use of antiembolism stockings if you note marking, blistering, or discoloration of the skin, especially over heels and bony prominences or if the patient experiences pain or discomfort. Notify the practitioner; a foot impulse device or a sequential compression device may be prescribed as an alternative to antiembolism stockings.[4]
■ Don't allow the stockings to roll or turn down at the top or toe *because the excess pressure could cause venous strangulation.* Have the patient wear the stockings in bed and during ambulation *to provide continuous protection against VTE.*
■ Be alert for an allergic reaction *because some patients can't tolerate the sizing in new stockings.* Laundering the stockings before applying them reduces the risk of an allergic reaction to sizing. Remove the stockings at least once daily *to bathe the skin and observe for irritation and breakdown.*
■ Using warm water and mild soap, wash the stockings when they become soiled. Keep a second pair handy *so that the patient can wear them while the other pair is being laundered.*
■ Don't elevate the patient's legs while he's wearing compression stockings *because of the risk of decreased circulation.*

Measuring for antiembolism stockings

Measure the patient carefully to ensure that his antiembolism stockings provide enough compression for adequate venous return. Measure both legs because if the right and left leg measure differently, you many need to order two different stocking sizes.[1]

To choose the correct knee-length stocking, measure the circumference of the calf at its widest point[2] (top left) and the leg length from the popliteal fold (bend of the knee) to the base of the heel (bottom left).[2]

To choose a thigh-length stocking, measure the calf as for a knee-length stocking and the thigh at its widest point (top right). Then measure leg length from the bottom of the heel to the gluteal fold (bottom right).

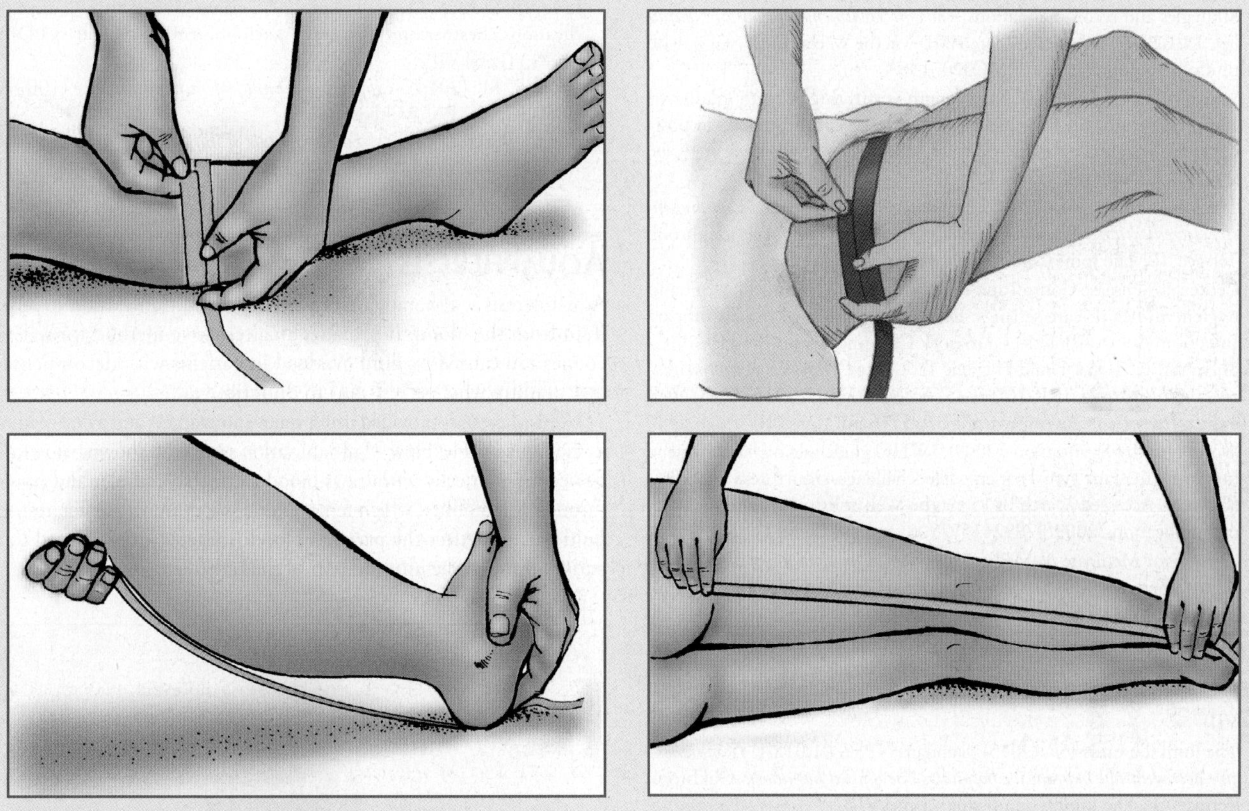

Patient teaching

If the patient will require antiembolism stockings after discharge, teach him or a family member how to apply them correctly and explain why he needs to wear them to increase compliance, which maximizes the effectiveness of treatment.[20] Advise them to follow the manufacturer's washing instructions. Inform them that, with proper care, stockings commonly last for 2 to 3 months before needing replacing.

Complications

Obstruction of arterial blood flow—characterized by cold and bluish toes, dusky toenail beds, decreased or absent pedal pulses, and leg pain or cramps—can result from application of antiembolism stockings. Less serious complications, such as an allergic reaction and skin irritation, can also occur.

Documentation

Record the date and time of stocking application, stocking style and size, the condition of the leg and foot before and after treatment, the condition of the toes during treatment, and any complications resulting from stocking use. Document stocking removal and the appearance of the patient's skin. Record any patient teaching and the patient's understanding of the teaching.

REFERENCES

1 Centers for Medicare & Medicaid Services, Department of Health and Human Services. (2012). "Hospital-acquired conditions" [Online]. Accessed March 2015 via the Web at http://www.cms.gov/Medicare/Medicare-Fee-for-Service-Payment/HospitalAcqCond/Hospital-Acquired_Conditions.html

2 Centers for Medicare & Medicaid Services, & The Joint Commission. (2014). "The specifications manual for national inpatient quality measures (version 4.3a)" [Online]. Accessed March 2015 via the Web at http://www.qualitynet.org/dcs/ContentServer?c=Page&pagename=QnetPublic%2FPage%2FQnetTier4&cid=1228773564870

3 Jarrett, N., et al. (2013). "Evidence-based guidelines for selected and previously considered hospital-acquired conditions: Final report" [Online]. Accessed March 2015 via the Web at http://www.cms.gov/Medicare/Medicare-Fee-for-Service-Payment/HospitalAcqCond/Downloads/Evidence-Based-Guidelines.pdf

4 Covidien. (2010). "T.E.D. anti-embolism stockings: Nursing procedure guide" [Online]. Accessed March 2015 via the Web at http://

www.covidien.com/imageServer.aspx/doc233679.pdf?contentID=28692&contenttype=application/pdf

5 National Institute for Health and Clinical Excellence. (2010). "Venous thromboembolism: Reducing the risk" [Online]. Accessed March 2015 via the Web at http://www.nice.org.uk/nicemedia/live/12695/47195/47195.pdf (Level VII)

6 Collins, L., & Seraj, S. (2010). Diagnosis and treatment of venous ulcers. *American Family Physician, 81,* 989–996. Accessed March 2015 via the Web at http://www.aafp.org/afp/2010/0415/p989.html

7 O'Meara, S., et al. (2012). Compression for venous leg ulcers. *Cochrane Database of Systematic Reviews, 2012*(11), CD000265. (Level I)

8 Kappelle, L. J. (2011). Preventing deep vein thrombosis after stroke: Strategies and recommendations. *Current Treatment Options in Neurology, 13,* 629–635. Accessed March 2015 via the Web at http://www.ncbi.nlm.nih.gov/pmc/articles/PMC3207135/

9 Sajid, M. S., et al. (2012). Knee length versus thigh length graduated compression stockings for prevention of deep vein thrombosis in postoperative surgical patients. *Cochrane Database of Systematic Reviews, 2012*(5), CD007162. (Level I)

10 The Joint Commission. (2015). Standard NPSG.07.01.01. *Comprehensive accreditation manual for hospitals: The official handbook.* Oakbrook Terrace, IL: The Joint Commission. (Level VII)

11 Centers for Disease Control and Prevention. (2002). Guideline for hand hygiene in health-care settings: Recommendations of the Healthcare Infection Control Practices Advisory Committee and the HICPAC/SHEA/APIC/IDSA Hand Hygiene Task Force. *MMWR Recommendations and Reports, 51*(RR-16), 1–45. Accessed March 2015 via the Web at http://www.cdc.gov/mmwr/pdf/rr/rr5116.pdf (Level II)

12 World Health Organization. (2009). "WHO guidelines on hand hygiene in health care: First global patient safety challenge, clean care is safer care" [Online]. Accessed March 2015 via the Web at http://whqlibdoc.who.int/publications/2009/9789241597906_eng.pdf (Level IV)

13 Centers for Medicare & Medicaid Services, Department of Health and Human Services. (2013). Condition of participation: Infection control. 42 C.F.R. § 482.42.

14 American Osteopathic Association. (2014). Standard 07.01.21. *Healthcare Facilities Accreditation Program: Accreditation requirements for acute care hospitals.* Chicago, IL: American Osteopathic Association. (Level VII)

15 The Joint Commission. (2015). Standard NPSG.01.01.01. *Comprehensive accreditation manual for hospitals: The official handbook.* Oakbrook Terrace, IL: The Joint Commission. (Level VII)

16 Centers for Medicare & Medicaid Services, Department of Health and Human Services. (2014). Condition of participation: Patient's rights. 42 C.F.R. § 482.13(c)(1).

17 Centers for Medicare & Medicaid Services, Department of Health and Human Services. (2014). Condition of participation: Medical record services. 42 C.F.R. § 482.24(b).

18 American Osteopathic Association. (2014). Standard 10.00.03. *Healthcare Facilities Accreditation Program: Accreditation requirements for acute care hospitals.* Chicago, IL: American Osteopathic Association. (Level VII)

19 Gee, E. (2011). Anti-embolism stockings. *Nursing Times, 107*(14), 18–19. Accessed March 2015 via the Web at http://www.nursingtimes.net/nursing-practice/clinical-zones/haematology/anti-embolism-stockings/5028392.article

20 Kanaan, A. O., et al. (2012). Evaluating the role of compression stockings in preventing post thrombotic syndrome: A review of the literature. *Thrombosis, 2012,* 694851. Accessed March 2015 via the Web at http://www.hindawi.com/journals/thromb/2012/694851/ (Level I)

ADDITIONAL REFERENCES

Craven, R. F., & Hirnle, C. J. (2012). *Fundamentals of nursing: Human health and function* (7th ed.). Philadelphia, PA: Lippincott Williams & Wilkins.

Duff, J., et al. (2011). Translating venous thromboembolism (VTE) prevention evidence into practice: A multidisciplinary evidence implementation project. *Worldviews on Evidence-Based Nursing, 8,* 30–39. (Level VI)

Guyatt, G. H., et al. (2012). Methodology for the development of antithrombotic therapy and prevention of thrombosis guidelines: Antithrombotic Therapy and Prevention of Thrombosis, 9th ed.: American College of Chest Physicians Evidence-Based Clinical Practice Guidelines. *Chest, 141,* 53S–70S. Accessed March 2015 via the Web at http://journal.publications.chestnet.org/pdfaccess.ashx?ResourceID=6568197&PDFSource=13 (Level VII)

James, A. (2011). Practice bulletin no. 123: Thromboembolism in pregnancy. *Obstetrics and Gynecology, 118,* 718–729. (Level VII)

Kahn, S. R., et al. (2012). Prevention of VTE in nonsurgical patients: Antithrombotic Therapy and Prevention of Thrombosis, 9th ed.: American College of Chest Physicians Evidence-Based Clinical Practice Guidelines. *Chest, 141,* 195S–226S. Accessed March 2015 via the Web at http://journal.publications.chestnet.org/pdfaccess.ashx?ResourceID=6568301&PDFSource=13 (Level VII)

Nettina, S. M. (2014). *Lippincott manual of nursing practice* (10th ed.). Philadelphia, PA: Wolters Kluwer.

Taylor, C. R., et al. (2011). *Fundamentals of nursing: The art and science of nursing care* (7th ed.). Philadelphia, PA: Lippincott Williams & Wilkins.

AQUAPHERESIS

Aquapheresis is a therapy that involves using ultrafiltration to remove fluid from the blood. It provides an alternative method for relieving congestion caused by fluid overload in patients with decompensated heart failure who are resistant to diuretics.[1]

Aquapheresis is provided using venovenous access and a device known as the Aquadex FlexFlow™ ultrafiltration system (as shown below). This device mechanically withdraws blood through a catheter and passes it through a hemofilter, which removes excess sodium and water, restoring fluid balance. After the patient's blood is filtered, it's returned to the patient through the infusion port of the catheter.

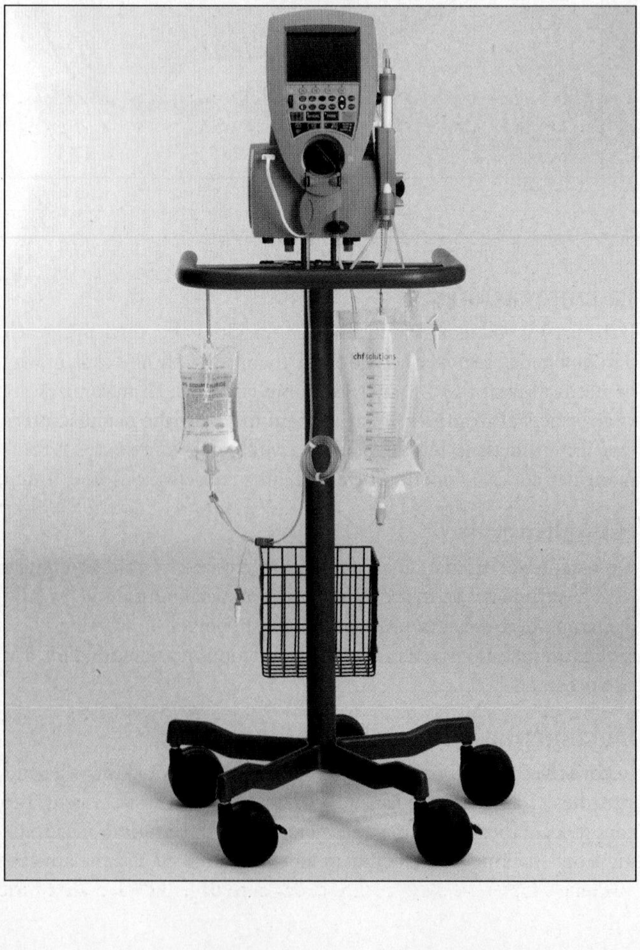

NURSING ALERT **Only individuals who have received specialized training in administering aquapheresis therapy are permitted to administer the therapy.[2]**

Equipment

Aquadex FlexFlow™ pump ■ sterile, disposable, single-use extracorporeal blood circuit set ■ scale ■ IV infusion pump (preferably a smart pump with dose-range alerts) ■ prescribed IV heparin bolus ■ heparin infusion ■ 500-mL IV bag of normal saline solution ■ 10-mL prefilled syringes containing preservative-free normal saline solution ■ graduated liquid waste receptacle ■ soap solution and cloth ■ lint-free cloth ■ gloves ■ sterile end caps ■ hospital-grade disinfectant pads (10% bleach solution, 95% isopropyl alcohol, or surface disinfectant) ■ venovenous access device (a #6 French dual-lumen extended-length peripheral catheter, a #5 French single-lumen extended-length peripheral catheter, and an 18G IV catheter, or a #7 or #8 French dual-lumen central venous access catheter).

Preparation of equipment

Before therapy begins, the practitioner inserts a venovenous access device. The catheter must be able to accommodate a blood flow of 10 to 40 mL/minute.[3,4]

Inspect the sterile packages *to make sure they're intact.* Don't use a blood circuit system that's damaged or that has kinks in the tubing. Follow sterile technique throughout the therapy.[3,4]

Implementation

- Verify the practitioner's order for aquapheresis in the patient's medical record, and make sure that diuretic and electrolyte replacement therapy has been discontinued before initiating therapy.
- Make sure that preprocedure laboratory test results are available and documented in the patient's medical record; report any abnormalities.
- Verify that written informed consent has been obtained and is documented in the patient's medical record.[5,6]
- Gather and prepare the equipment in the patient's room.
- Perform hand hygiene.[7,8,9,10,11]
- Confirm the patient's identity using at least two patient identifiers.[12]
- Explain the procedure to the patient *to allay his fears and promote cooperation.*
- Put on gloves.[13,14,15]
- Verify the patency of the access catheter by thoroughly disinfecting the access port and allowing it to dry, attaching a prefilled syringe containing preservative-free normal saline, aspirating for blood return, and then flushing the catheter.[16]

Priming the blood circuit

- Plug the power cord into a grounded electrical outlet.
- Press the ON/OFF key on the front panel. (See *A look at the aquapheresis circuit,* page 26.)
- Place the blood pump cartridge into the blood pump on the machine console and snap it into place. Then turn the knob clockwise until you hear a beep.
- Insert the ultrafiltrate cartridge in the side of the console and snap it into place. Then turn the knob clockwise until you hear a beep.
- Insert the tubing into the blood leak and air sensors.
- Put the pressure sensor cables into their proper connectors, located on the console.
- Insert the data key provided with the blood circuit system into the reader on the front of the console; *this data key facilitates many of the system's functions.*[3]
- Hang the empty ultrafiltrate collection bag on the machine's weight scale hook, and close the drain valve located at the bottom of the bag.
- Remove the end caps from the infusion tubing of the circuit and the priming adapter on the ultrafiltrate drainage bag, and then attach the circuit infusion tubing to the priming adapter on the ultrafiltrate drainage bag.
- Remove the end caps from the withdrawal tubing and the priming spike adapter, and then attach the withdrawal tubing to the withdrawal priming spike adapter.
- Spike the 500-mL priming bag of normal saline solution with the priming spike, and then hang the bag on the priming hook, making sure that the ultrafiltrate bag hangs freely.
- Open the clamps on the withdrawal tubing, infusion tubing, and ultrafiltrate bag priming adapter.
- Press the PRIME key and follow the onscreen instructions; priming should be completed and the system should be free from air in about 4 minutes.
- Empty the priming solution from the fluid collection bag before starting therapy. *Priming solution drains into the collection bag; emptying the collection bag ensures accuracy of the patient's output measurement.*
- Close the clamps on the blood circuit set, remove the end cap on the withdrawal catheter lumen, disconnect the withdrawal line from the IV spike, and connect the withdrawal line to the withdrawal catheter lumen.
- Remove the end cap from the infusion catheter lumen, disconnect the infusion line from the ultrafiltrate priming adapter, and connect the infusion line to the infusion catheter lumen.
- Trace the tubings from the patient to their points of origin *to make sure that you've attached them to the proper catheter lumens.*[17]
- Put sterile end caps on the normal saline solution priming spike and the ultrafiltrate priming adapter.

Beginning anticoagulant therapy

- Begin anticoagulant therapy at least 30 minutes before the procedure, as ordered, following safe medication administration practices. Typically, an IV bolus dose of heparin is given, followed by a continuous heparin infusion *to reduce the risk of clot formation within the system.*
- Avoid distractions and interruptions when preparing and administering medication *to prevent medication errors.*[18,19]
- Compare the medication label with the order in the patient's medical record.[20,21,22]
- Check the patient's medical record for an allergy or contraindication to the prescribed medication. If an allergy or contraindications exist, don't administer the medication; notify the practitioner.[20,21,22]
- Check the expiration date on the medication. If the medication is expired, return it to the pharmacy and obtain new medication.[20,21,22]
- Visually inspect the solution for particles or discoloration or other loss of integrity; don't administer the medication if integrity is compromised.[20,21,22]
- Discuss any unresolved concerns about the medication with the patient's practitioner.[20,22]
- If the patient is receiving the medication for the first time, teach him about potential adverse reactions, and discuss any other concerns related to the medication.[20,22]
- Verify that the medication is being administered at the proper time, in the prescribed dose, and by the correct route *to reduce the risk of medication errors.*[20,21,22]
- If your facility uses a bar code scanning system, scan your identification badge, the patient's identification bracelet, and the medication's bar code.

NURSING ALERT **Heparin, when administered IV, is considered a high-alert medication because it can cause significant patient harm when used in error.[23]**

- Before beginning the heparin infusion, have another nurse perform an independent double-check if required by your facility. (See *Double-checking high-alert medications,* page 27.)
- Compare the results of the independent double-check, if required. If no discrepancies exist, begin using the heparin (through the withdrawal

EQUIPMENT

A look at the aquapheresis circuit

Aquapheresis requires a circuit such as the one below to filter fluid and sodium from the blood of patients with fluid overload.

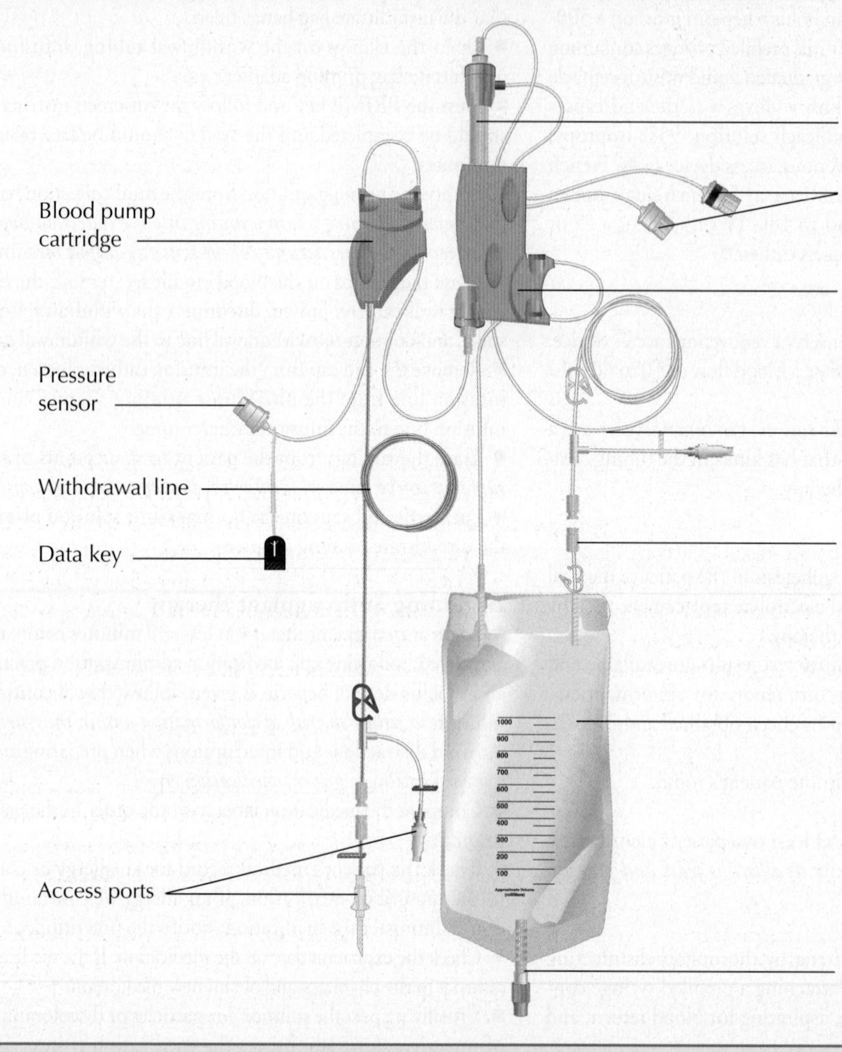

port of the access device). If discrepancies exist, rectify them before beginning the infusion.[24]

■ Make sure that the infusion pump alarm limits are set appropriately for the patient's correct condition and that the alarms are turned on, functioning properly, and audile to staff.[25,26,27]

Beginning aquapheresis therapy

■ Make sure the aquapheresis pump alarm limits are set appropriately for the patient's condition and that the alarms are turned in, functioning properly and audible to staff.[25,26,27]

■ Open the withdrawal and infusion tubing clamps.

■ Press the RUN key to begin therapy.[3]

■ If your unit has a hematocrit (HCT) monitor, make sure that the sensor clip is attached to the blood chamber on the blood circuit. Allow 5 to 10 minutes to elapse in the RUN mode *to complete the initial baseline measurement of the patient's HCT.* The text "Baselining" will appear; after "Baselining" is complete, press the HCT key and then set the HCT limit, using the up and down arrows. The HCT limit automatically restricts the fluid removal rate *to help prevent excessive volume depletion.*[4]

■ Set the blood flow rate by pressing the BLOOD FLOW key. Use the arrow keys to adjust the value. For a central venous catheter, begin the flow rate at 40 mL/minute. For a peripheral dual-lumen extended-length catheter, begin the flow rate at 25 mL/minute.

■ After the blood flow rate is stable, increase the rate in increments of 10 mL/hour until an adequate rate is determined. Use the arrow keys to adjust the rate. The average removal rate is 250 mL/hour. Patients in volume-sensitive states, such as those with right-sided heart failure, hepatic disease, or cardiogenic shock, usually require lower rates (50 to 100 mL/hr).[2,3]

■ Monitor the patient and the system for 10 minutes after beginning therapy. If after 10 minutes the system functions without alarming, secure the catheter.

■ Monitor the patient's vital signs every 15 minutes during the first hour of treatment and then hourly or more frequently as indicated by the patient's condition.[28,29]

■ Record intake and output hourly; include the ultrafiltrate in the patient's output volume.[3,28,29]
■ Monitor the system and respond to any alarms according to the manufacturer's guidelines. *The system has sensors to detect air bubbles in the blood circuit line, blood leaks in the ultrafiltrate line, and pressure in both lines.*[3]
■ Monitor the system for signs of clotting, such as frequent and unexpected infusion or withdrawal occlusions.[3]
■ Maintain the patient's fluid restriction.
■ Monitor the patient for signs of hypovolemia, such as tachycardia, hypotension, diminished urinary output, and elevations in blood urea nitrogen and creatinine levels.[30]
■ When the system alarms (indicating that the ultrafiltrate drainage bag is full), empty the bag into a liquid waste receptacle.[3]

Discontinuing aquapheresis therapy

■ Press the STOP key to stop the pumps.[3]
■ Clamp the withdrawal catheter extension tubing.
■ Disconnect the withdrawal blood circuit connection from the withdrawal catheter extension.
■ Flush the withdrawal catheter IV access and cap with preservative-free normal saline solution.
■ Clamp the infusion line.
■ Disconnect the infusion line.
■ Flush the infusion IV access and cap with preservative-free normal saline solution.
■ Return the HCT sensor to its dock on the back of the console.
■ Remove the blood circuit from the console by pressing the clips on the front and side cartridges and rotating the knobs while removing the tubing. Discard in an appropriate biohazard waste container.[3,31]
■ Power off the console by holding the ON/OFF key for 1 second.
■ Obtain the patient's weight.
■ Discard used supplies appropriately.[14]
■ Remove and discard your gloves.
■ Perform hand hygiene.[7,8,9,10,11]
■ Document the procedure.[32,33,34]

Cleaning the unit after each use

■ Put on clean gloves.[13,14]
■ Using a mild soap solution, clean the surface of the console.
■ Disinfect the console surfaces using 10% bleach solution, 95% isopropyl alcohol, or surface disinfectant. Apply the solution to a soft cloth to clean the console.[3,35]
■ Clean the tubing path through the air and blood leak detectors; use a flossing action to clean inside the detector with a lint-free cloth and warm water. Dry thoroughly.[3]
■ Remove the pumps, clean them, and reassemble them. Refer to the manual for instructions on removing and cleaning pumps. In some facilities, this is performed in the biomedical department.[3,35]
■ Remove and discard your gloves
■ Perform hand hygiene.[7,8,9,10,11]

Special considerations

■ The Joint Commission issued a sentinel event alert concerning medical device alarm safety *because alarm-related events have been associated with permanent loss of function or death.* Among the major contributing factors were improper alarm settings, alarm settings inappropriately turned off, and alarm signals not audible to staff. Make sure alarm limits are set appropriately and that alarms are turned on, functioning properly, and audible to staff. Follow facility guidelines for preventing alarm fatigue.[36]
■ Monitor partial thromboplastin time at intervals during therapy, as ordered or according to facility protocol. The recommended therapeutic range for therapy is 80 to 100 seconds.[2,29]

Double-checking high-alert medications[23]

If required by your facility, have another nurse perform an independent double-check of your preparation of a high-alert medication such as heparin *to ensure safe administration.* The second nurse must perform the following tasks:
■ Verify the patient's identity.
■ Make sure that the correct medication is being administered and is in the prescribed concentration.
■ Make sure that the medication's indication corresponds with the patient's diagnosis.
■ Verify that the dosage calculations are correct and that the dosing formula used to derive the final dose is correct.
■ Verify that the route of administration is safe and appropriate for the patient.
■ Make sure that pump settings are correct and that the infusion line is attached to the correct port.

■ Patients receiving warfarin (Coumadin) who have an International Normalized Ratio greater than 2 typically start on a continuous heparin infusion and aren't given an initial bolus of the drug. If heparin is contraindicated, argatroban may be prescribed.[3,37]
■ Aquapheresis can safely remove up to 500 mL or 1.1 lb (0.5 kg) of fluid per hour. The average treatment is 24 hours, with 6 L or 13.2 lb (6.0 kg) of fluid removed.[3]
■ Although patients can sit up in a chair and walk to the bathroom using the unit's battery backup, blood is pumped more efficiently through the filter with less patient movement, decreasing the length of the procedure.[3,23]
■ Magnetic resonance imaging (MRI) is contraindicated with the dual-lumen catheter *because the reinforcement coil may experience rotational or translational forces or temperature increases due to the magnetic field and pulsed radio-frequency fields.* Affix an AVOID MRI label to these catheters *to indicate this risk.*[24]
■ Adjust the ultrafiltration rates if the patient's blood pressure drops 10 mm Hg from baseline or if his heart rate is greater than 130 beats/minute after two consecutive measurements within 5 minutes. Obtain orders to reduce the ultrafiltration or briefly stop ultrafiltration *to allow the patient time to recover.*

Complications

An ultrafiltration alarm activates when ultrafiltrate pressure deviates from the usual range. This usually means clotting of the filter has occurred and requires that the filter be replaced. Contact the practitioner. If the practitioner wants to continue treatment, the procedure for replacement of the circuit and filter is located in the *Aquadex FlexFlow™ User's Guide.*[3]

Documentation

Record the date and time that therapy began; the reason for the therapy; the patient's weight before and after the treatment; vital signs and withdrawal, infusion, and ultrafiltrate pressures throughout the treatment; catheter access sites; initial Aquadex FlexFlow™ settings, changes made, and the reasons for such changes; intake and output; laboratory values, and the patient's tolerance to the procedure.

REFERENCES

1 De Maria, E., et al. (2010). Ultrafiltration for the treatment of diuretic-resistant, recurrent, acute decompensated heart failure: Experience in a single center. *Journal of Cardiovascular Medicine, 11,* 599–604.

2 *Dual lumen extended length catheter with coil reinforcement.* (2009). Brooklyn Park, MN: CHF Solutions, Inc.

3 *Aquadex FlexFlow™ user's guide.* (2007). Brooklyn Park, MN: CHF Solutions, Inc.

4 Gambro. (2011). "Aquadex FlexFlow™ details" [Online]. Accessed March 2015 via the Web at http://aquadex.gambro.com/en/aquadex/Our-Therapy/Product-Literature/Device-details/

5 The Joint Commission. (2015). Standard RI.01.03.01. *Comprehensive accreditation manual for hospitals: The official handbook.* Oakbrook Terrace, IL: The Joint Commission. (Level VII)

6 Centers for Medicare & Medicaid Services, Department of Health and Human Services. (2014). Condition of participation: Patient's rights. 42 C.F.R. § 482.13(b)(2).

7 The Joint Commission. (2015). Standard NPSG.07.01.01. *Comprehensive accreditation manual for hospitals: The official handbook.* Oakbrook Terrace, IL: The Joint Commission. (Level VII)

8 Centers for Disease Control and Prevention. (2002). Guideline for hand hygiene in health-care settings: Recommendations of the Healthcare Infection Control Practices Advisory Committee and the HICPAC/SHEA/APIC/IDSA Hand Hygiene Task Force. *MMWR Recommendations and Reports, 51*(RR-16), 1–45. Accessed March 2015 via the Web at http://www.cdc.gov/mmwr/pdf/rr/rr5116.pdf (Level II)

9 World Health Organization. (2009). "WHO guidelines on hand hygiene in health care: First global patient safety challenge, clean care is safer care" [Online]. Accessed March 2015 via the Web at http://whqlibdoc.who.int/publications/2009/9789241597906_eng.pdf (Level IV)

10 Centers for Medicare & Medicaid Services, Department of Health and Human Services. (2014). Condition of participation: Infection control. 42 C.F.R. § 482.42.

11 American Osteopathic Association. (2014). Standard 07.01.21. *Healthcare Facilities Accreditation Program: Accreditation requirements for acute care hospitals.* Chicago, IL: American Osteopathic Association. (Level VII)

12 The Joint Commission. (2015). Standard NPSG.01.01.01. *Comprehensive accreditation manual for hospitals: The official handbook.* Oakbrook Terrace, IL: The Joint Commission. (Level VII)

13 Siegel, J. D., et al. (2007). "2007 guideline for isolation precautions: Preventing transmission of infectious agents in healthcare settings" [Online]. Accessed March 2015 via the Web at http://www.cdc.gov/hicpac/pdf/isolation/Isolation2007.pdf (Level II)

14 Occupational Safety and Health Administration. (n.d.). "Bloodborne pathogens, standard number 1910.1030" [Online]. Accessed March 2015 via the Web at https://www.osha.gov/pls/oshaweb/owadisp.show_document?p_id=10051&p_table=STANDARDS

15 American Osteopathic Association. (2014). Standard 07.01.10. *Healthcare Facilities Accreditation Program: Accreditation requirements for acute care hospitals.* Chicago, IL: American Osteopathic Association. (Level VII)

16 Standard 45. Flushing and locking. Infusion nursing standards of practice. (2011). *Journal of Infusion Nursing, 34,* S59–S63. (Level VII)

17 U.S. Food and Drug Administration. (n.d.). "Look. Check. Connect. Safe medical device connections save lives" [Online]. Accessed March 2015 via the Web at http://www.fda.gov/downloads/MedicalDevices/Safety/AlertsandNotices/UCM134873.pdf

18 Westbrook, J., et al. (2010). Association of interruptions with an increased risk and severity of medication administration errors. *Archives of Internal Medicine, 170,* 683–690. (Level IV)

19 Institute for Safe Medication Practices. (2013). Side tracks on the safety express: Interruptions lead to errors and unfinished . . . Wait, what was I doing? *Nurse Advise-ERR, 11*(2), 1–4. Accessed March 2015 via the Web at https://www.ismp.org/Newsletters/acutecare/showarticle.aspx?id=37

20 The Joint Commission. (2015). Standard MM.06.01.01. *Comprehensive accreditation manual for hospitals: The official handbook.* Oakbrook Terrace, IL: The Joint Commission. (Level VII)

21 American Osteopathic Association. (2014). Standard 16.01.03. *Healthcare Facilities Accreditation Program: Accreditation requirements for acute care hospitals.* Chicago, IL: American Osteopathic Association. (Level VII)

22 Centers for Medicare & Medicaid Services, Department of Health and Human Services. (2014). Condition of participation: Preparation and administration of drugs. 42 C.F.R. § 482.23(c).

23 Institute for Safe Medication Practices. (2012). "ISMP's list of high-alert medications" [Online]. Accessed March 2015 via the Web at http://www.ismp.org/tools/highalertmedications.pdf

24 Institute for Safe Medication Practices. (2008). Conducting an independent double-check. *ISMP Medication Safety Alert! Nurse Advise-ERR, 6*(12), 1. Accessed March 2015 via the Web at http://www.ismp.org/newsletters/nursing/Issues/NurseAdviseERR200812.pdf

25 Graham, K. C., & Cvach, M. (2010). Monitor alarm fatigue: Standardizing use of physiological monitors and decreasing nuisance alarms. *American Journal of Critical Care, 19,* 28–37.

26 American Association of Critical-Care Nurses. (2013). "AACN practice alert: Alarm management" [Online]. Accessed March 2015 via the Web at http://www.aacn.org/wd/practice/docs/practicealerts/alarm-management-practice-alert.pdf (Level VII)

27 The Joint Commission. (2015). Standard NPSG.06.01.01. *Comprehensive accreditation manual for hospitals: The official handbook.* Oakbrook Terrace, IL: The Joint Commission. (Level VII)

28 The Joint Commission. (2015). Standard RC.02.01.01. *Comprehensive accreditation manual for hospitals: The official handbook.* Oakbrook Terrace, IL: The Joint Commission. (Level VII)

29 Wick, C., & Bakhai, A. (2012). Aquapheresis: A therapeutic option for fluid-overloaded patients. *British Journal of Cardiac Nursing, 7*(1), 20–24.

30 Mielniczuk, L. M., et al. (2010). Ultrafiltration in the management of acute decompensated heart failure. *Current Opinion in Cardiology, 25,* 155–160.

31 National Health Service, Purchasing and Supply Agency, Centre for Evidence-based Purchasing. (2008). *Evaluation report—CHF Solutions: Aquadex FlexFlow Ultrafiltration System (Report No. CEP 07017).* Newcastle upon Tyne, UK: Centre for Evidence-Based Purchasing.

32 The Joint Commission. (2015). Standard RC.01.03.01. *Comprehensive accreditation manual for hospitals: The official handbook.* Oakbrook Terrace, IL: The Joint Commission. (Level VII)

33 Centers for Medicare & Medicaid Services, Department of Health and Human Services. (2014). Condition of participation: Medical record services. 42 C.F.R. § 482.24(b).

34 American Osteopathic Association. (2014). Standard 10.00.03. *Healthcare Facilities Accreditation Program: Accreditation requirements for acute care hospitals.* Chicago, IL: American Osteopathic Association. (Level VII)

35 American Osteopathic Association. (2014). Standard 07.02.03. *Healthcare Facilities Accreditation Program: Accreditation requirements for acute care hospitals.* Chicago, IL: American Osteopathic Association. (Level VII)

36 The Joint Commission. (2013). "Sentinel event alert: Medical device alarm safety in hospitals" [Online]. Accessed March 2015 via the Web at http://www.jointcommission.org/assets/1/18/SEA_50_alarms_4_5_13_FINAL1.PDF (Level VII)

37 Costanzo, M. R. (2008). Ultrafiltration in the management of heart failure. *U.S. Cardiology: Touch Briefings, 5*(1), 66–69.

ADDITIONAL REFERENCES

Albert, N. M. (2012). Fluid management strategies in heart failure. *Critical Care Nurse, 32*(2), 20–34.

Bart, B. A., et al. (2012). Ultrafiltration in decompensated heart failure with cardiorenal syndrome. *New England Journal of Medicine, 367,* 2296–2304.

Felker, G. M., & Mentz, R. J. (2012). Diuretics and ultrafiltration in acute decompensated heart failure. *Journal of the American College of Cardiology, 59,* 2145–2153.

Fiaccadori, E., et al. (2011). Ultrafiltration in heart failure. *American Heart Journal, 161,* 439–449.

Peterangelo, M. (2009). Incorporating aquapheresis into therapy options for the treatment of volume overload: A CNS driven project. *Heart and Lung, 38,* 269–270.

Streets, K. W., & Vickers, S. M. (2012). Is this patient with heart failure a candidate for ultrafiltration? *Nursing 2012, 42*(6), 20–34.

ARTERIAL AND VENOUS SHEATH REMOVAL

The number of endovascular procedures performed by cardiologists and vascular surgeons has increased dramatically in the past decade. During such a procedure, the surgeon may place an arterial sheath, venous sheath, or both. Sheath removal can improve patient comfort and shorten the required time on bed rest, resulting in positive patient outcomes. However, sheath removal isn't without risks, so nurses assisting with the procedure must have appropriate training.

Manual compression can be used to help control bleeding following sheath removal, either alone or with a hemostasis pad. However, the nurse administering manual compression can experience fatigue and injury, and may develop carpal tunnel syndrome. Alternatively, devices can be used, including mechanical compression, collagen plug, staple-mediated closure, and percutaneous suture-mediated closure devices. Although mechanical compression techniques effectively prevent hematoma formation, the incidence of bleeding doesn't differ significantly for different methods of compression.[1] When using a plug-type device, staple-mediated closure device, or suture-mediated closure device, sheaths can be immediately removed after the procedure, regardless of the patient's coagulation status.

Equipment

Gloves ■ gown ■ mask and goggles or mask with face shield ■ electrocardiogram (ECG) monitor ■ blood pressure monitor ■ permanent marker ■ antiseptic solution (chlorhexidine or alcohol skin preparation) ■ sterile gauze ■ sterile gloves ■ hypoallergenic tape ■ fluid-impermeable pad ■ Optional: suture removal kit, sterile normal saline solution, transparent dressing, mechanical compression device, noninvasive hemostasis pad, prescribed local anesthetic (10 to 20 mL of 1% lidocaine),[2] prescribed analgesic, IV catheter insertion equipment.

Preparation of equipment

Administer an analgesic 20 to 30 minutes before the procedure, and assist with local anesthetic administration, as ordered, following safe medication administration practices *to promote patient comfort.*[2,3,4,5]

Perform hand hygiene[6,7,8,9,10,11,12] and then bring the equipment to the patient's bedside. Using sterile technique, open the gauze packages and place them within reach. If you're using a hemostasis pad, open it using sterile technique. (See the "Sterile technique, basic" procedure, page 715.)

Implementation

- Verify the practitioner's order for sheath removal.
- Before the procedure, review the patient's medical record *to assess for conditions that increase the patient's risk of bleeding* and check the patient's platelet count, prothrombin time, international normalized ratio, partial thromboplastin time, complete blood count, blood urea nitrogen and creatinine levels, and activated clotting time *to ensure that hemostasis can be achieved.*[3]

NURSING ALERT Keep in mind that patients receiving potent oral and IV antiplatelet and antithrombin medications who have such conditions as hypertension and renal dysfunction (defined as creatinine clearance of less than 60 mL/minute) are at increased risk for bleeding during percutaneous coronary intervention.[13]

- Gather and prepare the necessary equipment.
- Perform hand hygiene.[6,7,8,9,10,11,12]
- Confirm the patient's identity using at least two patient identifiers.[14]

Preparing for sheath removal

- Explain the procedure to the patient *to reduce anxiety and enhance cooperation.* Include anticipated postprocedure activity restrictions, discomfort caused by pressure to the site, and signs and symptoms to report.
- Make sure the patient is connected to the ECG monitor. Obtain the patient's vital signs and assess the ECG tracing on the monitor *to establish baselines.* Determine whether the patient's systolic blood pressure is less than 150 mm Hg *to facilitate homeostasis.* If the patient's blood pressure is elevated, notify the practitioner *because the practitioner may order medication to lower the patient's blood pressure before sheath removal to decrease postprocedure bleeding.*[3,13]
- Assess neurovascular status in the extremity distal to the sheath insertion site *to establish a baseline.*
- Mark the pulses distal to the sheath insertion site using a permanent marker *to facilitate finding the pulses.*
- Confirm that the patient has a patent IV catheter in place *in case emergency fluids or medications are required.* If not, insert one.[15] (See the "IV catheter insertion and removal" procedure, page 446.)
- Position the patient with the head of the bed flat *to promote hemostasis.*[3]
- Place the fluid-impermeable pad under the affected extremity *to keep the bed linens clean and to provide a place to set the sheath after removal.*
- If you're using a mechanical compression device, place it under the patient before sheath removal *to reduce patient movement and the risk of bleeding after sheath removal.*[3]
- If the sheath is sutured in place, open a suture removal kit using sterile technique.
- Perform hand hygiene.[6,7,8,9,10,11,12]
- Put on gloves and other personal protective equipment *to comply with standard precautions.*[16,17,18,19]
- Carefully remove the dressing covering the sheath insertion site.
- Clean the insertion site with the antiseptic solution.
- Remove and discard your gloves.[16,19]
- Perform hand hygiene.[6,7,8,9,10,11,12]
- Put on sterile gloves.[16,17,19]
- Remove the sutures, if present. (See the "Suture removal" procedure, page 731.)

Arterial sheath removal using manual or mechanical compression

- Locate the femoral pulse proximal to the insertion site *so that compression (manual or mechanical) can be properly positioned 1 to 2 cm above the insertion site.*[3]
- Hold the sheath with one hand while applying firm manual or mechanical pressure over the femoral artery with the other hand *to reduce bleeding.*
- Remove the sheath slowly while the patient exhales *to prevent the patient from bearing down during removal, which can cause a vasovagal response.* Continue to apply pressure manually or with the mechanical device.[3]

NURSING ALERT If you meet resistance while withdrawing he sheath, stop the procedure and notify the practitioner.[3]

- Apply continuous, firm pressure to the artery for approximately 20 minutes.[3] Ensure that the pressure is strong enough to stop the bleeding but not so strong that it obscures the pedal pulse. Continue to assess pulses distal to the insertion site; keep in mind that you might need a coworker to do this.

Arterial sheath removal using a noninvasive hemostasis pad with manual compression

- Apply pressure 1 to 2 cm proximal to the insertion site.[3]
- Place the pad directly over the insertion site.
- Remove the sheath slowly while the patient exhales *to prevent the patient from bearing down during removal, which can cause a vasovagal response.*
- Momentarily reduce proximal pressure to let a small amount of blood from the insertion site moisten the noninvasive hemostasis pad, and then reapply proximal pressure.[3]

■ After 3 to 4 minutes, slowly decrease pressure proximal to the insertion site while continuing to apply pressure to the insertion site for no less than 10 minutes. Continue to assess pulses distal to the insertion site; keep in mind that you might need a coworker to do this.[3]
■ Apply another sterile gauze pad over the hemostasis pad and cover the site with a transparent dressing *to reduce the risk of infection.*
■ Leave the hemostasis pad in place for 24 hours.
■ Remove manual pressure after hemostasis is achieved.

Venous sheath removal

■ Remove the venous sheath, if present, 5 to 10 minutes after removal of the arterial sheath *because pressure at the arterial site must be maintained for a longer time.*[3]
■ Apply pressure over the venous and arterial sites for 10 more minutes or until the bleeding stops.[3]
■ If a hemostasis pad is used, momentarily reduce proximal pressure *to let a small amount of blood from the insertion site moisten the noninvasive hemostasis pad,* and then reapply proximal pressure. After 3 to 4 minutes, slowly decrease pressure proximal to the insertion site while continuing to apply pressure to the insertion site for no less than 10 minutes. Then apply another sterile gauze pad over the hemostasis pad, cover the site with a transparent dressing, and leave it in place for 24 hours.
NURSING ALERT Avoid prolonged pressure on the femoral vein. Prolonged venous occlusion, especially with pressure devices, may cause venous thrombosis. Assess for neurovascular changes.[2]

Follow-up care

■ Apply sterile dressings to the arterial and venous insertion sites *to keep the areas clean and reduce the risk of infection.*[20,21]
■ Assess the patient's neurovascular status and vital signs as well as the insertion site in the affected limb every 15 minutes for 1 hour, every 30 minutes for the next hour, and then every hour for 4 hours *to detect signs of complications.*[3]
■ Instruct the patient to report any bleeding from the site, saturation of the dressing, or wetness or warmth on the groin or leg.
■ Tell the patient to report coolness, numbness, tingling, or pain in the affected extremity.
■ Keep the patient on bed rest for 2 but no longer than 6 hours when applying mechanical or manual pressure after arterial sheath removal *to reduce the complications of bed rest and back discomfort.*[3,22]
■ Keep the patient on bed rest for 1 to 4 hours when achieving hemostasis through percutaneous suture–mediated closure and hemostasis pads.
■ Keep the patient on bed rest for no more than 4 hours following venous sheath removal.
■ Discard used supplies in the appropriate receptacle.[16,17,19]
■ Remove and discard your gloves and other personal protective equipment, if worn.[16,19]
■ Perform hand hygiene.[6,7,8,9,10,11,12]
■ Perform a comprehensive pain assessment using techniques appropriate for the patient's age, conditions, and ability to understand.[23] Administer pain medication as ordered and indicated, using safe medication administration practices.[4,5]
■ Document the procedure.[24,25,26]

Special considerations

■ Remove the arterial sheath first *because you must apply pressure to the arterial site for a longer time than the venous site to achieve hemostasis. Doing so also enables you to use the venous line for IV fluids or medications as needed.*[3]
■ Some practitioners may prefer to use the radial artery for catheterizations. Because the radial artery is much smaller and located closer to the skin surface, internal bleeding is eliminated and any external bleeding can be easily compressed. After the catheter and sheath are removed from the radial artery, a compression device is placed around the wrist *to apply pressure.* Radial catheterization also eliminates the need for the patient to remain immobile. In general, patients find radial catheterization more comfortable than femoral catheterization *because they are able to sit up, walk, and eat immediately following removal.*[27]
■ If the patient is obese, you may need a second person to assist in holding back skin and abdominal folds.
■ In a patient with hypertension, you may need to apply pressure for a longer period of time *to ensure hemostasis.*
■ Read the manufacturer's instructions for correct use of mechanical compression devices. *Tissue damage can occur with incorrect use of the devices.*
■ If you can't stop the bleeding, notify the practitioner.

Patient teaching

Provide the patient and his family with written and oral discharge instructions. Tell the patient that he shouldn't lift anything heavier than 10 lb (4.5 kg) for 3 days and that he shouldn't drive or operate machinery for 24 hours. Tell him that he may remove the dressing and shower after 24 hours but that he shouldn't take a tub bath or swim until the skin is healed. After the initial 24 hours, the patient may clean the site with soap and water and apply a small adhesive bandage. Tell the patient to inspect the site daily and to notify his practitioner as soon as possible of any bleeding, redness, or discharge at the site or if he develops a fever.

Complications

The most common complication following sheath removal is bleeding, which occurs most commonly at the femoral artery access site. Retroperitoneal bleeding may also occur. Vascular complications include hematoma, pseudoaneurysm, arteriovenous fistula, embolus, and thrombus formation. Sensory or motor impairment may occur in the affected limb. Vasovagal complications may also occur.

Documentation

Record the date and time of sheath removal. Note whether an arterial sheath, a venous sheath, or both were removed and their locations. Record patient and family teaching about the removal procedure and activity restrictions following sheath removal as well as their understanding of the teaching. Note the patient's level of discomfort, using a 0 to 10 scale as well as the name, dose, route, and time of analgesics given. Document that laboratory values were checked before the sheath was removed and that they were within normal limits. Record vital signs, neurovascular status, and heart rhythm before sheath removal. State whether pulses distal to the sheath insertion sites were marked.

Note whether the patient has a patent IV line. Include that the patient was placed in a flat position for sheath removal. Describe the condition of the sheath insertion sites, noting redness, skin breakdown, drainage, bleeding, or hematoma formation. Note how many sutures were removed, if applicable. Explain any difficulties encountered during sheath removal. Record the type of hemostasis used and the time required for hemostasis to be achieved. Document the frequent of neurovascular, vital signs, and sheath removal site assessments. Note the patient's tolerance of the procedure.

Record complications, the time and name of the person notified, orders given, your interventions, and the patient's response to those interventions. Include the patient's position following sheath removal and the duration of bed rest.

REFERENCES

1 Benson, L. M., et al. (2005). Determining best practice: Comparison of three methods of femoral sheath removal after cardiac interventional procedures. *Heart and Lung, 34,* 115–121. (Level II)

2 Kern, M. J. (2012). *The interventional cardiac catheterization handbook* (3rd ed.). Philadelphia, PA: Saunders.
3 Lynn-McHale Wiegand, D. (Ed.). (2011). *AACN procedure manual for critical care* (6th ed.). St. Louis, MO: Saunders.
4 Centers for Medicare & Medicaid Services, Department of Health and Human Services. (2014). Condition of participation: Nursing services. 42 C.F.R. § 482.23(c).
5 American Osteopathic Association. (2014). Standard 16.01.03. *Healthcare Facilities Accreditation Program: Accreditation requirements for acute care hospitals.* Chicago, IL: American Osteopathic Association. (Level VII)
6 Centers for Disease Control and Prevention. (2002). Guideline for hand hygiene in health-care settings: Recommendations of the Healthcare Infection Control Practices Advisory Committee and the HICPAC/SHEA/APIC/IDSA Hand Hygiene Task Force. *MMWR Recommendations and Reports, 51*(RR-16), 1–45. Accessed March 2015 via the Web at http://www.cdc.gov/mmwr/pdf/rr/rr5116.pdf (Level II)
7 World Health Organization. (2009). "WHO guidelines on hand hygiene in health care: First global resident safety challenge, clean care is safer care" [Online]. Accessed March 2015 via the Web at http://whqlibdoc.who.int/publications/2009/9789241597906_eng.pdf (Level IV)
8 The Joint Commission. (2015). Standard NPSG.07.01.01. *Comprehensive accreditation manual for hospitals: The official handbook.* Oakbrook Terrace, IL: The Joint Commission. (Level VII)
9 Standard 19. Hand hygiene. Infusion nursing standards of practice. (2011). *Journal of Infusion Nursing, 34,* S26–S27. (Level VII)
10 Centers for Disease Control and Prevention. (2011). "Guidelines for the prevention of intravascular catheter-related infections" [Online]. Accessed March 2015 via the Web at http://www.cdc.gov/hicpac/pdf/guidelines/bsi-guidelines-2011.pdf (Level I)
11 Centers for Medicare & Medicaid Services, Department of Health and Human Services. (2014). Condition of participation: Infection control. 42 C.F.R. § 482.42.
12 American Osteopathic Association. (2014). Standard 07.01.21. *Healthcare Facilities Accreditation Program: Accreditation requirements for acute care hospitals.* Chicago, IL: American Osteopathic Association. (Level VII)
13 Merriweather, N., & Sulzbach-Hoke, L. M. (2012). Managing risk of complications at femoral vascular access sites in percutaneous coronary intervention. *Critical Care Nurse, 32*(5), 16–29. Accessed March 2015 via the Web at http://ccn.aacnjournals.org/content/32/5/16.full.pdf+html
14 The Joint Commission. (2015). Standard NPSG.01.01.01. *Comprehensive accreditation manual for hospitals: The official handbook.* Oakbrook Terrace, IL: The Joint Commission. (Level VII)
15 Standard 35. Vascular access site preparation and device placement. Infusion nursing standards of practice. (2011). *Journal of Infusion Nursing, 34,* S44–S46. (Level VII)
16 Siegel, J. D., et al. (2007). "2007 guideline for isolation precautions: Preventing transmission of infectious agents in healthcare settings" [Online]. Accessed March 2015 via the Web at http://www.cdc.gov/hicpac/pdf/isolation/Isolation2007.pdf (Level II)
17 Standard 18. Infection prevention. Infusion nursing standards of practice. (2011). *Journal of Infusion Nursing, 34,* S25–S26. (Level VII)
18 American Osteopathic Association. (2014). Standard 07.01.10. *Healthcare Facilities Accreditation Program: Accreditation requirements for acute care hospitals.* Chicago, IL: American Osteopathic Association. (Level VII)
19 Occupational Safety and Health Administration. (n.d.). "Bloodborne pathogens, standard number 1910.1030" [Online]. Accessed March 2015 via the Web at http://www.osha.gov/pls/oshaweb/owadisp.show_document?p_table=STANDARDS&p_id=10051 (Level VII)
20 Association of Professionals in Infection Control and Epidemiology. (2009). "An APIC guide 2009: Guide to the elimination of catheter-related bloodstream infections" [Online]. Accessed March 2015 via the Web at http://www.apic.org/Resource_/EliminationGuideForm/259c0594-17b0-459d-b395-fb143321414a/File/APIC-CRBSI-Elimination-Guide.pdf (Level IV)
21 Standard 46. Vascular access device site care and dressing changes. Infusion nursing standards of practice. (2011). *Journal of Infusion Nursing, 34,* S63–S64. (Level VII)
22 Walker, S., et al. (2008). Comparison of complications in percutaneous coronary intervention patients mobilized at 3, 4, and 6 hours after femoral arterial sheath removal. *Journal of Cardiovascular Nursing, 23,* 407–413. (Level II)
23 The Joint Commission. (2015). Standard PC.01.02.07. *Comprehensive accreditation manual for hospitals: The official handbook.* Oakbrook Terrace, IL: The Joint Commission. (Level VII)
24 The Joint Commission. (2015). Standard RC.01.03.01. *Comprehensive accreditation manual for hospitals: The official handbook.* Oakbrook Terrace, IL: The Joint Commission. (Level VII)
25 Centers for Medicare & Medicaid Services, Department of Health and Human Services. (2014). Condition of participation: Medical record services. 42 C.F. R. § 482.24(b).
26 American Osteopathic Association. (2014). Standard 10.00.03. *Healthcare Facilities Accreditation Program: Accreditation requirements for acute care hospitals.* Chicago, IL: American Osteopathic Association. (Level VII)
27 Balaji, N. R., & Shah, P. B. (2011). Radial artery catheterization. *Circulation, 124,* e407–e408. Accessed March 2015 via the Web at http://circ.ahajournals.org/content/124/16/e407.full.pdf+html

ADDITIONAL REFERENCES

Kordestani, S. S., et al. (2012). A randomized controlled trial on the hemostasis of femoral artery using topical hemostatic agent. *Clinical and Applied Thrombosis/Hemostasis, 18,* 501–505. (Level II)
Mego, D., et al. (2010). A poly-N-acetyl glucosamine hemostatic dressing for femoral artery access site hemostasis after percutaneous coronary intervention: A pilot study. *Journal of Invasive Cardiology, 22,* 35–39. (Level IV)
Sulzbach-Hoke, L. M., et al. (2010). Predictors of complications following sheath removal with percutaneous coronary intervention. *Journal of Cardiovascular Nursing, 25*(3), E1–E8. (Level VI)

ARTERIAL PRESSURE MONITORING

Arterial catheters provide direct arterial pressure monitoring, which permits continuous measurement of systolic, diastolic, and mean arterial pressures and allows for arterial blood sampling. Because direct measurement reflects systemic vascular resistance (SVR) as well as blood flow, it's generally more accurate than indirect methods (such as palpation and auscultation of Korotkoff [audible pulse] sounds), which are based on blood flow.

Direct monitoring is indicated when highly accurate or frequent blood pressure measurements are required, such as for patients with low cardiac output and high SVR. It can also be used for hospitalized patients who are obese or have severe edema—conditions that make indirect measurement difficult to perform—as well as for patients receiving titrated doses of vasoactive drugs and for those who require frequent blood sampling.

Arterial pressure monitoring is used in critical care settings. Catheter insertion, which can be performed at the beside under surgically sterile conditions, is performed by a practitioner. The catheter should be removed as soon as possible to decrease the risk of complications.[1]

A nurse caring for a patient undergoing arterial pressure monitoring must have an understanding of cardiac anatomy and physiology, the physiology of fluid and electrolyte balance, the pathophysiology of heart disease, and the hemodynamic alterations expected with cardiac interventions and surgery. Competence in setting up and maintaining arterial monitoring equipment, evaluating waveforms, and making clinical decisions about changes in a patient's therapy are also crucial. (See *Understanding an arterial waveform,* page 32.)

Understanding an arterial waveform

Normal arterial blood pressure produces a characteristic waveform, representing ventricular systole and diastole. The waveform has five distinct components: the anacrotic limb, the systolic peak, the dicrotic limb, the dicrotic notch, and end diastole.

The *anacrotic limb* marks the waveform's initial upstroke, which results as blood is rapidly ejected from the ventricle through the open aortic valve into the aorta. This rapid ejection causes a sharp rise in arterial pressure, which appears as the waveform's highest point, called the *systolic peak*.

As blood continues into the peripheral vessels, arterial pressure falls, and the waveform begins a downward trend. This part is called the *dicrotic limb*. Arterial pressure usually will continue to fall until pressure in the ventricle is less than pressure in the aortic root. When this occurs, the aortic valve closes. This event appears as a small notch (called the *dicrotic notch*) on the waveform's downside. When the aortic valve closes, diastole begins, progressing until the aortic root pressure gradually descends to its lowest point. On the waveform, this point is known as *end diastole*.

Normal arterial waveform

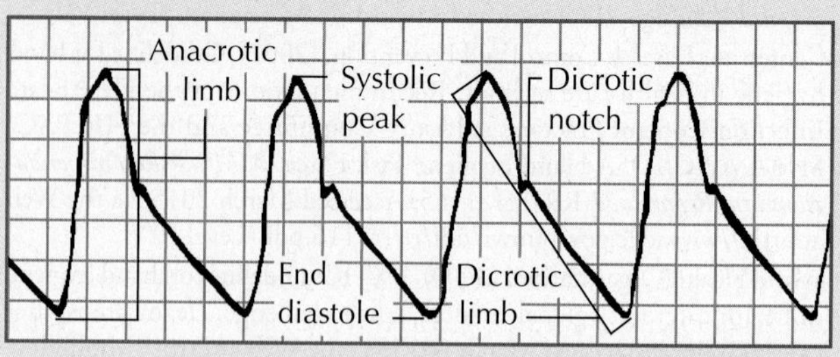

HOSPITAL-ACQUIRED CONDITION ALERT *Keep in mind that vascular catheter–associated infections are considered hospital-acquired conditions* because various best practices can reasonably prevent them. *Make sure to follow infection prevention practices, such as performing hand hygiene, using sterile technique, and properly preparing the insertion site, when assisting with arterial catheter insertion to reduce the risk of vascular catheter–associated infection.*[1,2]

A patient being monitored with an arterial pressure monitoring system can have blood samples for laboratory testing withdrawn from the arterial catheter. The arterial pressure monitoring system can be open or closed. An *open system* is one in which a collection tube holder is attached to the stopcock, withdrawing 5 mL of blood for waste, which is then discarded. A *closed system* has an attached reservoir that withdraws the waste; when all appropriate blood samples have been obtained, the blood in the reservoir can be returned to the patient.

According to the Centers for Disease Control and Prevention and the Infusion Nurses Society, the tubing and flush solution for an arterial line is considered a closed system and should be changed every 96 hours, immediately if contamination is suspected, or when the integrity of the product is compromised.[3] In some cases, however, you may need to change the flush solution more frequently due to use.

Removal of an arterial catheter should occur as soon as possible to decrease the risk of complications, such as thrombosis and infection.[1]

Equipment

For inserting a catheter

Gloves ▪ cap ▪ gown ▪ mask ▪ protective eyewear ▪ sterile gloves ▪ 16G to 20G catheter (the type and length depend on the patient's size and the insertion site, with a 20G catheter preferred for the radial artery site) ▪ preassembled preparation kit (if available) ▪ sterile drapes ▪ fluid-impermeable pad ▪ antiseptic solution (chlorhexidine [preferred] or tincture of iodine, povidone-iodine, or 70% alcohol if a contraindication to chlorhexidine exists)[3] ▪ prepared pressure transducer system ▪ ordered local anesthetic ▪ catheter securement device or sutures ▪ syringe and 21G to 25G 1″ (2.5-cm) needle ▪ IV pole ▪ tubing and medication labels ▪ site care kit ▪ padded arm board or limb splint ▪ leveling device or laser ▪ stethoscope and blood pressure cuff ▪ Optional: soap and water, clippers (for femoral artery insertion), portable ultrasound device, sterile probe cover, sterile ultrasound gel, sterile tape, soft limb restraint, sterile occlusive dressing, hypoallergenic tape.

For collecting a blood sample

Gloves ▪ collection tube holder or syringes of appropriate size and number for ordered laboratory tests ▪ needleless cannula ▪ labels ▪ laboratory biohazard bag ▪ needleless transfer device ▪ appropriate blood sample collection tubes ▪ disinfectant pad ▪ sterile, nonvented cap ▪ Optional: heparinized syringe or arterial blood gas kit, gown, mask and goggles or mask with face shield, laboratory request form.

For changing the tubing

Gloves ▪ gown ▪ mask ▪ protective eyewear ▪ fluid-impermeable pad ▪ preassembled arterial pressure tubing with flush device and disposable pressure transducer ▪ sterile gloves ▪ bag of IV flush solution (normal saline solution is recommended)[4] ▪ antiseptic solution swabs (preferably chlorhexidine) ▪ sterile occlusive dressing ▪ medication label ▪ pressure bag ▪ site care kit ▪ tubing labels.

For removing a catheter

Gloves ▪ sterile 4″ × 4″ (10-cm × 10-cm) gauze pads ▪ sterile suture removal kit ▪ dressing ▪ hypoallergenic tape ▪ Optional: mask, gown, protective eye wear, adhesive remover, sterile scissors, laboratory biohazard transport bag, sterile container, hemostatic pad, patch, or powder.

Preparation of equipment

Perform hand hygiene.[5,6,7] Set up and prime the monitoring system. (See the "Transducer system setup" procedure, page 780.) Use a closed flush system *to maintain patency of the pressure monitoring catheters.* Make sure you keep all parts of the pressure monitoring system sterile. Label all medications, medication containers, and other solutions on and off the sterile field.[8] When you've prepared the equipment, use the patient's individual vital sign parameters to guide you as you set the alarm limits on the bedside monitor.

Implementation

Inserting a catheter

- Gather and prepare the necessary equipment.
- Perform hand hygiene.[5,6,7]
- Confirm the patient's identity using at least two patient identifiers.[9]
- Position the patient for easy access to the catheter insertion site.
- Place a fluid-impermeable pad under the site.
- Put on a cap, a mask, gloves, and a gown and protective eye wear if needed.[9,10,11]

■ Obtain baseline data, including vital signs, level of consciousness, and hemodynamic parameters *to help identify acute changes.*
■ Make sure that informed consent has been obtained and is documented in the patient's medical record.[12]
■ Check the patient's history for any allergy or hypersensitivity to chlorhexidine or the ordered anesthetic.
■ Explain the procedure to the patient and his family, including the purpose of arterial pressure monitoring and the anticipated duration of catheter placement.
■ If the catheter will be inserted in the radial artery, perform an Allen test *to assess collateral circulation in the hand.*[13]
■ Conduct a time-out immediately before starting the procedure *to determine that the correct patient, site, positioning, and procedure are identified and to confirm, as applicable, that relevant information and necessary equipment are available.*[14]
■ If the intended site is visibly soiled, clean the area with soap and water before the practitioner prepares to site with antiseptic solution.[3] Then removes your gloves, perform hand hygiene, and put on a new pair of gloves.[5,6,7]
■ The practitioner wears a cap, mask, sterile gown, and sterile gloves during the procedure.[7] Make sure sterile technique is maintained throughout the procedure; voice your concerns if you notice a break in sterile technique.[5]
■ Using a preassembled preparation kit, the practitioner prepares and anesthetizes the insertion site. He cleans the area with chlorhexidine, allows it to dry, and then covers the surrounding area with a small, sterile fenestrated drape. (Maximal barrier protection should be used when inserting an axillary or femoral arterial catheter.)[2] The practitioner may use an ultrasound device with a sterile probe cover to locate the artery before insertion. The practitioner then inserts the catheter into the artery and attaches the catheter to the fluid-filled transducer tubing. During insertion, you may be required to assist with immobilizing the extremity and preparing the skin.
■ While the practitioner holds the catheter in place, activate the fast-flush release *to flush blood from the catheter.* After each fast-flush operation, observe the drip chamber *to verify that the continuous flush rate is as desired.* Watch for a waveform to appear on the bedside monitor.
■ The practitioner may suture the catheter in place, or secure it with a securement device. Cover the insertion site with a sterile occlusive dressing.
■ Immobilize the insertion site. With a radial or brachial site, use a padded arm board or limb splint that supports flexion of the joint *to maintain a functional position.*[15] With a femoral site, maintain the patient on bed rest, with the head of the bed raised no more than 30 degrees *to prevent the catheter from kinking.*
■ Level the zeroing stopcock of the transducer with the phlebostatic axis *because the phlebostatic axis reflects central arterial pressure.*[13]
■ Zero the system to atmospheric pressure *to prepare the monitoring system for accurate arterial pressure monitoring.*[1]
■ Obtain a manual blood pressure measurement and compare it with arterial blood pressure.[13]
■ Activate the monitor alarms as appropriate.
■ Remove and discard your personal protective equipment.
■ Perform hand hygiene.[5,6,7]
■ Run a waveform strip and document baseline data.[13]
■ Document the procedure.[16,17]

Collecting a blood sample

■ Perform hand hygiene.[5,6,7]
■ Confirm the patient's identity using at least two patient identifiers.[9]
■ Explain the procedure to the patient.
■ Put on gloves and other personal protective equipment as needed *to protect yourself from contact with bloodborne pathogens.*[12,13]
■ Position the patient for easy access to the catheter insertion site.
■ Assemble the equipment following sterile technique.
■ Locate the blood conservation reservoir and blood sampling port.
■ Trace the tubing from the patient to its point of origin *to make sure you're accessing the proper port.*
■ Temporarily silence the monitor alarms *to prevent unnecessary alarming that can contribute to alarm fatigue.*[18]

For an open monitoring system

■ Locate the blood sampling port of the stopcock nearest the patient on the arterial pressure monitoring system's tubing by tracing the tubing from the patient to its point of origin.[19]
■ Remove the nonvented cap from the stopcock (if a needleless cap isn't in place).
■ Thoroughly disinfect the stopcock port with a disinfectant pad using friction and then allow it to dry.[1,20]
■ Attach a cannula or adapter to the needleless blood collection tube holder.
■ Connect the needleless cannula or adapter with the needleless blood collection tube holder to the sampling port of the stopcock.
■ Turn off the stopcock to the flush solution.
■ Insert the labeled blood sample collection tube for the discard sample into the needleless blood collection tube holder. (This sample is discarded *because it's diluted with flush solution.*) Obtain a discard sample; in most cases, you'll withdraw 5 mL.
■ Insert each blood sample collection tube into the blood collection tube holder, keeping the stopcock turned off to the flush solution. Note that, because the blood collection tube holder is a nonvented system, no blood backflow from the patient will occur. Use the recommended order of draw to prevent tube additives from different tubes from mixing, *which may interfere with test results.*
■ After you've obtained blood for the final sample, turn off the stopcock to the needleless blood collection tube holder.
■ Activate the fast-flush release *to clear the tubing.*[13]
■ Turn off the stopcock to the patient, attach a labeled discard blood sample collection tube to the blood collection tube holder, and repeat the fast flush *to clear the stopcock port.*
■ Turn off the stopcock to the stopcock port, and remove the needleless cannula or adapter and the needleless blood collection tube holder.
■ Thoroughly disinfect the blood sampling port with a disinfectant pad using friction and allow it to dry.[20]
■ Place a new sterile, nonvented cap on the blood sampling port, if necessary.[13,20]

For a closed monitoring system

■ Locate the blood conservation reservoir and blood sampling port on the arterial pressure monitoring system's tubing by tracing the tubing from the patient to its point of origin.[19]
■ Turn the valve or stopcock off to the flush solution.
■ Open the valve or stopcock to the blood conservation reservoir.
■ Holding the blood conservation reservoir upright, slowly and gently pull back on the reservoir plunger until the reservoir fills with blood; this blood serves as discard blood. If you feel resistance, reposition the affected extremity and reattempt aspiration. If you still meet resistance, stop and notify the practitioner.[13]
■ Turn the one-way valve off to the reservoir by turning the handle perpendicular to the tubing *to ensure that the dead space volume remains in the reservoir.*[20]
■ Attach a needleless cannula to the needleless blood collection tube holder or syringe.[13]
■ Thoroughly disinfect the sampling port with an disinfectant pad using friction, and then allow it to dry.[1,20]

■ Access the blood sampling port using the needleless cannula with the attached needleless blood collection tube holder or syringe.[13]
■ If using the collection tube holder, attach the blood sample collection tubes and obtain the ordered samples. If using syringes, withdraw the appropriate volume of blood needed for the ordered samples.
■ When you have obtained the blood samples, remove the needleless cannula with the needleless blood collection tube holder or syringe.
■ Turn the valve to its original position, parallel to the tubing.
■ Open the valve to the discard blood and slowly and smoothly return the discard blood to the patient *to help decrease the risk of health-care acquired anemia.*[13]
■ Turn the valve to close the reservoir *to prevent the reservoir from becoming inadvertently activated.*
■ Open the valve or stopcock to the flush solution and activate the fast-flush device until the line is cleared of blood *to prevent clot formation.*[13]

Completing the procedure

■ Reactive the monitor alarms and check the monitor for the return of arterial waveform and pressure readings; make sure the alarm limits are appropriately set for the patient's current condition.[21] (See *Recognizing abnormal waveforms.*)
■ Label all blood sample collection tubes in the presence of the patient *to prevent mislabeling.*[14]
■ Send all samples to the laboratory in a laboratory transport bag with the appropriate documentation.
■ Remove and discard your gloves and other personal protective equipment if worn after the procedure.
■ Perform hand hygiene.[5,6,7]
■ Dispose of used supplies in appropriate containers.
■ Document the procedure.[16,17]

Changing the tubing

■ Perform hand hygiene.[5,6,7]
■ Confirm the patient's identify using at least two patient identifiers.[9]
■ Explain the procedure to the patient *to ensure cooperation.*
■ Position the patient for easy access to the catheter site.
■ Place a fluid-impermeable pad under the site.
■ Perform hand hygiene.[5,6,7]
■ Put on personal protective equipment, including a mask, a gown, gloves, and protective eyewear, as needed.[12,13]
■ Assemble the new pressure transducer system. (See the "Transducer system setup" procedure, page 780.)
■ Inflate the pressure bag to 300 mm Hg and check it for air leaks. Then release the pressure.
■ Prepare the IV flush solution and prime the pressure tubing and transducer system. If any additives were added, label the container with the date and time, the additive, and your initials.
■ Place the IV flush solution in the pressure bag. Apply 300 mm Hg of pressure to the system. Then hang the IV bag on a pole.[13]
■ Label all tubing with the date and time and your initials *to prevent an unintentional injection of drugs or other substances into the artery.*[19]
■ Remove the dressing from the catheter insertion site, taking care not to dislodge the catheter or cause vessel trauma.
■ Temporarily silence the monitor alarms.[13]
■ Turn off the flow clamp of the tubing segment that you'll change.
■ Disconnect the tubing from the catheter hub, taking care not to dislodge the catheter.
■ Immediately insert new tubing into the catheter hub. Trace the tubing from the patient to its point of origin *to make sure you've connected it to the proper port.*[19]
■ Secure the tubing *to prevent misconnections.*
■ Turn on the flow clamp.
■ Activate the transducer's fast-flush release *to clear the catheter of blood.*
■ Reactivate the monitor alarms.
■ Remove and discard your gloves, perform hand hygiene, and then put on sterile gloves.[5,6,7]
■ Clean the insertion site with an antiseptic swab (preferably chlorhexidine) and then allow it to dry.[1]
■ Apply an appropriate sterile occlusive dressing (transparent semipermeable dressing or gauze if the patient is diaphoretic or the site is oozing or bleeding) and label it with the date, the time, and your initials.[22]
■ Level the zeroing stopcock of the transducer with the phlebostatic axis *to reflect accurate central arterial pressure values,* and zero the system to atmospheric pressure.[13]
■ Remove and discard your glove, remove other personal protective equipment, and perform hand hygiene.[5,6,7]
■ Document the procedure.[16,17]

Removing a catheter

■ Verify the practitioner's order.
■ Check the patient's coagulation studies before catheter removal *to determine if you will need to hold pressure for a longer time in order to achieve hemostasis.*[13]
■ Gather all equipment.
■ Perform hand hygiene.[5,6,7]
■ Confirm the patient's identity using at least two patient identifiers.[9]
■ Explain the procedure to the patient.
■ Put on gloves and other personal protective equipment as needed *to comply with standard precautions.*[5,10]
■ Assist the patient to a sitting or recumbent position.[23,24]
■ Turn off the arterial monitoring alarms *to prevent nuisance alarms that contribute to alarm fatigue.*[13]
■ Turn off the flow clamp to the flush solution.[23,24]
■ Carefully remove the dressing over the insertion site *to prevent skin tearing or stripping.*[23,24] An adhesive remover may help with dressing removal.[23]

NURSING ALERT **Don't use scissors when removing arterial line dressings, tape, or the stabilization device to reduce the risk of severing the catheter or administration set or causing patient injury.**[25]

■ Remove the stabilization device. If sutures secured the catheter, remove them using a suture removal kit, and then carefully check that all sutures have been removed.[2,6,26]
■ Assess the catheter-skin junction for signs of infection, such as redness, swelling, and drainage from the insertion site.[13,27]
■ Turn the stopcock off to flush the solution.[13]
■ Apply pressure one to two finger widths above the insertion site with your nondominant hand *because the artery puncture site is above the catheter insertion site.*[13,27]
■ Apply a sterile gauze pad to the insertion site. With your dominant hand, slowly remove the catheter using gentle, even pressure.[1,27] Place the catheter tip on another sterile gauze pad.
■ Immediately after withdrawing the catheter, apply pressure to the site *to obtain hemostasis.*[13,27]
■ Maintain the pressure for at least 5 minutes until you achieve homeostasis. If necessary, apply a hemostatic pad, patch, or powder *to encourage clot formation.* Apply additional pressure if the site is femoral or if the patient has a coagulopathy or is receiving anticoagulants. Some facilities permit use of a compression device to apply pressure to a femoral site. (See the "Femoral compression" procedure, page 325.)
■ Apply a gauze pad and tape the dressing to the site. If the patient has fragile skin, use a dressing and tape specifically designed for fragile skin. Apply a pressure dressing to the site if necessary *to help prevent rebleeding in the patient who has a bleeding dyscrasia or who's receiving anticoagulant therapy.*
■ Assess the integrity of the removed catheter. Compare the length of the catheter with the original insertion length *to make sure you've removed*

Recognizing abnormal waveforms

Understanding a normal arterial waveform is relatively straightforward. However, an abnormal waveform is more difficult to decipher. Abnormal patterns and markings may provide important diagnostic clues to the patient's cardiovascular status, or they may simply signal trouble in the monitor. Use this chart to help you recognize and resolve waveform abnormalities.

ABNORMALITY	POSSIBLE CAUSES	NURSING INTERVENTIONS
Alternating high and low waves in a regular pattern 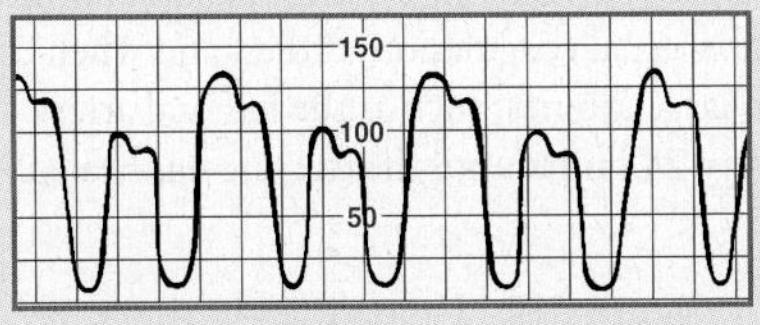	■ Ventricular bigeminy ■ Cardiac tamponade	■ Assess the patient's electrocardiogram *to confirm ventricular bigeminy.* The tracing should reflect premature ventricular contractions every second beat. ■ Assess the patient for signs and symptoms of cardiac tamponade, such as dyspnea, tachycardia, tachypnea, cool and clammy skin, pericardial friction rub, and diminished heart sounds.
Flattened waveform 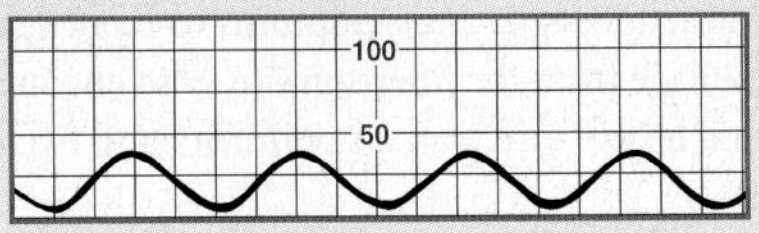	■ Overdamped waveform ■ Hypotensive patient	■ Perform the square wave test by activating and quickly releasing the fast-flush system. A sharp upstroke and then a return to baseline should appear on the monitor. Suspect an overdampened waveform if a slurred upstroke occurs at the beginning of the wave and if a loss of oscillations occurs after the initial downstroke. Check for kinks or obstructions in the line or tubing. Clear the line of air or blood. Repeat the square wave test *to verify an optimal waveform.* ■ If the square wave test indicates optimal waveform, assess and treat the patient for hypotension.
Slightly rounded waveform with consistent variations in systolic height 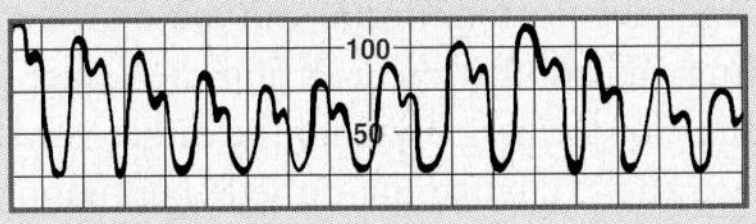	■ Patient on ventilator with positive end-expiratory pressure	■ Assess the patient's systolic blood pressure regularly. The difference between the highest and lowest systolic pressure reading should be less than 10 mm Hg. If the difference exceeds that amount, suspect pulsus paradoxus, possibly from cardiac tamponade.
Slow upstroke 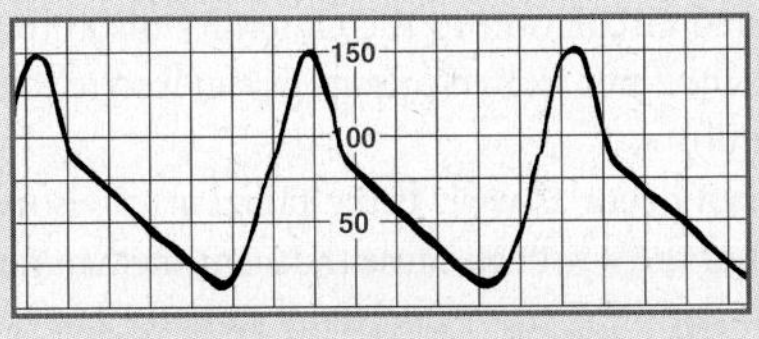	■ Aortic stenosis	■ Auscultate the patient's heart sounds for signs of aortic stenosis, such as a prolonged systolic ejection murmur and paradoxical splitting of the S2 heart sound. Also notify the practitioner, who will document suspected aortic stenosis in his notes.
Diminished amplitude on inspiration 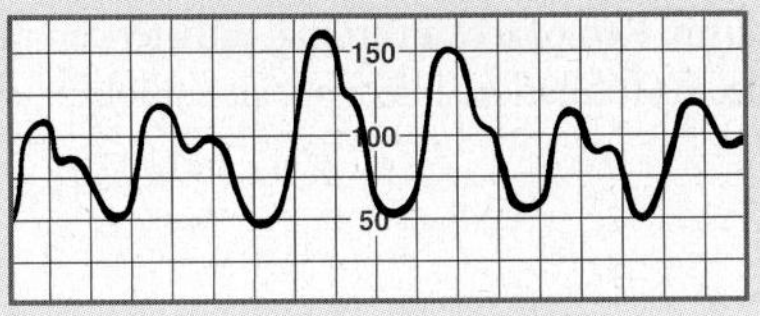	■ Pulsus paradoxus, possibly from cardiac tamponade, constrictive pericarditis, or lung disease	■ Note systolic pressure during inspiration and expiration. If inspiratory pressure is at least 10 mm Hg less than expiratory pressure, call the practitioner. ■ If you're also monitoring pulmonary artery pressure, observe for a diastolic plateau. This abnormal waveform occurs when the mean central venous pressure (right atrial pressure), mean pulmonary artery pressure, and mean pulmonary artery wedge pressure (pulmonary artery obstructive pressure) are within 5 mm Hg of one another.

the entire catheter.[27] If the catheter isn't intact, notify the practitioner immediately and monitor the patient closely for signs and symptoms of catheter embolism, such as dyspnea, cough, and chest pain.[27]

■ When bleeding is under control and if the practitioner has ordered a culture of the catheter tip, hold the catheter over the sterile container. Using sterile scissors, cut the tip so that it falls into the sterile container. Label the specimen in the presence of the patient *to prevent mislabeling* and place the container in a laboratory biohazard transport bag and send it to the laboratory.[28]

■ Discard used supplies in the appropriate receptacles.[29]

■ Remove and discard your gloves and any other personal protective equipment worn.

■ Perform hand hygiene.[5,6,7]

■ Inspect the site for bleeding and assess circulation in the extremity distal to the site by evaluating color, pulses, and sensation.[13] Repeat these assessments, as needed and ordered or as directed by your facility.

■ Perform hand hygiene.[5,6,7]

■ Document the procedure.[16,17]

Special considerations

Inserting a catheter

■ Be aware that several factors can lead to incorrect pressure readings, including a clotted catheter, loose connections, the addition of extra stopcocks or extension tubing, inadvertent entry of air into the system, and improper calibrating, leveling, or zeroing of the monitoring system. If the catheter lumen clots, the flush system may be improperly pressurized. Regularly assess the amount of flush solution in the IV bag, and maintain 300 mm Hg of pressure in the pressure bag.

■ Observing the pressure waveform on the monitor can enhance arterial pressure assessment. An abnormal waveform may reflect an arrhythmia (such as atrial fibrillation) or other cardiovascular problems, such as aortic stenosis, aortic insufficiency, pulsus alternans, or pulsus paradoxus.

■ Replace disposable or reusable transducers at 96-hour intervals. Replace other components of the system (including the tubing, the continuous-flush device, and flush solution) at the time the transducer is replaced.[1] Change the pressure tubing every 96 hours or immediately if contamination is suspected or the integrity of the system is compromised.[22]

■ Routine site care and dressing changes aren't performed on short peripheral catheters unless the dressing is soiled or no longer intact.[29]

■ Regularly assess the site for signs of infection, such as redness and swelling. Notify the practitioner immediately if you note such signs.

■ The Institute for Healthcare Improvement recommends using normal saline solution instead of a heparinized solution to flush the arterial line *to reduce the risk of medication errors associated with heparin, a high-alert medication.*[4]

Collecting a blood sample

■ Limit the number of times you enter the arterial pressure monitoring system by grouping blood draws, if possible, *to minimize the risk of infection.*

■ Always assess the arterial waveform before and after blood withdrawal *to ensure the system is operating properly.*

■ *To prevent health care–acquired anemia,* use the minimal amount of blood for discard.

■ *To detect health care–acquired anemia,* monitor hemoglobin level and hematocrit. Report decreasing levels to the practitioner.

■ Assess catheter necessity daily during multidisciplinary rounds, and discontinue the catheter as soon as it's no longer needed *to reduce the risk of infection.*

■ Be aware that erroneous pressure readings can result from a catheter that's clotted or positional, loose connections, the addition of extra stopcocks or extension tubing, inadvertent entry of air into the system, or improper calibration, leveling, or zeroing of the monitoring system. If the catheter lumen clots, the flush system may be improperly pressurized. Regularly assess the amount of flush solution in the IV bag, and maintain 300 mm Hg of pressure in the pressure bag.

Changing the tubing

■ Some facilities add 500 to 1,000 units of heparin to the flush bag *to help ensure a patent arterial line.* However, the Institute for Healthcare Improvement doesn't support its use as a flush solution *because it's a high-alert medication and therefore increases the risk of medication administration errors.*[4]

■ Observing the pressure waveform on the monitor can enhance assessment of arterial pressure. An abnormal waveform may reflect an arrhythmia (such as atrial fibrillation) or other cardiovascular problems, such as aortic stenosis, aortic insufficiency, pulsus alternans, or pulsus paradoxus.

■ Be aware that erroneous pressure readings can result from a catheter that's clotted or positional, loose connections, the addition of extra stopcocks or extension tubing, inadvertent entry of air into the system, or improper calibrating, leveling, or zeroing of the monitoring system. If the catheter lumen clots, the flush system may be improperly pressurized. Regularly assess the amount of flush solution in the IV bag, and maintain 300 mm Hg of pressure in the pressure bag.[22]

■ Replace arterial catheters only when there's a clinical indication to do so.[1]

■ Keep in mind that the risk of complications, such as thrombosis and infection, increases with the length of time the catheter is in place. Discontinue the catheter as soon as it's no longer needed *to reduce the risk of complications.*[13]

■ Assess the site for signs of infection, such as redness, swelling, and drainage. Notify the practitioner if you note such signs.

Removing a catheter

■ Be aware that you might need to apply direct pressure for a longer time *to achieve hemostasis* in patients receiving systemic heparin or thrombolytics, in patients with abnormal coagulation studies, and when catheters have been inserted in large arteries, such as the femoral artery.[13]

■ Change the dressing every 24 hours until the exit site has healed.

Patient teaching

Inserting a catheter

Teach the patient how to properly care for the arterial catheter, precautions for preventing infection, and signs and symptoms to report, such as pain, tenderness, and drainage from the insertion site. Also encourage the patient to make sure that health care workers perform hand hygiene before providing care.[29]

Removing a catheter

Teach the patient about reporting signs and symptoms of bleeding, infection, and phlebitis after catheter removal.

Complications

Arterial catheter insertion and pressure monitoring can cause such complications as arterial bleeding; infection at the insertion site, which can spread into the bloodstream; clot formation within the catheter, which can then be carried into the general circulation; catheter perforation of the vessel wall, which can be associated with excessive bleeding and extravasation of flush solution into the surrounding tissue; air embolism; arterial spasm; and impaired circulation to the extremity distal to the catheter insertion site, which, if not treated promptly, can lead to loss of tissue or, ultimately, the limb.

Other complications can occur as well. If the radial artery is used, prolonged hyperextension of the wrist can cause transient median nerve conduction deficits. Blood sampling from an arterial catheter can cause such complications as arterial bleeding, infection, air embolism, or arterial spasm; an arterial line tubing change may also result in arterial bleeding, infection, or air embolism. Removal of an arterial catheter can cause arterial bleeding and hematoma formation, infection, air embolism, arterial spasm, or thrombosis.

Documentation

If you assisted with insertion, record the date and time of insertion, assessment findings, the insertion site used, catheter size used, type of flush solution used, and the patient's response to the procedure. Document the color, warmth, sensation, and pulse strength of the extremity distal to the catheter insertion site before insertion, immediately after insertion, and at regular intervals as determined by your facility. Document alarm settings.

Record the patient's position for zeroing the transducer so that other health care team members can replicate the placement. Record the patient's manual blood pressure in comparison with the blood pressure obtained through the arterial catheter. Document dressing, tubing, and flush solution changes, when appropriate.

Document the date, time, and type of blood samples drawn, along with any laboratory test results (when available). Document the quality of the arterial waveform before specimen collection as well as any unexpected outcomes and interventions after specimen collection.

Record the date and time of a tubing change, the type of flush solution used, your assessment findings, and the patient's response to the procedure. Carefully document the amount of flush solution infused.

Document any patient teaching and the patient's understanding of your teaching.

REFERENCES

1 Centers for Disease Control and Prevention. (2011). "Guidelines for the prevention of intravascular catheter-related infections" [Online]. Accessed September 2014 via the Web at http://www.cdc.gov/hicpac/pdf/guidelines/bsi-guidelines-2011.pdf (Level I)

2 Jarrett, N., et al. (2013). "Evidence-based guidelines for selected and previously considered hospital-acquired conditions: Final report" [Online]. Accessed March 2015 via the Web at http://www.cms.gov/Medicare/Medicare-Fee-for-Service-Payment/HospitalAcqCond/Downloads/Evidence-Based-Guidelines.pdf

3 Standard 35. Vascular access site preparation and device placement. Infusion nursing standards of practice. (2011). *Journal of Infusion Nursing, 34,* S44–S46. (Level VII)

4 Institute for Healthcare Improvement. (2012). *How-to guide: Prevent harm from high-alert medications.* Cambridge, MA: Institutes for Healthcare Improvement. (Level VII)

5 The Joint Commission. (2015). Standard NPSG.07.01.01. *Comprehensive accreditation manual for hospitals: The official handbook.* Oakbrook Terrace, IL: The Joint Commission. (Level VII)

6 Centers for Disease Control and Prevention. (2002). Guideline for hand hygiene in health-care settings: Recommendations of the Healthcare Infection Control Practices Advisory Committee and the HICPAC/SHEA/APIC/IDSA Hand Hygiene Task Force. *MMWR Recommendations and Reports, 51* (RR-16), 1–45. Accessed March 2015 via the Web at http://www.cdc.gov/mmwr/pdf/rr/rr5116.pdf (Level II)

7 World Health Organization. (2009). "WHO guidelines on hand hygiene in health care: First global patient safety challenge, clean care is safer care" [Online]. Accessed March 2015 via the Web at http://whqlibdoc.who.int/publications/2009/9789241597906_eng.pdf (Level IV)

8 American Osteopathic Association. (2014). Standard 25.01.27. *Healthcare Facilities Accreditation Program: Accreditation requirements for acute care hospitals.* Chicago, IL: American Osteopathic Association. (Level VII)

9 The Joint Commission. (2015). Standard NPSG.01.01.01. *Comprehensive accreditation manual for hospitals: The official handbook.* Oakbrook Terrace, IL: The Joint Commission. (Level VII)

10 Siegel, J. D., et al. (2007). "2007 guideline for isolation precautions: Preventing transmission of infectious agents in healthcare settings" [Online]. Accessed June 2014 via the Web at http://www.cdc.gov/hicpac/pdf/isolation/Isolation2007.pdf (Level II)

11 American Osteopathic Association. (2014). Standard 07.01.10. *Healthcare Facilities Accreditation Program: Accreditation requirements for acute care hospitals.* Chicago, IL: American Osteopathic Association. (Level VII)

12 American Osteopathic Association. (2014). Standard 30.01.11. *Healthcare Facilities Accreditation Program: Accreditation requirements for acute care hospitals.* Chicago, IL: American Osteopathic Association. (Level VII)

13 Lynn-McHale Wiegand, D. (Ed.). (2011). *AACN procedure manual for critical care* (6th ed.). St. Louis, MO: Saunders.

14 The Joint Commission. (2015). Standard UP.01.01.01. *Comprehensive accreditation manual for hospitals: The official handbook.* Oakbrook Terrace, IL: The Joint Commission. (Level VII)

15 Standard 37. Joint stabilization. Infusion nursing standards of practice. (2011). *Journal of Infusion Nursing, 34,* S47–S48. (Level VII)

16 American Osteopathic Association. (2014). Standard 10.00.03. *Healthcare Facilities Accreditation Program: Accreditation requirements for acute care hospitals.* Chicago, IL: American Osteopathic Association. (Level VII)

17 Centers for Medicare & Medicaid Services, Department of Health and Human Services. (2014). Condition of participation: Nursing services. 42 C.F.R. § 482.24(b).

18 The Joint Commission. (2013). "Sentinel event alert: Medical device alarm safety in hospitals" [Online]. Accessed March 2015 via the Web at http://www.jointcommission.org/assets/1/18/SEA_50_alarms_4_5_13_FINAL1.PDF (Level VII)

19 U.S. Food and Drug Administration. (n.d.). "Look. Check. Connect. Safe medical device connections save lives" [Online]. Accessed March 2015 via the Web at http://www.fda.gov/downloads/MedicalDevices/Safety/AlertsandNotices/UCM134873.pdf

20 Standard 27. Needleless connectors. Infusion nursing standards of practice. (2011). *Journal of Infusion Nursing, 34*(Suppl. 1), S32–S33.

21 Graham, K. C., & Cvach, M. (2010). Monitor alarm fatigue: Standardizing use of physiological monitors and decreasing nuisance alarms. *American Journal of Critical Care, 19,* 28–37.

22 Standard 43. Administration set change. Infusion nursing standards of practice. (2011). *Journal of Infusion Nursing, 34*(Suppl. 1), S55–S57. (Level VII)

23 Infusion Nurses Society. (2011). *Policies and procedures for infusion nursing* (4th ed.). Boston, MA: Infusion Nurses Society.

24 Infusion Nurses Society. (2013). *Policies and procedures for infusion nursing of the older adult* (2nd ed.). Boston, MA: Infusion Nurses Society.

25 Standard 21. Scissors. Infusion nursing standards of practice. (2011). *Journal of Infusion Nursing, 34,* S27–S28. (Level VII)

26 Edwards Lifesciences. (2009). "Edwards TruWave disposable pressure transducer VAMP closed blood sampling systems" [Online]. Accessed March 2015 via the Web at http://ht.edwards.com/scin/edwards/sitecollectionimages/products/pressuremonitoring/truwaveb

27 Standard 44. Vascular access device removal. Infusion nursing standards of practice. (2011). *Journal of Infusion Nursing, 34,* S57–S59. (Level VII)

28 The Joint Commission. (2015). Standard NPSG.03.04.01. *Comprehensive accreditation manual for hospitals: The official handbook.* Oakbrook Terrace, IL: The Joint Commission. (Level VII)

29 Occupational Safety and Health Administration. (n.d.). "Bloodborne pathogens, standard number 1910.1030" [Online]. Accessed March 2015 via the Web at http://www.osha.gov/pls/oshaweb/owadisp.show_document?p_table=STANDARDS&p_id=10051

ADDITIONAL REFERENCE

Urden, L. D., et al. (2012). *Priorities in critical care nursing* (6th ed.). St. Louis, MO: Mosby.

ARTERIAL PUNCTURE FOR BLOOD GAS ANALYSIS

Obtaining an arterial blood sample requires percutaneous puncture of the brachial, radial, or femoral artery or withdrawal of a sample from an arterial line. After it's collected, the sample can be analyzed to determine arterial blood gas (ABG) values.

ABG analysis evaluates ventilation by measuring blood pH and the partial pressures of arterial oxygen ($Pa{O_2}$) and carbon dioxide ($Pa{CO_2}$). Blood pH measurement reveals the blood's acid-base balance, $Pa{O_2}$ indicates the amount of oxygen in the blood, and $Pa{CO_2}$ indicates the lungs' capacity to eliminate carbon dioxide. ABG samples can also be analyzed for total hemoglobin, oxygen content, saturation of dyshemoglobins, bicarbonate values, and base excess or deficit.[1]

Typically, ABG analysis is ordered when respiratory distress or failure is suspected. It's also performed during episodes of shock and after coronary artery bypass surgery, resuscitation from cardiac arrest, changes in respiratory therapy or status, and prolonged anesthesia.

Most ABG samples can be drawn by a respiratory therapist or specially trained nurse. Collection from the femoral artery, however, is usually performed by a practitioner. Before attempting a radial puncture,

Performing an Allen test

To perform an Allen test, rest the patient's arm on the mattress or bedside stand and support his wrist with a rolled towel. Then tell him to clench his fist. Using your index and middle fingers, press on the radial and ulnar arteries using firm pressure. Hold this position for a few seconds.

Without removing your fingers from the patient's arteries, ask him to unclench his fist and hold his hand in a relaxed position. The palm will be blanched *because pressure from your fingers has restricted the normal blood flow.*

Blanched palm

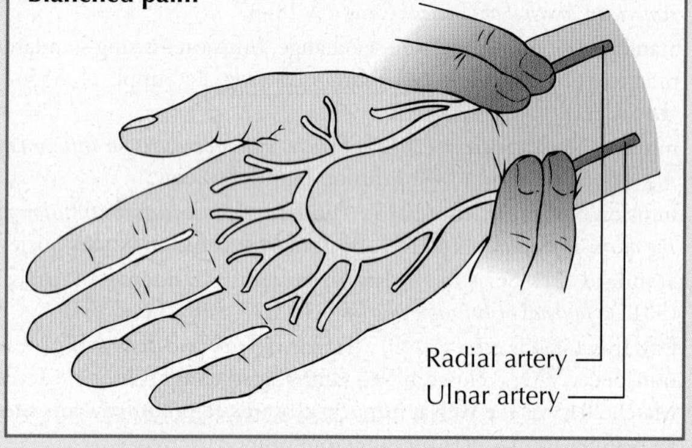

Release pressure on the patient's ulnar artery. The test is positive if his hand becomes flushed, *which indicates a patent ulnar artery,* and you can safely proceed with the radial artery puncture. The test is negative if his hand doesn't flush, indicating that blood flow is compromised. In that case, select another site for the puncture.

Flushed palm

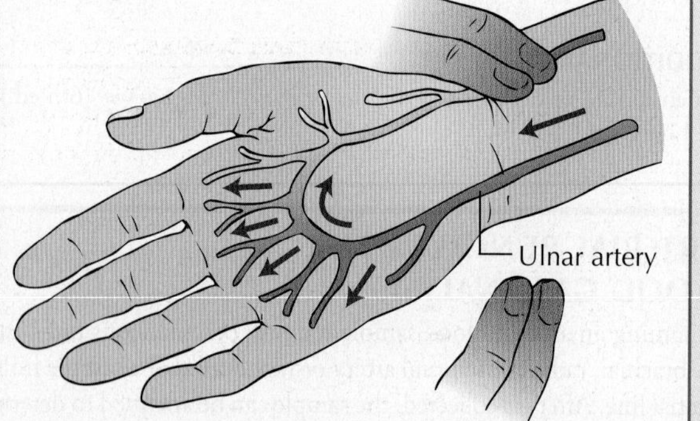

an Allen test should be performed *to assess for adequate circulation.* (See *Performing an Allen test.*)

Equipment

Preheparinized ABG plastic luer-lock syringe specially made for drawing blood for ABG analysis ■ 20G to 25G 1″ to 1½″ (2.5-cm to 3.8-cm) needle ■ gloves ■ 70% isopropyl alcohol pad or chlorhexidine solution pad[2,3,4] ■ two 2″ × 2″ (5-cm × 5-cm) gauze pads ■ rubber cap for syringe hub ■ laboratory biohazard transport bag ■ label ■ laboratory request form ■ small towel ■ adhesive bandage ■ Optional: Gown, mask and goggles with face shield, 1% lidocaine solution without epinephrine or eutectic mixture of local anesthetics cream, 1-mL syringe with 22G needle, 1-mL ampule of aqueous heparin (1:1,000), plastic bag, crushed ice.

Many health care facilities use a commercial ABG kit that contains some of the equipment listed above.

Preparation of equipment

If time allows, administer local anesthetic cream at least 1 hour before the procedure *because it requires at least 1 hour to achieve its effect.*

Open the ABG kit and remove the sample label and the plastic bag. If the syringe isn't heparinized, you will have to do so. To heparinize the syringe, first attach the 22G needle to the syringe. Then open the ampule of heparin. Draw all the heparin into the syringe *to prevent the sample from clotting.* Hold the syringe upright, and rotate the barrel while pulling the plunger back *to allow the heparin to coat the entire inside surface of the syringe.* Then slowly force the heparin toward the hub of the syringe, and expel all of the heparin.

Blood gases analysis should be performed within 10 minutes of obtaining the blood sample.[5] Fill a plastic bag with enough crushed ice to contain the syringe if you anticipate a delay in analysis.

Implementation

- Verify the practitioner's order.
- Review the patient's medical record for current anticoagulation therapy, clotting disorders, and pertinent laboratory values *to determine the patient's risk of prolonged bleeding after the procedure.* Discuss any concerns with the patient's practitioner.
- Perform hand hygiene.[6,7,8,9,10]
- Confirm the patient's identity using at least two patient identifiers.[11]
- Tell the patient you need to collect an arterial blood sample, and explain the procedure *to help ease anxiety and promote cooperation.* Tell him that the needle stick will cause some discomfort but that he must remain still during the procedure.
- Perform hand hygiene.[6,7,8,9,10]
- Put on gloves and a gown, mask and goggles, or a face shield with a mask, if exposure to blood is anticipated.[2,12,13]
- Place a rolled towel under the patient's wrist *for support.*
- Locate the artery, palpate it for a strong pulse, and perform an Allen test. If the test is negative, don't use the radial artery; instead, select another site.[3]
- Clean the intended puncture site with an antiseptic pad[2,3,4] using a back-and-forth motion while applying friction for 30 seconds according to the manufacturer's recommendation.[14]
- Allow the skin to dry.[13]
- If indicated, administer a local anesthetic to the puncture site. However, consider use of lidocaine carefully *because it delays the procedure, the patient may be allergic to the drug, and the resulting vasoconstriction may prevent successful puncture.*[15]
- Palpate the artery with the index and middle fingers of one hand while holding the syringe over the puncture site with the other hand. The puncture site should be between your index and middle fingers as they palpate the pulse.
- Hold the needle bevel up at a 30- to 60-degree angle. (See *Arterial puncture technique.*)
- Puncture the skin and the arterial wall in one motion, following the path of the artery.
- Watch for blood backflow in the syringe. Don't pull back on the plunger *because arterial blood should enter the syringe automatically.* Obtain 1 mL of blood.
- After collecting the sample, press a gauze pad firmly over the puncture site until the bleeding stops—at least 5 minutes. If the patient is receiving anticoagulant therapy or has a blood dyscrasia, apply pressure for 10 to 15 minutes; if necessary, ask a coworker to hold the gauze pad in place while you prepare the sample for transport to the laboratory. Don't ask

the patient to hold the pad *because failure to apply sufficient pressure can cause a large, painful hematoma to form, hindering future arterial punctures at that site.*

- Check the syringe for air bubbles. If any appear, remove them by holding the syringe upright and slowly ejecting some of the blood onto a 2″ × 2″ (5-cm × 5-cm) gauze pad *to prevent alteration of the test results.*[1]
- Use the syringe safety device to cover the needle, and then remove the needle and place a rubber cap directly on the syringe tip *to prevent the sample from leaking and to keep air out of the syringe.*
- Gently roll the syringe in your hands for 30 seconds *to mix the heparin, which prohibits the sample from clotting.*
- Label the syringe in the presence of the patient *to prevent mislabeling.*[11] Record on the label the patient's name or other patient identifier, birth date or age, room number, date and collection time, practitioner's name, test to be performed, clinical indication for the test, sample site, patient's respiratory rate, oxygen flow rate (if the patient is receiving supplemental oxygen), ventilator settings (if the patient is on the ventilator), and your signature.[1]
- Put the labeled sample in the laboratory biohazard transport bag. Attach a properly completed laboratory request form, and immediately send the sample to the laboratory.[1,16] If the sample can't be sent to the laboratory immediately, put it on ice.[14]
- When the site stops bleeding, apply a small adhesive bandage to the site.
- Monitor the patient's vital signs, and observe for signs of circulatory impairment, such as swelling, discoloration, pain, numbness, and tingling in the arm or leg. Also watch for bleeding at the puncture site.
- Discard used equipment in the appropriately.[17]
- Remove and discard your gloves and other personal protective equipment, if worn.
- Perform hand hygiene.[6,7,8,9,10]
- Document the procedure.[18,19,20]

Special considerations

- Chilling the sample extends the time to test the sample for up to 1 hour; if more than an hour has elapsed since collection, discard the sample.[3]
- If the patient is receiving oxygen, make sure this therapy has been underway for 20 to 30 minutes before collecting an arterial blood sample, if ordered. If the patient has received a nebulizer treatment, wait 20 minutes before collecting the sample. If the patient recently underwent suctioning or was placed on mechanical ventilation or if the fraction of inspired oxygen concentration has been changed, wait at least 15 minutes before collecting a blood sample.[14]
- Unless ordered, don't turn off existing oxygen therapy before collecting an arterial blood sample.
- Indicate on the laboratory request slip the amount and type of oxygen therapy the patient is receiving.
- If the patient isn't receiving oxygen, indicate that he's breathing room air.
- When filling out a laboratory request form for ABG analysis, include the patient's body temperature, activity level, and working diagnosis[1] *to help the laboratory staff calibrate the equipment and evaluate the results.*

Complications

If you use too much force when attempting to puncture an artery, the needle may touch the periosteum of the bone, causing the patient considerable pain, or you may advance the needle through the opposite wall of the artery. If this happens, slowly pull the needle back a short distance and check to see if you obtain blood return. If blood still fails to enter the syringe, withdraw the needle completely and attempt the puncture with a new needle and syringe. Don't make more than two attempts to withdraw blood from the same site. *Probing the artery may injure it and the radial nerve. Also, hemolysis will occur, altering test results.*

Arterial puncture technique

The angle of needle penetration in arterial blood gas sampling depends on which artery is being sampled. For the radial artery, which is used most often, the needle should enter bevel up at a 30- to 60-degree angle over the radial artery.

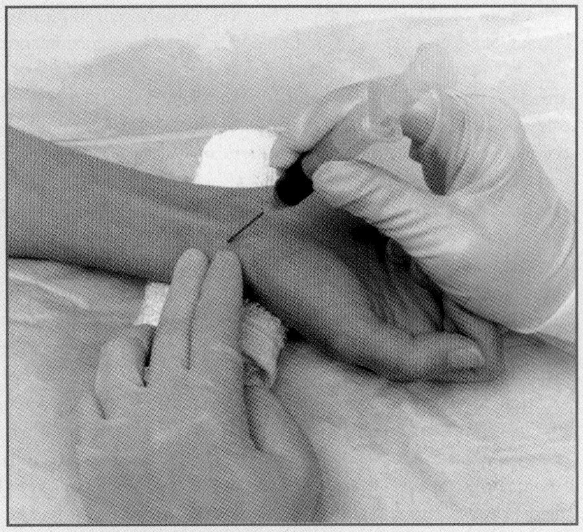

If arterial spasm occurs, blood won't flow into the syringe and you won't be able to collect the sample. If this happens, replace the needle with a smaller one and try the puncture again *because a smaller-bore needle is less likely to cause arterial spasm.*

Documentation

Record the results of the Allen test, the time the sample was drawn, the patient's temperature, the site of the arterial puncture, the amount of time that pressure was applied to the site to control bleeding, the name of the person drawing the sample, and the type and amount of oxygen therapy the patient was receiving.

REFERENCES

1 American Association for Respiratory Care (AARC). (2001). AARC clinical practice guideline: Blood gas analysis and hemoximetry: 2001 revision & update. *Respiratory Care, 46,* 498–505. Accessed March 2015 via the Web at http://www.rcjournal.com/cpgs/bgacpg-update.html (Level VII)

2 World Health Organization. (2010). "WHO guidelines on drawing blood: Best practices in phlebotomy" [Online]. Accessed March 2015 via the Web at http://whqlibdoc.who.int/publications/2010/9789241599221_eng.pdf (Level IV)

3 Kacmarek, R. M., et al. (2013). *Egan's fundamentals of respiratory care* (10th ed.). St Louis, MO: Mosby.

4 Centers for Disease Control and Prevention. (2011). "Guidelines for the prevention of intravascular catheter-related infections" [Online]. Accessed March 2015 via the Web at http://www.cdc.gov/hicpac/pdf/guidelines/bsi-guidelines-2011.pdf (Level I)

5 Lynn-McHale Wiegand, D. (Ed.). (2011). *AACN procedure manual for critical care* (6th ed.). St. Louis, MO: Saunders.

6 Centers for Disease Control and Prevention. (2002). Guideline for hand hygiene in health-care settings: Recommendations of the Healthcare Infection Control Practices Advisory Committee and the HICPAC/SHEA/APIC/IDSA Hand Hygiene Task Force. *MMWR Recommendations*

and Reports, 51(RR-16), 1–45. Accessed March 2015 via the Web at http://www.cdc.gov/mmwr/pdf/rr/rr5116.pdf (Level II)

7 The Joint Commission. (2015). Standard NPSG.07.01.01. *Comprehensive accreditation manual for hospitals: The official handbook.* Oakbrook Terrace, IL: The Joint Commission. (Level VII)

8 World Health Organization. (2009). "WHO guidelines on hand hygiene in health care: First global patient safety challenge, clean care is safer care" [Online]. Accessed March 2015 via the Web at http://whqlibdoc.who.int/publications/2009/9789241597906_eng.pdf (Level IV)

9 Centers for Medicare & Medicaid Services, Department of Health and Human Services. (2014). Condition of participation: Infection control. 42 C.F.R. § 482.42.

10 American Osteopathic Association. (2014). Standard 07.01.21. *Healthcare Facilities Accreditation Program: Accreditation requirements for acute care hospitals.* Chicago, IL: American Osteopathic Association. (Level VII)

11 The Joint Commission. (2015). Standard NPSG.01.01.01. *Comprehensive accreditation manual for hospitals: The official handbook.* Oakbrook Terrace, IL: The Joint Commission. (Level VII)

12 Siegel, J. D., et al. (2007). "2007 guideline for isolation precautions: Preventing transmission of infectious agents in healthcare settings" [Online]. Accessed March 2015 via the Web at http://www.cdc.gov/hicpac/pdf/isolation/Isolation2007.pdf (Level II)

13 American Osteopathic Association. (2014). Standard 07.01.10. *Healthcare Facilities Accreditation Program: Accreditation requirements for acute care hospitals.* Chicago, IL: American Osteopathic Association. (Level VII)

14 Fischbach, F., & Dunning, M. B. (2014). *A manual of laboratory and diagnostic tests* (9th ed.). Philadelphia, PA: Wolters Kluwer.

15 Aaron, S. D., et al. (2003). Topical tetracaine prior to arterial puncture: A randomized, placebo-controlled clinical trial. *Respiratory Medicine, 97,* 1195–1199. (Level II)

16 Knowles, T. P., et al. (2006). Effects of syringe material, sample storage time, and temperature on blood gases and oxygen saturation in arterialized human blood samples. *Respiratory Care, 51,* 732–736.

17 Occupational Safety and Health Administration. (n.d.). "Bloodborne pathogens, standard number 1910.1030" [Online]. Accessed March 2015 via the Web at http://www.osha.gov/pls/oshaweb/owadisp.show_document?p_table=STANDARDS&p_id=10051 (Level VII)

18 The Joint Commission. (2015). Standard RC.01.03.01. *Comprehensive accreditation manual for hospitals: The official handbook.* Oakbrook Terrace, IL: The Joint Commission. (Level VII)

19 Centers for Medicare & Medicaid Services, Department of Health and Human Services. (2014). Condition of participation: Medical record services. 42 C.F.R. § 482.24.

20 American Osteopathic Association. (2014). Standard 10.00.03. *Healthcare Facilities Accreditation Program: Accreditation requirements for acute care hospitals.* Chicago, IL: American Osteopathic Association. (Level VII)

ADDITIONAL REFERENCES

Johnson, K. L., et al. (2011). Effects of mean arterial pressure and needle size on arterial sampler filling time. *Respiratory Care, 56,* 456–459.

McCanny, P., et al. (2012). Venous vs arterial blood gases in the assessment of patients presenting with an exacerbation of chronic obstructive pulmonary disease. *American Journal of Emergency Medicine, 30,* 896–900.

Nettina, S. M. (2014). *Lippincott manual of nursing practice* (10th ed.). Philadelphia, PA: Wolters Kluwer.

Srisan, P., et al. (2011). Effects of temperature and time delay on arterial blood gas and electrolyte measurements. *Journal of the Medical Association of Thailand, 94,* S9–S14.

ASSESSMENT TECHNIQUES

A physical assessment involves four basic techniques: inspection, palpation, percussion, and auscultation. Performing these techniques correctly helps elicit valuable information about a patient's condition.

Inspection requires the use of vision to observe the details of the patient's appearance, behavior, and movement.[1] Special lighting and various equipment—such as an otoscope, a tongue blade, or an ophthalmoscope—may be used to enhance vision or examine an otherwise hidden area. Inspection begins during the first patient contact and continues throughout the assessment.

Palpation usually follows inspection, except when examining the abdomen or assessing infants and children. Palpation involves touching the body to determine the size, shape, and position of structures; to detect and evaluate temperature, pulsations, and other movement; and to elicit tenderness.

The four palpation techniques include light palpation, deep palpation, light ballottement, and deep ballottement. Ballottement is the technique used to evaluate a flowing or movable structure. It involves gently bouncing the structure by applying pressure against it and then waiting to feel it rebound. This technique may be used, for example, to check the position of an organ or a fetus.

Percussion involves quick, sharp tapping of the fingers or hands against body surfaces to produce sounds, detect tenderness, or assess reflexes. Percussing for sound helps locate organ borders, identify organ shape and position, and determine whether an organ is solid or filled with fluid or gas.

Organs and tissues produce sounds of varying loudness, pitch, and duration, depending on their density. For example, air-filled cavities such as the lungs produce markedly different sounds from those produced by the liver and other dense organs and tissues. Percussion techniques include indirect percussion, direct percussion, and blunt percussion.

Auscultation involves listening to various sounds of the body—particularly those produced by the heart, lungs, vessels, stomach, and intestines. Most auscultated sounds result from the movement of air or fluid through these structures.

Auscultation is usually performed after the other assessment techniques. When examining the abdomen, however, auscultation occurs after inspection but before percussion and palpation, which can alter bowel sounds. Auscultation is also best performed first on infants and young children, who may start to cry when palpated or percussed. Auscultation is most successful when performed in a quiet environment with a properly fitted stethoscope.

Equipment

Flashlight or gooseneck lamp ■ patient drape ■ stethoscope ■ hospital-grade disinfectant pad ■ Optional: gloves.

Implementation

- Gather all of the necessary equipment.
- Perform hand hygiene.[2,3,4,5,6,7]
- Put on gloves if needed *to comply with standard precautions.*[5,8]
- Confirm the patient's identity using at least two patient identifiers.[9]
- Provide privacy.
- Explain all aspects of the procedure to the patient.
- Ask the patient to undress, and then drape him appropriately.
- Make sure the room is warm and adequately lit *to make the patient comfortable and aid visual inspection.*
- Warm your hands and the stethoscope.

Inspection

- Use your eyes to observe the patient. Pay close attention to the details of his appearance, behavior, and movement, such as facial expressions, mood, physique, and conditioning.[1] Focus on areas related to the patient's chief complaint.
- To inspect a specific body area, first make sure the area is sufficiently exposed. Survey the entire area, noting key landmarks and checking its

Performing palpation

You should be familiar with four palpation techniques: light palpation, deep palpation, light ballottement, and deep ballottement. Remember to use the flattened finger pads for palpating tender tissues, feeling for crepitus (crackling) at the joints, and lightly probing the abdomen. Use the thumb and index finger for assessing hair texture, grasping tissues, and feeling for lymph node enlargement. Use the back, or dorsal, surface of the hand when feeling for warmth.

Light palpation

With the tips of two or three fingers held close together, press gently on the skin to a depth of ½″ to ¾″ (1 to 2 cm).[10] Use the lightest touch possible; too much pressure blunts your sensitivity.

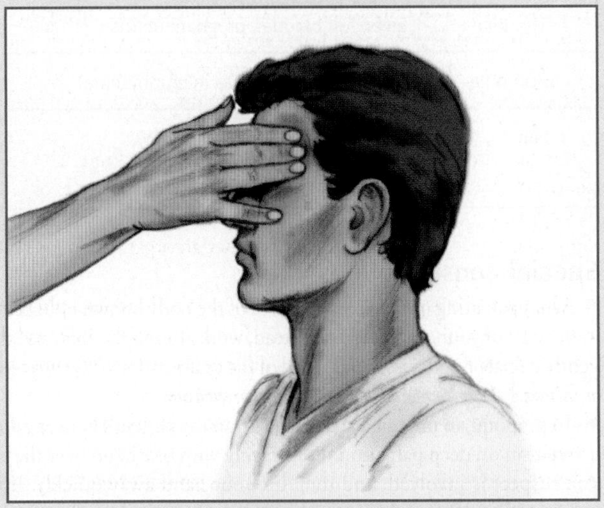

Light ballottement

Apply light, rapid pressure to the abdomen, moving from one quadrant to another. Keep your hand on the skin surface *to detect tissue rebound*.

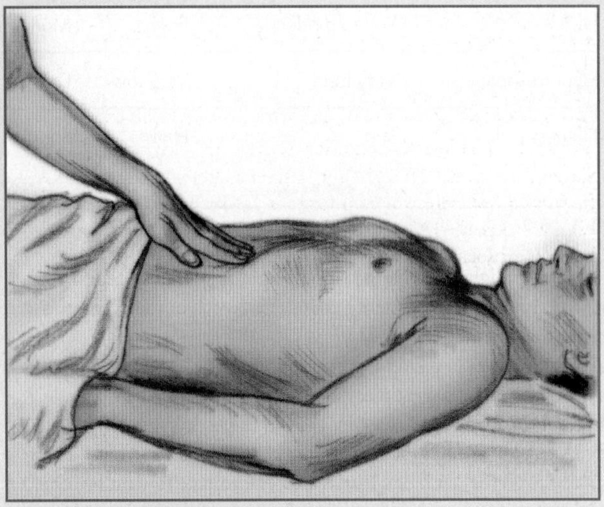

Deep palpation (bimanual palpation)

Place one hand on top of the other. Then press down about 1½″ to 2½″ (4 to 6 cm) with the fingertips of both hands.[10]

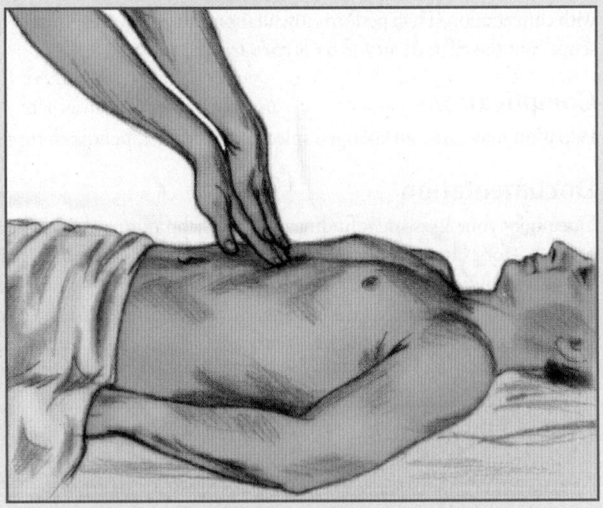

Deep ballottement

Apply abrupt, deep pressure on the patient's abdomen. Release the pressure completely, but maintain fingertip contact with the skin.

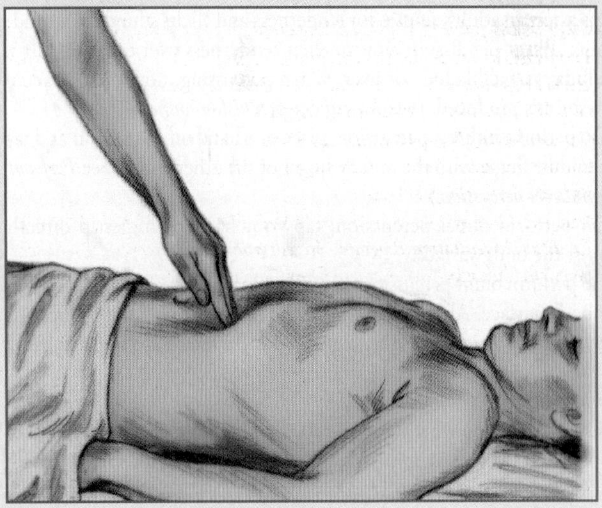

overall condition. Focus on specifics—color, shape, texture, size, and movement. Note unusual findings as well as predictable ones.

Palpation

■ Tell the patient what to expect, such as occasional discomfort as you apply pressure. Encourage the patient to relax *because muscle tension and guarding can interfere with performance and results of palpation.*

■ Provide just enough pressure to assess the tissue beneath one or both hands. Then release pressure and gently move to the next area, systematically covering the entire surface to be assessed. (See *Performing palpation.*)

■ To perform light palpation, depress the skin, indenting ½″ to ¾″ (1 to 2 cm). Use the lightest touch possible *because excessive pressure blunts your sensitivity.*[10]

■ If the patient tolerates light palpation and you need to assess deeper structures, palpate deeply by increasing your fingertip pressure, indenting the skin about 1½″ to 2½″ (4 to 6 cm). Place your other hand on top of the palpating hand *to control and guide your movements.*[10]

Identifying percussion sounds

Percussion produces sounds that vary according to the tissue being percussed. This chart lists important percussion sounds along with their characteristics and typical sources.

SOUND	INTENSITY	PITCH	DURATION	QUALITY	SOURCE
Resonance	Moderate to loud	Low	Long	Hollow	Normal lung
Tympany	Loud	High	Moderate	Drumlike	Gastric air bubble, intestinal air
Dullness	Soft to moderate	High	Moderate	Thudlike	Liver, full bladder, pregnant uterus
Hyperresonance	Very loud	Very low	Long	Booming	Hyperinflated lung (as in emphysema)
Flatness	Soft	High	Short	Flat	Muscle

- To perform light ballottement, apply light, rapid pressure from quadrant to quadrant on the patient's abdomen. Keep your hand on the skin *to detect tissue rebound.*
- To perform deeper ballottement, apply abrupt, deep pressure and then release it. Maintain fingertip contact.
- Use both hands (bimanual palpation) to trap a deep, underlying, hard-to-palpate organ (such as the kidney or spleen) or to fix or stabilize an organ (such as the uterus) with one hand while you palpate it with the other.

Percussion

- First, decide which of the percussion techniques best suits your assessment needs. Indirect percussion helps reveal the size and density of underlying thoracic and abdominal organs and tissues. Direct percussion helps assess an adult's sinuses for tenderness and elicits sounds in a child's thorax. Blunt percussion aims to elicit tenderness over organs, such as the kidneys, gallbladder, or liver. When percussing, note the characteristic sounds produced. (See *Identifying percussion sounds.*)
- To perform indirect percussion, place one hand on the patient and tap the middle finger with the middle finger of the other hand. (See *Performing indirect percussion.*)
- To perform direct percussion, tap your hand or fingertip directly against the body surface.
- To perform blunt percussion, strike the ulnar surface of your fist against the body surface. Alternatively, place the palm of one hand against the body, make a fist with the other hand, and strike the back of the first hand.

Auscultation

- First, determine whether to use the diaphragm or bell of the stethoscope. Use the diaphragm to detect high-pitched sounds, such as breath and bowel sounds. Keep in mind that bowel sounds shouldn't be described as absent until no sound is heard for 5 minutes.[11] Use the bell to detect lower-pitched sounds, such as heart and vascular sounds.
- Place the diaphragm or bell of the stethoscope over the appropriate area of the patient's body and place the earpieces in your ears.
- Listen intently to individual sounds, and try to identify their characteristics. Determine the intensity, pitch, and duration of each sound, and check the frequency of recurring sounds.
- Remove and discard your gloves if worn and perform hand hygiene.[2,3,4,6,7]
- Clean and disinfect your stethoscope using a disinfectant pad.[12,13]
- Perform hand hygiene.[2,3,4,6,7]
- Document the procedure.[14,15,16]

Special considerations

- Avoid palpating or percussing an area of the body known to be tender at the start of your examination. Instead, work around the area, and then gently palpate or percuss it at the end of the examination. *This progression minimizes the patient's discomfort and apprehension.*
- To pinpoint an inflamed area deep within the patient's body, perform a variation on deep palpation: Press firmly with one hand over the area you suspect is involved, and then lift your hand away quickly. If the patient reports that pain increases when you release the pressure, then you've identified rebound tenderness.

NURSING ALERT **Suspect peritonitis if you elicit rebound tenderness when examining the abdomen.**

- If you can't palpate because the patient fears pain, try distracting him with conversation. Then perform auscultation and gently press your stethoscope into the affected area *to try to elicit tenderness.*

Complications

Palpation may cause an enlarged spleen or infected appendix to rupture.

Documentation

Document your assessment findings and the technique used to elicit each finding—for example, "Right lower quadrant tenderness on deep palpation, no rebound tenderness." Indicate who you notified of any abnormal findings and the time of the notification. Document interventions required to treat those findings as well as the patient's response to them.

REFERENCES

1 Bickley, L. S. (2013). *Bates' guide to physical examination and history taking* (11th ed.). Philadelphia, PA: Lippincott Williams & Wilkins.

2 The Joint Commission. (2015). Standard NPSG.07.01.01. *Comprehensive accreditation manual for hospitals: The official handbook.* Oakbrook Terrace, IL: The Joint Commission. (Level VII)

3 Centers for Disease Control and Prevention. (2002). Guideline for hand hygiene in health-care settings: Recommendations of the Healthcare Infection Control Practices Advisory Committee and the HICPAC/SHEA/APIC/IDSA Hand Hygiene Task Force. *MMWR Recommendations and Reports, 51*(RR-16), 1–45. Accessed March 2015 via the Web at http://www.cdc.gov/mmwr/pdf/rr/rr5116.pdf (Level II)

4 World Health Organization. (2009). "WHO guidelines on hand hygiene in health care: First global patient safety challenge, clean care is safer care" [Online]. Accessed March 2015 via the Web at http://whqlibdoc.who.int/publications/2009/9789241597906_eng.pdf (Level IV)

Performing indirect percussion

To perform indirect percussion, use the middle finger of your nondominant hand as the pleximeter (the mediating device used to receive the taps) and the middle finger of your dominant hand as the plexor (the device used to tap the pleximeter). Place the pleximeter finger firmly against a body surface such as the upper back. With your wrist flexed loosely, use the tip of your plexor finger to deliver a crisp blow just beneath the distal joint of the pleximeter. Be sure to hold the plexor perpendicular to the pleximeter. Tap lightly and quickly, removing the plexor as soon as you have delivered each blow. Move your nondominant hand to cover the entire area to be percussed.

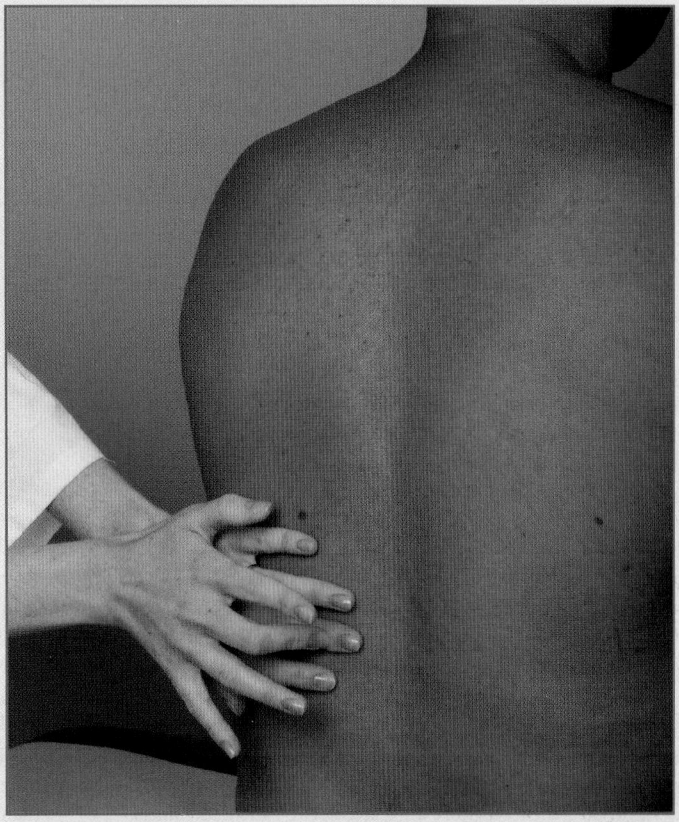

5 Siegel, J. D., et al. (2007). "2007 guideline for isolation precautions: Preventing transmission of infectious agents in healthcare settings" [Online]. Accessed March 2015 via the Web at http://www.cdc.gov/hicpac/pdf/isolation/Isolation2007.pdf (Level II)

6 Centers for Medicare & Medicaid Services, Department of Health and Human Services. (2014). Condition of participation: Infection control. 42 C.F.R. § 482.42.

7 American Osteopathic Association. (2014). Standard 07.01.21. *Healthcare Facilities Accreditation Program: Accreditation requirements for acute care hospitals.* Chicago, IL: American Osteopathic Association. (Level VII)

8 American Osteopathic Association. (2014). Standard 07.01.10. *Healthcare Facilities Accreditation Program: Accreditation requirements for acute care hospitals.* Chicago, IL: American Osteopathic Association. (Level VII)

9 The Joint Commission. (2015). Standard NPSG.01.01.01. *Comprehensive accreditation manual for hospitals: The official handbook.* Oakbrook Terrace, IL: The Joint Commission. (Level VII)

10 Jensen, S. (2011). *Nursing health assessment: A best practice approach.* Philadelphia, PA: Lippincott Williams & Wilkins.

11 Craven, H. (Ed.). (2009). *Core curriculum for medical-surgical nursing* (4th ed.). Pitman, NJ: Academy of Medical-Surgical Nurses.

12 Rutala, W. A., et al. (2008). "Guideline for disinfection and sterilization in healthcare facilities, 2008" [Online]. Accessed March 2015 via the Web at http://www.cdc.gov/hicpac/pdf/guidelines/Disinfection_Nov_2008.pdf (Level I)

13 American Osteopathic Association. (2014). Standard 07.02.03. *Healthcare Facilities Accreditation Program: Accreditation requirements for acute care hospitals.* Chicago, IL: American Osteopathic Association. (Level VII)

14 The Joint Commission. (2015). Standard RC.01.03.01. *Comprehensive accreditation manual for hospitals: The official handbook.* Oakbrook Terrace, IL: The Joint Commission. (Level VII)

15 Centers for Medicare & Medicaid Services, Department of Health and Human Services. (2014). Condition of participation: Medical record services. 42 C.F.R. § 482.24.

16 American Osteopathic Association. (2014). Standard 10.00.03. *Healthcare Facilities Accreditation Program: Accreditation requirements for acute care hospitals.* Chicago, IL: American Osteopathic Association. (Level VII)

ADDITIONAL REFERENCES

Craven, R. F., & Hirnle, C. J. (2012). *Fundamentals of nursing: Human health and function* (7th ed.). Philadelphia, PA: Lippincott Williams & Wilkins.

Jevon, P. (2006). Chest examination, part 1—Chest palpation. *Nursing Times, 102*(44), 26–27.

Jevon, P. (2006). Chest examination, part 2—Chest percussion. *Nursing Times, 102*(45), 26–27.

Jevon, P., & Cunnington, A. (2006). Chest examination, part 3—Chest auscultation. *Nursing Times, 102*(46), 26–27.

Nettina, S. M. (2014). *Lippincott manual of nursing practice* (10th ed.). Philadelphia, PA: Wolters Kluwer.

AUTOLOGOUS BLOOD COLLECTION, PREOPERATIVE

Preoperative autologous blood collection is the collection, processing, and storage of the patient's own blood before a scheduled procedure that's likely to cause significant bleeding.[1]

Autologous blood transfusion has several advantages over transfusion of blood from a blood bank. First, it minimizes the risk of infectious disease transmission (with the exception of bacterial sepsis) and alloimmunization of red cell, platelet, and leukocyte antigens. It also provides a source of blood for individuals who have rare blood types or antibodies that make it difficult to find compatible blood. Last, some individuals who refuse blood from donors because of religious or other beliefs may be willing to accept a transfusion of their own blood.[1]

Despite the advantages, there may be rare adverse effects associated with autologous blood transfusion, including septic transfusion reactions that can result from white blood cell cytokine release during storage. In addition, if the recipient is misidentified before transfusion, a hemolytic reaction may occur or the patient may be exposed to a transfusion-transmitted disease.[1,2]

Sepsis or suspected bacteremia is a contraindication to autologous collection. The practitioner may also prefer not to use blood from a patient who has an infectious disease or active infection. There are no specific age requirements; children younger than age 17 and elderly patients may participate. However, patients with other medical conditions may not be candidates for preoperative collection. The hemoglobin level of the patient should be 11 g/dL or higher, or the hematocrit, if used, should be 33% or higher. Moreover, if the patient weighs less than 110 lb (50 kg), it may be necessary to reduce the volume of blood obtained.[1]

Equipment

Gloves ▪ rubber ball ▪ 18G or 20G catheter and equipment for venipuncture ▪ blood collection bags ▪ consent form ▪ Optional: prescribed IV fluids, other personal protective equipment (mask, protective eyewear or mask with face shield, gowns or aprons).

Implementation

- Verify the practitioner's order for autologous blood collection.[1]
- Perform hand hygiene.[3,4,5,6,7,8]
- Confirm the patient's identity using at least two patient identifiers.[9]
- Explain the procedure to the patient. Make sure the patient understands that he may not receive his own blood exclusively if there's unexpected blood loss or an emergency need for more units than collected, or if fewer units were collected than desired. Also make sure he understands that a risk of certain adverse effects still exists with autologous blood transfusion. Explain that all collections should be completed more than 72 hours before the anticipated surgery or tranfusion.[1]
- Confirm that the written informed consent has been obtained and that the signed and witnessed form is in the patient's medical record.[1,10,11,12]
- *To prevent hypovolemia,* encourage the patient to drink plenty of fluids before collection. Explain that he may feel light-headed during the collection but that the problem can be treated.
- Verify that the patient's hemoglobin level is 11 g/dL or higher or, if hematocrit is used, 33% or higher.[1]
- Obtain and record vital signs before starting the collection *to provide a baseline.*[1]
- Help the patient into a supine position.
- Put on gloves and other personal protective equipment if needed *to comply with standard precautions.*[13,14,15,16]
- Prepare the collection bags according to the manufacturer's instructions.
- Prepare replacement IV fluids, if ordered.
- Select an appropriate IV catheter insertion site.[17]
- Prepare the patient's arm and IV catheter insertion site. Insert an 18G or 20G catheter.[18] (See the "IV catheter insertion and removal" procedure, page 446.)
- Connect the collecting system according to the manufacturer's instructions. Have the patient squeeze the rubber ball *to facilitate blood flow into the collecting bag.*
- Monitor the patient for adverse reactions.

NURSING ALERT Monitor the patient's vital signs closely for signs of hypotension during this process.[19]

- Administer replacement IV fluids, if ordered.
- When blood collection is complete, remove the IV catheter and perform site care.
- Recheck the patient's vital signs *to evaluate his response to the procedure.*
- Send a blood sample obtained from the patient to the laboratory to be checked for the patient's coagulation profile, hemoglobin, hematocrit, and calcium levels. Label the specimens in the presence of the patient *to prevent mislabeling.*[2,9]
- Clearly label the collection bag with the patient's name, at least two patient identifiers, and an AUTOLOGOUS BLOOD label. Make sure there's a mechanism to clearly determine the date of specimen collection and the identity of the person who collected the blood *to prevent blood administration errors.*[1]
- Send the blood to the blood bank.
- Discard all used supplies in appropriate receptacles.[13,14,20]
- Remove and discard your gloves and any other personal protective equipment worn.[13,14]
- Perform hand hygiene.[3,4,5,6,7,8]
- Document the procedure.[21,22,23,24]

Special considerations

- In the 4 to 6 weeks before surgery, the patient may be prescribed iron supplements *to prevent depletion of his iron stores.*[25]
- Monitor the patient closely during and after the collection. Although vasovagal reactions are usually mild and easy to treat, they can quickly progress to severe reactions, such as loss of consciousness and seizures.
- Have the patient remain supine for 10 minutes after the collection. If he feels light-headed or dizzy, advise him to sit down immediately and to lower his head between his knees. He may also lie down with his head lower than his body until his symptoms resolve.
- Instruct the patient to drink more fluids than usual for a few hours after the collection and to eat heartily at his next meal.
- Instruct the patient to monitor his IV site for a few hours after the collection. If some bleeding occurs, he should apply firm pressure for 5 to 10 minutes. If the bleeding continues, instruct him to notify his practitioner.
- The practitioner should order discontinuance of anticoagulation drugs before elective or nonemergent surgery.[2]

Complications

Preoperative collection may cause vasovagal reactions and hypovolemia.

Documentation

Document the time the collection began and ended, the amount of blood the patient donated, and his tolerance of the procedure. Note the condition of the IV site. Note that the blood sample was sent to the laboratory and that the blood was sent to the blood bank.

References

1 AABB. (2012). *Primer of blood administration.* Bethesda, MD: AABB. (Level VII)

2 American Society of Anesthesiologists. (2006). Practice guidelines for perioperative blood transfusion and adjuvant therapies: An updated report by the American Society of Anesthesiologists task force on perioperative blood transfusion and adjuvant therapies. *Anesthesiology, 105,* 198–208. Accessed March 2015 via the Web at http://journals.lww.com/anesthesiology/Fulltext/2006/07000/Practice_Guidelines_for_Perioperative_Blood.30.aspx (Level VII)

3 World Health Organization. (2009). "WHO guidelines on hand hygiene in health care: First global patient safety challenge, clean care is safer care" [Online]. Accessed March 2015 via the Web at http://whqlibdoc.who.int/publications/2009/9789241597906_eng.pdf (Level IV)

4 The Joint Commission. (2015). Standard NPSG.07.01.01. *Comprehensive accreditation manual for hospitals: The official handbook.* Oakbrook Terrace, IL: The Joint Commission. (Level VII)

5 Centers for Disease Control and Prevention. (2002). Guideline for hand hygiene in health-care settings: Recommendations of the Healthcare Infection Control Practices Advisory Committee and the HICPAC/SHEA/APIC/IDSA Hand Hygiene Task Force. *MMWR Recommendations and Reports, 51*(RR-16), 1–45. Accessed March 2015 via the Web at http://www.cdc.gov/mmwr/pdf/rr/rr5116.pdf (Level II)

6 Standard 19. Hand hygiene. Infusion nursing standards of practice. (2011). *Journal of Infusion Nursing, 34,* S26–S27. (Level VII)

7 Centers for Medicare & Medicaid Services, Department of Health and Human Services. (2014). Condition of participation: Infection control. 42 C.F.R. § 482.42.

8 American Osteopathic Association. (2014). Standard 07.01.21. *Healthcare Facilities Accreditation Program: Accreditation requirements for acute care hospitals.* Chicago, IL: American Osteopathic Association. (Level VII)

9 The Joint Commission. (2015). Standard NPSG.01.01.01. *Comprehensive accreditation manual for hospitals: The official handbook.* Oakbrook Terrace, IL: The Joint Commission. (Level VII)

10 The Joint Commission. (2015). Standard RI.01.03.01. *Comprehensive accreditation manual for hospitals: The official handbook.* Oakbrook Terrace, IL: The Joint Commission. (Level VII)

11 Centers for Medicare & Medicaid Services, Department of Health and Human Services. (2014). Condition of participation: Patient's rights. 42 C.F.R. § 482.13(b)(2).

12 American Osteopathic Association. (2014). Standard 15.01.11. *Healthcare Facilities Accreditation Program: Accreditation requirements for acute care hospitals.* Chicago, IL: American Osteopathic Association. (Level VII)

13 Occupational Safety and Health Administration. (n.d.). "Bloodborne pathogens, standard number 1910.1030" [Online]. Accessed March 2015 via the Web at http://www.osha.gov/pls/oshaweb/owadisp.show_document?p_table=STANDARDS&p_id=10051 (Level VII)

14 Siegel, J. D., et al. (2007). "2007 guidelines for isolation precautions: Preventing transmission of infectious agents in healthcare settings" [Online]. Accessed March 2015 via the Web at http://www.cdc.gov/hicpac/pdf/isolation/Isolation2007.pdf (Level II)

15 Standard 18. Infection prevention. Infusion nursing standards of practice. (2011). *Journal of Infusion Nursing, 34,* S25–S26. (Level VII)

16 American Osteopathic Association. (2014). Standard 07.01.10. *Healthcare Facilities Accreditation Program: Accreditation requirements for acute care hospitals.* Chicago, IL: American Osteopathic Association. (Level VII)

17 Standard 33. Site selection. Infusion nursing standards of practice. (2011). *Journal of Infusion Nursing, 34,* S40–S43. (Level VII)

18 Standard 57. Phlebotomy. Infusion nursing standards of practice. (2011). *Journal of Infusion Nursing, 34,* S77–S80. (Level VII)

19 John, T., et al. (2008). Blood conservation in a congenital cardiac surgery program. *AORN Journal, 87,* 1180–1190. (Level IV)

20 Standard 22. Safe handling and disposal of sharps, hazardous materials, and hazardous waste. Infusion nursing standards of practice. (2011). *Journal of Infusion Nursing, 34,* S28–S29. (Level VII)

21 The Joint Commission. (2015). Standard RC.01.03.01. *Comprehensive accreditation manual for hospitals: The official handbook.* Oakbrook Terrace, IL: The Joint Commission. (Level VII)

22 Standard 14. Documentation. Infusion nursing standards of practice. (2011). *Journal of Infusion Nursing, 34,* S20–S21. (Level VII)

23 Centers for Medicare & Medicaid Services, Department of Health and Human Services. (2014). Condition of participation: Medical record services. 42 C.F.R. § 482.24(b).

24 American Osteopathic Association. (2014). Standard 10.00.03. *Healthcare Facilities Accreditation Program: Accreditation requirements for acute care hospitals.* Chicago, IL: American Osteopathic Association. (Level VII)

25 Kapadia, B. H., et al. (2013). Preoperative blood management strategies for total knee arthroplasty. *Journal of Knee Surgery, 26,* 373–377. (Level V)

ADDITIONAL REFERENCES

AABB. (2013). *Standards for perioperative autologous blood collection and administration* (5th ed.). Bethesda, MD: ABBB.

Arya, R. C., et al. (2011). Blood component therapy: Which, when and how much. *Journal of Anaesthesiology and Clinical Pharmacology, 27,* 278–284. Accessed March 2015 via the Web at http://www.ncbi.nlm.nih.gov/pmc/articles/PMC3127320/

Chimutengwende-Gordon, M., et al. (2010). Perioperative blood transfusion: The role of allogenous and autologous transfusions, and pharmacological agents. *Journal of Perioperative Practice, 20,* 283–287.

Hinkle, J. L., & Cheever, K. H. (2014). *Brunner and Suddarth's textbook of medical-surgical nursing* (13th ed.). Philadelphia, PA: Wolters Kluwer.

Jakovina Blazekovic, C., et al. (2014). Pre-operative autologous blood donation versus no blood donation in total knee arthroplasty: A prospective randomised trial. *International Orthopaedics, 38,* 341–346. (Level II)

Liumbruno, G. M., et al. (2012). Autologous blood in obstetrics: Where are we going now? *Blood Transfusion, 10,* 125–147. Accessed March 2015 via the Web at http://www.ncbi.nlm.nih.gov/pmc/articles/PMC3320772/

Oz, B. S., et al. (2013). Comparison of results of autologous blood transfusion in open-heart surgery. *Cardiovascular Journal of Africa, 24,* 121–123. (Level IV)

AUTOLOGOUS BLOOD TRANSFUSION, PERIOPERATIVE

Perioperative autologous blood transfusion is the collection and reinfusion of the patient's own blood, which is collected intraoperatively from the operative site or from an extracorporeal circuit. One benefit of this procedure is that the patient can receive his own blood recovered from the operative field, minimizing the need for allogenic blood transfusion.[1,2] It may be used during vascular and orthopedic surgery because considerable bleeding may follow these surgeries, as well as in the treatment of traumatic injury.

Acute normovolemic hemodilution is another form of perioperative blood collection. It doesn't require the recovery of blood shed through suction, so it can be used in less vascular surgeries. In this procedure, units of the patient's blood are removed and stored in plastic blood collection bags in preparation for cardiopulmonary bypass or other surgery. After the blood is removed, the patient receives solutions containing crystalloid or colloid components or a combination of both to replace the removed blood, diluting the remaining cells in a larger volume of fluid; because of this, blood lost during surgery has a lower hematocrit. The patient's blood is then reinfused during surgery. This process helps to maintain the patient's red blood cell mass and provides viable platelets and clotting factors because the blood has been stored for only a few hours.[1]

Perioperative autologous blood transfusion is contraindicated when situations occur (such as trauma) that increase the risk of blood contamination with bacteria, tumor cells, or other harmful substances.[1]

Various types of devices can be used to retrieve blood from the operative site; apheresis devices are used prepare the components intraoperatively. (See *Autologous blood recovery systems,* page 46.) Follow the manufacturer's instructions for use when collecting, storing, and reinfusing the patient's blood.[1]

Equipment

Gloves ▪ mask with face shield or mask and goggles ▪ gown or apron ▪ data recording form ▪ preservative-free normal saline solution ▪ 10-mL syringe ▪ disinfectant pad (alcohol, tincture of iodine, or chlorhexidine-based) ▪ IV pole ▪ 250-mL bag of normal saline solution ▪ standard blood administration IV tubing set with gravity drip and microaggregate filter ▪ wall suction with pressure gauge, as needed ▪ autologous blood recovery system device with necessary supplies; for a Cell Saver® 5+ unit,

Autologous blood recovery systems

Autologous blood recovery systems are used in surgical procedures to salvage red blood cells (RBCs) when there's rapid bleeding or high-volume blood loss. Shed blood is collected and stored in a reservoir, where waste is separated from the healthy RBCs. The waste collects into a separate bag; healthy RBCs are then returned to the patient. This process can be performed in 3 to 7 minutes. In emergencies, the autologous blood recovery system can process up to 800 mL of blood each minute.

Advantages to autologous blood recovery systems include:

- up-to-date microprocessor and sensor technologies
- automated operation and manual operation options
- platelet sequestration
- RBC bags with integrated microaggregate filters
- features to ensure consistent processing and a high-quality blood product
- fast processing
- built-in safety features.

suction tubing and collection kit (an autotransfusion drain usually has stand-alone functioning).

Implementation

- Verify the practitioner's order for the rate of reinfusion and the amount of blood to be reinfused.
- Verify that consent for blood and blood product transfusion has been obtained and is in the patient's medical record.[3,4,5]
- Call the perfusionist to set up the autologous blood recovery system device and connect the tubing to the setup following the manufacturer's instructions. (Note that the person responsible for this step may vary by facility. The perioperative nurse or anesthesia care provider may set up the device in some facilities.)
- Perform hand hygiene.[6,7,8,9,10,11,12]
- Confirm the patient's identity using at least two patient identifiers.[13]
- Put on gloves and personal protective equipment *to comply with standard precautions.*[14,15,16]
- Make sure the collection chamber and the blood transfer bag are clearly marked with the patient's first and last name, identifying numbers, date and time of the collection initiation, and an AUTOLOGOUS BLOOD label. If applicable, include the time of, or condition for, expiration.[1,17]
- Obtain and record the patient's vital signs at an interval indicated by the patient's condition or at a frequency determined by your facility.
- Verify that the patient has a patent, acceptable venous access site available for blood administration. The access may be peripheral or central. Blood may be transfused via a 14G to 24G peripheral catheter.[18] (See the "Transfusion of blood and blood products" procedure, page 783.) *To assess patency,* aspirate the catheter for blood return using a 10-mL syringe, and then flush with preservative-free normal saline solution.[19]
- Insert one spike of the standard Y-type blood administration set into the 250-mL bag of normal saline solution. Close all clamps and hang the set on an IV pole.
- The anesthesia care provider, perioperative nurse, or perfusionist will start the shed blood collection according to the autologous blood recovery system device manufacturer's instructions. (Some devices process and centrifuge the blood automatically.)

NURSING ALERT **Monitor the patient's vital signs closely for signs of hypotension during this process.** ***Hypotension may occur as the result of hypovolemia.***[20]

- Monitor the status of the blood collection.
- When enough blood has been collected to reinfuse, spike the blood transfer bag with the open port of the standard blood administration IV set. Remove all air from the blood transfer bag. Hang it on the IV pole.
- Open the clamp from the normal saline solution and prime the filter and tubing *to remove all air from the tubing.* Close the clamp from the normal saline solution.
- Open the clamp from the blood transfer bag to the drip chamber of the blood administration set and prime the filter and tubing with blood *to remove all air from the tubing.*
- If you're using a postprocedure transfusion device, follow the manufacturer's instructions *to properly connect the device to the patient.* (Staff members should receive training on all transfusion devices before use.)
- Thoroughly disinfect the IV catheter hub with a disinfectant pad using friction and allow it to dry.[21]
- Attach the blood tubing to the venous access device and then trace the tubing from the patient to its point of origin before beginning the transfusion *to make sure it's connected to the proper port.*[22]
- Begin the reinfusion, as ordered.
- Monitor the patient throughout the procedure.[2]
- Make sure the reinfusion is completed in the surgery suite or postanesthesia care unit within the time period defined by the system used[1] or within your facility's recommended time frame.
- Record the patient's vital signs after the reinfusion is complete.
- Disconnect the blood collection setup from the patient's drains or have the anesthesia care provider, perioperative nurse, or perfusionist do so.
- Recheck the laboratory data for coagulation profile, hemoglobin, hematocrit, and calcium levels after the reinfusion is complete, or as the practitioner orders.
- Discard used supplies in appropriate receptacles.[14,15,23]
- Remove and discard your personal protective equipment[14,15,23] and perform hand hygiene.[6,7,8,9,10,11,12]
- Document the procedure.[24,25,26,27]

Special considerations

- If multiple units are to be reinfused, change the blood administration setup and filter after the completion of each unit or every 4 hours. If more than one unit can be infused within 4 hours, the administration set can be used for 4 hours.[17]
- You may need to replace clotting factors, fresh frozen plasma, or platelets if you're reinfusing large volumes of blood.
- Certain religious groups refuse blood transfusions because of their beliefs. However, many of these groups permit autologous blood transfusion if it's kept in a continuous closed circuit.[20]
- Frozen blood units usually expire after about 30 days. Once thawed, they are good for 24 hours.

Complications

There are more complications associated with the reinfusion of filtered, unwashed blood than with the transfusion of filtered, washed blood. These complications include fever, hypotension, myocardial infarction, infections, particulate and air embolism, and thrombocytopenia. Complications are more pronounced when the time from salvage to transfusion is greater than 6 hours.

Documentation

Document the time the collection began, the time the reinfusion started and ended, and the venous access site used for the reinfusion. Include the patient's vital signs before, during, and after reinfusion. Note the amount of blood collected, processed, and reinfused and the method used. Also document any postreinfusion laboratory studies obtained. Document the patient's tolerance of the procedure, any patient teaching, and the patient's understanding of your teaching.

REFERENCES

1 AABB. (2012). *Primer of blood administration.* Bethesda, MD: AABB. (Level VII)

2 American Society of Anesthesiologists. (2006). Practice guidelines for perioperative blood transfusion and adjuvant therapies: An updated report by the American Society of Anesthesiologists task force on perioperative blood transfusion and adjuvant therapies. *Anesthesiology, 105,* 198–208. Accessed March 2015 via the Web at http://journals.lww.com/anesthesiology/Fulltext/2006/07000/Practice_Guidelines_for_Perioperative_Blood.30.aspx (Level VII)

3 The Joint Commission. (2015). Standard RI.01.03.01. *Comprehensive accreditation manual for hospitals: The official handbook.* Oakbrook Terrace, IL: The Joint Commission. (Level VII)

4 Centers for Medicare & Medicaid Services, Department of Health and Human Services. (2014). Condition of participation: Patient's rights. 42 C.F.R. § 482.13(b)(2).

5 American Osteopathic Association. (2014). Standard 15.01.11. *Healthcare Facilities Accreditation Program: Accreditation requirements for acute care hospitals.* Chicago, IL: American Osteopathic Association. (Level VII)

6 The Joint Commission. (2015). Standard NPSG.07.01.01. *Comprehensive accreditation manual for hospitals: The official handbook.* Oakbrook Terrace, IL: The Joint Commission. (Level VII)

7 Centers for Disease Control and Prevention. (2002). Guideline for hand hygiene in health-care settings: Recommendations of the Healthcare Infection Control Practices Advisory Committee and the HICPAC/SHEA/APIC/IDSA Hand Hygiene Task Force. *MMWR Recommendations and Reports, 51*(RR-16), 1–45. Accessed March 2015 via the Web at http://www.cdc.gov/mmwr/pdf/rr/rr5116.pdf (Level II)

8 World Health Organization. (2009). "WHO guidelines on hand hygiene in health care: First global patient safety challenge, clean care is safer care" [Online]. Accessed March 2015 via the Web at http://whqlibdoc.who.int/publications/2009/9789241597906_eng.pdf (Level IV)

9 Recommended practice for hand hygiene in the perioperative setting. (2014). In R. Conner, et al. (Eds.), *Perioperative standards and recommended practices 2014.* Denver, CO: AORN, Inc. (Level VII)

10 Standard 19. Hand hygiene. Infusion nursing standards of practice. (2011). *Journal of Infusion Nursing, 34,* S26–S27. (Level VII)

11 Centers for Medicare & Medicaid Services, Department of Health and Human Services. (2014). Condition of participation: Infection control. 42 C.F.R. § 482.42.

12 American Osteopathic Association. (2014). Standard 07.01.21. *Healthcare Facilities Accreditation Program: Accreditation requirements for acute care hospitals.* Chicago, IL: American Osteopathic Association. (Level VII)

13 The Joint Commission. (2015). Standard NPSG.01.01.01. *Comprehensive accreditation manual for hospitals: The official handbook.* Oakbrook Terrace, IL: The Joint Commission. (Level VII)

14 Siegel, J. D., et al. (2007). "2007 guideline for isolation precautions: Preventing transmission of infectious agents in healthcare settings" [Online]. Accessed March 2015 via the Web at http://www.cdc.gov/hicpac/pdf/isolation/Isolation2007.pdf (Level II)

15 Occupational Safety and Health Administration (n.d.). "Bloodborne pathogens, standard number 1910.1030" [Online]. Accessed March 2015 via the Web at http://www.osha.gov/pls/oshaweb/owadisp.show_document?p_table=STANDARDS&p_id=10051

16 American Osteopathic Association. (2014). Standard 07.01.10. *Healthcare Facilities Accreditation Program: Accreditation requirements for acute care hospitals.* Chicago, IL: American Osteopathic Association. (Level VII)

17 The Joint Commission. (2015). Standard NPSG.01.03.01. *Comprehensive accreditation manual for hospitals: The official handbook.* Oakbrook Terrace, IL: The Joint Commission. (Level VII)

18 Standard 66. Transfusion therapy. Infusion nursing standards of practice. (2011). *Journal of Infusion Nursing, 34,* S93–S95. (Level VII)

19 Standard 45. Flushing and locking. Infusion nursing standards of practice. (2011). *Journal of Infusion Nursing, 34,* S59–S63. (Level VII)

20 John, T., et al. (2008). Blood conservation in a congenital cardiac surgery program. *AORN Journal, 87,* 1180–1190. (Level IV)

21 Standard 27. Needleless connectors. Infusion nursing standards of practice. (2011). *Journal of Infusion Nursing, 34,* S32–S33. (Level VII)

22 U.S. Food and Drug Administration. (n.d.). "Look. Check. Connect. Safe medical device connections save lives" [Online]. Accessed March 2015 via the Web at http://www.fda.gov/downloads/MedicalDevices/Safety/AlertsandNotices/UCM134873.pdf

23 Standard 22. Safe handling and disposal of sharps, hazardous materials, and hazardous waste. Infusion nursing standards of practice. *Journal of Infusion Nursing, 34,* S28–S29. (Level VII)

24 The Joint Commission. (2015). Standard RC.01.03.01. *Comprehensive accreditation manual for hospitals: The official handbook.* Oakbrook Terrace, IL: The Joint Commission. (Level VII)

25 Standard 14. Documentation. Infusion nursing standards of practice. (2011). *Journal of Infusion Nursing, 34,* S20–S21. (Level VII)

26 Centers for Medicare & Medicaid Services, Department of Health and Human Services. (2014). Condition of participation: Medical record services. 42 C.F.R. § 482.24(b).

27 American Osteopathic Association. (2014). Standard 10.00.03. *Healthcare Facilities Accreditation Program: Accreditation requirements for acute care hospitals.* Chicago, IL: American Osteopathic Association. (Level VII)

ADDITIONAL REFERENCES

AABB. (2013). *Standards for perioperative autologous blood collection and administration* (5th ed.). Bethesda, MD: AABB.

Anderson, L. (2010). Blood conservation in cardiac surgery. *Journal of Perioperative Practice, 20,* 436–439.

Chimutengwende-Gordon, M., et al. (2010). Perioperative blood transfusion: The role of allogenous and autologous transfusions, and pharmacological agents. *Journal of Perioperative Practice, 20,* 283–287.

Gee, A. O., et al. (2011). Autologous blood reinfusion in patients undergoing bilateral total hip arthroplasty. *Journal of Orthopaedic Surgery, 19,* 181–184. (Level IV)

Hanlon, L., et al. (2011). Comparison of cardiopulmonary complication rates in patients undergoing total knee arthroplasty and reinfusion of shed blood. *Orthopaedic Nursing, 30,* 307–311. (Level IV)

Hinkle, J. L., & Cheever, K. H. (2014). *Brunner and Suddarth's textbook of medical-surgical nursing* (13th ed.). Philadelphia, PA: Wolters Kluwer.

AUTOMATED EXTERNAL DEFIBRILLATION

Automated external defibrillators (AEDs) are commonly used to meet the need for early defibrillation, which is currently considered the most effective treatment for ventricular fibrillation (VF) and pulseless ventricular tachycardia. Some facilities now require every noncritical care unit to have an AED. These devices allow for early defibrillation in areas of a health care facility where staff members have no rhythm recognition skills and defibrillators aren't frequently used. When AEDs are used in health care facilities, first-responding staff members should have training to use the AED and have a goal of delivering the first shock within 3 minutes of the patients' collapse.[1,2] AEDs are also commonly used in such public places as shopping malls, sports stadiums, and airplanes. Instruction in using an AED is required as part of both basic life support (BLS) and advanced cardiac life support (ACLS) training, pediatric advanced life support training, and Heartsaver AED courses.

AEDs provide early defibrillation even when no health care provider is present. The AED interprets the victim's cardiac rhythm and gives the operator step-by-step directions on how to proceed if defibrillation is indicated. (See *Understanding an AED,* page 48.) Studies have shown that attempts to resuscitate victims of sudden cardiac arrest resulting from VF using public defibrillation equipment and administered by laypeople who are trained to use an AED have a survival rate of 41% to 74% when cardiopulmonary resuscitation (CPR) is initiated immediately and defibrillation occurs within 3 to 5 minutes.[1]

Understanding an AED

Each automated external defibrillator (AED) is equipped with a microcomputer that senses and analyzes a patient's heart rhythm at the push of a button. It then audibly or visually prompts the user to deliver a shock. AED models all have the same basic function, but each offers different operating options. For example, all AEDs communicate display directions via messages on a display screen, give voice commands, or both. Some AEDs simultaneously display a patient's heart rhythm.

All devices record the operator's interactions with the patient during defibrillation, either on a cassette tape or in a solid-state memory module. Some AEDs have an integral printer for immediate event documentation. The patient's practitioner may review the documented events. Local and state regulations govern who is responsible for collecting AED case data for reporting purposes.

There are two types of automated defibrillators: one with monophasic waveforms and one with biphasic waveforms. Monophasic waveform defibrillators were introduced first, and some are still in use today. The energy level on this type of device is usually preset by the manufacturer.

Biphasic waveforms are used in most AEDs. These devices are typically set to deliver escalating energy levels for the first three shocks and then, after the third shock, deliver subsequent shocks at the same energy as the third shock. Energy levels are commonly preconfigured at 120 to 200 joules.[1] The optimal energy level for a biphasic waveform defibrillator hasn't been determined. The optimal dose for each device that has proven most effective in eliminating ventricular fibrillation should be noted on the defibrillator.

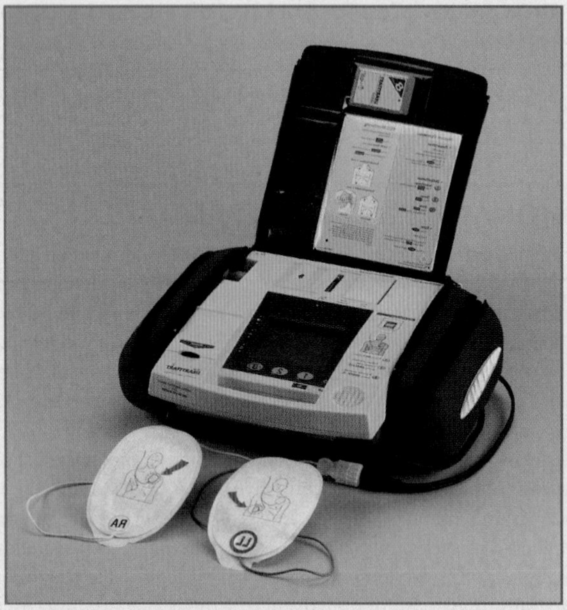

The 2010 American Heart Association guidelines for CPR and emergency cardiovascular care recommend rapid integration of CPR with the use of an AED, as follows:

- CPR should be initiated immediately, and then the AED should be used as soon as it's available.
- When two rescuers are available, one rescuer should begin CPR immediately while the second rescuer activates the emergency response system and prepares the defibrillator.
- CPR and defibrillation should be coordinated to minimize the time between stopping compressions and administering the shock.[2]
- First-responding personnel should receive AED training with the goal of delivering the first shock for any spontaneous cardiac arrest within 3 minutes of collapse.[2]
- An AED can be used for children ages 1 to 8; however, for this age-group, an AED with a pediatric dose attenuator system should be used, if available. If one isn't available, a standard AED can be used.
- If pediatric pads aren't available, adult pads can be used on a child. Place the pads at least 1″ (2.5 cm) apart, or use an anterior-posterior pad position.[3]
- An AED shouldn't be used for infants; instead, a manual defibrillator is preferred. However, if a manual defibrillator isn't available, an AED with a pediatric dose attenuator system may be used. If neither defibrillator is available, an AED without a dose attenuator may be used as a last resort.[1]

Equipment

AED ▪ two prepackaged, unopened AED electrodes ▪ gloves ▪ Optional: clippers.

Preparation of equipment

Verify that the AED is charging when not in use. Examine cables, connectors, and accessories for tears, cuts, and exposed wires, and replace as needed. Verify that the electrode pads are in sealed packages and haven't expired; obtain new ones if the integrity of the packaging is compromised or if the electrodes have expired.[4]

Implementation

- Gather and prepare the necessary equipment.
- Perform hand hygiene.[5,6,7,8,9]
- Put on gloves and follow standard precautions throughout the procedure.[10,11]
- After determining that the patient is unresponsive to questions and is apneic or only gasping, start CPR and follow BLS and ACLS protocols.[1]
- Ask a colleague to activate the emergency response system, bring the AED into the patient's room, and set it up as described below before the code team arrives.
- Turn on the AED and follow the visual or audible prompts.
- Open the foil packets containing the two electrode pads.
- Expose the patient's chest.
- Make sure the patient is in a dry environment and his chest is dry *because if personnel or the patient's skin cones in contact with water, personnel may receive a shock and the patient may receive skin burns during defibrillation.*[3]
- Remove metal objects that the patient may be wearing *because metal conducts electricity and could cause burns during defibrillation.*[3]
- Remove transdermal patches from the patient's chest (and back if using anterior-posterior placement) *because the medication may interfere with current conduction and produce burns.*[1,3]
- Remove the plastic backing film from the pads.
- Place one electrode pad on the right side of the patient's bare, dry chest just below the clavicle. Place the second electrode pad on the left side of the patient's bare, dry chest to the left of the heart's apex.[1] Depending on the manufacturer, images showing proper placement are located on the anterior surface of the pads.

NURSING ALERT **Don't interrupt CPR for electrode placement; even a few seconds of interruption can decrease coronary blood flow.**[2,12]

NURSING ALERT **Don't place the self-adhesive pads directly over an implantable cardioverter-defibrillator or implanted pacemaker; *this placement may damage the device.* Keep the electrodes about 3″ (7.6 cm) from the device, as recommended.**[3]

■ Attach one electrode pad to each electrode cable (if not already attached), and then connect the cable to the AED.
■ Next, use the machine to analyze the patient's heart rhythm. Ask everyone to stand clear, and press the ANALYZE button when the machine prompts you to do so. Be careful not to touch or move the patient while the AED is in analysis mode *because doing so may cause a delay in the AED's ability to analyze the rhythm.*[3] (If you get a CHECK ELECTRODES message, make sure the electrodes are correctly placed and the patient cable is securely attached; then press the ANALYZE button again.)
■ Wait for the AED to perform a self-test and analyze the patient's rhythm; when the patient needs a shock, the AED will prompt you with a STAND CLEAR message and emit a beep that changes into a steady tone as it's charging. If no shock is needed, the AED will display a NO SHOCK INDICATED message and prompt you to CHECK PATIENT.
■ When the AED is fully charged and prompts you to deliver a shock, make sure no one is touching the patient or his bed, and call out "Stand clear." Then press the SHOCK button on the AED. Most AEDs are ready to deliver a shock within 15 seconds (Note that some fully automated AEDS automatically deliver a shock within 15 seconds after analyzing the patient's rhythm.)
■ After the first shock, immediately continue CPR for about five cycles, beginning with chest compressions, for about 2 minutes. Don't delay compressions to recheck rhythm or pulse. After five cycles of CPR, the AED should analyze the rhythm again and deliver another shock, if indicated.[1]
■ If a nonshockable rhythm is detected, the AED should instruct you to resume CPR. Then continue the algorithm sequence until the code leader arrives.
■ After the code, remove and transcribe the AED's computer memory module or tape, or prompt the AED to print a rhythm strip with code data. Analyze and store the code data as directed by your facility.
■ Clean and disinfect the AED after use and replace electrodes.[13,14]
■ Remove and discard your gloves.[10]
■ Perform hand hygiene.[5,6,7,8,9]
■ Document the procedure.[15,16,17]

Special considerations

■ AEDs vary by manufacturer, so familiarize yourself with your facility's equipment.
■ AED operation should be checked at an interval established by your facility, typically after each use and every 8 hours.
■ Acceptable alternative electrode placement includes biaxillary positioning, with pads placed on the right and left lateral chest walls, or placement of one pad in the standard apical position, with the other pad on the right or left upper back.[1]
■ Excessive chest hair can interfere with optimal pad adhesion and may need to be removed. Use clippers to remove the hair, or rapidly remove an adhesive AED pad *to pull out the chest hair* and then apply a new one.[1]
■ After using an AED, give a summary to the code team leader that includes the patient's name, age, medical history, and chief complaint; what time you found the patient in cardiac arrest, started CPR, and applied the AED; the number of shocks the patient received; any time the patient regained a pulse; any postarrest care provided; and physical assessment findings.

Complications

Defibrillation can cause accidental electric shock to those providing care and skin burns to the patient. Radio-frequency (RF) interference may result in improper device operation, a distorted electrocardiogram (ECG), or failure to detect a shockable rhythm. Don't operate the device near cauterizers, diathermy equipment, cellular phones, or other potable and mobile RF communication equipment.

Documentation

Document the procedure, including the patient's ECG rhythm before and after defibrillation; the number of times defibrillation was performed; the energy used with each attempt; whether a pulse returned; the dosage, route, and time of drug administration; whether CPR was performed; how the patient's airway was maintained; and the patient's outcome. Record the patient's vital signs and your assessment findings.

REFERENCES

1 American Heart Association. (2010). 2010 American Heart Association guidelines for cardiopulmonary resuscitation and emergency cardiovascular care. *Circulation, 122,* S706–S719. (Level II)

2 American Heart Association. (2013). Strategies for improving survival after in-hospital cardiac arrest in the United States: 2013 consensus recommendations: A consensus statement from the American Heart Association. *Circulation, 127,* 1538–1563. (Level VII)

3 Lynn-McHale Wiegand, D. (Ed.). (2011). *AACN procedure manual for critical care* (6th ed.). St. Louis, MO: Saunders.

4 U.S. Food and Drug Administration. (2013). "Medical devices: Strategies for clinicians to maintain readiness of external defibrillators including AEDs" [Online]. Accessed March 2015 via the Web at http://www.fda.gov/MedicalDevices/ProductsandMedicalProcedures/CardiovascularDevices/ExternalDefibrillators/ucm233452.htm

5 World Health Organization. (2009). "WHO guidelines on hand hygiene in health care: First global patient safety challenge, clean care is safer care" [Online]. Accessed March 2015 via the Web at http://whqlibdoc.who.int/publications/2009/9789241597906_eng.pdf (Level IV)

6 The Joint Commission. (2015). Standard NPSG.07.01.01. *Comprehensive accreditation manual for hospitals: The official handbook.* Oakbrook Terrace, IL: The Joint Commission. (Level VII)

7 Centers for Disease Control and Prevention. (2002). Guideline for hand hygiene in health-care settings: Recommendations of the Healthcare Infection Control Practices Advisory Committee and the HICPAC/SHEA/APIC/IDSA Hand Hygiene Task Force. *MMWR Recommendations and Reports, 51*(RR-16), 1–45. Accessed March 2015 via the Web at http://www.cdc.gov/mmwr/pdf/rr/rr5116.pdf (Level II)

8 Centers for Medicare & Medicaid Services, Department of Health and Human Services. (2014). Condition of participation: Infection control. 42 C.F.R. § 482.42.

9 American Osteopathic Association. (2014). Standard 07.01.21. *Healthcare Facilities Accreditation Program: Accreditation requirements for acute care hospitals.* Chicago, IL: American Osteopathic Association. (Level VII)

10 Siegel, J. D., et al. (2007). "2007 guideline for isolation precautions: Preventing transmission of infectious agents in healthcare settings" [Online]. Accessed March 2015 via the Web at http://www.cdc.gov/hicpac/pdf/isolation/Isolation2007.pdf (Level II)

11 American Osteopathic Association. (2014). Standard 07.01.10. *Healthcare Facilities Accreditation Program: Accreditation requirements for acute care hospitals.* Chicago, IL: American Osteopathic Association. (Level VII)

12 Meaney, P. A. (2013). "CPR quality: Improving cardiac resuscitation outcomes both inside and outside the hospital: A consensus statement from the American Heart Association" [Online]. Accessed March 2015 via the Web at http://circ.ahajournals.org/content/early/2013/06/25/CIR.0b013e31829d8654 (Level II)

13 Rutala, W. A., et al. (2008). "Guideline for disinfection and sterilization in healthcare facilities, 2008" [Online]. Accessed March 2015 via the Web at http://www.cdc.gov/hicpac/pdf/guidelines/Disinfection_Nov_2008.pdf (Level I)

14 American Osteopathic Association. (2014). Standard 07.02.03. *Healthcare Facilities Accreditation Program: Accreditation requirements for acute care hospitals.* Chicago, IL: American Osteopathic Association. (Level VII)

15 The Joint Commission. (2015). Standard RC.01.03.01. *Comprehensive accreditation manual for hospitals: The official handbook.* Oakbrook Terrace, IL: The Joint Commission. (Level VII)

16 Centers for Medicare & Medicaid Services, Department of Health and Human Services. (2013). Condition of participation: Medical record services. 42 C.F.R. § 482.24(b).

17 American Osteopathic Association. (2014). Standard 10.00.03. *Healthcare Facilities Accreditation Program: Accreditation requirements for acute care hospitals.* Chicago, IL: American Osteopathic Association. (Level VII)

ADDITIONAL REFERENCES

Kette, F., et al. (2013). Electrical features of eighteen automated external defibrillators: A systematic evaluation. *Resuscitation, 84,* 1596–1603. (Level VI)

McDonald, D. D., et al. (2010). Motivating people to learn cardiopulmonary resuscitation and use of automated external defibrillators. *Journal of Cardiovascular Nursing, 25,* 69–74.

Nettina, S. M. (2014). *Lippincott manual of nursing practice* (10th ed.). Philadelphia, PA: Wolters Kluwer.

Starr, L. M. (2012). ACOEM position statement: Automated external defibrillation in the occupational setting. *Journal of Occupational and Environmental Medicine, 54,* 1170–1176. Accessed March 2015 via the Web at http://www.acoem.org/uploadedFiles/Public_Affairs/Policies_And_Position_Statements/Guidelines/Position_Statements/Automated%20External%20Defibrillation%20in%20Occup%20Setting.pdf (Level VII)

BACK CARE

Regular bathing and massage of a patient's neck, back, buttocks, and upper arms allows assessment of the patient's skin condition. Massage increases the blood supply to skin and muscles, promotes comfort and relaxation, and improves sleep.[1] However, massage is no longer recommended for bedridden patients at high risk for pressure ulcers,[2] and back massage is contraindicated in patients with rib or vertebral fractures, open wounds, stage I pressure ulcers, or burns.[1]

Equipment

Basin ■ skin cleaner ■ bath blanket ■ bath towel ■ washcloth ■ lotion with lanolin base ■ Optional: gloves (if the patient has open lesions or has been incontinent), gown, mask with face shield, goggles, bed linens.

Implementation

- Gather the equipment at the patient's bedside.
- Confirm the patient's identity using at least two patient identifiers.[3]
- Explain the procedure to the patient and provide privacy.[4] Ask him to tell you if you're applying too much or too little pressure.
- Fill the basin with warm water.
- Adjust the bed to a comfortable working height and lower the head of the bed, if allowed.
- Perform hand hygiene and put on gloves and other personal protective equipment, if needed, *to comply with standard precautions.*[5,6,7,8,9,10,11]
- Place the patient in the prone position, if possible, or on his side. Position him along the edge of the bed nearest you *to prevent back strain.*
- Untie the patient's gown, and expose his back, shoulders, and buttocks. Then drape the patient with a bath blanket *to prevent chills and minimize exposure.* Place a bath towel next to or under the patient's side *to protect bed linens from moisture.*
- Fold the washcloth around your hand to form a mitt *to prevent the loose ends of the cloth from dripping water onto the patient and to keep the cloth warm longer.* (See *Making a washcloth mitt.*) Then apply skin cleaner.
- Using long, firm strokes, bathe the patient's back, beginning at the neck and shoulders and moving downward to the buttocks. Rinse and dry this area well *because moisture trapped between the buttocks can cause chafing and predispose the patient to formation of pressure ulcers.* While giving back care, closely examine the patient's skin, especially the bony prominences of the shoulders, the scapulae, and the coccyx, for redness or abrasions.
- Pour a small amount of lotion into your palm. Rub your hands together *to warm and distribute the lotion.* Then apply the lotion to the patient's back, using long, firm strokes. *The lotion reduces friction, making back massage easier.*
- If permitted by the patient's condition, massage his back, beginning at the base of the spine and moving upward to the shoulders. For a relaxing effect, massage slowly; for a stimulating effect, massage quickly. Alternate the three basic strokes: effleurage, friction, and petrissage. (See *How to give a back massage.*) Add lotion as needed, keeping one hand on the patient's back *to avoid interrupting the massage.*
- Compress, squeeze, and lift the trapezius muscle *to help relax the patient.*
- Finish the massage by using long, firm strokes.
- Blot any excess lotion from the patient's back with a towel.
- Retie the patient's gown and straighten or change the bed linens as necessary.
- Return the bed to its original position, and make the patient comfortable.
- Empty and clean the basin, and store it with other supplies for single-patient use.
- Dispose of the bath blanket, towel, and washcloth in the appropriate receptacle.
- Remove and discard any gloves or other personal protective equipment worn, and return equipment to the appropriate storage area.
- Perform hand hygiene.[5,6,7,9,10]
- Document the procedure.[12,13,14]

Special considerations

- Before giving back care, assess the patient's body structure and skin condition, and tailor the duration and intensity of the massage accordingly. If you're giving back care at bedtime, have the patient ready for bed beforehand *so that the massage can help him fall asleep.*
- Use separate lotion for each patient *to prevent cross-contamination.* If the patient has oily skin, substitute a lotion of the patient's choice.
- When massaging the patient's back, stand with one foot slightly forward and your knees slightly bent *to allow effective use of your arm and shoulder muscles.*
- Don't massage the patient's legs unless ordered *because reddened legs can signal clot formation, and massage can dislodge the clot, causing an embolus.*
- Develop a turning schedule and give back care at each position change.

Documentation

Document back care in the patient's medical record. Record redness, abrasion, or change in skin condition in your notes.

REFERENCES

1 Craven, R. F., & Hirnle, C. J. (2012). *Fundamentals of nursing: Human health and function* (7th ed.). Philadelphia, PA: Lippincott Williams & Wilkins.

2 Wound, Ostomy and Continence Nurses Society (WOCN). (2010). *Guideline for prevention and management of pressure ulcers (WOCN clinical practice guideline no. 2).* Mount Laurel, NJ: WOCN. (Level V)

Making a washcloth mitt

To make a washcloth mitt, take a clean, dry washcloth and fold it in thirds lengthwise around your hand. Fold the top of the washcloth down and tuck it into the bottom of the mitt.

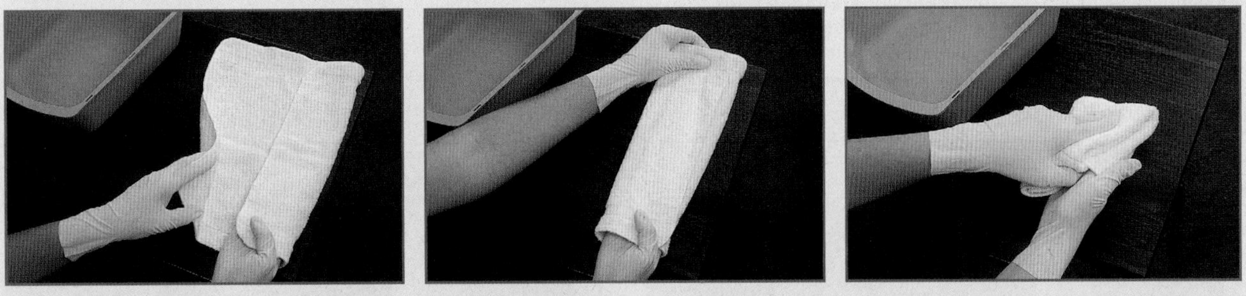

How to give a back massage

Three strokes commonly used when giving a back massage are effleurage, friction, and petrissage. Start with effleurage, go on to friction, and then to petrissage. Perform each stroke at least six times before moving on to the next; then repeat the whole series if desired. When performing effleurage and friction, keep your hands parallel to the vertebrae *to avoid tickling the patient.* For all three strokes, maintain a regular rhythm and steady contact with the patient's back *to help him relax.*

Effleurage
Using your palms, stroke from the buttocks up to the shoulders, over the upper arms, and back to the buttocks. Use slightly less pressure on the downward strokes.

Friction
Use circular thumb strokes to move from buttocks to shoulders; then, using a smooth stroke, return to the buttocks, as shown below.

Petrissage
Using your thumbs to oppose your fingers, knead and stroke half the back and upper arms, starting at the buttocks and moving toward the shoulder. Then knead and stroke the other half of the back, rhythmically alternating your hands.

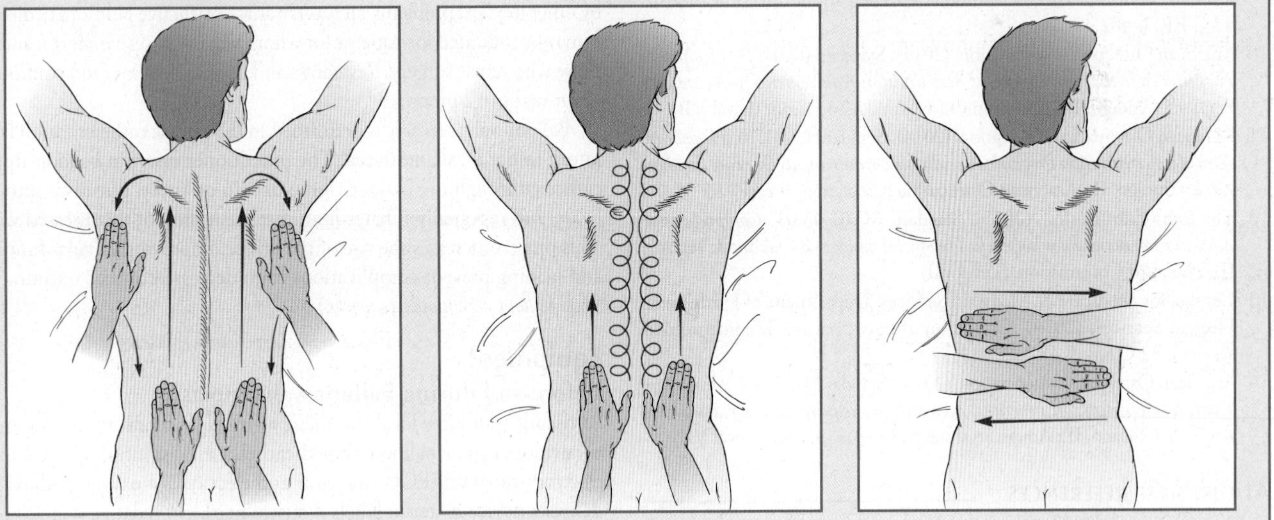

3 The Joint Commission. (2015). Standard NPSG.01.01.01. *Comprehensive accreditation manual for hospitals: The official handbook.* Oakbrook Terrace, IL: The Joint Commission. (Level VII)

4 American Hospital Association. (2003). "The patient care partnership: Understanding expectations, rights, and responsibilities" [Online]. Accessed March 2015 via the Web at http://www.aha.org/content/00-10/pcp_english_030730.pdf

5 The Joint Commission. (2015). Standard NPSG.07.01.01. *Comprehensive accreditation manual for hospitals: The official handbook.* Oakbrook Terrace, IL: The Joint Commission. (Level VII)

6 Centers for Disease Control and Prevention. (2002). Guideline for hand hygiene in health-care settings: Recommendations of the Healthcare Infection Control Practices Advisory Committee and the HICPAC/SHEA/APIC/IDSA Hand Hygiene Task Force. *MMWR Recommendations and Reports, 51*(RR-16), 1–45. Accessed March 2015 via the Web at http://www.cdc.gov/mmwr/pdf/rr/rr5116.pdf (Level II)

7 World Health Organization. (2009). "WHO guidelines on hand hygiene in health care: First global patient safety challenge, clean care is safer care" [Online]. Accessed March 2015 via the Web at http://whqlibdoc.who.int/publications/2009/9789241597906_eng.pdf (Level IV)

How balloon valvuloplasty works

In balloon valvuloplasty, the practitioner chooses an appropriate-sized balloon-tipped catheter. He may determine balloon size using this formula: Balloon size = patient's height (in cm) ÷10 + 10. Alternatively, he may directly measure the value diameter using two-dimensional echocardiography.[4,5] The practitioner then inserts the balloon-tipped catheter through the patient's femoral vein or artery, threads it into the heart, and locates the stenotic valve.

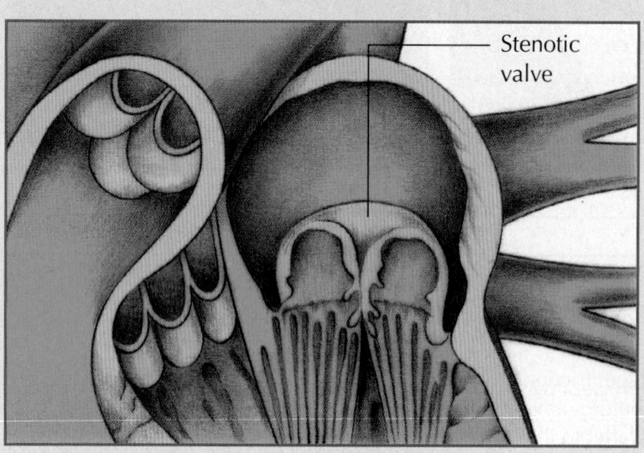

After locating the stenotic valve, the practitioner inflates the balloon, which increases the size of the valve opening.

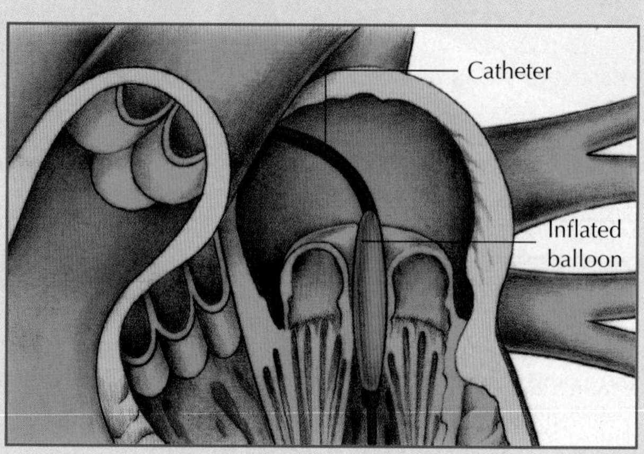

8 Siegel, J. D., et al. (2007). "2007 guideline for isolation precautions: Preventing transmission of infectious agents in healthcare settings" [Online]. Accessed March 2015 via the Web at http://www.cdc.gov/hicpac/pdf/isolation/Isolation2007.pdf (Level II)

9 Centers for Medicare & Medicaid Services, Department of Health and Human Services. (2014). Condition of participation: Infection control. 42 C.F.R. § 482.42.

10 American Osteopathic Association. (2014). Standard 07.01.21. *Healthcare Facilities Accreditation Program: Accreditation requirements for acute care hospitals.* Chicago, IL: American Osteopathic Association. (Level VII)

11 American Osteopathic Association. (2014). Standard 07.01.10. *Healthcare Facilities Accreditation Program: Accreditation requirements for acute care hospitals.* Chicago, IL: American Osteopathic Association. (Level VII)

12 The Joint Commission. (2015). Standard RC.01.03.01. *Comprehensive accreditation manual for hospitals: The official handbook.* Oakbrook Terrace, IL: The Joint Commission. (Level VII)

13 Centers for Medicare & Medicaid Services, Department of Health and Human Services. (2014). Condition of participation: Medical record services. 42 C.F.R. § 482.24.

14 American Osteopathic Association. (2014). Standard 10.00.03. *Healthcare Facilities Accreditation Program: Accreditation requirements for acute care hospitals.* Chicago, IL: American Osteopathic Association. (Level VII)

ADDITIONAL REFERENCES

Collinge, W., et al. (2013). Touch, caring, and cancer: Randomized controlled trial of a multimedia caregiver education program. *Supportive Care in Cancer, 21,* 1405–1414. (Level II)

Sefton, J. M., et al. (2012). Six weeks of massage therapy produces changes in balance, neurological, and cardiovascular measures in older persons. *International Journal of Therapeutic Massage & Bodywork, 5*(3), 28–40.

BALLOON VALVULOPLASTY CARE

Although surgery is the treatment of choice for valvular heart disease, balloon valvuloplasty is an alternative to valve replacement in patients with critical stenoses.[1] This technique enlarges the orifice of a heart valve that has been narrowed by a congenital defect, calcification, rheumatic fever, or aging. It evolved from percutaneous transluminal coronary angioplasty and uses the same balloon-tipped catheters for dilatation.

Balloon valvuloplasty was first successfully performed on pediatric patients, and then on elderly patients who had stenotic valves complicated by other medical problems such as chronic obstructive pulmonary disease. It may be indicated for patients for whom surgery poses a high risk and for those who refuse surgery. Restenosis and clinical deterioration commonly occur within 12 months.[2,3]

Balloon valvuloplasty is performed in the cardiac catheterization laboratory under local anesthesia. The practitioner inserts a balloon-tipped catheter through the patient's femoral vein or artery, threads it into the heart, and repeatedly inflates it against the leaflets of the diseased valve. This process increases the size of the orifice, improving valvular function and helping prevent complications from decreased cardiac output. (See *How balloon valvuloplasty works.*)

Equipment

Before and during balloon valvuloplasty

Antiseptic solution ▪ local anesthetic ▪ vital signs monitoring equipment ▪ valvuloplasty or balloon-tipped catheter ▪ IV solution and tubing ▪ electrocardiogram (ECG) monitor and electrodes ▪ oxygen and oxygen delivery device ▪ sterile labels ▪ sterile marker ▪ sedative ▪ emergency medications ▪ scissors ▪ heparin (or other anticoagulant) for injection[6] ▪ introducer kit for balloon catheter ▪ sterile gown ▪ sterile gloves ▪ gown ▪ gloves ▪ caps ▪ masks ▪ sterile drapes ▪ sterile dressings ▪ pulse oximeter ▪ IV catheter insertion equipment ▪ contrast medium ▪ Optional: suture material, clippers, prescribed antiplatelet and antithrombotic medications, pulmonary artery (PA) catheter, Doppler ultrasound blood flow detector.

After balloon valvuloplasty

Stethoscope ▪ automated blood pressure device or other blood pressure monitoring equipment ▪ pulse oximeter ▪ prescribed IV solution and administration set ▪ ECG monitor and electrodes ▪ PA monitoring system

▪ oxygen and oxygen delivery device ▪ prescribed medications ▪ emergency medications ▪ Doppler ultrasound blood flow detector ▪ programmable IV infusion pumps with dose-range alerts ▪ disinfectant pad ▪ Optional: compression device, supplies for arterial blood gas (ABG) analysis, gloves, gown, mask with face shield or mask and goggles, prescribed analgesic.

Implementation

Before balloon valvuloplasty

■ Conduct a preprocedure verification *to make sure that all relevant documentation, related information, and equipment are available and correctly identified to the patient's identifiers.*[7,8]

■ Verify that the laboratory and imaging studies have been completed, as ordered, and that the results are in the patient's medical record. Notify the practitioner of unexpected results. Ensure that the results of coagulation studies, complete blood count, serum electrolyte studies, and blood typing and crossmatching are available.[7,8]

■ Review baseline hemodynamic parameters and patient medications *for contraindications to the procedure.*[9,10]

■ Review the patient's medical record *to ensure that he isn't allergic to shellfish, iodine, or contrast media.*

■ Confirm that written informed consent has been obtained and is in the patient's medical record.[11,12,13]

■ Perform hand hygiene.[14,15,16,17,18]

■ Confirm the patient's identity using at least two patient identifiers.[19]

■ Reinforce the practitioner's explanation of the procedure, including its risks and alternatives, and answer the patient's questions.

■ Reassure the patient that, although he'll be awake during the procedure, he'll receive a sedative and a local anesthetic beforehand *so that he's comfortable.*

■ Tell the patient what to expect *to ease his anxiety and enhance cooperation.* For example, inform him that the hair in his groin area will be clipped and the skin cleaned with an antiseptic; that he'll feel a brief, stinging sensation when the local anesthetic is injected; and that he may feel pressure as the catheter moves along the vessel. Describe the warm, flushed feeling he's likely to experience from injection of the contrast medium.

■ Tell the patient that the procedure may last up to 4 hours and that he may feel discomfort from lying on a hard table for that long.

■ If the procedure isn't an emergency, confirm the patient's nothing-by-mouth status before the procedure; minimum fasting recommendations are 2 hours for clear liquids, 6 or more hours for a light meal or nonhuman milk, and 8 or more hours for fried or fatty foods or meat.[20]

■ Obtain vital *signs to serve as a baseline for comparison during and after the procedure.*

■ Perform a neurovascular assessment on all extremities. Assess the presence or absence and quality of all distal pulses. Assess faint or nonpalpable pulses using a Doppler ultrasound blood flow detector, as indicated. (See the "Doppler use" procedure, page 248.)[10]

■ Perform hand hygiene.[14,15,16,17,18]

■ Put on gloves *to comply with standard precautions.*[21,22]

■ Insert an IV catheter to provide access for medications. (See the "IV catheter insertion and removal" procedure, page 446.)

■ Clip hair from the insertion site, as needed; clean the sites with antiseptic solution.[23]

■ Have the patient void.

■ Administer an antiplatelet or antithrombotic agent, if ordered, following safe medication administration practices.[9,24,25]

NURSING ALERT *Aspirin reduces the frequency of ischemic complications after percutaneous coronary intervention (PCI). Although the minimum effective aspirin dosage before PCI hasn't been established, 325 mg of aspirin given at least 2 hours, and preferably 24 hours, before PCI is recommended.*[9]

■ Administer a sedative, as ordered, following safe medication administration practices.[24,25]

■ Remove and discard your gloves.[21]

■ Perform hand hygiene.[14,15,16,17,18]

■ Provide handoff communication regarding the patient's history, condition, and care to the nurse who will assume responsibility for the patient's care during the procedure and then give her the opportunity to ask questions. *Handoff communication between caregivers promotes patient safety and prevents errors.*[26]

■ Document the procedure.[27,28,29]

During balloon valvuloplasty

■ Ensure that you have received handoff communication from the person who was responsible for the patient's care before the procedure. Ask questions, if necessary, *to prevent errors.*[26]

■ Perform hand hygiene.[14,15,16,17,18]

■ Confirm the patient's identity using at least two patient identifiers.[19]

■ Put on a cap, a mask, a gown, and gloves.[21]

■ Attach the patient to the monitoring equipment. Make sure that the alarm limits are set appropriately for the patient's current condition and that the alarms are turned on, functioning properly, and audible to staff.[30,31,32,33]

■ Administer supplemental oxygen, as ordered.

■ The practitioner will put on a sterile gown and gloves, a mask, and a cap and will then open the sterile supplies. Assist as necessary.

■ Confirm that the correct procedure has been identified for the correct patient at the correct site.[7,8]

■ Label all medications, medication containers, and other solutions on and off the sterile field.[34,35]

■ The practitioner uses maximal barrier precautions and prepares and anesthetizes the catheter insertion site (usually at the femoral artery). He may insert a PA catheter if one isn't already in place.[36]

■ Conduct a time-out immediately before starting the procedure *to perform a final assessment that the correct patient, site, positioning, and procedure are identified and, as applicable, that all relevant information and necessary equipment are available.*[37]

■ The practitioner then inserts an introducer or a sheath into the site and threads a valvuloplasty or balloon-tipped catheter up into the heart.

■ The practitioner injects a contrast medium *to visualize the heart valves and assess the stenosis.* He also injects heparin or another anticoagulant[6] *to prevent the catheter from clotting.*[9,36,38]

■ Using low pressure, the practitioner repeatedly inflates the balloon on the valvuloplasty catheter for a short time, usually 15 to 30 seconds, gradually increasing the time and pressure. If these actions don't reduce the stenosis, the practitioner may use a larger balloon.

■ After completion of valvuloplasty, a series of angiograms is taken *to evaluate the effectiveness of the treatment.* Assist as necessary.

■ The practitioner may then suture the introducer or sheath in place *to allow the effects of the anticoagulant to wear off* and cover the insertion site with a sterile dressing, which is usually removed within 4 hours.

■ Remove and discard your gloves and perform hand hygiene.[14,15,16,17,18]

■ Continue to closely monitor the patient.

■ Document the procedure.[27,28,29]

After balloon valvuloplasty

■ Receive handoff communication from the person who was responsible for the patient's care during the procedure. Ask questions, if necessary, *to prevent errors in care that might occur with miscommunication.*[26]

■ Verify the practitioner's orders.

■ Perform hand hygiene.[14,15,16,17,18]

■ Put on gloves and other personal protective equipment as needed *to comply with standard precautions.*[21,22]

■ Confirm the patient's identity using at least two patient identifiers.[19]

■ Attach the patient to a continuous ECG monitor. Make sure that the alarm limits are set appropriately for the patient's current condition and that the alarms are turned on, functioning properly, and audible to staff.[30,31,32,33]

■ Obtain the patient's vital signs *to serve as a baseline for comparison,* and continue to monitor them frequently at an interval determined by your facility and the patient's condition; *there's no evidence-based research to indicate best practice for the frequency of vital signs monitoring.*[40]

■ Assess the sheath insertion site for bleeding, hematoma, and ecchymosis. If the sheath remains in place, refer to the "Arterial and venous sheath removal" procedure when removal is indicated. If the sheath was removed and a compression device remains in place over the insertion site, make sure that the device is applied properly.

■ For a patient is receiving IV heparin,[9] nitroglycerin, or another medicated infusion, administer the medication using a programmable IV infusion pump (preferably a smart pump with dose-range alerts)[41] *to prevent life-threatening dosing errors.* To do so, make sure that the infusion device alarm limits are set appropriately and that the alarms are turned on, functioning properly, and audible to staff.[30,31,32,33] Next, trace each tubing from the patient to its point of origin to make sure that it's attached to the correct port *to prevent dangerous misconnections.*[42] If required by your facility, have another nurse perform an independent double-check *to verify the patient's identity and to ensure that the correct medication is hanging in the prescribed concentration, that the medication's indication corresponds with the patient's diagnosis, that the dosage calculations are correct and the dosing formula used to derive the final dose is correct, that the route of administration is safe and proper for the patient, that the pump settings are correct, and that the infusion line is attached to the correct port.*[43,44] Compare the results of the independent double-check with the other nurse (if required) and, if no discrepancies exist, continue infusing the medication. If discrepancies exist, rectify them before continuing the infusion.[44]

■ Assess the patient's cardiac status *to obtain a baseline for comparison;* continue to monitor the patient's heart rate and rhythm, and auscultate regularly for murmurs, *which may indicate worsening valvular insufficiency.* Notify the practitioner if you detect a new or worsening murmur.

■ Assess the patient's respiratory status, including his oxygen saturation level, *to obtain a baseline for comparison;* continue to monitor respiratory status for changes *because changes in respiratory rate and pattern can be the first sign of a complication such as an embolism.* Monitor ABG results, as ordered.[10]

■ Monitor the patient's arterial pressure, pulmonary artery pressure, and other hemodynamic parameters as indicated.[10]

■ Continue to monitor the insertion site for bleeding and to assess peripheral pulses distal to the insertion site; also monitor the color, sensation, temperature, and capillary refill time of the affected extremity. Use a Doppler ultrasound blood flow detector to assess pedal pulses *because they may be difficult to assess, especially if the sheath remains in place.* Compare findings bilaterally.

■ Administer IV fluids, as prescribed, typically at a rate of at least 100 mL/hour, *to help the kidneys excrete the contrast medium used during the procedure.* Closely monitor intake and output and watch for signs of fluid overload, such as distended neck veins, atrial and ventricular gallops, dyspnea, pulmonary congestion, tachycardia, hypertension, and hypoxemia.

■ Assess for signs and symptoms of complications of the procedure, such as embolism (dyspnea, tachypnea, altered mental status, and tachycardia), hemorrhage (including retroperitoneal bleeding,)[10] myocardial ischemia (chest pain caused by obstruction of blood flow during valvuloplasty), and cardiac tamponade (decreased or absent peripheral pulses, pale or cyanotic skin, hypotension, and paradoxical pulse). Immediately report signs and symptoms of any of these complications.

■ Encourage the patient to perform deep-breathing exercises *to prevent atelectasis, which can occur with immobility.* Note that this step is especially important in elderly patients.

■ Keep the patient positioned with the affected leg straight and the head of bed elevated no more than 30 degrees *to prevent excessive hip flexion and to reduce the risk of vascular complications.*[45]

■ Perform a comprehensive pain assessment using techniques appropriate for the patient's age, condition, and ability to understand.[46]

■ Administer pain medications, as needed and prescribed, following safe medication administration practices.[24,25]

■ Assist the patient with meals, bedpan use, and position changes that are appropriate to his activity limitations.[45]

■ Discard used supplies in appropriate receptacles.[21]

■ Clean and disinfect your stethoscope using a disinfectant pad.[47,48]

■ Remove and discard any gloves or other personal protective equipment worn.[21]

■ Perform hand hygiene.[14,15,16,17,18]

■ Document the procedure.[27,28,29]

Special considerations

■ The Joint Commission issued a sentinel event alert concerning medical device alarm safety *because alarm-related events have been associated with permanent loss of function and death.* Among the major contributing factors were improper alarm settings, alarm settings inappropriately turned off, and alarm signals not audible to staff. Make sure that alarm limits are set appropriately and that alarms are turned on, functioning properly, and audible to staff. Follow facility guidelines for preventing alarm fatigue.[30]

■ Assess the patient's vital signs continually during the procedure,[39] especially for an aortic valvuloplasty. *During balloon inflation, the aortic outflow tract is completely obstructed, causing blood pressure to fall dangerously low.* Ventricular ectopy is also common during balloon positioning and inflation. Start treatment for ectopy when signs and symptoms develop or when ventricular tachycardia is sustained.

■ Carefully assess the patient's respiratory status; *changes in rate and pattern can be the first sign of a complication such as embolism.*

■ Assess the insertion site frequently throughout the procedure for bleeding, and monitor the International Normalized Ratio, prothrombin time, partial thromboplastin time and activated clotting time (especially if the patient is receiving heparin), and platelet count, as ordered.[6,10,36] Notify the practitioner of any critical test results within your facility's established time frame *so that the patient can be treated promptly.*[49]

■ Be aware that using heparin and a large-bore catheter can lead to arterial hemorrhage. Monitor the patient closely.

Complications

Severe complications, such as myocardial infarction or calcium emboli (embolization of debris released from the calcified valve), are rare. Other complications include bleeding or hematoma at the insertion site, arrhythmias, circulatory disorders distal to the insertion site, guide wire perforation of the ventricle leading to tamponade, disruption of the valve ring, restenosis of the valve, and valvular insufficiency, which can contribute to heart failure and reduced cardiac output. Infection and an allergic reaction to the contrast medium can also occur.

Documentation

Document vital signs, your assessments, diagnostic test results, any complications and interventions, and the patient's tolerance of the procedure. Document patient teaching and the patient's understanding of your teaching.

References

1 Bonow, R. O., et al. (2006). ACC/AHA 2006 guidelines for the management of patients with valvular heart disease: A report of the American College of Cardiology/American Heart Association Task Force on Practice Guidelines. *Journal of the American College of Cardiology, 48*(3), e1–e148. Accessed March 2015 via the Web at http://www.scahq.org/files/VHDFullText.pdf (Level VII)

2 Joint Task Force on the Management of Valvular Heart Disease of the European Society of Cardiology (ESC) and the European Association

for Cardio-Thoracic Surgery (EACTS). (2012). Guidelines on the management of valvular heart disease (version 2012). *European Heart Journal, 33,* 2451–2496. Accessed March 2015 via the Web at http://www.escardio.org/guidelines-surveys/esc-guidelines/GuidelinesDocuments/Guidelines_Valvular_Heart_Dis_FT.pdf (Level VII)

3 Fawzy, M. E., et al. (2009). Long-term (up to 18 years) clinical and echocardiographic results of mitral balloon valvuloplasty in 531 consecutive patients and predictors of outcome. *Cardiology, 113,* 213–221. (Level VI)

4 Nobuyoshi, M., et al. (2009). Percutaneous balloon mitral valvuloplasty: A review. *Circulation, 119,* e211–e219. Accessed March 2015 via the Web at http://circ.ahajournals.org/content/119/8/e211.full

5 Assadi, R. (2012). "Percutaneous mitral balloon valvuloplasty" [Online]. Accessed March 2015 via the Web at http://emedicine.medscape.com/article/1839677-overview

6 Merriweather, N., & Sulzbach-Hoke, L. M. (2012). Managing risk of complications at femoral vascular access sites in percutaneous coronary intervention. *Critical Care Nurse, 32*(5), 16–29. Accessed March 2015 via the Web at http://ccn.aacnjournals.org/content/32/5/16.full.pdf

7 The Joint Commission. (2015). Standard UP.01.01.01. *Comprehensive accreditation manual for hospitals: The official handbook.* Oakbrook Terrace, IL: The Joint Commission. (Level VII)

8 American Osteopathic Association. (2014). Standard 30.00.14. *Healthcare Facilities Accreditation Program: Accreditation requirements for acute care hospitals.* Chicago, IL: American Osteopathic Association. (Level VII)

9 Levine, G. N., et al. (2011). 2011 ACCF/AHA/SCAI guideline for percutaneous coronary intervention: A report of the American College of Cardiology Foundation/American Heart Association Task Force on Practice Guidelines and the Society for Cardiovascular Angiography and Interventions. *Circulation, 124,* e574–e651. Accessed March 2015 via the Web at http://circ.ahajournals.org/content/early/2011/11/07/CIR.0b013e31823ba622.full.pdf (Level VII)

10 Gulanick, M., & Meyers, J. L. (2013). *Nursing care plans: Diagnoses, interventions, and outcomes* (8th ed.). St. Louis, MO: Mosby.

11 The Joint Commission. (2015). Standard RI.01.03.01. *Comprehensive accreditation manual for hospitals: The official handbook.* Oakbrook Terrace, IL: The Joint Commission. (Level VII)

12 Centers for Medicare & Medicaid Services, Department of Health and Human Services. (2014). Condition of participation: Patient's rights. 42 C.F.R. § 482.13(b)(2).

13 American Osteopathic Association. (2014). Standard 30.01.11. *Healthcare Facilities Accreditation Program: Accreditation requirements for acute care hospitals.* Chicago, IL: American Osteopathic Association. (Level VII)

14 The Joint Commission. (2015). Standard NPSG.07.01.01. *Comprehensive accreditation manual for hospitals: The official handbook.* Oakbrook Terrace, IL: The Joint Commission. (Level VII)

15 Centers for Disease Control and Prevention. (2002). Guideline for hand hygiene in health-care settings: Recommendations of the Healthcare Infection Control Practices Advisory Committee and the HICPAC/SHEA/APIC/IDSA Hand Hygiene Task Force. *MMWR Recommendations and Reports, 51*(RR-16), 1–45. Accessed March 2015 via the Web at http://www.cdc.gov/mmwr/pdf/rr/rr5116.pdf (Level II)

16 World Health Organization. (2009). "WHO guidelines on hand hygiene in health care: First global patient safety challenge, clean care is safer care" [Online]. Accessed March 2015 via the Web at http://whqlibdoc.who.int/publications/2009/9789241597906_eng.pdf (Level IV)

17 Centers for Medicare & Medicaid Services, Department of Health and Human Services. (2014). Condition of participation: Infection control. 42 C.F.R. § 482.42.

18 American Osteopathic Association. (2014). Standard 07.01.21. *Healthcare Facilities Accreditation Program: Accreditation requirements for acute care hospitals.* Chicago, IL: American Osteopathic Association. (Level VII)

19 The Joint Commission. (2015). Standard NPSG.01.01.01. *Comprehensive accreditation manual for hospitals: The official handbook.* Oakbrook Terrace, IL: The Joint Commission. (Level VII)

20 American Society of Anesthesiologists. (2011). Practice guidelines for preoperative fasting and the use of pharmacologic agents to reduce the risk of pulmonary aspiration: Application to healthy patients undergoing elective procedures. *Anesthesiology, 114,* 495–511. (Level V)

21 Siegel, J. D., et al. (2007). "2007 guideline for isolation precautions: Preventing transmission of infectious agents in healthcare settings" [Online]. Accessed March 2015 via the Web at http://www.cdc.gov/hicpac/pdf/isolation/Isolation2007.pdf (Level II)

22 American Osteopathic Association. (2014). Standard 07.01.10. *Healthcare Facilities Accreditation Program: Accreditation requirements for acute care hospitals.* Chicago, IL: American Osteopathic Association. (Level VII)

23 The Joint Commission. (2015). Standard NPSG.07.05.01. *Comprehensive accreditation manual for hospitals: The official handbook.* Oakbrook Terrace, IL: The Joint Commission. (Level VII)

24 Centers for Medicare & Medicaid Services, Department of Health and Human Services. (2014). Condition of participation: Preparation and administration of drugs. 42 C.F.R. § 482.23(c).

25 American Osteopathic Association. (2014). Standard 16.01.03. *Healthcare Facilities Accreditation Program: Accreditation requirements for acute care hospitals.* Chicago, IL: American Osteopathic Association. (Level VII)

26 The Joint Commission. (2015). Standard PC.02.02.01. *Comprehensive accreditation manual for hospitals: The official handbook.* Oakbrook Terrace, IL: The Joint Commission. (Level VII)

27 The Joint Commission. (2015). Standard RC.01.03.01. *Comprehensive accreditation manual for hospitals: The official handbook.* Oakbrook Terrace, IL: The Joint Commission. (Level VII)

28 Centers for Medicare & Medicaid Services, Department of Health and Human Services. (2014). Condition of participation: Medical record services. 42 C.F.R. § 482.24(b).

29 American Osteopathic Association. (2014). Standard 10.00.03. *Healthcare Facilities Accreditation Program: Accreditation requirements for acute care hospitals.* Chicago, IL: American Osteopathic Association. (Level VII)

30 The Joint Commission. (2013). "Sentinel event alert: Medical device alarm safety in hospitals" [Online]. Accessed March 2015 via the Web at http://www.jointcommission.org/assets/1/18/SEA_50_alarms_4_5_13_FINAL1.PDF (Level VII)

31 The Joint Commission. (2015). Standard NPSG.06.01.01. *Comprehensive accreditation manual for hospitals: The official handbook.* Oakbrook Terrace, IL: The Joint Commission. (Level VII)

32 Graham, K. C., & Cvach, M. (2010). Monitor alarm fatigue: Standardizing use of physiological monitors and decreasing nuisance alarms. *American Journal of Critical Care, 19,* 28–37.

33 American Association of Critical-Care Nurses (AACN). (2013). "AACN practice alert: Alarm management" [Online]. Accessed March 2015 via the Web at http://www.aacn.org/wd/practice/docs/practicealerts/alarm-management-practice-alert.pdf (Level VII)

34 The Joint Commission. (2015). Standard NPSG.03.04.01. *Comprehensive accreditation manual for hospitals: The official handbook.* Oakbrook Terrace, IL: The Joint Commission. (Level VII)

35 American Osteopathic Association. (2014). Standard 25.01.27. *Healthcare Facilities Accreditation Program: Accreditation requirements for acute care hospitals.* Chicago, IL: American Osteopathic Association. (Level VII)

36 Agu, N. C., & Rao, P. S. (2012). Balloon aortic valvuloplasty. *Pediatrics & Therapeutics, S5,* 004. Accessed March 2015 via the Web at http://www.omicsonline.org/2161-0665/2161-0665-S5-003.pdf

37 The Joint Commission. (2015). Standard UP.01.03.01. *Comprehensive accreditation manual for hospitals: The official handbook.* Oakbrook Terrace, IL: The Joint Commission. (Level VII)

38 Ben-Dor, I., et al. (2010). Complications and outcome of balloon aortic valvuloplasty in high-risk or inoperable patients. *Journal of American College of Cardiology Interventions, 3,* 1150–1156. Accessed March 2015 via the Web at http://interventions.onlinejacc.org/article.aspx?articleid=1112045 (Level VI)

39 Mahmoud, S., et al. (2010). Blood pressure monitoring: A noble method for stepwise decision making in percutaneous mitral valvuloplasty. *Internet Journal of Cardiology, 8*, 2. Accessed March 2015 via the Web at http://ispub.com/IJC/8/2/7334 (Level VI)
40 American Society of PeriAnesthesia Nurses. (2015). *2015–2017 Perianesthesia nursing standards, practice recommendations and interpretive statements.* Cherry Hill, NJ: American Society of PeriAnesthesia Nurses. (Level VII)
41 The Joint Commission. (2015). Standard NPSG.03.05.01. *Comprehensive accreditation manual for hospitals: The official handbook.* Oakbrook Terrace, IL: The Joint Commission. (Level VII)
42 U.S. Food and Drug Administration. (n.d.). "Look. Check. Connect. Safe medical device connections save lives" [Online]. Accessed March 2015 via the Web at http://www.fda.gov/downloads/MedicalDevices/Safety/AlertsandNotices/UCM134873.pdf
43 Institute for Safe Medication Practices. (2012). "ISMP's list of high-alert medications" [Online]. Accessed March 2015 via the Web at http://www.ismp.org/tools/highalertmedications.pdf (Level VII)
44 Institute for Safe Medication Practices. (2008). Conducting an independent double-check. *ISMP Medication Safety Alert! Nurse Advise-ERR, 6*(12), 1. Accessed March 2015 via the Web at http://www.ismp.org/newsletters/nursing/Issues/NurseAdviseERR200812.pdf (Level VII)
45 Lynn-McHale Wiegand, D. (Ed.). (2011). *AACN procedure manual for critical care* (6th ed.). St. Louis, MO: Saunders.
46 The Joint Commission. (2015). Standard PC.01.02.07. *Comprehensive accreditation manual for hospitals: The official handbook.* Oakbrook Terrace, IL: The Joint Commission. (Level VII)
47 Rutala, W. A., et al. (2008). "Guideline for disinfection and sterilization in healthcare facilities, 2008" [Online]. Accessed March 2015 via the Web at http://www.cdc.gov/hicpac/pdf/guidelines/Disinfection_Nov_2008.pdf (Level I)
48 American Osteopathic Association. (2014). Standard 07.02.03. *Healthcare Facilities Accreditation Program: Accreditation requirements for acute care hospitals.* Chicago, IL: American Osteopathic Association. (Level VII)
49 The Joint Commission. (2015). Standard NPSG.02.03.01. *Comprehensive accreditation manual for hospitals: The official handbook.* Oakbrook Terrace, IL: The Joint Commission. (Level VII)

BARIATRIC BED USE

Obesity affects more than one-third of all Americans.[1] A patient is considered obese if his body mass index (BMI) is 30 kg/m^2 or greater.[1] Typical hospital beds are designed to hold patients who weigh up to 450 lb (204 kg) and don't have a wide abdominal girth. Bariatric beds are a recent addition to hospital equipment that are designed to accommodate larger patients. Various bariatric beds are available, ranging from beds that are simply larger versions of standard beds to beds with low-air-loss mattresses that provide pressure relief (as shown below).

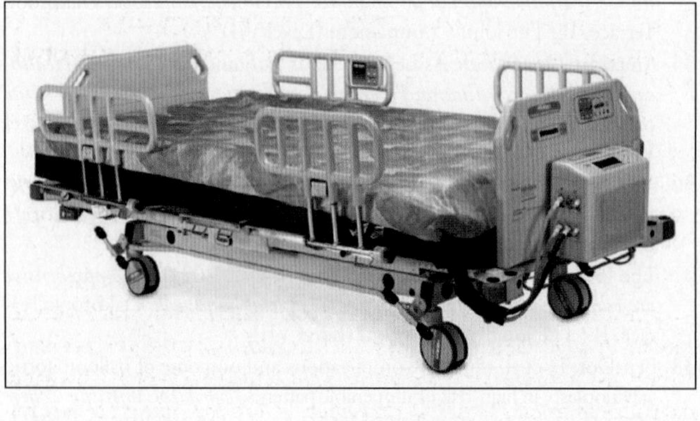

Bariatric beds provide more comfort for obese patients than standard-size beds. They help preserve self-esteem by providing these patients with a bed that easily fits their larger body size as well as special side rails that help them turn and reposition themselves. Bariatric beds allow caregivers to perform such routine care as boosting, turning, and transferring in and out of bed with greater ease and less risk of injury. Most bariatric beds have a built-in scale that allows the nurse to more easily weigh the patient. Some bariatric beds also convert to a cardiac chair.

Equipment

Bariatric bed ▪ Optional: overhead trapeze, special sheets.

Preparation of equipment

Obtain a bariatric bed from central supply or contact the company representative to have a bed delivered. Prepare the bed according to the manufacturer's guidelines. A company representative may be involved in the patient assessment *to ensure that the appropriate type and size of bed are provided.* Choose the appropriate type of mattress to meet your patient's needs. Specialized sheets may be necessary. Attach an overhead trapeze, if indicated.

Implementation

- Verify the practitioner's order for a bariatric bed.
- Perform hand hygiene.[2,3,4,5,6]
- Confirm the patient's identity using at least two patient identifiers.[7]
- Discuss the need for a specialized bed with the patient *so that he understands its benefits and therapeutic effects.*
- Consult with other health care team members, such as the doctor, surgical team members, physical therapist, occupational therapist, wound care specialist, and respiratory therapist, *to choose the appropriate type of bed for the patient's needs.*
- If the bed is rented, ask the company representative for an in-service appointment *so that all health care team members understand the bed's use and provide safe care.*
- Make sure that written instructions come with the bed, and keep them at the bedside.
- Provide the patient with product information, and orient him to the bed's functions and controls *so that the he understands its many features and safe use.*
- Perform hand hygiene.[2,3,4,5,6]
- Document the procedure.[8,9,10]

Special considerations

- Provide for other bariatric equipment, as needed, such as hospital gowns, commodes, wheelchairs, lifts, scales, and stretchers *for patient comfort and safety.*
- When sending the patient to other departments, call first to be sure they can accommodate a larger bed and are familiar with its use.

Documentation

Document the type of bed and the date and time of its delivery. Indicate that the representative oriented the staff how to safely use the bed. Document that the patient was oriented to safely use the bed and that he gave a return demonstration. Note if written information was given to the patient or left at the bedside. Also, record other equipment provided, such as an overhead trapeze or special sheets. Note the type of mattress on the bed. Document the patient's skin condition when placed on the bed. Record the patient's response to the bed.

REFERENCES

1 Ogden, C. L., et al. (2012). "Prevalence of obesity in the United States, 2009–2010 (NCHS Data Brief No. 82)" [Online]. Accessed March 2015 via the Web at http://www.cdc.gov/nchs/data/databriefs/db82.pdf
2 The Joint Commission. (2015). Standard NPSG.07.01.01. *Comprehensive accreditation manual for hospitals: The official handbook.* Oakbrook Terrace, IL: The Joint Commission. (Level VII)

3 Centers for Disease Control and Prevention. (2002). Guideline for hand hygiene in health-care settings: Recommendations of the Healthcare Infection Control Practices Advisory Committee and the HICPAC/SHEA/APIC/IDSA Hand Hygiene Task Force. *MMWR Recommendations and Reports, 51*(RR-16), 1–45. Accessed March 2015 via the Web at http://www.cdc.gov/mmwr/pdf/rr/rr5116.pdf (Level II)

4 World Health Organization. (2009). "WHO guidelines on hand hygiene in health care: First global patient safety challenge, clean care is safer care" [Online]. Accessed March 2015 via the Web at http://whqlibdoc.who.int/publications/2009/9789241597906_eng.pdf (Level IV)

5 Centers for Medicare & Medicaid Services, Department of Health and Human Services. (2014). Condition of participation: Infection control. 42 C.F.R. § 482.42.

6 American Osteopathic Association. (2014). Standard 07.01.21. *Healthcare Facilities Accreditation Program: Accreditation requirements for acute care hospitals.* Chicago, IL: American Osteopathic Association. (Level VII)

7 The Joint Commission. (2015). Standard NPSG.01.01.01. *Comprehensive accreditation manual for hospitals: The official handbook.* Oakbrook Terrace, IL: The Joint Commission. (Level VII)

8 The Joint Commission. (2015). Standard RC.01.03.01. *Comprehensive accreditation manual for hospitals: The official handbook.* Oakbrook Terrace, IL: The Joint Commission. (Level VII)

9 Centers for Medicare & Medicaid Services, Department of Health and Human Services. (2014). Condition of participation: Medical record services. 42 C.F.R. § 482.24.

10 American Osteopathic Association. (2014). Standard 10.00.03. *Healthcare Facilities Accreditation Program: Accreditation requirements for acute care hospitals.* Chicago, IL: American Osteopathic Association. (Level VII)

ADDITIONAL REFERENCE

Muir, M., & Archer-Heese, G. (2009). Essentials of a bariatric patient handling program. *Online Journal of Issues in Nursing, 14.* Accessed March 2015 via the Web at http://nursingworld.org/MainMenuCategories/ANAMarketplace/ANAPeriodicals/OJIN/TableofContents/Vol142009/No1Jan09/Bariatric-Patient-Handling-Program-.aspx

BED BATH

A complete bed bath cleans the patient's skin, stimulates circulation, provides mild exercise, and promotes comfort. Bathing also allows assessment of skin condition, joint mobility, and muscle strength. Depending on the patient's overall condition and duration of hospitalization, he may have a complete or partial bath daily. A partial bath, including hands, face, axillae, back, genitalia, and anal region, can replace a complete bath for the patient with dry, fragile skin or extreme weakness and can supplement a complete bath for the diaphoretic or incontinent patient.

Equipment

Bath blanket ▪ skin cleaner ▪ towels ▪ washcloths ▪ several pairs of gloves ▪ hospital-grade disinfectant ▪ bed linens ▪ Optional: personal protective equipment; basin; bedpan; urinal; deodorant; perineal pad; scrotal support; hypoallergenic moisturizing cream; no-rinse, pH-neutral skin cleaner; protective clothing for the patient (shirt with long sleeves, long pants, knee-high socks, shin and elbow guard pads); chlorhexidine-impregnated cloth; sealant; bath bag and warming unit; absorbent underpads or briefs.

Preparation of equipment

Adjust the temperature of the patient's room, and close any doors or windows *to prevent drafts and provide privacy.* Determine the patient's preference for skin cleaner and other hygiene aids *because some patients are allergic to soap or prefer bath oil or lotions.*

Bathing a patient at risk for skin tears[8]

Caring for a patient with fragile skin who's at risk for skin tears can pose a special challenge because mechanical trauma can result from even such routine care as bathing. When caring for the patient at risk, limit baths when possible; instead, as the patient's condition allows, encourage showering with warm, tepid water. When a bed bath is necessary, use a no-rinse, pH-neutral skin cleaner and use gentle technique during bathing. After bathing, allow the skin to remain damp, but not wet, and then hydrate the skin with a hypoallergenic moisturizer. Provide the patient with protective clothing, such as shirts with long sleeves, long pants, knee-high socks, or shin and elbow guard pads.

Implementation

- Gather the equipment on an overbed table or bedside stand.
- Perform hand hygiene.[1,2,3,4,5]
- Confirm the patient's identity using at least two patient identifiers.[6]
- Tell the patient you'll be giving him a bath, and provide privacy.[7]
- Offer him a bedpan or urinal, if needed.
- Help the patient into the supine position, if possible.
- If the patient's condition permits, encourage him to assist with bathing *to provide exercise and promote independence.*
- Fill the bath basin two-thirds full of tepid-to-warm water and bring it to the patient's bedside. Alternatively, use tepid-to-warm water directly from the patient's spigot.[8]
- Raise the patient's bed to a comfortable working height *to avoid back strain.*
- If the bed will be changed after the bath, remove the top linen. If not, fanfold it to the foot of the bed.
- Cover the patient with a bath blanket *to provide warmth and privacy.*
- Put on gloves and other personal protective equipment as needed *to comply with standard precautions.*[9]
- Remove the patient's gown and other articles, such as elastic stockings, elastic bandages, and restraints (as ordered).
- Place a towel under the patient's chin. Then wash the patient's face. Begin with the eyes, working from the inner to the outer canthus without soap. Use a separate section of the washcloth for each eye *to avoid spreading ocular infection.*
- If the patient can tolerates a skin cleaner, apply it to the cloth and wash the rest of his face, ears, and neck, using firm, gentle strokes. Rinse thoroughly *because residual soap can cause itching and dryness.* (See *Bathing a patient at risk for skin tears.*)
- Dry the area thoroughly, taking special care in skin folds and creases. Observe the skin for irritation, scaling, or other abnormalities.
- Turn down the bath blanket, and drape the patient's chest with a bath towel.
- Wash, rinse, and dry the chest and axillae, observing the patient's respirations throughout the procedure. Wash skin folds under the female patient's breasts by lifting each breast. Use firm strokes *to avoid tickling the patient.* If the patient tolerates deodorant, apply it. Replace the bath blanket to cover the patient's chest and axillae.
- Place a bath towel beneath the patient's arm farthest from you.
- Bathe the arm, using long, smooth strokes and moving from wrist to shoulder *to stimulate venous circulation.* If possible, soak the patient's hand in the basin *to remove dirt and soften the nails.* Observe the color of his hand and nail beds *to assess peripheral circulation.* Follow the same procedure for the other arm and hand.
- Turn down the bath blanket to expose the patient's abdomen and groin, keeping a bath towel across his chest *to prevent chills.* Bathe, rinse,

and dry the patient's abdomen and groin while checking for abdominal distention or tenderness. Then turn back the bath blanket to cover the patient's chest and abdomen.

■ Uncover the patient's leg farthest from you, and place a bath towel under it. Flex this leg and bathe it, moving from ankle to hip *to stimulate venous circulation.* Don't massage the leg, however, *to avoid dislodging any existing thrombus, possibly causing a pulmonary embolus.* Rinse and dry the leg.

■ If possible, place a basin on the patient's bed, flex the leg at the knee, and place the foot in the basin. Soak the foot, and then wash and rinse it thoroughly. Remove the foot from the basin, dry it, and clean the toenails. Observe the patient's skin condition and color during cleaning *to assess peripheral circulation.* Repeat the procedure for the other leg and foot.

■ Cover the patient with the bath blanket *to prevent chilling.* Then lower the bed and raise the side rails *to ensure patient safety while you change the bath water.*

■ Remove and discard your gloves and perform hand hygiene.[1,2,3,4,5,9,10]

■ Put on new gloves.[9,10]

■ Roll the patient on his side or stomach, place a towel beneath him, and cover him *to prevent chilling.*

■ Bathe, rinse, and dry his back and buttocks.

■ Bathe the anal area from front to back *to avoid contaminating the perineum.* Rinse and dry the area well.

■ Remove and discard your gloves.

■ After lowering the bed and raising the side rails *to ensure the patient's safety,* perform hand hygiene and change the bath water again.[1,2,3,4,5]

■ Put on new gloves.[9,10]

■ Turn the patient on his back and bathe the genital area thoroughly but gently, using a different section of the washcloth for each downward stroke. Bathe from front to back, avoiding the anal area. Rinse thoroughly and pat dry. Use a moisture barrier protectant on the skin, as needed *to protect and maintain intact skin.*[11]

■ If applicable, perform indwelling urinary catheter care. Apply perineal pads or scrotal supports as needed.

■ Remove and discard your gloves and perform hand hygiene.[1,2,3,4,5]

■ Apply a hypoallergenic moisturizing cream if needed to areas of dry skin *to prevent skin breakdown.*[12]

■ Dress the patient in a clean gown, and reapply any elastic bandages, elastic stockings, or restraints removed before the bath.

■ Put on gloves.[9,10]

■ Empty, clean, and disinfect the basin, using a hospital-grade disinfectant.

■ Remove and discard your gloves and perform hand hygiene.[1,2,3,4,5]

■ Put on new gloves.[9,10]

■ Remake the bed or change the linens, and remove the bath blanket.

■ Place a bath towel beneath the patient's head *to catch loose hair,* and then brush and comb the hair.

■ Return the bed to its original position and make the patient comfortable.

■ Carry soiled linens to the hamper with outstretched arms. *To avoid spreading microorganisms,* don't let soiled linens touch your clothing.

■ Remove and discard your gloves and any other personal protective equipment worn and perform hand hygiene.[1,2,3,4,5]

■ Document the procedure.[13,14,15]

Special considerations

■ In areas in your facility where central line–associated bloodstream infection rates are higher than desired, bathe patients daily who are older than age 2 months with a chlorhexidine-impregnated cloth according to the manufacturer's guidelines *to reduce the risk of central line–associated bloodstream infections.*[16,17,18]

■ Fold the washcloth around your hand to form a mitt while bathing the patient. *This technique keeps the cloth warm longer and avoids dribbling water on the patient from the cloth's loose ends.* Change the water as often as necessary *to keep it warm and clean.*

■ Carefully dry skin-fold areas, such as under breasts, in the groin area, and between fingers, toes, and buttocks. Separate skinfolds and apply a sealant *to prevent skin breakdown.*[11]

■ Use a bag bath (which contains 8 to 10 premoistened, disposable cloths that contain a no-rinse surfactant), if available, to bathe the patient. Before use, warm the cloths in a microwave or a special warming unit supplied by the manufacturer. Use a separate cloth to wash each part of the body. *A bag bath saves time compared with the conventional bed bath because no rinsing is required.*

■ *To improve circulation, maintain joint mobility, and preserve muscle tone,* move the body joints through their full range of motion during the bath.

■ If the patient is incontinent, use absorbent underpads or briefs to wick incontinence moisture away from the skin *because moisture trapped against the skin can cause maceration.*[11]

■ When bathing an older adult with dementia, focus on getting to know the person rather than just the task of bathing *to help reduce discomfort and anxiety.*[19,20]

Documentation

Record the date and time of the bed bath in the flowchart. Note the patient's tolerance of the bath, his range of motion, and his self-care abilities, and document any unusual findings.

References

1 The Joint Commission. (2015). Standard NPSG.07.01.01. *Comprehensive accreditation manual for hospitals: The official handbook.* Oakbrook Terrace, IL: The Joint Commission. (Level VII)

2 Centers for Disease Control and Prevention. (2002). Guideline for hand hygiene in health-care settings: Recommendations of the Healthcare Infection Control Practices Advisory Committee and the HICPAC/SHEA/APIC/IDSA Hand Hygiene Task Force. *MMWR Recommendations and Reports, 51*(RR-16), 1–45. Accessed March 2015 via the Web at http://www.cdc.gov/mmwr/pdf/rr/rr5116.pdf (Level II)

3 World Health Organization. (2009). "WHO guidelines on hand hygiene in health care: First global patient safety challenge, clean care is safer care" [Online]. Accessed March 2015 via the Web at http://whqlibdoc.who.int/publications/2009/9789241597906_eng.pdf (Level IV)

4 Centers for Medicare & Medicaid Services, Department of Health and Human Services. (2014). Condition of participation: Infection control. 42 C.F.R. § 482.42.

5 American Osteopathic Association. (2014). Standard 07.01.21. *Healthcare Facilities Accreditation Program: Accreditation requirements for acute care hospitals.* Chicago, IL: American Osteopathic Association. (Level VII)

6 The Joint Commission. (2015). Standard NPSG.01.01.01. *Comprehensive accreditation manual for hospitals: The official handbook.* Oakbrook Terrace, IL: The Joint Commission. (Level VII)

7 American Osteopathic Association. (2014). Standard 15.01.16. *Healthcare Facilities Accreditation Program: Accreditation requirements for acute care hospitals.* Chicago, IL: American Osteopathic Association. (Level VII)

8 LeBlanc, K., et al. (2013). International skin tear advisory panel: A tool kit to aid in the prevention, assessment, and treatment of skin tears using a simplified classification system. *Advances in Skin and Wound Care, 26,* 459–476. (Level VII)

9 Siegel, J. D., et al. (2007). "2007 guideline for isolation precautions: Preventing transmission of infectious agents in healthcare settings" [Online]. Accessed March 2015 via the Web at http://www.cdc.gov/hicpac/pdf/isolation/Isolation2007.pdf (Level II)

10 American Osteopathic Association. (2014). Standard 07.01.10. *Healthcare Facilities Accreditation Program: Accreditation requirements for acute care hospitals.* Chicago, IL: American Osteopathic Association. (Level VII)

11 Institute for Clinical Systems Improvement. (2012). "Health care protocol: Pressure ulcer prevention and treatment protocol (3rd ed.)" [Online]. Accessed March 2015 via the Web at https://www.icsi.org/_asset/6t7kxy/ (Level V)
12 Wound, Ostomy and Continence Nurses Society. (2010). "Guideline for prevention and management of pressure ulcers" [Online]. Accessed March 2015 via the Web at http://guideline.gov/content.aspx?id=23868
13 The Joint Commission. (2015). Standard RC.01.03.01. *Comprehensive accreditation manual for hospitals: The official handbook.* Oakbrook Terrace, IL: The Joint Commission. (Level VII)
14 Centers for Medicare & Medicaid Services, Department of Health and Human Services. (2014). Condition of participation: Medical record services. 42 C.F.R. § 482.24(b).
15 American Osteopathic Association. (2014). Standard 10.00.03. *Healthcare Facilities Accreditation Program: Accreditation requirements for acute care hospitals.* Chicago, IL: American Osteopathic Association. (Level VII)
16 Evans, H. L., et al. (2010). Effect of chlorhexidine whole-body bathing on hospital-acquired infections among trauma patients. *Archives of Surgery, 145,* 240–246.
17 Dixon, J. M., & Carver, R. L. (2010). Daily chlorhexidine gluconate bathing with impregnated cloths results in statistically significant reduction in central line-associated bloodstream infections. *American Journal of Infection Control, 38,* 817–821.
18 Marschall, J., et al. (2014). SHEA/IDSA practice recommendation: Strategies to prevent central line-associated bloodstream infections in acute care hospitals. *Infection Control and Hospital Epidemiology, 35,* 753–771. Accessed March 2015 via the Web at http://www.jstor.org/stable/10.1086/676533 (Level I)
19 Rader, J., et al. (2006). The bathing of older adults with dementia. *American Journal of Nursing, 106*(4), 40–48.
20 Konno, R., et al. (2013). "The best evidence for assisted bathing of older people with dementia: A comprehensive systematic review" [Online]. Accessed March 2015 via the Web at http://www.joannabriggslibrary.org/jbilibrary/index.php/jbisrir/article/view/607 (Level I)

ADDITIONAL REFERENCES

Craven, R. F., & Hirnle, C. J. (2012). *Fundamentals of nursing: Human health and function* (7th ed.). Philadelphia, PA: Lippincott Williams & Wilkins.
Coyer, F. M., et al. (2011). The provision of patient personal hygiene in the intensive care unit: A descriptive exploratory study of bed-bathing practice. *Australian Critical Care, 24,* 198–209.
Lopes, J. L., et al. (2013). Bed and shower baths: Comparing the perceptions of patients with acute myocardial infarction. *Journal of Clinical Nursing, 22,* 733–740. (Level VI)
Popovich, K. J., et al. (2012). Relationship between chlorhexidine gluconate skin concentration and microbial density on the skin of critically ill patients bathed daily with chlorhexidine gluconate. *Infection Control and Hospital Epidemiology, 33,* 889–896.
Rupp, M. E., et al. (2012). Effect of hospital-wide chlorhexidine patient bathing on healthcare-associated infections. *Infection Control and Hospital Epidemiology, 33,* 1094–1100.
Spencer, C., et al. (2013). Daily bathing with octenidine on an intensive care unit is associated with a lower carriage rate of methicillin-resistant *Staphylococcus aureus. Journal of Hospital Infection, 83,* 156–159. (Level VI)

BED EQUIPMENT, SUPPLEMENTAL

Certain equipment can promote a bedridden patient's comfort and help prevent pressure ulcers and other complications of immobility. Although recommended, pressure distribution devices should serve as adjuncts to—not replacement for—repositioning protocols.[1] A wood or hard plastic footboard helps prevent footdrop by maintaining proper alignment. It also raises bed linens off of the patient's feet. The foot cradle, a horizontal or arched bar over the end of the bed, keeps bed linens off of the patient's feet, preventing skin irritation and breakdown, especially in patients with peripheral vascular disease or neuropathy. A bed board, made of wood or wood covered with canvas, firms the mattress and is especially useful for the patient with spinal injuries. The metal basic frame and the metal trapeze (a triangular piece attached to this frame) allow the patient with arm mobility and strength to lift himself off the bed, facilitating bed making and bedpan positioning.

A vinyl water mattress exerts less pressure on the skin than a standard hospital mattress, helping to prevent or treat pressure ulcers. An alternating pressure pad (a vinyl pad divided into chambers filled with air or water and attached to an electric pump) serves the same purpose, but it also stimulates circulation by alternately inflating and deflating its chambers.

A reusable water mattress replaces the standard hospital mattress and rests on a sheet of heavy cardboard placed over the bedsprings; the smaller, less bulky disposable mattress rests on top of the standard hospital mattress. All supplemental bed equipment is optional, depending on the patient's needs. (See *Types of supplemental bed equipment,* page 60.)

Equipment

Footboard and cover ▪ drawsheet ▪ bath blanket ▪ foot cradle ▪ bed board ▪ basic frame with trapeze ▪ roller gauze ▪ water mattress ▪ stretcher ▪ alternating pressure pad ▪ pump and tubing ▪ footstool ▪ fluid-impermeable pad ▪ sandbag, bath blanket, or pillow ▪ Optional: safety pins, laundry bag, sheepskin, cloth and mild soap, towel.

The exact equipment needed depends on what supplemental bed equipment is being added to the patient's bed.

Preparation of equipment

If you're preparing a footboard for use, place a cover over it *to provide padding.* Alternatively, pad it with a folded drawsheet or bath blanket by bringing the top and side edges of the sheet or blanket to the back of the footboard, mitering the corners, and securing them at the center with safety pins. *Padding cushions the patient's feet against pressure from the hard footboard, helping to prevent skin irritation and breakdown.* Avoid wrinkles *to prevent skin irritation.*

If you're preparing to use a portable water mattress, check with the maintenance department before transferring the mattress *because its weight may rule out use on some electric beds.*

Make sure that all supplemental bed equipment is compatible with the bed frame, mattress, and rails *to ensure safety and prevent injury.*[2]

Implementation

- Perform hand hygiene.[3,4,5,6,7]
- Confirm the patient's identity using at least two patient identifiers.[8]
- Tell the patient what you're going to do, and describe the equipment.

Using a footboard

- Move the patient up in bed *to allow room for the footboard.*
- Loosen the top linens at the foot of the bed, and then fold them back over the patient *to expose his feet.*
- Lift the mattress at the foot of the bed.
- Place the lip of the footboard between the mattress and the bedsprings, or secure the footboard under both sides of the mattress.
- Adjust the footboard so that the patient's feet rest comfortably against it. If the footboard isn't adjustable, tuck a folded bath blanket between the board and the patient's feet.
- Unless the footboard has side supports, place a sandbag, a folded bath blanket, or a pillow alongside each foot *to maintain 90-degree foot alignment.*
- Fold the top linens over the footboard, tuck them under the mattress, and miter the corners.

Using a foot cradle

- Move the patient up in bed *to allow room for the foot cradle.*

EQUIPMENT

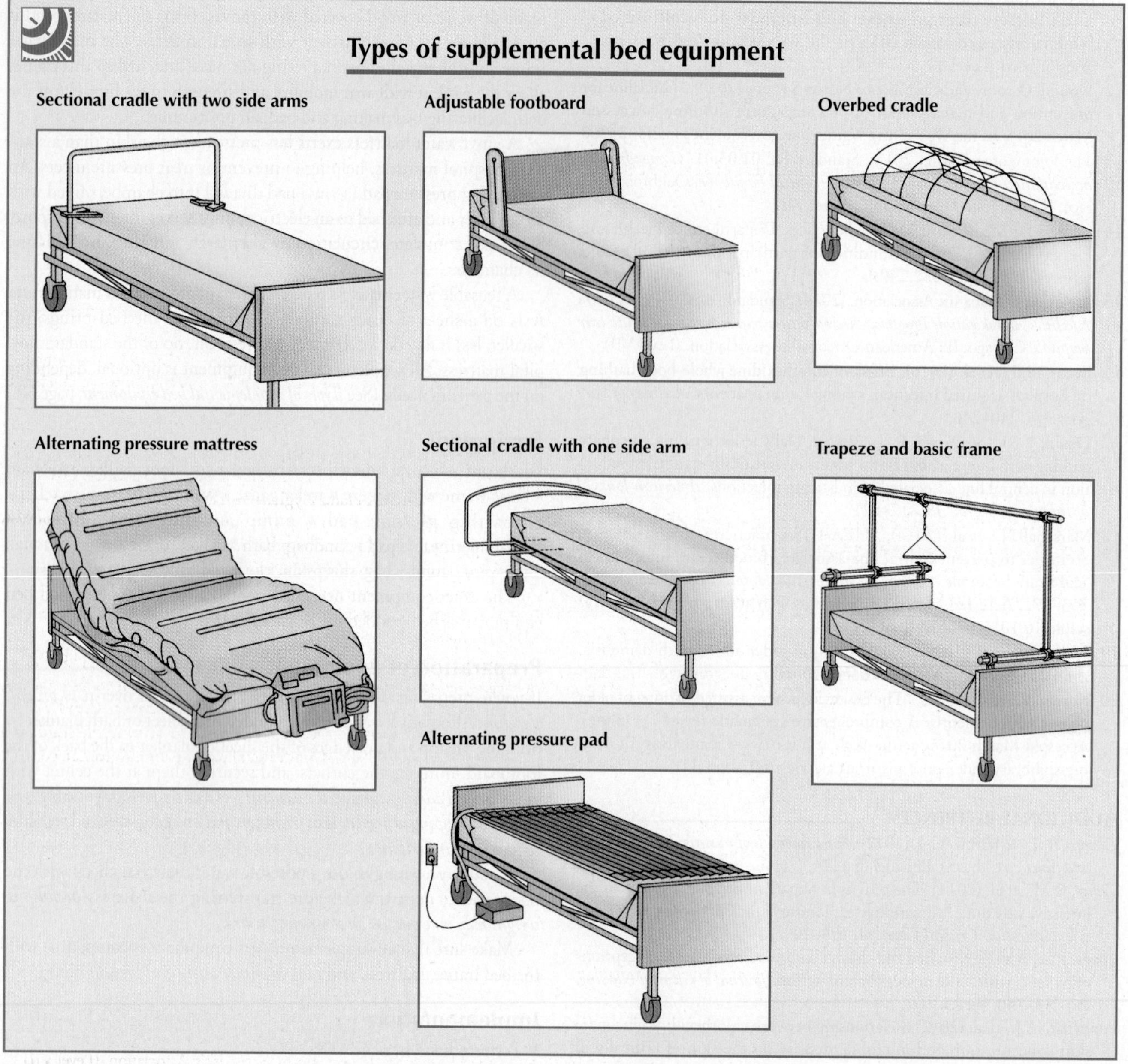

■ Loosen the top linens at the foot of the bed, and then fold them over the patient or to one side.
■ When using a one-piece cradle, place one side arm under the mattress, carefully extend the arch over the bed, and place the other side arm under the mattress on the opposite side. Adjust the tension rods *so that they rest securely over the edge of the mattress.*
■ When using a sectional cradle with two side arms, first place the side arms under the mattress. Secure the tension rods over the edge of the mattress. Then carefully place the arch over the bed and connect it to the side arms.
■ When using a sectional cradle with one side arm, connect the side arm and horizontal cradle bar before placement. Then place the side arm under the mattress on one side of the bed.
■ Cover the cradle with the top linens, tuck them under the mattress at the foot of the bed, and miter the corners.

Using a bed board

■ Transfer the patient from the bed to a stretcher or a chair. Obtain assistance if necessary.
■ Strip the linens from the bed. If you plan to reuse them, fold each piece neatly and hang it over the back of a chair. Otherwise, place soiled linens in a laundry bag.
■ If the bed board consists of wooden slats encased in canvas, lift the mattress at the head of the bed and center the board over the bedsprings *to prevent it from jutting out and causing accidental injury.* Unroll the slats to cover the bedsprings at the head of the bed. Then lift the mattress at the foot of the bed and unroll the remaining slats.
■ If the bed board consists of one solid or two hinged pieces of wood, lift the mattress on one side of the bed and center the board over the bedsprings.
■ After positioning the bed board, replace the linens.
■ Return the patient to bed.

Using a basic frame with trapeze

■ If an orthopedic technician isn't available to secure the frame and trapeze to the patient's bed, get assistance to attach these devices to the bed, as necessary. Hang the trapeze within the patient's easy reach *so he won't need to strain to reach it.*

Using a portable water mattress

- Ensure that the patient isn't prone to motion sickness *because the movement of the water in the mattress may cause nausea.*
- Obtain several coworkers to help transfer the mattress from the stretcher to the patient's bed *because the mattress is heavy and bulky.*
- Place a bottom sheet over the cover and tuck it in loosely.
- Place a sheepskin, fluid-impermeable pad, or drawsheet over the bottom sheet, as needed. Note that adding these items doesn't decrease the effectiveness of this mattress.
- Position the patient comfortably on the mattress
- Cover the patient with the top linens and tuck them in loosely.
- Check the water mattress daily *to ensure adequate flotation.* To do so, place your hand under the patient's thighs. If you can feel the bottom of the mattress, arrange to have water added.

Using an alternating pressure pad

- If possible, transfer the patient from the bed to a chair or stretcher. Get help, if necessary.
- Strip the linens from the bed.
- Inspect the plug and electrical cord of the alternating pressure pad for defects. Don't use the unit if it appears damaged.
- Unfold the pad on top of the mattress with the appropriate side facing up.
- Place the motor on a fluid-impermeable pad on the floor or on a footstool near the mattress outlets.
- Connect the tubing securely to the motor and to the mattress outlets.
- Plug the cord into an electrical outlet.
- Turn on the motor.
- After several minutes, observe the emptying and filling of the pad's chambers, and check the tubing for kinks *because they could interfere with the pad's function.*
- Place a bottom sheet over the pad and tuck it in loosely. *To avoid tube constriction,* don't miter the corner where the tubing is attached.
- Position the patient comfortably on the pad.
- Cover him with the top linens, and tuck them in loosely.
- If the pad becomes soiled, clean it with a damp cloth and mild soap, and then dry it well. *To avoid damaging the pad's surface,* don't use alcohol.
- When the patient no longer needs the pad or is discharged, turn off the motor, disconnect the tubing, and unplug the cord from the wall outlet. Remove the pad from the patient's bed, and fold and discard it. Inform the patient that the motor needed to power the pad can usually be rented from a surgical supply store. Explain to the patient or a caregiver how to operate the pad at home.
- Coil the tubing and electrical cord, and then strap them to the motor.
- Return the motor unit to the central supply department.

Completing the procedure

- Perform hand hygiene.[3,4,5,6,7]
- Document the procedure.[9,10,11]

Special considerations

- Place the patient in bed before positioning and securing an overbed or foot cradle *to ensure its proper placement and to prevent patient injury.* Similarly, remove the cradle before the patient gets out of bed. When turning or positioning the patient on his side, make sure the foot cradle's tension rod doesn't rest against his skin *because this may cause pressure and predispose him to skin breakdown.*
- Exercise caution when turning an obese patient on a water mattress *because turning displaces a large volume of water.* Keep the side rails raised during turning *to prevent falls.*
- Avoid placing excessive layers of drawsheets or fluid-impermeable pads between the alternating pressure pad and the patient *because these decrease the pad's effectiveness.* Avoid using pins and other sharp instruments near an alternating pressure pad or water mattress *to prevent accidental puncture.*

NURSING ALERT Because a plastic-covered mattress slides off a bed board easily, *make sure a coworker is standing on the opposite side of the bed when you're transferring the patient from stretcher to bed.*

Documentation

Record the type of supplemental bed equipment used, the time and date of use, and the patient's response to treatment.

REFERENCES

1 Wound, Ostomy and Continence Nurses Society (WOCN). (2010). *Guideline for prevention and management of pressure ulcers (WOCN clinical practice guideline no. 2).* Mount Laurel, NJ: WOCN. Accessed March 2015 via the Web at http://guideline.gov/content.aspx?id=23868 (Level I)

2 Todd, J. F. (2008). Waking up to hospital bed entrapment risks. *Nursing, 38*(1), 14–15.

3 The Joint Commission. (2015). Standard NPSG.07.01.01. *Comprehensive accreditation manual for hospitals: The official handbook.* Oakbrook Terrace, IL: The Joint Commission. (Level VII)

4 Centers for Disease Control and Prevention. (2002). Guideline for hand hygiene in health-care settings: Recommendations of the Healthcare Infection Control Practices Advisory Committee and the HICPAC/SHEA/APIC/IDSA Hand Hygiene Task Force. *MMWR Recommendations and Reports, 51*(RR-16), 1–45. Accessed March 2015 via the Web at http://www.cdc.gov/mmwr/pdf/rr/rr5116.pdf (Level II)

5 World Health Organization. (2009). "WHO guidelines on hand hygiene in health care: First global patient safety challenge, clean care is safer care" [Online]. Accessed March 2015 via the Web at http://whqlibdoc.who.int/publications/2009/9789241597906_eng.pdf (Level IV)

6 American Osteopathic Association. (2014). Standard 07.01.21. *Healthcare Facilities Accreditation Program: Accreditation requirements for acute care hospitals.* Chicago, IL: American Osteopathic Association. (Level VII)

7 Centers for Medicare & Medicaid Services, Department of Health and Human Services. (2014). Condition of participation: Infection control. 42 C.F.R. § 482.42.

8 The Joint Commission. (2015). Standard NPSG.01.01.01. *Comprehensive accreditation manual for hospitals: The official handbook.* Oakbrook Terrace, IL: The Joint Commission. (Level VII)

9 The Joint Commission. (2015). Standard RC.01.03.01. *Comprehensive accreditation manual for hospitals: The official handbook.* Oakbrook Terrace, IL: The Joint Commission. (Level VII)

10 Centers for Medicare & Medicaid Services, Department of Health and Human Services. (2014). Condition of participation: Medical record services. 42 C.F.R. § 482.24(b).

11 American Osteopathic Association. (2014). Standard 10.00.03. *Healthcare Facilities Accreditation Program: Accreditation requirements for acute care hospitals.* Chicago, IL: American Osteopathic Association. (Level VII)

ADDITIONAL REFERENCES

Craven, R. F., & Hirnle, C. J. (2012). *Fundamentals of nursing: Human health and function* (7th ed.). Philadelphia, PA: Lippincott Williams & Wilkins.

Taylor, C. R., et al. (2011). *Fundamentals of nursing: The art and science of nursing care* (7th ed.). Philadelphia, PA: Lippincott Williams & Wilkins.

BEDMAKING, OCCUPIED

For a bedridden patient, linen changes promote comfort and help prevent skin breakdown and health care–associated infection. Such changes require the use of side rails to prevent the patient from rolling out of bed and, depending on the patient's condition, the use of a turning sheet to move him from side to side.

Making an occupied bed may require more than one person. It also entails loosening the bottom sheet on one side and fanfolding it to the center of the mattress instead of loosening the bottom sheet on both sides and removing it, as in an unoccupied bed. Also, the foundation of the bed must be made before the top sheet is applied instead of both the

Making a traction bed

For a patient in traction, obtain help from a coworker to make the bed. Work from head to toe *to minimize the risk of traction misalignment.*

Preparation

■ Perform hand hygiene and follow standard precautions.[1,2,3,4,5]
■ Bring clean linens and arrange them in the order of use on the bedside stand or a chair.
■ Explain the procedure, provide privacy, and remove unnecessary furniture.

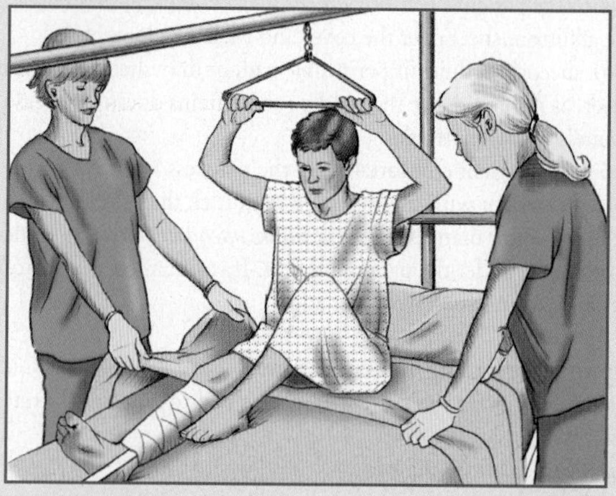

Changing the linens

■ Lower both side rails.
■ Stand near the headboard, opposite your coworker.
■ Gently pull the mattress to the head of the bed. Avoid sudden movements; *they can misalign traction and cause patient discomfort.*
■ Remove the pillow from the bed.
■ Loosen the bottom linens and roll them from the headboard toward the patient's head.
■ Remove the soiled pillowcase and replace it with a clean one.
■ Fold a clean bottom sheet crosswise and place the sheet across the head of the bed. Tell the patient to raise her head and upper shoulders by grasping the trapeze above the bed. With your coworker, quickly fanfold the bottom sheet from the head of the bed under the patient's shoulders so that it meets the soiled linen. Tuck at least 12″ (30.5 cm) of the bottom sheet under the head of the mattress. Miter the corners and tuck in the sides.
■ Tell the patient to raise her buttocks by grasping the trapeze (as shown on top right). As a team, move toward the foot of the bed and, in one movement, quickly and carefully roll soiled linens and clean linens under the patient.
■ Instruct the patient to release the trapeze and to rest. Place a pillow under her head for comfort.
■ If allowed, remove any pillows from under the patient's extremity. If pillow removal is contraindicated, continue to move linens toward the foot of the bed and under the patient's legs and traction while your coworker lifts the pillows and supports the patient's extremity.
■ Put soiled linens in a laundry bag or pillowcase.
■ Tuck the remaining loose linens securely under the mattress. *To ensure a tight-fitting bottom sheet,* have the patient raise herself off the bed by simultaneously grasping the trapeze and raising her buttocks while you pull the sheet tight. As needed, place a drawsheet or fluid-impermeable pad under her. Complete the bed making alone.
■ If the bottom sheet doesn't cover the foot of the mattress, cover it with a drawsheet. Miter its corners and tuck in the sides.
■ Replace the pillows under the patient's extremity, and then cover her with a clean top sheet. Fold over the top hem of the sheet approximately 8″ (20.5 cm). If one or both legs are in traction, fit the lower end of the sheet loosely over the traction apparatus; don't press on the traction ropes. To secure the sheet, tuck in the corner opposite the traction under the foot of the bed and miter the corner. Neatly tuck in the lower corner of the sheet on the traction side to expose the leg and foot.
■ If the traction equipment exposes the patient's sides, cover her with a drawsheet—not a full sheet or spread.
■ Lower the bed, but don't allow the traction weights to touch the floor. Raise the side rails to prevent falls. If allowed, leave one side rail down so the patient can reach the bedside stand.
■ Remove and discard your gloves, if worn.
■ Perform hand hygiene.[1,2,3]

foundation and top being made on one side before being completed on the other side. (See *Making a traction bed.*)

Equipment

Two sheets (one fitted, if available) ■ pillowcase ■ one or two drawsheets ■ spread ■ one or two bath blankets ■ laundry bag ■ Optional: comfort-enhancing device, fluid-impermeable pad, gloves, other personal protective equipment.

Preparation of equipment

Obtain clean linens, which should be folded in half lengthwise and then folded again. If the linens are folded incorrectly, refold them. The bottom sheet should be folded so the rough side of the hem is facedown when placed on the bed; *this helps prevent skin irritation caused by the rough hem edge rubbing against the patient's heels.* The top sheet should be folded similarly, so that the smooth side of the hem is face up when folded over the spread, giving the bed a finished appearance.

Implementation

■ Gather and prepare the equipment in the patient's room.
■ Perform hand hygiene and put on personal protective equipment as needed *to comply with standard precautions.*[1,2,3,4,5,6,7]
■ Confirm the patient's identity using at least two patient identifiers.[8]
■ Tell the patient you will be changing his bed linens. Explain how he can help if he's able, adjusting the plan according to his abilities and needs.
■ Provide privacy.[9]
■ Move furniture away from the bed *to ensure ample working space.*
■ Raise the side rail on the far side of the bed *to prevent falls.*
■ Adjust the bed to a comfortable working height *to prevent back strain.*
■ If permitted, lower the head of the bed *to ensure tight-fitting, wrinkle-free linens.*
■ When stripping the bed, watch for belongings among the linens.
■ Cover the patient with a bath blanket *to avoid exposure and provide warmth and privacy.*
■ Fanfold the top sheet and spread from beneath the bath blanket, and then bring them back over the blanket.
■ Loosen the top linens at the foot of the bed and remove them separately. If reusing the top linens, fold each piece and hang each piece over the back of the chair. Otherwise, place each piece in a laundry bag. *To avoid dispersing microorganisms,* don't fan the linens, hold them against your clothing, or place them on the floor.

■ If the mattress slid down when the head of the bed was raised, elicit the help of a coworker to pull it up again. *Adjusting the mattress after the bed is made loosens the linens.*
■ Roll the patient to the far side of the bed, and turn the pillow lengthwise under his head *to support his neck.* Ask him to help (if he can) by grasping the far side rail as he turns *so that he's positioned at the far side of the bed.*
■ Loosen the soiled bottom linens on the side of the bed nearest you. Then roll the linens toward the patient's back in the middle of the bed (as shown below).

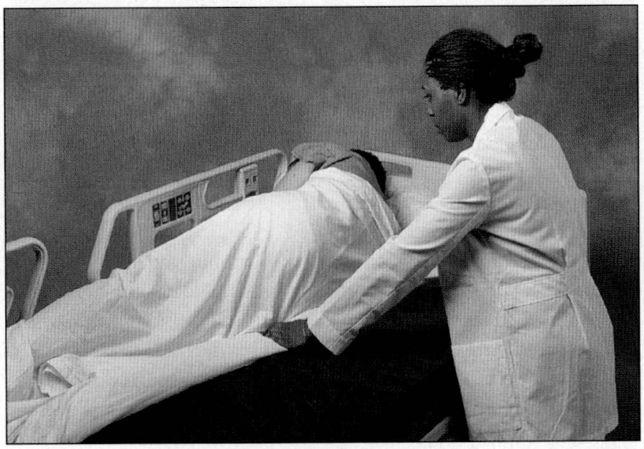

■ Place a clean bottom sheet on the bed, with its center fold in the middle of the mattress. For a fitted sheet, secure the top and bottom corners over the side of the mattress nearest you. For a flat sheet, place its end even with the foot of the mattress. Miter the top corner as you would for an unoccupied bed *to keep linens firmly tucked under the mattress, preventing wrinkling.*
■ Fanfold the remaining clean bottom sheet toward the patient, and place the drawsheet, if needed, about 15″ (38 cm) from the top of the bed, with its center fold in the middle of the mattress. Tuck in the entire edge of the drawsheet on the side nearest you. Fanfold the remaining drawsheet toward the patient (as shown below).

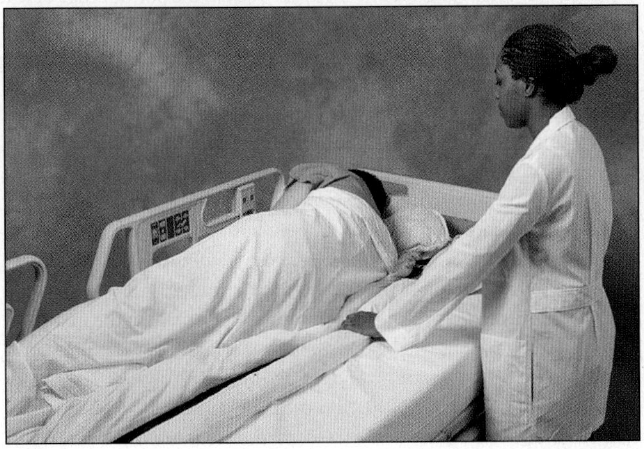

■ If necessary, position a fluid-impermeable pad on the drawsheet *to absorb excretions or surgical drainage,* and fanfold it toward the patient.
■ Raise the other side rail, and roll the patient to the clean side of the bed.
■ Move to the unfinished side of the bed and lower the side rail nearest you. Then loosen and remove the soiled bottom linens separately and place them in the laundry bag.
■ Pull the clean bottom sheet taut. Secure the fitted sheet or place the end of a flat sheet even with the foot of the bed, and miter the top corner. Pull the drawsheet taut and tuck it in. Unfold and smooth the fluid-impermeable pad, if used.
■ Assist the patient to the supine position if his condition permits.
■ Remove the soiled pillowcase, and place it in the laundry bag. Then slip the pillow into a clean pillowcase, tucking its corners well into the case *to ensure a smooth fit.* Place the pillow beneath the patient's head, with its seam toward the top of the bed *to prevent it from rubbing against the patient's neck, causing irritation.* Place the pillow's open edge away from the door *to give the bed a finished appearance.*
■ Unfold the clean top sheet over the patient with the rough side of the hem facing away from the bed *to avoid irritating the patient's skin.* Allow enough sheet to form a cuff over the spread.
■ Remove the bath blanket from beneath the sheet, and center the spread over the top sheet.
■ Tuck the top sheet and spread under the foot of the bed, and miter the bottom corners. Fold the top sheet over the spread *to give the bed a finished appearance.*
■ Make a 3″ (7.5-cm) toe pleat, or vertical tuck, in the top linens *to allow room for the patient's feet and to prevent pressure that can cause discomfort, skin breakdown, and footdrop.*
■ Raise the head of the bed to a comfortable position, make sure both side rails are raised, and then lower the bed and lock its wheels *to ensure the patient's safety.* Assess the patient's body alignment.
■ Place the call light within the patient's easy reach.
■ Remove the laundry bag from the room.
■ Remove and discard your gloves and any other personal protective equipment worn.
■ Perform hand hygiene *to prevent the spread of health care–associated infections.*[1,2,4,3,5,6]
■ Document the procedure, as applicable.[10,11,12]

Special considerations

■ Use a fitted sheet when available *because a flat sheet can slip out from under the mattress easily, especially if the mattress is plastic-coated.*
■ *To prevent the patient from sliding down in bed,* tuck a tightly rolled pillow under the top linens at the foot of the bed.
■ For a patient who is diaphoretic or bedridden, fold a bath blanket in half lengthwise and place it between the bottom sheet and the plastic mattress cover; *the blanket acts as a cushion and helps absorb moisture. To help prevent sheet burns on the heels and bony prominences,* center a bath blanket or sheepskin over the bottom sheet and tuck the blanket under the mattress.
■ If the patient can't help you move or turn him, devise a turning sheet *to facilitate bed making and repositioning.* To do this, first fold a drawsheet or bath blanket and place it under the patient's buttocks. Make sure the sheet extends from the shoulders to the knees *so that it supports most of the patient's weight.* Roll the sides of the sheet to form handles. Next, ask a coworker to help you lift and move the patient. With one person holding each side of the sheet, you can move the patient without wrinkling the bottom linens. If you can't get help and must turn the patient yourself, stand at the side of the bed. Turn the patient toward the rail and, if he's able, ask him to grasp the opposite rolled edge of the turning sheet. Pull the rolled edge carefully toward you and turn the patient.

Documentation

Although linen changes aren't usually documented, record the dates and times of linen changes in your notes for patients with incontinence, excessive wound drainage, pressure ulcers, or diaphoresis.

REFERENCES

1 The Joint Commission. (2015). Standard NPSG.07.01.01. *Comprehensive accreditation manual for hospitals: The official handbook.* Oakbrook Terrace, IL: The Joint Commission. (Level VII)
2 Centers for Disease Control and Prevention. (2002). Guideline for hand hygiene in health-care settings: Recommendations of the Healthcare

Infection Control Practices Advisory Committee and the HICPAC/SHEA/APIC/IDSA Hand Hygiene Task Force. *MMWR Recommendations and Reports, 51*(RR-16), 1–45. Accessed March 2015 via the Web at http://www.cdc.gov/mmwr/pdf/rr/rr5116.pdf (Level II)

3 World Health Organization. (2009). "WHO guidelines on hand hygiene in health care: First global patient safety challenge, clean care is safer care" [Online]. Accessed March 2015 via the Web at http://whqlibdoc.who.int/publications/2009/9789241597906_eng.pdf (Level IV)

4 Siegel, J. D., et al. (2007). "2007 guideline for isolation precautions: Preventing transmission of infectious agents in healthcare settings" [Online]. Accessed March 2015 via the Web at http://www.cdc.gov/hicpac/pdf/isolation/Isolation2007.pdf (Level II)

5 Centers for Medicare & Medicaid Services, Department of Health and Human Services. (2014). Condition of participation: Infection control. 42 C.F.R. § 482.42.

6 American Osteopathic Association. (2014). Standard 07.01.21. *Healthcare Facilities Accreditation Program: Accreditation requirements for acute care hospitals.* Chicago, IL: American Osteopathic Association. (Level VII)

7 American Osteopathic Association. (2014). Standard 07.01.10. *Healthcare Facilities Accreditation Program: Accreditation requirements for acute care hospitals.* Chicago, IL: American Osteopathic Association. (Level VII)

8 The Joint Commission. (2015). Standard NPSG.01.01.01. *Comprehensive accreditation manual for hospitals: The official handbook.* Oakbrook Terrace, IL: The Joint Commission. (Level VII)

9 American Osteopathic Association. (2014). Standard 15.01.16. *Healthcare Facilities Accreditation Program: Accreditation requirements for acute care hospitals.* Chicago, IL: American Osteopathic Association. (Level VII)

10 The Joint Commission. (2015). Standard RC.01.03.01. *Comprehensive accreditation manual for hospitals: The official handbook.* Oakbrook Terrace, IL: The Joint Commission. (Level VII)

11 Centers for Medicare & Medicaid Services, Department of Health and Human Services. (2014). Condition of participation: Medical record services. 42 C.F.R. § 482.24(b).

12 American Osteopathic Association. (2014). Standard 10.00.03. *Healthcare Facilities Accreditation Program: Accreditation requirements for acute care hospitals.* Chicago, IL: American Osteopathic Association. (Level VII)

ADDITIONAL REFERENCES

Bloomfield, J., et al. (2008). Recommended procedure for bedmaking in hospital. *Nursing Standard, 22*(23), 41–44.

Craven, R. F., & Hirnle, C. J. (2012). *Fundamentals of nursing: Human health and function* (7th ed.). Philadelphia, PA: Lippincott Williams & Wilkins.

Taylor, C., et al. (2011). *Fundamentals of nursing: The art and science of nursing care* (7th ed.). Philadelphia, PA: Lippincott Williams & Wilkins.

BEDMAKING, UNOCCUPIED

Although considered routine, daily changing and periodic straightening of bed linens promotes patient comfort and prevents skin breakdown. When preceded by hand hygiene, performed using clean technique, and followed by proper handling and disposal of soiled linens, this procedure helps control health care–associated infections.

Equipment

Two sheets (one fitted, if available) ▪ pillowcase ▪ bedspread ▪ laundry bag ▪ Optional: gloves, other personal protective equipment, fluid-impermeable pads, drawsheet.

Preparation of equipment

Obtain clean linens, which should be folded in half lengthwise and then folded again. If the linens are folded incorrectly, refold them. The bottom sheet should be folded so the rough side of the hem is facedown when placed on the bed; *this helps prevent skin irritation caused by the rough hem edge rubbing against the patient's heels.* The top sheet should be folded similarly, so that the smooth side of the hem is face up when folded over the spread, giving the bed a finished appearance.

Implementation

- Gather and prepare the equipment.
- Perform hand hygiene, bring clean linen to the bedside, and put on gloves and other personal protective equipment as needed *to comply with standard precautions.*[1,2,3,4,5,6,7]
- Confirm the patient's identity using at least two patient identifiers.[8]
- Tell the patient that you're going to change his bed. Help him to a chair if necessary.
- Move furniture away from the bed *to provide ample working space.*
- Lower the head of the bed and side rails *to make the mattress level and ensure tight-fitting, wrinkle-free linens.*
- Raise the bed to a comfortable working height *to prevent back strain.*
- When stripping the bed, watch for any belongings that may have fallen among the linens.
- Remove the pillowcase and place it in the laundry bag or in the middle of the bed. Set the pillow aside.
- Lift the mattress edge slightly and work around the bed, untucking the linens. If you plan to reuse the top linens, fold the top hem of the spread down to the bottom hem. Then pick up the hemmed corners, fold the spread into quarters, and hang it over the back of the chair. Do the same for the top sheet. Otherwise, carefully remove and place the top linens in the laundry bag or pillowcase. *To avoid spreading microorganisms,* don't fan the linens, hold them against your clothing, or place them on the floor.
- Remove the soiled bottom linens and place them in the laundry bag.
- If the mattress has slid downward, push it to the head of the bed. *Adjusting it after bed making loosens the linens.*
- Place the bottom sheet with its center fold in the middle of the mattress.
- For a fitted sheet, secure the top and bottom corners over the mattress corners on the side of the bed nearest you. For a flat sheet, align the end of the sheet with the foot of the mattress and miter the top corner *to keep the sheet firmly tucked under the mattress.* To miter the corner, first tuck the top end of the sheet evenly under the mattress at the head of the bed. Then lift the side edge of the sheet about 12″ (30.5 cm) from the mattress corner and hold it at a right angle to the mattress. Tuck in the bottom edge of the sheet hanging below the mattress. Finally, drop the top edge and tuck it under the mattress. (See *Making a mitered corner.*)
- After tucking under one side of the bottom sheet, place the drawsheet or fluid-impermeable pad (if either are needed) about 15″ (38 cm) from the top of the bed, with its center fold in the middle of the bed. Then tuck in the entire edge of the drawsheet on that side of the bed.
- Place the top sheet with its center fold in the middle of the bed and its wide hem even with the top of the bed. Position the rough side of the hem face up *so that the smooth side shows after folding.* Allow enough sheet at the top of the bed to form a cuff over the spread.
- Place the spread over the top sheet, with its center fold in the middle of the bed. (If the patient will be returning from surgery, use the alternative technique. [See *Making a surgical bed,* page 66.])
- Make a 3″ (7.6-cm) toe pleat, or vertical tuck, in the top linens *to allow room for the patient's feet and to prevent pressure that can cause discomfort, skin breakdown, and footdrop.*
- Tuck the top sheet and spread under the foot of the mattress. Then miter the bottom corners.
- Move to the opposite side of the bed and repeat the procedure.
- After fitting all corners of the bottom sheet or tucking them under the mattress, pull the sheet at an angle from the head toward the foot of the bed. *Doing so tightens the linens, making the bottom sheet taut and wrinkle-free and promoting patient comfort.*

Making a mitered corner

■ To make a mitered corner, after placing the sheet on the bed, grasp the side edge of the sheet and lift it up to form a triangle.

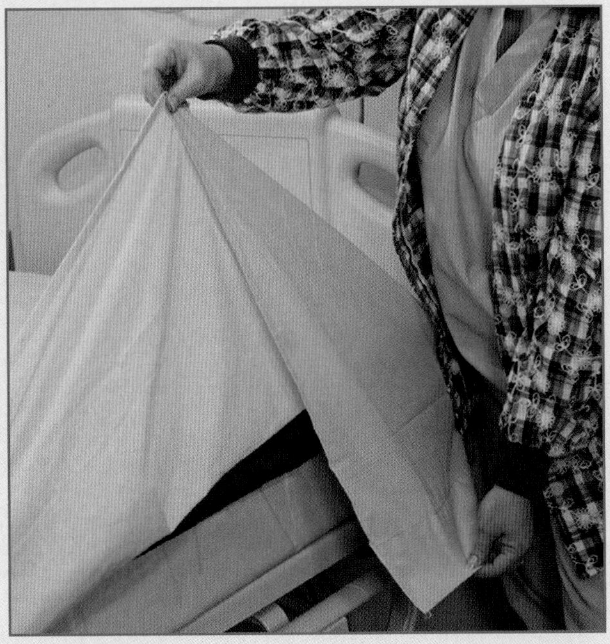

■ Then, place the sheet on the top of the bed, making a flat triangular fold.

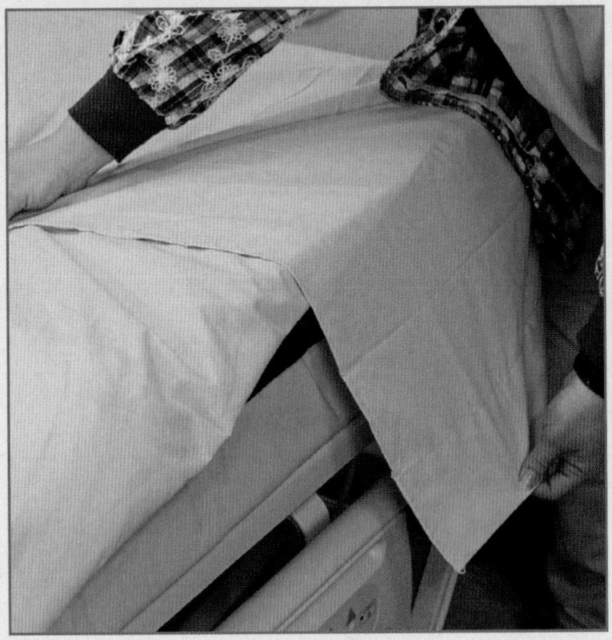

■ While holding the point of the triangle on the bed, tuck the sheet under the mattress.

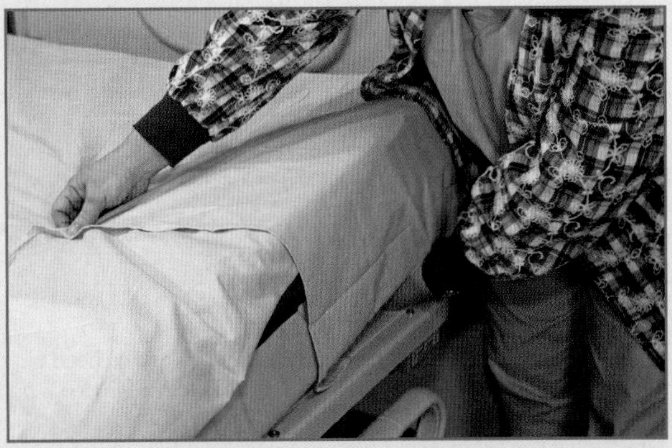

■ Take the triangular fold from the mattress and place it over the side of the mattress.

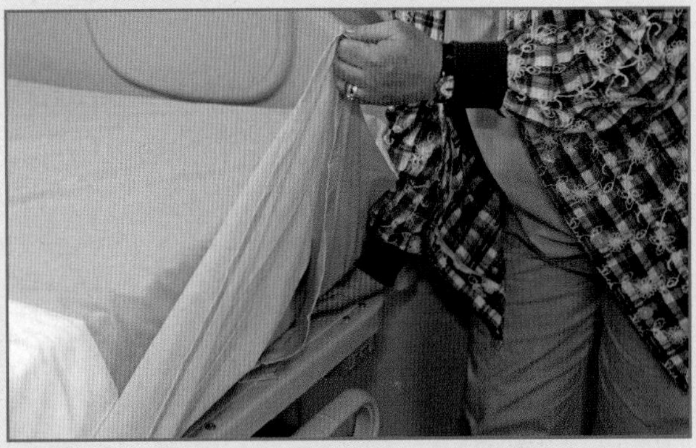

■ Tuck the remaining end of the triangular linen fold under the mattress.

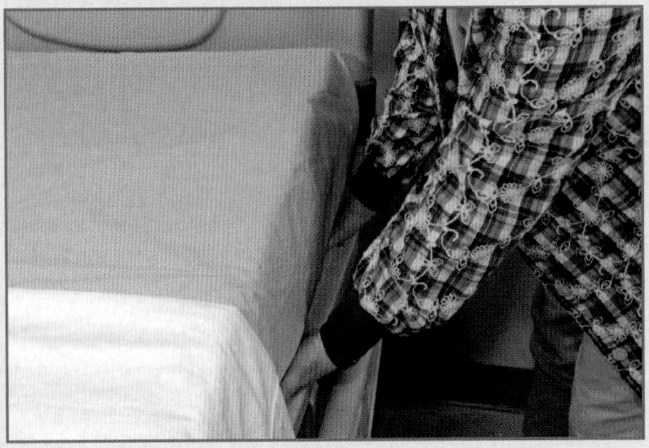

■ Fold the top sheet over the spread at the head of the bed *to form a cuff and to give the bed a finished appearance.* When making an open bed, fanfold the top linens to the foot of the bed. If a fluid-impermeable pad is needed, place it on top of the bottom sheets.

■ Slip the pillow into a clean case, tucking in the corners. Then place the pillow with its seam toward the top of the bed *to prevent it from rubbing against the patient's neck, causing irritation,* and its open edge facing away from the door *to give the bed a finished appearance.*

■ Lower the bed and lock its wheels *to ensure the patient's safety.*

■ Return furniture to its proper place.

■ Place the call light within the patient's easy reach.

■ Carry away soiled linens with outstretched arms *to avoid contaminating your uniform.*

■ After disposing of the linens, remove and discard your gloves and any other personal protective equipment worn.

Making a surgical bed

Preparation of a surgical bed permits easy patient transfer from surgery and promotes cleanliness and comfort. To make such a bed, take the following steps:

- Perform hand hygiene, bring clean linen to the bedside, and put on gloves, if needed.[1,2,3,5,6]
- Assemble linens as you would for making an unoccupied bed, including two clean sheets (one fitted, if available), a drawsheet, a bath blanket, a spread or sheet, a pillowcase, facial tissues, a trash bag, and fluid-impermeable pads. Raise the bed to a comfortable working height *to prevent back strain.*
- Slip the pillow into a clean pillowcase and place it on a nearby table or chair.
- Make the foundation of the bed using the bottom sheet and drawsheet.
- Place an open bath blanket about 15″ (38 cm) from the head of the bed with its center fold positioned in the middle of the bed. *The blanket warms the patient and counteracts the decreased body temperature caused by anesthesia.*
- Place a top sheet or spread on the bath blanket, and position it as you did the blanket. Then fold the blanket and sheet back from the top so that the blanket shows over the sheet. Similarly, fold the sheet and blanket up from the bottom (as shown in illustration 1).

1.

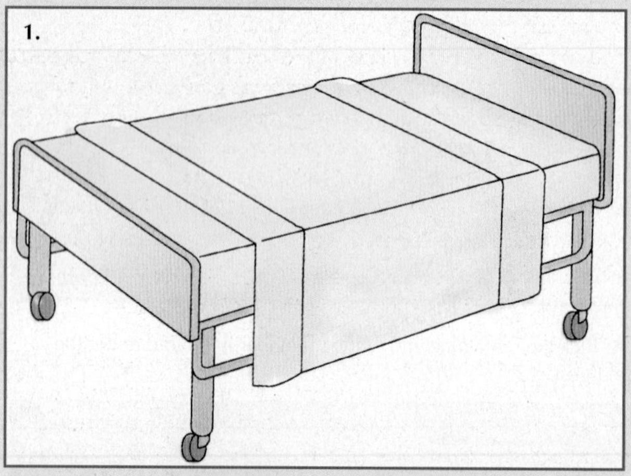

- On the side of the bed where you'll receive the patient, fold up the two outer corners of the sheet and blanket so they meet in the middle of the bed (as shown in illustration 2).
- Pick up the point hanging over this side of the bed and fanfold the linens back to the other side of the bed *so the linens won't interfere with patient transfer* (as shown in illustration 3).
- Raise the bed to the high position if you haven't already done so. Then lock the wheels and lower the side rails. Make sure the side rails work properly. Move the bedside stand and other objects out of the stretcher's path *to facilitate easy transfer when the patient arrives.*

2.

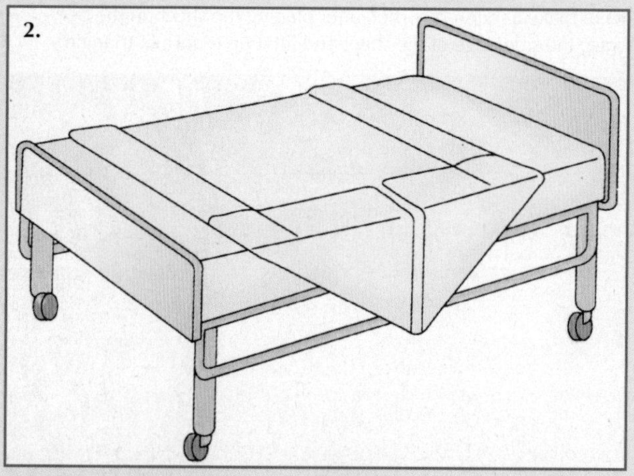

- After the patient is transferred to the bed, position the pillow for his comfort and safety. Cover him by pulling the top point of the sheet and blanket over him and opening the folds. After covering the patient, tuck in the linens at the foot of the bed and miter the corners.
- *To make the patient comfortable and to prevent unnecessary movement and linen changes,* try to anticipate and be ready for his special needs. For nausea, keep an emesis basin, facial tissues, and fluid-impermeable pads at the bedside. Also, remove all liquids from the bedside. If you expect bleeding or discharge, place one or more fluid-impermeable pads on the bed.
- Keep extra pillows handy *to elevate arms and legs and to promote circulation, thereby preventing edema.* If necessary, have IV equipment, suction apparatus, a roller for patient transfer, or other special equipment ready.

3.

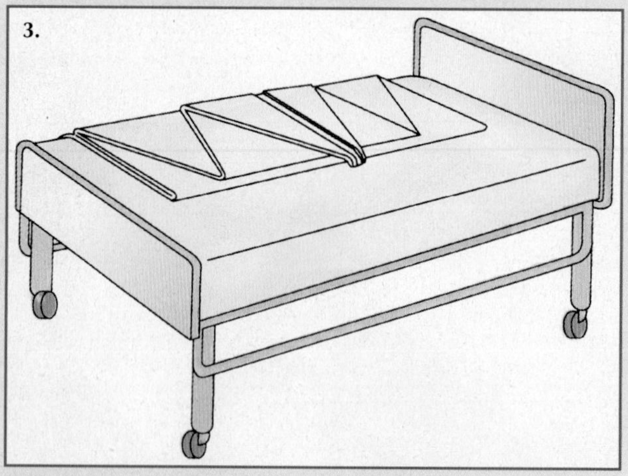

- Perform hand hygiene *to prevent the spread of microorganisms.*[1,2,3,5,6]
- Document the procedure as applicable.[9,10,11]

Special considerations

- Because a hospital mattress is usually covered with plastic *to protect it and to facilitate cleaning between patients,* a flat-bottom sheet tends to loosen and become untucked. Use a fitted sheet, if available.
- If a fitted sheet isn't available, consider tying the top corners of a flat sheet together under the top of the mattress *to prevent the sheet from becoming dislodged.*
- Place a bath blanket on top of the mattress, under the bottom sheet, helps *to absorb moisture and prevent dislodgment of the bottom sheet.*

Documentation

Although linen changes aren't usually documented, record their dates and times in your notes for patients with incontinence, excessive wound drainage, or diaphoresis.

REFERENCES

1 The Joint Commission. (2015). Standard NPSG.07.01.01. *Comprehensive accreditation manual for hospitals: The official handbook.* Oakbrook Terrace, IL: The Joint Commission. (Level VII)

2 Centers for Disease Control and Prevention. (2002). Guideline for hand hygiene in health-care settings: Recommendations of the Healthcare Infection Control Practices Advisory Committee and the HICPAC/SHEA/APIC/IDSA Hand Hygiene Task Force. *MMWR Recommendations and Reports, 51*(RR-16), 1–45. Accessed March 2015 via the Web athttp://www.cdc.gov/mmwr/pdf/rr/rr5116.pdf (Level II)

3 World Health Organization. (2009). "WHO guidelines on hand hygiene in health care: First global patient safety challenge, clean care is safer care" [Online]. Accessed March 2015 via the Web at http://whqlibdoc.who.int/publications/2009/9789241597906_eng.pdf (Level IV)

4 Siegel, J. D., et al. (2007). "2007 guideline for isolation precautions: Preventing transmission of infectious agents in healthcare settings" [Online]. Accessed March 2015 via the Web at http://www.cdc.gov/hicpac/pdf/isolation/Isolation2007.pdf (Level II)

5 Centers for Medicare & Medicaid Services, Department of Health and Human Services. (2014). Condition of participation: Infection control. 42 C.F.R. § 482.42.

6 American Osteopathic Association. (2014). Standard 07.01.21. *Healthcare Facilities Accreditation Program: Accreditation requirements for acute care hospitals.* Chicago, IL: American Osteopathic Association. (Level VII)

7 American Osteopathic Association. (2014). Standard 07.01.10. *Healthcare Facilities Accreditation Program: Accreditation requirements for acute care hospitals.* Chicago, IL: American Osteopathic Association. (Level VII)

8 The Joint Commission. (2015). Standard NPSG.01.01.01. *Comprehensive accreditation manual for hospitals: The official handbook.* Oakbrook Terrace, IL: The Joint Commission. (Level VII)

9 The Joint Commission. (2015). Standard RC.01.03.01. *Comprehensive accreditation manual for hospitals: The official handbook.* Oakbrook Terrace, IL: The Joint Commission. (Level VII)

10 Centers for Medicare & Medicaid Services, Department of Health and Human Services. (2014). Condition of participation: Medical record services. 42 C.F.R. § 482.24(b).

11 American Osteopathic Association. (2014). Standard 10.00.03. *Healthcare Facilities Accreditation Program: Accreditation requirements for acute care hospitals.* Chicago, IL: American Osteopathic Association. (Level VII)

ADDITIONAL REFERENCES

Bloomfield, J., et al. (2008). Recommended procedure for bedmaking in hospital. *Nursing Standard, 22*(23), 41–44.

Craven, R. F., & Hirnle, C. J. (2012). *Fundamentals of nursing: Human health and function* (7th ed.). Philadelphia, PA: Lippincott Williams & Wilkins.

Taylor, C., et al. (2011). *Fundamentals of nursing: The art and science of nursing care* (7th ed.). Philadelphia, PA: Lippincott Williams & Wilkins.

BEDPAN AND URINAL USE

Bedpans and urinals permit bedridden patients to eliminate and allow you to observe and measure their urine and stool accurately. Female patients use bedpans for defecation and urination; male patients use bedpans for defecation and urinals for urination. Either device should be offered frequently—before meals, visiting hours, morning and evening care, and treatments or procedures. Whenever possible, allow the patient privacy.

Equipment

Bedpan (either regular bedpan or fracture pan) or urinal with cover ■ toilet tissue ■ two washcloths ■ soap and water ■ two pairs of gloves ■ towel ■ fluid-impermeable pad ■ hospital-grade disinfectant ■ Optional: air freshener, cleaning wipes, bath blanket, small pillow.

Available in adult and pediatric sizes, a bedpan may be disposable or reusable (the latter can be sterilized). A fracture pan, a type of bedpan, is used when spinal injuries, body or leg casts, or other conditions prohibit or restrict turning the patient. Like a bedpan, the urinal may be disposable or reusable.

Preparation of equipment

Obtain the appropriate bedpan or urinal. For a thin patient, place a fluid-impermeable pad at the edge of the bedpan or use a fracture pan *to minimize pressure on the coccyx.*

Implementation

- Gather and prepare the equipment.
- Perform hand hygiene and put on gloves *to prevent contact with body fluids and to comply with standard precautions.*[1,2,3,4,5,6,7]
- Confirm the patient's identity using at least two patient identifiers.[8]
- Provide privacy.[9]
- Explain the procedure to the patient.

Placing a bedpan

- If allowed, elevate the head of the bed slightly *to prevent hyperextension of the spine when the patient raises the buttocks.*
- Rest the bedpan on the edge of the bed. Then, turn down the corner of the top linens and draw up the patient's gown. Ask him to raise his buttocks by flexing his knees and pushing down on his heels. While supporting the patient's lower back with one hand, center the curved, smooth edge of the bedpan beneath his buttocks.
- If the patient can't raise his buttocks, lower the head of the bed to horizontal and help the patient roll onto one side, with his buttocks toward you. Position the bedpan properly against his buttocks, and then help the patient roll back onto the bedpan. Once the patient is positioned comfortably, raise the head of the bed as indicated.
- After positioning the bedpan, elevate the head of the bed further to 30 degrees or higher, if allowed, until the patient is sitting erect. *This position, like the normal elimination posture, aids in defecation and urination.* (For information on another device that permits normal elimination posture, see *Using a commode,* page 68.)
- If elevating the head of the bed is contraindicated, tuck a small pillow or folded bath blanket under the patient's back *to cushion his sacrum against the edge of the bedpan and support his lumbar region.*
- If the patient can be left alone, place the bed in a low position and raise the side rails *to ensure his safety.* Place toilet tissue and the call light within the patient's reach, and instruct him to push the button after elimination. If the patient is weak or disoriented, remain with him.
- Before removing the bedpan, lower the head of the bed slightly. Then ask the patient to raise his buttocks off the bed. Support his lower back with one hand, and gently remove the bedpan with the other *to avoid skin injury caused by friction.* If the patient can't raise his buttocks, ask him to roll to the opposite side so that his buttocks are toward you while you assist with one hand. Hold the pan firmly with the other hand to avoid spills. Cover the bedpan and place it on the chair.
- Help clean the anal and perineal area, as necessary, *to prevent irritation and infection.* Turn the patient on his side, wipe carefully with toilet tissue, clean the area with a damp washcloth and soap or cleaning wipes, and dry well with a towel. Clean a female patient from front to back *to avoid introducing rectal contaminants into the vaginal or urethral openings.*

Using a commode

An alternative to a bedpan, a commode is a portable chair made of plastic or metal with a large opening in the center of the seat. It may have a bedpan or bucket that slides underneath the opening, or it may slide directly over the toilet, adding height to the standard toilet seat. Unlike a bedpan, a commode allows the patient to assume his normal elimination posture, which aids in defecation.

Before the patient uses it, inspect the commode's condition and make sure it's clean. Roll or carry the commode to the patient's room. Place it parallel and as close as possible to the patient's bed, and secure its brakes or wheel locks. If necessary, block its wheels with sandbags. Assist the patient onto the commode, provide toilet tissue, and place the call light within his reach. Instruct the patient to push the call light when he has finished.

If necessary, assist the patient with cleaning. Help him into bed and make him comfortable. Offer the patient soap, water, and a towel to wash his hands. Then close the lid of the commode or cover the bucket. Roll the commode or carry the bucket to the bathroom. If ordered, observe and measure the contents before disposal. Rinse and clean the bucket, and then spray or wipe the bucket and commode seat with disinfectant. Use an air freshener, if appropriate.

Placing a urinal

- Lift the corner of the top linens, hand the urinal to the patient, and allow him to position it.
- If the patient can't position the urinal himself, spread his legs slightly and hold the urinal in place *to prevent spills.*
- After the patient voids, carefully withdraw the urinal and close the lid or cover it.

After use of a bedpan or urinal

- Give the patient either a clean washcloth dampened with warm water and soap, or cleaning wipes, as well as a towel *to wash and dry his hands.* Check the bed linens for wetness or soiling, and straighten or change them, if needed. Make the patient comfortable. Place the bed in the low position and raise the side rails if appropriate.
- Take the bedpan or urinal to the bathroom or utility room. Observe the color, odor, amount, and consistency of its contents. If ordered, measure urine output or liquid stool, or obtain a specimen for laboratory analysis.
- Empty the bedpan or urinal into the toilet or designated waste area. Rinse it with water and clean it thoroughly, using a disinfectant solution. Dry, cover, and return it to the patient's bathroom for storage.
- Remove and discard your gloves and perform hand hygiene.[1,2,3,4,5,10]
- Use an air freshener, if necessary, *to eliminate offensive odors and minimize embarrassment.*
- Document the procedure.[11,12,13]

Special considerations

- Explain to the patient that drug treatment and changes in his environment, diet, and activities may disrupt his usual elimination schedule. Try to anticipate elimination needs, and offer the bedpan or urinal frequently *to help reduce embarrassment and minimize the risk of incontinence.*
- Don't place a bedpan or urinal on top of the bedside stand or overbed table *to avoid contaminating clean equipment and food trays.* Similarly, don't place it on the floor *to prevent the spread of microorganisms from the floor to the patient's bed linens when he uses the device.*
- If the patient feels pain during turning or feels uncomfortable on a standard bedpan, use a fracture pan. Unlike the standard bedpan, the fracture pan is slipped under the buttocks from the front rather than the side. Because it's shallower than the standard bedpan, you need only lift the patient slightly to position it. If the patient is obese or otherwise difficult to lift, ask a coworker to help you.
- If the patient has an indwelling urinary catheter in place, carefully position and remove the bedpan *to avoid tension on the catheter, which could dislodge it or irritate the urethra.* After the patient defecates, wipe, clean, and dry the anal region, taking care to avoid catheter contamination. If necessary, clean the urinary meatus.
- Don't leave the urinal, fracture pan, or regular bedpan in place for extended periods *to prevent skin breakdown.*

Documentation

Record the time, date, and type of elimination in the flowchart and the amount of urine output or liquid stool on the intake and output record, as needed. In your notes, document the amount, color, clarity, and odor of the urine or stool and the presence of blood, pus, or other abnormal characteristics in urine or stool. Document the condition of the perineum.

REFERENCES

1 The Joint Commission. (2015). Standard NPSG.07.01.01. *Comprehensive accreditation manual for hospitals: The official handbook.* Oakbrook Terrace, IL: The Joint Commission. (Level VII)

2 Siegel, J. D., et al. (2007). "2007 guideline for isolation precautions: Preventing transmission of infectious agents in healthcare settings" [Online]. Accessed March 2015 via the Web at http://www.cdc.gov/hicpac/pdf/isolation/Isolation2007.pdf (Level II)

3 Centers for Disease Control and Prevention. (2002). Guideline for hand hygiene in health-care settings: Recommendations of the Healthcare Infection Control Practices Advisory Committee and the HICPAC/SHEA/APIC/IDSA Hand Hygiene Task Force. *MMWR Recommendations and Reports, 51*(RR-16), 1–45. Accessed March 2015 via the Web at http://www.cdc.gov/mmwr/pdf/rr/rr5116.pdf (Level II)

4 World Health Organization. (2009). "WHO guidelines on hand hygiene in health care: First global patient safety challenge, clean care is safer care" [Online]. Accessed March 2015 via the Web at http://whqlibdoc.who.int/publications/2009/9789241597906_eng.pdf (Level IV)

5 Centers for Medicare & Medicaid Services, Department of Health and Human Services. (2014). Condition of participation: Infection control. 42 C.F.R. § 482.42.

6 American Osteopathic Association. (2014). Standard 07.01.21. *Healthcare Facilities Accreditation Program: Accreditation requirements for acute care hospitals.* Chicago, IL: American Osteopathic Association. (Level VII)

7 American Osteopathic Association. (2014). Standard 07.01.10. *Healthcare Facilities Accreditation Program: Accreditation requirements for acute care hospitals.* Chicago, IL: American Osteopathic Association. (Level VII)

8 The Joint Commission. (2015). Standard NPSG.01.01.01. *Comprehensive accreditation manual for hospitals: The official handbook.* Oakbrook Terrace, IL: The Joint Commission. (Level VII)

9 American Osteopathic Association. (2014). Standard 15.01.16. *Healthcare Facilities Accreditation Program: Accreditation requirements for acute care hospitals.* Chicago, IL: American Osteopathic Association. (Level VII)

10 American Osteopathic Association. (2014). Standard 07.01.21. *Healthcare Facilities Accreditation Program: Accreditation requirements for acute care hospitals.* Chicago, IL: American Osteopathic Association. (Level VII)

11 The Joint Commission. (2015). Standard RC.01.03.01. *Comprehensive accreditation manual for hospitals: The official handbook.* Oakbrook Terrace, IL: The Joint Commission. (Level VII)

12 Centers for Medicare & Medicaid Services, Department of Health and Human Services. (2014). Condition of participation: Medical record services. 42 C.F.R. § 482.24(b).

13 American Osteopathic Association. (2014). Standard 10.00.03. *Healthcare Facilities Accreditation Program: Accreditation requirements for acute care hospitals.* Chicago, IL: American Osteopathic Association. (Level VII)

ADDITIONAL REFERENCES

Craven, R. F., & Hirnle, C. J. (2012). *Fundamentals of nursing: Human health and function.* (7th ed.). Philadelphia, PA: Lippincott Williams & Wilkins.

Wound, Ostomy and Continence Nurses Society (WOCN). (2010). *Guideline for prevention and management of pressure ulcers.* Mount Laurel, NJ: WOCN. (Level VII)

BEDSIDE SPIROMETRY

Bedside spirometry uses portable equipment to measure forced vital capacity (FVC) and forced expiratory volume (FEV). These measurements, in turn, allow for the calculation of other pulmonary function indexes, such as timed forced expiratory flow rate. Depending on the type of spirometer used, bedside spirometry can also allow direct measurement of vital capacity (VC) and tidal volume.

Bedside spirometry identifies the presence and severity of airflow obstruction. It's recommended for use in patients with respiratory signs and symptoms to determine whether their signs and symptoms result from respiratory disease or other conditions.[1] Bedside spirometry can help diagnose chronic obstructive pulmonary disease by demonstrating obstructed airflow that isn't fully reversible.[1] It's also useful for evaluating a patient's preoperative anesthesia risk. Because the required breathing patterns can aggravate conditions such as bronchospasm, use of the bedside spirometer requires a review of the patient's history and close observation during testing.

Performing bedside spirometry requires proper education and training in the procedure to make sure that test results are accurate and aid in diagnosis.[2,3]

Equipment

Portable spirometer ▪ disposable mouthpiece ▪ stethoscope ▪ blood pressure monitoring equipment ▪ disinfectant pad ▪ scale ▪ stadiometer ▪ Optional: breathing tube, gloves, gown, mask, goggles, nose clip, bacteria filter.

Preparation of equipment

Review the manufacturer's instructions for assembly and use of the spirometer. If necessary, firmly insert the breathing tube *to ensure a tight connection.* If the tube comes preconnected, check the seals for tightness and the tubing for leaks. Insert the disposable mouthpiece and make sure that sure it's sealed tightly. Make sure that the unit has been calibrated according to the manufacturer's guidelines.

Implementation

▪ Review the patient's medical record *to confirm that his inhaled long-acting beta-adrenergic agonist bronchodilator and oral beta-adrenergic agonist medications were withheld before spirometry testing, as ordered.*[2,4]

NURSING ALERT *Oral and inhaled bronchodilators may be withheld from the patient before spirometry testing* **to establish baseline lung function and to optimally evaluate bronchodilator response.** *Be aware that the risk of bronchospasm is increased if these medications are withheld.*[5]

▪ Perform hand hygiene.[6,7,8,9,10]

▪ Confirm the patient's identity using at least two patient identifiers.[11]

▪ Explain the procedure to the patient. Emphasize that his cooperation is essential *to ensure accurate results.*

▪ Provide privacy.[12,13,14]

▪ Instruct the patient to remove or loosen bras, belts, and other constricting clothing *to prevent alteration of test results from restricted thoracic expansion and abdominal mobility.*

▪ Instruct the patient to void *to prevent abdominal discomfort.*

▪ Obtain the patient's weight and height without shoes *to calculate predicted lung volumes.*

▪ If the patient wears dentures that fit well, leave them in place *to promote a tight seal around the mouthpiece.* However, if the dentures fit poorly, have the patient remove them *to prevent incomplete closure of his mouth around the mouthpiece, which could allow air to leak around the mouthpiece.*

▪ If the patient smokes cigarettes, confirm that he hasn't smoked for at least 1 hour before the bedside spirometry procedure.[2]

▪ Perform hand hygiene.[6,7,8,9,10]

▪ Put on gloves and other personal protective equipment as needed *to comply with standard precautions.*[15,16]

▪ Enter the required information into the spirometer's computer system.[17]

▪ Obtain the patient's blood pressure, pulse, and respiratory rate, and auscultate his breath sounds *to serve as a baseline for comparison.*[2]

▪ Ensure that the patient is sitting straight in a chair or standing with his head slightly elevated, not looking down.

▪ If desired, allow the patient to practice the required breathing technique with the breathing tube unhooked. After practice, replace the tube and check the seal.

▪ Instruct the patient not to breathe through his nose. If the patient has difficulty complying, apply a nose clip.

▪ To measure VC, instruct the patient to inhale as deeply as possible, and then insert the mouthpiece so that his lips are sealed tightly around it *to prevent air leakage and to ensure an accurate digital readout or spirogram recording.*

▪ Tell him to exhale normally but completely and then remove the mouthpiece *to prevent recording his next inspiration.*

▪ Repeat the maneuver at least three times, allowing adequate rest (more than 1 minute) between each maneuver. Typically, no more than four maneuvers are required to achieve acceptable repeatability. *Acceptable repeatability is achieved when the difference between the largest and the next largest VC values for the maneuvers is 0.15 L or less.*[2,3]

▪ To measure FEV and FVC, adjust the spirometer settings to the appropriate mode according to the manufacturer's instructions.[17]

▪ Repeat the procedure followed for VC measurement, but instruct the patient to exhale as forcefully and completely as possible in one exhalation. Tell him when to start, and activate the spirometer's recorder at the same time. Coach the patient throughout inspiration and exhalation.

▪ Repeat the maneuver at least three times, allowing adequate rest (more than 1 minute) between each maneuver. Usually no more than eight maneuvers are required to achieve acceptable repeatability for FVC and FEV. *Acceptable repeatability is achieved when the difference between the largest and the next largest FVC and FEV values for the maneuvers is 0.15 L or less.*[2,3]

▪ Monitor the patient for increased shortness of breath, light-headedness, paroxysmal coughing, and chest pain.

▪ Compare VC values between the maneuvers.

NURSING ALERT *If any subsequent VC value is 20% lower than the original value and you're confident that there's no leak in the system, terminate the study* **because dangerous air trapping may result from forced exhalation.**

▪ After completing the procedure, generate a summary report from the spirometer's computer system.

▪ Obtain the patient's vital signs and assess his respiratory status *to make sure his condition is stable before leaving the patient's bedside.* Notify the practitioner of any changes in the patient's conditions.

▪ Discard the mouthpiece, and follow the manufacturer's instructions for cleaning and sterilizing the spirometer.[18]

▪ Remove and discard your gloves and any other personal protective equipment worn.[15,16]

▪ Perform hand hygiene.[6,7,8,9,10]

▪ Clean and disinfect your stethoscope using a disinfectant pad.[18]

▪ Perform hand hygiene.[6,7,8,9,10]

▪ Document the procedure.[19,20,21]

Special considerations

- Don't perform pulmonary function tests, including bedside spirometry, immediately after a large meal *because the patient may experience abdominal discomfort.*
- Encourage the patient to perform maximally during the test; *doing so may help him to exhale more forcefully.* If the patient coughs during expiration, wait until coughing subsides before repeating the measurement.
- Older adults patients with significant cognitive impairment and apraxia are less likely to perform spirometry correctly; however, advanced age alone shouldn't interfere with the ability to achieve accurate test results.[22]
- Patients as young as age 5 may be able to perform spirometry maneuvers well enough to produce accurate results. Some spirometry software manufacturers offer developmentally appropriate visual incentives to enhance test performance in children. Currently, newer methods of obtaining reliable pulmonary function tests in infants and toddlers are being used in some facilities.[23]
- Although FVC and VC are normally approximately equal, in patients with obstructive lung disease, FVC may be reduced but VC remains normal. In patients with restrictive lung disease, VC and FVC may be reduced.
- Although the reference data programmed in current spirometry software allows for automatic computation of predicted values, the interpretation of bedside spirometry results shouldn't rely on the software alone. Bedside spirometry results should be forwarded to the appropriate practitioner for interpretation.[3] If software isn't available, a properly trained practitioner can calculate predicted values and compare patient results with a reference table of predicted normal values *to aid in diagnosis.*[3]

Complications

Forced exhalation can cause dizziness or light-headedness, precipitate or worsen bronchospasm, rapidly increase exhaustion (possibly to the point where the patient requires mechanical support), and increase air trapping in a patient with emphysema.

Documentation

Record the date and time of the procedure; the patient's gender, age, height, and weight at the time of the testing; the patient's respiratory status before and after spirometry; any complications and nursing actions taken; and the patient's tolerance of the procedure.[2]

REFERENCES

1 Qaseem, A., et al. (2011). Diagnosis and management of stable chronic obstructive pulmonary disease: A clinical practice guideline update from the American College of Physicians, American College of Chest Physicians, American Thoracic Society, and European Respiratory Society. *Annals of Internal Medicine, 155,* 179–191. (Level VII)

2 Miller, M. R., et al. (2005). Series "ATS/ERS task force: Standardisation of lung function testing" Standardisation of spirometry. *European Respiratory Journal, 26,* 319–338. Accessed March 2015 via the Web at http://www.thoracic.org/statements/resources/pft/PFT2.pdf (Level VII)

3 Hill, S., & Winter, R. (2013). "A guide to performing quality assured diagnostic spirometry" [Online]. Accessed March 2015 via the Web at http://www.educationforhealth.org/data/files/resources/spirometry_guide_16-4-13.pdf

4 Jones, T. E., et al. (2013). Drugs potentially affecting the extent of airways reversibility on pulmonary function testing are frequently consumed despite guidelines. *International Journal of Chronic Obstructive Pulmonary Disease, 8,* 383–388. Accessed March 2015 via the Web at http://www.ncbi.nlm.nih.gov/pmc/articles/PMC3745286/

5 McCarthy, K. (2012). "Pulmonary function testing" [Online]. Accessed March 2015 via the Web at http://emedicine.medscape.com/article/303239-overview

6 The Joint Commission. (2015). Standard NPSG.07.01.01. *Comprehensive accreditation manual for hospitals: The official handbook.* Oakbrook Terrace, IL: The Joint Commission. (Level VII)

7 Centers for Disease Control and Prevention. (2002). Guideline for hand hygiene in health-care settings: Recommendations of the Healthcare Infection Control Practices Advisory Committee and the HICPAC/SHEA/APIC/IDSA Hand Hygiene Task Force. *MMWR Recommendations and Reports, 51*(RR-16), 1–45. Accessed March 2015 via the Web at http://www.cdc.gov/mmwr/pdf/rr/rr5116.pdf (Level II)

8 World Health Organization. (2009). "WHO guidelines on hand hygiene in health care: First global patient safety challenge, clean care is safer care" [Online]. Accessed March 2015 via the Web at http://whqlibdoc.who.int/publications/2009/9789241597906_eng.pdf (Level IV)

9 American Osteopathic Association. (2014). Standard 07.01.21. *Healthcare Facilities Accreditation Program: Accreditation requirements for acute care hospitals.* Chicago, IL: American Osteopathic Association. (Level VII)

10 Centers for Medicare & Medicaid Services, Department of Health and Human Services. (2014). Condition of participation: Infection control. 42 C.F.R. § 482.42.

11 The Joint Commission. (2015). Standard NPSG.01.01.01. *Comprehensive accreditation manual for hospitals: The official handbook.* Oakbrook Terrace, IL: The Joint Commission. (Level VII)

12 American Osteopathic Association. (2014). Standard 15.01.16. *Healthcare Facilities Accreditation Program: Accreditation requirements for acute care hospitals.* Chicago, IL: American Osteopathic Association. (Level VII)

13 The Joint Commission. (2015). Standard RI.01.01.01. *Comprehensive accreditation manual for hospitals: The official handbook.* Oakbrook Terrace, IL: The Joint Commission. (Level VII)

14 Centers for Medicare & Medicaid Services, Department of Health and Human Services. (2014). Condition of participation: Patient's rights. 42 C.F.R. § 482.13(c)(1).

15 American Osteopathic Association. (2014). Standard 07.01.10. *Healthcare Facilities Accreditation Program: Accreditation requirements for acute care hospitals.* Chicago, IL: American Osteopathic Association. (Level VII)

16 Siegel, J. D., et al. (2007). "2007 guideline for isolation precautions: Preventing transmission of infectious agents in healthcare settings" [Online]. Accessed March 2015 via the Web at http://www.cdc.gov/hicpac/pdf/isolation/Isolation2007.pdf (Level II)

17 CareFusion. (2010). "The spirometers of choice: Micro Medical™, MicroLab, and MicroLoop" [Online]. Accessed March 2015 via the Web at http://www.micromedical.co.uk/downloads/pdf/microlab_microloop.pdf

18 American Osteopathic Association. (2014). Standard 07.02.03. *Healthcare Facilities Accreditation Program: Accreditation requirements for acute care hospitals.* Chicago, IL: American Osteopathic Association. (Level VII)

19 The Joint Commission. (2015). Standard RC.01.03.01. *Comprehensive accreditation manual for hospitals: The official handbook.* Oakbrook Terrace, IL: The Joint Commission. (Level VII)

20 American Osteopathic Association. (2014). Standard 10.00.03. *Healthcare Facilities Accreditation Program: Accreditation requirements for acute care hospitals.* Chicago, IL: American Osteopathic Association. (Level VII)

21 Centers for Medicare & Medicaid Services, Department of Health and Human Services. (2014). Condition of participation: Medical record services. 42 C.F.R. § 482.24(b).

22 Haynes, J. M. (2014). Pulmonary function test quality in the elderly: A comparison with younger adults. *Respiratory Care, 59,* 16–21. Accessed March 2015 via the Web at https://www.aarc.org/education/webcast_central/archives/2014/01_10_2014_journal.pdf

23 Lesnick, B. L., & Davis, S. D. (2011). Infant pulmonary function testing: Overview of technology and practical considerations—new current procedural terminology codes effective 2010. *Chest, 139,* 1197–1202. Accessed March 2015 via the Web at http://www.ncbi.nlm.nih.gov/pmc/articles/PMC3198380/

Understanding biliary drainage catheter placement

The biliary drainage catheter is inserted in the common bile duct, anchored to the abdominal wall, and connected to a closed drainage system.

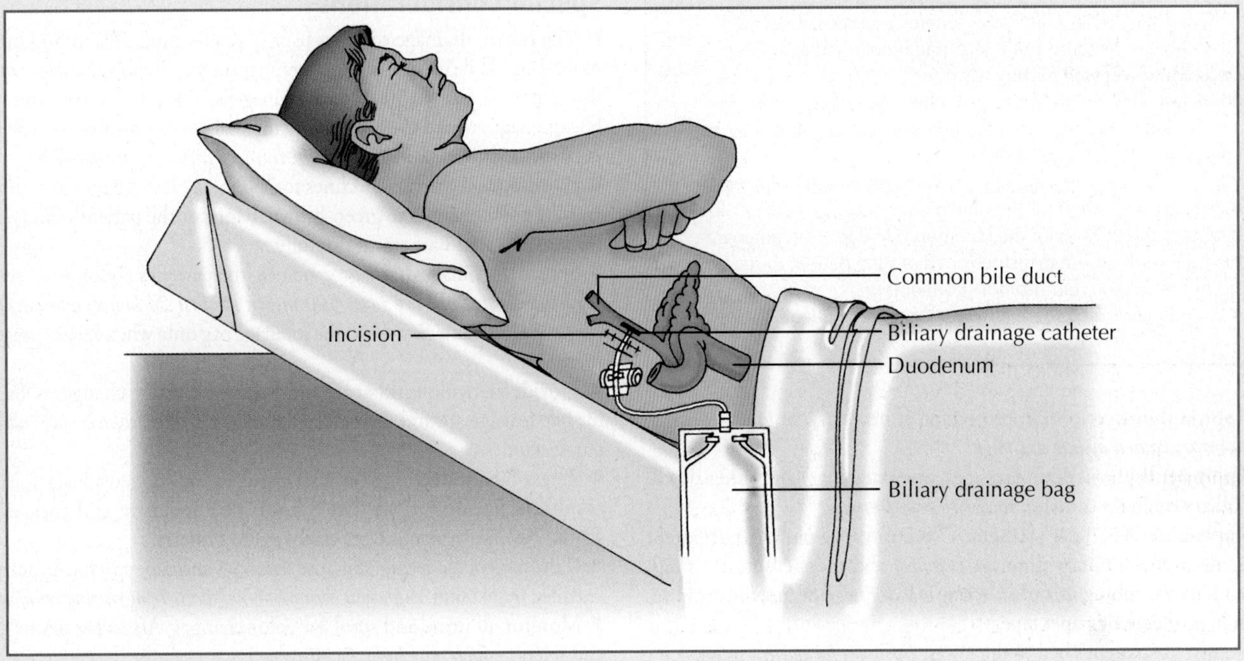

BILIARY DRAINAGE CATHETER CARE

The biliary drainage catheter (also called a *T tube*) may be inserted in the common bile duct after cholecystectomy, choledochostomy, or liver transplant and during treatment for cholelithiasis to promote biliary drainage.

The practitioner inserts the biliary drainage catheter into the common bile duct and draws the long end through the incision. The catheter is then connected to a closed drainage system. (See *Understanding biliary drainage catheter placement.*) The catheter typically remains in place postoperatively for between 7 and 14 days—potentially longer after a liver transplant. Biliary drainage catheter dressings are changed routinely, as ordered, to prevent infection and skin excoriation from bile.

Equipment

Gloves ▪ sterile gloves ▪ sterile drape ▪ sterile 4″ × 4″ (10-cm × 10-cm) gauze pads ▪ normal saline solution ▪ prescribed antiseptic cleaning agent ▪ two sterile basins ▪ sterile precut drain dressings ▪ hypoallergenic paper tape ▪ Optional: prescribed pain medication, gown, protective eyewear, transparent dressing, skin protectant, clamp or stopcock, thermometer, stethoscope, graduated collection container.

Implementation

- Verify the practitioner's order.
- Check the patient's medical recorder for a history of allergies.
- Gather and prepare the equipment
- Perform hand hygiene.[1,2,3,4,5]
- Confirm the patient's identity using at least two patient identifiers.[6]
- Provide privacy.[7,8]
- Explain the procedure to the patient *to decrease anxiety and ensure cooperation.*

Changing the dressing

- Perform a comprehensive pain assessment using techniques appropriate for the patient's age, condition, and ability to understand.[9] Before the dressing change, administer pain medications, as needed and ordered, following safe medication practices.[10,11,12]
- Raise the bed to a comfortable working height, and position the patient *to allow clear access to the dressing.*
- Put on gloves and other personal protective equipment as needed *to comply with standard precautions.*[13,14,15]
- Without dislodging the biliary drainage catheter, carefully remove the old dressing *to prevent skin stripping or tearing.*[16]
- Dispose of the old dressing in the appropriate receptacle.
- Remove and discard your gloves.[13,14,15]
- Perform hand hygiene.[1,2,3,4,5]
- Create a sterile field using a sterile drape. Open the sterile packages, and place each item on the sterile field. Pour the prescribed antiseptic cleaning agent into a sterile basin and the normal saline solution into another sterile basin.
- Put on sterile gloves and follow strict sterile technique *to prevent contamination of the incision.*[13,14,15]
- Inspect the incision and biliary drainage catheter insertion site for signs and symptoms of infection, such as redness, edema, warmth, tenderness, induration, and skin excoriation. Also assess the catheter and site for wound dehiscence or evisceration, if applicable.
- Use a sterile 4″ × 4″ (10-cm × 10-cm) gauze pad soaked in the prescribed antiseptic cleaning agent to clean and remove dried matter or bile drainage from around the biliary drainage catheter. Starting always at the catheter insertion site, gently wipe outward in a continuous circular motion *to prevent recontamination of the catheter insertion site.*
- Use a sterile 4″ × 4″ (10-cm × 10-cm) gauze pad soaked in normal saline solution to rinse the area. Dry the area with another sterile 4″ × 4″ (10-cm × 10-cm) gauze pad.

TROUBLESHOOTING

Managing biliary drainage catheter obstruction

If the patient's biliary drainage catheter becomes obstructed after cholecystectomy, notify the practitioner and take these steps while you wait for him to arrive:
- Unclamp the biliary drainage catheter (if it was clamped 1 hour before or after a meal), and connect the catheter to a closed gravity-drainage system.
- Inspect the catheter carefully *to detect any kinks or obstructions.*
- Prepare the patient for possible biliary drainage catheter irrigation or direct X-ray of the common bile duct (cholangiography). Describe these measures briefly to the patient *to reduce his apprehension and promote cooperation.*
- Provide encouragement and support to the patient.

- Apply a thin layer of skin protectant, if necessary, *to protect the skin from injury caused by bile drainage.*
- Apply sterile precut drain dressings, one extending from either side of the biliary drainage catheter, *to absorb bile drainage.*
- Apply a sterile 4″ × 4″ (10-cm × 10-cm) gauze pad or transparent dressing over the biliary drainage catheter and the incision dressings. Don't kink the tubing *to avoid blocking bile drainage.* Secure the dressings with hypoallergenic paper tape.
- Return the patient's bed to the lowest position *for patient safety.*

Emptying the drainage bag

- Put on gloves as needed *to comply with standard precautions.*[13,14,15]
- Place the graduated collection container under the outlet valve of the drainage bag.
- Supporting the biliary drainage bag *to prevent traction on the biliary drainage catheter and accidental removal,*[17] open the outlet valve, empty the bag's contents completely into the container, and close the valve, without contaminating the valve, tubing, or clamp (if used).
- Wipe the end of the outlet valve with a clean gauze pad *to remove residual drainage that may remain after closing.*
- Carefully measure and record the character, color, and amount of drainage.
- Check bile drainage amounts regularly *to ensure patient comfort and safety.*
- Obtain the patient's vital signs; monitor intake and output; and assess for such signs and symptoms of obstructed bile flow as chills; fever; tachycardia; nausea; right-upper-quadrant fullness and pain; jaundice; dark, foamy urine; and clay-colored stools. Report any such signs or symptoms to the practitioner immediately.

Clamping the tube

- Put on gloves as needed *to comply with standard precautions.*[13,14,15]
- Occlude the biliary drainage catheter with a clamp, or close the stopcock, if present. *Clamping the tube 1 hour before and after meals diverts bile back to the duodenum to aid digestion.*
- Monitor the patient's response to having the catheter clamped.
- Supporting the biliary drainage bag *to prevent traction on the catheter and accidental removal,* unclamp the biliary drainage catheter or open the stopcock as ordered.[17]
- Check bile drainage amounts regularly, and empty the drainage bag into a graduated collection container for measurement, as needed, *to ensure patient comfort and safety.*

Completing the procedure

- Dispose of used equipment and materials appropriately.
- Remove and discard your gloves,[13,14,15] and perform hand hygiene.[1,2,3,4,5]
- Document the procedure.[18,19,20]

Special considerations

- The biliary drainage catheter usually drains from 300 to 500 mL of blood-tinged bile in the first 24 hours after surgery. Report drainage within that time that exceeds 500 mL; if drainage is 50 mL or less or if you note bile drainage around the tube, notify the practitioner *because the tube may be obstructed.* (See *Managing biliary drainage catheter obstruction.*)
- Bile drainage typically declines to 200 mL or less 4 days after surgery and the color changes to green-brown. Monitor the patient's fluid, electrolyte, and acid-base status carefully.
- Secure the biliary drainage system at the patient's abdominal level *to prevent excessive bile loss (over 500 mL in the first 24 hours) and backflow contamination.* Bile flows into the drainage bag only when biliary pressure increases.
- Provide meticulous skin care and frequent dressing changes. Observe for bile leakage around the biliary drainage catheter, *which may indicate obstruction.*
- Assess biliary drainage catheter patency and catheter insertion site condition hourly for the first 8 hours postoperative and then every 4 hours until the practitioner removes the catheter.
- If the patient has fragile skin, use dressings and tape specifically formulated for fragile skin *to prevent skin stripping and tearing during removal.*[17]
- Monitor all urine and stool for color changes. Assess for icteric skin and sclera, *which may indicate jaundice.*

Patient teaching

Inform the patient that loose bowel movements commonly occur in the first few weeks after surgery. Teach him how to care for the biliary drainage catheter at home, including providing meticulous skin care and dressing changes. Also inform the patient about the signs and symptoms of catheter and biliary obstruction that he should report to the practitioner. Teach him how to manage the catheter when turning, walking, and performing activities of daily living. Caution him that he should avoid direct pulling or traction on the catheter[17] and that bile stains clothing.

Complications

Obstructed bile flow, skin excoriation or breakdown, catheter dislodgment, drainage reflux, and infection are the most common complications related to biliary drainage catheters.

Documentation

Record the appearance of the dressing and surrounding skin. Record the color, character, and volume of bile collected. Keep a precise record of the patient's temperature and the amount and frequency of urination and bowel movements. Document any patient teaching provided and the patient's understanding of your teaching.

REFERENCES

1 Centers for Disease Control and Prevention. (2002). Guideline for hand hygiene in health-care settings: Recommendations of the Healthcare Infection Control Practices Advisory Committee and the HICPAC/SHEA/APIC/IDSA Hand Hygiene Task Force. *MMWR Recommendations and Reports, 51*(RR-16), 1–45. Accessed May 2015 via the Web at http://www.cdc.gov/mmwr/pdf/rr/rr5116.pdf (Level II)

2 The Joint Commission. (2015). Standard NPSG.07.01.01. *Comprehensive accreditation manual for hospitals: The official handbook.* Oakbrook Terrace, IL: The Joint Commission. (Level VII)

3 World Health Organization. (2009). "WHO guidelines on hand hygiene in health care: First global patient safety challenge, clean care is safer care"

[Online]. Accessed May 2015 via the Web at http://whqlibdoc.who.int/publications/2009/9789241597906_eng.pdf (Level IV)
4 American Osteopathic Association. (2014). Standard 07.01.21. *Healthcare Facilities Accreditation Program: Accreditation requirements for acute care hospitals.* Chicago, IL: American Osteopathic Association. (Level VII)
5 Centers for Medicare & Medicaid Services, Department of Health and Human Services. (2014). Condition of participation: Infection control. 42 C.F.R. § 482.42.
6 The Joint Commission. (2015). Standard NPSG.01.01.01. *Comprehensive accreditation manual for hospitals: The official handbook.* Oakbrook Terrace, IL: The Joint Commission. (Level VII)
7 American Osteopathic Association. (2014). Standard 15.01.16. *Healthcare Facilities Accreditation Program: Accreditation requirements for acute care hospitals.* Chicago, IL: American Osteopathic Association. (Level VII)
8 Centers for Medicare & Medicaid Services, Department of Health and Human Services. (2014). Condition of participation: Patient's rights. 42 C.F.R. § 482.13(c)(1).
9 The Joint Commission. (2015). Standard PC.01.02.07. *Comprehensive accreditation manual for hospitals: The official handbook.* Oakbrook Terrace, IL: The Joint Commission. (Level VII)
10 The Joint Commission. (2015). Standard MM.06.01.01. *Comprehensive accreditation manual for hospitals: The official handbook.* Oakbrook Terrace, IL: The Joint Commission. (Level VII)
11 American Osteopathic Association. (2014). Standard 16.01.03. *Healthcare Facilities Accreditation Program: Accreditation requirements for acute care hospitals.* Chicago, IL: American Osteopathic Association. (Level VII)
12 Centers for Medicare & Medicaid Services, Department of Health and Human Services. (2014). Condition of participation: Nursing services. 42 C.F.R. § 482.23(c).
13 Siegel, J. D., et al. (2007). "2007 guideline for isolation precautions: Preventing transmission of infectious agents in healthcare settings" [Online]. Accessed May 2015 via the Web at http://www.cdc.gov/hicpac/pdf/isolation/Isolation2007.pdf (Level II)
14 Occupational Safety and Health Administration. (n.d.). "Bloodborne pathogens, standard number 1910.1030" [Online]. Accessed May 2015 via the Web at https://www.osha.gov/pls/oshaweb/owadisp.show_document?p_table=STANDARDS&p_id=10051 (Level VII)
15 American Osteopathic Association. (2014). Standard 07.01.10. *Healthcare Facilities Accreditation Program: Accreditation requirements for acute care hospitals.* Chicago, IL: American Osteopathic Association. (Level VII)
16 LeBlanc, K., et al. (2013). International skin tear advisory panel: A tool kit to aid in the prevention, assessment, and treatment of skin tears using a simplified classification system. *Advances in Skin and Wound Care, 26,* 459–476. (Level IV)
17 LeMone, P., et al. (2011). *Medical-surgical nursing: Critical thinking in patient care, Vol. 1* (5th ed.). Cranbury, NJ: Prentice Hall.
18 The Joint Commission. (2015). Standard RC.01.03.01. *Comprehensive accreditation manual for hospitals: The official handbook.* Oakbrook Terrace, IL: The Joint Commission. (Level VII)
19 American Osteopathic Association. (2014). Standard 10.00.03. *Healthcare Facilities Accreditation Program: Accreditation requirements for acute care hospitals.* Chicago, IL: American Osteopathic Association. (Level VII)
20 Centers for Medicare & Medicaid Services, Department of Health and Human Services. (2014). Condition of participation: Medical record services. 42 C.F.R. § 482.24(b).

BINDER APPLICATION

Binders are lengths of cloth or elasticized material that encircle the chest, abdomen, or groin to provide support, keep dressings in place (especially for patients allergic to tape), reduce edema, and decrease tension on wounds and suture lines. Binders also promote early mobilization, increase patient comfort, and can hasten the healing process.[1] When properly used postoperatively, abdominal binders don't adversely impede lung function.[1] Elasticized abdominal binders are typically fastened with Velcro.

Equipment

Tape measure ■ binder of appropriate size and type ■ safety pins ■ dressing materials ■ Optional: gloves, 4″ × 4″ (10-cm × 10-cm) gauze pads.

Commercial elastic binders are now commonly used instead of standard cotton straight and Scultetus binders that require pins. Disposable T-binders are available, and scrotal supports typically replace binders for male patients, except after abdominal-perineal resection.

Preparation of equipment

Measure the area that the binder must fit, and obtain the proper size and type of binder from the central supply department.

Implementation

■ Verify the practitioner's order.
■ Gather and prepare the necessary equipment.
■ Perform hand hygiene.[2,3,4,5,6]
■ Confirm the patient's identity using at least two patient identifiers.[7]
■ Provide privacy.[8]
■ Explain the procedure to the patient *to promote cooperation and reduce anxiety.*
■ Put on gloves as needed *to comply with standard precautions.*[9,10,11]
■ Raise the patient's bed to a comfortable working height *to avoid muscle strain when applying the binder.* If the side rails on the bed are raised, lower the side rail on the side of the bed where you're working.
■ Place the patient in the supine position with his head slightly elevated and his knees slightly flexed *to decrease tension on the abdomen.*
■ Assess the patient's condition.
■ Remove and discard the dressing.
■ Assess the wound or suture line, as appropriate.
■ Remove and discard your gloves if worn,[9,10,11] perform hand hygiene,[2,3,4,5,6] and put on new gloves as needed.[9,10,11]
■ Cover the wound with a new sterile dressing.

Applying a straight abdominal binder

■ Accordion-fold half of the binder, slip it under the patient, and pull it through from the other side. Make sure the binder is straight, free of wrinkles, and evenly distributed under the patient. Its lower edge should extend well below the hips.
■ Overlap one side snugly onto the other (as shown below).

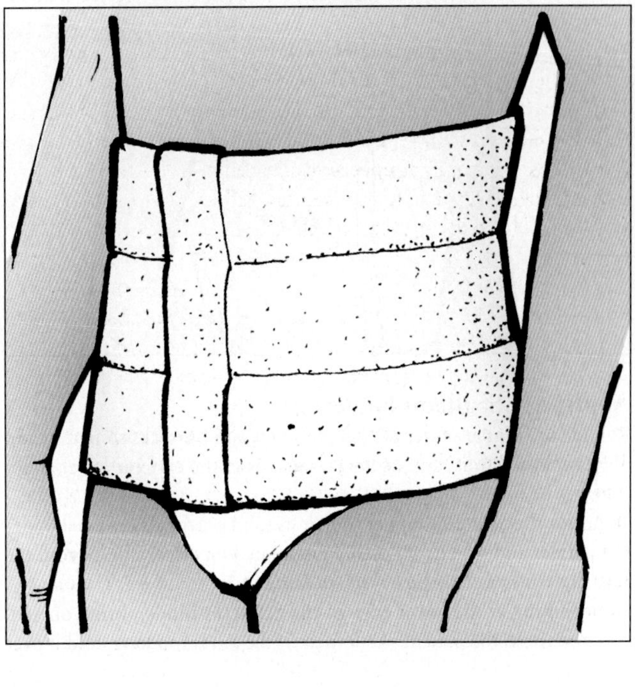

■ Starting at the lower edge, close the Velcro closure. *Fastening the abdominal binder from the lower edge upward in postsurgical application helps to relieve gravitational pull on the wound.*
■ Insert one finger under the binder's edge *to ensure a snug fit that's still loose enough to avoid impaired circulation and respiration as well as patient discomfort.* Avoid making the binder too tight around the diaphragm *because it may interfere with breathing.*
■ *For maximum support,* wrap the binder so that it applies even pressure across the body section. Eliminate all wrinkles, and avoid placing pressure over bony prominences.

Applying a breast binder

■ Wash and thoroughly dry under pendulous breasts. Place 4″ × 4″ (10-cm × 10-cm) gauze pads under breasts, as necessary, *to prevent skin irritation.*
■ Slip the binder under the patient's chest so that its lower edge aligns with the waist.
■ Straighten the binder *to distribute it evenly on either side.*
■ Position the binder so that the patient's nipples are centered in the breast tissue. *This position ensures proper breast alignment and support and produces faster tissue involution.*
■ *For maximum support,* wrap the binder so that it applies even pressure across the body section. Eliminate all wrinkles, and avoid placing pressure over bony prominences.
■ Pull the binder's edges snugly together and begin closing the Velcro closures upward from the waist.
■ Adjust the shoulder straps to fit properly and secure them with the Velcro fasteners (as shown below).
■ Ask the patient if the binder feels comfortable. Explain that it may feel tight initially but should feel comfortable shortly. Make adjustments, as needed. Instruct the patient to notify the nurse immediately if the binder feels too tight or too loose or comes apart.

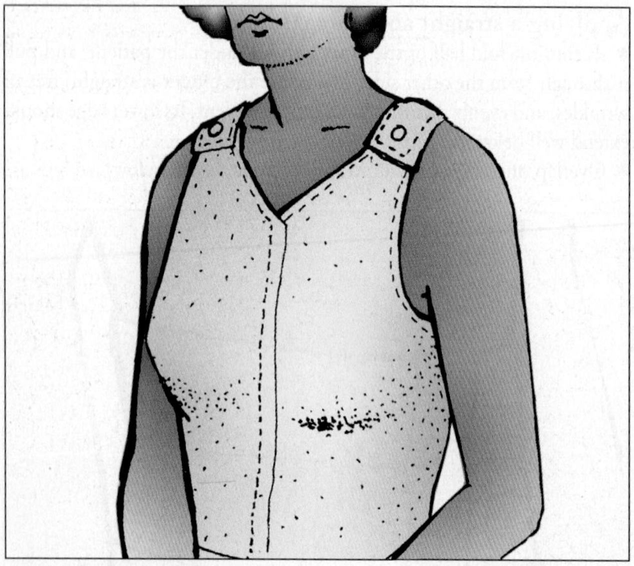

Applying a Scultetus binder

■ Slide the binder under the patient's hips and buttocks so that its top aligns with the waist and its lowest tail crosses the extreme lower abdomen.
■ Adjust the Scultetus binder so that its solid portion is centered under the patient and its tails are evenly distributed on either side. Spread the tails out flat *so you can pick them up easily.*
■ Beginning at the lower edge of the Scultetus binder, bring one tail straight across the patient's abdomen. If the tail is too long, fold it over flat at the end. Hold this tail snugly in place as you bring the opposite tail across on top of it, overlapping the first tail's upper half and continuing with succeeding tail pieces.

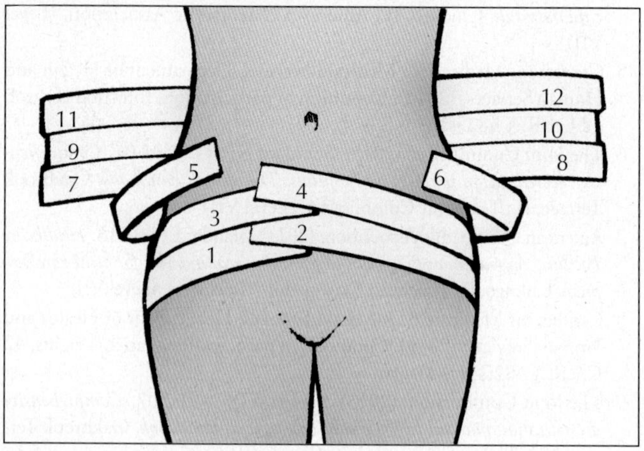

■ Secure the top strap with the Velcro fasteners.

Applying a T-binder

■ Slip the T-binder under the patient's waist, with its tails extending below the buttocks. Smooth the waistband and tails *to remove twists, which can chafe the patient's skin.*
■ Pull the waistband snugly into position at the patient's waistline or lower across the abdomen.
■ Fasten the Velcro closure.
■ Bring the free tail up between the patient's legs over the dressing or perineal pad.
■ For a female patient, bring the single tail up to the center of the waist, loop it behind and over the waistband, and secure it to the waistband with the Velcro closures.

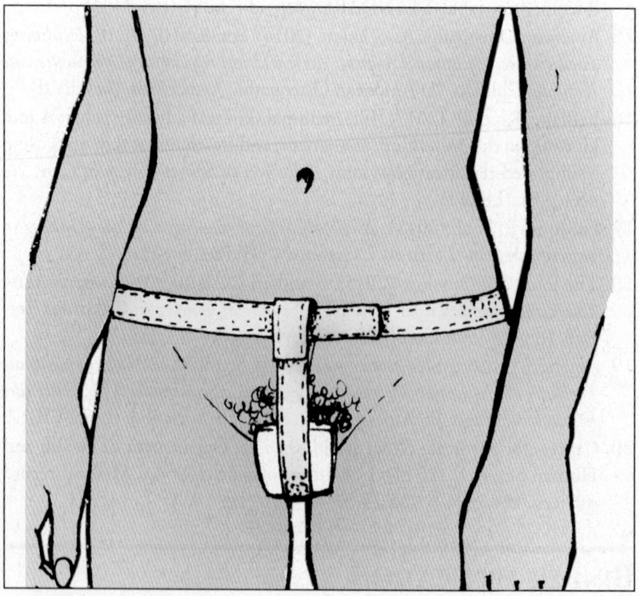

■ For a male patient, bring the two tails up on either side of the penis *to provide even support for the testes.* Loop the ends behind and over the waistband on either side of the midline, and fasten them to the waistband by closing the Velcro closures.

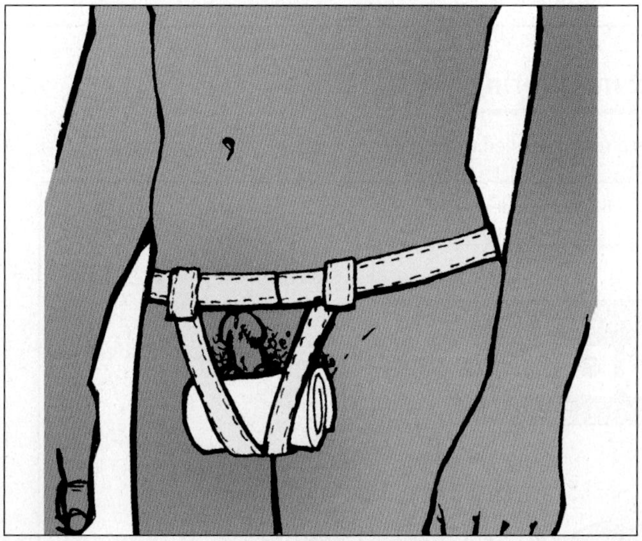

■ *For maximum support,* wrap the binder so that it applies even pressure across the body section. Eliminate all wrinkles and avoid placing pressure over bony prominences.

■ Tell the patient to call for assistance before voiding or defecating *to unfasten and reapply the binder.*

Completing the application of any binder

■ Ask the patient if the binder feels comfortable. Tell him that it may feel tight initially but should feel comfortable shortly. Instruct the patient to notify you immediately if the binder feels too tight or too loose or comes apart.

■ Return the bed to its lowest position *for patient safety.*

■ If the patient can ambulate, ask him to do so *to evaluate the fit of the binder.*

■ Remove and discard your gloves if worn.[9,10,11]

■ Perform hand hygiene.[2,3,4,5,6]

■ Document the procedure.[12,13,14]

Special considerations

■ Be careful not to compress any tubes, drains, or catheters and not to position them so that they are working against gravity.

■ Make sure that binder placement doesn't interfere with elimination.

■ Observe the patient and check binder placement every 4 hours, and as needed. Check the skin for color, palpate it for warmth, check pulses, and assess for tingling or numbness. Check respiratory status, and encourage coughing, deep breathing, and incentive spirometry, if ordered.[1,15]

■ Assess the patient's lower extremities for color, pulses, and edema. Encourage movement of the patient's feet and legs *to prevent deep vein thrombosis.*[16]

■ Reapply the binder when a dressing needs changing, when the binder becomes loose or too tight, and at other times according to the practitioner's orders. When changing the binder, observe the skin for signs of irritation. Provide appropriate skin care before reapplying the binder.

Patient teaching

If the patient will need a binder after discharge, teach him and a family member how to remove it, inspect the skin, bathe the area, and reapply the binder. Tell the patient and family member where to purchase binders and how to care for them. For a patient with cancer, the American Cancer Society may provide assistance in obtaining binders. If commercially manufactured binders are unavailable, advise the patient and family that a clean towel or sheeting material can be used instead. Periodically reinforce previous teaching and instructions.

Complications

Irritation of the underlying skin can result from perspiration or friction.

Documentation

Record the date and time of binder application, reapplication, and removal; binder type and location; purpose of application; skin condition before and after application; dressing changes or skin care; complications; the patient's tolerance of the treatment; and any patient teaching provided.

REFERENCES

1 Cheifetz, O., et al. (2010). The effect of abdominal support on functional outcomes in patients following major abdominal surgery: A randomized controlled trial. *Physiotherapy Canada, 62,* 242–253. Accessed March 2015 via the Web at http://www.ncbi.nlm.nih.gov/pmc/articles/PMC2909864/ (Level II)

2 Centers for Disease Control and Prevention. (2002). Guideline for hand hygiene in health-care settings: Recommendations of the Healthcare Infection Control Practices Advisory Committee and the HICPAC/SHEA/APIC/IDSA Hand Hygiene Task Force. *MMWR Recommendations and Reports, 51*(RR-16), 1–45. Accessed March 2015 via the Web at http://www.cdc.gov/mmwr/pdf/rr/rr5116.pdf (Level II)

3 The Joint Commission. (2015). Standard NPSG.07.01.01. *Comprehensive accreditation manual for hospitals: The official handbook.* Oakbrook Terrace, IL: The Joint Commission. (Level VII)

4 World Health Organization. (2009). "WHO guidelines on hand hygiene in health care: First global patient safety challenge, clean care is safer care" [Online]. Accessed March 2015 via the Web at http://whqlibdoc.who.int/publications/2009/9789241597906_eng.pdf (Level IV)

5 Centers for Medicare & Medicaid Services, Department of Health and Human Services. (2014). Condition of participation: Infection control. 42 C.F.R. § 482.42.

6 American Osteopathic Association. (2014). Standard 07.01.21. *Healthcare Facilities Accreditation Program: Accreditation requirements for acute care hospitals.* Chicago, IL: American Osteopathic Association. (Level VII)

7 The Joint Commission. (2015). Standard NPSG.01.01.01. *Comprehensive accreditation manual for hospitals: The official handbook.* Oakbrook Terrace, IL: The Joint Commission. (Level VII)

8 American Osteopathic Association. (2014). Standard 15.01.16. *Healthcare Facilities Accreditation Program: Accreditation requirements for acute care hospitals.* Chicago, IL: American Osteopathic Association. (Level VII)

9 Siegel, J. D., et al. (2007). "2007 guideline for isolation precautions: Preventing transmission of infectious agents in healthcare settings" [Online]. Accessed March 2015 via the Web at http://www.cdc.gov/hicpac/pdf/isolation/Isolation2007.pdf (Level II)

10 Occupational Safety and Health Administration. (n.d.). "Bloodborne pathogens, standard number 1910.1030" [Online]. Accessed March 2015 via the Web at http://www.osha.gov/pls/oshaweb/owadisp.show_document?p_table=STANDARDS&p_id=10051 (Level VII)

11 American Osteopathic Association. (2014). Standard 07.01.10. *Healthcare Facilities Accreditation Program: Accreditation requirements for acute care hospitals.* Chicago, IL: American Osteopathic Association. (Level VII)

12 The Joint Commission. (2015). Standard RC.01.03.01. *Comprehensive accreditation manual for hospitals: The official handbook.* Oakbrook Terrace, IL: The Joint Commission. (Level VII)

13 Centers for Medicare & Medicaid Services, Department of Health and Human Services. (2014). Condition of participation: Medical record services. 42 C.F.R. § 482.24(b).

14 American Osteopathic Association. (2014). Standard 10.00.03. *Healthcare Facilities Accreditation Program: Accreditation requirements for acute care hospitals.* Chicago, IL: American Osteopathic Association. (Level VII)

15 Restrepo, R. D., et al. (2011). AARC clinical practice guideline: Incentive spirometry: 2011. *Respiratory Care, 56,* 1600–1604. Accessed March 2015 via the Web at http://rc.rcjournal.com/contents/56/10/1600.full.pdf+html (Level VII)

16 Toft, M. H., et al. (2008). Haemodynamic and respiratory effects of an abdominal compression binder. *Clinical Physiology and Functional Imaging, 28,* 398–402. (Level II)

EQUIPMENT

Bispectral index monitoring

Bispectral index monitoring consists of a monitor and cable connected to a sensor applied to the patient's forehead (as shown below).

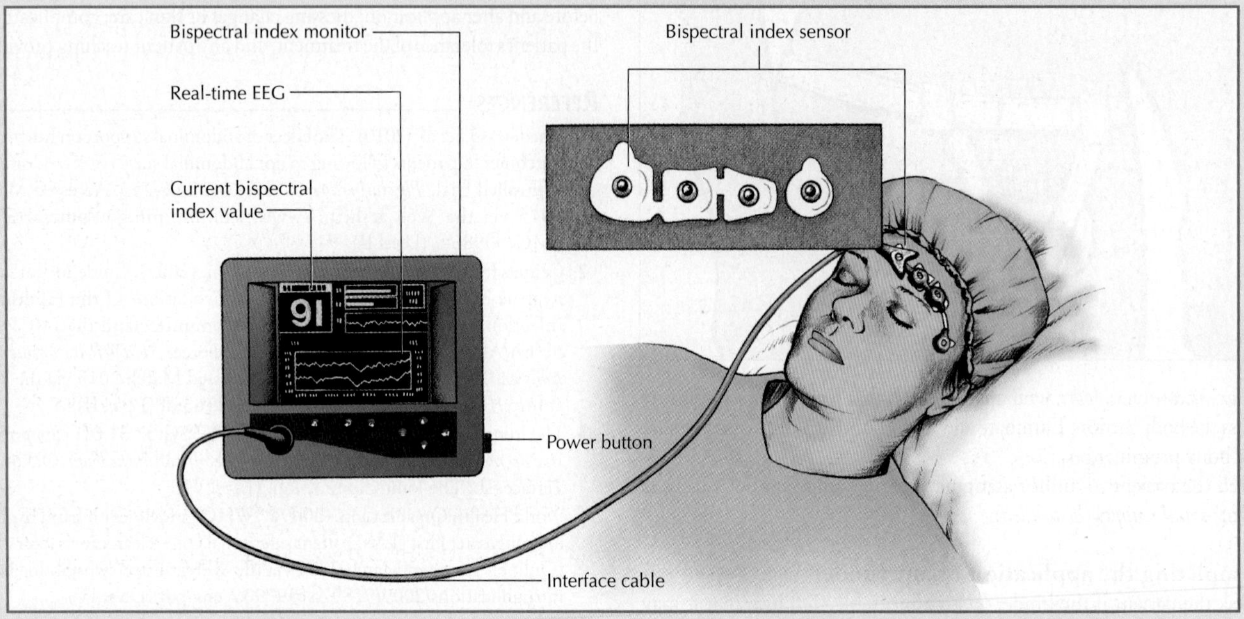

BISPECTRAL INDEX MONITORING

Bispectral index monitoring involves the use of an electronic device that converts EEG waves into a number. This number, statistically derived from raw EEG data, indicates the depth or level of a patient's sedation and provides a direct measure of the effects of sedatives and anesthetics on the brain. Unlike reliance on subjective assessments and vital signs, bispectral index monitoring provides objective, reliable data on which to base care decisions, thus minimizing the risks of oversedation and undersedation. When used appropriately, bispectral index monitoring can decrease the total amount of sedation needed to keep a patient adequately sedated.[1,2]

The bispectral index monitor is attached to a sensor applied to the patient's forehead. The sensor obtains information about the patient's electrical brain activity and then translates this information into a number from 0 (indicating no brain activity) to 100 (indicating a patient who's awake and alert). On the critical care unit and in the operating room, bispectral index monitoring is used to assess sedation when the patient is receiving mechanical ventilation or neuromuscular blockers or during barbiturate coma or bedside procedures.[3]

Equipment

Bispectral index monitor and cable ▪ bispectral index sensor ▪ alcohol pad ▪ gauze pad ▪ soap and water ▪ Optional: gloves.

Implementation

- Gather the necessary equipment.
- Place the bispectral index monitor close to the patient's bed, and plug the power cord into the wall outlet.
- Turn on the monitor to allow it to initiate a self-test according to the manufacturer's instructions *to ensure that the equipment is functioning properly.*[4]
- Perform hand hygiene.[5,6,7,8,9]
- Put on gloves as needed *to comply with standard precautions.*[10,11]
- Confirm the patient's identity using at least two patient identifiers.[12]
- Explain the procedure and rationale to the patient and his family. (See *Bispectral index monitoring.*)
- Provide privacy.[13,14,15]
- Clean the patient's forehead with soap and water and allow it to dry. If necessary, wipe the forehead with an alcohol pad and then dry it with a gauze pad *to ensure that the skin is oil-free.*[4]
- Open the sensor package and apply the sensor to the patient's forehead. Position the circle labeled "1" midline, approximately 2″ (about 5 cm) above the bridge of the nose.[4]
- Position the circle labeled "3" vertically on the right or left temple area, at the level of the outer canthus of the eye, between the corner of the eye and the patient's hairline.
- Ensure that the circle labeled "4" and the line below it are parallel to the eye on the appropriate side.
- Position the circle labeled "2" between the circles labeled "1" and "4."
- Apply gentle but firm pressure around the edges of the sensor, including the areas in between the numbered circles, *to ensure proper adhesion.*
- Press firmly on each of the numbered circles for about 5 seconds *to ensure that the electrodes adhere to the skin.*[4]
- Connect the sensor to the interface cable and monitor.
- Watch the monitor for information related to impedance (electrical resistance) testing.

NURSING ALERT *Be aware that, for the monitor to display a reading, impedance values must be below a specified threshold. If they aren't, be vprepared to troubleshoot sensor problems.* (*See* Troubleshooting sensor problems.)

- Select a smoothing rate (the time during which data is analyzed for calculation of the bispectral index; usually 15 or 30 seconds) using the ADVANCE SETUP button.

- Read and record the bispectral index value.
- Check the sensor site. Change the sensor every 24 hours or more frequently as needed *to ensure adequate electrical contact.*[4]
- Remove and discard your gloves, if worn.
- Perform hand hygiene.[5,6,7,8,9]
- Document the procedure.[16,17,18]

Special considerations

- Always evaluate the bispectral index value in light of other patient assessment findings. Don't rely on the bispectral index value alone.[2] (See *Interpreting bispectral index values.*)
- Keep in mind that movement may occur with low bispectral index values. Be alert for artifacts that could falsely elevate bispectral index values.

NURSING ALERT ***Bispectral index values may be elevated*** **because of muscle shivering, tightening, or twitching, or with the use of electromechanical devices either with the patient or in close proximity to the patient, the bispectral index monitor, or the sensor.** ***Interpret the bispectral index value cautiously in these situations.***[2]

- Anticipate the need to adjust the dosage of sedation based on the patient's bispectral index value.[2]
- Minimize patient position changes during bispectral index monitoring. Studies have shown that changing a patient's position during monitoring can significantly affect the bispectral values.[2,19]

NURSING ALERT ***Keep in mind that a decrease in stimulation, increased sedation, recent administration of a neuromuscular blocking agent or analgesia, or hypothermia may decrease the bispectral index, indicating the need for a decrease in sedative agents. Pain may cause an elevated bispectral index, indicating a need for an increase in sedation.***[2]

Documentation

Document initiation of bispectral index monitoring, including the baseline bispectral index value and location of the sensor. Record assessment findings with the bispectral index value to provide a clear overall picture of the patient's condition.

Record any increases or decreases in bispectral index values, along with actions instituted based on values and any changes in sedative agents administered.

REFERENCES

1 Olson, D. M., et al. (2009). A randomized evaluation of bispectral index-augmented sedation assessment in neurological patients. *Neurocritical Care, 11,* 20–27. (Level III)

2 Kelly, S. D. (2010). *Monitoring consciousness using the bispectral index during anesthesia: A pocket guide for clinicians* (2nd ed.). Boulder, CO: Covidien.

3 Goodwin, H., et al. (2012). 'Cooperative sedation': Optimizing comfort while maximizing systemic and neurological function. *Critical Care, 16*(2), 217. Accessed March 2015 via the Web at http://www.ncbi.nlm.nih.gov/pmc/articles/PMC3681362/pdf/cc11231.pdf

4 Lynn-McHale Wiegand, D. (Ed.). (2011). *AACN procedure manual for critical care* (6th ed.). St. Louis, MO: Saunders.

5 Centers for Disease Control and Prevention. (2002). Guideline for hand hygiene in health-care settings: Recommendations of the Healthcare Infection Control Practices Advisory Committee and the HICPAC/SHEA/APIC/IDSA Hand Hygiene Task Force. *MMWR Recommendations and Reports, 51*(RR-16), 1–45. Accessed March 2015 via the Web at http://www.cdc.gov/mmwr/pdf/rr/rr5116.pdf (Level II)

6 World Health Organization (2009). "WHO guidelines on hand hygiene in health care: First global patient safety challenge, clean care is safer care" [Online]. Accessed March 2015 via the Web at http://whqlibdoc.who.int/publications/2009/9789241597906_eng.pdf (Level IV)

TROUBLESHOOTING

Troubleshooting sensor problems

When initiating bispectral index monitoring, be aware that the monitor may display messages that indicate a problem. The chart below highlights these messages and offers possible solutions.

MESSAGE	POSSIBLE SOLUTIONS
High impedance message	Check sensor adhesion; reapply firm pressure to each of the numbered circles on the sensor for 5 seconds; if the message continues, check the connection between the sensor and the monitor; if necessary, apply a new sensor.
Noise message	Remove possible pressure on the sensor; investigate possible electrical interference from equipment.
Lead-off message	Check sensor for electrode displacement or lifting; reapply with firm pressure or, if necessary, apply a new sensor.

Interpreting bispectral index values

Use the following guidelines to interpret your patient's bispectral index value:

BISPECTRAL INDEX		
100	Awake	
80	Light to moderate sedation	Light hypnotic state
70	Deep sedation (low probability of explicit recall)	Light hypnotic state
60	General anesthesia (low probability of consciousness)	Moderate hypnotic state
40	Deep hypnotic state	
0	Flat-line EEG	

7 The Joint Commission. (2015). Standard NPSG.07.01.01. *Comprehensive accreditation manual for hospitals: The official handbook.* Oakbrook Terrace, IL: The Joint Commission. (Level VII)
8 American Osteopathic Association. (2014). Standard 07.01.21. *Healthcare Facilities Accreditation Program: Accreditation requirements for acute care hospitals.* Chicago, IL: American Osteopathic Association. (Level VII)
9 Centers for Medicare & Medicaid Services, Department of Health and Human Services. (2014). Condition of participation: Infection control. 42 C.F.R. § 482.42.
10 Siegel, J. D., et al. (2007). "2007 guideline for isolation precautions: Preventing transmission of infectious agents in healthcare settings" [Online]. Accessed March 2015 via the Web at http://www.cdc.gov/hicpac/pdf/isolation/Isolation2007.pdf (Level II)
11 American Osteopathic Association. (2014). Standard 07.01.10. *Healthcare Facilities Accreditation Program: Accreditation requirements for acute care hospitals.* Chicago, IL: American Osteopathic Association. (Level VII)
12 The Joint Commission. (2015). Standard NPSG.01.01.01. *Comprehensive accreditation manual for hospitals: The official handbook.* Oakbrook Terrace, IL: The Joint Commission. (Level VII)
13 Centers for Medicare & Medicaid Services, Department of Health and Human Services. (2014). Condition of participation: Patient's rights. 42 C.F.R. § 482.13(c)(1).
14 The Joint Commission. (2015). Standard RI.01.01.01. *Comprehensive accreditation manual for hospitals: The official handbook.* Oakbrook Terrace, IL: The Joint Commission. (Level VII)
15 American Osteopathic Association. (2014). Standard 15.01.16. *Healthcare Facilities Accreditation Program: Accreditation requirements for acute care hospitals.* Chicago, IL: American Osteopathic Association. (Level VII)
16 The Joint Commission. (2015). Standard RC.01.03.01. *Comprehensive accreditation manual for hospitals: The official handbook.* Oakbrook Terrace, IL: The Joint Commission. (Level VII)
17 Centers for Medicare & Medicaid Services, Department of Health and Human Services. (2014). Condition of participation: Medical record services. 42 C.F.R. § 482.24(b).
18 American Osteopathic Association. (2014). Standard 10.00.03. *Healthcare Facilities Accreditation Program: Accreditation requirements for acute care hospitals.* Chicago, IL: American Osteopathic Association. (Level VII)
19 Kaki, A. M., & Almarakbi, W. A. (2009). Does patient position influence the reading of the bispectral index monitor? *Anesthesia and Analgesia, 109,* 1843–1846. (Level VI)

Additional references

American Association of Neuroscience Nurses. (2010). *Core curriculum for neuroscience nursing* (5th ed.). Glenview, IL: American Association of Neuroscience Nurses.
Anderson, J., et al. (2010). Bispectral index monitoring to facilitate early extubation following cardiovascular surgery. *Clinical Nurse Specialist: The Journal for Advanced Nursing Practice, 24,* 140–148.
Quiraishi, S. A., et al. (2011). Bispectral index monitoring in the management of sedation in an intensive care unit patient with locked-in syndrome. *American Journal of Critical Care, 20,* 487–490.

Bladder ultrasonography

Urine retention, a potentially life-threatening condition, may result from neurologic or psychological disorders or obstruction of urine flow. It's also a common complication of some types of surgery.[1] Medications such as anticholinergics, antihistamines, and antidepressants, and analgesia (especially spinal and epidural) may also cause urine retention. Traditionally, the amount of urine retained in the bladder was measured by urinary catheterization, which placed the patient at risk for catheter-associated urinary tract infection. Bladder ultrasonography is a noninvasive method of assessing bladder volume with a lower risk of urinary tract infection.

HOSPITAL-ACQUIRED CONDITION ALERT *Keep in mind that a catheter-associated urinary tract infection is considered a hospital-acquired condition* because it can be reasonably prevented using best practices. *Use bladder ultrasonography (instead of catheterization) to assess bladder volume, as indicated,* to reduce the risk of catheter-associated urinary tract infections.[2,3,4,5,6]

Equipment

Bladder ultrasonography unit with probe ■ ultrasonic transmission gel ■ gauze pads ■ disinfectant pad ■ Optional: washcloth, gloves.

Implementation

- Verify the practitioner's order.
- Perform hand hygiene.[7,8,9,10,11]
- Confirm the patient's identity using at least two patient identifiers.[12]
- Bring the bladder ultrasonography unit to the bedside.
- Explain the procedure to the patient *to help reduce anxiety.*
- Provide privacy.[13,14,15]
- If this is a postvoiding scan, ask the patient to void; assist as necessary.
- Position the patient in the supine position with the head resting on a pillow *to prevent tightening of abdominal muscles, which may prevent scanning.*
- Perform hand hygiene.[7,8,9,10,11]
- Put on gloves as needed *to comply with standard precautions.*[16,17]
- Clean the rounded end of the ultrasonography probe with a disinfectant pad following the manufacturer's instructions.[18,19]
- Expose the patient's suprapubic area.
- Turn on the bladder ultrasonography unit by pressing the POWER button, and then select the proper examination mode *to ensure the accuracy of your scan.*
- Place ultrasonic transmission gel on the end of the probe *to promote an airtight seal for optimal sound wave transmission.*
- Tell the patient that the gel will feel cold when placed on the abdomen.
- Locate the symphysis pubis, and place the probe about 1″ (2.5 cm) superior to the symphysis pubis.
- Locate the icon (a rough figure of a patient) on the probe and make sure the head of the icon points toward the head of the patient.
- Press the SCAN button, marked with a sound-wave pattern, *to activate the scan.* Hold the probe steady until you hear the beep.
- Look at the aiming icon and the screen, which displays the bladder position and volume. Reposition the probe, and scan until the bladder is centered in the aiming screen. The largest measurement will be saved.
- Press DONE when finished.
- The bladder ultrasonography unit will display the measured urine volume and the longitudinal and horizontal axis scans.
- Press PRINT to obtain a hard copy of your results.
- Turn off the unit. Use a gauze pad to clean the gel off the probe.
- Using a gauze pad or washcloth, remove the gel from the patient's skin.
- Remove and discard your gloves, if worn.[16,17]
- Perform hand hygiene.[7,8,9,10,11]
- Clean and disinfect the unit, including the probe, using a disinfectant according to the scanner manufacturer's instructions.[18,19]
- Perform hand hygiene.[7,8,9,10,11]
- Notify the practitioner of the scan results, as indicated.[20]
- Document the procedure.[21,22,23]

Special considerations

- Some scanners require you to choose a sex. If a female patient has had a hysterectomy, select male.[20]
- If the postvoid residual volume (PRV) is more than 50% of the voided volume, the PRV is more than 600 mL, or the patient is uncomfortable and hasn't voided for longer than 5 hours, the practitioner may order catheterization. (See the "Indwelling urinary catheter insertion", and the "Intermittent urinary catheterization" procedures, pages 394, 409.)[20]
- Be aware that high PVR recorded by a bladder ultrasound scanner should correlate closely with the volume resulting from catheterization.

Any discrepancy in PVR volume between these two methods may indicate cystic or pelvic issues, which can cause falsely elevated PRV volumes.[24]

- In obsess patients or when there is an organ shift, the bladder may not be located in the usual position.[25]

Documentation

Record the patient's name, the date, and the time on the printout, and attach the printout to the patient's medical record. In the patient's medical record, also document the procedure, voided volume (if applicable), bladder scan urine volume, intermittent catheterization volume (if applicable), and the practitioner who was notified of the results, as well as whether it was a prevoid or postvoid scan.[25] Also document any treatment provided and the patient's response to the treatment.

REFERENCES

1 Griesdale, D. E., et al. (2011). Risk factors for urinary retention after hip or knee replacement: A cohort study. *Canadian Journal of Anaesthesia, 58,* 1097–1104. (Level VI)

2 Jarrett, N., et al. (2013). "Evidence-based guidelines for selected and previously considered hospital-acquired conditions: Final report" [Online]. Accessed March 2015 via the Web at http://www.cms.gov/Medicare/Medicare-Fee-for-Service-Payment/HospitalAcqCond/Downloads/Evidence-Based-Guidelines.pdf

3 Lo, E., et al. (2014). SHEA/IDSA practice recommendation: Strategies to prevent catheter-associated urinary tract infections in acute care hospitals: 2014 update. *Infection Control and Hospital Epidemiology, 35,* 464–479. Accessed March 2015 via the Web at http://www.jstor.org/stable/pdfplus/10.1086/675718.pdf?acceptTC=true&jpdConfirm=true (Level I)

4 Association of Professionals in Infection Control and Epidemiology (APIC). (2014). "APIC implementation guide: Guide to preventing catheter-associated urinary tract infections" [Online]. Accessed March 2015 via the Web at http://apic.org/Resource_/EliminationGuideForm/6473ab9b-e75c-457a-8d0f-d57d32bc242b/File/APIC_CAUTI_web_0603.pdf (Level IV)

5 American Osteopathic Association. (2014). Standard 07.01.02. *Healthcare Facilities Accreditation Program: Accreditation requirements for acute care hospitals.* Chicago, IL: American Osteopathic Association. (Level VII)

6 The Joint Commission. (2015). Standard NPSG.07.06.01. *Comprehensive accreditation manual for hospitals: The official handbook.* Oakbrook Terrace, IL: The Joint Commission. (Level VII)

7 The Joint Commission. (2015). Standard NPSG.07.01.01. *Comprehensive accreditation manual for hospitals: The official handbook.* Oakbrook Terrace, IL: The Joint Commission. (Level VII)

8 World Health Organization. (2009). "WHO guidelines on hand hygiene in health care: First global patient safety challenge, clean care is safer care" [Online]. Accessed March 2015 via the Web at http://whqlibdoc.who.int/publications/2009/9789241597906_eng.pdf (Level IV)

9 Centers for Disease Control and Prevention. (2002). Guideline for hand hygiene in health-care settings: Recommendations of the Healthcare Infection Control Practices Advisory Committee and the HICPAC/SHEA/APIC/IDSA Hand Hygiene Task Force. *MMWR Recommendations and Reports, 51*(RR-16), 1–45. Accessed March 2015 via the Web at http://www.cdc.gov/mmwr/pdf/rr/rr5116.pdf (Level II)

10 American Osteopathic Association. (2014). Standard 07.01.21. *Healthcare Facilities Accreditation Program: Accreditation requirements for acute care hospitals.* Chicago, IL: American Osteopathic Association. (Level VII)

11 Centers for Medicare & Medicaid Services, Department of Health and Human Services. (2014). Condition of participation: Infection control. 42 C.F.R. § 482.42.

12 The Joint Commission. (2015). Standard NPSG.01.01.01. *Comprehensive accreditation manual for hospitals: The official handbook.* Oakbrook Terrace, IL: The Joint Commission. (Level VII)

13 American Osteopathic Association. (2014). Standard 15.01.16. *Healthcare Facilities Accreditation Program: Accreditation requirements for acute care hospitals.* Chicago, IL: American Osteopathic Association. (Level VII)

14 The Joint Commission. (2015). Standard RI.01.01.01. *Comprehensive accreditation manual for hospitals: The official handbook.* Oakbrook Terrace, IL: The Joint Commission. (Level VII)

15 Centers for Medicare & Medicaid Services, Department of Health and Human Services. (2014). Condition of participation: Patient's rights. 42 C.F.R. § 482.13(c)(1).

16 Siegel, J. D., et al. (2007). "2007 guideline for isolation precautions: Preventing transmission of infectious agents in healthcare settings" [Online]. Accessed March 2015 via the Web at http://www.cdc.gov/hicpac/pdf/isolation/Isolation2007.pdf (Level II)

17 American Osteopathic Association. (2014). Standard 07.01.10. *Healthcare Facilities Accreditation Program: Accreditation requirements for acute care hospitals.* Chicago, IL: American Osteopathic Association. (Level VII)

18 Rutala, W. A., et al. (2008). "Guideline for disinfection and sterilization in healthcare facilities, 2008" [Online]. Accessed March 2015 via the Web at http://www.cdc.gov/hicpac/pdf/guidelines/Disinfection_Nov_2008.pdf (Level I)

19 American Osteopathic Association. (2014). Standard 07.02.03. *Healthcare Facilities Accreditation Program: Accreditation requirements for acute care hospitals.* Chicago, IL: American Osteopathic Association. (Level VII)

20 Agency for Clinical Innovation and the Urology Nursing Working Group. (2013). "Clinical guideline: Non real time bladder scanner" [Online]. Accessed March 2015 via the Web at http://www.aci.health.nsw.gov.au/__data/assets/pdf_file/0019/191062/ACI_Bladder_Scanner_Jan13.pdf (Level VII)

21 The Joint Commission. (2015). Standard RC.01.03.01. *Comprehensive accreditation manual for hospitals: The official handbook.* Oakbrook Terrace, IL: The Joint Commission. (Level VII)

22 American Osteopathic Association. (2014). Standard 10.00.03. *Healthcare Facilities Accreditation Program: Accreditation requirements for acute care hospitals.* Chicago, IL: American Osteopathic Association. (Level VII)

23 Centers for Medicare & Medicaid Services, Department of Health and Human Services. (2014). Condition of participation: Medical record services. 42 C.F.R. § 482.24(b).

24 Alagiakrishnan, K., & Valpreda, M. (2009). Ultrasound bladder scanner presents falsely elevated postvoid residual volumes. Canadian Family Physician, 55, 163–164. Accessed March 2015 via the Web at http://www.cfp.ca/content/55/2/163.full.pdf+html

25 Cowie, B. G. (2012). "Canadian Nurse Continence Advisors Association: Best practices: Bladder scan" [Online]. Accessed March 2015 via the Web at http://www.cnca.ca/pdf/Cowie%20-%20Bladder_Scan_07_Sept_12.pdf (Level VII)

ADDITIONAL REFERENCES

Dicuio, M., et al. (2010). Is it possible to predict post-residual voided urine by bladder scan before uroflowmetry—A useful and timesaving test to reduce the number of non-evaluable uroflow measurements? *Archives of Italian Urology and Andrology, 82,* 100–104.

Palese, A., et al. (2010). The effectiveness of the ultrasound bladder scanner in reducing urinary tract infections: A meta-analysis. *Journal of Clinical Nursing, 19,* 2970–2979. (Level I)

BLOOD CULTURE SAMPLE COLLECTION

Blood, which is normally bacteria-free, is susceptible to infection through intravascular catheters as well as from thrombophlebitis, infected shunts, or bacterial endocarditis due to prosthetic heart valve replacements. Bacteria may also invade the vascular system from local tissue infections through the lymphatic system and the thoracic duct.

Blood cultures detect bacterial invasion in the blood (bacteremia) and the systemic spread of such an infection (septicemia) through the bloodstream. Blood culture sample collection involves collecting a venous blood sample by venipuncture at the patient's bedside and transferring the sample into two bottles, one containing an anaerobic medium and the other, an aerobic medium. The bottles undergo incubation, which encourages organisms present in the sample to grow in the media. Blood cultures allow identification of about 67% of pathogens within 24 hours and up to 90% within 72 hours. If possible, blood cultures should be collected before starting antimicrobial

Collecting blood culture samples from a central venous access catheter

If the patient has no obvious source of infection and you suspect a catheter-related bloodstream infection, withdraw one set of samples from the distal lumen of the catheter and one set of samples peripherally.[3] If you need to obtain two sets from the central venous access catheter, withdraw two blood samples through different lumens, if available.[3,4] If only one lumen is available, withdraw two separate samples through the same lumen on separate occasions.[4]

Implementation

- Verify the practitioner's orders.
- Gather the appropriate equipment.
- Check the expiration dates on the culture bottles and replace outdated bottles.
- Perform hand hygiene and put on gloves.[7,8,9,10,11]
- Confirm the patient's identity using at least two patient identifiers.[12]
- Tell the patient you need to collect a series of blood samples *to check for infection.*
- Turn off all infusions for 3 to 5 minutes, depending on the patient's condition.[3]
- Clamp the catheter *to prevent accidental exposure to blood and to reduce the risk of air embolism.*[13]
- Change the needleless injection cap of the lumen you'll be using to obtain the blood culture specimen *to reduce the risk of contamination and false-positive results.*[2,3,13,14]
- Thoroughly disinfect the needleless connector with an antiseptic pad using friction.[15] Allow it to dry.
- Connect the empty syringe to the catheter, release the clamp, and withdraw 10 to 20 mL of blood.[1] Don't discard this first-drawn blood; this is the blood sample that you'll be injecting into the culture bottle.[2,13]
- Clamp the catheter and remove the syringe.
- Thoroughly disinfect the injection cap with an antiseptic pad using friction.[15] Allow it to dry.
- Connect the syringe with preservative-free normal saline solution, open the clamp, flush the device, and close the clamp according to the type of needleless connector used.[13,14]
- Clean the diaphragm tops of the culture bottles with an alcohol pad.[1]
- Inject the blood into each bottle using a needleless transfer device, dividing it between the two bottles.[1]
- Label the culture bottles with the patient's name and identification number, the date and time of specimen collection, and the contents of the culture bottles in the presence of the patient *to prevent mislabeling.*[12,13,14]
- Discard used supplies in the appropriate containers.[10]
- Remove and discard your gloves and perform hand hygiene.[7,8,9,11]
- Place the samples in a laboratory biohazard transport bag and, along with the laboratory request form, immediately send them to the laboratory.
- Perform hand hygiene.[7,8,9,11]
- Document the procedure.[16,17]

therapy because antimicrobial therapy may interfere with bacterial growth.[1,2,3]

Ideally, you should obtain blood specimens for culture from two to four blood draws from separate venipuncture sites, not through a vascular catheter. Perform these blood draws simultaneously or over a short period (within a few hours).[4,5,6] Although blood culture specimens collected from central venous catheters are associated with higher false-positive rates, you may do so if you suspect a catheter-related bloodstream infection.[3] (See *Collecting blood culture samples from a central venous access catheter.*) If you suspect such an infection, withdraw one set of blood cultures through the device and one set from a separate venipuncture. Blood cultures from both the catheter and venipuncture should be positive for the same organism, with associated clinical signs and symptoms and no other recognized source. A positive culture from the device only most likely stems from a contaminant and the patient shouldn't receive treatment.[1]

Equipment

Tourniquet ▪ gloves ▪ antiseptic pad (chlorhexidine-based, tincture of iodine, or alcohol) ▪ alcohol pad ▪ 20-mL syringes (one syringe for each set of cultures) ▪ 20G 1½″ (3.8-cm) needles ▪ blood culture bottles (aerobic and anaerobic) ▪ laboratory request form ▪ laboratory biohazard transport bag ▪ 2″ × 2″ (5-cm × 5-cm) sterile gauze pads ▪ small adhesive bandages ▪ labels ▪ needleless transfer devices.

Preparation of equipment

Check the expiration dates on the culture bottles and replace outdated bottles.

Implementation

- Verify the practitioner's order.
- Gather and prepare the appropriate equipment.
- Perform hand hygiene and put on gloves.[7,8,9,10,11,18,19]
- Confirm the patient's identity using at least two patient identifiers.[12]
- Tell the patient that you need to collect a series of blood samples *to check for infection.* Explain the procedure *to ease his anxiety and promote cooperation.* Explain that the procedure usually requires two blood samples collected from two different sites.
- Apply a tourniquet 2″ (5 cm) proximal to the area chosen for the venipuncture. (See the "Venipuncture" procedure, page 821.)
- Clean the venipuncture site with an antiseptic pad such as chlorhexidine, and allow it to dry.[2,3,13]
- Perform a venipuncture, drawing 10 to 20 mL of blood.[1]
- Remove the tourniquet. Apply pressure to the venipuncture site using a sterile 2″ × 2″ (5-cm × 5-cm) gauze pad. Then cover the site with a small adhesive bandage.
- Disinfect the diaphragm tops of the culture bottles with an alcohol pad.[1]
- Divide the blood by injecting the appropriate amount into each culture bottle using a needleless transfer device *to ensure the most accurate test results.*[1]
- Label the culture bottles with the patient's name and identification number, the date and time of the specimen collection, and the contents of the culture bottles in the presence of the patient *to prevent mislabeling.*[12,13]
- Discard syringes and needles in the appropriate containers.[10]
- Remove and discard your gloves and perform hand hygiene.[7,8,9,11]
- Place the sample in a laboratory biohazard transport bag and, along with the laboratory request form, immediately send them to the laboratory.
- Perform hand hygiene.[7,8,9,11,18]
- Document the procedure.[16,17,20]

Special considerations

- If a patient presents with severe sepsis, obtain blood cultures before administering antimicrobial therapy if doing so won't cause a significant delay (greater than 45 minutes) in starting therapy. Obtain at least two sets of blood cultures (aerobic and anaerobic bottles), with at least one drawn percutaneously and one drawn through each vascular access device, unless the device was inserted within the past 48 hours.[21]

Complications

The most common complication of venipuncture is the formation of a hematoma. Improper technique may cause false-positive results, leading to inappropriate antimicrobial use.

Documentation

Record the date and time of blood sample collection, the name of the test, the amount of blood collected, the number of bottles used, the patient's temperature, and any adverse reactions to the procedure.

References

1 Septimus, E. (2012). "Get smart for healthcare: Clinician guide" [Online]. Accessed March 2015 via the Web at http://www.cdc.gov/getsmart/healthcare/learn-from-others/resources/clinician-guide.html

2 Standard 49. Infection. Infusion nursing standards of practice. (2011). *Journal of Infusion Nursing, 34,* S68–S69. (Level I)

3 Halm, M., et al. (2011). Blood cultures and central catheters: Is the "easiest way" best practice? *American Journal of Critical Care, 20,* 335–338.

4 Centers for Disease Control and Prevention. (2013). "Device-associated module: Central line–associated bloodstream infection (CLABSI) event" [Online]. Accessed March 2015 via the Web at http://www.cdc.gov/nhsn/pdfs/pscmanual/4psc_clabscurrent.pdf

5 Clinical and Laboratory Standards Institute (CLSI). (2007). *Principles and procedure for blood cultures: Approved guideline (CLSI document M47-A).* Wayne, PA: Clinical and Laboratory Standards Institute.

6 Baron, E. J., et al. (2005). *Cumitech 1C: Blood cultures IV.* Washington, DC: ASM Press.

7 The Joint Commission. (2015). Standard NPSG.07.01.01. *Comprehensive accreditation manual for hospitals: The official handbook.* Oakbrook Terrace, IL: The Joint Commission. (Level VII)

8 Centers for Disease Control and Prevention. (2002). Guideline for hand hygiene in health-care settings: Recommendations of the Healthcare Infection Control Practices Advisory Committee and the HICPAC/SHEA/APIC/IDSA Hand Hygiene Task Force. *MMWR Recommendations and Reports, 51*(RR-16), 1–45. Accessed March 2015 via the Web at http://www.cdc.gov/mmwr/pdf/rr/rr5116.pdf (Level II)

9 World Health Organization. (2009). "WHO guidelines on hand hygiene in health care: First global patient safety challenge, clean care is safer care" [Online]. Accessed March 2015 via the Web at http://whqlibdoc.who.int/publications/2009/9789241597906_eng.pdf (Level IV)

10 Occupational Safety and Health Administration. (n.d.). "Bloodborne pathogens, standard number 1910.1030" [Online]. Accessed March 2015 via the Web at http://www.osha.gov/pls/oshaweb/owadisp.show_document?p_table=STANDARDS&p_id=10051 (Level VII)

11 Centers for Medicare & Medicaid Services, Department of Health and Human Services. (2014). Condition of participation: Infection control. 42 C.F.R. § 482.42.

12 The Joint Commission. (2015). Standard NPSG.01.01.01. *Comprehensive accreditation manual for hospitals: The official handbook.* Oakbrook Terrace, IL: The Joint Commission. (Level VII)

13 Infusion Nurses Society. (2011). *Policies and procedures for infusion nursing* (4th ed.). Boston, MA: Infusion Nurses Society.

14 Infusion Nurses Society. (2013). *Policies and procedures for infusion nursing of the older adult* (2nd ed.). Boston, MA: Infusion Nurses Society.

15 Centers for Disease Control and Prevention. (2011). "Guidelines for the prevention of intravascular catheter-related infections" [Online]. Accessed March 2015 via the Web at http://www.cdc.gov/hicpac/pdf/guidelines/bsi-guidelines-2011.pdf (Level I)

16 The Joint Commission. (2015). Standard RC.01.03.01. *Comprehensive accreditation manual for hospitals: The official handbook.* Oakbrook Terrace, IL: The Joint Commission. (Level VII)

17 Centers for Medicare & Medicaid Services, Department of Health and Human Services. (2014). Condition of participation: Medical record services. 42 C.F.R. § 482.24(b).

18 American Osteopathic Association. (2014). Standard 07.01.21. *Healthcare Facilities Accreditation Program: Accreditation requirements for acute care hospitals.* Chicago, IL: American Osteopathic Association. (Level VII)

19 American Osteopathic Association. (2014). Standard 07.01.10. *Healthcare Facilities Accreditation Program: Accreditation requirements for acute care hospitals.* Chicago, IL: American Osteopathic Association. (Level VII)

20 American Osteopathic Association. (2014). Standard 10.00.03. *Healthcare Facilities Accreditation Program: Accreditation requirements for acute care hospitals.* Chicago, IL: American Osteopathic Association (Level VII)

21 Dellinger, R. P. (2013). Surviving sepsis campaign: International guidelines for management of severe sepsis and septic shock: 2012. *Critical Care Medicine, 41,* 580–637. (Level I)

Additional references

Craven, R. F., & Hirnle, C. J. (2012). *Fundamentals of nursing: Human health and function* (7th ed.). Philadelphia, PA: Lippincott Williams & Wilkins.

Fischbach, F., & Dunning, M. B. (2014). *A manual of laboratory and diagnostic tests* (9th ed.). Philadelphia, PA: Wolters Kluwer.

Institute for Healthcare Improvement. (2013). "Timing of blood cultures" [Online]. Accessed March 2015 via the Web at http://www.ihi.org/knowledge/Pages/Measures/TimingofBloodCultures.aspx

Standard 57. Phlebotomy. Infusion nursing standards of practice. (2011). *Journal of Infusion Nursing, 34,* S78–S79. (Level VII)

Blood glucose monitoring

Blood glucose meters measure blood glucose concentrations. A drop of blood is placed on a blood glucose test strip either before or after the strip is inserted into the meter, depending on the type of blood glucose meter used. A portable blood glucose meter provides quantitative measurements that compare in accuracy with other laboratory tests. Most meters store successive test results electronically to help determine glucose patterns. If a glucose result doesn't correlate with the patient's clinical condition, the result should be confirmed through conventional laboratory sampling of plasma glucose.[1]

For a patient who's receiving nutrition, the timing of glucose monitoring should match carbohydrate intake. For a patient who isn't receiving nutrition, blood glucose monitoring should be performed every 4 to 6 hours. More frequent monitoring, ranging from every 30 minutes to every 2 hours, is required for a patient receiving an IV insulin infusion.[1]

In a hospitalized patient, hyperglycemia is defined as any blood glucose level greater than 140 mg/dL (7.8 mmol/L). Levels significantly and persistently higher than this may require treatment. Hypoglycemia is defined as a blood glucose level less than 70 mg/dL (3.9 mmol/L); cognitive impairment commonly occurs at around 50 mg/dL (2.8 mmol/L). Early recognition and treatment of moderate to mild hypoglycemia (between 40 and 69 mg/dL [2.2 and 3.8 mmol/L]) can prevent a patient from deteriorating to severe hypoglycemia.[1]

The Centers for Disease Control and Prevention recommends that, whenever possible, blood glucose meters shouldn't be shared. If a device must be shared, it should be cleaned and disinfected after every use, following the manufacturer's instructions, *to prevent carryover of blood and infectious agents.* If the manufacturer doesn't specify how the device should be cleaned and disinfected, then it shouldn't be shared. Single-use, auto-disabling fingerstick devices should also be used *to prevent the spread of bloodborne pathogens.*[1,2,3]

Equipment

Gloves ■ portable blood glucose meter ■ alcohol pads ■ disinfectant pads ■ gauze pads ■ single-use, auto-disabling lancet[4] ■ blood glucose test strips ■ Optional: small adhesive bandage; barcode scanner; warm, moist compresses; soap; water; towel.

Preparation of equipment

Check the expiration date on the test strips. Make sure that the cap on the vial of strips is properly secured, and observe the strip for discoloration. *Strips are sensitive to light and humidity and may become inactivated.* Calibrate and run the blood glucose meter with a quality-control test following the manufacturer's instructions *to ensure accurate test results.* Most hospital-based glucose meters must have quality-control tests performed every 24 hours. Follow the manufacturer's instructions for calibration.

Before testing, turn on the meter. If appropriate, ensure that the code strip number on the test strip matches the code number on the meter. Enter your operator identification and password, if required. Enter and then confirm the patient's identification information, either manually or by using a barcode scanner, if available; if the patient information has already been entered by another user, confirm it.

Implementation

- Verify the practitioner's order.
- Gather and prepare the appropriate equipment
- Perform hand hygiene and put on gloves.[5,6,7,8,9,10,11]
- Confirm the patient's identity using at least two patient identifiers.[12]
- Explain the procedure to the patient.
- Select the puncture site—usually the fingertip in adults.[13] Some devices allow for collection from alternative sites; consult the manufacturer's instructions.
- If necessary, dilate the capillaries by applying warm, moist compresses to the area for about 10 minutes.
- If the patient is able, have her wash her hands with soap and water and then dry them *to remove any sugar may remain on her skin after exposure to sugar-containing products.*[14] If the patient can't wash her hands, clean the intended puncture site with an alcohol pad and allow it to dry completely *because alcohol may interfere with test results if not permitted to dry completely* (as shown below).[13]

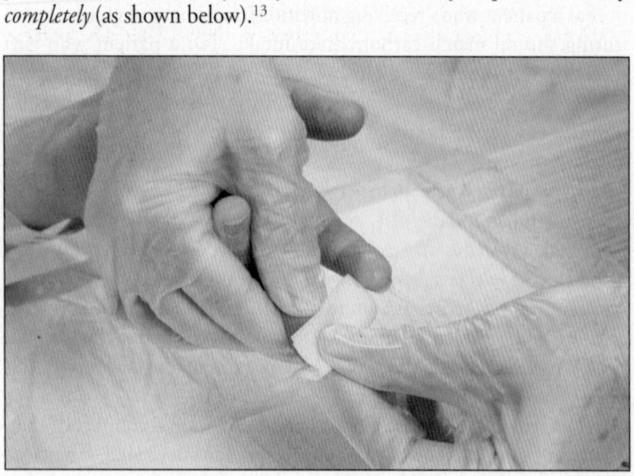

- Insert the test strip into the blood glucose meter, according to the manufacturer's instructions.

Alternatively, some meters require that you insert the test strip after applying the blood sample (as shown on top right).

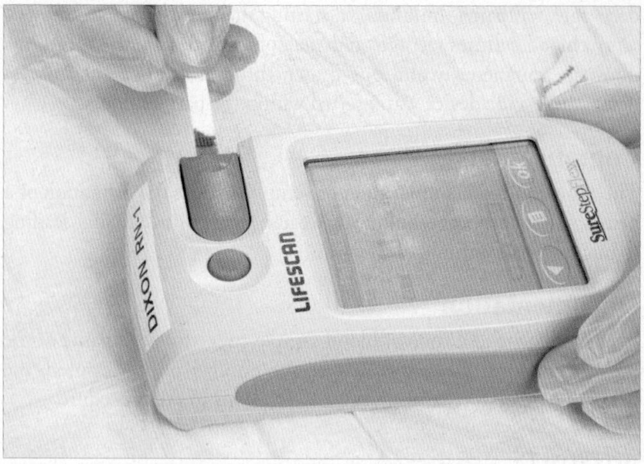

- To collect a sample from the fingertip, use a single-use, auto-disabling lancet on the side of the patient's fingertip perpendicular to the lines of the fingerprints.[2,13] Puncture the skin with a quick, continuous, and deliberate stroke (as shown below) *to achieve a good flow of blood and to prevent the need to repeat the puncture.*[13]

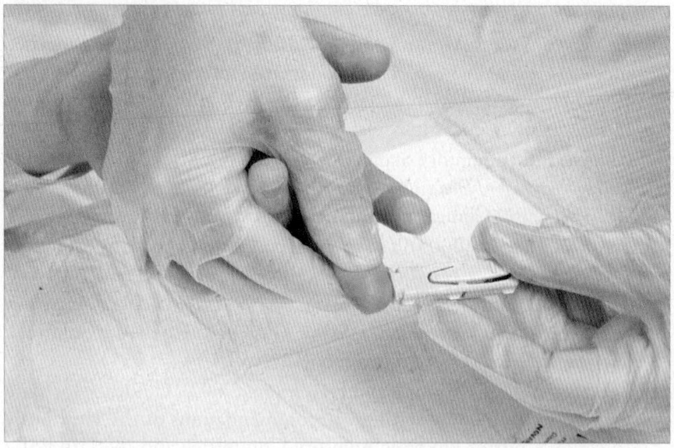

- If required by your facility, wipe away the first drop of blood using a gauze pad *because it may be contaminated with tissue, fluid, or debris.*[13]
- Touch a drop of blood to the test area of the test strip; make sure the entire test area is covered. Some meters require a hanging drop; refer to the manufacturer's instructions for use. Don't squeeze the patient's finger too tightly *because doing so may dilute the specimen with plasma.*[13]
- After collecting the blood sample, apply firm pressure to the puncture site *to stop the bleeding.*
- Read the digital display on the blood glucose meter when the alarm sounds.
- Discard the lancet in a puncture-resistant sharps container.[2,8]
- Remove the test strip and dispose of it properly.[8]
- After bleeding has stopped, you may apply a small adhesive bandage to the puncture site, if necessary.
- Remove and discard your gloves, and perform hand hygiene.[5,6,7,9]

NURSING ALERT ***If you obtain an extremely low or high blood glucose meter result, obtain a serum blood glucose level immediately to confirm the result.***

- Clean and disinfect the blood glucose meter with a disinfectant pad, following the blood glucose meter manufacturer's instructions.[1,2,15] *Contaminated blood glucose monitoring equipment increases the risk of infection by such bloodborne pathogens as hepatitis B, hepatitis C, and human immunodeficiency viruses.*[1,2,16]
- Perform hand hygiene.[5,6,7,9,17]
- Report critical test results to the practitioner within the time period specified by your facility *to prevent treatment delays.*[10]
- Document the procedure.[18,19,20]

Oral and IV glucose tolerance tests

For monitoring trends in glucose metabolism, two tests may offer benefits over testing blood with test strips.

Oral glucose tolerance test

The most sensitive test for detecting borderline diabetes mellitus, the oral glucose tolerance test (OGTT) measures carbohydrate metabolism after ingestion of a challenge dose of glucose. The body absorbs this dose rapidly, causing plasma glucose levels to rise and peak within 30 minutes to 1 hour. The pancreas responds by secreting insulin, causing glucose levels to return to normal within 2 to 3 hours. During this period, plasma and urine glucose levels are monitored *to assess insulin secretion and the body's ability to metabolize glucose.*

Although you may not collect the blood and urine specimens (usually five of each) required for this test, you will be responsible for preparing the patient for the test and monitoring his physical condition during the test.

Begin by explaining the OGTT to the patient. Then, tell the patient to maintain a high-carbohydrate diet for 3 days and to fast for 10 to 16 hours before the test, as ordered. The patient must not smoke, drink coffee or alcohol, or exercise strenuously for 8 hours before or during the test. Inform him that he'll then receive a challenge dose of 100 g of carbohydrate (usually a sweetened carbonated beverage or gelatin).

Inform the patient who will perform the venipunctures and when, and explain that the needle punctures and the pressure of the tourniquet may cause slight discomfort. Reassure the patient that collecting each blood sample usually takes less than 3 minutes. As ordered, withhold drugs that may affect test results. Remind him to save the first urine specimen voided after waking on the day of the test.

During the test period, watch for signs and symptoms of hypoglycemia—weakness, restlessness, nervousness, hunger, and sweating—and report these to the practitioner immediately. Encourage the patient to drink plenty of water *to promote adequate urine excretion*. Provide a bedpan, urinal, or specimen container when necessary.

IV glucose tolerance test

This test may be chosen for patients who can't absorb an oral dose of glucose—for example, those with malabsorption disorders or short-bowel syndrome or those who have had a gastrectomy. This test measures blood glucose after an IV infusion of 50% glucose over 3 or 4 minutes. Blood samples are then drawn after 30 minutes, 1 hour, 2 hours, and 3 hours. After an immediate glucose peak of 300 to 400 mg/dL (16.7 to 22.2 mmol/L) accompanied by glycosuria, the normal glucose curve falls steadily, reaching fasting levels within 1 to 1¼ hours. Failure to achieve fasting glucose levels within 2 to 3 hours typically confirms diabetes.

Special considerations

- Don't select cold, cyanotic, or swollen puncture sites *to ensure an adequate blood sample.* If you can't obtain a capillary sample, perform a venipuncture and place a large drop of venous blood on the test strip. If you want to test blood from a refrigerated sample, allow the blood to return to room temperature before testing it.
- *To help detect abnormal glucose metabolism and diagnose diabetes mellitus,* the practitioner may order other blood glucose tests. (See *Oral and IV glucose tolerance tests.*)
- Store the test strips away from heat and humidity *because these conditions can affect the accuracy of the results.*

Patient teaching

Teach the patient who will be performing blood glucose monitoring at home the proper use of the lancet and portable blood glucose meter, as necessary. Also teach the importance of washing the hands with soap and water, drying them, and then using the first drop of blood for self-monitoring of blood glucose level. If handwashing isn't possible and the patient's hands aren't visibly soiled or exposed to sugar-containing products, advise the patient to use the second drop of blood after wiping away the first drop.[14] Provide the patient with written instructions.

Documentation

Record the date and the time of testing and results in the patient's medical records. Document the date, the time, and the name of the practitioner notified of the test results, if necessary. Record any prescribed interventions and the patient's response to those interventions. Document teaching provided to the patient and family and their comprehension of the teaching.

REFERENCES

1 American Diabetes Association. (2013). Standards of medical care in diabetes—2013. *Diabetes Care, 36,* S11–S66. Accessed March 2015 via the Web at http://care.diabetesjournals.org/content/36/Supplement_1/S11.full (Level VII)

2 Centers for Disease Control and Prevention. (2012). "Infection prevention during blood glucose monitoring and insulin administration" [Online]. Accessed March 2015 via the Web at http://www.cdc.gov/injectionsafety/blood-glucose-monitoring.html#Best

3 Klonoff, D. C., & Perz, J. F. (2010). Assisted monitoring of blood glucose: Special safety needs for a new paradigm in testing glucose. *Journal of Diabetes Science and Technology, 4,* 1027–1031.

4 U.S. Food and Drug Administration. (2010). "Use of fingerstick devices on more than one person poses risk for transmitting bloodborne pathogens: Initial communication: Update 11/29/2010" [Online]. Accessed March 2015 via the Web at http://www.fda.gov/MedicalDevices/Safety/AlertsandNotices/ucm224025.htm.

5 The Joint Commission. (2015). Standard NPSG.07.01.01. *Comprehensive accreditation manual for hospitals: The official handbook.* Oakbrook Terrace, IL: The Joint Commission. (Level VII)

6 Centers for Disease Control and Prevention. (2002). Guideline for hand hygiene in health-care settings: Recommendations of the Healthcare Infection Control Practices Advisory Committee and the HICPAC/SHEA/APIC/IDSA Hand Hygiene Task Force. *MMWR Recommendations and Reports, 51*(RR-16), 1–45. Accessed March 2015 via the Web at http://www.cdc.gov/mmwr/pdf/rr/rr5116.pdf (Level II)

7 World Health Organization. (2009). "WHO guidelines on hand hygiene in health care: First global patient safety challenge, clean care is safer care" [Online]. Accessed March 2015 via the Web at http://whqlibdoc.who.int/publications/2009/9789241597906_eng.pdf (Level IV)

8 Occupational Safety and Health Administration. (n.d.). "Bloodborne pathogens, standard number 1910.1030" [Online]. Accessed March 2015 via the Web at http://www.osha.gov/pls/oshaweb/owadisp.show_document?p_table=STANDARDS&p_id=10051 (Level VII)

9 Centers for Medicare & Medicaid Services, Department of Health and Human Services. (2014). Condition of participation: Infection control. 42 C.F.R. § 482.42.

10 The Joint Commission. (2015). Standard NPSG.02.03.01. *Comprehensive accreditation manual for hospitals: The official handbook.* Oakbrook Terrace, IL: The Joint Commission. (Level VII)

11 American Osteopathic Association. (2014). Standard 07.01.10. *Healthcare Facilities Accreditation Program: Accreditation requirements for acute*

care hospitals. Chicago, IL: American Osteopathic Association. (Level VII)

12 The Joint Commission. (2015). Standard NPSG.01.01.01. *Comprehensive accreditation manual for hospitals: The official handbook.* Oakbrook Terrace, IL: The Joint Commission. (Level VII)

13 World Health Organization. (2010). "WHO guidelines on drawing blood: Best practices in phlebotomy" [Online]. Accessed March 2015 via the Web at http://www.who.int/injection_safety/phleb_final_screen_ready.pdf

14 Hortensius, J., et al. (2011). Self-monitoring of blood glucose: The use of the first or the second drop of blood. *Diabetes Care, 34,* 556–560. Accessed March 2015 via the Web at http://care.diabetesjournals.org/content/34/3/556.full (Level II)

15 Rutala, W. A., et al. (2008). "Guideline for disinfection and sterilization in healthcare facilities, 2008" [Online]. Accessed March 2015 via the Web at http://www.cdc.gov/hicpac/pdf/guidelines/Disinfection_Nov_2008.pdf (Level I)

16 American Osteopathic Association. (2014). Standard 07.02.03. *Healthcare Facilities Accreditation Program: Accreditation requirements for acute care hospitals.* Chicago, IL: American Osteopathic Association. (Level VII)

17 American Osteopathic Association. (2014). Standard 07.01.21. *Healthcare Facilities Accreditation Program: Accreditation requirements for acute care hospitals.* Chicago, IL: American Osteopathic Association. (Level VII)

18 The Joint Commission. (2015). Standard NPSG.01.01.01. *Comprehensive accreditation manual for hospitals: The official handbook.* Oakbrook Terrace, IL: The Joint Commission. (Level VII)

19 Centers for Medicare & Medicaid Services, Department of Health and Human Services. (2014). Condition of participation: Medical record services. 42 C.F.R. § 482.24(b).

20 American Osteopathic Association. (2014). Standard 07.01.10. *Healthcare Facilities Accreditation Program: Accreditation requirements for acute care hospitals.* Chicago, IL: American Osteopathic Association. (Level VII)

Additional references

Craven, R. F., & Hirnle, C. J. (2012). *Fundamentals of nursing: Human health and function* (7th ed.). Philadelphia, PA: Lippincott Williams & Wilkins.

Goldstein, D. E., et al. (2004). Tests of glycemia in diabetes. *Diabetes Care, 27,* S91–S93.

Blood pressure assessment

Defined as the lateral force exerted by blood on the arterial walls, blood pressure depends on the force of ventricular contractions, arterial wall elasticity, peripheral vascular resistance, and blood volume and viscosity. Systolic, or maximum, pressure occurs during left ventricular contraction and reflects the integrity of the heart, arteries, and arterioles. Diastolic, or minimum, pressure occurs during left ventricular relaxation and directly indicates blood vessel resistance.

Pulse pressure, the difference between systolic and diastolic pressures, varies inversely with arterial elasticity. Rigid vessels, incapable of distention and recoil, produce high systolic pressure and low diastolic pressure. Normally, systolic pressure exceeds diastolic pressure by about 40 mm Hg. Narrowed pulse pressure—a difference of less than 30 mm Hg—occurs when systolic pressure falls and diastolic pressure rises. These changes reflect reduced stroke volume, increased peripheral resistance, or both. Widened pulse pressure—a difference of more than 50 mm Hg between systolic and diastolic pressures—occurs when systolic pressure rises and diastolic pressure remains constant, or when systolic pressure rises and diastolic pressure falls. These changes reflect increased stroke volume, decreased peripheral resistance, or both.

Frequent blood pressure measurement is critical after serious injury, surgery, or anesthesia and during any illness or condition that threatens cardiovascular stability. (Frequent measurement may be performed with an automated vital signs monitor.) Regular measurement is indicated for patients with a history of hypertension or hypotension, and annual screening is recommended for all adults.

To measure blood pressure in the upper arm, use the auscultatory or oscillatory method. If you can't use the upper arm or if the maximum-sized blood pressure cuff doesn't properly fit, you can measure blood pressure in the forearm; if you can't use the arms at all, measure blood pressure in the calf or thigh. To obtain a baseline measurement, measure blood pressure in both arms. If there's a significant difference in blood pressure between the arms, use the arm with the higher pressure, and continue to monitor blood pressure in the same arm, using the same device *to ensure accurate measurement.*[1]

The "2014 Evidence-Based Guidelines for the Management of High Blood Pressure in Adults: Report of the Panel Members Appointed to the Eighth Joint National Committee (JNC8)" recommends treating hypertensive patients aged 60 years or older to achieve a blood pressure goal of less than 150/90 mm Hg; for patients ages 30 to 59 years, the panel recommends treatment to achieve a diastolic blood pressure goal of less than 90 mm Hg. Because there's insufficient evidence for a systolic goal in patients younger than age 60 or a diastolic goal in patients younger than age 30, the panel recommends a treatment goal for these patients of less than 140/90 mm Hg, based solely on expert opinion.[2]

Equipment

Aneroid sphygmomanometer ■ stethoscope ■ hospital-grade disinfectant pads ■ Optional: automated vital signs monitor.

A sphygmomanometer consists of an inflatable compression cuff linked to a manual air pump and an aneroid gauge. Use a recently calibrated aneroid gauge.[3] To obtain an accurate reading, you can rest the gauge in any position, but view it directly from the front.

Cuffs come in sizes ranging from newborn to extra-large adult. Disposable cuffs and thigh cuffs are available. Use an appropriate-sized cuff and follow the manufacturer's instructions for proper fit and placement.[1]

An automated vital signs monitor is a noninvasive device that measures pulse rate, systolic and diastolic pressures, and mean arterial pressure at preset intervals. (See *Using an electronic vital signs monitor.*)

Preparation of equipment

Carefully choose a cuff of appropriate size for the patient; the bladder should encircle at least 80% of the upper arm.[1,4] *An excessively narrow cuff may cause a falsely high pressure reading; an excessively wide one, a falsely low reading.*[5] (For information on other situations that can cause false-high or false-low readings, see *Correcting problems of blood pressure measurement,* page 86.) If you aren't using your own stethoscope, disinfect the earpieces with a disinfectant pad before placing them in your ears *to avoid cross-contamination.*[6]

To use an automated vital signs monitor, collect the monitor, dual air hose, and pressure cuff. Then make sure the monitor unit is firmly positioned near the patient's bed.

Implementation

- Gather and prepare the appropriate equipment.
- Perform hand hygiene.[7,8,9,10,11]
- Confirm the patient's identity using at least two patient identifiers.[12]
- Have the patient rest for at least 5 minutes before measuring his blood pressure. Make sure he hasn't smoked or had caffeine for at least 30 minutes.
- Tell the patient that you're going to measure his blood pressure.
- Place the patient in the supine position, or have him sit erect during blood pressure measurement in the upper arms. If the patient is sitting erect, make sure his back and arms are supported, his legs are uncrossed,

EQUIPMENT

Using an electronic vital signs monitor

An electronic vital signs monitor allows you to track a patient's vital signs continually, without having to reapply a blood pressure cuff each time. In addition, the patient won't need an invasive arterial line to gather similar data.

Some automated vital signs monitors are lightweight and battery-operated and can be attached to an IV pole for continuous monitoring, even during patient transfers. Make sure you know the capacity of the monitor's battery and plug the machine in whenever possible *to keep it charged.* Regularly calibrate the monitor *to ensure accurate readings.*

Before using any monitor, check its accuracy. Oscillatory devices should meet the Association for the Advancement of Medical Instrumentation standards when compared with the auscultatory method.[1] Determine the patient's pulse rate and blood pressure manually, using the same arm you'll use for the monitor cuff. Compare your results when you get initial readings from the monitor. If the results differ, call your supply department or the manufacturer's representative.

Check the manufacturer's guidelines *because most automated monitoring devices are intended for serial monitoring only and may be inaccurate for a one-time measurement.*

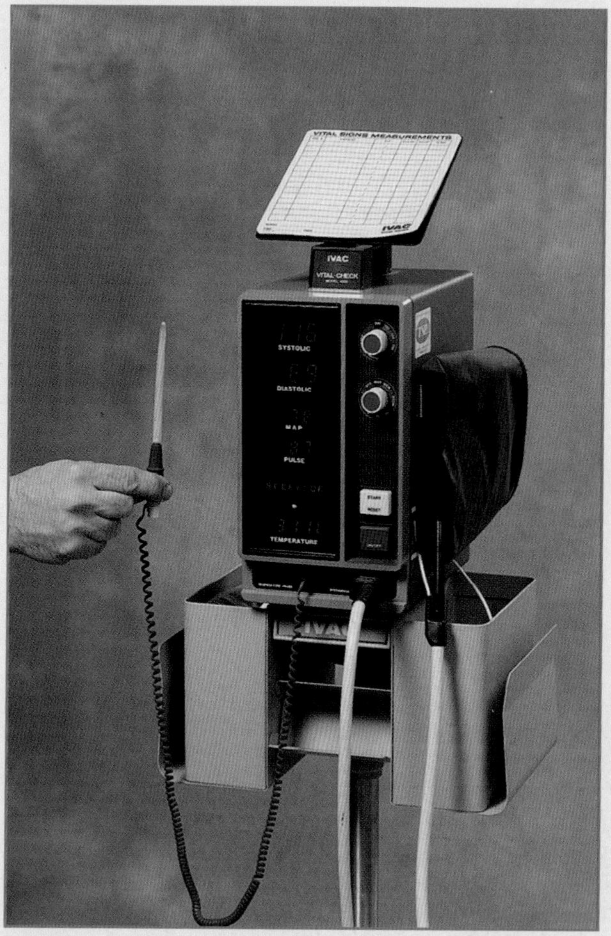

Preparing the device

- Explain the procedure to the patient. Describe the alarm system *so he won't be frightened if it's triggered.*
- Make sure the power switch is off. Then plug the monitor into a properly grounded wall outlet.
- Secure the dual air hose to the front of the monitor.
- Connect the pressure cuff's tubing into the other ends of the dual air hose, and tighten connections *to prevent air leaks.* Keep the air hose away from the patient *to avoid accidental dislodgment.*
- Squeeze all air from the cuff and wrap it loosely around the patient's arm about 3/4" to 1" (2 to 2.5 cm) above the antecubital fossa. Never apply the cuff to a limb that has an IV catheter in place. Position the cuff's "artery" arrow over the palpated brachial artery. Then secure the cuff for a snug fit.[1]

Selecting parameters

- When you turn on the monitor, it will default to a manual mode. (In this mode, you can obtain vital signs yourself before switching to the automatic mode.) Press the AUTO/MANUAL button to select the automatic mode. The monitor will give you baseline data for the pulse rate, systolic and diastolic pressures, and mean arterial pressure.
- Compare your previous manual results with these baseline data. If they match, you're ready to set the alarm parameters. Press the SELECT button to blank out all displays except systolic pressure.
- Use the HIGH and LOW limit buttons to set the specific parameters for systolic pressure. (These limits range from a high of 240 mm Hg to a low of 0 mm Hg.) You'll also do this three more times for mean arterial pressure, pulse rate, and diastolic pressure. After you've set the parameters for diastolic pressure, press the SELECT button again to display all current data. Even if you forget to do this last step, the monitor will automatically display current data 10 seconds after you set the last parameters.

Collecting data

- You also need to program the monitor according to the desired frequency. Press the SET button until you reach the desired time interval in minutes. If you've chosen the automatic mode, the monitor will display a default cycle time of 3 minutes. A 1-minute interval between inflations of the cuff is necessary *to avoid venous congestion.*[1] You can override the default cycle time to set the interval you prefer.
- You can obtain a set of vital signs at any time by pressing the START button.
- Pressing the CANCEL button will stop the interval and deflate the cuff.
- You can retrieve stored data by pressing the PRIOR DATA button. The monitor will display the last data obtained, along with the time elapsed since then. Scrolling backward, you can retrieve data from the previous 99 minutes.
- Make sure that the patient's vital signs are documented frequently on a vital sign assessment sheet.

and both feet are on the floor *because crossing the legs may increase blood pressure.*[1,2,13,14,15] His arm should be extended at heart level (the phlebostatic axis, fourth intercostal space, halfway between the anterior and posterior diameter of the chest) and well supported.[1] *If the artery is below heart level, you may get a false-high reading.*[16]

- Make sure the patient is relaxed and comfortable when you measure his blood pressure *so it stays at its normal level.*
- Remain quiet during blood pressure measurement and instruct the patient to do the same *because systolic and diastolic blood pressure increase with talking.*[1]

TROUBLESHOOTING

Correcting problems of blood pressure measurement

REACTION AND CAUSES	NURSING ACTIONS
FALSE-HIGH READING	
Cuff too small	Make sure the cuff bladder length is 80% of the arm circumference and the width is at least 40% of arm circumference (a length-to-width ratio of 2:1).
Cuff wrapped too loosely, reducing its effective width	Tighten the cuff.
Slow cuff deflation, causing venous congestion in the arm or leg	Never deflate the cuff more slowly than 2 mm Hg/heartbeat.
Poorly timed measurement (after patient has eaten, ambulated, appeared anxious, or flexed arm muscles)	Postpone blood pressure measurement or help the patient relax before taking pressures.
FALSE-LOW READING	
Incorrect position of arm or leg	Make sure the arm or leg is level with the patient's heart.
Failure to notice auscultatory gap (sound fades out for 10 to 15 mm Hg, then returns)	Estimate systolic pressure by palpation before actually measuring it. Then check this pressure against the measured pressure.
Inaudible low-volume sounds	Before reinflating the cuff, instruct the patient to raise the arm or leg to decrease venous pressure and amplify low-volume sounds. After inflating the cuff, tell the patient to lower the arm or leg. Then deflate the cuff and listen. If you still fail to detect low-volume sounds, document the palpated systolic pressure.

- Wrap the deflated cuff snugly around the patient's upper arm. (See *Positioning the blood pressure cuff.*)
- If a conventional cuff won't fit the patient's arm properly, measure blood pressure using the forearm, but keep in mind that forearm and upper arm blood pressure measurements aren't interchangeable. If you can't use either upper arm or forearm, consider measuring blood pressure in the calf or thigh. In adults, calf blood pressure should be used only if the upper arms aren't accessible or if the proper size cuff isn't available.[1]
- To obtain a forearm blood pressure, apply the appropriate-sized cuff and position it midway between the elbow and the wrist; position the arm at heart level.[1]

NURSING ALERT *Don't apply a blood pressure cuff over a peripherally inserted central venous or midline catheter; apply the cuff distal to the insertion site. Don't measure blood pressure in an extremity with deep vein thrombosis, grafts, or ischemic changes; with a peripheral IV catheter while fluid is infusing; that has an incision or other trauma; that's affected by lymphedema after mastectomy or lumpectomy* (because doing so can further compromise lymphatic circulation and worsen edema); *or that has an arteriovenous fistula or hemodialysis shunt* (because blood flow through the vascular device might become compromised.)[1]

- If you're using the calf for blood pressure measurement, place the patient in the supine position and then apply an appropriate-sized cuff. Position the lower edge of the cuff about 1″ (2.5 cm) above the malleoli. Keep in mind that calf pressures aren't interchangeable with upper arm pressures.[1]
- If you're using the thigh for blood pressure measurement, place the patient in the prone position; if the patient can't tolerate prone positioning, place him in the supine position with his knee slightly bent. Apply an appropriate-sized cuff over the lower third of the patient's thigh so that the lower edge of the cuff is about ¾″ to 1″ (2 to 2.5 cm) above the popliteal fossa (as shown on top right).[1]

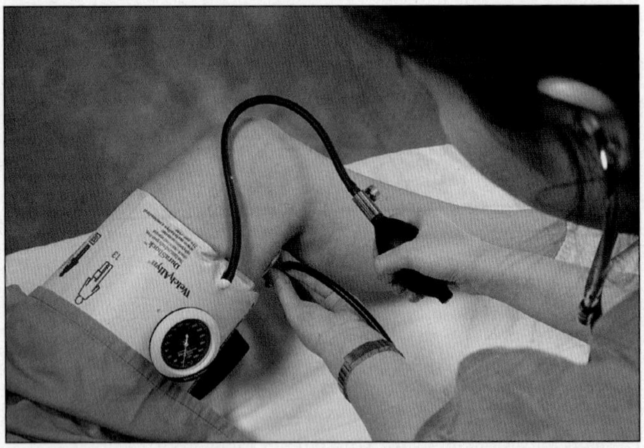

- If necessary, connect the appropriate tube to the rubber bulb of the air pump and the other tube to the gauge.
- Determine how high to pump the blood pressure cuff by estimating the systolic blood pressure by palpation. As you feel the radial artery with the fingers of one hand, inflate the cuff until the radial pulse disappears. Read this pressure on the gauge and add 30 mm Hg to it.[4] Use this sum as the target inflation *to prevent discomfort from overinflation.* Deflate the cuff. If you're using the calf, palpate either the dorsalis pedis or posterior tibial arteries; if you're using the thigh, palpate the popliteal artery.[1]
- If you're using the patient's upper arm, locate the brachial artery by palpation. If you're using the patient's calf, palpate either the dorsalis pedis or posterior tibial arteries; if you're using the patient's thigh, palpate the popliteal artery.[1] Center the bell of the stethoscope over the part of the artery where you detect the strongest beats, and hold it in place with

one hand. *The bell of the stethoscope transmits low-pitched arterial blood sounds more effectively than does the diaphragm.*

■ Using the thumb and index finger of your other hand, turn the thumbscrew on the rubber bulb of the air pump clockwise to close the valve.

■ Pump up the cuff to the predetermined level.

■ Insert the stethoscope earpieces into your ears.

■ Carefully open the valve of the air pump, and then slowly deflate the cuff—no faster than 3 mm Hg/second.[4] While releasing air, watch the mercury column or aneroid gauge and auscultate for the sound over the artery.

■ When you hear the first beat or clear tapping sound, note the pressure on the column or gauge; this is the systolic pressure. (The beat or tapping sound is the first of five Korotkoff sounds. The second sound resembles a murmur or swish; the third sound, crisp tapping; the fourth sound, a soft, muffled tone; and the fifth, the point at which sound disappears.)

■ Continue to release air gradually while auscultating for the sound over the artery.

■ Note the pressure when the sound disappears; this is the diastolic pressure—the fifth Korotkoff sound.

■ After you hear the last Korotkoff sound, deflate the cuff slowly for at least another 10 mm Hg *to ensure that no further sounds are audible.*

■ Rapidly deflate the cuff. Record the pressure, wait 2 minutes, and then repeat the procedure. Average the two readings. If there is more than a 5 mm Hg difference between the first and second readings, take the average of two or more readings.[4,5]

■ Remove the cuff.

■ Assess the patient's skin integrity under the blood pressure cuff.[1]

■ If the cuff isn't dedicated for single-patient use, clean and disinfect it with a disinfectant pad.[6,17]

■ Clean and disinfect your stethoscope using an disinfectant pad.[6,17]

■ Dispose of waste in the appropriate receptacle.

■ Perform hand hygiene.[7,8,9,10,11]

■ Document the procedure.[18,19,20]

Special considerations

■ Unstable patients as well as those receiving blood transfusions or oral or IV medication to stabilize blood pressure may require frequent blood pressure readings.

■ If you can't auscultate blood pressure, you may estimate systolic pressure. To do this, first palpate the brachial or radial pulse. Then inflate the cuff until you no longer detect the pulse. Slowly deflate the cuff and, when you detect the pulse again, record the pressure as the palpated systolic pressure.

■ Patients with aortic dissection, congenital heart disease, coarctation of the aorta, peripheral vascular disease, or unilateral neurologic or musculoskeletal abnormalities may demonstrate an interarm difference in blood pressure. If you detect an interarm difference in blood pressure, use the arm with the higher pressure.[1]

■ Prolonged use of automated electronic blood pressure devices and frequent blood pressure measurement can cause excessive venous pressure and tissue ischemia.[1]

■ Excessive patient movement caused by restlessness or shivering can interfere with the detection of cardiac oscillations, leading to erroneous readings.[1]

■ If the patient is crying or anxious, delay blood pressure measurement, if possible, until the patient becomes calm *to avoid falsely elevated readings.*

■ Occasionally, blood pressure must be measured in both arms or with the patient in two different positions (such as lying and standing or sitting and standing). In such cases, observe and record any significant difference between the two readings and record the blood pressure as well as the extremity and position used.

Positioning the blood pressure cuff

Wrap the cuff snugly around the patient's upper forearm so that the end of the cuff is 3/4″ to 1″ (2 to 2.5 cm) above the antecubital fossa *to allow for placement of your stethoscope.* Align the cuff to make sure that the mark on the cuff for "artery" is positioned over the artery.[1]

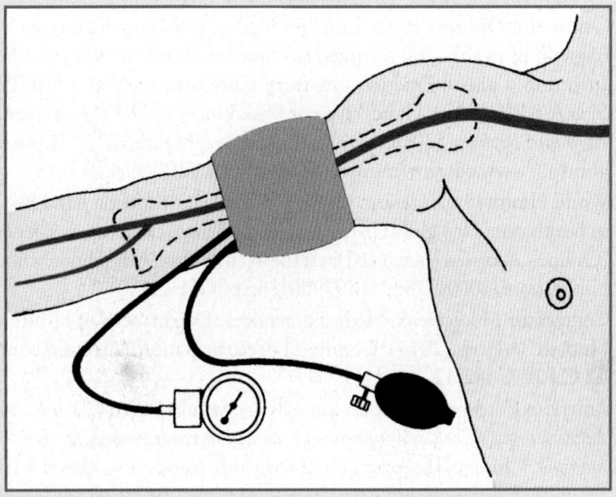

■ Measure the blood pressure of patients taking antihypertensive medications while they're in a sitting position *to ensure accurate measurements.*

Complications

Improper technique can cause inaccurate readings, which can lead to unnecessary or inadequate treatment. Measuring blood pressure on the same arm as an arteriovenous fistula or hemodialysis shunt can compromise blood flow through the vascular device.[1]

Documentation

In the patient's medical record, record blood pressure as systolic over diastolic pressure, such as 120/78 mm Hg. Document an auscultatory gap, if present. If required by your facility, document blood pressures on a graph, using dots or checkmarks. Also, document the extremity used and the patient's position. Include patient teaching about lifestyle modifications, drug therapy, and follow-up care. Record the name of any practitioner notified about blood pressure results, prescribed interventions, and the patient's response to those interventions.

REFERENCES

1 American Association of Critical-Care Nurses (AACN). (2010). "AACN practice alert: Noninvasive blood pressure monitoring" [Online]. Accessed March 2015 via the Web at http://www.aacn.org/WD/Practice/Docs/PracticeAlerts/NIBP%20Monitoring%2004-2010%20final.pdf (Level VII)

2 James, P.A., et al. (2013). "2014 evidence-based guideline for the management of high blood pressure in adults: Report from the panel members appointed to the Eighth Joint National Committee (JNC 8)" [Online]. Accessed March 2015 via the Web at http://jama.jamanetwork.com/article.aspx?articleid=1791497 (Level II)

3 Canzanello, V. J., et al. (2001). Are aneroid sphygmomanometers accurate in hospital and clinic settings? *Archives of Internal Medicine, 161,* 729–731. (Level VI)

4 Pickering, T. G., et al. (2005). Recommendations for blood pressure measurement in humans and experimental animals: Part 1: Blood pressure measurement in humans: A statement for professionals from the Subcommittee of Professional and Public Education of the American

Heart Association Council on High Blood Pressure Research. *Hypertension, 45,* 142–161. (Level I)
5 Lockwood, C., et al. (2004). Vital signs. *JBI Reports, 2,* 207–230.
6 Rutala, W. A., et al. (2008). "Guideline for disinfection and sterilization in healthcare facilities, 2008" [Online]. Accessed March 2015 via the Web at http://www.cdc.gov/hicpac/pdf/guidelines/Disinfection_Nov_2008.pdf (Level I)
7 The Joint Commission. (2015). Standard NPSG.07.01.01. *Comprehensive accreditation manual for hospitals: The official handbook.* Oakbrook Terrace, IL: The Joint Commission. (Level VII)
8 Centers for Disease Control and Prevention. (2002). Guideline for hand hygiene in health-care settings: Recommendations of the Healthcare Infection Control Practices Advisory Committee and the HICPAC/SHEA/APIC/IDSA Hand Hygiene Task Force. *MMWR Recommendations and Reports, 51*(RR-16), 1–45. Accessed March 2015 via the Web at http://www.cdc.gov/mmwr/pdf/rr/rr5116.pdf (Level II)
9 World Health Organization. (2009). "WHO guidelines on hand hygiene in health care: First global patient safety challenge, clean care is safer care" [Online]. Accessed March 2015 via the Web at http://whqlibdoc.who.int/publications/2009/9789241597906_eng.pdf (Level IV)
10 Centers for Medicare & Medicaid Services, Department of Health and Human Services. (2014). Condition of participation: Infection control. 42 C.F.R. § 482.42.
11 American Osteopathic Association. (2014). Standard 07.01.21. *Healthcare Facilities Accreditation Program: Accreditation requirements for acute care hospitals.* Chicago, IL: American Osteopathic Association. (Level VII)
12 The Joint Commission. (2015). Standard NPSG.01.01.01. *Comprehensive accreditation manual for hospitals: The official handbook.* Oakbrook Terrace, IL: The Joint Commission. (Level VII)
13 Foster-Fitzpatrick, L., et al. (1999). The effects of crossed leg on blood pressure measurement. *Nursing Research, 48,* 105–108. (Level III)
14 Keele-Smith, R., & Price-Daniel, C. (2001). Effects of crossing legs on blood pressure measurement. *Clinical Nursing Research, 10,* 202–213.
15 Pinar, R., et al. (2004). Effects of crossed leg on blood pressure. *Blood Pressure, 13,* 252–254. (Level III)
16 Mourad, A., et al. (2003). Arm position and blood pressure: A risk factor for hypertension? *Journal of Human Hypertension, 17,* 389–395. (Level III)
17 American Osteopathic Association. (2014). Standard 07.02.03. *Healthcare Facilities Accreditation Program: Accreditation requirements for acute care hospitals.* Chicago, IL: American Osteopathic Association. (Level VII)
18 The Joint Commission. (2015). Standard RC.01.03.01. *Comprehensive accreditation manual for hospitals: The official handbook.* Oakbrook Terrace, IL: The Joint Commission. (Level VII)
19 Centers for Medicare & Medicaid Services, Department of Health and Human Services. (2014). Condition of participation: Medical record services. 42 C.F.R. § 482.24.
20 American Osteopathic Association. (2014). Standard 10.00.03. *Healthcare Facilities Accreditation Program: Accreditation requirements for acute care hospitals.* Chicago, IL: American Osteopathic Association. (Level VII)

ADDITIONAL REFERENCES

Craven, R. F., & Hirnle, C. J. (2012). *Fundamentals of nursing: Human health and function* (7th ed.). Philadelphia, PA: Lippincott Williams & Wilkins.
Lawson, L. (2011). Severely elevated blood pressure: When is it an emergency? *Journal of Cardiovascular Nursing, 26,* 519–523.
Phillips, R. A. (2012). Controversies in blood pressure goal guidelines and masked hypertension. *Annals of the New York Academy of Sciences, 1254,* 115–122.

BODY JEWELRY REMOVAL

Piercings and body jewelry may be present on virtually any body part. The most common sites are the ears, nose, tongue, eyebrows, lips, and umbilicus. Less common sites include the nipples and genitals.

Depending on the risk to the patient and the medical interventions to be performed, the practitioner may order body jewelry removed *to reduce the risk of such complications as electrical burns, aspiration, and pressure or tissue injures.*[1,2,3] However, urgent medical care should never be delayed while attempting to remove body jewelry.

During the process of helping a patient to remove body jewelry or of removing it from an unconscious patient, make sure that the patient isn't harmed and the patient's dignity is preserved. Also, take steps to avoid damaging the body jewelry during the removal process and to retain the jewelry for reinsertion later.

Equipment

Gloves ■ antiseptic solution ■ personal belongings envelope ■ Optional: ring-opening or ring-spreading pliers, ring forceps, ball-grabber, bead tweezer, lubricating gel, Food and Drug Administration (FDA)–approved inert plastic radiolucent retainer, microbore extension tubing, thick suture material, epidural catheter, sterile dressing.

Implementation

■ Verify the practitioner's order for body jewelry removal, and review the patient's medical record for scheduled diagnostic tests or surgical procedures.
■ If required by your facility, ensure that written consent to remove the body jewelry has been obtained and included in the patient's medical record.[4,5]
■ Perform hand hygiene.[6,7,8,9,10]
■ Confirm the patient's identity using at least two patient identifiers.[11]
■ Ask the patient whether he's wearing body jewelry, especially jewelry that isn't readily visible. If the patient is unconscious, ask the patient's family members about known body jewelry and note the presence of body jewelry during the physical examination.
■ Explain to the patient the reason why the body jewelry has to be removed, and encourage him to ask questions as needed.
■ Determine the type of body jewelry to be removed.
■ Ask the patient how long he has had the piercings and whether retainers are required to maintain their patency.
■ Gather the appropriate equipment.
■ Perform hand hygiene and put on gloves.[6,7,8,9,10,12,13]
■ Ask the patient to remove the jewelry himself, if he can; offer to assist as needed.
■ If the patient is unconscious, remove the jewelry, following the proper technique for the type of jewelry or body piercing present.[14] (See *Removing body jewelry.*)

NURSING ALERT *When removing jewelry from the nostril, nasal septum, cheek, tongue, or lip, use special care to prevent the jewelry from slipping into the airway* because this may result in aspiration.

■ Assess the skin at the body piercing site for signs of infection (redness, swelling, purulent drainage) *because jewelry harbors microorganisms that may become entrapped in area skin. Body jewelry removal provides an opportunity to effectively remove microorganisms from the piercing site.*
■ Clean all open wounds, and apply a sterile dressing, if needed.
■ If needed, help the patient insert a retainer (or insert one on an unconscious patient) *to maintain patency of the piercing.*
■ Clean soiled body jewelry with antiseptic solution *because all piercings should be considered contaminated with body fluids.*
■ Place the body jewelry in a personal belongings envelope that's labeled with the patient's name and identification number; give the envelope to a family member or secure it as directed by your facility.
■ Remove and discard your gloves and perform hand hygiene.[6,7,8,9,10]
■ Document the procedure.[15,16,17]

Special considerations

■ If the patient refuses to remove the jewelry, notify the practitioner *so that the risks of proceeding with any scheduled procedures can be reevaluated.*
■ Gloves can provide additional traction and grip when removing body jewelry.

Removing body jewelry

JEWELRY TYPE	JEWELRY DESCRIPTION	REMOVAL TOOLS	REMOVAL TECHNIQUE
Barbell (straight, curved, or circular) 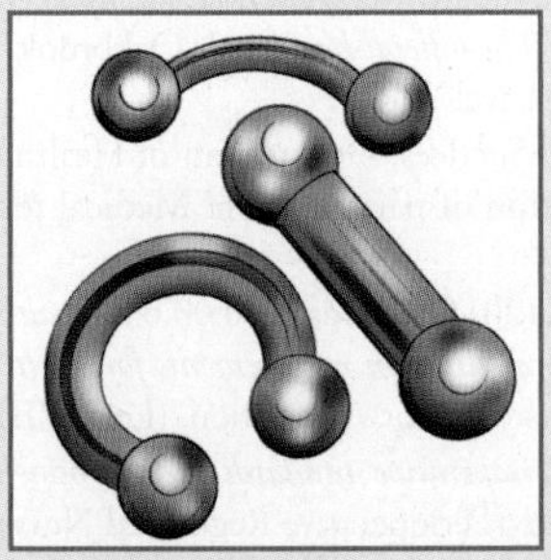	Straight, curved, or circular post with balls on the ends; one or both of the balls unscrew from the rod	■ Gloves ■ Ball grabber ■ Bead tweezer ■ Ring forceps	■ Grasp the removable ball with the ball grabber, bead tweezer, or ring forceps while holding the opposite end still, and turn the ball counterclockwise to loosen it. ■ After loosening the ball, fully unscrew it by hand and pull the open end of the post toward the side of the stationary ball to remove it. ■ Use caution when pulling the post through the body part *to prevent injury from any screw threads on the end of the post.*
Captive bead ring (also called ball closure ring) 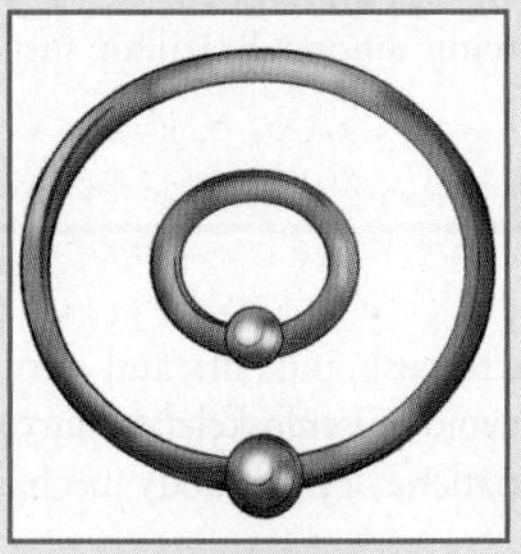	Sphere (or other shape) held in place by the tension of the ring	■ Gloves ■ Ring-opening or ring-spreading pliers	■ Insert ring-opening or ring-spreading pliers into the middle of the ring, and slowly pry the ring open. ■ Remove the ball; then remove the ring. ■ Use care when removing the ball, *which can fall when separated from the ring.*
Labret or Monroe 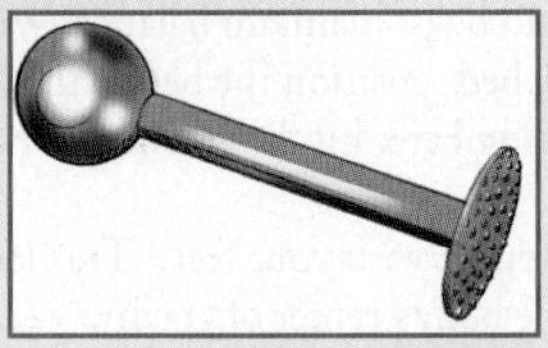	Straight barbell with one flat end resembling the head of a nail; the ball may be attached to the post with either internal or external threading	■ Gloves ■ Ball grabber ■ Bead tweezers ■ Tongue stabilizer or ring forceps	■ Stabilize the stud with the bead tweezers, and rotate the ball counterclockwise. ■ Use caution when pulling the post through the body part *to prevent injury from any screw threads on the end of the post.*
Tunnel 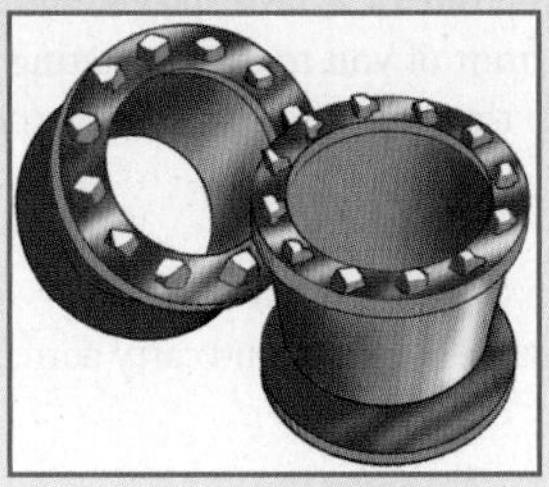	Large, round tube usually held in place with an O-ring; the tunnel may be flared on one end	■ Gloves ■ Lubricating gel	■ If the tunnel has an O-ring, slide it off and remove the tube. ■ If the tunnel has a flared outer edge held in place by the surface tension of the skin, use gentle traction and lubricating gel during removal. ■ If the tunnel consists of two separate pieces screwed together, grasp each half (front and back) and rotate counterclockwise to separate.

■ Body jewelry located on the patient's face, eyebrows, nose, or mouth should be removed while the patient is sitting upright *to minimize the risk of aspiration.*

■ For procedures requiring electrocauterization, metal body jewelry located between the active and dispersive electrodes should be removed *to minimize the risk of burns in the operating room.*[18]

■ Body jewelry located near the surgical site should be removed preoperatively and before the skin is prepped *because jewelry harbors microorganisms.*[18]

■ Removing jewelry from a piercing that isn't completely healed or well established (which can take 6 to 12 months for some piercings) may result in rapid closure of the piercing, making reinsertion difficult or impossible. A commercially available, FDA-approved inert plastic retainer may be inserted through a piercing to replace metal body jewelry. Alternatively, if such a retainer isn't available, microbore extension tubing, thick suture material, or an epidural catheter may be threaded through the piercing and secured *so that the hole doesn't close.*

Complications

Body jewelry removed from a piercing site may have rough, burred edges that may damage tissue during removal, creating a source for possible infection. Infection may also occur as a result of an incompletely healed piercing. Removing tongue jewelry can result in tissue trauma and create airway management problems.

Aspiration may occur during intubation if body jewelry located in and around the mouth loosens and dislodges.

NURSING ALERT *Don't delay emergency intubation for the purpose of attempting to remove body jewelry.*

Burns may result if metal body jewelry heats up as a result of exposure to electrical currents during electrocauterization in the operating room. Pressure injuries may result if an unconscious patient is positioned on a body part with body jewelry in place. Traumatic injury may occur if body jewelry accidentally becomes entangled in bedding or caught on equipment.

Documentation

Record patient teaching provided, any questions asked by the patient, and your responses to such questions. Document whether you or the patient removed the body jewelry, the type of body jewelry removed and its location on the body, the condition of the skin at the piercing site, any drainage noted at the piercing site, the disposition of the body jewelry, and measures taken to prevent closure and infection at the site.

REFERENCES

1 DeBoer, S., et al. (2008). Body piercing and airway management: Photo guide to tongue jewelry removal techniques. *AANA Journal, 76,* 19–23.

2 DeBoer, S., et al. (2006). Managing body jewelry in emergency situations: Misconceptions, patient care, and removal techniques. *Journal of Emergency Nursing, 32,* 159–164.

3 DeBoer S., et al. (2008). Puncturing myths about body piercing and tattooing. *Nursing2008, 38*(11), 50–54.

4 The Joint Commission. (2015). Standard RI.01.03.01. *Comprehensive accreditation manual for hospitals: The official handbook.* Oakbrook Terrace, IL: The Joint Commission. (Level VII)

5 Centers for Medicare & Medicaid Services, Department of Health and Human Services. (2014). Condition of participation: Patient's rights. 42 C.F.R. § 482.13(b).

6 Centers for Disease Control and Prevention. (2002). Guideline for hand hygiene in health-care settings: Recommendations of the Healthcare Infection Control Practices Advisory Committee and the HICPAC/SHEA/APIC/IDSA Hand Hygiene Task Force. *MMWR Recommendations and Reports, 51*(RR-16), 1–45. Accessed March 2015 via the Web at http://www.cdc.gov/mmwr/pdf/rr/rr5116.pdf (Level II)

7 The Joint Commission. (2015). Standard NPSG.07.01.01. *Comprehensive accreditation manual for hospitals: The official handbook.* Oakbrook Terrace, IL: The Joint Commission. (Level VII)

8 World Health Organization. (2009). "WHO guidelines on hand hygiene in health care: First global patient safety challenge, clean care is safer care" [Online]. Accessed March 2015 via the Web at http://whqlibdoc.who.int/publications/2009/9789241597906_eng.pdf. (Level IV)

9 Centers for Medicare & Medicaid Services, Department of Health and Human Services. (2014). Condition of participation: Infection control. 42 C.F.R. § 482.42.

10 American Osteopathic Association. (2014). Standard 07.01.21. *Healthcare Facilities Accreditation Program: Accreditation requirements for acute care hospitals.* Chicago, IL: American Osteopathic Association. (Level VII)

11 The Joint Commission. (2015). Standard NPSG.01.01.01. *Comprehensive accreditation manual for hospitals: The official handbook.* Oakbrook Terrace, IL: The Joint Commission. (Level VII)

12 Siegel, J. D., et al. (2007). "2007 guideline for isolation precautions: Preventing transmission of infectious agents in healthcare settings" [Online]. Accessed March 2015 via the Web at http://www.cdc.gov/hicpac/pdf/isolation/Isolation2007.pdf (Level II)

13 American Osteopathic Association. (2014). Standard 07.01.10. *Healthcare Facilities Accreditation Program: Accreditation requirements for acute care hospitals.* Chicago, IL: American Osteopathic Association. (Level VII)

14 Perioperative Patient Safety Subcommittee of the Committee on Clinical, Administrative, Professional and Emergency Services. (2006). "Guidelines for caring for patients with body jewelry/piercings in the operating room and procedure areas" [Online]. Accessed March 2014 via the Web at http://www.mchc.com/EWEB/upload/Piercing_Guide.pdf

15 The Joint Commission. (2015). Standard RC.01.03.01. *Comprehensive accreditation manual for hospitals: The official handbook.* Oakbrook Terrace, IL: The Joint Commission. (Level VII)

16 Centers for Medicare & Medicaid Services, Department of Health and Human Services. (2014). Condition of participation: Medical record services. 42 C.F.R. § 482.24.

17 American Osteopathic Association. (2014). Standard 10.00.03. *Healthcare Facilities Accreditation Program: Accreditation requirements for acute care hospitals.* Chicago, IL: American Osteopathic Association. (Level VII)

18 Conner, R., et al. (Eds.). (2013). *Perioperative standards and recommended practice.* Denver, CO: Association of Perioperative Registered Nurses.

ADDITIONAL REFERENCES

Armstrong, M. L., et al. (2006). Genital piercings: What is known and what people with genital piercings tell us. *Urologic Nursing, 26,* 173–179.

Diccini, S., et al. (2009). Body piercing among Brazilian surgical patients. *AORN Journal, 89,*161–165.

BODY MECHANICS

Many patient care activities require you to push, pull, lift, and carry. By using proper body mechanics, you can avoid musculoskeletal injury and fatigue and reduce the risk of injuring patients. Proper body mechanics can be summed up in three principles:

- Keep a low center of gravity by flexing your hips and knees instead of bending at the waist. This position distributes weight evenly between the upper and lower body and helps maintain balance. When providing patient care to a patient in bed, position the bed at the correct height (waist level when providing care; hip level when moving the patient).[1]
- Maintain a wide, stable base of support with your feet.[1] This tactic provides lateral stability and lowers the body's center of gravity.
- Maintain proper body alignment and keep your body's center of gravity directly over the base of support by moving your feet rather than twisting and bending at the waist. Keep the back, neck, pelvis, and feet aligned. Keep your work directly in front of you to avoid rotating the spine. When caring for a patient, keep the patient as close to your body as possible to minimize reaching.[1]

Implementation

Follow the directions below to push, pull, stoop, lift, and carry correctly.

Pushing and pulling correctly

- Stand close to the object, and place one foot slightly ahead of the other, as in a walking position. Tighten your leg muscles and set your pelvis by simultaneously contracting the abdominal and gluteal muscles.
- To push, place your hands on a stable part of the object and flex your elbows. Lean into the object by shifting weight from your back leg to your front leg, and apply smooth, continuous pressure (as shown on next page, top left).

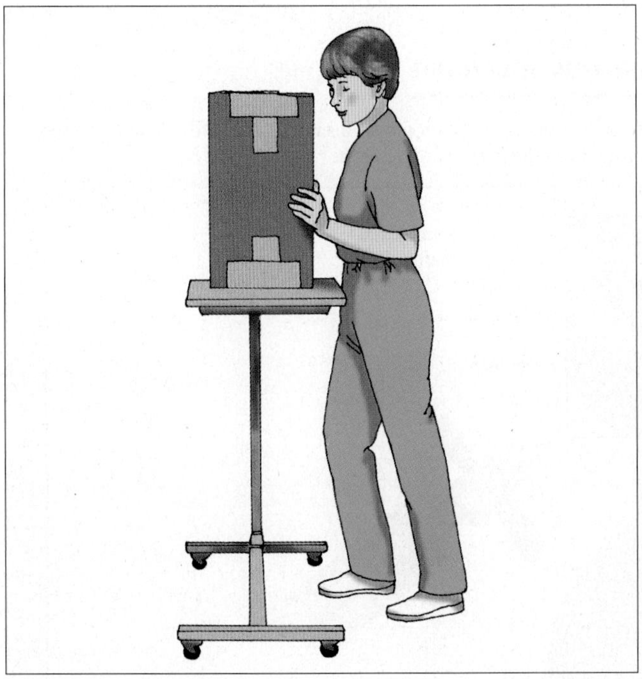

■ To pull, grasp the object and flex your elbows. Lean away from the object by shifting weight from your front leg to your back leg. Pull smoothly, avoiding sudden, jerky movements.

■ After you've started to move the object, keep it in motion; *stopping and starting uses more energy.*

Stooping correctly

■ Stand with your feet 10″ to 12″ (25.5 to 30.5 cm) apart and one foot slightly ahead of the other *to widen the base of support.*

■ Lower yourself by flexing your knees, and place more weight on your front foot than on your back foot. Keep your upper body straight by not bending at the waist (as shown below).

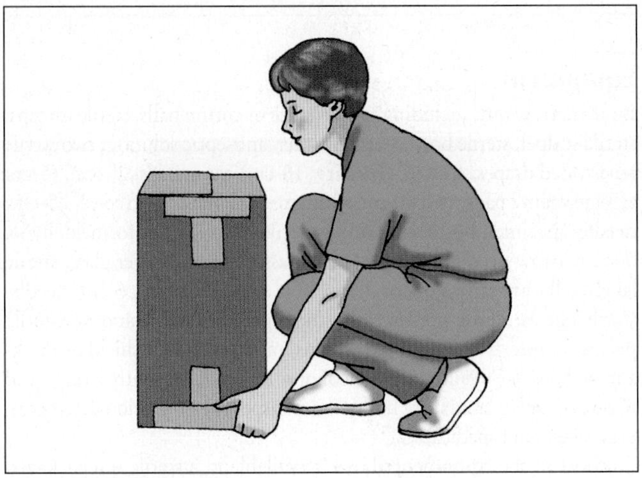

■ To stand up again, straighten your knees and keep your back straight.

Lifting and carrying correctly

■ Assume the stooping position directly in front of the object *to minimize back flexion and avoid spinal rotation when lifting.*

■ Grasp the object, and tighten your abdominal muscles.

■ Stand up by straightening your knees, using your leg and hip muscles. Always keep your back straight *to maintain a fixed center of gravity.* Keep the weight of the object as close to your body as possible (as shown below).

■ Carry the object close to your body at waist height—near the body's center of gravity—*to avoid straining your back muscles.*

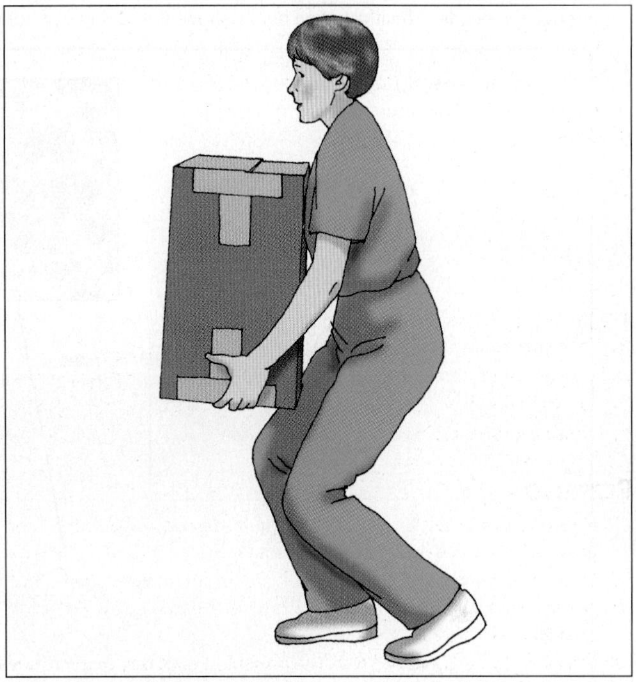

Special considerations

■ Wear shoes with low heels, flexible nonslip soles, and closed backs *to promote correct body alignment, promote proper body mechanics, and prevent accidents.*

■ When possible, pull rather than push an object *because the elbow flexors are stronger than the extensors.* Pulling an object allows the use of hip and leg muscles and avoids the use of lower back muscles.

■ When doing heavy lifting or moving, remember to use assistive or mechanical devices, if available, or obtain assistance from coworkers; know your limitations and use sound judgment.
Mechanical and other assistive devices have been shown to significantly decrease the incidences of low back injury in nursing personnel.[2,3]

References

1 Waters, T. R., et al. (2009). "Safe patient handling training for schools of nursing" [Online]. Accessed March 2015 via the Web at http://www.cdc.gov/niosh/docs/2009-127/pdfs/2009-127.pdf (Level VII)

2 Collins, J. W., & Owen, B. D. (1996). NIOSH research initiatives to prevent back injuries to nursing assistants, aides, and orderlies in nursing homes. *American Journal of Industrial Medicine, 29,* 421–424.

3 Vieira, E. R., et al. (2006). Low back problems and possible improvements in nursing jobs. *Journal of Advanced Nursing, 55,* 79–89.

Additional references

American Nurses Association. (n.d.). "Safe patient handling and mobility: Interprofessional national standards" [Online]. Accessed March 2015 via the Web at http://nursingworld.org/Safe-Patient-Handling-and-Mobility

Collins, J. W., et al. (2004). An evaluation of a "best practices" musculoskeletal injury prevention program in nursing homes. *Injury Prevention, 10,* 206–211. Accessed March 2014 via the Web at http://injuryprevention.bmj.com/content/10/4/206.full.pdf+html

Craven, R. F., & Hirnle, C. J. (2012). *Fundamentals of nursing: Human health and function* (7th ed.). Philadelphia, PA: Lippincott Williams & Wilkins.

Obtaining a bone marrow specimen

Aspiration removes cells through a needle inserted into the marrow cavity of the bone; a biopsy removes a small, solid core of marrow tissue through the needle. The illustration below shows the removal of bone marrow from the posterior iliac crest.

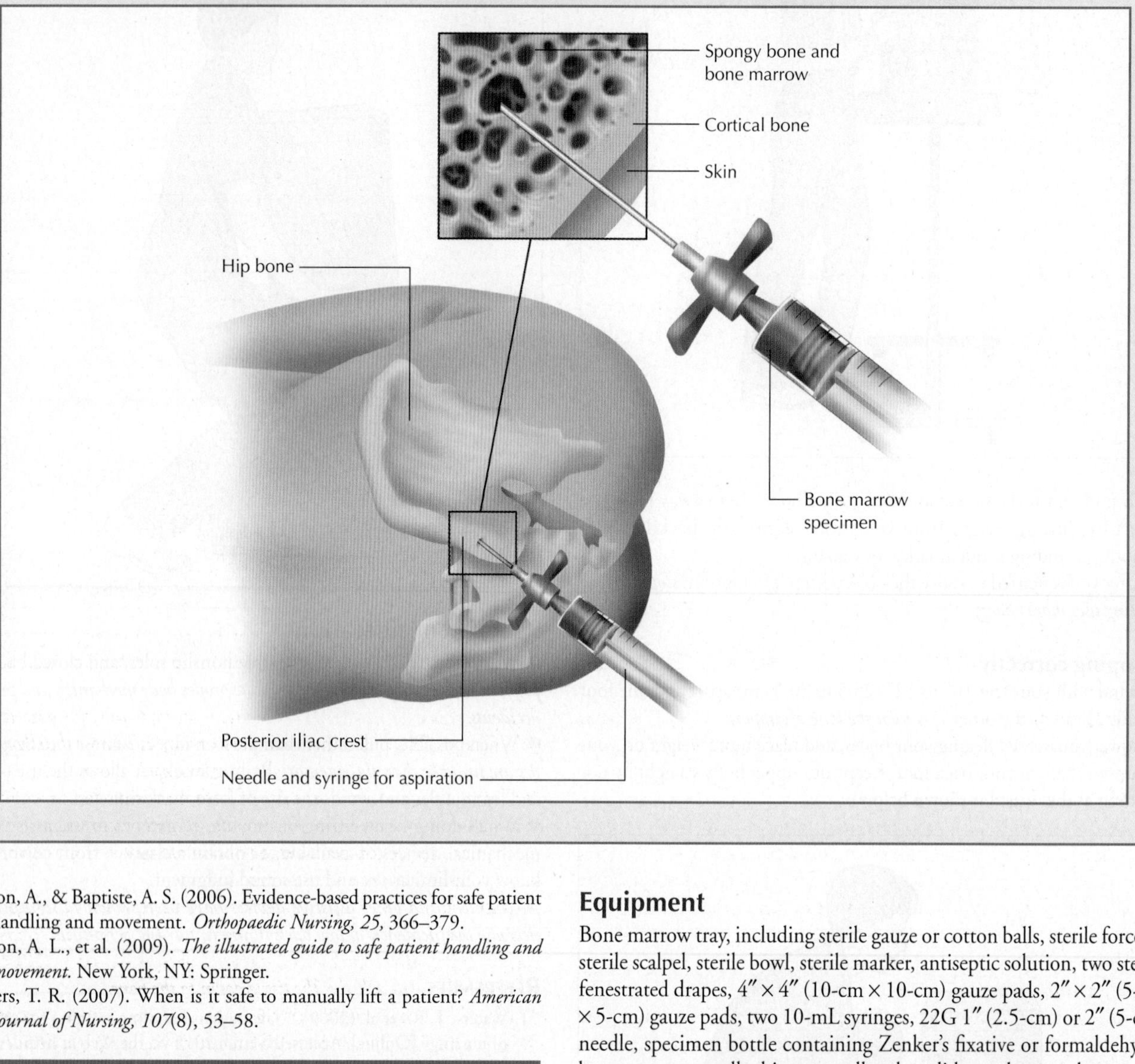

Nelson, A., & Baptiste, A. S. (2006). Evidence-based practices for safe patient handling and movement. *Orthopaedic Nursing, 25,* 366–379.

Nelson, A. L., et al. (2009). *The illustrated guide to safe patient handling and movement.* New York, NY: Springer.

Waters, T. R. (2007). When is it safe to manually lift a patient? *American Journal of Nursing, 107*(8), 53–58.

Bone marrow aspiration and biopsy

Bone marrow is the major site of blood cell formation. A practitioner may obtain a bone marrow specimen by aspiration or needle biopsy. The specimen enables evaluation of overall blood composition, blood elements, precursor cells, and abnormal or malignant cells. (See *Obtaining a bone marrow specimen.*)

Aspiration helps diagnose leukemia, anemia, and other blood disorders. In this procedure, the practitioner removes cells through a needle inserted into the marrow cavity of the bone. In a needle biopsy, the practitioner removes a small, solid core of marrow tissue through the needle.

A doctor, an advanced practice nurse, or another specially trained practitioner can perform both procedures, usually at the same time, to stage the disease and monitor the patient's response to treatment. However, bone marrow biopsy is contraindicated in patients with severe bleeding disorders.

Equipment

Bone marrow tray, including sterile gauze or cotton balls, sterile forceps, sterile scalpel, sterile bowl, sterile marker, antiseptic solution, two sterile fenestrated drapes, 4″ × 4″ (10-cm × 10-cm) gauze pads, 2″ × 2″ (5-cm × 5-cm) gauze pads, two 10-mL syringes, 22G 1″ (2.5-cm) or 2″ (5-cm) needle, specimen bottle containing Zenker's fixative or formaldehyde, bone marrow needle, biopsy needle, glass slides and cover glass, sterile labels, adhesive tape, 26G or 27G, ½″ (1.3-cm) to ⅝″ (1.6-cm) needle, sterile gloves, sterile pressure dressing ■ gloves ■ sterile and nonsterile personal protective equipment (gowns, masks with face shield or masks and goggles) ■ 70% isopropyl alcohol ■ 1% lidocaine with syringe and needle ■ labels ■ laboratory biohazard transport bag ■ Optional: sedative, prescribed pain medication.

Most of the equipment above is available in a sterile, prepackaged tray. Familiarize yourself with your facility's tray and obtain any additional equipment needed.

Implementation

- Verify the practitioner's order.
- Gather the appropriate equipment.
- Confirm that written informed consent has been obtained is in the patient's medical record.[1,2,3]
- Check the patient's history for hypersensitivity to the local anesthetic.

Common sites for bone marrow aspiration and biopsy

The posterior superior iliac crest is the preferred site for aspiration *because the risk of pain is decreased, accessibility is increased, and no vital organs or vessels are nearby.* The patient is placed either in the lateral position with one leg flexed, or in the prone position. The anterior iliac crest may be used with a patient who can't lie prone or when the posterior iliac crest is unapproachable or not available because of infection, injury, or morbid obesity. This location is generally not preferred, however, *because of its dense cortical layer, which makes obtaining specimens more difficult, necessitates smaller specimens, and increases the risk of pain.*

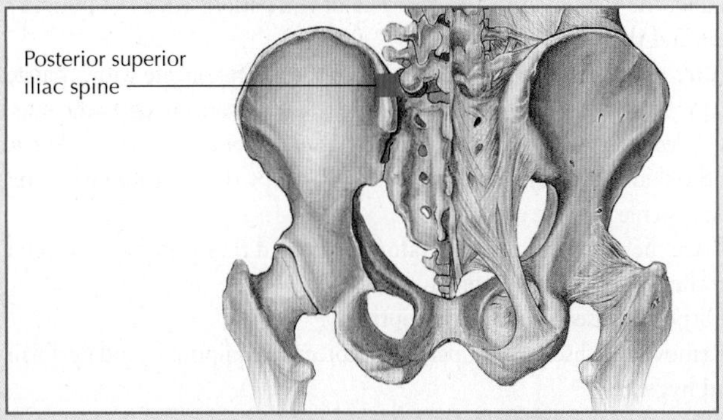

The spinous process of the third or fourth lumbar vertebra is the preferred site if multiple punctures are necessary or marrow is absent at other sites. The patient sits on the edge of the bed, leaning over the bedside stand.

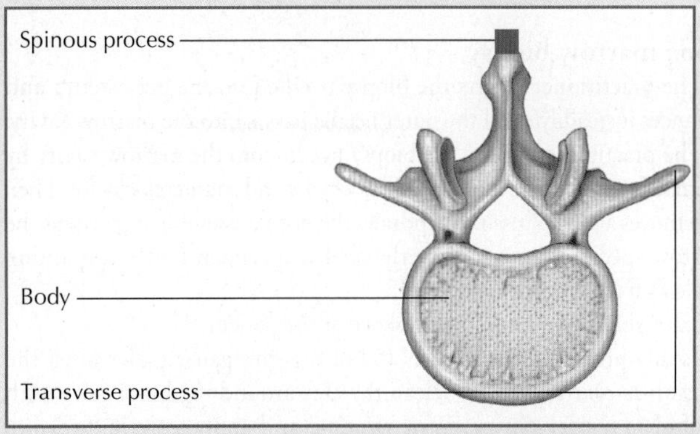

■ Conduct a preprocedure verification *to make sure that all relevant documentation, information, and equipment are available and correctly identified to the patient's identifiers.*[4,5]

■ Perform hand hygiene.[6,7,8,9,10]

■ Confirm the patient's identity by using at least two patient identifiers.[11]

■ Tell the patient that the practitioner will collect a bone marrow specimen, and explain the procedure *to ease his anxiety and ensure cooperation.* Tell him which bone will be aspirated. Inform him that he'll receive a local anesthetic and feel heavy pressure from insertion of the biopsy or aspiration needle, as well as a brief pulling sensation. Tell him the practitioner may make a small incision *to avoid tearing the skin.*

■ If the patient has osteoporosis, tell him that the needle pressure may be minimal; if he has osteopetrosis, inform him that a drill may be needed.

■ Inform the patient that the procedure normally takes about 20 minutes and that more than one marrow specimen may be required.

■ Verify that the practitioner has marked the aspiration site with his initials or another unambiguous mark as determined by your facility.[5,12]

■ Administer a sedative as ordered, following safe medication administration practices.[13,14,15]

■ Perform hand hygiene and put on personal protective equipment.[6,7,8,9,10,16,17]

■ The practitioner performs hand hygiene and puts on sterile gloves and personal protective equipment.

■ Prepare the sterile field, open the prepackaged tray, and prepare the supplies.

■ Label all medications, medication containers, and other solutions on and off the sterile field.[18,19]

■ Position the patient according to the selected puncture site and instruct him to remain as still as possible. (See *Common sites for bone marrow aspiration and biopsy.*)

■ Using sterile forceps and sterile gauze or cotton balls, the practitioner cleans the puncture site with antiseptic solution and allows it to dry; then the practitioner covers the area with sterile drapes.

■ Conduct a time-out immediately before starting the procedure *to ensure that the correct patient, site, positioning, and procedure are identified and that, as applicable, all relevant information and necessary equipment are available during and after the procedure.*[20]

■ To anesthetize the site, the practitioner infiltrates it with 1% lidocaine, using a 26G or 27G ½″ to ⅝″ (1.3-cm to 1.6-cm) needle to inject a small amount intradermally and then a larger 22G 1″ or 2″ (2.5-cm to 5-cm) needle *to anesthetize the tissue down to the bone.*

■ When the needle tip reaches the bone, the practitioner anesthetizes the periosteum by injecting a small amount of lidocaine in a circular area about ¾″ (2 cm) in diameter. The practitioner should withdraw the needle from the periosteum after each injection.

■ After allowing about 1 minute for the lidocaine to take effect, the practitioner may use a scalpel to make a small stab incision in the patient's skin to accommodate the bone marrow needle. *This technique avoids pushing skin into the bone marrow and also helps avoid unnecessary skin tearing to help reduce the risk of infection.*

Bone marrow aspiration

■ The practitioner inserts the bone marrow needle and lodges it firmly in the bone cortex. If the patient feels sharp pain instead of pressure when the needle first touches bone, the practitioner probably inserted the needle outside the anesthetized area. If this happens, the practitioner should withdraw the needle slightly and moved to the anesthetized area.

■ The practitioner advances by applying an even, downward force with the heel of his hand or the palm, while twisting the needle back and forth slightly. A crackling sensation means that the needle has entered the marrow cavity.

- Next, the practitioner removes the inner cannula, attaches the syringe to the needle, aspirates the required specimen (usually 3 to 5 mL), and withdraws the needle. The practitioner places the specimen on a glass slide and covers it with the cover glass.
- Label the specimen in the presence of the patient with the patient's name and the date.[11]
- After needle removal, apply pressure to the aspiration site with a gauze pad for 5 minutes *to control bleeding* while an assistant prepares the marrow slides. Then clean the area with alcohol *to remove the antiseptic solution,* dry the skin thoroughly with a 4″ × 4″ (10-cm × 10-cm) gauze pad, and apply a sterile pressure dressing.
- Place the specimen in a laboratory biohazard transport bag and send it to the laboratory immediately.
- Dispose of used supplies appropriately.[21]
- Remove and discard your personal protective equipment, and perform hand hygiene.[6,7,8,9]
- Document the procedure.[22,23,24]

Bone marrow biopsy

- The practitioner inserts the biopsy needle into the periosteum and advances it steadily until the outer needle passes into the marrow cavity.
- The practitioner directs the biopsy needle into the marrow cavity by alternately rotating the inner needle clockwise and counterclockwise. Then he removes a plug of tissue, withdraws the needle assembly, and expels the marrow specimen into a properly labeled specimen bottle containing Zenker's fixative or formaldehyde.
- Label the specimen in the presence of the patient.[11]
- Firmly press a sterile 2″ × 2″ (5-cm × 5-cm) gauze pad against the incision *to control bleeding,* clean the area around the biopsy site with alcohol *to remove the antiseptic solution,* and apply a sterile pressure dressing.
- Dispose of used supplies appropriately.[21]
- Place the specimen in a biohazard transport bag and send it to the laboratory,
- Remove and discard your personal protective equipment, and perform hand hygiene.[6,7,8,9,10]
- Document the procedure.[22,23,24]

Special considerations

- Faulty needle placement may yield too little aspirate. If no specimen is produced, the needle must be withdrawn from the bone (but not from the overlying soft tissue), the stylet replaced, and the needle inserted into a second site within the anesthetized field.
- If the patient has received sedation, caution him about safety concerns and driving restrictions. Monitor the patient according to facility protocol.
- Bone marrow specimens shouldn't be collected from irradiated areas *because radiation may have altered or destroyed the marrow.*
- Before discharge, apply pressure to the puncture site until there's no further bleeding noted. Direct, firm pressure over the biopsy site can be supplemented by having the patient lie supine.

Patient teaching

Instruct the patient to leave the sterile dressing in place for 24 to 48 hours, depending on the practitioner's orders. Advise the patient to avoid tub baths, hot tubs, swimming pools, and whirlpool baths for 48 hours after the procedure *to allow the biopsy site adequate time to heal.* Tell the patient that he may experience mild to moderate discomfort at the site for 24 to 48 hours. He may take analgesics as needed; however, instruct him to avoid aspirin and nonsteroidal anti-inflammatory drugs for 24 to 48 hours *to minimize the risk of bleeding from the site.* Instruct the patient to call the practitioner if he experiences bleeding or fever after discharge.

Complications

Bleeding and infection are potentially life-threatening complications of aspiration or biopsy at any site. Complications of sternal needle puncture are uncommon but include puncture of the heart and major vessels, causing severe hemorrhage; puncture of the mediastinum, causing mediastinitis or pneumomediastinum; and puncture of the lung, causing pneumothorax.

If a hematoma occurs around the puncture site, apply warm soaks. Give analgesics for site pain or tenderness.

Documentation

Document the time and date, the location, and the patient's tolerance of the procedure. Note the amount and color of marrow aspirated, laboratory tests ordered, and time the specimen was sent. Chart the patient's vital signs, pain level, complications, and type of dressing applied. Also document patient teaching.

REFERENCES

1 The Joint Commission. (2015). Standard RI.01.03.01. *Comprehensive accreditation manual for hospitals: The official handbook.* Oakbrook Terrace, IL: The Joint Commission. (Level VII)

2 American Osteopathic Association. (2014). Standard 15.01.11. *Healthcare Facilities Accreditation Program: Accreditation requirements for acute care hospitals.* Chicago, IL: American Osteopathic Association. (Level VII)

3 Centers for Medicare & Medicaid Services, Department of Health and Human Services. (2014). Condition of participation: Patient's rights. 42 C.F.R. § 482.13(b)(2).

4 The Joint Commission. (2015). Standard UP.01.01.01. *Comprehensive accreditation manual for hospitals: The official handbook.* Oakbrook Terrace, IL: The Joint Commission. (Level VII)

5 American Osteopathic Association. (2014). Standard 30.00.14. *Healthcare Facilities Accreditation Program: Accreditation requirements for acute care hospitals.* Chicago, IL: American Osteopathic Association. (Level VII)

6 Centers for Disease Control and Prevention. (2002). Guideline for hand hygiene in health care settings: Recommendations of the Healthcare Infection Control Practices Advisory Committee and the HICPAC/SHEA/APIC/IDSA Hand Hygiene Task Force. *MMWR Recommendations and Reports, 51*(RR-16), 1–45. Accessed March 2015 via the Web at http://www.cdc.gov/mmwr/pdf/rr/rr5116.pdf (Level II)

7 The Joint Commission. (2015). Standard NPSG.07.01.01. *Comprehensive accreditation manual for hospitals: The official handbook.* Oakbrook Terrace, IL: The Joint Commission. (Level VII)

8 World Health Organization. (2009). "WHO guidelines on hand hygiene in health care: First global patient safety challenge, clean care is safer care" [Online]. Accessed March 2015 via the Web at http://whqlibdoc.who.int/publications/2009/9789241597906_eng.pdf (Level IV)

9 Centers for Medicare & Medicaid Services, Department of Health and Human Services. (2014). Condition of participation: Infection control. 42 C.F.R. § 482.42.

10 American Osteopathic Association. (2014). Standard 07.01.21. *Healthcare Facilities Accreditation Program: Accreditation requirements for acute care hospitals.* Chicago, IL: American Osteopathic Association. (Level VII)

11 The Joint Commission. (2015). Standard NPSG.01.01.01. *Comprehensive accreditation manual for hospitals: The official handbook.* Oakbrook Terrace, IL: The Joint Commission. (Level VII)

12 The Joint Commission. (2015). Standard UP.01.02.01. *Comprehensive accreditation manual for hospitals: The official handbook.* Oakbrook Terrace, IL: The Joint Commission. (Level VII)

13 Talamo, G., et al. (2010). Oral administration of analgesia and anxiolysis for pain associated with bone marrow biopsy. *Supportive Care in Cancer, 18,* 301–305.

14 The Joint Commission. (2015). Standard MM.06.01.01. *Comprehensive accreditation manual for hospitals: The official handbook.* Oakbrook Terrace, IL: The Joint Commission. (Level VII)

15 Centers for Medicare & Medicaid Services, Department of Health and Human Services. (2014). Condition of participation: Nursing services. 42 C.F.R. § 482.23 (c).
16 Siegel, J. D., et al. (2007). "2007 guideline for isolation precautions: Preventing transmission of infectious agents in healthcare settings" [Online]. Accessed March 2015 via the Web at http://www.cdc.gov/hicpac/pdf/isolation/Isolation2007.pdf (Level II)
17 American Osteopathic Association. (2014). Standard 07.01.10. *Healthcare Facilities Accreditation Program: Accreditation requirements for acute care hospitals.* Chicago, IL: American Osteopathic Association. (Level VII)
18 The Joint Commission. (2015). Standard NPSG.03.04.01. *Comprehensive accreditation manual for hospitals: The official handbook.* Oakbrook Terrace, IL: The Joint Commission. (Level VII)
19 American Osteopathic Association. (2014). Standard 25.01.27. *Healthcare Facilities Accreditation Program: Accreditation requirements for acute care hospitals.* Chicago, IL: American Osteopathic Association. (Level VII)
20 The Joint Commission. (2015). Standard UP.01.03.01. *Comprehensive accreditation manual for hospitals: The official handbook.* Oakbrook Terrace, IL: The Joint Commission. (Level VII)
21 Occupational Safety and Health Administration. (n.d.). "Bloodborne pathogens, standard number 1910.1030" [Online]. Accessed March 2015 via the Web at http://www.osha.gov/pls/oshaweb/owadisp.show_document?p_table=STANDARDS&p_id=10051 (Level VII)
22 The Joint Commission. (2015). Standard RC.01.03.01. *Comprehensive accreditation manual for hospitals: The official handbook.* Oakbrook Terrace, IL: The Joint Commission. (Level VII)
23 Centers for Medicare & Medicaid Services, Department of Health and Human Services. (2014). Condition of participation: Medical record services. 42 C.F.R. § 482.24.
24 American Osteopathic Association. (2014). Standard 10.00.03. *Healthcare Facilities Accreditation Program: Accreditation requirements for acute care hospitals.* Chicago, IL: American Osteopathic Association. (Level VII)

ADDITIONAL REFERENCES

Beattie, S. (2007). Bone marrow aspiration and biopsy. *RN, 70,* 41–43.
Lynn-McHale Wiegand, D. (Ed.). (2011). *AACN procedure manual for critical care* (6th ed.). Philadelphia, PA: Saunders.
Nettina, S. M. (2014). *Lippincott manual of nursing practice* (10th ed.). Philadelphia, PA: Wolters Kluwer.

BRAIN TISSUE OXYGEN MONITORING AND CARE

Brain tissue oxygen ($PbtO_2$) monitoring is used to measure oxygen delivery to the cerebral tissue and to identify cerebral ischemia and hypoxia in patients with traumatic brain injury, stroke, or aneurysm or traumatic subarachnoid hemorrhage or in other patients at risk for secondary brain injury. Secondary brain injury typically results when complications, such as elevated intracranial pressure (ICP), shivering, agitation, seizures, fever, hypotension, hypovolemia, anemia, and hypoxia, cause cerebral hypoxia. Cerebral hypoxia, in turn, can lead to cerebral ischemia.

$PbtO_2$ monitoring is achieved using a $PbtO_2$ probe that's inserted through an intracranial bolt or tunneled under the scalp using a probe guide and trocar. When used with an intracranial bolt, the system measures ICP, brain tissue temperature, and $PbtO_2$ saturation. By detecting early changes in ICP and $PbtO_2$, this system allows treatment interventions to be performed before secondary brain injury occurs.[1] Contraindications of $PbtO_2$ monitoring include anticoagulation therapy, insertion site infection, and coagulopathy.

The normal value for $PbtO_2$ ranges between 20 and 35 mm Hg.[2] Decreased $PbtO_2$ values occur when there's an increased oxygen demand or a decrease in oxygen delivery.[2] Increased $PbtO_2$ values occur when there's increased oxygen delivery or decreased oxygen demand.[2]

Equipment

$PbtO_2$ monitor ■ monitor-to-patient connecting cables ■ $PbtO_2$ probe ■ cardiopulmonary monitor ■ blood pressure monitoring device ■ thermometer ■ Optional: sedatives, neuromuscular blocking agents, other medications as prescribed,[3] cooling devices as ordered,[3] gloves, cap, gown, goggles or mask with face shield.

Preparation of equipment

If the $PbtO_2$ monitor you're using isn't self-calibrating, calibrate the unit according to the manufacturer's instructions *because failure to calibrate the device can lead to false readings.*

Implementation

- Verify the practitioner's order.
- Perform hand hygiene *to reduce the transmission of microorganisms.*[4,5,6,7,8]
- Confirm the patient's identity using at least two patient identifiers.[9]
- Ensure that the patient and his family members understand the procedure. Answer any questions *to evaluate their understanding of the information provided.*
- Put on personal protective equipment as needed *to comply with standard precautions.*[10,11]
- Assess the patient's ICP (see the "Intracranial pressure monitoring" procedure, page 424), neurologic status, vital signs, and $PbtO_2$ every 15 minutes until the patient's condition stabilizes, then hourly or at an interval determined by your facility *to obtain a baseline and for ongoing assessment.*[2,12] Ensure that all monitor alarm limits are set appropriately for the patient's current condition and that the alarms are turned on, functioning properly, and audible to staff.[13,14,15,16]
- Perform an oxygen challenge test, as ordered, if the $PbtO_2$ reading is unexpectedly low or if you question the $PbtO_2$ probe's accuracy. This can be done by setting the fraction of inspired oxygen on the ventilator at 100% for 2 to 5 minutes; if the probe is accurate, the $PbtO_2$ value will be increased.[2,3,17]
- Maintain the $PbtO_2$ value between 20 and 35 mm Hg, or as ordered by the practitioner.[2]
- Obtain the patient's temperature every 1 to 2 hours and compare it with the cerebral temperature.[2] Institute cooling measures, as indicated and ordered by the practitioner, *to reduce metabolic demand resulting from hyperthermia.*[3]

NURSING ALERT ***The use of noninvasive and invasive cooling measures may result in patient shivering, which can increase skeletal muscle oxygen consumption and reduce valuable cerebral oxygen reserves. A sedative and neuromuscular blocking agent may be required to maintain hypothermia and minimize systemic oxygen consumption.***[3]

- Administer and titrate the patient's sedative and neuromuscular blocking agent as ordered, following safe medication administration practices.[18,19,20] Maintain target sedation levels *to avoid oversedation.*[3,21] Remember that a patient receiving a neuromuscular blocking agent requires close observation *because of the inability to breathe on his own or communicate.*
- Administer other medications as prescribed; antipyretics and anti-inflammatory agents may be prescribed *to reduce hyperthermia.*[3]
- Remove and discard any personal protective equipment worn.[10,11]
- Perform hand hygiene.[4,5,6,7,8]
- Document the procedure.[22,23,24]

Special considerations

- The Joint Commission has issued a sentinel event alert concerning medical device alarm safety *because alarm-related events have been associated with permanent loss of function or death.* Among the major contributing factors were improper alarm settings, alarm settings inappropriately turned off, and alarm signals not audible to staff. Make sure that alarm limits are set appropriately and that alarms are turned on, functioning properly, and audible to staff. Follow facility guidelines for preventing alarm fatigue.[13]

■ $PbtO_2$ probes are compatible with magnetic resonance imaging (MRI) scanners not equipped with fiber-optic ICP devices. Follow the manufacturer's guidelines regarding MRI compatibility with the $PbtO_2$ probe. As directed, disconnect all cables and patient monitoring devices from the probe before entering the MRI environment *to avoid serious patient injury.*[25]

■ For most patients, the goal is to achieve a $PbtO_2$ value of greater than 20 mm Hg.[3]

■ $PbtO_2$ probes may remain in place for 5 to 7 days; check the manufacturer's guidelines.[2]

Complications

Possible complications of $PbtO_2$ monitoring include infection, cerebrospinal fluid leak, and bleeding.

Documentation

Document neurologic assessment findings; vital signs; ICP; temperature; teaching provided to the patient and his family and their understanding of the teaching; the patient's tolerance of the procedure; insertion site assessment; and any unexpected complications or outcomes if applicable. Record $PbtO_2$ readings at least every hour.

REFERENCES

1 Wilensky, E. M., et al. (2005). Brain tissue oxygen practice guidelines using the LICOX® CMP monitoring system. *Journal of Neuroscience Nursing, 37,* 277–288.

2 Lynn-McHale Wiegand, D. (Ed.). (2011). *AACN procedure manual for critical care* (6th ed.). St. Louis, MO: Saunders.

3 Cecil, S., et al. (2011). Traumatic brain injury: Advanced multimodal neuromonitoring from theory to clinical practice. *Critical Care Nurse, 31*(2), 25–36. Accessed March 2015 via the Web at http://www.aacn.org/WD/CETests/Media/C112.pdf

4 Centers for Disease Control and Prevention. (2002). Guideline for hand hygiene in health-care settings: Recommendations of the Healthcare Infection Control Practices Advisory Committee and the HICPAC/SHEA/APIC/IDSA Hand Hygiene Task Force. *MMWR Recommendations and Reports, 51*(RR-16), 1–45. Accessed March 2015 via the Web at http://www.cdc.gov/mmwr/pdf/rr/rr5116.pdf (Level II)

5 The Joint Commission. (2015). Standard NPSG.07.01.01. *Comprehensive accreditation manual for hospitals: The official handbook.* Oakbrook Terrace, IL: The Joint Commission. (Level VII)

6 World Health Organization. (2009). "WHO guidelines on hand hygiene in health care: First global patient safety challenge, clean care is safer care" [Online]. Accessed March 2015 via the Web at http://whqlibdoc.who.int/publications/2009/9789241597906_eng.pdf (Level IV)

7 American Osteopathic Association. (2014). Standard 07.01.21. *Healthcare Facilities Accreditation Program: Accreditation requirements for acute care hospitals.* Chicago, IL: American Osteopathic Association. (Level VII)

8 Centers for Medicare & Medicaid Services, Department of Health and Human Services. (2014). Condition of participation: Infection control. 42 C.F.R. § 482.42.

9 The Joint Commission. (2015). Standard NPSG.01.01.01. *Comprehensive accreditation manual for hospitals: The official handbook.* Oakbrook Terrace, IL: The Joint Commission. (Level VII)

10 Siegel, J. D., et al. (2007). "2007 guideline for isolation precautions: Preventing transmission of infectious agents in healthcare settings" [Online]. Accessed March 2015 via the Web at http://www.cdc.gov/hicpac/pdf/isolation/Isolation2007.pdf (Level II)

11 American Osteopathic Association. (2014). Standard 07.01.10. *Healthcare Facilities Accreditation Program: Accreditation requirements for acute care hospitals.* Chicago, IL: American Osteopathic Association. (Level VII)

12 American Association of Neuroscience Nurses (AANN). (2011). *Care of the patient undergoing intracranial pressure monitoring/external ventricular drainage or lumbar drainage: AANN clinical practice guideline series.* Glenview, IL: AANN. Accessed March 2015 via the Web at http://www.aann.org/uploads/AANN11_ICPEVDnew.pdf (Level VII)

13 The Joint Commission. (2013). "Sentinel event alert: Medical device alarm safety in hospitals" [Online]. Accessed March 2015 via the Web at http://www.jointcommission.org/assets/1/18/SEA_50_alarms_4_5_13_FINAL1.PDF (Level VII)

14 The Joint Commission. (2015). Standard NPSG.06.01.01. *Comprehensive accreditation manual for hospitals: The official handbook.* Oakbrook Terrace, IL: The Joint Commission. (Level VII)

15 American Association of Critical-Care Nurses (AACN). (2013). "AACN practice alert: Alarm management" [Online]. Accessed March 2015 via the Web at http://www.aacn.org/wd/practice/docs/practicealerts/alarm-management-practice-alert.pdf (Level VII)

16 Graham, K. C., & Cvach, M. (2010). Monitor alarm fatigue: Standardizing use of physiological monitors and decreasing nuisance alarms. *American Journal of Critical Care, 19,* 28–37.

17 Martini, R. P., et al. (2013). Targeting brain tissue oxygenation in traumatic brain injury. *Respiratory Care, 58,* 162–172. Accessed March 2015 via the Web at http://rc.rcjournal.com/content/58/1/162.full.pdf

18 American Osteopathic Association. (2014). Standard 16.01.03. *Healthcare Facilities Accreditation Program: Accreditation requirements for acute care hospitals.* Chicago, IL: American Osteopathic Association. (Level VII)

19 Centers for Medicare & Medicaid Services, Department of Health and Human Services. (2014). Condition of participation: Nursing services. 42 C.F.R. § 482.23(c).

20 The Joint Commission. (2015). Standard MM.06.01.01. *Comprehensive accreditation manual for hospitals: The official handbook.* Oakbrook Terrace, IL: The Joint Commission. (Level VII)

21 Grap, M. J., et al. (2012). Sedation in adults receiving mechanical ventilation: Physiological and comfort outcomes. *American Journal of Critical Care, 21,* e53–e64. Accessed March 2015 via the Web at http://www.aacn.org/wd/Cetests/media/A1221033.pdf

22 The Joint Commission. (2015). Standard RC.01.03.01. *Comprehensive accreditation manual for hospitals: The official handbook.* Oakbrook Terrace, IL: The Joint Commission. (Level VII)

23 American Osteopathic Association. (2014). Standard 10.00.03. *Healthcare Facilities Accreditation Program: Accreditation requirements for acute care hospitals.* Chicago, IL: American Osteopathic Association. (Level VII)

24 Centers for Medicare & Medicaid Services, Department of Health and Human Services. (2014). Condition of participation: Medical record services. 42 C.F.R. § 482.24(b).

25 Integra NeuroSciences. (2006). "MRI safety fact sheet: Licox® IT2 complete brain oxygen and temperature tunneling probe kit" [Online]. Accessed March 2015 via the Web at http://www.integralife.com/products%2Fpdfs%2FMRI_Safety.pdf

ADDITIONAL REFERENCES

Chen, H. I., et al. (2011). Detection of cerebral compromise with multimodality monitoring in patients with subarachnoid hemorrhage. *Neurosurgery, 69,* 53–63.

Dengler, J., et al. (2011). Cerebral tissue oxygenation measured with two different probes: Challenges and interpretation. *Intensive Care Medicine, 37,* 1809–1815.

Fuchs, H., et al. (2012). Brain oxygenation monitoring during neonatal resuscitation of very low birth weight infants. *Journal of Perinatology, 32,* 356–362.

Keddie, S., & Rohman, L. (2012). Reviewing the reliability, effectiveness and applications of Licox in traumatic brain injury. *Nursing in Critical Care, 17,* 204–212.

Nanqunoori, R., et al. (2012). Brain tissue oxygen-based therapy and outcome after severe traumatic brain injury: A systematic literature review. *Neurocritical Care, 17,* 131–138.

Brain tissue oxygen monitoring systems

Brain tissue oxygen ($PbtO_2$) can be monitored using a tunneled system or a bolt system.

Tunneled system

With the *tunneled system,* shown below, an oxygen catheter probe is tunneled under the scalp using a probe guide and trocar. It may be inserted during a cranial procedure at the margins of an existing bone flap or it may be inserted through a burr hole.

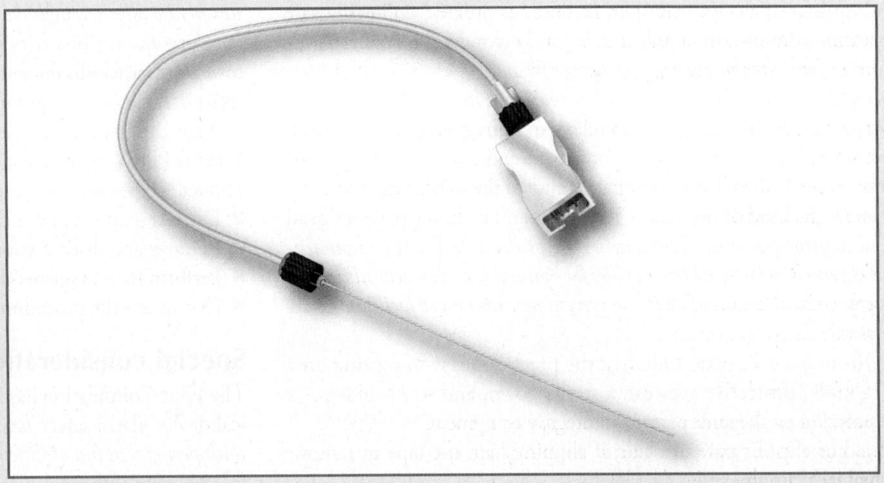

Bolt system

A *bolt system,* shown below, is inserted through a burr hole and has the capability of monitoring $PbtO_2$, brain tissue temperature, and intracranial pressure.

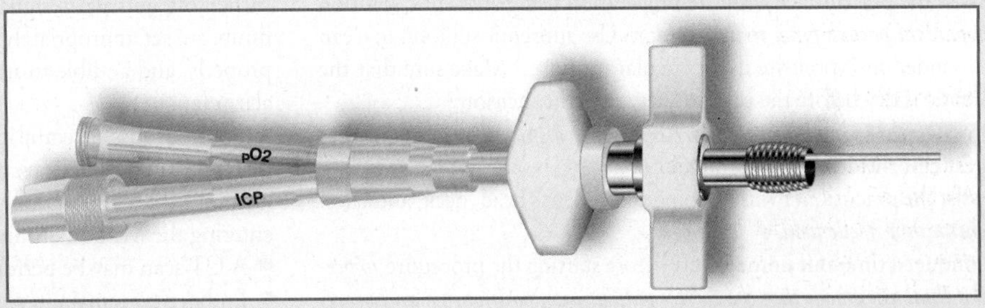

Brain tissue oxygen monitoring device, insertion, assisting

Brain tissue oxygen ($PbtO_2$) monitoring is used to measure oxygen delivery to the cerebral tissue and identify cerebral ischemia and hypoxia in patients with traumatic brain injury, stroke, or aneurysmal or traumatic subarachnoid hemorrhage as well as in those at risk for secondary brain injury. Secondary brain injury commonly results when such complications as elevated intracranial pressure (ICP), shivering, agitation, seizures, fever, hypotension, hypovolemia, anemia, and hypoxia lead to cerebral hypoxia. In turn, cerebral hypoxia can cause cerebral ischemia.

$PbtO_2$ monitoring is used in conjunction with ICP monitoring to detect early changes in ICP and $PbtO_2$ so that treatment interventions can be performed before secondary brain injury occurs.[1] Contraindications to $PbtO_2$ monitoring include anticoagulation therapy, insertion site infection, and coagulopathy.[2]

In this procedure, the practitioner inserts a $PbtO_2$ probe through an intracranial bolt that he then inserts through a burr hole. Alternatively, he may tunnel the probe under the scalp using a probe guide and trocar (See *Brain tissue oxygen monitoring systems.*) When used with an intracranial bolt, the system measures ICP, $PbtO_2$, and brain tissue temperature.[3] The practitioner determines the insertion method and placement location after studying a computed tomography (CT) scan of the patient's brain and considering the patient's diagnosis.[2] Normal values for $PbtO_2$ range from 20 to 35 mm Hg.[2]

Equipment

Sterile gloves, gowns, and drapes ■ goggles and mask or mask and face shield ■ cap ■ antiseptic solution ■ 4″ × 4″ (10-cm × 10-cm) gauze ■ $PbtO_2$ monitor ■ monitor-to-patient connecting cables ■ cranial access tray ■ $PbtO_2$ probe ■ tape ■ sterile gauze dressing ■ intracranial bolt system ■ sterile occlusive dressing ■ transparent adhesive dressing ■ cardiopulmonary monitor ■ pulse oximeter and probe ■ blood pressure monitoring equipment ■ prescribed sedative ■ prescribed analgesia ■ Optional: clippers, arm board, towels, washcloths.

Preparation of equipment

Gather the $PbtO_2$ monitor and plug it into AC wall outlet. Next, attach the cables to the $PbtO_2$ monitor. Some monitors and cables are color-coded.

Implementation

- Verify the practitioner's orders.
- Gather the appropriate equipment.
- Confirm that written informed consent has been obtained and is in the patient's medical record.[4,5,6]
- Conduct a preprocedure verification *to make sure that all relevant documentation, related information, and equipment are available and correctly identified to the patient's identifiers.*[7,8]
- Verify that the laboratory and imaging studies have been completed, as ordered, and that the results are in the patient's medical record. Notify the practitioner of any unexpected results.
- Perform hand hygiene *to reduce the transmission of microorganisms.*[9,10,11,12,13]
- Confirm the patient's identity using at least two patient identifiers.[14]
- Ensure that the patient, as appropriate, and his family understand the procedure. Answer any questions *to evaluate their understanding of the information provided.*

■ Verify that the practitioner has marked the insertion site using an unambiguous mark according to the method determined by your facility.[15]
■ Assess the patient's neurologic status before insertion *so that you can recognize any changes during and after insertion of the PbtO$_2$ proble.*[2]
■ Administer analgesia, sedation, or both, as ordered, following safe medication administration practices, before beginning the insertion procedure *to facilitate the insertion process.*[16,17,18]
■ Keep the door to the room closed *to maintain sterility.*[19]
■ Prepare the equipment, being careful not to contaminate the sterile field. Label all medications, medication containers, and other solutions on and off the sterile field while maintaining sterility of the sterile field.[20,21]
■ Elevate the head of the bed to 30 degrees and place the patient's head in the neutral position. *This position helps decrease ICP by promoting jugular venous outflow, which provides for optimal insertion accessibility.*[2,19]
■ Immobilize the patient's head *to prevent movement and facilitate device insertion.*[19]
■ Perform hand hygiene and assist the practitioner with putting on a cap, a mask, protective eyewear, a sterile gown, and sterile gloves, as necessary. Put on the same personal protective equipment.[9,10,11,12,13,19,22,23]
■ Braid or clip the patient's hair; if clipping hair, use tape to remove residual hair clippings.[19]
■ Assist the practitioner with site preparation using antiseptic solution *to prepare the patient for a sterile procedure.* Use antiseptic solution to clean the intended insertion site using circular motion.[19] Make sure that the antiseptic is dry before the practitioner starts the incision.[2]
NURSING ALERT *Use of chlorhexidine is disputed* because studies suggest chlorhexidine is neurotoxic.[2]
■ Assist the practitioner with draping the patient's head, neck, and chest *to maintain a sterile field.*[2,19]
■ Conduct a time-out immediately before starting the procedure *to perform a final assessment that the correct patient, site, positioning, and procedure are identified and that all relevant information and necessary equipment are available.*[19,24]
■ Assist the practitioner with opening sterile trays, packaged probes, and other equipment *to help maintain a sterile environment and provide efficiency.*[2]
■ Turn on the PbtO$_2$ monitor and follow the manufacturer's guidelines *to prepare the monitor.*[2]
■ If you are using a Licox monitor, place the smart card into the card slot located on the front of the monitor. *This monitor requires the smart card numbers to match those on the oxygen probe that the practitioner will insert.*[2]
■ During insertion, continually monitor the patient's heart rate and rhythm, respiratory rate, and pulse oximetry, and frequently monitor blood pressure. Perform neurologic assessments every 15 minutes *to ensure prompt recognition and treatment of neurologic changes.*[2,19]
■ Assist the practitioner with intracranial bolt insertion, which may be inserted before the P$_{bt}$O$_2$ probe is inserted. (See the "Intracranial pressure monitoring" procedure, page 424.)
■ Assist the practitioner with the oxygen and temperature probe insertions.
■ After the practitioner inserts the oxygen and temperature probes, connect them to the monitor cables.
■ Look at the monitor for temperature and PbtO$_2$ values. *Temperature values will be accurate, but PbtO$_2$ values may take as long as 2 hours to be accurate as brain tissue settles after the trauma of probe placement.*[2]
■ Depending on the beside monitor, you may be able to use a cable to capture the values from the PbtO$_2$ monitor to the bedside monitor *to allow integration between monitoring systems.*
■ Make sure that all monitor alarm limits are set appropriately for the patient's current condition and that the alarms are turned on, functioning properly, and audible to staff.[25,26,27,28]
■ Apply a sterile occlusive dressing at the insertion site *to prevent an infection.*
■ Secure the PbtO$_2$ monitor cables *to prevent tension at the insertion site.*[2] Anchor cables from the patient's head and shoulder with a transparent adhesive dressing. *It's important to make sure that the entire setup is supported but to also allow enough slack for the patient to be turned and moved.* You may use an arm board *to support and secure the cables*[2] and also place towels or washcloths under the setup *for support.* Make sure that the cables aren't dragging on the ground.
■ After the brain tissue has adjusted to device insertion, maintain the patient's PbtO$_2$ value between 20 and 35 mm Hg or as ordered by the practitioner.[2,29] (See Brain tissue oxygen monitoring and care, page 95.)
■ Discard used supplies in the appropriate containers.[22,23]
■ Remove and discard your personal protective equipment.[22,23]
■ Perform hand hygiene.[9,10,11,12,13]
■ Document the procedure.[30,31,32]

Special considerations

The Joint Commission has issued a sentinel event alert concerning medical device alarm safety *because alarm-related events have been associated with permanent loss of function or death.* Among the major contributing factors were improper alarm settings, alarm settings inappropriately turned off, and alarm signals not audible to staff. Make sure that alarm limits are set appropriately and that alarms are turned on, functioning properly, and audible to staff. Follow facility guidelines for preventing alarm fatigue.[28]
■ PbtO$_2$ probes are compatible with magnetic resonance imaging (MRI) machines unless they have a fiber-optic ICP device. As directed, disconnect all cables and patient monitoring devices from the probe before entering the MRI environment *to avoid serious patient injury.*[33]
■ A CT scan may be performed to confirm catheter placement.[19]
■ Probes may remain in place for 5 to 7 days. Check the manufacturer's guidelines.[2]

Complications

Possible complications include infection, cerebrospinal fluid leak, and bleeding.

Documentation

Document neurologic assessments, ICP, vital signs (including temperature), pulse oximetry, and medications administered. Note teaching provided to the patient, as appropriate, and to his family, and their understanding of the teaching. Document the patient's tolerance of the procedure, insertion site assessment, and any unexpected complications or outcomes. Record PbtO$_2$ readings at least every hour.

References

1 Wilensky, E. M., et al. (2005). Brain tissue oxygen practice guidelines using the LICOX® CMP monitoring system. *Journal of Neuroscience Nursing, 37,* 278–288.
2 Lynn-McHale Wiegand, D. (Ed.). (2011). *AACN procedure manual for critical care* (6th ed.). St. Louis, MO: Saunders.
3 Fischbach, F. T., & Dunning, M. B. (2014). *A manual of laboratory and diagnostic tests* (9th ed.). Philadelphia, PA: Wolters Kluwer.
4 The Joint Commission. (2015). Standard RI.01.03.01. *Comprehensive accreditation manual for hospitals: The official handbook.* Oakbrook Terrace, IL: The Joint Commission. (Level VII)
5 Centers for Medicare & Medicaid Services, Department of Health and Human Services. (2014). Condition of participation: Patient's rights. 42 C.F.R. § 482.13.
6 American Osteopathic Association. (2014). Standard 15.01.11. *Healthcare Facilities Accreditation Program: Accreditation requirements for acute care hospitals.* Chicago, IL: American Osteopathic Association. (Level VII)

7 The Joint Commission. (2015). Standard UP.01.01.01. *Comprehensive accreditation manual for hospitals: The official handbook.* Oakbrook Terrace, IL: The Joint Commission. (Level VII)

8 American Osteopathic Association. (2014). Standard 30.00.14. *Healthcare Facilities Accreditation Program: Accreditation requirements for acute care hospitals.* Chicago, IL: American Osteopathic Association. (Level VII)

9 Centers for Disease Control and Prevention. (2002). Guideline for hand hygiene in health-care settings: Recommendations of the Healthcare Infection Control Practices Advisory Committee and the HICPAC/SHEA/APIC/IDSA Hand Hygiene Task Force. *MMWR Recommendations and Reports, 51*(RR-16), 1–45. Accessed March 2015 via the Web at http://www.cdc.gov/mmwr/pdf/rr/rr5116.pdf (Level II)

10 The Joint Commission. (2015). Standard NPSG.07.01.01. *Comprehensive accreditation manual for hospitals: The official handbook.* Oakbrook Terrace, IL: The Joint Commission. (Level VII)

11 World Health Organization. (2009). "WHO guidelines on hand hygiene in health care: First global patient safety challenge, clean care is safer care" [Online]. Accessed March 2015 via the Web at http://whqlibdoc.who.int/publications/2009/9789241597906_eng.pdf (Level IV)

12 Centers for Medicare & Medicaid Services, Department of Health and Human Services. (2014). Condition of participation: Infection control. 42 C.F.R. § 482.42.

13 American Osteopathic Association. (2014). Standard 07.01.21. *Healthcare Facilities Accreditation Program: Accreditation requirements for acute care hospitals.* Chicago, IL: American Osteopathic Association. (Level VII)

14 The Joint Commission. (2015). Standard NPSG.01.01.01. *Comprehensive accreditation manual for hospitals: The official handbook.* Oakbrook Terrace, IL: The Joint Commission. (Level VII)

15 The Joint Commission. (2015). Standard UP.01.02.01. *Comprehensive accreditation manual for hospitals: The official handbook.* Oakbrook Terrace, IL: The Joint Commission. (Level VII)

16 Centers for Medicare & Medicaid Services, Department of Health and Human Services. (2014). Condition of participation: Nursing services. 42 C.F.R. § 482.23(c).

17 The Joint Commission. (2015). Standard MM.06.01.01. *Comprehensive accreditation manual for hospitals: The official handbook.* Oakbrook Terrace, IL: The Joint Commission. (Level VII)

18 American Osteopathic Association. (2014). Standard 16.01.03. *Healthcare Facilities Accreditation Program: Accreditation requirements for acute care hospitals.* Chicago, IL: American Osteopathic Association. (Level VII)

19 American Association of Neuroscience Nurses (AANN). (2011). *Care of the patient undergoing intracranial pressure monitoring/external ventricular drainage or lumbar drainage: AANN clinical practice guideline series.* Glenview, IL: AANN. Accessed March 2015 via the Web at http://www.aann.org/uploads/AANN11_ICPEVDnew.pdf (Level V)

20 The Joint Commission. (2015). Standard NPSG.03.04.01. *Comprehensive accreditation manual for hospitals: The official handbook.* Oakbrook Terrace, IL: The Joint Commission. (Level VII)

21 American Osteopathic Association. (2014). Standard 25.01.27. *Healthcare Facilities Accreditation Program: Accreditation requirements for acute care hospitals.* Chicago, IL: American Osteopathic Association. (Level VII)

22 Siegel, J. D., et al. (2007). "2007 guideline for isolation precautions: Preventing transmission of infectious agents in healthcare settings" [Online]. Accessed March 2015 via the Web at http://www.cdc.gov/hicpac/pdf/isolation/Isolation2007.pdf (Level II)

23 American Osteopathic Association. (2014). Standard 07.01.10. *Healthcare Facilities Accreditation Program: Accreditation requirements for acute care hospitals.* Chicago, IL: American Osteopathic Association. (Level VII)

24 The Joint Commission. (2015). Standard UP.01.03.01. *Comprehensive accreditation manual for hospitals: The official handbook.* Oakbrook Terrace, IL: The Joint Commission. (Level VII)

25 Graham, K. C., & Cvach, M. (2010). Monitor alarm fatigue: Standardizing use of physiological monitors and decreasing nuisance alarms. *American Journal of Critical Care, 19*, 28–37.

26 American Association of Critical-Care Nurses (AACN). (2013). "AACN practice alert: Alarm management" [Online]. Accessed March 2015 via the Web at http://www.aacn.org/wd/practice/docs/practicealerts/alarm-management-practice-alert.pdf (Level VII)

27 The Joint Commission. (2015). Standard NPSG.06.01.01. *Comprehensive accreditation manual for hospitals: The official handbook.* Oakbrook Terrace, IL: The Joint Commission. (Level VII)

28 The Joint Commission. (2013). "Sentinel event alert: Medical device alarm safety in hospitals" [Online]. Accessed March 2015 via the Web at http://www.jointcommission.org/assets/1/18/SEA_50_alarms_4_5_13_FINAL1.PDF (Level VII)

29 Cecil, S., et al. (2011). Traumatic brain injury: Advanced multimodal neuromonitoring from theory to clinical practice. *Critical Care Nurse, 31*(2), 25–36. Accessed March 2015 via the Web at http://www.aacn.org/WD/CETests/Media/C112.pdf

30 The Joint Commission. (2015). Standard RC.01.03.01. *Comprehensive accreditation manual for hospitals: The official handbook.* Oakbrook Terrace, IL: The Joint Commission. (Level VII)

31 Centers for Medicare & Medicaid Services, Department of Health and Human Services. (2014). Condition of participation: Medical record services. 42 C.F.R. § 482.24(b).

32 American Osteopathic Association. (2014). Standard 10.00.03. *Healthcare Facilities Accreditation Program: Accreditation requirements for acute care hospitals.* Chicago, IL: American Osteopathic Association. (Level VII)

33 Integra NeuroSciences. (2006). "MRI safety fact sheet: Licox® IT2 complete brain oxygen and temperature tunneling probe kit" [Online]. Accessed March 2015 via the Web at http://www.integralife.com/products%2Fpdfs%2FMRI_Safety.pdf

ADDITIONAL REFERENCES

Chen, H. I., et al. (2011). Detection of cerebral compromise with multimodality monitoring in patients with subarachnoid hemorrhage. *Neurosurgery, 69*, 53–63.

Dengler, J., et al. (2011). Cerebral tissue oxygenation measured by two different probes: Challenges and interpretation. *Intensive Care Medicine, 37*, 1809–1815.

Fuchs, H., et al. (2012). Brain oxygenation monitoring during neonatal resuscitation of very low birth weight infants. *Journal of Perinatology, 32*, 356–362.

Keddie, S., & Rohman, L. (2012). Reviewing the reliability, effectiveness and applications of Licox in traumatic brain injury. *Nursing in Critical Care, 17*, 704–712.

Nanqunoori, R., et al. (2012). Brain tissue oxygen-based therapy and outcome after severe traumatic brain injury: A systematic literature review. *Neurocritical Care, 17*, 131–138. (Level I)

BRONCHOSCOPY, ASSISTING

Bronchoscopy is an invasive procedure that's used to diagnose and manage various inflammatory, infectious, and malignant diseases of the airways and lungs.[1] The procedure involves using a flexible fiberoptic scope connected to a light source to visualize the upper and lower airways. (See *Features of the bronchoscope,* page 100.) Bronchoscopy may be used for the retrieval of tissue specimens, cell washings, bronchoalveolar lavage, coagulation, or the laser removal of abnormal tissue.[1]

Bronchoscopy is indicated for various diagnostic and therapeutic purposes. However, it should be performed only when the relative benefits outweigh the risks. (See *Indications for bronchoscopy,* page 101.)[1]

Bronchoscopy is contraindicated in patients with severe refractory hypoxemia, hemodynamic instability, and coagulopathy or bleeding diathesis that can't be corrected.[1]

To assists the practitioner during a bronchoscopy, you must have knowledge of the technique, the purpose of the procedure, and associated complications. Your responsibilities may include patient preparation and monitoring, handling specimens, and postprocedure care and monitoring.[1]

Features of the bronchoscope

A bronchoscope has four channels, as shown in the inset below: two light channels (A), which provide a light source; one visualizing channel (B) to see through; and one open channel (C), which accommodates biopsy forceps, a cytology brush, suction apparatus, a lavage device, anesthetic, or oxygen. The bronchoscope can be inserted through the nose, mouth, or tracheostomy into the bronchi.

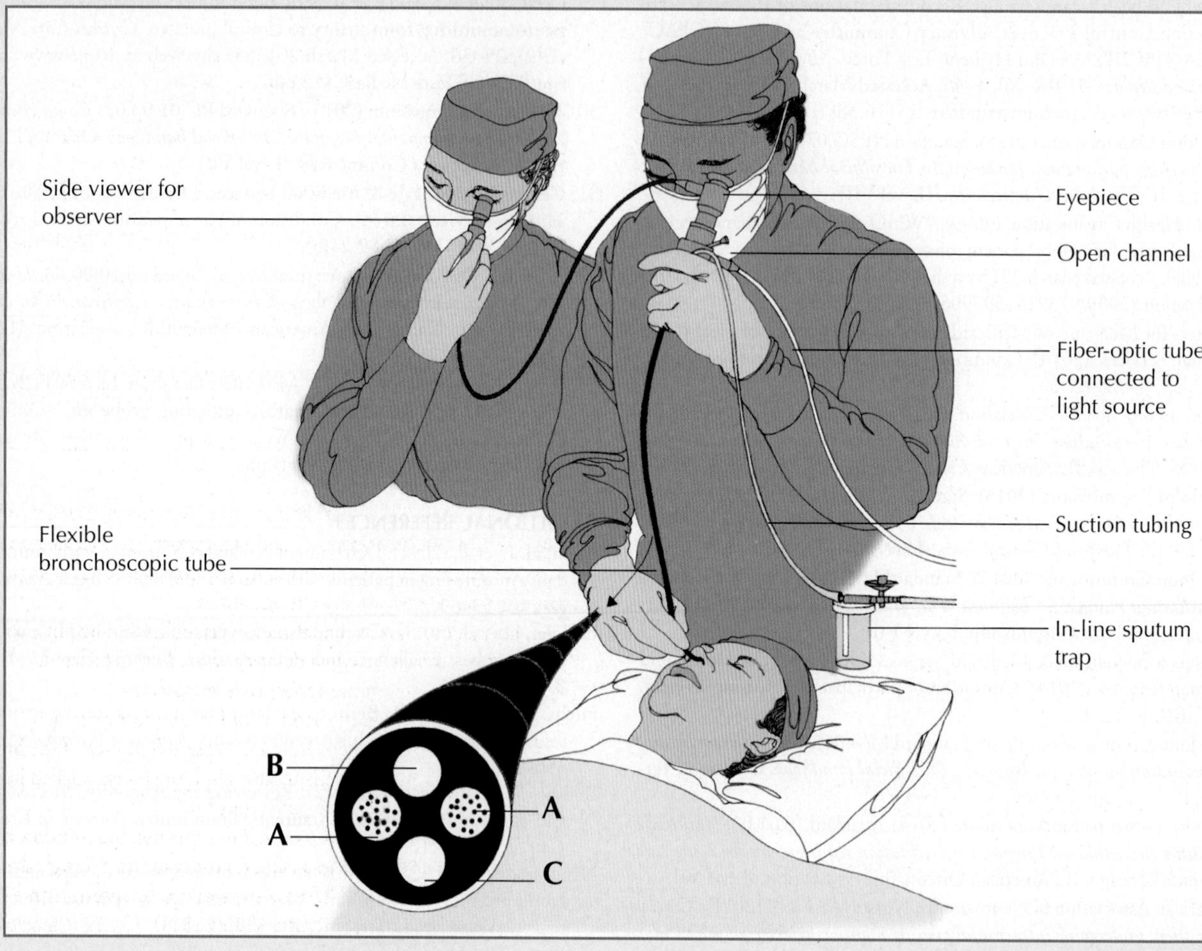

Equipment

Bronchoscope ▪ suction apparatus ▪ specimen containers ▪ labels ▪ cytology brush ▪ biopsy forceps ▪ water-soluble lubricant ▪ sterile gauze sponges ▪ topical anesthetic (viscous lidocaine, 1% lidocaine, and 1% lidocaine with epinephrine) ▪ syringes (5 mL, 10 mL, and 30 mL) ▪ pulse oximeter ▪ nebulizer equipment or atomizer with mask ▪ cardiac monitor ▪ blood pressure monitor ▪ oxygen delivery equipment ▪ emergency equipment (crash cart with cardiac medications, defibrillator, handheld resuscitation bag with mask, intubation equipment) ▪ personal protective equipment (gown, gloves, mask and goggles or mask with face shield) ▪ 150-mL bottle of normal saline solution ▪ prescribed sedative and its reversal agent ▪ laboratory biohazard transport bag ▪ watertight polyethylene bag ▪ oral care supplies ▪ disinfectant ▪ soft, lint-free, disposable cloth or sponge ▪ enzymatic detergent solution ▪ Optional: bite block, ventilator, capnography monitoring equipment, IV insertion equipment, endotracheal tube adapter, prescribed medications, N-95 particulate respirator or powered air purifying respirator.

Preparation of equipment

Prepare intubation equipment if endotracheal intubation is necessary. Apply water-soluble lubricant to the gauze sponges for lubricating the bronchoscope. Fill syringes with normal saline solution and according to the practitioner's preference. Label all medications appropriately *to prevent medication errors.*[2] Set up and test suction apparatus and make sure it's functioning properly. Fill specimen containers with normal saline solution. Make sure other emergency equipment, such as a crash cart with defibrillator and cardiac medications, are readily available *in case complications arise.*[1]

Implementation

- Verify practitioner's orders.
- Gather and prepare the equipment.
- Confirm that written informed consent has been obtained and in the patient's medical record.[3,4,5]
- Conduct a preprocedure verification *to make sure that all relevant documentation, related information, and equipment are available and correctly identified to the patient's identifiers.*[6,7]
- Perform hand hygiene.[8,9,10,11,12]
- Confirm the patient's identity using at least two patient identifiers.[13]
- Confirm the patient' nothing-by-mouth status before the procedure; minimum fasting recommendations include 2 hours for clear liquids, 6 or more hours for a light meal or milk, and 8 hours or more for fried

or fatty foods or meat. If the need for bronchoscopy is emergent, collaborate with the practitioner *to compare the risks and benefits of the procedure, considering the amount and type of fluids or solids ingested.*[14]

■ Make sure that the patient and his family understand the procedure; answer any questions they may have *to evaluate their understanding of information previously given.*

■ Make sure that the patient has patent IV access. Insert an IV catheter, if the patient doesn't already have one in place. (See the "IV catheter insertion and removal" procedure, page 446.)

■ Make sure that a sedative was administered 30 to 45 minutes before the procedure.[1]

■ Perform hand hygiene.[8,9,10,11,12]

■ Put on gloves and other personal protective equipment, including a gown, a mask (a fit-tested N-95 particulate respirator or powered air purifying respirator if *Mycobacterium tuberculosis,* severe acute respiratory syndrome (SARS), or avian or pandemic influenza viruses are suspected or conformed), and goggles or mask with face shield.[15,16]

■ Make sure the patient is attached to a cardiac monitor, pulse oximeter, blood pressure monitor, and capnography (if needed).[17,18] Make sure that alarm limits are set according to the patient's current condition and that the alarms are turned on, functioning properly, and audible to staff.[18,19,20]

■ Remove the patient's eyeglasses and any removable devices from the patient's mouth, such as dentures, partial plates, or retainers, if applicable.

■ Provide oral care *to avoid introducing microorganisms from the patient's mouth into the airway during the procedure.*[21]

■ Obtain the patient's vital signs, and assess his level of consciousness (LOC), breath sounds, cardiac rhythm, oxygen saturation level, and end-tidal carbon dioxide ($ETCO_2$) *to serve as a baseline for comparison during and after the procedure.* If the patient is receiving mechanical ventilation, also assess his ventilation parameters, such as tidal volume, peak inspiratory pressure, and inspiratory flow, *to evaluate his response to the procdure.*[1]

■ Position the patient in a semi-recumbent or supine position.[22]

■ Conduct a time-out immediately before the procedure *to ensure that the correct patient, site, positioning, and procedure are identified and that all relevant information and necessary equipment are available.*[23]

■ Administer oxygen therapy, as ordered, *to prevent hypoxia.*

■ Administer moderate sedation, as ordered, following safe medication administration practices *to relieve the patient's anxiety and promote cooperation.* (See the "Moderate sedation" procedure, page 505.)

■ If the patient is intubated, insert a bite block *to prevent the patient from biting down on the endotracheal tube during the procedure.*

■ Hand the bronchoscope to the practitioner and turn on its light source. Assist with lubricating the bronchoscope, as needed.[1]

■ The practitioner sprays a local anesthetic into the patient's mouth and throat.

■ The practitioner introduces the bronchoscope through the patient's mouth, nose, tracheostomy, or endotracheal tube adapter. When the bronchoscope is just above the vocal cords, lidocaine is flushed through the inner channel of the scope to the vocal cords *to anesthetize deeper areas.*

■ The practitioner inspects the trachea and bronchi, observes the color of the mucosal lining, and notes masses or inflamed areas. The practitioner may use biopsy forceps *to remove a tissue specimen from a suspect area,* a cytology brush *to obtain cells from the surface of a lesion,* or a suction apparatus *to remove foreign bodies or mucus plugs.*

■ Assist the practitioner with lavage, if necessary, *to remove thickened secretions.* Record the lavage volumes delivered and retrieved.[1]

■ Assist with specimen collection. Place the specimens in appropriate containers and then label the specimen containers in the presence of the patient *to prevent mislabeling.*[13]

■ Assess the patient's vital signs, LOC, subjective response to the procedure (pain, discomfort, dyspnea), breath sounds, cardiac rhythm, oxygen saturation level, and $ETCO_2$. If the patient is intubated, monitor tidal volume, peak inspiratory pressure, and inspiratory flow. Continuously monitor the patient until he returns to his presedation LOC. Inform the practitioner immediately of any abnormalities.[1]

■ Maintain the patient's oxygen saturation (as monitored by pulse oximetry), as ordered. Increase oxygen delivery, if needed, as ordered.

■ Discard used supplies in the appropriate receptacles.[24]

■ Clean the bronchoscope and send it for formal reprocessing.

■ Start mechanical cleaning by wiping the external surface of the bronchoscope with a soft, lint-free, disposable cloth or sponge soaked in the freshly prepared enzymatic detergent solution.[25,26,27]

■ Insert the distal portion of the bronchoscope into the solution container and use the suction device to suction the solution through the air, water, and biopsy channels. Alternate suctioning the solution and suctioning air until the return solution is visibly clean. Then flush or blow air through the channels, according to the bronchoscope manufacturer's instructions.[25,26,27]

■ Detach the bronchoscope from the light source and suction setup. If it's a video bronchoscope, attach the protective video cap to the device.[25]

■ Place the bronchoscope in a container for transportation to the reprocessing area. If the reprocessing area is adjacent to the area where the bronchoscope was used, an open container is sufficient; if the reprocessing area is distant, use a fully enclosed, labeled container or watertight polyethylene bag for transportation.[25,26,27]

■ Clean and disinfect all furniture and equipment used during the procedure *to prevent transmission of microorganisms.*[25,27]

■ Remove and discard your personal protective equipment, and perform hand hygiene.[8,9,10,11]

■ Document the procedure.[28,29,30]

Indications for bronchoscopy[1]

Bronchoscopy helps diagnose and treat conditions that may affect the patient's airway. Bronchoscopy may be used to:

■ evaluate persistent atelectasis or pulmonary infiltrates
■ evaluate recurrent pneumonia
■ assess upper airway patency
■ assess upper airway function
■ investigate the cause of hemoptysis, unexplained cough, dyspnea, localized wheezing, or stridor
■ obtain lower respiratory tract secretions, cell washings, and biopsies for histologic and microbiological evaluation
■ determine the extent and location of injury from toxic inhalation or aspiration
■ evaluate problems associated with endotracheal or tracheostomy tubes
■ assist with difficult intubation or percutaneous tracheotomy
■ determine whether mucus plugs are responsible for lobar or segmental atelectasis
■ perform balloon dilatation to treat tracheobronchial stenosis
■ remove abnormal endobronchial tissue or foreign material.

Special considerations

■ The Joint Commission issued a sentinel event alert concerning medical device alarm safety *because alarm-related events have been associated with permanent loss of function or death.* Among the major contributing factors were improper alarm settings, alarm settings inappropriately turned off, and alarm signals not audible to staff. Make sure alarm limits are set appropriately and that alarms are turned on, functioning properly, and audible to staff. Follow facility guidelines for preventing alarm fatigue.[31]

■ In addition to standard precautions, institute airborne precautions if a mycobacterial infection is suspected or confirmed. (See the "Airborne precautions" procedure, page 10.) If SARS or avian or pandemic influenza are suspected or confirmed, institute both airborne and contact precautions.[15]

■ After the procedure, if the patient is conscious, position him in the semi-Fowler position *to prevent aspiration.* If the patient is unconscious, position him on one side with the head of the bed slightly elevated. Encourage him to expectorate saliva instead of swallowing it. Notify the practitioner if the patient develops fever, chest pain, discomfort, shortness of breath, abnormal breath sounds, or hemoptysis.[1]

■ If a transbronchial biopsy was performed, arrange for a chest X-ray 1 hour after the procedure, as ordered, *to determine whether a pneumothorax is present.*

■ A patient with respiratory failure who can't breathe adequately by himself may need to be intubated and placed on mechanical ventilation during the procedure.

Complications

Complications include bleeding, respiratory depression, airway obstruction, cardiopulmonary arrest, arrhythmia, esophageal fistula, and pneumothorax. Other adverse events may include hypoxemia, hypercapnia, bronchospasm, hypotension, laryngospasm, bradycardia, epistaxis, and hemoptysis.[1,32] Transbronchial biopsies are associated with hemorrhage and pneumothorax.

NURSING ALERT ***The risk of complications is higher in patients with coagulopathy, refractory hypoxemia, and unstable hemodynamic status, but the procedure may still be performed if the benefits outweigh the risks.***[1]

Documentation

Record the date, time, and duration of the procedure. Also document vital signs before, during, and after the procedure. Include any preprocedure activities, such as teaching provided to the patient and family and their understanding of your teaching. Document all assessment findings before and during the procedure and any medications administered and the patient's response to them. Document the patient's response to the procedure. After the procedure, document the patient's LOC, airway patency, respiratory rate and depth, pulse oximetry levels, and whether supplemental oxygen was used.

REFERENCES

1 American Association for Respiratory Care. (2007). "AARC clinical practice guideline: Bronchoscopy assisting—2007 revision & update" [Online]. Accessed March 2015 via the Web at http://www.rcjournal.com/cpgs/pdf/bronchoscopy_assisting.pdf (Level VII)

2 American Osteopathic Association. (2014). Standard 25.01.18. *Healthcare Facilities Accreditation Program: Accreditation requirements for acute care hospitals.* Chicago, IL: American Osteopathic Association. (Level VII)

3 American Osteopathic Association. (2014). Standard 15.01.11. *Healthcare Facilities Accreditation Program: Accreditation requirement for acute care hospitals.* Chicago, IL: American Osteopathic Association. (Level VII)

4 The Joint Commission. (2015). Standard RI.01.03.01. *Comprehensive accreditation manual for hospitals: The official handbook.* Oakbrook Terrace, IL: The Joint Commission. (Level VII)

5 Centers for Medicare & Medicaid Services, Department of Health and Human Services. (2014). Condition of participation: Patient's rights. 42 C.F.R. § 482.13(b)(2).

6 The Joint Commission. (2015). Standard UP.01.01.01. *Comprehensive accreditation manual for hospitals: The official handbook.* Oakbrook Terrace, IL: The Joint Commission. (Level VII)

7 American Osteopathic Association. (2014). Standard 30.00.14. *Healthcare Facilities Accreditation Program: Accreditation requirements for acute care hospitals.* Chicago, IL: American Osteopathic Association. (Level VII)

8 Centers for Disease Control and Prevention. (2002). Guideline for hand hygiene in health-care settings: Recommendations of the Healthcare Infection Control Practices Advisory Committee and the HICPAC/SHEA/APIC/IDSA Hand Hygiene Task Force. *MMWR Recommendations and Reports, 51*(RR-16), 1–45. Accessed March 2015 via the Web at http://www.cdc.gov/mmwr/pdf/rr/rr5116.pdf (Level II)

9 The Joint Commission. (2015). Standard NPSG.07.01.01. *Comprehensive accreditation manual for hospitals: The official handbook.* Oakbrook Terrace, IL: The Joint Commission. (Level VII)

10 World Health Organization. (2009). "WHO guidelines on hand hygiene in health care: First global patient safety challenge, clean care is safer care" [Online]. Accessed March 2015 via the Web at http://whqlibdoc.who.int/publications/2009/9789241597906_eng.pdf (Level IV)

11 Centers for Medicare & Medicaid Services, Department of Health and Human Services. (2014). Condition of participation: Infection control. 42 C.F.R. § 482.42.

12 American Osteopathic Association. (2014). Standard 07.01.21. *Healthcare Facilities Accreditation Program: Accreditation requirements for acute care hospitals.* Chicago, IL: American Osteopathic Association. (Level VII)

13 The Joint Commission. (2015). Standard NPSG.01.01.01. *Comprehensive accreditation manual for hospitals: The official handbook.* Oakbrook Terrace, IL: The Joint Commission. (Level VII)

14 American Society of Anesthesiologists. (2011). "Practice guidelines for preoperative fasting and the use of pharmacologic agents to reduce the risk of pulmonary aspiration: Application to healthy patients undergoing elective procedures" [Online]. Accessed March 2015 via the Web at http://journals.lww.com/anesthesiology/Fulltext/2011/03000/Practice_Guidelines_for_Preoperative_Fasting_and.13.aspx (Level V)

15 Siegel, J. D., et al. "2007 guideline for isolation precautions: Preventing transmission of infectious agents in healthcare settings" [Online]. Accessed March 2015 via the Web at http://www.cdc.gov/hicpac/pdf/isolation/Isolation2007.pdf (Level II)

16 American Osteopathic Association. (2014). Standard 07.01.10. *Healthcare Facilities Accreditation Program: Accreditation requirements for acute care hospitals.* Chicago, IL: American Osteopathic Association. (Level VII)

17 Kacmarek, R. M., et al. (2013) *Egan's fundamentals of respiratory care* (10th ed.). St. Louis, MO: Mosby.

18 The Joint Commission. (2015). Standard NPSG.06.01.01. *Comprehensive accreditation manual for hospitals: The official handbook.* Oakbrook Terrace, IL: The Joint Commission. (Level VII)

19 American Association of Critical-Care Nurses. (2013). "AACN practice alert: Alarm management" [Online]. Accessed March 2015 via the Web at http://www.aacn.org/wd/practice/docs/practicealerts/alarm-management-practice-alert.pdf (Level VII)

20 Graham, K. C., & Cvach, M. (2010). Monitor alarm fatigue: Standardizing use of physiological monitors and decreasing nuisance alarms. *American Journal of Critical Care, 19,* 28–37.

21 Jelic, S., et al. (2008). Clinical review: Airway hygiene in the intensive care unit. *Critical Care, 12,* 209.

22 van Zwam, J. P., et al. (2010). Flexible bronchoscopy in supine or sitting position: A randomized prospective analysis of safety and patient comfort. *Journal of Bronchology and Interventional Pulmonology, 17,* 29–32. (Level II)

23 The Joint Commission. (2015). Standard UP.01.03.01. *Comprehensive accreditation manual for hospitals: The official handbook.* Oakbrook Terrace, IL: The Joint Commission. (Level VII)

24 Occupational Safety and Health Administration. (n.d.). "Bloodborne pathogens, standard number 1910.1030" [Online]. Accessed March 2015 via the Web at http://www.osha.gov/pls/oshaweb/owadisp.show_document?p_table=STANDARDS&p_id=10051 (Level VII)

25 Rutala, W. A., et al. (2008). "Guideline for disinfection and sterilization in healthcare facilities, 2008" [Online]. Accessed March 2015 via the Web at http://www.cdc.gov/hicpac/pdf/guidelines/Disinfection_Nov_2008.pdf (Level I)

26 Mehta, A. C., et al. (2005). American College of Chest Physicians and American Association for Bronchoscopy [corrected] consensus statement: Prevention of flexible bronchoscopy-associated infection. *Chest, 128,* 1742–1755.

27 American Osteopathic Association. (2014). Standard 07.02.03. *Healthcare Facilities Accreditation Program: Accreditation requirements for acute care hospitals.* Chicago, IL: American Osteopathic Association. (Level VII)

28 The Joint Commission. (2015). Standard RC.01.03.01. *Comprehensive accreditation manual for hospitals: The official handbook.* Oakbrook Terrace, IL: The Joint Commission. (Level VII)

29 Centers for Medicare & Medicaid Services, Department of Health and Human Services. (2014). Condition of participation: Medical record services. 42 C.F.R. § 482.24(b).

30 American Osteopathic Association. (2014). Standard 10.00.03. *Healthcare Facilities Accreditation Program: Accreditation requirements for acute care hospitals.* Chicago, IL: American Osteopathic Association. (Level VII)

31 The Joint Commission. (2013). "Sentinel event alert: Medical device alarm safety in hospitals" [Online] Accessed March 2015 via the Web at http://www.jointcommission.org/assets/1/18/SEA_50_alarms_4_5_13_FINAL1.PDF (Level VII)

32 Jin, F., et al. (2008). Severe complications of bronchoscopy. *Respiration, 76,* 429–433. (Level V)

ADDITIONAL REFERENCES

Diaz-Guzman, E., et al. (2009). Safety of diagnostic bronchoscopy in patients with pulmonary hypertension. *Respiration, 77,* 292–297.

Kvale, P. A. (2006). Chronic cough due to lung tumors: ACCP evidence-based clinical practice guidelines. *Chest, 129,* 147S–153S. (Level V)

Tomaske, M., et al. (2006). Anesthesia and periinterventional morbidity of rigid bronchoscopy for tracheobronchial foreign body diagnosis and removal. *Pediatric Anesthesia, 16,* 123–129.

BUCCAL AND SUBLINGUAL DRUG ADMINISTRATION

Certain drugs are given buccally or sublingually to prevent their destruction or transformation in the stomach or small intestine. These drugs act quickly because the oral mucosa's thin epithelium and abundant vasculature allow direct absorption into the bloodstream. Most drugs administered by this route reach peak levels in 10 to 15 minutes of administration—typically much faster than when those same drugs are swallowed.[1]

Other benefits of buccal and sublingual administration include ease of administration in patients who refuse to swallow a tablet, such as pediatric, geriatric, and psychiatric patients; convenience of drug administration; and accurate dosing compared with liquid formulations. Because sublingual and buccal administration interferes with eating, drinking, and talking, long-term administration by these routes may be undesirable. Buccal and sublingual drugs shouldn't be administered to uncooperative or unconscious patients, and they may be inappropriate for use in patients with dry mouth, oral cavity injuries, or cognitive impairment.[2]

Drugs given buccally include nitroglycerin and methyltestosterone; drugs given sublingually include ergotamine tartrate, isosorbide dinitrate, fentanyl, nitroglycerin, and some benzodiazepines.[3]

Equipment

Patient's medication and medical record ▪ prescribed medication ▪ gloves.

Implementation

- Avoid distractions and interruptions when preparing and administering medications *to prevent medication administration errors.*[4,5]
- Verify the practitioner's order.
- Compare the medication label with the order in the patient's medication record.[6,7,8]
- Check the patient's medical record for an allergy or a contraindication to the prescribed medication. If an allergy or contraindication exists, don't administer the medication; instead, notify the practitioner.[6,7,8]
- Check the expiration date on the medication. If the medication is expired, return it to the pharmacy and obtain a new medication.[6,7,8]
- Visually inspect the medication for any loss of integrity; don't administer the medication if it's integrity is compromised.[6,7,8]
- Discuss any unresolved concerns about the medication with the patient's practitioner.[6,7,8]
- Perform hand hygiene.[9,10,11,12,13]
- Put on gloves.[14,15]
- Confirm the patient's identity using at least two patient identifiers.[8,16]
- If the patient is receiving the medication for the first time, teach him about potential adverse reactions and discuss other concerns related to the medication.[6,7,8]
- Verify that the medication is being administered at the proper time, in the prescribed dose, and by the correct route *to reduce the risk of medication errors.*[6,7,8]
- If your facility uses a bar code scanning system, scan your identification badge, the patient's identification bracelet, and the medication's bar code.
- Assist the patient to a sitting position *to avoid aspiration of medication.*
- Assess the patient's buccal or sublingual mucosa for redness or altered integrity. If the integrity of the mucosa is compromised, don't proceed with the medication administration. Instead, notify the practitioner.
- For buccal administration, place the tablet in the buccal pouch, between the cheek and gum. For sublingual administration, place the tablet under the patient's tongue. (See *Placing drugs in the oral mucosa,* page 104.)
- Instruct the patient to keep the medication in place until it dissolves completely *to ensure absorption.*
- Caution him against chewing the tablet or touching it with his tongue *to prevent accidental swallowing.*
- If a sublingual spray is ordered, have the patient open his mouth for administration. Remind him not to breathe while the medication is being sprayed.
- Remove and discard your gloves.[14]
- Perform hands hygiene.[9,10,11,12,13]
- Document the procedure.[17,18,19]

Special considerations

- Don't give liquids to a patient who's receiving buccal medication *because some buccal tablets can take up to 1 hour to be absorbed.* Tell the patient not to rinse his mouth until the tablet has been absorbed.
- Tell the patient with angina to wet the nitroglycerin tablet with saliva and to keep it under his tongue until it has been fully absorbed.
- If the patient smokes, advise him not to smoke before the drug has dissolved *because nicotine's vasoconstrictive effects slow absorption.*

Patient teaching

Teach the patient about the medication, dosing, correct administration technique, and any adverse reactions and when to report them to the practitioner.

Complications

Some buccal medications may irritate the mucosa. Alternate sides of the mouth for repeat doses *to prevent continuous irritation of the same site.* Sublingual medications, such as nitroglycerin, may cause a tingling sensation under the tongue. If the patient finds this sensation bothersome, try placing the drug in the buccal pouch instead.

Documentation

Record the name of the medication, the dose and route, the date and time, and patient's reaction, if any.[17] Note down any adverse reactions, prescribed interventions if necessary, and the patient's response to your interventions. Document any patient teaching and the patient's understanding of the teaching.

Placing drugs in the oral mucosa

Buccal and sublingual administration routes allow some drugs, such as nitroglycerin and methyltestosterone, to enter the bloodstream rapidly without being degraded in the GI tract. To give a drug buccally, insert it between the patient's cheek and teeth (as shown below). Ask her to close her mouth and hold the tablet against her cheek until the tablet is absorbed.

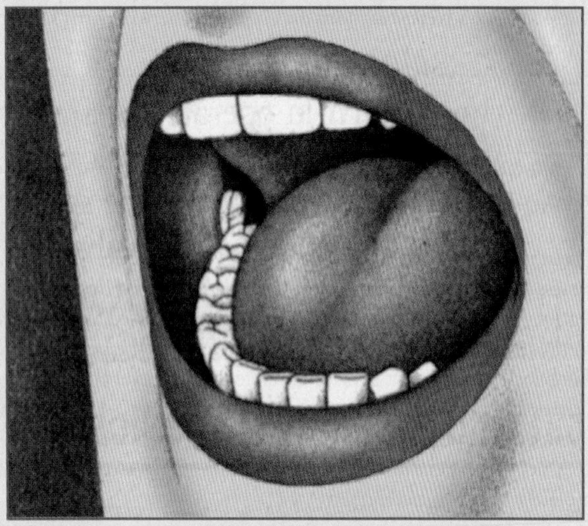

To give a drug sublingually, place it under the patient's tongue (as shown below), and ask her to leave it there until it's dissolved.

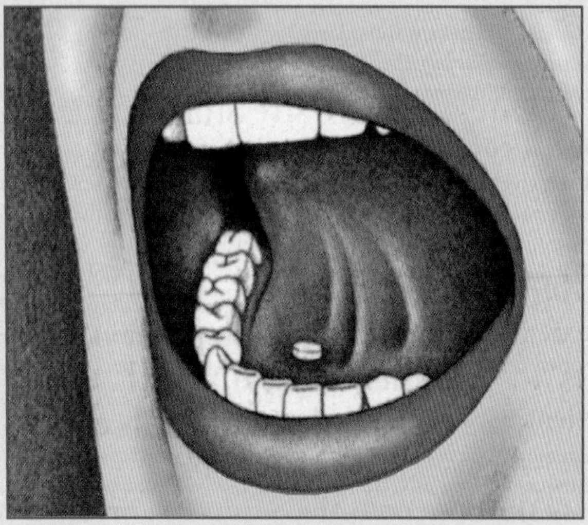

References

1 Narang, N., & Sharma, J. (2011). Sublingual mucosa as a route for systemic drug delivery. *International Journal of Pharmacy and Pharmaceutical Sciences, 3*(2), 18–22. Accessed March 2015 via the Web at http://www.ijppsjournal.com/Vol3Suppl2/1092.pdf

2 Nibha, K. P., & Pancholi, S. S. (2012). An overview on: Sublingual route for systemic drug delivery. *International Journal of Research in Pharmaceutical and Biomedical Sciences, 3,* 913–923. Accessed March 2015 via the Web at http://www.ijrpbsonline.com/files/73-32115.pdf

3 Gupta, S., et al. (2011). Is premedication with midazolam more effective by the sublingual than the oral route? *Anesthesia Essays and Researches, 5,* 43–47. (Level II)

4 Westbrook, J., et al. (2010). Association of interruptions with an increased risk and severity of medication administration errors. *Archives of Internal Medicine, 170,* 683–690. (Level IV)

5 Institute for Safe Medication Practices. (2013). Side tracks on the safety express: Interruptions lead to errors and unfinished . . . Wait, what was I doing? *Nurse Advis-ERR, 11*(2), 1–4. Accessed March 2015 via the Web at https://www.ismp.org/Newsletters/acutecare/showarticle.aspx?id=37

6 The Joint Commission. (2015). Standard MM.06.01.01. *Comprehensive accreditation manual for hospitals: The official handbook.* Oakbrook Terrace, IL: The Joint Commission. (Level VII)

7 Centers for Medicare & Medicaid Services, Department of Health and Human Services. (2014). Condition of participation: Nursing services. 42 C.F.R. § 482.23(c).

8 American Osteopathic Association. (2014). Standard 16.01.03. *Healthcare Facilities Accreditation Program: Accreditation requirements for acute care hospitals.* Chicago, IL: American Osteopathic Association. (Level VII)

9 The Joint Commission. (2015). Standard NPSG.07.01.01. *Comprehensive accreditation manual for hospitals: The official handbook.* Oakbrook Terrace, IL: The Joint Commission. (Level VII)

10 Centers for Disease Control and Prevention. (2002). Guideline for hand hygiene in health-care settings: Recommendations of the Healthcare Infection Control Practices Advisory Committee and the HICPAC/SHEA/APIC/IDSA Hand Hygiene Task Force. *MMWR Recommendations and Reports, 51*(RR-16), 1–45. Accessed March 2015 via the Web at http://www.cdc.gov/mmwr/pdf/rr/rr5116.pdf (Level II)

11 World Health Organization. (2009). "WHO guidelines on hand hygiene in health care: First global patient safety challenge, clean care is safer care" [Online]. Accessed March 2015 via the Web at http://whqlibdoc.who.int/publications/2009/9789241597906_eng.pdf (Level IV)

12 Centers for Medicare & Medicaid Services, Department of Health and Human Services. (2014). Condition of participation: Infection control. 42 C.F.R. § 482.42.

13 American Osteopathic Association. (2014). Standard 07.01.21. *Healthcare Facilities Accreditation Program: Accreditation requirements for acute care hospitals.* Chicago, IL: American Osteopathic Association. (Level VII)

14 Siegel, J. D., et al. (2007). "2007 guideline for isolation precautions: Preventing transmission of infectious agents in healthcare settings" [Online]. Accessed March 2015 via the Web at http://www.cdc.gov/hicpac/pdf/isolation/Isolation2007.pdf (Level II)

15 American Osteopathic Association. (2014). Standard 07.01.10. *Healthcare Facilities Accreditation Program: Accreditation requirements for acute care hospitals.* Chicago, IL: American Osteopathic Association. (Level VII)

16 The Joint Commission. (2015). Standard NPSG.01.01.01. *Comprehensive accreditation manual for hospitals: The official handbook.* Oakbrook Terrace, IL: The Joint Commission. (Level VII)

17 The Joint Commission. (2015). Standard RC.01.03.01. *Comprehensive accreditation manual for hospitals: The official handbook.* Oakbrook Terrace, IL: The Joint Commission. (Level VII)

18 Centers for Medicare & Medicaid Services, Department of Health and Human Services. (2014). Condition of participation: Medical record services. 42 C.F.R. § 482.24(b).

19 American Osteopathic Association. (2014). Standard 10.00.03. *Healthcare Facilities Accreditation Program: Accreditation requirements for acute care hospitals.* Chicago, IL: American Osteopathic Association. (Level VII)

Additional references

Craven, R. F., & Hirnle, C. J. (2012). *Fundamentals of nursing: Human health and function* (7th ed.). Philadelphia, PA: Lippincott Williams & Wilkins.

Nettina, S. M. (2014). *Lippincott manual of nursing practice* (10th ed.). Philadelphia, PA: Wolters Kluwer.

Patel, V. F., et al. (2011). Advances in oral transmucosal drug delivery. *Journal of Controlled Release, 153,* 106–116.

Rauck, R., et al. (2012). Efficacy and safety of fentanyl sublingual spray for the treatment of breakthrough cancer pain: A randomized, double-blind, placebo-controlled study. *Current Medical Research and Opinion, 28,* 859–870. (Level II)

Senel, S., et al. (2012). Recent developments in buccal and sublingual delivery systems. *Expert Opinion on Drug Delivery, 9,* 615–628.

Burn care at the scene

By acting promptly when a burn injury occurs, you can improve a patient's chance of uncomplicated recovery. Emergency care at the scene should include steps to stop the burn from worsening; assessment of the patient's circulation, airway, and breathing (CAB); a call for help from an emergency medical team; and emotional and physiologic support for the patient.

Stop the burning process

- If the victim is on fire, tell him to fall to the ground and roll to put out the flames. (*If he panics and runs, air will fuel the flames, worsening the burn and increasing the risk of inhalation injury.*) Or, if you can, wrap the victim in a blanket or other large covering *to smother the flames and protect the burned area from dirt.* Keep his head outside the blanket *so that he doesn't breathe toxic fumes.* As soon as the flames are out, unwrap the patient *so that the heat can dissipate.*
- Cool the burned area with any nonflammable liquid *to decrease pain and stop the burn from growing deeper or larger.*
- If possible, remove any potential sources of heat, such as jewelry, belt buckles, and some types of clothing. *In addition to adding to the burning process, these items may cause constriction as edema develops.* If the patient's clothing adheres to his skin, don't try to remove it. Rather, cut around it.
- Cover the wound with a clean, dry, sheet or other smooth, non-fuzzy material.

Assess the damage

- Assess the patient's CAB, and perform cardiopulmonary resuscitation, if necessary. Then check for other serious injuries, such as fractures, spinal cord injury, lacerations, blunt trauma, and head contusions.
- Estimate the extent and depth of the burns. If flames caused the burns and the injury occurred in a closed space, assess for signs of inhalation injury: singed nasal hairs, burns on the face or mouth, soot-stained sputum, coughing or hoarseness, wheezing, or respiratory distress. Also assess for signs of carbon monoxide poisoning: dizziness, nausea, headache, and seizures.
- Call for help as quickly as possible. Send someone to contact the emergency medical service (EMS).
- If the patient is conscious and alert, try to get a brief medical history as soon as possible.
- Reassure the patient that help is on the way. Provide emotional support by staying with him, answering questions, and explaining what's being done for him.
- When help arrives, give the EMS a report on the patient's status.

Taylor, C., et al. (2011). *Fundamentals of nursing: The art and science of nursing care* (7th ed.). Philadelphia, PA: Lippincott Williams & Wilkins.

BURN CARE

The goals of burn care are to maintain the patient's physiologic stability, repair skin integrity, prevent infection, and promote maximal functioning and psychosocial health. Competent care immediately after a burn occurs can dramatically improve the success of overall treatment. (See *Burn care at the scene.*)

Every burn victim should be evaluated initially as a trauma patient. Focus on the primary trauma survey, while maintaining the patient's circulation, airway, and breathing. When the burn is caused by a chemical agent, the priority is to remove the offending agent and irrigate the affected area with water. After the primary trauma survey, do a head-to-toe assessment, followed by efforts to stop the burn and contain the injury.

Burn severity is determined by the depth and extent of the burn in conjunction with other factors, such as age, complications, coexisting illnesses, and the possibility of abuse. (See *Estimating burn surfaces in adults and children* and *Evaluating burn severity,* pages 106, 107.)

To promote stability, you'll need to carefully monitor the patient's respiratory status, especially if he has suffered smoke inhalation. Be aware that a patient with partial- to full-thickness burns involving more than 20% of his total body surface area usually needs fluid resuscitation, which aims to support the body's compensatory mechanisms without overwhelming them.[1] Expect to give fluids (for instance, a crystalloid solution such as lactated Ringer solution[2]) to keep the patient's urine output at 0.5 to 1 mL/kg/hour for children and 1 to 1.5 mL/kg/hour for adults, and expect to monitor blood pressure and heart rate.[1] You'll also need to control body temperature because skin loss interferes with temperature regulation. Use warm fluids, heat lamps, and hyperthermia blankets, as appropriate, to keep the patient's temperature above 97°F (36.1°C), if possible. Additionally, you'll frequently review laboratory values such as serum electrolyte levels to detect early changes in the patient's condition.

Infection can increase wound depth, cause rejection of skin grafts, slow healing, worsen pain, prolong hospitalization, and even lead to death. To help prevent infection, dress the burn site as ordered, monitor and rotate IV lines regularly, and carefully assess the burn extent, body system functions, and the patient's emotional status.

Early positioning after a burn is extremely important to prevent contractures. Careful positioning and regular exercise for burned extremities help maintain joint function and minimize deformity. When the extremities aren't being exercised, they should be maintained in maximal extension, using splints, if necessary. Focus particular attention on the patient's hands and neck because they are the most prone to rapid contracture. (See *Positioning the burn patient to prevent deformity,* page 108.)

An *escharotomy* is usually performed within the first 24 hours of the burn injury.[3] This procedure releases the constricting necrotic skin (eschar) and allows the body tissue and organs to maintain normal perfusion and function. *Debridement* of the wound, a procedure that removes loose necrotic tissue, is performed 2 to 7 days after the burn injury.[3] Debridement cleans the surfaces of the wound, allowing the wound to heal more quickly. *Burn wound excision* is a procedure that removes all necrotic tissue and prepares the wound surface for closure using wound care (such as topical antimicrobials or biological or synthetic wound covers), grafting, or flap closure. These procedures are usually used only on deep partial-thickness or full-thickness burns.[3]

The use of sterile or clean technique for wound care depends on the patient's immune status, whether the wound is chronic or acute, the type of wound, the wound's location and depth, and the wound-healing environment.[4,5] Burns are considered acute wounds.[3] For acute burns, use sterile technique and wear a gown, a cap, and a mask whenever the burn wound is exposed.[6,7] Wear a clean gown when applying dressings.[7] Wear clean gloves to remove a soiled dressing and to clean the wound; wear sterile gloves to apply topical agents and inner dressings.[7] Wear sterile gloves to perform sharp bedside debridement.[5] Further research is needed to determine which wound cleaning and dressing products optimize healing.[8] Most wounds require dressing changes one to three times per day.[3]

A patient may have multiple burn wounds at different stages of healing. Appropriate care requires multiple treatment modalities and daily evaluation.[3]

Estimating burn surfaces in adults and children

You need to use different formulas to compute burned body surface area (BSA) in adults and children because the proportion of BSA varies with growth.

Rule of Nines

You can quickly estimate the extent of an adult patient's burn by using the Rule of Nines. This method quantifies BSA in percentages, either in fractions of nine or in multiples of nine. To use this method, mentally assess your patient's burns using the body chart shown below. Add the corresponding percentages for each body section burned. Use the total—a rough estimate of burn extent—to calculate initial fluid replacement needs.

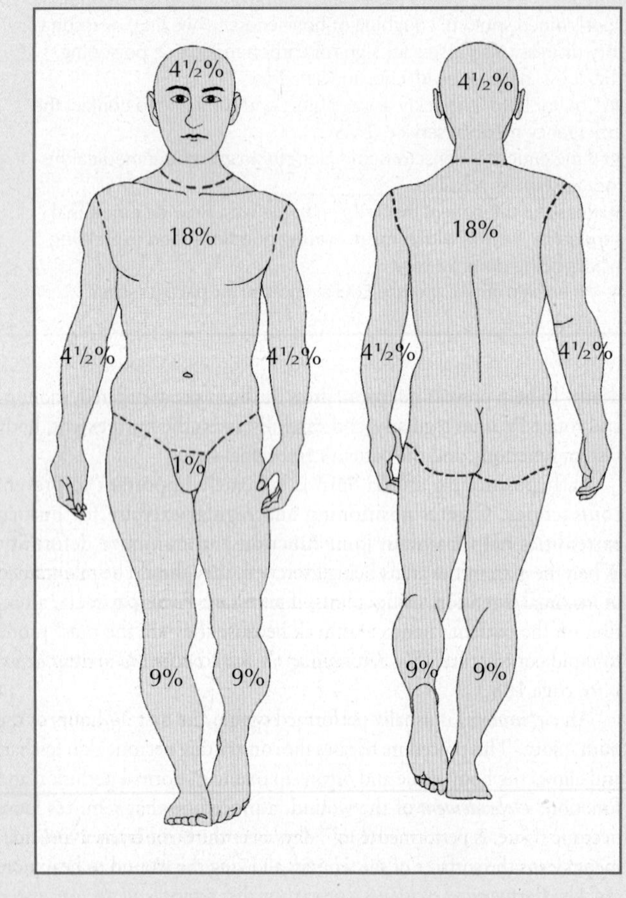

Lund and Browder chart

The Rule of Nines isn't accurate for infants and children because their body shapes differ from those of adults. An infant's head, for example, accounts for about 17% of his total BSA, compared with 7% for an adult. Instead, use the Lund and Browder chart shown here.

Percentage of burned body surface by age

At birth	0 to 1 yr	1 to 4 yrs	5 to 9 yrs	10 to 15 yrs	Adult
A: Half of head					
9½%	8½%	6½%	5½%	4½%	3½%
B: Half of thigh					
2¾%	3¼%	4%	4¼%	4½%	4¾%
C: Half of leg					
2½%	2½%	2¾%	3%	3¼%	3½%

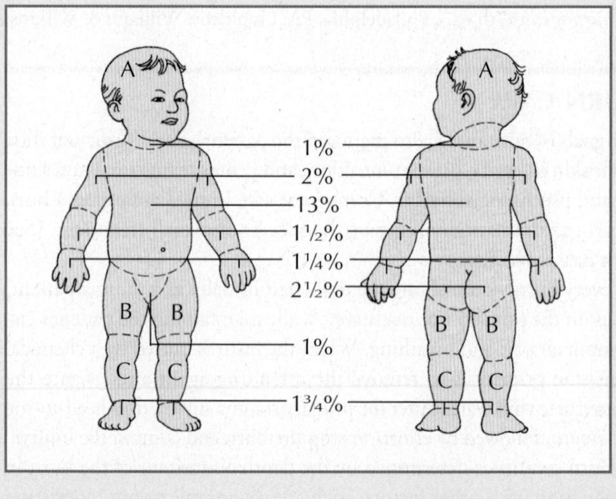

Equipment

Normal saline solution ■ sterile bowl ■ sterile scissors ■ sterile tissue forceps ■ prescribed topical medication ■ prescribed pain medication ■ sterile tongue depressor ■ sterile cotton-tipped applicator or eye dropper ■ sterile burn gauze ■ sterile roller gauze ■ elastic netting or tape ■ sterile 4″ × 4″ (10-cm × 10-cm) gauze pads ■ gloves ■ sterile gloves ■ gowns ■ mask ■ cap ■ heat lamps ■ impervious plastic trash bag ■ cotton bath blanket ■ Optional: hair clippers, specialty vest dressing, splint, tracheostomy ties, eye pads, moisture chambers for eyes.

A sterile field is required, and all equipment and supplies used in the dressing should be sterile.

Preparation of equipment

Warm normal saline solution by immersing unopened bottles in warm water. Gather equipment on the dressing table. Make sure the treatment area has adequate light *to allow accurate wound assessment.* Open equipment packages using sterile technique. Arrange supplies on a sterile field in order of use.

Implementation

- Verify the practitioner's orders.
- Gather the appropriate equipment.
- Perform hand hygiene.[9,10,11]
- Confirm the patient's identity using at least two patient identifiers.[12]
- Perform a comprehensive pain assessment using techniques appropriate for the patient's age, condition, and ability to understand.[13]
- Administer an analgesic, as prescribed, *to increase the patient's comfort and tolerance levels.* Oral analgesics should be given at an appropriate time before the procedure, depending on the medication's onset and peak of action. An IV analgesic may be given immediately before the procedure.
- Explain the procedure to the patient and provide privacy.

Evaluating burn severity[1]

To judge a burn's severity, assess its depth and extent as well as the presence of other factors.

Superficial or epidermal (first-degree) burn

Does the burned area appear pink or red with minimal edema? Is the area sensitive to touch and temperature changes? If so, the patient most likely has a superficial or epidermal (first-degree) burn affecting only the epidermal skin layer (shown below).

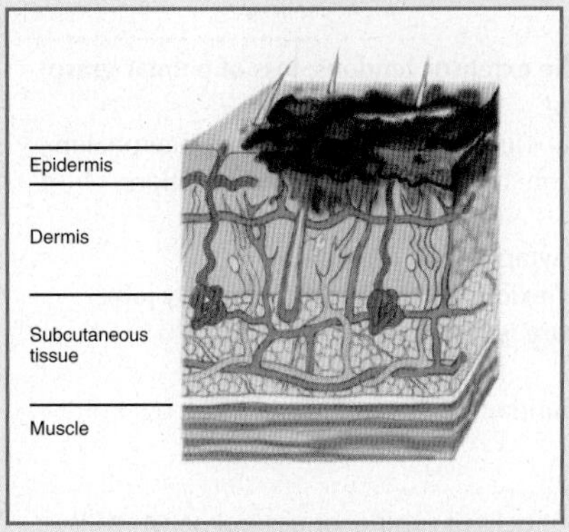

Partial-thickness (second-degree) burn

Does the burned area appear pink or red, with a mottled appearance? Do red areas blanch when you touch them? Does the skin have large, thick-walled blisters with subcutaneous edema? Does touching the burn cause severe pain? Is the hair still present? If so, the patient most likely has a partial-thickness (second-degree) burn (shown below), affecting the epidermal and dermal layers.

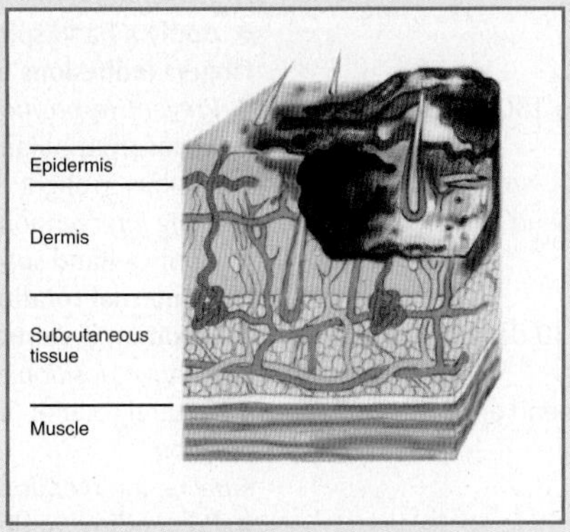

Full-thickness (third-degree) burn

Does the burned area appear red, waxy white, brown, or black? Does red skin remain red with no blanching when you touch it? Is the skin leathery with extensive subcutaneous edema? Is the skin insensitive to touch? Does the hair fall out easily? If so, the patient most likely has a full-thickness (third-degree) burn that affects all skin layers (shown below).

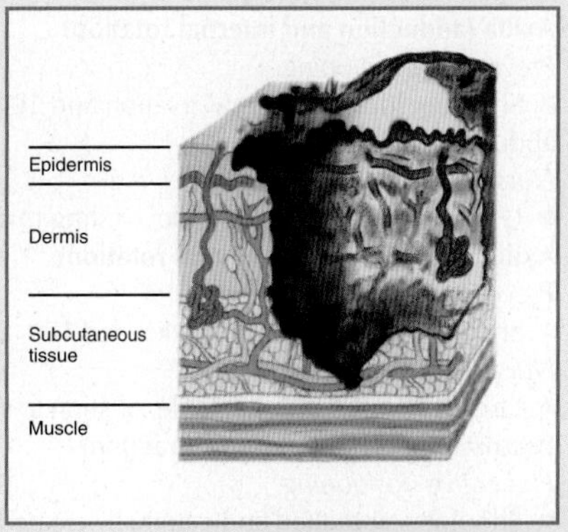

- Turn on overhead heat lamps *to keep the patient warm.* Make sure that they don't overheat the patient. Cover the patient with a cotton bath blanket *to prevent chilling.*
- Prepare the sterile field and supplies using sterile technique. Pour warmed normal saline solution into the sterile bowl in the sterile field.
- Perform hand hygiene and put on a cap, a mask, a gown, and gloves.[9,10,11,14,7]
- Remove old dressings, if present, and clean the wound with sterile gauze pads and normal saline solution, removing exudate and crusts as necessary with the sterile forceps and sterile scissors.
- *Because soiled dressings harbor infectious microorganisms,* dispose of the dressings carefully in the impervious plastic trash bag.[15]
- Assess the wound for color, size, odor, depth, drainage, bleeding, cellulitis, epithelial budding, eschar separation, peripheral pulses, and sensation.[16]
- Remove and discard your gloves and gown.
- Perform hand hygiene and put on a clean gown and sterile gloves.[7,9,10,11,14]

Providing arm and leg care

- Wrap the burn gauze once around the patient's arm or leg, overlapping the edges slightly, until the wound is covered.
- Wrap from the distal area to the proximal area *to stimulate circulation.*
- Apply a dry roller gauze dressing and secure it with elastic netting or tape.

Providing hand and foot care

- Wrap each finger or toe individually with a single layer of a 4″ × 4″ (10-cm × 10-cm) gauze pad, or place gauze between the toes, as appropriate.
- Place the patient's hand in a functional position and secure this position with a dressing.
- Apply splints as ordered.

Providing chest, abdomen, and back care

- Apply prescribed medication to the wound using the sterile tongue depressor; follow safe medication administration practices.
- Cover the entire burn area with sheets of burn gauze.
- Wrap the area with roller gauze or apply a specialty vest dressing.
- Secure the dressing with elastic netting or tape.
- Make sure the dressing doesn't restrict the patient's respiratory function.

Providing facial care

- If the patient has scalp burns, clip the hair around the burn, as ordered. Clip other hair until it's about 2″ (5 cm) long *to prevent contamination of burned scalp areas.*
- Remove facial hair daily if it comes in contact with burned areas.
- Typically, facial burns are managed with milder topical agents (such as triple antibiotic ointment) and are left open to air. If dressings are required, make sure they don't cover the patient's eyes, nostrils, or mouth.

Providing ear care

- Clip the hair around the affected ear.
- Place a layer of 4″ × 4″ (10-cm × 10-cm) gauze behind the auricle *to prevent webbing.*
- Apply the prescribed topical medication to 4″ × 4″ (10-cm × 10-cm) gauze pads, and place the pads over the burned area or leave open to air, as ordered. Before securing the dressing with a roller bandage, position the patient's ears normally *to avoid damaging the auricular cartilage.*
- Assess the patient's hearing ability.

Providing eye care

- Note that cleaning of the area should be done as needed *to remove crusts and drainage.*

Positioning the burn patient to prevent deformity

For each of the potential deformities listed below, you can use the corresponding positioning and interventions to help prevent the deformity.

Neck (flexion contracture of neck)
Preventive positioning
■ Extension
Nursing interventions
■ Remove pillow from bed.

Neck (extensor contracture of neck)
Preventive positioning
■ Prone with head slightly raised
Nursing interventions
■ Place pillow or rolled towel under upper chest to flex cervical spine, or apply cervical collar.

Axilla (adduction and internal rotation)
Preventive positioning
■ Shoulder joint in external rotation and 100- to 130-degree abduction
Nursing interventions
■ Use an IV pole, bedside table, or sling to suspend arm.

Axilla (adduction and external rotation)
Preventive positioning
■ Shoulder joint in forward flexion and 100- to 130-degree abduction
Nursing interventions
■ Use an IV pole, bedside table, or sling to suspend arm.

Pectoral region (shoulder protraction)
Preventive positioning
■ Shoulders abducted and externally rotated
Nursing interventions
■ Remove pillow from bed.

Chest or abdomen (kyphosis)
Preventive positioning
■ Shoulders abducted and externally rotated with hips neutral (not flexed)
Nursing interventions
■ Use no pillow under head or legs.

Lateral trunk (scoliosis)
Preventive positioning
■ Supine; affected arm abducted
Nursing interventions
■ Put pillows or blanket rolls at sides.

Elbow (flexion and pronation)
Preventive positioning
■ Arm extended and supinated
Nursing interventions
■ Use an elbow splint, arm board, or bedside table.

Wrist (flexion)
Preventive positioning
■ Splint in 15-degree extension
■ *Nursing interventions*
■ Apply a hand splint.

Wrist (extension)
Preventive positioning
■ Splint in 15-degree flexion
Nursing interventions
■ Apply a hand splint.

Fingers (adhesions of the extensor tendons; loss of palmar grasp)
■ *Preventive positioning*
■ Metacarpophalangeal joints in maximum flexion; interphalangeal joints in slight flexion; thumb in maximum abduction
Nursing interventions
■ Apply a hand splint; wrap fingers separately.

Hip (internal rotation, flexion, and adduction; possibly joint subluxation if contracture is severe)
Preventive positioning
■ Neutral rotation and abduction; maintain extension by prone position
Nursing interventions
■ Put a pillow under buttocks (if supine) or use trochanter rolls or knee or long leg splints.

Knee (flexion)
Preventive positioning
■ Extension maintained.
Nursing interventions
■ Use a knee splint with no pillows under legs.

Ankle (plantar flexion if foot muscles are weak or their tendons are divided)
Preventive positioning
■ 90-degree dorsiflexion
Nursing interventions
■ Use a footboard or ankle splint.

■ After cleaning, administer ordered eye ointment or drops using a sterile cotton-tipped applicator or eyedropper and using safe medication administration practices *to keep the eyes moist.* Use moisture chambers as needed, especially if the patient can't close his eyes completely.

■ Close the patient's eyes before applying eye pads *to prevent corneal abrasion.* Don't apply topical ointments near the eyes without a practitioner's order.

Providing nasal care

■ Check the patient's nostrils for inhalation injury: inflamed mucosa, singed vibrissae, and soot.

■ Apply the prescribed ointments using a sterile tongue depressor; use safe medication administration practices.

■ If the patient has a nasogastric tube, use tracheostomy ties to secure the tube. Check the ties frequently for tightness resulting from swelling of facial tissue. Clean the area around the tube, as needed.

Completing burn care

■ Dispose of equipment and supplies appropriately.[15]

■ Remove and discard your gloves and other personal protective equipment, and perform hand hygiene.[9,10,11]

■ Document the procedure.[17,18]

Special considerations

■ *To prevent cross-contamination,* clean and dress the cleanest areas first and the dirtiest or most contaminated areas last. Make sure you remove and discard your gloves, perform hand hygiene, and put on new gloves each time you move from one area to another. *To help prevent excessive pain or cross-contamination,* you may need to perform the dressing in stages *to avoid exposing all wounds at the same time.*

■ Thorough assessment and documentation of the wound's appearance are essential *to detect infection and other complications.* A purulent wound or green-gray exudate indicates infection, an overly dry wound suggests dehydration, and a wound with a swollen, red edge suggests cellulitis. Suspect a fungal infection if the wound is white and powdery. Healthy granulation tissue appears clean, pinkish, faintly shiny, and free of exudate.

PATIENT TEACHING

Successful burn self-care after discharge

You can help the patient make a successful transition from the health care facility to home by encouraging him to follow the wound care and self-care guidelines below.

- *To enhance healing,* instruct the patient to eat well-balanced meals with adequate carbohydrates and proteins, to eat between-meal snacks, and to include at least one protein source in each meal and snack. Tell him to avoid tobacco, alcohol, and caffeine *because they constrict peripheral blood flow.*
- Advise the patient to wash new skin with mild soap and water. *To prevent excessive skin dryness,* instruct him to use a lubricating lotion and to avoid lotions containing alcohol or perfume. Caution the patient to avoid bumping or scratching regenerated skin tissue.
- Recommend nonrestrictive, nonabrasive clothing, which should be laundered in a mild detergent. Advise the patient to wear protective clothing during cold weather *to prevent frostbite.*
- Warn the patient not to expose new skin to strong sunlight and always to use a sunblock with a sun protection factor of 20 or higher. Also, tell him not to expose new skin to irritants, such as paint, solvent, strong detergents, and antiperspirants. Recommend cool baths or ice packs *to relieve itching.*
- *To minimize scar formation,* the patient may need to wear a pressure garment—usually for 23 hours a day for 6 months to 1 year. Instruct him to remove it only during daily hygiene. Suspect that the garment is too tight if it causes cold, numbness, or discoloration in the fingers or toes or if its seams and zippers leave deep, red impressions for more than 10 minutes after the garment is removed.
- Restoring function to the burned area is a major goal for a patient with a burn. Tell the patient to follow the exercise regimen prescribed by the physical and occupational therapist and to go to follow-up visits with his practitioner.[3]

- *Blisters protect underlying tissue,* so leave them intact unless they impede joint motion, become infected, or cause patient discomfort. If ordered, they can be debrided with sterile forceps or in the shower.
- Keep in mind that the patient with healing burns has increased nutritional needs. He'll require extra protein and carbohydrates *to accommodate an almost doubled basal metabolism.*
- If you must manage a burn with topical medications, exposure to air, and no dressing, watch for such problems as wound adherence to bed linens, poor drainage control, and partial loss of topical medications.

Patient teaching

Begin discharge planning as soon as the patient enters the facility *to help him (and his family) make a smooth transition from facility to home. To encourage therapeutic compliance,* prepare him to expect scarring, teach him wound management and pain control, and urge him to follow the prescribed exercise regimen. Provide encouragement and emotional support, and urge the patient to join a burn survivor support group. Also, teach the family or caregivers how to encourage, support, and provide care for the patient. (See *Successful burn self-care after discharge.*)

Complications

Infection is the most common burn complication.

Documentation

Record the date and time of all care provided. Describe wound condition, special dressing-change techniques, topical medications administered, positioning of the burned area, and the patient's tolerance of the procedure. Record the preprocedure pain medication administered and its effectiveness. Note patient teaching provided and the patient's response to instruction.

REFERENCES

1 Pham, T. N. (2008). American Burn Association practice guidelines: Burn shock resuscitation. *Journal of Burn Care & Research, 29,* 257–266. (Level VII)

2 Perel, P., et al. (2013). Colloids versus crystalloids for fluid resuscitation in critically ill patients. *Cochrane Database of Systematic Reviews, 2013*(4), CD000567. (Level I)

3 Kagan, R. J., et al. (2013). Surgical management of the burn wound and use of skin substitutes: An expert panel white paper. *Journal of Burn Care & Research, 34,* e60–e79. (Level VII)

4 Australian Wound Management Association, Inc. (2010). "Standards for wound management" [Online]. Accessed March 2015 via the Web at http://www.awma.com.au/publications/2011_standards_for_wound_management_v2.pdf (Level VII)

5 Wound, Ostomy and Continence Nurses Society (WOCN) Wound Committee and the Association for Professionals in Infection Control and Epidemiology, Inc. (APIC) 2000 Guidelines Committee. (2000, updated 2011). Clean vs. sterile dressing techniques for management of chronic wounds: A fact sheet. *Journal of Wound, Ostomy and Continence Nursing, 39*(Suppl. 2), S30–S34. (Level VII)

6 Weber, J., et al. (2004). Infection control in burn patients. *Burns, 30*(8), A16–A24.

7 Knighton, J. (n.d.). "Wound management: Wound care for the adult burn patient" [Online]. Accessed March 2015 via the Web at http://burnresource.com/pdfs/wound_management.pdf

8 Hayek, S. et al. (2010). Burn wound cleansing—A myth or a scientific practice. *Annals of Burns and Fire Disasters, 23,* 19–24.

9 The Joint Commission. (2015). Standard NPSG.07.01.01. *Comprehensive accreditation manual for hospitals: The official handbook.* Oakbrook Terrace, IL: The Joint Commission. (Level VII)

10 World Health Organization. (2009). "WHO guidelines on hand hygiene in health care: First global patient safety challenge, clean care is safer care" [Online]. Accessed March 2015 via the Web at http://whqlibdoc.who.int/publications/2009/9789241597906_eng.pdf (Level IV)

11 Centers for Disease Control and Prevention. (2002). Guideline for hand hygiene in health-care settings: Recommendations of the Healthcare Infection Control Practices Advisory Committee and the HICPAC/SHEA/APIC/IDSA Hand Hygiene Task Force. *MMWR Recommendations and Reports, 51*(RR-16), 1–45. Accessed March 2015 via the Web at http://www.cdc.gov/mmwr/pdf/rr/rr5116.pdf (Level II)

12 The Joint Commission. (2015). Standard NPSG.01.01.01. *Comprehensive accreditation manual for hospitals: The official handbook.* Oakbrook Terrace, IL: The Joint Commission. (Level VII)

13 The Joint Commission. (2015). Standard PC.01.02.07. *Comprehensive accreditation manual for hospitals: The official handbook.* Oakbrook Terrace, IL: The Joint Commission. (Level VII)

14 Siegel, J. D., et al. (2007). "2007 guideline for isolation precautions: Preventing transmission of infectious agents in healthcare settings" [Online]. Accessed March 2015 via the Web at http://www.cdc.gov/hicpac/pdf/isolation/Isolation2007.pdf (Level II)

15 Occupational Safety and Health Administration. (n.d.). "Bloodborne pathogens, standard number 1910.1030" [Online]. Accessed March 2015 via the Web at http://www.osha.gov/pls/oshaweb/owadisp.show_document?p_table=STANDARDS&p_id=10051 (Level VII)

16 Lynn-McHale Wiegand, D. (Ed.). (2011). *AACN procedure manual for critical care* (6th ed.). St. Louis, MO: Saunders.

17 The Joint Commission. (2015). Standard RC.01.03.01. *Comprehensive accreditation manual for hospitals: The official handbook.* Oakbrook Terrace, IL: The Joint Commission. (Level VII)

18 Centers for Medicare & Medicaid Services, Department of Health and Human Services. (2014). Condition of participation: Medical record services. 42 C.F.R. § 482.24(b).

Additional references

Committee on Organization and Delivery of Burn Care, American Burn Association. (2006). Practice guidelines for burn care, 2006. *Journal of Burn Care & Research, 27,* 437–438.

Fahlstrom, K., et al. (2013). Implementation of a nurse-driven burn resuscitation protocol: A quality improvement project. *Critical Care Nurse, 33*(1), 25–35.

Lipley, N. (2007). New guidelines for managing patients with burns. *Emergency Nurse, 14*(10), 3.

Rowley-Conwy, G. (2010). Infection prevention and treatment in patients with major burn injuries. *Nursing Standard, 25*(7), 51–58.

Tengvall, O. M., et al. (2006). Differences in pain patterns for infected and non-infected patients with burn injuries. *Pain Management Nursing, 7,* 176–182.

World Health Organization. (2007). "Management of burns" [Online]. Accessed March 2015 via the Web at http://www.who.int/surgery/publications/Burns_management.pdf (Level VII)

Burn dressing application, biological and synthetic

Biological dressings provide a temporary protective covering for burn wounds and for clean granulation tissue. They also temporarily secure fresh skin grafts and protect graft donor sites. In common use are three organic materials—pigskin, cadaver skin, and amniotic membrane—and one synthetic material, Biobrane. (See *Comparing biological and synthetic dressings.*) Besides stimulating new skin growth, these dressings act like normal skin: They reduce heat loss, block infection, and minimize fluid, electrolyte, and protein losses.[1]

Amniotic membrane or fresh cadaver skin is usually applied to the patient in the operating room, although it may be applied in a treatment room or at the bedside. Pigskin and Biobrane may be applied in either the operating or a treatment room. Before applying a biological or synthetic dressing, the wound must be cleaned and debrided. The frequency of dressing changes depends on the type of wound and the dressing's specific function.

The use of sterile or clean technique for wound care depends on the patient's immune status, the wound status (chronic or acute), the type of wound, its location and depth, and the wound healing environment.[4,5] Burns are considered acute wounds.[2] For acute burns, use sterile technique and wear a gown, a cap, and a mask whenever the burn wound is exposed.[6,7] Wear a clean gown when applying dressings.[6] Wear clean gloves to remove a soiled dressing and to clean the wound, and wear sterile gloves to apply topical agents and inner dressings.[2,6] Wear sterile gloves when performing sharp bedside debridement.[5]

Equipment

Cap ▪ mask ▪ two pairs of sterile gloves ▪ gown ▪ biological or synthetic dressing ▪ normal saline solution ▪ sterile basin ▪ Xeroflo gauze ▪ roller gauze dressing ▪ nonadhesive dressing ▪ elastic netting or tape ▪ sterile 4″ × 4″ (10-cm × 10-cm) gauze pads ▪ Optional: prescribed analgesic, sterile forceps, sterile scissors, sterile hemostat.

Preparation of equipment

Place the biological dressing in the sterile basin containing sterile normal saline solution (or open the Biobrane package). Using sterile technique, open the sterile dressing packages. Arrange the equipment on the dressing cart and keep the cart readily accessible. Make sure the treatment area has adequate light *to allow accurate wound assessment and dressing placement.*

Implementation

- Verify the practitioner's order.
- Perform hand hygiene.[8,9,10]
- Confirm the patient's identity using at least two patient identifiers.[11]
- If this is the patient's first treatment, explain the procedure *to allay his fears and promote cooperation.* Provide privacy.
- Perform a comprehensive pain assessment using techniques appropriate for the patient's age, condition, and ability to understand.[12]
- If ordered, administer an analgesic following safe medication administration practices *to increase the patient's comfort and tolerance levels.* Oral analgesics should be given at an appropriate time before the procedure, depending on the medication's onset and peak of action. An IV analgesic may be given immediately before the procedure.
- Provide a warm environment.[13]
- Perform hand hygiene and put on a cap, a mask, a gown, and sterile gloves.[5,6,8,9,10,14]
- Assess the burn wound, noting the color, size, odor, and depth of the wound as well as the presence of drainage, bleeding, edema, and eschar. Monitor for cellulitis in the surrounding tissue.[13]
- Clean and debride the wound *to reduce bacteria.*[13,15] (See the "Sharp debridement" procedure, page 692.)
- Remove and discard your gloves. Perform hand hygiene and put on a fresh pair of sterile gloves.[5,6,8,9,10,14]
- Place the dressing directly on the wound surface. Apply pigskin, dermal (shiny) side down; apply Biobrane, nylon-backed (dull) side down.[3] Roll the dressing directly onto the skin, if applicable. Place the dressing strips so that the edges touch but don't overlap. Use sterile forceps, if necessary. Smooth the dressing. Eliminate folds and wrinkles by rolling out the dressing with the hemostat handle, the forceps handle, or your dominant hand *to cover the wound completely and ensure adherence.*
- Use the scissors to trim the dressing around the wound *so that the dressing fits the wound without overlapping adjacent areas.*
- Place Xeroflo gauze directly over an allograft, pigskin graft, or amniotic membrane. Place a few layers of sterile 4″ × 4″ (10-cm × 10-cm) gauze on top *to absorb exudate,* and wrap with a roller gauze dressing. Secure the dressing with tape or elastic netting. During daily dressing changes, the dressing will be removed down to the Xeroflo gauze, and the sterile 4″ × 4″ (10-cm × 10-cm) gauze will be replaced after the Xeroflo gauze is inspected for drainage, adherence, and signs of infection.
- Place a nonadhesive dressing (such as Exu-Dry) over the Biobrane *to absorb drainage and provide stability.* Wrap the dressing with a roller gauze dressing, and secure it with tape or elastic netting. For the first 24 hours, keep the outer dressing in place and don't get it wet. After 24 hours, the dressing will be removed down to the Biobrane during daily dressing changes and you'll inspect the site for signs of infection. After the Biobrane adheres (usually in 2 to 3 days), it doesn't need to be covered with a dressing.[3]
- Position the patient comfortably, elevating the area if possible *to reduce edema, which may prevent the biological dressing from adhering.*
- Reassess the patient's pain and respond appropriately.[12]
- Discard used equipment and supplies in the appropriate receptacles.[16]
- Remove and discard your gloves and personal protective equipment.
- Perform hand hygiene.[8,9,10]
- Document the procedure.[17,18]

Special considerations

- Handle a biological or synthetic dressing as little as possible.

Comparing biological and synthetic dressings

Type	Description and uses	Nursing considerations
Cadaver (allograft)	▪ Obtained at autopsy up to 24 hours after death ▪ Applied in the operating room or at the bedside to debrided, clean wounds ▪ Available as fresh cryopreserved homografts in tissue banks nationwide ▪ Provides protection, especially to granulation tissue after escharotomy ▪ May be used in some patients as a test graft for autografting ▪ Covers excised wounds immediately ▪ Used most frequently for burns when autograft skin isn't available[2]	▪ Observe for exudate. ▪ Watch for signs of rejection. ▪ Keep in mind that the gauze dressing may be removed every 8 hours to observe the graft.
Pigskin (heterograft or xenograft)	▪ Applied in the operating room or at the bedside ▪ Comes fresh or frozen in rolls or sheets ▪ Can cover and protect debrided, untidy wounds; mesh autografts; clean (eschar-free) partial-thickness burns; and exposed tendons	▪ Reconstitute frozen form with normal saline solution 30 minutes before use. ▪ Watch for signs of rejection. ▪ Cover with gauze dressing or leave exposed to air, as ordered.
Amniotic membrane (homograft)	▪ Available from the obstetric department ▪ Must be sterile and come from an uncomplicated birth; serologic tests must be done ▪ Bacteriostatic condition doesn't require antimicrobials ▪ May be used to protect partial-thickness burns or (temporarily) granulation tissue before autografting ▪ Applied by the practitioner to clean wounds only	▪ Change the membrane every 48 hours. ▪ Cover the membrane with a gauze dressing or leave it exposed, as ordered. ▪ If you apply a gauze dressing, change it every 48 hours.
Biobrane (biosynthetic membrane)	▪ Comes in sterile, prepackaged sheets in various sizes and in glove form for hand burns ▪ Used to cover donor graft sites, superficial partial-thickness burns, debrided wounds awaiting autograft, and meshed autografts ▪ Reduces pain ▪ Applied by the nurse	▪ Apply taut against the skin. ▪ Leave the membrane in place until the tissue underneath is healed, typically 7 to 14 days.[3] ▪ Don't use this dressing for preparing a granulation bed for subsequent autografting.

Patient teaching

Instruct the patient or caregiver to assess the site daily for signs of complications, such as infection, swelling, blisters, drainage, and separation. Make sure the patient knows who to contact if these complications develop.

Complications

Infection can develop under a biological or synthetic dressing. Observe the wound carefully during dressing changes for signs of infection. If wound drainage appears purulent, remove the dressing, clean the area with normal saline solution or another prescribed cleaning solution as ordered, and apply a fresh biological or synthetic dressing.

Documentation

Record the time and date of dressing changes. Note areas of application, the quality of adherence, and purulent drainage or other signs of infection. Also describe the patient's tolerance of the procedure.

References

1 Bezuhly, M., & Fish, J. S. (2012). Acute burn care. *Plastic and Reconstructive Surgery, 130,* 349e–358e.

2 Kagan, R. J., et al. (2013). Surgical management of the burn wound and use of skin substitutes: An expert panel white paper. *Journal of Burn Care & Research, 34,* e60–e79.

3 Smith & Nephew. (n.d.). "Biobrane: Biosynthetic wound dressing, instructions for use" [Online]. Accessed March 2015 via the Web at http://www.smith-nephew.com/uk/products/wound_management/product-search/biobrane/

4 Australian Wound Management Association. (2010). "Standards for wound management" [Online]. Accessed March 2015 via the Web at http://www.awma.com.au/publications/2011_standards_for_wound_management_v2.pdf (Level VII)

5 Wound, Ostomy and Continence Nurses Society (WOCN) Wound Committee and the Association for Professionals in Infection Control and Epidemiology, Inc. (APIC) 2000 Guidelines Committee. (2000, updated 2011). Clean vs. sterile dressing techniques for management of chronic wounds: A fact sheet. *Journal of Wound, Ostomy, and Continence Nursing, 39*(Suppl. 2), S30–S34. (Level VII)

6 Knighton, J. (n.d.). "Wound management: Wound care for the adult burn patient" [Online]. Accessed March 2015 via the Web at http://burnresource.com/pdfs/wound_management.pdf

7 Weber, J., et al. (2004). Infection control in burn patients. *Burns, 30*(8), A16–A24.

8 The Joint Commission. (2015). Standard NPSG.07.01.01. *Comprehensive accreditation manual for hospitals: The official handbook.* Oakbrook Terrace, IL: The Joint Commission. (Level VII)

9 Centers for Disease Control and Prevention. (2002). Guideline for hand hygiene in health-care settings: Recommendations of the Healthcare Infection Control Practices Advisory Committee and the HICPAC/SHEA/APIC/IDSA Hand Hygiene Task Force. *MMWR Recommendations and Reports, 51*(RR-16), 1–45. Accessed March 2015 via the Web at http://www.cdc.gov/mmwr/pdf/rr/rr5116.pdf (Level II)

10 World Health Organization. (2009). "WHO guidelines on hand hygiene in health care: First global patient safety challenge, clean care is safer care"

[Online]. Accessed March 2015 via the Web at http://whqlibdoc.who.int/publications/2009/9789241597906_eng.pdf (Level IV)

11 The Joint Commission. (2015). Standard NPSG.01.01.01. *Comprehensive accreditation manual for hospitals: The official handbook.* Oakbrook Terrace, IL: The Joint Commission. (Level VII)

12 The Joint Commission. (2015). Standard PC.01.02.07. *Comprehensive accreditation manual for hospitals: The official handbook.* Oakbrook Terrace, IL: The Joint Commission. (Level VII)

13 Lynn-McHale Wiegand, D. (Ed.). (2011). *AACN procedure manual for critical care* (6th ed.). St. Louis, MO: Saunders.

14 Siegel, J. D., et al. (2007). "2007 guideline for isolation precautions: Preventing transmission of infectious agents in healthcare settings" [Online]. Accessed March 2015 via the Web at http://www.cdc.gov/hicpac/pdf/isolation/Isolation2007.pdf (Level II)

15 Verger, J. T., & Lebet, R. M. (Eds.). (2008). *AACN procedure manual for pediatric acute and critical care.* St. Louis, MO: Saunders.

16 Occupational Safety and Health Administration. (n.d.). "Bloodborne pathogens, standard number 1910.1030" [Online]. Accessed March 2015 via the Web at http://www.osha.gov/pls/oshaweb/owadisp.show_document?p_table=STANDARDS&p_id=10051 (Level VII)

17 The Joint Commission. (2015). Standard RC.01.03.01. *Comprehensive accreditation manual for hospitals: The official handbook.* Oakbrook Terrace, IL: The Joint Commission. (Level VII)

18 Centers for Medicare & Medicaid Services, Department of Health and Human Services. (2012). Condition of participation: Medical record services. 42 C.F.R. § 482.24(b).

Additional references

Andonovska, D., et al. (2008). The advantages of the application of amnion membrane in the treatment of burns. *Prilozi, 29*(1), 183–198.

Damanhuri, M., et al. (2011). Advances in tissue-engineered skin substitutes. *Wounds International, 2*(1). Accessed March 2015 via the Web at http://www.woundsinternational.com/product-reviews/advances-in-tissue-engineered-skin-substitutes/page-1

Ermolov, A. S., et al. (2008). The use of bioactive wound dressing, stimulating epithelial regeneration of IIIa-degree burn wounds. *Bulletin of Experimental Biology and Medicine, 146,*153–157.

Kesting, M. R., et al. (2008). The role of allogenic amniotic membrane in burn treatment. *Journal of Burn Care & Research, 29,* 907–916.

Lineen, E., & Namias, N. (2008). Biologic dressing in burns. *Journal of Craniofacial Surgery, 19,*923–928.

Pham, C., et al. (2007). Bioengineered skin substitutes for the management of burns: A systematic review. *Burns, 33,* 946–957. (Level I)

C

Canes

Indicated for the patient with one-sided weakness or injury, occasional loss of balance, or increased joint pressure, a cane provides balance and support for walking and reduces fatigue and strain on weight-bearing joints. Available in various sizes, the cane should extend from the greater trochanter to the floor and have a rubber tip to prevent slipping. Canes are contraindicated for the patient with bilateral weakness; such a patient should use crutches or a walker.

Equipment

Rubber-tipped cane ■ Optional: gait belt.

Although wooden canes are available, three types of aluminum canes are used most frequently. The standard aluminum cane (used by the patient who needs only slight assistance with walking) provides the least support. The T-handle cane (used by the patient with hand weakness) has a straight-shaped handle with grips and a bent shaft. It provides greater stability than the standard cane. Three- or four-pronged (quad) canes are used by the patient with poor balance or one-sided weakness and an inability to hold onto a walker with both hands. The base of these types of canes splits into three or four short, splayed legs and provides greater stability than a standard cane but considerably less than a walker.

Preparation of equipment

Ask the patient to hold the cane on the uninvolved side 6″ (15 cm) from the base of the little toe. If the cane is made of aluminum, adjust its height by pushing in the metal button on the shaft and raising or lowering the shaft; if it's wood, the rubber tip can be removed and excess length sawed off. The handle of the cane should be level with the greater trochanter to allow approximately 30-degree flexion at the elbow. If the cane is too short, the patient will have to drop his shoulder to lean on it; if it's too long, he'll have to raise his shoulder and will have difficulty supporting his weight.

Implementation

- Perform hand hygiene.[1,2,3,4,5]
- Confirm the patient's identity using at least two patient identifiers.[6]
- Tell the patient to hold the cane on the uninvolved side[7] *to promote a reciprocal gait pattern and to distribute weight away from the involved side.*
- Instruct the patient to hold the cane close to his body *to prevent leaning* and to move the cane forward 4″ to 8″ (10 to 20 cm) and simultaneously move the involved leg forward, followed by the uninvolved leg.
- Encourage the patient to keep the stride length of each leg and the timing of each step (cadence) equal.
- Demonstrate the technique for the patient.
- Have the patient return the demonstration, and provide additional teaching as needed.

Negotiating stairs

- Instruct the patient to always use a railing, if present, when going up or down stairs. Tell him to hold the cane with the other hand (as shown below). To ascend stairs, tell the patient to lead with the uninvolved leg and follow with the involved leg; to descend, tell him to lead with the involved leg and follow with the uninvolved one. Help the patient remember by telling him to use this mnemonic device: "Up with the good; down with the bad."

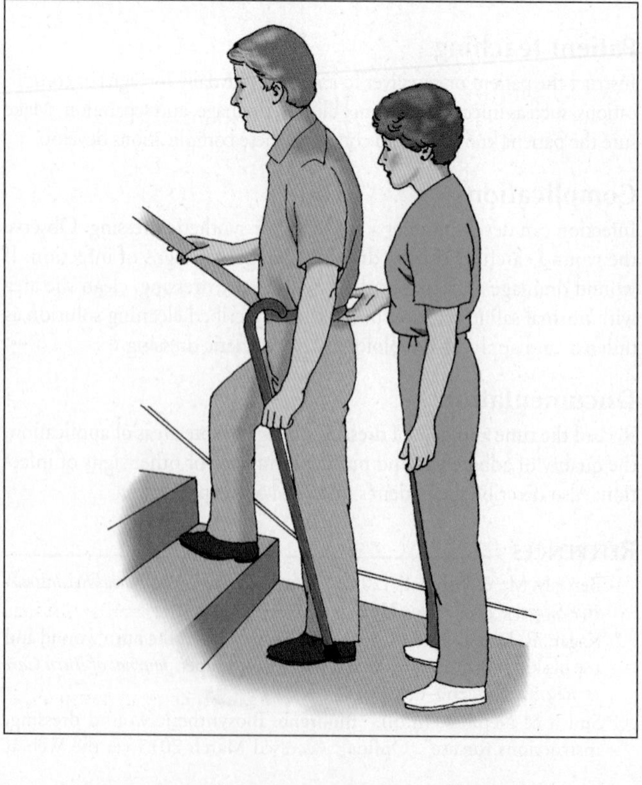

■ To negotiate stairs without a railing, tell the patient to use the walking technique to ascend and descend the stairs. Thus, to ascend stairs, tell the patient to hold the cane on the uninvolved side, step with the uninvolved leg, advance the cane, and then move the involved leg. To descend, he should hold the cane on the uninvolved side, lead with the cane, then advance the involved leg and then, finally, the uninvolved leg.
■ Remind the patient always to move the cane just before moving the involved leg in all stair use regardless of direction.

Using a chair

■ To teach the patient to sit down, stand by his affected side and tell him to place the backs of his legs against the edge of the chair seat. Then tell him to move the cane out from his side and to reach back with both hands to grasp the chair's armrests. Supporting his weight on the armrests, he can then lower himself onto the seat. While he's seated, he should keep the cane hooked on the armrest or the chair back.
■ To teach the patient to get up, stand by his affected side and tell him to unhook the cane from the chair and hold it in his stronger hand as he grasps the armrests. Then tell him to move his uninvolved foot slightly forward, to lean slightly forward, and to push against the armrests to raise himself upright (as shown below).

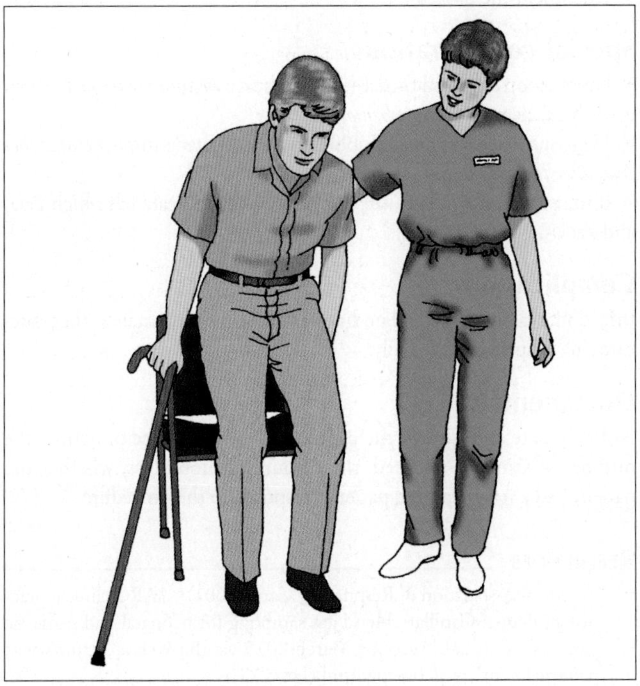

■ Instruct the patient not to lean on the cane when sitting or rising from the chair *to prevent falls.*
■ Supervise the patient each time he gets into or out of a chair until you're both certain he can do it alone.
■ Perform hand hygiene.[1,2,3,4,5]
■ Document the procedure.[8,9,10]

Special considerations

■ *To prevent falls during the learning period,* guard the patient carefully by standing behind him slightly to his stronger side and putting one foot between his feet and your other foot to the outside of the uninvolved leg. If necessary, use a gait belt.
■ Coordinate practice sessions in the physical therapy department, if necessary.

Patient teaching

Instruct the patient and his family to assess the patient's home environment for safety concerns. Tell them to secure or remove loose rugs, electrical cords, and clutter from the floor. Instruct the patient to use safety bars and a raised toilet seat in the bathroom and a nonskid mat in the bathtub. Recommend that the patient use a fanny pack or backpack to carry items around the house and keep personal items close by.[7] Also recommend that he wear nonskid slippers or shoes with rubber soles and replace the tip of his cane when it's worn out.

Complications

A poorly fitted cane or unclear instructions can cause the patient to lose his balance and fall.

Documentation

Record the type of cane used, the amount of guarding required, the distance walked, and the patient's understanding and tolerance of cane walking.

REFERENCES

1 The Joint Commission. (2015). Standard NPSG.07.01.01. *Comprehensive accreditation manual for hospitals: The official handbook.* Oakbrook Terrace, IL: The Joint Commission. (Level VII)
2 Centers for Disease Control and Prevention. (2002). Guideline for hand hygiene in health-care settings: Recommendations of the Healthcare Infection Control Practices Advisory Committee and the HICPAC/SHEA/APIC/IDSA Hand Hygiene Task Force. *HMMWR Recommendations and Reports, 51*(RR-16), 1–45. Accessed March 2015 via the Web at http://www.cdc.gov/mmwr/pdf/rr/rr5116.pdf (Level II)
3 World Health Organization. (2009). "WHO guidelines on hand hygiene in health care: First global patient safety challenge, clean care is safer care" [Online]. Accessed March 2015 via the Web at http://whqlibdoc.who.int/publications/2009/9789241597906_eng.pdf (Level IV)
4 Centers for Medicare & Medicaid Services, Department of Health and Human Services. (2014). Condition of participation: Infection control. 42 C.F.R. § 482.42.
5 American Osteopathic Association. (2014). Standard 07.01.21. *Healthcare Facilities Accreditation Program: Accreditation requirements for acute care hospitals.* Chicago, IL: American Osteopathic Association. (Level VII)
6 The Joint Commission. (2015). Standard NPSG.01.01.01. *Comprehensive accreditation manual for hospitals: The official handbook.* Oakbrook Terrace, IL: The Joint Commission. (Level VII)
7 American Academy of Orthopaedic Surgeons. (2007). "How to use crutches, canes, and walkers" [Online]. Accessed March 2015 via the Web at http://orthoinfo.aaos.org/topic.cfm?topic=a00181
8 The Joint Commission. (2015). Standard RC.01.03.01. *Comprehensive accreditation manual for hospitals: The official handbook.* Oakbrook Terrace, IL: The Joint Commission. (Level VII)
9 American Osteopathic Association. (2014). Standard 10.00.03. *Healthcare Facilities Accreditation Program: Accreditation requirements for acute care hospitals.* Chicago, IL: American Osteopathic Association.
10 Centers for Medicare & Medicaid Services, Department of Health and Human Services. (2014). Condition of participation: Medical record services. 42 C.F.R. § 482.24.

ADDITIONAL REFERENCES

Allet, L., et al. (2009). Effect of different walking aids on walking capacity of patients with poststroke hemiparesis. *Archives of Physical Medicine and Rehabilitation, 90*(8), 1408–1413.
Craven, R. F., & Hirnle, C. J. (2009). *Fundamentals of nursing: Human health and function* (6th ed.). Philadelphia, PA: Lippincott Williams & Wilkins.
Demers, L., et al. (2008). Tracking mobility-related assistive technology in an outcomes study. *Assistive Technology, 20*(2), 73–83.

CAPILLARY BLOOD GAS SAMPLING

Arterial blood gas (ABG) analysis evaluates ventilation by measuring blood pH and the partial pressures of arterial oxygen (Pao_2) and carbon dioxide ($Paco_2$). Blood pH measurement reveals the blood's acid-base balance. Pao_2 indicates the amount of oxygen that the lungs deliver to the blood, and $Paco_2$ indicates the lungs' capacity to eliminate carbon dioxide. ABG samples can also be analyzed for oxygen content and saturation and for bicarbonate values.

An alternative to ABG sampling, capillary blood gas sampling is used to help monitor a patient's respiratory status. The procedure can be performed in the presence of hypothermia and hypoperfusion (provided that hypertension isn't present) and can be easier to perform than ABG sampling in these situations. It involves a simple fingerstick and is less painful than an arterial puncture.

Capillary blood must be collected in special balanced-heparin capillary blood gas collection tubes. The laboratory should receive the sample within 15 minutes of collection;[1] a delay may alter the results because of cellular metabolism or hemolysis.

Equipment

Single use, auto-disabling sterile lancet (1.5 mm in depth) ▪ alcohol pad ▪ 2″ × 2″ (5-cm × 5-cm) sterile gauze pads ▪ gloves ▪ preheparinized glass capillary tube ▪ warming supplies (such as a chemical warmer or a warm cloth that's less than 109°F [42.8°C]) ▪ sealing clay, wax sealer, or cap ▪ sample collection label ▪ laboratory biohazard transport bag ▪ Optional: topical anesthetic cream, small adhesive bandage.

Implementation

- Verify the practitioner's order.
- Gather the necessary supplies.
- Perform hand hygiene.[2,3,4,5,6]
- Confirm the patient's identity using at least two patient identifiers.[7]
- Explain the procedure to the patient, allowing him to ask questions and express anxiety as needed *to promote better understanding of what is to be done.*
- Select the capillary puncture site. Either the earlobe or the finger is the preferred site in adults.[8] Select a site on the second or third finger, using the side of the finger, parallel to the side edges of the nail.[8] Avoid the finger's tip or pad *to prevent additional discomfort.*

NURSING ALERT *Avoid using extremities with impaired circulation or localized infection.*

- Apply a topical anesthetic if indicated and time allows *to decrease discomfort.*

NURSING ALERT *Don't use lidocaine or prilocaine if the patient is receiving methemoglobin-inducing agents, such as sulfonamides and acetaminophen,* because a risk of methemoglobinemia exists.

- Apply the warming device to the puncture site for 5 to 10 minutes *to increase blood flow and reduce hemolysis and bruising.* Don't use products warmed in a microwave *because uneven heating by the microwave presents a burn risk.*
- Perform hand hygiene and put on gloves.[2,3,4,5,9,10]
- Remove the warming device from the puncture site.
- If topical anesthetic cream was used, remove it before cleaning the puncture site.
- Clean the puncture site with an alcohol pad and allow it to dry completely *because alcohol may interfere with test results if not permitted to dry completely.*[8]
- Place the extremity in a dependent position and grasp it firmly.
- To perform the puncture, use a single-use, auto-disabling lancet *to prevent transmission of bloodborne pathogens.*[11] Puncture the skin with a quick, continuous, and deliberate stroke *to achieve good flow of blood and to prevent the need to repeat the puncture.*[8]
- If required by your facility, wipe the first drop of blood away with a sterile gauze pad *because residual alcohol or tissue fluids may contaminate the blood gas sample.*[8,12]
- Hold the capillary tube horizontally *to fill it by capillary action and to prevent air entrapment.* Avoid squeezing the finger too tightly *because doing so may dilute the specimen with plasma and increases the possibility of hemolysis.*[8]
- Fill the entire tube with blood and seal it.
- Apply firm pressure to the puncture site with a sterile gauze pad *to stop the bleeding.*[8]

NURSING ALERT *If the patient has a hematologic disorder or is receiving certain medications, such as warfarin, heparin, or aspirin, he may have a prolonged clotting time.*

- Label the sample in the presence of the patient *to prevent mislabeling.*[7]
- Properly dispose of contaminated equipment. Place the lancet in a sharps container and blood-soaked gauze in a biohazard bag.[13]
- Remove and discard your gloves, and perform hand hygiene.[2,3,4,5,6]
- Place the sample in a laboratory biohazard transport bag and send it to the laboratory immediately.
- Evaluate the puncture site for evidence of continued bleeding. Apply a small adhesive bandage, if necessary.
- Keep the wound clean and dry.
- Perform hand hygiene.[2,3,4,5,6]
- Document the procedure.[14,15,16]

Special considerations

- Never scoop up blood from the patient's skin *because it may be partially coagulated, which can cause hemolysis.*
- Make sure there are no air bubbles in the collected sample *because they may alter the test results.*
- If the patient has a fever, the test results may indicate false-high Pao_2 and $Paco_2$.

Complications

Infection, scarring, calcified nodules, or bruising may occur at the puncture site. Inspect the site daily.

Documentation

Note the date and time of the procedure, the site of the puncture, the number of samples obtained, the amount of blood loss, whether the patient had a fever, and the patient's response to the procedure.

REFERENCES

1 American Association of Respiratory Care. (2001). "AARC clinical practice guideline: Capillary blood gas sampling for neonatal and pediatric patients" [Online]. Accessed March 2015 via the Web at http://www.rcjournal.com/cpgs/cbgscpg.html (Level VII)

2 Centers for Disease Control and Prevention. (2002). Guideline for hand hygiene in health-care settings: Recommendations of the Healthcare Infection Control Practices Advisory Committee and the HICPAC/SHEA/APIC/IDSA Hand Hygiene Task Force. *MMWR Recommendations and Reports, 51*(RR-16), 1–45. Accessed March 2015 via the Web at http://www.cdc.gov/mmwr/pdf/rr/rr5116.pdf (Level II)

3 The Joint Commission. (2015). Standard NPSG.07.01.01. *Comprehensive accreditation manual for hospitals: The official handbook.* Oakbrook Terrace, IL: The Joint Commission. (Level VII)

4 World Health Organization. (2009). "WHO guidelines on hand hygiene in health care: First global patient safety challenge, clean care is safer care" [Online]. Accessed March 2015 via the Web at http://whqlibdoc.who.int/publications/2009/9789241597906_eng.pdf (Level IV)

5 Centers for Medicare & Medicaid Services, Department of Health and Human Services. (2014). Condition of participation: Infection control. 42 C.F.R. § 482.42.

6 American Osteopathic Association. (2014). Standard 07.01.21. *Healthcare Facilities Accreditation Program: Accreditation requirements for acute care hospitals.* Chicago, IL: American Osteopathic Association. (Level VII)
7 The Joint Commission. (2015). Standard NPSG.01.01.01. *Comprehensive accreditation manual for hospitals: The official handbook.* Oakbrook Terrace, IL: The Joint Commission. (Level VII)
8 World Health Organization. (2010). "WHO guidelines of drawing blood: Best practices in phlebotomy" [Online]. Accessed March 2015 via the Web at http://www.who.int/injection_safety/phleb_final_screen_ready.pdf
9 Siegel, J. D., et al. (2007). "2007 guideline for isolation precautions: Preventing transmission of infectious agents in healthcare settings" [Online]. Accessed March 2015 via the Web at http://www.cdc.gov/hicpac/pdf/isolation/Isolation2007.pdf (Level II)
10 American Osteopathic Association. (2014). Standard 07.01.10. *Healthcare Facilities Accreditation Program: Accreditation requirements for acute care hospitals.* Chicago, IL: American Osteopathic Association. (Level VII)
11 Centers for Disease Control and Prevention. (2011). "CDC clinical reminder: Use of fingerstick devices on more than one person poses risk for transmitting bloodborne pathogens" [Online]. Accessed March 2015 via the Web at http://www.cdc.gov/injectionsafety/Fingerstick-DevicesBGM.html
12 Fischbach, F., & Dunning, M. B. (2014). *A manual of laboratory and diagnostic tests* (9th ed.). Philadelphia, PA: Wolters Kluwer.
13 Occupational Safety and Health Administration. (n.d.). "Bloodborne pathogens, standard number 1910.1030" [Online]. Accessed March 2015 via the Web at http://www.osha.gov/pls/oshaweb/owadisp.show_document?p_table=STANDARDS&p_id=10051 (Level VII)
14 The Joint Commission. (2015). Standard RC.01.03.01. *Comprehensive accreditation manual for hospitals: The official handbook.* Oakbrook Terrace, IL: The Joint Commission. (Level VII)
15 Centers for Medicare & Medicaid Services, Department of Health and Human Services. (2014). Condition of participation: Medical record services. 42 C.F.R. § 482.24(b).
16 American Osteopathic Association. (2014). Standard 10.00.03. *Healthcare Facilities Accreditation Program: Accreditation requirements for acute care hospitals.* Chicago, IL: American Osteopathic Association. (Level VII)

ADDITIONAL REFERENCES

Craven, R. F., Hirnle, C. J. (2012). *Fundamentals of nursing: Human health and function* (7th ed.). Philadelphia, PA: Lippincott Williams & Wilkins.
Zavorsky, G. S., et al. (2007). Arterial versus capillary blood gases: A meta-analysis. *Respiratory Physiology & Neurobiology, 155,* 268–279. (Level I)

CARBON MONOXIDE OXIMETRY

Intermittent or continuous carbon monoxide oximetry can be performed noninvasively with a lightweight, portable display unit that's connected to a sensor probe placed on the adult patient's fingertip or an infant's foot. The sensor probe collects data about the patient's carboxyhemoglobin saturation and sends that information to the oximeter, which then displays the calculated data in the form of a percentage. A carboxyhemoglobin saturation level greater than 3% for nonsmokers and 10% to 15% for smokers indicates exposure to exogenous carbon monoxide.[1]

Carbon monoxide levels can be increased as a result of chronic exposure to cigarette smoke or from acute episodes, such as from exposure to a combustion heater and inadequate ventilation of natural gas, fire, or vehicle exhaust. However, carbon monoxide poisoning is commonly misdiagnosed because the initial signs and symptoms—fatigue, shortness of breath, mild headache, and nausea—are similar to those of a viral-related illness. Severe signs and symptoms include dizziness, increasingly acute headaches, weakness, drowsiness, and nausea accompanied by vomiting. Carbon monoxide poisoning can result in long-term neurologic damage, psychiatric and cardiovascular disorders, and death.

Carbon monoxide poisoning is typically diagnosed using the patient's history, physical examination findings, and laboratory test results that reveal an elevated carbon monoxide level. Recent studies show that carbon monoxide oximetry can also be useful for first-line screening[2] and to monitor carbon monoxide trends.[3] However, further study is needed to confirm the accuracy of these findings.[1]

Equipment

Noninvasive pulse carbon monoxide oximeter ■ appropriate sensor (according to the patient's age, weight, digit size, and the anticipated duration of monitoring)[4] ■ flow sheet for recording data ■ disinfectant pads ■ Optional: nail clippers, nail polish remover, batteries, connecting cable.

Preparation of equipment

Plug the carbon monoxide oximeter into an electrical source, and then turn on the unit. Plug the cable into the oximeter unit. Select a sensor that's compatible with the particular device and appropriate for the patient, and connect it to the cable.[4] If using a portable, handheld carbon monoxide oximeter, ensure that the unit is charged; replace the batteries as needed according to the manufacturer's instructions. Attach an appropriate patient sensor to the carbon monoxide oximeter.[4] Calibrate the carbon monoxide oximeter, if required, following the manufacturer's instructions.

Implementation

■ Verify the practitioner's order for pulse carbon monoxide oximetry.
■ Gather and prepare the appropriate equipment.
■ Review the patient's medical record for current illnesses and any history of carbon monoxide exposure.
■ Perform hand hygiene.[5,6,7,8,9]
■ Confirm the patient's identity using at least two patient identifiers.[10]
■ Explain the procedure to the patient, and answer any questions.
■ Select a finger for the test. Although the index finger is commonly used, you may use a smaller finger if the patient's fingers are too large for the equipment. Select one that appears to be adequately perfused. If possible, don't choose a finger in the hand of an arm being used for blood pressure monitoring.[11]

NURSING ALERT *If you're testing a neonate or small infant, wrap the probe around the foot with the light beams and detectors aligned opposite each other. For a large infant, use a probe that fits on the great toe and secure it to the foot.*

■ Make sure the patient isn't wearing false fingernails or nail polish *to enhance the accuracy of the measurement.* Remove nail polish and other substances that might interfere with the transmission of light between the sensor's source light source and the detector.[4,11]
■ Clean the patient's finger and fingernail with a disinfectant pad, and allow it to dry.[11]
■ Place the sensor probe on the patient's finger, making sure the light source and the detector are aligned opposite each other.[4] If the patient has long fingernails, position the probe perpendicular to the finger, if possible, or clip the fingernail.
■ Position the patient's hand at heart level *to eliminate venous pulsations and to promote accurate readings.*
■ Look at the display panel on the carbon monoxide oximeter; the perfusion indicator should begin registering a pulse. Adjust the sensor and sensitivity, as needed, to achieve an adequate pulse display *because, without a pulse, signal readings are erroneous.*[11]
■ During oximetry, determine whether blood flow to the site is adequate by assessing the patient's pulse rate and capillary refill time. If it isn't, loosen restraints, remove tight-fitting clothes, take off a blood pressure cuff, or check arterial and IV lines, as appropriate. If none of these interventions works, you may need to use an alternate site.[4]
■ Wait the time recommended by the manufacturer before obtaining the reading.
■ Monitor the patient's carbon monoxide level and pulse rate on the display screen, and then obtain readings for both.

■ Press the SPCO key *to obtain carbon monoxide reading.* Confirm the value as needed by placing the sensor on another finger and obtain a reading.
■ For continuous monitoring, set the alarm limits appropriately for the patient's current condition and make sure the alarms are turned on, functioning properly, and audible to staff.[12,13,14,15] Reposition reusable sensors at least every 4 hours; if using adhesive sensors, inspect the application site at least every 8 hours unless otherwise directed, and reapply sensors to different sites as needed.[4] Keep the monitoring site clean and dry, and make sure that the skin doesn't become irritated from the sensor.
■ Report critical test results to the practitioner within the time frame established by your facility *to prevent life-threatening treatment delays.*[16]
■ Record all measurements in the patient's medical record.
■ Perform hand hygiene.[5,6,7,8,9]
■ When monitoring is complete, clean and disinfect the oximeter, cable, and sensor (if not disposable) and the cable (as applicable) according to the manufacturer's instructions.[17,18]
■ Perform hand hygiene.[5,6,7,8,9]
■ Document the procedure.[19,20,21]

Special considerations

■ Low carbon monoxide levels don't rule out exposure, especially if the patient has already received 100% oxygen or if significant time has elapsed since exposure. In addition to carbon monoxide oximetry, monitor the patient's clinical status and other laboratory parameters, such as arterial or venous blood gas values.[22]
■ Individuals who chronically smoke may have mildly elevated carbon monoxide levels as high as 10%. Persistence of fetal hemoglobin may also falsely elevate levels.[1,22]
■ The Joint Commission issued a sentinel event alert concerning medical device alarm safety *because alarm-related events have been associated with permanent loss of function and death.* Among the major contributing factors were improper alarm settings, inappropriately turned off alarms, and alarm signals that were not audible to staff. Make sure that alarm limits are appropriately set and that alarms are turned on, functioning properly, and audible to staff. Follow facility guidelines for preventing alarm fatigue.[15]

Documentation

Document the date and time that you attached the oximeter unit to the patient. Record the initial percentage of carboxyhemoglobin registered as well as pulse rate and oxygen saturation level. Record the date, time, and name of the practitioner notified of abnormal results, if applicable; the prescribed interventions; and the patient's response to those interventions. Also document patient teaching provided, questions asked by the patient, and your responses.

REFERENCES

1 Clardy, P. F., et al. Carbon monoxide poisoning. (2014). In: *UpToDate,* Traub, S. J., et al. (Eds.). Accessed March 2015 via the Web at http://www.uptodate.com/contents/search

2 Sebbane, M., et al. (2013). Emergency department management of suspected carbon monoxide poisoning: Role of pulse co-oximetry. *Respiratory Care, 58,* 1614–1620. Accessed March 2015 via the Web at http://rc.rcjournal.com/content/early/2013/03/19/respcare.02313.full.pdf+html (Level VI)

3 Park, Y. H., et al. (2012). The accuracy of noninvasive hemoglobin monitoring using the Radical-7 Pulse CO-Oximeter in children undergoing neurosurgery. *Anesthesia and Analgesia, 115,* 1302–1307. (Level VI)

4 Masimo Corporation. (2011). "Rad-57 operator's manual: Masimo Rainbow SET: Signal extraction pulse CO-oximeter" [Online]. Accessed March 2015 via the Web at http://www.masimo.com/pdf/rad-57/LAB5813D.pdf

5 The Joint Commission. (2015). Standard NPSG.07.01.01. *Comprehensive accreditation manual for hospitals: The official handbook.* Oakbrook Terrace, IL: The Joint Commission. (Level VII)

6 Centers for Disease Control and Prevention. (2002). Guideline for hand hygiene in health-care settings: Recommendations of the Healthcare Infection Control Practices Advisory Committee and the HICPAC/SHEA/APIC/IDSA Hand Hygiene Task Force. *MMWR Recommendations and Reports, 51*(RR-16), 1–45. Accessed March 2015 via the Web at http://www.cdc.gov/mmwr/pdf/rr/rr5116.pdf (Level VII)

7 World Health Organization. (2009). "WHO guidelines on hand hygiene in health care: First global patient safety challenge, clean care is safer care" [Online]. Accessed March 2015 via the Web at http://whqlibdoc.who.int/publications/2009/9789241597906_eng.pdf (Level IV)

8 American Osteopathic Association. (2014). Standard 07.01.21. *Healthcare Facilities Accreditation Program: Accreditation requirements for acute care hospitals.* Chicago, IL: American Osteopathic Association. (Level VII)

9 Centers for Medicare & Medicaid Services, Department of Health and Human Services. (2014). Condition of participation: Infection control. 42 C.F.R. § 482.42.

10 The Joint Commission. (2015). Standard NPSG.01.01.01. *Comprehensive accreditation manual for hospitals: The official handbook.* Oakbrook Terrace, IL: The Joint Commission. (Level VII)

11 World Health Organization. (2011). "Pulse oximetry training manual" [Online]. Accessed March 2015 via the Web at http://www.who.int/patientsafety/safesurgery/pulse_oximetry/who_ps_pulse_oxymetry_training_manual_en.pdf?ua=1 (Level VII)

12 The Joint Commission. (2015). Standard NPSG.06.01.01. *Comprehensive accreditation manual for hospitals: The official handbook.* Oakbrook Terrace, IL: The Joint Commission. (Level VII)

13 Graham, K. C., & Cvach, M. (2010). Monitor alarm fatigue: Standardizing use of physiological monitors and decreasing nuisance alarms. *American Journal of Critical Care, 19,* 28–37.

14 American Association of Critical-Care Nurses. (2013). "AACN practice alert: Alarm management" [Online]. Accessed March 2015 via the Web at http://www.aacn.org/wd/practice/docs/practicealerts/alarm-management-practice-alert.pdf (Level VII)

15 The Joint Commission. (2013). "Sentinel event alert: Medical device alarm safety in hospitals" [Online]. Accessed March 2015 via the Web at http://www.jointcommission.org/assets/1/18/SEA_50_alarms_4_5_13_FINAL1.PDF (Level VII)

16 The Joint Commission. (2015). Standard NPSG.02.03.01. *Comprehensive accreditation manual for hospitals: The official handbook.* Oakbrook Terrace, IL: The Joint Commission. (Level VII)

17 American Osteopathic Association. (2014). Standard 07.02.03. *Healthcare Facilities Accreditation Program: Accreditation requirements for acute care hospitals.* Chicago, IL: American Osteopathic Association. (Level VII)

18 Rutala, W. A., et al. (2008). "Guideline for disinfection and sterilization in healthcare facilities, 2008" [Online]. Accessed March 2015 via the Web at http://www.cdc.gov/hicpac/pdf/guidelines/Disinfection_Nov_2008.pdf (Level I)

19 The Joint Commission. (2015). Standard RC.01.03.01. *Comprehensive accreditation manual for hospitals: The official handbook.* Oakbrook Terrace, IL: The Joint Commission. (Level VII)

20 American Osteopathic Association. (2014). Standard 10.00.03. *Healthcare Facilities Accreditation Program: Accreditation requirements for acute care hospitals.* Chicago, IL: American Osteopathic Association. (Level VII)

21 Centers for Medicare & Medicaid Services, Department of Health and Human Services. (2014). Condition of participation: Medical record services. 42 C.F.R. § 482.24(b).

22 Shochat, G. N. (2012). "Carbon monoxide toxicity" [Online]. Accessed March 2015 via the Web at http://emedicine.medscape.com/article/819987-overview

ADDITIONAL REFERENCE

Roth, D., et al. (2011). Victim of carbon monoxide poisoning identified by carbon monoxide oximetry. *Journal of Emergency Medicine, 40,* 640–642.

CARDIAC MONITORING

Because it allows continuous observation of the heart's electrical activity, cardiac monitoring is used in patients with conduction disturbances or in those at risk for life-threatening arrhythmias. To reduce the number of false alarms that can contribute to alarm fatigue, only those patients with clinical indications for monitoring should receive cardiac monitoring.[1,2]

Like other forms of electrocardiography, cardiac monitoring uses electrodes placed on the patient's chest to transmit electrical signals that are converted into a tracing of cardiac rhythm on an oscilloscope.

Two types of monitoring may be performed: hardwire or telemetry. In hardwire monitoring, the patient is connected to a monitor at the bedside. The rhythm display appears at the bedside, but it may also be transmitted to a console at a remote location. Telemetry uses a small transmitter connected to the patient to send electrical signals to another location, where they're displayed on a monitor screen. Battery powered and portable, telemetry frees the patient from cumbersome wires and cables and lets him be comfortably mobile. Telemetry is especially useful for monitoring arrhythmias that occur during sleep, rest, exercise, or stressful situations.

Regardless of the type, cardiac monitors can display the patient's heart rate and rhythm, produce a printed record of cardiac rhythm, and sound an alarm if the patient's heart rate rises above or falls below specified limits. Monitors also recognize and count abnormal heartbeats as well as changes. For example, ST-segment monitoring helps detect myocardial ischemia, electrolyte imbalance, coronary artery spasm, and hypoxic events. The ST segment represents early ventricular repolarization, and any changes in this waveform component reflect alterations in myocardial oxygenation.[3] Any monitoring lead that views an ischemic heart region will reveal ST-segment changes. The monitor's software establishes a template of the patient's normal QRST pattern from the selected leads; then the monitor displays ST-segment changes. Some monitors display such changes continuously; others, only on command. (See *Lead selection.*)

One application of bedside cardiac monitoring is a reduced-lead continuous 12-lead electrocardiogram (ECG) system (EASI system). This system uses an advanced algorithm and only five electrodes placed on the torso to derive a 12-lead ECG. The system allows all 12 leads to be simultaneously displayed and recorded. (See *Understanding the EASI system,* page 118.)

Lead selection

Select the best monitoring leads for arrhythmia identification; display two leads when possible.[4]

CLINICAL CONCERN	LEAD
Bundle branch block	V_1 or V_6
Ischemia based on the area of infarction or site of percutaneous coronary intervention	
Anterior	V_3, V_4
Septal	V_1, V_2
Lateral	I, aV_L, V_5, V_6
Inferior	II, III, aV_F
Right ventricle	V_{4R}
Junctional rhythm with retrograde P waves	II
Optimal view of atrial activity	I, II, or Lewis lead (positive and negative electrodes at the second and fourth intercostal spaces at the right sternal border)
Ventricular ectopy, wide complex tachycardia	V_1 (may use V_6 along with V_1)
Ventricular pacing	V_1 or II

Equipment

Cardiac monitor ▪ lead wires ▪ patient cable ▪ disposable pregelled electrodes (the number varies from three to five, depending on patient's needs) ▪ washcloth, soap, and water ▪ 4″ × 4″ (10-cm × 10-cm) gauze pads ▪ Optional: clippers, gloves.

For telemetry

Transmitter ▪ transmitter pouch ▪ telemetry battery pack, leads, and electrodes.

Preparation of equipment

Plug the cardiac monitor into an electrical outlet and turn it on *to warm up the unit while you prepare the equipment and the patient.* Insert the cable into the appropriate socket in the monitor. Connect the leadwires to the cable. In some systems, the leadwires are permanently secured to the cable. Each leadwire should indicate the location for attachment to the patient: right arm (RA), left arm (LA), right leg (RL), left leg (LL), and chest (C). This designation should appear on the leadwire, if it's permanently connected, or at the connection of the leadwires and cable to the patient. Then connect an electrode to each of the leadwires, carefully checking that each leadwire is in its correct outlet.

For telemetry monitoring, insert a new battery into the transmitter.[5] Match the poles on the battery with the polar markings on the transmitter case. Test the battery's charge and test the unit by pressing the button at the top of the unit; *this ensures that the battery is operational.* If the leadwires aren't permanently affixed to the telemetry unit, attach them securely. If they must be attached individually, connect each one to the correct outlet.

Implementation

- Perform hand hygiene.[6,7,8,9,10]
- Confirm the patient's identity using at least two patient identifiers.[11]
- Provide privacy.[12,13]
- Explain the procedure to the patient.
- Put on gloves if necessary *to comply with standard precautions.*[14,15]
- Assist the patient to the supine position and expose his chest.[5]
- Determine electrode positions on the patient's chest based on the system and lead you're using. (See *Positioning monitoring leads,* page 119.)
- If necessary, clip the hair in an area around each electrode site *to ensure good skin contact with the electrodes.*[3,5]
- Clean the electrode area with soap and water and dry it completely *to enable adequate transmission of electrical impulses.*[1] Don't use alcohol to prepare the sites *because it can dry out the patient's skin.*[1]
- Roughen the skin at the intended sites with a washcloth, a gauze pad, or the sandpaper on the electrode *to remove part of the stratum corneum or outer layer of the dermis to facilitate transmission of the electrical signals.*[1]
- Remove the backing from the pregelled electrode. Check the gel for moistness. If the gel is dry, discard it and replace it with a fresh electrode.[5]

Understanding the EASI system

The five-lead EASI (reduced-lead continuous 12-lead electrocardiogram [ECG]) configuration gives a three-dimensional view of the electrical activity of the heart from the frontal, horizontal, and sagittal planes to provide 12 leads of information. A mathematical calculation in the electronics of the monitoring system is applied to the information, creating a derived 12-lead ECG. Electrode placement for the EASI system is as follows:

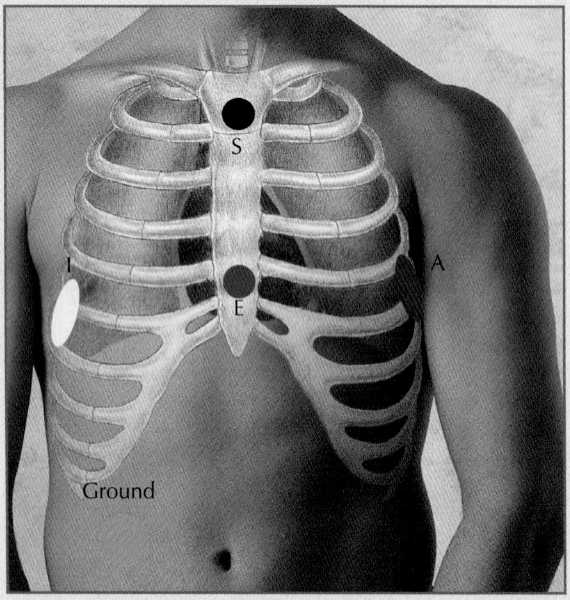

E lead	lower part of the sternum at the level of the fifth intercostal space
A lead	left midaxillary line at the level of the fifth intercostal space
S lead	upper part of the sternum
I lead	right midaxillary line at the level of the fifth intercostal space
Ground	anywhere on the torso

■ Apply the electrode to the appropriate site by pressing one side of the electrode against the patient's skin, pulling gently, and then pressing the other side against the skin. Press your fingers in a circular motion around the electrode *to fix the gel and stabilize the electrode.* Avoid pressing directly on the gel pad *to prevent spreading of the gel and loss of adhesion and transmission.*[5] Repeat this procedure for each electrode.

For hardwire monitoring

■ When all the electrodes are in place, attach the leadwires and check for a tracing on the cardiac monitor. Assess the quality of the ECG. (See *Identifying cardiac monitor problems,* page 120.)

■ *To verify that each beat is being detected by the monitor,* compare the digital heart rate display with your count of the patient's heart rate.

■ If necessary, adjust the size and position of the rhythm tracing on the recording paper following the manufacturer's instructions.

For telemetry monitoring

■ Attach an electrode to the end of each leadwire.

■ Place the transmitter in the pouch. Tie the pouch strings around the patient's neck and waist, making sure that the pouch fits snugly without causing him discomfort. If no pouch is available, place the transmitter in the patient's bathrobe pocket. Some patient gowns have a built-in pocket *to hold the transmitter and make movement easier.*[5]

■ Check the patient's waveform for clarity, position, and size. Adjust the gain and baseline, as needed. (If necessary, ask the patient to remain resting or sitting in his room while you locate his ECG pattern at the central station.)

Completing the procedure

■ Select the best monitoring leads for arrhythmia identification; display two leads when possible. Use lead II to evaluate atrial activity and measure heart rate and use lead V_1 if available to assess for a wide QRS complex. A five-lead monitoring system is required to monitor V leads; use MCL_1 if a five-lead monitoring system isn't available.[4]

■ Set the upper and lower limits of the heart rate alarm, taking into consideration the patient's current heart rate and clinical condition.[16] Turn on alarms and make sure they're functioning properly and audible to staff.[1,17,18,19] If your system has an arrhythmia and pacemaker recognition system, follow the manufacturer's directions *to set individual parameters and to activate the alarm.*

■ To obtain a rhythm strip, press the RECORD key on the bedside monitor or at the central station. Label or make sure that the strip is labeled with the patient's name, identification number, date, time, and lead(s) recorded. Also measure and record the PR interval, QRS duration, and QT interval.

■ Identify and document the rhythm. Place the rhythm strip in the appropriate location in the patient's medical record.[20]

■ Discard the used supplies in the appropriate receptacle.[14]

■ Remove and discard your gloves if worn.[14]

■ Perform hand hygiene.[6,7,8,9,10]

■ Document the procedure.[20,21,22]

Special considerations

■ The Joint Commission has issued a sentinel event alert concerning medical device alarm safety *because alarm-related events have been associated with permanent loss of function or death.* Among the major contributing factors were improper alarm settings, alarm settings inappropriately turned off, and alarm signals not audible to staff. Make sure that alarm limits are set appropriately and that alarms are turned on, functioning properly, and audible to staff.

■ Monitor the ECG pattern continually for arrhythmias, along with the patient's response to any rhythm or heart rate change, and intervene appropriately. Obtain a rhythm strip when any rhythm change occurs.[5]

■ In patients at high risk for torsades de points, measure QT interval and calculate QT_C (QT interval corrected for heart rate) using a consistent lead. A QT_C greater than 0.5 second is dangerously prolonged and associated with torsades de points. Patients at risk include those who are taking antiarrhythmics, antibiotics, antipsychotics, and other medications that prolong QT_C and those with severe bradycardia, hypokalemia, hypomagnesemia, or drug overdose.[4]

■ Ensure proper electrode placement every shift *to ensure accurate interpretation of cardiac rhythm.*[23]

■ Make sure that all electrical equipment and outlets are grounded *to avoid electric shock and interference (artifacts).* Also ensure that the patient is clean and dry[23] *to prevent electric shock.*

■ Avoid opening the electrode packages until just before using *to prevent the gel from drying out.*

Positioning monitoring leads

The illustrations below show the electrode placement for a five-lead system and a three-lead system. *Proper lead placement is necessary for accurate arrhythmia identification.*[4] The angle of Louis, or sternal angle, is a clinical landmark formed by the junction of the manubrium and the sternum.

Five-lead system

In the five-lead system, the electrode positions generally remain constant. *To select the leads you want to monitor,* simply use the lead selection button at the central station or on the bedside monitor.

In the five-lead system (shown at right):

- Place the right arm (RA) electrode near the right shoulder, close to the junction of the right arm and torso.
- Place the left arm (LA) electrode near the left shoulder, close to the junction of the left arm and torso.
- Place the right leg (RL) electrode below the level of the lowest rib on the right abdominal area.
- Place the left leg (LL) electrode below the level of the lowest rib on the left abdominal area.
- Place the chest (C) electrode in the fourth intercostal space to the right of the sternum for V_1 **or** in the fifth intercostal space in the left midaxillary line for V_6.[5]

Note: The chest electrode can be placed in any of the standard V_1 to V_6 locations, but V_1 and then V_6 are generally selected because of their value in arrhythmia monitoring.

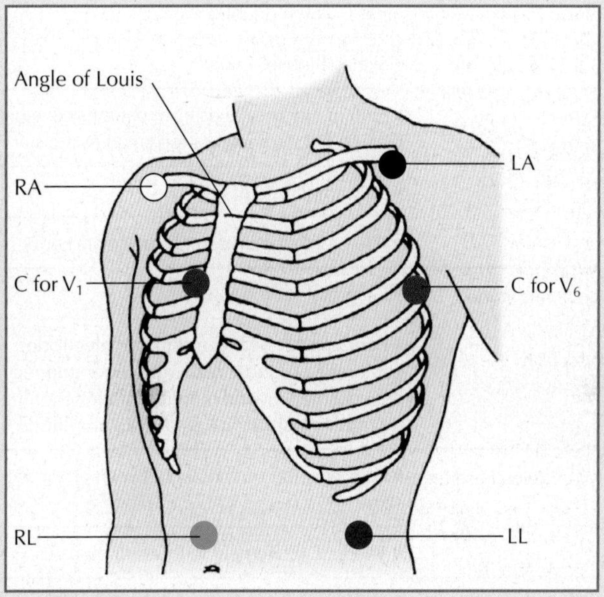

Three-lead system

In the three-lead system, the electrodes may need to change position. The first choice of leads to be monitored is modified chest lead 1 (MCL_1), followed by modified chest lead 6 (MCL_6), and then lead II.

For MCL_1 or MCL_6, in the three-lead system (shown below on left):

- Place the RA electrode near the left shoulder, close to the junction of the left arm and torso.[5]
- Place the LA electrode in the fourth intercostal space to the right of the sternum.[5]
- Place the LL electrode in the fifth intercostal space in the left midaxillary line.[5]
- Select lead I on the monitor to obtain MCL_1 and lead II to obtain MCL_6.[5]

For lead II in the three-lead system (shown below on right):

- Place the RA electrode near the right shoulder, close to the junction of the right arm and torso.
- Place the LA electrode near the left shoulder, close to the junction of the left arm and torso.
- Place the LL electrode below the level of the lowest rib on the left abdominal area.
- Select lead II on the monitor.

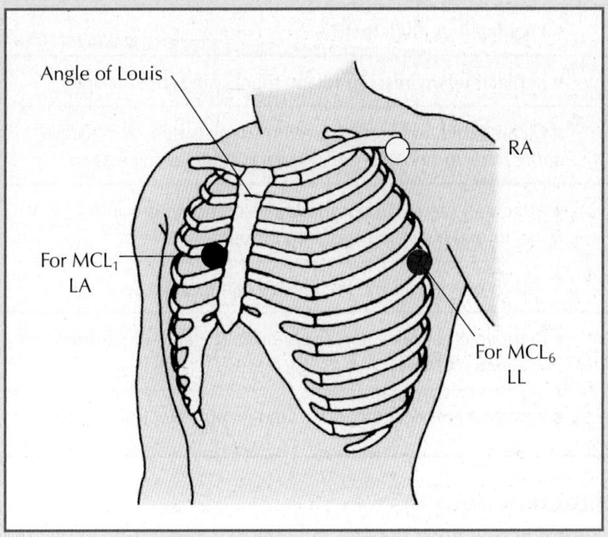

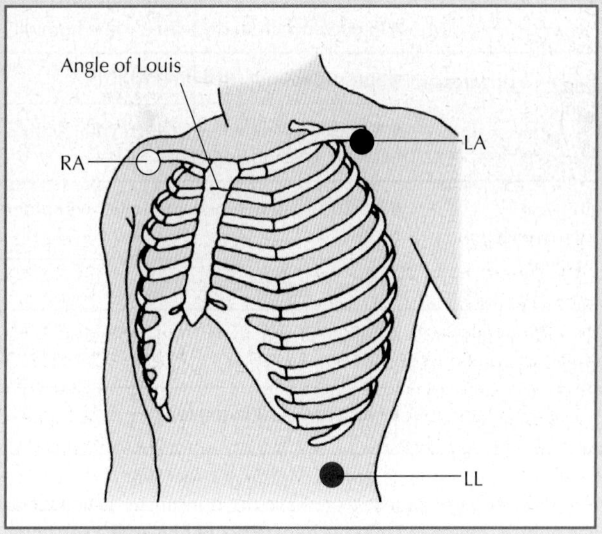

- Avoid placing the electrodes on bony prominences, hairy areas, areas where defibrillator pads will be placed, or areas for chest compression.[23]
- Assess the electrode sites for signs of irritation or sensitivity reaction. Change and reposition the electrodes daily or more often if needed.[1,24]
- If the patient is being monitored by telemetry, show him how the transmitter works. If applicable, show him the button that will produce a recording of his ECG at the central station. Teach him how to push the button whenever he has symptoms *so that the central console will print a*

TROUBLESHOOTING

Identifying cardiac monitor problems

PROBLEM	POSSIBLE CAUSES	SOLUTIONS
False–high-rate alarm	■ Monitor interpreting large T waves as QRS complexes, which doubles the rate	■ Reposition electrodes to lead where QRS complexes are taller than T waves. Decrease gain, if necessary.
	■ Skeletal muscle activity	■ Place electrodes away from major muscle masses.
False–low-rate alarm	■ Shift in electrical axis from patient movement, making QRS complexes too small to register	■ Reapply electrodes. Set gain so height of complex is greater than 1 millivoltage.
	■ Low amplitude of QRS	■ Increase gain.
	■ Poor contact between electrode and skin	■ Reapply electrodes.
Low amplitude	■ Gain dial set too low	■ Increase gain.
	■ Poor contact between skin and electrodes; dried gel; broken or loose leadwires; poor connection between patient and monitor; malfunctioning monitor; physiologic loss of QRS amplitude	■ Check connections on all leadwires and monitoring cable. Replace electrodes as necessary.
Wandering baseline	■ Poor position or contact between electrodes and skin	■ Reposition or replace electrodes.
	■ Thoracic movement with respirations	■ Reposition electrodes.
Artifact (waveform interference)	■ Patient having seizures, chills, or anxiety	■ Notify practitioner and treat patient as ordered. Keep patient warm and reassure him.
	■ Patient movement	■ Help patient relax.
	■ Electrodes applied improperly	■ Check electrodes and reapply, if necessary.
	■ Static electricity	■ Make sure cables don't have exposed connectors. Change patient's static-causing gown or pajamas.
	■ Electrical short circuit in leadwires or cable	■ Replace broken equipment. Use stress loops when applying leadwires.
	■ Interference from decreased room humidity	■ Regulate humidity to 40%.
Broken leadwires or cable	■ Stress loops not used on leadwires	■ Replace leadwires and retape them using stress loops.
	■ Cables and leadwires cleaned with alcohol or acetone, causing brittleness	■ Clean cable and leadwires with soapy water. *Don't allow cable ends to become wet.* Replace cable as necessary.
60-cycle interference (fuzzy baseline)	■ Electrical interference from other equipment in room	■ Attach all electrical equipment to common ground. Check plugs to make sure prongs aren't loose.
	■ Patient's bed improperly grounded	■ Attach bed ground to the room's common ground.
Skin excoriation under electrode	■ Patient allergic to electrode adhesive	■ Remove electrodes and apply nonallergenic electrodes and nonallergenic tape.
	■ Electrode on skin too long	■ Remove electrode, clean site, and reapply electrode at new site.

rhythm strip. Tell the patient to remove the transmitter if he takes a shower or bath. However, stress the importance of him letting you know before he removes the unit.

Complications

Complications include skin irritation or sensitivity to the electrode adhesive or gel.

Documentation

Record in your notes the date and time that monitoring begins and the monitoring lead used. Note any patient and family teaching and their understanding of your teaching. Document a rhythm strip at least every shift and with any changes in the patient's condition (or as directed by your facility). Make sure that the strip is labeled with the patient's name and identification number as well as the date, time, lead(s) recorded, appropriate measurements, and rhythm interpretation.

REFERENCES

1 American Association of Critical-Care Nurses. (2013). "AACN practice alert: Alarm management" [Online]. Accessed March 2015 via the Web at http://www.aacn.org/wd/practice/docs/practicealerts/alarm-management-practice-alert.pdf (Level VII)

2 Funk, M., et al. (2010). Unnecessary arrhythmia monitoring and underutilization of ischemia and QT interval monitoring in current clinical practice: Baseline results of the practical use of the latest standards for electrocardiography trial. *Journal of Electrocardiology, 43,* 542–547.

3 American Heart Association. (2004). AHA scientific statement: Practice standards for electrocardiographic monitoring in hospital settings. *Circulation, 110,* 2721–2746. Accessed March 2015 via the Web at http://circ.ahajournals.org/content/110/17/2721.long (Level VII)

4 American Association of Critical Care Nurses. (2008). "Practice alert: Dysrhythmia monitoring" [Online]. Accessed March 2015 via the Web at http://www.aacn.org/WD/Practice/Docs/PracticeAlerts/Dysrhythmia_Monitoring_04-2008.pdf (Level VII)

5 Lynn-McHale Wiegand, D. (Ed.). (2011). *AACN procedure manual for critical care* (6th ed.). St. Louis, MO: Saunders.

6 Centers for Disease Control and Prevention. (2002). Guideline for hand hygiene in health-care settings: Recommendations of the Healthcare Infection Control Practices Advisory Committee and the HICPAC/SHEA/APIC/IDSA Hand Hygiene Task Force. *MMWR Recommendations and Reports, 51*(RR-16), 1–45. Accessed March 2015 via the Web at http://www.cdc.gov/mmwr/pdf/rr/rr5116.pdf (Level II)

7 The Joint Commission. (2015). Standard NPSG.07.01.01. *Comprehensive accreditation manual for hospitals: The official handbook.* Oakbrook Terrace, IL: The Joint Commission. (Level VII)

8 World Health Organization. (2009). "WHO guidelines on hand hygiene in health care: First global patient safety challenge, clean care is safer care" [Online]. Accessed March 2015 via the Web at http://whqlibdoc.who.int/publications/2009/9789241597906_eng.pdf (Level IV)

9 Centers for Medicare & Medicaid Services, Department of Health and Human Services. (2014). Condition of participation: Infection control. 42 C.F.R. § 482.42.

10 American Osteopathic Association. (2014). Standard 07.01.21. *Healthcare Facilities Accreditation Program: Accreditation requirements for acute care hospitals.* Chicago, IL: American Osteopathic Association. (Level VII)

11 The Joint Commission. (2015). Standard NPSG.01.01.01. *Comprehensive accreditation manual for hospitals: The official handbook.* Oakbrook Terrace, IL: The Joint Commission. (Level VII)

12 Centers for Medicare & Medicaid Services, Department of Health and Human Services. (2014). Condition of participation: Patient's rights. 42 C.F.R. § 482.13(c)(1).

13 American Osteopathic Association. (2014). Standard 15.01.16. *Healthcare Facilities Accreditation Program: Accreditation requirements for acute care hospitals.* Chicago, IL: American Osteopathic Association. (Level VII)

14 Siegel, J. D., et al. (2007). "2007 guideline for isolation precautions: Preventing transmission of infectious agents in healthcare settings" [Online]. Accessed March 2015 via the Web at http://www.cdc.gov/hicpac/pdf/isolation/Isolation2007.pdf (Level II)

15 American Osteopathic Association. (2014). Standard 07.01.10. *Healthcare Facilities Accreditation Program: Accreditation requirements for acute care hospitals.* Chicago, IL: American Osteopathic Association. (Level VII)

16 Bell, L., & Cox, B. (2008). Monitoring clinical alarms. *American Journal of Critical Care, 17,* 44.

17 The Joint Commission. (2013). "Sentinel event alert: Medical device alarm safety in hospitals" [Online]. Accessed March 2015 via the Web at http://www.jointcommission.org/assets/1/18/SEA_50_alarms_4_5_13_FINAL1.PDF (Level VII)

18 The Joint Commission. (2015). Standard NPSG.06.01.01. *Comprehensive accreditation manual for hospitals: The official handbook.* Oakbrook Terrace, IL: The Joint Commission. (Level VII)

19 Graham, K. C., & Cvach, M. (2010). Monitor alarm fatigue: Standardizing use of physiological monitors and decreasing nuisance alarms. *American Journal of Critical Care, 19,* 28–34.

20 The Joint Commission. (2015). Standard RC.01.03.01. *Comprehensive accreditation manual for hospitals: The official handbook.* Oakbrook Terrace, IL: The Joint Commission. (Level VII)

21 Centers for Medicare & Medicaid Services, Department of Health and Human Services. (2014). Condition of participation: Medical record services. 42 C.F.R. § 482.24(b).

22 American Osteopathic Association. (2014). Standard 10.00.03. *Healthcare Facilities Accreditation Program: Accreditation requirements for acute care hospitals.* Chicago, IL: American Osteopathic Association. (Level VII)

23 Melendez, L. A., & Pino, R. M. (2012). Electrocardiogram interference: A thing of the past? *Biomedical Instrumentation and Technology, 46,* 470–477. (Level VI)

24 Cvach, M. M., et al. (2010). Daily electrode change and effect on cardiac monitor alarms: An evidence-based approach. *Journal of Nursing Care Quality, 28,* 265–271.

ADDITIONAL REFERENCES

Bonzheim, K. A., et al. (2011). Communication strategies and timeliness of response to life critical telemetry alarms. Telemedicine Journal and E-Health, 17, 241–246. Accessed March 2015 via the Web at http://www.ncbi.nlm.nih.gov/pmc/articles/PMC3136730/ (Level VI)

Lazzara, P. B., et al. (2010). The evolution of a centralized telemetry program. *Nursing Management, 41*(11), 51–54.

CARDIAC OUTPUT MEASUREMENT

Cardiac output—the amount of blood ejected by the heart in 1 minute—helps evaluate cardiac function. The most widely used method of calculating this measurement is the bolus thermodilution technique. This technique evaluates the cardiac status of critically ill patients and those suspected of having cardiac disease.

To measure cardiac output using the bolus thermodilution technique, a quantity of solution colder than the patient's blood is injected into the right atrium through the proximal port on a pulmonary artery (PA) catheter. This indicator solution mixes with the blood as it travels through the right ventricle into the PA (as shown below). A thermistor on the catheter registers the change in temperature of the flowing blood. A computer then plots the temperature change over time as a curve and calculates flow based on the area under the curve.

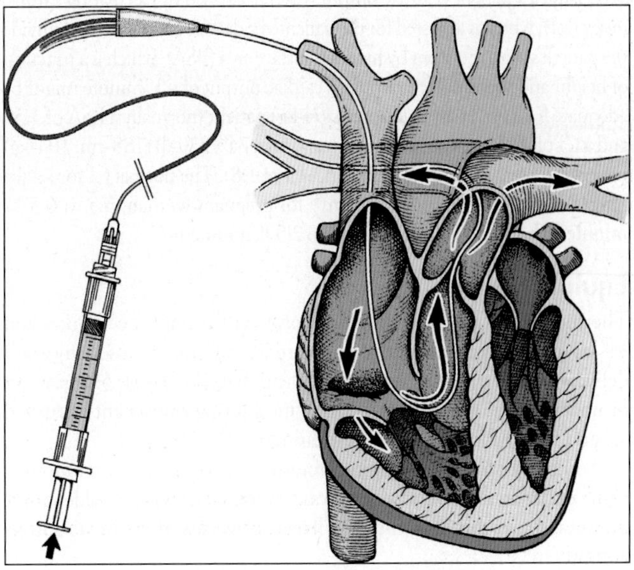

Depending on the patient's status and your facility's preference, iced or room-temperature injectant may be used. Although iced injectant may provide a stronger signal because it's colder, room-temperature injectant is more convenient and generally provides equally accurate measurements.

EQUIPMENT

Cardiac output setup

The photo below shows you how a cardiac output setup should look when it's put together correctly and completely.

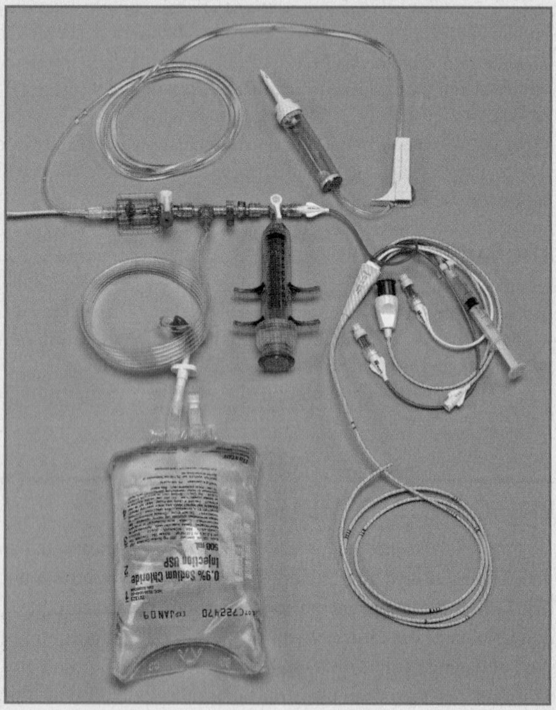

However, iced injectant may be more accurate in hypothermic patients or when smaller volumes of injectant must be used (3 to 5 mL), as in patients with volume restrictions.

The normal range for cardiac output is 4 to 8 L/minute.[1] However, the adequacy of a patient's cardiac output is better assessed by calculating cardiac index (CI), which is adjusted for the patient's body size. To calculate CI, divide the patient's cardiac output by his body surface area (BSA), which is a function of height and weight. For example, a cardiac output of 4 L/minute might be adequate for a 65″, 120-lb (165-cm, 54-kg) patient (normally a BSA of 1.59 and a CI of 2.5) but would be inadequate for a 74″, 230-lb (188-cm, 104-kg) patient (normally a BSA of 2.26 and a CI of 1.8). The normal CI for adults ranges from 2.5 to 4.2 L/minute/m^2; for pregnant women, 3.5 to 6.5 L/minute/m^2; and for elderly adults, 2 to 2.5 L/minute/m^2.

Equipment

Thermodilution PA catheter in position ▪ cardiac output computer and cables (or a module for the bedside cardiac monitor) ▪ closed injectant delivery system ▪ 10-mL syringe ▪ 500-mL bag of dextrose 5% in water or normal saline solution ▪ vital signs monitoring equipment ▪ crushed ice and water (for iced-injectant measurement).

Some bedside cardiac monitors measure cardiac output continuously, using either an invasive or a noninvasive method. If your bedside monitor doesn't have this capability, you'll need a free-standing cardiac output computer.

Preparation of equipment

Perform hand hygiene.[2,3,4,5,6] Assemble the equipment at the patient's bedside. Maintain sterile technique throughout equipment preparation.[1] Insert the closed injectant system tubing into the 500-mL bag of IV solution. Connect the 10-mL syringe to the system tubing, and prime the tubing with IV solution until it's free of air. Then clamp the tubing. (See *Cardiac output setup.*)

After clamping the tubing, connect the primed system to the stopcock of the proximal injectant lumen of the PA catheter.

If using iced injectant, place the coiled segment into a clean container and add crushed ice and water to cover the entire coil. Let the solution cool for 15 to 20 minutes. If using room-temperature injectant, connect the primed system to the stopcock of the proximal injectant lumen of the PA catheter. Next, connect the temperature probe from the cardiac output computer to the closed injectant system's flow-through housing device. Connect the cardiac output computer cable to the thermistor connector on the PA catheter and verify the blood temperature reading. Lastly, turn on the cardiac output computer and enter the correct computation constant, as provided by the catheter's manufacturer. The constant is determined by the volume and temperature of the injectant as well as the size and type of catheter. The patient's height and weight are also factored into the calculation.

Implementation

- Perform hand hygiene.[2,3,4,5,6]
- Confirm the patient's identity using at least two patient identifiers.[7]
- Explain to the patient that the procedure will help determine how well his heart is pumping and that he'll feel no discomfort.
- Obtain the patient's vital signs, and assess his respiratory and cardiovascular status, including cardiac rhythm. Monitor for signs and symptoms of inadequate perfusion, including restlessness, fatigue, changes in level of consciousness, decreased capillary refill time, diminished peripheral pulses, oliguria, and pale, cool skin.[1]
- Make sure the patient is in a comfortable, supine position with the head of the bed elevated no more than 20 degrees. If the patient's condition prevents this position, use consistent positioning *to ensure consistent cardiac output measurement.*[1] Tell him not to move during the procedure *because movement can cause an error in measurement.*[8]
- If the proximal port is being used for an infusion, flush the port with normal saline solution at an appropriate rate *to clear the line of infusing medication without administering a bolus of medication to the patient.* If able, restrict infusions delivered through the introducer or other central lines *because measurements obtained during administration of other infusions may be elevated by as much as 40%.*
- If using iced injectant, note the temperature of the injectant on the computer or monitor screen; *the injectant temperature should be at least 10° F (5.6° C) less than the patient's core temperature.*[5]
- Verify the presence of a PA waveform and observe the patient's heart rate and cardiac rhythm on the cardiac monitor; *a rapid heart rate or an arrhythmia may decrease cardiac output and lead to varying cardiac output measurements.*[1]
- Turn the stopcock, unclamp the injectant IV tubing (as shown below), and withdraw exactly 10 mL of solution into the syringe. Reclamp the tubing.[1]

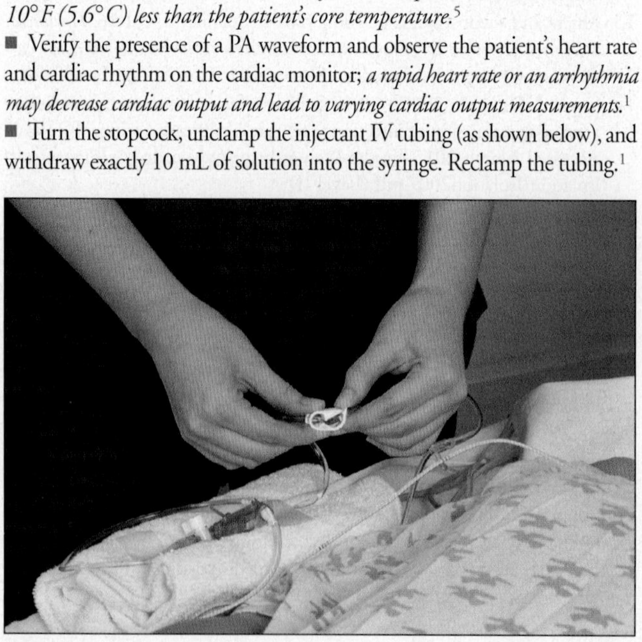

- Turn the stopcock at the catheter injectant lumen *to open a fluid path between the injectant lumen of the PA catheter and syringe.*
- Press the START button on the cardiac output computer, or wait for the INJECT message to flash.
- Observe for a steady baseline temperature before injecting the solution *because an abnormal baseline may increase variability in cardiac output measurement.*[1]
- Inject the solution smoothly within 4 seconds at end expiration *to decrease variation in cardiac output measurements caused by the respiratory cycle* (as shown below).[1] Make sure fluid doesn't leak at the connectors.[1]

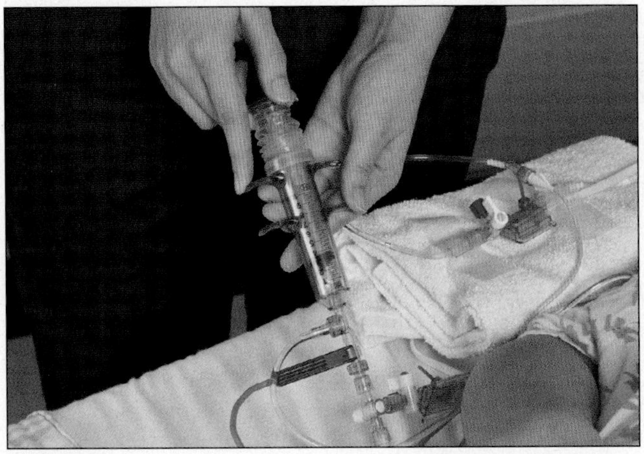

- If available, analyze the contour of the thermodilution curve on a strip chart recorder for a rapid upstroke and a gradual, smooth return to baseline. (See *Analyzing thermodilution curves,* page 124.)
- Repeat these steps up to five times, waiting 1 minute between injections. Compute the average of three measurements that are within 10% of the median value, and record the patient's cardiac output.[1]
- Return the stopcock to its original position, and make sure the injectant delivery system tubing is clamped (as shown below).[1]
- Restart medication infusions, as necessary.[1]
- Verify the presence of a PA waveform on the cardiac monitor.[1]
- Make sure the clamp on the injectant bag is secured *to prevent inadvertent delivery of the injectant to the patient.*[1]

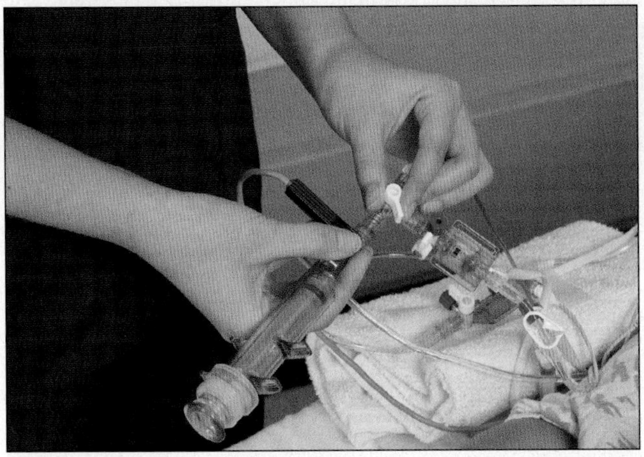

- Assess the patient's respiratory and cardiovascular status, including cardiac rhythm after the procedure, and compare your findings with baseline findings *to evaluate the patient's hemodynamic status.*[1]
- Position the patient for comfort.
- Discard used supplies in the appropriate recptacles.[9,10]
- Perform hand hygiene.[2,3,4,5,6]
- Record the fluid volume injected for cardiac output measurements in the patient's intake and output record.
- Document the procedure.[11,12,13]

Special considerations

- Certain factors can affect the accuracy and reproducibility of bolus thermodilution cardiac output values, including variations in injectant temperatures or volumes, rapid volume infusions during bolus injections, respiratory cycle influences, an inaccurate computation constant, and thermal instability after cardiopulmonary bypass.[14]
- Handle the injectant solution as little as *possible to avoid thermal indicator variations, which may alter cardiac output values.*[1]

Complications

Complications from cardiac output measurement are rare but may include bradycardia and other hemodynamic changes.

Documentation

Document the patient's cardiac output, CI, and other hemodynamic values as well as his vital signs at the time of measurement. Note the patient's position during measurement and any other complications, such as bradycardia or hemodynamic changes. Record the date, time, and name of the practitioner notified of any abnormal results; prescribed interventions; and the patient's response to those interventions. Document any patient teaching provided and the patient's understanding of the teaching.

References

1 Lynn-McHale Wiegand, D. (Ed.). (2011). *AACN procedure manual for critical care* (6th ed.). St. Louis, MO: Saunders.

2 The Joint Commission. (2015). Standard NPSG.07.01.01. *Comprehensive accreditation manual for hospitals: The official handbook.* Oakbrook Terrace, IL: The Joint Commission. (Level VII)

3 World Health Organization. (2009). "WHO guidelines on hand hygiene in health care: First global patient safety challenge, clean care is safer care" [Online]. Accessed March 2015 via the Web at http://whqlibdoc.who.int/publications/2009/9789241597906_eng.pdf (Level IV)

4 Centers for Disease Control and Prevention. (2002). Guideline for hand hygiene in health-care settings: Recommendations of the Healthcare Infection Control Practices Advisory Committee and the HICPAC/SHEA/APIC/IDSA Hand Hygiene Task Force. *MMWR Recommendations and Reports, 51*(RR-16), 1–45. Accessed March 2015 via the Web at http://www.cdc.gov/mmwr/pdf/rr/rr5116.pdf (Level II)

5 Centers for Medicare & Medicaid Services, Department of Health and Human Services. (2014). Condition of participation: Infection control. 42 C.F.R. § 482.42.

6 American Osteopathic Association. (2014). Standard 07.01.21. *Healthcare Facilities Accreditation Program: Accreditation requirements for acute care hospitals.* Chicago, IL: American Osteopathic Association. (Level VII)

7 The Joint Commission. (2015). Standard NPSG.01.01.01. *Comprehensive accreditation manual for hospitals: The official handbook.* Oakbrook Terrace, IL: The Joint Commission. (Level VII)

8 Giuliano, K. K., et al. (2003). Backrest angle and cardiac output measurement in critically ill patients. *Nursing Research, 52,* 242–248. (Level VI)

9 Occupational Safety and Health Administration. (n.d.). "Bloodborne pathogens, standard number 1910.1030" [Online]. Accessed March 2015 via the Web at http://www.osha.gov/pls/oshaweb/owadisp.show_document?p_table=STANDARDS&p_id=10051 (Level VII)

10 Siegel, J. D., et al. (2007). "2007 guideline for isolation precautions: Preventing transmission of infectious agents in healthcare settings" [Online]. Accessed March 2015 via the Web at http://www.cdc.gov/hicpac/pdf/isolation/Isolation2007.pdf (Level II)

11 The Joint Commission. (2015). Standard RC.01.03.01. *Comprehensive accreditation manual for hospitals: The official handbook.* Oakbrook Terrace, IL: The Joint Commission. (Level VII)

Analyzing thermodilution curves

The thermodilution curve provides valuable information about cardiac output, injection technique, and equipment problems. When studying the curve, keep in mind that the area under the curve is inversely proportionate to the cardiac output: The smaller the area under the curve, the higher the cardiac output; the larger the area under the curve, the lower the cardiac output.

In addition to providing a record of cardiac output, the curve may indicate problems related to technique, such as erratic or slow injectant instillations, or other problems, such as respiratory variations or electrical interference. The curves below correspond to those typically seen in clinical practice.

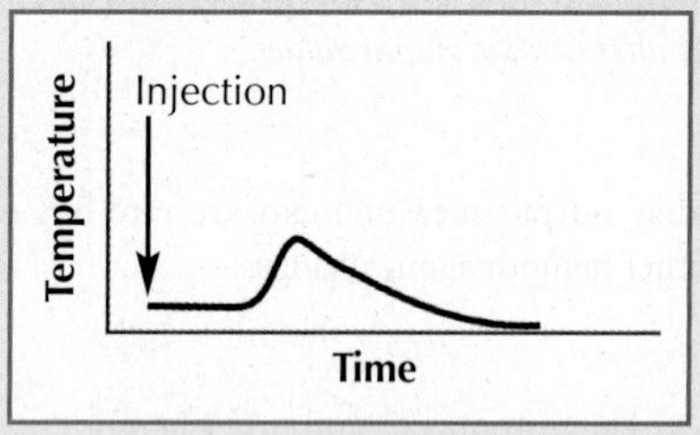

Normal thermodilution curve

With an accurate monitoring system and a patient who has adequate cardiac output, the thermodilution curve begins with a smooth, rapid upstroke and is followed by a smooth, gradual downslope. The curve shown at left indicates that the injectant instillation time was within the recommended 4 seconds and that the temperature curve returned to baseline.

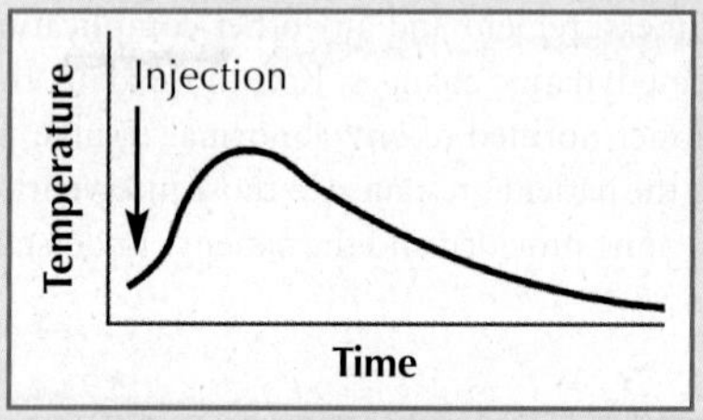

Low cardiac output curve

A thermodilution curve representing low cardiac output shows a rapid, smooth upstroke (from proper injection technique). However, because the heart is ejecting blood less efficiently from the ventricles, the injectant warms slowly and takes longer to be ejected. Consequently, the curve takes longer to return to baseline. This slow return produces a larger area under the curve, corresponding to low cardiac output.

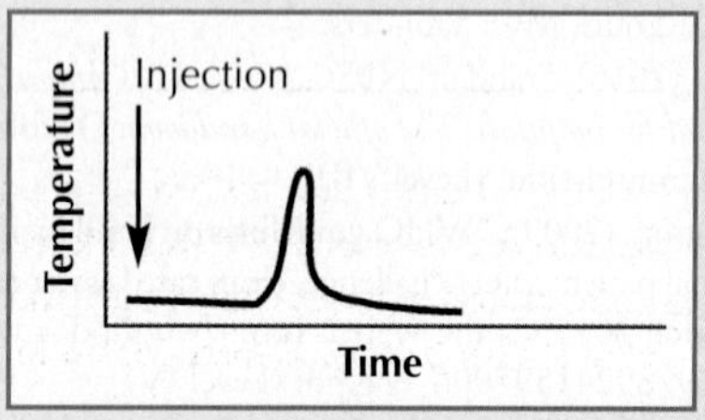

High cardiac output curve

As with a low cardiac output curve, the thermodilution curve representing high cardiac output has a rapid, smooth upstroke from proper injection technique. However, because the ventricles are ejecting blood too forcefully, the injectant moves through the heart quickly and the curve returns to baseline more rapidly. The smaller area under the curve suggests higher cardiac output.

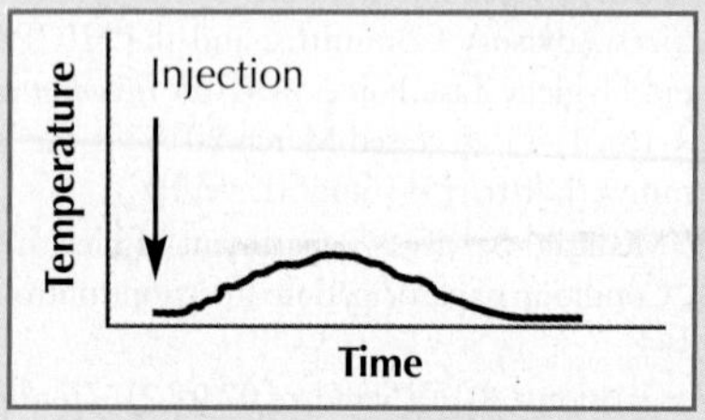

Curve reflecting poor technique

A curve reflecting poor technique results from an uneven and too-slow (taking more than 4 seconds) administration of injectant. The uneven and slower-than-normal upstroke and the larger area under the curve erroneously indicate low cardiac output. A kinked catheter, unsteady hands during the injection, or improper placement of the injectant lumen in the introducer sheath may also cause this type of curve.

12 Centers for Medicare & Medicaid Services, Department of Health and Human Services. (2014). Condition of participation: Medical record services. 42 C.F.R. § 482.24(b).

13 American Osteopathic Association. (2014). Standard 10.00.03. *Healthcare Facilities Accreditation Program: Accreditation requirements for acute care hospitals.* Chicago, IL: American Osteopathic Association. (Level VII)

14 McGee, W. T., et al. (2010). Edward's critical care education: Quick guide to cardiopulmonary care (2nd ed.). Accessed March 2015 via the Web at http://ht.edwards.com/scin/edwards/sitecollectionimages/products/mininvasive/ewquic

Additional references

Ball, T. R., et al. (2013). Accuracy of noninvasive estimated continuous cardiac output (esCCO) compared to thermodilution cardiac output: A pilot study in cardiac patients. *Journal of Cardiothoracic and Vascular Anesthesia, 27,* 1128–1132. (Level IV)

Sakka, S. G., et al. (2012). The transpulmonary thermodilution technique. *Journal of Clinical Monitoring and Computing, 26,* 347–353.

Walsh, E., et al. (2010). Iced vs. room-temperature injectates for cardiac index measurement during hypothermia and normothermia. *American Journal of Critical Care, 19,* 365–372. Accessed March 2015 via the Web at http://ajcc.aacnjournals.org/content/19/4/365.full.pdf (Level VI)

Cardiopulmonary resuscitation, adult

Cardiopulmonary resuscitation (CPR) seeks to restore and maintain the patient's respirations and circulation after his heartbeat and breathing have stopped. The ultimate goal of the resuscitation process is to return a patient to his previous quality of life and functional state. CPR is a basic life support (BLS) procedure performed on victims of cardiac arrest. It should be performed according to the 2010 American Heart Association (AHA) guidelines.[1]

Studies show that early CPR can improve a patient's likelihood of survival. Chest compressions are particularly important because perfusion during CPR depends on them. To prevent a delay in chest compressions, the AHA changed the sequence of CPR in the 2010 guidelines from "A-B-C" (airway, breathing, and compressions) to "C-A-B" (compressions, airway, and breathing), which gives the highest priority to chest compressions when resuscitating a patient in cardiac arrest.[1]

High-quality CPR is important not only at the onset of resuscitation but throughout the resuscitation process. Key components of high-quality CPR are minimizing chest compression interruptions, providing compressions of adequate rate and depth, avoiding leaning between compressions, and avoiding excessive ventilation.[2] Integrating defibrillation and other advanced cardiac life support (ACLS) measures into the resuscitation process minimizes interruptions in CPR.[1]

Equipment

Backboard or other firm surface ▪ automated external defibrillator (AED) ▪ Optional: barrier mask with one-way valve, gloves, other personal protective equipment.

Implementation

Guidelines for performing CPR vary depending on whether CPR is being performed by one or two rescuers.

One-person CPR

- The following illustrated instructions provide a step-by-step guide for CPR as currently recommended by the AHA. (See *The AHA BLS algorithm,* page 126.)
- As a sole rescuer, you will determine unresponsiveness, check for breathing, activate the emergency response system, check for a pulse, and begin chest compressions.[1]
- Assess the patient *to determine if he's unconscious* (as shown below). Tap him on the shoulder and shout, "Are you alright?" *This helps ensure that you don't begin CPR on a conscious person.* While checking for responsiveness, check to see if the patient is apneic or only gasping (as opposed to breathing regularly). If the patient is unresponsive and apneic or only gasping, assume that he's in cardiac arrest.[1]

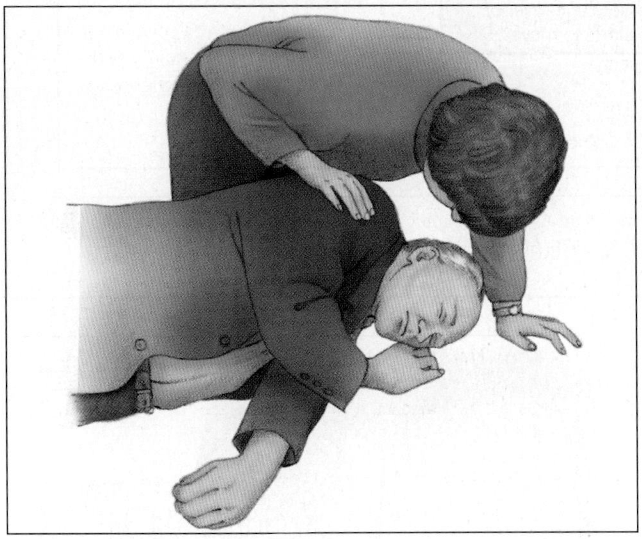

- Immediately call out for help and have someone activate the emergency response system or call a code.[1]
- Send someone to get the AED. If no one is available, get the AED and return to the patient.[1]
- Put on gloves as well as other personal protective equipment as needed and available *to comply with standard precautions and to prevent exposure to potentially infectious blood and body fluids.*[3,4]
- Place the patient in the supine position on a firm surface, such as a backboard or the floor; if the patient is on an air-filled mattress, deflate the mattress *to maximize the effectiveness of chest compressions.* When moving him, roll his head and torso as a unit (as shown below); avoid twisting or pulling his neck, shoulders, or hips. Don't delay the initiation of CPR to place the patient on a backboard.[1]

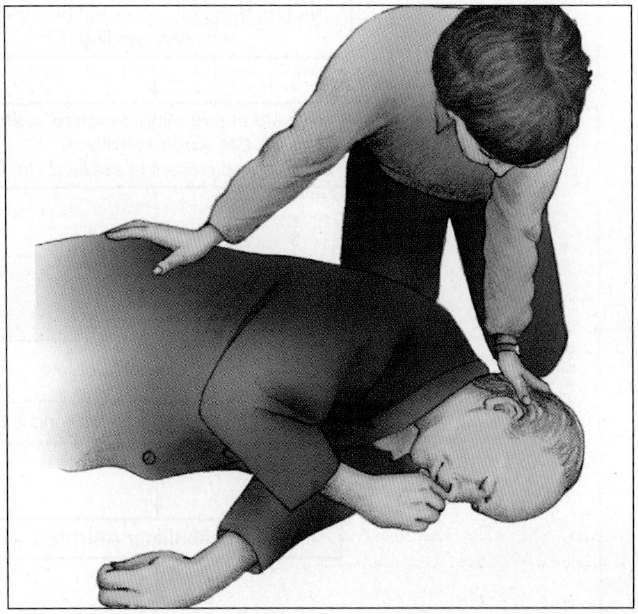

- Kneel beside the patient's chest or stand beside his bed at his chest. Palpate the carotid artery that's closest to you. To do this, place your index and middle fingers in the groove between the trachea and the sternocleidomastoid muscle (as shown below). Palpate for no longer than 10 seconds.[1]

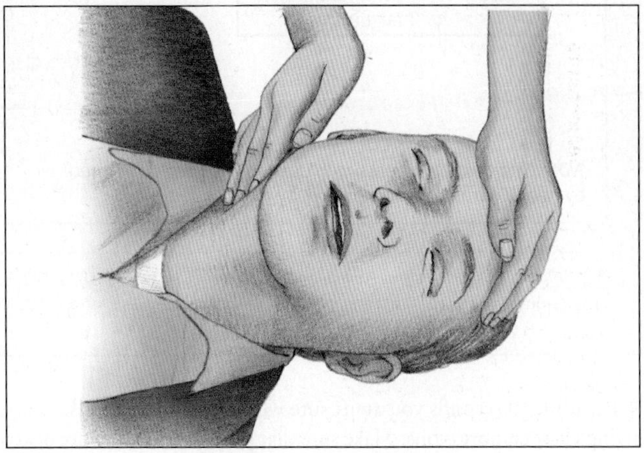

- If you detect a strong, easily palpable pulse, don't begin chest compressions. Instead, if the patient requires ventilator support, perform rescue breathing by giving the patient 10 to 12 breaths/minute (1 breath every 5 to 6 seconds). Give each breath over 1 second, regardless of whether there's an advanced airway in place; each breath should cause visible chest rise.[1,2] Avoid excessive ventilation by giving breaths at a rate less than 12 per minute; *this minimizes the impact of positive-pressure ventilation on blood flow.*[2]

The AHA BLS algorithm[1]

The following algorithm shows the steps to follow when cardiac arrest is suspected in an adult patient.

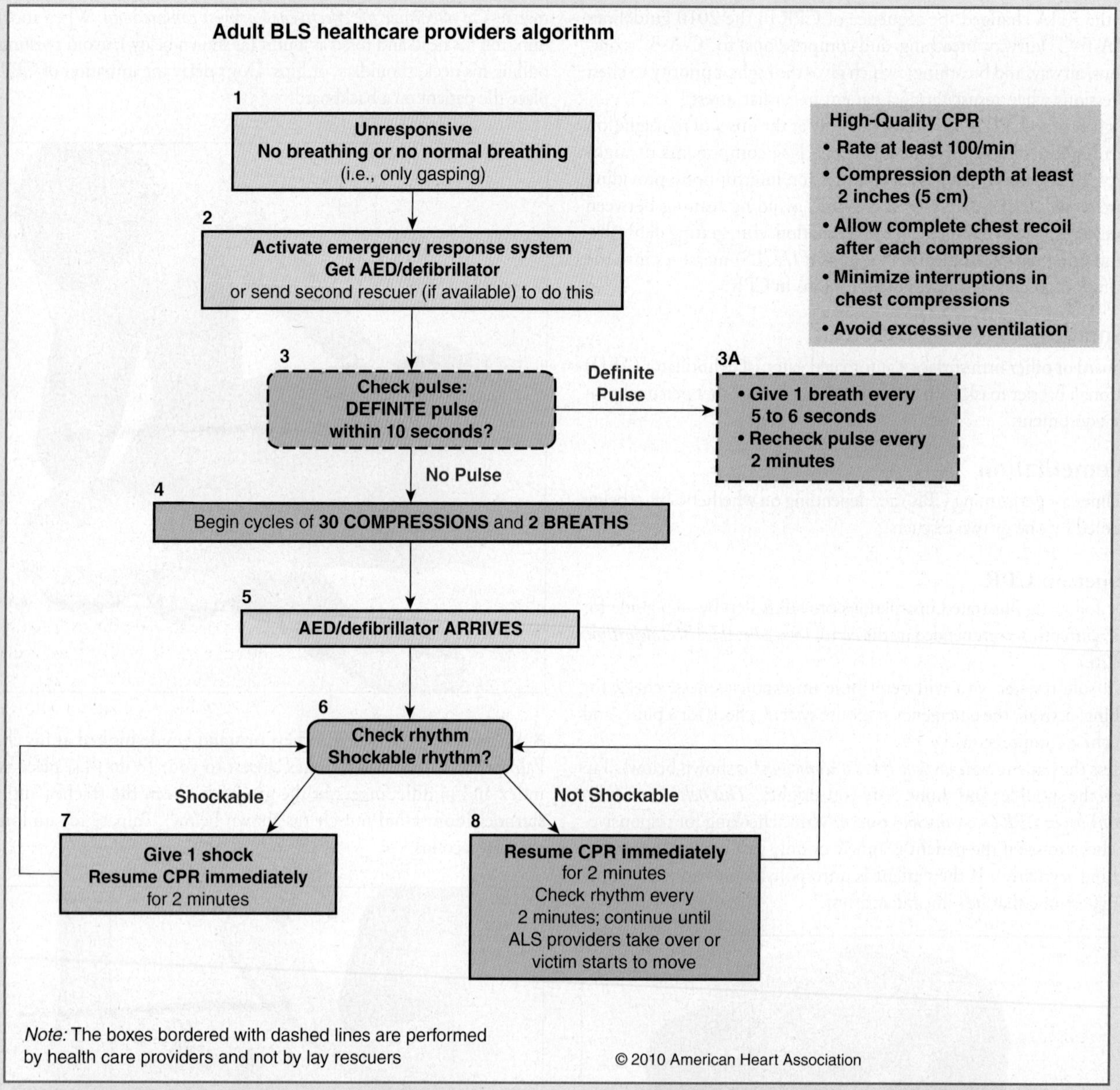

Reprinted with permission. American Heart Association. (2010). 2010 American Heart Association guidelines for cardiopulmonary resuscitation and emergency cardiovascular care, part 4: CPR overview. *Circulation, 122* (Suppl. 3), S676–684. © 2010 American Heart Association.

■ If within 10 seconds you aren't sure whether you feel a pulse, start giving chest compressions. Make sure that your knees or feet are apart *to provide a wide base of support.* Place the heel of one hand on the center of the patient's chest (over the lower half of the sternum) and the heel of the other hand on top of the first so that your hands are overlapped and parallel (as shown at right).[1]

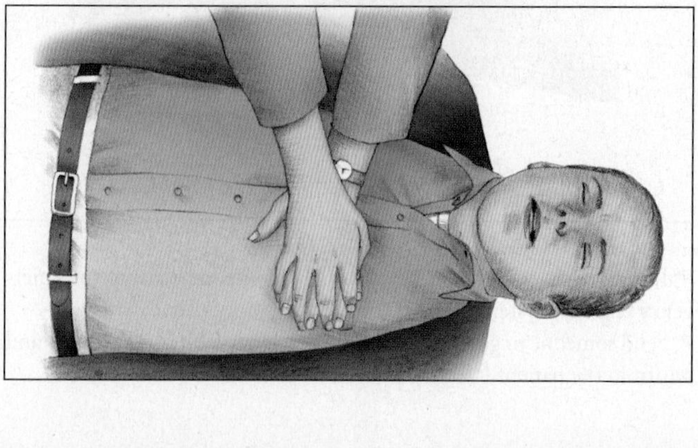

■ With your elbows locked, arms straight, and shoulders directly over your hands (as shown below), give compressions. Using the weight of your upper body, compress the patient's chest at least 2″ (5 cm), keeping chest compression and chest recoil durations equal. Allow the chest to completely recoil after each chest compression *so the heart can adequately refill with blood.*[1] Avoid leaning over the patient's chest, *which could prevent the chest from recoiling completely.*[2]

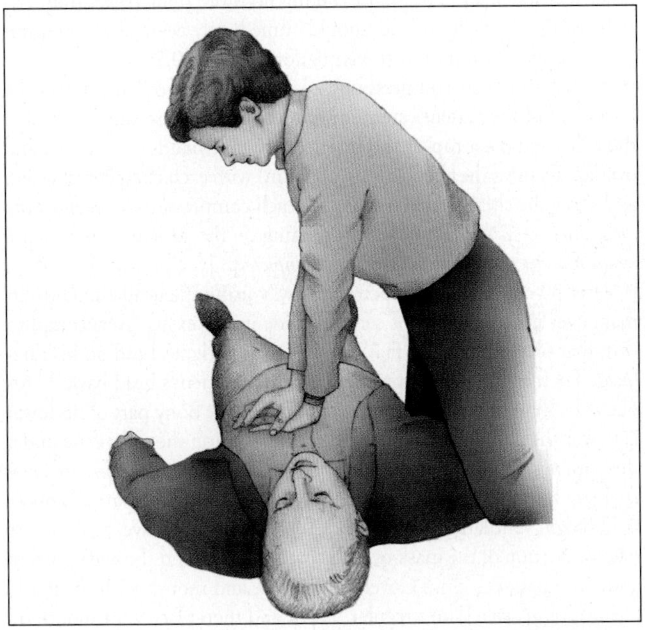

■ Give 30 compressions at a rate of 100 to 120 compressions per minute, pushing hard and fast.[2] After administering 30 compressions, open the patient's airway and give 2 ventilations. If the patient doesn't appear to have a cervical spine injury, use the head-tilt–chin-lift maneuver *to open his airway.*[1] To accomplish this, first place your hand that's closer to the patient's head on his forehead. Then apply enough pressure to tilt the patient's head back. Next, place the fingertips of your other hand under the bony part of his lower jaw near the chin; avoid placing your fingertips on the soft tissue under the patient's chin *because you may inadvertently obstruct the airway you're trying to open.* At the same time, keep his mouth partially open (as shown below).

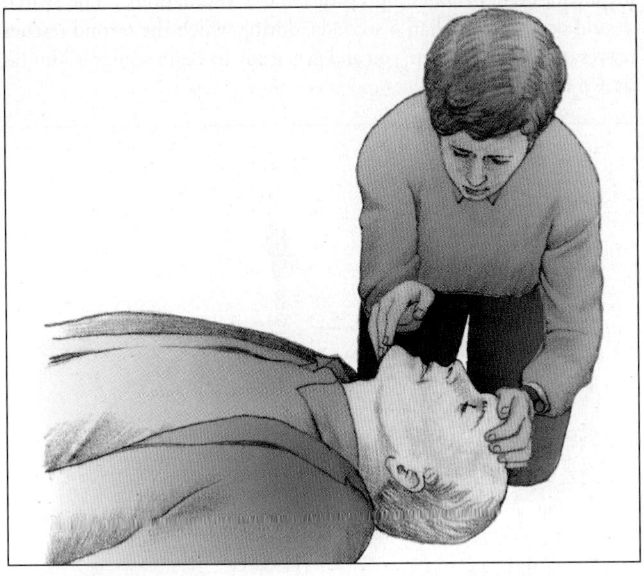

■ If you suspect a neck injury, use the jaw-thrust maneuver.[1] To perform this maneuver, kneel at the patient's head with your elbows on the ground. Rest your thumbs on his lower jaw near the corners of the mouth, pointing your thumbs toward his feet. Then place your fingertips around the lower jaw. To open the airway, lift the lower jaw with your fingertips (as shown below).

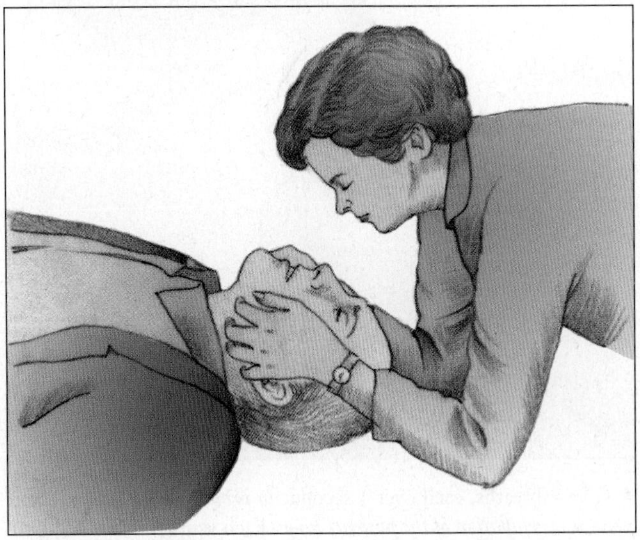

■ To begin ventilations using a mask with a one-way valve, position the narrow portion of the mask over the patient's nose and the wide portion above the patient's chin. Covering the nose and mouth with the mask, create a tight seal. Take a regular breath and place your mouth on the mouthpiece. Keep in mind that a handheld resuscitation bag and mask is recommended only when a second rescuer arrives; it isn't recommended for use by a lone rescuer.[1]

■ Alternatively, to begin ventilations using mouth-to-mouth rescue breathing, pinch the patient's nostrils shut with the thumb and index finger of the hand you've had on his forehead (as shown below).

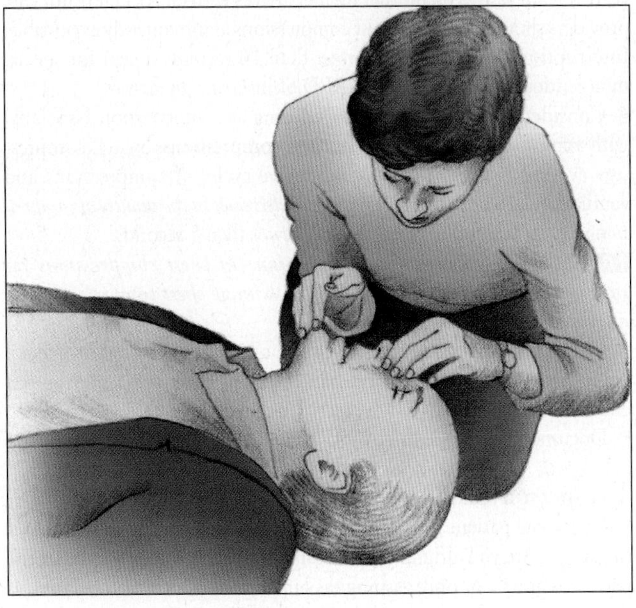

■ Take a regular breath and place your mouth over the patient's mouth, creating a tight seal (as shown on next page, top left).

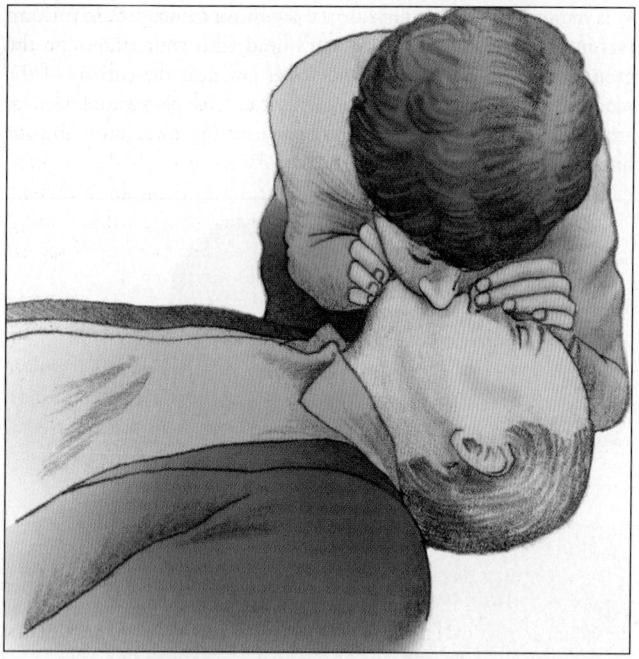

■ Give 2 breaths, each over 1 second, *to promote oxygenation and to prevent overinflation of the patient's lungs.* Each ventilation should have enough volume to produce visible chest rise *to ensure adequate ventilation.*[1,2]

■ If the first ventilation isn't successful, reposition the patient's head and try again *because the most common cause of ventilation difficulty is an improperly opened airway.*[1] If you're still unsuccessful, he may have a foreign body airway obstruction. (See the "Foreign-body airway obstruction and management" procedure, page 329.)

■ Give 30 chest compressions at a rate of approximately 100 to 120 per minute.[2] Push hard and fast. Open the airway and give 2 ventilations. Then find the proper hand position again and deliver 30 more compressions. Continue chest compressions until the emergency medical service (EMS) team arrives or another rescuer arrives with an AED. Health care providers should interrupt chest compressions as infrequently as possible. Interruptions should last no longer than 10 seconds except for special interventions, such as using the AED or inserting an airway.[1]

■ Consider switching compressors during any intervention associated with appropriate interruptions in chest compressions. Switch compressors every 2 minutes (or after about five cycles of compressions and ventilations at a ratio of 30:2) *to prevent decreases in the quality of compressions.* Try to accomplish the switch in fewer than 5 seconds.

NURSING ALERT *Avoid interruptions in chest compressions for interventions such as pulse checks to maximize chest compression time and improve tissue oxygenation.*[2]

■ Remove and discard your gloves and any other personal protective equipment worn[3] and perform hand hygiene when resuscitation has ended.[5,6,7,8,9]

■ Document the procedure.[10,11,12]

Two-person CPR

■ Check the patient for response by tapping him on the shoulder and shouting, "Are you alright?" At the same time, check to see whether the patient is apneic or only gasping (as opposed to breathing regularly). If the patient is unresponsive and apneic or only gasping, assume he's in cardiac arrest.

■ Put on gloves and other personal protective equipment as needed and available *to comply with standard precautions and to prevent exposure to potentially infectious blood and body fluids.*[3,4]

■ Place the patient in the supine position on a firm surface, such as a backboard or the floor; if the patient is on an air-filled mattress, deflate the mattress *to maximize the effectiveness of chest compressions.* When moving the patient, roll his head and torso as a unit; avoid twisting or pulling the neck, shoulders, or hips.

■ If the patient is unresponsive and apneic or only gasping, one rescuer should activate EMS and get an AED or other defibrillator, while the other rescuer checks for a pulse, taking no more than 10 seconds. If a pulse isn't present, this rescuer should immediately begin chest compressions, using a compression-to-ventilation ratio of 30:2.

■ To perform chest compressions, place the heel of one hand over the lower half of the patient's sternum (middle of the chest) and the heel of the other hand on top of the first so that your hands are parallel and overlap. Depress the chest at least 2″ (5 cm) with each chest compression and allow the chest to fully recoil after each compression *so the heart can adequately refill with blood.*[1] Avoid leaning on the patient's chest, *which could prevent the chest from recoiling completely.*[2]

■ After 30 compressions, open the airway using the head-tilt–chin-lift maneuver if no evidence of cervical spine injury exists. To accomplish this, first place your hand that's closer to the patient's head on his forehead. Then apply enough pressure to tilt the patient's head back. Next, place the fingertips of your other hand under the bony part of his lower jaw near the chin; avoid placing your fingertips on the soft tissue under the patient's chin *because you may inadvertently obstruct the airway you're trying to open.* At the same time, keep the patient's mouth partially open.

■ To begin ventilations using a mask with a one-way valve, position the narrow portion of the mask over the patient's nose and the wide portion above the patient's chin. Covering the nose and mouth with the mask, create a tight seal. Take a regular breath and then place your mouth on the mouthpiece and perform 2 ventilations. Alternatively, to begin ventilations using mouth-to-mouth rescue breathing, pinch the patient's nostrils shut with the thumb and index finger of the hand you've had on his forehead. Take a regular breath and place your mouth over the patient's mouth, creating a tight seal, and perform 2 ventilations.[1] Each ventilation should have enough volume to produce a minimal chest rise *to ensure adequate ventilation.*[1,2]

■ If the EMS team haven't arrived after five cycles of 30 compressions to 2 ventilations (about 2 minutes), tell the second rescuer to repeat the call for help.

■ If the second rescuer is another health care professional, the two of you can perform two-person CPR. He should start assisting after you've finished a cycle of 30 compressions and 2 ventilations.[1] The switch should occur in less than 5 seconds, during which the second rescuer moves into place opposite you and gets ready to begin compressions (as shown below).[1]

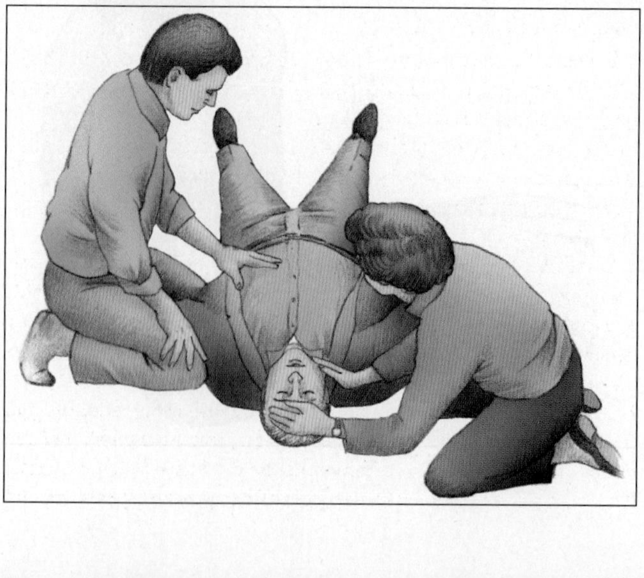

■ The second rescuer should begin delivering compressions (as shown below). The compressor (at this point, the second rescuer) should count out loud so the ventilator can anticipate when to give ventilations. The rescuers should deliver 30 cycles of compressions (100 to 120 compressions per minute)[2] and 2 ventilations; the first rescuer should deliver ventilations during pauses in compressions and deliver each breath over 1 second.[1] Avoid excessive ventilation by giving breaths at a rate of less than 12 per minute *to minimize the impact of positive-pressure ventilation on blood flow.*[2]

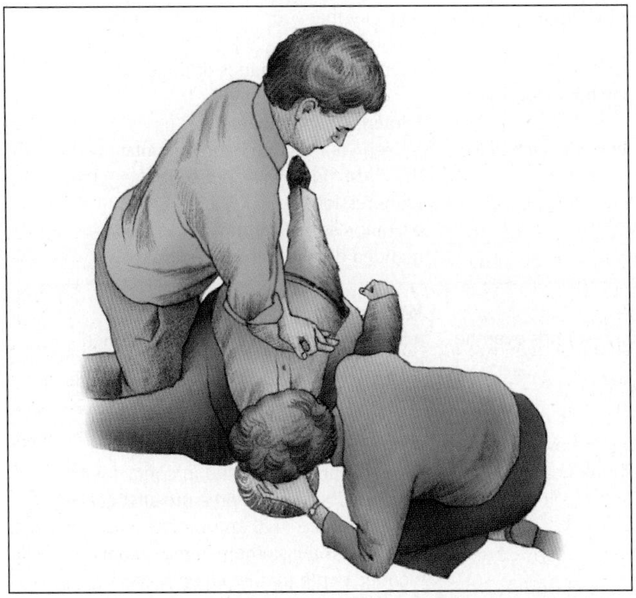

■ The compressor role should switch after five cycles of compressions and ventilations *to prevent rescuer fatigue and a subsequent decrease in compression quality;* the switch should occur in less than 5 seconds.[1] Chest compressions shouldn't be interrupted for longer than 10 seconds unless such specific interventions such as defibrillation or advanced airway placement are necessary.[1]

NURSING ALERT *Avoid interruptions to chest compressions such as pulse checks to maximize chest compression time and improve tissue oxygenation.*[2]

■ Both rescuers should continue administering CPR until the EMS team arrives or until normal breathing and effective circulation return.[1]

■ Remove and discard your gloves and any other personal protective equipment worn[3] and perform hand hygiene when resuscitation has ended.[5,6,7,8,9]

■ Document the procedure.[10,11,12]

Special considerations

■ Evidence for an optimum compression rate suggests a target of 100 to 120 compressions per minute. Rates above or below this target range appear to reduce survival to discharge.[2]

■ If hemodynamic monitoring, such as arterial or central venous catheter monitoring or capnography, are in place, they should be used to monitor the patient's response to CPR and the effectiveness of resuscitation efforts.[2]

■ Some health care professionals are hesitant to give mouth-to-mouth rescue breaths. For this reason, the AHA recommends that all health care professionals learn how to use disposable airway equipment.[1] When using a barrier device, the rescuer should not delay chest compressions while setting up the device.[1]

■ Bag-and-mask ventilation can be delivered with room air or oxygen, but supplemental oxygen (in a concentration greater than 40% and at a minimum flow rate of 10 L/minute) should be used when available. Bag-and-mask ventilation is most effective when provided by two trained and experienced rescuers. One rescuer should open the patient's airway and seal the mask to the patient's face while the other rescuer squeezes the bag and delivers the ventilations.[1]

■ After an advanced airway is in place, the compressing rescuer should give continuous chest compressions at a rate of 100 to 120 per minute[2] without pauses for ventilation. The rescuer delivering ventilation can provide a breath every 6 to 8 seconds (which yields 8 to 10 breaths/minute).[1]

■ Give the patient's family the option of remaining at the bedside during resuscitation *because doing so helps meet the psychosocial needs of the patient and family in a time of crisis.*[13]

Complications

CPR can cause certain complications—especially if the compressor doesn't place her hands properly on the sternum. These complications include fractured ribs, a lacerated liver, and punctured lungs. Gastric distention, a common complication, results from giving too much air during ventilation. (See *Potential hazards of CPR,* page 130.)

Documentation

Whenever you perform CPR, document why you initiated it, whether the victim suffered from cardiac or respiratory arrest, when you found the victim and started CPR, and the duration of CPR. Note the patient's response, any complications, and interventions to correct complications.

If the victim also received ACLS measures, document which interventions were performed, who performed them, when they were performed, and what equipment was used.

REFERENCES

1 American Heart Association. (2010). 2010 American Heart Association guidelines for cardiopulmonary resuscitation and emergency cardiovascular care. *Circulation, 122,* S685–S705. (Level II)

2 American Heart Association. (AHA). (2013). "AHA consensus statement: Cardiopulmonary resuscitation quality: Improving cardiac resuscitation outcomes both inside and outside the hospital" [Online]. Accessed March 2015 via the Web at http://circ.ahajournals.org/content/128/4/417.full (Level VII)

3 Siegel, J. D., et al. (2007). "2007 guideline for isolation precautions: Preventing transmission of infectious agents in healthcare settings" [Online]. Accessed March 2015 via the Web at http://www.cdc.gov/hicpac/pdf/isolation/Isolation2007.pdf (Level II)

4 American Osteopathic Association. (2014). Standard 07.01.10. *Healthcare Facilities Accreditation Program: Accreditation requirements for acute care hospitals.* Chicago, IL: American Osteopathic Association. (Level VII)

5 World Health Organization. (2009). "WHO guidelines on hand hygiene in health care: First global patient safety challenge, clean care is safer care" [Online]. Accessed March 2015 via the Web at http://whqlibdoc.who.int/publications/2009/9789241597906_eng.pdf (Level IV)

6 The Joint Commission. (2015). Standard NPSG.07.01.01. *Comprehensive accreditation manual for hospitals: The official handbook.* Oakbrook Terrace, IL: The Joint Commission. (Level VII)

7 Centers for Disease Control and Prevention. (2002). Guideline for hand hygiene in health-care settings: Recommendations of the Healthcare Infection Control Practices Advisory Committee and the HICPAC/SHEA/APIC/IDSA Hand Hygiene Task Force. *MMWR Recommendations and Reports, 51*(RR-16), 1–45. Accessed March 2015 via the Web at http://www.cdc.gov/mmwr/pdf/rr/rr5116.pdf (Level II)

8 Centers for Medicare & Medicaid Services, Department of Health and Human Services. (2014). Condition of participation: Infection control. 42 C.F.R. § 482.42.

9 American Osteopathic Association. (2014). Standard 07.01.21. *Healthcare Facilities Accreditation Program: Accreditation requirements for acute care hospitals.* Chicago, IL: American Osteopathic Association. (Level VII)

10 The Joint Commission. (2015). Standard RC.01.03.01. *Comprehensive accreditation manual for hospitals: The official handbook.* Oakbrook Terrace, IL: The Joint Commission. (Level VII)

Potential hazards of CPR

Cardiopulmonary resuscitation (CPR) can cause various complications, including injury to bones and vital organs. This chart describes the causes of CPR hazards and lists preventive steps.

HAZARD	CAUSES	ASSESSMENT FINDINGS	PREVENTIVE MEASURES
Sternum and rib fractures	■ Osteoporosis ■ Malnutrition ■ Improper hand placement	■ Paradoxical chest movement ■ Chest pain or tenderness that increases with inspiration ■ Crepitus ■ Palpation of movable bony fragments over the sternum ■ On palpation, sternum feels unattached to surrounding ribs	***While performing CPR:*** ■ Ensure that your hands are positioned properly. ■ Don't rest your hands or fingers on the patient's ribs. ■ Interlock your fingers. ■ Keep your bottom hand in contact with the chest, but release pressure after each compression. ■ Compress the sternum at the recommended depth for the patient's age.
Pneumothorax, hemothorax, or both	■ Lung puncture from fractured rib	■ Chest pain and dyspnea ■ Decreased or absent breath sounds over the affected lung ■ Tracheal deviation from midline ■ Hypotension ■ Hyperresonance to percussion over the affected area, along with shoulder pain	***While performing CPR:*** ■ Ensure that your hands are positioned properly. ■ Don't rest your hands or fingers on the patient's ribs. ■ Interlock your fingers. ■ Keep your bottom hand in contact with the chest, but release pressure after each compression. ■ Compress the sternum at the recommended depth for the patient's age.
Injury to the heart and great vessels (pericardial tamponade, atrial or ventricular rupture, vessel laceration, cardiac contusion, punctures of the heart chambers)	■ Improperly performed chest compressions ■ Transvenous or transthoracic pacing attempts ■ Central line placement during resuscitation ■ Intracardiac drug administration	■ Jugular vein distention ■ Muffled heart sounds ■ Pulsus paradoxus ■ Narrowed pulse pressure ■ Electrical alternans (decreased electrical amplitude of every other QRS complex) ■ Adventitious heart sounds ■ Hypotension ■ Electrocardiogram changes (arrhythmias, ST-segment elevation, T-wave inversion, and marked decrease in QRS voltage)	■ Perform chest compressions properly.
Organ laceration (primarily liver and spleen)	■ Forceful compression ■ Sharp edge of a fractured rib or xiphoid process	■ Persistent right upper quadrant tenderness (liver injury) ■ Persistent left upper quadrant tenderness (splenic injury) ■ Increasing abdominal girth	***While performing CPR:*** ■ Ensure that your hands are positioned properly. ■ Don't rest your hands or fingers on the patient's ribs. ■ Interlock your fingers. ■ Keep your bottom hand in contact with the chest, but release pressure after each compression. ■ Compress the sternum at the recommended depth for the patient's age.
Aspiration of stomach contents	■ Gastric distention and an elevated diaphragm from high ventilatory pressures	■ Fever, hypoxia, and dyspnea ■ Auscultation of wheezes and crackles ■ Increased white blood cell count ■ Changes in color and odor of lung secretions	■ Intubate early. ■ Insert a nasogastric tube and apply suction, if gastric distention is marked.

11 Centers for Medicare & Medicaid Services, Department of Health and Human Services. (2014). Condition of participation: Medical record services. 42 C.F.R. § 482.24(b).

12 American Osteopathic Association. (2014). Standard 10.00.03. *Healthcare Facilities Accreditation Program: Accreditation requirements for acute care hospitals.* Chicago, IL: American Osteopathic Association. (Level VII)

13 American Association of Critical-Care Nurses. (2010). "AACN practice alert: Family presence during resuscitation and invasive procedures" [Online]. Accessed March 2015 via the Web at http://www.aacn.org/wd/practice/docs/practicealerts/family%20presence%2004-2010%20final.pdf (Level VII)

ADDITIONAL REFERENCES

Carpico, B., & Jenkins, P. (2011). Resuscitation review to improve nursing performance during cardiac arrest. *Journal for Nurses in Staff Development, 27,* 7–12. (Level VI)

McDonald, D. D., et al. (2010). Motivating people to learn cardiopulmonary resuscitation and use of automated external defibrillators. *Journal of Cardiovascular Nursing, 25,* 69–74. (Level II)

Nettina, S. M. (2014). *Lippincott manual of nursing practice* (10th ed.). Philadelphia, PA: Wolters Kluwer.

Reynolds, J. C., et al. (2012). Cardiopulmonary resuscitation update. *Emergency Medicine Clinics of North America, 30,* 35–49.

CARDIOPULMONARY RESUSCITATION, CHILD

An adult who needs cardiopulmonary resuscitation (CPR) typically suffers from a primary cardiac disorder or an arrhythmia that has stopped the heart. A child who needs CPR typically suffers from hypoxia caused by respiratory difficulty or respiratory arrest.

Most pediatric crises requiring CPR are preventable. They include motor vehicle accidents, drowning, burns, smoke inhalation, falls, poisoning, suffocation, and choking (typically from inhaling a balloon, small object, or food, such as hot dogs, rounded candies, nuts, and grapes).[1] Other causes of cardiopulmonary arrest in children include laryngospasm and edema from upper respiratory infections and sudden infant death syndrome.

The goal of CPR is the return of spontaneous circulation.[1] However, CPR techniques differ depending on whether the patient is an adult, a child, or an infant. For CPR purposes, the American Heart Association (AHA) defines a patient by age. An infant is younger than age 1; a child is age 1 to puberty.[1]

Survival chances improve the sooner CPR begins and the faster advanced life-support systems are implemented. However, before beginning CPR on a child, you must first determine whether the child's respiratory distress results from a mechanical obstruction or an infection, such as epiglottiditis or croup. These latter conditions require immediate medical attention, not CPR. CPR is appropriate only when the child isn't breathing or is only gasping (as opposed to breathing regularly).[1]

Chest compressions are particularly important because perfusion of vital organs during CPR depends on them. To prevent a delay in chest compressions, the AHA changed the sequence of CPR in the 2010 guidelines from "A-B-C" (airway, breathing, and compressions) to "C-A-B" (compressions, airway, and breathing), which gives the highest priority to chest compressions when resuscitating a patient in cardiac arrest.[1]

High-quality CPR is important not only at the outset of resuscitation, but throughout the entire resuscitation process. Key components of high-quality CPR are minimizing chest compression interruptions, providing compressions of adequate rate and depth, avoiding leaning between compressions, and avoiding excessive ventilation.[2]

Equipment

Backboard or other firm surface ▪ automated external defibrillator (AED) (preferably with pediatric attenuator for children younger than age 8) or defibrillator ▪ Optional: barrier mask with one-way valve, gloves, other personal protective equipment.

Implementation

▪ To assess responsiveness, gently tap the child and ask loudly, "Are you okay?" Call the child's name if you know it *to elicit a response.*[1]

▪ If the child is conscious but has difficulty breathing, help her into a position that best eases her breathing—if she hasn't naturally assumed this position.

▪ Call for help *to alert others and to enlist the help of emergency medical services (EMS).* If you're alone and the child isn't breathing or is only gasping, perform CPR for five cycles (2 minutes) before calling for help. A single cycle for a lone rescuer is 30 chest compressions and 2 breaths.[1]

▪ Put on gloves and other personal protective equipment as needed and available *to comply with standard precautions and to prevent exposure to potentially infectious blood and body fluids.*[3,4]

▪ Place the child in the supine position on a firm surface, such as a backboard or the floor.[1] *The surface should provide the resistance needed for adequate chest compressions.* When moving the child, roll her head and torso as a unit (as shown below) *to avoid twisting or pulling her neck, shoulders, or hips.* Don't delay the initiation of CPR to obtain and position a backboard.

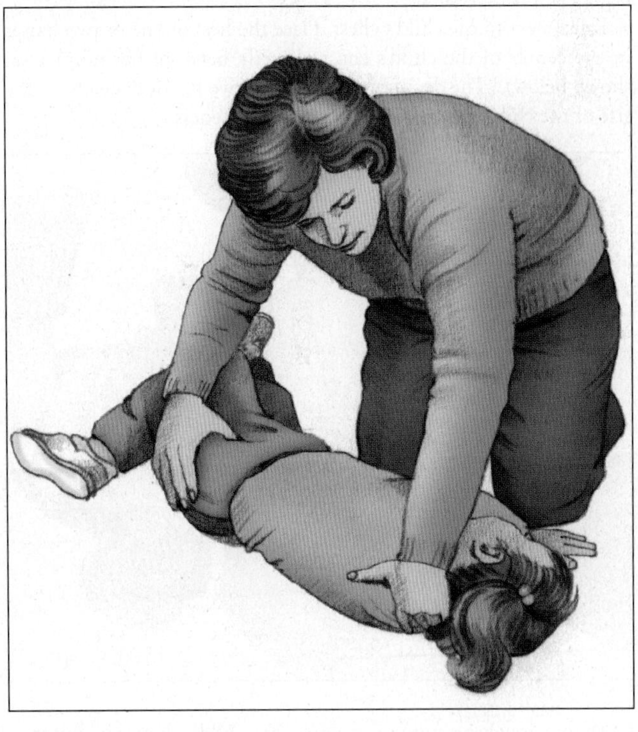

Restoring circulation

▪ Assess circulation by palpating the carotid or femoral artery for a pulse.[1]

▪ Locate the carotid artery with two or three fingers of one hand. *To palpate the carotid artery,* place your fingers in the center of the child's neck on the side closest to you, and slide your fingers into the groove formed by the trachea and the sternocleidomastoid muscles (as shown on next page, top left). *To palpate the femoral* artery, place your fingers in the center of the child's groin, just below the inguinal ligament. Palpate the artery for no more than 10 seconds *to confirm the child's pulse status.*[1]

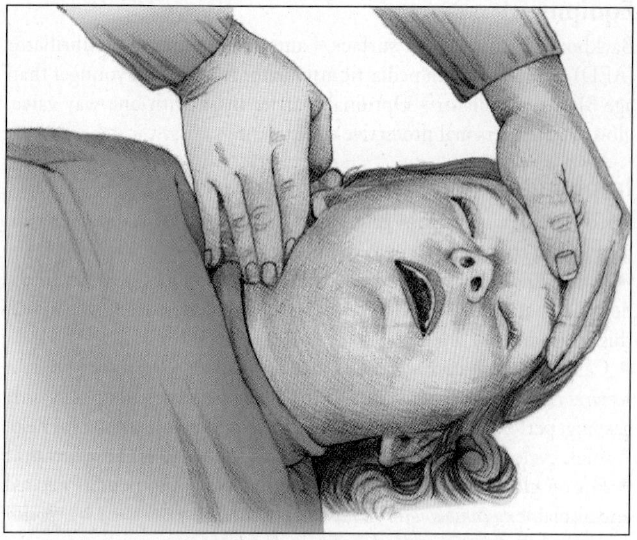

■ If you feel the child's pulse, continue rescue breathing, giving 1 breath every 3 to 5 seconds (12 to 20 breaths/minute). Reassess the pulse about every 2 minutes, but spend no more than 10 seconds doing so.[1]
■ If you can't feel a pulse or the pulse is less than 60 beats/minute and the child has signs of poor perfusion, such as pallor, cyanosis, or mottling, begin chest compressions.[1]
■ Kneel next to the child's chest. Place the heel of one or two hands in the center of the child's chest, directly between her nipples (as shown below).[1] The decision to use one or two hands depends on the size of the child and the compressor's effectiveness.

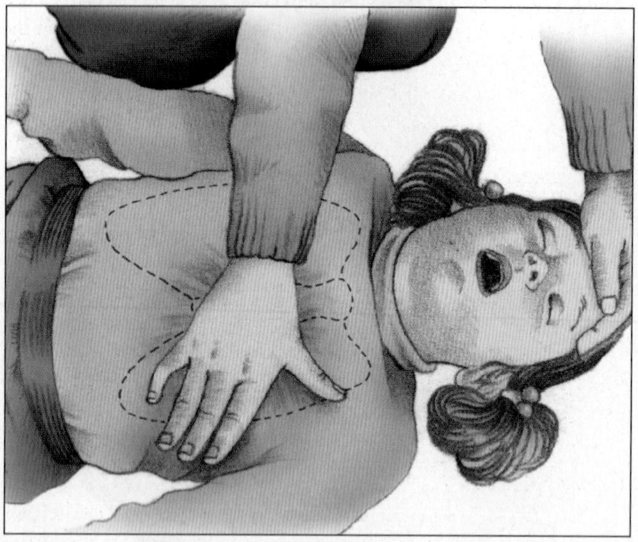

■ Apply enough pressure to compress the child's chest downward at least a third the depth of the anterior-posterior dimensions of the chest,[2] which corresponds to approximately 2″ (5 cm) in most children. Allow the chest to completely recoil after each compression. Deliver cycles of 30 compressions and 2 breaths.[1]

NURSING ALERT *During pediatric CPR, incomplete chest wall recoil is common, particularly when rescuers become fatigued; incomplete recoil is associated with higher intrathoracic pressures and significantly decreased venous return, coronary perfusion, blood flow, and cerebral perfusion.*[1]

Establishing a patent airway

■ Kneel or stand beside the child's shoulder. Place one hand on the child's forehead and gently lift her chin with your other hand *to open her airway* using the head-tilt–chin-lift maneuver (as shown below). Don't place your fingers on the soft neck tissue *to avoid obstructing the airway.* Never let the child's mouth close completely.

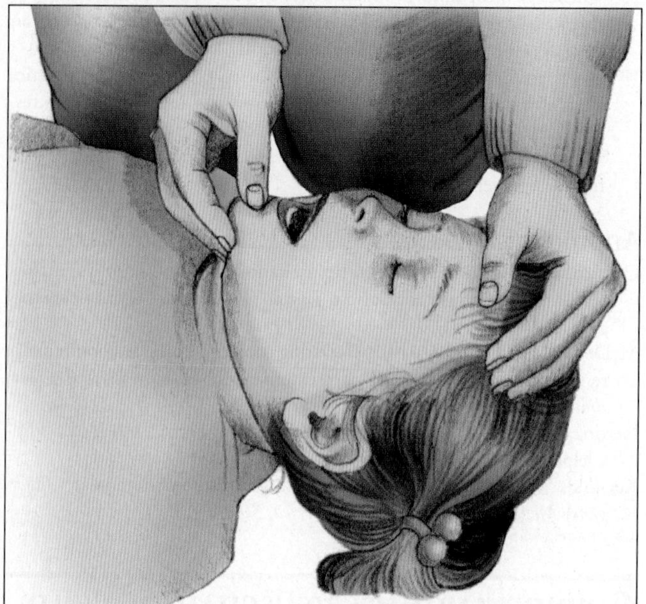

■ If there's evidence of trauma that suggests a spinal injury, use the jaw-thrust maneuver to open the child's airway *to keep from moving the child's neck.*[1] To do this, kneel beside the child's head. With your elbows on the ground, rest your thumbs at the corners of the child's mouth and place two or three fingers of each hand under the lower jaw. Lift the jaw upward.
■ While maintaining an open airway, place your ear near the child's mouth and nose *to evaluate her breathing status* (as shown below).[1] Look for chest movement and scan the child for breathing.

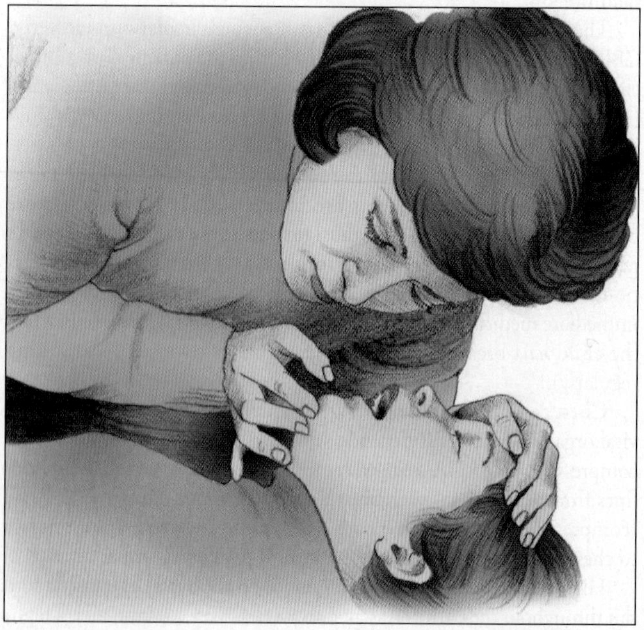

■ If the child is breathing, maintain an open airway and monitor respirations.

Restoring ventilation

■ If the child isn't breathing, maintain the open airway position. To begin ventilations using a mask with a one-way valve, position the narrow portion of the mask over the child's nose and the wide portion above the child's chin. Covering the nose and mouth with the mask, create a tight seal. Take a regular breath and place your mouth on the mouthpiece. Alternatively, to begin ventilations using mouth-to-mouth rescue breathing, pinch the child's nostrils shut with the thumb and index finger of the hand you've had on her forehead (as shown below). Take a regular breath and place your mouth over the child's mouth, creating a tight seal. Keep in mind that a handheld resuscitation bag and mask is recommended only when a second rescuer arrives; it isn't recommended for use by a lone rescuer.

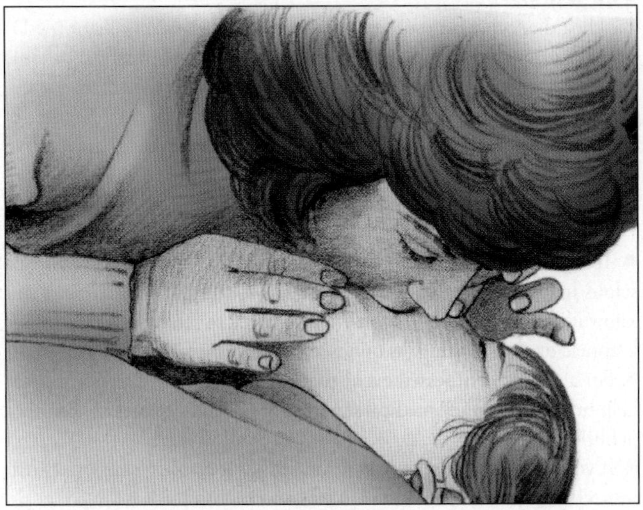

■ Give 2 slow breaths (1 second/breath), pausing between each one.[1]

■ If your first attempt at ventilation fails to restore the child's breathing, reposition the child's head *to open the airway,* and try again. In an unresponsive child, the tongue may obstruct the airway. Ensure that breaths are effective by watching for the chest to rise. If the chest doesn't rise, reposition the head, make a better mouth-to-mouth seal, and breathe again.

■ Continue rescue breathing with 1 breath every 3 to 5 seconds (12 to 20 breaths/minute) if you can detect a pulse and the pulse is greater than 60 beats/minute. If you can't detect a pulse, continue cycles of 30 compressions to 2 ventilations.

NURSING ALERT *Avoid interruptions to chest compressions such as pulse checks* to maximize chest compression time and improve tissue oxygenation.[2]

NURSING ALERT *Excessive ventilation is harmful and should be avoided.[2] Use only the force and tidal volume necessary to just make the chest rise. Give each breath slowly, lasting approximately 1 second, and watch for chest rise. If the chest doesn't rise, reopen the airway, verify that the seal is tight between your mouth and the face or the mask and the face (or between the bag and the advanced airway), and reattempt ventilation.*[1]

■ If you're still alone after five cycles (2 minutes) of CPR, call EMS, get an AED or other defibrillator if appropriate, and check the child's cardiac rhythm *to detect whether a shockable rhythm is present.* If a shockable rhythm is present, deliver a shock. Resume CPR for 2 minutes, beginning with chest compressions, immediately after the shock is delivered.[1]

■ When a second rescuer arrives, continue with two-person CPR. (See "Two-person CPR" in the "Cardiopulmonary resuscitation, adult" procedure, page 128.)

■ Remove and discard your gloves and any other personal protective equipment worn.[3]

■ Perform hand hygiene.[5,6,7,8,9]

■ Document the procedure.[10,11,12]

Special considerations

■ Some health care professionals hesitate to give mouth-to-mouth rescue breaths. For this reason, the AHA recommends that all health care professionals learn how to use disposable airway equipment.[1] When using a barrier device, the rescuer shouldn't delay chest compressions while setting up the device.[1]

■ Because effective bag-and-mask ventilation requires complex steps, it isn't recommended for a lone rescuer during CPR. Instead, mouth-to-barrier device techniques can be used. Bag-and-mask ventilation can be provided effectively during two-person CPR.[1]

■ A child's tongue can easily block her small airway. If this occurs, simply opening the airway may eliminate the obstruction.

■ When performing chest compressions, take care to ensure smooth motions. Keep your fingers off—and the heel of your hand on—the child's chest at all times. Also, time your motions so that the compression and relaxation phases are equal *to promote effective compressions.*

■ If a child is having difficulty breathing and a parent or guardian is present, find out whether the child recently had a fever or an upper respiratory tract infection. If so, suspect epiglottitis. In this instance, don't attempt to manipulate the airway *because laryngospasm can occur and completely obstruct the airway.* Allow the child to assume a comfortable position, and monitor her breathing until assistance arrives.

■ Give the child's parents or guardian the option of remaining at the bedside during resuscitation *because doing so helps meet the psychosocial needs of the child and family.*[13]

Complications

CPR can cause complications, including fractured ribs, a lacerated liver, and punctured lungs, if the compressor doesn't place her hands on the sternum properly. Gastric distention, a common complication, results from giving too much air during ventilation.

Documentation

Document all of the events of resuscitation and the names of the individuals who were present. Record whether the child suffered cardiac or respiratory arrest. Note the location where the arrest occurred, the time CPR began, the duration of the procedure, and the outcome. Document any complications—for example, a fractured rib, a bruised mouth, or gastric distention—as well as actions taken to correct them.

If the child received pediatric advanced life support, document which interventions were performed, who performed them, when they were performed, and what equipment was used.

REFERENCES

1 American Heart Association. (2010). 2010 American Heart Association guidelines for cardiopulmonary resuscitation and emergency cardiovascular care. *Circulation, 122,* S862–S875. (Level II)

2 American Heart Association. (AHA). (2013). "AHA consensus statement: Cardiopulmonary resuscitation quality: Improving cardiac resuscitation outcomes both inside and outside the hospital" [Online]. Accessed March 2015 via the Web at http://circ.ahajournals.org/content/128/4/417.full (Level VII)

3 Siegel, J. D., et al. (2007). "2007 guideline for isolation precautions: Preventing transmission of infectious agents in healthcare settings" [Online]. Accessed March 2015 via the Web at http://www.cdc.gov/hicpac/pdf/isolation/Isolation2007.pdf (Level II)

4 American Osteopathic Association. (2014). Standard 07.01.10. *Healthcare Facilities Accreditation Program: Accreditation requirements for acute care hospitals.* Chicago, IL: American Osteopathic Association. (Level VII)

5 World Health Organization. (2009). "WHO guidelines on hand hygiene in health care: First global patient safety challenge, clean care is safer care" [Online]. Accessed March 2015 via the Web at http://whqlibdoc.who.int/publications/2009/9789241597906_eng.pdf (Level IV)
6 The Joint Commission. (2015). Standard NPSG.07.01.01. *Comprehensive accreditation manual for hospitals: The official handbook.* Oakbrook Terrace, IL: The Joint Commission. (Level VII)
7 Centers for Disease Control and Prevention. (2002). Guideline for hand hygiene in health-care settings: Recommendations of the Healthcare Infection Control Practices Advisory Committee and the HICPAC/SHEA/APIC/IDSA Hand Hygiene Task Force. *MMWR Recommendations and Reports, 51*(RR-16), 1–45. Accessed March 2015 via the Web at http://www.cdc.gov/mmwr/pdf/rr/rr5116.pdf (Level II)
8 Centers for Medicare & Medicaid Services, Department of Health and Human Services. (2014). Condition of participation: Infection control. 42. C.F.R. § 482.42.
9 American Osteopathic Association. (2014). Standard 07.01.21. *Healthcare Facilities Accreditation Program: Accreditation requirements for acute care hospitals.* Chicago, IL: American Osteopathic Association. (Level VII)
10 The Joint Commission. (2015). Standard RC.02.01.01. *Comprehensive accreditation manual for hospitals: The official handbook.* Oakbrook Terrace, IL: The Joint Commission. (Level VII)
11 Centers for Medicare & Medicaid Services, Department of Health and Human Services. (2014). Condition of participation: Medical record services. 42 C.F.R. § 482.24(b).
12 American Osteopathic Association. (2014). Standard 10.00.03. *Healthcare Facilities Accreditation Program: Accreditation requirements for acute care hospitals.* Chicago, IL: American Osteopathic Association. (Level VII)
13 American Association of Critical-Care Nurses. (2010). "AACN practice alert: Family presence during resuscitation and invasive procedures" [Online]. Accessed March 2015 via the Web at http://www.aacn.org/wd/practice/docs/practicealerts/family%20presence%2004-2010%20final.pdf (Level VII)

ADDITIONAL REFERENCES

Kleinman, M. E., et al. (2010). Pediatric basic and advanced life support: 2010 international consensus on cardiopulmonary resuscitation and emergency cardiovascular care science with treatment recommendations. *Circulation, 122,* S466–S515. Accessed March 2015 via the Web at http://pediatrics.aappublications.org/content/126/5/e1261.full.pdf (Level II)

Lubrano, R., et al. (2012). How the newly introduced compression, airway, and breathing sequence affects the training in pediatric cardiopulmonary resuscitation. *American Journal of Emergency Medicine, 30,* 371–372.

CARDIOPULMONARY RESUSCITATION, INFANT

An adult who needs cardiopulmonary resuscitation (CPR) typically suffers from a primary cardiac disorder or an arrhythmia that has stopped the heart. An infant who needs CPR typically suffers from hypoxia caused by respiratory difficulty or respiratory arrest.

In infants, the leading causes of cardiopulmonary arrest are congenital malformations, complications of prematurity, and sudden infant death syndrome.[1] Other causes of cardiopulmonary arrest in infants include laryngospasm and edema from upper respiratory infections and choking. Liquids are the most common cause of choking in infants.[1]

The goal of CPR is the return of spontaneous circulation.[1] However, CPR techniques differ depending on whether the patient is an adult, a child, or an infant. For CPR purposes, the American Heart Association (AHA) defines a patient by age. An infant is younger than age 1; a child is age 1 to puberty.[1]

Survival chances improve the sooner CPR begins and the faster advanced life-support systems are implemented. CPR is appropriate only when the infant isn't breathing or is only gasping (as opposed to breathing regularly).[1] Chest compressions are particularly important because perfusion to vital organs during CPR depends on them. To prevent a delay in chest compressions, the AHA changed the sequence of CPR in the 2010 guidelines from "A-B-C" (airway, breathing, and compressions) to "C-A-B" (compressions, airway, and breathing), which gives the highest priority to chest compressions when resuscitating a patient in cardiac arrest.[1]

High-quality CPR is important not only at the onset of resuscitation, but throughout the entire resuscitation process. Key components of high-quality CPR are minimizing chest compression interruptions, providing compressions of adequate rate and depth, avoiding leaning between compressions, and avoiding excessive ventilation.[2]

Equipment

Backboard or other firm surface ■ automated external defibrillator (AED) or defibrillator (a manual device is preferred in infants with a shockable rhythm; if a manual device isn't available, a device with a pediatric attenuator is preferred; if neither is available, an AED without a dose attenuator may be used) ■ Optional: gloves, other personal protective equipment.

Implementation

- To assess responsiveness, gently tap the foot of the apparently unconscious infant and say loudly, "Are you okay?" Call out his name if you know it. While assessing responsiveness, check to see whether the infant is apneic or only gasping (as opposed to breathing regularly).[1]
- For a sudden, witnessed event that causes unresponsiveness, call for help or call emergency medical services (EMS) and get an AED or other defibrillator.
- If you witnessed the event that caused nonresponsiveness, perform resuscitation measures for 2 minutes and then call for help. Move an uninjured infant close to a telephone, or make sure you have a cell phone or other telephone nearby, if necessary.[1]
- Put on gloves and other personal protective equipment as needed *to comply with standard precautions and to prevent exposure to potentially infections blood and body fluids.*[3,4]
- Place the infant supine on a firm surface.[2]

Restoring heartbeat and circulation

- Assess the infant's pulse by palpating the brachial artery, located inside the infant's upper arm between the elbow and the shoulder (as shown below).[1] Take no more than 10 seconds to try to find a pulse. If you find a pulse and the pulse is greater than or equal to 60 beats/minute, continue rescue breathing but don't initiate chest compressions.[1]

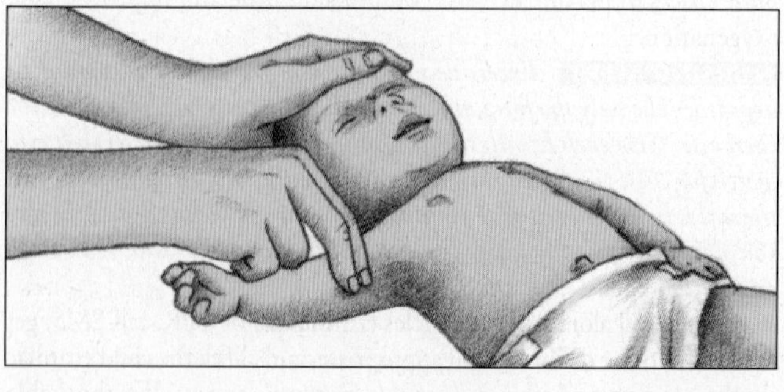

- Begin chest compressions if you find no pulse or the pulse rate is less than 60 beats/minute and the infant shows signs of poor perfusion, such as pallor, cyanosis, or mottling. Place two fingers on the sternum just below the nipple line (as shown on next page, top left). Use these two fingers to depress the sternum at least a third of the depth of the chest at 100 compressions per minute.[1] When performing chest compressions, take care to ensure smooth motions. Keep your fingers on the infant's chest at all times. Time your motions so that the compression and relaxation phases are equal *to promote effective compressions.*

NURSING ALERT *During pediatric CPR, incomplete chest wall recoil is common, particularly when rescuers become fatigued. Incomplete recoil during CPR is associated with higher intrathoracic pressures and significantly decreased venous return, coronary perfusion, blood flow, and cerebral perfusion.*[1]

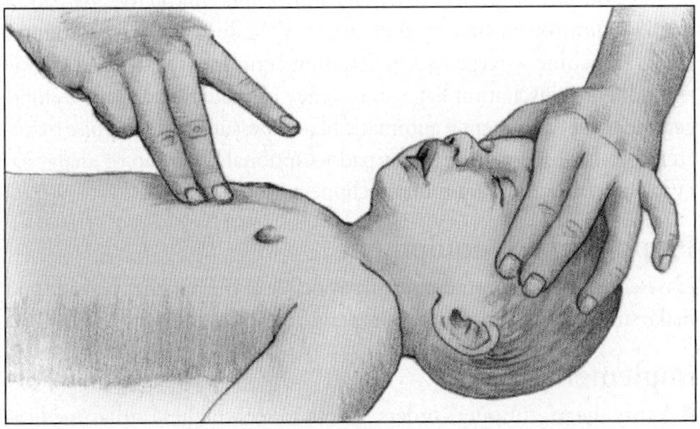

Restoring ventilation

- Complete 30 compressions, open the airway, and give 2 breaths.
- Open the airway using the head-tilt–chin-lift maneuver, unless contraindicated by trauma. If spinal injury is suspected, use the jaw-thrust maneuver. Don't hyperextend the infant's neck.
- To begin ventilations using a mask with a one-way valve, position the narrow portion of the mask over the infant's nose and the wide portion above the infant's chin. Covering the nose and mouth with the mask, create a tight seal. Take a regular breath and place your mouth on the mouthpiece. Alternatively, take a breath and tightly seal your mouth over the infant's nose and mouth (as shown below).[1]

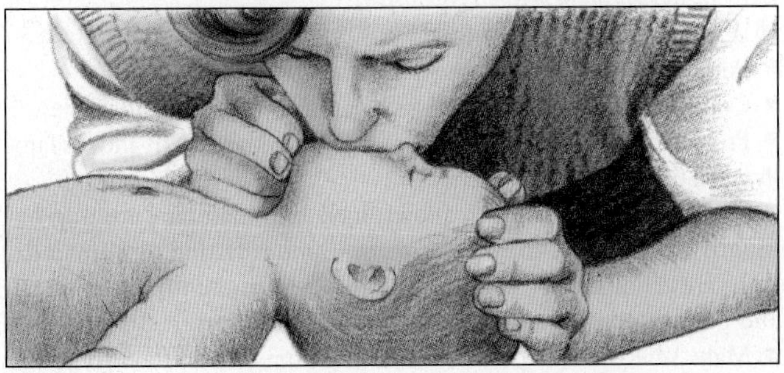

- Deliver 2 breaths. If the infant's chest rises and falls, then the amount of air is probably adequate. If the chest doesn't rise, reposition the head, make a better seal, and try again.[1] Avoid excessive ventilation.[2]
- After 2 minutes of CPR, activate the emergency response system if you're still alone, and obtain an AED or defibrillator.
- Check the infant's cardiac rhythm with the AED or defibrillator. If a shockable rhythm is present, deliver a shock, as indicated.[1]
- Resume CPR with cycles of 30 compressions to 2 ventilations until the EMS team arrives or the infant begins breathing spontaneously.[1]

NURSING ALERT *Avoid interruptions to chest compressions such as pulse checks* to maximize chest compression time and improve tissue oxygenation.[2]

- Continue to monitor the infant if pulse and respirations return.
- Remove and discard your gloves and any other personal protective equipment worn.[3]
- Perform hand hygiene.[5,6,7,8,9]
- Document the procedure.[10,11,12]

Special considerations

- The AHA recommends that all health care professionals learn how to use disposable airway equipment.[1] When using a barrier device, the rescuer shouldn't delay chest compressions while setting up the device.[1]

Because effective bag-and-mask ventilation requires complex steps, it isn't recommended for a lone rescuer performing CPR. During CPR, the lone rescuer should use mouth-to-barrier device techniques for ventilation. Bag-and-mask ventilation can be provided effectively during two-person CPR.[1]

- If two rescuers are available, the two thumb–encircling hands technique is preferred for chest compressions. Place your hands around the infant's chest with your fingers around the thorax and your thumbs together on the lower half of the sternum.[1] Compress the sternum with your thumbs and squeeze your fingers for counterpressure. Use a compression-to-ventilation ratio of 15 to 2.[1]
- An infant's tongue can easily block his small airway. If this occurs, simply opening the airway may eliminate the obstruction.
- If the infant has breathing difficulty and a parent or guardian is present, find out whether the infant recently had a fever or an upper respiratory tract infection. If so, suspect epiglottitis. In this instance, don't attempt to manipulate the airway *because laryngospasm may occur and completely obstruct the airway.* Allow the infant to assume a comfortable position, and monitor his breathing until additional assistance arrives.
- Give the infant's parents or guardian the option of remaining at the bedside during resuscitation *because doing so helps meet the psychosocial needs of the infant and family in a time of crisis.*[13]

Complications

CPR can cause complications, including fractured ribs, a lacerated liver, and punctured lungs, if the compressor doesn't place the fingers on the sternum properly. Gastric distention, a common complication, results from giving too much air during ventilation.

Documentation

Document all of the events of resuscitation and the names of the individuals who were present. Record whether the infant suffered cardiac or respiratory arrest. Note the location where the arrest occurred, the time CPR began, how long the procedure continued, and the outcome. Document any complications—for example, a fractured rib, a bruised mouth, or gastric distention—as well as actions taken to correct them.

If the infant received pediatric advanced life support, document which interventions were performed, who performed them, when they were performed, and what equipment was used.

REFERENCES

1 American Heart Association. (2010). 2010 American Heart Association guidelines for cardiopulmonary resuscitation and emergency cardiovascular care. *Circulation, 122,* S862–S875. (Level II)

2 American Heart Association (AHA). (2013). "AHA consensus statement: Cardiopulmonary resuscitation quality: Improving cardiac resuscitation outcomes both inside and outside the hospital" [Online]. Accessed March 2015 via the Web at http://circ.ahajournals.org/content/128/4/417.full (Level VII)

3 Siegel, J. D., et al. (2007). "2007 guideline for isolation precautions: Preventing transmission of infectious agents in healthcare settings" [Online]. Accessed March 2015 via the Web at http://www.cdc.gov/hicpac/pdf/isolation/Isolation2007.pdf (Level II)

4 American Osteopathic Association. (2014). Standard 07.01.10. *Healthcare Facilities Accreditation Program: Accreditation requirements for acute care hospitals.* Chicago, IL: American Osteopathic Association. (Level VII)

5 The Joint Commission. (2015). Standard NPSG.07.01.01. *Comprehensive accreditation manual for hospitals: The official handbook.* Oakbrook Terrace, IL: The Joint Commission. (Level VII)

6 World Health Organization. (2009). "WHO guidelines on hand hygiene in health care: First global patient safety challenge, clean care is safer care" [Online]. Accessed March 2015 via the Web at http://whqlibdoc.who.int/publications/2009/9789241597906_eng.pdf (Level IV)
7 Centers for Disease Control and Prevention. (2002). Guideline for hand hygiene in health-care settings: Recommendations of the Healthcare Infection Control Practices Advisory Committee and the HICPAC/SHEA/APIC/IDSA Hand Hygiene Task Force. *MMWR Recommendations and Reports, 51*(RR-16), 1–45. Accessed March 2015 via the Web at http://www.cdc.gov/mmwr/pdf/rr/rr5116.pdf (Level II)
8 Centers for Medicare & Medicaid Services, Department of Health and Human Services. (2014). Condition of participation: Infection control. 42. C.F.R. § 482.42.
9 American Osteopathic Association. (2014). Standard 07.01.21. *Healthcare Facilities Accreditation Program: Accreditation requirements for acute care hospitals.* Chicago, IL: American Osteopathic Association. (Level VII)
10 The Joint Commission. (2015). Standard RC.02.01.01. *Comprehensive accreditation manual for hospitals: The official handbook.* Oakbrook Terrace, IL: The Joint Commission. (Level VII)
11 Centers for Medicare & Medicaid Services, Department of Health and Human Services. (2014). Condition of participation: Medical record services. 42. C.F.R. § 482.24(b).
12 American Osteopathic Association. (2014). Standard 10.00.03. *Healthcare Facilities Accreditation Program: Accreditation requirements for acute care hospitals.* Chicago, IL: American Osteopathic Association. (Level VII)
13 American Association of Critical-Care Nurses. (2010). "AACN practice alert: Family presence during resuscitation and invasive procedures" [Online]. Accessed March 2015 via the Web at http://www.aacn.org/wd/practice/docs/practicealerts/family%20presence%2004-2010%20final.pdf (Level VII)

ADDITIONAL REFERENCES

Bowden, V. R., & Greenberg, C. S. (2012). *Pediatric nursing procedures* (3rd ed.). Philadelphia, PA: Lippincott Williams & Wilkins.
Matshes, E. W., & Lew, E. O. (2010). Two-handed cardiopulmonary resuscitation can cause rib fractures in infants. *American Journal of Forensic Medicine and Pathology, 31,* 303–307.

CARDIOVERSION, SYNCHRONIZED

Synchronized cardioversion delivers an electrical charge to the myocardium that's timed with the QRS complex. This charge causes immediate depolarization, interrupting reentry circuits and allowing the sinoatrial node to resume control. Synchronizing the electrical charge with the QRS complex prevents delivery during the relative refractory period of the cardiac cycle, when a shock could lead to ventricular fibrillation.[1]

Synchronized cardioversion is the treatment of choice for arrhythmias, such as unstable supraventricular tachycardia due to reentry, unstable atrial flutter, unstable atrial fibrillation, or unstable monomorphic ventricular tachycardia with a pulse that doesn't respond to vagal maneuvers (Valsalva maneuver or carotid sinus massage) or drug therapy.[1] The procedure can be elective or urgent depending on the patient's tolerance of the arrhythmia.[1] For example, if the patient is hemodynamically stable, the procedure is commonly elective, allowing for time to assess the patient's cardiac and metabolic status to determine whether there's a reversible cause that can be treated. If the patient is unstable (altered mental status, shock or hypotension, and chest pain), immediate cardioversion is necessary.[2]

Contraindications to synchronized cardioversion include tachycardia related to digoxin toxicity, sinus tachycardia, and multifocal atrial tachycardia. Because atrial fibrillation increases the risk of stroke, cardioversion is contraindicated in patients with atrial fibrillation who aren't receiving anticoagulation, unless transesophageal imaging is performed to rule out thrombus formation.[3,4] Anticoagulation therapy is recommended for 3 weeks before elective cardioversion to convert hemodynamically stable atrial fibrillation to normal sinus rhythm.[5]

Practitioners using synchronized cardioversion should adhere to the 2010 American Heart Association guidelines.[1]

Equipment

Cardioverter-defibrillator ■ self-adhesive cardioversion-defibrillation pads or anterior, posterior, or transverse paddles and conductive gel pads ■ cardiac monitor with recording system ■ 12-lead electrocardiogram (ECG) machine ■ oxygen administration equipment ■ artificial airway ■ handheld resuscitation bag ■ emergency cardiac medications ■ emergency pacing equipment ■ automatic blood pressure device ■ pulse oximeter ■ stethoscope ■ disinfectant pad ■ Optional: sedation or analgesia, IV catheter insertion equipment, clippers, gloves.

Preparation of equipment

Have emergency equipment readily available at the patient's bedside and make sure that it's functioning properly.

Implementation

■ Verify the practitioner's orders. Check to see whether cardiac medications have been prescribed for administration before the procedure.
■ Check the patient's medical record for recent serum potassium and magnesium levels and arterial blood gas results. Also check the most recent digoxin level if ordered. *Electrolyte imbalances, acid-base disturbances, and digoxin toxicity increase the risk of arrhythmias.*[5] Notify the practitioner of critical test results within your facility's established time frame *so that the patient can be treated promptly.*[6]
■ Confirm that written informed consent is obtained and that the consent is included in the patient's medical record.[5,7,8,9]
■ Gather the appropriate equipment.
■ Conduct a preprocedure verification *to make sure that all relevant documentation, related information, and equipment are available and correctly identified to the patient's identifiers.*[10]
■ Perform hand hygiene.[11,12,13,14,15]
■ Put on gloves if needed *to comply with standard precautions.*[16,17]
■ Confirm the patient's identity using at least two patient identifiers.[18]
■ Provide privacy and explain the procedure to the patient and his family *to allay their fears and anxiety.*[19,20]
■ If the patient's condition allows, have him maintain nothing-by-mouth status before the procedure; minimum fasting recommendations are 2 hours for clear liquids, 6 hours or more for a light meal, and 8 hours or more for fried or fatty foods or meat.[21]
■ Make sure that the patient is attached to a cardiac monitor, pulse oximeter, and automatic blood pressure device. Make sure that the alarm limits are set appropriately for the patient's current condition and that the alarms are turned on, functioning properly, and audible to staff.[22,23,24,25]
■ Obtain the patient's vital signs and oxygen saturation level, and assess his neurologic, cardiovascular, and respiratory status *to determine whether immediate cardioversion is necessary.*[2,5]
■ If the patient's oxygenation is inadequate or if he shows signs of labored breathing, notify the practitioner and administer supplemental oxygen, as prescribed.[2]
■ Make sure that the patient has patent IV access; if he doesn't, insert an IV catheter. (See the "IV catheter insertion and removal" procedure, page 446.)
■ Obtain a 12-lead ECG *to better define the patient's heart rhythm and to serve as a baseline for comparison.* If the patient is unstable, don't delay immediate cardioversion to obtain the ECG.[2,5]
■ Administer cardiac medications if prescribed following safe medication administration practices.[26,27]

■ Remove all metal objects from the patient *because metal conducts electricity and could cause burns during cardioversion.*[5]

■ If the patient has dentures, a partial plate, or another oral prosthesis, determine whether the device supports airway patency or has the potential to obstruct it. Remove the device if it increases the risk of airway obstruction.[5]

■ Make sure that the patient is in a dry environment and that his chest is dry *because if the rescuer or patient comes in contact with water, a conductor of electricity, the rescuer can receive a shock and the patient can receive skin burns.*[5]

■ Place the patient in the supine position *to provide access to the patient's chest during the procedure.*[5]

■ If necessary, clip hair from the patient's chest *to make sure that the electrodes adhere properly.*[5]

■ Remove transdermal medication patches from the patient's chest if present, or make sure that the cardioversion-defibrillation pads or paddles don't touch the patches during the procedure *to prevent a chest burn during cardioversion.*[5]

■ If the patient isn't already receiving supplemental oxygen, consider preoxygenate him before cardioversion *to promote myocardial oxygenation and to reduce the risk of cerebral and cardiac complications.*[5]

■ A specially trained health care provider will administer moderate sedation or anesthesia if time allows and the patient's condition permits.

■ Monitor the patient's heart rate, blood pressure, and respiratory rate *to promptly detect changes in the patient's condition and prevent treatment delays.*

■ Conduct a time-out before starting the procedure, if the patient's condition allows, *to perform a final assessment ensuring that the correct patient, site, positioning, and procedure are identified and, as applicable, that all relevant information and necessary equipment are available.*[28]

■ Turn on the cardioverter-defibrillator.[5]

■ Attach the patient to the monitoring leadwires on the cardioverter-defibrillator *because the device must be able to sense the R wave to provide synchronized cardioversion.*[5]

■ Apply the self-adhesive cardioversion-defibrillation pads according to the manufacturer's directions; if you're using anterolateral placement, place one pad at the heart's apex just left of the nipple at the midaxillary line and the other pad just below the right clavicle to the right of the sternum. Alternatively, remove the paddles from the machine. Place the paddles and the conductive gel pads using anterolateral placement.[1,5] Alternative pad positions, including anteroposterior, anterior–left infrascapular, and anterior–right infrascapular, can also be used depending on the patient's individual characteristics.[1]

NURSING ALERT To decrease transthoracic resistance, *avoid placing the self-adhesive cardioversion-defibrillation pads or paddles over a female patient's breast.*[5]

■ Turn on the ECG recording device to obtain a continuous printout *to document the patient's response to cardioversion.*[5]

■ Push the SYNC button *to synchronize the machine with the patient's QRS complex.* Assess the cardioverter-defibrillator waveform and make sure that the SYNC button flashes with each of the patient's QRS complexes; listen for audible beeps. *Synchronization with the patient's QRS complex prevents the random discharge of electrical charges, which may cause ventricular fibrillation.*[5]

■ Set the energy level to the prescribed dose. Advanced cardiac life support protocols call for an initial shock of 50 to 100 joules for a patient with unstable supraventricular tachycardia, 120 to 200 joules for a patient with atrial fibrillation, 50 to 100 joules for a patient with atrial flutter, and 100 joules for a patient with monomorphic ventricular tachycardia with a pulse.[1]

■ Make sure that everyone stands clear from contact with the patient and his bed *to prevent conduction of electrical current to health care workers.*[15]

■ Charge the cardioverter-defibrillator.

■ Disconnect the oxygen source before cardioversion *to decrease the risk of combustion in the presence of electrical current.*[5]

■ Confirm that all personnel are clear of the patient and his bed. If you're using cardioversion-defibrillation pads, push the discharge button. Alternatively, if you're using paddles, apply firm pressure (approximately 25 to 30 lb [11.3 to 13.6 kg])[29] to each paddle against the patient's chest wall, push the discharge button, and wait for the energy to be discharged. Keep in mind that the machine has to synchronize the discharge with the QRS complex.

NURSING ALERT *Don't touch the bed, the patient, or any equipment attached to the patient while cardioversion is being administered* to prevent transfer of the electrical current to caregivers.

■ Assess the patient's cardiac rhythm on the monitor.

■ If the arrhythmia fails to convert after the initial shock, repeat the procedure, increasing the energy dose in a stepwise fashion[1] or as instructed by the practitioner. Check that the synchronization mode is active after each cardioversion attempt *because many defibrillators automatically default to the unsynchronized mode.*

■ When the patient's rhythm converts, monitor his vital signs, oxygen saturation level, and cardiovascular, neurologic, and respiratory status *to evaluate his response to the procedure.*[5] Make sure you reconnect the patient to the oxygen source as appropriate.

■ Turn off the continuous ECG recording device.

■ Obtain a follow-up 12-lead ECG, as ordered.

■ Inspect the patient's chest for electrical burns; treat burns as needed and prescribed.[5]

■ Perform a comprehensive pain assessment using techniques appropriate for the patient's age, condition, and ability to understand.[30] Administer analgesia as ordered and indicated using safe medication administration practices.[26,27]

■ Discard used supplies in the appropriate receptacles.[16]

■ Remove and discard your gloves if worn.[16]

■ Perform hand hygiene.[11,12,13,14,15]

■ Clean and disinfect your stethoscope using a disinfectant pad.[31,32]

■ Clean and disinfect the cardioverter-defibrillator and make sure that it's ready for reuse.[5,31,32]

■ Perform hand hygiene.[11,12,13,14,15]

■ Document the procedure.[33,34,35]

Special considerations

■ Be aware that synchronized cardioversion must sense the R wave to deliver the current outside of the heart's vulnerable period. Make sure that the synchronization markers are clearly visible on the monitor and that their location is consistent from beat to beat. If necessary, adjust the lead or size settings *to yield the best display.*[36]

■ If the patient has a permanent pacemaker or an implantable cardioverter-defibrillator, don't place the pads or paddles over the device *because doing so can impair current flow to the patient's heart and damage the device.*[5]

■ The Joint Commission has issued a sentinel event alert concerning medical device alarm safety *because alarm-related events have been associated with permanent loss of function or death.* Among the contributing factors are improper alarm settings, alarm settings inappropriately turned off, and alarm signals not audible to staff. Make sure that alarm limits are set appropriately and that alarms are turned on, functioning properly, and audible to staff. Follow facility guidelines for preventing alarm fatigue.[22]

Complications

Common complications following synchronized cardioversion are skin burns, pulmonary edema, hypotension, embolism, and transient harmless arrhythmias, such as atrial, ventricular, and junctional premature beats. Serious ventricular arrhythmias such as ventricular fibrillation can also occur; however, this type of arrhythmia is more likely to result from high amounts of electrical energy, digoxin toxicity, severe heart disease, electrolyte imbalances, or improper synchronization with the R wave.

Documentation

Document the procedure, including the voltage delivered with each attempt, rhythm strips before and after the procedure, medications administered, and the patient's tolerance of the procedure. Note any emergency interventions required and the patient's response to these interventions. Record the patient's vital signs and your assessment findings. Document any patient teaching and the patient's understanding of the teaching.

REFERENCES

1 American Heart Association. (2010). 2010 American Heart Association guidelines for cardiopulmonary resuscitation and emergency cardiovascular care. *Circulation, 122,* S706–S719. (Level II)

2 American Heart Association. (2010). 2010 American Heart Association guidelines for cardiopulmonary resuscitation and emergency cardiovascular care. *Circulation, 122,* S729–S776. (Level II)

3 Beinart, S. C. (2013). "Synchronized electrical cardioversion" [Online]. Accessed March 2015 via the Web at http://emedicine.medscape.com/article/1834044-overview

4 Marchiondo, K. (2007). Transesophageal imaging and interventions: Nursing implications. *Critical Care Nurse, 27*(2), 25–36. (Level V)

5 Lynn-McHale Wiegand, D. (Ed.). (2011). *AACN procedure manual for critical care* (6th ed.). St. Louis, MO: Saunders.

6 The Joint Commission. (2015). Standard NPSG.02.03.01. *Comprehensive accreditation manual for hospitals: The official handbook.* Oakbrook Terrace, IL: The Joint Commission. (Level VII)

7 The Joint Commission. (2015). Standard RI.01.03.01. *Comprehensive accreditation manual for hospitals: The official handbook.* Oakbrook Terrace, IL: The Joint Commission. (Level VII)

8 Centers for Medicare & Medicaid Services, Department of Health and Human Services. (2014). Condition of participation: Patient's rights. 42 C.F.R. § 482.13(b)(2).

9 American Osteopathic Association. (2014). Standard 30.01.11. *Healthcare Facilities Accreditation Program: Accreditation requirements for acute care hospitals.* Chicago, IL: American Osteopathic Association. (Level VII)

10 The Joint Commission. (2015). Standard UP.01.01.01. *Comprehensive accreditation manual for hospitals: The official handbook.* Oakbrook Terrace, IL: The Joint Commission. (Level VII)

11 The Joint Commission. (2015). Standard NPSG.07.01.01. *Comprehensive accreditation manual for hospitals: The official handbook.* Oakbrook Terrace, IL: The Joint Commission. (Level VII)

12 Centers for Disease Control and Prevention. (2002). Guideline for hand hygiene in health-care settings: Recommendations of the Healthcare Infection Control Practices Advisory Committee and the HICPAC/SHEA/APIC/IDSA Hand Hygiene Task Force. *MMWR Recommendations and Reports, 51*(RR-16), 1–45. Accessed March 2015 via the Web at http://www.cdc.gov/mmwr/pdf/rr/rr5116.pdf (Level II)

13 World Health Organization. (2009). "WHO guidelines on hand hygiene in health care: First global patient safety challenge, clean care is safer care" [Online]. Accessed March 2015 via the Web at http://whqlibdoc.who.int/publications/2009/9789241597906_eng.pdf (Level IV)

14 Centers for Medicare & Medicaid Services, Department of Health and Human Services. (2014). Condition of participation: Infection control. 42 C.F.R. § 482.42.

15 American Osteopathic Association. (2014). Standard 07.01.21. *Healthcare Facilities Accreditation Program: Accreditation requirements for acute care hospitals.* Chicago, IL: American Osteopathic Association. (Level VII)

16 Siegel, J. D., et al. (2007). "2007 guideline for isolation precautions: Preventing transmission of infectious agents in healthcare settings" [Online]. Accessed March 2015 via the Web at http://www.cdc.gov/hicpac/pdf/isolation/Isolation2007.pdf (Level II)

17 American Osteopathic Association. (2014). Standard 07.01.10. *Healthcare Facilities Accreditation Program: Accreditation requirements for acute care hospitals.* Chicago, IL: American Osteopathic Association. (Level VII)

18 The Joint Commission. (2015). Standard NPSG.01.01.01. *Comprehensive accreditation manual for hospitals: The official handbook.* Oakbrook Terrace, IL: The Joint Commission. (Level VII)

19 Centers for Medicare & Medicaid Services, Department of Health and Human Services. (2014). Condition of participation: Patient's rights. 42 C.F.R. § 482.13(c)(1).

20 American Osteopathic Association. (2014). Standard 15.01.16. *Healthcare Facilities Accreditation Program: Accreditation requirements for acute care hospitals.* Chicago, IL: American Osteopathic Association. (Level VII)

21 American Society of Anesthesiologists. (2011). Practice guidelines for preoperative fasting and the use of pharmacologic agents to reduce the risk of pulmonary aspiration: Application to healthy patients undergoing elective procedures. *Anesthesiology, 114,* 495–511. (Level VII)

22 The Joint Commission. (2013). "Sentinel event alert: Medical device alarm safety in hospitals" [Online]. Accessed March 2015 via the Web at http://www.jointcommission.org/assets/1/18/SEA_50_alarms_4_5_13_FINAL1.PDF (Level VII)

23 The Joint Commission. (2015). Standard NPSG.06.01.01. *Comprehensive accreditation manual for hospitals: The official handbook.* Oakbrook Terrace, IL: The Joint Commission. (Level VII)

24 Graham, K. C. & Cvach, M. (2010). Monitor alarm fatigue: Standardizing use of physiological monitors and decreasing nuisance alarms. *American Journal of Critical Care, 19,* 28–37.

25 American Association of Critical-Care Nurses. (2013). "AACN practice alert: Alarm management" [Online]. Accessed March 2015 via the Web at http://www.aacn.org/wd/practice/docs/practicealerts/alarm-management-practice-alert.pdf (Level VII)

26 Centers for Medicare & Medicaid Services, Department of Health and Human Services. (2014). Condition of participation: Nursing services. 42 C.F.R. § 482.23(c).

27 American Osteopathic Association. (2014). Standard 16.01.03. *Healthcare Facilities Accreditation Program: Accreditation requirements for acute care hospitals.* Chicago, IL: American Osteopathic Association. (Level VII)

28 The Joint Commission. (2015). Standard UP.01.03.01. *Comprehensive accreditation manual for hospitals: The official handbook.* Oakbrook Terrace, IL: The Joint Commission. (Level VII)

29 McKean, S. C., et al. (Eds.). (2012). *Principles and practice of hospital medicine.* New York, NY: McGraw Hill.

30 The Joint Commission. (2015). Standard PC.01.02.07. *Comprehensive accreditation manual for hospitals: The official handbook.* Oakbrook Terrace, IL: The Joint Commission. (Level VII)

31 Rutala, W. A., et al. (2008). "Guideline for disinfection and sterilization in healthcare facilities, 2008" [Online]. Accessed March 2015 via the Web at http://www.cdc.gov/hicpac/pdf/guidelines/Disinfection_Nov_2008.pdf (Level I)

32 American Osteopathic Association. (2014). Standard 07.02.3. *Healthcare Facilities Accreditation Program: Accreditation requirements for acute care hospitals.* Chicago, IL: American Osteopathic Association. (Level VII)

33 The Joint Commission. (2015). Standard RC.01.03.01. *Comprehensive accreditation manual for hospitals: The official handbook.* Oakbrook Terrace, IL: The Joint Commission. (Level VII)

34 Centers for Medicare & Medicaid Services, Department of Health and Human Services. (2014). Condition of participation: Medical record services. 42 C.F.R. § 482.24(b).

35 American Osteopathic Association. (2014). Standard 10.00.03. *Healthcare Facilities Accreditation Program: Accreditation requirements for acute care hospitals.* Chicago, IL: American Osteopathic Association. (Level VII)

36 ZOLL Medical Corporation. (2010). "Zoll M series operator's guide" [Online]. Accessed March 2015 via the Web at http://www.zoll.com/medical-products/product-manuals/

Elements of a nursing diagnosis

The following summary presents the key elements of a nursing diagnosis.

Human response or problem

After analyzing the patient's condition, choose a diagnostic label from a facility-sanctioned list or create a label specific to the patient. For consistency, most facilities use NANDA-I's list of nursing diagnoses. An example of a diagnostic label is *Excess fluid volume.*

Related factors

The second part of the nursing diagnosis lists factors that seem to influence the patient in a way that pertains to the diagnostic label. Connect these factors to the diagnostic label with the phrase *related to* or the abbreviation *R/T*. The previous example could read, *Excess fluid volume R/T increased sodium intake.*[1]

Defining characteristics

To complete the nursing diagnosis, list defining characteristics, which are signs and symptoms uncovered during assessment that help define the diagnostic label. You may list them beneath the diagnosis and related factors. Or you may add them to the diagnostic statement and connect them with the phrase *as evidenced by* or the abbreviation *AEB*. The example could read, *Excess fluid volume R/T increased sodium intake AEB edema, weight gain over a short period of time, dyspnea on exertion, and S_3 heart sounds.*[1]

ADDITIONAL REFERENCES

Chen, W. S., et al. (2013). Comparison of pharmacological and electrical cardioversion in permanent atrial fibrillation after prosthetic cardiac valve replacement: A prospective randomized trial. *Journal of International Medical Research, 41,* 1067–1073. (Level II)

Hardin, S. R., & Kaplow, R. (2010). *Cardiac surgery essentials for critical care nursing.* Sudbury, MA: Jones & Bartlett.

Knight, B. P. Cardioversion for specific arrhythmias. (2014). In *UpToDate,* Page, R. L. & Downey, B. C. (Eds.). Accessed March 2015 via the Web at http://www.uptodate.com/contents/search

CARE PLAN PREPARATION

A care plan directs the patient's nursing care from admission to discharge. This written action plan is based on nursing diagnoses that have been formulated after reviewing assessment findings, and it embodies the components of the nursing process: assessment, diagnosis, planning, implementation, and evaluation. (See *Elements of a nursing diagnosis.*) The care plan consists of three parts: *goals* or *expected outcomes,* which describe behaviors or results to be achieved within a specified time; appropriate *nursing actions* or *interventions* needed to achieve these goals; and *evaluations of the established goals.*

A nursing care plan should be written for each patient, preferably within 24 hours of admission. It's usually started by the patient's primary nurse or the nurse who admits the patient. If the care plan contains more than one nursing diagnosis, assign priority to each diagnosis and implement those with the highest priority first.[1] Update and revise the plan throughout the patient's stay, based on the patient's response.[2,3] The document becomes part of the permanent patient record.[4]

Some health care facilities use standardized care plans that can be modified to serve many patients. Others use computer programs to facilitate development of nursing care plans.

A nursing care plan serves as a database for planning assignments, giving change-of-shift reports, conferring with the practitioner or other members of the health care team, planning patient discharge, and documenting patient care. In addition, the care plan can be used as a management tool to determine staffing needs and assignments.

Equipment

Nursing care plan form or care plan in electronic format ■ patient's medical record.

Implementation

- Review the patient's medical record, especially the nursing assessment completed on admission. Review diagnostic test results, the medical plan, and other information that may affect patient care. If the patient has just been admitted, complete a nursing history and physical assessment and add it to the patient's record.
- Perform hand hygiene.[5,6,7,8,9]
- Confirm the patient's identity by using at least two patient identifiers.[10]
- Obtain from the patient any additional subjective or objective information needed to complete your assessment.
- Based on an analysis of the data, determine which nursing diagnoses will guide your patient care.[2] Address all of the patient's significant needs when determining nursing diagnoses.
- Work with the patient to identify individualized short-term and long-term goals (expected outcomes) for each nursing diagnosis. Short-term goals can be achieved quickly; long-term goals take more time to achieve and usually involve prevention, patient teaching, and rehabilitation. A correctly written outcome expresses the desired patient behavior, the criteria for measurement, and the appropriate time and conditions under which the behavior will occur. For example, an outcome containing all these elements might read: "By Monday, using crutches, Mary Ballin will be able to walk to the end of the hall and back." *Expected outcomes serve as the basis for evaluating the effectiveness of your nursing interventions.*
- Select interventions that will help the patient achieve the stated outcome for each nursing diagnosis. Include specific information, such as the frequency or particular intervention technique. *Outcomes establish criteria against which you'll judge further nursing actions.* (See *Tips for writing an effective patient care plan,* page 140.)
- Evaluate the patient's progress and revise the care plan as appropriate.[2,3]
- Perform hand hygiene.[5,6,7,8,9]
- Complete documentation of the care plan.[4,11,12,13]

Special considerations

- If you don't have an electronic medical record, fill out the nursing care plan in ink *because the document is part of the permanent medical record.* If you must revise your plan as the patient's condition changes, fill out a new care plan and add it to the medical record.
- Sign and date the care plan whenever you make new entries *to keep the plan current and to maintain accountability for planning the patient's care.*
- Customize a standardized care plan *to avoid "standardizing" the patient's care and to allow you to address the patient's individual concerns.*
- Long-term goals may not be met during hospitalization, so your planning should address postdischarge and home care needs. Interventions may include coordinating home care services.
- The nursing care plan may be a part of a multidisciplinary plan of care, such as a critical pathway. Critical pathways address standardized desired outcomes of care for a specific treatment or diagnosis.

Tips for writing an effective patient care plan

How do you write a care plan that's realistic, accurate, and helpful? Here are some guidelines.

Be systematic

Avoid setting an initial outcome that's impossible to achieve. For example, suppose the outcome for a newly admitted patient with a stroke was "Patient will ambulate without assistance." Although this outcome is certainly appropriate in the long term, several short-term outcomes such as "Patient maintains joint range-of-motion" need to be achieved first.

Be realistic

The nursing intervention should match staff resources and capabilities. For example, "Passive range-of-motion exercises to all extremities every 2 hours" may not be reasonable given the unit's staffing pattern and care requirements. The goals you set to correct a patient's problem should reflect what is reasonably possible in your setting—for example, "Passive range-of-motion exercises with a.m. care, p.m. care, and once at night."

Be clear

Remember, you'll use goals to evaluate the effectiveness of the care plan, so it's important to express them clearly.

Be specific

"Give plenty of fluids" doesn't indicate much; the directive is nonspecific. In contrast, an intervention that says "Encourage fluids—1,000 mL/day shift, 1,000 mL/evening shift, 500 mL/night shift" allows another nurse to carry out the intervention with some assurance of having done what you ordered.

Be brief

An intervention that says "Follow turning schedule posted at bedside" is more readable and useful than having the entire schedule written on the nursing plan.

Documentation

Documentation of the patient's progress (or lack of it) is required by The Joint Commission and other regulatory agencies that monitor health care quality.[2] Document all pertinent nursing diagnoses, expected outcomes, nursing interventions, and evaluations of expected outcomes. Write the care plan clearly and concisely so that other members of the health care team can understand it.

References

1 Herdman, T. H. (Ed.). (2012). *NANDA international nursing diagnoses: Definitions and classifications, 2012-2014.* Oxford: Wiley-Blackwell.

2 The Joint Commission. (2015). Standard PC.01.03.01. *Comprehensive accreditation manual for hospitals: The official handbook.* Oakbrook Terrace, IL: The Joint Commission. (Level VII)

3 Centers for Medicare & Medicaid Services, Department of Health and Human Services. (2014). Condition of participation: Nursing services. 42 C.F.R. § 482.23(b)(4).

4 The Joint Commission. (2015). Standard RC.02.01.01. *Comprehensive accreditation manual for hospitals: The official handbook.* Oakbrook Terrace, IL: The Joint Commission. (Level VII)

5 The Joint Commission. (2015). Standard NPSG.07.01.01. *Comprehensive accreditation manual for hospitals: The official handbook.* Oakbrook Terrace, IL: The Joint Commission. (Level VII)

6 World Health Organization. (2009). "WHO guidelines on hand hygiene in health care: First global patient safety challenge, clean care is safer care" [Online]. Accessed March 2015 via the Web at http://whqlibdoc.who.int/publications/2009/9789241597906_eng.pdf (Level IV)

7 Centers for Disease Control and Prevention. (2002). Guideline for hand hygiene in health-care settings: Recommendations of the Healthcare Infection Control Practices Advisory Committee and the HICPAC/SHEA/APIC/IDSA Hand Hygiene Task Force. *MMWR Recommendations and Reports, 51*(RR-16), 1–45. Accessed March 2015 via the Web at http://www.cdc.gov/mmwr/pdf/rr/rr5116.pdf (Level II)

8 Centers for Medicare & Medicaid Services, Department of Health and Human Services. (2014). Condition of participation: Infection control. 42 C.F.R. § 482.42.

9 American Osteopathic Association. (2014). Standard 07.01.21. *Healthcare Facilities Accreditation Program: Accreditation requirements for acute care hospitals.* Chicago, IL: American Osteopathic Association. (Level VII)

10 The Joint Commission. (2015). Standard NPSG.01.01.01. *Comprehensive accreditation manual for hospitals: The official handbook.* Oakbrook Terrace, IL: The Joint Commission. (Level VII)

11 The Joint Commission. (2015). Standard RC.01.03.01. *Comprehensive accreditation manual for hospitals: The official handbook.* Oakbrook Terrace, IL: The Joint Commission. (Level VII)

12 Centers for Medicare & Medicaid Services, Department of Health and Human Services. (2014). Condition of participation: Medical record services. 42 C.F.R. § 482.24.

13 American Osteopathic Association. (2014). Standard 10.00.03. *Healthcare Facilities Accreditation Program: Accreditation requirements for acute care hospitals.* Chicago, IL: American Osteopathic Association. (Level VII)

Additional references

American Nurses Association. (2010). *Nursing: Scope and standards of practice* (2nd ed.). Washington, DC: American Nurses Association.

Carpenito-Moyet, L. J. (2013). *Nursing diagnosis: Application to clinical practice* (14th ed.). Philadelphia, PA: Lippincott Williams & Wilkins.

Clemnow, R. (2006). Care plans as the main focus of nursing handover: Information exchange model. *Journal of Clinical Nursing, 15,* 1463–1465.

CAST APPLICATION

A cast is a hard mold that encases a body part, usually an extremity, to provide immobilization of bones and surrounding tissue. It can be used to treat injuries (including fractures), correct orthopedic conditions (such as deformities), or promote healing after general or plastic surgery, amputation, or nerve and vascular repair. (See *Types of cylindrical casts.*)

Casts may be constructed of cotton-polyester, plaster, fiberglass, or other synthetic materials. Typically a practitioner applies a cast and a nurse prepares the patient and the equipment and assists during the procedure. With special preparation, a nurse or other health care practitioner may apply or change a standard cast, but an orthopedist must reduce and set the fracture.

Contraindications for casting may include the presence of skin disease, peripheral vascular disease, diabetes mellitus, an open or draining wounds, extreme edema, and susceptibility to skin breakdown. These aren't strict contraindications; the practitioner must weigh the potential risks and benefits for each patient.

EQUIPMENT

Types of cylindrical casts

Made of cotton-polyester, fiberglass, plaster, or other synthetic material, casts may be applied almost anywhere on the body—to support a single finger or the entire body. Common casts are shown below.

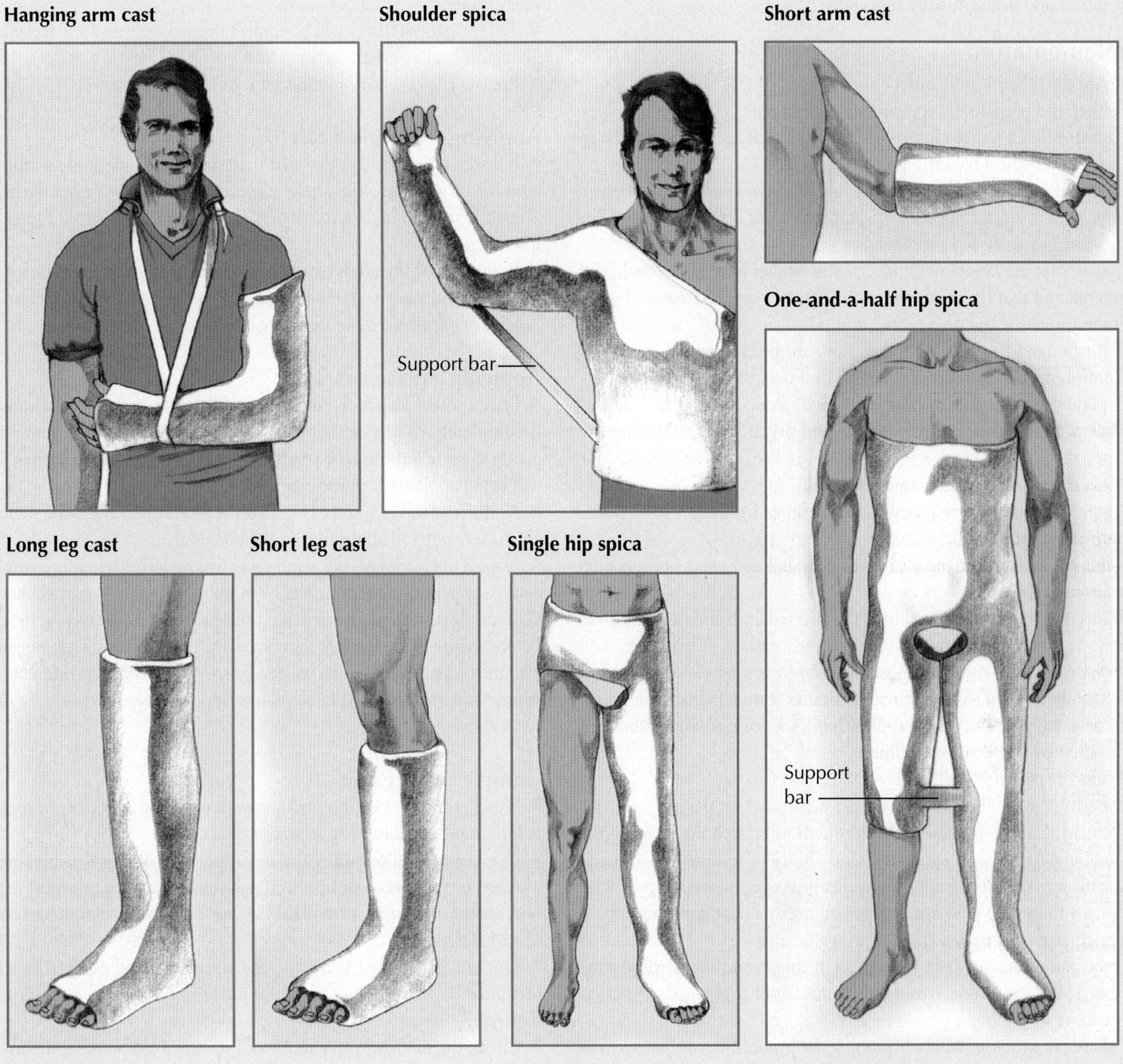

Equipment

Tubular stockinette ▪ casting material ▪ bucket of cold water ▪ sink equipped with a plaster trap ▪ fluid-impermeable pads ▪ cotton undercast padding ▪ two pairs of rubber gloves ▪ prescribed pain medication ▪ thermometer ▪ blood pressure cuff and manometer ▪ stethoscope ▪ disinfectant pad ▪ adhesive tape or moleskin ▪ pillows or a bath blanket ▪ Optional: plaster splints, sponge or felt padding, local anesthetic, suture material, dressing, cast stand, fan.

Preparation of equipment

Gather the tubular stockinette and cast material. Tubular stockinettes range from 2″ to 12″ (5 cm × 30.5 cm) wide; plaster rolls range from 2″ to 6″ (5 cm to 15 cm) wide; and plaster splints range from 3″ to 6″ (7.6 cm to 15 cm) wide. Put on rubber gloves.

For a cotton-polyester or fiberglass cast

Gently squeeze the packaged casting material *to make sure the envelopes don't have any air leaks. Humid air penetrating the packaging can cause the casting material to fail.* To prepare the casting material, follow the manufacturer's directions for the appropriate water temperature to use. Place the equipment so that it's easily accessible during the procedure. Remove and discard your gloves and perform hand hygiene.[1,2,3]

For a plaster cast

Gently squeeze the packaged casting material *to make sure envelopes don't have any air leaks. Humid air leaking into the envelope can cause the plaster to become stale, which could make it set too quickly, form lumps, fail to bond with lower layers, or set as a soft, friable mass.*

Follow the manufacturer's instructions for water temperature when preparing plaster. Using water that's room temperature or slightly warmer is advised *because it allows the cast to set in about 7 minutes without excessive exothermia.* (Cold water retards the rate at which setting occurs and may be used to facilitate molding of difficult casts. Warm water speeds the rate of cast setting and raises the temperature of the skin under the cast.) Place equipment so that it's easily accessible. Remove and discard your gloves and perform hand hygiene.[1,2,3]

Implementation

- Verify the practitioner's order.
- Gather and prepare the appropriate equipment.
- Confirm that a written informed consent has been obtained and is in the patient's medical record.[4,5]
- Conduct a preprocedure verification *to make sure that all relevant documentation, related information, and equipment are available and correctly identified to the patient identifiers.*[6]

Verify that the laboratory and imaging studies have been completed as ordered and that the results are in the patient's medical record. Notify the practitioner of any unexpected results.[6]

- Perform hand hygiene and follow standard precautions.[1,2,3,7]
- Confirm the patient's identity using at least two patient identifiers.[8]
- Explain the procedure *to allay the patient's fears.*
- Make sure that the extremity is clean and dry; if it isn't, clean and dry it.[9]
- Mark the procedure site if indicated.[10]
- Cover the appropriate parts of the patient's bedding with a fluid-impermeable pad.
- Remove jewelry from the limb to be casted. *Jewelry may interfere with circulation to the limb.*
- Assess the condition of the skin of the affected limb and note any areas of abnormal color, ecchymosis, open wounds, rashes, or irritation. *This will make it easier to evaluate any patient complaints after the cast is applied.*
- Assess the patient's baseline neurovascular status. Palpate the pulses and assess temperature, color, capillary refill, motion, sensation, and pain in the affected and unaffected limbs.
- Assess the patient's vital signs.
- Determine when the patient was last medicated for pain.
- Perform a comprehensive pain assessment using techniques appropriate for the patient's age, condition, and ability to understand. Provide medication as ordered using safe medication administration practices. Perform a follow-up pain assessment and notify the practitioner if pain isn't adequately controlled.[11]
- If the patient has an open wound, assist the practitioner with administering a local anesthetic, closing the wound, and applying dressings, as needed.
- Conduct a time-out before beginning the procedure *to perform a final assessment that the correct patient, site, positioning, and procedure are identified and, as applicable, that all relevant information and necessary equipment are available.*[12]
- Perform hand hygiene and put on rubber gloves.[1,2,3,7]
- Help the practitioner position the limb, as ordered. (The limb may be cast in a position of comfort, flexion, or extension.)[9]
- Support the limb in the prescribed position while the practitioner applies the tubular stockinette and cotton undercast padding. The stockinette should extend beyond the ends of the cast *to pad the edges.*[9] (If the patient has an open wound or a severe contusion, the practitioner may not use a stockinette.) Next, the practitioner applies four layers of cotton undercast padding to the limb *to reduce the risk of cast saw burns during cast removal.* The padding should be an appropriate width for the size of the patient, and the practitioner should wrap it from distal to proximal. The practitioner should place extra padding over bony prominences *to prevent skin breakdown.*[9]

Applying a cotton-polyester cast

- Open the casting materials one roll at a time *because cotton and polyester casting must be applied within 3 minutes. Humidity in the air hardens the tape.*
- Immerse the roll in cold water, and squeeze it four times *to ensure uniform saturation.*
- Remove the material from the bucket dripping wet and hand it to the practitioner.
- Tell the patient that it will be applied immediately and will feel warm, giving off heat as it sets.
- Prepare the necessary number of rolls in similar fashion.

Applying a fiberglass cast

- If water-activated fiberglass cast material is being used, use a minimal amount of water *to initiate the chemical reaction that causes the cast to harden. Using too much water makes the cast difficult to apply.* Open one roll at a time.
- If light-cured fiberglass cast material is being used, you can unroll the material more slowly. *This material remains soft and malleable until it's exposed to ultraviolet light, which sets it.*

Applying a plaster cast

- Place a roll of plaster casting on its end in the bucket of water. Immerse it completely. When air bubbles stop rising from the roll, remove it, gently squeeze out the excess water, and hand it to the practitioner, who will begin applying it to the extremity.
- As the first roll is applied, prepare a second roll in the same manner. Try to stay one roll ahead during the procedure.
- As each roll is applied, the practitioner will smooth it to remove wrinkles and to spread the plaster into the cloth webbing, emptying air pockets. If plaster splints are used, they will be applied to the middle layers of the cast. Before wrapping the last roll, the ends of the tubular stockinette are pulled over the cast edges to create a padded end. *This prevents cast crumbling and reduces skin irritation.* The final roll is wrapped *to keep the ends of the stockinette in place.*

Completing the cast

- "Petal" the edges of the cast *to reduce roughness and cushion pressure points, as needed.* (See *How to petal a cast.*)
- Use a cast stand or your palm to support the cast in the therapeutic position until it becomes firm to touch (usually within minutes) *to prevent indentation in the cast.* Place the cast on a firm, smooth surface to continue drying.[9]
- Promote drying by leaving the cast uncovered and exposed to air; if permitted by your facility, fans can be used *to increase airflow, which speeds the drying process.*[9]
- Check the neurovascular status of the casted limb and compare the findings bilaterally. Palpate the patient's pulses and assess the color, temperature, capillary refill, motion, and sensation of the limbs bilaterally.
- *To facilitate venous return and reduce edema,* elevate the limb above the level of the heart using pillows or bath blankets.
- Arrange for an X-ray of the limb *to ensure proper positioning,* if ordered.
- Remove and discard your gloves and perform hand hygiene.[1,2,3]
- Clean and disinfect your stethoscope with a disinfectant pad.[13]
- Perform hand hygiene.[1,2,3]
- Document the procedure.[14,15]

Special considerations

- A cotton-polyester cast dries soon after application. During this drying period, the cast must be properly positioned *to prevent a surface depression that could cause pressure areas or dependent edema.* Assess the patient's neurovascular status, monitor drainage, and check the condition of the cast periodically.

- After the cast dries completely, it looks shiny and no longer feels damp or soft. Monitor any drainage, prevent skin breakdown near the cast, and prevent complications due to immobility.
- Patient teaching must begin immediately after the cast is applied and should continue until the patient or caregiver can effectively care for the cast.
- Never use the bed or table to support the cast as it sets *because molding can occur and cause pressure necrosis in the underlying tissue.*
- If a cast is applied after surgery or traumatic injury, remember that the most accurate way to assess for excessive bleeding is to monitor vital signs. *You can't use the amount of blood that you see on the cast as a way of telling if the patient is bleeding. A visible spot of blood on the cast can be misleading: one drop of blood can produce a circle 3″ (7.6 cm) in diameter.*
- Casts may need to be opened to assess underlying skin or pulses or to relieve pressure in a specific area. In a windowed cast, a specific area is cut out *to allow inspection of the underlying skin or relieve pressure.* A bivalved cast is split medially and laterally, creating anterior and posterior sections. One of the sections may be removed to prevent pressure while the remaining section maintains the immobilization.
- The practitioner usually removes the cast with the assistance of a nurse. (See the "Cast removal" procedure, page 144.) Tell the patient that when the cast is removed, his casted limb will appear thinner with less muscle tone than his contralateral limb. His skin will also appear yellow or gray in color from the accumulated dead skin and oils from glands near the skin surface. Reassure the patient that with good care and exercise his limb will return to normal.

Patient teaching

Sometime before discharge, teach the patient how to care for his cast. Tell him to keep the casted limb elevated for the first 24 to 72 hours above the level of his heart *to minimize swelling.*[16] If his leg is casted, he can keep it elevated by lying supine with his leg on top of pillows. If his arm is casted, he should keep his hand and elbow higher than his shoulder. In addition, tell him to place ice in a dry plastic bag and then wrap it loosely around the cast at the injury site.[16]

Instruct the patient to call the practitioner if he can't move his fingers or toes; if he has numbness or tingling in the casted limb; if he has increased pain, burning, stinging or a feeling that the cast is too tight; or if he has swelling below the cast.[16] Advise him to maintain muscle strength by continuing any recommended exercises. If he has signs and symptoms of infection (such as fever, unusual pain, or a foul odor from the cast), if he has any questions about his cast care, or if the cast loosens, cracks, or breaks, advise him to call his practitioner.

Tell the patient to keep the cast dry. *Moisture can weaken or destroy it.* If the practitioner approves, the patient may cover his cast with a plastic bag or waterproof cast cover for showering or bathing.[9]

Urge the patient not to insert anything (such as an object or powder) into the cast to relieve itching. *Foreign matter can damage the skin and cause infection.* Tell him to tap a pen on the outside of the cast instead or use a hair dryer on a cool setting to blow cool air into the cast.[9] Warn him not to damage any area of the cast or bear weight on it unless his practitioner approves.

If the patient must use crutches, instruct him to remove throw rugs and other obstacles from his environment *to reduce his risk of falling.* If the patient's cast is on his dominant arm, he may need help performing activities of daily living.

Complications

The complications associated with improper cast application include compartment syndrome, palsy, paresthesia, ischemia, ischemic myositis, pressure necrosis, deep vein thrombosis, and misalignment or nonunion of the fracture.

How to petal a cast

Rough cast edges can be cushioned by petaling them with adhesive tape or moleskin. To do so, first cut several 4″ × 2″ (10- × 5-cm) strips. Round off one end of each strip *to keep it from curling.* Then, making sure the rounded end of the strip is on the outside of the cast, tuck the straight end just inside the cast edge.

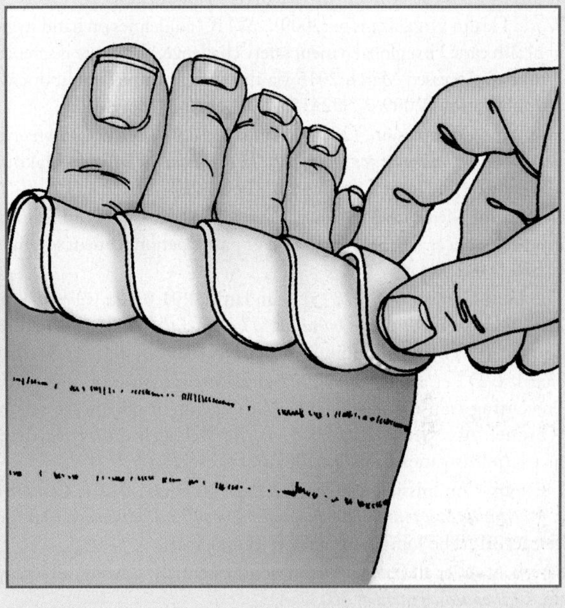

Smooth the moleskin with your finger until you're sure it's secured inside and out. Repeat the procedure, overlapping the moleskin pieces until you've gone all the way around the cast edge.

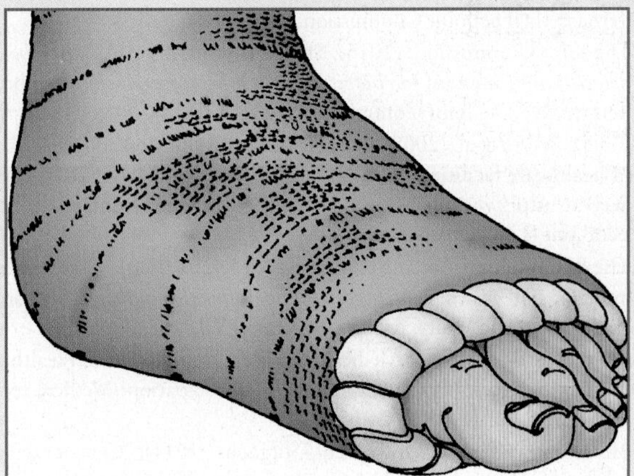

Documentation

Record the date and time of the cast application and assessment of the limb, both before and after the cast was applied. Note any open wounds or abnormal skin. Record neurovascular assessments before and after cast application, and compare them with assessments of the unaffected limb. Note the location of any special devices, such as felt pads or plaster splints. Document any teaching performed.

REFERENCES

1 The Joint Commission. (2015). Standard NPSG.07.01.01. *Comprehensive accreditation manual for hospitals: The official handbook.* Oakbrook Terrace, IL: The Joint Commission. (Level VII)

2 Centers for Disease Control and Prevention. (2002). Guideline for hand hygiene in health-care settings: Recommendations of the Healthcare Infection Control Practices Advisory Committee and the HICPAC/SHEA/APIC/IDSA Hand Hygiene Task Force. *MMWR Recommendations and Reports, 51*(RR-16), 1–45. Accessed March 2015 via the Web at http://www.cdc.gov/mmwr/pdf/rr/rr5116.pdf (Level II)

3 World Health Organization. (2009). "WHO guidelines on hand hygiene in health care: First global patient safety challenge, clean care is safer care" [Online]. Accessed March 2015 via the Web at http://whqlibdoc.who.int/publications/2009/9789241597906_eng.pdf (Level IV)

4 The Joint Commission. (2015). Standard RI.01.03.01. *Comprehensive accreditation manual for hospitals: The official handbook.* Oakbrook Terrace, IL: The Joint Commission. (Level VII)

5 Centers for Medicare & Medicaid Services, Department of Health and Human Services. (2014). Condition of participation: Patient's rights. 42 C.F.R. § 482.13.

6 The Joint Commission. (2015). Standard UP.01.01.01. *Comprehensive accreditation manual for hospitals: The official handbook.* Oakbrook Terrace, IL: The Joint Commission. (Level VII)

7 Siegel, J. D., et al. (2007). "2007 guideline for isolation precautions: Preventing transmission of infectious agents in healthcare settings" [Online]. Accessed March 2015 via the Web at http://www.cdc.gov/hicpac/pdf/isolation/Isolation2007.pdf (Level II)

8 The Joint Commission. (2015). Standard NPSG.01.01.01. *Comprehensive accreditation manual for hospitals: The official handbook.* Oakbrook Terrace, IL: The Joint Commission. (Level VII)

9 Satryb, S. A., et al. (2011). Orthopaedic essentials: Casting, all wrapped up. *Orthopaedic Nursing, 30,* 37–41.

10 The Joint Commission. (2015). Standard UP.01.02.01. *Comprehensive accreditation manual for hospitals: The official handbook.* Oakbrook Terrace, IL: The Joint Commission. (Level VII)

11 The Joint Commission. (2015). Standard PC.01.02.07. *Comprehensive accreditation manual for hospitals: The official handbook.* Oakbrook Terrace, IL: The Joint Commission. (Level VII)

12 The Joint Commission. (2015). Standard UP.01.03.01. *Comprehensive accreditation manual for hospitals: The official handbook.* Oakbrook Terrace, IL: The Joint Commission. (Level VII)

13 Rutala, W. A., et al. (2008). "Guideline for disinfection and sterilization in healthcare facilities, 2008" [Online]. Accessed March 2015 via the Web at http://www.cdc.gov/hicpac/pdf/guidelines/Disinfection_Nov_2008.pdf (Level I)

14 The Joint Commission. (2015). Standard RC.01.03.01. *Comprehensive accreditation manual for hospitals: The official handbook.* Oakbrook Terrace, IL: The Joint Commission. (Level VII)

15 Centers for Medicare & Medicaid Services, Department of Health and Human Services. (2014). Condition of participation: Medical record services. 42 C.F.R. § 482.24(b).

16 American Academy of Orthopaedic Surgeons. (2011). "Care of casts and splints" [Online]. Accessed March 2015 via the Web at http://orthoinfo.aaos.org/topic.cfm?topic=A00095

17 Rasul, A. T. (2013). "Acute compartment syndrome" [Online]. Accessed March 2015 via the Web at http://emedicine.medscape.com/article/307668-overview#aw2aab6b2b6

ADDITIONAL REFERENCE

Nettina, S. M. (2014). *Lippincott manual of nursing practice* (10th ed.). Philadelphia, PA: Wolters Kluwer.

CAST REMOVAL

Typically, a cast is removed when a fracture heals or requires further manipulation. Less common indications include cast damage, a pressure ulcer under the cast, excessive drainage or bleeding, and a constrictive cast.

Equipment

Cast spreader ■ cast saw with vacuum attachment ■ cast scissors ■ washcloth ■ towel ■ soap and water ■ Optional: hearing protection, gloves, goggles, masks.

Preparation of equipment

The cast saw may be loud enough to require the use of hearing protection for the patient and staff members present during the cast removal, according to Occupational Safety and Health Administration (OSHA) standards.[1] Follow the manufacturer's directions for use.

Implementation

- Verify the practitioner's order.
- Gather the equipment.
- Perform hand hygiene.[2,3,4]
- Confirm the patient's identity using at least two patient identifiers.[5]
- Explain the procedure to the patient. Explain that the cast saw uses an oscillating blade that won't cut the skin.[6] Tell him that he will feel some heat and vibration when the cast is split with the cast saw[7] and instruct him to report any discomfort or excessive heat during the procedure. Emphasize that he must remain still.
- Have the staff and the patient put on hearing-protective equipment and goggles, masks, and gloves, if needed.[8]
- Monitor that patient's anxiety level as the cast is removed.
- Assist the practitioner as needed when the cast is removed. First, one side of the cast is cut and then the other (as shown below). The cast is then opened with a spreader. Cast scissors are used to cut through the cast padding.
- Support the extremity and examine the skin.[6]

Gently wash and dry the skin that was under the cast *to remove the accumulated dead skin.*

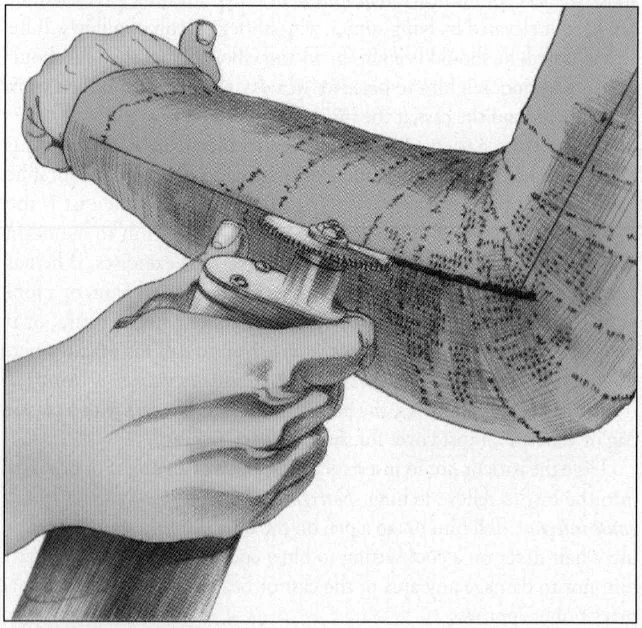

- Remove and discard your personal protective equipment, if worn, and perform hand hygiene.[2,3,4]
- Document the procedure.[9,10]

Special considerations

If the cast saw doesn't have a vacuum attachment to dispose of the cast dust during removal, the staff and patient should wear masks and eye protection during the procedure *to prevent inhalation of particulate cast material.*

Patient teaching

Explain to the patient that when the padding is cut, he will see discolored skin and signs of poor muscle tone. Tell him to avoid rubbing or scratching the skin *because doing so can damage the newly exposed skin.*[6] Teach him how to perform skin care after the cast is removed.

Complications

The practitioner may accidentally injure the patient's skin with the cast saw, scissors, or spreader.

Documentation

Assess the neurovascular integrity of the limb before cast removal. Document the date and time of removal and the patient's tolerance of the procedure. Note the neurovascular assessment and condition of the patient's skin after the cast is removed. Note any complications from the procedure and nursing actions taken.

REFERENCES

1 Occupational Safety and Health Administration. (2008). "Occupational noise exposure standard 1910.95" [Online]. Accessed March 2015 via the Web at https://www.osha.gov/pls/oshaweb/owadisp.show_document?p_table=standards&p_id=9735
2 The Joint Commission. (2015). Standard NPSG.07.01.01. *Comprehensive accreditation manual for hospitals: The official handbook.* Oakbrook Terrace, IL: The Joint Commission. (Level VII)
3 Centers for Disease Control and Prevention. (2002). Guideline for hand hygiene in health-care settings: Recommendations of the Healthcare Infection Control Practices Advisory Committee and the HICPAC/SHEA/APIC/IDSA Hand Hygiene Task Force. *MMWR Recommendations and Reports, 51*(RR-16), 1–45. Accessed March 2015 via the Web at http://www.cdc.gov/mmwr/pdf/rr/rr5116.pdf (Level II)
4 World Health Organization. (2009). "WHO guidelines on hand hygiene in health care: First global patient safety challenge, clean care is safer care" [Online]. Accessed March 2015 via the Web at http://whqlibdoc.who.int/publications/2009/9789241597906_eng.pdf (Level IV)
5 The Joint Commission. (2015). Standard NPSG.01.01.01. *Comprehensive accreditation manual for hospitals: The official handbook.* Oakbrook Terrace, IL: The Joint Commission. (Level VII)
6 Satryb, S. A., et al. (2011). Orthopaedic essentials: Casting, all wrapped up. Orthopaedic Nursing, 30, 37–41.
7 American Academy of Orthopaedic Surgeons. (2011). "Care of casts and splints" [Online]. Accessed March 2015 via the Web at http://orthoinfo.aaos.org/topic.cfm?topic=A00095
8 Siegel, J. D., et al. "2007 guideline for isolation precautions: Preventing transmission of infectious agents in healthcare settings" [Online]. Accessed March 2015 via the Web at http://www.cdc.gov/hicpac/pdf/isolation/Isolation2007.pdf (Level II)
9 The Joint Commission. (2015). Standard RC.01.03.01. *Comprehensive accreditation manual for hospitals: The official handbook.* Oakbrook Terrace, IL: The Joint Commission. (Level VII)
10 Centers for Medicare & Medicaid Services, Department of Health and Human Services. (2014). Condition of participation: Medical record services. 42 C.F.R. § 482.24(b).

ADDITIONAL REFERENCE

Nettina, S. M. (2014). *Lippincott manual of nursing practice* (10th ed.). Philadelphia, PA: Wolters Kluwer.

CENTRAL VENOUS ACCESS CATHETER

A central venous access catheter is a sterile catheter that's inserted through a large vein, such as the subclavian or internal jugular vein, to provide access to the central veins. The catheter is made of polyurethane or silicone rubber. Catheters impregnated with antiseptics (such as chlorhexidine) and antimicrobials (such as silver, carbon, platinum, minocycline, and rifampin) are recommended for patients whose catheter is expected to remain in place for longer than 5 days to reduce the risk for vascular catheter–associated infection.[1] Power injectable catheters are also available to enable power injection of contrast media in patients who require computed tomography and other testing. A practitioner inserts a central venous catheter through a large vein, such as the subclavian or jugular vein, and places the tip of the catheter in the superior vena cava. (See *Central venous access catheter pathways.*)

By providing access to the central veins, central venous therapy offers several benefits. It allows monitoring of central venous pressure, which indicates blood volume or pump efficiency, and permits aspiration of blood samples for diagnostic tests. It also allows for the administration of IV fluids (in large amounts if necessary) in emergencies, when decreased peripheral circulation makes peripheral vein access difficult, when prolonged IV therapy reduces the number of accessible peripheral

Central venous access catheter pathways

The illustrations below show two common pathways for central venous access catheter insertion. Typically, a central venous access catheter is inserted in the subclavian vein or the internal jugular vein. The catheter typically terminates in the superior vena cava. The subclavian site is preferred over the internal jugular site in adults to reduce the risk of infection;[1,6] however, in patients with advanced kidney disease and in those receiving hemodialysis, the subclavian site should be avoided to prevent subclavian vein stenosis.[1]

Insertion: Subclavian vein
Termination: Superior vena cava

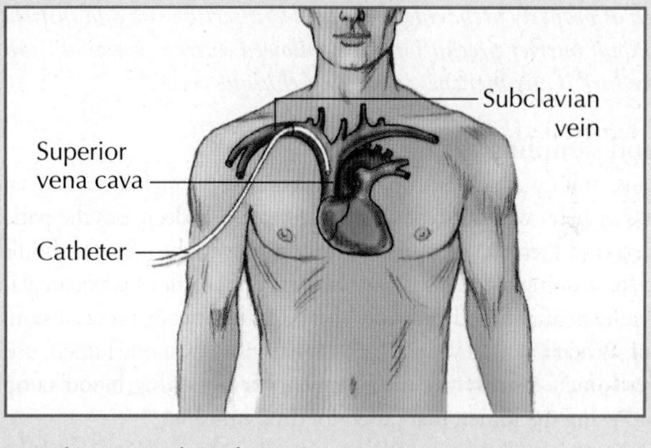

Insertion: Internal jugular vein
Termination: Superior vena cava

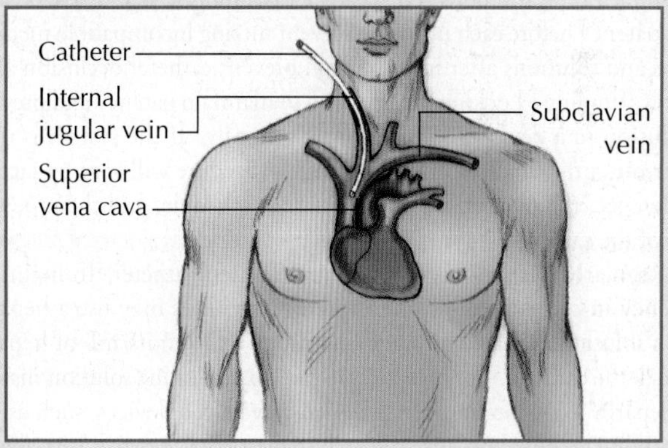

veins, when solutions must be diluted (for large fluid volumes or irritating or hypertonic fluids such as total parenteral nutrition solutions), and when a patient requires long-term venous access. Because multiple blood samples can be drawn through it without repeated venipuncture, a central venous access catheter decreases the patient's anxiety and preserves peripheral veins.

Central venous therapy increases the risk of complications, such as pneumothorax, vascular catheter–associated infection, sepsis, thrombus formation, and vessel and adjacent organ perforation (all life-threatening conditions). Because of age-related changes in the immune system, older adults are more susceptible to infection than are younger adults. Remote infections may also increase the risk of vascular catheter–associated bloodstream infection in older adults.[2]

HOSPITAL-ACQUIRED CONDITION ALERT *Keep in mind that a vascular catheter–associated infection is considered a hospital-acquired condition because it can be reasonably prevented using a variety of best practices. Make sure that infection-prevention techniques (such as properly preparing the intended insertion site and instituting maximal barrier precautions) are followed during insertion; stop the procedure if any breaches in sterile technique occur.*[3,4,5]

Blood sampling

Because multiple blood samples can be drawn through a central venous access catheter without repeated venipuncture, it decreases the patient's anxiety and preserves peripheral veins. However, the catheter should be used for drawing blood only when necessary. If you don't adequately flush the catheter after blood withdrawal, a thrombotic catheter occlusion can occur. When a central venous catheter has more than one lumen, use the larger lumen, usually the distal lumen, for obtaining blood samples. Avoid using the lumen that's used for drug infusion.

Flushing and locking

Flushing a central venous access catheter is a routine step to assess catheter patency before each infusion, prevent mixing incompatible medications and solutions after infusion, and prevent catheter occlusion after blood sampling.[7] Locking is performed to maintain patency and prevent occlusion in a device that's used intermittently.[7] If the system is used intermittently, the flushing and locking procedure will vary by facility preference, the medication administration schedule, and the type and size of the catheter.

Regularly flush all lumens of a multilumen catheter. To maintain patency in catheters used intermittently, facilities may use a heparin flush solution available in prefilled syringes of 10 units/mL of heparin to lock the catheter. Use preservative-free normal saline solution instead of heparin to maintain patency in two-way valved devices, such as the Groshong catheter, because research suggests that heparin isn't always needed to maintain patency.

The recommended frequency for flushing and locking central venous access catheters varies. When no therapy is being infused, follow these guidelines:

- Flush nontunneled, nonvalved catheters at least every 24 hours. If required by your facility, you may also heparin lock the catheter with 5 mL of 10 units/mL heparin.[7,8]
- Flush nontunneled, valved catheters at least weekly. If required by your facility, you may also heparin lock the catheter with 5 mL of 10 units/mL heparin.[7,8]
- Flush tunneled, nonvalved catheters at least weekly. If required by your facility, you may also heparin lock the catheter with 5 mL of 10 units/mL heparin.[7,8]
- Flush tunneled, valved catheters at least weekly. If required by your facility, you may also heparin lock the catheter with 5 mL of 10 units/mL heparin.[7,8]

The flushing volume should be at least twice the internal volume of the central venous access catheter; a larger volume may be necessary if the catheter was used for blood sampling or transfusion. The syringe size used for flushing varies according to the catheter manufacturer's instructions, although most manufacturers require a minimum of a 10-mL syringe.[6]

Changing the dressing

Despite the various designs and applications of central venous access devices, certain aspects of dressing changes apply to all device types. The sterility and integrity of the device must be maintained at all times to reduce the risk of vascular catheter–associated infection.

Transparent semipermeable dressings should be changed at least every 7 days, and gauze dressings should be changed every 2 days.[9,10] Either dressing should be changed immediately if the dressing becomes damp, loosened, or visibly soiled.[1,9,11]

Removing a central venous access catheter

Removal of a central venous access catheter requires sterile technique and is usually performed by a practitioner or nurse, either at the end of therapy or at the onset of complications. Check with your facility and your state's nurse practice act to determine whether removing a catheter is in your scope of practice.

If the central venous access catheter was inserted in an emergency situation, remove it as soon as possible, but not longer than 48 hours after insertion.[12] Assess catheter necessity daily during multidisciplinary rounds, and remove the catheter as soon as it's no longer needed; *this reduces the risk of central line–related bloodstream infection.*[1,11,12,13,14,15] Consider the patient's condition and therapy, catheter position, and catheter function when deciding whether to remove the catheter. If you suspect or confirm a central line–related bloodstream infection, base the decision to remove or salvage the catheter on blood culture results, the patient's condition, available vascular access sites, the effectiveness of antimicrobial therapy, and the practitioner's direction.[12]

Equipment

For insertion of a central venous access catheter

Facility-approved disinfectant ▪ insertion checklist ▪ sterile gloves ▪ sterile gowns ▪ caps ▪ masks ▪ blanket ▪ fluid-impermeable pad ▪ large sterile drape ▪ antiseptic solution (chlorhexidine-based preferred; tincture of iodine, povidone-iodine, or alcohol if chlorhexidine is contraindicated) ▪ alcohol pads ▪ preservative-free normal saline solution flushes ▪ ultrasound device with sterile probe cover ▪ sterile ultrasound gel ▪ 3-mL syringe with 25G 1" (2.5-cm) needle ▪ 1% or 2% injectable lidocaine ▪ catheter securement device or suture material and suture kit (sterile scissors, hemostat, and needle holder) ▪ two central venous access catheters (antimicrobial impregnated, if indicated) ▪ sterile needleless connectors ▪ IV solution with administration set ▪ infusion pump (preferably a smart pump with dose-range alerts) ▪ sterile marker ▪ sterile labels ▪ sterile transparent semipermeable dressing ▪ sign ▪ Optional: skin preparation kit, cardiac monitor, pulse oximeter, sterile towel, antiseptic soap.

The type of catheter selected depends on the type of therapy to be used. (See *Guide to central venous access catheters.*)

Use an all-inclusive insertion kit or cart that contains all of the necessary components for maintaining sterile technique during catheter insertion *to reduce the risk of catheter-related bloodstream infection.*[1,11,12,13,14,15]

For blood sampling from a central venous access catheter

Gloves ▪ 10-mL prefilled syringes of preservative-free normal saline solution ▪ antiseptic pads (alcohol, tincture of iodine, or chlorhexidine-based) ▪ appropriate-size syringes or needleless blood collection tube holder ▪ blood collection tubes ▪ labels ▪ laboratory request forms ▪ laboratory biohazard transport bag ▪ Optional: prefilled syringe containing locking

EQUIPMENT

Guide to central venous access catheters

TYPE	DESCRIPTION	INDICATIONS	ADVANTAGES AND DISADVANTAGES	NURSING CONSIDERATIONS
Short-term single-lumen catheter	■ Polyurethane or silicone rubber ■ About 8″ (20.5 cm) long ■ Lumen gauge varies ■ Percutaneously placed 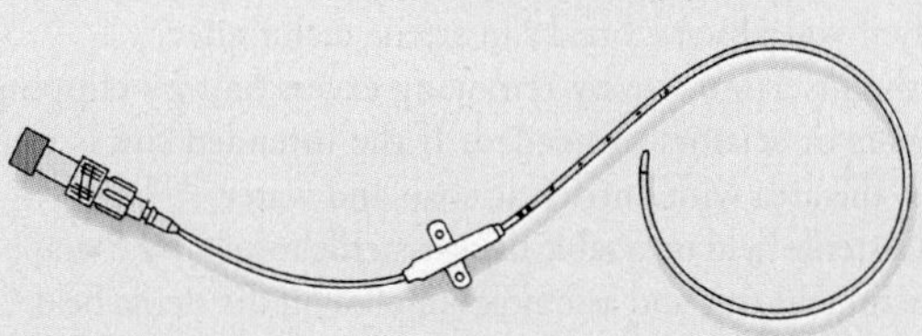	■ Short-term central venous access ■ Emergency access ■ Patient who needs only one lumen	***Advantages*** ■ Easily inserted at bedside ■ Easily removed ■ Stiffness aids central venous pressure monitoring ***Disadvantages*** ■ Limited functions	■ Assess frequently for signs of infection and catheter patency.
Short-term multilumen catheter	■ Polyurethane or silicone rubber ■ Two, three, or four lumens exiting at ¾″ (2-cm) intervals ■ Lumen gauges vary ■ Percutaneously placed 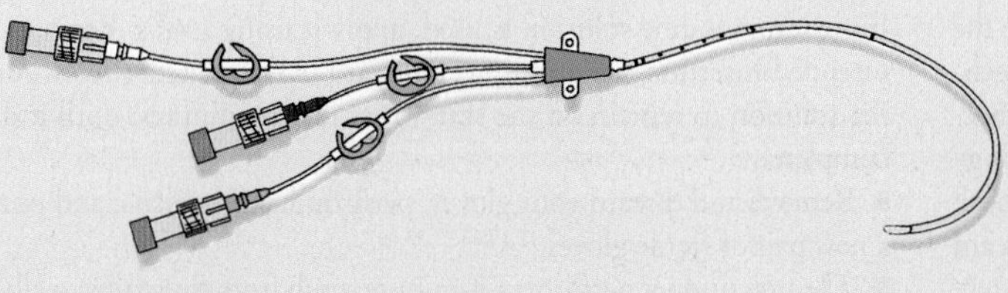	■ Short-term central venous access ■ Patient with limited insertion sites who requires multiple infusions	***Advantages*** ■ Easily inserted at bedside ■ Easily removed ■ Stiffness aids central venous pressure monitoring ■ Allows infusion of multiple (even incompatible) solutions through the same catheter ***Disadvantages*** ■ Limited functions	■ Know gauge and purpose of each lumen. ■ During dressing changes, assess the external length of the catheter *to detect catheter migration.*
Short-term power-injector catheter	■ Polyurethane or similar materials ■ One, two, or three lumens ■ Lumen gauges vary ■ Percutaneously placed 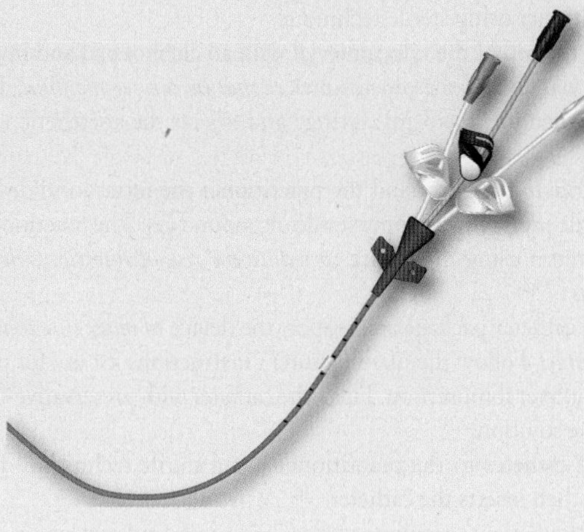	■ Short-term central venous access ■ Patient who requires contrast media for testing ■ Patient with limited insertion sites who requires IV fluids, blood products, parenteral nutrition, blood withdrawal, or central venous pressure monitoring	***Advantages*** ■ Allows power injection of contrast media ■ Easily inserted at bedside ■ Easily removed ***Disadvantages*** ■ None	■ Don't use a syringe smaller than 10 mL to flush the device. ■ During dressing changes, assess the external length of the catheter *to detect catheter migration.*

solution, mask with face shield or mask and goggles, blood transfer unit, needleless connector.

For flushing and locking a central venous access catheter

Gloves ■ prefilled 10-mL syringe with preservative-free normal saline solution ■ antiseptic pads (alcohol, tincture of iodine, or chlorhexidine-based) ■ Optional: prefilled syringe with heparin lock solution.

For changing the dressing on a central venous access catheter

Antiseptic solution (chlorhexidine preferred;[9] tincture of iodine, povidone-iodine, or alcohol if the patient is sensitive to chlorhexidine) ■ sterile transparent semipermeable dressing or sterile 4″ × 4″ (10-cm × 10-cm) gauze pads ■ skin preparation solution (as needed to facilitate dressing adherence) ■ catheter securement device, sterile tape, or adhesive strips ■ gloves ■ mask ■ label ■ sterile disposable tape measure ■ Optional: chlorhexidine-impregnated sponge dressing, adhesive remover, dressings and tape specially formulated for fragile skin.

Commercially prepared central venous access device dressing change kits that include most of the equipment needed are available and are recommended.[2,10]

For changing a needleless connector on a central venous access catheter

Gloves ▪ antiseptic pads (alcohol, tincture of iodine, chlorhexidine-based) ▪ sterile needleless connector ▪ prefilled syringe containing preservative-free normal saline solution ▪ Optional: padded clamp.

For removing a central venous access catheter

Gloves ▪ sterile suture removal set ▪ sterile 2″ × 2″ (5-cm × 5-cm) gauze pads ▪ tape (paper or silicone tape for frail skin)[16] ▪ sterile transparent semipermeable dressing ▪ petroleum-based ointment ▪ equipment for monitoring vital signs ▪ Optional: labeled specimen container; protective eyewear; adhesive remover; sterile scissors and forceps; hemostatic pad, patch, or powder

Preparation of equipment

Gather all necessary equipment. Before insertion of a central venous access catheter, confirm catheter type and size with the practitioner; usually, a 14G or 16G catheter is selected. Set up equipment for insertion, dressing change, and line removal, using strict sterile technique. Perform hand hygiene *to prevent the spread of microorganisms.*[1,17,18,19,20,21,22,23] Set up the IV solution and prime the administration set using strict sterile technique.[21] Attach the tubing to the infusion pump, and recheck all connections *to make sure they're tight.*[24] As ordered, notify the radiology department that a chest X-ray will be needed *to confirm placement.* Check all expiration dates, and inspect packages for any tears. Label the discard blood collection tube or the discard syringe *to prevent confusing it with the actual specimen.*

Implementation

For all procedures

- Gather the appropriate equipment.
- Confirm the patient's identity using at least two patient identifiers.[25]
- Explain the procedure to the patient.

Assisting with inserting a central venous access catheter

- Verify the practitioner's order.
- Confirm that written informed consent has been obtained, if necessary, and that the consent form is in the patient's medical record.[25,26,27]
- Check the patient's history for hypersensitivity to latex or to the local anesthetic.
- Conduct a preprocedure verification *to make sure that all relevant documentation, related information, and equipment are available and correctly identified to the patient's identifiers.*[28,29]
- Confirm the patient's identify using at least two patient identifiers.[30]
- Provide the patient with information that addresses the rationale for device insertion, the insertion process, expected dwell time, care and maintenance of the device, and signs and symptoms of complications that should be reported.[31]
- Close the door to the room and place a sign on the door that reads "Sterile Procedure in Progress—Do Not Enter."[2,10]
- Attach the patient to a cardiac monitor and pulse oximeter, if available. Make sure that the alarm limits are set appropriately for the patient's current condition and that the alarms are turned on, functioning properly, and audible to staff.[32,33,34,35]
- Put on a cap and mask.[2,10]
- Perform hand hygiene.[1,17,18,19,20,21,22,23]
- Disinfect the work area (such as an overbed table) with a facility-approved disinfectant, and then allow it to dry completely.[2,10]
- Elevate the bed to a comfortable working level *to avoid back strain.*
- Place the patient in the Trendelenburg position *to dilate the veins and to reduce the risk of air embolism.*
- For subclavian vein insertion, place a rolled blanket lengthwise between the patient's shoulders *to increase venous distention.* For jugular vein insertion, place a rolled blanket under the opposite shoulder *to extend the patient's neck, making anatomic landmarks more visible.* Place a fluid-impermeable pad under the patient *to prevent the bed from being soiled.*
- Use an insertion checklist *to help comply with infection prevention and safety practices during insertion.*[1,11,13,14,15] Stop the procedure immediately if you observe breaks in sterile technique.[7]
- Prepare the insertion site by removing excess hair by clipping it with a clippers or scissors, if needed. If the intended site is visibly soiled, clean the area with antiseptic soap and water.[2,10,31]
- Establish a sterile field on a table using a sterile towel or the wrapping from the instrument tray and assemble supplies on the sterile field.[2,10]
- Label all medications, medication containers, and other solutions on and off the sterile field.[36,37]
- Perform hand hygiene.[1,17,18,19,20,21,22,23]
- Put on a sterile gown and sterile gloves *to comply with maximal barrier precautions.*[1,38,39]
- Prepare the insertion site with a chlorhexidine sponge[1,6,15,31] using a vigorous side-to-side motion for 30 seconds; allow the area to air-dry.[1,10] If povidone-iodine solution is used, apply it using swabs. Begin at the intended insertion site and move outward in concentric circles. Allow the solution to remain on the skin for at least 2 minutes, until it dries completely.[2,10]
- Remove and discard your gloves, perform hand hygiene, and put on a new pair of sterile gloves.[17,19,20,23,38,39]
- The practitioner performs a 3-minute scrub from fingertips to elbows and then puts on a cap, a mask, a sterile gown, and sterile gloves.[2,10]
- He drapes the patient with a large, full-body sterile drape *to create a sterile field and to comply with maximal barrier precautions.*[1,15]
- Conduct a time-out before beginning the procedure *to verify the correct patient, procedure, and positioning.*[40]
- Open the packaging of the 3-mL syringe and 25G needle and hand it to the practitioner using sterile technique.
- Disinfect the top of the lidocaine vial with an alcohol pad and invert it. Turn the vial toward the practitioner *so that he can see the fluid.* The practitioner then fills the 3-mL syringe and injects the anesthetic into the site.
- Using sterile technique, hand the practitioner the ultrasound device with the sterile probe cover. Apply sterile ultrasound gel. The practitioner locates the vessel using the device t*o reduce the risk of insertion-related complications.*[1,10,31]
- Open the catheter package and inspect the device *to make sure that its integrity is intact.* Follow the manufacturer's instructions for use for preparing the catheter for insertion. Flush the catheter with preservative-free normal saline solution.[2,10]
- Hand the catheter to the practitioner using sterile technique. The practitioner then inserts the catheter.[2,10]
- Monitor the patient's respiratory rate, heart rate, and oxygen saturation level during the procedure. If cardiac monitoring is available, monitor for arrhythmias while the guide wire and catheter are advanced.[41]
- After the catheter is inserted and advanced to the desired tip location, the practitioner aspirates each lumen for blood return.[2,10]
- Flush the catheter with preservative-free normal saline solution, observing for complications.[2,10]
- Attach primed sterile needleless connectors to the catheter lumens.[2,10]
- The practitioner secures the catheter with a catheter securement device or sutures the catheter in place.[42]

ELDER ALERT *Central venous access catheters can be secured with sterile surgical strips, sterile tape, sterile manufactured securement devices, or sutures. Keep in mind that adhesive-backed tape and securement devices can cause tearing of an older adult's skin if removed improperly. An older adult can also develop sensitivities to adhesives, causing redness, itching, and rash, which can cause catheter dislodgment if the patient rubs, scratches, or pulls at the adhesive device.*[2] *Use nontraumatic tape and ensure proper adhesive removal as needed* to prevent skin stripping and tearing.[16]

- Use antiseptic solution *to remove dried blood, which can harbor microorganisms.*
- Apply a chlorhexidine-impregnated sponge dressing if required by your facility *to reduce the risk of central line–related bloodstream infection.*[1,9]
- Apply a sterile transparent semipermeable dressing (as shown below).[1,6] Expect some serosanguineous drainage during the first 24 hours.[9]

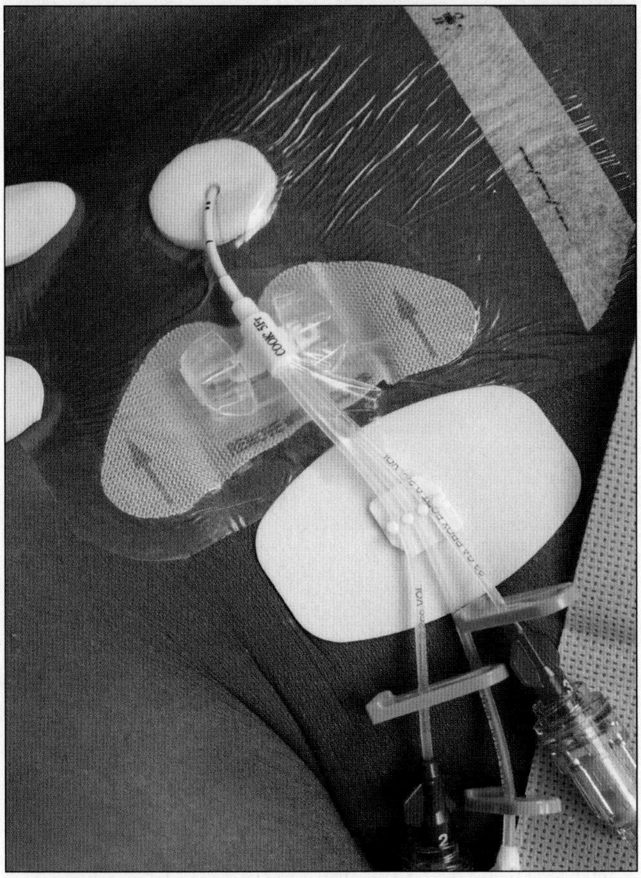

- Label the dressing with the date, the time, and your initials.[9]
- Place the patient in a comfortable position, return the bed to the lowest height, and reassess his status.
- After an X-ray confirms correct catheter placement in the superior vena cava, initiate IV therapy, if ordered.[31]
- Clamp the catheter or ask the patient to perform the Valsalva maneuver while you attach the IV tubing. *The Valsalva maneuver increases intrathoracic pressure, reducing the possibility of an air embolus.* Keep in mind that the Valsalva maneuver is contraindicated in patients with increased intracranial pressure. Alternatively, lock the device, if ordered.
- Trace the tubing from the patient to its point of origin *to make sure that it's connected to the proper port.*[24,43]
- Make sure that the infusion pump alarm limits are set according to the patient's current condition and that the alarms are turned on, functioning properly, and audible to staff.[32,33,34]

Blood sampling using a central venous access catheter

- Verify the practitioner's order.
- Perform hand hygiene.[1,17,18,19,20,21,22,23]
- Put on gloves; also put on goggles and a mask or face shield if splashing is likely *to comply with standard precautions.*[21,38,39,44]
- Expose the central venous tunneled catheter.
- Stop any running infusions, including those running through another lumen of the catheter.[2,10]
- Thoroughly disinfect the needleless connector with an antiseptic pad using friction, and allow it to dry.[2,10,15]
- Maintaining the sterility of the syringe tip, attach the syringe containing preservative-free normal saline solution to the needleless connector and aspirate for blood return. If you can't obtain a blood return, have the patient change position, cough, move his arm above his head, or take a deep breath and hold it momentarily.[2,10,50] Notify the practitioner if troubleshooting is ineffective.
- Flush the catheter with preservative-free normal saline solution.[50]
- Clamp the catheter lumen, thoroughly disinfect the needleless connector with an antiseptic pad using friction, and allow it to dry.[2,10]

Using the blood collection tube holder method

- Attach the blood collection tube holder with needleless adapter to the needleless connector, release the clamp, and engage the labeled discard blood collection tube to aspirate 4 to 5 mL of blood.[2,10]
- Clamp the catheter, remove the labeled discard blood collection tube from the needleless blood collection tube holder, and discard it in the appropriate receptacle.[44,45]
- Insert another blood collection tube into the needleless blood collection holder using the correct order of draw.[2] Unclamp the catheter and obtain the samples, as ordered; repeat the steps as necessary until you've obtained all of the samples.
- Clamp the catheter and remove the needleless blood collection tube holder.

Using the syringe method

- Attach the labeled discard syringe to the catheter, release the clamp, and gently withdraw 4 to 5 mL of blood for the discard sample.[2]
- Clamp the catheter, remove the labeled discard syringe, and then discard it in the appropriate receptacle.[38,44,45]
- Thoroughly disinfect the needleless connector using friction, allow it to dry, connect an empty syringe to the needleless connector, release the clamp, and withdraw the blood sample.
- Repeat as necessary until you've obtained all blood samples.
- Clamp the catheter and remove the syringe.
- Transfer blood samples from the syringe or syringes to the appropriate blood specimen tubes.[2]

Completing a blood specimen collection by either method

- *To make sure that tube additives are properly mixed with the blood sample,* carefully invert each tube the appropriate number of times as indicated by the tube's additive. Don't shake the collection tubes; *vigorous shaking may causing foaming and hemolysis.*[52,53,54]
- Thoroughly disinfect the needleless connector with an antiseptic pad using friction, and then allow it to dry.[2,10,15,51]
- Maintaining the sterility of the syringe tip, connect the syringe with preservative-free normal saline solution.[2,7,10]
- Open the clamp and flush the catheter with preservative-free normal saline solution, and then clamp the catheter.[2,10]
- Change the needleless connector according to the manufacturer's instructions if the integrity of the device is compromised, you suspect compromise, or there's blood or debris in the connector.[2,10,51]

- Continue the patient's prescribed continuous IV infusion. If the patient doesn't have a continuous infusion prescribed, proceed with locking the device, if required by your facility.
- Thoroughly disinfect the needleless connector with an antiseptic pad using friction and allow it to dry.[2,10]
- While maintaining the sterility of the syringe tip, attach the syringe of locking solution to the needleless connector and unclamp the device.[2,10]
- Slowly inject the solution into the catheter.[2,10]
- Clamp the device following the sequence required for the specific type of needleless connector used. For a positive-pressure needleless connector, clamp the catheter after disconnecting the syringe. For a negative-pressure needleless connector, clamp the catheter while maintaining pressure on the syringe plunger and then disconnect the syringe. For a neutral needleless connector, clamp the catheter before or after disconnecting the syringe.[2,10]
- Label the sample collection tubes in the presence of the patient *to prevent mislabeling.*[30]
- Place the collection tubes in a laboratory biohazard transport bag[38] and send them to the laboratory with a completed laboratory request form, if required.

Flushing a central venous access catheter

- Verify the practitioner's order.
- Perform hand hygiene[1, 17,18,19,20,21,22,23] and put on gloves. [21,38,39,44]
- Thoroughly disinfect the needleless connector with an antiseptic pad using friction (as shown below), and then allow it to dry.[1,2,10,51]

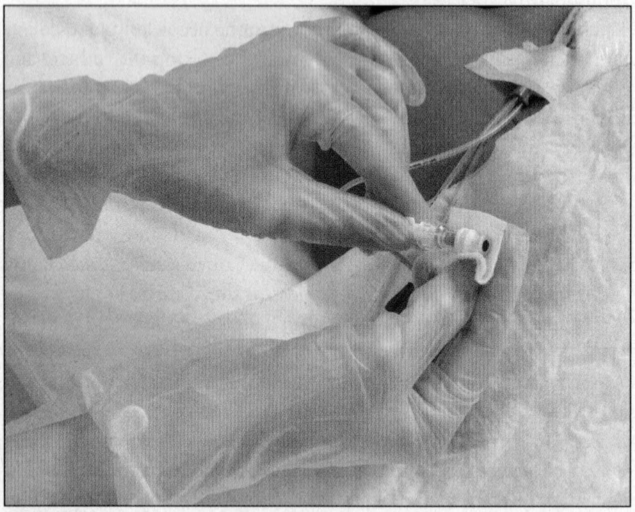

- While maintaining sterility of the syringe tip, attach a prefilled syringe containing preservative-free normal saline solution to the needleless connector (use a 10-mL syringe to assess vascular access device patency *to prevent catheter damage;* alternatively, use a smaller flush syringe that's designed to generate lower amounts of pressure), unclamp the catheter, and slowly aspirate until you obtain a brisk, positive blood return (as shown on top right) *to confirm the patency of the access device.*[2,7,10] If you don't obtain a blood return, notify the patient's practitioner *because the catheter tip might have migrated*; arrange for a chest X-ray as ordered *to verify placement.*[8]

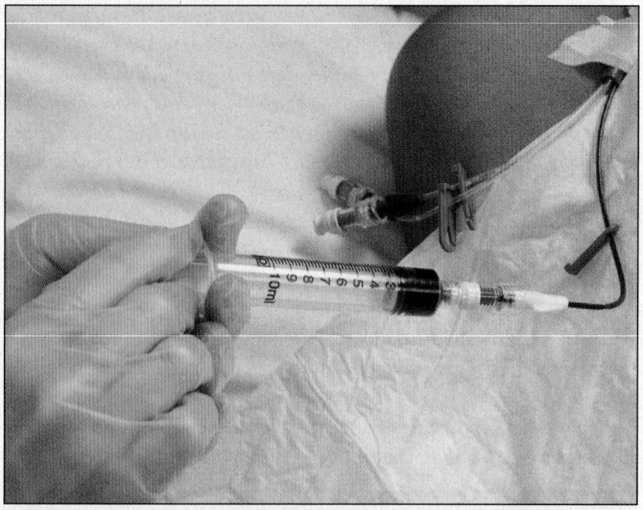

- Slowly inject preservative-free normal saline solution into the central venous access catheter, noting any resistance during injection (as shown below). If you note resistance, stop the injection; don't inject against resistance. Further evaluate the device if you're unable to flush it freely.[2,10]

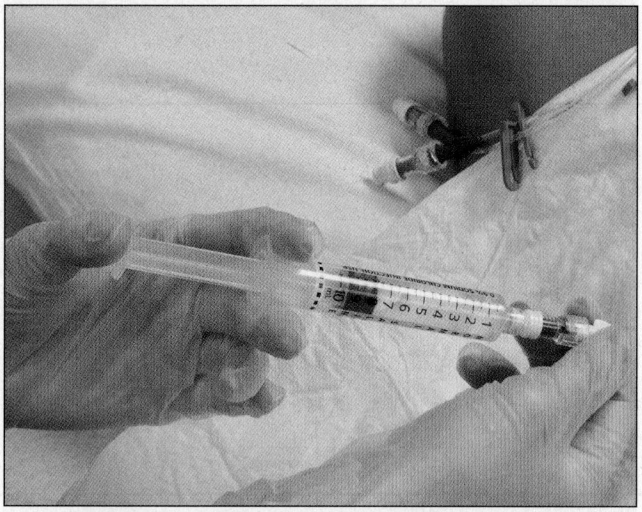

- Remove and discard the syringe in an appropriate container.[2,10]
- Administer the prescribed IV fluid or proceed with locking the device, if indicated.[2,10]

Locking a central venous access catheter

- Thoroughly disinfect the needleless connector with an antiseptic pad using friction, and then allow it to dry.[1,2,10,51]
- While maintaining sterility of the syringe tip, attach the syringe containing the locking solution to the needleless connector.[2,10]
- Slowly inject the locking solution into the central venous access catheter.[2,10]
- After locking the catheter, follow a clamping sequence to reduce blood reflux based on the type of needleless connector: For a positive-pressure needleless connector, clamp the catheter after disconnecting the syringe.[2,10] For a negative-pressure needleless connector, maintain pressure on the syringe while clamping the catheter.[2,10] For a neutral needleless connector, clamp the catheter before or after disconnecting the syringe.[2,10,49]

Changing a needleless connector on a central venous access catheter

- Verify the practitioner's order.
- Perform hand hygiene.[1,17,18,19,20,21,22,23]

■ Open the needleless connector package using sterile technique, and inspect the integrity of the device.[55,56]
■ Attach the prefilled syringe to the new needleless connector using sterile technique. Prime the needleless connector with preservative-free normal saline solution *to purge the needleless connector of air.*[2,10,55,56] Tap the needleless connector while priming *to purge all of the air.*[56] Leave the syringe in place.
■ Close the clamp between the connector and the catheter *to prevent air from entering the catheter, which could cause air embolism.*[57]
■ Remove the existing needleless connector.[2,10]
■ Thoroughly disinfect the catheter hub with an antiseptic pad using friction, and then allow it to dry.[1,2,20,51]
■ Remove the protective cover from the new needleless connector.[56]
■ Attach the new primed needleless connector to the catheter hub (as shown below). Rotate the device to tighten it, taking care not to overtighten.[56]

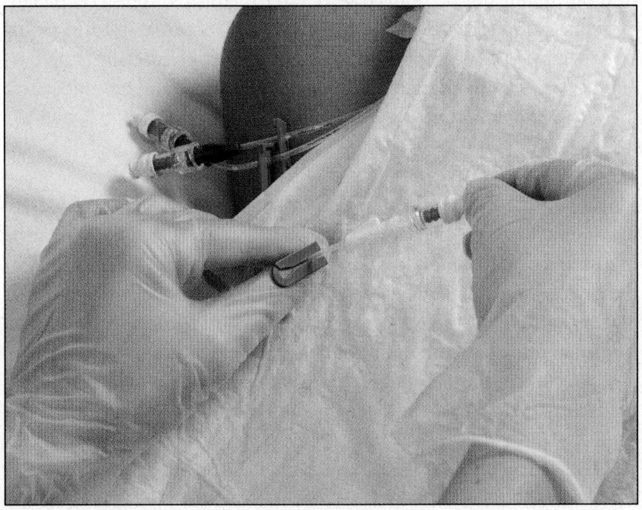

■ Unclamp the catheter, aspirate for blood return, and flush the catheter with the attached normal saline solution. Lock the catheter, if appropriate.
NURSING ALERT *If you don't get blood return or if resistance occurs during flushing, stop and evaluate the cause.*[7]
■ Clamp the catheter and remove the syringe in the sequence appropriate for the device, according to the manufacturer's instructions. For a positive-pressure needleless connector, clamp after the syringe is disconnected.[2,10] For a negative-pressure needleless connector, maintain pressure on the syringe plunger while closing the clamp.[2,10] For a neutral needleless connector, clamp before or after disconnecting the syringe.[2,10]

Changing the dressing on a central venous access catheter

■ Review the patient's medical record for information related to the central venous access device.
■ Determine the date of the last dressing change.
■ Perform hand hygiene.[1,17,18,19,20,21,22,23]
■ Put on a mask.[2,10]
■ Assemble the supplies on a sterile field.[2,10]
■ Put on gloves.
■ Remove the existing dressing by lifting the edge of the dressing at the catheter hub and gently pulling the dressing perpendicular to the skin toward the insertion site *to prevent catheter dislodgment and tearing or stripping of fragile skin.*[2,10] If necessary, use a nonacetone adhesive remover to remove adhesive from the patient's skin *because a product containing acetone can harm the catheter.* Discard the dressing in an appropriate receptacle.
■ If a chlorhexidine-impregnated sponge dressing was used to provide sustained antimicrobial action at the insertion site, remove and discard it in an appropriate receptacle.
■ Remove the catheter securement device, and discard it.[2,10]
■ If applicable, place a chlorhexidine-impregnated sponge dressing at the catheter base.1,9,11,13 *To facilitate future removal,* position the chlorhexidine-impregnated sponge dressing with the catheter resting on or near the radial slit of the dressing. The edges of the slit must touch *to maximize antimicrobial action.*
NURSING ALERT *Don't use chlorhexidine-impregnated sponge dressings on patients younger than age 2 months or on patients who are sensitive to chlorhexidine* because the dressing has constant contact with the skin.[1,9,11,13]
■ Apply a sterile transparent semipermeable dressing over the insertion site. Alternatively, apply a sterile 4″ × 4″ (10-cm × 10-cm) gauze dressing.[1,9,11,13] If the patient has fragile skin, use dressings and tape specially formulated for fragile skin *to prevent skin stripping and tearing during removal.*[16]
■ Label the dressing with the date, the time, and your initials.[2,9,10]

Removing a central venous access catheter

■ Verify the practitioner's order.
■ Perform hand hygiene.[1,17,18,19,20,21,22,23]
■ Teach the patient how to perform the Valsalva maneuver; if the Valsava maneuver is contraindicated, tell the patient to exhale during the procedure *to prevent air embolism.*[2,10]
■ Put on gloves and protective eyewear (if needed).[1,38,39]
■ Discontinue IV fluid administration and clamp the IV tubing.[2,10]
■ Position the patient so that the insertion site is at or below the level of the heart *to prevent an air embolism.*[2,12]
■ Remove and discard the old dressing.[2,10]
ELDER ALERT *Remove tape and other adhesive materials carefully* to avoid skin injury, including tearing and bruising. *Use an adhesive remover if necessary* to help the removal process.[10]
■ Remove the catheter securement device or sutures if present.[2,10]
■ Inspect the site for signs of infection, such as redness, swelling, or drainage.[2]
■ Apply a sterile gauze pad to the insertion site. With your dominant hand, slowly remove the catheter using gentle, even pressure.[2,10]
■ Have the patient perform the Valsalva maneuver (unless contraindicated) or exhale as you withdraw the last catheter segment from the vein *to prevent an air embolism.*[2,57]
■ If you meet resistance as you remove the catheter, don't forcibly remove it. Notify the practitioner immediately to discuss options for successful removal.[2,10,12]
■ Apply immediate pressure to the insertion site with the sterile gauze pad until hemostasis is achieved (a minimum of 30 seconds).[1,12] A hemostatic patch, pad, or powder may be needed *to potentiate clot formation.*[12]
■ Inspect the catheter tip and measure the length of the *catheter to ensure that the catheter has been completely removed.*[12] If you suspect that the catheter hasn't been completely removed, notify the practitioner immediately and monitor the patient for signs of distress.
■ Apply petroleum-based ointment to the exit site; then cover it with a sterile gauze pad and a transparent semipermeable dressing to seal the skin-to-vein tract and to decrease the risk of air embolism.[2,10,12]
■ Label the dressing with the date, the time, and your initials.[9]
■ Change the dressing every 24 hours until healing has occurred.[2]
■ Dispose of the IV tubing and used equipment properly.
■ Encourage the patient to remain recumbent or in a sitting position for at least 30 minutes after device removal.[2,10]

After the procedure

- After all procedures, dispose of all used supplies in the appropriate receptacles.[38,44,45]
- Remove and discard your gloves, goggles, and mask or face shield, if worn.[38,44,45]
- Perform hand hygiene.[1,17,18,19,20,21,22,23]
- Document the procedure.[46,47,48,49]

Special considerations

- Bathe the patient daily using a chlorhexidine wash *to reduce the risk of central line–associated bloodstream infection.*[1]
- The Joint Commission issued a sentinel event alert concerning medical device alarm safety *because alarm-related events have been associated with permanent loss of function and death.* Among the major contributing factors were improper alarm settings, inappropriately turned off alarms, and alarm signals that were not audible to staff. Make sure that alarm limits are appropriately set and that alarms are turned on, functioning properly, and audible to staff. Follow facility guidelines for preventing alarm fatigue.[35]
- After insertion, watch for signs and symptoms of pneumothorax, such as shortness of breath, uneven chest movement, tachycardia, and chest pain. Notify the practitioner immediately if such signs and symptoms appear.
- Replace dressings according to the type of dressing used: Change transparent semipermeable dressings at least every 7 days and gauze dressings every 2 days. Remove the existing dressing, clean the catheter-skin junction with an antiseptic solution, replace the stabilization device (if used), and apply a sterile dressing.[1,9]
- Change the tubing no more frequently than every 96 hours and immediately upon suspected contamination or when the integrity of the product or system has been compromised.[1,58] Change tubing used for continuous lipid administration every 24 hours.[1,58] When lipids are administered intermittently, change tubing with each new container.[58]
- Change the solution every 24 hours or at an interval determined by your facility while the central venous access catheter is in place.
- Use sterile technique when performing dressing, tubing, and solution changes for a central venous access catheter. (See "Changing the dressing on a central venous access catheter," page 151.)
- Assess the site for signs and symptoms of infection, such as discharge, inflammation, and tenderness.
- *To prevent an air embolism,* close the catheter clamp, or have the patient perform the Valsalva maneuver or exhale each time the catheter hub is open to air.
- Teach the patient and his family about measures to prevent central line–related bloodstream infection, including the importance of hand hygiene. Encourage them to remind staff members who fail to comply.[15]
- Routinely evaluate catheter necessity and discontinue catheter use as soon as it's no longer needed *to reduce the risk of central line–associated bloodstream infection.*[11]
- Routinely flush the access device after blood sampling, before and after medication administration, with discontinuation of an infusion, and when the catheter isn't in use.[2,10]
- When a medication is incompatible with preservative-free normal saline solution, flush the device with dextrose 5% in water and then follow by flushing with preservative-free normal saline solution, heparin flush solution, or both. Dextrose 5% in water should be flushed from the catheter *because it provides nutrients for biofilm growth,*[7] *which increases the risk of central line–associated bloodstream infection.*
- Visually inspect or palpate the catheter-site junction through the intact dressing daily *to assess for signs of infection.*[9]
- Notify the IV therapy team if available or the patient's practitioner immediately if you identify problems with the central venous access device.
- If fasting was required for an ordered test, confirm that the patient has fasted.[50] *Some tests require other dietary restrictions,* so verify that such restrictions were implemented, if applicable.
- Use the minimal amount of discard blood *to help prevent nosocomial anemia.*[50]
- Group multiple blood draws together whenever possible *to reduce the number of times the system is entered and to minimize the risk of infection.*[50]
- Be aware of the type of solution infusing through the catheter and any effects it may have on laboratory test results. Temporarily stop infusions if drawing blood through a multilumen central venous access catheter, or flush the line with preservative-free normal saline solution before drawing a discard sample.[50]

Complications

Complications can occur at any time during infusion therapy. Traumatic complications such as pneumothorax typically occur on catheter insertion but might not be noticed until after the procedure is completed. Systemic complications such as sepsis typically occur later during infusion therapy. Other complications include phlebitis (especially in peripheral central venous therapy), thrombus formation, and air embolism. (See *Risks of central venous therapy.*)

Documentation

Document the specific site preparation; infection prevention and safety measures followed; type, length, and gauge of the catheter; date and time of insertion; number and location of insertion attempts; functionality of the device; local anesthetic used; condition of the site; type of securement device; and type of dressing applied. Also note patient teaching performed and the patient's understanding of that teaching.[47]

Document the date and time, the amount and type of flush solution used, the patency of the catheter, and any complications that occur.

REFERENCES

1 Centers for Disease Control and Prevention. (2011). "Guidelines for the prevention of intravascular catheter-related infections" [Online]. Accessed March 2015 via the Web at http://www.cdc.gov/hicpac/pdf/guidelines/bsi-guidelines-2011.pdf

2 Infusion Nurses Society. (2013). *Policies and procedures for infusion nursing of the older adult* (2nd ed.). Boston, MA: Infusion Nurses Society.

3 Jarrett, N. M., et al. (2014). "Evidence-based guidelines for selected, candidate, and previously considered hospital-acquired conditions: Final report" [Online]. Accessed March 2015 via the Web at http://www.cms.gov/Medicare/Medicare-Fee-for-Service-Payment/HospitalAcqCond/Downloads/Evidence-Based-Guidelines.pdf

4 American Osteopathic Association. (2014). Standard 07.01.02. *Healthcare Facilities Accreditation Program: Accreditation requirements for acute care hospitals.* Chicago, IL: American Osteopathic Association. (Level VII)

5 American Osteopathic Association. (2014). Standard 07.01.19. *Healthcare Facilities Accreditation Program: Accreditation requirements for acute care hospitals.* Chicago, IL: American Osteopathic Association. (Level VII)

6 Rupp, S. M., et al. (2012). Practice guidelines for central venous access: A report by the American Society of Anesthesiologists Task Force on Central Venous Access. *Anesthesiology, 116,* 539–573. (Level VII)

7 Standard 45. Flushing and locking. Infusion nursing standards of practice. (2011). *Journal of Infusion Nursing, 34,* S59–S63. (Level VII)

8 Infusion Nurses Society. (2012). "INS infusion spotlight: Flushing and locking" [Online]. Accessed March 2015 via the Web at http://www.ins1.org/files/public/09_12_Infusion_Spotlight.pdf

9 Standard 46. Vascular access device site care and dressing changes. Infusion nursing standards of practice. (2011). *Journal of Infusion Nursing, 34,* S63–S64. (Level VII)

10 Infusion Nurses Society. (2011). *Policies and procedures for infusion nursing* (4th ed.). Boston, MA: Infusion Nurses Society.

Risks of central venous therapy

Signs and symptoms	Possible causes	Nursing interventions	Prevention
Infection			
■ Redness, warmth, tenderness, or swelling at the insertion or exit site ■ Possible exudate of purulent material ■ Local rash or pustules ■ Fever, chills, and malaise ■ Leukocytosis ■ Nausea and vomiting	■ Failure to maintain sterile technique during catheter insertion or care ■ Failure to comply with dressing change protocol ■ Wet or soiled dressing remaining on the site ■ Immunosuppression ■ Irritated suture line ■ Contaminated catheter or solution ■ Frequent opening of the catheter or long-term use of a single IV access site	■ Monitor temperature frequently. ■ Monitor vital signs closely. ■ Culture the site. ■ Re-dress using sterile technique. ■ Treat systemically with antibiotics or antifungals, depending on culture results and the practitioner's order. ■ Assist with catheter removal, if ordered ■ Collect peripheral blood cultures, as ordered (recommended). ■ If the catheter is removed, culture its tip. ■ Document interventions.[46, 47]	■ Maintain sterile technique. Use sterile gloves, masks, and gowns when appropriate.[39] ■ Observe dressing-change protocols. ■ Change a wet, soiled, or loosened dressing immediately.[58] ■ Examine solutions for cloudiness and turbidity before infusing; check fluid containers for leaks. ■ Use a 0.2-micron filter (or a 1.2-micron filter for 3-in-1 total parenteral nutrition solutions). ■ Keep the system closed as much as possible.
Pneumothorax, hemothorax, chylothorax, or hydrothorax			
■ Decreased breath sounds on affected side ■ With hemothorax, decreased hemoglobin level because of blood pooling ■ Abnormal chest X-ray	■ Repeated or long-term use of the same vein ■ Preexisting cardiovascular disease ■ Lung puncture by the catheter during insertion or exchange over a guide wire ■ Large blood vessel puncture with bleeding inside or outside the lung ■ Lymph node puncture with leakage of lymph fluid ■ Infusion of solution into the chest area through an infiltrated catheter	■ Notify the practitioner. ■ Remove the catheter or assist with removal if necessary. ■ Administer oxygen as ordered. ■ Set up and assist with chest tube insertion. ■ Document interventions.[46,47]	■ Position the patient head down with a rolled towel between his scapulae *to dilate and expose the internal jugular or subclavian vein as much as possible during catheter insertion.* ■ Assess for early signs of fluid infiltration (swelling in the shoulder, neck, chest, and arm). ■ Ensure that the patient is immobilized and prepared for insertion. Active patients may need to be sedated or taken to the operating room.
Air embolism			
■ Sudden onset of dyspnea ■ Breathlessness ■ Tachyarrhythmias ■ Weak pulse ■ Increased central venous pressure ■ Hypotension ■ Chest pain ■ Jugular vein distention ■ Wheezing ■ Altered mental status ■ Altered speech ■ Numbness ■ Paralysis ■ Loss of consciousness ■ Continued coughing[28]	■ Intake of air into the central venous system during catheter insertion or tubing changes, or inadvertent opening, cutting, or breaking of the catheter	■ Clamp, fold, or close the existing catheter or occlude the insertion site immediately.[51] ■ Place the patient in a left lateral decubitus position, if not contraindicated by other conditions.[51] ■ Administer oxygen. ■ Notify the practitioner. ■ Document the patient's condition and your interventions.[46,47]	■ Purge all air from the administration sets and add-on devices before starting an infusion. ■ Teach the patient to perform the Valsalva maneuver during catheter insertion and tubing changes, if not contraindicated by his condition.[57] ■ Use air-eliminating filters. ■ Use an infusion device with air detection capability. ■ Trace the tubing from the patient to its point of origin *to prevent misconnections.* ■ Position the patient so that the insertion site is at or below heart level when changing administration sets or needleless connectors.[57] ■ Use luer-lock tubing and secure all connections.[58]

(continued)

Risks of central venous therapy *(continued)*

Signs and symptoms	Possible causes	Nursing interventions	Prevention
Thrombosis			
■ Edema at puncture site ■ Erythema ■ Ipsilateral swelling of arm, neck, and face ■ Pain along vein ■ Fever, malaise ■ Chest pain ■ Dyspnea ■ Cyanosis	■ Sluggish flow rate ■ Composition of catheter material (polyvinyl chloride catheters are more thrombogenic) ■ Hematopoietic status of patient ■ Preexisting limb edema ■ Infusion of irritating solutions	■ Notify the practitioner. ■ Remove the catheter, if ordered. ■ Administer anticoagulant therapy, as prescribed. ■ Verify thrombosis with diagnostic studies. ■ Apply warm, wet compresses locally. ■ Don't use the limb on the affected side for subsequent venipuncture. ■ Document interventions.[46,47]	■ Encourage early mobilization of the affected extremity. ■ Maintain a steady flow rate with an infusion pump, or flush the catheter at regular intervals. ■ Use catheters made of less thrombogenic materials *to prevent thrombosis.* ■ Dilute irritating solutions. ■ Use a 0.2-micron filter for infusions.

11 Marschall, J., et al. (2014). SHEA/IDSA practice recommendation: Strategies to prevent central line–associated bloodstream infections in acute care hospitals. *Infection Control and Hospital Epidemiology, 35,* 753–771. Accessed March 2015 via the Web at http://www.jstor.org/stable/10.1086/676533 (Level I)

12 Standard 44. Vascular access device removal. Infusion nursing standards of practice. (2011). *Journal of Infusion Nursing, 34,* S57–S59. (Level VII)

13 Association of Professionals in Infection Control and Epidemiology (APIC). (2009). "An APIC guide 2009: Guide to the elimination of catheter-related bloodstream infections" [Online]. Accessed March 2015 via the Web at http://www.apic.org/Resource_/EliminationGuideForm/259c0594-17b0-459d-b395-fb143321414a/File/APIC-CRBSI-Elimination-Guide.pdf (Level IV)

14 Institute for Healthcare Improvement. (2012). *How-to-guide: Prevent central line–associated bloodstream infections.* Cambridge, MA: Institute for Healthcare Improvement. (Level V)

15 The Joint Commission. (2015). Standard NPSG.07.04.01. *Comprehensive accreditation manual for hospitals: The official handbook.* Oakbrook Terrace, IL: The Joint Commission. (Level VII)

16 LeBlanc, K., et al. (2013). International Skin Tear Advisory Panel: A tool kit to aid in the prevention, assessment, and treatment of skin tears using a simplified classification system. *Advances in Skin & Wound Care, 26,* 459–476.

17 The Joint Commission. (2015). Standard NPSG.07.01.01. *Comprehensive accreditation manual for hospitals: The official handbook.* Oakbrook Terrace, IL: The Joint Commission. (Level VII)

18 Standard 19. Hand hygiene. Infusion nursing standards of practice. (2011). *Journal of Infusion Nursing, 34,* S26–S27. (Level VII)

19 Centers for Disease Control and Prevention. (2002). Guideline for hand hygiene in health-care settings: Recommendations of the Healthcare Infection Control Practices Advisory Committee and the HICPAC/SHEA/APIC/IDSA Hand Hygiene Task Force. *MMWR Recommendations and Reports, 51*(RR-16), 1–45. Accessed March 2015 via the Web at http://www.cdc.gov/mmwr/pdf/rr/rr5116.pdf (Level II)

20 World Health Organization. (2009). "WHO guidelines on hand hygiene in health care: First global patient safety challenge, clean care is safer care" [Online]. Accessed March 2015 via the Web at http://whqlibdoc.who.int/publications/2009/9789241597906_eng.pdf (Level IV)

21 Standard 18. Infection prevention. Infusion nursing standards of practice. (2011). *Journal of Infusion Nursing, 34,* S25–S26. (Level IV)

22 Centers for Medicare & Medicaid Services, Department of Health and Human Services. (2014). Condition of participation: Infection control. 42 C.F.R. § 482.42.

23 American Osteopathic Association. (2014). Standard 07.01.21. *Healthcare Facilities Accreditation Program: Accreditation requirements for acute care hospitals.* Chicago, IL: American Osteopathic Association. (Level VII)

24 U.S. Food and Drug Administration. (n.d.). "Look. Check. Connect. Safe medical device connections save lives" [Online]. Accessed March 2015 via the Web at http://www.fda.gov/downloads/MedicalDevices/Safety/AlertsandNotices/UCM134873.pdf

25 Centers for Medicare & Medicaid Services, Department of Health and Human Services. (2014). Condition of participation: Patient's rights. 42 C.F.R. § 482.13(b).

26 American Osteopathic Association. (2014). Standard 15.01.11. *Healthcare Facilities Accreditation Program: Accreditation requirements for acute care hospitals.* Chicago, IL: American Osteopathic Association. (Level VII)

27 Standard 12. Informed consent. Infusion nursing standards of practice. (2011). *Journal of Infusion Nursing, 34,* S17–S18. (Level VII)

28 The Joint Commission. (2015). Standard UP.01.01.01. *Comprehensive accreditation manual for hospitals: The official handbook.* Oakbrook Terrace, IL: The Joint Commission. (Level VII)

29 American Osteopathic Association. (2014). Standard 30.00.14. *Healthcare Facilities Accreditation Program: Accreditation requirements for acute care hospitals.* Chicago, IL: American Osteopathic Association. (Level VII)

30 The Joint Commission. (2015). Standard NPSG.01.01.01. *Comprehensive accreditation manual for hospitals: The official handbook.* Oakbrook Terrace, IL: The Joint Commission. (Level VII)

31 Standard 35. Vascular access site preparation and device placement. Infusion nursing standards of practice. (2011). *Journal of Infusion Nursing, 34,* S44–S45. (Level VII)

32 Graham, K. C., & Cvach, M. (2010). Monitor alarm fatigue: Standardizing use of physiological monitors and decreasing nuisance alarms. *American Journal of Critical Care, 19,* 28–37.

33 American Association of Critical-Care Nurses (AACN). (2013). "AACN practice alert: Alarm management" [Online]. Accessed March 2015 via the Web at http://www.aacn.org/wd/practice/docs/practicealerts/alarm-management-practice-alert.pdf (Level VII)

34 The Joint Commission. (2015). Standard NPSG.06.01.01. *Comprehensive accreditation manual for hospitals: The official handbook.* Oakbrook Terrace, IL: The Joint Commission. (Level VII)

35 The Joint Commission. (2013). "Sentinel event alert: Medical device alarm safety in hospitals" [Online]. Accessed March 2015 via the Web at http://www.jointcommission.org/assets/1/18/SEA_50_alarms_4_5_13_FINAL1.PDF (Level VII)

36 The Joint Commission. (2015). Standard NPSG.03.04.01. *Comprehensive accreditation manual for hospitals: The official handbook.* Oakbrook Terrace, IL: The Joint Commission. (Level VII)
37 American Osteopathic Association. (2014). Standard 25.01.27. *Healthcare Facilities Accreditation Program: Accreditation requirements for acute care hospitals.* Chicago, IL: American Osteopathic Association. (Level VII)
38 Siegel, J. D., et al. (2007). "2007 guideline for isolation precautions: Preventing transmission of infectious agents in healthcare settings" [Online]. Accessed March 2015 via the Web at http://www.cdc.gov/hicpac/pdf/isolation/Isolation2007.pdf (Level II)
39 American Osteopathic Association. (2014). Standard 07.01.10. *Healthcare Facilities Accreditation Program: Accreditation requirements for acute care hospitals.* Chicago, IL: American Osteopathic Association. (Level VII)
40 The Joint Commission. (2015). Standard UP.01.03.01. *Comprehensive accreditation manual for hospitals: The official handbook.* Oakbrook Terrace, IL: The Joint Commission. (Level VII)
41 Lynn-McHale Wiegand, D. (Ed.). (2011). *AACN procedure manual for critical care* (6th ed.). St. Louis, MO: Saunders.
42 Standard 36. Vascular access device stabilization. Infusion nursing standards of practice. (2011). *Journal of Infusion Nursing, 34,* S46–S47. (Level VII)
43 Standard 61. Parenteral medication and solution administration. Infusion nursing standards of practice. (2011). *Journal of Infusion Nursing, 34,* S86–S87.
44 Occupational Safety and Health Administration. (n.d.). "Bloodborne pathogens, standard number 1910.1030" [Online]. Accessed March 2015 via the Web at http://www.osha.gov/pls/oshaweb/owadisp.show_document?p_table=STANDARDS&p_id=10051 (Level VII)
45 Standard 22. Safe handling and disposal of sharps, hazardous materials, and hazardous waste. Infusion nursing standards of practice. (2011). *Journal of Infusion Nursing, 34,* S28–S29. (Level VII)
46 The Joint Commission. (2015). Standard RC.01.03.01. *Comprehensive accreditation manual for hospitals: The official handbook.* Oakbrook Terrace, IL: The Joint Commission. (Level VII)
47 Standard 14. Documentation. Infusion nursing standards of practice. (2011). *Journal of Infusion Nursing, 34,* S20–S21. (Level VII)
48 Centers for Medicare & Medicaid Services, Department of Health and Human Services. (2014). Condition of participation: Medical record services. 42 C.F.R. § 482.24.
49 American Osteopathic Association. (2014). Standard 10.00.03. *Healthcare Facilities Accreditation Program: Accreditation requirements for acute care hospitals.* Chicago, IL: American Osteopathic Association. (Level VII)
50 Standard 57. Phlebotomy. Infusion nursing standards of practice. (2011). *Journal of Infusion Nursing, 34,* S77–S79. (Level VII)
51 Standard 27. Needleless connectors. Infusion nursing standards of practice. (2011). *Journal of Infusion Nursing, 34,* S32–S33. (Level VII)
52 Becton, Dickinson and Company. (2012). "BD Vacutainer® evacuated blood collection system: For *in vitro* diagnostic use" [Online]. Accessed March 2015 via the Web at http://www.bd.com/vacutainer/pdfs/VDP40161.pdf
53 Becton, Dickinson and Company. (2010). "BD vacutainer® order of draw for multiple tube collections" [Online]. Accessed March 2015 via the Web at http://www.bd.com/vacutainer/pdfs/plus_plastic_tubes_wallchart_orderofdraw_VS5729.pdf
54 Johnson, L. (2013). "National Center for Competency Testing: Phlebotomy order of draw: Who, what, when, where, why, & how" [Online]. Accessed March 2015 via the Web at http://www.ncctinc.com/documents/Phlebotomy%20Order%20of%20Draw.pdf
55 CareFusion. (2010). "SmartSite® needle-free valve user's manual" [Online]. Accessed March 2015via the Web at http://www.carefusion.com/pdf/Infusion/clinical_documentation/faq_tip_sheets/IV1372-SSusers guide.pdf
56 CareFusion. (2012). "MaxPlus® clear needleless connector: Quick reference guide" [Online]. Accessed March 2015via the Web at http://www.carefusion.com/pdf/Infusion/MaxPlus_Clear_In-Service_Poster-MX2989-ML3126.pdf
57 Standard 50. Air embolism. Infusion nursing standards of practice. (2011). *Journal of Infusion Nursing, 34,* S69–S70. (Level VII)
58 Standard 43. Administration set change. Infusion nursing standards of practice. (2011). *Journal of Infusion Nursing, 34,* S55–S57. (Level VII)

CENTRAL VENOUS PRESSURE MONITORING

With central venous pressure (CVP) monitoring, the practitioner inserts a catheter through a vein and advances until its tip lies in or near the right atrium. Because no major valves lie at the junction of the vena cava and right atrium, pressure at end diastole reflects back to the catheter. When connected to a monitoring system, the catheter measures CVP—an index of right ventricular function.

CVP monitoring helps to assess cardiac function, evaluate venous return to the heart, and indirectly gauge how well the heart is pumping. The central venous (CV) line also provides access to a large vessel for rapid, high-volume fluid administration and allows frequent blood withdrawal for laboratory samples. (See "Blood sampling using a central venous access catheter" in the "Central venous access catheter" procedure, page 149.)

CVP monitoring can be done intermittently or continuously. The catheter is inserted percutaneously or using a cutdown method. Typically, a single-lumen CVP line is used for intermittent pressure readings. To measure a patient's volume status, a disposable plastic water manometer or transducer is attached between the IV line and the central venous catheter with a three- or four-way stopcock. CVP is recorded in centimeters of water (cm H_2O) or millimeters of mercury (mm Hg), read from manometer markings.

Normal CVP ranges from 5 to 10 cm H_2O or 2 to 6 mm Hg.[1] Changes in preload status are reflected in CVP readings. Any condition that alters venous return, circulating blood volume, or cardiac performance may affect CVP. If circulating volume increases, such as with enhanced venous return to the heart from fluid overload, heart failure, and positive-pressure breathing, CVP rises. If circulating volume decreases, such as with reduced venous return from hypovolemia secondary to dehydration, interstitial fluid shift or hemorrhage, and negative pressure breathing, CVP drops.

Equipment

Leveling device ▪ IV pole ▪ IV solution ▪ gloves and other personal protective equipment ▪ Optional: dressing materials.

For CVP measurement with a water manometer

Disposable CVP manometer set ▪ additional stopcock (to attach the CVP manometer to the catheter) ▪ IV drip chamber and tubing ▪ tape ▪ dressing materials ▪ Optional: extension tubing.

For CVP measurement with a transducer

Pressure-monitoring kit with disposable pressure transducer ▪ bedside pressure module ▪ pressure bag ▪ IV pole with transducer mount ▪ continuous IV flush solution.

Implementation

- Gather the necessary equipment.
- Perform hand hygiene.[2,3,4,5,6,7]
- Put on gloves and other personal protective equipment as needed,[8,9]
- Confirm the patient's identity using at least two patient identifiers.[10]
- Explain the procedure to the patient *to reduce his anxiety and enhance cooperation.*

Measuring CVP with a water manometer

- Connect the IV solution to the IV tubing and the manometer. Prime the IV tubing and manometer setup. Make sure all air bubbles are removed from tubing. Attach the water manometer to an IV pole or place it next to the patient's chest.
- Assist the practitioner as he inserts the CV catheter, if necessary. (See "Assisting with inserting a central venous access catheter" in the "Central venous access catheter" procedure, page 148.)
- Connect the IV tubing to the CV catheter. Trace the tubing from the patient to its point of origin *to make sure that it's attached to the correct port.*[11]

Measuring CVP with a water manometer

To ensure accurate central venous pressure (CVP) readings, make sure that the manometer base is aligned with the patient's right atrium (the zero reference point). The manometer set usually contains a leveling rod to allow you to determine this alignment quickly.

After adjusting the manometer's position, examine the three-way stopcock. By turning it to any position shown below, you can control the direction of fluid flow. Four-way stopcocks are also available.

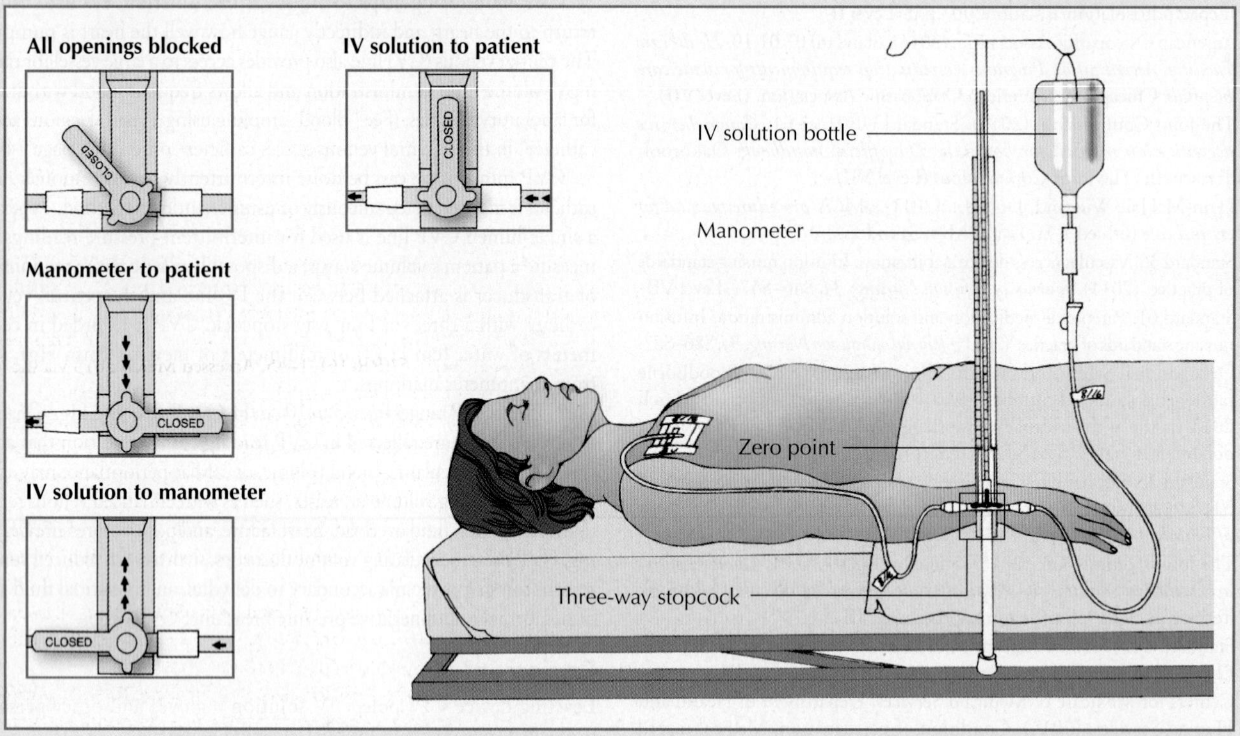

■ With the CV catheter in place, position the patient with the head of the bed between 0 and 45 degrees with the bed in its lowest position.[1] Align the base of the manometer with the zero reference point using a leveling device and secure the manometer in place. *Because CVP reflects right atrial pressure,* align the right atrium (the zero reference point) with the zero mark on the manometer. To find the right atrium, locate the fourth intercostal space at the midaxillary line. Mark the appropriate place on the patient's chest *so that all subsequent recordings will be made using the same location.*

■ When the head of the bed is elevated, the phlebostatic axis remains constant, but the midaxillary line changes. Use the same degree of elevation for all subsequent measurements. (See *Measuring CVP with a water manometer.*)

■ Typically, markings on the manometer range from –2 to 38 cm H_2O (–1.5 to 28 mm Hg). *However, because manufacturer's markings may differ,* read the directions before setting up the manometer and obtaining readings.

■ Turn the stopcock off to the patient and slowly fill the manometer with IV solution until the fluid level is 10 to 20 cm H_2O higher than the patient's expected CVP value. Don't overfill the tube *because fluid that spills over the top can become a source of contamination.*

Intermittent CVP readings using a water manometer

■ Turn the stopcock off to the IV solution and open to the patient. The fluid level in the manometer will drop. When the fluid level comes to rest, it will fluctuate slightly with respirations. Expect it to drop during inspiration and to rise during expiration.

■ Record CVP at the end of expiration, when intrathoracic pressure has a negligible effect and the fluctuation is at its highest point.[1] Depending on the type of water manometer used, note the value either at the bottom of the meniscus or at the midline of the small floating ball.

■ After you've obtained the CVP value, turn the stopcock to resume the IV infusion. Adjust the IV drip rate, as required.

■ Place the patient in a comfortable position.

■ Remove and discard any personal protective equipment worn.[8]

■ Perform hand hygiene.[2,3,4,5,6,7]

■ Document the procedure.[12,13,14]

Continuous CVP readings using a water manometer

■ Make sure the stopcock is turned so that the IV solution port, CVP column port, and patient port are open. Be aware that with this stopcock position, infusion of the IV solution increases CVP. Therefore, expect higher readings than those taken with the stopcock turned off to the IV solution.

■ If the IV solution infuses at a constant rate, CVP will change as the patient's condition changes, although the initial reading will be higher. Assess the patient closely for changes.

■ Record CVP values at appropriate intervals.

■ Remove and discard any personal protective equipment worn.[8]

■ Perform hand hygiene.[2,3,4,5,6,7]

■ Document the procedure.[12,13,14]

Measuring CVP with transducer

■ Set up a pressure transducer system. (See the "Transducer system setup" procedure, page 780.)

■ Make sure the CV catheter or the proximal lumen of a pulmonary artery catheter is attached to the system. (If the patient has a CV catheter with multiple lumens, the distal port is dedicated to continuous CVP monitoring, and the other lumens are used for fluid administration.) Trace the tubing from the patient to its point of origin *to make sure that it's connected to the proper port.*[11]
■ Position the patient with the head of the bed between 0 and 60 degrees.[1,15]
■ Locate the level of the right atrium by identifying the midaxillary point at the fourth intercostal space. Mark this location on the patient's skin *to use for all subsequent readings.*[1,15]
■ Zero the transducer, leveling the transducer air-fluid interface stopcock with the right atrium.
■ Perform a square waveform test (dynamic response test) *to verify the accuracy of the pressure monitoring system.*[1,15]
■ Read the CVP value by measuring the mean of the *a* wave at end-expiration.[1] (See *Interpreting CVP measurements,* page 158.) The monitor will also provide a value on the digital display. Make sure the patient is still when the reading is taken *to prevent artifact.* (See *Identifying hemodynamic pressure-monitoring problems,* page 159.)
■ Remove and discard your personal protective equipment.[8]
■ Perform hand hygiene.[2,3,4,5,6,7]
■ Document the procedure.[12,13,14]

Special considerations

■ As ordered, obtain chest X-rays following insertion and daily if needed and ordered *to check catheter placement.*
■ To care for the insertion site, change a gauze dressing every 48 hours and a transparent semipermeable dressing at least every 7 days. Change either dressing immediately if it becomes soiled, damp, or loosened.[16,17]
■ Perform hand hygiene before performing dressing changes and use sterile technique and sterile gloves when re-dressing the site.[2,3,4,5,7,8,9] When removing the old dressing and securement device, observe for signs of infection, such as redness, and note any patient complaints of tenderness. Clean the catheter-skin junction with an antiseptic solution and replace securement device. Then apply a chlorhexidine-impregnated sponge dressing, if indicated by your facility, and cover the site with a sterile gauze dressing or a transparent semipermeable dressing.[17]
■ After the initial CVP reading, reevaluate readings frequently *to establish a baseline for the patient.* Experts recommend obtaining readings at 15-, 30-, and 60-minute intervals *to establish a baseline.* If the patient's CVP fluctuates by more than 2 cm H_2O (1.5 mm Hg), suspect a change in his clinical status and report this finding to the practitioner.

HOSPITAL-ACQUIRED CONDITION ALERT *Keep in mind that the Centers for Medicare & Medicaid Services has added vascular catheter-associated infections to their list of hospital-acquired conditions that have payment implications. Use evidence-based practices to reduce the risk of these infections.*[18]

■ Change the IV flush solution, pressure tubing, and the IV tubing every 96 hours or immediately if you suspect contamination or a compromise of the integrity of the product or system. Label the IV solution, tubing, and dressing with the date, the time, and your initials.[16,19]
■ Assess catheter necessity daily during multidisciplinary rounds; the catheter should be removed as soon as it's no longer needed *to reduce the risk for central line–related bloodstream infection.*[20,21,22]

Complications

Complications of CVP monitoring include pneumothorax (which typically occurs upon catheter insertion), sepsis, thrombus, vessel or adjacent organ puncture, and air embolism.

Documentation

Document all dressing, tubing, and solution changes; the condition of the site; and site care given. Record the patient's CVP readings, the practitioner notified, prescribed interventions, and the patient's response. Document the patient's tolerance of the procedure, the date and time of catheter removal, and the type of dressing applied. Note the condition of the catheter insertion site and whether a culture specimen was collected. Note any complications and actions taken. Document any patient teaching provided and the patient's understanding of your teaching.

REFERENCES

1 Lynn-McHale Wiegand, D. (Ed.). (2011). *AACN procedure manual for critical care* (6th ed.). St. Louis, MO: Saunders.
2 The Joint Commission. (2015). Standard NPSG.07.01.01. *Comprehensive accreditation manual for hospitals: The official handbook.* Oakbrook Terrace, IL: The Joint Commission. (Level VII)
3 Centers for Disease Control and Prevention. (2002). Guideline for hand hygiene in health-care settings: Recommendations of the Healthcare Infection Control Practices Advisory Committee and the HICPAC/SHEA/APIC/IDSA Hand Hygiene Task Force. *MMWR Recommendations and Reports, 51*(RR-16), 1–45. Accessed March 2015 via the Web at http://www.cdc.gov/mmwr/pdf/rr/rr5116.pdf (Level II)
4 World Health Organization. (2009). "WHO guidelines on hand hygiene in health care: First global patient safety challenge, clean care is safer care" [Online]. Accessed March 2015 via the Web at http://whqlibdoc.who.int/publications/2009/9789241597906_eng.pdf (Level IV)
5 Centers for Medicare & Medicaid Services, Department of Health and Human Services. (2014). Condition of participation: Infection control. 42 C.F.R. § 482.42.
6 The Joint Commission. (2015). Standard NPSG.07.04.01. *Comprehensive accreditation manual for hospitals: The official handbook.* Oakbrook Terrace, IL: The Joint Commission. (Level VII)
7 American Osteopathic Association. (2014). Standard 07.01.21. *Healthcare Facilities Accreditation Program: Accreditation requirements for acute care hospitals.* Chicago, IL: American Osteopathic Association. (Level VII)
8 Siegel, J. D., et al. (2007). "2007 guideline for isolation precautions: Preventing transmission of infectious agents in healthcare settings" [Online]. Accessed March 2015 via the Web at http://www.cdc.gov/hicpac/pdf/isolation/Isolation2007.pdf (Level II)
9 American Osteopathic Association. (2014). Standard 07.01.10. *Healthcare Facilities Accreditation Program: Accreditation requirements for acute care hospitals.* Chicago, IL: American Osteopathic Association. (Level VII)
10 The Joint Commission. (2015). Standard NPSG.01.01.01. *Comprehensive accreditation manual for hospitals: The official handbook.* Oakbrook Terrace, IL: The Joint Commission. (Level VII)
11 U.S. Food and Drug Administration. (n.d.). "Look. Check. Connect. Safe medical device connections save lives" [Online]. Accessed March 2015 via the Web at http://www.fda.gov/downloads/MedicalDevices/Safety/AlertsandNotices/UCM134873.pdf
12 The Joint Commission. (2015). Standard RC.01.03.01. *Comprehensive accreditation manual for hospitals: The official handbook.* Oakbrook Terrace, IL: The Joint Commission. (Level VII)
13 Centers for Medicare & Medicaid Services, Department of Health and Human Services. (2014). Condition of participation: Medical record services. 42 C.F.R. § 482.24(b).
14 American Osteopathic Association. (2014). Standard 10.00.03. *Healthcare Facilities Accreditation Program: Accreditation requirements for acute care hospitals.* Chicago, IL: American Osteopathic Association. (Level VII)
15 American Association of Critical-Care Nurses (AACN). (2009). "AACN practice alert: Pulmonary artery/central venous pressure measurement" [Online]. Accessed March 2015 via the Web at http://www.aacn.org/wd/practice/docs/pap-measurement.pdf (Level VII)
16 Centers for Disease Control and Prevention. (2011). "Guidelines for the prevention of intravascular catheter-related infections" [Online]. Accessed March 2015 via the Web at http://www.cdc.gov/hicpac/pdf/guidelines/bsi-guidelines-2011.pdf (Level I)

Interpreting CVP measurements

A pressure transducer set produces an intermittent or continuous waveform and readout that's displayed on the patient's bedside monitor, along with the patient's electrocardiogram (ECG) and other tracings. This method allows you to continually monitor for acute or gradual changes.

When using a pressure transducer set, make sure the central venous catheter or the proximal lumen of a pulmonary artery catheter is attached to the system and that the patient is still when the reading is taken *to prevent artifact*.

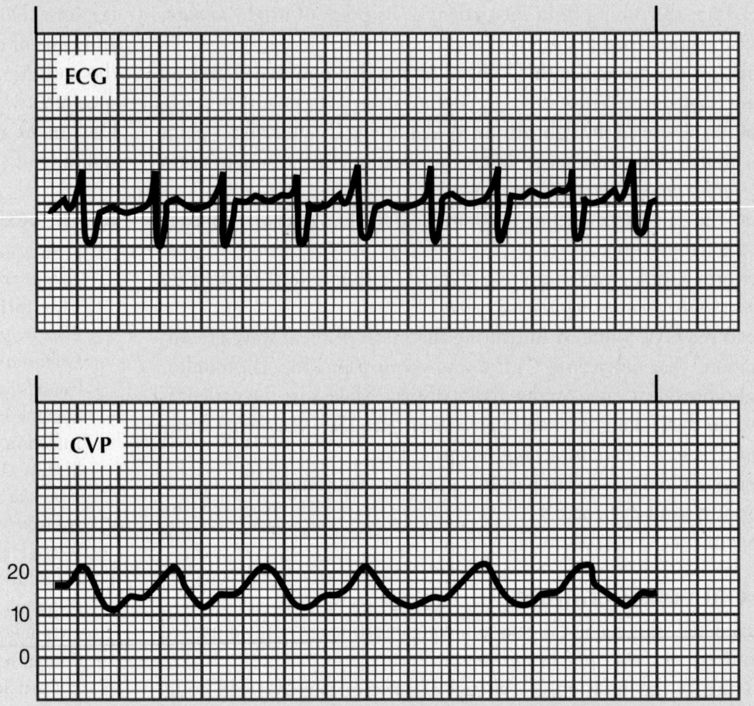

There are three waves to be aware of when interpreting a central venous pressure (CVP) waveform: the *a*, *c*, and *v* waves. Understanding how these waves relate to cardiac function is necessary to accurately interpret the CVP waveform.

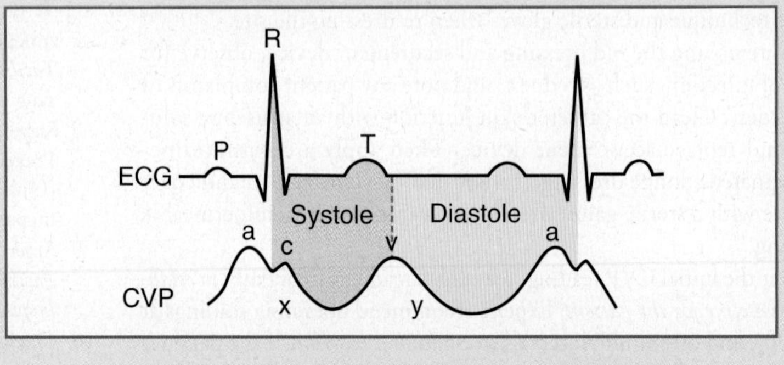

A wave (atrial contraction)

The most prominent wave is the *a* wave, which results from atrial contraction at end-diastole. As the right atria contracts, it forces blood into the right ventricle, causing a rise in pressure. This rise in pressure travels through the central line to the transducer and is represented by a positive inflection on the CVP waveform. When compared with the ECG waveform produced at the same time, the *a* wave on the CVP occurs after the P wave. To measure CVP, or right atrial pressure, measure the mean of the *a* wave at end-expiration.[1]

C wave (closure of the tricuspid valve)

Isovolumic right ventricular contraction, which closes the tricuspid valve and causes it to bow back toward the right atrium in early systole, produces a transient increase in atrial pressure. This increase in pressure is represented by the *c* wave on the waveform. The *c* wave, also a positive inflection on the CVP waveform, follows the onset of the QRS complex on the ECG.

V wave (ventricular contraction)

The last atrial pressure peak is the *v* wave, caused by a combination of atrial filling and ventricular contraction during late systole while the tricuspid valve remains closed. The *v* wave peaks just after the T wave on the ECG.

17 Standard 46. Vascular access device site care and dressing changes. Infusion nursing standards of practice. (2011). *Journal of Infusion Nursing, 34*, S63–S64. (Level VII)

18 Centers for Medicare & Medicaid Services, Department of Health and Human Services. (2014). "Hospital-acquired conditions" [Online]. Accessed March 2015 via the Web at http://www.cms.gov/Medicare/Medicare-Fee-for-Service-Payment/HospitalAcqCond/Hospital-Acquired_Conditions.html

19 Standard 43. Administration set change. Infusion nursing standards of practice. (2011). *Journal of Infusion Nursing, 34*, S55–S57. (Level VII)

20 Association of Professionals in Infection Control and Epidemiology (APIC). (2009). "An APIC guide 2009: Guide to the elimination of catheter-related

TROUBLESHOOTING

Identifying hemodynamic pressure-monitoring problems

Problem	Possible causes	Nursing interventions
No waveform	■ Power supply turned off	■ Check the power supply.
	■ Monitor screen pressure range set too low	■ Raise the monitor screen pressure range, if necessary. ■ Rebalance and recalibrate the equipment.
	■ Loose connection in line	■ Tighten loose connections.
	■ Transducer not connected to amplifier ■ Stopcock off to patient	■ Check and tighten the connection ■ Position the stopcock correctly.
	■ Catheter occluded or out of blood vessel	■ Use the fast-flush valve *to flush the line,* or try to aspirate blood from the catheter. If the line remains blocked, notify the practitioner and prepare to replace the line.[1]
Drifting waveforms	■ Improper warm-up	■ Allow the monitor and transducer to warm up for 10 to 15 minutes.
	■ Electrical cable kinked or compressed	■ Place the monitor's cable where it can't be stepped on or compressed.
	■ Temperature change in room air or IV flush solution	■ Routinely zero and calibrate the equipment 30 minutes after setting it up *to allow IV fluid to warm to room temperature.*
Line fails to flush	■ Stopcocks positioned incorrectly	■ Make sure stopcocks are positioned correctly.
	■ Inadequate pressure from pressure bag	■ Make sure the pressure bag gauge reads 300 mm Hg.
	■ Kink in pressure tubing	■ Check the pressure tubing for kinks.
	■ Blood clot in catheter	■ Try to aspirate the clot with a syringe. If the line still won't flush, notify the practitioner and prepare to replace the catheter, if necessary. *Important:* Never use a syringe to flush a hemodynamic catheter.
Artifact (waveform interference)	■ Patient movement	■ Wait until the patient is quiet before taking a reading.
	■ Electrical interference	■ Make sure electrical equipment is connected and grounded correctly.
	■ Catheter fling (tip of pulmonary artery [PA] catheter moving rapidly in large blood vessel in heart chamber)	■ Notify the practitioner, who may try to reposition the catheter.
False-high readings	■ Transducer balancing port positioned below patient's right atrium	■ Position the balancing port level with the patient's right atrium.
	■ Flush solution flow rate too fast	■ Check the flush solution flow rate. Maintain it at 3 to 4 mL/hour.
	■ Air in system	■ Remove air from the lines and the transducer.
	■ Catheter fling (tip of PA catheter moving rapidly in large blood vessel or heart chamber)	■ Notify the practitioner, who may try to reposition the catheter.
False-low readings	■ Transducer balancing port positioned above patient's right atrium	■ Position the balancing port level with the patient's right atrium.
	■ Transducer imbalance	■ Make sure the transducer's flow system isn't kinked or occluded, and rebalance and recalibrate the equipment.
	■ Loose connection	■ Tighten loose connections.

(continued)

TROUBLESHOOTING

Identifying hemodynamic pressure-monitoring problems *(continued)*

PROBLEM	POSSIBLE CAUSES	NURSING INTERVENTIONS
Damped waveform	■ Air bubbles	■ Secure all connections. ■ Remove air from the lines and the transducer. ■ Check for and replace cracked equipment.
	■ Blood clot in catheter	■ Try to aspirate the clot with a syringe. If the line still won't flush, notify the practitioner and prepare to replace the catheter, if necessary. *Important:* Never use a syringe to flush a hemodynamic catheter.
	■ Blood flashback in line	■ Make sure stopcock positions are correct; tighten loose connections and replace cracked equipment; flush the line with the fast-flush valve; replace the transducer dome if blood backs up into it.
	■ Incorrect transducer position	■ Make sure the transducer is kept at the level of the right atrium at all times. *Improper levels give false-high or false-low pressure readings.*
	■ Arterial catheter out of blood vessel or pressed against vessel wall	■ Reposition the catheter if it's against the vessel wall. ■ Try to aspirate blood *to confirm proper placement in the vessel.* If you can't aspirate blood, notify the practitioner and prepare to replace the line. Notify the practitioner immediately if you note bloody drainage at the insertion site; the catheter may be displaced.

bloodstream infections" [Online]. Accessed March 2015 via the Web at http://www.apic.org/Resource_/EliminationGuideForm/259c0594-17b0-459d-b395-fb143321414a/File/APIC-CRBSI-Elimination-Guide.pdf (Level IV)

21 Institute for Health Care Improvement. (2012). *How-to guide: Prevent central line-associated bloodstream infections.* Cambridge, MA: Institute for Healthcare Improvement. (Level VII)

22 Marschall, J., et al. (2014). SHEA/IDSA practice recommendation: Strategies to prevent central line-associated bloodstream infections in acute care hospitals. *Infection Control and Hospital Epidemiology, 35,* 753–771. Accessed Month Year via the Web at http://www.jstor.org/stable/10.1086/676533 (Level I)

CEREBROSPINAL FLUID DRAINAGE MANAGEMENT

Cerebrospinal fluid (CSF) drainage aims to reduce CSF pressure to the desired level and then to maintain it at that level. CSF drainage techniques fall into two categories: internal and external. Internal drainage devices, or shunts, are surgically implanted devices that divert CSF to the abdomen or heart when proper CSF absorption is impaired or obstructed, such as with hydrocephalus. External drainage is indicated when a temporary diversion of the CSF is needed; it's commonly used to manage increased intracranial pressure (ICP) and to promote spinal cord or cerebral dura mater healing after traumatic injury or surgery. In this case, and depending on the indication and the desired outcome, CSF can be externally drained through a catheter and a closed drainage collection system from either the lateral ventricle (ventriculostomy) or the lumbar subarachnoid space.

Therapeutic uses for external CSF drainage include ICP monitoring via the ventriculostomy; direct instillation of medications, contrast media, or air for diagnostic radiology; and aspiration of CSF for laboratory analysis. (See *CSF drainage.*)

This procedure focuses on external ventricular drainage management.

Equipment

External ventricular drainage set (includes drainage tubing and sterile drainage bag) ■ paper tape ■ IV pole ■ vital signs monitoring equipment ■ Optional: gloves, other personal protective equipment, sterile connector device, facility-approved antiseptic, sterile specimen container, laboratory transport bag, prescribed analgesics, sterile gloves, mask.

Preparation of equipment

After the practitioner inserts the catheter (see the "Ventricular drain insertion, assisting" procedure, page 828), connect the ICP monitoring system and external drainage system to the distal tip of the catheter. Trace the tubing from the patient to its point of origin *to ensure that the tubing is connected to the correct port.* Secure the connection points with paper tape or a sterile connector device.[1,2] Place the collection system, including the drip chamber and drainage bag, on an IV pole. Level the system at the level ordered by the practitioner.[3] A computed tomography scan may be performed *to confirm catheter placement.*[2]

Implementation

- Perform hand hygiene.[4,5,6,7,8]
- Confirm the patient's identity using at least two patient identifiers.[9]
- Explain the procedure to the patient and his family *to allay their fear and anxiety.*
- Put on gloves and other personal protective equipment as needed *to comply with standard precaustions.*[10,11,12]
- Check the patient's positioning *to ensure that the drip chamber of the ICP monitoring system is located at the ordered reference level.*[2]

■ Trace the drainage tubing from the patient to its point of origin *to ensure you're accessing the correct tubing.* Make sure that the drainage tubing is labeled clearly *so that staff members don't mistake it for IV tubing.*[1,2]
■ Assess frequently that the ventricular drain is leveled appropriately if the patient is active or moving around in bed *to prevent overdrainage or underdrainage.* The flow rate of CSF drainage is regulated by raising the pressure level on the drip chamber above the foramen of Monro, which is the zero reference level.[2,3]
■ Ensure that the CSF drainage system is clamped or open appropriately, according to the practitioner's order. Depending on the patient's condition, the practitioner may keep the ventricular drain stopcock set as "off" to the drain and "open" to the transducer for continuous ICP monitoring. When ICP reaches a predetermined pressure, he may order the stopcock "open" to drain CSF for a short period. Alternately, the practitioner may order continuous drainage with intermittent stopcock closings for ICP readings.[2]
■ Check the CSF drainage system for patency, as needed, by lowering the entire system briefly to assess the drip rate into the drip chamber.[2]
■ Perform a neurologic assessment and obtain the patient's vital signs hourly, or more frequently if the patient's condition warrants. Assess for signs and symptoms of increased ICP, including decreased level of consciousness, nausea, vomiting, headache, lethargy, and agitation.[2,3]
■ Obtain mean hourly ICP, and notify the practitioner immediately if ICP exceeds the established parameter; if no parameter has been established, notify the practitioner if ICP rises above 20 mm Hg. Assess ICP in relation to the patient's mean arterial pressure *to provide an indicator of the patient's cerebral perfusion pressure.*[2]

NURSING ALERT ***To obtain accurate ICP and waveform readings, set the stopcock as "off" to the drain and "open" to the transducer.*** **The ventricular drainage system can drain CSF or monitor ICP; it can't perform both functions at the same time.**[2]

■ Assess the CSF drainage volume, color, and clarity, and notify the practitioner if the appearance or volume changes.[2,3]
■ Assess the CSF drainage system at least every 4 hours, or more frequently if the patient's condition warrants; begin the inspection at the insertion site and continue along the entire drainage system. Check for cracks in the system or fluid leaking from the insertion site, and assess the condition of the dressing *to decrease the risk of infection and overdrainage.*[13,14]
■ Remove and discard any other personal protective equipment worn.[10,11,12]
■ Perform hand hygiene.[4,5,6,7,8]
■ Document the procedure.[15,16,17]

CSF drainage

Cerebrospinal fluid (CSF) drainage aims to control intracranial pressure (ICP) during treatment for traumatic injury or other conditions that cause a rise in ICP. A ventricular drain using a closed drainage system is detailed below.

Ventricular drain

To insert a ventricular drain, the practitioner makes a burr hole in the patient's skull and inserts the catheter into the ventricle. The distal end of the catheter is connected to a closed drainage system.

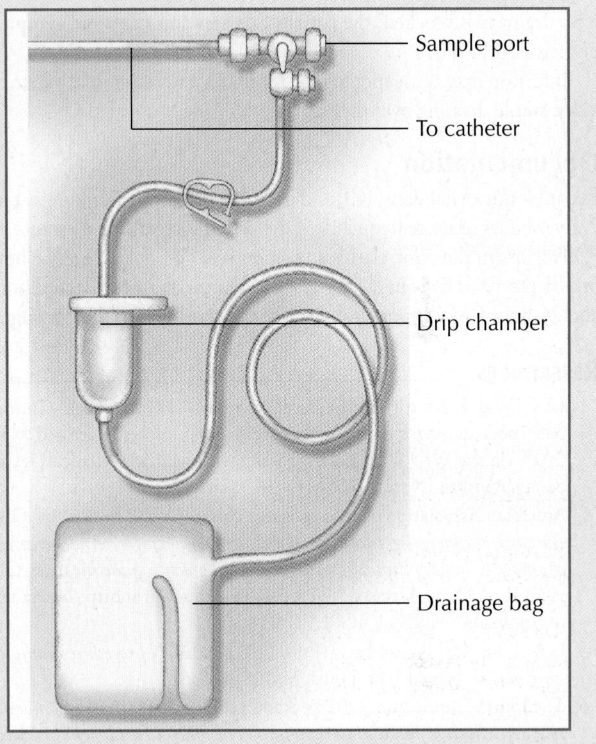

Special considerations

■ Change the drainage bag when it becomes nearly (about three-quarters) full. Use sterile technique and wear sterile gloves and a mask when changing the bag *to reduce the risk of infection.*[2,10,11,12]
■ If the catheter is open to drainage, maintain a continual hourly output of CSF *to prevent overdrainage or underdrainage.* Overdrainage may occur if the drip chamber is placed too far below the catheter insertion site. Underdrainage may reflect kinked tubing, catheter displacement, clot formation, or a drip chamber placed higher than the catheter insertion site.[2]
■ If a CSF specimen is needed for laboratory analysis, use strict sterile technique when accessing the external drainage system. Perform hand hygiene, put on a mask and sterile gloves, and set up a sterile field. Scrub the access port for 3 minutes with povidone-iodine (or other facility-approved antiseptic) and allow it to dry. Obtain the CSF specimen, label the specimen container in the presence of the patient, place it in a laboratory transport bag, and send it to the laboratory.[2,10,11,12]
■ Monitor ICP waveforms *to detect changes in the waveform* and troubleshoot when necessary. (See the "Intracranial pressure monitoring" procedure, page 424.)[2]
■ A patient may experience a chronic headache during continuous CSF drainage. Reassure the patient that this isn't unusual; administer analgesics, as ordered and needed, following safe medication administration practices.
■ Transferring a patient away from the patient floor to perform tests and procedures is discouraged *to prevent catheter dislodgment.* Check for the option of performing such tests and procedures at the patient's bedside. If a patient must be transported, keep the drainage system upright and aligned with the patient.[14]
■ Follow strict sterile technique when connecting tubing, flushing the system, obtaining specimens from the drainage system, and changing the dressing.[2,3]

Patient teaching

Teach the patient and his family members about the reason for the drain. Explain to the patient and his family that his activity level must be restricted during CSF drainage. The patient may not sit up, stand, or walk when the drain is open and he must ask for assistance with movement. The CSF drainage system must be turned off when the patient is repositioned or transferred. Instruct the patient to avoid straining, coughing, and sneezing during CSF drainage.

Complications

Signs of overdrainage of CSF include headache, tachycardia, diaphoresis, and nausea. Acute CSF overdrainage may result in collapsed ventricles, tentorial herniation, and medullary compression.[14]

NURSING ALERT *If CSF drainage accumulates too rapidly, clamp the system, notify the practitioner immediately, and perform a complete neurologic assessment* **because this complication constitutes a potential neurosurgical emergency.**[14]

Cessation of drainage may indicate clot formation. If you can't quickly identify the cause of the obstruction, notify the practitioner. If CSF drainage is blocked, the patient may develop signs and symptoms of increased ICP.

Infection may cause meningitis. Maintain a sterile closed system and a dry, sterile dressing over the site.

Documentation

Record routine vital signs, ICP, and neurologic assessment findings at least every 4 hours or more frequently if the patient's condition warrants it.

Document the color, clarity, and amount of CSF at least every 8 hours, or as determined by your facility or the patient's condition. Record hourly and 24-hour CSF output, and describe the condition of the dressing.

References

1 U.S. Food and Drug Administration. (n.d.). "Look. Check. Connect. Safe medical device connections save lives" [Online]. Accessed March 2015 via the Web at http://www.fda.gov/downloads/MedicalDevices/Safety/AlertsandNotices/UCM134873.pdf

2 American Association of Neuroscience Nurses (AANN). (2011). *Care of the patient undergoing intracranial pressure monitoring/external ventricular drainage or lumbar drainage: AANN clinical practice guideline series.* Glenview, IL: AANN. Accessed March 2015 via the Web at http://www.aann.org/uploads/AANN11_ICPEVDnew.pdf

3 Lynn-McHale Wiegand, D. (Ed.). (2011). *AACN procedure manual for critical care* (6th ed.). St. Louis, MO: Saunders.

4 The Joint Commission. (2015). Standard NPSG.07.01.01. *Comprehensive accreditation manual for hospitals: The official handbook.* Oakbrook Terrace, IL: The Joint Commission. (Level VII)

5 Centers for Disease Control and Prevention. (2002). Guideline for hand hygiene in health-care settings: Recommendations of the Healthcare Infection Control Practices Advisory Committee and the HICPAC/SHEA/APIC/IDSA Hand Hygiene Task Force. *MMWR Recommendations and Reports, 51*(RR-16), 1–45. Accessed March 2015 via the Web at http://www.cdc.gov/mmwr/pdf/rr/rr5116.pdf (Level II)

6 World Health Organization. (2009). "WHO guidelines on hand hygiene in health care: First global patient safety challenge, clean care is safer care" [Online]. Accessed March 2015 via the Web at http://whqlibdoc.who.int/publications/2009/9789241597906_eng.pdf (Level IV)

7 American Osteopathic Association. (2014). Standard 07.01.21. *Healthcare Facilities Accreditation Program: Accreditation requirements for acute care hospitals.* Chicago, IL: American Osteopathic Association. (Level VII)

8 Centers for Medicare & Medicaid Services, Department of Health and Human Services. (2014). Condition of participation: Infection control. 42 C.F.R. § 482.42.

9 The Joint Commission. (2015). Standard NPSG.01.01.01. *Comprehensive accreditation manual for hospitals: The official handbook.* Oakbrook Terrace, IL: The Joint Commission. (Level VII)

10 Siegel, J. D., et al. (2007). "2007 guideline for isolation precautions: Preventing transmission of infectious agents in healthcare settings" [Online]. Accessed March 2015 via the Web at http://www.cdc.gov/hicpac/pdf/isolation/Isolation2007.pdf (Level II)

11 American Osteopathic Association. (2014). Standard 07.01.10. *Healthcare Facilities Accreditation Program: Accreditation requirements for acute care hospitals.* Chicago, IL: American Osteopathic Association. (Level VII)

12 The Joint Commission. (2015). Standard IC.02.01.01. *Comprehensive accreditation manual for hospitals: The official handbook.* Oakbrook Terrace, IL: The Joint Commission. (Level VII)

13 Bader, M. K., & Littlejohns, L. R. (Eds.). (2010). *AANN core curriculum for neuroscience nursing* (5th ed.). Glenview, IL: American Association of Neuroscience Nurses.

14 Medtronic, Inc. (2013). "Duet external drainage and monitoring system" [Online]. Accessed March 2015 via the Web at http://manuals.medtronic.com/wcm/groups/mdtcom_sg/@emanuals/@era/@st/documents/documents/contrib_088173.pdf

15 The Joint Commission. (2015). Standard RC.01.03.01. *Comprehensive accreditation manual for hospitals: The official handbook.* Oakbrook Terrace, IL: The Joint Commission. (Level VII)

16 American Osteopathic Association. (2014). Standard 10.00.03. *Healthcare Facilities Accreditation Program: Accreditation requirements for acute care hospitals.* Chicago, IL: American Osteopathic Association. (Level VII)

17 Centers for Medicare & Medicaid Services, Department of Health and Human Services. (2014). Condition of participation: Medical record services. 42 C.F.R. § 482.24(b).

Additional reference

Hickey, J.V. (20147). *The clinical practice of neurological and neurosurgical nursing* (6th ed.). Philadelphia, PA: Wolters Kluwer.

Cervical collar application

A cervical collar may be used for an acute injury (such as strained cervical muscles) or a chronic condition (such as arthritis or cervical metastasis). A cervical collar may augment such splinting devices as a spine board to prevent potential cervical spine fracture or spinal cord damage after an acute injury.

Designed to hold the neck straight with the chin slightly elevated and tucked in, the collar immobilizes the cervical spine, decreases muscle spasms, and reduces pain; it also prevents further injury and promotes healing. As symptoms of an acute injury subside, the patient may gradually discontinue wearing the collar, alternating periods of wear with increasing periods of removal, until he no longer needs the collar.

This procedure focuses on patients with nonacute injuries or chronic conditions.

Equipment

Cervical collar in the appropriate size ■ Optional: cotton (for padding). (See *Types of cervical collars.*)

Implementation

- Verify the practitioner's order.
- Gather the equipment.
- Perform hand hygiene.[1,2,3]
- Confirm the patient's identity using at least two patient identifiers.[4]
- Explain the procedure to the patient.
- Check the patient's neurovascular status before application.
- Instruct the patient to position his head slowly to face directly forward.
- With the patient upright (if possible) and facing forward, measure the height needed for the collar by measuring from the bottom of the patient's chin to the top of his sternum.
- Measure the circumference of the patient's neck.
- Select the appropriate collar by applying the patient's measurements to the manufacturer's size chart.
- Place the cervical collar in front of the patient's neck *to ensure that the size is correct.*
- Fit the collar snugly around the neck and attach the Velcro fasteners or buckles at the back of his neck.

- Check the patient's airway and neurovascular status *to ensure that the collar isn't too tight.*
- Perform hand hygiene.[1,2,3]
- Document the procedure.[5,6]

Special considerations

- For a sprain or a potential cervical spine fracture, make sure the collar isn't too high in front *because this may hyperextend the neck.* In a neck sprain, such hyperextension may cause ligaments to heal in a shortened position. In a potential cervical spine fracture, hyperextension may cause serious neurologic damage.
- If the patient complains of pressure, the collar may be too tight. Remove and reapply it. If the patient complains of skin irritation or friction, the collar itself may be irritating him. Apply protective cotton padding between the irritated skin and the collar.

Patient teaching

Teach the patient how to apply the collar and how to do a neurovascular check. Have the patient demonstrate how to apply the collar after you have instructed him. Some collars are complex and the patient (or caregiver) may need to practice if he will be responsible for application. If indicated, advise sleeping without a pillow.

Complications

Hard cervical collars can cause pain, breathing restriction, tissue ischemia, and an increased risk of aspiration.[7]

Documentation

Note the type and size of the cervical collar and the time and date of application. Record the results of neurovascular checks. Document patient comfort, the collar's snugness, and all patient instructions provided.

REFERENCES

1 The Joint Commission. (2015). Standard NPSG.07.01.01. *Comprehensive accreditation manual for hospitals: The official handbook.* Oakbrook Terrace, IL: The Joint Commission. (Level VII)

2 Centers for Disease Control and Prevention. (2002). Guideline for hand hygiene in health-care settings: Recommendations of the Healthcare Infection Control Practices Advisory Committee and the HICPAC/SHEA/APIC/IDSA Hand Hygiene Task Force. *MMWR Recommendations and Reports, 51*(RR-16), 1–45. Accessed March 2015 via the Web at http://www.cdc.gov/mmwr/pdf/rr/rr5116.pdf (Level II)

3 World Health Organization. (2009). "WHO guidelines on hand hygiene in health care: First global patient safety challenge, clean care is safer care" [Online]. Accessed March 2015 via the Web at http://whqlibdoc.who.int/publications/2009/9789241597906_eng.pdf (Level IV)

4 The Joint Commission. (2015). Standard NPSG.01.01.01. *Comprehensive accreditation manual for hospitals: The official handbook.* Oakbrook Terrace, IL: The Joint Commission. (Level VII)

5 The Joint Commission. (2015). Standard RC.01.03.01. *Comprehensive accreditation manual for hospitals: The official handbook.* Oakbrook Terrace, IL: The Joint Commission. (Level VII)

6 Centers for Medicare & Medicaid Services, Department of Health and Human Services. (2014). Condition of participation: Medical record services. 42 C.F.R. § 482.24(b).

7 Muzin, S., et al. (2008). When should a cervical collar be used to treat neck pain? *Current Reviews in Musculoskeletal Medicine, 1,* 114–119. Accessed March 2015 via the Web at http://www.ncbi.nlm.nih.gov/pmc/articles/PMC2684205/

EQUIPMENT

Types of cervical collars

Cervical collars are used to support an injured or weakened cervical spine and to maintain alignment during healing.

Made of rigid plastic, a molded cervical collar holds the patient's neck firmly, keeping it straight, with her chin slightly elevated and tucked in.

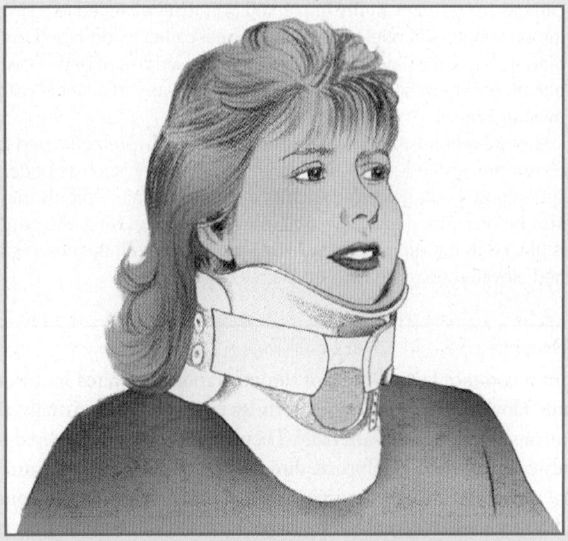

The soft cervical collar, made of spongy foam, provides gentler support and reminds the patient to avoid cervical spine motion.

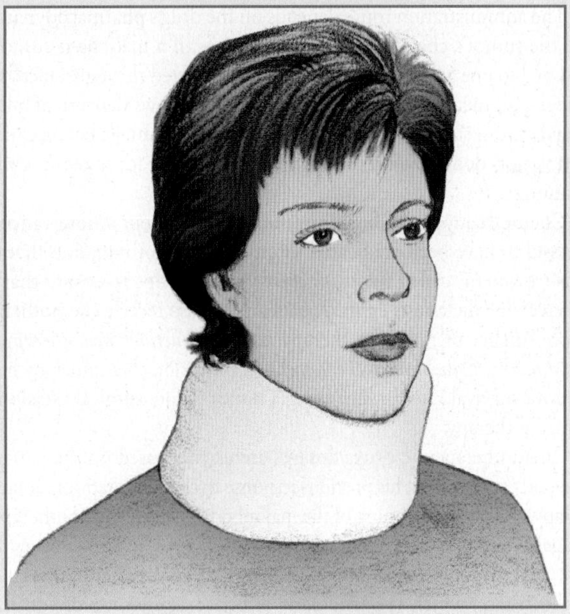

CHEMOTHERAPEUTIC DRUG ADMINISTRATION

Administration of chemotherapeutic drugs requires skills in addition to those used when giving other drugs.[1] For example, some drugs require specialized equipment or must be given through an unusual route. Others become unstable over time, and some must be protected from light. Chemotherapeutic drug dosages must also be exact to avoid possibly fatal complications. For these reasons, only a practitioner or registered nurse who has completed competency training in administration and safe handling of chemotherapeutic drugs may administer them.[2]

Chemotherapeutic drugs may be administered through a number of routes. Intravascular IV administration (using peripheral or central veins),

Intraperitoneal chemotherapy: An alternative approach

Intraperitoneal chemotherapy is used to treat ovarian cancer that has spread within the peritoneal cavity *because much higher concentrations of the drug can be delivered directly to the peritoneal cavity when compared with the IV route of administration.*[3]

Typically, intraperitoneal chemotherapy is administered through a single-lumen implanted port that's connected to a silicone peritoneal catheter, or through a fully implanted port that's attached to a single-lumen venous silicone catheter. Peritoneal catheters designed for dialysis have been associated with an increased risk of bowel complications when used to administer chemotherapy in patients with ovarian cancer.[3]

Before administrations, the patient is typically premedicated for chemotherapy-induced nausea with an antiemetic such as ondansetron and a corticosteroid such as dexamethasone. Opioids may also be prescribed *to relieve abdominal cramping.* Next, the patient is placed in the supine or semi-Fowler position with the head of the bed elevated no more than 30 degrees.[3]

The peritoneal port is accessed using a 19G or 20G 1″ to 2″ (2.5- to 5-cm) right-angled noncoring needle: patency is verified.[2,3] Chemotherapy is infused as rapidly as possible by gravitational flow;[3] an in-line fluid warmer is used to warm the solution to body temperature *to prevent abdominal cramping.* After the chemotherapy is infused, 1 L of warmed normal saline solution may be infused *to help distribute the medication.*

Stop the infusion if the patient becomes too uncomfortable. After the chemotherapy is infused, have the patient change position every 10 to 15 minutes for 1 to 2 hours *to help disperse the medication around the peritoneal cavity.*[2,3] Ninety percent of the administered chemotherapy drugs are absorbed within 4 hours of administration.[4]

After administering the chemotherapy drug, flush the port and catheter according to facility guidelines, remove the needle, and apply an occlusive dressing; the dressing can be safely removed after 12 hours.[3]

the most commonly used route of administration, is covered in this procedure. However, chemotherapeutic drugs may also be given orally, subcutaneously, IM, or intra-arterially. They may also be administered into a body cavity or the pleural space, through an Ommaya reservoir into the spinal canal, or through a device implanted in a vein or subcutaneously.

Intraperitoneal chemotherapy, in addition to IV chemotherapy, is an option for treating advanced ovarian cancer. It may also be used to treat malignant peritoneal mesothelioma, appendiceal malignancy, peritoneal carcinomatosis, and peritoneal dissemination from pancreatic cancer. (See *Intraperitoneal chemotherapy: An alternative approach.*)

The administration route depends on the drug's pharmacodynamics and the tumor's characteristics. For example, if a malignant tumor is confined to one area, the drug may be administered through a localized, or regional, method. Regional administration allows delivery of a high drug dose directly to the tumor—a significant advantage because many solid tumors don't respond to drug levels that are safe for systemic administration.

Chemotherapy may be administered to a patient whose cancer is believed to have been eradicated through surgery or radiation therapy. This treatment, called *adjuvant chemotherapy,* helps to ensure that no undetectable metastasis exists. A patient may also receive chemotherapy before surgery or radiation therapy, called *induction chemotherapy* (or *neoadjuvant* or *synchronous chemotherapy.*) Induction chemotherapy helps improve survival rates by shrinking a tumor before surgical excision or radiation therapy.

Chemotherapeutic drugs dosages are usually based on the patient's total body surface area, his previous response to chemotherapy or radiation therapy, and the functioning of the major body systems. Chemotherapeutic agents generally prove more effective when given in higher doses, but their adverse effects often limit the dosage. An exception to this rule is methotrexate, which is particularly effective against rapidly growing tumors but also toxic to normal tissues that rapidly grow and divide. Practitioners have discovered that they can give a large dose of methotrexate to destroy cancer cells and then, before the drug has had a chance to permanently damage vital organs, give a dose of folinic acid antidote. This antidote stops the effects of methotrexate, preserving normal tissue.

If the patient is pregnant, the practitioner and other members of the health care team should collaborate with the patient's obstetric team before starting chemotherapy. Chemotherapy is contraindicated during the first trimester and isn't recommended after 35 weeks' gestation to avoid delivery during a period of bone marrow suppression.[4]

Equipment

Material safety data sheet (MSDS) for the prescribed chemotherapy drug ▪ prescribed chemotherapy drug ▪ antiseptic pad ▪ administration set ▪ prescribed IV solution ▪ needleless luer-lock connectors ▪ syringes of preservative-free normal saline flush solution ▪ infusion pump (preferably a smart pump with dose-range alerts) ▪ low-pressure, flow-control infusion device (for vesicant administration) ▪ powder-free chemotherapy gloves ▪ nonlinting, nonabsorbent disposable gown ▪ face shield ▪ goggles ▪ chemotherapy sharps container ▪ hazardous-waste container approved for cytotoxic waste ▪ labels ▪ scale ▪ stethoscope ▪ thermometer ▪ automated blood pressure device or sphygmomanometer ▪ chemotherapy spill kit ▪ detergent ▪ extravasation equipment ▪ emergency equipment ▪ fluid-impermeable pad ▪ Optional: aluminum foil or brown paper bag, noncoring needle, IV insertion equipment, gauze pads, other prescribed medications, National Institute for Occupational Safety and Health (NIOSH)–approved respirator mask, booties, transport bag.

Preparation of equipment

Gather the appropriate equipment. Make sure that a chemotherapy spill kit, extravasation equipment, and emergency equipment are readily available. Make sure that the emergency equipment is functioning properly.

The pharmacy may prepare the medication for you. If you must prepare the medication, wash your hands with soap and water and put on personal protective equipment (a gown, two pairs of gloves, a face shield and goggles if splashing is likely, and a NIOSH-approved respirator mask if aerosolization is possible). Use a closed-system device and prepare the medication in a biological safety cabinet following appropriate safety standards. Cap the end of the primed administration tubing or the luer-lock end of the syringe. Label the medication with the patient's full name and second identifier, complete generic medication name, route of administration, total dose to be given, total volume required to administer the dosage, date and time of preparation, date and time of administration, and date and time of expiration (when a syringe is not for immediate use).[2] Place a warning on the medication *to indicate that it's a cytotoxic medication.* Wipe the outside of the solution container or syringe with moist gauze and then place it in a sealable bag for transport, making sure not to contaminate the outside of the transport bag. Label the outside of the bag *to indicate that its contents are hazardous.* Discard material that has come in contact with the cytotoxic medication in a waste container designed for cytotoxic waste. Use detergent and water to wash surfaces that have come in contact with the medication.

Remove and discard your gown and outer gloves. Remove and discard your inner gloves. Wash your hands with soap and water.[2,4,5]

Implementation

- Avoid distractions and interruptions when preparing and administering the medication *to prevent medication administration errors.*[6,7]
- Review the patient's medical record for initial cancer diagnosis and staging or current cancer status; recent treatments, including surgery, radiation therapy, hormone therapy, chemotherapy, and complementary therapy; medical, psychiatric, and surgical history; allergic or hypersensitivity reactions; patient understanding of chemotherapy treatment; pregnancy and reproductive status, including last menstrual period, if applicable; physical examination results, including assessment of organ function appropriate for the planned treatment regimen.[2,4]
- Review an accurate list of all the patient's medications and supplements.[4]
- Read the practitioner's order and make sure that it includes the patient's full name and a second patient identifier; the date; the diagnosis; any allergies; the regimen name and cycle number; the name of the medication ordered; the dose; the patient's height, weight, and any other variables used to calculate the dose;[1] the method for dose calculation; the route of administration; the frequency or dates of administration; supportive care measures, such as premedications for hypersensitivity and nausea (if necessary); treatment criteria; the sequence of medication administration; and the protocol name or number.[2,4]
- In collaboration with the patient's multidisciplinary team, review the patient's laboratory test results, specifically complete blood count, blood urea nitrogen level, platelet count, urine creatinine level, and liver function study results.[1]
- Review the patient's height, weight, and body surface area.[1]
- Verify that the prescribed medication dose is appropriate for the patient, diagnosis, and treatment plan. If you have concerns, consult with the prescribing practitioner or the pharmacist.[11,12,13]
- Have a second qualified health care worker independently verify the chemotherapy order before medication preparation, confirming the two patient identifiers, medication name, dose, medication volume, route of administration, calculation for dosing, and treatment cycle and day of cycle.[2,4]
- Familiarize yourself with the information contained within the MSDS specific to the prescribed drug.[1,14]
- Gather and prepare the appropriate equipment.
- Prepare the medication or obtain it from the pharmacy.
- When you receive the drug from the pharmacy, compare the medication label with the order in the patient's medical record.[11,12,13] Make sure that it's properly labeled with the patient's full name and a second identifier, full generic drug name, drug administration route, total dose to be given, total volume required to administer the dose, date of administration, and date and time of preparation and expiration. The container should also contain a label that clearly identifies the drug as hazardous.[2]
- If you must prepare the drug yourself, make sure you properly label it. (See the "Chemotherapeutic drug preparation and handling" procedure, page 169.)
- Check the expiration date on the medication. If the medication is expired, return it to the pharmacy and obtain new medication.[11,12,13]
- Visually inspect the solution for particles, discoloration, and other signs of loss of integrity; don't administer the medication if its integrity is compromised.[11,12,13]
- Wash your hands with soap and water.[15,16,17,18,19]
- Confirm the patient's identity using at least two patient identifiers.[20]
- Confirm that the patient received written educational material appropriate for his reading level and understanding and that the material includes information about his diagnosis, chemotherapy plan, possible long- and short-term adverse effects, risks associated with the regimen, reportable signs and symptoms, monitoring, sexual relations, contraception, special precautions, and follow-up care.[2,4]
- Review with the patient his current medications, including over-the-counter medications and complementary and alternative therapies; notify the practitioner of any changes.[2,11]
- Verify allergies, previous reactions, and treatment-related toxicities with the patient.[2,4]
- Administer any prescribed premedications following safe medication administration practices.[12,13]
- Ask the patient about any psychosocial concerns or cultural or spiritual issues that may affect treatment, and take action as indicated.[2]
- Assess the patient's clinical and performance status.[2]
- Obtain the patient's vital signs and current weight.[4]
- Recalculate the dose as ordered using the patient's body surface area, and check your calculations against the written order.[1]
- Determine the best site to administer the drug. When selecting the site, consider drug compatibilities, frequency of administration, and the vesicant and irritant potential of the drug; *continuous vesicant infusions shouldn't be administered through a peripheral IV catheter because of the risk of extravasation.*[14] (See *Classifying chemotherapeutic drugs.*) Use a central venous access catheter or implanted access device to administer a vesicant drug that will be infusing for longer than 30 minutes.[4]
- If a central venous access catheter or implanted port isn't available and the drug must be given through a peripheral IV catheter, avoid using a site that's more than 24 hours old[4] and assess the site for signs of inflammation or infiltration; if the integrity of the IV site is uncertain, insert a new IV catheter at another site.[4]
- To identify an administration site, examine the patient's veins, starting with his hand and proceeding to his forearm. Veins of choice are pliable and smooth; large veins of the forearm are preferred.[4] Select the smallest gauge and shortest catheter needed to accommodate the prescribed therapy, and avoid using of steel needles.[4,21] (See the "IV catheter insertion and removal" procedure, page 446.)

NURSING ALERT *If you're using a topical anesthetic before peripheral IV insertion, use one with a short duration of action* because longer-acting

Classifying chemotherapeutic drugs

To administer chemotherapy safely, you need to know each drug's potential for damaging tissue. In this regard, chemotherapeutic drugs are classified as vesicants, nonvesicants, or irritants.

Vesicants
- dactinomycin
- daunorubicin
- docetaxel
- doxorubicin
- epirubicin
- idarubicin
- mechlorethamine
- mitomycin
- mitoxantrone
- paclitaxel
- vinblastine
- vincristine sulfate PFS
- vinorelbine

Nonvesicants
- asparaginase
- cyclophosphamide
- cytarabine
- floxuridine
- fluorouracil

Irritants
- bleomycin
- carboplatin
- carmustine
- dacarbazine
- etoposide
- gemcitabine
- ifosfamide
- irinotecan
- melphalan
- streptozocin
- topotecan

Safe handling of chemotherapeutic agents

When preparing and administering chemotherapeutic agents, safe handling and personal protection must be strictly enforced to prevent accidental exposure to cytotoxic drugs. The National Institute for Occupational Safety and Health (NIOSH) recommends reducing exposure risk by using the following personal protective equipment.[5,23]

Gowns

- Use a disposable, lint-free gown made of polyethylene-coated materials; it should have long sleeves with tight-fitting cuffs. The gown shouldn't have seams or closures that could permit drugs to pass through it.
- Dispose of your gown after each use; *reusing a gown increases the risk of exposure to hazardous drugs.*
- Wear a gown whenever splashing or spilling is possible, such as when compounding drugs and administering them.
- Don't wear your gown outside the compounding or administration area *to avoid contaminating other areas with the hazardous drug.*
- If gown permeation information isn't available, change your gown every 2 to 3 hours or immediately if a spill or splash occurs.[4,5,23]

Gloves

- Use powder-free chemotherapy gloves.
- Wash your hands thoroughly with soap and water before putting on and after taking off gloves.
- Inspect gloves for defects before use.
- Remove and discard your gloves every 30 minutes; remove and discard them immediately if they become damaged and when contact with the drug is known or suspected.
- Wear two pairs of gloves when compounding, administering, and disposing of hazardous drugs. Wear the inner glove under the gown cuff and the outer glove over the cuff. Place gloves with long cuffs over the cuff of the gown *to protect the wrist and forearm.*
- Turn gloves inside-out when removing them *so that contaminated surfaces don't touch uncontaminated surfaces.*
- Wear sterile chemotherapy gloves when compounding sterile preparations.[4,5,23]

Face shield and goggles

- Wear a face shield and goggles whenever splashing is likely; *face shields alone don't provide adequate eye and face protection.*
- Wear a face shield and goggles when compounding a drug outside of the biological safety cabinet (BSC) or isolator (for example, in the operating room), working at or above eye level, cleaning a BSC or isolator, or cleaning a spill.

Respirators

- Use a NIOSH-approved, full-face-piece chemical cartridge-type respirator for large spills, such as when an IV bag breaks, a line disconnects and leaks, or known or suspected airborne exposure to vapors or gases occurs.[4,5,23]
- Consider all personal protective equipment worn when handling hazardous drugs as contaminated with hazardous drugs; contain and dispose of used personal protective equipment in a hazardous-waste container.
- According to NIOSH, cytotoxic drugs, including oral drugs that must be compounded or crushed, should be prepared in a primary engineering control (PEC), such as a BSC or a compounding sterile containment isolator. The PEC should provide vertical laminar airflow, eliminate exhaust with a high-efficiency particulate air (HEPA) filter (ideally, it should be vented outside), and have a continuously running blower. The room in which a BSC is located should be in a buffer area with negative pressure and be restricted to authorized personnel. Use of a PEC doesn't eliminate the need for personal protective equipment to prevent inhalation, direct skin contact, and direct eye contact.[4]
- Use tubing and syringes with luer-lock connectors. Spike IV bags and prime tubing with a compatible IV solution before adding the cytotoxic drug. Apply a label that reads CYTOTOXIC AGENT or a similar distinct warning, and wipe the outside of the container with moist gauze before placing it in a sealable bag for transport. Select a transport bag that can contain spillage if dropped. Label the outermost part of the bag *to indicate that the contents are hazardous.* Make sure that whoever transports the drug has access to a spill kit and knows how to use it.[4]
- Storage and labeling of chemotherapeutic agents should follow the facility's pharmacy guidelines. *To prevent accidental ingestion of cytotoxic agents,* never eat, drink, smoke, chew gum, apply cosmetics, or store food in areas where chemotherapy is prepared or administered. In addition, all personnel handling chemotherapeutic agents should have specific instructions related to hazardous waste and spill precautions.

topical anesthetics such as eutectic mixture of local anesthetics (EMLA) cream (lidocaine 2.5% and prilocaine 2.5%) may mask changes in sensation at the IV site that signal possible vesicant extravasation.[22]

- Wash your hands with soap and water.[15,16,17,18,19]
- Put on necessary protective equipment (two pairs of gloves, a gown, a face shield and goggles if splashing is likely, and a respirator, if necessary). Make sure your inner glove cuff is worn under the gown cuff and the outer glove cuff extends over the gown cuff *to fully protect your skin.* Inspect your gloves *to make sure they're physically intact.*[5,14] (See *Safe handling of chemotherapeutic agents.*) Wear personal protective equipment through all stages of handling and administering the drug. Change your gloves every 30 minutes. If a drug spill occurs or your gloves become punctured or torn, remove them immediately, wash your hands with soap and water, and then put on new gloves.[4]
- Establish blood return and patency regardless of the access type *to prevent extravasation injury.*[1,4]

NURSING ALERT *Don't test vein patency with a chemotherapeutic drug.* If the vein isn't patent, severe tissue damage can result. *Use preservative-free normal saline solution (or, less commonly, a dextrose 5% solution if the medication is incompatible with normal saline solution)* to assess patency and flush the IV device.[22,24]

- If your facility uses a bar code scanning system, scan your identification badge, the patient's identification bracelet, and the medication's bar code, as indicated by your facility's system.
- Thoroughly disinfect the injection port with an antiseptic pad using friction, and then allow it to dry.[25]
- If you're administering the drug by piggyback or short-term infusion, trace the tubing from the patient to its point of origin and then attach the tubing to the appropriate injection port using a needleless luer-lock connector. If you're administering by continuous infusion, trace the tubing from the patient to its point of origin and attach the tubing directly to the IV catheter or into a compatible line of maintenance IV solution. *Trace the tubing to make sure that you're connecting the tubing to the correct port before beginning the infusion.*[26] Secure all connections with luer-lock devices. If you're administering the drug by IV injection, refer to the practitioner's orders and pharmacy guidelines for recommended IV injection rates, diluents, and other drug-specific details.[4]

■ Use an electronic infusion pump for specific types of antineoplastic drugs and for all continuous infusions. When administering a vesicant, use a low-pressure, flow-control infusion device *to minimize pressure on the vein.*[1,4]
■ Have another individual who's qualified to prepare or administer chemotherapy perform an independent double-check to verify the patient's identity and make sure that the correct drug is prepared in the prescribed concentration and volume, the drug hasn't expired, the drug's indication corresponds with the patient's diagnosis, the dosage calculations are correct and the dosing formula used to derive the final dose is correct, the route of administration is safe and proper for the patient, the drug's integrity is intact, the infusion pump settings are correct, and the infusion line is attached to the correct port (if applicable) *to reduce the risk of medication errors.* Both you and the other qualified individual involved in the independent double-check should sign your names in the patient's medical record *to indicate that the verification took place.*[1,2,4,27]
■ Compare the results of the independent double-check. If discrepancies exist, rectify them before administering the drug.[27]
■ Begin administration as prescribed. Make sure that the administration tubing is clearly labeled *to alert staff members that a hazardous drug is being administered through the designated line.*[28]
■ During IV administration, closely monitor the patient for signs and symptoms of a hypersensitivity reaction (agitation, chest tightness, shortness of breath, hypotension, rash, itching, facial edema, light-headedness, dizziness, and abdominal cramping) or extravasation (swelling, redness, stinging, burning or pain at the access site, loss of blood return from the device, and IV flow rate slowing or stoppage).[4]
■ When administering a vesicant drug by short-term infusion using a peripheral vein, stay with the patient during the infusion. Monitor the site for extravasation and verify blood return every 5 to 10 minutes. When administering a vesicant by IV injection, verify blood return every 2 to 5 mL. When administering a vesicant through a central venous access device or implanted port, check for blood return periodically.[4]
■ After administration, place a fluid-impermeable pad underneath the connection site between the access device and administration tubing *to absorb drug droplets that may spill.* Disconnect the tubing from the access site, and then remove the IV container with the tubing attached; don't remove the spike from the IV container or reuse the tubing.[4]
■ Dispose of the IV container, tubing, and fluid-impermeable pad in a hazardous-waste receptacle. Dispose of syringes in a chemotherapy sharps container.[4,5]
■ Verify catheter patency[1] and then flush the catheter with a compatible IV solution.[4,24]
■ Lock the venous access device.[24]
■ Clean and decontaminate surfaces that might have come in contact with the drug.[4,5]
■ Remove and discard your personal protective equipment in a hazardous-waste receptacle. Remove and discard your gown and outer gloves first. Then remove and discard your inner gloves.[4,5]
■ Wash your hands with soap and water.[4,5,15,16,17,18,19]
■ Document the procedure.[29,30,31]

Special considerations

■ Be aware that verbal orders aren't permitted for chemotherapy agents, except to hold or stop chemotherapy administration.[2,4]
■ Monitor the patient's cumulative chemotherapy dose *to make sure that the drug is discontinued if the maximum lifetime dose is achieved.*[1]
■ Be aware that each chemotherapy agent has unique adverse effects. Assess and monitor the patient for anticipated adverse effects for the agent administered. Treatment-related toxicities should be evaluated, graded, and documented using standard definitions and criteria.[2]

Managing extravasation

Extravasation—the infiltration of a vesicant drug into the surrounding tissue—can result from a punctured vein or leakage around a venipuncture site. If vesicant drugs or fluids extravasate, blistering, peeling and sloughing of the skin, tissue necrosis; damage to tendons, nerves and joints; functional and sensory impairment of the affected area; and disfigurement can occur.[4,32]

Extravasation of vesicant drugs requires emergency treatment.[32] Essential steps include the following:
■ Immediately stop administering the vesicant and other IV fluids infusing through the access device.[4,32]
■ Disconnect the IV tubing from the access device, but don't remove the device or noncoring needle.[4,32]
■ Attempt to aspirate residual vesicant from the access device or noncoring needle using a small syringe (3 mL).[4,32]
■ Notify the practitioner.[4,32]
■ Remove the peripheral IV catheter or noncoring needle after the treatment plan has been determined.[4,32]
■ Use a standardized scale to assess and document the extent of the extravasation.[32]
■ Estimate the amount of solution that has escaped into the tissue based on the rate of injection or infusion and the length of time since your last assessment.[32]
■ Treat the site as prescribed; treatment may include elevating the extremity, cold or heat application, and antidote administration.[4,32]
■ Surgical intervention may be necessary in some cases.

■ If some of the chemotherapy drug comes in contact with your skin, thoroughly wash the involved area with soap (not a germicidal agent) and water. If eye contact occurs, flood the eye with water or saline solution for at least 15 minutes while holding the eyelid open. Obtain a medical evaluation as soon as possible after accidental exposure.[4]
■ If a spill occurs, use a chemotherapy spill kit to clean the area. Post a sign to warn others. Wear all personal protective equipment (double gloves, a gown, face shield or goggles, booties, and a respirator if aerosolization is possible) when cleaning the spill. Report and document the spill appropriately.[4]
■ If you suspect extravasation, stop the infusion immediately,[32] leave the IV catheter in place, and notify the practitioner. (See *Managing extravasation.*)
■ During infusion, some drugs need protection from direct sunlight *to avoid possible drug breakdown.* In this case, cover the container with a brown paper bag or aluminum foil.

Patient teaching

Before a patient begins a chemotherapy regimen, provide written or electronic information about his diagnosis, the goals of therapy, the planned schedule and duration of chemotherapy, the possible short- and long-term adverse effects, and regimen- or drug-specific signs and symptoms that require medical attention. The information should include emergency contact information for the practice or organization, signs and symptoms that should trigger a call, and the person who should be called. Also provide a plan for monitoring and follow-up care. Make sure that the materials provided are appropriate for the patient or caregiver's reading and comprehension level.[2]

Tell the patient that for the first 48 hours after receiving a dose of chemotherapy, when he voids, he should close the lid and flush the toilet at least two times. Teach the patient and his family how to handle contaminated bed linens and clothing. Suggest that, while wearing gloves, they place contaminated items in a pillowcase and then machine wash them twice in hot water with regular detergent separately from other household items. Have them dispose of used gloves in an appropriately labeled hazardous-waste container.[4]

Complications

Common adverse effects of chemotherapy are nausea and vomiting, ranging from mild to debilitating. Bone marrow suppression, another major complication, can lead to neutropenia and thrombocytopenia. Other adverse effects include intestinal irritation, stomatitis, pulmonary fibrosis, cardiotoxicity, nephrotoxicity, neurotoxicity, hearing loss, anemia, alopecia, urticaria, radiation recall (if drugs are given with, or soon after, radiation therapy), anorexia, esophagitis, diarrhea, and constipation.

IV administration of chemotherapeutic drugs can also lead to phlebitis; cellulitis; thrombosis; extravasation causing blistering, peeling, and sloughing of the skin; tissue necrosis; damage to tendons, nerves, and joints; functional and sensory impairment of the affected area; and disfigurement.

Documentation

Facilities commonly require nursing documentation on a chemotherapy flow sheet. Document according to your facility's documentation system. Record any premedication administered before the procedure. Document the location and description of the access site and verification of blood return. Also record the drugs, dosages, route of administration, sequence of drug administration, needle type and size used, amount and type of flushing solution, and the site's condition after treatment. Document any adverse reactions, the patient's tolerance of the treatment, teaching provided to the patient and family, and their understanding of that teaching. Record any treatment required after chemotherapy administration.

REFERENCES

1 Standard 62. Antineoplastic therapy. Infusion nursing standards of practice. (2011). *Journal of Infusion Nursing, 34,* S87–S89. (Level VII)

2 Neuss, M. N., et al. (2013). "2013 updated American Society of Clinical Oncology/Oncology Nursing Society chemotherapy administration safety standards including standards for the safe administration and management of oral chemotherapy" [Online]. Accessed March 2015 via the Web at http://www.asco.org/sites/www.asco.org/files/oral_standards_jop_article.pdf (Level VII)

3 Hinkle, J. L., & Cheever, K. H. (2014). *Brunner & Suddarth's textbook of medical-surgical nursing* (13th ed.). Philadelphia, PA: Wolters Kluwer.

4 Polovich, M., et al. (Eds.). (2014). *Chemotherapy and biotherapy guidelines and recommendations for practice* (4th ed.). Pittsburgh, PA: Oncology Nursing Society.

5 National Institute for Occupational Safety and Health (NIOSH). (2004). "NIOSH alert: Preventing occupational exposures to antineoplastic and other hazardous drugs in health care settings" [Online]. Accessed March 2015 via the Web at http://www.cdc.gov/niosh/docs/2004-165/pdfs/2004-165.pdf (Level VII)

6 Westbrook, J., et al. (2010). Association of interruptions with an increased risk and severity of medication administration errors. *Archives of Internal Medicine, 170,* 683–690. (Level IV)

7 Institute for Safe Medication Practices. (2013). Side tracks on the safety express: Interruptions lead to errors and unfinished . . . Wait, what was I doing? *Nurse Advise-ERR, 11*(2), 1–4. Accessed March 2015 via the Web at https://www.ismp.org/Newsletters/acutecare/showarticle.aspx?id=37

8 American Osteopathic Association. (2014). Standard 15.01.11. *Healthcare Facilities Accreditation Program: Accreditation requirements for acute care hospitals.* Chicago, IL: American Osteopathic Association. (Level VII)

9 The Joint Commission. (2015). Standard RI.01.03.01. *Comprehensive accreditation manual for hospitals: The official handbook.* Oakbrook Terrace, IL: The Joint Commission. (Level VII)

10 Centers for Medicare & Medicaid Services, Department of Health and Human Services. (2014). Condition of participation: Patient's rights. 42 C.F.R. § 482.13(b)(2).

11 The Joint Commission. (2015). Standard MM.06.01.01. *Comprehensive accreditation manual for hospitals: The official handbook.* Oakbrook Terrace, IL: The Joint Commission. (Level VII)

12 Centers for Medicare & Medicaid Services, Department of Health and Human Services. (2014). Condition of participation: Nursing services. 42 C.F.R. § 482.23(c).

13 American Osteopathic Association. (2014). Standard 16.01.03. *Healthcare Facilities Accreditation Program: Accreditation requirements for acute care hospitals.* Chicago, IL: American Osteopathic Association. (Level VII)

14 Occupational Safety and Health Administration (OSHA). (1999). "OSHA technical manual: Controlling occupational exposure to hazardous drugs" [Online]. Accessed March 2015 via the Web at http://www.osha.gov/dts/osta/otm/otm_vi/otm_vi_2.html (Level I)

15 The Joint Commission. (2015). Standard NPSG.07.01.01. *Comprehensive accreditation manual for hospitals: The official handbook.* Oakbrook Terrace, IL: The Joint Commission. (Level VII)

16 Centers for Disease Control and Prevention. (2002). Guideline for hand hygiene in health-care settings: Recommendations of the Healthcare Infection Control Practices Advisory Committee and the HICPAC/SHEA/APIC/IDSA Hand Hygiene Task Force. *MMWR Recommendations and Reports, 51*(RR-16), 1–45. Accessed March 2015 via the Web at http://www.cdc.gov/mmwr/pdf/rr/rr5116.pdf (Level II)

17 World Health Organization. (2009). "WHO guidelines on hand hygiene in health care: First global patient safety challenge, clean care is safer care" [Online]. Accessed March 2015 via the Web at http://whqlibdoc.who.int/publications/2009/9789241597906_eng.pdf (Level IV)

18 Centers for Medicare & Medicaid Services, Department of Health and Human Services. (2014). Condition of participation: Infection control. 42 C.F.R. § 482.42.

19 American Osteopathic Association. (2014). Standard 07.01.21. *Healthcare Facilities Accreditation Program: Accreditation requirements for acute care hospitals.* Chicago, IL: American Osteopathic Association. (Level VII)

20 The Joint Commission. (2015). Standard NPSG.01.01.01. *Comprehensive accreditation manual for hospitals: The official handbook.* Oakbrook Terrace, IL: The Joint Commission. (Level VII)

21 Standard 32. Vascular access device selection. Infusion nursing standards of practice. (2011). *Journal of Infusion Nursing, 34,* S37–S40. (Level VII)

22 Schulmeister, L. (2010). Preventing and managing vesicant chemotherapy extravasations. *Journal of Supportive Oncology, 8,* 212–215. Accessed March 2015 via the Web at http://www.oncologypractice.com/jso/journal/articles/0805212.pdf

23 National Institute for Occupational Safety and Health (NIOSH). (2008). "Workplace solutions: Personal protective equipment for health care workers who work with hazardous drugs" [Online]. Accessed March 2015 via the Web at http://www.cdc.gov/niosh/docs/wp-solutions/2009-106/pdfs/2009-106.pdf (Level VII)

24 Standard 45. Flushing and locking. Infusion nursing standards of practice. (2011). *Journal of Infusion Nursing, 34,* S59–S63. (Level VII)

25 Standard 27. Needleless connectors. Infusion nursing standards of practice. (2011). *Journal of Infusion Nursing, 34,* S32–S33. (Level VII)

26 U.S. Food and Drug Administration. (n.d.). "Look. Check. Connect. Safe medical device connections save lives" [Online]. Accessed March 2015 via the Web at http://www.fda.gov/downloads/MedicalDevices/Safety/AlertsandNotices/UCM134873.pdf

27 Institute for Safe Medication Practices. (2008). Conducting an independent double-check. *ISMP Medication Safety Alert! Nurse Advise-ERR, 6*(12), 1. Accessed March 2015 via the Web at http://www.ismp.org/newsletters/nursing/Issues/NurseAdviseERR200812.pdf (Level VII)

28 Institute for Safe Medication Practices. (2012). "ISMP's list of high-alert medications" [Online]. Accessed March 2015 via the Web at http://www.ismp.org/tools/highalertmedications.pdf (Level VII)

29 The Joint Commission. (2015). Standard RC.01.03.01. *Comprehensive accreditation manual for hospitals: The official handbook.* Oakbrook Terrace, IL: The Joint Commission. (Level VII)

30 Centers for Medicare & Medicaid Services, Department of Health and Human Services. (2014). Condition of participation: Medical record services. 42 C.F.R. § 482.24(b).
31 American Osteopathic Association. (2014). Standard 10.00.03. *Healthcare Facilities Accreditation Program: Accreditation requirements for acute care hospitals.* Chicago, IL: American Osteopathic Association. (Level VII)
32 Standard 48. Infiltration and extravasation. Infusion nursing standards of practice. (2011). *Journal of Infusion Nursing, 34,* S66–S68. (Level VII)

ADDITIONAL REFERENCES

Beatty, K., et al. (2011). Advances in oncology care: Targeted therapies. *AACN Advanced Critical Care, 22,* 323–334.
Bertoglio, S., et al. (2012). Efficacy of normal saline versus heparinized saline solution for locking catheters of totally implantable long-term central vascular access devices in adult cancer patients. *Cancer Nursing, 35*(4), E35–E42. (Level IV)
Camp-Sorrell, M., & Camp-Sorrell, D. (2010). *Access device guidelines: Recommendations for nursing practice and education* (3rd ed.). Pittsburgh, PA: Oncology Nursing Society. (Level VII)
Schulmeister, L. (2011). Extravasation management: Clinical update. *Seminars in Oncology Nursing, 27,* 82–90.

CHEMOTHERAPEUTIC DRUG PREPARATION AND HANDLING

Nurses should take extra care when preparing chemotherapeutic drugs, both for the patient's safety and for their own. Patients who receive chemotherapeutic drugs risk teratogenic, mutagenic, and carcinogenic effects,[1] but the people who prepare and handle the drugs are at risk as well. According to the Occupational Safety and Health Administration (OSHA), no acceptable levels of exposure have been determined for these drugs and some drugs exhibit toxicity at low doses;[1] because of this, the goal is to prevent or minimize workplace exposure.

OSHA, the National Institute for Occupational Safety and Health (NIOSH), the American Society of Health System Pharmacists, and the Oncology Nursing Society have established guidelines for handling and administering chemotherapeutic drugs. These guidelines are strongly recommended; adhering to them will reduce the risk of contamination to both yourself and your environment.

The use of proper personal protective equipment is essential.[2] Personal protective equipment must include chemotherapy-resistant gowns and gloves, which should be worn when handling, preparing, and priming administration sets; administering or disposing of chemotherapeutic agents; cleaning up spills; and handling excreta.[3] Gowns should be lint-free, have a full front and back closure, and have elastic or knit cuffs. They should be worn once and discarded appropriately; they should never be worn for multiple patients or worn multiple times for the same patient. Hanging up a used gown is prohibited. Double-gloving is recommended, and gloves need to be replaced every 30 minutes, when visibly contaminated, and after each individual patient contact. A face mask and goggles should also be worn when splashing is likely.[4] A face mask and a NIOSH-approved respirator should be worn when cleaning up chemotherapy spills. Surgical masks shouldn't be used because they aren't effective against aerosolization of chemotherapeutic drugs.

All health care workers who handle chemotherapeutic drugs must be properly educated and trained.[2,5] A requirement of such training involves learning how to reduce exposure when handling the drugs.[6] A second requirement states that the drugs should be prepared in a class II biological safety cabinet.[6]

OSHA guidelines further recommend that chemotherapeutic drugs be mixed in a properly enclosed and ventilated work area and that respiratory and skin protection be worn.[6] Smoking, drinking, applying cosmetics, and eating where these drugs are prepared, stored, or used should be strictly prohibited, and sterile technique should be used while mixing these drugs.

Gloves, gowns, syringes or vials, and other materials that have been used in chemotherapeutic preparation and administration present a possible source of exposure or injury to the facility's staff members, patients, and visitors; using properly labeled, sealed, and covered containers, handled only by trained and protected personnel, should be routine practice.[6] Spills also present a hazard, and all employees should be familiar with appropriate spill procedures for their own protection.[6]

Equipment

Material safety data sheet (MSDS) for each prescribed chemotherapy drug ▪ prescribed drug or drugs ▪ patient's medication record ▪ nonlinting, nonabsorbent disposable gown ▪ powder-free chemotherapy gloves ▪ face shield ▪ goggles ▪ NIOSH-approved respirator mask (if aerosolization is likely) ▪ plastic absorbent pad ▪ sterile gauze pads ▪ hazardous-waste container ▪ IV solution ▪ compatibility reference source ▪ medication labels ▪ class II biological safety cabinet ▪ disposable towel ▪ syringes and needles of various sizes with luer-lock connectors ▪ IV tubing with luer-lock fittings ▪ infusion pump (preferably a smart pump with dose-range alerts)[2] ▪ chemotherapy spill kit ▪ Optional: booties, closed system transfer devices.

Preparation of equipment

Make sure that a chemotherapy spill kit is readily available.

Implementation

- Be familiar with the information contained within the MSDS for each prescribed chemotherapy drug.[2,6]
- Gather the appropriate equipment.
- Verify the practitioner's written order,[2] and have a second practitioner who's qualified to prepare or administer chemotherapy verify the order independently.[5] Keep in mind that verbal orders aren't permitted for chemotherapeutic agents, except to hold or stop administrion.[2,3,5]
- Confirm that the practitioner has obtained written informed consent from the patient and that the consent is in the patient's medical record.[5,7,8,9]
- Wash your hands with soap and water.[3,10,11,12,13,14]
- Put on personal protective equipment (two pairs of gloves, a gown, a face shield [when splashing is possible], and a respirator, if necessary).[4] Make sure your inner glove cuff is worn under the gown cuff and the outer glove cuff extends over the gown cuff *to fully protect your skin.* Inspect your gloves *to make sure they're physically intact.*[3,4]
- When working with chemotherapeutic drugs, change your gloves every 30 minutes. If you spill a drug solution on your gloves or puncture or tear a glove, remove your gloves immediately. Wash your hands with soap and water before putting on new gloves and any time you remove your gloves.[3,4,6,10,11,12,13,14]
- Maintain sterile technique when compounding these hazardous drugs.[15,16,17]
- Wear personal protective equipment and take care when unpacking chemotherapy vials *to reduce exposure. The exteriors of chemotherapy vials have been found to be contaminated upon arrival from the manufacturers.*[3,4]
- Prepare the drugs in a class II biological safety cabinet.[4,6] Leave the hood blower turned on 24 hours per day, 7 days per week.[3]
- Before you prepare the drug (and after you finish), clean the internal surfaces of the cabinet with 70% alcohol and a disposable towel. Discard the towel in a hazardous-waste container approved for cytotoxic waste.[6]
- Cover the work surface with a clean plastic absorbent pad *to minimize contamination by droplets or spills.* Change the pad at the end of the shift or whenever a spill occurs.[6]
- Consider all of the equipment used in drug preparation, as well as any unused drug, as hazardous waste.[4,6] Dispose of all equipment appropriately.

- Always work below eye level *to prevent accidental exposure to the eyes.*[3]
- Prepare the drug according to current product instructions, paying attention to compatibility, stability, and reconstitution technique.
- Label the prepared drug with the patient's name and a second identifier; drug's full generic name; drug administration route; total dose to be administered; total volume required to administer the dosage; date of administration; date and time of drug expiration; and special handling instructions as appropriate.[5] Also label all chemotherapeutic drugs with a hazardous-drug label, such as one that states CYTOTOXIC AGENT.[4,6]
- Prime all IV bags with a compatible fluid before adding the chemotherapeutic drug.[3]
- Wipe the exterior of the IV bag or syringe with sterile gauze before placing it in a sealed bag for transport.[3]
- Clean and decontaminate all work surfaces that may have come in contact with the hazardous drug.[3]
- Remove and discard your personal protective equipment before leaving the work area.[4,18]
- Wash your hands with soap and water.[3,10,11,12,13,14]
- Put on protective equipment (two pairs of gloves, a gown, a face shield [when splashing is possible], and a respirator, if necessary). Make sure your inner glove cuff is worn under the gown cuff and the outer glove cuff extends over the gown cuff *to fully protect your skin.* Inspect your gloves *to make sure they're physically intact.*[3,4]
- Confirm the patient's identity using at least two patient identifiers.[19]

NURSING ALERT *Chemotherapy drugs are considered high-alert medications* because they can cause significant patient harm when used in error. *Before administering the drug, have another individual who's qualified to prepare or administer chemotherapy perform an independent double-check.*[5,20]

- Have a second individual who's qualified to prepare or administer chemotherapy perform an independent double-check to verify the patient's identity and to make sure that the correct drug is prepared in the prescribed concentration and volume; the drug hasn't expired; the drug's indication corresponds with the patient's diagnosis; the dosage calculations are correct and the dosing formula used to derive the final dose is correct; the route of administration is safe and proper for the patient; the drug's integrity is intact; the infusion pump settings are correct; and the infusion line is attached to the correct port (if applicable) *to reduce the risk of medication errors.* Both you and the other practitioner involved in the independent double-check should sign your names in the patient's medical record *to indicate that the verification took place.*[2,5,21]
- After comparing results of the independent double-check with the other individual, if discrepancies exist, rectify them before administering the drug.
- Confirm with the patient his planned treatment before drug administration.[5]
- Place a plastic absorbent pad under the infusion site *to absorb any medication spillage.*
- Consider all of the equipment used in drug preparation, as well as any unused drug, as hazardous waste.[3]
- Place all chemotherapeutic waste products in a hazardous-waste container.[3,6]
- After drug administration, remove the intact IV container and tubing. Don't remove the spike from the IV container or reuse the tubing.
- Discard the solution container and IV tubing in a hazardous-waste container.[3,6]
- Remove and discard your personal protective equipment appropriately. Remove and discard your outer gloves and gown first. Then remove your inner gloves.[3]
- Wash your hands with soap and water.[3,10,11,12,13,14]
- Document the procedure.[22,23,24]

Special considerations

- Use resources to evaluate the hazard potential of the prescribed drug,[1] including the drug's MSDS; product labeling approved by the U.S. Food and Drug Administration (FDA); special health warnings from drug manufacturers, the FDA, and other professional organizations; reports and case studies published in medical and other professional health care journals; and evidence-based recommendations from other institutions that meet the criteria defining hazardous drugs.
- Take precautions to reduce your exposure to chemotherapeutic drugs. *Systemic absorption can occur through ingestion of contaminated materials, contact with the skin, or inhalation.* You can inhale a drug without realizing it, such as while opening a vial, clipping a needle, expelling air from a syringe, or discarding excess drug. You can also absorb a drug from handling contaminated stools or body fluids.[25]
- Use only syringes and IV sets that have luer-lock fittings.
- Note that gloves, gowns, syringes or vials, and other materials that have been used in chemotherapeutic preparation and administration present a source of contamination to the facility's staff members, patients, visitors, and environment; using properly labeled, sealed, and enclosed containers for discarded equipment handled only by trained and protected personnel should be routine practice.[4]
- If some of the drug comes in contact with your skin, wash the involved area thoroughly with soap (not a germicidal agent) and water. If eye contact occurs, flood the eye with water or saline solution for at least 15 minutes while holding the eyelid open. Obtain a medical evaluation as soon as possible after accidental exposure.[3]
- If a spill occurs, use a chemotherapeutic spill kit to clean the area. Wear all personal protective equipment (double gloves and a gown), including a respirator mask, goggles, and booties. Post a sign to warn others. Follow you facility's guidelines for hazardous spills. Report and document the spill as directed by your facility.[3,4]
- Don't place any food or drinks in the same refrigerator as chemotherapeutic drugs.[4] For accidental ingestion, don't induce vomiting unless indicated by the MSDS. Seek emergency treatment.[3]
- Become familiar with drug excretion patterns, and use chemotherapeutic-resistant personal protective equipment (double gloves, a gown, and a face shield) when handling a chemotherapy patient's body fluids and excreta for the first 48 hours after the patient receives chemotherapy.[3]
- Provide male patients with a urinal with a tight-fitting lid.
- Before flushing the toilet, place a waterproof pad over the toilet bowl *to prevent splashing.*
- Wear chemotherapy-resistant gloves and a gown when handling linens soiled with body fluids. Place soiled linens in isolation linen bags designated for separate laundering.
- Note that women who are pregnant, trying to conceive, or breastfeeding shouldn't be exposed to chemotherapeutic drugs.[2,3,6,26]

Patient teaching

Before a patient starts chemotherapy, provide him with written information about his diagnosis, the goal of therapy, the duration of chemotherapy (including the drugs he will receive and the schedule), possible short- and long-term adverse effects, drug-specific risks that require the practitioner to be notified, and follow-up.[5] When teaching a patient about handling chemotherapeutic drugs, discuss appropriate safety measures. If the patient will be receiving chemotherapy at home, teach him how to dispose of contaminated equipment. Tell the patient and his family to wear gloves whenever handling chemotherapy equipment or contaminated linens or gowns and pajamas. Instruct them to place soiled linens in a separate, washable pillowcase and to launder the pillowcase twice, with the soiled linens inside, separately from other linens.

When providing home care, empty waste products into the toilet close to the water *to minimize splashing.* Close the lid and flush at least two times.

All materials used for treatment should be placed in a leak-proof container and taken to a designated disposal area. The patient or his family should make arrangements with either a health care facility or private company for pickup and proper disposal of contaminated waste.

Complications

Long-term or chronic effects of chemotherapeutic drug exposure that have been identified include damage to the liver, kidneys, bone marrow, lungs, and heart; infertility (temporary and permanent); effects on reproduction and the developing fetus in pregnant women; hearing impairment; and cancer.[4] Direct exposure to these drugs may burn and damage the skin.

Documentation

Document each incidence of exposure according to your facility's guidelines.

REFERENCES

1 National Institute for Occupational Safety and Health (NIOSH). (2012). "NIOSH list of antineoplastic and other hazardous drugs in healthcare settings 2012 [NIOSH Publication Number 2012-150]" [Online]. Accessed March 2015 via the Web at http://www.cdc.gov/niosh/docs/2012-150/pdfs/2012-150.pdf

2 Standard 62. Antineoplastic therapy. Infusion nursing standards of practice. (2011). *Journal of Infusion Nursing, 34,* S87–S89. (Level VII)

3 Polovich, M., et al. (Eds.). (2014). *Chemotherapy and biotherapy guidelines and recommendations for practice* (4th ed.). Pittsburgh, PA: Oncology Nursing Society.

4 National Institute for Occupational Safety and Health (NIOSH). (2004). "NIOSH alert: Preventing occupational exposure to antineoplastic and other hazardous drugs in health care settings" [Online]. Accessed March 2015 via the Web at http://www.cdc.gov/niosh/docs/2004-165/pdfs/2004-165.pdf (Level VII)

5 Neuss, M. N., et al. (2013). "2013 Updated American Society of Clinical Oncology/Oncology Nursing Society chemotherapy administration safety standards including standards for the safe administration and management of oral chemotherapy" [Online]. Accessed March 2015 via the Web at http://www.asco.org/sites/www.asco.org/files/oral_standards_jop_article.pdf (Level VII)

6 Occupational Safety & Health Administration. (1999). "OSHA technical manual: Controlling occupational exposure to harmful drugs" [Online]. Accessed March 2015 via the Web at http://www.osha.gov/dts/osta/otm/otm_vi/otm_vi_2.html (Level I)

7 The Joint Commission. (2015). Standard RI.01.03.01. *Comprehensive accreditation manual for hospitals: The official handbook.* Oakbrook Terrace, IL: The Joint Commission. (Level VII)

8 Centers for Medicare & Medicaid Services, Department of Health and Human Services. (2014). Condition of participation: Patient's rights. 42 C.F.R. § 482.13(b)(2).

9 American Osteopathic Association. (2014). Standard 15.01.11. *Healthcare Facilities Accreditation Program: Accreditation requirements for acute care hospitals.* Chicago, IL: American Osteopathic Association. (Level VII)

10 Centers for Disease Control and Prevention. (2002). Guideline for hand hygiene in health-care settings: Recommendations of the Healthcare Infection Control Practices Advisory Committee and the HICPAC/SHEA/APIC/IDSA Hand Hygiene Task Force. *MMWR Recommendations and Reports, 51*(RR-16), 1–45. Accessed March 2015 via the Web at http://www.cdc.gov/mmwr/pdf/rr/rr5116.pdf (Level II)

11 The Joint Commission. (2015). Standard NPSG.07.01.01. *Comprehensive accreditation manual for hospitals: The official handbook.* Oakbrook Terrace, IL: The Joint Commission. (Level VII)

12 World Health Organization. (2009). "WHO guidelines on hand hygiene in health care: First global patient safety challenge, clean care is safer care" [Online]. Accessed March 2015 via the Web at http://whqlibdoc.who.int/publications/2009/9789241597906_eng.pdf (Level IV)

13 Centers for Medicare & Medicaid Services, Department of Health and Human Services. (2014). Condition of participation: Infection control. 42 C.F.R. § 482.42.

14 American Osteopathic Association. (2014). Standard 07.01.21. *Healthcare Facilities Accreditation Program: Accreditation requirements for acute care hospitals.* Chicago, IL: American Osteopathic Association. (Level VII)

15 The Joint Commission. (2015). Standard MM.05.01.07. *Comprehensive accreditation manual for hospitals: The official handbook.* Oakbrook Terrace, IL: The Joint Commission. (Level VII)

16 Centers for Medicare & Medicaid Services, Department of Health and Human Services. (2014). Condition of participation: Nursing services. 42 C.F.R. § 482.23(c).

17 American Osteopathic Association. (2014). Standard 16.01.03. *Healthcare Facilities Accreditation Program: Accreditation requirements for acute care hospitals.* Chicago, IL: American Osteopathic Association. (Level VII)

18 Siegel, J. D., et al. (2007). "2007 guideline for isolation precautions: Preventing transmission of infectious agents in healthcare settings" [Online]. Accessed March 2015 via the Web at http://www.cdc.gov/hicpac/pdf/isolation/Isolation2007.pdf (Level II)

19 The Joint Commission. (2015). Standard NPSG.01.01.01. *Comprehensive accreditation manual for hospitals: The official handbook.* Oakbrook Terrace, IL: The Joint Commission. (Level VII)

20 Institute for Safe Medication Practices. (2012). "ISMP's list of high-alert medications" [Online]. Accessed March 2015 via the Web at http://www.ismp.org/tools/highalertmedications.pdf (Level VII)

21 Institute for Safe Medication Practices. (2008). Conducting an independent double-check. *ISMP Medication Safety Alert! Nurse Advise-ERR, 6*(12), 1. Accessed March 2015 via the Web at http://www.ismp.org/newsletters/nursing/Issues/NurseAdviseERR200812.pdf (Level VII)

22 The Joint Commission. (2015). Standard RC.01.03.01. *Comprehensive accreditation manual for hospitals: The official handbook.* Oakbrook Terrace, IL: The Joint Commission. (Level VII)

23 Centers for Medicare & Medicaid Services, Department of Health and Human Services. (2014). Condition of participation: Medical record services. 42 C.F.R. § 482.24(b).

24 American Osteopathic Association. (2014). Standard 10.00.03. *Healthcare Facilities Accreditation Program: Accreditation requirements for acute care hospitals.* Chicago, IL: American Osteopathic Association. (Level VII)

25 Elshamy, K., et al. (2010). Health hazards among oncology nurses exposed to chemotherapy drugs. *African Journal of Haematology/Oncology, 1,* 70–78. Accessed March 2015 via the Web at http://www.afjho.com/index.php/AJOHAO/article/download/20/32 (Level VI)

26 Lawson, C. C., et al. (2012). Occupational exposures among nurses and risk of spontaneous abortion. *American Journal of Obstetrics and Gynecology, 206,* 327.e1–327.e8. (Level IV)

ADDITIONAL REFERENCE

American Society of Health System Pharmacists. (2006). "ASHP Guidelines on handling hazardous drugs." *Drug Distribution and Control: Preparation and Handling Guidelines, 63,* 1172–1193 [Online]. Accessed March 2015 via the Web at http://www.ashp.org/s_ashp/docs/files/BP07/Prep_Gdl_HazDrugs.pdf

CHEST PHYSIOTHERAPY

Chest physiotherapy includes postural drainage, chest percussion and vibration, and coughing and deep-breathing exercises. Together, these techniques mobilize secretions, help to reexpand alveoli, and promote efficient use of respiratory muscles.

Postural drainage performed in conjunction with percussion and vibration encourages peripheral pulmonary secretions to mobilize into the major bronchi or trachea and is accomplished by sequential repositioning of the patient. Secretions usually drain best with the patient positioned so that the bronchi are perpendicular to the floor, such as with the semi- or high-Fowler position. Lower and middle lobe bronchi usually empty best with the patient in the head-down position; upper lobe bronchi, in the head-up position. (See *Positioning patients for postural drainage,* page 172.)

Positioning patients for postural drainage

The following illustrations show the various postural drainage positions and the areas of the lungs affected by each. Before beginning, assess whether the patient can tolerate the recommended positioning; once the patient is positioned, perform ongoing assessments *to determine continued tolerance.*

Lower lobes: Posterior basal segments

Elevate the foot of the bed 30 degrees. Have the patient lie prone with his head lowered. Position pillows under his chest and abdomen. Percuss his lower ribs on both sides of his spine.

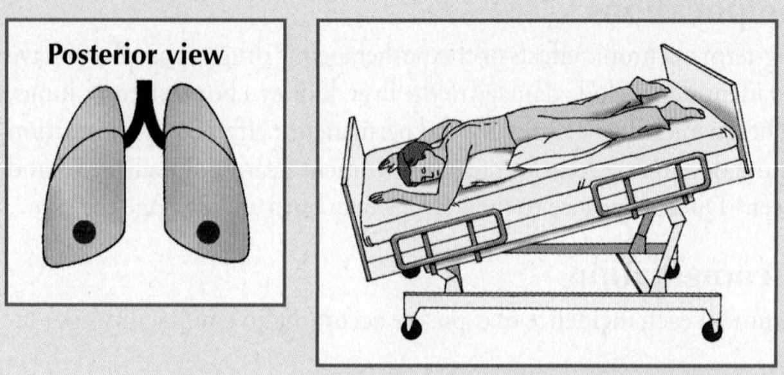

Lower lobes: Lateral basal segments

Elevate the foot of the bed 30 degrees. Instruct the patient to lie on his abdomen with his head lowered and his upper leg flexed over a pillow *for support.* Then have him rotate a quarter turn upward. Percuss his lower ribs on the uppermost portion of his lateral chest wall.

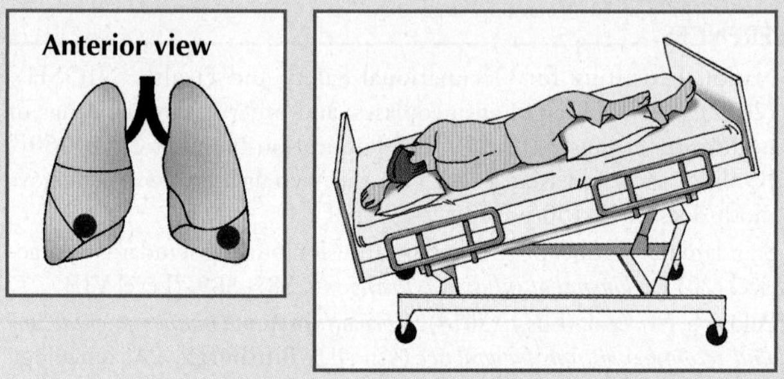

Lower lobes: Anterior basal segments

Elevate the foot of the bed 30 degrees. Instruct the patient to lie on his side with his head lowered. Then place pillows under his head and between his knees. Percuss with a slightly cupped hand over the lower ribs just beneath the axilla. If an acutely ill patient has trouble breathing in this position, adjust the bed to an angle he can tolerate. Then begin percussion.

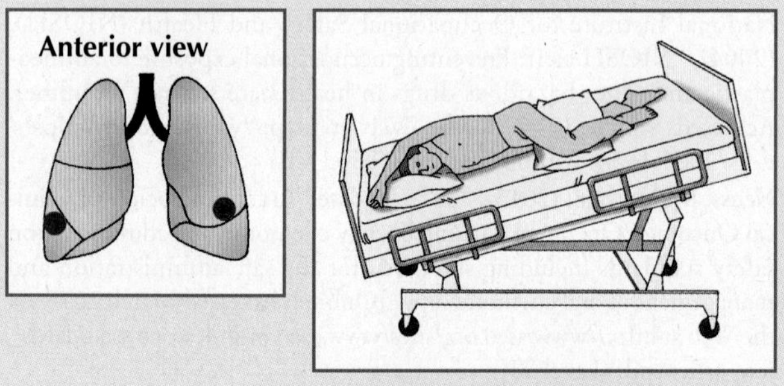

Lower lobes: Superior segments

With the bed flat, have the patient lie on his abdomen. Place two pillows under his hips. Percuss on both sides of his spine at the lower tip of his scapulae.

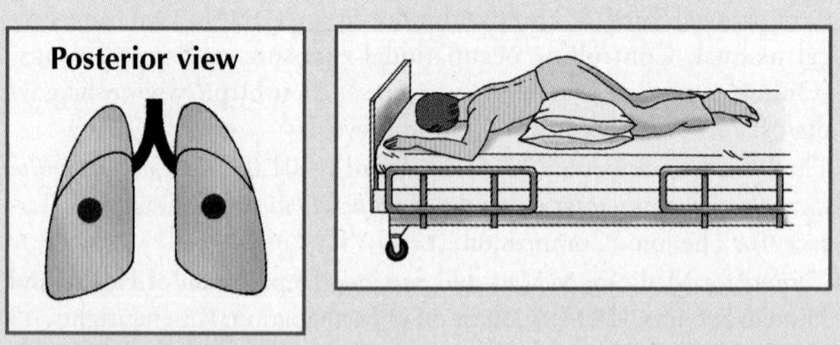

Right middle lobe: Medial and lateral segments

Elevate the foot of the bed 15 degrees. Have the patient lie on his left side with his head down and his knees flexed. Then have him rotate a quarter turn backward. Place a pillow beneath him. Percuss with your hand moderately cupped under the right nipple. For a female patient, cup your hand so that its heel is under the armpit and your fingers extend forward beneath the breast.

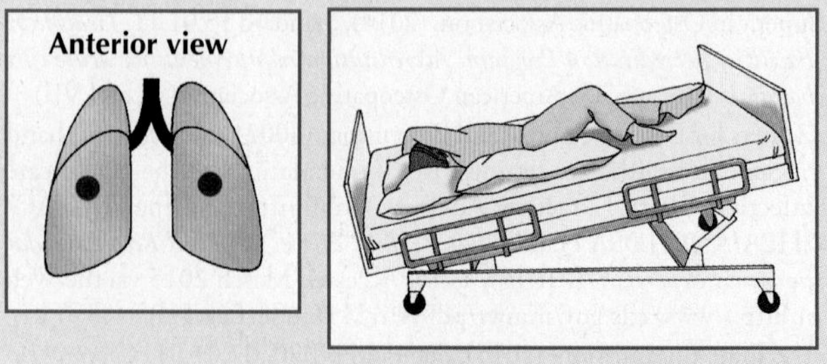

(continued)

Positioning patients for postural drainage *(continued)*

Left upper lobe: Superior and inferior segments, lingular portion

Elevate the foot of the bed 15 degrees. Have the patient lie on his right side with his head down and knees flexed. Then have him rotate a quarter turn backward. Place a pillow behind him, from shoulders to hips. Percuss with your hand moderately cupped over his left nipple. For a female patient, cup your hand so that its heel is beneath the armpit and your fingers extend forward beneath the breast.

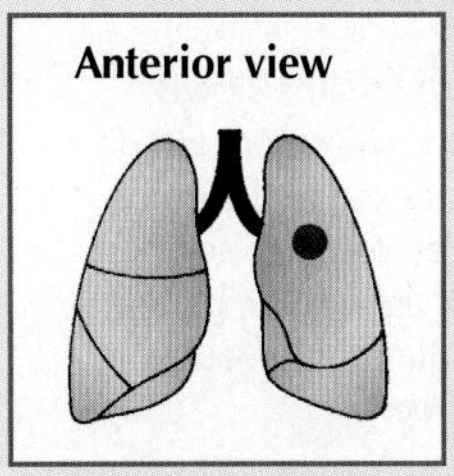

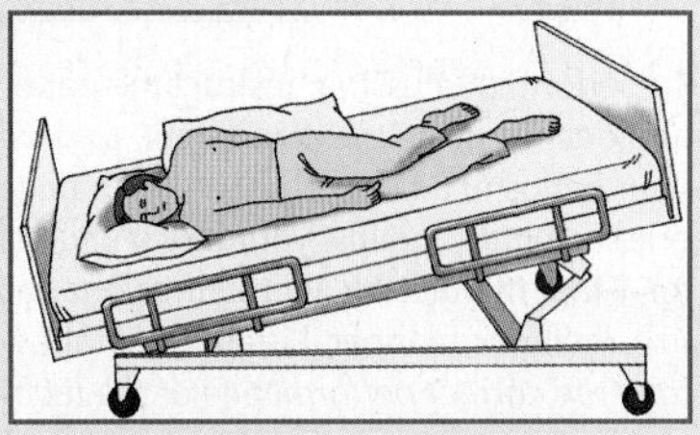

Upper lobes: Anterior segments

Make sure the bed is flat. Have the patient lie on his back with a pillow folded under his knees. Then have him rotate slightly away from the side being drained. Percuss between his clavicle and nipple.

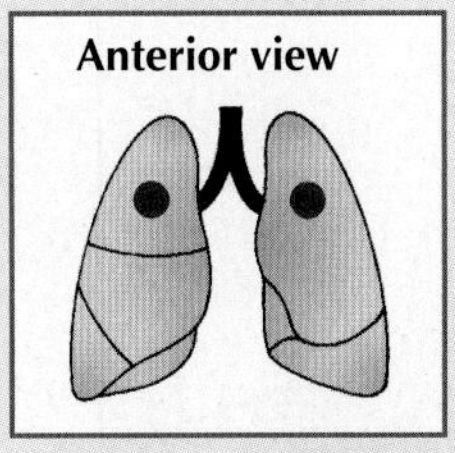

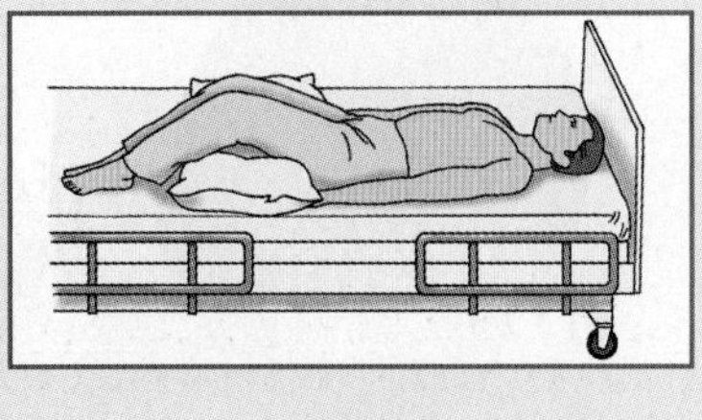

Upper lobes: Apical segments

Keep the bed flat. Have the patient lean back at a 30-degree angle against you and a pillow. Percuss with a cupped hand between his clavicles and the top of each scapula.

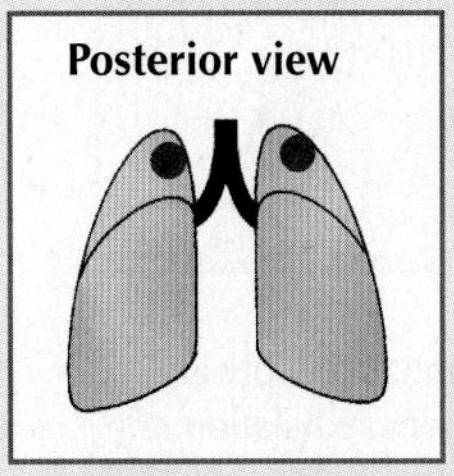

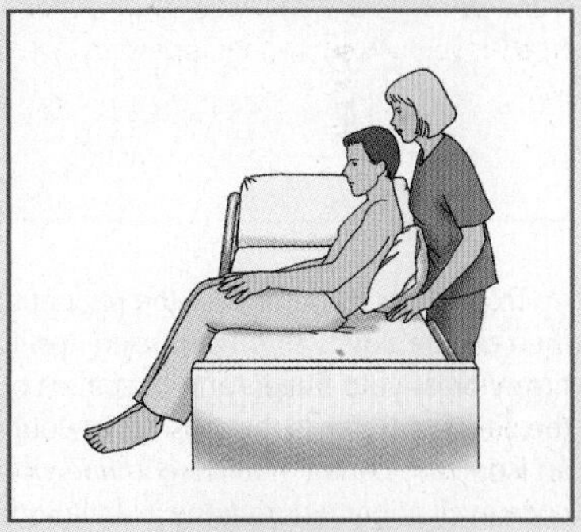

Upper lobes: Posterior segments

Keep the bed flat. Have the patient lean over a pillow at a 30-degree angle. Percuss and clap his upper back on each side.

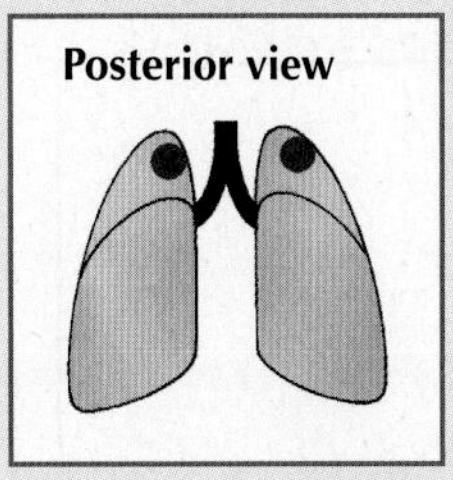

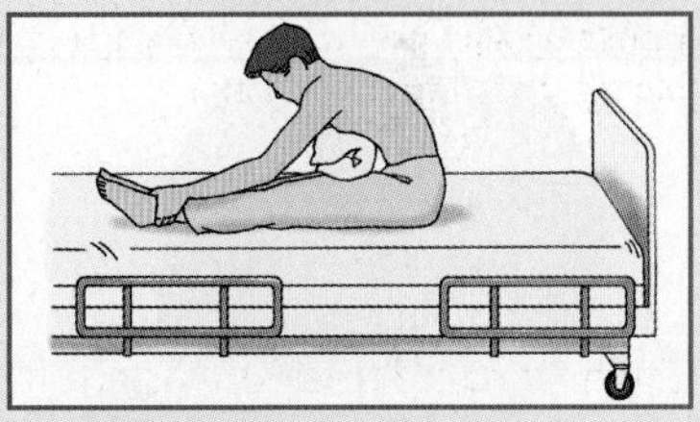

Percussing the chest with cupped hands mechanically dislodges thick, tenacious secretions from the bronchial walls. Vibration can be used with percussion to enhance secretion mobility or as an alternative to it in a patient who is frail, in pain, or recovering from thoracic surgery or trauma. Percussion and vibration can also be performed using a mechanical device.

Candidates for chest physiotherapy include patients who produce large amounts of sputum, such as those with bronchiectasis and cystic fibrosis.[1] The procedure hasn't proved effective in treating patients with status asthmaticus, pneumonia,[2] or acute exacerbations of chronic bronchitis when the patient has scant secretions and is being mechanically ventilated. Chest physiotherapy has little value for treating patients with stable, chronic bronchitis and, although some evidence suggests benefits, chest physiotherapy isn't recommended for routine postoperative care.[1]

Contraindications to chest physiotherapy include active pulmonary bleeding with hemoptysis, a posthemorrhage stage, hemodynamic instability, fractured ribs or an unstable chest wall, increased intracranial pressure (ICP), lung contusions, pulmonary tuberculosis, untreated pneumothorax, acute asthma or bronchospasm, lung abscess or tumor, bony metastasis, head injury, and recent myocardial infarction. Chest physiotherapy isn't recommended for patients with chronic obstructive pulmonary disease because it can cause bronchoconstriction.[3]

Equipment

Stethoscope ■ pillows or folded towels ■ adjustable hospital bed ■ gloves ■ facial tissues ■ suction equipment ■ oral care supplies ■ facility-approved disinfectant ■ no-touch receptacle[4] ■ Optional: sterile specimen container, gown, mask, face shield or protective eyewear, prescribed medications, tilt table, postural drainage table, supplemental oxygen, laboratory transport bag.

Preparation of equipment

Gather the equipment at the patient's bedside. Set up suction equipment and test its function.

Implementation

- Verify the practitioner's order.
- Perform hand hygiene.[5,6,7,8,9]

Performing percussion and vibration

To perform percussion, instruct the patient to breathe slowly and deeply, using the diaphragm, *to promote relaxation*. Hold your hands in a cupped shape, with fingers flexed and thumbs pressed tightly against your index fingers. Percuss each segment for 1 to 2 minutes by alternating your hands against the patient in a rhythmic manner. Listen for a hollow sound on percussion *to verify correct performance of the technique*.

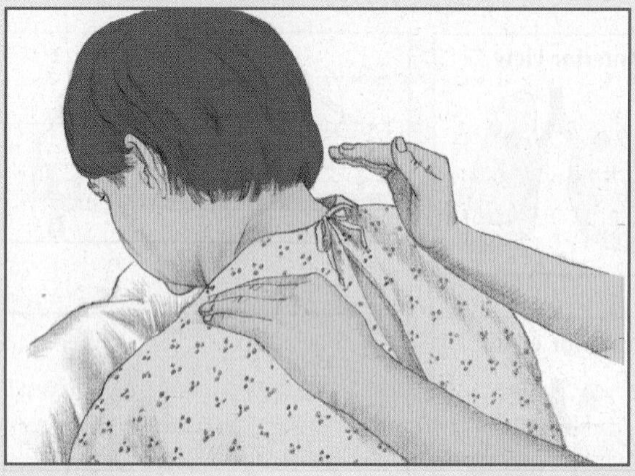

To perform vibration, ask the patient to inhale deeply and then exhale slowly through pursed lips. During exhalation, firmly press your fingers and the palms of your hands against the chest wall. Tense the muscles of your arms and shoulders in an isometric contraction *to send fine vibrations through the chest wall*. Vibrate during five exhalations over each chest segment.

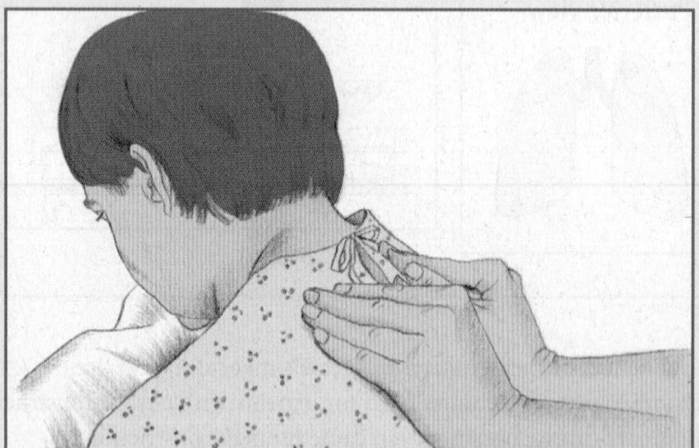

- Confirm the patient's identity using at least two patient identifiers.[10]
- Explain the procedure to the patient.
- Provide privacy.[11,12,13]
- Put on gloves and other personal protective equipment as needed *to comply with standard precautions.*[14,15]
- Auscultate the patient's breath sounds *to determine baseline respiratory status.*
- Perform a comprehensive pain assessment using techniques appropriate for the patient's age, condition, and ability to understand.[16] If needed, administer pain medication before the procedure, as ordered, following safe medication practices.[17,18,19]
- Position the patient as ordered. In generalized disease, drainage usually begins with the lower lobes, continues with the middle lobes, and ends with the upper lobes. In localized disease, drainage begins with the affected lobes and then proceeds to the other lobes *to avoid spreading the disease to uninvolved areas.*

NURSING ALERT ***Take the necessary precautions to prevent patient falls throughout positioning.***[20,21]

- Instruct the patient to remain in each position for 3 to 15 minutes. During this time, perform percussion and vibration as ordered. (See *Performing percussion and vibration.*)
- After postural drainage, percussion, or vibration, instruct the patient to deep breathe and cough *to remove loosened secretions.* Hand the patient a facial tissue and tell him to inhale deeply through his nose and then exhale in three short huffs. Tell him to inhale deeply again, cover his mouth and nose with the tissue, and cough and expectorate through a slightly open mouth into the tissue; three consecutive coughs are highly effective. Alternatively, if a sputum specimen is necessary, have the patient expectorate into a sterile specimen container. Label the specimen in the presence of the patient *to prevent mislabeling.*[10] Send the specimen to the laboratory in a laboratory transport bag.
- Have the patient perform coughing exercises for about 1 minute and then rest for 2 minutes. Gradually progress to a 10-minute exercise period four times daily. Try to schedule the last session just before bedtime *to help maximize the patient's oxygenation while he's sleeping.*
- If the patient's cough is ineffective, suction the patient.
- Monitor the patient's response to the treatment. Be alert for significant color changes, particularly if the patient becomes dusky, *which may indicate poor oxygenation.*
- Provide a no-touch receptacle for the patient to dispose of the used tissues.[4]
- Have the patient perform hand hygiene.[14,15]
- Reassess and respond to the patient's pain, as necessary.[16,22]
- Provide oral hygiene *because secretions may have a foul taste or a stale odor.* (See the "Oral care" procedure, page 560.)
- Auscultate the patient's breath sounds and compare your findings with the baseline findings *to evaluate the effectiveness of therapy.*
- Remove and discard gloves and any other personal protective equipment worn.[14]
- Perform hand hygiene.[6,7,8,9]
- Disinfect your stethoscope using a facility-approved disinfectant pad.[23,24]
- Perform hand hygiene.[5,6,7,8,9]
- Document the procedure.[25,26,27]

Special considerations

- *For optimal effectiveness and safety,* modify chest physiotherapy according to the patient's condition. For example, initiate or increase the flow of supplemental oxygen, if indicated. If the patient tires quickly during therapy, shorten the sessions *because fatigue leads to shallow respirations and increased hypoxia.*
- Maintain adequate hydration in the patient receiving chest physiotherapy *to prevent mucus dehydration and promote easier mobilization of secretions.* Avoid performing postural drainage immediately before or within 1½ hours after meals *to avoid nausea, vomiting, and aspiration of food or vomitus.*
- *Because chest percussion can induce bronchospasm,* any adjunct treatment (for example, intermittent positive-pressure breathing or aerosol or nebulizer therapy) should precede chest physiotherapy.
- Refrain from percussing over the spine, liver, kidneys, and spleen *to avoid injury to the spine or internal organs.* Also avoid performing percussion on bare skin or the female patient's breasts.
- Percuss over soft clothing (but not over buttons, snaps, or zippers), or place a thin towel over the area. Remove jewelry that might scratch or bruise the patient.

Complications

During postural drainage in head-down positions, pressure on the diaphragm by abdominal contents can impair respiratory excursion and lead to hypoxia. The head-down position can also lead to increased ICP, precluding the use of chest physiotherapy in a patient with head injury, elevated ICP, or acute neurologic impairment. Vigorous percussion or vibration can cause rib fracture, especially in a patient with osteoporosis. In an emphysematous patient with blebs, coughing could lead to pneumothorax.

Documentation

Record the date and time of chest physiotherapy. Note the positions used for secretion drainage and the length of time each was maintained. Note which chest segments were percussed or vibrated. Record the color, amount, odor, and viscosity of any secretions produced and the presence of any blood. Record any complications, nursing actions taken, and the patient's response to those actions. Also document the patient's tolerance of the procedure.

REFERENCES

1 Strickland, S. L., et al. (2013). AARC clinical practice guideline: Effectiveness of nonpharmacologic airway clearance therapies in hospitalized patients. *Respiratory Care, 58,* 2187–2193. Accessed March 2015 via the Web at http://rc.rcjournal.com/content/58/12/2187.full (Level VII)

2 Yang, M., et al. (2013). Chest physiotherapy for pneumonia in adults. *Cochrane Database of Systematic Reviews, 2013,* CD006338.

3 Stoller, J. K. Management of exacerbations of chronic obstructive pulmonary disease. (2014). In: *UpToDate,* Barnes, P. J., & Hollingsworth, H. (Eds.). Accessed March 2015 via the Web at http://www.uptodate.com/contents/search

4 Centers for Disease Control and Prevention. (2012). "Respiratory hygiene/cough etiquette in healthcare settings" [Online]. Accessed March 2015 via the Web at http://www.cdc.gov/flu/professionals/infectioncontrol/resphygiene.htm

5 The Joint Commission. (2015). Standard NPSG.07.01.01. *Comprehensive accreditation manual for hospitals: The official handbook.* Oakbrook Terrace, IL: The Joint Commission. (Level VII)

6 Centers for Disease Control and Prevention. (2002). Guideline for hand hygiene in health-care settings: Recommendations of the Healthcare Infection Control Practices Advisory Committee and the HICPAC/SHEA/APIC/IDSA Hand Hygiene Task Force. *MMWR Recommendations and Reports, 51*(RR-16), 1–45. Accessed March 2015 via the Web at http://www.cdc.gov/mmwr/pdf/rr/rr5116.pdf (Level II)

7 World Health Organization. (2009). "WHO guidelines on hand hygiene in health care: First global patient safety challenge, clean care is safer care" [Online]. Accessed March 2015 via the Web at http://whqlibdoc.who.int/publications/2009/9789241597906_eng.pdf (Level IV)

8 Centers for Medicare & Medicaid Services, Department of Health and Human Services. (2014). Condition of participation: Infection control. 42 C.F.R. § 482.42.

9 American Osteopathic Association. (2014). Standard 07.01.21. *Healthcare Facilities Accreditation Program: Accreditation requirements for acute care hospitals.* Chicago, IL: American Osteopathic Association. (Level VII)

10 The Joint Commission. (2015). Standard NPSG.01.01.01. *Comprehensive accreditation manual for hospitals: The official handbook.* Oakbrook Terrace, IL: The Joint Commission. (Level VII)

11 American Osteopathic Association. (2014). Standard 15.01.16. *Healthcare Facilities Accreditation Program: Accreditation requirements for acute care hospitals.* Chicago, IL: American Osteopathic Association. (Level VII)

12 The Joint Commission. (2015). Standard RI.01.01.01. *Comprehensive accreditation manual for hospitals: The official handbook.* Oakbrook Terrace, IL: The Joint Commission. (Level VII)

13 Centers for Medicare & Medicaid Services, Department of Health and Human Services. (2014). Condition of participation: Patient's rights. 42 C.F.R. § 482.13(c)(1).

14 Siegel, J. D., et al. (2007). "2007 guideline for isolation precautions: Preventing transmission of infectious agents in healthcare settings" [Online]. Accessed March 2015 via the Web at http://www.cdc.gov/hicpac/pdf/isolation/Isolation2007.pdf (Level II)

15 American Osteopathic Association. (2014). Standard 07.01.10. *Healthcare Facilities Accreditation Program: Accreditation requirements for acute care hospitals.* Chicago, IL: American Osteopathic Association. (Level VII)

16 The Joint Commission. (2015). Standard PC.01.02.07. *Comprehensive accreditation manual for hospitals: The official handbook.* Oakbrook Terrace, IL: The Joint Commission. (Level VII)

17 The Joint Commission. (2015). Standard MM.06.01.01. *Comprehensive accreditation manual for hospitals: The official handbook.* Oakbrook Terrace, IL: The Joint Commission. (Level VII)

18 Centers for Medicare & Medicaid Services, Department of Health and Human Services. (2014). Condition of participation: Nursing services. 42 C.F.R. § 482.23(c).

19 American Osteopathic Association. (2014). Standard 16.01.03. *Healthcare Facilities Accreditation Program: Accreditation requirements for acute care hospitals.* Chicago, IL: American Osteopathic Association. (Level VII)

20 Ganz, D. A., et al. (2013). *Preventing falls in hospitals: A toolkit for improving quality of care* (AHRQ publication no. 13-0015-EF). Rockville, MD: Agency for Healthcare Research and Quality. (Level VII)

21 The Joint Commission. (2015). Standard PC.01.02.08. *Comprehensive accreditation manual for hospitals: The official handbook.* Oakbrook Terrace, IL: The Joint Commission. (Level VII)

22 American Osteopathic Association. (2014). Standard 16.02.05. *Healthcare Facilities Accreditation Program: Accreditation requirements for acute care hospitals.* Chicago, IL: American Osteopathic Association. (Level VII)

23 Rutala, W. A., et al. (2008). "Guideline for disinfection and sterilization in healthcare facilities, 2008" [Online]. Accessed March 2015 via the Web at http://www.cdc.gov/hicpac/pdf/guidelines/Disinfection_Nov_2008.pdf (Level I)

24 American Osteopathic Association. (2014). Standard 07.02.03. *Healthcare Facilities Accreditation Program: Accreditation requirements for acute care hospitals.* Chicago, IL: American Osteopathic Association. (Level VII)

25 The Joint Commission. (2015). Standard RC.01.03.01. *Comprehensive accreditation manual for hospitals: The official handbook.* Oakbrook Terrace, IL: The Joint Commission. (Level VII)

26 Centers for Medicare & Medicaid Services, Department of Health and Human Services. (2014). Condition of participation: Medical record services. 42 C.F.R. § 482.24(b).

27 American Osteopathic Association. (2014). Standard 10.00.03. *Healthcare Facilities Accreditation Program: Accreditation requirements for acute care hospitals.* Chicago, IL: American Osteopathic Association. (Level VII)

ADDITIONAL REFERENCES

Esguerra-Gonzalez, A., et al. (2013). Pain after lung transplant: High frequency chest wall oscillation vs chest physiotherapy. *American Journal of Critical Care, 22,* 115–125. Accessed March 2015 via the Web at http://www.aacn.org/wd/Cetests/media/a132223.pdf

Flude, L. J., et al. (2012). Chest physiotherapy techniques in bronchiectasis. *Clinics in Chest Medicine, 33,* 351–361.

Nettina, S. M. (2014). *Lippincott manual of nursing practice* (10th ed.). Philadelphia, PA: Wolters Kluwer.

Taylor, C., et al. (2015). *Fundamentals of nursing: The art and science of nursing care* (8th ed.). Philadelphia, PA: Lippincott Williams & Wilkins.

Yang, M., et al. (2010). Chest physiotherapy for pneumonia in adults. *Cochrane Database of Systematic Reviews, 2,* CD006338.

CHEST TUBE DRAINAGE SYSTEM MONITORING AND CARE

Maintaining and troubleshooting a patient's chest tube keeps the chest tube functioning properly and prevents infection. As part of this process, the nurse is responsible for making respiratory and thoracic assessments, obtaining vital signs that reflect effectiveness of therapy or impending complications, and knowing the appropriate interventions to perform in response to changes in the patient's therapy.

Equipment

Vital signs monitoring equipment ▪ stethoscope ▪ pulse oximeter and probe ▪ gloves ▪ sterile gloves ▪ single-use, disposable, sterile chest tube drainage collection unit ▪ sterile water ▪ suction source ▪ suction connection tubing ▪ two sterile 4″ × 4″ (10-cm × 10-cm) drain dressings ▪ sterile 4″ × 4″ (10-cm × 10-cm) or 2″ × 2″ (5-cm × 5-cm) gauze pads ▪ sterile petroleum gauze ▪ 3″ to 4″ (7.6- to 10-cm) sturdy elastic tape ▪ 1″ (2.5-cm) adhesive tape for connections ▪ two rubber-tipped clamps for each chest tube inserted ▪ disinfectant pad ▪ Optional: sterile nonadherent gauze, sterile transparent dressing with a one-way valve, needle and syringe or needless syringe, Kelly clamps, container of normal saline solution, mask, goggles, mask with face shield.

Implementation

- Review the practitioner's orders regarding chest tube care.
- Perform hand hygiene.[1,2,3,4,5]
- Confirm the patient's identity using at least two patient identifiers.[6]
- Explain the procedure to the patient.
- Perform a comprehensive pain assessment using techniques appropriate for the patient's age, condition, and ability to understand. Administer ordered pain medication, as needed, following safe medication administration practices.[7,8,9,10] *Relieving the patient's pain promotes comfort, which facilitates deep breathing, coughing, and range-of-motion (ROM) exercises.*
- Maintain sterile technique and wear appropriate personal protective equipment *to comply with standard precautions* whenever you make changes in the system or alter any of the connections *to avoid introducing pathogens into the pleural space.*[11,12,13,14,15]

Providing routine care for all drainage systems

- Repeatedly note the character, consistency, and amount of drainage in the drainage collection chamber. Notify the practitioner immediately of a sudden decrease in drainage or the presence of frank bloody drainage.[16]
- Mark the drainage level by writing the time and date at the drainage level on the drainage collection chamber at an interval determined by your facility or the patient's condition.
- Observe the integrity of the drainage tubing and chest tube every 2 to 4 hours as well as with a change in the patient's condition *to ensure that the system is intact, with no air leaks, and to help prevent kinks or clots from forming.*[11]
- Periodically check that the air vent in the system is working properly (if applicable). *Occlusion of the air vent results in a buildup of pressure in the system that could cause the patient to develop a tension pneumothorax.*
- Coil the system's tubing and secure it to the edge of the bed. Make sure the tubing remains at the level of the patient. Avoid creating dependent loops, kinks, or pressure on the tubing *because fluid-filled dependent loops can rapidly change pleural pressures, resulting in dramatically decreased drainage.*[17] Avoid lifting the drainage system above the patient's chest *because fluid may flow back into the pleural space.*[11,16]
- Keep two rubber-tipped clamps at the bedside *to clamp the chest tube to help locate an air leak in the system or if the commercially prepared system cracks.*

NURSING ALERT *Never clamp the tube to get the patient out of bed or during transportation of the patient.* Whenever the chest tube is clamped, air or fluid can't escape from the pleural space, which puts the patient at risk for a tension pneumothorax.[11]

- Encourage the patient to cough frequently and breathe deeply *to help drain the pleural space and expand the lungs.*[11]
- Instruct the patient to sit upright *for optimal lung expansion* and to splint the insertion site while coughing *to minimize pain.*
- Check the rate and quality of the patient's respirations and auscultate his lungs periodically *to assess air exchange in the affected lung.*[11] *Diminished or absent breath sounds may indicate that the lung hasn't reexpanded.*
- Tell the patient to immediately report any breathing difficulty. Notify the practitioner immediately if the patient develops cyanosis, decreased oxygen saturation, rapid or shallow breathing, subcutaneous emphysema, chest pain, or excessive bleeding.
- Check the chest tube dressing at least every 8 hours. Palpate the area surrounding the dressing for crepitus or subcutaneous emphysema, *which indicates that air is leaking into the subcutaneous tissue surrounding the insertion site.* Change the dressing when soiled or according to the practitioner's order or at an interval determined by your facility.[11] (See *Changing a chest tube dressing.*)
- Replace the chest tube drainage system as ordered or as needed. (See *Replacing the chest tube drainage system,* page 178.) Notify the practitioner if you must change the device because of a leak.
- Encourage active (or assist with passive) ROM exercises for the patient's arm or the affected side. Usually, the thoracotomy patient will splint his arm *to decrease his discomfort.*[11]
- Remind the ambulatory patient to keep the drainage system below the level of the chest tube *to facilitate gravity drainage*[22] and to be careful not to disconnect the tubing *to maintain the water seal.*
- Troubleshoot the system as needed when problems arise. (See *Troubleshooting chest tubes,* page 179.) *Early and prompt attention to system difficulties will minimize the patient's complications.*

Additional steps for a water-seal–wet suction system

- Check the water-seal level every shift and maintain the proper level *to ensure proper use of the system and to maintain the patient's safety.*
- Check for fluctuations in the water-seal chamber as the patient breathes. *Normal fluctuations of 2″ to 4″ (about 5 to 10 cm) reflect pressure changes in the pleural space during respiration.* To check for fluctuation when a suction system is being used, momentarily disconnect the suction system *so that the air vent is opened* and observe for fluctuation.
- Check for intermittent bubbling in the water-seal chamber. *This bubbling occurs normally when the system is removing air from the pleural cavity.* If bubbling isn't readily apparent during quiet breathing, have the patient take a deep breath or cough. *Absence of bubbling indicates that the pleural space has sealed.*[11]
- Check the water level in the suction-control chamber. Detach the chamber or bottle from the suction source; when bubbling ceases, observe the water level. If necessary, add sterile water to bring the level to the 20-cm line or to the ordered level.
- Check for gentle bubbling in the suction-control chamber, *which indicates the proper suction level.*

Additional steps for a water-seal–dry suction system

- Check the water-seal level every shift and maintain the proper level *to ensure that the system is being used properly and to maintain the patient's safety.*
- Check for fluctuation in the water-seal chamber as the patient breathes. *Normal fluctuations of 2″ to 4″ (about 5 to 10 cm) reflect pressure changes in the pleural space during respiration.* To check for fluctuation when a suction system is being used, momentarily disconnect the suction system *so that the air vent is opened* and observe for fluctuation.
- Check for intermittent bubbling in the water-seal chamber. *This bubbling occurs normally when the system is removing air from the pleural cavity.* If bubbling isn't readily apparent during quiet breathing,

have the patient take a deep breath or cough. *Absence of bubbling indicates that the pleural space has sealed.*[11]

■ Check that the rotary dry suction control dial is turned to the ordered suction mark, usually −20 cm, and verify that the appropriate indicator is present, indicating that the system has applied the desired amount of suction. In some models, an orange float appears in an indicator window. Other models indicate delivery of the correct amount of suction when the bellows reach the calibrated triangular mark in the suction monitor bellows window. Always refer to the manufacturer's instructions.

Additional steps for a dry seal–dry suction system

■ Check the air-leak monitor for right-to-left bubbling and fluctuation every shift (or more often as symptoms warrant). *Fluctuation of water in the air-leak monitor chamber is a normal reflection of pressure changes in the pleural cavity during respirations. Bubbling indicates that air is leaving the system and is normal for the patient with a pneumothorax, but it could indicate an air leak.*

■ Check that the rotary dry suction control dial is turned to the ordered suction mark, usually −20 cm suction, and verify that the appropriate indicator is present, indicating the system has applied the desired amount of suction. In some models, an orange float appears in an indicator window. Other models indicate delivery of the correct amount of suction when the bellows reach the calibrated triangular mark in the suction monitor bellows window. Always refer to the manufacturer's instructions.

Special considerations

■ Instruct staff members and visitors to avoid touching the equipment *to prevent complications from separated connections.*

■ No clear evidence exists regarding optimal suction pressure. Research has shown that, in routine cases, limited or no suction results in reduced chest tube dwell time and shorter stays in the health care facility.[17]

■ If the system cracks, clamp the chest tube momentarily with the two rubber-tipped clamps at the bedside (placed there at the time of tube insertion). Place the clamps close to each other near the insertion site; they should face in opposite directions *to provide a more complete seal.* Observe the patient for altered respirations while the tube is clamped. Then replace the damaged equipment. (Prepare the new unit before clamping the tube.)

■ For the patient on a ventilator with positive end-expiratory pressure (PEEP), continuous bubbling typically occurs *because PEEP maintains positive pressure in the alveoli, resulting in air continually flowing through the lungs.* However, lack of continuous bubbling for patients on PEEP is normal.

NURSING ALERT ***Don't strip a chest drain (occluding the chest tube with one hand while quickly squeezing and moving the other hand down the tube to move fluid down the tube into the drainage chamber)*** **because stripping can cause intraluminal pressures to rise to a dangerously high level, which may convert a simple pneumothorax to life-threatening pneumothorax and cause tissue trauma and unnecessary discomfort.**[17] ***Don't milk, fanfold, or tap the chest drain*** **because it hasn't been demonstrated that such manipulations improve fluid drainage from the chest.**

■ Remember that routine clamping of the chest tube isn't recommended *because of the risk of tension pneumothorax.*

■ During patient transport, keep the chest tube drainage system below chest level. Don't clamp the chest tube during transport.

■ If you hear air leaking from the site, tape the dressing on only two or three sides *to allow air to escape and to prevent a tension pneumothorax.* Closely monitor the patient and prepare for insertion of a new chest tube.

Complications

Complications of chest tube drainage system monitoring and care include accidental tube dislodgment, infection, pain, air leak from the

Changing a chest tube dressing

Change the dressings around the chest tube according to the practitioner's orders if permitted by your facility. Follow these steps:

■ Perform hand hygiene.[1,2,3,4,5]

■ Put on gloves and other personal protective equipment if needed.[12,15]

■ Confirm the patient's identity using at least two patient identifiers.[6]

■ Explain the procedure to the patient.

■ Remove the dressings around the chest tube insertion site and dispose of them in the appropriate receptacle.[18] Examine the site for signs of infection or subcutaneous emphysema.

■ Remove and discard your gloves[12,15] and perform hand hygiene.[1,2,3,4,5]

■ Open the packages containing the petroleum gauze, 4″ × 4″ (10-cm × 10-cm) drain dressings, and gauze pads (although no clear evidence supports the best type of dressing to apply to the chest tube insertion site.)[17]

■ Put on sterile gloves.[12,15]

■ Place the petroleum gauze and two 4″ × 4″ (10-cm × 10-cm) drain dressings around the insertion site, one from the top and the other from the bottom (as shown below), *to seal the insertion site from any air entry or escape.*[11]

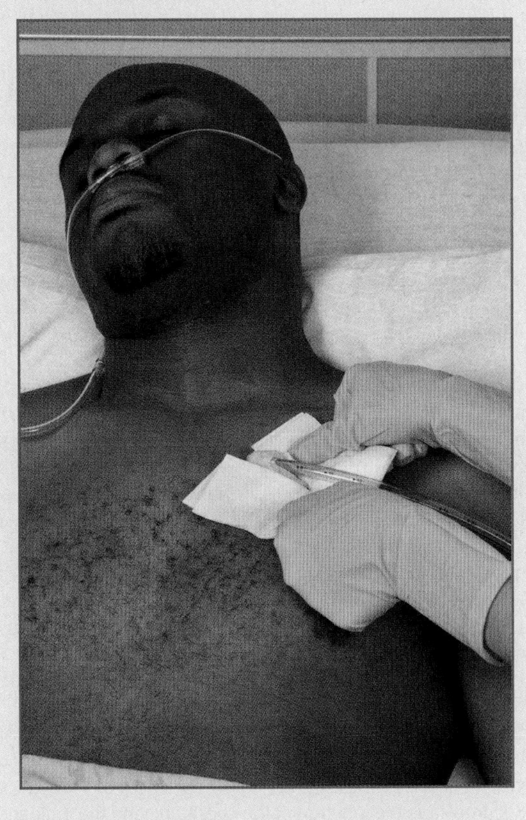

■ Place several 4″ × 4″ (10-cm × 10-cm) gauze pads on top of the drain dressings.[11]

■ Tape the dressings, covering them completely *to form an occlusive dressing.*

■ Mark the dressing with the date, the time, and your initials.

■ Dispose of used supplies in the appropriate receptacle.

■ Remove and discard your gloves and any other personal protective equipment worn.[12,15]

■ Perform hand hygiene.[1,2,3,4,5]

■ Document the procedure.[19,20]

Replacing the chest tube drainage system

In certain circumstances, you may need to replace the chest tube drainage system. Follow these steps for replacement:

- Gather the necessary supplies.
- Perform hand hygiene.[1,2,3,4,5]
- Confirm the patient's identity using at least two patient identifiers.[6]
- Explain the procedure to the patient.
- Open a new, single-use, sterile chest drainage unit.
- If you're using a chest drainage system that has a water seal, fill the water-seal chamber with sterile water to the specified level, according to the manufacturer's instructions.
- If you're using a dry-seal chest drainage system, fill the air-leak monitor with sterile water to the specified level, according to the manufacturer's instructions.
- If you're using a wet suction chest drainage system, fill the suction-control chamber with sterile water to 20 cm H_2O or as ordered by the practitioner. *The addition of suction (usually 20 cm H_2O) increases the negative intrapleural pressure and helps overcome air leakage by improving the rate of airflow out of the patient and improving fluid removal.* If you're using a dry suction chest drainage system, turn the rotary dry suction control dial to the ordered suction mark, usually –20 cm.
- Maintain a sterile patient connection tube with the cap in place *to enable later connection of the chest tube catheter to the chest tube drainage system collection device after removal of the existing device.*
- Place the chest tube drainage system at the bedside in the upright position, at least 1′ (30 cm) below the patient's chest. *To avoid accidentally knocking over the device,* hang it on the bed frame with the hangers provided or secure it according to the manufacturer's instructions.[21] Ensure that the device is ready when you remove the existing device.
- Put on gloves and other personal protective equipment if needed.[12,15]
- If using suction, turn off the suction to the current drainage system.
- Undo the tape on the connections from the existing chest tube drainage system to the chest tube catheter *to allow access to the chest tube catheter for drainage device replacement.*
- Briefly cross-clamp the chest tube catheter with two gauze-wrapped Kelly clamps (to avoid ripping or tearing the catheter) about 1½″ to 2½″ (4 cm to 6.5 cm) from the insertion site *to minimize dead space and stop air from entering or exiting the catheter.*
- Instruct the patient to perform the Valsalva maneuver *to force air out of the pleural space and keep air from entering while you switch the tubing.* If the patient can't perform the maneuver, make the system switch at the end of exhalation if the patient is breathing spontaneously or the end of inspiration of a machine-generated breath.[22]
- Using sterile technique, disconnect the old drainage system and connect the new one.
- Remove the clamp or clamps and instruct the patient to breathe normally *to allow fluid and air removal to begin again.*
- Secure the chest tube and drainage tube so that there's no tension pulling on the insertion site *to help prevent accidental tube dislodgment.*
- Securely tape the junction of the chest tube and the drainage tube *to prevent dangerous disconnections.*

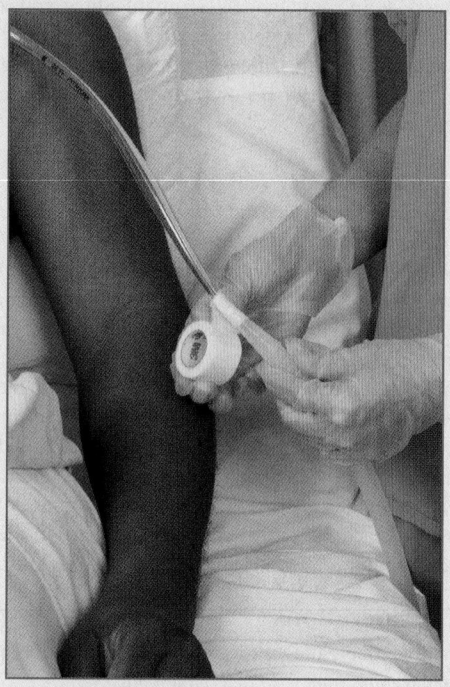

- Dispose of equipment and waste in the appropriate receptacle.[18]
- Remove and discard your gloves and any other personal protective equipment worn.[12,15]
- Perform hand hygiene.[1,2,3,4,5]
- Make sure that all clamps are open and that the drainage tubing has a straight flow to the chest tube drainage collection device and has no dependent loops or kinks.
- Make sure that the chest tube drainage system is correctly connected to the patient's chest tube; then, if appropriate, connect the suction tubing to the drainage system and the suction regulator.
- If you're using a wet suction chest drainage system, adjust the suction until gentle bubbling appears in the suction control chamber. If you're using a dry suction chest drainage system, adjust the suction regulator and verify that the appropriate indicator is present, indicating that the system has applied the desired amount of suction. Verify suction operation according to the manufacturer's instructions.
- Check the status of the drainage tubing.
- Reassess the patient after the procedure. Obtain vital signs and assess skin color, perfusion, level of consciousness, oxygen requirements, hemodynamic stability, comfort and pain levels, and respiratory rate, pattern, and effort *to identify the patient's response to and tolerance of the procedure.*
- Perform hand hygiene.[1,2,3,4,5]
- Clean and disinfect your stethoscope using a disinfectant pad.[23,24]
- Perform hand hygiene.[1,2,3,4,5]
- Document the procedure.[19,20]

insertion site, tubing disconnection, and chest tube occlusion with subsequent tension pneumothorax.

Documentation

Routine care

Record the date and time thoracic drainage began, the type of system used, the amount of suction applied to the pleural cavity, presence or absence of bubbling or fluctuation in the water-seal or air-leak monitor chamber (if applicable), initial amount and type of drainage, and the patient's respiratory status.

At the end of each shift, record the frequency of system inspection; amount, color, and consistency of drainage; presence or absence of bubbling or fluctuation in the water-seal or air-leak monitor chamber (if applicable); the patient's respiratory status; condition of the chest dressings; if

TROUBLESHOOTING

Troubleshooting chest tubes

Use this table to determine possible causes of and interventions for common chest tube problems.

PROBLEM	POSSIBLE CAUSES	INTERVENTION
Water level in the water-seal chamber not rising and falling with breathing	Clot in chest tubing or patient's chest	If available, incorporate an active chest tube clearance device into the drainage system *to prevent clot formation.*[17,25] Avoid fluid-filled dependent loops in the drainage tubing; if unable to maintain, lift and drain the tubing every 15 minutes.[17] Stripping and milking the tubing aren't recommended *because detrimental changes in intrathoracic pressure can result.*[17]
	Dependent loop or kink in patient's tube with fluid occlusion	Straighten the catheter and tubing along its length to its connection with the collection device.
	Dislodgment of catheter from patient	If the chest tube accidentally dislodges and the patient has an air leak from the chest tube, immediately cover the site with a sterile dressing and tape it on three sides, allowing air to escape on the fourth side *to reduce the risk of tension pneumothorax.*[22] Alternatively, cover the site with a sterile transparent dressing with a one-way valve, if available.[26] If there was no air leak present in your previous assessment, place a sterile transparent dressing over the site and monitor the patient closely for signs and symptoms of respiratory distress.[22] Stay with the patient and have a colleague call the practitioner immediately. Assess for signs and symptoms of tension pneumothorax (hypotension; distended jugular veins; absent or decreased breath sounds; tracheal shift; hypoxemia; weak, rapid pulse; dyspnea; tachypnea; diaphoresis; and chest pain). Then ask your colleague to gather the equipment needed to reinsert the chest tube.
	Disconnection of patient's tube from chest tube connector	Keep rubber-tipped clamps at the bedside.[16] If the drainage system cracks or a tube disconnects, clamp the chest tube momentarily as close to the insertion site as possible. Alternately, you can clamp the chest tube with a gauze-wrapped Kelly clamp *to prevent puncturing or tearing the tube. Because no air or liquid can escape from the pleural space while the tube is clamped,* observe the patient closely for signs and symptoms of tension pneumothorax while the clamp is in place. As an alternative to clamping the tube, you can submerge the distal end of the tube in a container of normal saline solution *to create a temporary water seal* while you replace the drainage system. Notify the practitioner immediately.
	Closed clamp to the patient's chest tube	Clamp only when indicated; otherwise, leave tube open.
	Chest drainage tubing not positioned sufficiently below the patient's chest	Lower the chest tube *to enable gravity drainage.*
	In-line connectors not properly secured, allowing for an air leak	Make sure that inline connectors are properly secured and sealed at all times; check for loose connections periodically.
Constant bubbling in the water-seal chamber	Air leak	*To determine the source of an air leak (patient or catheter connection),* momentarily clamp the chest tube close to the chest drain and observe the water seal. If the bubbling stops, the air leak may be from the catheter connections or the patient's chest. Check the catheter connections and the patient's dressing for a partially withdrawn catheter. If the catheter is dislodged, follow the procedure for a dislodged catheter, described above. If bubbling continues after temporarily clamping the patient's tube, there's a system leak, which requires system replacement.

(continued)

TROUBLESHOOTING

Troubleshooting chest tubes *(continued)*

Problem	Possible causes	Intervention
Overfilled water-seal level (water above ¾" [2-cm] limit line) or overfilled suction-control chamber	Too much water in the chamber	Press and hold the negative-pressure relief valve at the top of the chest drainage system *to vent excess negative pressure in the water-seal chamber.* Release the valve when the level of the water returns to the ¾" (2-cm) mark. *To remove water from the suction-control chamber,* insert a syringe and withdraw excess.
Not enough water in the water-seal or suction-control chamber	Evaporation, underfilling, or spillage	Add additional sterile water to the suction-control chamber by temporarily turning off the suction source, removing the rubber stopper, and adding sterile water to the desired level. You may add additional sterile water to the water-seal chamber with a syringe by quickly and temporarily clamping the patient's tube and injecting water to the desired level.
Suction-control chamber isn't bubbling or is bubbling too vigorously	Possible disconnection of suction source or too much suction-source pressure in the system	Make sure that the suction tubing is connected and the suction source is turned on. A constant, gentle bubbling is normal. Adjust the suction-control source for gentle bubbling.
Chest drainage system accidentally knocked over	Human error	Set the system upright and check the fluid levels in the water-seal and suction-control chambers for proper volumes and adjust them accordingly. Most units have a baffle system that prevents fluids from mixing between chambers, allowing for proper function after setting upright again.
Patient being transported or leaving the unit	As the situation indicates	Don't clamp the catheter tubing; disconnect the suction tubing from the suction source. The system continues to collect fluid (by gravity) or air (by water seal). Keep the collection system below the level of the chest tube at all time *to facilitate drainage.*[22]
Specimen collection required	Practitioner's orders for laboratory analysis	After disinfecting the tube collection site, remove fluid with a needle and syringe from the self-sealing portion of the drainage tubing or with a needleless syringe from the needleless site of the drainage tubing.

pain medication was administered; any complications and nursing actions taken; and any patient teaching provided.

Dressing change

Record the date, time, and reasons for changing the dressing. Document your assessment findings before and after the procedure and the patient's response to the procedure. Record the condition of the insertion site, the patient's respiratory status and vital signs, and any teaching provided.

Drainage system collection device change

Record the date, time, and reasons for changing the chest tube drainage system. Document your assessment findings before and after the procedure and the patient's response to the procedure. Note the type of drainage system used, the amount of suction applied to the pleural cavity (if applicable), the presence or absence of bubbling or fluctuation in the water-seal or air-leak monitor chamber (if applicable), the patient's respiratory status, and the amount, color, and consistency of drainage. Record the patient's respiratory status and vital signs, the amount of drainage and its color and consistency, and any teaching provided.

References

1 Centers for Disease Control and Prevention. (2002). Guideline for hand hygiene in health-care settings: Recommendations of the Healthcare Infection Control Practices Advisory Committee and the HICPAC/SHEA/APIC/IDSA Hand Hygiene Task Force. *MMWR Recommendations and Reports, 51*(RR-16), 1–45. Accessed March 2015 via the Web at http://www.cdc.gov/mmwr/pdf/rr/rr5116.pdf (Level II)

2 The Joint Commission. (2015). Standard NPSG.07.01.01. *Comprehensive accreditation manual for hospitals: The official handbook.* Oakbrook Terrace, IL: The Joint Commission. (Level VII)

3 World Health Organization. (2009). "WHO guidelines on hand hygiene in health care: First global patient safety challenge, clean care is safer care" [Online]. Accessed March 2015 via the Web at http://whqlibdoc.who.int/publications/2009/9789241597906_eng.pdf (Level IV)

4 American Osteopathic Association. (2014). Standard 07.01.21. *Healthcare Facilities Accreditation Program: Accreditation requirements for acute care hospitals.* Chicago, IL: American Osteopathic Association. (Level VII)

5 Centers for Medicare & Medicaid Services, Department of Health and Human Services. (2014). Condition of participation: Infection control. 42 C.F.R. § 482.42.

6 The Joint Commission. (2015). Standard NPSG.01.01.01. *Comprehensive accreditation manual for hospitals: The official handbook.* Oakbrook Terrace, IL: The Joint Commission. (Level VII)

7 The Joint Commission. (2015). Standard PC.01.02.07. *Comprehensive accreditation manual for hospitals: The official handbook.* Oakbrook Terrace, IL: The Joint Commission. (Level VII)

8 American Osteopathic Association. (2014). Standard 16.01.03. *Healthcare Facilities Accreditation Program: Accreditation requirements for acute care hospitals.* Chicago, IL: American Osteopathic Association. (Level VII)

9 The Joint Commission. (2015). Standard MM.06.01.01. *Comprehensive accreditation manual for hospitals: The official handbook.* Oakbrook Terrace, IL: The Joint Commission. (Level VII)
10 Centers for Medicare & Medicaid Services, Department of Health and Human Services. (2014). Condition of participation: Nursing services. 42 C.F.R. § 482.23(c).
11 Lynn-McHale Wiegand, D. (Ed.). (2011). *AACN procedure manual for critical care* (6th ed.). St. Louis, MO: Saunders.
12 Siegel, J. D., et al. (2007). "2007 guideline for isolation precautions: Preventing transmission of infectious agents in healthcare settings" [Online]. Accessed March 2015 via the Web at http://www.cdc.gov/hicpac/pdf/isolation/Isolation2007.pdf (Level II)
13 Centers for Disease Control and Prevention. (2004). Guidelines for preventing health-care-associated pneumonia, 2003: Recommendations of CDC and the Healthcare Infection Control Practices Advisory Committee. *MMWR Recommendations and Reports, 53*(RR-3), 1–32. Accessed March 2015 via the Web at http://www.cdc.gov/mmwr/pdf/rr/rr5303.pdf (Level II)
14 Centers for Medicare & Medicaid Services & The Joint Commission. (2014). "The specifications manual for national hospital inpatient quality measures" [Online]. Accessed March 2015 via the Web at http://www.qualitynet.org/dcs/ContentServer?c=Page&pagename=QnetPublic%2FPage%2FQnetTier4&cid=1228773564870
15 American Osteopathic Association. (2014). Standard 07.01.10. *Healthcare Facilities Accreditation Program: Accreditation requirements for acute care hospitals.* Chicago, IL: American Osteopathic Association. (Level VII)
16 Rajan, C. S. (2013). "Tube thoracostomy management" [Online]. Accessed March 2015 via the Web at http://emedicine.medscape.com/article/1503275-overview
17 American Association of Critical Care Nurses. (2013). "Evidence-based care of patients with chest tubes" [Online]. Accessed March 2015 via the Web at http://www.atriummed.com/EN/chest_drainage/Documents/Evidence-Based%20Care%20of%20Patients%20With%20Chest%20Tubes%20Complete.pdf (Level VII)
18 Occupational Safety and Health Administration. (n.d.). "Bloodborne pathogens, standard number 1910.1030" [Online]. Accessed March 2015 via the Web at http://www.osha.gov/pls/oshaweb/owadisp.show_document?p_table=STANDARDS&p_id=10051 (Level VII)
19 The Joint Commission. (2015). Standard RC.01.03.01. *Comprehensive accreditation manual for hospitals: The official handbook.* Oakbrook Terrace, IL: The Joint Commission. (Level VII)
20 Centers for Medicare & Medicaid Services, Department of Health and Human Services. (2014). Condition of participation: Medical record services. 42 C.F.R. § 482.24(b).
21 Atrium Medical Corporation. (2012). "A personal guide to managing chest drainage" [Online]. Accessed March 2015 via the Web at http://www.atriummed.com/EN/Chest_Drainage/Documents/BlueHandbook342263L.pdf
22 Carroll, P. (2011). "Managing chest drainage" [Online]. Accessed March 2015 via the Web at http://www.atriummed.com/EN/Chest_Drainage/Documents/continuing%20education%202010%20Online.pdf
23 Rutala, W. A., et al. (2008). "Guideline for disinfection and sterilization in healthcare facilities, 2008" [Online]. Accessed March 2015 via the Web at http://www.cdc.gov/hicpac/pdf/guidelines/Disinfection_Nov_2008.pdf (Level I)
24 American Osteopathic Association. (2014). Standard 07.02.03. *Healthcare Facilities Accreditation Program: Accreditation requirements for acute care hospitals.* Chicago, IL: American Osteopathic Association. (Level VII)
25 Perrault, L. P., et al. (2012). The PleuraFlow active chest tube clearance system: Initial clinical experience in adult cardiac surgery. *Innovations, 7,* 354–358.
26 Durai, R., et al. (2010). Managing a chest tube and drainage system. *AORN Journal, 91,* 275–280. Accessed March 2015 via the Web at http://isgweb.aorn.org/ISGWeb/downloads/CEA10006-9943.pdf

ADDITIONAL REFERENCE

Nettina, S. M. (2014). *Lippincott manual of nursing practice* (10th ed.). Philadelphia, PA: Wolters Kluwer.

CHEST TUBE DRAINAGE SYSTEM SETUP

Chest tube drainage uses gravity and, sometimes, suction to restore negative pressure and remove material that collects in the pleural cavity. The disposable drainage system combines drainage collection, a wet or dry seal, and suction control. The seal in the drainage system allows air and fluid to escape from the pleural cavity but doesn't allow air to reenter. Patient safety features on the device include a pressure relief valve and an air-leak indicator. There are three types of chest tube drainage systems: a water-seal–wet suction system, a water-seal–dry suction system, and a dry seal–dry suction system.

A practitioner may order chest tube drainage to remove accumulated air, fluids (blood, pus, chyle, and serous fluids), or solids (blood clots) from the pleural cavity; to restore negative pressure in the pleural cavity; or to reexpand a partially or totally collapsed lung.

Equipment

Single-use, disposable, sterile chest drainage collection unit (water-seal–wet suction system, water-seal–dry suction system, or dry seal–dry suction system) ▪ sterile water or normal saline solution ▪ gloves ▪ suction source ▪ suction-control device ▪ suction connection tubing ▪ tape ▪ Optional: sterile occlusive dressing, sterile occlusive dressing with one-way valve, two rubber-tipped clamps, needle and syringe, padded clamps.

Implementation

- Verify the practitioner's order *to determine the type of drainage system to be used and other procedural details.*
- Gather the necessary supplies.
- Perform hand hygiene.[1,2,3,4,5]
- Confirm the patient's identity using at least two patient identifiers.[6]
- Explain the procedure to the patient.
- Put on gloves *to comply with standard precautions.*[7,8]
- Maintain sterile technique throughout the procedure and whenever you make changes in the system or alter connections *to avoid introducing pathogens into the pleural space.*
- Open the single-use, sterile chest drainage unit. Use the unit's floor stand to set the unit on the floor or use the hangers to hang it level on the bed below the level of the patient's chest tube.[9,10]

Water-seal–wet suction system

- Use sterile water to fill the water-seal chamber to the specified level according to the manufacturer's instructions. The water-seal chamber acts as a one-way valve to allow air to pass out of the lung, move down through a narrow channel, and bubble out through the bottom of the water seal.
- Fill the suction-control chamber with sterile water or normal saline solution to the prescribed level (usually 10 to 20 cm H_2O).
- After the practitioner inserts the chest tube, trace the chest tube from the point of origin[11] and connect the patient's chest tube to the chest tube drainage system. (See the "Chest tube insertion, assisting" procedure, page 184.)
- Secure the connection with tape *to ensure that the system remains airtight.*[12]
- Connect the suction tubing to the drainage system and the suction regulator (as shown on next page, top left).

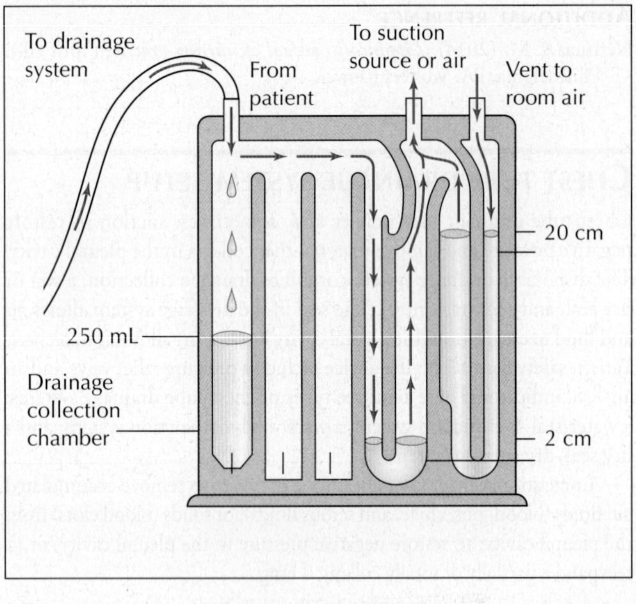

■ Adjust the suction until gentle bubbling appears in the suction-control chamber. *The addition of suction increases the negative intrapleural pressure and helps overcome air leakage by improving the rate of airflow out of the patient and improving fluid removal.*

Water-seal–dry suction system

■ Use sterile water to fill the water-seal chamber to the specified level according to the manufacturer's instructions. The water-seal chamber acts as a one-way valve to allow air to pass out of the lung, move down through a narrow channel, and bubble out through the bottom of the water seal.

■ If the practitioner orders suction, turn the rotary dry suction control dial to the ordered suction mark, usually –20 cm.

■ After the practitioner inserts the chest tube, trace the chest tube from the point of origin,[11] connect the patient's chest tube to the chest tube drainage system, and secure the connection with tape *to ensure the system remains airtight.* [12]

■ Connect the suction tubing to the drainage system and adjust the suction regulator. Verify suction operation according to the manufacturer's instructions. An indicator appears when the desired negative pressure is achieved. In some models, an orange float appears in an indicator window. Other models indicate delivery of the correct amount of suction when the bellows reach the calibrated triangular mark in the suction monitor bellows window (as shown on top right). *The addition of suction increases the negative intrapleural pressure and helps overcome air leakage by improving the rate of airflow out of the patient and improving fluid removal.*

Dry seal–dry suction system

■ Use sterile water to fill the air-leak monitor chamber to the specified level according to the manufacturer's instructions.

■ If the practitioner orders suction, turn the rotary dry suction control dial to the ordered suction mark, usually –20 cm.

■ After the practitioner inserts the chest tube, trace the chest tube from the point of origin,[11] connect the patient's chest tube to the chest tube drainage system, and secure the connection with tape *to ensure the system remains airtight.* (See the "Chest tube insertion, assisting" procedure, page 184.)[12]

■ Connect the suction tubing to the drainage system and adjust the suction regulator. Verify suction operation according to the manufacturer's instructions. An indicator appears when the desired negative pressure is achieved. In some models, an orange float appears in an indicator window. Other models indicate delivery of the correct amount of suction when the bellows reach the calibrated triangular mark in the suction monitor bellows window (as shown below). *The addition of suction increases the negative intrapleural pressure and helps overcome air leakage by improving the rate of airflow out of the patient and improving fluid removal.*

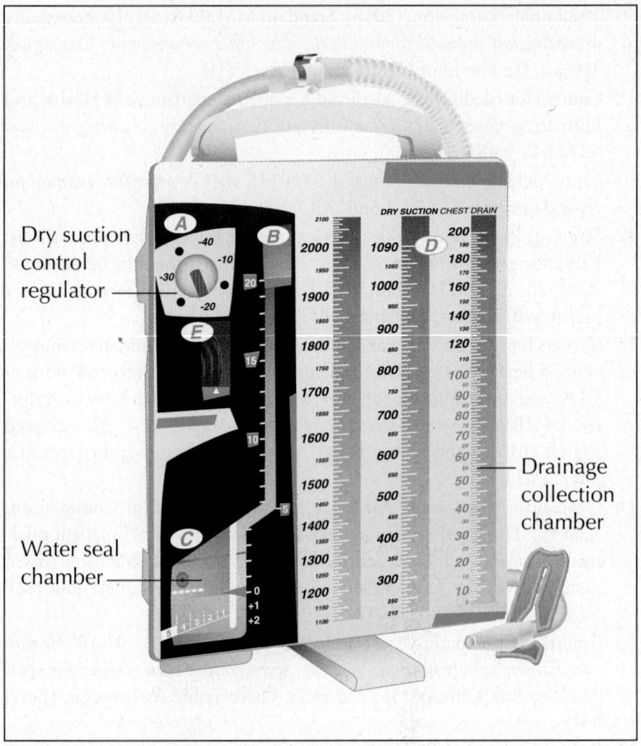

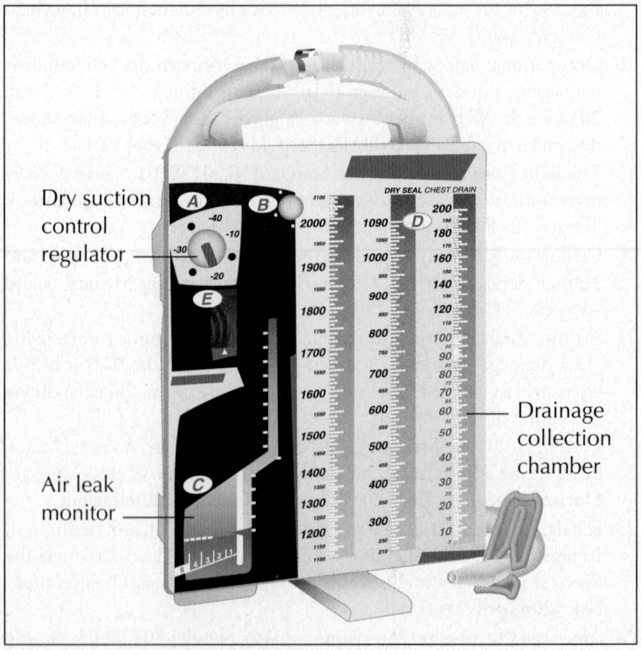

For all drainage systems

■ Place the drainage system at the bedside below the patient's chest tube in the upright position.[9,10] *Placement of the device below chest enables gravity—in addition to negative pressure—to drain the tube for optimal results. To avoid accidentally knocking over the device,* hang it on the bed frame with the hangers provided or by secure it according to the manufacturer's instructions.[9,13]

■ Remove and discard your gloves.[7,8]

- Perform hand hygiene.[1,2,3,4,5]
- Document the procedure.[14,15,16]

Special considerations

- Don't overfill the water-seal chamber. *A fluid level greater than 2 cm makes breathing more difficult.* If you accidentally overfill the chamber, aspirate the excess water with a needle and syringe. Many models have a grommet to access the water-seal chamber.[13]
- Some systems have a stopcock that can be gradually closed *to limit the suction flow into the drainage* system. If the patient's chest tube is to gravity drainage, leave the stopcock in the ON or OPEN position.[13]
- No clear evidence exists regarding the optimal amount of suction pressure. Research has shown that, in routine cases, limited or no suction results in reduced chest tube dwell time and shorter stays in the health care facility.[17]
- Don't at any time block the pressure relief valve, which is usually located on the top of the unit.[13]
- If excessive continuous bubbling is present in the water-seal chamber, especially if you're using suction, rule out a leak in the drainage system. Try to locate the leak by cross-clamping the tube momentarily at various points along its length. (The bubbling will stop when a clamp is placed between the air leak and the water seal.) Begin clamping at the tube's proximal end and work down toward the drainage system, paying special attention to the seal around the connections. If a connection is loose, push it back together and tape it securely. If you clamp along the tube's entire length and the bubbling doesn't stop, the drainage system may be cracked and need replacement.
- If the chest tube and drainage system become disconnected, you can create a temporary water seal by immersing the end of the chest tube into a bottle of sterile water *to prevent pneumothorax.*[9]
- If the chest tube accidentally pulls out and the patient had an air leak from the chest tube, immediately cover the site with a sterile dressing and tape it on three sides, allowing air to escape on the fourth side *to reduce the risk of tension pneumothorax.*[9] Alternately, cover the site with a sterile occlusive dressing with a one-way valve, if available.[18] If your previous assessment didn't detect an air leak, place a sterile occlusive dressing over the site and monitor the patient closely for signs of respiratory distress.[9] Stay with the patient and have a colleague call the practitioner immediately. Assess the patient for signs and symptoms of tension pneumothorax, including hypotension; distended jugular veins; absent or decreased breath sounds; tracheal shift; hypoxemia; weak, rapid pulse; dyspnea; tachypnea; diaphoresis; and chest pain. Then have your colleague gather the equipment needed to reinsert the chest tube.
- Instruct staff members and visitors to avoid touching the equipment *to prevent complications from separated connections.*
- To attach a new drainage system when the existing one is full, briefly cross-clamp the chest tube with two padded clamps close to the insertion site and, using sterile technique, disconnect the old drainage system.[12] Then connect the new drainage system and remove the clamps.

Complications

Complications associated with chest tube drainage setup include infection, accidental chest tube dislodgement, pain, air leak from the insertion site, and tubing disconnection.

Documentation

Record the date and time that chest tube drainage began, the type of drainage system used, the amount of suction applied to the pleural cavity (if applicable), the presence or absence of bubbling or fluctuation in the water-seal chamber (if applicable), the patient's respiratory status, and the initial amount, color, and consistency of drainage. Also document any teaching provided to the patient.

REFERENCES

1 Centers for Disease Control and Prevention. (2002). Guideline for hand hygiene in health-care settings: Recommendations of the Healthcare Infection Control Practices Advisory Committee and the HICPAC/SHEA/APIC/IDSA Hand Hygiene Task Force. *MMWR Recommendations and Reports, 51*(RR-16), 1–45. Accessed March 2015 via the Web at http://www.cdc.gov/mmwr/pdf/rr/rr5116.pdf (Level II)

2 The Joint Commission. (2015). Standard NPSG.07.01.01. *Comprehensive accreditation manual for hospitals: The official handbook.* Oakbrook Terrace, IL: The Joint Commission. (Level VII)

3 World Health Organization. (2009). "WHO guidelines on hand hygiene in health care: First global patient safety challenge, clean care is safer care" [Online]. Accessed March 2015 via the Web at http://whqlibdoc.who.int/publications/2009/9789241597906_eng.pdf (Level IV)

4 American Osteopathic Association. (2014). Standard 07.01.21. *Healthcare Facilities Accreditation Program: Accreditation requirements for acute care hospitals.* Chicago, IL: American Osteopathic Association. (Level VII)

5 Centers for Medicare & Medicaid Services, Department of Health and Human Services. (2014). Condition of participation: Infection control. 42 C.F.R. § 482.42.

6 The Joint Commission. (2015). Standard NPSG.01.01.01. *Comprehensive accreditation manual for hospitals: The official handbook.* Oakbrook Terrace, IL: The Joint Commission. (Level VII)

7 Siegel, J. D., et al. (2007). "2007 guideline for isolation precautions: Preventing transmission of infectious agents in healthcare settings" [Online]. Accessed March 2015 via the Web at http://www.cdc.gov/hicpac/pdf/isolation/Isolation2007.pdf (Level II)

8 American Osteopathic Association. (2014). Standard 07.01.10. *Healthcare Facilities Accreditation Program: Accreditation requirements for acute care hospitals.* Chicago, IL: American Osteopathic Association. (Level VII)

9 Carroll, P. (2011). "Managing chest drainage" [Online]. Accessed March 2015 via the Web at http://www.atriummed.com/EN/Chest_Drainage/Documents/continuing%20education%202010%20Online.pdf

10 Rajan, C. S. (2013). "Tube thoracostomy management" [Online]. Accessed March 2015 via the Web at http://emedicine.medscape.com/article/1503275-overview

11 U.S. Food and Drug Administration. (n.d.). "Look. Check. Connect. Safe medical device connections save lives" [Online]. Accessed March 2015 via the Web at http://www.fda.gov/downloads/MedicalDevices/Safety/AlertsandNotices/UCM134873.pdf

12 Lynn-McHale Wiegand, D. (Ed.). (2011). *AACN procedure manual for critical care* (6th ed.). St. Louis, MO: Saunders.

13 Atrium Medical Corporation. (2012). "A personal guide to managing chest drainage" [Online]. Accessed March 2015 via the Web at http://www.atriummed.com/EN/Chest_Drainage/Documents/BlueHandbook342263L.pdf

14 The Joint Commission. (2015). Standard RC.01.03.01. *Comprehensive accreditation manual for hospitals: The official handbook.* Oakbrook Terrace, IL: The Joint Commission. (Level VII)

15 American Osteopathic Association. (2014). Standard 10.00.03. *Healthcare Facilities Accreditation Program: Accreditation requirements for acute care hospitals.* Chicago, IL: American Osteopathic Association. (Level VII)

16 Centers for Medicare & Medicaid Services, Department of Health and Human Services. (2014). Condition of participation: Medical record services. 42 C.F.R. § 482.24(b).

17 American Association of Critical Care Nurses. (2013). "Evidence-based care of patients with chest tubes" [Online]. Accessed March 2015 via the Web at http://www.atriummed.com/EN/chest_drainage/Documents/Evidence-Based%20Care%20of%20Patients%20With%20Chest%20Tubes%20Complete.pdf (Level VII)

18 Durai, R., et al. (2010). Managing a chest tube and drainage system. *AORN Journal, 91,* 275–280. Accessed March 2015 via the Web at http://isgweb.aorn.org/ISGWeb/downloads/CEA10006-9943.pdf

ADDITIONAL REFERENCE

Nettina, S. M. (2014). *Lippincott manual of nursing practice* (10th ed.). Philadelphia, PA: Wolters Kluwer.

Chest tube insertion, assisting

The pleural space normally contains a thin layer of lubricating fluid that allows the visceral and parietal pleura to move without friction during respiration. An excess of fluid (hemothorax or pleural effusion), air (pneumothorax), or both in this space alters intrapleural pressure and causes partial or complete lung collapse.

Chest tube insertion allows drainage of air or fluid from the pleural space. Usually performed by a practitioner with a nurse assisting, this procedure requires sterile technique. The insertion site varies, depending on the patient's condition. For pneumothorax, the second to third intercostal space is the usual site because air rises to the top of the intrapleural space. For hemothorax or pleural effusion, the fourth to sixth intercostal spaces are common sites because fluid settles to the lower levels of the intrapleural space. For removal of air and fluid, a chest tube is inserted into a high and a low site.

After insertion, the practitioner connects one or more chest tubes to a thoracic drainage system that removes air, fluid, or both from the pleural space and prevents backflow into that space, promoting lung reexpansion.

Equipment

Vital signs monitoring equipment ■ lidocaine local anesthetic (0.5% or 1%) ■ sterile gowns ■ sterile gloves ■ masks ■ caps ■ eye goggles or face mask with eye shield ■ antiseptic wipes ■ rolled towels or blanket ■ sterile drapes ■ chlorhexidine-based antiseptic swabs ■ sterile syringes (assortment of sizes: 3 mL, 5 mL, and tuberculin) ■ 22G and 25G needles ■ sterile chest tube tray, which includes hemostats, forceps, trocar, scalpel, Kelly clamps, scissors, skin expanders, and sponges ■ sterile chest tube catheter (#16 to #20 French catheter for air or serous fluid; #28 to #40 French catheter for blood, pus, or thick fluid) ■ suture material (usually #2-0 to #3-0 silk with cutting needle) ■ sterile petroleum gauze ■ two sterile 4″ × 4″ (10-cm × 10-cm) drain dressings ■ sterile 4″ × 4″ (10-cm × 10-cm) or 2″ × 2″ (5-cm × 5-cm) gauze pads ■ 3″ to 4″ (7.6- to 10-cm) sturdy elastic tape ■ 1″ (2.5-cm) adhesive tape for connections ■ two rubber-tipped clamps for each chest tube inserted ■ sterile chest tube drainage system with tubing and connector ■ sterile marker ■ sterile labels ■ prescribed sedation ■ prescribed pain medication ■ stethoscope ■ disinfectant pad ■ Optional: suction source, suction-control device, suction connection tubing, sterile nonadherent gauze, transparent dressing, sterile water, Y connector.

Prepackaged sterile chest tube trays are commercially available and contain most of the equipment listed.

Preparation of equipment

Check the expiration date on the sterile packages, and inspect for tears. Then gather all equipment in the patient's room. Set up the drainage system according to the manufacturer's instructions. (See the "Chest tube drainage system setup" procedure, page 181.) Place the system next to the patient's bed below chest level *to facilitate drainage.*[1] Label all medications, medication containers, and other solutions on and off the sterile field.[2,3]

Implementation

■ Verify the order for chest tube insertion and the number and sizes of chest tubes needed.[4]

■ Make sure that a signed informed consent form is in the patient's medical record unless the procedure is an emergency.[5,6,7]

■ Conduct a preprocedure verification *to make sure that all relevant documentation, related information, and equipment are available and correctly identified to the patient's identifiers.*[4,8]

■ Review the patient's medical record for a history of chronic lung disease, spontaneous pneumothorax, and pulmonary disease or procedures that may have included the need for chest tube placement.

■ Perform hand hygiene.[9,10,11,12,13]

■ Confirm the patient's identity using at least two patient identifiers.[6,14]

■ Provide privacy.[15,16,17]

■ Explain the procedure to the patient *to allay his anxiety and promote cooperation with the procedure.*

■ Verify that the practitioner has marked the insertion site with his initials or with another unambiguous mark designated by your facility's policy before the procedure is performed.[18]

■ Confirm that the correct procedure has been identified for the correct patient at the correct site.[4,8]

■ Assess the patient for signs and symptoms of respiratory distress, including tachypnea, decreased or absent breath sounds, dyspnea, cyanosis, asymmetrical chest expansion, anxiety, restlessness, shortness of breath, tachycardia, hypotension, arrhythmias, and sudden sharp chest pain.

■ Obtain the patient's baseline data, including vital signs, skin color, perfusion, level of consciousness, oxygen requirements, hemodynamic stability, and respiratory rate, pattern, and effort *to help identify and document acute changes that may occur during and after the procedure.*

■ Administer sedation and pain medication as ordered, following safe medication practices.[19,20,21] The practitioner may request sedation (benzodiazepines) and opioid analgesia *to reduce pain and to help the patient remain calm.*

■ Position the patient for chest tube insertion. (Typically, the practitioner places the chest tube in the midaxillary to anterior axillary line.) It's easiest to lay the patient in the supine position, using rolled towels or a blanket to slightly rotate the upper body in a side-lying position, with the arm of the affected side raised above the head.

■ Perform hand hygiene[9,10,11,12,13] and put on sterile gloves and attire, including eyewear, *to maintain standard precautions and infection protection practices for a sterile surgical procedure.*[22,23]

■ Conduct a time-out immediately before starting the procedure *to perform a final assessment that the correct patient, site, positioning, and procedure are identified and that, as applicable, all relevant information and necessary equipment are available during and after the procedure.*[24]

■ If the patient can cooperate, ask the patient to take a deep breath just before tube insertion. *A deep breath displaces the diaphragm downward, minimizing the risk of injury.*

■ Assist the practitioner, as needed, with the procedure, while continually assessing the patient for vital sign changes. (See *Inserting the chest tube.*)

■ Remove and discard your gloves.[22,23]

■ Perform hand hygiene.[9,10,11,12,13]

■ Open the packages containing the petroleum gauze, 4″ × 4″ (10-cm × 10-cm) drain dressings, and gauze pads (although no clear evidence supports the best type of dressing to apply to the chest tube insertion site).[25]

■ Put on new sterile gloves.[22,23]

■ Place petroleum gauze around the chest tube, and then place two 4″ × 4″ (10-cm × 10-cm) drain dressings around the insertion site, one from the top and the other from the bottom (as shown on next page, top left), *to seal the insertion site from any air entry or escape.*

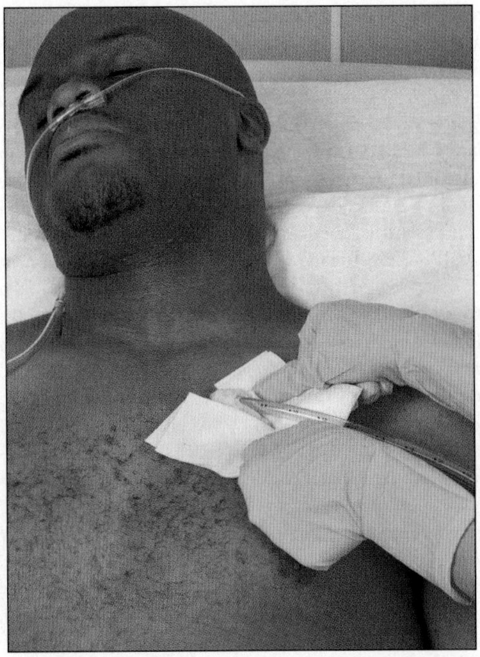

■ Place several 4″ × 4″ (10-cm × 10-cm) gauze pads on top of the drain dressings.
■ Tape the dressings, covering them completely *to form an occlusive dressing.*
■ Write the date, the time, and your initials on the dressing.
■ Secure the chest tube and drainage tube so that there's no tension pulling on the insertion site *to help prevent accidental tube dislodgment.*[26]
■ Securely tape the junction of the chest tube and the drainage tube (as shown below) *to prevent their separation.*[26]

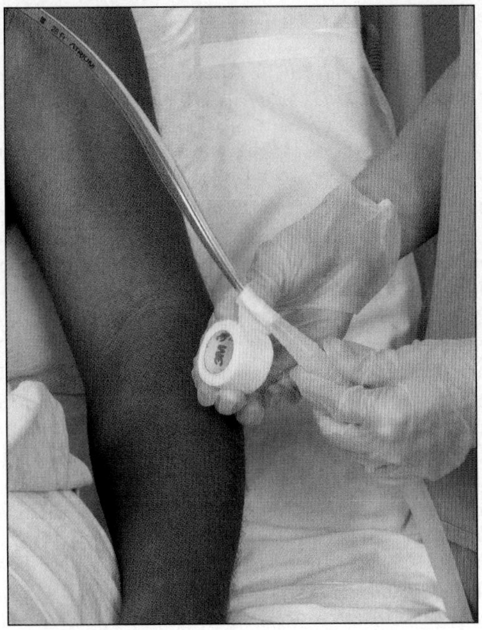

■ Secure the chest tube drainage system according to the manufacturer's instructions *to keep the drainage system from tipping over.*[27]
■ Dispose of equipment and waste in the appropriate biohazard receptacles.[28]
■ Remove and discard your gloves and other personal protective equipment[22,23] and perform hand hygiene.[9,10,11,12,13]
■ Ensure that all clamps are open and that the drainage tubing has a straight flow to the chest tube drainage collection system and has no dependent loops or kinks *because fluid-filled dependent loops can rapidly change pleural pressure, resulting in dramatically decreased drainage.*[29]
■ Ensure that the chest tube drainage system is correctly connected to the patient's chest tube; then, if ordered, connect the suction tubing to the drainage system and the suction regulator.
■ Adjust the suction until gentle bubbling appears in the suction-control chamber of a wet suction system or that the appropriate indicator appears when the dry suction system achieves the desired negative pressure.
■ Check the status of the drainage tubing.
■ Reassess the patient after the procedure.[30] Obtain vital signs and assess skin color, perfusion, level of consciousness, oxygen requirements, hemodynamic stability, comfort level, pain level, and respiratory rate, pattern, and effort *to identify the patient's tolerance of the procedure and response to chest tube placement.*
■ Arrange for a portable chest X-ray, as ordered, *to check tube position, air or fluid evacuation, and lung reexpansion.*[26]
■ Monitor the patient's vital signs at an interval determined by your facility or as indicated by the patient's condition. Auscultate his breath sounds at least every 4 hours *to assess air exchange in the affected lung. Diminished or absent breath sounds indicate that the lung hasn't reexpanded.*
■ Record the type, color, and amount of drainage in the drainage collection chamber. Notify the practitioner immediately of a sudden decrease in drainage or the presence of frank bloody drainage.[1]
■ Mark the drainage level on the disposable chest drainage collection device at an interval determined by your facility or as indicated by the patient's condition.
■ Perform hand hygiene.[9,10,11,12,13]
■ Clean and disinfect your stethoscope using a disinfectant pad.[31,32]

Inserting the chest tube

Chest tube insertion involves these steps:
■ The practitioner puts on a cap, a mask, eye protection, a sterile gown, and sterile gloves and prepares a sterile field using sterile drapes.
■ The practitioner prepares the insertion site using chlorhexidine-based antiseptic swabs. After the antiseptic dries completely, the practitioner drapes the patient, leaving the insertion site exposed.
■ The nurse disinfects the rubber stopper of the lidocaine vial with an antiseptic pad. Then she inverts the bottle and holds it for the practitioner to withdraw the anesthetic.
■ The practitioner injects a local anesthetic at the site *to reduce the pain of the procedure* and waits for the anesthetic to take effect.
■ The practitioner makes a skin incision about 1″ (2.5-cm) long and then inserts a hemostat through the opening *to enter the pleural space.* Typically, when the pleural space is entered, you'll see a return of pleural contents, confirming penetration.
■ The practitioner spreads the hemostat open slightly *to enlarge the opening enough to accommodate the chest tube.*
■ Using his finger, the practitioner creates a track for the chest tube. He then clamps the chest tube with the hemostat and inserts them through the incision, guiding the hemostat and tube along his inserted finger.
■ The practitioner removes the hemostat and immediately connects the chest tube to the drainage system.
■ The nurse assists the practitioner in attaching the disposable sterile chest tube drainage system to the chest tube, using a Y-connector if placing more than one chest tube.
■ The practitioner sutures the chest tube securely into place and wraps sterile petroleum gauze around the chest tube where it enters the chest.

- Perform hand hygiene.[9,10,11,12,13]
- Document the procedure.[33,34,35]

Special considerations

NURSING ALERT *Don't strip a chest drain (occluding the chest tube with one hand while quickly squeezing and moving the other hand down the tube to move fluid down the tube into the drainage chamber)* because intraluminal pressures can rise dangerously high, which may convert a simple pneumothorax to life-threatening pneumothorax and cause tissue trauma and unnecessary discomfort. *Don't milk, fanfold, or tap the chest drain* because it hasn't been demonstrated that such manipulations improve fluid drainage from the chest.[29]

NURSING ALERT *Drain large effusions slowly* because rapid removal (removal of more than 1 L of pleural fluid) during the first 30 minutes after chest tube insertion may cause post-thoracentesis pulmonary edema.[36]

- Routine clamping of the chest tube isn't recommended *because of the risk of tension pneumothorax.*
- During patient transport, keep the chest tube drainage system below chest level.[1] Don't clamp the chest tube during transport.
- Keep a rubber-tipped clamp, sterile dressing, and tape at the bedside *in case of accidental dislodgement.*[1]
- If you hear air leaking from the site, tape the dressing on three sides *to allow air to escape and to prevent a tension pneumothorax.* Notify the practitioner. Closely monitor the patient and prepare for insertion of a new chest tube.

Complications

Complications of chest tube insertion include bleeding if a vessel is inadvertently nicked during the insertion process, subcutaneous emphysema from air leaking into the pleural space, and infection.

Documentation

Record the date and time of chest tube insertion, who inserted the tube, the insertion site, the size of the chest tube used, medications given, the chest tube drainage system used, the presence of drainage and bubbling, associated complications and nursing actions taken, and patient teaching provided. Document your assessment findings before and after the procedure and the patient's response to the procedure. Record the patient's respiratory status and vital signs as well as amount of drainage and its color and consistency every 2 to 4 hours.

REFERENCES

1 Rajan, C. S. (2013). "Tube thoracostomy management" [Online]. Accessed March 2015 via the Web at http://emedicine.medscape.com/article/1503275-overview

2 The Joint Commission. (2015). Standard NPSG.03.04.01. *Comprehensive accreditation manual for hospitals: The official handbook.* Oakbrook Terrace, IL: The Joint Commission. (Level VII)

3 American Osteopathic Association. (2014). Standard 25.01.27. *Healthcare Facilities Accreditation Program: Accreditation requirements for acute care hospitals.* Chicago, IL: American Osteopathic Association. (Level VII)

4 The Joint Commission. (2015). Standard UP.01.01.01. *Comprehensive accreditation manual for hospitals: The official handbook.* Oakbrook Terrace, IL: The Joint Commission. (Level VII)

5 The Joint Commission. (2015). Standard RI.01.03.01. *Comprehensive accreditation manual for hospitals: The official handbook.* Oakbrook Terrace, IL: The Joint Commission. (Level VII)

6 American Osteopathic Association. (2014). Standard 15.01.11. *Healthcare Facilities Accreditation Program: Accreditation requirements for acute care hospitals.* Chicago, IL: American Osteopathic Association. (Level VII)

7 Centers for Medicare & Medicaid Services, Department of Health and Human Services. (2014). Condition of participation: Patient's rights. 42 C.F.R. § 482.13

8 American Osteopathic Association. (2014). Standard 30.00.14. *Healthcare Facilities Accreditation Program: Accreditation requirements for acute care hospitals.* Chicago, IL: American Osteopathic Association. (Level VII)

9 Centers for Disease Control and Prevention. (2002). Guideline for hand hygiene in health-care settings: Recommendations of the Healthcare Infection Control Practices Advisory Committee and the HICPAC/SHEA/APIC/IDSA Hand Hygiene Task Force. *MMWR Recommendations and Reports, 51*(RR-16), 1–45. Accessed March 2015 via the Web at http://www.cdc.gov/mmwr/pdf/rr/rr5116.pdf (Level II)

10 The Joint Commission. (2015). Standard NPSG.07.01.01. *Comprehensive accreditation manual for hospitals: The official handbook.* Oakbrook Terrace, IL: The Joint Commission. (Level VII)

11 World Health Organization. (2009). "WHO guidelines on hand hygiene in health care: First global patient safety challenge, clean care is safer care" [Online]. Accessed March 2015 via the Web at http://whqlibdoc.who.int/publications/2009/9789241597906_eng.pdf (Level IV)

12 American Osteopathic Association. (2014). Standard 07.01.21. *Healthcare Facilities Accreditation Program: Accreditation requirements for acute care hospitals.* Chicago, IL: American Osteopathic Association. (Level VII)

13 Centers for Medicare & Medicaid Services, Department of Health and Human Services. (2014). Condition of participation: Infection control. 42 C.F.R. § 482.42.

14 The Joint Commission. (2015). Standard NPSG.01.01.01. *Comprehensive accreditation manual for hospitals: The official handbook.* Oakbrook Terrace, IL: The Joint Commission. (Level VII)

15 American Osteopathic Association. (2014). Standard 15.01.16. *Healthcare Facilities Accreditation Program: Accreditation requirements for acute care hospitals.* Chicago, IL: American Osteopathic Association. (Level VII)

16 Centers for Medicare & Medicaid Services, Department of Health and Human Services. (2014). Condition of participation: Patient's rights. 42 C.F.R. § 482.13(c)(1).

17 The Joint Commission. (2015). Standard RI.01.01.01. *Comprehensive accreditation manual for hospitals: The official handbook.* Oakbrook Terrace, IL: The Joint Commission. (Level VII)

18 The Joint Commission. (2015). Standard UP.01.02.01. *Comprehensive accreditation manual for hospitals: The official handbook.* Oakbrook Terrace, IL: The Joint Commission. (Level VII)

19 American Osteopathic Association. (2014). Standard 16.01.03. *Healthcare Facilities Accreditation Program: Accreditation requirements for acute care hospitals.* Chicago, IL: American Osteopathic Association. (Level VII)

20 Centers for Medicare & Medicaid Services, Department of Health and Human Services. (2014). Condition of participation: Nursing services. 42 C.F.R. § 482.23(c).

21 The Joint Commission. (2015). Standard MM.06.01.01. *Comprehensive accreditation manual for hospitals: The official handbook.* Oakbrook Terrace, IL: The Joint Commission. (Level VII)

22 Siegel J. D., et al. (2007). "2007 guideline for isolation precautions: Preventing transmission of infectious agents in healthcare settings" [Online]. Accessed March 2015 via the Web at http://www.cdc.gov/hicpac/pdf/isolation/Isolation2007.pdf (Level II)

23 American Osteopathic Association. (2014). Standard 07.01.10. *Healthcare Facilities Accreditation Program: Accreditation requirements for acute care hospitals.* Chicago, IL: American Osteopathic Association. (Level VII)

24 The Joint Commission. (2015). Standard UP.01.03.01. *Comprehensive accreditation manual for hospitals: The official handbook.* Oakbrook Terrace, IL: The Joint Commission. (Level VII)

25 Durai, R., et al. (2010). Managing a chest tube and drainage system. *AORN Journal, 91,* 275–280. Accessed March 2015 via the Web at http://isgweb.aorn.org/ISGWeb/downloads/CEA10006-9943.pdf

26 Lynn-McHale Wiegand, D. (Ed.). (2011). *AACN procedure manual for critical care* (6th ed.). St. Louis, MO: Saunders.

27 Atrium Medical Corporation. (2012). "A personal guide to managing chest drainage" [Online]. Accessed March 2015 via the Web at http://www.atriummed.com/EN/Chest_Drainage/Documents/BlueHandbook342263L.pdf

28 Occupational Safety and Health Administration. (n.d.). "Bloodborne pathogens, standard number 1910.1030" [Online]. Accessed March 2015 via the Web at http://www.osha.gov/pls/oshaweb/owadisp.show_document?p_table=STANDARDS&p_id=10051 (Level VII)
29 American Association of Critical Care Nurses. (2013). "Evidence-based care of patients with chest tubes" [Online]. Accessed March 2015 via the Web at http://www.atriummed.com/EN/chest_drainage/Documents/Evidence-Based%20Care%20of%20Patients%20With%20Chest%20Tubes%20Complete.pdf (Level VII)
30 The Joint Commission. (2015). Standard PC.01.02.05. *Comprehensive accreditation manual for hospitals: The official handbook.* Oakbrook Terrace, IL: The Joint Commission. (Level VII)
31 Rutala, W. A., et al. (2008). "Guideline for disinfection and sterilization in healthcare facilities, 2008" [Online]. Accessed March 2015 via the Web at http://www.cdc.gov/hicpac/pdf/guidelines/Disinfection_Nov_2008.pdf (Level I)
32 American Osteopathic Association. (2014). Standard 07.02.03. *Healthcare Facilities Accreditation Program: Accreditation requirements for acute care hospitals.* Chicago, IL: American Osteopathic Association. (Level VII)
33 The Joint Commission. (2015). Standard RC.01.03.01. *Comprehensive accreditation manual for hospitals: The official handbook.* Oakbrook Terrace, IL: The Joint Commission. (Level VII)
34 American Osteopathic Association. (2014). Standard 10.00.03. *Healthcare Facilities Accreditation Program: Accreditation requirements for acute care hospitals.* Chicago, IL: American Osteopathic Association. (Level VII)
35 Centers for Medicare & Medicaid Services, Department of Health and Human Services. (2014). Condition of participation: Medical record services. 42 C.F.R. § 482.24(b).
36 Huggins, J. T., & Doelken, P. Large volume thoracentesis. (2014). In: *UpToDate,* Sahn, S. (Ed.). Accessed March 2015 via the Web at http://www.uptodate.com/contents/search

ADDITIONAL REFERENCE

Nettina, S. M. (2014). *Lippincott manual of nursing practice* (10th ed.). Philadelphia, PA: Wolters Kluwer.

CHEST TUBE REMOVAL, ASSISTING

The pleural space normally contains a thin layer of lubricating fluid that allows the visceral and parietal pleura to move without friction during respiration. Excess fluid, air, or both in this space alters intrapleural pressure and causes partial or complete lung collapse. A chest tube allows drainage of the air or fluid from the pleural space and enables lung reexpansion and the restoration of negative pressure to the pleural space.

After the patient's lung has reexpanded and any drainage has been controlled, the practitioner may order you to clamp a chest tube or discontinue suction, with the tube left to water-seal drainage for several hours before removal to assess patient tolerance. This waiting period allows time to observe the patient for signs and symptoms of respiratory distress, an indication that air or fluid remains trapped in the pleural space. The practitioner may also order a chest X-ray before removal to ensure lung expansion.

Chest tube removal usually happens as soon as it's no longer clinically indicated to prevent infection along the tube tract.[1] Chest tube removal is the responsibility of the doctor, nurse practitioner, advance practice nurse, or physician's assistant, according to scope of practice.

Equipment

Gloves ▪ sterile gloves ▪ goggles ▪ masks ▪ gowns ▪ two rubber-tipped chest tube clamps (two per chest tube) ▪ prescribed medication ▪ suture removal kit ▪ fluid-impermeable pad ▪ sterile petroleum gauze ▪ 4″ × 4″ (10-cm × 10-cm) sterile gauze dressings ▪ tape ▪ antiseptic swabs ▪ vital signs monitoring equipment ▪ stethoscope ▪ disinfectant pad ▪ Optional: prescribed pain medication.

Implementation

- Verify the practitioner's order for chest tube removal.
- Gather the appropriate equipment.
- Perform hand hygiene.[2,3,4,5,6]
- Confirm the patient's identity using at least two patient identifiers.[7]
- Explain the procedure to the patient *to ensure his cooperation and decrease anxiety.*
- Provide privacy.[8,9,10]
- Premedicate the patient, as ordered, following safe medication administration practices *to reduce the patient's discomfort.*[11,12,13]
- Obtain vital signs and perform a respiratory assessment.
- Perform hand hygiene and put on goggles, a mask, a gown, and gloves.[2,3,4,5,6,14,15]
- Place the patient in the semi-Fowler position or on his unaffected side *to enhance access to the insertion site.*[1]
- Place a fluid-impermeable pad under the affected side *to protect the linens from drainage and to provide a place to put the chest tube after removal.*
- Prepare the suture removal kit and a sterile airtight dressing with petroleum gauze and 4″ × 4″ (10-cm × 10-cm) sterile gauze dressings *so that the practitioner can cover the insertion site with it immediately after quickly and smoothly removing the chest tube.*[1]
- The practitioner performs hand hygiene and puts on goggles, a mask, a gown, and sterile gloves.[15]
- If instructed by the practitioner, remove the existing chest tube dressings and discard them appropriately.[16] Be careful not to dislodge the chest tube prematurely.
- Assist the practitioner as needed with cleaning the area around the tubes with an antiseptic swab and removing the sutures.[1]
- Trace the chest tube from the point of origin to the patient *to make sure that you're removing the proper tube.*[17] Clamp the chest tube catheter (if not already done) with two clamps *to minimize dead space and stop air from entering or exiting catheter.*[1]
- Assist the practitioner as necessary. The practitioner will instruct the patient to perform the Valsalva maneuver by exhaling and bearing down *to increase intrathoracic pressure and prevent air from entering the pleural space as he removes the chest tube* and covers the insertion site with the airtight dressing.[1]
- Help secure the dressing with tape. Make it as airtight as possible *to seal the insertion site from air entry.*[1]
- Instruct the patient to breathe normally.
- Mark the dressing with the date, the time, and your initials.
- Dispose of equipment and waste in an appropriate receptacle.[16]
- Remove and discard your gloves and other personal protective equipment[14,15] and perform hand hygiene.[2,3,4,5,6]
- Closely monitor the patient after the procedure *to determine the patient's response to and tolerance of the procedure.*
- Obtain vital signs, including respiratory rate, pattern, and effort. Monitor the patient's color, perfusion, level of consciousness, oxygen requirements, and hemodynamic stability. Assess the patient carefully for signs and symptoms of pneumothorax, subcutaneous emphysema, or infection.
- Obtain a chest X-ray, as ordered, *to ensure lung expansion.*[1]

NURSING ALERT *Notify the practitioner immediately if the patient develops acute respiratory distress* because such distress may indicate the need for a new chest tube.

- Position the patient for comfort.
- Encourage coughing and deep breathing. (See *Instructions for coughing and deep breathing,* page 188.)
- Assess the chest tube site and dressing for drainage and re-dress as needed or ordered.
- Perform a comprehensive pain assessment using techniques appropriate for the patient's age, condition, and ability to understand.[18]

PATIENT TEACHING

Instructions for coughing and deep breathing

Coughing or "huffing" helps break up secretions in the lungs for suctioning or expectorating mucus. Deep-breathing exercises help to expand the lungs and force better distribution of the air into all areas. The patient may initially need to lie down to do these exercises, but eventually he can do them while sitting upright, and then while walking.

Coughing

Help the patient to a sitting position. For a controlled cough, the patient purses his lips and takes a deep breath. He should hold the breath for several seconds and then briefly and gently cough twice. For huffing, the patient purses his lips and takes a deep breath. After holding his breath for several seconds, he exhales, using his stomach muscles to push out the air. The vocal chords remain open so that the cough has almost a whispery sound. Coughing and huffing are repeated several times per day, as needed.

Deep-breathing exercises

The patient starts by taking a deep breath through the nose, and then purses his lips as if to whistle. He then exhales the air slowly through pursed lips. The exhalation should take twice as long as the inhalation. For example, the patient may start by inhaling for 2 seconds and then exhaling for 4 seconds. After taking several deep breaths, he should breathe at a normal rhythm and then begin another cycle of deep breathing.

Usually, the patient will perform coughing and deep-breathing exercises together. To do this, first tell the patient to breathe in deeply through his nose and then exhale in three short huffs. Then have him inhale deeply again and cough through a slightly open mouth. Three consecutive coughs are highly effective. An effective cough sounds deep, low, and hollow; an ineffective cough is high-pitched. If possible, have the patient perform this exercise for about 1 minute and then rest for 2 minutes.

- Administer pain medication, as needed and prescribed, following safe medication administration practices.[11,12,13]
- Clean and disinfect your stethoscope using a disinfectant pad.[19,20]
- Perform hand hygiene.[2,3,4,5,6]
- Document the procedure.[21,22,23]

Special considerations

- The practitioner may elect to physiologically simulate tube removal by clamping the chest tube for 4 to 6 hours[24] or by placing the tube in a temporary water seal to remove suction for 6 to 24 hours[1] before removing the tube *to evaluate the patient's tolerance and to confirm that pneumothorax hasn't recurred.*

Complications

Complications of chest tube removal include infection at the site, tension pneumothorax, and redevelopment of the pneumothorax, hemothorax, or chylothorax (lymphatic fluid [chyle] in the pleural space) that was present before tube placement.

Documentation

Record the date and time of chest tube removal, your preparation procedures, the patient's vital signs and respiratory status, medications given and their effectiveness, and the patient's tolerance of the procedure. Document the condition of the insertion site, complications and nursing actions taken, and any teaching provided.

REFERENCES

1 Lynn-McHale Wiegand, D. (Ed.). (2011). *AACN procedure manual for critical care* (6th ed.). St. Louis, MO: Saunders.

2 Centers for Disease Control and Prevention. (2002). Guideline for hand hygiene in health-care settings: Recommendations of the Healthcare Infection Control Practices Advisory Committee and the HICPAC/SHEA/APIC/IDSA Hand Hygiene Task Force. *MMWR Recommendations and Reports, 51*(RR-16), 1–45. Accessed March 2015 via the Web at http://www.cdc.gov/mmwr/pdf/rr/rr5116.pdf (Level II)

3 The Joint Commission. (2015). Standard NPSG.07.01.01. *Comprehensive accreditation manual for hospitals: The official handbook.* Oakbrook Terrace, IL: The Joint Commission. (Level VII)

4 World Health Organization. (2009). "WHO guidelines on hand hygiene in health care: First global patient safety challenge, clean care is safer care" [Online]. Accessed March 2015 via the Web at http://whqlibdoc.who.int/publications/2009/9789241597906_eng.pdf (Level IV)

5 Centers for Medicare & Medicaid Services, Department of Health and Human Services. (2014). Condition of participation: Infection control. 42 C.F.R. § 482.42.

6 American Osteopathic Association. (2014). Standard 07.01.21. *Healthcare Facilities Accreditation Program: Accreditation requirements for acute care hospitals.* Chicago, IL: American Osteopathic Association. (Level VII)

7 The Joint Commission. (2015). Standard NPSG.01.01.01. *Comprehensive accreditation manual for hospitals: The official handbook.* Oakbrook Terrace, IL: The Joint Commission. (Level VII)

8 Centers for Medicare & Medicaid Services, Department of Health and Human Services. (2014). Condition of participation: Patient's rights. 42 C.F.R. § 482.13(c)(1).

9 The Joint Commission. (2015). Standard RI.01.01.01. *Comprehensive accreditation manual for hospitals: The official handbook.* Oakbrook Terrace, IL: The Joint Commission. (Level VII)

10 American Osteopathic Association. (2014). Standard 15.01.16. *Healthcare Facilities Accreditation Program: Accreditation requirements for acute care hospitals.* Chicago, IL: American Osteopathic Association. (Level VII)

11 Centers for Medicare & Medicaid Services, Department of Health and Human Services. (2014). Condition of participation: Nursing services. 42 C.F.R. § 482.23(c).

12 The Joint Commission. (2015). Standard MM.06.01.01. *Comprehensive accreditation manual for hospitals: The official handbook.* Oakbrook Terrace, IL: The Joint Commission. (Level VII)

13 American Osteopathic Association. (2014). Standard 16.01.03. *Healthcare Facilities Accreditation Program: Accreditation requirements for acute care hospitals.* Chicago, IL: American Osteopathic Association. (Level VII)

14 American Osteopathic Association. (2014). Standard 07.01.10. *Healthcare Facilities Accreditation Program: Accreditation requirements for acute care hospitals.* Chicago, IL: American Osteopathic Association. (Level VII)

15 Siegel J. D., et al. (2007). "2007 guideline for isolation precautions: Preventing transmission of infectious agents in healthcare settings" [Online]. Accessed March 2015 via the Web at http://www.cdc.gov/hicpac/pdf/isolation/Isolation2007.pdf (Level II)

16 Occupational Safety and Health Administration. (n.d.). "Bloodborne pathogens, standard number 1910.1030" [Online]. Accessed March 2015 via the Web at http://www.osha.gov/pls/oshaweb/owadisp.show_document?p_table=STANDARDS&p_id=10051 (Level VII)

17 U.S. Food and Drug Administration. (n.d.). "Look. Check. Connect. Safe medical device connections save lives" [Online]. Accessed March 2015 via the Web at http://www.fda.gov/downloads/MedicalDevices/Safety/AlertsandNotices/UCM134873.pdf

18 The Joint Commission. (2015). Standard PC.01.02.07. *Comprehensive accreditation manual for hospitals: The official handbook.* Oakbrook Terrace, IL: The Joint Commission. (Level VII)

19 Rutala, W. A., et al. (2008). "Guideline for disinfection and sterilization in healthcare facilities, 2008" [Online]. Accessed March 2015 via the Web at http://www.cdc.gov/hicpac/pdf/guidelines/Disinfection_Nov_2008.pdf (Level I)

20 American Osteopathic Association. (2014). Standard 07.02.03. *Healthcare Facilities Accreditation Program: Accreditation requirements for acute care hospitals.* Chicago, IL: American Osteopathic Association. (Level VII)

21 The Joint Commission. (2015). Standard RC.01.03.01. *Comprehensive accreditation manual for hospitals: The official handbook.* Oakbrook Terrace, IL: The Joint Commission. (Level VII)

22 Centers for Medicare & Medicaid Services, Department of Health and Human Services. (2014). Condition of participation: Medical record services. 42 C.F.R. § 482.24(b).

23 American Osteopathic Association. (2014). Standard 10.00.03. *Healthcare Facilities Accreditation Program: Accreditation requirements for acute care hospitals.* Chicago, IL: American Osteopathic Association. (Level VII)

24 Doelken, P. Placement and management of thoracostomy tubes. (2012). In *UpToDate,* Sahn, S. A., et al. (Eds.). Accessed March 2015 via the Web at http://www.uptodate.com/contents/search

ADDITIONAL REFERENCE

Nettina, S. M. (2014). *Lippincott manual of nursing practice* (10th ed.). Philadelphia, PA: Wolters Kluwer.

CLAVICLE STRAP APPLICATION

Also called a *figure-eight strap,* a clavicle strap reduces and immobilizes fractures of the clavicle. It does this by elevating, extending, and supporting the shoulders in position for healing, known as the *position of attention.* A commercially available figure-eight strap or a 4″ (10-cm) elastic bandage may serve as a clavicle strap. (See *Types of clavicle straps.*) This strap is contraindicated for an uncooperative patient. Clavicle straps are typically worn for 4 to 8 weeks.

Equipment

Figure-eight clavicle strap or 4″ (10-cm) elastic bandage ■ tape ■ cotton batting or padding ■ powder or cornstarch ■ marking pen ■ Optional: scissors, safety pins, analgesics.

Implementation

- Verify the practitioner's order.
- Gather the equipment.
- Perform hand hygiene.[1,2,3]
- Confirm the patient's identity using at least two patient identifiers.[4]
- Explain the procedure to the patient and provide privacy.
- Help the patient take off his shirt or cut off the shirt if movement is too painful.
- *Assess the arm's neurovascular integrity* by palpating skin temperature; observing the color and temperature of the hand and fingers; palpating the radial, ulnar, and brachial pulses bilaterally; and then comparing the affected with the unaffected side. Ask the patient about any numbness or tingling distal to the injury, and assess his motor function.
- Perform a comprehensive pain assessment using techniques appropriate for the patient's age, condition, and ability to understand.[5]
- Administer analgesics as ordered following safe medication administration practices.[6] Perform a follow-up pain assessment and notify the practitioner if the pain isn't adequately controlled.[5]
- Demonstrate how to assume the position of attention. Instruct the patient to sit upright and assume this position gradually *to minimize pain.*
- Gently apply powder or cornstarch, as appropriate, to the axillae and shoulder area *to reduce friction from the clavicle strap.* You can use cornstarch if the patient is allergic to powder.

EQUIPMENT

Types of clavicle straps

Clavicle straps provide support to the shoulder *to help heal a fractured clavicle.* These straps are available ready-made. They can also be made from a bandage.

Commercially made clavicle straps have a short back panel and long straps that extend around the patient's shoulders and axillae. They have Velcro pads or buckles on the ends *for easy fastening.*

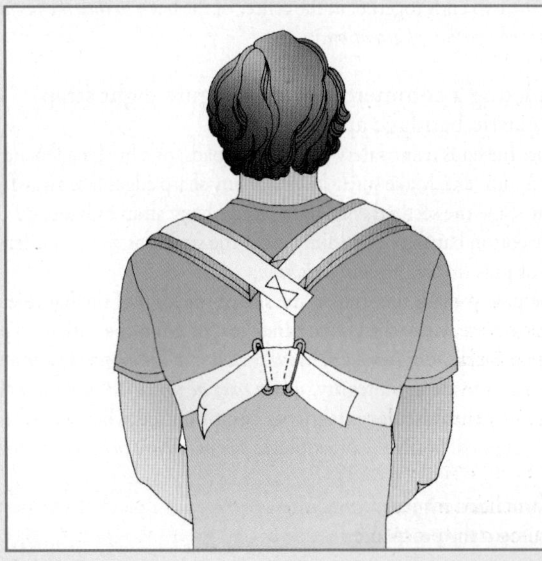

When making a clavicle strap with a wide elastic bandage, start in the middle of the patient's back. After wrapping the bandage around the shoulders, fasten the ends with safety pins.

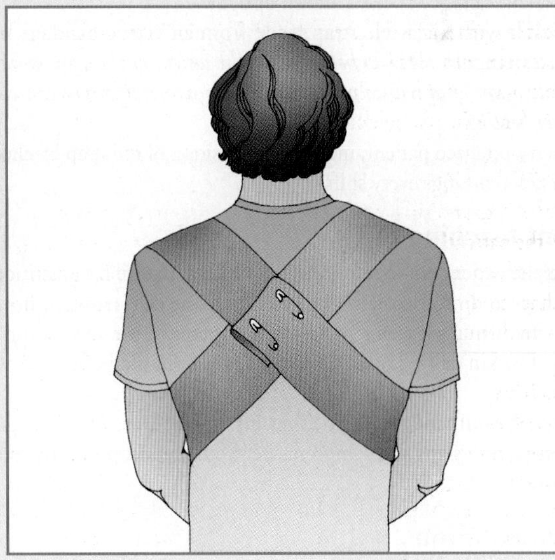

Applying a commercially made figure-eight strap

- Place the apex of the triangle between the scapulae and drape the straps over the shoulders. Bring the strap with the Velcro or buckle end under one axilla and through the loop; then pull the other strap under the other axilla and through the loop.
- Gently adjust the straps *so that they support the shoulders in the position of attention.*

- Bring the straps back under the axillae toward the anterior chest, making sure they maintain the position of attention.

Applying a 4″ (10-cm) elastic bandage strap

- Roll both ends of the elastic bandage toward the middle, leaving 12″ to 18″ (30.5 to 45.7 cm) unrolled.
- Place the unrolled portion diagonally across the patient's back, from right shoulder to left axilla.
- Bring the lower end of the bandage under the left axilla and back over the left shoulder; loop the upper end over the right shoulder and under the axilla.
- Pull the two ends together at the center of the back *so that the bandage supports the position of attention.*

Completing a commercially made figure-eight strap or an elastic bandage application

- Secure the ends using safety pins, Velcro pads, or a buckle, depending on the equipment. Make sure a buckle or any sharp edges face away from the skin. Tape the secured ends to the underlying strap or bandage.
- Place cotton batting or padding under the straps, as well as under the buckle or pins, *to prevent skin irritation.*
- Use a pen to mark the strap at the site of the loop of the figure-eight strap, or the site where the elastic bandage crosses on the patient's back. *If the strap loosens, this mark helps you tighten it to the original position.*
- Assess neurovascular integrity, *which may be impaired by a strap that's too tight.* If neurovascular integrity is compromised when the strap is correctly applied, notify the practitioner. *He may want to change the treatment.*
- Perform hand hygiene.[1,2,3]
- Document the procedure.[7,8]

Special considerations

- If possible, perform the procedure with the patient standing. However, this may not be feasible *because the pain from the fracture can cause syncope.* If the patient can't stand, have him sit upright.
- An adult with a clavicle strap made from an elastic bandage may require a triangular sling *to help support the weight of the arm, enhance immobilization, and reduce pain. Inadequate immobilization can cause improper healing.*
- For a hospitalized patient, monitor the position of the strap by checking the pen markings every shift.

Patient teaching

Instruct the patient not to remove the clavicle strap until his practitioner orders him to do so. Explain that, with help, he can maintain proper hygiene by lifting segments of the strap to remove the cotton and by washing his skin daily. Explain that fresh cotton should be applied after cleaning.

Teach the outpatient how to assess his own neurovascular integrity and to recognize signs and symptoms he should report promptly to the practitioner.

Documentation

In the appropriate section of the emergency department medical record, record the date and time of strap application, type of clavicle strap, type of padding used, bilateral neurovascular integrity before and after the procedure, analgesics administered, and instructions to the patient.

REFERENCES

1 World Health Organization. (2009). "WHO guidelines on hand hygiene in health care: First global patient safety challenge, clean care is safer care" [Online]. Accessed December 2013 via the Web at http://whqlibdoc.who.int/publications/2009/9789241597906_eng.pdf (Level IV)

2 Centers for Disease Control and Prevention. (2002). Guideline for hand hygiene in health-care settings: Recommendations of the Healthcare Infection Control Practices Advisory Committee and the HICPAC/SHEA/APIC/IDSA Hand Hygiene Task Force. *MMWR Recommendations and Reports, 51*(RR-16), 1–45. Accessed March 2015 via the Web at http://www.cdc.gov/mmwr/pdf/rr/rr5116.pdf (Level II)

3 The Joint Commission. (2015). Standard NPSG.07.01.01. *Comprehensive accreditation manual for hospitals: The official handbook.* Oakbrook Terrace, IL: The Joint Commission. (Level VII)

4 The Joint Commission. (2015). Standard NPSG.01.01.01. *Comprehensive accreditation manual for hospitals: The official handbook.* Oakbrook Terrace, IL: The Joint Commission. (Level VII)

5 The Joint Commission. (2015). Standard PC.01.02.07. *Comprehensive accreditation manual for hospitals: The official handbook.* Oakbrook Terrace, IL: The Joint Commission. (Level VII)

6 The Joint Commission. (2015). Standard MM.06.01.01. *Comprehensive accreditation manual for hospitals: The official handbook.* Oakbrook Terrace, IL: The Joint Commission. (Level VII)

7 The Joint Commission. (2015). Standard RC.01.03.01. *Comprehensive accreditation manual for hospitals: The official handbook.* Oakbrook Terrace, IL: The Joint Commission. (Level VII)

8 Centers for Medicare & Medicaid Services, Department of Health and Human Services. (2014). Condition of participation: Medical record services. 42 C.F.R. § 482.24(b).

ADDITIONAL REFERENCES

American Academy of Orthopaedic Surgeons. (2011). "Clavicle fracture (broken collarbone)" [Online]. Accessed March 2015 via the Web at http://orthoinfo.aaos.org/topic.cfm?topic=a00072

McKee, M. D., et al. (2007). Nonoperative treatment compared with plate fixation of displaced midshaft clavicular fractures. A multicenter, randomized clinical trial. *Journal of Bone and Joint Surgery, 89,* 1–10. (Level II)

CLOSED-WOUND DRAIN MANAGEMENT

Closed-wound drains are typically inserted during surgery in anticipation of substantial postoperative drainage. Studies show improved patient outcomes when they're inserted during clean surgical cases.[1,2] A closed-wound drain, commonly used after joint replacements and thyroid, breast, axillary, and abdominal procedures, prevents exudate from accumulating.[3]

The drain is usually emptied every 4 to 8 hours. Jackson-Pratt and Hemovac closed drainage systems are used most commonly. (See *Types of closed drainage systems.*)

A closed-wound drain consists of perforated tubing connected to a portable vacuum unit. The distal end of the tubing lies within the wound and usually leaves the body from a site other than the primary suture line to preserve the integrity of the surgical wound. The tubing exit site is treated as an additional surgical wound; the drain is usually sutured to the skin.

If the wound produces heavy drainage, the closed-wound drain may be left in place for longer than 1 week. Drainage must be emptied and measured frequently to maintain maximum suction and prevent strain on the suture line.

Equipment

Graduated cylinder ■ antiseptic pads ■ gloves ■ fluid-impermeable pad ■ Optional: gown, mask with face shield, mask, goggles, sterile laboratory container, label, antiseptic cleaning agent or antimicrobial swabs, sterile gauze pads, laboratory biohazard transport bag.

Implementation

- Verify the practitioner's order.
- Gather the appropriate equipment.
- Perform hand hygiene.[4,5,6]

■ Confirm the patient's identity using at least two patient identifiers.[7]
■ Explain the procedure to the patient and provide privacy.
■ Put on gloves and other personal protective equipment if appropriate.[8]
■ Assess the patient's condition.
■ *Protect the patient's linens* by placing a fluid-impermeable pad under the drain.
■ Unclip the vacuum unit from the patient's bed or gown.
■ *Release the vacuum* by removing the spout plug on the collection chamber. The container expands completely as it draws in air.
■ Empty the unit's contents into a graduated cylinder and note the amount and appearance of the drainage.
■ If diagnostic tests will be performed on the fluid specimen, pour the drainage directly into a sterile laboratory container, note the amount and appearance, and label the specimen in the presence of the patient *to avoid mislabeling.* Place the specimen into a laboratory biohazard transport bag, and send it to the laboratory.
■ Use an antiseptic pad to clean the unit's spout and plug.
■ *To reestablish the vacuum that creates the drain's suction power,* fully compress the vacuum unit. With one hand holding the compressed unit *to maintain the vacuum,* replace the spout plug with your other hand (as shown below).

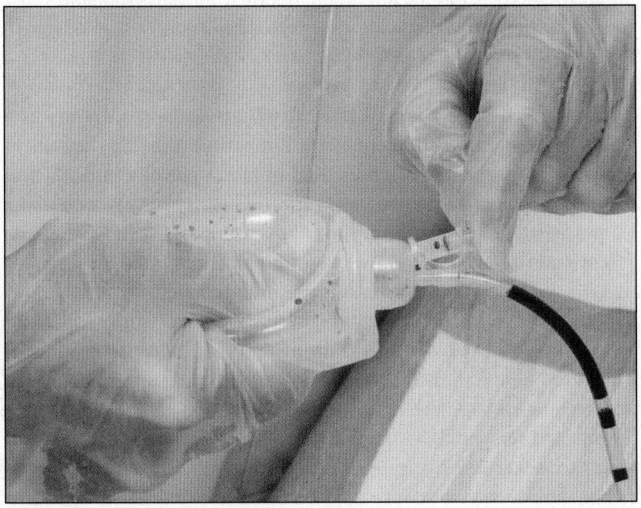

■ Check the patency of the equipment. Make sure the tubing is free of twists, kinks, and leaks *because the drainage system must be airtight to work properly.* The vacuum unit should remain compressed when you release manual pressure; *rapid reinflation indicates an air leak.* If this occurs, recompress the unit and make sure the spout plug is secure.
■ Secure the vacuum unit to the patient's gown. Fasten it below wound level *to promote drainage.* Don't apply tension on drainage tubing when fastening the unit *to prevent possible dislodgment.*
■ Observe the sutures that secure the drain to the patient's skin; look for signs of pulling or tearing and for swelling or infection of surrounding skin. Gently clean the sutures with sterile gauze pads soaked in an antiseptic cleaning agent or with an antimicrobial swab, if ordered.
■ Properly dispose of drainage and solutions, and clean or dispose of soiled equipment and supplies.
■ Remove and discard your gloves and any other personal protective equipment worn, and perform hand hygiene.[4,5,6]
■ Document the procedure.[9,10]

Special considerations

■ Check the drain frequently *to make sure suction is maintained.* Empty the drain and measure its contents every 4 to 8 hours or more often according to the patient's condition and the amount of drainage. *Removing excess drainage maintains maximum suction and avoids straining the drain's suture line.*
■ Empty the drain and measure its contents before the patient ambulates *to prevent the weight of drainage from pulling on the drain as the patient ambulates.*
■ If the patient has more than one closed drain, number the drains *so you can record drainage from each site.*

NURSING ALERT ***Be careful not to mistake chest tubes for closed-wound drains*** **because the vacuum of a chest tube should never be released.**

EQUIPMENT

Types of closed drainage systems

There are two common types of closed drainage systems. The Jackson-Pratt drain, which is typically used with breast and abdominal surgery, collects exudate in a bulblike device.

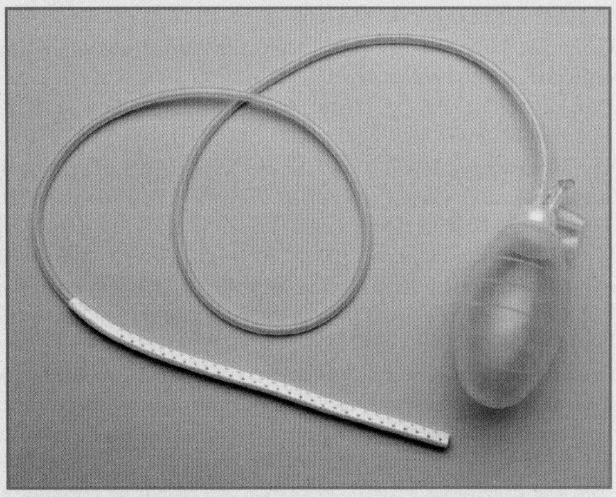

The Hemovac drain is used when blood drainage is expected after surgery, such as in abdominal and orthopedic surgeries.

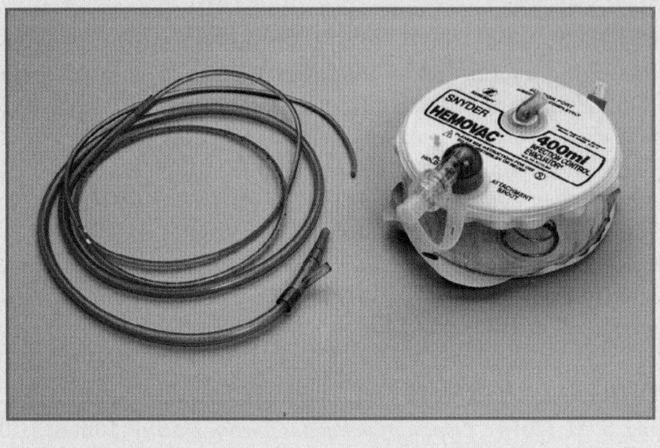

Complications

Occlusion of the tubing by fibrin, clots, or other particles can reduce or obstruct drainage. Infection may develop at the tubing exit site. Other complications include breakage of the drain, difficulty in removal, inadvertent removal, pain, a puckering scar, and visceral perforation.[3]

Documentation

Record the date and time you empty the drain, the appearance of the drain site and the presence of swelling or other signs of infection, equipment malfunction and consequent nursing actions, and the patient's tolerance of the treatment. On the intake and output sheet, record drainage color, consistency, type, and amount. If the patient has more than one closed-wound drain, number the drains and record the information above separately for each drainage site.

References

1 Corion, L. U., et al. (2009). Draining after breast reduction: A randomised controlled inter-patient study. *Journal of Plastic, Reconstructive and Anesthetic Surgery, 62,* 865–868. (Level II)

2 Gaines, R. J., & Dunbar, R. P. (2008). The use of surgical drains in orthopedics. *Orthopedics, 31,* 702–705.

3 Durai, R., & Ng, P. C. H. (2010). Surgical vacuum drains: Types, uses, and complications. *AORN Journal, 91,* 266–271.

4 The Joint Commission. (2015). Standard NPSG.07.01.01. *Comprehensive accreditation manual for hospitals: The official handbook.* Oakbrook Terrace, IL: The Joint Commission. (Level VII)

5 World Health Organization. (2009). "WHO guidelines on hand hygiene in health care: First global patient safety challenge, clean care is safer care" [Online]. Accessed March 2015 via the Web at http://whqlibdoc.who.int/publications/2009/9789241597906_eng.pdf (Level IV)

6 Centers for Disease Control and Prevention. (2002). Guideline for hand hygiene in health-care settings: Recommendations of the Healthcare Infection Control Practices Advisory Committee and the HICPAC/SHEA/APIC/IDSA Hand Hygiene Task Force. *MMWR Recommendations and Reports, 51*(RR-16), 1–45. Assessed March 2015via the Web at http://www.cdc.gov/mmwr/pdf/rr/rr5116. pdf (Level II)

7 The Joint Commission. (2015). Standard NPSG.01.01.01. *Comprehensive accreditation manual for hospitals: The official handbook.* Oakbrook Terrace, IL: The Joint Commission. (Level VII)

8 Siegel, J. D., et al. (2007). "2007 guideline for isolation precautions: Preventing transmission of infectious agents in healthcare settings" [Online]. Accessed March 2015 via the Web at http://www.cdc.gov/hicpac/pdf/isolation/Isolation2007.pdf (Level II)

9 The Joint Commission. (2015). Standard RC.01.03.01. *Comprehensive accreditation manual for hospitals: The official handbook.* Oakbrook Terrace, IL: The Joint Commission. (Level VII)

10 Centers for Medicare & Medicaid Services, Department of Health and Human Services. (2014). Condition of participation: Medical record services. 42 C.F.R. § 482.24(b).

Additional reference

Nettina, S. M. (2014). *Lippincott manual of nursing practice* (10th ed.). Philadelphia, PA: Wolters Kluwer.

Code management

The goals of any code are to restore the patient's spontaneous heartbeat and respirations and to prevent hypoxic damage to the brain and other vital organs. Fulfilling these goals requires a team approach. Ideally, the team should consist of health care workers trained in advanced cardiac life support (ACLS), although health care workers trained in basic life support (BLS) may also be a part of the team. Sponsored by the American Heart Association (AHA), the ACLS course incorporates BLS skills with advanced resuscitation techniques. BLS and ACLS should be performed according to the 2010 AHA guidelines.

Because ventricular fibrillation commonly precedes sudden cardiac arrest, initial resuscitative efforts should focus on early cardiopulmonary resuscitation (CPR), rapid recognition of arrhythmias and, when indicated, defibrillation. If monitoring equipment isn't available, perform BLS measures.

A code may be called for patients with absent pulse, apnea or inadequate breathing, ventricular fibrillation, pulseless ventricular tachycardia, pulseless electrical activity, or asystole. Family members may be present during a code if your facility's policy supports it. The Emergency Nurses Association and the American Association of Critical Care Nurses support the option of family presence during invasive procedures and CPR.[1]

According to the *2010 AHA Guidelines for CPR and Emergency Cardiovascular Care,* ACLS interventions build on the foundation of BLS, which includes immediate recognition and activation of the emergency response system, early high-quality CPR, and rapid defibrillation to increase the patient's chance of survival. The recommended priority of the 2010 AHA guidelines is performing high-quality CPR chest compressions of adequate rate and depth that allow complete chest recoil after each compression with minimal interruptions in addition to avoiding excessive ventilation.[2]

To prevent a delay in chest compressions, the AHA changed the sequence of CPR in the 2010 guidelines from "A-B-C" (airway, breathing, and compressions) to "C-A-B" (compressions, airway, and breathing), which gives the highest priority to chest compressions when resuscitating a patient in cardiac arrest. In addition to high-quality CPR, the only rhythm-specific therapy known to increase survival is defibrillation. As such, defibrillation remains of primary importance in the CPR cycle when a rhythm check reveals ventricular fibrillation or pulseless ventricular tachycardia. Establishing vascular access, administering medications, and inserting an advanced airway are important, but these measures shouldn't cause significant interruptions in CPR or delay defibrillation.[2]

Equipment

Oral, nasal, and endotracheal (ET) airways ▪ one-way valve masks ▪ oxygen source ▪ oxygen flowmeter ▪ intubation supplies ▪ handheld resuscitation bag with mask ▪ suction supplies ▪ gloves ▪ cardiac arrest board ▪ peripheral IV supplies (14G and 18G peripheral IV catheters) ▪ IV administration sets (macrodrip and microdrip) ▪ IV fluids (dextrose 5% in water [D_5W], normal saline solution, and lactated Ringer solutions) ▪ electrocardiogram (ECG) monitor and leads ▪ cardioverter-defibrillator ▪ self-adhesive defibrillator pads and cable or prepackaged gelled conduction pads ▪ emergency medications (adenosine, amiodarone, atropine, calcium, diltiazem, dobutamine, dopamine, epinephrine, isoproterenol, lidocaine, magnesium sulfate, procainamide, sotalol, vasopressin, and verapamil) ▪ Optional: transcutaneous pacemaker, transvenous pacemaker, mask, goggles or mask with face shield, gown, end-tidal carbon dioxide detector, continuous quantitative waveform capnography, esophageal detector, intraosseous (IO) infusion supplies, ECG electrodes, automated external defibrillator, central venous access catheter insertion supplies, tape or securement device.

Preparation of equipment

Because effective emergency care depends on reliable and accessible equipment, the equipment, as well as the personnel, must be ready for a code at any time. You also should be familiar with the cardiac drugs you may have to administer during a code. (See *Common emergency cardiac drugs.*)

Always be aware of your patient's code status as defined by the practitioner's orders, the patient's advance directives, and family wishes. If the practitioner has ordered a "no code," make sure the practitioner has written and signed the order. If possible, have the patient or a responsible family member cosign the order.[3]

For some patients, you may need to consider whether the family wishes to be present during a code. If they do want to be present, see if another nurse or clergy member can remain with them.

Implementation

- Put on gloves and other personal protective equipment as needed *to comply with standard precautions.*[5,6,7]
- If you're the first to arrive at the scene of a code, tap the patient on the shoulder and shout, "Are you all right?" If the patient is unresponsive,

Common emergency cardiac drugs

You may be called on to administer several cardiac drugs during a code. This chart lists the most common emergency cardiac drugs, along with their actions, indications, and dosages.

DRUG	ACTIONS	INDICATIONS	TYPICAL ADULT DOSAGE
adenosine	■ Slows conduction through atrioventricular (AV) node; may interrupt reentry through AV node ■ Shortens duration of atrial action potential during supraventricular tachycardia	■ Stable narrow complex regular tachycardia ■ Unstable narrow complex regular tachycardia ■ Stable regular monomorphic wide complex tachycardia	■ Initially, give 6 mg rapid IV push over 1 to 3 seconds; if conversion hasn't occurred within 2 minutes, you may administer 12 mg by rapid IV push. ■ Reduce initial dose to 3 mg when administered through a central venous catheter in patients receiving dipyridamole or carbamazepine and in heart transplant recipients. ■ Follow each dose with a 20-mL saline flush.[2] ■ *Caution:* Note that slower-than-recommended administration decreases the drug's effectiveness. ■ Avoid use in patients with asthma.[2]
amiodarone	■ Thought to prolong refractory period and action potential duration	■ Cardiac arrest caused by persistent ventricular tachycardia (VT) or ventricular fibrillation (VF) ■ Stable irregular narrow complex tachycardia (atrial fibrillation) ■ Stable regular narrow complex tachycardia	■ For cardiac arrest, administer 300 mg IV push or intraosseously (IO); repeat 150 mg IV push in 3 to 5 minutes. Dilute in 20 to 30 mL of dextrose 5% in water (D_5W). Maximum dose: 2.2 g IV/24 hour.[2] ■ For narrow complex tachycardia, administer 150 mg over 10 minutes, followed by 1 mg/minute infusion for 6 hours, and then 0.5 mg/minute.[2]
atropine	■ Accelerates AV conduction and heart rate by blocking vagal nerve	■ Symptomatic bradycardia	■ Administer 0.5 mg IV push repeated every 3 to 5 minutes until the heart rate reaches 60 beats/minute; can give up to 3 mg total.[2] ■ *Caution:* Atropine is no longer recommended for use during pulseless electrical activity (PEA) or asystole, and it's ineffective for type 2 AV block and new third-degree wide-complex AV block; it may cause paradoxical bradycardia in patients with these conditions.[4]
diltiazem	■ Slows AV node conduction and increases AV node refractoriness	■ Stable narrow complex tachycardia ■ Atrial fibrillation or atrial flutter with rapid ventricular response	■ Initially, administer 15 to 20 mg (0.25 mg/kg) IV over 2 minutes, followed by 20 to 25 mg (0.35 mg/kg) IV in 15 minutes, if needed. ■ Maintenance is 5 to 15 mg/hour titrated to ventricular response.[2]
dobutamine	■ Increases myocardial contractility without raising oxygen demand	■ Heart failure ■ Cardiogenic shock after cardiac arrest	■ Administer 5 to 10 mcg/kg/minute by continuous IV infusion. ■ Titrate as needed to optimize blood pressure, cardiac output, and systemic perfusion.[2]
dopamine	■ Produces inotropic effect, increasing cardiac output, blood pressure, and renal perfusion	■ Symptomatic bradycardia associated with hypotension (except when caused by hypovolemia)	■ Administer a continuous IV infusion at 2 to 20 mcg/kg/minute. (*Note:* Always dilute and give IV drip, never IV push. Titrate to patient response.) ■ *Caution:* Don't administer in the same IV line with alkaline solutions.[2]

(continued)

Common emergency cardiac drugs *(continued)*

Drug	Actions	Indications	Typical adult dosage
epinephrine	■ Increases heart rate, peripheral resistance, and blood flow to heart (enhancing myocardial and cerebral oxygenation) ■ Strengthens myocardial contractility ■ Increases coronary perfusion pressure during cardiopulmonary resuscitation	■ VF ■ Pulseless VT ■ PEA ■ Asystole ■ Severe hypotension (secondary agent) ■ Symptomatic bradycardia	■ Initially, administer 10 mL of 1:10,000 solution (1 mg) IV push or IO; you may repeat every 3 to 5 minutes, as needed. After each dose, flush 20 mL of IV fluid if administered peripherally.[2] ■ Administer 2 to 2½ times the IV dose given endotracheally if no IV line is available.[2] (*Note:* 1:1,000 solution contains 1 mg/mL, so it must be diluted in 9 mL of normal saline solution to provide 1 mg/10 mL.)[2] ■ For hypotension, administer 1 mg/500 mL of D_5W by continuous infusion; titrate to the desired effect (2 to 10 mcg/minute).[2] ■ *Caution:* Don't administer in the same IV line with alkaline solutions.
isoproterenol	■ Enhances automaticity and accelerates conduction ■ Increases heart rate and cardiac contractility, but exacerbates ischemia and arrhythmias in patients with ischemic heart disease	■ Symptomatic bradycardia unresponsive to atropine (while awaiting pacemaker insertion) ■ Torsades de pointes (polymorphic VT) when accompanied by bradycardia ■ Brugada syndrome	■ Administer a continuous IV infusion at 2 to 10 mcg/minute, titrated according to heart rate and rhythm response.[2] Monitor heart rate and blood pressure carefully; doses that increase heart rate to greater than 130 beats/minute may induce ventricular arrhythmias. ■ *Caution:* Avoid use in patients with torsades de pointes associated with familial long QT syndrome.[2]
lidocaine	■ Depresses automaticity and conduction of ectopic impulses in ventricles, especially in ischemic tissue ■ Raises fibrillation threshold, especially in an ischemic heart	■ Cardiac arrest from VF or VT when amiodarone isn't available	■ Initially, administer 1 to 1.5 mg/kg IV push or IO; you may follow this with a 0.5 to 0.75 mg/kg bolus dose every 5 to 10 minutes, up to a total of 3 mg/kg.[2] ■ Maintenance is a continuous IV infusion of 2 g/500 mL of D_5W at 1 to 4 mg/minute *to prevent recurrence of lethal arrhythmias*.[2]
magnesium sulfate	■ Mechanism of action unclear but may help in cardiac arrest associated with refractory VT or VF	■ Cardiac arrest associated with torsades de pointes ■ Torsades de pointes associated with a long QT interval ■ Cardiac arrest and severe cardiotoxicity caused by hypomagnesemia	■ For cardiac arrest associated with torsades de pointes, administer 1 to 2 g IV in 10 mL of D_5W.[2] ■ For torsades de pointes without cardiac arrest, administer 1 to 2 g in 50 to 100 mL of D_5W over 15 minutes.[2] ■ For cardiac arrest and severe cardiotoxicity caused by hypomagnesemia, administer 1 to 2 g IV push in 10 mL of D_5W.[2]
procainamide	■ Depresses automaticity and conduction ■ Prolongs refraction in atria and ventricles	■ Premature ventricular contractions ■ Stable monomorphic VT ■ Supraventricular arrhythmias	■ Administer 20 to 50 mg/minute IV infusion up to a total of 17 mg/kg, followed by a maintenance dose of 1 to 4 mg/minute by IV infusion. ■ Administration is limited by the need for slow infusion.
sotalol	■ Depresses sinus heart rate ■ Slows conduction through the AV node ■ Prolongs the monophasic action potential	■ Spontaneously hemodynamically stable sustained monomorphic VT	■ Administer 1.5 mg/kg IV over 5 minutes or less.[2] ■ *Caution*: Avoid use in patients with prolonged QT interval.
vasopressin	■ Causes peripheral vasoconstriction	■ Cardiac arrest	■ Administer 40 units IV or IO as a single dose, one time only; may replace the first or second dose of epinephrine.[2]
verapamil	■ Slows conduction through AV node ■ Causes vasodilation ■ Produces negative inotropic effect on heart, depressing myocardial contractility	■ Paroxysmal supraventricular tachycardia with narrow QRS complex and rate control in atrial fibrillation	■ Initially, administer 2.5 to 5 mg IV push over 2 minutes (over 3 minutes in older adults). Repeat dose of 5 to 10 mg every 15 to 30 minutes, if needed to a total dose of 20 mg. ■ Monitor electrocardiogram and blood pressure.[2] ■ *Caution:* Don't use drug to treat preexcited atrial fibrillation or flutter.[2]

check to see if the patient is apneic or is only gasping (as opposed to breathing regularly).[2]

■ If the patient is unresponsive and apneic or is only gasping, assume that he is in cardiac arrest and immediately activate the emergency response system.[2]

■ Take no longer than 10 seconds to check for a pulse; if you don't feel a pulse within that time, begin chest compressions. Depress the adult sternum at least 2″ (5 cm), allowing the chest to completely recoil after each compression *so that the heart can adequately fill with blood.*[8] Avoid leaving over the patient's chest, *which could prevent the chest from recoiling completely.*[9] Perform 30 compressions at a rate of 100 to 120 compressions per minute, followed by 2 breaths.[9] Each breath should have enough volume to produce a minimal chest rise *to ensure adequate ventilation.*[8,9]

■ After a second person arrives with the defibrillator and other emergency equipment, have that person place the cardiac arrest board under the patient (or, if the patient is on an air-filled mattress, make sure that it's deflated) and then assist with CPR.[2]

■ The second person should get into position on the other side of the patient and be ready to begin chest compressions after you complete five cycles of compressions and ventilations at a ratio of 30:2. The switch should take fewer than 5 seconds *because interruptions in chest compressions can compromise vital organ perfusion.* The compressor should be relieved every 2 minutes *to prevent rescuer fatigue that could lead to inadequate compression rates or depth.*[2]

■ Have the nurse assigned to the patient relate the patient's medical history and describe the events leading to cardiac arrest.

■ A third person, either a nurse certified in BLS or a respiratory therapist, will then attach the handheld resuscitation bag to the oxygen source.

■ Ideally, a fourth person will be available to open the patient's airway and seal the mask to the patient's face. After the mask is in place, the other person will squeeze the resuscitation bag to deliver 2 ventilations (each over 1 second) during a brief pause after 30 compressions. Both people will watch for the chest to rise. If a fourth person isn't available, the third person will open the patient's airway, seal the mask to the patient's face using one hand and then, with the other hand, squeeze the resuscitation bag to deliver 2 ventilations during a brief pause after 30 compressions.[2]

■ When the ACLS-trained nurse arrives, she'll expose the patient's chest and apply the self-adhesive defibrillation pads *to obtain a quick look at the patient's cardiac rhythm.* Alternatively, she'll apply prepackaged defibrillator pads and then apply the paddles to the patient's chest *to obtain a quick cardiac rhythm.* If the patient is in ventricular fibrillation or pulseless ventricular tachycardia, ACLS protocol calls for defibrillation as soon as possible with 360 joules (monophasic) or 120 to 200 joules (biphasic) according to the manufacturer's recommendations. Then resume CPR immediately. Don't do a rhythm check at this time. Do it after five cycles of CPR; if you detect a rhythm, perform a pulse check. The ACLS-trained nurse will act as code leader until the practitioner arrives.[2]

■ If not already in place, apply ECG electrodes and attach the patient to the defibrillator's cardiac monitor. Avoid placing electrodes on bony prominences or hairy areas. Also avoid the areas where the defibrillator pads will be placed and where chest compressions will be given. If you're using hands-free defibrillator pads, you'll need to apply ECG electrodes or attach them to the defibrillator *because these pads detect the patient's rhythm in a manner similar to an automated external defibrillator.*

■ After five cycles of CPR, check the patient's rhythm and give another shock at the same or higher rate if using a biphasic defibrillator, or at the same rate if using a monophasic defibrillator, if necessary.[2]

■ As CPR and defibrillation continue, you or an ACLS-trained nurse will then start two peripheral IV lines with large-bore IV catheters; alternatively, IO access may be established if peripheral access isn't readily available.[2] Avoid interrupting chest compressions for IV or IO insertion. When inserting a peripheral IV catheter, use only a large vein, such as the antecubital vein, *to allow for rapid fluid administration and to prevent drug extravasation.*

■ As soon as the IV catheter is in place, begin an infusion of normal saline solution or lactated Ringer solution *to help prevent circulatory collapse;* although D_5W continues to be an acceptable alternative, the latest ACLS guidelines encourage the use of normal saline solution or lactated Ringer solution *because D_5W can produce hyperglycemic effects during cardiac arrest.*[2]

■ While one nurse obtains access for parenteral medications, another nurse will set up portable or wall-suction equipment and suction the patient's oral secretions, as necessary, *to maintain an open airway.*

■ The ACLS-trained nurse will then prepare and administer emergency cardiac drugs, as needed.[10,11] (See *AHA algorithm,* page 196.) Administer medications according to the AHA algorithm immediately after a rhythm check. *The AHA algorithm shows the timing of drug administration and shock administration.*[2] Keep in mind that drugs administered through a central venous access device reach the myocardium more quickly than those administered through a peripheral line. Drugs administered peripherally should be followed by a 20-mL bolus of IV fluid *to facilitate the flow of the drug to central circulation.*[2]

■ If IV or IO access can't be established, you may administer medications such as epinephrine, lidocaine, and vasopressin through an ET tube during cardiac arrest. The optimal dose of most drugs given by this route is unknown, but typically the dose is 2 to 2½ times the recommended IV dose. To administer through an ET tube, dilute the drugs in 5 to 10 mL of normal saline solution or sterile water and then instill them into the patient's ET tube. *Studies have shown that dilution with sterile water, instead of normal saline solution, may improve absorption of epinephrine and lidocaine.* Afterward, ventilate the patient manually *to improve absorption by distributing the drug throughout the bronchial tree.*[2]

■ The ACLS-trained nurse will also prepare for and assist with ET intubation or other advanced airway placement. Compression interruption should be minimized during advanced airway placement.[2]

■ Suction the patient as needed. After the patient has been intubated, ET tube placement should be confirmed with a clinical assessment and using a device such as an end-tidal carbon dioxide detector, continuous quantitative waveform capnography, or an esophageal detector; the continuous quantitative waveform capnography is the recommended device.[2] Assessment includes visualization of chest expansion, auscultation for equal breath sounds, and auscultation for absent breath sounds over the epigastrium. When the tube is correctly positioned, tape it securely with tape or a commercial device. *To serve as a reference,* mark the point on the tube that's level with the patient's lips. Document the tube location on the code record.[2]

■ After the ET tube is inserted, the nurse performing chest compressions should deliver 100 to 120 compressions per minute continuously without pauses for ventilations;[9] the nurse delivering ventilations should administer 1 breath every 6 to 8 seconds (8 to 10 breaths/minute) *to avoid excessive ventilations, minimizing the impact of positive-pressure ventilation on blood flow.*[2,9]

■ Meanwhile, other team members should keep a written record of the events. Other duties include prompting participants about when to perform certain activities (such as when to check a pulse or take vital signs), overseeing the effectiveness of CPR, and keeping track of the time between therapies. Each team member should know what the other participant's role is *to prevent duplicating effort.* Lastly, someone from the team should make sure that the primary nurse's other patients are reassigned to another nurse.

■ Remove and discard your gloves and any other personal protective equipment worn.[5,6]

■ Perform hand hygiene.[12,13,14,15,16]

■ Document the procedure.[17,18,19]

AHA algorithm[2]

This American Heart Association (AHA) algorithm shows the guidelines for treating an adult in cardiac arrest.

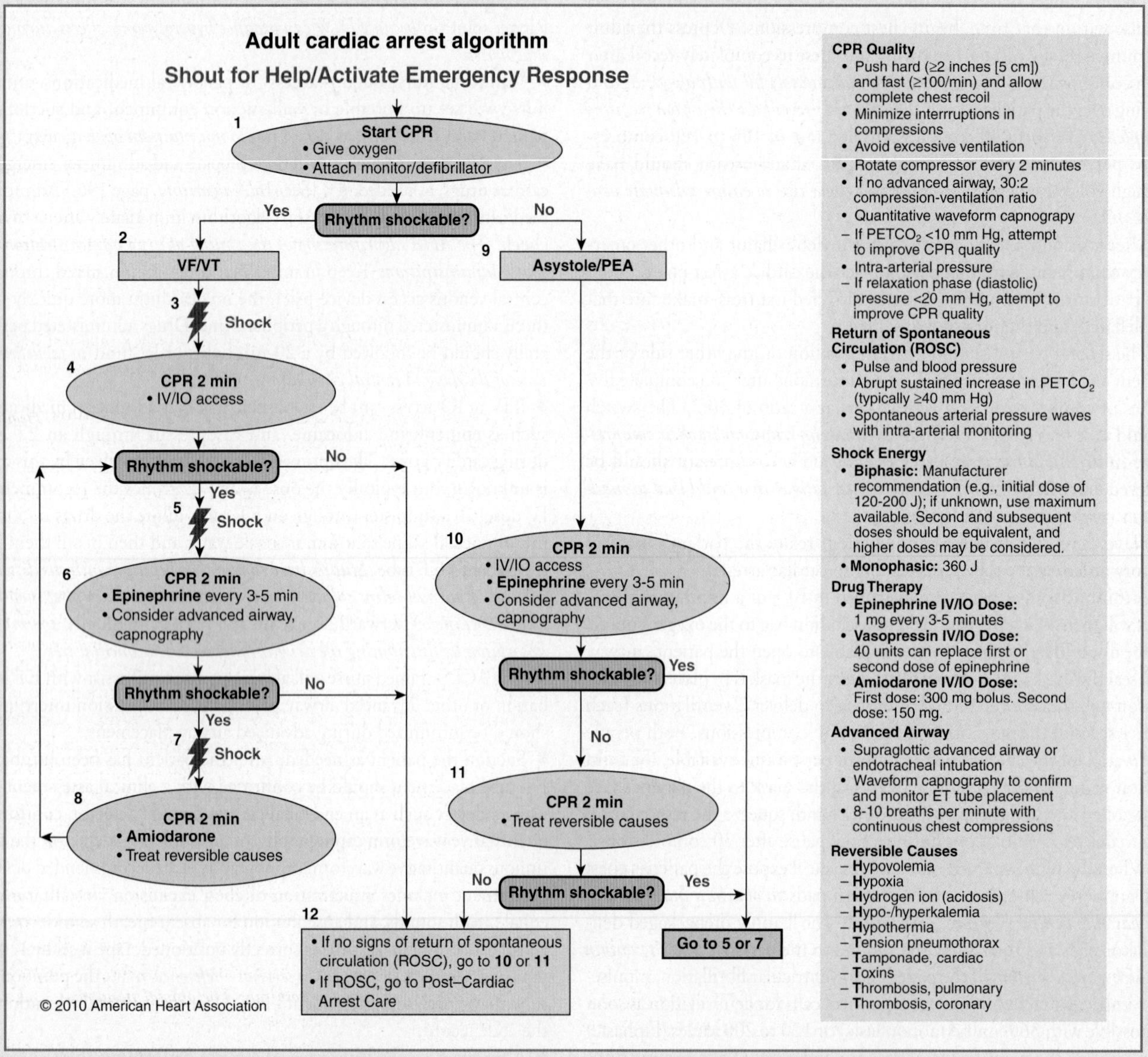

Reprinted with permission. American Heart Association. (2010). 2010 American Heart Association guidelines for cardiopulmonary resuscitation and emergency cardiovascular care, part 8: Adult advanced cardiovascular live support. *Circulation, 122* (Suppl. 3), S729–767. © 2010 American Heart Association.

Special considerations

- Evidence for an optimum compression rate suggests a target of 100 to 120 compressions per minute. Rates above or below this target range appear to reduce survival to discharge.[9]
- If hemodynamic monitoring, such as arterial or central venous catheters or capnography, are in place, they should be used to monitor the patient's response to CPR and the effectiveness of resuscitation efforts.[9]
- If defibrillator gel pads aren't available, a conductive gel must be placed on defibrillator paddles before use. Place the gel on one paddle, and rub the two paddles together to spread the gel evenly between them. Ensure that the surface of the paddle is completely covered.
- If family members are at the facility during the code, have someone, such as a clergy member or social worker, remain with them. Keep family members informed of the patient's status.
- If the family isn't at the facility, contact them as soon as possible. Encourage them not to drive to the facility, but offer to call someone who can give them a ride.
- When the patient's condition has stabilized, assess his level of consciousness, breath sounds, heart sounds, peripheral perfusion, bowel sounds, and urine output. Also take vital signs every 15 minutes and monitor cardiac rhythm continuously.[2]
- *Because therapeutic hypothermia is the only intervention demonstrated to improve neurologic recovery,* it should be considered for any patient who can't follow verbal commands after return of spontaneous circulation.[2]

■ Make sure that the patient receives an adequate supply of oxygen, whether through a mask or a ventilator.[2] Titrate inspired oxygen to the lowest level required to achieve an arterial oxygen saturation of 94% or higher *to avoid potential oxygen toxicity.*[2]

■ Check the infusion rates of all IV fluids, and use infusion pumps (preferably smart pumps with dose-range alerts) to deliver vasoactive drugs. Make sure that infusion pump alarm limits are set appropriately for the patient's current condition and that alarms are turned on, functioning properly, and audible to staff.[20,21,22]

■ *To evaluate the effectiveness of fluid therapy,* insert an indwelling catheter if the patient doesn't already have one, or use a bladder scanner to measure the volume of urine in the bladder. Also insert a nasogastric tube *to relieve or prevent gastric distention.*

■ If appropriate, reassure the patient and explain what's happening. Allow the patient's family to visit as soon as possible.

■ If the patient dies, notify family members and allow them to see the patient as soon as possible.

■ *To make sure that the code team performs optimally,* schedule a time to review the code.

Complications

Even when performed correctly, CPR can cause fractured ribs, liver laceration, lung puncture, and gastric distention. Defibrillation can cause electric shock. Emergency intubation can result in esophageal or tracheal laceration, subcutaneous emphysema, or accidental right mainstem bronchus intubation. (Decreased or absent breath sounds on the left side of the chest and normal breath sounds on the right may signal accidental right mainstem bronchus intubation.)

Documentation

During the code, document the events in as much detail as possible. Note whether the arrest was witnessed or unwitnessed, the time of the arrest, the time CPR was begun, the time the ACLS-trained nurse arrived, and the total resuscitation time. Also document the number of defibrillations, the times they were performed, the joule level, the patient's cardiac rhythm before and after defibrillation, and whether or not the patient had a pulse.

Document all drug therapy, including dosages, routes of administration, and patient response. Record all procedures, such as peripheral and central line insertion, pacemaker insertion, and ET tube insertion, noting the time performed and the patient's tolerance of the procedure. Also keep track of all arterial blood gas and laboratory results.

Record whether the patient is transferred to another unit or facility, along with his condition at the time of transfer and whether his family was notified. Lastly, document any complications and the measures taken to correct them. When your documentation is complete, have the practitioner and ACLS nurse review and then sign the document.

REFERENCES

1 Emergency Nurses Association. (2010). "Position statement: Family presence during invasive procedures and resuscitation in the emergency department" [Online]. Accessed March 2015 via the Web at http://www.ena.org/SiteCollectionDocuments/Position%20Statements/FamilyPresence.pdf (Level VII)

2 American Heart Association. (2010). 2010 American Heart Association guidelines for cardiopulmonary resuscitation and emergency cardiovascular care. *Circulation, 122,* S729–S767. (Level II)

3 The Joint Commission. (2015). Standard RI.01.02.01. *Comprehensive accreditation manual for hospitals: The official handbook.* Oakbrook Terrace, IL: The Joint Commission. (Level VII)

4 Field, J. M., et al. (2009). *The textbook of emergency cardiovascular care and CPR.* Philadelphia, PA: Lippincott Williams & Wilkins.

5 Siegel, J. D., et al. (2007). "2007 guideline for isolation precautions: Preventing transmission of infectious agents in healthcare settings" [Online]. Accessed March 2015 via the Web at http://www.cdc.gov/hicpac/pdf/isolation/Isolation2007.pdf (Level II)

6 Occupational Safety and Health Administration. (n.d.). "Bloodborne pathogens, standard number 1910.1030" [Online]. Accessed March 2015 via the Web at http://www.osha.gov/pls/oshaweb/owadisp.show_document?p_table=STANDARDS&p_id=10051 (Level VII)

7 American Osteopathic Association. (2014). Standard 07.01.10. *Healthcare Facilities Accreditation Program: Accreditation requirements for acute care hospitals.* Chicago, IL: American Osteopathic Association. (Level VII)

8 American Heart Association. (2010). 2010 American Heart Association guidelines for cardiopulmonary resuscitation and emergency cardiovascular care. *Circulation, 122,* S676–S684. (Level II)

9 American Heart Association. (AHA). (2013). "AHA consensus statement: Cardiopulmonary resuscitation quality: Improving cardiac resuscitation outcomes both inside and outside the hospital" [Online]. Accessed March 2015 via the Web at http://circ.ahajournals.org/content/128/4/417.full (Level VII)

10 Centers for Medicare & Medicaid Services, Department of Health and Human Services. (2014). Condition of participation: Nursing services. 42 C.F.R. § 482.23(c).

11 American Osteopathic Association. (2014). Standard 16.01.03. *Healthcare Facilities Accreditation Program: Accreditation requirements for acute care hospitals.* Chicago, IL: American Osteopathic Association. (Level VII)

12 The Joint Commission. (2015). Standard NPSG.07.01.01. *Comprehensive accreditation manual for hospitals: The official handbook.* Oakbrook Terrace, IL: The Joint Commission. (Level VII)

13 Centers for Disease Control and Prevention. (2002). Guideline for hand hygiene in health-care settings: Recommendations of the Healthcare Infection Control Practices Advisory Committee and the HICPAC/SHEA/APIC/IDSA Hand Hygiene Task Force. *MMWR Recommendations and Reports, 51*(RR-16), 1–45. Accessed March 2015 via the Web at http://www.cdc.gov/mmwr/pdf/rr/rr5116.pdf (Level II)

14 World Health Organization. (2009). "WHO guidelines on hand hygiene in health care: First global patient safety challenge, clean care is safer care" [Online]. Accessed March 2015 via the Web at http://whqlibdoc.who.int/publications/2009/9789241597906_eng.pdf (Level IV)

15 Centers for Medicare & Medicaid Services, Department of Health and Human Services. (2014). Condition of participation: Infection control. 42 C.F.R. § 482.42.

16 American Osteopathic Association. (2014). Standard 07.01.21. *Healthcare Facilities Accreditation Program: Accreditation requirements for acute care hospitals.* Chicago, IL: American Osteopathic Association. (Level VII)

17 The Joint Commission. (2015). Standard RC.01.03.01. *Comprehensive accreditation manual for hospitals: The official handbook.* Oakbrook Terrace, IL: The Joint Commission. (Level VII)

18 Centers for Medicare & Medicaid Services, Department of Health and Human Services. (2014). Condition of participation: Medical record services. 42 C.F.R. § 482.24(b).

19 American Osteopathic Association. (2014). Standard 10.00.03. *Healthcare Facilities Accreditation Program: Accreditation requirements for acute care hospitals.* Chicago, IL: American Osteopathic Association. (Level VII)

20 The Joint Commission. (2015). Standard NPSG.06.01.01. *Comprehensive accreditation manual for hospitals: The official handbook.* Oakbrook Terrace, IL: The Joint Commission. (Level VII)

21 Graham, K. C., & Cvach, M. (2010). Monitor alarm fatigue: Standardizing use of physiological monitors and decreasing nuisance alarms. *American Journal of Critical Care, 19,* 28–37.

22 American Association of Critical-Care Nurses. (2013). "AACN practice alert: Alarm management" [Online]. Accessed March 2015 via the Web at http://www.aacn.org/wd/practice/docs/practicealerts/alarm-management-practice-alert.pdf (Level VII)

Reducing pain with ice massage

Normally, ice shouldn't be applied directly to a patient's skin *because it risks damaging the skin surface and underlying tissues.* However, when carefully performed, this technique—called ice massage—may help patients tolerate brief, painful procedures such as bone marrow aspiration, catheterization, chest tube removal, injection into joints, lumbar puncture, and suture removal.

Prepare for ice massage by gathering the ice, a porous covering to hold it in (if desired), and a cloth for wiping water from the patient as the ice melts. One option for the ice is to freeze water in a paper cup ahead of time and then remove the paper from half the cup, exposing the ice you'll use for the procedure.

Just before the procedure begins, rub the ice over the appropriate area *to numb it.* Assess the site frequently; stop rubbing immediately if you detect signs of tissue intolerance.

As you begin the procedure, rub the ice over a point near but not at the site. *This action distracts the patient from the procedure itself and gives him another stimulus to concentrate on.* If the procedure lasts longer than 10 minutes or if you think tissue damage may occur, move the ice to a different site and continue massage.

If you know in advance that the procedure probably will last longer than 10 minutes, massage the site intermittently—2 minutes of massage alternating with a rest period until the skin regains its normal color. Alternatively, you can divide the area into several sites and apply ice to each one for several minutes at a time.

COLD APPLICATION

The application of cold constricts blood vessels; inhibits local circulation, suppuration, and tissue metabolism; relieves vascular congestion; slows bacterial activity in infections; reduces body temperature; and may act as a temporary anesthetic during brief, painful procedures. (See *Reducing pain with ice massage.*) Cold helps decrease edema by decreasing capillary permeability and causing vasoconstriction. Because treatment with cold also relieves inflammation, reduces edema, and slows bleeding, it may provide effective initial treatment after eye injuries, strains, sprains, bruises, muscle spasms, and burns. Also referred to as *cryotherapy,* cold therapy is typically used to relieve pain following certain surgical procedures, including arthroscopy.[1,2]

Cold can be applied in dry or moist forms, but ice shouldn't be placed directly on a patient's skin because it may further damage tissue. Moist application is more penetrating than dry application because moisture facilitates conduction. Devices for applying cold include ice bags or collars, K pads (which can produce cold or heat), and chemical cold packs and ice packs. Devices for applying moist cold include cold compresses for small body areas and cold packs for large areas.

Cold treatments should be used cautiously on patients with impaired circulation, on children, and on elderly or arthritic patients because of the risk of ischemic tissue damage.

Equipment

Patient thermometer ■ towel ■ adhesive tape or roller gauze ■ Optional: gloves.

For an ice bag or collar

Ice bag or collar ■ tap water ■ crushed ice ■ absorbent, protective cloth covering.

For a K pad

K pad and control unit ■ distilled water ■ temperature-adjustment key ■ absorbent, protective cloth covering.

For a chemical cold pack

Single-use pack for applying dry cold ■ cloth covering.

For a cold compress or pack

Basin of ice ■ container of tap water ■ bath thermometer ■ compress material (4″ × 4″ [10-cm × 10-cm] gauze pads or washcloths) or pack material (towels or flannel) ■ fluid-impermeable pad ■ waterproof covering.

Preparation of equipment

For an ice bag or collar

Select a device of the correct size, fill it with cold tap water, and check for leaks. Then empty the device and fill it about halfway with crushed ice. *Using small pieces of ice helps the device mold to the patient's body.* Squeeze the device *to expel air that might reduce conduction.* Fasten the cap and wipe any moisture from the outside of the device. Wrap the bag or collar in a cloth covering, and secure the cover with tape or roller gauze. *The protective cover prevents tissue trauma and absorbs condensation.*

For a K pad

Make sure the K pad provides cold therapy. Check the cord for damage. Then fill the control unit two-thirds full with distilled water or to the level recommended by the manufacturer. Don't use tap water *because it leaves mineral deposits in the unit.* Check for leaks, and then tilt the unit several times *to clear the pad's tubing of air.* Tighten the cap. After ensuring that the hoses between the control unit and pad are free of tangles, place the unit on the bedside table, slightly above the patient *so gravity can assist water flow.* If the central supply department hasn't preset the temperature, use the temperature-adjustment key to adjust the control unit to the lowest temperature. Cover the pad with an absorbent, protective cloth and secure the cover with tape or roller gauze. Plug in the unit and turn it on. Allow the pad to cool for 2 minutes before placing it on the patient.

For a chemical cold pack

If you choose one of the lightweight plastic packs that contains a chemical that turns cold when activated, select a pack of the appropriate size and follow the manufacturer's directions (striking, squeezing, or kneading) *to activate the cold-producing chemicals.* Make certain that the container hasn't been broken during activation. Alternatively, you may choose a reusable sealed cold pack that's filled with an alcohol-based solution and stored frozen; for this type of pack, keep in mind that you may disinfect the exterior of the pack after use and refreeze it for use again. For either chemical cold pack, wrap the pack in a cloth covering and secure the cover with tape or roller gauze.

For a cold compress or pack

Cool a container of tap water by placing it in a basin of ice or by adding ice to the water. Using a bath thermometer for guidance, adjust the water temperature to 59°F (15°C) or as ordered. Immerse the compress material or pack material in the water.

Implementation

- Select and prepare the appropriate cold device.
- Perform hand hygiene.[3,4,5,6,7]
- Confirm the patient's identity using at least two patient identifiers.[8]
- Explain the procedure to the patient.
- Provide privacy.[9,10]
- Make sure the room is warm and free from drafts.
- Put on gloves if needed *to comply with standard precautions.*[11,12]

PATIENT TEACHING

Using cold for a muscle sprain

For each application, instruct the patient to obtain enough crushed ice to cover the painful area, place it in a plastic bag, and place the bag inside a pillowcase or large piece of cloth, as shown at right.

For later applications, the patient may want to fill a paper cup with water, stand a tongue blade in the cup, and place it in the freezer. After the water freezes, he can peel the paper off the ice and hold it with the protruding handle. If he chooses this method, tell him to first cover the area with a cloth *because applying ice directly to the skin can cause frostbite or cold shock.*

Instruct the patient to rub the ice over the painful area for the specified treatment time. Warn him that although ice eases pain in a joint that has begun to stiffen, he shouldn't let the analgesic effect encourage overuse of the joint.

After 24 to 72 hours, when heat and swelling have subsided or when cold no longer helps, the patient should switch to heat application, as directed. (See the "Heat application" procedure, page 348.)

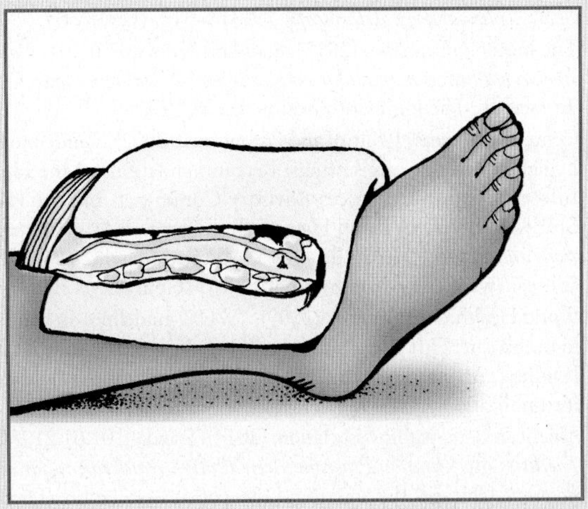

- Record the patient's temperature, pulse, and respirations *to serve as a baseline for comparison.*
- Expose only the treatment site *to avoid chilling the patient.*

Applying an ice bag or collar, a K pad, or a chemical cold pack

- Place the covered cold device on the treatment site and begin timing the application.
- Observe the site frequently for signs of tissue intolerance, such as blanching, mottling, cyanosis, maceration, and blisters. Also, be alert for shivering and complaints of burning or numbness. If these signs or symptoms develop, discontinue treatment and notify the practitioner.
- Refill or replace the cold device as necessary *to maintain the correct temperature.* Change the protective cover if it becomes wet.
- Remove the device after the prescribed treatment period (usually 30 minutes).

Applying a cold compress or pack

- Place a fluid-impermeable pad under the site.
- Remove the compress or pack from the water, and wring it out *to prevent dripping.*
- Apply the compress or pack to the treatment site and begin timing the application.
- Cover the compress or pack with a waterproof covering *to provide insulation and to keep the surrounding area dry.* Secure the covering with tape or roller gauze *to prevent it from slipping.*
- Assess the application site frequently for signs of tissue intolerance, and note any complaints of burning or numbness. If these issues develop, discontinue treatment and notify the practitioner.
- Change the compress or pack as needed *to maintain the correct temperature.*
- Remove it after the prescribed treatment period (usually 20 minutes).

Concluding all cold applications

- Dry the patient's skin and re-dress the treatment site according to the practitioner's orders.
- Position the patient comfortably
- Assess the patient's temperature, pulse, and respirations and compare them with baselines *to determine the patient's tolerance of the procedure.*
- Properly dispose of liquids and soiled materials.
- If treatment will be repeated, clean and store the equipment in the patient's room, out of his reach; otherwise, return it to storage.
- Perform hand hygiene.[3,4,5,6,7]
- Document the procedure.[13,14,15]

Special considerations

- Apply cold immediately after an injury *to minimize edema.* Although colder temperatures can be tolerated for a longer time when the treatment site is small, don't continue any application for longer than 1 hour *to avoid reflex vasodilation.* The application of temperatures below 59°F (15°C) also causes local reflex vasodilation.
- Use sterile technique when applying cold to an open wound or to a lesion that may open during treatment *to prevent wound contamination.* Also, maintain sterile technique during eye treatment, with separate sterile equipment for each eye *to prevent cross-contamination.*

Patient teaching

- Teach the patient how to apply cold for a muscle sprain so he can properly do so when he returns home if appropriate. (See *Using cold for a muscle sprain.*)
- Avoid securing cooling devices with pins *because an accidental puncture could allow extremely cold fluids to leak out and burn the patient's skin.*
- If the patient is unconscious, anesthetized, neurologically or cognitively impaired, or otherwise insensitive to cold, stay with him throughout the treatment and check the application site frequently for complications.

Complications

Hemoconcentration may cause thrombi. Intense cold may cause pain, burning, or numbness.

Documentation

Record the time, date, and duration of cold application; the type of device used (ice bag or collar, K pad, chemical cold pack, or cold compress or pack); the application site; the temperature or temperature setting; the patient's temperature, pulse, and respirations before and after application; skin appearance before, during, and after application; signs of complications; and the patient's tolerance of treatment. Document any patient teaching provided and the patient's understanding of that teaching.

REFERENCES

1 Fang, L., et al. (2012). The effects of cryotherapy in relieving postarthroscopy pain. *Journal of Clinical Nursing, 21*, 636–643. (Level VI)

2 Meyer-Marcotty, M., et al. (2011). Standardized combined cryotherapy and compression using Cryo/Cuff after wrist arthroscopy. *Knee Surgery, Sports Traumatology, Arthroscopy, 19*, 314–319. (Level VI)

3 The Joint Commission. (2015). Standard NPSG.07.01.01. *Comprehensive accreditation manual for hospitals: The official handbook.* Oakbrook Terrace, IL: The Joint Commission. (Level VII)

4 Centers for Disease Control and Prevention. (2002). Guideline for hand hygiene in health-care settings: Recommendations of the Healthcare Infection Control Practices Advisory Committee and the HICPAC/SHEA/APIC/IDSA Hand Hygiene Task Force. *MMWR Recommendations and Reports, 51*(RR-16), 1–45. Accessed March 2015 via the Web at http://www.cdc.gov/mmwr/pdf/rr/rr5116.pdf (Level II)

5 World Health Organization. (2009). "WHO guidelines on hand hygiene in health care: First global patient safety challenge, clean care is safer care" [Online]. Accessed March 2015 via the Web at http://whqlibdoc.who.int/publications/2009/9789241597906_eng.pdf (Level IV)

6 American Osteopathic Association. (2014). Standard 07.01.21. *Healthcare Facilities Accreditation Program: Accreditation requirements for acute care hospitals.* Chicago, IL: American Osteopathic Association. (Level VII)

7 Centers for Medicare & Medicaid Services, Department of Health and Human Services. (2014). Condition of participation: Infection control. 42 C.F.R. § 482.42.

8 The Joint Commission. (2015). Standard NPSG.01.01.01. *Comprehensive accreditation manual for hospitals: The official handbook.* Oakbrook Terrace, IL: The Joint Commission. (Level VII)

9 Centers for Medicare & Medicaid Services, Department of Health and Human Services. (2014). Condition of participation: Patient's rights. 42 C.F.R. § 482.13(c)(1).

10 American Osteopathic Association. (2014). Standard 15.01.16. *Healthcare Facilities Accreditation Program: Accreditation requirements for acute care hospitals.* Chicago, IL: American Osteopathic Association. (Level VII)

11 American Osteopathic Association. (2014). Standard 07.01.10. *Healthcare Facilities Accreditation Program: Accreditation requirements for acute care hospitals.* Chicago, IL: American Osteopathic Association. (Level VII)

12 Siegel, J. D., et al. (2007). "2007 guideline for isolation precautions: Preventing transmission of infectious agents in healthcare settings" [Online]. Accessed March 2015 via the Web at http://www.cdc.gov/hicpac/pdf/isolation/Isolation2007.pdf (Level II)

13 The Joint Commission. (2015). Standard RC.01.03.01. *Comprehensive accreditation manual for hospitals: The official handbook.* Oakbrook Terrace, IL: The Joint Commission. (Level VII)

14 American Osteopathic Association. (2014). Standard 10.00.03. *Healthcare Facilities Accreditation Program: Accreditation requirements for acute care hospitals.* Chicago, IL: American Osteopathic Association. (Level VII)

15 Centers for Medicare & Medicaid Services, Department of Health and Human Services. (2014). Condition of participation: Medical record services. 42 C.F.R. § 482.24(b).

ADDITIONAL REFERENCES

Chailler, M., et al. (2010). Cold therapy for the management of pain associated with deep breathing and coughing post-cardiac surgery. *Canadian Journal of Cardiovascular Nursing, 20*(2), 18–24. (Level II)

Craven, R. F., & Hirnle, C. J. (2012). *Fundamentals of nursing: Human health and function* (7th ed.). Philadelphia, PA: Lippincott Williams & Wilkins.

Garra, G., et al. (2010). Heat or cold packs for neck and back strain: A randomized controlled trial of efficacy. *Academic Emergency Medicine, 17*, 484–489. (Level II)

Nettina, S. M. (2014). *Lippincott manual of nursing practice* (10th ed.). Philadelphia, PA: Wolters Kluwer.

Quinn, E. (2013). "RICE is best for soft tissue injuries" [Online]. Accessed March 2015 via the Web at http://sportsmedicine.about.com/cs/rehab/a/rice.htm

COLOSTOMY AND ILEOSTOMY CARE

A patient with an ascending, transverse, or descending colostomy or an ileostomy must wear an external pouch to collect emerging fecal matter, which may be watery, pasty, or formed, depending on location of the stoma. Besides collecting waste matter, the pouch helps to control odor and protect the stoma and peristomal skin. Most disposable pouching systems can be used for 3 to 7 days;[1] however, single-use, closed-end pouches should be changed more frequently.

All pouching systems need to be changed immediately if a leak develops, and every pouch needs emptying when it's one-third to one-half full. The patient with an ileostomy may need to empty his pouch four or five times daily.

The best time to change the pouching system is when the bowel is least active, usually in the morning before breakfast. After a few months, most patients can predict the best changing time.

The selection of a pouching system should take into consideration which system provides the best adhesive seal and skin protection for the individual patient. The type of pouch selected also depends on the stoma's location and structure, abdominal contours, availability of supplies, wear time, consistency of output, personal preference, patient or caregiver ability to manage the stoma, and cost.[2]

Equipment

For appliance care

Pouching system ■ pen ■ scissors ■ stoma measuring guide ■ plastic bag ■ water ■ washcloth and towel ■ soft cloth or gauze ■ gloves ■ facility-approved ostomy skin assessment tool[2,3,4,5] ■ Optional: stoma paste or moldable barrier ring, closure clamp, paper tape, clippers, liquid skin sealant, pouch deodorant.

Pouching systems may be disposable or reusable, drainable or closed-ended, and one-piece or two-piece. (See *Comparing ostomy pouching systems.*)

For pouch emptying

Bedpan, toilet, or measuring device ■ gloves ■ tissue ■ Optional: pouch deodorant, facility-approved stomal skin assessment tool.[2,3,4,5]

Implementation

- Gather the appropriate equipment.
- Perform hand hygiene.[6,7,8,9,10]
- Put on gloves *to comply with standard precautions.*[11,12]
- Confirm the patient's identity using at least two patient identifiers.[13]
- Explain the procedure to the patient *to decrease anxiety and ensure cooperation.* As you perform each step, explain what you are doing and why *because the patient will eventually need to perform the procedure.*
- Provide privacy and emotional support.[14,15,16]

Fitting the skin barrier and pouch

- For a pouch with an attached skin barrier (one-piece pouch), measure the stoma with the measuring guide. Select the opening size that matches the stoma.
- For an adhesive-backed pouch with a separate skin barrier (two-piece pouch), measure the stoma with the measuring guide and select the opening that matches the stoma. Trace the selected size opening onto the paper back of the skin barrier's adhesive side. Cut out the opening. If the pouch has precut openings, which can be handy for a round stoma, select an opening that's 1/8″ (0.3 cm) larger than the stoma. If the pouch comes without an opening, cut the hole 1/8″ (0.3 cm) wider than the measured tracing (although many pouching systems can now be fit up to the stoma edge without risk of trauma to the stoma). The cut-to-fit system works best for

Comparing ostomy pouching systems

Manufactured in many shapes and sizes, ostomy pouches are fashioned for comfort, safety, and easy application. For example, a disposable, closed-end pouch may meet the needs of a patient who irrigates the ostomy, who wants added security, or who wants to discard the pouch after each bowel movement. Another patient may prefer a reusable, drainable pouch. Some commonly available pouches are described below.

Disposable pouches

The patient who must empty the pouch often (because of diarrhea or a new colostomy or ileostomy) may prefer a one-piece, drainable, disposable pouch with a closure clamp attached to a skin barrier (as shown below). These transparent or opaque, odor-proof plastic pouches come with attached adhesive backing. Some pouches have microporous adhesive or belt tabs. The bottom opening allows for easy draining. This pouch may be used permanently or temporarily, until stoma size stabilizes.

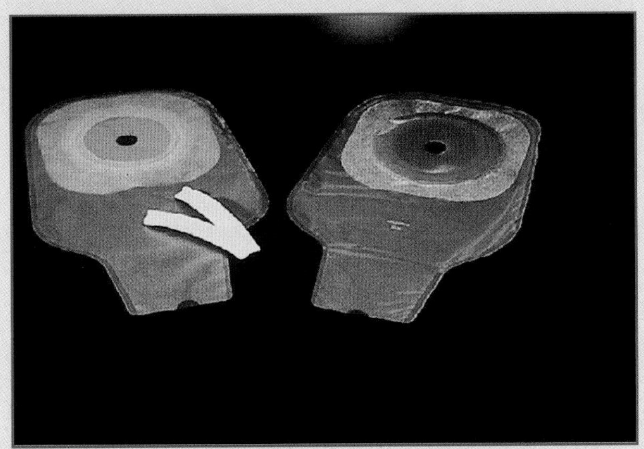

Also disposable and also made of transparent or opaque odor-proof plastic, a one-piece, disposable, closed-end pouch may come with a filter. A patient with a regular bowel elimination pattern may choose this style for additional security and confidence.

A two-piece, drainable, disposable pouch with separate skin barrier (as shown below) permits more frequent pouch changes. Also made of transparent or opaque odor-proof plastic, this style comes with belt tabs and usually snaps to the skin barrier with a flange mechanism. Newer, two-piece pouches have an adhesive coupling. The pouch sticks to the wafer, allowing greater flexibility and comfort.

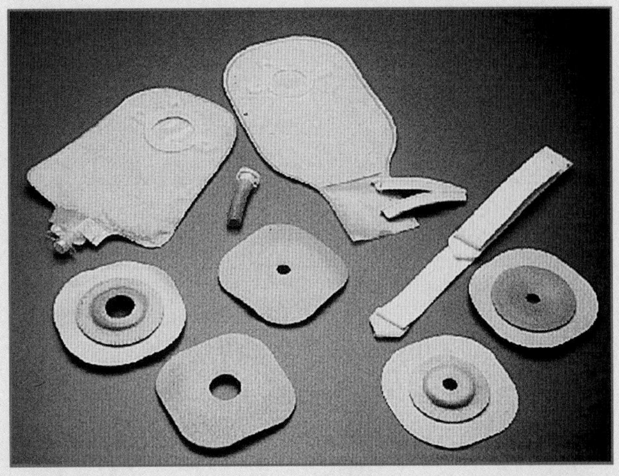

Reusable pouches

Typically manufactured from sturdy, opaque, hypoallergenic plastic, the reusable pouch comes with a separate custom-made faceplate and O-ring. The device has a 1- to 3-month life span, depending on how frequently the patient empties the pouch. Reusable equipment may benefit a patient who needs a firm faceplate or who wishes to minimize cost.

an irregularly shaped stoma. (See *Applying a skin barrier and pouch,* page 202.)

Applying or changing the pouch

■ Empty, remove, and discard the old pouch, if applicable (as shown below).

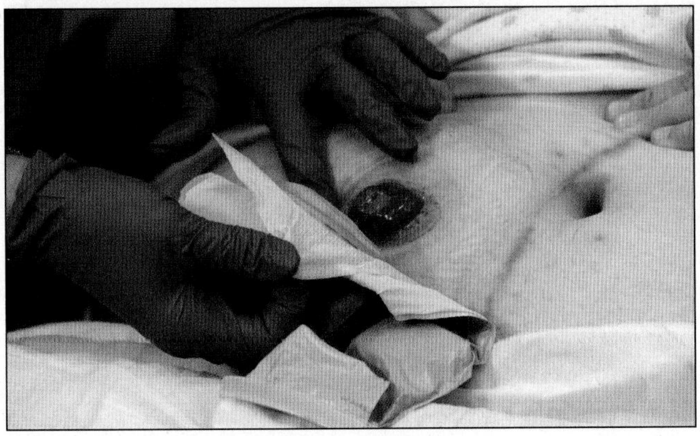

■ Wipe the stoma and peristomal skin gently with a soft cloth or gauze (as shown below).

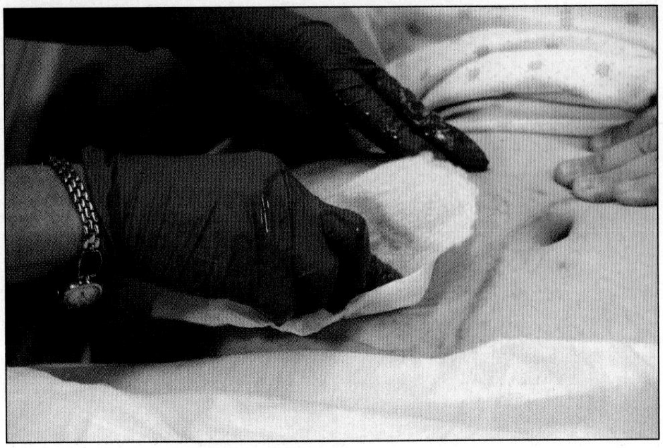

■ Carefully wash with water and dry the peristomal skin by patting gently. Allow the skin to dry thoroughly. Inspect the peristomal skin and stoma (as shown on page 203, top left). If necessary, clip surrounding hair (in a direction away from the stoma) *to promote a better seal and avoid skin irritation from hair pulling against the adhesive.*

Applying a skin barrier and pouch

Fitting a skin barrier and ostomy pouch properly can be done in a few steps. Shown below is a two-piece pouching system with flanges.

1. Measure the stoma using a measuring guide.

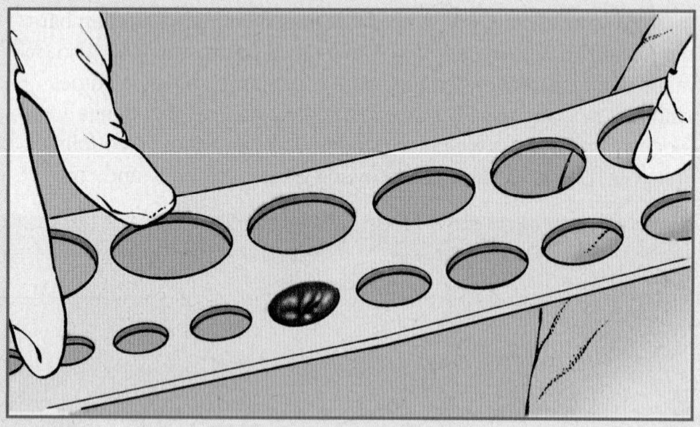

2. Trace the appropriate circle carefully on the back of the skin barrier.

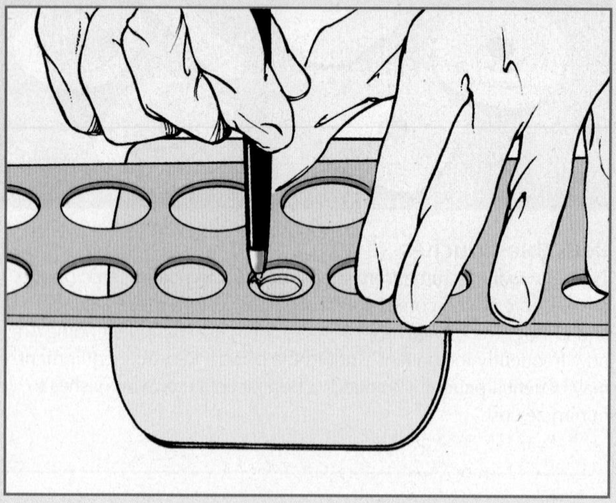

3. Cut the circular opening in the skin barrier (or cut the opening to reflect the configuration of the stoma if it's not circular). Smooth any rough edges with your finger.

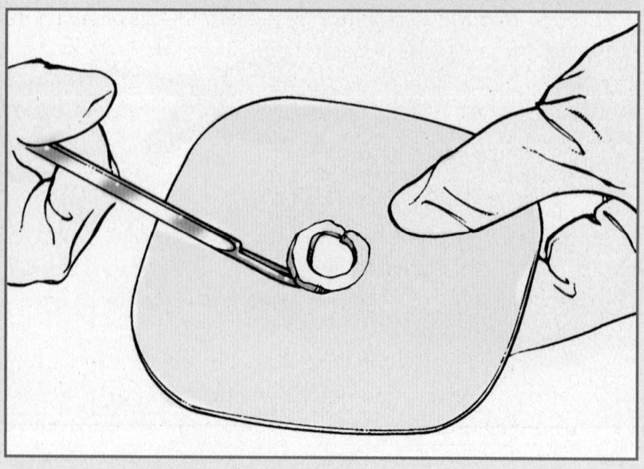

4. Remove the backing from the skin barrier and apply barrier paste or moldable barrier ring, as needed, along the edge of the circular opening.

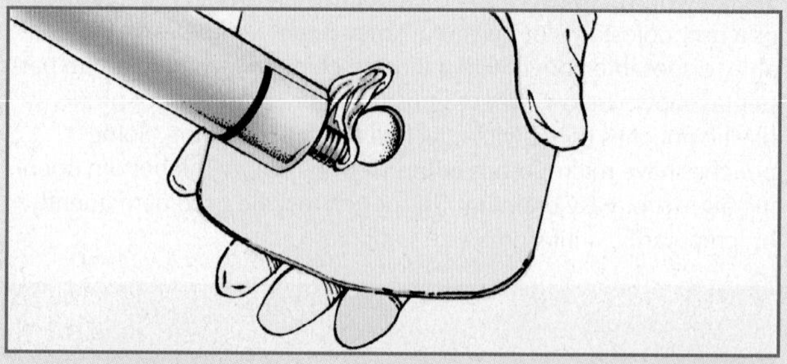

5. Center the skin barrier over the stoma, adhesive side down, and gently press it to the skin. When using a two-piece system, gently press the pouch opening onto the ring until it snaps into place. When using a two-piece adhesive coupling device, line up the adhesive portion of the pouch to the "landing zone" of the wafer. Press together *for adhesion*. The pouches used in a two-piece system can be attached to the wafer before application and applied like a one-piece system if the patient is still experiencing incisional discomfort. Other two-piece systems have a floating flange that allows the user to insert the fingers underneath *so that snapping the flange to the pouch doesn't exert pressure.*

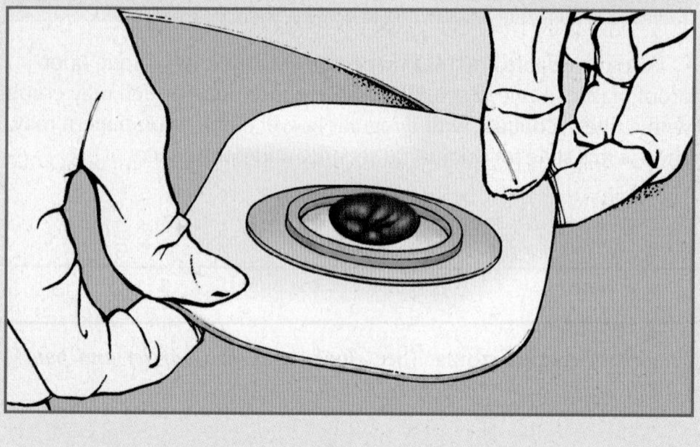

6. Close the bottom of the pouch by folding the end upward and using the clip that comes with the product or close the integrated closure system.

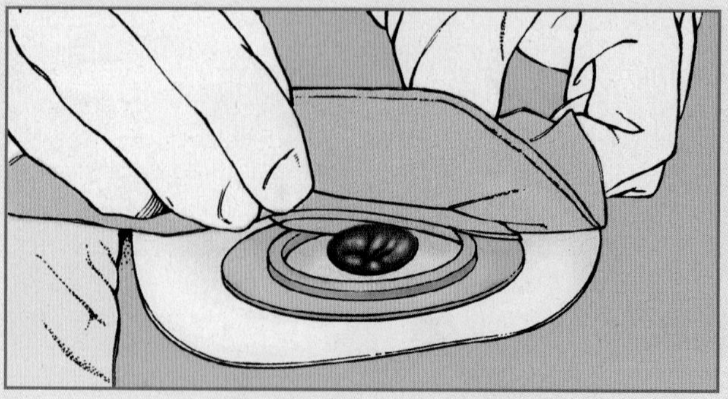

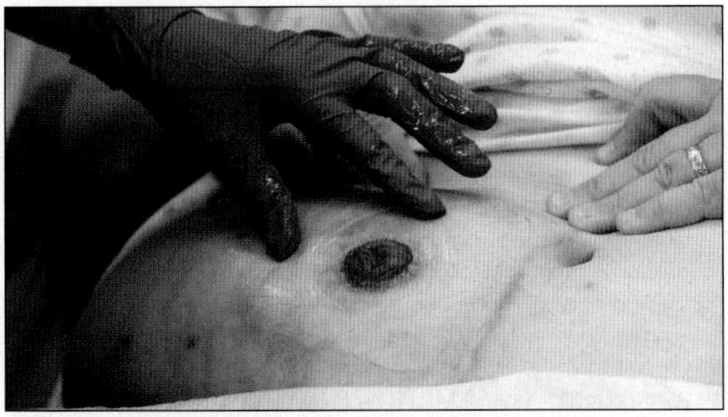

■ You may want to apply a ring of stoma paste or a molded barrier ring around the opening on the back of the skin barrier (depending on the type of stoma, abdominal contours, and effluent) *to provide extra skin protection and a better seal to prevent leakage.*
■ If applying a two-piece appliance with a separate skin barrier, peel off the paper backing of the prepared skin barrier, center the barrier over the stoma, and press gently *to ensure adhesion.*
■ For a pouching system with flanges, align the lip of the pouch flange with the bottom edge of the skin barrier flange. Gently press around the circumference of the pouch flange, beginning at the bottom, until the pouch securely adheres to the barrier flange. (The pouch will click into its secured position.) Holding the barrier against the skin, gently pull on the pouch *to confirm the seal between flanges.*
■ Encourage the patient to stay quietly in position for about 5 minutes *to improve adherence. The patient's body warmth helps to improve adherence and soften a rigid skin barrier.*
■ Leave a bit of air in the pouch *to allow drainage to fall to the bottom.*
■ Apply the closure clamp, if necessary.

Emptying the pouch
■ Tilt the bottom of the pouch upward and remove the closure clamp or undo the integrated closure system (as shown below).

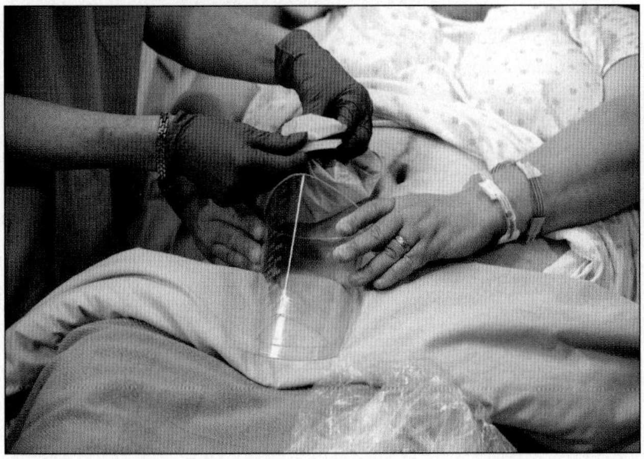

■ Turn up a cuff on the lower end of the pouch; allow it to drain into the toilet, bedpan, or measuring device (as shown on top right).
■ Wipe the bottom of the pouch.
■ Instill pouch deodorant, if desired.

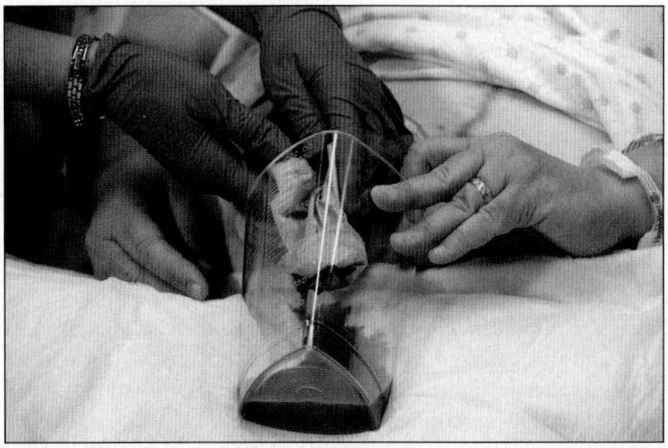

■ Reapply the closure clamp or secure the integrated closure system (as shown below).

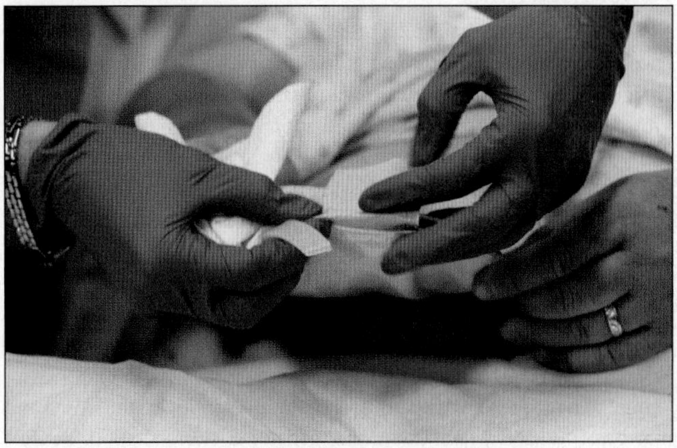

■ Discard the fecal material and clean the bedpan or measuring container appropriately.[11,12]

Completing the procedure
■ Remove and discard your gloves.[11,12]
■ Perform hand hygiene.[6,7,8,9,10]
■ Document the procedure.[17,18,19]

Special considerations
■ When caring for a stoma during the immediate postoperative period, select an appliance with a larger opening, adjust the size of the appliance skin barrier by cutting a larger opening, or cut radial slits in the skin barrier *to allow for flexibility because a newly created stoma may become edematous over the first 24 to 48 hours.* Use a sealant *to protect skin integrity around the opening.* Adjust the size of the opening as stomal swelling subsides. Avoid cutting the opening too big after the initial postoperative period *to prevent peristomal skin complications.*[2]
■ Between 6 and 8 weeks after surgery, the stoma will shrink to its permanent size. At that point, pattern-making preparations will be unnecessary unless the patient gains weight, has additional surgery, or injures the stoma.
■ Use commercial pouch deodorants, if desired, although, most pouches are odor-free; odor should only be evident when you empty the pouch or if it leaks. Before discharge, suggest that, if desired, the patient avoid odor-causing foods, such as fish, eggs, onions, and garlic.
■ If the patient wears a reusable pouching system, suggest obtaining two or more systems *so the patient can wear one while the other dries after cleaning with soap and water or a commercially prepared cleaning solution.*

■ Most ostomy product manufacturers will provide a patch test, if requested, *to determine whether the patient has an allergy to a specific ostomy appliance care product.*[3]

■ If necessary, release flatus by tilting the pouch bottom upward, releasing the clamp, and expelling the flatus.

■ Never make a pinhole in a pouch to release gas. *This destroys the odor-proof seal.*

■ Remove the pouching system if the patient reports pain or irritation at the peristomal site. Inspect the peristomal skin and stoma. Use a facility-approved assessment tool *to objectively identify and track changes in peristomal skin.* Use the tool to assess for discoloration, erosion, and tissue overgrowth.[2,3,4,5] Observe for signs of mechanical, chemical, allergic, infectious, or disease-related complications (which may be linked to preexisting skin conditions, such as psoriasis, eczema, or seborrheic dermatitis).[4] Notify the practitioner or a WOCN of changes, as needed.

Patient teaching

After performing and explaining the procedure to the patient and caregiver, encourage the patient's increasing involvement in self-care. Before discharge, make sure that the patient and family can care for the ostomy. Provide written instructions and information about obtaining replacement equipment. Offer the patient and caregiver a pamphlet or video instructions related to ostomy care. Make sure that the patient or caregiver feels comfortable calling the practitioner, nurse, or WOCN to ask questions or discuss problems. Refer the patient to a local ostomy group. Provide counseling on nutrition, clothing, medications, body image, psychosocial issues, interpersonal relationships, and possible complications.[1,3]

Complications

Failure to fit the pouch properly over the stoma can injure the stoma and may cause leakage, which can induce peristomal skin irritation. Be alert for a possible allergic reaction to adhesives and other ostomy products.

Documentation

Record the date and time of the pouching system change or emptying; note the character of drainage, including color, amount, type, and consistency. Also describe the appearance of the stoma and the peristomal skin using a facility-approved assessment tool if possible.[2,3,4,5] Document any patient teaching provided. Record the patient's response to self-care, and evaluate the learning progress.

References

1 Wound, Ostomy and Continence Nurses Society. (2010). *Management of the patient with a fecal ostomy: Best practice guideline for clinicians.* Mount Laurel, NJ: Wound, Ostomy, and Continence Nurses Society. (Level VII)

2 Australian Association of Stomal Therapy Nurses, Inc. (AASTN). (2013). "Clinical guidelines for stomal therapy nursing practice" [Online]. Accessed March 2015 via the Web at http://www.stomaltherapy.com/documents/AASTN_Guidelines_book_2013.pdf (Level VII)

3 Jordan, R., & Christian, M. (2013). Understanding periostomal skin complications. *Wound Care Advisor, 2*(2), 36–41. Accessed March 2015 via the Web at http://woundcareadvisor.com/wp-content/uploads/2013/05/Understanding_M-J13.pdf

4 Jemec, G. B., et al. (2011). Assessing peristomal skin changes in ostomy patients: Validation of the Ostomy Skin Tool. *British Journal of Dermatology, 164,* 330–335. (Level II)

5 Haugen, H., & Ratliff, C. R. (2013). Tools for assessing peristomal skin complications. *Journal of Wound, Ostomy and Continence Nursing, 40,* 131–134.

6 Centers for Disease Control and Prevention. (2002). Guideline for hand hygiene in health-care settings: Recommendations of the Healthcare Infection Control Practices Advisory Committee and the HICPAC/SHEA/APIC/IDSA Hand Hygiene Task Force. *MMWR Recommendations and Reports, 51*(RR-16), 1–45. Accessed March 2015 via the Web at http://www.cdc.gov/mmwr/pdf/rr/rr5116.pdf (Level II)

7 The Joint Commission. (2015). Standard NPSG.07.01.01. *Comprehensive accreditation manual for hospitals: The official handbook.* Oakbrook Terrace, IL: The Joint Commission. (Level VII)

8 World Health Organization. (2009). "WHO guidelines on hand hygiene in health care: First global patient safety challenge, clean care is safer care" [Online]. Accessed March 2015 via the Web at http://whqlibdoc.who.int/publications/2009/9789241597906_eng.pdf (Level IV)

9 American Osteopathic Association. (2014). Standard 07.01.21. *Healthcare Facilities Accreditation Program: Accreditation requirements for acute care hospitals.* Chicago, IL: American Osteopathic Association. (Level VII)

10 Centers for Medicare & Medicaid Services, Department of Health and Human Services. (2014). Condition of participation: Infection control. 42 C.F.R. § 482.42.

11 Siegel, J. D., et al. (2007). "2007 guideline for isolation precautions: Preventing transmission of infectious agents in healthcare settings" [Online]. Accessed March 2015 via the Web at http://www.cdc.gov/hicpac/pdf/isolation/Isolation2007.pdf (Level II)

12 American Osteopathic Association. (2014). Standard 07.01.10. *Healthcare Facilities Accreditation Program: Accreditation requirements for acute care hospitals.* Chicago, IL: American Osteopathic Association. (Level VII)

13 The Joint Commission. (2015). Standard NPSG.01.01.01. *Comprehensive accreditation manual for hospitals: The official handbook.* Oakbrook Terrace, IL: The Joint Commission. (Level VII)

14 American Osteopathic Association. (2014). Standard 15.01.16. *Healthcare Facilities Accreditation Program: Accreditation requirements for acute care hospitals.* Chicago, IL: American Osteopathic Association. (Level VII)

15 Centers for Medicare & Medicaid Services, Department of Health and Human Services. (2014). Condition of participation: Patient's rights. 42 C.F.R. § 482.13(c)(1).

16 The Joint Commission. (2015). Standard RI.01.01.01. *Comprehensive accreditation manual for hospitals: The official handbook.* Oakbrook Terrace, IL: The Joint Commission. (Level VII)

17 Occupational Safety and Health Administration. (n.d.). "Bloodborne pathogens, standard number 1910.1030" [Online]. Accessed March 2015 via the Web at https://www.osha.gov/pls/oshaweb/owadisp.show_document?p_id=10051&p_table=STANDARDS (Level VII)

18 The Joint Commission. (2015). Standard RC.01.03.01. *Comprehensive accreditation manual for hospitals: The official handbook.* Oakbrook Terrace, IL: The Joint Commission. (Level VII)

19 American Osteopathic Association. (2014). Standard 10.00.03. *Healthcare Facilities Accreditation Program: Accreditation requirements for acute care hospitals.* Chicago, IL: American Osteopathic Association. (Level VII)

20 Centers for Medicare & Medicaid Services, Department of Health and Human Services. (2014). Condition of participation: Medical record services. 42 C.F.R. § 482.24(b).

Additional references

Doubleman, J. (2013). Ostomy 101: Colostomy, ileostomy, and urostomy. *Wound Care Advisor, 2*(2), 31–36. Accessed March 2015 via the Web at http://woundcareadvisor.com/wp-content/uploads/2013/03/Ost_M-A13.pdf

Doughty, D. B., & Landmann, R. G. Management of patients with a colostomy or ileostomy. (2013). In: *UpToDate,* Weiser, M., & Duda, R. B. (Eds.). Accessed March 2015 via the Web at http://www.uptodate.com/contents/search

Nettina, S. M. (2014). *Lippincott manual of nursing practice* (10th ed.). Philadelphia, PA: Wolters Kluwer.

Taylor, C., et al. (2015). *Fundamentals of nursing: The art and science of nursing care* (8th ed.). Philadelphia, PA: Wolters Kluwer.

Colostomy irrigation

Colostomy irrigation involves instilling warm water (irrigant) into the colon via a descending or sigmoid colostomy stoma. The warm water helps to stimulate bowel peristalsis and trains the bowel to empty at this specific time. The goal of irrigation is to prevent the passage of feces or flatus between irrigations. This can be achieved when irrigation is performed once a day or every other day in select patients. The surgeon typically determines whether a patient is a candidate for colostomy irrigation.[1] Colostomy irrigation may also be used to empty the large bowel before diagnostic testing (such as colonoscopy) or colon surgery.[1]

Although colostomy irrigation may begin as soon as bowel function resumes, most practitioners recommend waiting until bowel movements are more predictable. After colostomy irrigation is initiated, it may take 4 to 6 weeks before bowel emptying becomes regulated. Colostomy irrigation is most effective when performed 1 hour after a meal and at the same time each day.[1,2]

Colostomy irrigation is contraindicated in patients with bowel disease, irritable bowel syndrome, hernia, severe heart or kidney disease, an ascending or transverse colostomy, or an ileostomy.[1,2]

Equipment

Colostomy irrigation set (irrigation drain or sleeve, ostomy belt, water-soluble lubricant, drainage pouch clamp, irrigation bag with clamp, tubing, cone tip, clip) ▪ 1L (1 qt) tap water irrigant warmed to about 105°F (40.6°C) ▪ IV pole or wall hook ▪ washcloth ▪ towel ▪ water ▪ ostomy appliance ▪ gloves ▪ facility-approved ostomy skin assessment tool[3,4,5,6] ▪ Optional: fluid-impermeable pad, bedpan, chair, graduated measuring container, small dressing or bandage, stoma cap, soft silicone catheter.

Preparation of equipment

Depending on the patient's condition, colostomy irrigation may be performed using a bedpan or in the bathroom using a chair and the toilet.

Set up the irrigation bag, tubing, and cone tip. If irrigation will take place with the patient in bed, place the bedpan beside the bed and elevate the head of the bed between 45 and 90 degrees, if allowed. If irrigation will take place in the bathroom, have the patient sit on the toilet or on a chair facing the toilet, whichever he finds more comfortable.

Fill the irrigation bag with warmed tap water. Hang the bag on the IV pole or wall hook. The bottom of the bag should be at the patient's shoulder level *to prevent the fluid from entering the bowel too quickly.* Most irrigation sets also have a clamp that regulates the flow rate.

Prime the tubing with irrigant *to prevent air from entering the colon and possibly causing cramps and gas pains.*

Implementation

- Perform hand hygiene.[7,8,9,10,11]
- Confirm the patient's identity using at least two patient identifiers.[12]
- Explain every step of the procedure to the patient *because he'll eventually be irrigating the colostomy himself.*
- Provide privacy.[13,14,15]
- If the patient is in bed, place a fluid-impermeable pad under him *to protect the sheets or chair surface from soiling.*
- Put on gloves *to comply with standard precautions.*[16,17]
- Remove the ostomy appliance if the patient uses one.
- Place the irrigation sleeve over the stoma. If the sleeve doesn't have an adhesive backing, secure the sleeve with an ostomy belt. If the patient has a two-piece pouching system with flanges, snap off the pouch and save it. Snap on the irrigation sleeve.
- Place the open-ended bottom of the irrigation sleeve in the bedpan, toilet, or appropriate measuring container *to promote drainage by gravity.*
- Lubricate your gloved small finger with water-soluble lubricant and insert the finger into the stoma. If you're teaching the patient, have him do this step *to determine the bowel angle at which to insert the cone safely.* Expect the stoma to tighten when the finger enters the bowel and then to relax in a few seconds.
- Lubricate the cone with water-soluble lubricant *to prevent it from irritating the mucosa.*
- Insert the cone into the top opening of the irrigation sleeve and then into the stoma. Angle the cone to match the bowel angle. Insert it gently but snugly; never force it in place.
- Instruct the patient to take slow, deep breaths *to relax the abdominal muscles.*[18]
- Unclamp the irrigation tubing and allow the water to flow slowly. If you don't have a clamp to control the irrigant's flow rate, pinch the tubing *to control the flow.* The water should enter the colon over 5 to 10 minutes.
- Explain to the patient that he may experience a sensation of fullness or bloating during the instillation.[18] If he reports cramping, slow or stop the flow, keep the cone in place, and have him take a few deep breaths until the cramping stops. *Cramping during irrigation may result from a bowel that's ready to empty, water that's too cold, a rapid flow rate, or air in the tubing.*
- After 15 minutes, close the bottom of the irrigation sleeve with the clip provided in the irrigation kit. *The initial return of water and stool occurs within 15 minutes after irrigation.*[18] Have the patient remain stationary for 15 or 20 minutes *to allow the initial effluent to drain.*
- If the patient is ambulatory, encourage him to perform activities of daily living during the next 30 to 45 minutes *to stimulate peristalsis and evacuation of stool.*[1] Alternatively, if the patient is nonambulatory, instruct him to massage his abdomen or lean forward *to stimulate peristalsis and evacuation of stool.*[1,18]
- After 45 minutes, empty the contents of the irrigation sleeve into the bedpan, toilet, or appropriate measuring container.
- Measure output, as ordered; subtract the amount of irrigant used from the total amount of effluent *to determine the amount of effluent.*
- Remove the irrigation sleeve.
- Using a washcloth and water, gently clean the area around the stoma. Rinse it, and then dry the area thoroughly with a clean towel.
- Inspect the peristomal skin and stoma. Use a facility-approved assessment tool if available *to objectively identify and track changes in peristomal skin.* Use the tool to assess for discoloration, erosion, and tissue overgrowth.[3,4,5,6] Observe for signs of mechanical, chemical, allergic, infectious, or disease-related complications (which may be linked to preexisting skin conditions, such as psoriasis, eczema, or seborrheic dermatitis). Notify the practitioner or a wound-ostomy-continence nurse of changes, as needed.
- Apply a clean ostomy appliance. (See the "Colostomy and ileostomy care" procedure, page 200.) If the patient has a regular bowel elimination pattern, he may prefer a small dressing, bandage, or commercial stoma cap.
- Discard a disposable irrigation sleeve in the appropriate receptacle.[16,17] Rinse a reusable irrigation sleeve with mild soap and water and hang it to dry along with the irrigation bag, tubing, and cone.[18,19]
- Remove and discard your gloves.[16,17]
- Perform hand hygiene.[7,8,9,10,11]
- Document the procedure.[20,21,22]

Special considerations

- Irrigating a colostomy to establish a regular bowel elimination pattern doesn't work for all patients. If the bowel continues to move between irrigations, try decreasing the volume of irrigant. *Increasing the irrigant won't help because it serves only to stimulate peristalsis.* Keep a record of results. Also consider irrigating every other day.
- Irrigation may help to regulate bowel function in patients with a descending or sigmoid colostomy *because this is the bowel's stool storage area.* However, a patient with an ascending or transverse colostomy won't benefit from irrigation. Also, a patient with a descending or sigmoid colostomy who's missing part of the ascending or transverse colon may not be able to irrigate successfully *because his ostomy may function like an ascending or transverse colostomy.*

- If diarrhea develops, discontinue irrigations until stools form again. Keep in mind that irrigation alone won't achieve regularity for the patient. He must also observe a complementary diet and exercise regimen.
- If the patient has a strictured stoma that prohibits cone insertion, remove the cone from the irrigation tubing and replace it with a soft silicone catheter. Angle the catheter gently 2″ to 4″ (5 to 10 cm) into the bowel *to instill the irrigant.* Don't force the catheter into the stoma, and don't insert it further than the recommended length *because you may perforate the bowel.*

Patient teaching

After explaining the procedure to, and performing the procedure on, the patient, encourage the patient's increasing involvement in self-care. Discuss with the patient his bathroom setup, how to hang the irrigation bag, and how to manage all of the equipment to avoid spills. Also discuss how to avoid excessive tiredness during the procedure. If the patient will use reusable irrigation bags, teach him to discard the bags after 1 month (or sooner if an odor is detected). Teach the patient to monitor his diet to determine whether certain foods are interfering with the irrigation outcomes. Offer written instructions and information on obtaining replacement equipment.

Complications

Bowel perforation may result if a catheter is incorrectly inserted into the stoma. Fluid and electrolyte imbalances may result from using too much irrigant.

Documentation

Record the date and time of irrigation and the type and amount of irrigant. Note the stoma's color and the character of drainage, including the color, consistency, and amount. Record any patient teaching. Describe teaching content and the patient's response to self-care instruction. Evaluate the patient's learning progress.

REFERENCES

1 Wound, Ostomy and Continence Nurses Society. (2010). *Management of the patient with a fecal ostomy: Best practice guideline for clinicians.* Mount Laurel, NJ: Wound, Ostomy and Continence Nurses Society. (Level VII)

2 Williams, J. (2011). Principles and practice of colostomy irrigation. *Gastrointestinal Nursing, 9*(9), 15–16.

3 Haugen, H., & Ratliff, C. R. (2013). Tools for assessing peristomal skin complications. *Journal of Wound, Ostomy and Continence Nursing, 40,* 131–134.

4 Jemec, G. B., et al. (2011). Assessing peristomal skin changes in ostomy patients: Validation of the Ostomy Skin Tool. *British Journal of Dermatology, 164,* 330–335. (Level II)

5 Jordan, R., & Christian, M. (2013). Understanding periostomal skin complications. *Wound Care Advisory, 2*(2), 36–41. Accessed March 2015 via the Web at http://woundcareadvisor.com/wp-content/uploads/2013/05/Understanding_M-J13.pdf

6 Australian Association of Stomal Therapy Nurses, Inc. (AASTN). (2013). "Clinical guidelines for stomal therapy nursing practice" [Online]. Accessed March 2015 via the Web at http://www.stomaltherapy.com/documents/AASTN_Guidelines_book_2013.pdf (Level VII)

7 The Joint Commission. (2015). Standard NPSG.07.01.01. *Comprehensive accreditation manual for hospitals: The official handbook.* Oakbrook Terrace, IL: The Joint Commission. (Level VII)

8 Centers for Disease Control and Prevention. (2002). Guideline for hand hygiene in health-care settings: Recommendations of the Healthcare Infection Control Practices Advisory Committee and the HICPAC/SHEA/APIC/IDSA Hand Hygiene Task Force. *MMWR Recommendations and Reports, 51*(RR-16), 1–45. Accessed March 2015 via the Web at http://www.cdc.gov/mmwr/pdf/rr/rr5116.pdf (Level II)

9 World Health Organization. (2009). "WHO guidelines on hand hygiene in health care: First global patient safety challenge, clean care is safer care" [Online]. Accessed March 2015 via the Web at http://whqlibdoc.who.int/publications/2009/9789241597906_eng.pdf (Level IV)

10 American Osteopathic Association. (2014). Standard 07.01.21. *Healthcare Facilities Accreditation Program: Accreditation requirements for acute care hospitals.* Chicago, IL: American Osteopathic Association. (Level VII)

11 Centers for Medicare & Medicaid Services, Department of Health and Human Services. (2014). Condition of participation: Infection control. 42 C.F.R. § 482.42.

12 The Joint Commission. (2015). Standard NPSG.01.01.01. *Comprehensive accreditation manual for hospitals: The official handbook.* Oakbrook Terrace, IL: The Joint Commission. (Level VII)

13 American Osteopathic Association. (2014). Standard 15.01.16. *Healthcare Facilities Accreditation Program: Accreditation requirements for acute care hospitals.* Chicago, IL: American Osteopathic Association. (Level VII)

14 The Joint Commission. (2015). Standard RI.01.01.01. *Comprehensive accreditation manual for hospitals: The official handbook.* Oakbrook Terrace, IL: The Joint Commission. (Level VII)

15 Centers for Medicare & Medicaid Services, Department of Health and Human Services. (2014). Condition of participation: Patient's rights. 42 C.F.R. § 482.13(c)(1).

16 Siegel, J. D., et al. (2007). "2007 guideline for isolation precautions: Preventing transmission of infectious agents in healthcare settings" [Online]. Accessed March 2015 via the Web at http://www.cdc.gov/hicpac/pdf/isolation/Isolation2007.pdf (Level II)

17 American Osteopathic Association. (2014). Standard 07.01.10. *Healthcare Facilities Accreditation Program: Accreditation requirements for acute care hospitals.* Chicago, IL: American Osteopathic Association. (Level VII)

18 Memorial Sloan Kettering Cancer Center™. (2013). "Patient and caregiver education: Irrigating your sigmoid or descending colostomy" [Online]. Accessed March 2015 via the Web at http://www.mskcc.org/printpdf/cancer-care/patient-education/resources/colostomy-irrigation-instructions-sigmoid-descending-colostomy?inline=1

19 American Osteopathic Association. (2014). Standard 07.02.03. *Healthcare Facilities Accreditation Program: Accreditation requirements for acute care hospitals.* Chicago, IL: American Osteopathic Association. (Level VII)

20 The Joint Commission. (2015). Standard RC.01.03.01. *Comprehensive accreditation manual for hospitals: The official handbook.* Oakbrook Terrace, IL: The Joint Commission. (Level VII)

21 American Osteopathic Association. (2014). Standard 10.00.03. *Healthcare Facilities Accreditation Program: Accreditation requirements for acute care hospitals.* Chicago, IL: American Osteopathic Association. (Level VII)

22 Centers for Medicare & Medicaid Services, Department of Health and Human Services. (2014). Condition of participation: Medical record services. 42 C.F.R. § 482.24(b).

CONTACT LENS CARE

Illness or emergency treatment may require that you insert or remove and store a patient's contact lenses. Proper handling and lens care techniques help prevent eye injury and infection as well as lens loss or damage. Appropriate lens-handling techniques depend in large part on what type of lenses the patient wears. Although most patients can remove their own contact lenses, you should be able to remove the lenses if the patient can't. Patients may present to the emergency department because of difficulty removing their own lenses or with acute ophthalmologic complications associated with contact lens use. Assess a patient with an altered mental status to determine whether he's wearing contact lenses, and then remove them if present.

All contact lenses float on the corneal tear layer. Soft lenses typically have diameters larger than the cornea; rigid lenses typically have diameters smaller than the cornea. Because they're larger and more pliable, soft lenses tend to mold themselves more closely to the eye for a more stable fit than rigid lenses.

Modes of lens wear vary widely. Although most patients remove and clean their lenses daily, some wear lenses overnight or for several days (sometimes up to a month) without removing them for cleaning. Still other patients wear disposable lenses, which means that they replace old lenses with new ones at regular intervals (a few days to a few months), possibly without removing them for cleaning between replacements.

Keep in mind that handling contact lenses improperly can provide a direct source of contamination or injury to the eye.

Equipment

Powder-free gloves ■ towel ■ lens storage case or two small medicine cups (labeled left and right) ■ sterile normal saline solution or soaking solution if available ■ Optional: patient's own equipment for contact lens care (surfactant solution and enzyme agent), flashlight, rigid contact lens remover, adhesive tape.

Preparation of equipment

If a commercial lens storage case isn't available, place enough sterile normal saline solution into two small medicine cups *to submerge a lens in each one. To avoid confusing the left and right lenses,* which may have different prescriptions, mark one cup "L" and the other cup "R" and place the corresponding lens in each cup.

Implementation

- Gather the appropriate equipment.
- Perform hand hygiene.[1,2,3,4,5]
- Confirm the patient's identity using at least two patient identifiers.[6]
- Determine whether the patient wears soft or rigid contact lenses. *Rigid lenses are smaller in diameter than the cornea, and smaller than soft contact lenses.*
- Explain the procedure to the patient.
- Put on gloves *to help prevent ocular infection.*[7,8]

Inserting soft lenses

- Place a towel on the patient's chest.
- *To see if the lens is inside out,* bend it between your thumb and index finger or fill it with saline or soaking solution. If the lens tends to roll inward or the edge points slightly inward, it's oriented correctly. If the edge points outward or the lens tends to collapse over your fingertip, it's probably inside out and should be reversed.
- Wet the lens with fresh normal saline solution and rub it gently between your thumb and index finger, or place it on your palm and rub it with your opposite index finger. Rinse well.
- Place the lens, convex side down, on the tip of the index finger of your dominant hand.
- Instruct the patient to gaze upward slightly.
- Confirm that you have the correct lens for the correct eye, separate the eyelids with your other thumb and index finger, and place the lens on the sclera, just below the cornea. Then, slide the lens gently upward with your finger until it centers on the cornea.
- Using the same procedure, insert the opposite lens.

Inserting rigid lenses

- Wet one lens with solution and gently rub it between your thumb and index finger, or place it on your palm and rub it with your opposite index finger. Rinse well with the solution, leaving a small amount in the lens.
- Place the lens, convex side down, on the tip of the index finger of your dominant hand.
- Instruct the patient to gaze upward slightly.
- After confirming you have the correct lens for the correct eye, separate the eyelids with your other thumb and index finger and gently place the lens directly on the cornea. You don't need to press it to the eye *because the tear film will attract it naturally at the first touch.*
- Using the same procedure, insert the opposite lens.

Removing soft lenses

- Place the patient in the supine position *to prevent the lens from popping out onto the floor, risking loss or damage.*
- Examine the eye and cornea with a flashlight if needed, and ensure that the correct lens is present and centered on the cornea before attempting to remove it. *Attempting to remove a contact lens that isn't there may result in a corneal abrasion.*[9]
- If the patient is wearing soft contact lenses, add a few drops of normal saline solution to each eye 5 to 10 minutes before removal *to hydrate the soft lenses, making removal easier.*[9]
- Using your nondominant hand, raise the patient's upper eyelid and hold it against the orbital rim.
- Lightly place the forefinger of your other hand on the lens and move it down onto the sclera below the cornea.
- Pinch the lens between your forefinger and thumb; it should pop off (as shown below).

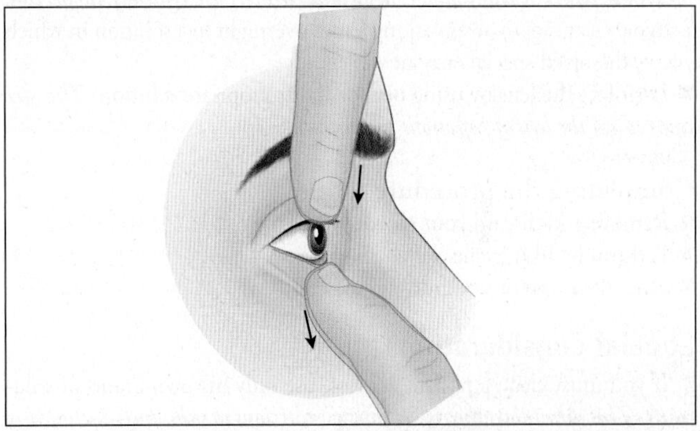

- After removal, place the lens in the proper well of the storage case (marked "L" or "R") with enough of the appropriate storage solution to cover it.[10] Alternatively, place the lens in a labeled medicine cup with solution, and secure adhesive tape over the top of the cup *to prevent loss of the lens.*
- Remove and care for the other lens using the same technique.

Removing rigid lenses

- Before removing a lens, place the patient in the supine position *to prevent the lens from popping out onto the floor, risking loss or damage.*
- Examine the patient's eye and cornea with a flashlight if needed, and ensure that the contact lens is present and centered on the cornea before attempting to remove it. *Attempting to remove a contact lens that isn't there may result in a corneal abrasion.*[9]
- Place one thumb against the patient's upper eyelid and the other thumb against the lower eyelid.
- Move the eyelids toward each other while gently pressing inward against the eye *to trap the lens edge and break the suction.* Extract the lens from the patient's eyelashes.
- Depending on the lens type and thickness, it may pop out when the suction breaks. You may want to try to break the suction with one hand while cupping the other hand below the patient's eye *to catch the lens as it falls.*
- Sometimes the lens will pop out on its own if you ask the patient to blink after stretching the corner of the eyelids toward the temporal bone, thus tightening the lid edges against the globe of the eye.
- If the lens doesn't pop out on its own, use a rigid contact lens remover to carefully remove the lens. Moisten the remover's suction cup with normal saline solution, and then gently touch it to the center of the contact lens. Make sure to apply it directly to the lens, not the eye. After the suction cup attaches to the lens, gently twist the lens off the eye. Then carefully slide the lens off of the suction cup *because pulling the lens directly off of the suction cup may cause the lens to warp.*

■ After removal, place the lens in the proper well of the storage case (marked "L" or "R") with enough of the appropriate storage solution to cover it.[10] Alternatively, place the lens in a labeled medicine cup with solution, and secure adhesive tape over the top of the cup *to prevent loss of the lens.*
■ Remove and care for the opposite lens using the same technique.

Cleaning and disinfecting lenses

■ *Because lens-cleaning steps vary with lens type and with each manufacturer's and practitioner's instructions,* ask the patient to guide you step-by-step through his normal cleaning routine.
■ If the patient can't tell you how to clean his lenses properly, remember that all lens types require two steps: cleaning and disinfection.
■ Clean the lens by rubbing it with a surfactant solution *to remove most surface deposits.* For most patients, especially those who wear soft lenses, the cleaning step may also include use of an enzyme agent *to remove protein deposits against which surfactant cleaners are typically ineffective.* Enzyme cleaning involves soaking lenses overnight in a solution in which you've dissolved special enzyme tablets.
■ Disinfect the lens by using heat or the appropriate solution. *This step aims to rid the lens of infectious organisms.*

Completing the procedure

■ Remove and discard your gloves.[7]
■ Perform hand hygiene.[1,2,3,4,5]
■ Document the procedure.[11,12,13]

Special considerations

■ If you must clean a patient's lenses, use only his own brand of solutions. *This minimizes the risk of allergic reactions to substances included in other solution brands.* Never touch the nozzle of a solution bottle to the lens, your fingers, or anything else *to avoid contaminating the solution in the bottle.*
■ If the patient's eyes appear dry or you have trouble moving the lens on the eye, instill several drops of sterile normal saline solution and wait a few minutes before trying again to remove the lens *to prevent corneal damage.* If you still can't remove the lens easily, notify the practitioner.
■ Don't instill eye medication while the patient is wearing lenses. *The lenses could trap the medication, possibly causing eye irritation or lens damage.*
■ Don't allow soft lenses, which are 40% to 60% water, to dry out. If they do, soak them in sterile normal saline solution and they may return to their natural shape.
■ If an unconscious patient is admitted to the emergency department, check for contact lenses by opening each eyelid and searching with a small flashlight. If you detect lenses, remove them immediately *because tears can't circulate freely beneath the lenses with eyelids closed, possibly leading to corneal oxygen depletion or infection.*
■ If the patient has had a serious eye injury while wearing a contact lens and globe perforation is suspected, don't attempt to remove the lens; instead, the patient should be referred to an ophthalmologist. Place an eye shield (not a pad) over the *eye to minimize or prevent pressure on the globe.*[9]
■ If the patient can't provide adequate care for his lenses during hospitalization, encourage him to send them home with a family member. If you aren't sure how to care for the lenses in the interim, store them in sterile normal saline solution until a family member can take them home.

Patient teaching

Advise contact lens wearers to carry appropriate identification *to speed lens removal and ensure proper care in an emergency.*

Complications

The main risk of contact lens removal is corneal abrasion. You can minimize the risk of corneal abrasion by ensuring that the contact lens is centered on the cornea and following the methods described above. More significant complications are likely to result from contact lenses left in the eyes for prolonged periods and can be especially serious in patients with a reduced level of consciousness. Complications of contact lens wear include lens deposits, allergic conjunctivitis, giant papillary conjunctivitis, peripheral corneal infiltrates, microbial keratitis, and corneal neovascularization. All types of contact lenses reduce the amount of oxygen that reaches the cornea. Oxygenation is reduced further if the patient wears contact lenses when his eyes are closed.[9]

Documentation

Record eye condition before and after removal of lenses; the time of lens insertion, removal, and cleaning; the location of stored lenses; and, if applicable, the removal of lenses from the facility by a family member.

REFERENCES

1 The Joint Commission. (2015). NPSG.07.01.01. *Comprehensive accreditation manual for hospitals: The official handbook.* Oakbrook Terrace, IL: The Joint Commission. (Level VII)

2 Centers for Disease Control and Prevention. (2002). Guideline for hand hygiene in health-care settings: Recommendations of the Healthcare Infection Control Practices Advisory Committee and the HICPAC/SHEA/APIC/IDSA Hand Hygiene Task Force. *MMWR Recommendations and Reports, 51*(RR-16), 1–45. Accessed March 2015 via the Web at http://www.cdc.gov/mmwr/pdf/rr/rr5116.pdf (Level II)

3 World Health Organization. (2009). "WHO guidelines on hand hygiene in health care: First global patient safety challenge, clean care is safer care" [Online]. Accessed March 2015 via the Web at http://whqlibdoc.who.int/publications/2009/9789241597906_eng.pdf (Level IV)

4 Centers for Medicare & Medicaid Services, Department of Health and Human Services. (2014). Condition of participation: Infection control. 42 C.F.R. § 482.42.

5 American Osteopathic Association. (2014). Standard 07.01.21. *Healthcare Facilities Accreditation Program: Accreditation requirements for acute care hospitals.* Chicago, IL: American Osteopathic Association. (Level VII)

6 The Joint Commission. (2015). NPSG.01.01.01. *Comprehensive accreditation manual for hospitals: The official handbook.* Oakbrook Terrace, IL: The Joint Commission. (Level VII)

7 Siegel, J. D., et al. (2007). "2007 guideline for isolation precautions: Preventing transmission of infectious agents in healthcare settings" [Online]. Accessed March 2015 via the Web at http://www.cdc.gov/hicpac/pdf/isolation/Isolation2007.pdf (Level II)

8 American Osteopathic Association. (2014). Standard 07.01.10. *Healthcare Facilities Accreditation Program: Accreditation requirements for acute care hospitals.* Chicago, IL: American Osteopathic Association. (Level VII)

9 Tatham, A., et al. (2012). "Contact lens removal" [Online]. Accessed March 2015 via the Web at http://emedicine.medscape.com/article/1413506-overview#a01

10 Weissman, B. A., et al. (2006). "Optometric clinical practice guideline: Care of the contact lens patient (2nd ed.)" [Online]. Accessed March 2015 via the Web at http://www.aoa.org/documents/cpg-19.pdf (Level VII)

11 The Joint Commission. (2015). Standard RC.01.03.01. *Comprehensive accreditation manual for hospitals: The official handbook.* Oakbrook Terrace, IL: The Joint Commission. (Level VII)

12 Centers for Medicare & Medicaid Services, Department of Health and Human Services. (2014). Condition of participation: Medical record services. 42 C.F.R. § 482.24(b).

13 American Osteopathic Association. (2014). Standard 10.00.03. *Healthcare Facilities Accreditation Program: Accreditation requirements for acute care hospitals.* Chicago, IL: American Osteopathic Association. (Level VII)

CONTACT PRECAUTIONS

Contact precautions are used to prevent the spread of microorganisms by direct or indirect contact with the patient or the patient's environment. (See *Conditions requiring contact precautions,* page 210.) Effective contact precautions require a single room, if possible, and the use of gloves and gowns by anyone having contact with the patient, the patient's support equipment, or items that have come in contact with the patient or the patient's environment.[1] Proper hand hygiene and handling and disposal of articles that have come in contact with the patient and his environment are essential.[1]

Equipment

Contact precautions sign ▪ gloves ▪ plastic bags ▪ additional supplies needed for patient care, such as a thermometer, stethoscope, blood pressure cuff, and clean dressings.

Preparation of equipment

Keep all contact precaution supplies outside the patient's room in a wall- or door-mounted cabinet, a cart, or an anteroom.

Implementation

- Place a contact precautions sign outside the patient's door, as required by your facility, *to notify anyone entering the room of the situation.*[1,8,9,10]
- Perform hand hygiene.[9,11,12,13,14]
- Put on a gown and gloves before entering the patient's room. Instruct any visitors to do the same according to your facility's policy. (See the "Isolation garb use" procedure, 441.)[1,15]
- Confirm the patient's identity using at least two patient identifiers.[16]
- Situate the patient in a single room with private toilet facilities and an anteroom, if possible. If necessary, two patients with the same infection may share a room; however, consult with your facility's infection preventionist before placing two patients together.[1]
- Explain isolation procedures to the patient and his family *to ease patient anxiety and promote cooperation.*
- Always change gloves after contact with a contaminated body site or contact with body fluids, excretions, mucous membranes, nonintact skin, and wound dressings.[1] Perform hand hygiene after removing used gloves and before putting on new gloves.[9,11,12,13,14]
- Handle all items that have come in contact with the patient as you would for a patient on standard precautions.[1]
- Limit the patient's movement from the room. If the patient must be moved, cover any infected areas with clean dressings.[1] Notify the receiving department or area of the patient's isolation precautions *so that the precautions will be maintained and the patient can be returned to the room promptly.*
- Teach the patient and his family about the importance of hand hygiene[9,11,12,13,14] in preventing the spread of infection and about other measures to prevent the spread of multidrug-resistant organisms.[4,17]
- Remove and discard your gown and gloves before leaving the room.[1]
- Perform hand hygiene after leaving the patient's room.[9,11,12,13,14]
- Document the procedure.[18,19,20]

Special considerations

- Clean and disinfect equipment that must be used for different patients in between each patient use according to your facility's policy *to prevent cross-contamination.* If *Clostridium difficile* is confirmed or suspected after cleaning, consider using an Environmental Protection Agency–registered disinfectant that has a sporicidal claim or a sodium hypochlorite solution for disinfection. Notify environmental services after the patient is discharged and have them clean and disinfect the room.[1,2,9,21,22,23]
- Try to dedicate certain reusable equipment (thermometer, stethoscope, blood pressure cuff) for the patient in contact precautions *to reduce the risk of transmitting infection to other patients.*[1]
- Results of several studies concerning the benefits of a single-patient room to prevent transmission of *C. difficile* are inconclusive. Some studies have shown that being in the same room with a colonized or infected adult patient isn't necessarily a risk factor for transmission. Patient factors play a key role in determining the risk of transmission. The need for a single-patient room, private bathroom, or both for any patient should be determined on a case-by-case basis.[1,2]

Complications

Social isolation is a complication of contact precautions.

Documentation

Record the need for contact precautions on the nursing care plan and as otherwise indicated by your facility. Document initiation and maintenance of the precautions, the patient's tolerance of the procedure, and any patient or family teaching provided and their understanding of your teaching. Also document the date contact precautions were discontinued.

REFERENCES

1 Siegel, J. D., et al. (2007). "2007 guideline for isolation precautions: Preventing transmission of infectious agents in healthcare settings" [Online]. Accessed March 2015 via the Web at http://www.cdc.gov/hicpac/pdf/isolation/Isolation2007.pdf (Level II)

2 Centers for Disease Control and Prevention. (2012). "Frequently asked questions about *Clostridium difficile* for healthcare providers" [Online]. Accessed March 2015 via the Web at http://www.cdc.gov/HAI/organisms/cdiff/cdiff_faqs_HCP.html

3 Cohen, S. H., et al. (2010). Clinical practice guidelines for *Clostridium difficile* infection in adults: 2010 update by the Society for Healthcare Epidemiology (SHEA) and the Infectious Disease Society of America (IDSA). *Infection Control and Hospital Epidemiology, 31,* 431–455. (Level VII)

4 The Joint Commission. (2015). Standard NPSG.07.03.01. *Comprehensive accreditation manual for hospitals: The official handbook.* Oakbrook Terrace, IL: The Joint Commission. (Level VII)

5 Dubberke, E. R., & Gerding, D. N. (2011). "Rationale for hand hygiene recommendations after caring for a patient with *Clostridium difficile* infection" [Online]. Accessed March 2015 via the Web at http://www.shea-online.org/Portals/0/CDI%20hand%20hygiene%20Update.pdf (Level VII)

6 Centers for Disease Control and Prevention. (2005). Guidelines for preventing the transmission of *Mycobacterium tuberculosis* in health care settings, 2005. *MMWR Recommendations and Reports, 54*(RR-17), 1–140. Accessed March 2015 via the Web at http://www.cdc.gov/mmwr/PDF/rr/rr5417.pdf (Level VII)

7 Hall, A. J., et al. (2011). Updated norovirus outbreak management and disease prevention guidelines. *MMWR Recommendations and Reports, 60*(RR-03), 1–15. Accessed March 2015 via the Web at http://www.cdc.gov/mmwr/preview/mmwrhtml/rr6003a1.htm?s_cid=rr6003a1_w (Level VII)

8 The Joint Commission. (2015). Standard IC.02.01.01. *Comprehensive accreditation manual for hospitals: The official handbook.* Oakbrook Terrace, IL: The Joint Commission. (Level VII)

9 Centers for Medicare & Medicaid Services, Department of Health and Human Services. (2014). Condition of participation: Infection control. 42 C.F.R. § 482.42.

10 American Osteopathic Association. (2014). Standard 07.01.10. *Healthcare Facilities Accreditation Program: Accreditation requirements for acute care hospitals.* Chicago, IL: American Osteopathic Association. (Level VII)

11 The Joint Commission. (2015). Standard NPSG.07.01.01. *Comprehensive accreditation manual for hospitals: The official handbook.* Oakbrook Terrace, IL: The Joint Commission. (Level VII)

12 World Health Organization. (2009). "WHO guidelines on hand hygiene in health care: First global patient safety challenge, clean care is safer care"

(*Text continues on page 213*)

Conditions requiring contact precautions[1]

The Centers for Disease Control and Prevention recommends contact precautions for patients who are infected or colonized (positive for the microorganism without clinical signs or symptoms of infection) with epidemiologically important organisms that can be transmitted by direct or indirect contact.

CONDITION	PRECAUTIONARY PERIOD	SPECIAL CONSIDERATIONS (IF APPLICABLE)
Abscess, major draining	■ Duration of illness or until drainage stops or can be contained by a dressing	■ Droplet precautions should be added for the first 24 hours of appropriate antibiotic therapy if invasive group A streptococcal disease is suspected.
Acute viral (acute hemorrhagic) conjunctivitis	■ Duration of illness	
Adenovirus gastroenteritis, diapered or incontinent patient	■ Duration of illness or a duration that's appropriate to control a facility outbreak	
Adenovirus pneumonia	■ Duration of illness	■ Droplet precautions should also be instituted. ■ Precautions should be extended in immunocompromised patients *because viral shedding is prolonged.*
Avian influenza	■ For 14 days after onset of signs and symptoms or until an alternate diagnosis is confirmed	■ Airborne precautions should also be implemented. ■ Eye protection should be worn by individuals within 3″ (1 M) of the patient.
Bronchiolitis	■ Duration of illness	
Burkholderia cepacia pneumonia in a patient with cystic fibrosis	■ Unknown	■ Contact precautions should also be instituted for patients with cystic fibrosis whose respiratory tracts are colonized with bacteria. ■ Exposure to other patients with cystic fibrosis should be avoided.
Campylobacter species gastroenteritis, diapered or incontinent patient	■ Duration of illness or a duration that's appropriate to control a facility outbreak	
Cholera gastroenteritis, diapered or incontinent patient	■ Duration of illness or a duration that's appropriate to control a facility outbreak	
Clostridium difficile gastroenteritis	■ Duration of illness	■ Discontinue the antibiotic the patient was previously exposed to.[2,3] ■ Environmental cleaning and disinfection should be done consistently; consider using an Environmental Protection Agency (EPA)–registered disinfectant that has a sporicidal claim or a sodium hypochlorite solution.[2,3] ■ Consistently use gloves *to help prevent the spread of* C. difficile *spores via the hands of health care workers.* ■ After removing gloves, perform hand hygiene. *Because alcohol doesn't kill* C. difficile *spores,* using either regular or antimicrobial soap and water for hand hygiene is more effective than using alcohol-based hand sanitizers at removing spores; however, *to help ensure compliance with hand hygiene,* alcohol-based hand rubs can be used. In the event of an outbreak, consider using soap and water rather than hand sanitizers.[2,3,4,5]
Cryptosporidium species gastroenteritis, diapered or incontinent patient	■ Duration of illness or a duration that's appropriate to control a facility outbreak	
Diphtheria, cutaneous	■ Until two cultures (obtained 24 hours apart) are negative	

Conditions requiring contact precautions[1] *(continued)*

CONDITION	PRECAUTIONARY PERIOD	SPECIAL CONSIDERATIONS (IF APPLICABLE)
Escherichia coli gastroenteritis (0157:H7 and other shiga toxin–producing strains, other species), diapered or incontinent patient	■ Duration of illness or a duration that's appropriate to control a facility outbreak	
Enteroviral infection, diapered or incontinent patient	■ Duration of illness	
Giardia lamblia gastroenteritis, diapered or incontinent patient	■ Duration of illness or a duration that's appropriate to control a facility outbreak	
Hepatitis type A	■ Duration of hospitalization in infants and children younger than age 3 years ■ For 2 weeks after the onset of signs and symptoms in children ages 3 to 14 years ■ For 1 week after the onset of signs and symptoms in children older than age 14 years	
Hepatitis type E, diapered or incontinent patient	■ Duration of illness	
Herpes simplex, neonatal	■ Until lesions are dry and crusted ■ For asymptomatic, exposed neonates, until cultures obtained at 24 and 36 hours of age are negative; incubation required for 48 hours	
Herpes zoster, disseminated disease or localized disease in an immunocompromised patient	■ Duration of illness or until disseminated disease is ruled out in an immunocompromised patient	■ Airborne precautions should also be implemented. ■ Susceptible health care workers shouldn't enter the room if immune staff members are available.
Human metapneumovirus	■ Duration of illness	■ Wear masks according to standard precautions.
Impetigo	■ For 24 hours after initiation of effective therapy	
Monkeypox	■ Until lesions are crusted	■ Airborne precautions should also be implemented until monkeypox is confirmed and smallpox is ruled out.
Multidrug-resistant organism (MDRO) infection or colonization (such as with methicillin-resistant *Staphylococcus aureus,* vancomycin-resistant enterococcus, vancomycin intermediate-resistant *S. aureus,* vancomycin-resistant *S. aureus,* extended beta-lactamase producers, resistant *Streptococcus pneumonia,* and carbapenem-resistant *Enterobacteriaceae*)	■ Duration specified by your facility's infection control program, which is based on local, state, regional, and national recommendations	■ Following standard precautions only may be permitted in some areas.[4] ■ For guidance concerning new or emerging MDROs, consult your state or local health department.

(continued)

Conditions requiring contact precautions[1] *(continued)*

CONDITION	PRECAUTIONARY PERIOD	SPECIAL CONSIDERATIONS (IF APPLICABLE)
Mycobacterium tuberculosis, draining extrapulmonary lesion	■ Until patient improves clinically and drainage has stopped or until three consecutive drainage cultures test negative	■ Airborne precautions should also be implemented.[6] ■ Active pulmonary tuberculosis should be ruled out.
Norovirus gastroenteritis, diapered or incontinent patient	■ Duration of illness or a period following recovery while patient is still shedding the virus at high levels (usually 24 to 72 hours)[7]	■ Those who clean areas that are heavily contaminated with feces or vomitus should wear a mask. ■ Environmental cleaning and disinfection should be done consistently, with special attention given to restrooms and high-touch surfaces, such as door knobs and hand rails; a hypochlorite solution or an EPA-approved product effective against norovirus should be used.[7] ■ In some situations in health care facilities, isolation of exposed and potentially incubating patients may also be necessary.[7]
Parainfluenza virus infection, infant or young child	■ Duration of illness	■ Viral shedding may be prolonged in immunocompromised patients. ■ Antigen testing to determine when contact precautions can be discontinued may be unreliable.
Pediculosis (head lice infestation)	■ For 4 hours after the initiation of effective therapy	
Poliomyelitis	■ Duration of illness	
Pressure ulcer; major, draining	■ Duration of illness ■ Until drainage stops or wound drainage can be contained	
Respiratory syncytial virus infection; infant, young child, or immunocompromised adult	■ Duration of illness	■ Viral shedding may be prolonged in immunocompromised patients. ■ Antigen testing to determine when contact precautions can be discontinued may be unreliable. ■ Wear a mask according to standard precautions.
Ritter's disease (staphylococcal scaled skin syndrome)	■ Duration of illness	■ Health care workers may be a source of nursery or neonatal intensive care unit outbreaks.
Rotavirus gastroenteritis	■ Duration of illness	■ Environmental cleaning and disinfection should be done consistently. ■ Soiled diapers should be changed and disposed of frequently. ■ Viral shedding may be prolonged in children and the elderly.
Rubella, congenital syndrome	■ Until the child is 1 year old or until nasopharyngeal and urine cultures are repeatedly negative after age 3 months	
Salmonella species gastroenteritis, diapered or incontinent patient	■ Duration of illness or a duration that's appropriate to control a facility outbreak	
Scabies	■ For 24 hours following initiation of effective therapy	
Severe acute respiratory syndrome	■ Duration of illness plus 10 days after fever resolves (provided respiratory signs and symptoms have improved or resolved)	■ Airborne precautions should also be implemented.
Shigella species gastroenteritis, diapered or incontinent patient	■ Duration of illness or a duration that's appropriate to control a facility outbreak	

C

Conditions requiring contact precautions[1] *(continued)*

Condition	Precautionary period	Special considerations (if applicable)
Staphylococcus aureus enterocolitis, diapered or incontinent children	■ Duration of illness	
Staphylococcus aureus–infected draining major skin wound or burn	■ Duration of illness	
Streptococcus group A–infected draining major skin wound or burn	■ For 24 hours following initiation of effective therapy	■ Droplet precautions should also be initiated.
Vaccinia, eczema; fetal, generalized, or progressive	■ Until lesions are dry and crusted and scabs are separated	
Vaccinia blepharitis or conjunctivitis with copious drainage	■ Until drainage ceases	
Vibrio parahaemolyticus gastroenteritis, diapered or incontinent patient	■ Duration of illness or a duration that's appropriate to control a facility outbreak	
Yersinia enterocolitica gastroenteritis, diapered or incontinent patient	■ Duration of illness or a duration that's appropriate to control a facility outbreak	
Zoster (chickenpox, disseminated zoster, or localized zoster in an immunodeficient patient)	■ Until all lesions are crusted; requires airborne precautions	

[Online]. Accessed March 2015 via the Web at http://whqlibdoc.who.int/publications/2009/9789241597906_eng.pdf (Level IV)

13 Centers for Disease Control and Prevention. (2002). Guideline for hand hygiene in health-care settings: Recommendations of the Healthcare Infection Control Practices Advisory Committee and the HICPAC/SHEA/APIC/IDSA Hand Hygiene Task Force. *MMWR Recommendations and Reports, 51*(RR-16), 1–45. Accessed March 2015 via the Web at http://www.cdc.gov/mmwr/pdf/rr/rr5116.pdf (Level II)

14 American Osteopathic Association. (2014). Standard 07.01.21. *Healthcare Facilities Accreditation Program: Accreditation requirements for acute care hospital.* Chicago, IL: American Osteopathic Association. (Level VII)

15 Siegel, J. D., et al. (2006). "Management of multidrug-resistant organisms in healthcare settings, 2006" [Online]. Accessed March 2015 via the Web at http://www.cdc.gov/hicpac/pdf/MDRO/MDROGuideline2006.pdf (Level VII)

16 The Joint Commission. (2015). Standard NPSG.01.01.01. *Comprehensive accreditation manual for hospitals: The official handbook.* Oakbrook Terrace, IL: The Joint Commission. (Level VII)

17 American Osteopathic Association. (2014). Standard 07.01.02. *Healthcare Facilities Accreditation Program: Accreditation requirements for acute care hospitals.* Chicago, IL: American Osteopathic Association. (Level VII)

18 The Joint Commission. (2015). Standard RC.01.03.01. *Comprehensive accreditation manual for hospitals: The official handbook.* Oakbrook Terrace, IL: The Joint Commission. (Level VII)

19 Centers for Medicare & Medicaid Services, Department of Health and Human Services. (2014). Condition of participation: Medical record services. 42 C.F.R. § 482.24(b).

20 American Osteopathic Association. (2014). Standard 10.00.03. *Healthcare Facilities Accreditation Program: Accreditation requirements for acute care.* Chicago, IL: American Osteopathic Association. (Level VII)

21 Rutala, W. A., et al. (2008). "Guideline for disinfection and sterilization in healthcare facilities, 2008" [Online]. Accessed March 2015 via the Web at http://www.cdc.gov/hicpac/pdf/guidelines/Disinfection_Nov_2008.pdf (Level I)

22 The Joint Commission. (2015). Standard IC.02.02.02. *Comprehensive accreditation manual for hospitals: The official handbook.* Oakbrook Terrace, IL: The Joint Commission. (Level VII)

23 American Osteopathic Association. (2014). Standard 07.02.03. *Healthcare Facilities Accreditation Program: Accreditation requirements for acute care hospitals.* Chicago, IL: American Osteopathic Association. (Level VII)

Additional references

Almaguer-Leyva, M., et al. (2013). Hand hygiene compliance in patients under contact precautions and in general hospital population. *American Journal of Infection Control, 41,* 976–978. (Level VI)

Behta, M., et al. (2011). Documentation of contact precautions in an electronic record. *Journal of Nursing Care Quality, 26,* 252–259. (Level VI)

Centers for Disease Control and Prevention. (2013). "2012 CRE ToolKit—Guidance for control of carbapenem-resistant Enterobacteriaceae (CRE)" [Online]. Accessed March 2015 via the Web at http://www.cdc.gov/hai/organisms/cre/cre-toolkit/f-level-prevention.html (Level VII)

Jessee, M. A., & Mion, L. C. (2013). Is evidence guiding practice? Reported versus observed adherence to contact precautions: A pilot study. *American Journal of Infection Control, 41,* 965–970. (Level VI)

Mehrotra, P., et al. (2013). Effects of contact precautions on patient perception of care and satisfaction: A prospective cohort study. *Infection Control and Hospital Epidemiology, 34,* 1087–1093. (Level IV)

CONTINENT ILEOSTOMY CARE

An alternative to conventional ileostomy, a continent, or pouch, ileostomy (also called a *Koch ileostomy* or an *ileal pouch*) features an internal reservoir fashioned from the terminal ileum. This procedure may be used for a patient who requires proctocolectomy for chronic ulcerative colitis or multiple polyposis. Other patients may have a traditional ileostomy converted to a continent ileostomy. This procedure is contraindicated in Crohn disease or gross obesity. Patients who need emergency surgery and those who can't care for the pouch are also unlikely to have this procedure.

The length of preoperative hospitalization varies with the patient's condition. Nursing responsibilities include providing bowel preparation, antibiotic therapy, and emotional support. After surgery, nursing responsibilities include ensuring patency of the drainage catheter, assessing GI function, caring for the stoma and peristomal skin, managing pain resulting from surgery, and, if necessary, providing perineal skin care.

Patient teaching on pouch intubation and drainage usually begins soon after surgery. Continuous drainage is maintained for about 2 to 6 weeks to allow the suture lines to heal. During this period, a drainage catheter is attached to low intermittent suction. After the suture line heals, the patient learns how to drain the pouch himself.

Equipment

Leg drainage bag ▪ bedside drainage bag ▪ normal saline solution or water ▪ 50-mL catheter-tip syringe ▪ continent ileostomy catheter ▪ 4″ × 4″ × 1″ (10-cm × 10-cm × 2.5-cm) foam dressing and Montgomery straps ▪ precut drain dressing ▪ gloves ▪ water-soluble lubricant ▪ graduated container ▪ skin sealant ▪ preoperative checklist ▪ vital signs monitor ▪ blood glucose monitoring equipment ▪ pulse oximeter and probe ▪ Optional: IV insertion equipment, prescribed antibiotics, prescribed bowel preparation, disposable clippers, chlorhexidine, other prescribed medications, pneumatic compression system, end-tidal carbon dioxide monitor, facility-approved sedation scale, supplemental oxygen administration supplies, commercial catheter securement device.

Implementation

Preoperative care

- Verify the practitioner's orders regarding preoperative care.
- Review the patient's medical record for his medical and surgical history, a reconciled list of current medications, any allergies, and risk factors that increase the patient's risk of adverse reactions to medications, including age, altered liver and kidney function, a history of sleep apnea, weight (obese patients may be at increased risk of apnea; thin patients may be more sensitive to dose levels of medication), asthma, a history of smoking, drug-drug interactions, and first-time medication use.[1]
- Gather the appropriate supplies.
- Confirm that the practitioner has obtained written informed consent and that the consent is in the patient's medical record.[2,3,4]
- Perform a preprocedure verification *to make sure that all relevant documentation, related information, and equipment are available and correctly identified with the patient's identifiers.*[5,6]
- Verify that all laboratory and imaging studies are complete, as ordered, and that the results are in the patient's medical record. Notify the practitioner of any unexpected results.[5,6]
- Perform hand hygiene.[7,8,9,10,11]
- Confirm the patient's identity using at least two patient identifiers.[12]
- Obtain a health history, including previous surgery, skin condition, history of multiple drug–resistant organisms, external or implanted medical devices, sensory limitations, and home use of noninvasive positive-pressure ventilation or apnea monitors.[13]
- Obtain a pain and analgesic history; ask about measures that have been effective in relieving or controlling pain in the past. Also ask about expectations for controlling pain after surgery. *By obtaining a thorough pain history preoperatively, the health care team may be able to better control pain postoperatively.*[13]
- Perform educational, socioeconomic, cultural, and spiritual assessments *to determine the patient's level of understanding about the surgical procedure and whether he has special needs while in the facility.*[13,14]
- Assess for mobility limitations and disabilities, including mental and physical impairments, *which may require the use of additional equipment or supplies.* Assess and address the patient's safety needs, including the risk of falling, and implement fall-prevention interventions as needed.[13,14,15]
- Assess the patient's risk of postoperative nausea and vomiting (PONV) *so that the practitioner can consider PONV prophylaxis to decrease postoperative discomfort.* Consider the patient's history of PONV, the duration of surgery, and the type of surgery being performed in your assessment.[13]
- Assess the patient's cognitive, mental, and cardiopulmonary status; skin condition; functional and sensory limitations; and use of any hearing or visual aids and assistive or prosthetic devices.[14]
- Obtain other assessment data pertinent to the surgical procedure. (See the "Preoperative care" procedure, page 628.)[13]
- Reinforce and, if necessary, supplement the practitioner's explanation of a continent ileostomy and its implications for the patient.
- If a wound-ostomy-continence nurse (WOCN) is available at your facility, reinforce her preoperative teaching, which should include anatomy and physiology of the GI tract, the details of the procedure, demonstration of ostomy appliances, expected lifestyle changes, and measures to prepare psychologically for the procedure.[16] (See *Understanding pouch construction.*)
- Assess patient and family attitudes related to the operation and to the forthcoming changes in the patient's body image.[14]
- Provide encouragement and support.
- Make sure the stoma site is marked preoperatively *to reduce the incidence of complications and improve self-care.*[16,17]
- Teach the patient how to use a 0-to-10 pain scale to rate and report pain and discuss such analgesic tools and methods as patient-controlled analgesia.[18]
- Administer the prescribed bowel preparation, as ordered.
- Monitor and control the patient's blood glucose level, as ordered, *to reduce the risk of surgical site infection.*[19]
- Don't remove hair unless it will interfere with the surgical procedure. If hair removal is necessary, remove it before the patient enters the operating room by clipping; don't use a razor.[19]

Instruct the patient (assisting, as needed) to perform two preoperative baths or showers with chlorhexidine, as ordered, *to reduce the number of microorganisms on the skin, which reduces the risk of subsequent contamination of the surgical wound.*[20]

- If the patient was receiving a beta-adrenergic blocker before surgery, collaborate with the patient's practitioner *to make sure he receives it during the perioperative period, as appropriate.*[21]
- Administer venous thromboembolism (VTE) prophylaxis, as ordered.[15,21,22] Intermittent pneumatic compression is recommended for patients at low risk for VTE; for patients at moderate risk for VTE who aren't at risk for major bleeding complications, unfractionated heparin, low-molecular-weight heparin, or intermittent pneumatic compression is recommended; for patients at high risk for VTE who aren't at high risk for major bleeding complications, unfractionated heparin, low-molecular-weight heparin, and mechanical prophylaxis with elastic stockings or intermittent pneumatic compression is recommended.[23]
- Complete a surgical safety checklist to ensure compliance with best practices to improve surgical patient safety.[19]
- Make sure the patient has patent IV access; insert a new IV catheter, as ordered, if necessary. (See the "IV catheter insertion and removal, page 446".)
- Administer antibiotics, as ordered, following safe medication administration practices. The patient should receive prophylactic antibiotics

1 hour before surgical incision (2 hours are permitted for the administration of vancomycin and fluoroquinolones) *to reduce the risk of surgical site infection.*[1,21,24,25]

■ Maintain nothing-by-mouth status, as ordered. Minimum fasting recommendations include 2 hours for clear liquids, 6 or more hours for a light meal or nonhuman milk, and 8 hours or more for fried or fatty foods or meat.[26]

■ Maintain normothermia (95.9°F [35.5°C] or higher) during the perioperative period *because preoperative and intraoperative warming reduces the risk of surgical site infection and intraoperative blood loss.*[19]

■ Provide hand-off communication to the person who'll be assuming care of the patient during the procedure; allow time for questions.[27]

■ Perform hand hygiene.[7,8,9,10,11]

■ Document the procedure.[28,29,30]

Postoperative care

■ Receive hand-off communication from the person who was responsible for the patient's care; ask questions as necessary *to prevent patient care errors during transitions in care.*[27]

■ Verify the practitioner's orders regarding postoperative care.

■ Gather the appropriate equipment.

■ Perform hand hygiene.[7,8,9,10,11]

■ Put on gloves as needed for care.[31,32]

■ Confirm the patient's identity using at least two patient identifiers.[12]

■ Provide privacy.[33,34,35]

■ Explain the procedure to the patient.

■ Perform a comprehensive postoperative assessment. (See the "Postoperative care" procedure, page 624.)

Administer supplemental oxygen, as needed and prescribed. *Supplemental oxygen administration is recommended during and following surgical procedures involving mechanical ventilation to optimize tissue oxygenation and subsequently reduce the risk of surgical site infection.*[19]

■ Administer pain medication, as needed and ordered, following safe medication administration practices. If the medication is administered using an infusion device, verify proper programming of the device before administration. Advise the patient and his family to notify a staff member promptly of any changes that might be a reaction to the medication.[1] Reassess the patient's pain level after administration *to evaluate the effectiveness of therapy;* respond as necessary.[1,25]

NURSING ALERT *If the patient is receiving opioids to treat pain, keep in mind that these medications can cause oversedation and respiratory compromise. Failure to recognize and respond to progressive signs of respiratory compromise (somnolence, a decreased respiratory rate and oxygen saturation level) can lead to respiratory depression and death.*[1]

■ Monitor the patient's vital signs, oxygen saturation level by pulse oximetry, end-tidal carbon dioxide (if needed and available), respiratory status, and sedation level (using a facility-approved sedation scale) at a frequency determined by your facility and the patient's condition. Monitor the patient closely *to determine whether administered medications are achieving their therapeutically intended benefit and to promptly identify and respond to adverse effects of the medication.*

■ Notify the practitioner of changes in the patient's condition.[3]

■ Attach the drainage catheter emerging from the ileostomy to continuous gravity drainage or low intermittent suction, as ordered.

■ Trace all tubing from the patient to their point of origin *to make sure they're attached to the proper ports.*[1,36]

■ Encourage early ambulation *to prevent VTE.*[23] A leg drainage bag may be attached to the patient's thigh during ambulation. Continue other prescribed methods of VTE prophylaxis.[23]

■ Ensure discontinuation of prophylactic antibiotics within 24 hours of the end of surgery.[19,21,22]

■ Irrigate the ileostomy catheter with 30 mL of normal saline solution, as ordered and needed, *to prevent catheter obstruction and allow fluid return by gravity.* During the early postoperative period, keep the pouch empty; drainage will be serosanguineous.

■ Monitor the patient's intake and output and electrolyte levels (as ordered) *to assess for fluid and electrolyte imbalances.*[1]

■ If the patient required an indwelling urinary catheter for surgery and it wasn't removed in the postanesthesia care unit, remove it as soon as it's no longer needed *to reduce the risk of catheter-associated urinary tract infection.* Unless required by the patient's condition, you should remove the catheter by postoperative day 1 or 2. (The day of surgery is considered day 0.)[21]

■ Check the ileostomy catheter frequently after the patient begins eating solid food *to ensure that neither mucus nor undigested food particles block the catheter.*

■ If the patient complains of abdominal cramps, distention, and nausea—signs and symptoms of bowel obstruction—the ileostomy catheter may be clogged. Gently irrigate with 20 to 30 mL of water or normal saline solution until the ileostomy catheter drains freely. Then move the ileostomy catheter slightly or rotate it gently *to help clear the obstruction.* Finally, try milking the catheter. If these measures fail, notify the practitioner.

Understanding pouch construction

Depending on the patient and related factors during intestinal surgery, the practitioner may construct a pouch to collect fecal matter internally. To make such a pouch, the practitioner loops about 12″ (30.5 cm) of ileum and sutures the inner sides together.

He opens the loop with a U-shaped cut and seams the inside to create a smooth lining. Then he fashions a nipple or valve between what is becoming the pouch and what will be the stoma. He folds the open ileum over, sews the pouch closed, and fixes the pouch to the abdominal wall.

Because the pouch holds fecal matter in reserve, the patient benefits from not having to change and empty ostomy equipment. Instead, the patient empties and irrigates the pouch as needed by inserting a catheter though the stoma and into the pouch.

Initially after surgery, the nurse performs this procedure until the patient is able to do it.

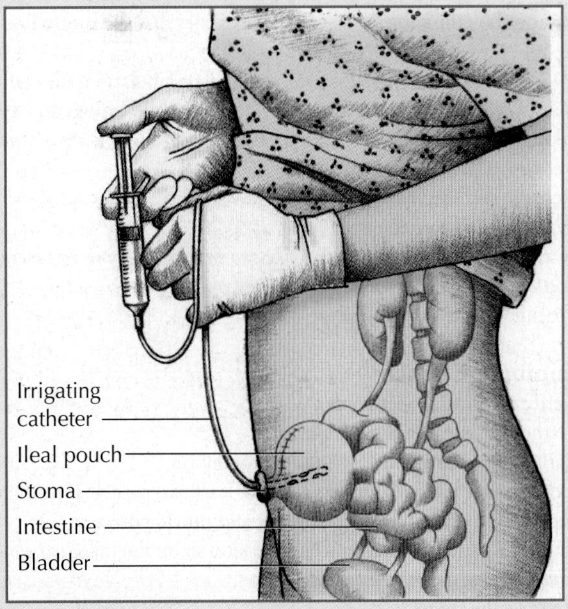

- Provide stoma and peristomal skin care.
- Remove the dressing, gently clean the peristomal area with water, and pat dry.
- Inspect the peristomal skin and stoma. Use a facility-approved assessment tool if available. Inspect the stoma frequently for color, edema, and bleeding. *Normally pink to red, a stoma that turns dark red or blue-red may have a compromised blood supply.* Observe for signs of mechanical, chemical, allergic, infectious, or disease-related complications *to objectively identify and track changes in peristomal skin.* Notify the practitioner or your facility's WOCN with problems, as needed.[37,38,39,40]
- Use a skin sealant around the stoma *to prevent skin irritation.*
- Apply a new stoma dressing. One technique involves slipping a precut drain dressing around the catheter *to cover the stoma.* Cut a hole slightly larger than the lumen of the catheter in the center of a 4″ × 4″ × 1″ (10-cm × 10-cm × 2.5-cm) piece of foam. Disconnect the catheter from the drainage bag and insert the distal end of the catheter through the hole in the foam. Slide the foam pad onto the dressing. Secure the foam in place with Montgomery straps. Secure the catheter by wrapping the strap ties around it or by using a commercial catheter securement device. Then reconnect the catheter to the drainage bag. (The drainage catheter will be removed by the surgeon when he determines that the suture line has healed.)
- *To reduce discomfort from gas pain,* encourage ambulation. Also tell the patient to chew food well, limit conversation while eating, and avoid drinking from a straw *to decrease the possibility of swallowing air, which can cause gas pain.*
- Remove and discard your gloves.[31,32]
- Perform hand hygiene.[7,8,9,10,11]
- If available, consult with a WOCN *to provide ongoing postoperative education.*[16]
- Document the procedure.[28,29,30]

Draining the pouch

- Verify the practitioner's order.
- Gather the appropriate equipment.
- Perform hand hygiene[7,8,9,10] and put on gloves.[31]
- Confirm the patient's identity using at least two patient identifiers.[12]
- Explain the procedure to the patient and provide privacy.
- Have the patient with a pouch conversion sit on the toilet *to help him feel more at ease during the procedure.*
- Remove the stoma dressing.
- Encourage the patient to relax his abdominal muscles *to allow the catheter to slide easily into the pouch.*
- Lubricate the drainage catheter tip with the water-soluble lubricant and insert it with a steady, gentle pressure and a slight twisting motion into the stoma. Gently push the catheter downward. (The direction of insertion may vary depending on the patient.)
- When the drainage catheter reaches the nipple valve of the internal pouch or reservoir (after about 2″ to 2½″ [5 cm to 6.5 cm]), you'll feel resistance. Instruct the patient to take a deep breath as you exert gentle pressure on the catheter to insert it through the valve. If this fails, have the patient lie in the supine position and rest for a few minutes. Then, with the patient still supine, try to insert the catheter again. You can also try using a smaller catheter.
- Gently advance the catheter to the suture marking made by the surgeon.
- Let the pouch drain completely, which usually takes 5 to 10 minutes. With thick drainage or a clogged catheter, the process may take 30 minutes.
- If the tube clogs, irrigate with 30 mL of water or normal saline using the 50-mL catheter-tip syringe. You can also rotate and milk the tube. If these steps fail, remove, rinse, and reinsert the catheter.
- Remove the catheter after completing drainage.
- Measure the output, subtracting the amount of irrigant used.
- Rinse the catheter thoroughly with warm water.
- Clean the peristomal area and apply a fresh stoma dressing.
- Remove and discard your gloves.[31]
- Perform hand hygiene.[7,8,9,10]
- Document the procedure.[28,29,30]

Special considerations

- Encourage the patient to refrain from smoking for 30 days before the procedure *to reduce the risk of surgical site infection.*[19,41,42,43]
- Never aspirate fluid from the catheter *because the resulting negative pressure may damage inflamed tissue.*
- The first few times you intubate the pouch, the patient may be tense, making insertion difficult. Encourage relaxation. *To shorten drainage time,* have the patient cough, press gently on his abdomen over the pouch, or suddenly tighten his abdominal muscles and then relax them.

Patient teaching

Make sure the patient can properly intubate and drain the pouch himself. Provide the patient with the appropriate equipment. If the postoperative drainage catheter is still in place, teach the patient how to care for it properly. Make sure the patient has a pouch-draining schedule, and give him appropriate pamphlets or video instructions on pouch care. Make sure he feels comfortable calling the practitioner, nurse, or WOCN to ask questions or discuss problems. Tell the patient where to obtain supplies. Refer the patient to a local ostomy group. Provide counseling on nutrition, clothing, medications, body image, psychological and social issues, interpersonal relationships, and possible complications.[16]

Complications

Common postoperative complications include obstruction, fistula, pouch perforation, nipple valve dysfunction, abscesses, diarrhea, skin irritation, stenosis of the stoma, and bacterial overgrowth in the pouch.

Documentation

Record the date, the time, and all aspects of preoperative and postoperative care. Include the condition of the stoma and peristomal skin, diet, medications, intubations, patient teaching, and discharge planning.

References

1 Centers for Medicare & Medicaid Services, Department of Health and Human Services. (2014). Condition of participation: Nursing services. 42 C.F.R. § 482.23(c).
2 The Joint Commission. (2015). Standard RI.01.03.01. *Comprehensive accreditation manual for hospitals: The official handbook.* Oakbrook Terrace, IL: The Joint Commission. (Level VII)
3 Centers for Medicare & Medicaid Services, Department of Health and Human Services. (2014). Condition of participation: Patient's rights. 42 C.F.R. § 482.13.
4 American Osteopathic Association. (2014). Standard 30.01.11. *Healthcare Facilities Accreditation Program: Accreditation requirements for acute care hospitals.* Chicago, IL: American Osteopathic Association. (Level VII)
5 The Joint Commission. (2015). Standard UP.01.01.01. *Comprehensive accreditation manual for hospitals: The official handbook.* Oakbrook Terrace, IL: The Joint Commission. (Level VII)
6 American Osteopathic Association. (2014). Standard 30.00.14. *Healthcare Facilities Accreditation Program: Accreditation requirements for acute care hospitals.* Chicago, IL: American Osteopathic Association. (Level VII)
7 The Joint Commission. (2015). Standard NPSG.07.01.01. *Comprehensive accreditation manual for hospitals: The official handbook.* Oakbrook Terrace, IL: The Joint Commission. (Level VII)
8 Centers for Disease Control and Prevention. (2002). Guideline for hand hygiene in health-care settings: Recommendations of the Healthcare

Infection Control Practices Advisory Committee and the HICPAC/SHEA/APIC/IDSA Hand Hygiene Task Force. *MMWR Recommendations and Reports, 51*(RR-16), 1–45. Accessed March 2015 via the Web at http://www.cdc.gov/mmwr/pdf/rr/rr5116.pdf (Level II)

9 World Health Organization. (2009). "WHO guidelines on hand hygiene in health care: First global patient safety challenge, clean care is safer care" [Online]. Accessed March 2015 via the Web at http://whqlibdoc.who.int/publications/2009/9789241597906_eng.pdf (Level IV)

10 Centers for Medicare & Medicaid Services, Department of Health and Human Services. (2014). Condition of participation: Infection control. 42 C.F.R. § 482.42.

11 American Osteopathic Association. (2014). Standard 07.01.21. *Healthcare Facilities Accreditation Program: Accreditation requirements for acute care hospitals.* Chicago, IL: American Osteopathic Association. (Level VII)

12 The Joint Commission. (2015). Standard NPSG.01.01.01. *Comprehensive accreditation manual for hospitals: The official handbook.* Oakbrook Terrace, IL: The Joint Commission. (Level VII)

13 American Society of PeriAnesthesia Nurses. (2012). *2012-2014 Perianesthesia nursing standards, practice recommendations and interpretive statements.* Cherry Hill, NJ: American Society of PeriAnesthesia Nurses. (Level VII)

14 The Joint Commission. (2010). *Advancing effective communication, cultural competence and patient- and family-centered care: A roadmap for hospitals.* Oakbrook Terrace, IL: The Joint Commission.

15 American Osteopathic Association. (2014). Standard 16.02.02. *Healthcare Facilities Accreditation Program: Accreditation requirements for acute care hospitals.* Chicago, IL: American Osteopathic Association. (Level VII)

16 Wound, Ostomy and Continence Nurses Society. (2010). *Management of the patient with a fecal ostomy: Best practice guideline for clinicians.* Mount Laurel, NJ: Wound, Ostomy and Continence Nurses Society. (Level VII)

17 The Joint Commission. (2015). Standard UP.01.02.01. *Comprehensive accreditation manual for hospitals: The official handbook.* Oakbrook Terrace, IL: The Joint Commission. (Level VII)

18 American Society of Anesthesiologists, Committee on Standards and Practice Parameters. (2012). Practice guidelines for acute pain management in the perioperative setting: An updated report by the American Society of Anesthesiologists Task Force on Acute Pain Management. *Anesthesiology, 116,* 248–273. Accessed March 2015 via the Web at http://journals.lww.com/anesthesiology/Fulltext/2012/02000/Practice_Guidelines_for_Acute_Pain_Management_in.11.asp (Level VII)

19 Anderson, D. J., et al. (2014). SHEA/IDSA practice recommendation: Strategies to prevent surgical site infections in acute care hospitals: 2014 update. *Infection Control and Hospital Epidemiology, 35,* 605–627. Accessed March 2015 via the Web at http://www.jstor.org/stable/10.1086/676022 (Level I)

20 Recommended practices for preoperative patient skin antisepsis. (2014). In R. Conner, et al. (Eds.), *Perioperative standards and recommended practices 2014.* Denver, CO: AORN, Inc. (Level VII)

21 Centers for Medicare & Medicaid Services and The Joint Commission. (2013). "The specifications manual for national hospital inpatient quality measures (version 4.3b)" [Online]. Accessed March 2015 via the Web at http://www.qualitynet.org/dcs/ContentServer?c=Page&pagename=QnetPublic%2FPage%2FQnetTier4&cid=1228773564870

22 Institute for Healthcare Improvement. (2012). *How-to guide: Prevent surgical site infections.* Cambridge, MA: Institute for Healthcare Improvement. (Level VII)

23 Guyatt, G. H., et al. (2012). Antithrombotic therapy and prevention of thrombosis: American College of Chest Physicians evidence-based clinical practice guidelines (9th ed.). *Chest, 141,* 2S–70S.

24 Bratzler, D. W., et al. (2013). American Society of Health-System Pharmacists report: Clinical practice guidelines for antimicrobial prophylaxis in surgery. *American Journal of Health System Pharmacists, 70,* 195–283.

25 American Osteopathic Association. (2014). Standard 16.01.03. *Healthcare Facilities Accreditation Program: Accreditation requirements for acute care hospitals.* Chicago, IL: American Osteopathic Association. (Level VII)

26 American Society of Anesthesiologists. (2011). Practice guidelines for preoperative fasting and the use of pharmacologic agents to reduce the risk of pulmonary aspiration: Application to healthy patients undergoing elective procedures. *Anesthesiology, 114,* 495–511. (Level V)

27 The Joint Commission. (2015). Standard PC.02.02.01. *Comprehensive accreditation manual for hospitals: The official handbook.* Oakbrook Terrace, IL: The Joint Commission. (Level VII)

28 The Joint Commission. (2015). Standard RC.01.03.01. *Comprehensive accreditation manual for hospitals: The official handbook.* Oakbrook Terrace, IL: The Joint Commission. (Level VII)

29 Centers for Medicare & Medicaid Services, Department of Health and Human Services. (2014). Condition of participation: Medical record services. 42 C.F.R. § 482.24(b).

30 American Osteopathic Association. (2014). Standard 10.00.03. *Healthcare Facilities Accreditation Program: Accreditation requirements for acute care hospitals.* Chicago, IL: American Osteopathic Association. (Level VII)

31 Siegel, J. D., et al. (2007). "2007 guideline for isolation precautions: Preventing transmission of infectious agents in healthcare settings" [Online]. Accessed March 2015 via the Web at http://www.cdc.gov/hicpac/pdf/isolation/Isolation2007.pdf (Level II)

32 American Osteopathic Association. (2014). Standard 07.01.10. *Healthcare Facilities Accreditation Program: Accreditation requirements for acute care hospitals.* Chicago, IL: American Osteopathic Association. (Level VII)

33 Centers for Medicare & Medicaid Services, Department of Health and Human Services. (2014). Condition of participation: Patient's rights. 42 C.F.R. § 482.13(c)(1).

34 The Joint Commission. (2015). Standard RI.01.01.01. *Comprehensive accreditation manual for hospitals: The official handbook.* Oakbrook Terrace, IL: The Joint Commission. (Level VII)

35 American Osteopathic Association. (2014). Standard 15.01.16. *Healthcare Facilities Accreditation Program: Accreditation requirements for acute care hospitals.* Chicago, IL: American Osteopathic Association. (Level VII)

36 U.S. Food and Drug Administration. (n.d.). "Look. Check. Connect. Safe medical device connections save lives" [Online]. Accessed March 2015 via the Web at http://www.fda.gov/downloads/MedicalDevices/Safety/AlertsandNotices/UCM134873.pdf

37 Haugen, H., & Ratliff, C. R. (2013). Tools for assessing peristomal skin complications. *Journal of Wound, Ostomy and Continence Nursing, 40,* 131–134.

38 Jemec, G. B., et al. (2011). Assessing peristomal skin changes in ostomy patients: Validation of the Ostomy Skin Tool. *British Journal of Dermatology, 164,* 330–335. (Level II)

39 Jordan, R., & Christian, M. (2013). Understanding periostomal skin complications. *Wound Care Advisory, 2*(2), 36–41. Accessed March 2015 via the Web at http://woundcareadvisor.com/wp-content/uploads/2013/05/Understanding_M-J13.pdf

40 Australian Association of Stomal Therapy Nurses, Inc. (2013). "Clinical guidelines for stomal therapy nursing practice" [Online]. Accessed March 2015 via the Web at http://www.stomaltherapy.com/documents/AASTN_Guidelines_book_2013.pdf (Level VII)

41 Hawn, M. T., et al. (2011). The attributable risk of smoking on surgical complications. *Annals of Surgery, 245,* 914–920.

42 Sharma, A., et al. (2013). Tobacco smoking and postoperative outcomes after colorectal surgery. *Annals of Surgery, 258,* 296–300.

43 Mangram, A. J., et al. (1999). Hospital Infection Control Practices Advisory Committee: Guideline for prevention of surgical site infection. *Infection Control and Hospital Epidemiology, 20,* 250–278. (Level V)

ADDITIONAL REFERENCE

Nettina, S. M. (2014). *Lippincott manual of nursing practice* (10th ed.). Philadelphia, PA: Wolters Kluwer.

How peritoneal dialysis works

Peritoneal dialysis works through a combination of diffusion and osmosis.

Diffusion

In diffusion, particles move through a semipermeable membrane from an area of high-solute concentration to an area of low-solute concentration. In peritoneal dialysis, the water-based dialysate being infused contains glucose, sodium chloride, calcium, magnesium, acetate or lactate, and no waste products. Therefore, the waste products and excess electrolytes in the blood cross through the semipermeable peritoneal membrane into the dialysate. Removing the waste-filled dialysate and replacing it with fresh solution keeps the waste concentration low and encourages further diffusion.

Osmosis

In osmosis, fluids move through a semipermeable membrane from an area of low-solute concentration to an area of high-solute concentration. In peritoneal dialysis, dextrose is added to the dialysate to give it a higher solute concentration than the blood, creating a high osmotic gradient. Water migrates from the blood through the peritoneal membrane at the beginning of each infusion, when the osmotic gradient is highest.

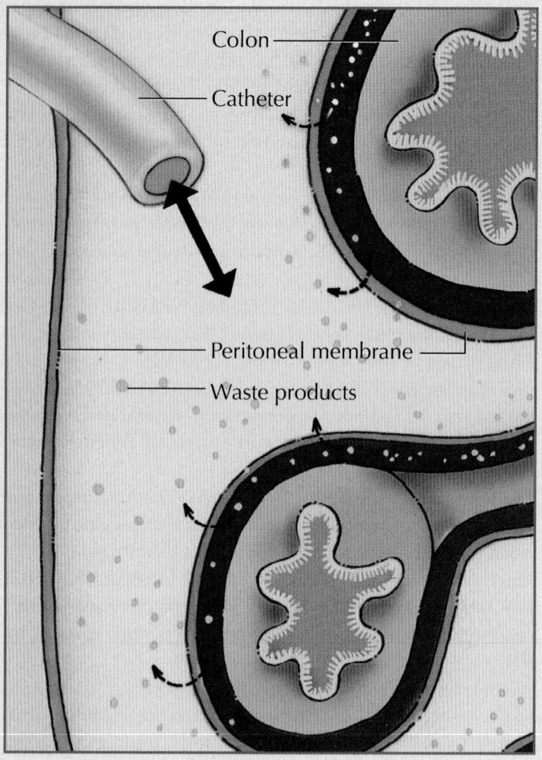

CONTINUOUS AMBULATORY PERITONEAL DIALYSIS

Continuous ambulatory peritoneal dialysis (CAPD) requires insertion of a permanent peritoneal catheter (such as a Tenckhoff catheter) to circulate dialysate continuously in the peritoneal cavity. Inserted under a local anesthetic, the catheter is sutured in place and its distal portion is tunneled subcutaneously to the skin surface. There it serves as a port for the dialysate solution, which flows in and out of the peritoneal cavity by gravity. (See *How peritoneal dialysis works.*)

CAPD is used most commonly for patients with stage 5 (end-stage) kidney disease who are looking for an alternative to hemodialysis. It can also be used in patients with vascular access issues, chronic heart failure, and ischemic heart disease.[1] This procedure can be a welcome alternative to hemodialysis because it gives the patient more independence, requires less travel for treatments, and results in more stable fluid and electrolyte levels than conventional hemodialysis.[2] Because the patient can resume normal daily activities between solution changes, CAPD helps promote independence and a return to a near-normal lifestyle. It also costs less than hemodialysis.

Conditions that may prohibit CAPD include recent abdominal surgery, abdominal adhesions, an infected abdominal wall, diaphragm tears, ileus, and respiratory insufficiency.

There are two methods of administering CAPD: the manual exchange method and the continuous-cycle method. This procedure covers the manual exchange method. Manual exchanges typically take about 30 minutes each and are required about four times a day. The continuous-cycle method is an automated system available for home use. (See *Continuous-cycle peritoneal dialysis.*) Patients or family members can learn to perform either method of CAPD administration with appropriate training.

Equipment

Scale ▪ vital sign monitoring equipment.

For dialysate draining, flushing, and infusing

Prescribed dialysate solution double-bag set (preattached dialysate solution bag, drainage collection bag, and CAPD administration set [Y-set]) ▪ heating pad or commercial warmer ▪ three face masks ▪ IV pole ▪ sterile 4″ × 4″ (10-cm × 10-cm) gauze pads ▪ sterile basin ▪ antiseptic solution ▪ sterile gloves ▪ sterile drapes ▪ fluid-impermeable pad ▪ Optional: transfer set change kit with patient connector, sterile caps or commercially prepared sterile caps with prefilled antiseptic, sterile swabs, specimen container or sterile culture tube with transport medium, prescribed medication, sterile syringes, antiseptic pads, graduated cylinder.

For catheter dressing changes

Sterile drapes ▪ sterile 4″ × 4″ (10-cm × 10-cm) gauze pads ▪ dressing ▪ two masks ▪ sterile basin ▪ hypoallergenic tape or catheter securement device ▪ antiseptic solution ▪ sterile gloves ▪ sterile cap ▪ Optional: commercially prepared sterile cap with prefilled antiseptic, prescribed antibiotic ointment.

All equipment used for CAPD must be kept sterile. Commercially prepared sterile CAPD kits are available.

NURSING ALERT *The most common serious complication associated with CAPD is peritonitis.* To prevent peritonitis, *the use of a double-bag exchange system is recommended. Also avoid manual spiking; if spiking is required, use a connect assist device.*[3,4]

Preparation of equipment

Warm the dialysate solution before instillation using a heating pad or manufacturer-supplied commercial warming device. The dialysate solution should feel warm to the touch on the inner wrist. *To measure the temperature of the solution,* fold the solution bag over an electronic thermometer probe. The temperature should measure no higher than 98.6°F (37°C). Avoid overheating. Invert the bag several times *for even heat distribution.*[5]

Implementation

- Review the patient's medical record for primary kidney disease and other comorbid conditions, response to previous peritoneal dialysis treatments, medication history, and pertinent laboratory test results.[6]
- Avoid distractions and interruptions when preparing and administering medication, including dialysate solution, *to prevent administration errors.*[7,8]
- Verify the practitioner's order for the prescribed dialysate solution, dwell times, and exchange frequency.[9,10,11]
- Gather the appropriate equipment.
- Compare the dialysate solution label with the order in the patient's medical record.[9,10,11]
- Check the patient's medical record for an allergy or contraindication to the prescribed dialysate solution or its additives. If an allergy or contraindication exists, don't administer the dialysate solution; instead, notify the practitioner.[9,10,11]
- Check the expiration date on the dialysate solution. If the dialysate solution has expired, return it to the pharmacy and obtain a new dialysate solution.[9,10,11]
- Inspect the dialysate solution visually for particles, discoloration, or other signs of loss of integrity; don't administer the dialysate solution if its integrity has been compromised.[9,10,11]
- Discuss any unresolved concerns about the dialysate solution with the patient's practitioner.
- Gather the appropriate equipment.
- Perform hand hygiene.[12,13,14,15,16]
- Confirm the patient's identity using at least two patient identifiers.[9,10,11,17]
- Explain the procedure to the patient.
- Provide privacy.[18,19,20]
- Obtain the patient's baseline vital signs.
- Weigh the patient *to establish a baseline weight.* Weigh him at the same time each day *to help monitor fluid balance.*
- Instruct the patient to void, if he's able.[21]

Draining the dialysate

- Perform hand hygiene.[12,13,14,15,16]
- Confirm the patient's identity using at least two patient identifiers.[17]
- For a patient with a newly implanted catheter, place him in the supine position.[6]
- Prepare the sterile field by placing a sterile drape on a dry surface near the patient. Take care to maintain the drape's sterility.
- Place a sterile basin on the sterile field. Place four sterile gauze pads in the sterile basin, and saturate them with the antiseptic solution. Place the remaining gauze pads on the sterile field.[22]
- Put on gloves and a mask, and provide a mask for the patient.[22,23]
- Hang the dialysate solution bag on an IV pole, and place the drainage collection bag on a fluid-impermeable pad on the floor.[24]
- Verify that a transfer set is attached to the catheter. If not, apply a transfer set using sterile technique, and verify that the clamp is closed. *A transfer set acts as an extension of the peritoneal catheter, preventing contamination and facilitating sterile connections and disconnections.*
- Carefully remove the dressing covering the peritoneal catheter and discard it.[22] Don't touch the catheter or the skin. Check the skin integrity at the catheter exit site, and assess for signs of infection, such as purulent drainage, redness, or edema. If drainage is present, obtain a specimen using a sterile swab, put it in a specimen container or a sterile culture tube with transport medium, label the specimen in the presence of the patient *to prevent mislabeling,*[17] and notify the practitioner.
- Palpate the catheter exit site and subcutaneous tunnel route for tenderness or pain. If these symptoms occur, notify the practitioner.

NURSING ALERT ***If the patient has drainage, tenderness, or pain, don't proceed with the infusion without specific orders.***

- Remove and discard your gloves.[22,23]
- Perform hand hygiene.[12,13,14,15,16]
- Put on sterile gloves.[25]
- Using one of the antiseptic-soaked gauze pads, scrub the transfer set-cap connection for 1 minute.[25] Discard the used gauze pad.
- Wrap another antiseptic-soaked gauze pad around the distal end of the transfer set-cap connection, and leave it in place for 3 to 5 minutes *to reduce the transmission of microorganisms.*[25] Alternatively, if a commercially prepared antiseptic cap is in place, remove it from the end of the transfer set.
- Trace the tubing from the double-bag Y-set to the transfer set *to make sure that you're connecting the tubing to the correct port.*[26] Attach the double-bag Y-set connector to the transfer set.[24,25] Secure the luer-lock connector tightly.
- Confirm that the clamp on the drain line of the double-bag Y-set is open and that the clamp on the fill line of the double-bag Y-set is closed.
- Open the transfer set clamp *to drain effluent.*[24]
- Remove and discard the patient's mask.
- Observe the outflow of the previous peritoneal dialysis cycle *to ensure that the fluid has drained completely before beginning another dialysate solution infusion.* Note the clarity, color, and odor of the outflow. *Cloudy effluent may indicate peritonitis.*[24,27]
- Monitor the patient's vital signs during outflow of the dialysate solution *to assess for signs of hypovolemia (hypotension and tachycardia)*; notify the practitioner if such signs occur.[25]
- After draining has been completed, clamp the drain line of the double-bag Y-set and close the transfer set clamp.[24]
- Weigh or measure the effluent as required.
- Discard used supplies in the appropriate receptacles.[22,23]
- Remove and discard your gloves and mask.[22,23]
- Perform hand hygiene.[12,13,14,15,16]

EQUIPMENT

Continuous-cycle peritoneal dialysis

Continuous-cycle peritoneal dialysis (CCPD), which is an automated continuous-cycle system, makes continuous ambulatory peritoneal dialysis easier for the patient. CCPD can be performed while the patient is awake or asleep. The system runs the dialysis treatment automatically until all the dialysate solution is infused. The system controls the cycles—draining the solution, refilling the solution, and monitoring the dwell time. In the morning, clean dialysate solution is left in the peritoneal cavity after the patient disconnects from the machine.[2] *Because the system remains closed throughout the treatment,* the risk of contamination is decreased. The system's alarms warn about general system, dialysate solution, and patient problems.

The cycler can be set to an intermittent or continuous dialysate schedule at home or in a health care facility. The patient typically initiates CCPD at bedtime and undergoes three to seven exchanges, depending on patient's treatment regimen.

The continuous cycler follows the same aseptic care and maintenance procedures as the manual method.

Flushing and infusing the dialysate

- After draining has been completed, perform hand hygiene.[12,13,14,15,16]
- Confirm the patient's identity using at least two patient identifiers.[17]
- Put on gloves.[22,23]
- Break the seal or frangible pin on the dialysate solution bag.[24]
- Open the clamp on the double-bag Y-set fill line, open the clamp on the Y-set drain line for 5 seconds *to flush fresh dialysate solution into the drainage collection bag,* and close the clamp on the drain line immediately after flushing *to avoid draining too much dialysate solution.*[24]
- Open the transfer set clamp *to allow dialysate solution to enter the peritoneal cavity.*[24] After the dialysate solution has filled the peritoneal cavity, clamp the fill line on the double-bag Y-set and close the clamp on the transfer set.[24]
- Monitor the patient's vital signs *for evidence of fluid overload.* Also assess the patient for decreased breath sounds, increased dyspnea, peripheral edema, and ascites. Notify the practitioner if these signs are present.
- Discard used supplies in the appropriate receptacles.[22,23]
- Remove and discard your gloves and mask.[22,23]

Changing the catheter dressing

- Perform hand hygiene.[12,13,14,15,16]
- Put on a mask, and provide one for the patient.[22,23]
- Set up a sterile field next to the patient by covering a clean, dry surface with a sterile drape. Maintain the drape's sterility. Place all equipment on the sterile field. Place 4″ × 4″ (10-cm × 10-cm) gauze pads in the basin, and saturate them with antiseptic solution.[25] Open the 4″ × 4″ (10-cm × 10-cm) gauze pads to be used as the dressing, and place them onto the sterile field.[25]
- Put on sterile gloves.[25]
- Disconnect the double-bag Y-set connector from the transfer set.[24]
- Use a sterile gauze pad to hold the transfer set off the patient's skin *to prevent contamination.*
- If required by your facility, disinfect the end of the transfer set. *Some facilities don't require disinfection of the catheter if a new sterile cap is attached to the transfer set.*[25]
- Pick up the new sterile cap, and attach it to the transfer set using sterile technique.[24,25]
- Using the antiseptic-soaked gauze pads, clean the catheter and exit site junction (following the antiseptic manufacturer's instructions) and then allow them to air-dry.[25]
- Apply an antibiotic ointment to the catheter exit site, if ordered.[21,28]
- Apply a new dressing to the catheter site.
- Secure the catheter and transfer set to the patient's abdomen using hypoallergenic tape or other securement device *to prevent accidental dislodgment.*[25,29]
- Instruct the patient that he may resume activities during the prescribed dialysate solution dwell time (usually 4 to 6 hours).
- Remove and discard the patient's mask.[22,23]
- Discard used supplies in the appropriate receptacles.[22,23]
- Remove and discard your gloves and mask.[22,23]
- Perform hand hygiene.[12,13,14,15,16]
- Document the procedure.[30,31,32]

Special considerations

- Medications, such as insulin or antibiotics, may be added to the dialysate solution. Follow the practitioner's order and safe medication administration practices when adding medication to the dialysate solution, if unable to have it prepared by the pharmacy.[10,33,34] *To ensure effective treatment,* confirm that the prescribed drug is compatible with the dialysate solution and its container.[35]
- If inflow and outflow are slow or absent, check the tubing for kinks. Raising the dialysate solution or repositioning the patient may increase the inflow rate. Applying manual pressure to the lateral aspects of the patient's abdomen may also help increase drainage.
- Repeat the procedure for the prescribed number of exchanges.
- Once-weekly sterile dressing changes are recommended until the patient's catheter exit site is healed (which may take up to 6 weeks). More frequent dressing changes may be needed if the dressing becomes soiled or if the patient experiences excessive sweating.[29]
- As clinically indicated and ordered, obtain a residual urine or effluent sample for analysis *to measure urea and creatinine clearance levels for monitoring the efficacy of dialysis.*[21,36]
- Some patient transfer sets are equipped with an adapter that allows the user to choose DRAIN or FILL when performing an exchange. Always follow the manufacturer's instructions for use.[24]

Patient teaching

Teach the patient and his family members how to use sterile technique throughout the procedure, especially for cleaning and dressing changes, *to prevent complications such as peritonitis.* Stress the importance of good hand-washing technique *to reduce the risk of infection.* Provide additional training to the patient and his family members, as needed, *because doing so helps reduce the risk of peritonitis.*[3]

Teach the patient and his family members the signs and symptoms of peritonitis—cloudy drainage, fever, and abdominal pain and tenderness—and stress the importance of notifying the practitioner immediately if such signs or symptoms occur.

Review with the patient and his family members catheter insertion site care, including cleaning, dressing changes, and application of antibiotic ointment as ordered.[21,28] Also tell them to call the practitioner if redness and drainage occur at the catheter insertion site *because these are signs of infection.*

Instruct the patient to record his weight and blood pressure daily and to check regularly for swelling of the extremities. Teach him to keep an accurate record of intake and output.

Complications

Peritonitis is the most frequent complication of CAPD. Although treatable, it can permanently scar the peritoneal membrane, decreasing its permeability and reducing the efficiency of dialysis. Untreated peritonitis can cause septicemia and death.

Excessive fluid loss may result from a concentrated (4.25%) dialysate solution, improper or inaccurate monitoring of inflow and outflow, or inadequate oral fluid intake. Excessive fluid retention may result from improper or inaccurate monitoring of inflow and outflow as well as from excessive salt or oral fluid intake.

Leaks, obstructions, and hernias may result from placement and location of the peritoneal catheter.[28]

Documentation

Record the type and amount of dialysate instilled and returned for each exchange, the time and duration of the exchange, and any medication added. Note the color, clarity, and odor of the returned exchange dialysate, and check it for mucus, pus, and blood. Document any discrepancy between fluid intake and output, as well as any signs of fluid imbalance, such as weight changes, decreased breath sounds, increased dyspnea, peripheral edema, ascites, and changes in skin turgor. Record the patient's weight, blood pressure, and pulse rate after his last fluid exchange for the day.

References

1 National Kidney Foundation. (2006). "Clinical practice guidelines for peritoneal dialysis adequacy, 2006 update" [Online]. Accessed March

2015 via the Web at http://www.kidney.org/sites/default/files/docs/12-50-0210_jag_dcp_guidelines-pd_oct06_sectionb_ofc.pdf (Level I)
2 American Association of Kidney Patients. (2014). "The facts about peritoneal dialysis" [Online]. Accessed March 2015 via the Web at https://www.aakp.org/education/resourcelibrary/dialysis-resources/item/the-facts-of-peritoneal-dialysis.html
3 Piraino, B., et al. (2011). ISPD position statement on reducing the risks of peritoneal dialysis-related infections. *Peritoneal Dialysis International, 31,* 614–630. (Level V)
4 Chaudhary, K., et al. (2010). Peritoneal dialysis first: Rationale. *Clinical Journal of the American Society of Nephrology, 6,* 447–456. Accessed March 2015 via the Web at http://cjasn.asnjournals.org/content/6/2/447.full
5 BC Renal. (2014). "Warming peritoneal dialysis solutions" [Online]. Accessed March 2015 via the Web at http://www.bcrenalagency.ca/sites/default/files/documents/files/Warming%20Peritoneal%20Dialysis%20Solutions.pdf
6 Gomez, N. J. (Ed.). (2011). *Nephrology nursing scope and standards of practice* (7th ed.). Pitman, NJ: American Nephrology Nurses' Association. (Level VII)
7 Westbrook, J., et al. (2010). Association of interruptions with an increased risk and severity of medication administration errors. *Archives of Internal Medicine, 170,* 683–690.
8 Institute for Safe Medication Practices. (2012). Side tracks on the safety express: Interruptions lead to errors and unfinished . . . Wait, what was I doing? *Nurse Advise-ERR, 11*(2), 1–4. Accessed March 2015 via the Web at https://www.ismp.org/Newsletters/acutecare/showarticle.aspx?id=37
9 American Osteopathic Association. (2014). Standard 16.01.03. *Healthcare Facilities Accreditation Program: Accreditation requirements for acute care hospitals.* Chicago, IL: American Osteopathic Association. (Level VII)
10 Centers for Medicare & Medicaid Services, Department of Health and Human Services. (2014). Condition of participation: Nursing services. 42 C.F.R. § 482.23(c).
11 The Joint Commission. (2015). Standard MM.06.01.01. *Comprehensive accreditation manual for hospitals: The official handbook.* Oakbrook Terrace, IL: The Joint Commission. (Level VII)
12 The Joint Commission. (2015). Standard NPSG.07.01.01. *Comprehensive accreditation manual for hospitals: The official handbook.* Oakbrook Terrace, IL: The Joint Commission. (Level VII)
13 Centers for Disease Control and Prevention. (2002). Guideline for hand hygiene in health-care settings: Recommendations of the Healthcare Infection Control Practices Advisory Committee and the HICPAC/SHEA/APIC/IDSA Hand Hygiene Task Force. *MMWR Recommendations and Reports, 51*(RR-16), 1–45. Accessed March 2015 via the Web at http://www.cdc.gov/mmwr/pdf/rr/rr5116.pdf (Level II)
14 World Health Organization. (2009). "WHO guidelines on hand hygiene in health care: First global patient safety challenge, clean care is safer care" [Online]. Accessed March 2015 via the Web at http://whqlibdoc.who.int/publications/2009/9789241597906_eng.pdf (Level IV)
15 American Osteopathic Association. (2014). Standard 07.01.21. *Healthcare Facilities Accreditation Program: Accreditation requirements for acute care hospitals.* Chicago, IL: American Osteopathic Association. (Level VII)
16 Centers for Medicare & Medicaid Services, Department of Health and Human Services. (2014). Condition of participation: Infection control. 42 C.F.R. § 482.42.
17 The Joint Commission. (2015). Standard NPSG.01.01.01. *Comprehensive accreditation manual for hospitals: The official handbook.* Oakbrook Terrace, IL: The Joint Commission. (Level VII)
18 The Joint Commission. (2015). Standard RI.01.01.01. *Comprehensive accreditation manual for hospitals: The official handbook.* Oakbrook Terrace, IL: The Joint Commission. (Level VII)
19 American Osteopathic Association. (2014). Standard 15.01.16. *Healthcare Facilities Accreditation Program: Accreditation requirements for acute care hospitals.* Chicago, IL: American Osteopathic Association. (Level VII)
20 Centers for Medicare & Medicaid Services, Department of Health and Human Services. (2014). Condition of participation: Patient's rights. 42 C.F.R. § 482.13(c)(1).
21 Woodrow, G., & Davies, S. (2010). *Clinical practice guidelines: Peritoneal dialysis, 2009-2012.* (5th ed.). Hampshire, UK: UK Renal Association [Online]. Accessed March 2015 via the Web at http://www.renal.org/docs/default-source/guidelines-resources/Peritoneal_Dialysis_FINAL_DRAFT_-_09_May_2010.pdf?sfvrsn=0 (Level VII)
22 Siegel, J. D., et al. (2007). "2007 guideline for isolation precautions: Preventing transmission of infectious agents in healthcare settings" [Online]. Accessed March 2015 via the Web at http://www.cdc.gov/hicpac/pdf/isolation/Isolation2007.pdf (Level II)
23 American Osteopathic Association. (2014). Standard 07.01.10. *Healthcare Facilities Accreditation Program: Accreditation requirements for acute care hospitals.* Chicago, IL: American Osteopathic Association. (Level VII)
24 Baxter P. D. (2007). "Ultrabag aseptic exchange procedure" [Online]. Accessed March 2015 via the Web at http://www.capd.org.tw/4_2/UltraBagusa.pdf
25 Lynn-McHale Wiegand, D. (Ed.). (2011). *AACN procedure manual for critical care* (6th ed.). St. Louis, MO: Saunders.
26 U.S. Food and Drug Administration. (n.d.). "Look. Check. Connect. Safe medical device connections save lives" [Online]. Accessed March 2015 via the Web at http://www.fda.gov/downloads/MedicalDevices/Safety/AlertsandNotices/UCM134873.pdf
27 Lemone, P., et al. (2011). *Medical-surgical nursing: Critical thinking in client care.* Upper Saddle River, NJ: Pearson.
28 Burkart, J. M. Patient information: Peritoneal dialysis (Beyond the basics.). (2014). In: *UpToDate,* Golper, T. A., & Sheridan, A. M. (Eds.). Accessed March 2015 via the Web at http://www.uptodate.com/contents/search
29 Warady, B., et al. (2012). Consensus guidelines for the prevention and treatment of catheter-related infections and peritonitis in pediatric patients receiving peritoneal dialysis: 2012 update. *Peritoneal Dialysis International, 32*(Suppl. 2), 32–86. Accessed March 2015 via the Web at http://www.ncbi.nlm.nih.gov/pmc/articles/PMC3524923/
30 The Joint Commission. (2015). Standard RC.01.03.01. *Comprehensive accreditation manual for hospitals: The official handbook.* Oakbrook Terrace, IL: The Joint Commission. (Level VII)
31 American Osteopathic Association. (2014). Standard 10.00.03. *Healthcare Facilities Accreditation Program: Accreditation requirements for acute care hospitals.* Chicago, IL: American Osteopathic Association. (Level VII)
32 Centers for Medicare & Medicaid Services, Department of Health and Human Services. (2014). Condition of participation: Medical record services. 42 C.F.R. § 482.24(b).
33 American Osteopathic Association. (2014). Standard 16.01.03. *Healthcare Facilities Accreditation Program: Accreditation requirements for acute care hospitals.* Chicago, IL: American Osteopathic Association. (Level VII)
34 The Joint Commission. (2015). Standard MM.06.01.01. *Comprehensive accreditation manual for hospitals: The official handbook.* Oakbrook Terrace, IL: The Joint Commission. (Level VII)
35 de Vin, F., et al. (2009). Intraperitoneal administration of drugs in peritoneal dialysis patients: A review of compatibility and guidance for clinical use. *Peritoneal Dialysis International, 29*(1), 5–15. Accessed March 2015 via the Web at http://www.pdiconnect.com/content/29/1/5.full
36 Burkart, J. M., & Henrich, W. L. Adequacy of peritoneal dialysis. (2014). In: *UpToDate,* Golper, T. A., & Sheridan, A. M. (Eds.). Accessed March 2015 via the web at http://www.uptodate.com/contents/search

ADDITIONAL REFERENCE

Nettina, S. M. (2014). *Lippincott manual of nursing practice* (10th ed.). Philadelphia, PA: Wolters Kluwer.

CONTINUOUS BLADDER IRRIGATION

Continuous bladder irrigation can help prevent urinary tract obstruction after prostate or bladder surgery by flushing out small blood clots.[1] It may also be used to treat an irritated, inflamed, or infected bladder lining.

Continuous bladder irrigation requires the placement of a triple-lumen indwelling urinary catheter. One lumen controls balloon inflation, a second lumen allows irrigant inflow, and a third allows irrigant

EQUIPMENT

Setup for continuous bladder irrigation

In continuous bladder irrigation, a triple-lumen indwelling urinary catheter is inserted through the patient's urethra and advanced to the bladder. The urinary catheter allows irrigation solution to flow into the bladder through one lumen and flow out through a second lumen, as shown in the inset. The third lumen is used to inflate the balloon that holds the urinary catheter in place in the patient's bladder.

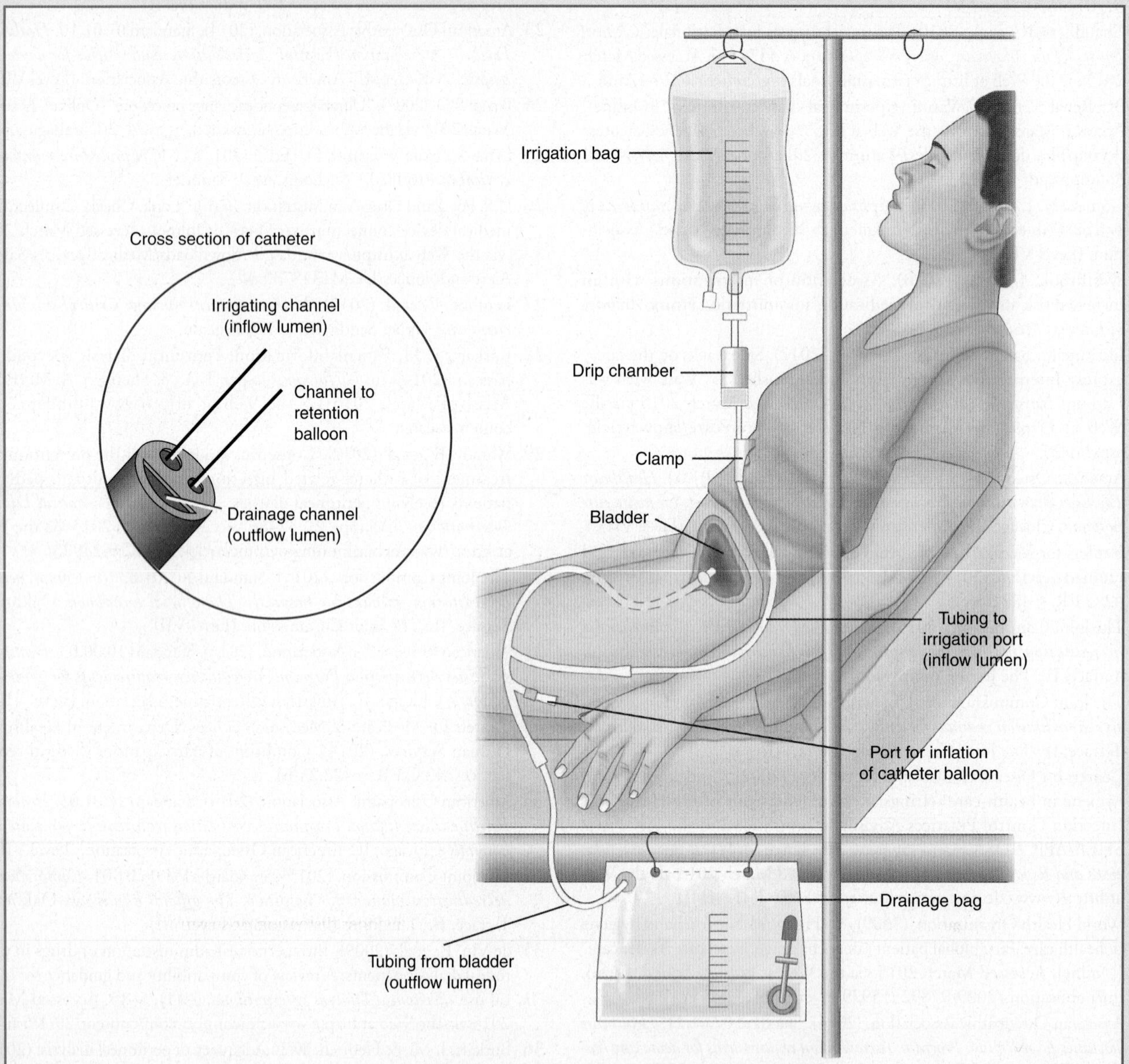

outflow. The continuous flow of irrigation solution through the bladder creates a mild tamponade that may help prevent venous hemorrhage. (See *Setup for continuous bladder irrigation.*) Although the catheter is inserted while the patient is in the operating room after prostate or bladder surgery, it may be inserted at the bedside if the patient's isn't undergoing surgery.

Unless specified otherwise, the patient should remain on bed rest throughout continuous bladder irrigation to avoid kinking, dislodging, or pulling on the catheter, which increase the risk of catheter-associated urinary tract infection (CAUTI). The urinary catheter should be removed as soon as it's no longer needed to reduce the risk of CAUTI.[1,2,3]

HOSPITAL-ACQUIRED CONDITION ALERT *The Centers for Medicare & Medicaid Services has identified CAUTI as a hospital-acquired condition* because it can be prevented reasonably using a variety of best practices. *Follow CAUTI prevention practices (including performing hand hygiene before and after urinary catheter manipulation; maintaining a sterile, continuously closed drainage system; maintaining an unobstructed urine flow; emptying the collection bag regularly; replacing the urinary catheter and collection system using sterile technique when disconnection, leakage, or breaks in sterile technique occur; and discontinuing the urinary catheter as soon as it's no longer clinically indicated) when caring for the patient with an indwelling urinary catheter* to reduce the risk of CAUTI.[2,4,5,6,7,8,9]

Equipment

Prescribed sterile irrigation solution ▪ sterile tubing for use with bladder irrigation system ▪ drainage bag and tubing ▪ gloves ▪ antiseptic pad ▪ IV pole ▪ vital signs monitoring equipment ▪ Optional: gown, goggles.[10]

Normal saline solution is usually prescribed for continuous bladder irrigation after prostate or bladder surgery. Large volumes of irrigating solution are usually required during the first 24 to 48 hours after prostate or bladder surgery *to prevent hemorrhage and blockage.* The irrigation solution may also contain an antibiotic.

Preparation of equipment

Ensure that the irrigation solution is at room temperature *to prevent bladder spasm.*

Implementation

- Avoid distractions and interruptions when preparing and administering the irrigation solution *to prevent administration errors.*[11,12]
- Verify the practitioner's order in the patient's medical record.[13,14,15]
- Gather the prescribed irrigation solution and supplies.
- Compare the label on the irrigation solution with the order in the patient's medical record.
- Check the patient's medical record for allergies or contraindications to the prescribed irrigation solution. If an allergy or a contraindication exists, don't administer the solution; instead, notify the practitioner.[13,14,15]
- Check the expiration date on the irrigation solution. If the solution has expired, obtain a new supply of the irrigation solution.[13,14,15]
- Inspect the irrigation solution visually for particles, discoloration, or other loss of integrity; don't administer the solution if its integrity has been compromised.[13,14,15]
- Perform hand hygiene.[16,17,18,19,20]
- Confirm the patient's identity using at least two patient identifiers.[21]
- Assemble all equipment at the patient's bedside.
- Provide privacy.[22,23,24]
- Explain the procedure to the patient *to allay any fears.*
- If the patient is receiving the irrigation solution for the first time, teach about potential adverse reactions and address any other concerns related to the solution.[13,14,15]
- Insert the spike of the tubing into the container of irrigating solution bag.
- Squeeze the drip chamber on the spike of the tubing.
- Open the flow clamp and prime the tubing *to remove air, which could cause bladder distention.* Then close the clamp.
- Hang the bag of irrigation solution on the IV pole.
- Perform hand hygiene.[16,17,18,19,20]
- Put on gloves and, if needed, a gown and goggles *to comply with standard precautions.*[1,10,25,26]
- Clean the opening to the inflow lumen of the urinary catheter with the antiseptic pad and allow it to dry.[2,4,10]
- Insert the distal end of the tubing securely into the inflow lumen of the urinary catheter. Trace the tubing from the patient to its point of origin *to make sure you've attached it to the proper port.*[27]
- Secure the urinary catheter properly *to prevent movement and urethral tension, which increase the risk of CAUTI.*[1,2,3,4]
- Ensure that the urinary catheter's outflow lumen is attached securely to the drainage bag tubing *to maintain a closed system, preventing disconnections that increase the risk of CAUTI.*
- Open the flow clamp under the bag of irrigation solution, and set the drip rate as ordered.
- *To prevent air from entering the system,* don't allow the irrigation solution bag to empty completely before replacing it.
- Keep the drainage bag below the level of the bladder at all times *to prevent backflow of urine into the bladder, which increases the risk of CAUTI.*[1,2,4] Don't place the drainage bag on the floor.[1,2,3]
- Maintain the urinary catheter and drainage bag tubing free from kinking.[2,3]
- Empty the drainage bag regularly, using a separate collection container for each patient.[1,2,3] Use sterile technique, avoid splashing, and prevent contact of the drainage spigot with the nonsterile collecting container *to avoid the risk of contamination.*[1,2,3,4]
- Measure the outflow volume accurately. It should equal or, allowing for urine production, exceed the inflow volume slightly. If the inflow volume exceeds the outflow volume postoperatively, suspect bladder rupture at the suture lines or renal damage, and notify the practitioner immediately.
- Assess the outflow drainage for changes in appearance and for blood clots, especially if continuous bladder irrigation is being performed postoperatively to control bleeding. If the drainage is bright red, the irrigation solution usually should be infused rapidly (with the flow clamp wide open) until the drainage clears. Notify the practitioner immediately if you suspect hemorrhage. If the drainage is clear, the solution is usually given at a rate of 40 to 60 drops/minute. The practitioner typically specifies the rate for irrigation solutions containing an antibiotic.
- Monitor vital signs as often as required by the patient's condition, increasing the frequency if the patient becomes unstable.
- Monitor urine output, assess the patient for abdominal pain, and palpate for bladder distention as indicated. Notify the practitioner of abnormal findings.
- Check the inflow and outflow tubing periodically for kinks *to make sure the solution is running freely, without obstruction, which reduces the risk of CAUTI.*[1,2,4]
- Remove and discard your gloves and any other personal protective equipment worn.[25,26]
- Perform hand hygiene.[16,17,18,19,20]
- Document the procedure.[28,29,30]

Special considerations

- Don't clean the periurethral area with an antiseptic pad; instead, clean the meatal surface during routine hygiene *to reduce the risk of CAUTI.*[1,2,3,5]
- Encourage oral fluid intake of 2 to 3 L/day unless contraindicated by another medical condition.

Complications

Interruptions in a continuous bladder irrigation system can predispose the patient to infection. Obstruction in the urinary catheter's outflow lumen can cause bladder distention or spasm.

Documentation

Each time a container of irrigation solution is emptied, record the date, time, and amount of fluid given on the intake and output record. Record the time and amount of fluid each time you empty the drainage bag. Note the appearance of the drainage and any complaints expressed by the patient. Note the patient's tolerance of the procedure.

REFERENCES

1 Centers for Disease Control and Prevention. (2009). "Guideline for the prevention of catheter-associated urinary tract infections" [Online]. Accessed March 2015 via the Web at http://www.cdc.gov/hicpac/pdf/CAUTI/CAUTIguideline2009final.pdf (Level I)

2 Lo, E., et al. (2014). SHEA/IDSA practice recommendation: Strategies to prevent catheter-associated urinary tract infections in acute care hospitals: 2014 update. *Infection Control and Hospital Epidemiology, 35,* 464–479. Accessed March 2015 via the Web at http://www.jstor.org/stable/pdfplus/10.1086/675718.pdf?acceptTC=true&jpdConfirm=true (Level I)

3 Association of Professionals in Infection Control and Epidemiology (APIC). (2014). "APIC Implementation Guide: Guide to preventing catheter-associated urinary tract infections" [Online]. Accessed March 2015 via the Web at http://apic.org/Resource_/EliminationGuideForm/6473ab9b-e75c-457a-8d0f-d57d32bc242b/File/APIC_CAUTI_web_0603.pdf (Level IV)

4 The Joint Commission. (2015). Standard NPSG.07.06.01. *Comprehensive accreditation manual for hospitals: The official handbook.* Oakbrook Terrace, IL: The Joint Commission. (Level VII)

5 Seckel, M. A. (2013). Maintaining urinary catheters: What does the evidence say? *Nursing, 43*(2), 63–65.

6 Society of Urologic Nurses and Associates. (2010). "Clinical practice guidelines: Prevention and control of catheter-associated urinary tract infection (CAUTI)" [Online]. Accessed March 2015 via the Web at http://www.suna.org/sites/default/files/download/cautiGuideline.pdf (Level VII)

7 Centers for Medicare & Medicaid Services, Department of Health and Human Services. (2014). "Hospital-acquired conditions" [Online]. Accessed March 2015 via the Web at http://www.cms.gov/Medicare/Medicare-Fee-for-Service-Payment/HospitalAcqCond/Hospital-Acquired_Conditions.html

8 Jarrett, N., et al. (2013). "Evidence-based guidelines for selected and previously considered hospital-acquired conditions: Final report" [Online]. Accessed March 2015 via the Web at http://www.cms.gov/Medicare/Medicare-Fee-for-Service-Payment/HospitalAcqCond/Downloads/Evidence-Based-Guidelines.pdf

9 American Osteopathic Association. (2014). Standard 07.01.17. *Healthcare Facilities Accreditation Program: Accreditation requirements for acute care hospitals.* Chicago, IL: American Osteopathic Association. (Level VII)

10 ACI Urology Network—Nursing. (2012). "Bladder irrigation: Guidelines" [Online]. Accessed March 2015 via the Web at http://www.aci.health.nsw.gov.au/__data/assets/pdf_file/0007/165589/Bladder-Irrigation-Toolkit.pdf (Level VII)

11 Westbrook, J., et al. (2010). Association of interruptions with an increased risk and severity of medication administration errors. *Archives of Internal Medicine, 170,* 683–690. (Level IV)

12 Institute for Safe Medication Practices. (2012). Side tracks on the safety express: Interruptions lead to errors and unfinished . . . Wait what was I doing? Nurse Advise-ERR, 11(2), 1–4.

13 The Joint Commission. (2015). Standard MM.06.01.01. *Comprehensive accreditation manual for hospitals: The official handbook.* Oakbrook Terrace, IL: The Joint Commission. (Level VII)

14 Centers for Medicare & Medicaid Services, Department of Health and Human Services. (2014). Condition of participation: Nursing services. 42 C.F.R. § 482.23(c).

15 American Osteopathic Association. (2014). Standard 16.01.03. *Healthcare Facilities Accreditation Program: Accreditation requirements for acute care hospitals.* Chicago, IL: American Osteopathic Association. (Level VII)

16 The Joint Commission. (2015). Standard NPSG.07.01.01. *Comprehensive accreditation manual for hospitals: The official handbook.* Oakbrook Terrace, IL: The Joint Commission. (Level VII)

17 Centers for Disease Control and Prevention. (2002). Guidelines for hand hygiene in health-care settings: Recommendations of the Healthcare Infection Control Practices Advisory Committee and the HICPAC/SHEA/APIC/IDSA Hand Hygiene Task Force. *MMWR Recommendations and Reports, 51*(RR-16), 1–45. Accessed March 2015 via the Web at http://www.cdc.gov/mmwr/pdf/rr/rr5116.pdf (Level II)

18 World Health Organization. (2009). "WHO guidelines on hand hygiene in health care: First global patient safety challenge, clean care is safer care" [Online]. Accessed March 2015 via the Web at http://whqlibdoc.who.int/publications/2009/9789241597906_eng.pdf (Level IV)

19 Centers for Medicare & Medicaid Services, Department of Health and Human Services. (2014). Condition of participation: Infection control. 42 C.F.R. § 482.42.

20 American Osteopathic Association. (2014). Standard 07.01.21. *Healthcare Facilities Accreditation Program: Accreditation requirements for acute care hospitals.* Chicago, IL: American Osteopathic Association. (Level VII)

21 The Joint Commission. (2015). Standard NPSG.01.01.01. *Comprehensive accreditation manual for hospitals: The official handbook.* Oakbrook Terrace, IL: The Joint Commission. (Level VII)

22 Centers for Medicare & Medicaid Services, Department of Health and Human Services. (2014). Condition of participation: Patient's rights. 42 C.F.R. § 482.13(c)(1).

23 The Joint Commission. (2015). Standard RI.01.01.01. *Comprehensive accreditation manual for hospitals: The official handbook.* Oakbrook Terrace, IL: The Joint Commission. (Level VII)

24 American Osteopathic Association. (2014). Standard 15.01.16. *Healthcare Facilities Accreditation Program: Accreditation requirements for acute care hospitals.* Chicago, IL: American Osteopathic Association. (Level VII)

25 Siegel, J. D., et al. (2007). "2007 guideline for isolation precautions: Preventing transmission of infectious agents in healthcare settings" [Online]. Accessed March 2015 via the Web at http://www.cdc.gov/hicpac/pdf/isolation/Isolation2007.pdf (Level II)

26 American Osteopathic Association. (2014). Standard 07.01.10. *Healthcare Facilities Accreditation Program: Accreditation requirements for acute care hospitals.* Chicago, IL: American Osteopathic Association. (Level VII)

27 U.S. Food and Drug Administration. (n.d.). "Look. Check. Connect. Safe medical device connections save lives" [Online]. Accessed March 2015 via the Web at http://www.fda.gov/downloads/MedicalDevices/Safety/AlertsandNotices/UCM134873.pdf

28 The Joint Commission. (2015). Standard RC.01.03.01. *Comprehensive accreditation manual for hospitals: The official handbook.* Oakbrook Terrace, IL: The Joint Commission. (Level VII)

29 Centers for Medicare & Medicaid Services, Department of Health and Human Services. (2014). Condition of participation: Medical record services. 42 C.F.R. § 482.24(b).

30 American Osteopathic Association. (2014). Standard 10.00.03. *Healthcare Facilities Accreditation Program: Accreditation requirements for acute care hospitals.* Chicago, IL: American Osteopathic Association. (Level VII)

ADDITIONAL REFERENCE

Hinkle, J. L., & Cheever, K. H. (2014). *Brunner & Suddarth's textbook of medical-surgical nursing* (13th ed.). Philadelphia, PA: Wolters Kluwer.

CONTINUOUS PASSIVE MOTION DEVICE USE

A continuous passive motion (CPM) device is commonly used after joint surgery—particularly after total knee arthroplasty. The device increases range of motion in the joint as the flexion and extension settings are adjusted during therapy. It minimizes the negative effects of immobility because of increased circulation from the passive movement of the limb. The device also stimulates healing within the articular cartilage and reduces adhesions and swelling.

The practitioner determines the amount of flexion and extension of the joint and the cycle rate (the number of revolutions per minute) as well as the length of time it should be used.

Although the CPM device is usually used on the knee, it may be appropriate for other joints as well.

Equipment

CPM device ■ single-patient-use soft-goods kit ■ tape measure ■ goniometer ■ Optional: gloves, prescribed analgesic.

Implementation

- Verify the practitioner's order.
- Gather the appropriate equipment.
- Apply the soft-goods padding to the CPM device.
- Perform hygiene and follow standard precaustions.[1,2,3,4]
- Confirm the patient's identity using at least two patient identifiers.[5]
- Explain the procedure to the patient *to reduce anxiety and encourage compliance.*

- Perform a comprehensive pain assessment using techniques appropriate for the patient's age, condition, and ability to understand.[6]
- Administer a prescribed analgesic, if needed, following safe medication administration practices.[7] Allow time for the full effect of the analgesic to occur before starting the machine. Perform a follow-up pain assessment and notify the practitioner if pain isn't adequately controlled.[6]
- Provide privacy. Place the bed at a comfortable working height.
- Determine the distance between the patient's gluteal crease and the popliteal space using the measuring tape.
- Measure the length of the patient's lower leg from his knee to ¼″ (0.6 cm) beyond the bottom of his foot.
- Adjust the thigh length and footplate position on the CPM machine based on your measurements.
- Position the patient in the middle of the bed.
- Support the affected extremity, elevating it *to allow placement of the padded CPM device on the bed.* Gently lower the leg onto the device (as shown below).

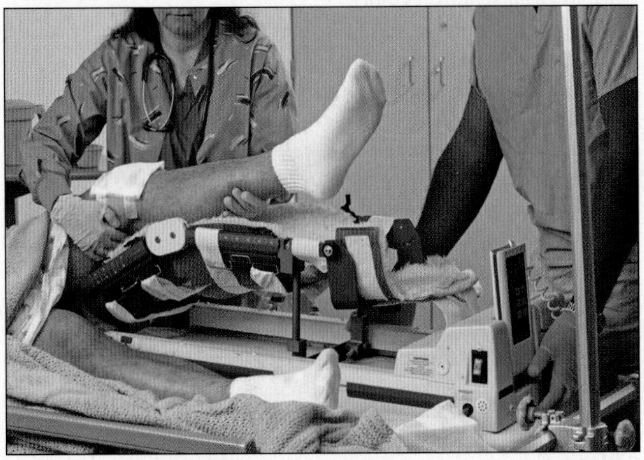

- Make sure the patient's knee is resting at the hinged joint of the CPM machine and that his leg is slightly abducted.
- Adjust the footplate to maintain a neutral position for the patient's foot (as shown below). Assess the patient's position to make sure the leg isn't internally or externally rotated *to prevent injury.*

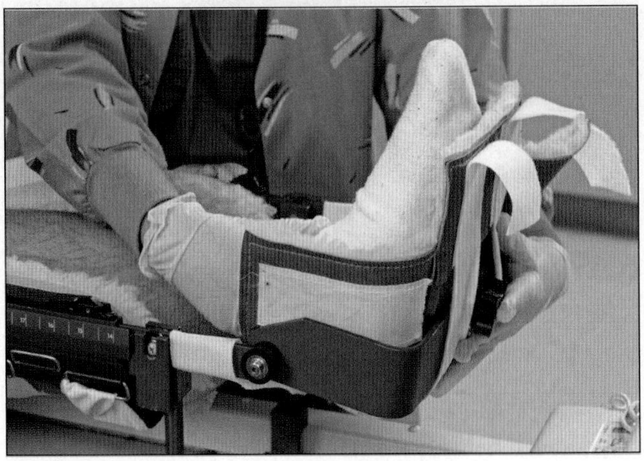

- Secure the restraining straps under the CPM device and around the patient's leg *to hold the leg in position.* Check that two fingers fit between the strap and the patient's leg (as shown on top right) *to prevent injury from excessive pressure from the strap.*

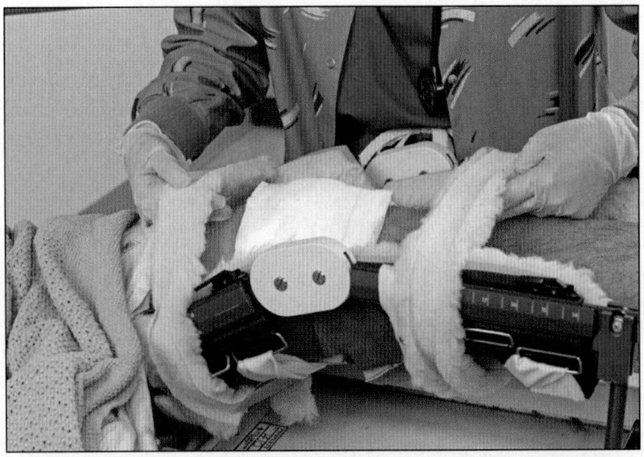

- Turn the unit on at the main power switch and set the controls to the level prescribed by the practitioner.
- Teach the patient how to use the STOP/GO button.
- Set the device to ON and start the therapy by pressing the GO button. Monitor the patient and the device through the first few cycles. Verify the angle of flexion when the device reaches its greatest height by measuring with a goniometer (as shown below) *to ensure the device is set to the prescribed parameters.*

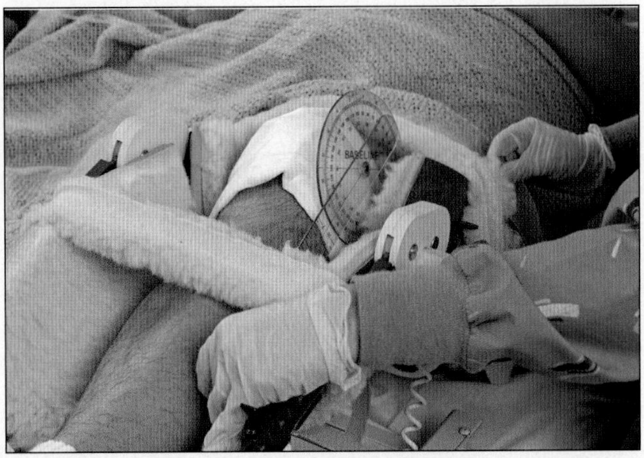

- Return the bed to the lowest position *for patient safety.* Make sure the call light and other necessary items are within easy reach of the patient.
- Check the patient's level of comfort frequently and perform skin and neurovascular assessments at least every 8 hours or more frequently for a patient with increased vascular risks.
- Remove and discard your gloves, if worn, and perform hand hygiene.[1,2,4]
- Document the procedure.[8]

Special considerations

- The use of the CPM device is in addition to physical therapy during the rehabilitation process.
- Encourage the patient to use the CPM device as prescribed *to promote healing and function of the joint.*

Patient teaching

Instruct the patient how to use the device and patient controls. Make the patient aware of setting changes and the goals of CPM therapy. Teach the patient to report signs and symptoms of neurovascular impairment, such as numbness or tingling, sudden pain, or coolness of the affected limb.

Documentation

Record settings and the patient's tolerance of the CPM device. Note the patient's skin and incision condition and your neurovascular assessment. Document your pain assessment, nursing actions taken, and outcomes. Also record any patient teaching provided and the patient's response to the teaching.

References

1 The Joint Commission. (2015). Standard NPSG.07.01.01. *Comprehensive accreditation manual for hospitals: The official handbook.* Oakbrook Terrace, IL: The Joint Commission. (Level VII)
2 Centers for Disease Control and Prevention. (2002). Guideline for hand hygiene in health-care settings: Recommendations of the Healthcare Infection Control Practices Advisory Committee and the HICPAC/SHEA/APIC/IDSA Hand Hygiene Task Force. *MMWR Recommendations and Reports, 51*(RR-16), 1–45. Accessed March 2015 via the Web at http://www.cdc.gov/mmwr/pdf/rr/rr5116.pdf (Level II)
3 Siegel, J. D., et al. (2007). "2007 guideline for isolation precautions: Preventing transmission of infectious agents in healthcare settings" [Online]. Accessed March 2015 via the Web at http://www.cdc.gov/hicpac/pdf/isolation/Isolation2007.pdf (Level II)
4 World Health Organization. (2009). "WHO guidelines on hand hygiene in health care: First global patient safety challenge, clean care is safer care" [Online]. Accessed March 2015 via the Web at http://whqlibdoc.who.int/publications/2009/9789241597906_eng.pdf (Level IV)
5 The Joint Commission. (2015). Standard NPSG.01.01.01. *Comprehensive accreditation manual for hospitals: The official handbook.* Oakbrook Terrace, IL: The Joint Commission. (Level VII)
6 The Joint Commission. (2015). Standard PC.01.02.07. *Comprehensive accreditation manual for hospitals: The official handbook.* Oakbrook Terrace, IL: The Joint Commission. (Level VII)
7 The Joint Commission. (2015). Standard MM.06.01.01. *Comprehensive accreditation manual for hospitals: The official handbook.* Oakbrook Terrace, IL: The Joint Commission. (Level VII)
8 The Joint Commission. (2015). Standard RC.01.03.01. *Comprehensive accreditation manual for hospitals: The official handbook.* Oakbrook Terrace, IL: The Joint Commission. (Level VII)

Continuous positive airway pressure use

Continuous positive airway pressure (CPAP) provides constant pressure into the airways to help hold the airway open, mobilize secretions, treat atelectasis and, generally, ease the work of breathing. It's also used to treat chronic obstructive sleep apnea. CPAP keeps the entire airway open, from the nares to the alveoli, increasing functional residual capacity and improving gas exchange.

Although intubated patients may also receive CPAP through a ventilator, the procedure discussed here focuses on nonintubated patients who receive CPAP through a high-flow generating system, which can be used in the health care facility or at home and can reduce or eliminate the need for intubation. Many patients are started on CPAP in the health care facility and then continue therapy at home.

Although CPAP has traditionally been administered through a face mask, other, more comfortable methods include nasal pillows and the nasal mask.

Because of increased thoracic pressure, CPAP is contraindicated in patients with increased intracranial pressure, hemodynamic instability, or recent facial, oral, or skull trauma. CPAP is also contraindicated in patients with untreated penumothorax.[1]

Equipment

Nasal mask, nasal pillows, or face mask (properly sized) ▪ permanent marker ▪ CPAP machine ▪ oxygen delivery tubing ▪ washcloth ▪ water ▪ facility-approved disinfectant ▪ Optional: oxygen source, pulse oximeter, gloves, mask, goggles, gown, mask with face shield, skin barrier.[2]

Preparation of equipment

In most facilities, a respiratory therapist assumes the responsibility for setting up and administering CPAP. If a respiratory therapist isn't available and you must set up a CPAP machine, follow the manufacturer's instructions. Position the CPAP machine so that the tubing easily reaches the patient, and plug in the machine. Don't plug the CPAP machine into an outlet with another plug in it, and don't use an extension cord to reach the outlet. Connect the oxygen delivery tubing to the air outlet valve on the CPAP unit, if ordered.

Implementation

- Verify the practitioner's order.
- Notify the respiratory therapist (if available in your facility) of the CPAP order.
- Gather and prepare the appropriate equipment.
- Perform hand hygiene[3,4,5,6,7] and put on personal protective equipment as needed *to comply with standard precaustions.*[8,9]
- Confirm the patient's identity using at least two patient identifiers.[10]
- Explain the procedure to the patient and answer any questions *to decrease anxiety and increase compliance.*
- Provide privacy.[11,12,13]
- Have the patient wash his face with a washcloth and water *to remove facial oils and help achieve a better fit.*
- Check the nasal mask, nasal pillows, or face mask *to make sure that the cushioning isn't hard or broken.* If it is, replace it.

Applying a nasal mask

- Place the nasal mask so that the longer straps are located at the top of the mask (as shown below).

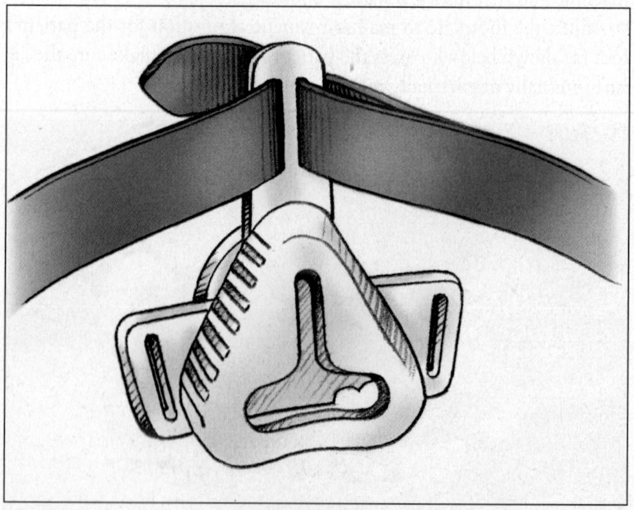

- Make sure that the Velcro is facing away from you, and thread the four tabs through the slots on the sides and top of the mask (as shown on next page, top left).

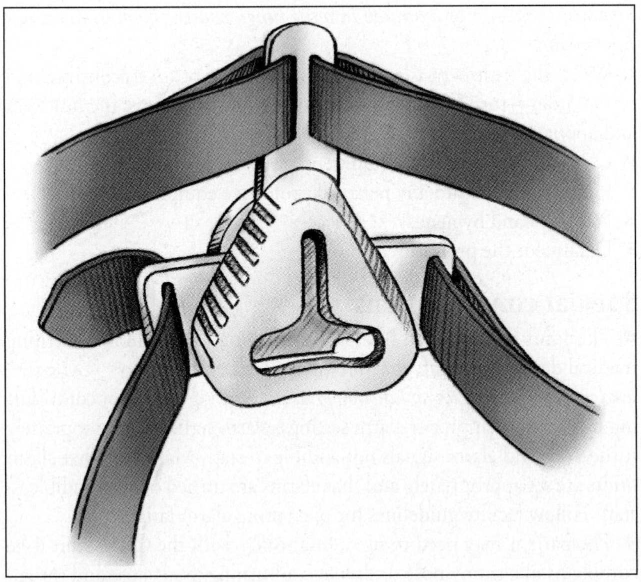

- Pull the straps through the slots and fasten them using the Velcro.
- Place the mask over the patient's nose and position the headgear over the patient's head.
- Gradually tighten all the straps on the mask until a seal is obtained. The mask doesn't have to be very tight to fit correctly—it just has to have a seal (as shown below).

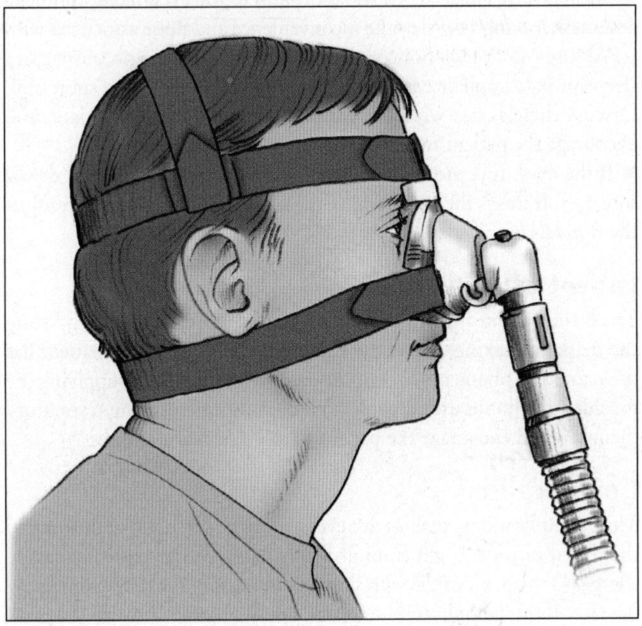

- Use the permanent marker to mark the straps with the final position *to eliminate having to fit the mask each time the patient wears it.*

Applying nasal pillows

- Insert the nasal pillows into the shell, making sure they fit correctly and that there's no air leaking around them (as shown on top right).

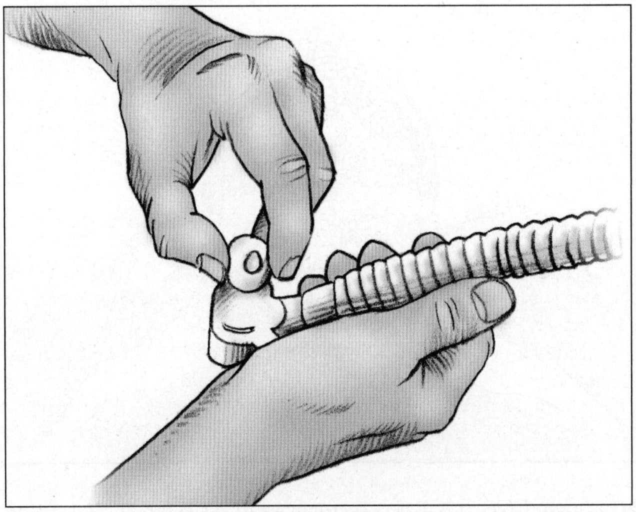

- Place the headgear around the patient's head and use the Velcro straps *to achieve the proper fit.* After the straps are in the correct place, remove the headgear without undoing the straps.
- Attach the nasal pillows to the headgear by wrapping the Velcro around the tubing, leaving room for rotation (as shown below).

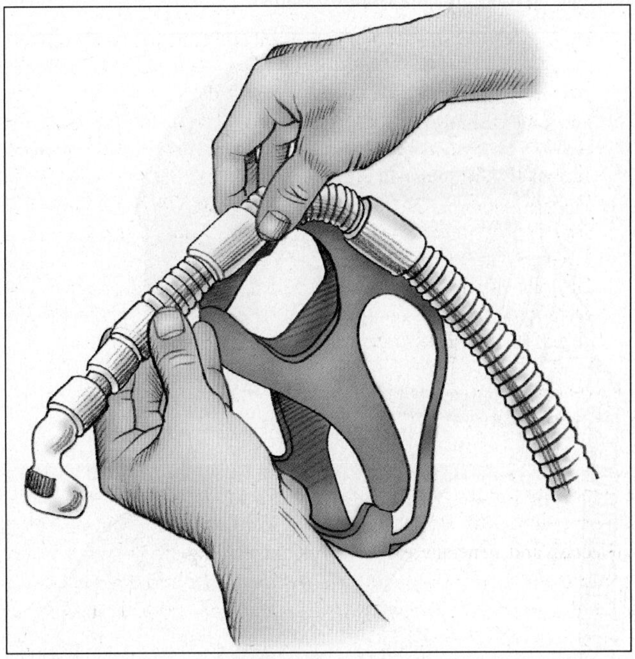

- Place the completely assembled headgear back on the patient and position the nasal pillows comfortably.
- Attach the shell strap across the shell and adjust the tension of the strap until there's a seal in both nostrils (as shown on next page, top left).

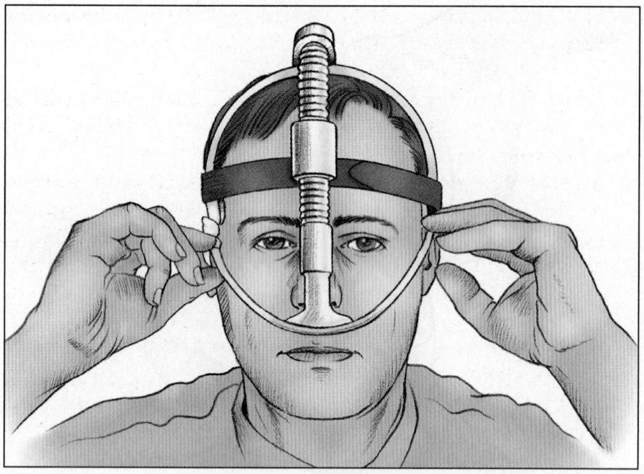

■ Be careful not to block the exhalation port on the backside of the shell.

Applying a face mask

■ Hold the mask against the patient's face and position the headgear over his head.

■ Using the Velcro straps, adjust the straps (as with the nasal mask) until there are no leaks present (as shown below).

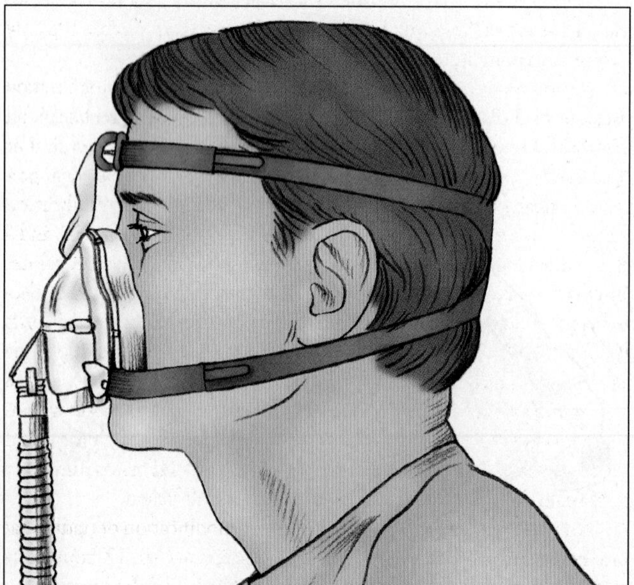

■ Connect the flexible tubing to the mask.

Administering CPAP

■ After the administration device is correctly fitted on the patient, turn on the pressure generator.

■ Turn on the CPAP unit before turning on the oxygen flow to the ordered level. Make sure the alarm limits are set appropriately for the patient's current condition and that the alarms are turned on, functioning properly, and audible to staff.[14,15,16]

■ If ordered, monitor the patient's pulse oximetry during the treatment.

■ As ordered and tolerated, provide a CPAP mask break every 4 hours. Check strap tension and skin integrity beneath and around the mask regularly *to prevent device-related skin breakdown.*[2]

■ Provide frequent oral care. (See the "Oral care" procedure, page 560.) *CPAP may cause dry mouth; the oropharynx may become colonized with organisms that can be aspirated into the lungs, causing hospital-associated pneumonia.*[17]

■ When the treatment is over—in the morning or on discontinuation of the order—turn off the pressure generator and remove the headgear and appliance from the patient.

■ Clean and disinfect the equipment and store it properly.[18,19]

■ Remove and discard any personal protective equipment[8,9] worn.

■ Perform hand hygiene.[3,4,5,6,7]

■ Document the procedure.[20,21,22]

Special considerations

■ The Joint Commission has issued a sentinel event alert concerning medical device alarm safety *because alarm-related events have been associated with permanent loss of function or death.* Among the major contributing factors were improper alarm settings, alarm settings inappropriately turned off, and alarm signals not audible to staff. Make sure that alarm limits are set appropriately and that alarms are turned on and audible to staff. Follow facility guidelines for preventing alarm fatigue.[14]

■ The patient may need to use a humidifier with the CPAP unit if he complains of a runny nose or dryness or burning in his nose and throat. Discuss this option with the practitioner and obtain an order for humidification.

■ Always make sure there's air coming out of the unit when the power is turned on.

■ *Because CPAP administered via a mask can cause nausea and vomiting,* it shouldn't be used in a patient who's unresponsive or at risk for aspiration.

■ Such adverse effects of CPAP as dryness of the eyes, nasal stuffiness, and mask leaking as well as the inconvenience and noise associated with CPAP use can lead to noncompliance.[23] For patients with obstructive sleep apnea, compliance is important for the treatment to be successful. Discuss these issues with the patient, intervene as appropriate, and encourage the patient to report persistent adverse effects.

■ If the mask isn't properly fitted, the patient may complain of dry or sore eyes. If this is the case, remove the mask and headgear and readjust them *to minimize leaks.*

Patient teaching

Teach the patient how to use the machine at home, including fitting the mask and taking care of the equipment. Make sure the patient has the name and phone number of the company that will be supplying the machine for home use. Provide a contact number for the respiratory therapist, and encourage the patient to call if he has questions.

Complications

Most complications, such as dry eyes, runny or dry nose, or burning in the throat or nose, result from ill-fitting masks. Some patients may be allergic to the mask or develop skin irritation from the mask contacting the face. If this complication happens, apply a barrier between the mask and the skin.

CPAP also potentially causes decreased cardiac output due to increased intrathoracic pressure. Other complications include nosebleeds, abdominal bloating, headaches, and nightmares.

Documentation

Document the CPAP settings, the length of time the patient was on CPAP, how the patient tolerated CPAP, and if there were any complications. Also record any patient teaching provided.

References

1 Wilkins, R. L., et al. (2012). *Egan's fundamentals of respiratory care* (10th ed.). St. Louis, MO: Mosby.

2 Walden, C., et al. (2013). "Getting in step: Partnering with respiratory therapy to reduce device related pressure ulcers" [Online]. Accessed March 2015 via the Web at http://www.serwocn.org/2013Conference/images/posters/2013%20Poster%2015%20-%20SE%20Regional%20WOCN%208-30-13.pdf
3 The Joint Commission. (2015). Standard NPSG.07.01.01. *Comprehensive accreditation manual for hospitals: The official handbook.* Oakbrook Terrace, IL: The Joint Commission. (Level VII)
4 Centers for Disease Control and Prevention. (2002). Guideline for hand hygiene in health-care settings: Recommendations of the Healthcare Infection Control Practices Advisory Committee and the HICPAC/SHEA/APIC/IDSA Hand Hygiene Task Force. *MMWR Recommendations and Reports, 51*(RR-16), 1–45. Accessed March 2015 via the Web at http://www.cdc.gov/mmwr/pdf/rr/rr5116.pdf (Level II)
5 World Health Organization. (2009). "WHO guidelines on hand hygiene in health care: First global patient safety challenge, clean care is safer care" [Online]. Accessed March 2015 via the Web at http://whqlibdoc.who.int/publications/2009/9789241597906_eng.pdf (Level IV)
6 Centers for Medicare & Medicaid Services, Department of Health and Human Services. (2014). Condition of participation: Infection control. 42 C.F.R. § 482.42.
7 American Osteopathic Association. (2014). Standard 07.01.21. *Healthcare Facilities Accreditation Program: Accreditation requirements for acute care hospitals.* Chicago, IL: American Osteopathic Association. (Level VII)
8 Siegel, J. D., et al. (2007). "2007 guideline for isolation precautions: Preventing transmission of infectious agents in healthcare settings" [Online]. Accessed March 2015 via the Web at http://www.cdc.gov/hicpac/pdf/isolation/Isolation2007.pdf (Level II)
9 American Osteopathic Association. (2014). Standard 07.01.10. *Healthcare Facilities Accreditation Program: Accreditation requirements for acute care hospitals.* Chicago, IL: American Osteopathic Association. (Level VII)
10 The Joint Commission. (2015). Standard NPSG.01.01.01. *Comprehensive accreditation manual for hospitals: The official handbook.* Oakbrook Terrace, IL: The Joint Commission. (Level VII)
11 Centers for Medicare & Medicaid Services, Department of Health and Human Services. (2014). Condition of participation: Patient's rights. 42 C.F.R. § 482.13(c)(1).
12 The Joint Commission. (2015). Standard RI.01.01.01. *Comprehensive accreditation manual for hospitals: The official handbook.* Oakbrook Terrace, IL: The Joint Commission. (Level VII)
13 American Osteopathic Association. (2014). Standard 15.01.16. *Healthcare Facilities Accreditation Program: Accreditation requirements for acute care hospitals.* Chicago, IL: American Osteopathic Association. (Level VII)
14 The Joint Commission. (2013). "Sentinel event alert: Medical device alarm safety in hospitals" [Online]. Accessed March 2015 via the Web at http://www.jointcommission.org/assets/1/18/SEA_50_alarms_4_5_13_FINAL1.PDF (Level VII)
15 The Joint Commission. (2015). Standard NPSG.06.01.01. *Comprehensive accreditation manual for hospitals: The official handbook.* Oakbrook Terrace, IL: The Joint Commission. (Level VII)
16 American Association of Critical-Care Nurses. (2013). "AACN practice alert: Alarm management" [Online]. Accessed March 2015 via the Web at http://www.aacn.org/wd/practice/docs/practicealerts/alarm-management-practice-alert.pdf (Level VII)
17 Centers for Disease Control and Prevention. (2004). Guidelines for preventing health-care-associated pneumonia, 2003: Recommendations of CDC and the Healthcare Infection Control Practices Advisory Committee. *MMWR Recommendations and Reports, 53*(RR-3), 1–32. Accessed March 2015 via the Web at http://www.cdc.gov/mmwr/pdf/rr/rr5303.pdf (Level II)
18 Rutala, W. A., et al. (2008). "Guideline for disinfection and sterilization in healthcare facilities, 2008" [Online]. Accessed March 2015 via the Web at http://www.cdc.gov/hicpac/pdf/guidelines/Disinfection_Nov_2008.pdf (Level I)
19 American Osteopathic Association. (2014). Standard 07.02.03. *Healthcare Facilities Accreditation Program: Accreditation requirements for acute care hospitals.* Chicago, IL: American Osteopathic Association. (Level VII)
20 The Joint Commission. (2015). Standard RC.01.03.01. *Comprehensive accreditation manual for hospitals: The official handbook.* Oakbrook Terrace, IL: The Joint Commission. (Level VII)
21 Centers for Medicare & Medicaid Services, Department of Health and Human Services. (2014). Condition of participation: Medical record services. 42 C.F.R. § 482.24(b).
22 American Osteopathic Association. (2014). Standard 10.00.03. *Healthcare Facilities Accreditation Program: Accreditation requirements for acute care hospitals.* Chicago, IL: American Osteopathic Association. (Level VII)
23 Weaver, T. Adherence with continuous positive airway pressure (CPAP). (2013). In: *UpToDate,* Basner, R. C., & Eichler, A. F. (Eds.). Accessed March 2015 via the Web at http://www.uptodate.com/contents/search

ADDITIONAL REFERENCE

Nettina, S. M. (2014). *Lippincott manual of nursing practice* (10th ed.). Philadelphia, PA: Wolters Kluwer.

CONTINUOUS RENAL REPLACEMENT THERAPY

Continuous renal replacement therapy (CRRT) is an extracorporeal purification therapy used to treat patients with acute kidney injury. Unlike the more traditional hemodialysis, CRRT is administered around the clock, providing patients with continuous therapy and sparing them the destabilizing hemodynamic and electrolytic changes characteristic of traditional hemodialysis. For patients who can't tolerate traditional hemodialysis—such as those who have hypotension—CRRT is often the only choice of treatment.

The techniques used vary in complexity. Slow continuous ultrafiltration uses arteriovenous access and the patient's blood pressure to circulate blood through a hemofilter. Because the goal of this therapy is the removal of fluids, the patient doesn't receive replacement fluids, which can help prevent or treat fluid overload.[1] Continuous venovenous hemofiltration (CVVH) uses a double-lumen catheter to provide access to a vein, and a pump moves blood through the hemofilter. This process removes solutes and fluids primarily by convection. Replacement fluids help maintain electrolyte and acid-base balance.[1] Continuous venovenous hemodialysis (CVVHD) uses a double-lumen catheter to provide access to a vein while a pump moves dialysate solution concurrently with blood flow. This process continuously removes fluid and solutes primarily by diffusion. Continuous venovenous hemodiafiltration (CVVHDF) combines the equipment and fluid and solute removal processes of CVVH and CVVHD to continuously remove fluids and solutes by both convection and diffusion.

Slow extended daily dialysis (SLEDD) is a modification of traditional intermittent hemodialysis. SLEDD usually occurs in 6- to 12-hour treatments, administered 5 to 7 days each week. The blood flow rates range from 100 to 250 mL/minute, resulting in an extended dialysis time, decreased solute rate, and ultrafiltration.

CVVH, CVVHD, CVVHDF, or SLEDD is used instead of continuous arteriovenous hemofiltration (CAVH) to treat critically ill patients. CVVH in particular has several advantages over CAVH: it doesn't require arterial access, it's appropriate for patients with low mean arterial pressures, and it has a better solute clearance.

Before the procedure, the practitioner inserts a double-lumen vascular access catheter; the internal jugular vein is the preferred insertion site. The practitioner should avoid the subclavian site in patients with advanced kidney disease to prevent subclavian stenosis and the femoral insertion site because of its association with an increased risk of infection.[2]

HOSPITAL-ACQUIRED CONDITION ALERT ***Keep in mind that a vascular catheter–associated infection is considered a hospital-acquired condition*** **because the use of various prevention techniques (such as performing hand hygiene, properly preparing the access site, and maintaining sterile technique) when accessing the patient's double-lumen catheter can reasonably prevent it.**[2,3,4,5,6]

Equipment

CRRT equipment (pump or other CCRT device, tubing with hemofilter) ■ preservative-free normal saline solution or other flush solution ■ prescribed dialysate solution ■ prescribed replacement solution ■ gloves ■ mask with face shield or mask and goggles ■ gown ■ antiseptic solution ■ sterile gauze pads ■ sterile syringes (10 mL) ■ sterile drape ■ sterile container ■ tape ■ infusion pump ■ cardiac monitor ■ blood pressure monitoring device ■ pulse oximeter and probe ■ scale ■ Optional: occlusive dressing for catheter insertion sites, supplies for blood sampling, prescribed medications, prescribed IV fluids, anticoagulant infusion, infusion pump (preferably a smart pump with dose-range alerts), anticoagulant antagonist, hemodynamic monitoring equipment, extra mask, extra blankets or warming blanket.

Preparation of equipment

Check the sterility of the hemofilter and blood tubing. Prime the CRRT circuit and set up the CRRT device or pump following the manufacturer's instructions. Make sure that the CRRT device is plugged into an outlet that has an emergency power source. Ensure that the equipment, including the blood pumps, pressure monitors, and air alert detector and pressure and safety alarms, is functioning properly. Make sure that the return osmosis water system has been tested and meets requirements.[7] (*See Setup for CVVH.*)

Implementation

■ Review and verify the practitioner's CRRT treatment orders, including modality, vascular access site and type, type of CRRT device and pump, type of hemofilter, blood pump speed, anticoagulant therapy (drug dose, infusion rate, associated laboratory tests, and anticoagulant monitoring parameters), replacement fluid (if necessary), hourly ultrafiltration rate, hourly net fluid goals, dialysate solution rate (if necessary), vital signs and hemodynamic parameter frequency, and laboratory results (including parameters for electrolyte repletion and critical values that require nephrologist notification).[7]

■ Review the patient's medical records for a completed medical history of the patient's health, current diseases, current therapy and medications, diagnostic tests, family and social history, and allergies.[7]

■ Confirm that the practitioner has obtained written informed consent and that the consent is in the patient's medical record.[8,9,10]

■ Verify that laboratory studies (electrolyte levels, coagulation studies, complete blood count, blood urea nitrogen, and creatinine studies) are complete, as ordered, and that the results are in the patient's medical record. Notify the practitioner of any unexpected results.

■ If the practitioner didn't insert the vascular access catheter using fluoroscopy, confirm that he verified vascular access catheter tip placement before use.[7]

■ Gather and prepare the necessary equipment.

■ If prescribed, compare the replacement fluid with the practitioner's order and make sure that the solution is sterile.[7]

■ Verify the dialysate and bicarbonate mixtures with the practitioner's order. Make sure that the solutions are clearly labeled with the date and time of expiration.[7] If the solutions are expired, return them to the pharmacy and obtain new solutions.[11,12,13]

■ Visually inspect the solutions for particles, discoloration, or other loss of integrity; don't administer the solutions if their integrity is compromised.[11,12,13]

■ Perform hand hygiene.[14,15,16,17,18]

■ Confirm the patient's identity using at least two patient identifiers.[19]

■ Explain the procedure to the patient.

■ Make sure that the patient is attached to a cardiac monitor, blood pressure monitoring device, and pulse oximeter *to closely monitor him for changes in his condition.* Make sure that the alarm limits are set appropriately for the patient's current condition and that the alarms are turned on, functioning properly, and audible to staff.[20,21,22]

■ Obtain vital signs *to serve as a baseline for comparison.*[7]

■ Assess the patient's cardiac, pulmonary, neuromuscular, GI, renal, hematologic, integumentary, immunologic, and psychosocial status.[7]

■ Assess the integrity of the vascular access catheter. Assess the insertion site for redness, swelling, discoloration, bruising, drainage, bleeding, and evidence of catheter migration.[7]

■ Obtain the patient's weight *to serve as a baseline for evaluating the effectiveness of therapy.*[7]

■ Notify the practitioner of any assessment findings that require an alteration in the patient's treatment plan.[7]

■ Position the patient *for comfort.*[7]

■ Put on gloves, a gown, and a mask and goggles or a face shield.[23,24] Have the patient put on a mask if possible.[7]

■ Make sure that the CRRT device is set up and functioning properly, and that the pressure monitors, air alert detector, and pressure safety alarms are set, turned on, functioning properly, and audible to staff.[7,20,22]

■ Prepare a sterile field. Place a sterile drape under the venous access catheter.

■ Thoroughly clean and disinfect the catheter hub with a facility-approved antiseptic (chlorhexidine or povidone-iodine) and allow it to dry. (Povidone-iodine must be dry for 2 minutes.)[27]

■ Attach a sterile 10-mL syringe to the arterial port and open the clamp. Withdraw the locking solution while minimizing the amount of blood withdrawn.[7] Close the clamp. Discard the waste syringe in the appropriate receptacle. Repeat this process for the venous port.[25]

■ Attach a 10-mL syringe containing preservative-free normal saline flush solution to the arterial port. Open the clamp and flush with 10 mL of normal saline flush *solution to assess catheter patency and integrity.*[7] Close the clamp and repeat this process for the venous port of the access catheter.

■ If catheter patency is compromised, assess for mechanical or thrombotic obstruction. If you suspect thrombotic obstruction, institute thrombolytic therapy as ordered or according to your facility's protocol.[7]

■ Using sterile technique, disconnect the cap from the arterial side of the primed tubing. Trace the tubing from the patient to the point of origin and then, using sterile technique, connect the arterial line to the hemofilter setup.[26] Repeat this process for the venous side and secure both connections.[7]

■ Keep the vascular access device and connections visible at all times *to promptly detect misconnections.*[7]

■ If your facility uses a bar code scanning system, scan your identification badge, the patient's identification bracelet, and the dialysate fluid's bar code, as indicated by your facility's bar code system.

NURSING ALERT *Dialysate is considered a high-alert medication* because it can cause significant harm when used in error.[27]

■ If required by your facility, have another nurse perform an independent double-check of the dialysate *to verify the patient's identity and to make sure that the correct dialysate is hanging in the prescribed concentration, the medication's indication corresponds with the patient's diagnosis, the dosage calculations are correct, the dosing formula used to derive the final dose is correct, the route of administration is safe and proper for the patient, the pump settings are correct, and the infusion lines are attached to the correct ports.*[28] Rectify any inconsistencies before beginning treatment.

■ Open the clamps on the arterial and venous tubing. Turn on the hemofilter and monitor the blood flow rate through the circuit. Start the flow rate at half the prescribed rate (or as directed by your facility), assess the patient's response, and then increase it to the prescribed rate.[7]

■ Remove the patient's mask if worn.

■ Administer an anticoagulant, as indicated and prescribed, following safe medication administration practices. Have another nurse perform an independent double-check if required by your facility. Tailor administration to the patient's response and the practitioner-ordered parameters.[7,11,12,13,29]

EQUIPMENT

Setup for CVVH

You'll typically perform continuous renal replacement therapy using continuous venovenous hemofiltration (CVVH). For this technique, the practitioner inserts a special catheter into a large vein, such as the internal jugular vein. He then attaches tubing with a hemofilter to the catheter and uses an external pump *to move blood through the system.* The patient's venous blood moves through the arterial lumen to the pump, which then pushes the blood through the catheter to the hemofilter. The hemofilter removes fluid and toxic solutes (ultrafiltrate) from the patient's blood and drains them into a collection device. It doesn't remove blood cells *because they are too large to pass through the filter.* As the blood exits the hemofilter, the pump then pushes it through the venous lumen back to the patient.

Several components of the pump provide safety mechanisms. Pressure monitors on the pump maintain the blood flow through the circuit at a constant rate. An air detector traps air bubbles before the blood returns to the patient. A venous filter collects any blood clots that may be in the blood. A blood-leak detector signals when blood is present in the dialysate. A venous clamp operates if it detects air in the circuit or if there is any disconnection in the blood line.

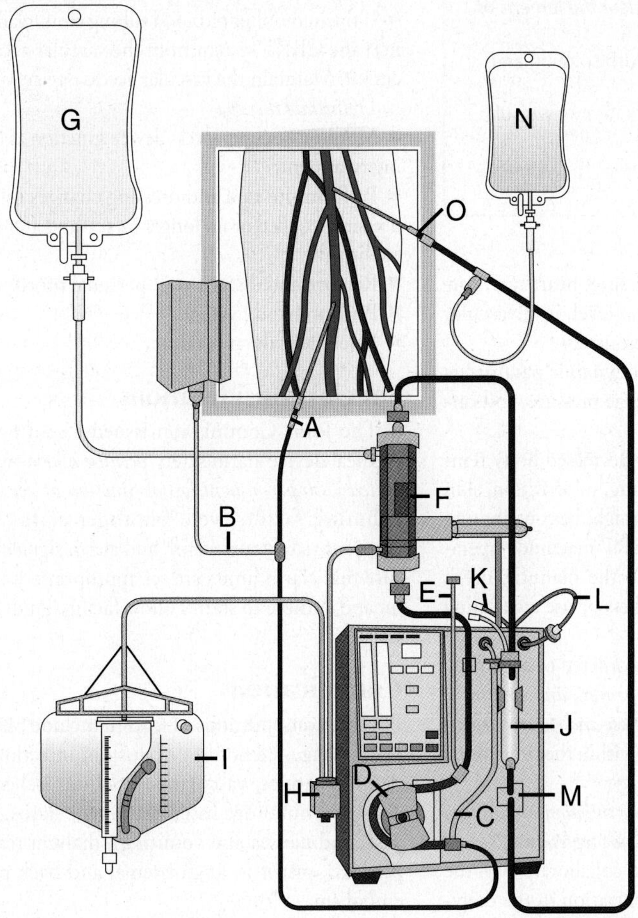

KEY:

A. Blood exiting the body
B. Heparin infusion
C. Arterial pressure monitor (prefilter pressure)
D. Blood pump
E. Saline infusion line (saline not shown here)
F. Filter
G. Dialysate
H. Blood leak detector
I. Graduated collection device
J. Air and foam detector
K. Syringe line
L. Venous pressure monitor (postfilter pressure)
M. Clamp
N. Replacement fluid
O. Blood returns to body

- Begin administering the dialysate at the prescribed rate, and start the ultrafiltration process, as indicated by the type of machine used.[7]
- Secure the hemofilter and all line connections using appropriate securement devices; keep the connections visible *to detect dangerous disconnections promptly.*[7]
- Closely monitor the patient's response to the initiation of therapy; changes in heart rate and rhythm, blood pressure, and physical condition, such as dizziness or increased anxiety, may occur.[7] Watch for signs and symptoms of dialyzer or hemofilter reaction (hypotension, pruritus, back pain, angioedema, arrhythmia, and anaphylaxis).[7]
- Monitor and record the blood flow rate and ultrafiltration flow rate at least hourly. Record changes that occur as a result of the practitioner's order or the patient's response to treatment.[7]

Reacting in an emergency[7]

If a situation arises that requires emergency intervention, such as a circuit leak, hemofilter rupture, clotting, circuit disconnection, or dialyzer or hemofilter reaction, or if the patient's condition suddenly deteriorates, follow these steps:

- Stop the continuous renal replacement therapy (CRRT) machine's blood pump as well as the other pumps and CRRT infusions.
- Clamp and disconnect the blood lines; avoid returning the blood to the patient.
- Thoroughly disinfect the catheter hub using a disinfectant (2% chlorhexidine or povidone-iodine) and allow it to dry.
- Flush each lumen of the vascular access catheter with 10 mL of preservative-free normal saline solution *to clear the lumens of blood.*
- Lock each lumen with a facility-approved flush solution and then cap them using a sterile cap.
- Continue to monitor the patient's status and laboratory test results.
- Discard the CRRT system in the appropriate contaminated-waste container.

- Monitor the patient's temperature, blood pressure, heart rate, cardiac rhythm, respiratory status, oxygen saturation level, intravascular and extravascular fluid status, and level of consciousness.
- Assess central venous pressure and other hemodynamic parameters (pulmonary artery pressure, pulmonary artery wedge pressure, and cardiac output and index) if available.[7]
- If the patient exhibits signs and symptoms of decreased body temperature, such as hemodynamic instability, shivering, piloerection, skin pallor, coolness, or cyanosis, assess for factors that might be contributing to a decrease in core temperature. Adjust the CRRT machine's operational temperature as ordered and according to the manufacturer's instructions. Provide the patient with extra blankets or use a warming blanket if indicated.[7]
- Obtain blood samples for laboratory testing, as ordered or according to protocol, *to monitor blood glucose, blood urea nitrogen, and creatinine levels; coagulation and hematologic status; and acid-base and electrolyte balance.* Report critical test results to the practitioner within the time frame established by your facility *to prevent treatment delays.*[29,30]
- Adjust dialysate fluids, if used, *to correct electrolyte imbalances.* Administer intermittent electrolyte infusions, as ordered, *for repletion.*[7]
- If the patient's blood glucose levels are elevated, collaborate with the patient's practitioner to adjust the glucose concentration in the dialysate solution, modify the replacement fluid composition if possible and appropriate, or administer insulin, as prescribed, following safe medication administration practices.[7,11,12,13]
- Monitor the patient for signs and symptoms of dialysis disequilibrium syndrome (although rare with CRRT), such as headache, nausea, vomiting, hypertension, decreased sensorium, seizures, and coma.[7]
- Inspect the ultrafiltrate during the procedure. It should remain clear yellow with no gross blood. *Pink-tinged or bloody ultrafiltrate may signal a membrane leak in the hemofilter, which permits bacterial contamination and possible exsanguination.* If you observe this sign, stop the treatment. (See *Reacting in an emergency.*)[7] Prepare a new system to restart therapy, as indicated.
- Calculate the volume of required replacement fluid every hour, as ordered. Infuse the prescribed amount and type of replacement fluid through the infusion pump into the arterial side of the circuit *to achieve the planned fluid balance.*

NURSING ALERT *The practitioner prescribes the targeted net fluid loss.* To calculate the volume of replacement fluid to administer, *first determine the patient's total fluid loss in the previous hour. Add the total fluid amount in the collection device in the past hour to any other fluid losses (such as blood loss, emesis, or nasogastric drainage); the sum is the total fluid loss. From the total fluid loss, subtract the patient's fluid intake from the past hour; then subtract the net fluid loss prescribed by the practitioner.* This calculation will give you the volume of replacement fluid to infuse.

- Flush the CRRT circuit with the prescribed volume of normal saline solution at the prescribed interval and as needed *to maintain patency.* Be sure to include the flush solution in the patient's hourly fluid intake.[7]
- Assess the CRRT circuit and hemofilter for signs of altered patency, such as arterial and venous pressure changes, dark fibers in the hemofilter, changes in transmembrane pressure, separation of formed cells and serum in the tubing, or a decrease in hemofilter temperature. If you note such signs, prepare for a system change, as necessary.[7]
- If the hemofilter or blood tubing clots, clamp the blood lines, disconnect the CRRT system from the vascular access device, and discard the circuit. Maintain the vascular access device *to maintain patency until you can reinitiate therapy.*
- Monitor vascular access device function at least every 30 minutes during treatment.[7]
- Perform site care and dressing changes using sterile technique if the dressing is soiled or no longer intact[2] and at intervals determined by your facility.[2,3,4,5,6,7]
- Remove and discard your personal protective equipment.[23,24]
- Perform hand hygiene.[14,15,16,17,18]
- Document the procedure.[31,32,33]

Special considerations

- The Joint Commission issued a sentinel event alert concerning medical device alarm safety *because alarm-related events have been associated with permanent loss of function or death.* Among the major contributing factors were improper alarm settings, alarm settings inappropriately turned off, and alarm signals not audible to staff. Make sure that alarm limits are set appropriately and that alarms are turned on and audible to staff. Follow facility guidelines for preventing alarm fatigue.[20]

Complications

Possible complications of CRRT include bleeding from catheter sites, hemorrhage, hemofilter occlusion, infection, hypothermia, unstable hemodynamics, vascular access limb ischemia, thrombosis, dialysis disequilibrium (decreased neurologic status, seizure activity, hypertension, and nausea and vomiting), dialyzer reaction (hypotension, anaphylaxis, pruritus, angioedema, and back pain), hypoxemia, and air embolism.

Documentation

Record the time the treatment began and ended; fluid balance information; neurologic, respiratory, and hemodynamic assessment findings; vital signs; times of dressing changes; medications given; the patient's tolerance of the procedure; any complications noted; and nursing actions taken and the patient's response to those actions.

REFERENCES

1 Baxter. (2014). "Continuous renal replacement therapy" [Online]. Accessed March 2015 via the Web at http://www.baxter.com/healthcare_professionals/therapies/renal/acute_kidney_treatment/continuous_renal_replacement_therapy.html#crrt_treatments

2 Centers for Disease Control and Prevention. (2011). "Guidelines for the prevention of intravascular catheter-related infections" [Online]. Accessed March 2015 via the Web at http://www.cdc.gov/hicpac/pdf/guidelines/bsi-guidelines-2011.pdf (Level I)

3 American Osteopathic Association. (2014). Standard 07.01.19. *Healthcare Facilities Accreditation Program: Accreditation requirements for acute care hospitals.* Chicago, IL: American Osteopathic Association. (Level VII)
4 American Osteopathic Association. (2014). Standard 07.01.02. *Healthcare Facilities Accreditation Program: Accreditation requirements for acute care hospitals.* Chicago, IL: American Osteopathic Association. (Level VII)
5 Jarrett, N., et al. (2013). "Evidence-based guidelines for selected and previously considered hospital-acquired conditions: Final report" [Online]. Accessed March 2015 via the Web at http://www.cms.gov/Medicare/Medicare-Fee-for-Service-Payment/HospitalAcqCond/Downloads/Evidence-Based-Guidelines.pdf
6 The Joint Commission. (2015). Standard NPSG.07.04.01. *Comprehensive accreditation manual for hospitals: The official handbook.* Oakbrook Terrace, IL: The Joint Commission. (Level VII)
7 Gomez, N. (Ed.). (2011). *Nephrology nursing scope and standards of practice* (7th ed.). Pitman, NJ: American Nephrology Nurses' Association.
8 The Joint Commission. (2015). Standard RI.01.03.01. *Comprehensive accreditation manual for hospitals: The official handbook.* Oakbrook Terrace, IL: The Joint Commission. (Level VII)
9 Centers for Medicare and & Medicaid Services, Department of Health and Human Services. (2014). Condition of participation: Patient's rights. 42 C.F.R. § 482.13.
10 American Osteopathic Association. (2014). Standard 15.01.11. *Healthcare Facilities Accreditation Program: Accreditation requirements for acute care hospitals.* Chicago, IL: American Osteopathic Association. (Level VII)
11 The Joint Commission. (2015). Standard MM.06.01.01. *Comprehensive accreditation manual for hospitals: The official handbook.* Oakbrook Terrace, IL: The Joint Commission. (Level VII)
12 American Osteopathic Association. (2014). Standard 16.01.03. *Healthcare Facilities Accreditation Program: Accreditation requirements for acute care hospitals.* Chicago, IL: American Osteopathic Association. (Level VII)
13 Centers for Medicare & Medicaid Services, Department of Health and Human Services. (2014). Condition of participation: Nursing services. 42 C.F.R. § 482.23(c).
14 The Joint Commission. (2015). Standard NPSG.07.01.01. *Comprehensive accreditation manual for hospitals: The official handbook.* Oakbrook Terrace, IL: The Joint Commission. (Level VII)
15 Centers for Disease Control and Prevention. (2002). Guideline for hand hygiene in health-care settings: Recommendations of the Healthcare Infection Control Practices Advisory Committee and the HICPAC/SHEA/APIC/IDSA Hand Hygiene Task Force. *MMWR Recommendations and Reports, 51*(RR-16), 1–45. Accessed March 2015 via the Web at http://www.cdc.gov/mmwr/pdf/rr/rr5116.pdf (Level II)
16 World Health Organization. (2009). "WHO guidelines on hand hygiene in health care: First global patient safety challenge, clean care is safer care" [Online]. Accessed March 2015 via the Web at http://whqlibdoc.who.int/publications/2009/9789241597906_eng.pdf (Level IV)
17 Centers for Medicare & Medicaid Services, Department of Health and Human Services. (2014). Condition of participation: Infection control. 42 C.F.R. § 482.42.
18 American Osteopathic Association. (2014). Standard 07.01.21. *Healthcare Facilities Accreditation Program: Accreditation requirements for acute care hospitals.* Chicago, IL: American Osteopathic Association. (Level VII)
19 The Joint Commission. (2014). Standard NPSG.01.01.01. *Comprehensive accreditation manual for hospitals: The official handbook.* Oakbrook Terrace, IL: The Joint Commission. (Level VII)
20 The Joint Commission. (2013). "Sentinel event alert: Medical device alarm safety in hospitals" [Online]. Accessed March 2015 via the Web at http://www.jointcommission.org/assets/1/18/SEA_50_alarms_4_5_13_FINAL1.PDF (Level VII)
21 American Association of Critical-Care Nurses (AACN). (2013). "AACN practice alert: Alarm management" [Online]. Accessed March 2015 via the Web at http://www.aacn.org/wd/practice/docs/practicealerts/alarm-management-practice-alert.pdf (Level VII)
22 Graham, K. C., & Cvach, M. (2010). Monitor alarm fatigue: Standardizing use of physiological monitors and decreasing nuisance alarms. *American Journal of Critical Care, 19,* 28–37.
23 Siegel, J. D., et al. (2007). "2007 guideline for isolation precautions: Preventing transmission of infectious agents in healthcare settings" [Online]. Accessed March 2015 via the Web at http://www.cdc.gov/hicpac/pdf/isolation/Isolation2007.pdf (Level II)
24 American Osteopathic Association. (2014). Standard 07.01.10. *Healthcare Facilities Accreditation Program: Accreditation requirements for acute care hospitals.* Chicago, IL: American Osteopathic Association. (Level VII)
25 Occupational Safety and Health Administration. (n.d.). "Bloodborne pathogens, standard number 1910.1030" [Online]. Accessed March 2015 via the Web at http://www.osha.gov/pls/oshaweb/owadisp.show_document?p_table=standards&p_id=10051 (Level VII)
26 U.S. Food and Drug Administration. (n.d.). "Look. Check. Connect. Safe medical device connections save lives" [Online]. Accessed March 2015 via the Web at http://www.fda.gov/downloads/MedicalDevices/Safety/AlertsandNotices/UCM134873.pdf
27 Institute for Safe Medication Practices. (2014). "ISMP list of high-alert medications in acute care settings" [Online]. Accessed March 2015 via the Web at http://www.ismp.org/tools/highalertmedications.pdf (Level VII)
28 Institute for Safe Medication Practices. (2008). Conducting an independent double-check. *ISMP Medication Safety Alert! Nurse Advise-ERR, 6*(12), 1. Accessed March 2015 via the Web at http://www.ismp.org/newsletters/nursing/Issues/NurseAdviceERR200812.pdf (Level VII)
29 The Joint Commission. (2015). Standard NPSG.03.05.01. *Comprehensive accreditation manual for hospitals: The official handbook.* Oakbrook Terrace, IL: The Joint Commission. (Level VII)
30 The Joint Commission. (2015). Standard NPSG.02.03.01. *Comprehensive accreditation manual for hospitals: The official handbook.* Oakbrook Terrace, IL: The Joint Commission. (Level VII)
31 The Joint Commission. (2015). Standard RC.01.03.01. *Comprehensive accreditation manual for hospitals: The official handbook.* Oakbrook Terrace, IL: The Joint Commission. (Level VII)
32 American Osteopathic Association. (2014). Standard 10.00.03. *Healthcare Facilities Accreditation Program: Accreditation requirements for acute care hospitals.* Chicago, IL: American Osteopathic Association. (Level VII)
33 Centers for Medicare & Medicaid Services, Department of Health and Human Services. (2014). Condition of participation: Medical record services. 42 C.F.R. § 482.24(b).

CREDÉ MANEUVER

When lower motor neuron damage impairs the voiding reflex, the bladder may become flaccid or areflexic. Because the bladder fails to contract properly, urine collects inside it, causing distention and increasing the risk of infection. The Credé maneuver—application of manual pressure over the lower abdomen—promotes complete emptying of the bladder. After appropriate instruction, the patient can perform the maneuver himself, unless he can't reach his lower abdomen or lacks sufficient strength and dexterity.

Bladder expression using the Credé maneuver was historically used in an attempt to promote continence and ensure adequate bladder evacuation. This maneuver is no longer recommended for patients with a spinal cord injury because it raises pressure against a closed bladder outlet, increasing the risk of reflux, hernia, rectogenital prolapse, and hemorrhoids.[1] Because of the high pressure that may be created during this procedure, it's potentially hazardous for patients with neurogenic lower urinary tract dysfunction.[2]

Equipment

Gloves ▪ bedpan, urinal, or bedside commode ▪ Optional: ultrasound bladder scanner.

Implementation

- Gather the appropriate equipment.
- Perform hand hygiene.[3,4,5,6,7]
- Confirm the patient's identity using at least two patient identifiers.[8]
- Explain the procedure to the patient.

Performing the Credé maneuver

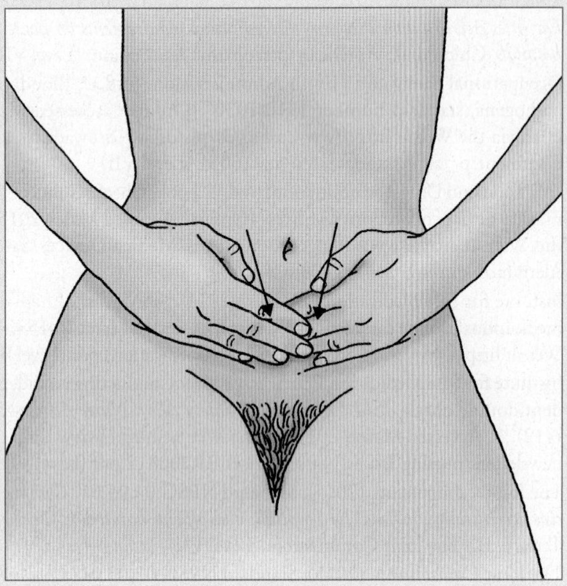

■ Put on gloves as needed *to comply with standard precautions.*[10,11]

■ If allowed and if the patient is on bedrest, place the patient in the Fowler position and place the bedpan or urinal. Alternatively, if the patient's condition permits, assist him onto the bedside commode. A male patient may benefit from standing, if possible.

■ Place your hands flat on the patient's abdomen just below the umbilicus. Ask the female patient to bend forward from the hips. Then firmly stroke downward toward the bladder about six times *to stimulate the voiding reflex.*

NURSING ALERT *Any method of assisted bladder emptying should be used very cautiously.*[2]

■ Place one hand on top of the other above the pubic arch. Press firmly inward and downward *to compress the bladder and expel residual urine.* (See *Performing the Credé maneuver.*)

■ Remove and discard your gloves, if worn,[10] and perform hand hygiene.[3,4,5,6,7]

■ Document the procedure.[12,13,14]

Special considerations

■ Some facilities require a practitioner's order for performance of the Credé maneuver. This procedure shouldn't be performed on patients with normal bladder tone or who experience bladder spasms.

■ An ultrasound bladder scanner, if available, may be used to document urine volume before and after the procedure.

■ After the patient has learned the procedure and can use it successfully, measuring the expelled urine may not be necessary. The patient may then use the maneuver to void directly into the toilet.

Patient teaching

Explain to the patient that the Credé maneuver is a simple exercise that can be done at home. Tell the patient that he can start a stream of urine from his bladder by performing this easy-to-do maneuver. Tell the male patient to void directly into the toilet from a standing position if possible. The female patient should sit on the toilet as she normally would.

Show the female patient how to lean forward, bending at the hips, *to increase pressure on the bladder.* Have the patient place one hand on top of the other in a return demonstration. Explain that the stroking movement compresses the bladder and expels urine.

Complications

Increasing pressures may raise the risk of reflux and associated complications, hernia, rectogenital prolapse, and hemorrhoids. In one study of spinal cord–injured patients who had been practicing the Credé maneuver to expel urine for more than 20 years, urologic complications included 93.2% of the population experiencing 100 mL or more of residual urine, 35.1% developing hydronephrosis, 31.3% experiencing urinary lithiasis, and 16.2% developing renal damage.[15]

Documentation

Record the date and time of the procedure, the amount and characteristics of urine expelled, and the patient's tolerance of the procedure. Document any patient teaching performed.

REFERENCES

1 Fonte, N. (2008). Urological care of the spinal cord–injured patient. *Journal of Wound, Ostomy and Continence Nursing, 35,* 323–331. (Level V)

2 Pannek, J., et al. (2011). "Guidelines on neurogenic lower urinary tract dysfunction" [Online]. Accessed March 2015 via the Web at http://www.uroweb.org/gls/pdf/17_Neurogenic%20LUTS.pdf (Level VII)

3 The Joint Commission. (2015). Standard NPSG.07.01.01. *Comprehensive accreditation manual for hospitals: The official handbook.* Oakbrook Terrace, IL: The Joint Commission. (Level VII)

4 Centers for Disease Control and Prevention. (2002). Guideline for hand hygiene in health-care settings: Recommendations of the Healthcare Infection Control Practices Advisory Committee and the HICPAC/SHEA/APIC/IDSA Hand Hygiene Task Force. *MMWR Recommendations and Reports, 51*(RR-16), 1–45. Accessed March 2015 via the Web at http://www.cdc.gov/mmwr/pdf/rr/rr5116.pdf (Level II)

5 World Health Organization. (2009). "WHO guidelines on hand hygiene in health care: First global patient safety challenge, clean care is safer care" [Online]. Accessed March 2015 via the Web at http://whqlibdoc.who.int/publications/2009/9789241597906_eng.pdf (Level IV)

6 Centers for Medicare & Medicaid Services, Department of Health and Human Services. (2014). Condition of participation: infection control. 42 C.F.R. § 482.42.

7 American Osteopathic Association. (2014). Standard 07.01.21. *Healthcare Facilities Accreditation Program: Accreditation requirements for acute care hospitals.* Chicago, IL: American Osteopathic Association. (Level VII)

8 The Joint Commission. (2015). Standard NPSG.01.01.01. *Comprehensive accreditation manual for hospitals: The official handbook.* Oakbrook Terrace, IL: The Joint Commission. (Level VII)

9 American Osteopathic Association. (2014). Standard 15.01.16. *Healthcare Facilities Accreditation Program: Accreditation requirements for acute care hospitals.* Chicago, IL: American Osteopathic Association. (Level VII)

10 Siegel, J. D., et al. (2007). "2007 guideline for isolation precautions: Preventing transmission of infectious agents in healthcare settings" [Online]. Accessed March 2015 via the Web at http://www.cdc.gov/hicpac/pdf/isolation/Isolation2007.pdf (Level II)

11 American Osteopathic Association. (2014). Standard 07.01.10. *Healthcare Facilities Accreditation Program: Accreditation requirements for acute care hospitals.* Chicago, IL: American Osteopathic Association. (Level VII)

12 The Joint Commission. (2015). Standard RC.01.03.01. *Comprehensive accreditation manual for hospitals: The official handbook.* Oakbrook Terrace, IL: The Joint Commission. (Level VII)

13 Centers for Medicare & Medicaid Services, Department of Health and Human Services. (2014). Condition of participation: Medical services record. 42 C.F.R. § 482.24(b).

14 American Osteopathic Association. (2014). Standard 10.00.03. *Healthcare Facilities Accreditation Program: Accreditation requirements for acute care hospitals.* Chicago, IL: American Osteopathic Association. (Level VII)

15 Chang, S. M., et al. (2000). Urologic status of 74 spinal cord injury patients from the 1976 Tangshan earthquake, and managed for 20 years using the Credé maneuver. *Spinal Cord, 38,* 552–554. (Level VI)

CRICOTHYROTOMY, ASSISTING

When endotracheal intubation or a tracheotomy can't be performed quickly and other nonsurgical methods have failed to establish an airway, an emergency cricothyrotomy may be necessary.[1] This rarely performed procedure involves puncturing the trachea through the cricothyroid membrane.

Usually, your role will be to assist the doctor or other specially trained practitioner responsible for airway management.[2] Ideally, cricothyrotomy is performed using sterile technique; however, sterile technique may not be possible in an emergency.

Equipment

For scalpel or needle cricothyrotomy

■ Sterile gloves ■ personal protective equipment (face mask, eye protection, gown) ■ antiseptic cleaning solution ■ sterile 4″ × 4″ (10-cm × 10-cm) gauze pads ■ sterile drape ■ sterile towels ■ tape ■ oxygen source ■ oxygen delivery equipment[3] ■ blood pressure cuff and manometer ■ pulse oximeter ■ end-tidal carbon dioxide detector ■ stethoscope ■ disinfectant pad ■ Optional: ultrasound equipment, 1% lidocaine, syringe, needle.[1]

For scalpel cricothyrotomy

Scalpel ■ #6 or smaller tracheostomy tube (if available) ■ Trousseau dilator[1] (if available) ■ tracheal hook[1] ■ handheld resuscitation bag or T tube and wide-bore oxygen tubing.

For needle cricothyrotomy

14G (or larger) through-the-needle or over-the-needle catheter ■ 10-mL syringe ■ tape ■ IV extension tubing ■ hand-operated release valve or pressure-regulating adjustment valve.

Preparation of equipment

Have one person stay with the patient while another collects the necessary equipment. Prepare a sterile field with the sterile drape. Pour antiseptic solution onto gauze pads. Open sterile packages and prepare the practitioner's supplies, as needed.

Implementation

■ Perform hand hygiene.[4,5,6,7,8]
■ Put on sterile gloves and personal protective equipment.[9,10]
■ Confirm the patient's identity using at least two patient identifiers.[11]
■ Place the patient in the supine position.
■ Hyperextend the patient's neck *to expose the area of the incision site. If there's a risk of cervical neck injury,* maintain the patient's neck in the neutral position.[1]
■ Administer oxygen by the most effective delivery route (blow by, nasal cannula, facemask, hand-held resuscitation bag, or T-tube).[3]
■ The practitioner cleans the patient's neck with antiseptic cleaning solution, following the manufacturer's instructions, and allows it to dry.
■ Assist with draping the patient's neck with sterile towels.
■ The practitioner locates the precise insertion site by sliding his thumb and fingers down to the thyroid gland. He'll know he's located its outer borders when the space between his fingers and thumb widens.
■ The practitioner assesses for hematomas, which may displace the trachea to the unaffected side.
■ The practitioner then moves his fingers across the center of the gland, over the anterior edge of the cricoid ring (as shown on top right).

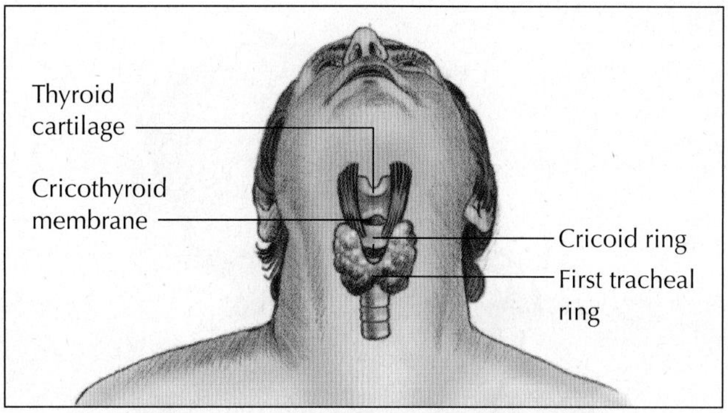

Using a scalpel

■ Hand the practitioner a scalpel so that he can make a horizontal incision, less than ½″ (1.3 cm) long, in the cricothyroid membrane just above the cricoid ring.
■ The practitioner inserts a Trousseau dilator *to prevent tissue from closing around the incision.* If a dilator isn't available, he inserts the handle of the scalpel and rotates it 90 degrees (as shown below).

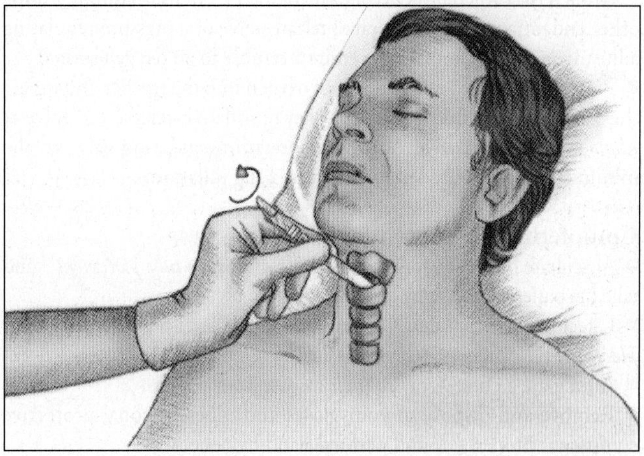

■ The practitioner inserts a tracheal hook into the opening, allowing for passage of an appropriately sized cuffed tracheostomy tube.[1] If a small tracheostomy tube (#6 or smaller) is available, he inserts it into the opening and secures it *to help maintain a patent airway.* If a tracheostomy tube isn't available, he may tape the dilator or scalpel handle in place until a tracheostomy tube is available.
■ If the patient can breathe spontaneously, attach a humidified oxygen source to the tracheostomy tube with a T tube; if he can't, attach a handheld resuscitation bag. You'll need to inflate the cuff of the tracheostomy tube with a syringe *to provide positive-pressure ventilation.*

Using a needle

■ Attach a 10-mL syringe to a 14G (or larger) through-the-needle or over-the-needle catheter. Hand the through-the-needle or over-the-needle catheter to the practitioner, who inserts it into the cricothyroid membrane just above the cricoid ring.
■ The practitioner directs the catheter downward at a 45-degree angle (as shown on next page, top left) to the trachea *to avoid damaging the vocal cords.* He maintains negative pressure by pulling back the syringe plunger as he advances the catheter. He'll know the catheter has entered the trachea when air enters the syringe.

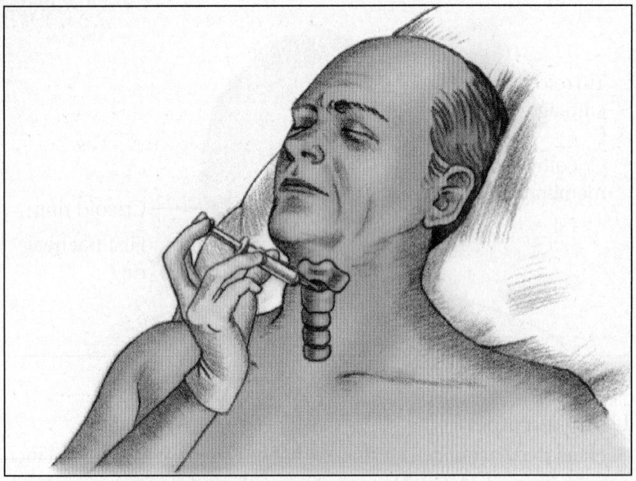

■ When the catheter reaches the trachea, the practitioner advances it and removes the needle and syringe.

■ Tape the catheter in place.

Attach the catheter hub to one end of the IV extension tubing. At the other end, attach a hand-operated release valve or a pressure-regulating adjustment valve. Connect the entire assembly to an oxygen source.

■ Press the release valve to introduce oxygen into the trachea and inflate the lungs. When you can see that they're inflated, release the valve *to allow passive exhalation.* Adjust the pressure-regulating valve to the minimum pressure needed for adequate lung inflation.

Completing the procedure

■ Auscultate bilaterally for breath sounds *to confirm tube placement*[12] and take the patient's vital signs.

■ Check the patient's end-tidal carbon dioxide level *to verify correct tube placement.*[12]

■ Anticipate a chest X-ray *to evaluate tube placement.*

■ Remove and dispose of your gloves and other personal protective equipment properly[9,10] and perform hand hygiene.[4,5,6,7,8]

■ Clean and disinfect your stethoscope using a disinfectant pad.[13,14]

■ Perform hand hygiene.[4,5,6,7,8]

■ Document the procedure.[15,16,17]

Special considerations

PEDIATRIC ALERT ***Scalpel cricothyrotomy isn't recommended for children younger than age 12*** **because it could damage the cricoid cartilage—the only circumferential support to the upper trachea.**

■ Monitor the patient's heart rate, blood pressure, respiratory rate, and oxygen saturation level throughout the procedure.[2]

■ Check for bleeding at the insertion site; subcutaneous emphysema or inadequate ventilation, *which may indicate tube displacement or an air leak;* and tracheal or vocal cord damage.

■ Whenever possible, use ultrasound equipment *to visualize the patient's anatomy* before starting the procedure.

■ If time allows and your facility indicates that cricothyrotomy falls within universal protocol guidelines, follow the necessary steps, including conducting a time-out immediately before starting the procedure, *to ensure that the correct patient, site, positioning, and procedure are identified and that (as applicable) all relevant information and necessary equipment are available.*[18,19,20]

Complications

Hemorrhage, perforation of the thyroid or esophagus, and subcutaneous or mediastinal emphysema may occur from this procedure. Infection may occur several days after the procedure.

Documentation

Document the date, time, and circumstances requiring the procedure and the patient's vital signs. Note whether the patient initiated spontaneous respirations after the procedure. Record how much and by what method oxygen was delivered. If any procedures (such as endotracheal intubation) were performed after the airway was established, note them.

REFERENCES

1 Markowitz, J. E. (2013). "Surgical airway techniques" [Online]. Accessed March 2015 via the Web at http://emedicine.medscape.com/article/80241-overview#a01

2 Bair, A. E. Emergent surgical cricothyrotomy (cricothyroidotomy). (2012). In: *UpToDate,* Wolfson, A. B., & Grayzel, J. (Eds.). Accessed March 2015 via the Web at http://www.uptodate.com/contents/search

3 American Society of Anesthesiologists Task Force. (2013). Practice guidelines for management of the difficult airway: An updated report by the American Society of Anesthesiologists Task Force on Management of a Difficult Airway. *Anesthesiology, 118*(2), 251–270. (Level VII)

4 The Joint Commission. (2015). Standard NPSG.07.01.01. *Comprehensive accreditation manual for hospitals: The official handbook.* Oakbrook Terrace, IL: The Joint Commission. (Level VII)

5 Centers for Disease Control and Prevention. (2002). Guideline for hand hygiene in health-care settings: Recommendations of the Healthcare Infection Control Practices Advisory Committee and the HICPAC/SHEA/APIC/IDSA Hand Hygiene Task Force. *MMWR Recommendations and Reports, 51*(RR-16), 1–45. Accessed March 2015 via the Web at http://www.cdc.gov/mmwr/pdf/rr/rr5116.pdf (Level II)

6 World Health Organization. (2009). "WHO guidelines on hand hygiene in health care: First global patient safety challenge, clean care is safer care" [Online]. Accessed March 2015 via the Web at http://whqlibdoc.who.int/publications/2009/9789241597906_eng.pdf (Level IV)

7 Centers for Medicare & Medicaid Services, Department of Health and Human Services. (2014). Condition of participation: Infection control. 42 C.F.R. § 482.42.

8 American Osteopathic Association. (2014). Standard 07.01.21. *Healthcare Facilities Accreditation Program: Accreditation requirements for acute care hospitals.* Chicago, IL: American Osteopathic Association. (Level VII)

9 Siegel, J. D., et al. (2007). "2007 guideline for isolation precautions: Preventing transmission of infectious agents in healthcare settings" [Online]. Accessed March 2015 via the Web at http://www.cdc.gov/hicpac/pdf/isolation/Isolation2007.pdf (Level II)

10 American Osteopathic Association. (2014). Standard 07.01.10. *Healthcare Facilities Accreditation Program: Accreditation requirements for acute care hospitals.* Chicago, IL: American Osteopathic Association. (Level VII)

11 The Joint Commission. (2015). Standard NPSG.01.01.01. *Comprehensive accreditation manual for hospitals: The official handbook.* Oakbrook Terrace, IL: The Joint Commission. (Level VII)

12 Lynn-McHale Wiegand, D. (Ed.). *AACN procedure manual for critical care* (6th ed.). St. Louis, MO: Saunders.

13 Rutala, W. A., et al. (2008). "Guideline for disinfection and sterilization in healthcare facilities, 2008" [Online]. Accessed March 2015 via the Web at http://www.cdc.gov/hicpac/pdf/guidelines/Disinfection_Nov_2008.pdf (Level I)

14 American Osteopathic Association. (2015). Standard 07.02.03. *Healthcare Facilities Accreditation Program: Accreditation requirements for acute care hospitals.* Chicago, IL: American Osteopathic Association. (Level VII)

15 The Joint Commission. (2015). Standard RC.01.03.01. *Comprehensive accreditation manual for hospitals: The official handbook.* Oakbrook Terrace, IL: The Joint Commission. (Level VII)

16 Centers for Medicare & Medicaid Services, Department of Health and Human Services. (2014). Condition of participation: Medical record services. 42 C.F.R. § 482.24(b).

17 American Osteopathic Association. (2014). Standard 10.00.03. *Healthcare Facilities Accreditation Program: Accreditation requirements for acute care hospitals.* Chicago, IL: American Osteopathic Association. (Level VII)

18 The Joint Commission. (2015). Standard UP.01.01.01. *Comprehensive accreditation manual for hospitals: The official handbook.* Oakbrook Terrace, IL: The Joint Commission. (Level VII)

Fitting a patient for a crutch

To measure for an axillary crutch, position the crutch so that it extends from a point 4″ to 6″ (10 to 15 cm) to the side and 4″ to 6″ (10 to 15 cm) in front of the patient's feet to 1″ to 1½″ (2.5 to 4 cm) below the axilla.

Adjust the handgrips so that the patient's elbows are flexed at a 30-degree angle[1] and the wrists are at a 15-degree angle when he's standing with the crutches in the resting position. The handgrips should be even with the top of the hip line. Check that the vinyl padding on the arm cuffs, the rubber handgrips, and the rubber tips at the end of the crutches are placed securely.

To fit a forearm crutch, have the patient flex his elbow so the crease in his wrist is at his hip. Then measure his forearm from 3″ (7.5 cm) below the elbow (A) and add the distance between his wrist and the floor (B). This is the total length (C).

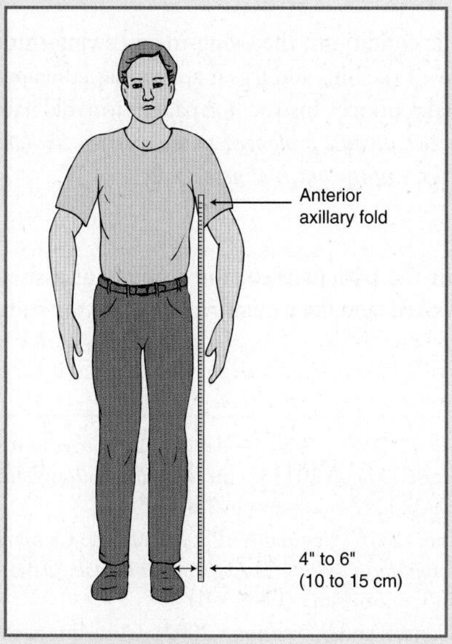

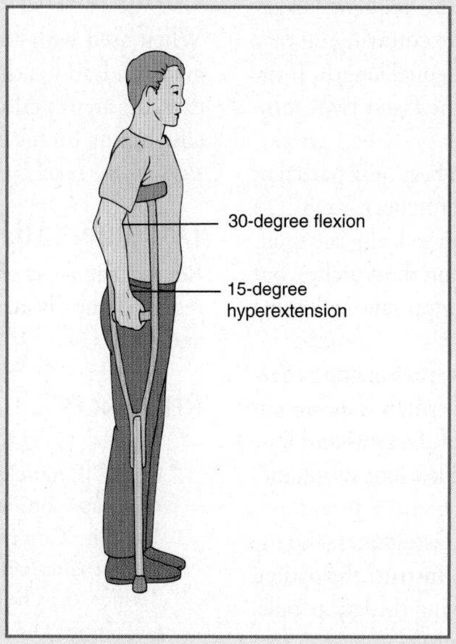

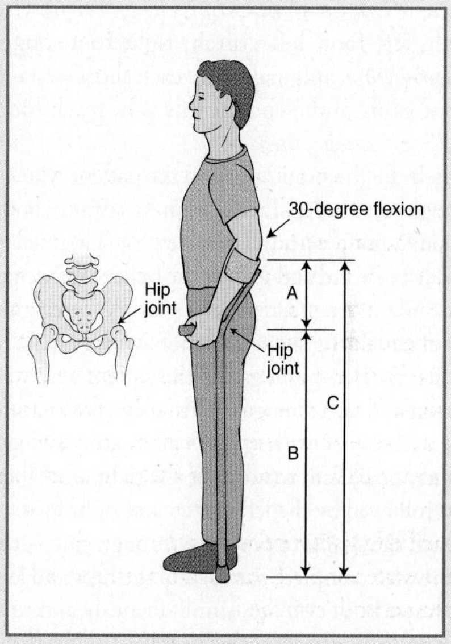

19 The Joint Commission. (2015). Standard UP.01.03.01. *Comprehensive accreditation manual for hospitals: The official handbook.* Oakbrook Terrace, IL: The Joint Commission. (Level VII)

20 American Osteopathic Association. (2014). Standard 30.00.14. *Healthcare Facilities Accreditation Program: Accreditation requirements for acute care hospitals.* Chicago, IL: American Osteopathic Association. (Level VII)

ADDITIONAL REFERENCE

Walls, R., & Murphy, M. (Eds.). (2012). *Manual of emergency airway management* (4th ed.). Philadelphia, PA: Lippincott Williams & Wilkins.

CRUTCH USE

Crutches remove weight from one or both legs, enabling the patient to support himself with his hands and arms. Typically prescribed for the patient with lower-extremity injury or weakness or one who has had a surgical procedure on the lower limbs, crutches require balance, stamina, and upper-body strength for successful use.[1] Crutch selection and walking gait depend on the patient's condition. The patient who can't use crutches may be able to use a walker.

Two types of crutches are currently in use: axillary and forearm (nonaxillary) crutches. Patients with a sprain, strain, or cast should use axillary crutches, which are made of standard aluminum or wood. The primary advantage of axillary crutches is that they allow the transfer of 80% of a person's body weight. Forearm crutches provide better trunk support than forearm crutches, but they require stamina and upper-body strength.

Forearm (nonaxillary) crutches, such as aluminum or platform forearm crutches, allow the transfer of 40% to 50% of the patient's body weight, providing stability and moderate support. Forearm crutches are indicated for patients with generalized weakness in the lower extremities, such as those with paraplegia or cerebral palsy. An aluminum forearm crutch has a collar that fits around the patient's forearm and a horizontal handgrip that provides support. A wooden forearm crutch resembles a wooden axillary crutch that ends proximally, with a closed leather band that can be situated around the proximal portion of the patient's forearm. A platform forearm crutch is indicated for patients with painful wrist and hand conditions (such as arthritis), weak handgrip because of pain and deformities of the hands and wrists, and elbow contractures. A platform is placed on the top level of the crutch, a vertical handgrip is placed at the distal end of the platform, and Velcro straps are applied around the patient's forearm.

Equipment

Crutches with appropriate padding, handgrips, and rubber suction tips ■ Optional: gait belt, full-length mirror.

Preparation of equipment

After choosing the appropriate crutches, adjust their height with the patient standing or, if necessary, recumbent. (See *Fitting a patient for a crutch.*)

Implementation

- Consult with the patient's practitioner and physical therapist *to coordinate rehabilitation orders and teaching.*

- Determine the patient's weight-bearing status *to help determine which gait to teach the patient.*
- Perform hand hygiene.[2,3,4,5,6]
- Confirm the patient's identity using at least two patient identifiers.[7]
- Explain the procedure to the patient.
- Place a gait belt around the patient's waist, if necessary, *to help prevent falls.* Tell the patient to position the crutches and to shift his weight from side to side.
- Place the patient in front of a full-length mirror, if available, *to facilitate learning and coordination.*
- Teach the four-point gait to the patient who can bear weight on both legs. Although this is the safest gait *because three points are always in contact with the floor,* it requires greater coordination than others *because it requires constant shifting of weight.* Use this sequence: right crutch, left foot, left crutch, right foot. Suggest counting *to help develop rhythm,* and make sure each short step is of equal length. If the patient gains proficiency at this gait, teach him the faster two-point gait. (See *Crutch gaits.*)
- Teach the three-point gait to the patient who can bear only partial or no weight on one leg. Instruct him to advance both crutches 6″ to 8″ (15 to 20 cm) along with the involved leg. Then tell him to bring the unaffected leg forward and to bear the bulk of his weight on the crutches, but some of it on the affected leg, if possible. Stress the importance of taking steps of equal length and duration, with no pauses.
- Teach the two-point gait to the patient with weak legs but good coordination and arm strength. This is the most natural crutch-walking gait *because it mimics walking,* with alternating swings of the arms and legs. Instruct the patient to advance the right crutch and left foot simultaneously, followed by the left crutch and right foot.
- Teach the swing-to or swing-through gaits—the fastest ones—to the patient with complete paralysis of the hips and legs. Instruct the patient to advance both crutches simultaneously and to swing the legs parallel to (swing-to) or beyond the crutches (swing-through).
- To teach the patient to get up from a chair, tell him to hold both crutches in one hand, with the tips resting firmly on the floor. He should then push up from the chair with his free hand, supporting himself with the crutches.
- To sit down, the patient reverses the process: Tell him to support himself with the crutches in one hand and to lower himself with the other.
- To teach the patient to ascend stairs using the three-point gait, tell him to lead with the unaffected (good) leg and to follow with both the crutches and the affected (bad) leg. To descend stairs he should lead with the crutches and the affected (bad) leg and follow with the unaffected (good) leg. He may find it helpful to remember the phrase, "up with the good; down with the bad."
- Have the patient provide return demonstrations using the appropriate gait, using a chair, and negotiating stairs.
- Perform hand hygiene.[2,3,4,5,6]
- Document the procedure.[8,9,10]

Special considerations

- Consult with the physical therapy department *because at a minimum, gait training should include aerobic conditioning exercises, coordination and balancing exercises, and range-of-motion and muscle strengthening of both the upper and lower limbs.*[1] Also, teach the patient two gaits if possible—one fast and one slow—*so that he can alternate between them to prevent excessive muscle fatigue and so he can adjust more easily to various walking conditions.*
- Encourage the patient to remove rugs and clutter from the floor *to decrease the risk of falls.*
- Have the patient wear a tennis shoe or other flat rubber-soled shoe on the foot *to prevent slipping.*
- Instruct the patient not to move too fast or to swing his leg too far forward *because this could cause a loss of balance.*
- Check the wing nuts or locking mechanisms on the crutches daily *to make sure they're tightened securely.*

Patient teaching

Instruct the patient to contact his practitioner with questions about how to use the crutches or if the crutches don't fit, break, or are lost. Tell the patient to notify his practitioner if he develops blisters, rashes, or painful calluses or if his skin breaks down on his hands, forearms, or underarms. He should seek care immediately if he experiences sudden numbness of his hands or arms.

Complications

When used with chronic conditions, the swing-to and swing-through gaits can lead to atrophy of the hips and legs if appropriate therapeutic exercises aren't performed routinely. Instruct the patient to avoid habitually leaning on his crutches *because prolonged pressure on the axillae can damage the brachial nerves, causing brachial nerve palsy.*

Documentation

Record the type of gait the patient used, the amount of assistance required, the distance walked, and the patient's tolerance of the crutches and gait.

REFERENCES

1 Kedlaya, D., & Kuang, T. (2013). "Assistive devices to improve independence" [Online]. Accessed March 2015 via the Web at http://emedicine.medscape.com/article/325247-overview#aw2aab6b3

2 The Joint Commission. (2015). Standard NPSG.07.01.01. *Comprehensive accreditation manual for hospitals: The official handbook.* Oakbrook Terrace, IL: The Joint Commission. (Level VII)

3 Centers for Disease Control and Prevention. (2002). Guideline for hand hygiene in health-care settings: Recommendations of the Healthcare Infection Control Practices Advisory Committee and the HICPAC/SHEA/APIC/IDSA Hand Hygiene Task Force. *MMWR Recommendations and Reports, 51*(RR-16), 1–45. Accessed March 2015 via the Web at http://www.cdc.gov/mmwr/pdf/rr/rr5116.pdf (Level II)

4 World Health Organization. (2009). "WHO guidelines on hand hygiene in health care: First global patient safety challenge, clean care is safer care" [Online]. Accessed March 2015 via the Web at http://whqlibdoc.who.int/publications/2009/9789241597906_eng.pdf (Level IV)

5 Centers for Medicare & Medicaid Services, Department of Health and Human Services. (2014). Condition of participation: Infection control. 42 C.F.R. § 482.42.

6 American Osteopathic Association. (2014). Standard 07.01.21. *Healthcare Facilities Accreditation Program: Accreditation requirements for acute care hospitals.* Chicago, IL: American Osteopathic Association. (Level VII)

7 The Joint Commission. (2015). Standard NPSG.01.01.01. *Comprehensive accreditation manual for hospitals: The official handbook.* Oakbrook Terrace, IL: The Joint Commission. (Level VII)

8 The Joint Commission. (2015). Standard RC.01.03.01. *Comprehensive accreditation manual for hospitals: The official handbook.* Oakbrook Terrace, IL: The Joint Commission. (Level VII)

9 Centers for Medicare & Medicaid Services, Department of Health and Human Services. (2014). Condition of participation: Medical record services. 42 C.F.R. § 482.24(b).

10 American Osteopathic Association. (2014). Standard 10.00.03. *Healthcare Facilities Accreditation Program: Accreditation requirements for acute care hospitals.* Chicago, IL: American Osteopathic Association. (Level VII)

Crutch gaits

This is a guide for using the four-point, three-point, and two-point swing-to or swing-through gaits. Start at the bottom and move upward. *Note:* Shaded areas indicate weight bearing.

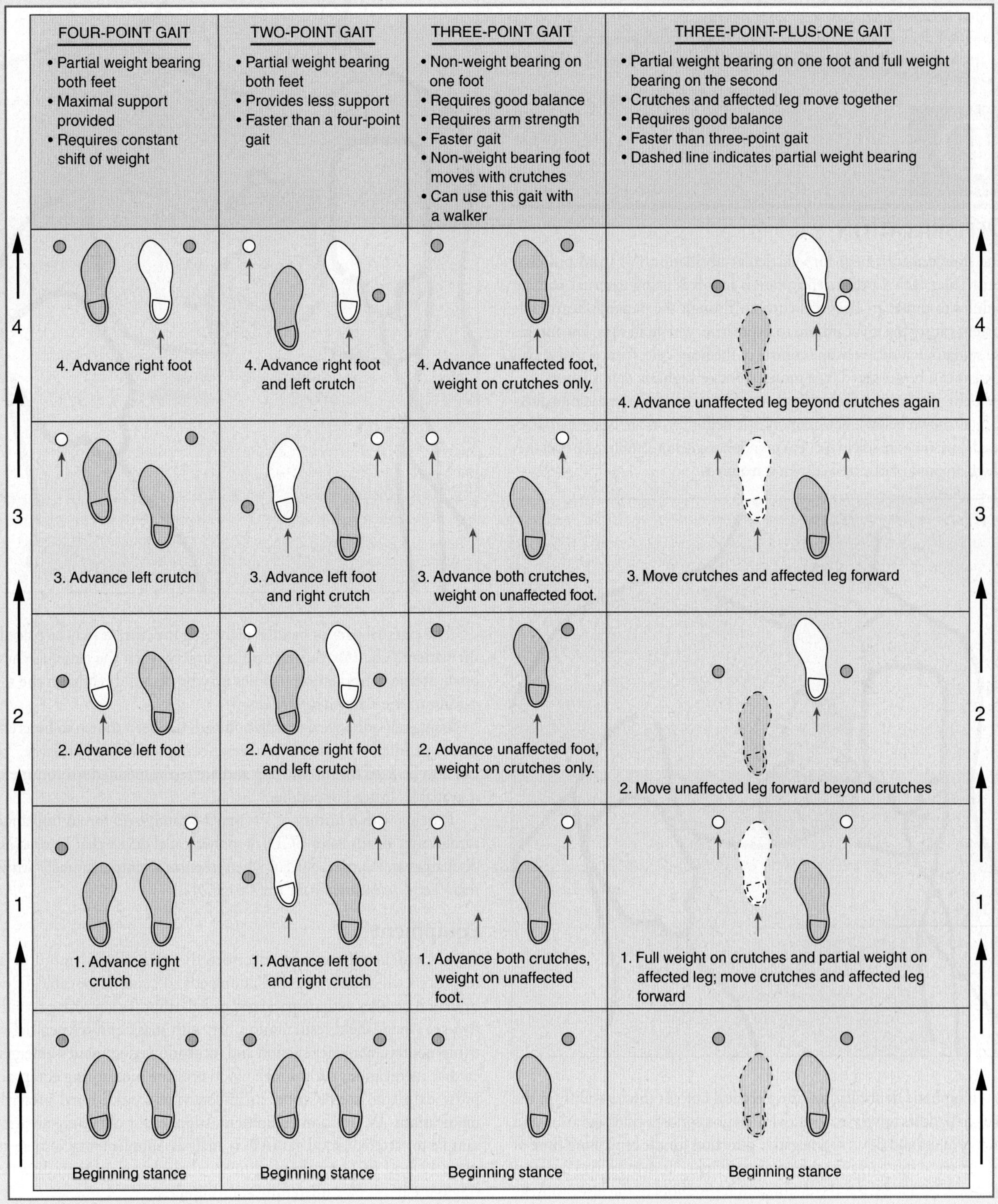

ADDITIONAL REFERENCES

Borrelli, J., & Haslach, H. W. (2013). Experimental characterization of axillary/underarm interface pressure in swing-through crutch walking. *Journal of Rehabilitation Research and Design, 50,* 423–436. (Level VI)

Craven, R. F., & Hirnle, C. J. (2012). *Fundamentals of nursing: Human health and function* (7th ed.). Philadelphia, PA: Lippincott Williams & Wilkins.

Edelstein, J. E. (2013). Assistive devices for ambulation. *Physical Medicine and Rehabilitation Clinics of North America, 24,* 291–303. (Level V)

Westerhoff, P., et al. (2012). In vivo measurement of shoulder joint loads during walking with crutches. *Clinical Biomechanics, 27,* 711–718. (Level VI)

D

DEFIBRILLATION

The standard treatment for ventricular fibrillation (VF) and pulseless ventricular tachycardia, defibrillation involves using external pads or paddles to direct an electrical current through the patient's heart. The current causes the myocardium to depolarize, which, in turn, encourages the sinoatrial node to resume control of the heart's electrical activity. This current can be delivered by a monophasic or biphasic defibrillator.

Defibrillators with monophasic waveforms deliver current in one direction (as shown below). Few monophasic defibrillators are being manufactured, but some are still in use. For monophasic defibrillation to be effective, a high amount of electrical current is required.

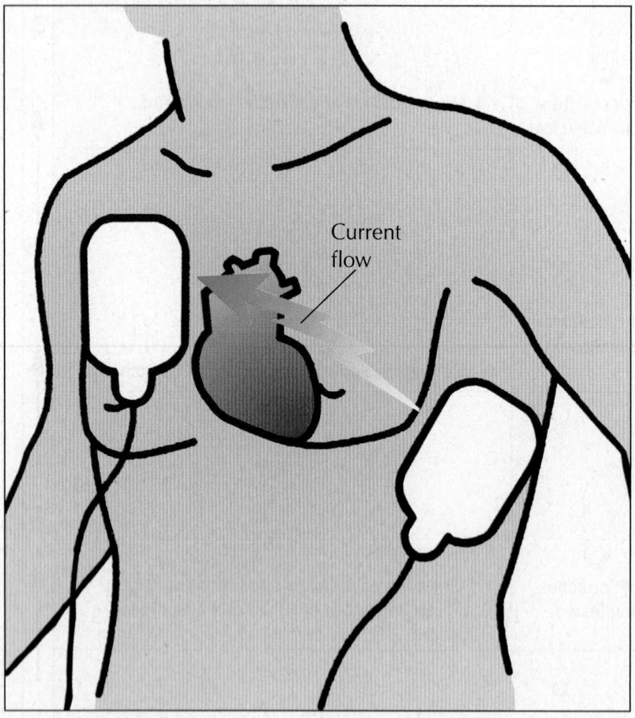

In biphasic defibrillation, the electrical current discharged from the pads or paddles travels in a positive direction for a specified duration and then reverses and flows in a negative direction for the remaining time of the electrical discharge (as shown on top right). It delivers two currents of electricity and lowers the defibrillation threshold of the heart muscle, making it possible to successfully defibrillate VF with smaller amounts of energy. The biphasic defibrillator can adjust for differences in impedance or the resistance of the current through the chest. This helps reduce the number of shocks needed to terminate VF. Biphasic technology uses lower energy levels and fewer shocks, which reduces the damage to the myocardial muscle. Biphasic defibrillators, when used at the clinically appropriate energy level, may be used for defibrillation and, when placed in the synchronized mode, may be used for synchronized cardioversion.

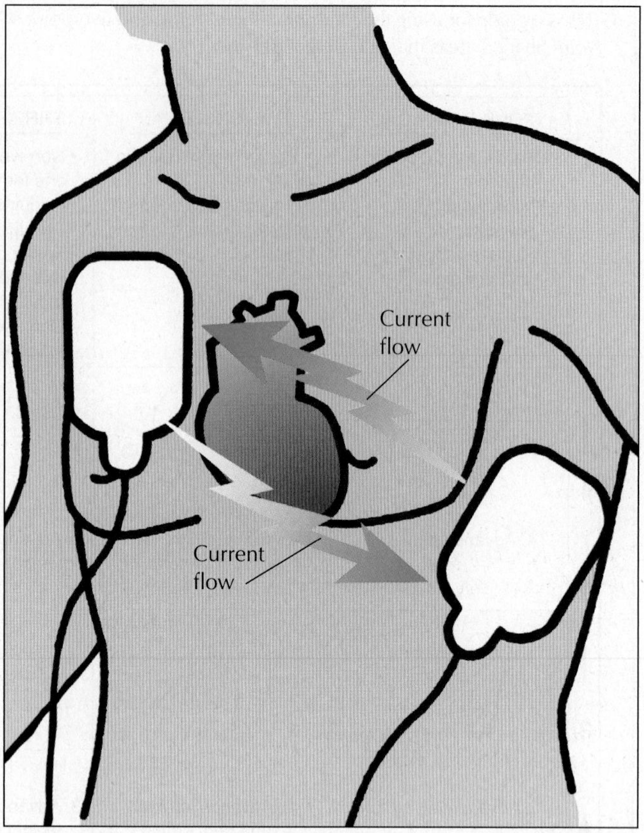

The external pads or paddles delivering the current may be placed on the patient's chest or, during cardiac surgery when the patient's chest is open, sterile defibrillation paddles may be placed directly on the myocardium. (See *Using a defibrillator.*)

Using self-adhesive defibrillation pads has been shown to be as effective as paddles, with the advantage of being convenient and safe. They can also be used for monitoring and are recommended for routine use, if available, instead of paddles.[3]

Patients with a history of VF may be candidates for an implantable cardioverter-defibrillator (ICD), a sophisticated device that automatically discharges an electrical current when it senses a ventricular tachyarrhythmia. (See *Understanding the ICD,* page 242.)

Equipment

Gloves ▪ defibrillator with electrocardiogram (ECG) monitor and recorder ▪ self-adhesive defibrillation pads and connector cable, or defibrillation paddles with prepackaged gelled defibrillation pads or conductive gel ▪ hand-held resuscitation bag with mask and oxygen delivery equipment ▪ emergency suction and intubation equipment ▪ emergency cardiac medications ▪ Optional: blood pressure monitoring equipment, pulse oximeter, stethoscope, disinfectant pad, additional prescribed medications, IV infusion equipment, supplies for obtaining an arterial sample for arterial blood gas (ABG) analysis, supplemental oxygen supplies, 12-lead ECG machine, clippers or electric razor with disposable single-use head, IV catheter insertion supplies.

Preparation of equipment

Make sure the defibrillation pads or paddles are connected to the defibrillator and that the defibrillator battery is adequately charged or the defibrillator electrical cord is plugged into the wall. Keep the defibrillation pads in their packages before use *to prevent the conductive gel from drying out.* Ensure that resuscitation equipment and medications are immediately available.

Implementation

- Perform hand hygiene.[4,5,6,7,8]
- Confirm the patient's identity using at least two patient identifiers.[9]
- If time allows, make sure the patient and family understand the procedure.
- Put on gloves and follow standard precautions throughout the procedure.[10,11]
- Assess the patient to determine that he's unresponsive and not breathing or only gasping.[2]
- If the patient is unresponsive and not breathing or only gasping, call for help and then take up to 10 seconds to attempt to feel for a pulse (carotid or femoral). If you're alone and don't feel a pulse or you're unsure whether you feel a pulse, begin chest compressions. After 30 compressions, open the patient's airway using a head tilt–chin lift maneuver and give two breaths. If there's evidence of trauma that suggests spinal injury, use a jaw thrust maneuver to open the airway. Continue cardiopulmonary resuscitation (CPR) until the defibrillator and emergency equipment arrive.[2]
- Make sure that the patient is in a dry environment and that his chest is dry *because if a staff member or the patient comes into contact with water, the staff member may receive a shock and the patient may receive skin burns.*[3]
- Remove metallic objects that the patient may be wearing *because metal conducts electricity and could cause burns during defibrillation.*[3]
- Remove transdermal medication patches from the patient's chest (and back if using anterior-posterior placement) *because the medication may interfere with current medications and produce burns.*[2,3]

NURSING ALERT *When performing defibrillation, don't place the self-adhesive pads or paddles directly over an ICD or implanted pacemaker.* This placement may damage the device.[3]

Defibrillation using self-adhesive defibrillation pads

- Expose the patient's chest and apply the self-adhesive defibrillation pads. For anterolateral placement, position one pad to the right of the upper sternum, just below the right clavicle, and the other over the fifth or sixth intercostal space at the left anterior axillary line (as shown below). For anteroposterior placement, position the anterior pad directly over the heart at the precordium, to the left of the lower sternal border (as shown on next page, middle left). Place the posterior pad under the patient's body beneath the heart and immediately below the scapula (but not on the vertebral column) (as shown on next page, bottom left). *Defibrillation occurs when an electrical current passes through the cardiac muscle to restore a single source of impulse production. Appropriate pad positioning maximizes the flow of electrical current through the heart.*[3]

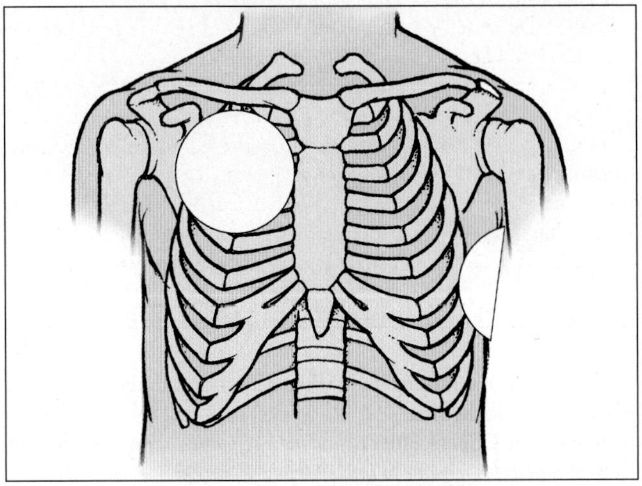

Using a defibrillator

Because ventricular fibrillation leads to death if not corrected, the success of defibrillation depends on early recognition and quick treatment of this arrhythmia.[2] In addition to treating ventricular fibrillation, defibrillation may also be used to treat ventricular tachycardia that doesn't produce a pulse.[3] To allow you to treat patients as quickly as possible, familiarize yourself with the defibrillator available at your facility. Use the defibrillators below as a guide to the parts of a defibrillator.

Defibrillator with self-adhesive defibrillation pads

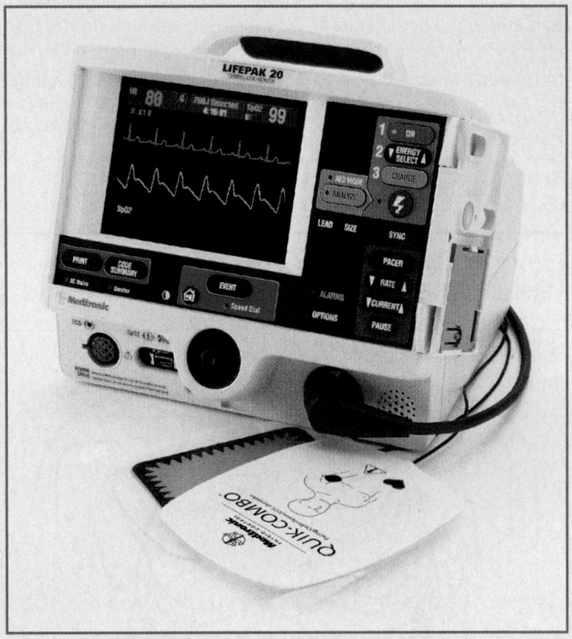

Defibrillator with paddles

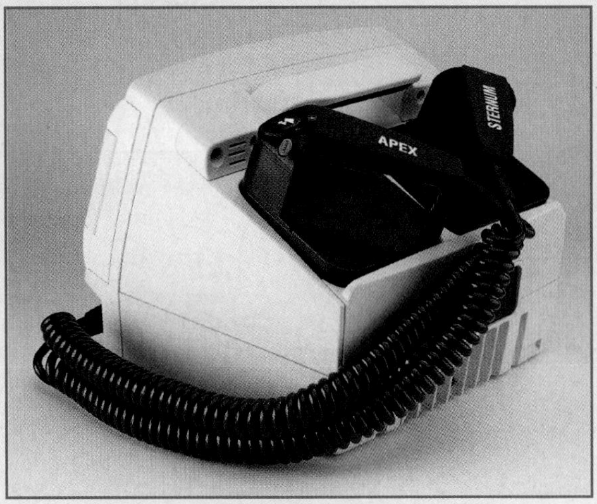

Understanding the ICD

The implantable cardioverter-defibrillator (ICD) has a programmable pulse generator and lead system that monitors the heart's activity, detects ventricular bradyarrhythmias and tachyarrhythmias, and responds to each with different interventions. These interventions include antitachycardia pacing, cardioversion, defibrillation, and bradycardia pacing. Some ICDs can be programmed to pace both the atrium and ventricle or both ventricles (cardiac resynchronization therapy). Some models can also detect and correct atrial arrhythmias.

Implantation is similar to implantation of a permanent pacemaker. The cardiologist positions the lead or leads in the endocardium of the right ventricle (and the right atrium if both chambers require pacing) and then connects the other end to the generator (about the size of a wallet), which is implanted in the right or left upper chest near the collarbone. New, smaller devices can be installed through the blood vessels. These newer devices can also store information related to the arrhythmic event and perform electrophysiology testing.

Anterolateral placement

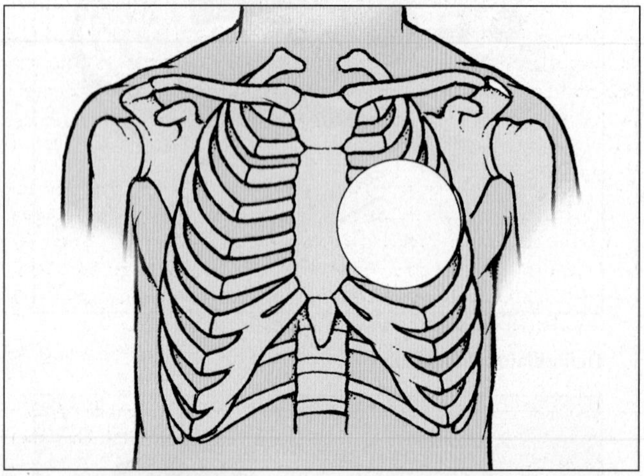

Anterior placement

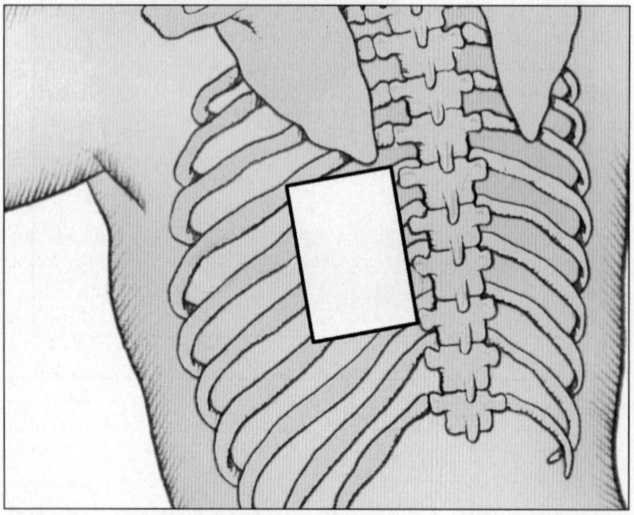

Posterior placement

■ Turn on the defibrillator and, if performing external defibrillation using a biphasic defibrillator, use clinically appropriate energy levels (usually 120 to 200 joules) following the manufacturer's recommended dose.[2] If you're using a monophasic defibrillator, set the energy level for 360 joules for an adult patient.

■ Connect the monitoring leads of the defibrillator to the patient *to assess his cardiac rhythm.*

■ Turn on the ECG recorder *to provide a visual recording of the patient's ECG as well as his response to interventions.*[3]

■ Charge the self-adhesive defibrillator pads by pressing the appropriate button on the defibrillator.

■ Reassess the patient's cardiac rhythm.

■ Disconnect the oxygen source during actual defibrillation *to decrease the chance of combustion caused by arcing of the electrical current in the presence of oxygen.*[3]

■ If the patient remains in VF or pulseless ventricular tachycardia, say "all clear" or use similar wording three times and visually verify that all staff members are clear of the patient and the bed before discharging the electrical current. *Electrical current can be conducted from the patient to anyone in contact with the patient.*[3]

Defibrillation using defibrillator paddles

■ If the defibrillator can monitor the patient's rhythm using the paddles, turn on the defibrillator, expose the patient's chest, and place the gelled defibrillation pads on the patient's chest. For anterolateral placement, position one gelled defibrillation pad to the right of the upper sternum, just below the right clavicle, and the other over the fifth or sixth intercostal space at the left anterior axillary line. For anteroposterior placement, position the anterior gelled defibrillation pad directly over the heart at the precordium to the left of the lower sternal border. Place the posterior gelled defibrillation pad under the patient's body beneath the heart and immediately below the scapula (but not on the vertebral column). *Defibrillation occurs when an electrical current passes through the cardiac muscle to restore a single source of impulse production. Appropriate positioning of the pads maximizes the flow of electrical current through the heart.*[3]

■ Press the paddles firmly against the patient's chest on top of the gelled defibrillation pads using about 25 lb (11 kg) of pressure *to quickly view the cardiac rhythm.*[12]

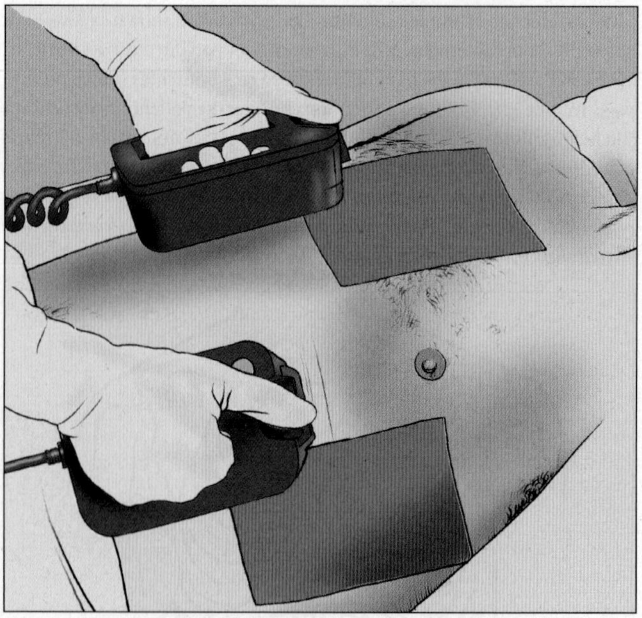

■ Connect the monitoring leads of the defibrillator to the patient, and assess his cardiac rhythm.

■ Turn on the ECG recorder *to provide a visual recording of the patient's ECG as well as his response to interventions.*

- Charge the paddles by pressing the charge buttons, located either on the defibrillator or on the paddles themselves.
- Reassess the patient's cardiac rhythm.
- Disconnect the oxygen source during actual defibrillation *to decreases the risk of combustion caused by arcing of the electrical current in the presence of oxygen.*
- If the patient remains in VF or pulseless ventricular tachycardia, instruct all staff members to stand clear of the patient and the bed. Visually verify all staff members are clear of the patient and the bed before discharging the current. *Electrical current can be conducted from the patient to anyone in contact with the patient.*
- Discharge the current by pressing both paddle charge buttons simultaneously, maintaining 25 lb (11 kg) of pressure on both paddles.[12] *Using this pressure decreases transthoracic resistance.* Hold until the defibrillator delivers the electrical current.[3]

Completing the procedure

- Resume CPR immediately, beginning with chest compressions, giving five cycles. *Defibrillation is more likely to be effective if followed immediately with a cycle of chest compressions and with minimal interruption in chest compressions.*[2]
- Reassess the patient's cardiac rhythm.
- If the patient remains in VF or pulseless ventricular tachycardia, prepare to defibrillate a second time. Reset the energy level defibrillator to 360 joules (or the biphasic energy equivalent) and continue CPR while the defibrillator is charging. Announce that you're preparing to defibrillate, and follow the procedure described above.[3]
- Resume CPR immediately, starting with chest compressions, and complete five cycles.[2]
- Reassess the patient. If the patient remains in VF or pulseless ventricular tachycardia and defibrillation is again necessary, reset the energy level to 360 joules for the monophasic defibrillator (or the biphasic energy equivalent). Then follow the same procedure as before.
- Resume CPR immediately, starting with chest compressions, and give five cycles.[2]
- If defibrillation restores a normal rhythm, check the patient's central and peripheral pulses and obtain a blood pressure reading and heart rate. Assess the patient's respiratory status, level of consciousness, cardiac rhythm, breath sounds, skin color, and urine output. Obtain baseline ABG levels and a 12-lead ECG. Provide supplemental oxygen and ventilation, and insert an IV catheter (if not already in place) and administer medications, as needed and ordered, following safe medication administration practices.[13,14,15] Check the patient's chest for electrical burns and treat them, as ordered. Also prepare the defibrillator for immediate reuse.
- Discard all supplies, remove and discard your gloves, and perform hand hygiene.[4,5,6,7,8,10]
- Provide support and information to the patient's family, as needed. After resuscitation, inform the patient about what happened, if appropriate.
- Clean and disinfect your stethoscope, if used, suing a disinfectant pad.[16,17]
- Perform hand hygiene.[4,5,6,7,8]
- Document the procedure.[18,19,20]

Special considerations

- Additional defibrillation should be done 30 seconds to 1 minute after administering medications.
- Check defibrillator operation regularly (usually once per shift), as determined by your facility.
- If gelled definrillation pads aren't available, defibrillator paddles require that a conductive gel be placed on the paddles before use. Place the gel on one paddle, and rub the two paddles together *to spread the gel evenly between them.* Ensure that the surface of the paddle is completely covered.
- Defibrillation can be affected by several factors, including paddle size and placement, condition of the patient's myocardium, duration of the arrhythmia, chest resistance, and the number of countershocks.[1]
- Don't place the pad or paddle over a female patient's breast. Instead, place the apex of the pad or paddle at the fifth to sixth intercostal space, with the middle of the pad or paddle at the midaxillary line.
- Family members of the patient undergoing resuscitation should be given the option to remain at the bedside during resuscitation *because it helps meet the psychosocial needs of the patient and his family in a time of crisis.*[21]
- If the patient has a hairy chest, remove the hair from necessary locations for pad or paddle placement. *Chest hair can increase transthoracic impedance.*

Complications

Defibrillation can cause accidental electrical shock to those providing care. Using dry self-adhesive defibrillation pads or applying an insufficient amount of conductive medium can lead to skin burns.

Documentation

Document the procedure, including the patient's ECG rhythm both before and after defibrillation; the number of times defibrillation was performed; the energy used with each attempt; whether a pulse returned; the dosage, route, and time of drug administration; whether CPR was performed; how the airway was maintained; and the patient's outcome. Record the patient's vital signs and your assessment findings. Document any patient or family teaching and their comprehension of your teaching.

REFERENCES

1 Chan, P. S., et al. (2008). Delayed time to defibrillation after in-hospital cardiac arrest. *New England Journal of Medicine, 358,* 9–17. (Level VI)

2 American Heart Association. (2010). 2010 American Heart Association guidelines for cardiopulmonary resuscitation and emergency cardiovascular care. *Circulation, 122,* S685–S719. (Level II)

3 Lynn-McHale Wiegand, D. (Ed.). (2011). *AACN procedure manual for critical care* (6th ed.). St. Louis, MO: Saunders.

4 The Joint Commission. (2015). Standard NPSG.07.01.01. *Comprehensive accreditation manual for hospitals: The official handbook.* Oakbrook Terrace, IL: The Joint Commission. (Level VII)

5 World Health Organization. (2009). "WHO guidelines on hand hygiene in health care: First global patient safety challenge, clean care is safer care" [Online]. Accessed March 2015 via the Web at http://whqlibdoc.who.int/publications/2009/9789241597906_eng.pdf (Level IV)

6 Centers for Disease Control and Prevention. (2002). Guideline for hand hygiene in health-care settings: Recommendations of the Healthcare Infection Control Practices Advisory Committee and the HICPAC/SHEA/APIC/IDSA Hand Hygiene Task Force. *MMWR Recommendations and Reports, 51*(RR-16), 1–45. Accessed March 2015 via the Web at http://www.cdc.gov/mmwr/pdf/rr/rr5116.pdf (Level II)

7 Centers for Medicare & Medicaid Services, Department of Health and Human Services. (2014). Condition of participation: Infection control. 42 C.F.R. § 482.42.

8 American Osteopathic Association. (2014). Standard 07.01.21. *Healthcare Facilities Accreditation Program: Accreditation requirements for acute care hospitals.* Chicago, IL: American Osteopathic Association. (Level VII)

9 The Joint Commission. (2015). Standard NPSG.01.01.01. *Comprehensive accreditation manual for hospitals: The official handbook.* Oakbrook Terrace, IL: The Joint Commission. (Level VII)

10 Siegel, J. D., et al. (2007). "2007 guideline for isolation precautions: Preventing transmission of infectious agents in healthcare settings" [Online]. Accessed March 2015 via the Web at http://www.cdc.gov/hicpac/pdf/isolation/Isolation2007.pdf (Level II)

11 American Osteopathic Association. (2014). Standard 07.01.10. *Healthcare Facilities Accreditation Program: Accreditation requirements for acute care hospitals.* Chicago, IL: American Osteopathic Association. (Level VII)
12 Woods, S. L., et al. (2010). *Cardiac nursing* (6th ed.). Philadelphia, PA: Lippincott Williams & Wilkins.
13 American Osteopathic Association. (2014). Standard 16.01.03. *Healthcare Facilities Accreditation Program: Accreditation requirements for acute care hospitals.* Chicago, IL: American Osteopathic Association. (Level VII)
14 Centers for Medicare & Medicaid Services, Department of Health and Human Services. (2014). Condition of participation: Preparation and administration of drugs. 42 C.F.R. § 482.23(c).
15 The Joint Commission. (2015). Standard MM.06.01.01. *Comprehensive accreditation manual for hospitals: The official handbook.* Oakbrook Terrace, IL: The Joint Commission. (Level VII)
16 Rutala, W. A., et al. (2008). "Guideline for disinfection and sterilization in healthcare facilities, 2008" [Online]. Accessed March 2015 via the Web at http://www.cdc.gov/hicpac/pdf/guidelines/Disinfection_Nov_2008.pdf (Level I)
17 American Osteopathic Association. (2014). Standard 07.01.10. *Healthcare Facilities Accreditation Program: Accreditation requirements for acute care hospitals.* Chicago, IL: American Osteopathic Association. (Level VII)
18 The Joint Commission. (2015). Standard RC.01.03.01. *Comprehensive accreditation manual for hospitals: The official handbook.* Oakbrook Terrace, IL: The Joint Commission. (Level VII)
19 American Osteopathic Association. (2014). Standard 10.00.03. *Healthcare Facilities Accreditation Program: Accreditation requirements for acute care hospitals.* Chicago, IL: American Osteopathic Association. (Level VII)
20 Centers for Medicare & Medicaid Services, Department of Health and Human Services. (2014). Condition of participation: Medical record services. 42 C.F.R. § 482.24(b).
21 American Association of Critical-Care Nurses (AACN). (2010). "AACN practice alert: Family presence during resuscitation and invasive procedures" [Online]. Accessed March 2015 via the Web at http://www.aacn.org/wd/practice/docs/practicealerts/family%20presence%2004-2010%20final.pdf

ADDITIONAL REFERENCE

Nettina, S. M. (2014). *Lippincott manual of nursing practice* (10th ed.). Philadelphia, PA: Wolters Kluwer.

DISCHARGE

Although discharge from a health care facility is usually considered routine, effective discharge requires careful planning and continuing assessment of the patient's needs during his hospitalization. Ideally, discharge planning begins shortly after admission.[1,2,3,4] Discharge planning aims to teach the patient and his family about his illness and its effect on his lifestyle, to provide instructions for home care, to communicate dietary or activity instructions, and to explain the purpose, adverse effects, and scheduling of drug treatment.[3,4] It can also include arranging for transportation, follow-up care if necessary, and coordination of outpatient or home health care services.

Equipment

Wheelchair, unless the patient leaves by ambulance ▪ patient's medical record ▪ patient instruction sheet ▪ appropriate forms and written information ▪ discharge summary sheet ▪ plastic bag or patient's suitcase for personal belongings ▪ equipment for vital signs measurement ▪ hospital-grade disinfectant.

Implementation

- Perform hand hygiene.[5,6,7,8,9]
- Confirm the patient's identity using at least two patient identifiers.[10]
- Inform the patient's family of the time and date of discharge as soon as it's known. If the patient's family can't arrange transportation, notify the social services department. (Always confirm arranged transportation on the day of discharge.)[2,3,4]
- Obtain a written discharge order from the practitioner. If the patient discharges himself against medical advice, obtain the appropriate form. (See *Dealing with a discharge against medical advice.*)[3]
- If the patient requires home medical care, confirm arrangements with the appropriate facility department or community agency.[4,11]
- Review the patient's discharge care plan, initiated on admission and modified during his hospitalization, with the patient and his family.[1,3,4] List prescribed drugs on the patient instruction sheet along with the dosage, prescribed time schedule, and adverse reactions that he should report to the practitioner.[12,13] Ensure that the drug schedule is consistent with the patient's lifestyle *to prevent improper administration and to promote patient compliance.* Remind the patient to discard old medication lists when he returns home.
- Review procedures the patient or his family will perform at home. If necessary, demonstrate these procedures, provide written instructions, and check performance with a return demonstration.[3,4]
- List dietary and activity instructions on the patient instruction sheet, if applicable, and review the reasons for them. If the practitioner orders bed rest, make sure the patient's family can provide daily care and will obtain necessary equipment.[3,4]
- Check with the practitioner about the patient's next office appointment; if the practitioner hasn't yet done so, inform the patient of the date, time, and location. If scheduling is your responsibility, make an appointment with the practitioner, outpatient clinic, physical therapy, X-ray department, or other health services, as needed. If the patient can't arrange transportation to these appointments, notify the social services department.[2,3,4]
- Retrieve the patient's valuables from the facility's safe and review each item with him. Then obtain the patient's signature *to verify receipt of his valuables.*
- Instruct the patient to give a list of medications to his practitioner; to update the information when medications are discontinued, dosages are changed, or new medications (including over-the-counter products) are added; and carry a medication list that contains all of this information at all times in the event of an emergency.[12,13]
- Obtain from the pharmacy any drugs the patient brought with him. Return these to the patient if drug therapy is unchanged. If giving a new prescription, provide an explanation of the indications, dosage, schedule, and adverse effects.[12]
- Provide the patient (and his family as needed) with written information on the medications he should be taking upon discharge.[12]
- If the patient is being discharged to another facility, such as an assisted-living or long-term care facility, or if the patient will be followed up at home by a home care agency, make sure that the reconciled list of the patient's medications is communicated to the next practitioner who will be caring for the patient and that the communication is documented in the patient's medical record *to reduce the risk of transition-related medication events.* If the next practitioner is unknown, make sure that the list is given to the patient or, if appropriate, his family.[2,4,11,12]
- Ask the patient, responsible family member, or caregiver to verbalize their understanding of the discharge instructions.
- Have the patient, responsible family member, or caregiver sign the discharge instruction sheet attesting to receipt of the information.
- Sign and date the form as required by your facility and give the original to the patient, responsible family member, or caregiver.
- If appropriate, perform hand hygiene,[5,6,7,8] obtain the patient's vital signs, and record them on the discharge summary form. Notify the practitioner if any signs are abnormal, such as an elevated temperature. *If necessary, the practitioner may alter the patient's discharge plan.*
- Before the patient is discharged, perform a physical assessment. If you detect abnormal signs or if the patient develops new symptoms, notify the practitioner and delay discharge until he has seen the patient.

Dealing with a discharge against medical advice

Occasionally, the patient or his family may demand discharge against medical advice (AMA). If this situation occurs, notify the practitioner immediately. If the practitioner fails to convince the patient to remain in the facility, he'll ask the patient to sign an AMA form releasing the facility from legal responsibility for any medical problems the patient may experience after discharge.

If the practitioner isn't available, discuss the discharge form with the patient and obtain his signature. If the patient refuses to sign the AMA form, don't detain him. *Detaining him violates his legal rights.* After the patient leaves, document the incident thoroughly in your notes, complete an incident report according to facility policy, and notify the practitioner.

Adapted from Videbeck, S. L. (2014). *Psychiatric-mental health nursing* (6th ed.). Philadelphia, PA: Wolters Kluwer.

PATIENT TEACHING

Discharge teaching goals

Your discharge teaching should aim to ensure that the patient:
- understands his illness
- understands and can manage medications, schedules, and information
- carefully follows his diet
- manages his activity level
- understands his treatments
- recognizes his need for rest
- knows about possible complications
- knows when and where to seek follow-up care
- is aware of available community resources as needed.

Remember that your discharge teaching must include the patient's family or other caregivers *to ensure that the patient receives proper home care.*[2,3]

- Ensure that all devices, such as IV catheters, indwelling urinary catheters, and drains that have been discontinued by the ordering practitioner, have been properly removed before *discharge to avoid potential complications.*
- Help the patient get dressed if necessary.
- Collect the patient's personal belongings from his room, compare them with the admission inventory of belongings, and help place them in his suitcase or a plastic bag.
- After checking the room for misplaced belongings, help the patient into the wheelchair, and escort him to the exit; if the patient is leaving by ambulance, help him onto the stretcher.
- After the patient has left the area, strip the bed linens and notify the housekeeping staff that the room is ready for cleaning.
- Clean and disinfect reusable equipment using a hospital-grade disinfectant.[14,15]
- Perform hand hygiene.[5,6,7,8,9]
- Document the procedure.[16,17,18]

Special considerations

- Whenever possible, involve the patient's family in discharge planning *so they can better understand and perform patient care procedures.*[2,3,4]

Patient teaching

Patient teaching provides patients and their caregivers with the knowledge and skills that they need to manage their health care need when they are discharged. (See *Discharge teaching goals.*)

Documentation

Although your facility determines the extent and form of discharge documentation, you'll usually record the time and date of discharge; vital signs, physical assessment results if applicable, and any devices that remain in the patient and that have been removed; family members or caregivers present for teaching; details of instructions given to the patient, including medications, activity, diet, treatments, and the use of medical equipment; signs and symptoms to report to the practitioner; and the date, time, and locations of follow-up appointments.[17,19]

REFERENCES

1 The Joint Commission. (2015). Standard PC.04.01.01. *Comprehensive accreditation manual for hospitals: The official handbook.* Oakbrook Terrace, IL: The Joint Commission. (Level VII)

2 The Joint Commission. (2015). Standard PC.04.01.03. *Comprehensive accreditation manual for hospitals: The official handbook.* Oakbrook Terrace, IL: The Joint Commission. (Level VII)

3 The Joint Commission. (2015). Standard PC.04.01.05. *Comprehensive accreditation manual for hospitals: The official handbook.* Oakbrook Terrace, IL: The Joint Commission. (Level VII)

4 Centers for Medicare & Medicaid Services, Department of Health and Human Services. (2014). Condition of participation: Discharge planning. 42 C.F.R. § 482.43.

5 The Joint Commission. (2015). Standard NPSG.07.01.01. *Comprehensive accreditation manual for hospitals: The official handbook.* Oakbrook Terrace, IL: The Joint Commission. (Level VII)

6 Centers for Disease Control and Prevention. (2002). Guideline for hand hygiene in health-care settings: Recommendations of the Healthcare Infection Control Practices Advisory Committee and the HICPAC/SHEA/APIC/IDSA Hand Hygiene Task Force. *MMWR Recommendations and Reports, 51*(RR-16), 1–45. Accessed March 2015 via the Web at http://www.cdc.gov/mmwr/pdf/rr/rr5116.pdf (Level II)

7 World Health Organization. (2009). "WHO guidelines on hand hygiene in health care: First global patient safety challenge, clean care is safer care" [Online]. Accessed March 2015 via the Web at http://whqlibdoc.who.int/publications/2009/9789241597906_eng.pdf (Level IV)

8 Centers for Medicare & Medicaid Services, Department of Health and Human Services. (2014). Condition of participation: Infection control. 42 C.F.R. § 482.42.

9 American Osteopathic Association. (2014). Standard 07.01.21. *Healthcare Facilities Accreditation Program: Accreditation requirements for acute care hospitals.* Chicago, IL: American Osteopathic Association. (Level VII)

10 The Joint Commission. (2015). Standard NPSG.01.01.01. *Comprehensive accreditation manual for hospitals: The official handbook.* Oakbrook Terrace, IL: The Joint Commission. (Level VII)

11 The Joint Commission. (2015). Standard PC.04.02.01. *Comprehensive accreditation manual for hospitals: The official handbook.* Oakbrook Terrace, IL: The Joint Commission. (Level VII)

12 The Joint Commission. (2015). Standard NPSG.03.06.01. *Comprehensive accreditation manual for hospitals: The official handbook.* Oakbrook Terrace, IL: The Joint Commission. (Level VII)

13 American Osteopathic Association. (2014). Standard 25.02.13. *Healthcare Facilities Accreditation Program: Accreditation requirements for acute care hospitals.* Chicago, IL: American Osteopathic Association. (Level VII)

14 Rutala, W. A., et al. (2008). "Guideline for disinfection and sterilization in healthcare facilities, 2008" [Online]. Accessed March 2015 via the Web at http://www.cdc.gov/hicpac/pdf/guidelines/Disinfection_Nov_2008.pdf (Level I)

15 American Osteopathic Association. (2014). Standard 07.02.03. *Healthcare Facilities Accreditation Program: Accreditation requirements for acute care hospitals.* Chicago, IL: American Osteopathic Association. (Level VII)

16 The Joint Commission. (2015). Standard RC.01.03.01. *Comprehensive accreditation manual for hospitals: The official handbook.* Oakbrook Terrace, IL: The Joint Commission. (Level VII)

17 Centers for Medicare & Medicaid Services, Department of Health and Human Services. (2014). Condition of participation: Medical record services. 42 C.F.R. § 482.24(b).

18 American Osteopathic Association. (2014). Standard 10.00.03. *Healthcare Facilities Accreditation Program: Accreditation requirements for acute care hospitals.* Chicago, IL: American Osteopathic Association. (Level VII)

19 The Joint Commission. (2015). Standard RC.02.04.01. *Comprehensive accreditation manual for hospitals: The official handbook.* Oakbrook Terrace, IL: The Joint Commission. (Level VII)

ADDITIONAL REFERENCE

Videbeck, S. L. (2014). *Psychiatric-mental health nursing* (6th ed.). Philadelphia, PA: Wolters Kluwer.

DOCUMENTATION

Documentation is the process of preparing a complete record of a patient's care and is a vital tool for communication among health care team members. Accurate, detailed documentation shows the extent and quality of the care that nurses provide, the outcomes of that care, and treatment and education that the patient still needs. Thorough, accurate documentation decreases the potential for miscommunication and errors.

Documentation is a valuable method for demonstrating that the nurse has applied nursing knowledge, skills, and judgment according to professional nursing standards. In a court of law, the patient's health record serves as the legal record of the care provided to that patient. Accrediting agencies and risk managers use the medical record to evaluate the quality of care a patient receives. Insurance companies use documentation systems to verify the care received. Nursing documentation in the medical record may also be used for research and education as well as for quality improvement programs.

Equipment

Medical record (electronic or written) ▪ pen with black or blue ink, if using a written medical record.

Preparation of equipment

Various systems are available for documentation. Because each documentation system follows specific policies and procedures for charting, you should familiarize yourself with the requirements of each system. (See *Comparing charting systems.*)

Implementation

- Understand your state's nurse practice act and make sure your documentation reflects the state's laws governing the scope of nursing practice.[1]

Paper-based documentation

- Write legibly *because illegible entries can result in misinterpretation of information and possible patient harm.*
- Use ink *because the medical record is a permanent document and ink can't be erased.*
- Sign all entries using your first and last name and title *to clearly identify who wrote the entry.*[2,3,4,5]
- When signing your initials on a form, use your full signature in the appropriate place on the form *to identify yourself as the care provider.*[2,3,4,5]
- Stamp each sheet of the medical record with the patient's identifying information *to avoid documenting on the wrong patient or mistaking the patient for another.*
- If you make an error, draw a single line through the mistake and make a notation, such as "documentation error," and initial it along with the date and time, as required by your facility. Then, record the correct entry. Don't use correction fluid, erasures, or entries between lines.
- Don't leave blank lines within and between entries. Draw a line through the blank line *to ensure that no further entries may be made.*
- Document chronologically, using the correct time and date. Avoid block documentation, *which is vague, implies inattention to the patient, and makes it hard to determine when specific events occurred.*[4,5,6]
- When documentation continues from one page to the next, sign the bottom of the first page. At the top of the next page, write the date, the time, and "continued from previous page."
- Document the time as required by your facility using 24-hour military time or including "a.m." or "p.m."
- If you need to add a late entry, such as an event that you forgot to document earlier or when the medical record wasn't available, add the entry on the next available line and label it as a "late entry" *to show it's out of sequence.* Then record the date and time of the entry as well as the date and time when the entry should have been made.

Computer-based documentation

- Specifically state in the body of your note the time that events occurred and action was taken *because most computer systems record the date and time that entries are made, which may not reflect when the care was actually provided.*[4,5,7]
- Document time as required by your facility, using either 24-hour military time or including "a.m." or "p.m."
- Make sure that no one else can read the screen, and log off when you are finished documenting. Never share your password with anyone else.[4,5,7]
- Know that most software programs establish an electronic signature based on your personal user password.[2,3,4,5]
- Follow your facility's guidelines for correcting errors, such as documenting on the wrong chart.

Completing the procedure

- Document information as soon as possible *to ensure the accuracy of the information and to reflect ongoing care. Delayed documentation increases the potential for omissions, error, and inaccuracy due to memory lapse.*[4,5,7]
- Document only care, treatments, and medications that have actually been provided or administered; never chart in advance.[4,5,7]
- Describe observations and behaviors of the patient rather than label the patient. Don't offer opinions or use subjective statements or judgments.
- Use correct spelling and grammar in your entries *because misspelled words and poor grammar look unprofessional and can lead to errors.*
- Use only approved abbreviations. (See *Abbreviations to avoid,* page 248.)[8]

Special considerations

- Maintain the confidentiality of the medical record at all times. Keep the medical record closed when not in use and store it in a secure place.
- Never tamper with documentation or any part of the clinical record; tampering includes adding to a clinical note at a later date without indicating that it's a late entry, inserting inaccurate information in the record, purposely omitting information, rewriting or altering the documentation, destroying clinical record notes or other documentation, or adding to someone else's notes without indicating your identity and the date.
- If information listed on a form doesn't apply to your patient, write "N/A" (not applicable) rather than leaving the space blank. *This notation shows that you read the question and that it doesn't apply rather than that you forgot to gather the data. It also prevents someone else from adding the information later.*

Comparing charting systems

System	Useful settings	Parts of record	Assessment	Care plan	Outcomes and evaluations	Progress notes format
Narrative	■ Acute care ■ Long-term care ■ Home care ■ Ambulatory care	■ Progress notes ■ Flow sheets to supplement care plan	■ Initial: history and admission form ■ Ongoing: progress notes	■ Care plan	■ Progress notes ■ Discharge summaries	■ Narration at time of entry
Problem-oriented medical record (POMR)	■ Acute care ■ Long-term care ■ Home care ■ Rehabilitation ■ Mental health facilities	■ Database ■ Care plan ■ Problem list ■ Progress notes ■ Discharge summary	■ Initial: database and care plan ■ Ongoing: progress notes	■ Database ■ Nursing care plan based on problem list	■ Progress notes (section E of SOAPIE and SOAPIER)	■ SOAP, SOAPIE, SOAPIER (acronym for subjective, objective, assessment, plan, intervention, evaluation, revision)
Problem-intervention-evaluation (PIE)	■ Acute care	■ Assessment flow sheets ■ Progress notes ■ Problem list	■ Initial: assessment form ■ Ongoing: assessment form every shift	■ None; included in progress notes (section P)	■ Progress notes (section E of PIE)	■ Problem ■ Intervention ■ Evaluation
FOCUS	■ Acute care ■ Long-term care	■ Progress notes ■ Flow sheets ■ Checklists	■ Initial: patient history and admission assessment ■ Ongoing: assessment form	■ Nursing care plan based on problems or nursing diagnoses	■ Progress notes	■ Data ■ Action ■ Response
Charting by exception (CBE)	■ Acute care ■ Long-term care	■ Care plan ■ Flow sheets, including patient-teaching records and patient-discharge notes ■ Graphic record ■ Progress notes	■ Initial: database assessment sheet ■ Ongoing: nursing and medical order flow sheets	■ Nursing care plan based on nursing diagnoses	■ Progress notes (section E of CBE)	■ SOAPIE or SOAPIER
Flow sheet, assessment, concise, timely (FACT)	■ Acute care ■ Long-term care	■ Assessment sheet ■ Flow sheets ■ Progress notes	■ Initial: baseline assessment ■ Ongoing: flow sheets and progress notes	■ Nursing care plan based on nursing diagnoses	■ Flow sheets	■ Data ■ Action ■ Response
Core	■ Acute care ■ Long-term care	■ Kardex ■ Flow sheets ■ Progress notes	■ Initial: baseline assessment ■ Ongoing: progress notes	■ Care plan	■ Progress notes (section E of DAE)	■ Data ■ Action ■ Evaluation
Computerized	■ Acute care ■ Long-term care ■ Home care ■ Ambulatory care	■ Progress notes ■ Flow sheets ■ Nursing care plan ■ Database ■ Teaching plan	■ Initial: baseline assessment ■ Ongoing: progress notes	■ Database ■ Care plan	■ Outcome-based care plan	■ Evaluative statements ■ Expected outcomes ■ Learning outcomes

Documentation

Document the patient's vital signs, your assessment findings, the patient's care plan, your interventions, the patient's response to your interventions, and patient and family teaching According to your facility's documentation system.

REFERENCES

1 Anders, J., & Daly, T. (2009). "The crucial role of the nurse in EHR implementation" [Online]. Accessed March 2015 via the Web at http://www.healthleadersmedia.com/content/242945.pdf

Abbreviations to avoid[8]

To reduce the risk of medical errors, The Joint Commission has created a "Do Not Use" list of abbreviations. The list applies to all orders and medication-related documentation that's handwritten, part of a free-text computer entry, or on preprinted forms.

ABBREVIATION	POTENTIAL PROBLEM	PREFERRED TERM
U (for "unit")	Mistaken as zero, four, or cc.	Write "unit."
IU (for "international unit")	Mistaken as IV (intravenous) or 10 (ten).	Write "international unit."
Q.D., Q.O.D, QD, QOD, q.d., q.o.d., qd, qod (Latin abbreviations for "once daily" and "every other day")	Mistaken for each other. The period after the "Q" can be mistaken for an "I" and the "O" can be mistaken for "I."	Write "daily" and "every other day."
Trailing zero (X.0 mg) (Note: Prohibited only for medication-related notations); lack of leading zero (.X mg)	Decimal point is missed.	Never write a zero by itself after a decimal point (X mg), and always use a zero before a decimal point (0.X mg).
MS MSO4 MgSO4	Confused for one another. Can mean "morphine sulfate" or "magnesium sulfate."	Write "morphine sulfate" or "magnesium sulfate."

2 The Joint Commission. (2015). Standard RC.01.02.01. *Comprehensive accreditation manual for hospitals: The official handbook.* Oakbrook Terrace, IL: The Joint Commission. (Level VII)

3 Centers for Medicare & Medicaid Services, Department of Health and Human Services. (2014). Condition of participation: Nursing services. 42 C.F.R. § 482.23

4 Centers for Medicare & Medicaid Services, Department of Health and Human Services. (2014). Condition of participation: Medical record services. 42 C.F.R. § 482.24(b).

5 American Osteopathic Association. (2014). Standard 10.00.03. *Healthcare Facilities Accreditation Program: Accreditation requirements for acute care hospitals.* Chicago, IL: American Osteopathic Association. (Level VII)

6 The Joint Commission. (2015). Standard RC.01.01.01. *Comprehensive accreditation manual for hospitals: The official handbook.* Oakbrook Terrace, IL: The Joint Commission. (Level VII)

7 The Joint Commission. (2015). Standard RC.01.03.01. *Comprehensive accreditation manual for hospitals: The official handbook.* Oakbrook Terrace, IL: The Joint Commission. (Level VII)

8 The Joint Commission. (2015). Standard IM.02.02.01. *Comprehensive accreditation manual for hospitals: The official handbook.* Oakbrook Terrace, IL: The Joint Commission. (Level VII)

ADDITIONAL REFERENCES

Collins, S. A., et al. (2013). Relationship between nursing documentation and patients' mortality. *American Journal of Critical Care, 22,* 306–313. (Level VI)

The Joint Commission. (2013). "Facts about the official 'Do Not Use' List" [Online]. Accessed March 2015 via the Web at http://www.jointcommission.org/assets/1/18/Do_Not_Use_List.pdf

The Joint Commission. (2015). Standard IM.02.01.03. *Comprehensive accreditation manual for hospitals: The official handbook.* Oakbrook Terrace, IL: The Joint Commission. (Level VII)

Kelley, T. F., et al. (2011). Electronic nursing documentation as a strategy to improve quality of patient care. *Journal of Nursing Scholarship, 43,* 154–162. (Level V)

Kirkendall, E. S., et al. (2013). Transitioning from a computerized provider order entry and paper documentation system to an electronic health record: Expectations and experiences of hospital staff. *International Journal of Medical Informatics, 82,* 1037–1045. (Level IV)

Yee, T., et al. (2012). The influence of integrated electronic medical records and computerized nursing notes on nurses' time spent in documentation. *Computers, Informatics, Nursing, 30,* 287–292. (Level VI)

DOPPLER USE

More sensitive than palpation for determining pulse rate, the Doppler ultrasound blood flow detector is especially useful when a pulse is faint or weak. Unlike palpation, which detects arterial wall expansion and retraction, this instrument detects the motion of red blood cells (RBCs). Doppler ultrasound is also commonly used to measure blood pressure in low-flow states, to evaluate lower extremity peripheral perfusion, and to asses fetal heart sounds after the first trimester of pregnancy.[1,2,3,4]

Equipment

Doppler ultrasound blood flow detector ▪ coupling or transmission gel ▪ soft cloth ▪ hospital-grade disinfectant.

Implementation

- Gather the necessary equipment
- Perform hand hygiene.[5,6,7,8,9]
- Confirm the patient's identity using at least two patient identifiers.[10]
- Explain the procedure to the patient.
- Apply a small amount of coupling or transmission gel (not water-soluble lubricant) to the ultrasound probe.
- Position the probe on the skin directly over the selected artery.
- When using a Doppler model with a speaker, turn on the instrument and set the volume control to the lowest setting. If your model doesn't have a speaker, plug in the earphones and slowly raise the volume.
- *To obtain the best signal,* tilt the probe 45 degrees from the artery, making sure to put gel between the skin and the probe.[11] Slowly move the probe in a circular motion *to locate the center of the artery and the Doppler signal*—a pulsatile hissing noise that occurs as blood flows through the artery with each heartbeat. Avoid moving the probe rapidly *because doing so creates interference and distorts the signal.*
- Count the number of signals for 60 seconds *to determine the pulse rate.*

■ After you've measured the pulse rate, turn off the device.
■ Wipe the gel from the patient and the probe using a soft cloth, and then clean and disinfect the probe and unit following the manufacturer's instructions.[11,12,13] Don't immerse the probe or bump it against a hard surface.
■ Perform hand hygiene.[5,6,7,8,9]
■ Document the procedure.[14,15,16]

Special considerations

■ A Doppler ultrasound stethoscope is basically a stethoscope fitted with an audio unit, volume control, and transducer, which amplifies the movement of RBCs.
■ Complete Doppler ultrasound assessment requires listening to and interpreting various signals transmitted from the Doppler probe. An experienced Doppler user can recognize the characteristic sounds of open and obstructed arteries. Doppler sounds vary in pitch (frequency) with the velocity of blood flow.[17]

Documentation

Record the location and quality of the pulse as well as the pulse rate and time of measurement. Document patient teaching performed and the patient's comprehension of that teaching.

REFERENCES

1 Hotoleanu, C., et al. (2010). Correlations between clinical probability and Doppler ultrasound results in the assessment of deep venous thrombosis. *Medical Ultrasonography, 12,* 17–21. Accessed March 2015 via the Web at http://www.medultrason.ro/assets/Magazines/Medultrason-2010-vol12-no1/04Hotoleanu.pdf
2 Chesbro, S. B., et al. (2011). Reliability of Doppler and stethoscope methods of determining systolic blood pressures: Considerations for calculating an ankle-brachial index. *Journal of the National Medical Association, 103,* 863–869. (Level VI)
3 Calabia, J., et al. (2011). Doppler ultrasound in the measurement of pulse wave velocity: Agreement with the Complior method. *Cardiovascular Ultrasound, 9*(1), 13–18. Accessed March 2015 via the Web at http://www.cardiovascularultrasound.com/content/pdf/1476-7120-9-13.pdf (Level VI)
4 Jezewski, J., et al. (2011). A novel technique for fetal heart rate estimation from Doppler ultrasound signal. *Biomedical Engineering Online, 10,* 92.
5 The Joint Commission. (2015). Standard NPSG.07.01.01. *Comprehensive accreditation manual for hospitals: The official handbook.* Oakbrook Terrace, IL: The Joint Commission. (Level VII)
6 Centers for Disease Control and Prevention. (2002). Guideline for hand hygiene in health-care settings: Recommendations of the Healthcare Infection Control Practices Advisory Committee and the HICPAC/SHEA/APIC/IDSA Hand Hygiene Task Force. *MMWR Recommendations and Reports, 51*(RR-16), 1–45. Accessed March 2015 via the Web at http://www.cdc.gov/mmwr/pdf/rr/rr5116.pdf (Level II)
7 World Health Organization. (2009). "WHO guidelines on hand hygiene in health care: First global patient safety challenge, clean care is safer care" [Online]. Accessed March 2015 via the Web at http://whqlibdoc.who.int/publications/2009/9789241597906_eng.pdf (Level IV)
8 American Osteopathic Association. (2014). Standard 07.01.21. *Healthcare Facilities Accreditation Program: Accreditation requirements for acute care hospitals.* Chicago, IL: American Osteopathic Association. (Level VII)
9 Centers for Medicare & Medicaid Services, Department of Health and Human Services. (2014). Condition of participation: Infection control. 42 C.F.R. § 482.42.
10 The Joint Commission. (2015). Standard NPSG.01.01.01. *Comprehensive accreditation manual for hospitals: The official handbook.* Oakbrook Terrace, IL: The Joint Commission. (Level VII)
11 Summit Doppler Systems. (n.d.). "LifeDop ABI vascular system: User manual" [Online]. Accessed March 2015 via the Web at http://www.summitdoppler.com/site/files/969/108804/373733/512490/LifeDop_ABI_Manual_-_AB_&_AC_Models.pdf
12 Rutala, W. A., et al. (2008). "Guideline for disinfection and sterilization in healthcare facilities, 2008" [Online]. Accessed March 2015 via the Web at http://www.cdc.gov/hicpac/pdf/guidelines/Disinfection_Nov_2008.pdf (Level I)
13 American Osteopathic Association. (2014). Standard 07.02.03. *Healthcare Facilities Accreditation Program: Accreditation requirements for acute care hospitals.* Chicago, IL: American Osteopathic Association. (Level VII)
14 The Joint Commission. (2015). Standard RC.01.03.01. *Comprehensive accreditation manual for hospitals: The official handbook.* Oakbrook Terrace, IL: The Joint Commission. (Level VII)
15 American Osteopathic Association. (2014). Standard 10.00.03. *Healthcare Facilities Accreditation Program: Accreditation requirements for acute care hospitals.* Chicago, IL: American Osteopathic Association. (Level VII)
16 Centers for Medicare & Medicaid Services, Department of Health and Human Services. (2014). Condition of participation: Medical record services. 42 C.F.R. § 482.24(b).
17 Beldon, P. (2010). Performing a Doppler assessment: The procedure. *Wound Essentials, 5,* 87–90. Accessed March 2015 via the Web at http://www.wounds-uk.com/pdf/content_9496.pdf

DROPLET PRECAUTIONS

Droplet precautions prevent infectious pathogens from traveling from the respiratory tract of an infectious person to the mucous membranes of a susceptible host.[1] These pathogens, which are carried by respiratory droplets, spread when an infected individual coughs, sneezes, or talks during such procedures as suctioning or endotracheal intubation. (See *Conditions requiring droplet precautions,* page 250.)

Ideally, a patient requiring droplet precautions should be placed in a single-patient room.[1] People having direct contact with the patient and those who will be within 3′ (1 M) of him should wear a surgical mask covering their nose and mouth. When exposure to a highly virulent pathogen is likely, it may be prudent to wear a mask when within 6′ to 10′ (2 to 3 M) of the patient or upon entering the patient's room.[1]

As a general precaution, instruct anyone who enters your health care facility with signs of a respiratory infection (such as cough, congestion, rhinorrhea, or increased respiratory secretions) to cover his mouth and nose with a tissue when coughing and have him dispose of soiled tissues promptly.[2] Have him wear a surgical mask, if tolerated, and instruct him to perform hand hygiene after contact with respiratory secretions.[1] If possible, separate him by at least 3′ (0.9 M) from other people in common waiting areas to prevent the spread of infection.[1] These actions can help prevent the spread of infectious pathogens until appropriate isolation precautions are established.

PEDIATRIC ALERT *When handling infants or young children who require droplet precautions, you may also need to institute contact precautions and wear gloves and a* gown to prevent soiling of clothing from nasal and oral secretions.

Equipment

Mask ■ tissues ■ droplet precautions sign ■ hospital-grade disinfectant ■ Optional: gowns, gloves, no-touch tissue disposal receptacle.

Preparation of equipment

Keep all droplet precaution supplies outside the patient's room in a cart or anteroom.

Implementation

■ Put a droplet precautions sign at the patient's door *to notify anyone entering the room of the situation.*[4,5,6]
■ Perform hand hygiene.[5,7,8,9,10]
■ Put on a gown, if necessary, *to comply with standard precautions.*[1]

Conditions requiring droplet precautions[1]

These conditions require droplet precautions because they can be transmitted via respiratory droplets from infectious patients.

Condition	Precautionary period	Special considerations (as applicable)
Adenovirus infection in infants and young children	▪ For duration of illness	▪ Institute contact precautions in addition to droplet precautions. ▪ Prolonged viral shedding occurs in immunocompromised patients.
Diphtheria (pharyngeal)	▪ Until antibiotics are completed and two cultures taken at least 24 hours apart are negative	
Haemophilus influenzae type b disease, including epiglottitis, meningitis, pneumonia, and sepsis	▪ Until 24 hours after initiation of effective therapy	
Influenza (seasonal)	▪ For 5 days after onset of signs and symptoms ▪ For duration of illness in immunocompromised patients	▪ Viral shedding is prolonged in immunocompromised patients.
Mumps	▪ For 9 days after onset of swelling[3]	▪ Susceptible health care workers shouldn't provide care if immune caregivers are available.
Mycoplasma pneumoniae infection	▪ For duration of illness	
Neisseria meningitidis disease, including meningitis, pneumonia, and sepsis	▪ Until 24 hours after initiation of effective therapy	▪ Household contacts should receive postexposure prophylactic antibiotic therapy. ▪ Health care workers exposed to respiratory secretions should receive postexposure prophylactic antibiotic therapy. ▪ Postexposure vaccine may be given to control outbreaks.
Parvovirus B19 (erythema infectiosum)	▪ For duration of hospitalization for chronic disease that occurs in immunocompromised patients ▪ For 7 days in patients with transient aplastic crisis or red-cell crisis	▪ Duration of precautions for immunosuppressed patients with persistently positive polymerase chain reaction is unknown, but transmission has occurred.
Pertussis (whooping cough)	▪ Until 5 days after initiation of effective therapy	▪ Household contacts should receive postexposure prophylaxis. ▪ Health care workers with prolonged exposure to respiratory secretions should receive postexposure prophylaxis.
Pneumonic plague	▪ Until 48 hours after initiation of effective therapy	▪ Exposed health care workers should receive postexposure prophylactic antibiotics.
Rhinovirus	▪ For duration of illness	▪ Also institute contact precautions if contact with copious moist secretions is likely.
Rubella (German measles)	▪ Until 7 days after onset of rash	▪ Susceptible health care workers shouldn't enter the room if immune caregivers are available. ▪ Administer vaccine to nonpregnant susceptible individuals within 3 days of exposure. ▪ Place exposed susceptible patients on droplet precautions.

(continued)

Conditions requiring droplet precautions[1] *(continued)*

CONDITION	PRECAUTIONARY PERIOD	SPECIAL CONSIDERATIONS (AS APPLICABLE)
Severe acute respiratory distress syndrome	■ For duration of illness plus 10 days after resolution of fever	■ Airborne precautions are preferred. ■ Institute contact precautions in addition to airborne or droplet precautions. ■ Wear eye protection. ■ Vigilant environmental disinfection is required.
Streptococcal group A disease, including pharyngitis (in infants and young children), pneumonia, serious invasive wounds, and scarlet fever (in infants and young children)	■ Until 24 hours after initiation of effective therapy	■ Also institute contact precautions if skin lesions are present.
Viral hemorrhagic infection (Ebola, Lassa, Marburg, and Crimean-Congo hemorrhagic fever viruses)	■ For duration of illness	■ Also institute contact precautions. ■ Wear eye protection. ■ Handle wastes appropriately. ■ Use an N-95 (or higher) respirator mask when performing aerosol-generating procedures. ■ Make sure public health officials are notified if Ebola is suspected.

■ Just before entering the patient's room, put on a mask and secure the ties or elastic band at the middle of the back of your head and neck. Fit the flexible metal nose strip to your nose bridge so it fits firmly but comfortably. Make sure the mask fits snugly to your face and below your chin.[1]
■ Put on gloves, if necessary, *to comply with standard precautions.*[1]
■ Confirm the patient's identity using at least two patient identifiers.[11]
■ Situate the patient in a single room with private toilet facilities and an anteroom if possible. If necessary, two patients with the same infection may share a room if approved by your facility's infection preventionist.[1]
■ Explain isolation procedures to the patient and his family *to ease patient anxiety and promote cooperation.*
■ If the patient is wearing a mask during transport to the room, remove his mask once he reaches his room and discard it in the appropriate receptacle.
■ Instruct the patient to cover his nose and mouth with a facial tissue while coughing or sneezing, dispose of the tissue immediately,[2] and then perform hand hygiene *to prevent the spread of infectious droplets.*[5,7,8,9,10]
■ Provide the patient with a no-touch receptacle for tissue disposal if available.
■ Remove your gloves and gown (if worn), and mask in the anteroom or, if an anteroom isn't available, at the patient's doorway just before leaving the room. To remove your mask, untie the strings or remove the elastic bands and dispose of the mask, handling it by the strings or elastic bands only *because the front of the mask is considered contaminated.*[1]
■ Perform hand hygiene.[5,7,8,9,10]
■ Clean and disinfect equipment that isn't dedicated for single-patient use with a hospital-grade disinfectant after use *to prevent the spread of infection to other patients.*[5,12,13,14]
■ Perform hand hygiene.[5,7,8,9,10]
■ Document the procedure.[15,16,17]

Special considerations

■ Make sure all visitors wear masks when in close proximity to the patient (within 3′ [0.9 M]) and, if necessary, gowns and gloves.[1]
■ If the patient must leave the room for essential procedures, make sure he wears a surgical mask over his nose and mouth and instruct the patient to use respiratory hygiene and proper cough etiquette.[1] Notify the receiving department or area of the patient's isolation precautions *so that the precautions will be maintained and the patient can be returned to the room promptly.*
■ *Because pathogens in respiratory droplets don't remain infectious over long distances (they generally drop to the ground within 3′ [0.9 M]),* special air handling and ventilation systems and an airborne infection isolation room with negative airflow aren't necessary.[1]
■ Perform hand hygiene, as indicated, during patient care.[5,7,8,9,10]
■ It isn't necessary for health care workers to wear masks when transporting a patient on droplet precautions *because the patient is wearing one.*[1]
■ Single-patient rooms are preferred for patients who require droplet precautions. However, when transmission continues after implementing routine infection control measures, consider creating patient and staff member cohorts. Consult with your infection preventionist before cohorting patients or staff members.[1]

Complications

Social isolation is a complication of droplet precautions.

Documentation

Record the need for droplet precautions on the nursing care plan and as otherwise indicated by your facility. Document initiation and maintenance of the precautions, the patient's compliance with droplet precautions, any patient or family teaching performed, and their understanding of the teaching. Also document the date and time droplet precautions were discontinued.

REFERENCES

1 Siegel, J. D., et al. (2007). "2007 guideline for isolation precautions: Preventing transmission of infectious agents in healthcare settings" [Online]. Accessed March 2015 via the Web at http://www.cdc.gov/hicpac/pdf/isolation/Isolation2007.pdf (Level II)

2 Centers for Disease Control and Prevention. (2009, updated 2012). "Respiratory hygiene/cough etiquette in healthcare settings" [Online]. Accessed March 2015 via the Web at http://www.cdc.gov/flu/professionals/infectioncontrol/resphygiene.htm (Level VII)

3 Centers for Disease Control and Prevention. (2008). "Updated recommendations for isolation of persons with mumps" [Online]. Accessed March 2015 via the Web at http://www.cdc.gov/mmwr/preview/mmwrhtml/mm5740a3.htm (Level VII)

4 The Joint Commission. (2015). Standard IC.02.01.01. *Comprehensive accreditation manual for hospitals: The official handbook.* Oakbrook Terrace, IL: The Joint Commission. (Level VII)

5 Centers for Medicare & Medicaid Services, Department of Health and Human Services. (2014). Condition of participation: Infection control. 42 C.F.R. § 482.42.

6 American Osteopathic Association. (2014). Standard 07.01.10. *Healthcare Facilities Accreditation Program: Accreditation requirements for acute care hospitals.* Chicago, IL: American Osteopathic Association. (Level VII)

7 The Joint Commission. (2015). Standard NPSG.07.01.01. *Comprehensive accreditation manual for hospitals: The official handbook.* Oakbrook Terrace, IL: The Joint Commission. (Level VII)

8 Centers for Disease Control and Prevention. (2002). Guideline for hand hygiene in health-care settings: Recommendations of the Healthcare Infection Control Practices Advisory Committee and the HICPAC/SHEA/APIC/IDSA Hand Hygiene Task Force. *MMWR Recommendations and Reports, 51*(RR-16), 1–45. Accessed March 2015 via the Web at http://www.cdc.gov/mmwr/pdf/rr/rr5116.pdf (Level II)

9 World Health Organization. (2009). "WHO guidelines on hand hygiene in health care: First global patient safety challenge, clean care is safer care" [Online]. Accessed March 2015 via the Web at http://whqlibdoc.who.int/publications/2009/9789241597906_eng.pdf (Level IV)

10 American Osteopathic Association. (2014). Standard 07.01.21. *Healthcare Facilities Accreditation Program: Accreditation requirements for acute care hospitals.* Chicago, IL: American Osteopathic Association. (Level VII)

11 The Joint Commission. (2015). Standard NPSG.01.01.01. *Comprehensive accreditation manual for hospitals: The official handbook.* Oakbrook Terrace, IL: The Joint Commission. (Level VII)

12 Rutala, W. A., et al. (2008). "Guideline for disinfection and sterilization in healthcare facilities, 2008" [Online]. Accessed March 2015 via the Web at http://www.cdc.gov/hicpac/pdf/guidelines/Disinfection_Nov_2008.pdf (Level I)

13 The Joint Commission. (2015). Standard IC.02.02.01. *Comprehensive accreditation manual for hospitals: The official handbook.* Oakbrook Terrace, IL: The Joint Commission. (Level VII)

14 American Osteopathic Association. (2014). Standard 07.02.03. *Healthcare Facilities Accreditation Program: Accreditation requirements for acute care hospitals.* Chicago, IL: American Osteopathic Association. (Level VII)

15 The Joint Commission. (2015). Standard RC.01.03.01. *Comprehensive accreditation manual for hospitals: The official handbook.* Oakbrook Terrace, IL: The Joint Commission. (Level VII)

16 Centers for Medicare & Medicaid Services, Department of Health and Human Services. (2014). Condition of participation: Medical record services. 42 C.F.R. § 482.24(b).

17 American Osteopathic Association. (2014). Standard 10.00.03. *Healthcare Facilities Accreditation Program: Accreditation requirements for acute care hospitals.* Chicago, IL: American Osteopathic Association. (Level VII)

ADDITIONAL REFERENCE

Craven, R. F., & Hirnle, C. J. (2012). *Fundamentals of nursing: Human health and function* (7th ed.). Philadelphia, PA: Lippincott Williams & Wilkins.

DRUG AND ALCOHOL SPECIMEN COLLECTION

Drug and alcohol specimen collection is performed to identify a patient's drug or alcohol use for several reasons, including obtaining evidence for a possible criminal charges after an accident, helping to determine a cause of death, and screening for employment suitability or adherence to an ongoing drug addiction rehabilitation program. It's also used to establish a differential diagnosis for a patient who's experiencing an altered mental state or has such signs and symptoms as slurred speech, dizziness, confusion, blurred vision, anxiety, hallucinations, memory impairment, lack of muscle coordination, or hyperthermia. The collection method and source of the specimens vary, based on the reason for testing. Because of the variability in local and state laws, nurses must strictly follow all facility guidelines.

Drug testing that's performed to determine employment suitability and rehabilitation program adherence usually involves a urine sample collected under highly controlled conditions. Although collection requirements may vary slightly, depending on the employer and type of employment or rehabilitation program, most include a designated collection site, security for the collection site, use of authorized personnel, privacy during collection, integrity and identity of the specimen, and chain-of-custody documentation. Some rehabilitation programs and employment circumstances may require the specimen collection to be observed. Testing is usually limited to five drug types: marijuana, cocaine, opiates, amphetamines, and phencyclidine (PCP). In the case of employment screening, if the results of the initial test are positive, a confirmatory test is performed using gas chromatography–mass spectrometry.

Depending on the reason for collection and your state laws, you should ensure that informed consent has been obtained from the patient or a family member before obtaining the sample. Consent may not be required if it's an emergency, if results will be used only for a differential diagnosis in an acute crisis, or if the patient is not in a condition to grant permission. In a criminal case, a law enforcement officer can't order blood to be drawn and doesn't have the legal right to grant permission if the patient refuses consent.

Blood samples, when needed, are collected in 10-mL gray-top blood collection tubes that contain a preservative (100 mg of sodium fluoride) *to help prevent deterioration of the specimen,* including changes in alcohol concentration and the breakdown of cocaine, and an anticoagulant (20 mg of potassium oxalate) *to prevent the sample from clotting.* The integrity and identity of the specimen must be maintained and, if indicated, chain-of-custody documentation preserved.

In general, prescription and over-the-counter drugs can be detected in blood within 4 to 24 hours and in urine for 2 to 4 days. Detection times for alcohol and other drugs vary. (See *Drug detection times.*)

This procedure focuses on drug and alcohol specimen collection for medicolegal reasons. When specimens are collected for a patient who's experiencing an altered mental state or other signs and symptoms, be sure to use the appropriate collection tubes. (See the "Venipuncture" procedure, page 821.)

Equipment

Gloves ▪ Optional: LIMITED ACCESS signs, shipping containers (if samples are to be sent to an outside laboratory), sphygmomanometer, stethoscope, thermometer, pulse oximeter.

Urine sample

Urine collection cup with temperature measurement device attached in sealed covering ▪ 90-mL plastic, screw-top specimen container in sealed covering ▪ adhesive label ▪ plastic sealable bag ▪ absorbent material ▪ chain-of-custody labels ▪ chain-of-custody form with multiple copies ▪ bluing agent for toilet water ▪ Optional: digital thermometer.

Blood sample

Two 10-mL gray-top blood tubes containing sodium fluoride and potassium oxalate with adhesive labels ▪ needleless blood collection tube holder ▪ venipuncture supplies ▪ nonalcohol swab (povidone-iodine) ▪ 2″ × 2″ (5-cm × 5-cm) sterile gauze pads ▪ evidence seals ▪ padded transport box ▪ biohazard laboratory transport bag ▪ chain-of-custody labels ▪ chain-of-custody form with multiple copies ▪ evidence tape ▪ Optional: soap and water.

Note: Prepackaged blood and urine collection kits for such specimens are commercially available and contain everything necessary to collect and preserve the chain of custody for the specimens.

Drug detection times

DRUG	BLOOD	URINE
Amphetamines	1 to 3 days	Typically, 1 to 5 days (sometimes longer)
Cocaine	5 to 6 hours in refrigerated blood (will break down in unrefrigerated blood)	12 hours
Cocaine metabolite	Varies	2 to 4 days
Ethanol	3 to 12 hours	3 to 12 hours
Marijuana	Infrequent user: 1 to 4 hours Frequent user: 3 to 6 hours	Not found in urine
Marijuana metabolite	Infrequent user: typically, 2 to 3 days (sometimes longer) Frequent user: 2 or more weeks	Infrequent user: 2 weeks Frequent user: 3 to 6 weeks
Opiates	1 to 4 hours	3 to 4 days
Phencyclidine (PCP)	1 to 3 days	Typically, 3 to 7 (sometimes longer)

Preparation of equipment

Make sure that access to collection materials and specimens is adequately restricted. Make sure that LIMITED ACCESS signs are posted in the specimen collection area *to ensure patient privacy during the specimen collection process.*

Implementation

- Verify the practitioner's order for drug and alcohol specimen collection.
- If required, verify that informed consent has been obtained and is included in the patient's medical record.[1,2,3]
- Perform hand hygiene.[4,5,6,7,8]
- Confirm the patient's identity using at least two patient identifiers.[9]
- Provide privcy.[10]
- Explain the appropriate procedure to the patient, allowing him to ask questions as needed.
- Assess the patient's level of consciousness and behavior.
- If applicable, obtain the patient's vital signs, including heart rate, respiratory rate, blood pressure, temperature, and pulse oximetry.
- Obtain a thorough current and past medication history that includes prescription and nonprescription drugs and herbal supplements.

Urine sample collection

- Prepare the collection site by turning off the water supply or securing water sources.[11]
- Add bluing agent to the toilet and water tank *to prevent undetected specimen dilution by the donor.*[11]
- Remove the waste container, soap dispenser, and any unnecessary items from the bathroom.[11]
- Perform hand hygiene.[4,5,6,7,8]
- Put on gloves.[12,13]
- Gather the necessary supplies or prepackaged urine collection kit.
- Instruct the patient to remove any unnecessary outer clothing, such as a coat, hat, or extra shirt. If the patient refuses to remove a head covering based on religious practices, he may be exempt unless the collector has a visual indicator that the patient may be concealing something under the covering. Keep personal items such as a briefcase or purse with the patient's outer clothing.
- Instruct the patient to empty his pockets into a lockable cabinet or box, and have him turn his pockets inside out *to ensure that they're emptied and that he doesn't have anything that could be used to adulterate the specimen.*
- Have the patient wash and dry his hands.
- Provide the patient with the sealed collection kit or container, and have him unwrap or break the seal on the kit or collection container.
- If direct observation isn't mandated for specimen collection, have the patient enter the bathroom and instruct him to provide a urine specimen of at least 30 mL into the collection cup, to not flush the toilet, to not wash his hands until told to do so after delivering the specimen to you and watching the specimen being sealed with the labels, and to immediately leave the bathroom with the specimen and hand it to you when he's finished urinating.
- If direct observation is mandated, observe the patient during the collection procedure.
- If the patient has a medical condition that requires an indwelling urinary catheter or an external urine collection bag, collect a fresh specimen. Instruct the patient to empty his urine collection bag in the bathroom and then show you the empty bag, drink sufficient fluid to provide a specimen, and pour the urine from the bag into the collection container in the privacy of the bathroom when at least 30 mL of urine has been collected.[11]
- Check the specimen's temperature by reading the temperature strip, and note it on the chain-of-custody form.
- Check the specimen volume *to ensure that the specimen contains the required amount of urine.*
- Open the sealed screw-top specimen container and transfer the urine into the container.
- Label the specimen container with the patient's name and identification number and the date and time in the presence of the patient *to prevent mislabeling.*[9]
- Complete the required information on the chain-of-custody seal, initial the seal, have the patient initial the seal, and place it over the top of the specimen container.[11]
- Turn the water on and allow the patient to wash his hands.
- Complete the chain-of-custody form and have the patient sign the form.[11]

- Give the patient a copy of the chain-of-custody form.
- Place the specimen, absorbent material, and completed chain-of-custody form in the plastic sealable shipping bag.
- Seal the bag in the presence of the patient.
- Remove and discard your gloves.[12]
- Perform hand hygiene.[4,5,6,7,8]
- Place the specimen in a secure refrigerator if it won't be immediately transported to the laboratory.
- Make sure the person who removes the specimen for transport signs the chain-of-custody form. Retain a copy and place it in the patient's medical record.
- Document the procedure.[14,15,16]

Blood sample collection

- Perform hand hygiene.[4,5,6,7,8]
- Put on gloves.[12,13]
- Gather the necessary supplies or prepackaged blood collection kit.
- If applicable, ensure that the collection is observed by the law enforcement officer as required by your facility and state law.
- Choose a venipuncture site. The most common sites are the veins in the antecubital space of the arms; however, if the patient has scarring in this area from self-injected drugs, you may need to find an alternate venipuncture site.
- Clean the skin at the venipuncture site with a nonalcohol swab such as povidone-iodine. If a nonalcohol swab isn't available, use a gauze pad with a solution of soap and water, making sure that the soap doesn't contain any alcohol.
- Use proper venipuncture technique to collect the blood sample. (See the "Venipuncture" procedure, page 821.)
- Fill the collection tubes completely *to minimize the air space above the specimen, which can change the testing results.*
- Slowly invert the tubes completely at least five times *to ensure proper mixing of the additives.* Don't shake them vigorously.
- Label the specimen tubes with the patient's name and identification number and the date and time in the presence of the patient *to prevent mislabeling.*[9] Obtain the officer's initials on the tubes, if applicable.
- Complete the required information on the evidence seals, initial the seals, and have the patient initial the seals.
- Place a completed evidence seal across the top of each tube.
- Complete the chain-of-custody labels and form, and have the patient sign the form.
- Place the tubes into a padded transport box and then into a biohazard laboratory transport bag.[17]
- Seal the bag with the chain-of-custody and evidence labels.
- Remove and discard your gloves.[12]
- Perform hand hygiene.[5,6,7,8]
- Attach the chain-of-custody form.

NURSING ALERT *Make sure you complete all of the above steps in full view of the patient and, if applicable, the appropriate law enforcement officer.*

- Place the specimen in a secure refrigerator if it won't be immediately transported to the laboratory.
- Perform hand hygiene.[4,5,6,7,8]
- Make sure the person who removes the specimen for transport signs the chain-of-custody form. Retain a copy and place it in the patient's medical record.
- Document the procedure.[14,15,16]

Special considerations

- Consent must be obtained if your state law doesn't cover the specimen collection.
- If the specimen is being collected for a law enforcement agency, make sure that an officer has notified the patient of his rights and explained the procedure before you obtain the sample.
- If the patient is a minor, permission must be obtained from the parent or legal guardian, unless state laws supersede it.
- Temperature strips attached to urine collection containers allow temperature certification between 90°F and 100°F (32.2°C and 37.8°C), which are acceptable under most standards. However, some testing standards require that the urine's temperature be taken with a digital thermometer and be between 96°F and 99°F (35.6°C and 37.2°C).
- If the specimen volume is inadequate, discard any specimen collected and the specimen collection container used for that attempt, have the patient sit in a waiting area where you can continuously observe him, and provide the patient with up to 40 ounces of water to drink (which should be evenly spread out over a 3-hour period or until he can provide an adequate specimen). Instruct the patient to tell you when he feels he can provide the specimen. If, after 3 hours, the patient can't provide a specimen, the collection should be terminated and you should notify the person who requested the test.

Complications

If specimen collection is performed with no subsequent medical follow-up, serious medical conditions may be overlooked, causing the patient to experience adverse effects. Mishandling of the specimen or improper documentation of the chain of custody may lead to the evidence being inaccurate or inadmissible in court.

There are many ways for patients to circumvent testing: adding adulterants to urine at the time of testing, diluting urine through excessive water ingestion, consuming substances that interfere with testing, and substituting a clean urine sample. Appropriate collection techniques and tests of specimen integrity can reduce the risk of tampering.[18]

Documentation

Record the date and time, what test is being performed, the reason for the test, and the type of specimen that was obtained. Note whether a law enforcement officer was present for the specimen collection, including the agency he represented and his badge number. Document that the chain of custody was preserved.

REFERENCES

1 The Joint Commission. (2015). Standard RI.01.03.01. *Comprehensive accreditation manual for hospitals: The official handbook.* Oakbrook Terrace, IL: The Joint Commission. (Level VII)

2 Centers for Medicare & Medicaid Services, Department of Health and Human Services. (2014). Condition of participation: Patient's rights. 42 C.F.R. § 482.13(b)(2).

3 American Osteopathic Association. (2014). Standard 15.01.11. *Healthcare Facilities Accreditation Program: Accreditation requirements for acute care hospitals.* Chicago, IL: American Osteopathic Association. (Level VII)

4 Centers for Disease Control and Prevention. (2002). Guideline for hand hygiene in health care settings: Recommendations of the Healthcare Infection Control Practices Advisory Committee and the HICPAC/SHEA/APIC/IDSA Hand Hygiene Task Force. *MMWR Recommendations and Reports, 51*(RR-16), 1–45. Accessed March 2015 via the Web at http://www.cdc.gov/mmwr/pdf/rr/rr5116.pdf (Level II)

5 The Joint Commission. (2015). Standard NPSG.07.01.01. *Comprehensive accreditation manual for hospitals: The official handbook.* Oakbrook Terrace, IL: The Joint Commission. (Level VII)

6 World Health Organization. (2009). "WHO guidelines on hand hygiene in health care: First global patient safety challenge, clean care is safer care" [Online]. Accessed March 2015 via the Web at http://whqlibdoc.who.int/publications/2009/9789241597906_eng.pdf (Level IV)

7 Centers for Medicare & Medicaid Services, Department of Health and Human Services. (2014). Condition of participation: Infection control. 42 C.F.R. § 482.42.

8 American Osteopathic Association. (2014). Standard 07.01.21. *Healthcare Facilities Accreditation Program: Accreditation requirements for acute care hospitals.* Chicago, IL: American Osteopathic Association. (Level VII)

D

Five stages of dying

According to Elisabeth Kübler-Ross, author of *On Death and Dying,* the dying patient may progress through five psychological stages in preparation for death. Although each patient experiences these stages differently, and not necessarily in this order, understanding them will help you meet your patient's needs.

Denial

When the patient first learns of his terminal illness, he may refuse to accept the diagnosis. He may experience physical signs and symptoms similar to a stress reaction—shock, fainting, pallor, sweating, tachycardia, nausea, and GI disorders. During this stage, be honest with the patient but not blunt or callous. Maintain communication with him so he can discuss his feelings when he accepts the reality of death. Don't force the patient to confront this reality.

Anger

After the patient stops denying his impending death, he may show deep resentment toward those who will live on after he dies—to you, to the facility staff, and to his own family. Although you may instinctively draw back from the patient or even resent this behavior, remember that he is dying and has a right to be angry. After you accept his anger, you can help him find different ways to express it and can help his family to understand it.

Bargaining

Although the patient acknowledges his impending death, he may attempt to bargain for more time with God or fate. He will probably strike this bargain secretly. If he does confide in you, listen.

Depression

In this stage, the patient may first experience regrets about his past and then grieve about his current condition. He may withdraw from his friends, his family, his practitioner, and you. He may suffer from anorexia, increased fatigue, or self-neglect. You may find him sitting alone, in tears. Accept the patient's sorrow, and listen. Provide comfort by touch, as appropriate. Resist the temptation to make optimistic remarks or cheerful small talk.

Acceptance

The patient who reaches this last stage accepts the inevitability and imminence of his death—without emotion. The patient may simply desire the quiet company of a family member or friend. If, for some reason, a family member or friend can't be present, stay with the patient to satisfy his final need. Remember, however, that many patients die before reaching this stage.

9 The Joint Commission. (2015). Standard NPSG.01.01.01. *Comprehensive accreditation manual for hospitals: The official handbook.* Oakbrook Terrace, IL: The Joint Commission. (Level VII)

10 American Osteopathic Association. (2014). Standard 15.01.16. *Healthcare Facilities Accreditation Program: Accreditation requirements for acute care hospitals.* Chicago, IL: American Osteopathic Association. (Level VII)

11 U.S. Department of Transportation, Office of Drug and Alcohol Policy and Compliance. (2010). "Urine specimen collection guidelines" [Online]. Accessed March 2015 via the Web at http://www.dot.gov/sites/dot.dev/files/docs/ODAPC%20Urine_Specimen_Collection_Guidelines_Octobe_1_2010.pdf (Level VII)

12 Siegel, J. D., et al. (2007). "2007 guideline for isolation precautions: Preventing transmission of infectious agents in healthcare settings" [Online]. Accessed March 2015 via the Web at http://www.cdc.gov/hicpac/pdf/isolation/Isolation2007.pdf (Level II)

13 American Osteopathic Association. (2014). Standard 07.01.10. *Healthcare Facilities Accreditation Program: Accreditation requirements for acute care hospitals.* Chicago, IL: American Osteopathic Association. (Level VII)

14 The Joint Commission. (2015). Standard RC.01.03.01. *Comprehensive accreditation manual for hospitals: The official handbook.* Oakbrook Terrace, IL: The Joint Commission. (Level VII)

15 Centers for Medicare & Medicaid Services, Department of Health and Human Services. (2014). Condition of participation: Medical record services. 42 C.F.R. § 482.24(b).

16 American Osteopathic Association. (2014). Standard 10.00.03. *Healthcare Facilities Accreditation Program: Accreditation requirements for acute care hospitals.* Chicago, IL: American Osteopathic Association. (Level VII)

17 Occupational Safety and Health Administration. (n.d.). "Bloodborne pathogens, standard number 1910.1030" [Online]. Accessed March 2015 via the Web at http://www.osha.gov/pls/oshaweb/owadisp.show_document?p_table=STANDARDS&p_id=10051 (Level VII)

18 Standridge, J. B., et al. (2010). Urine drug screening: A valuable office procedure. *American Family Physician, 81,* 635–640. (Level VII)

Additional reference

Phan, H. M., et al. (2012). Drug testing in the workplace. *Pharmacotherapy: The Journal of Human Pharmacology and Drug Therapy, 32,* 649–656.

Dying patient care

Death may be defined as either irreversible cessation or circulatory and respiratory functions or irreversible cessation of all functions of the entire brain, including the brain stem.[1] Signs and symptoms of impending death vary and may include confusion; decreased level of consciousness; irregular or decreased respirations that may be accompanied by rattling and gurgling sounds; weak or erratic pulse; decreased blood pressure; decreased socialization or social withdrawal; pale, mottled, cyanotic, diaphoretic, or cool skin; bowel and bladder incontinence; involuntary movements; and loss of reflexes in the extremities.

A patient needs intensive physical support and emotional comfort as he approaches death. Emotional support for a dying patient and his family most commonly entails reassurance; your physical presence helps ease fear and loneliness. More intense emotional support is important at much earlier stages, especially for patients with long-term progressive illnesses who can work through the stages of dying. (See *Five stages of dying.*)

Respect the patient's wishes about extraordinary means of supporting life. The patient may have a current, signed advance directive. This document, legally binding in most states, declares the patient's wishes for end-of-life care should he be unable to make decisions for himself. (See the "Advance directives" procedure, page 7.)

Equipment

Clean bed linens ■ clean gowns ■ gloves ■ water-filled basin ■ soap ■ washcloth ■ towels ■ lotion ■ fluid-impermeable pads ■ oral care supplies ■ petroleum jelly ■ protective barrier cream ■ sponge-tipped swab ■ suction equipment, as necessary ■ Optional: indwelling urinary catheter, prescribed medications, suction equipment, vital signs measurement equipment.

Implementation

- Verify the presence of a current, signed advance directive in the patient's medical record. Obtain one from the patient's family members

Understanding organ and tissue donation

A federal regulation was enacted in 1998 and revised in 2004 that requires facilities to report any person whose death is imminent or who has died in the health care facility to a regional organ procurement organization in a timely manner.[6] This regulation was enacted so that no potential donor is missed. The regulation ensures that the family of every potential donor will understand the option to donate. According to the American Medical Association, about 25 kinds of organs and tissues are transplanted. Although donor organ requirements vary, the typical donor must be between ages of newborn and 60 years and free from transmissible disease. Tissue donations are less restrictive, and some tissue banks will accept skin from donors up to age 75.

Collection of most organs, such as the heart, liver, kidney, or pancreas, requires that the patient be pronounced brain dead and kept physically alive until the organs are harvested. Tissue, such as eyes, skin, bone, and heart valves, may be taken after death. Contact your regional organ procurement organization for specific organ donation criteria or to identify a potential donor. If you don't know the regional organ procurement organization in your area, call the United Network for Organ Sharing at 804-782-4800.

if indicated; offer information on advance directives as requested and required by your facility.[2,3]

- Clarify and communicate goals of treatment and the patient's values with the patient's family and multidisciplinary team.
- Gather equipment at the patient's bedside, as needed.

Meeting physical needs

- Perform hand hygiene.[4,5,6,7,8]
- Confirm the patient's identity using at least two patient identifiers.[9]
- Put on new gloves[10,11] and perform hand hygiene[4,5,6,7,8] whenever moving from a contaminated to a clean area during patient care.
- Obtain vital signs and perform assessments, as indicated.
- Perform a comprehensive pain assessment using techniques appropriate for the patient's age, condition, and ability to understand. Administer pain medications, as needed and prescribed, using safe medication administration practices.[12]
- Use nonpharmacologic pain management strategies, such as guided imagery, massage, and progressive relaxation, as adjuvant therapy.
- When the patient's vision and hearing start to fail, turn his head toward the light and speak to him from near the head of the bed. *Because hearing may be acute despite loss of consciousness,* avoid whispering or speaking inappropriately about the patient in his presence.
- Monitor skin integrity carefully and reposition the patient in bed at least every 2 hours *because sensation, reflexes, and mobility diminish first in the legs and gradually in the arms.* Avoid shearing forces and use left sheets for repositioning. Make sure the bed sheets cover him loosely *to reduce discomfort caused by pressure on arms and legs.*
- Change the bed linens and the patient's gown as needed. Provide skin care during gown changes
- Adjust the room temperature for patient comfort, if necessary.
- Observe for incontinence or anuria, the result of diminished neuromuscular control, decreased renal function, constipation, or diarrhea. If necessary, obtain an order to catheterize the patient, or place fluid-impermeable pads beneath the patient's buttocks. Provide perineal care using soap, a water-filled basin, a washcloth, and towels *to prevent irritation.* Apply a protective barrier cream as indicated.
- Elevate the head of the bed *to decrease respiratory resistance.* Provide gentle suction of the patient's oropharynx as indicated *to remove thick, copious secretions.* As the patient's condition deteriorates, he may breathe mostly through his mouth.
- Offer fluids, frequently and respectfully; don't force the patient to take fluids.
- Provide oral care frequently, taking care to lubricate the patient's lips and mouth with petroleum jelly and a sponge-tipped swab *to counteract dryness.*
- Provide eye care using artificial tears or ophthalmic saline solution, if ordered, *to prevent corneal ulceration, which can cause blindness and prevent the use of these tissues for transplantation after the patient dies.*
- Reassess the patient's pain and respond appropriately.[12]
- Discard used supplies in the appropriate receptacles.[10]
- Remove and discard your gloves.[10]
- Perform hand hygiene.[4,5,6,7,8]

Meeting emotional needs

- Fully explain all care and treatments to the family and patient even if he's unconscious *because his hearing may be intact.* Answer any questions as candidly as possible while remaining sensitive and respectful.
- Allow the patient and his family to express their feelings, which may range from anger to loneliness. Take time to talk with the patient and his family. Sit near the head of the bed, and avoid looking rushed or unconcerned.
- Assure the family that care will continue before, during, and after the withdrawal of life-sustaining measures as indicated, regardless of the outcome.
- Encourage appropriate affection among the patient and family members, and provide for privacy and confidentiality.
- Appreciate cultural, spiritual, and religious traditions related to the dying process.
- Notify family members, if they're absent, when the patient wishes to see them. Let the patient and his family discuss death at their own pace.
- Offer to contact a member of the clergy, palliative care team, hospice, or social services department if appropriate.
- Document the procedure.[13,14,15]

Special considerations

- If family members remain with the patient, show them the location of bathrooms, lounges, and cafeterias. Explain the patient's needs, treatments, and care plan to them. If appropriate, offer to teach them specific skills so that they can take part in nursing care. Emphasize that their efforts are important and effective. As the patient's death approaches, give them emotional support.
- Teach the family about signs and symptoms of impending death.
- Collaborate with the multidisciplinary team *to determine whether procedures and unnecessary medications can be discontinued;* necessary medications should be administered by an alternative route when the by-mouth route becomes difficult.
- Family dynamics and cultural, religious, and spiritual beliefs may all affect the grieving experience. Matters commonly expressed and discussed include questions about an afterlife, unresolved social or emotional issues, and financial concerns.
- Respect the patient's and family's wishes regarding complementary and alternative medicine; refer to the National Institutes of Health's National Center for Complementary and Alternative Medicine as requested.
- At an appropriate time, discuss with the patient's family whether they have considered organ and tissue donation. Explain the process and obtain consents as indicated. Check the patient's records *to determine whether he has completed an organ donor card.* (See *Understanding organ and tissue donation.*)

Documentation

Record changes in the patient's vital signs and general status. Document end-of-life care discussions and choices made and advance directives formulated. Obtain all necessary signatures, consents, and required copies. Note the times of cardiac arrest and the end of respiration, and notify the practitioner when these occur.

REFERENCES

1 The President's Commission for the Study of Ethical Problems in Medicine and Biomedical and Behavioral Research. (1981). "Defining death: Medical, legal, and ethical issues in the determination of death" [Online]. Accessed March 2015 via the Web at http://bioethics.georgetown.edu/pcbe/reports/past_commissions/defining_death.pdf (Level VII)

2 The Joint Commission. (2015). Standard RI.01.05.01. *Comprehensive accreditation manual for hospitals: The official handbook.* Oakbrook Terrace, IL: The Joint Commission. (Level VII)

3 Centers for Medicare & Medicaid Services, Department of Health and Human Services. (2014). Condition of participation: Patient's rights. 42 C.F.R. § 482.13(b)(3).

4 The Joint Commission. (2015). Standard NPSG.07.01.01. *Comprehensive accreditation manual for hospitals: The official handbook.* Oakbrook Terrace, IL: The Joint Commission. (Level VII)

5 Centers for Disease Control and Prevention. (2002). Guideline for hand hygiene in health-care settings: Recommendations of the Healthcare Infection Control Practices Advisory Committee and the HICPAC/SHEA/APIC/IDSA Hand Hygiene Task Force. *MMWR Recommendations and Reports, 51*(RR-16), 1–45. Accessed March 2015 via the Web at http://www.cdc.gov/mmwr/pdf/rr/rr5116.pdf (Level II)

6 World Health Organization. (2009). "WHO guidelines on hand hygiene in health care: First global patient safety challenge, clean care is safer care" [Online]. Accessed March 2015 via the Web at http://whqlibdoc.who.int/publications/2009/9789241597906_eng.pdf (Level IV)

7 Centers for Medicare & Medicaid Services, Department of Health and Human Services. (2014). Condition of participation: Infection control. 42 C.F.R. § 482.42.

8 American Osteopathic Association. (2014). Standard 07.01.21. *Healthcare Facilities Accreditation Program: Accreditation requirements for acute care hospitals.* Chicago, IL: American Osteopathic Association. (Level VII)

9 The Joint Commission. (2015). Standard NPSG.01.01.01. *Comprehensive accreditation manual for hospitals: The official handbook.* Oakbrook Terrace, IL: The Joint Commission. (Level VII)

10 Siegel, J. D., et al. (2007). "2007 guideline for isolation precautions: Preventing transmission of infectious agents in healthcare settings" [Online]. Accessed March 2015 via the Web at http://www.cdc.gov/hicpac/pdf/isolation/Isolation2007.pdf (Level II)

11 American Osteopathic Association. (2014). Standard 07.01.10. *Healthcare Facilities Accreditation Program: Accreditation requirements for acute care hospitals.* Chicago, IL: American Osteopathic Association. (Level VII)

12 The Joint Commission. (2015). Standard PC.01.02.07. *Comprehensive accreditation manual for hospitals: The official handbook.* Oakbrook Terrace, IL: The Joint Commission. (Level VII)

13 The Joint Commission. (2015). Standard RC.01.03.01. *Comprehensive accreditation manual for hospitals: The official handbook.* Oakbrook Terrace, IL: The Joint Commission. (Level VII)

14 Centers for Medicare & Medicaid Services, Department of Health and Human Services. (2014). Condition of participation: Medical record services. 42 C.F.R. § 482.24(b).

15 American Osteopathic Association. (2014). Standard 10.00.03. *Healthcare Facilities Accreditation Program: Accreditation requirements for acute care hospitals.* Chicago, IL: American Osteopathic Association. (Level VII)

16 Centers for Medicare & Medicaid Services, Department of Health and Human Services. (2014). Condition of participation: Organ, tissue, and eye procurement. 42 C.F.R. § 482.45.

17 American Osteopathic Association. (2014). Standard 14.00.01. *Healthcare Facilities Accreditation Program: Accreditation requirements for acute care hospitals.* Chicago, IL: American Osteopathic Association. (Level VII)

ADDITIONAL REFERENCES

Atwood, D., et al. (2012). Organ donation considerations. *Nursing Management, 43*(6), 22–27.

Craven, R. F., & Hirnle, C. J. (2012). *Fundamentals of nursing: Human health and function* (7th ed.). Philadelphia, PA: Lippincott Williams & Wilkins.

Curtis, J. R., et al. (2012). Effects of a quality-improvement intervention on end-of-life care in the intensive care unit: A randomized trial. *American Journal of Respiratory and Critical Care Medicine, 183,* 348–355. (Level II)

Lynn, P. (2011). *Taylor's handbook of clinical nursing skills.* Philadelphia, PA: Lippincott Williams & Wilkins.

Mak, Y. M., et al. (2013). Experiences and perceptions of nurses caring for dying patients and families in the acute medical admission setting. *International Journal of Palliative Nursing, 19,* 423–431. (Level VI)

Taylor, C., et al. (2011). *Fundamentals of nursing: The art and science of nursing care* (7th ed.). Philadelphia, PA: Lippincott Williams & Wilkins.

EARDROP INSTILLATION

Eardrops treat infection and inflammation, soften cerumen for later removal, produce local anesthesia, or facilitate removal of an insect or other foreign body trapped in the ear.

Instillation of eardrops is usually contraindicated if the patient has a perforated eardrum but it may be permitted with certain medications and adherence to sterile technique. Other conditions may also prohibit instillation of certain medications into the ear. For example, instillation of drops containing hydrocortisone is contraindicated if the patient has herpes, another viral infection, or a fungal infection.

Equipment

Prescribed eardrops ■ light source ■ facial tissues ■ Optional: gloves, cotton-tipped applicator, cotton ball, irrigant.

Preparation of equipment

Before administration, allow the medication to reach room temperature, or warm the solution by gently rotating the container in your hands. *Instilling cold eardrop can cause dizziness and nausea.*

Implementation

- Avoid distractions and interruptions when preparing and administering the medication *to prevent medication errors.*[1,2]
- Verify the practitioner's order.[3,4,5]
- Compare the medication label with the order in the patient's medical record and verify that the medication is correct.[3,4,5]
- Check the patient's medical record for an allergy or a contraindication to the prescribed medication.[3,4,5] If an allergy or other contraindication exists, don't administer the medication; instead, notify the practitioner.
- Check the expiration date on the medication.[3,4,5] If the medication is expired, return it to the pharmacy and obtain new medication.
- Visually inspect the medication for particles, discoloration, or other signs of loss of integrity; don't administer the medication if its integrity is compromised.[3,4,5]
- Discuss any unresolved concerns about the medication with the patient's practitioner.[3,4,5]
- Perform hand hygiene.[6,7,8,9,10]
- Confirm the patient's identity using at least two patient identifiers.[11]
- If the patient is receiving the medication for the first time, teach him about potential adverse effects and discuss any other concerns related to the medications.[3,4,5]

Positioning the patient for eardrop instillation

Before instilling eardrops, have the patient lie on his side. Then straighten the patient's ear canal *to help the medication reach the eardrum.* For an adult, gently pull the auricle up and back; for an infant or young child, gently pull down and back (as shown below).

Adult

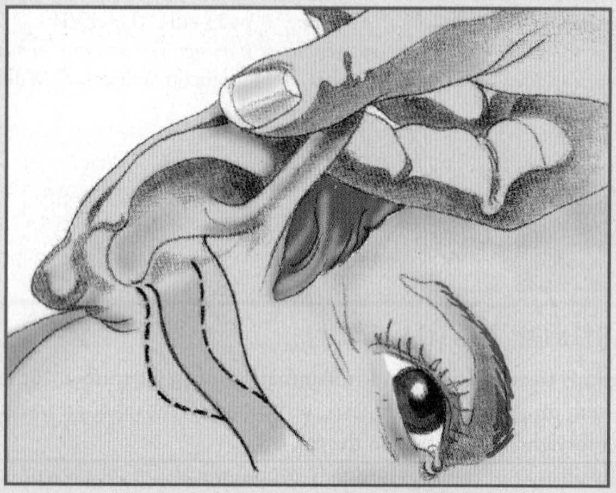

Child

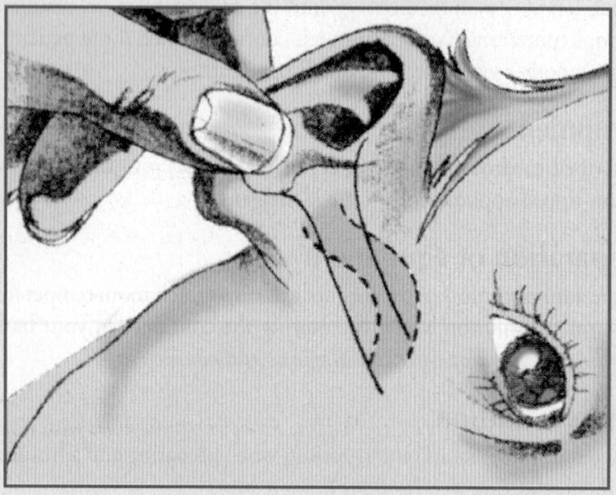

- Verify the medication is being administered at the proper time, in the prescribed dose, and by the correct route *to reduce the risk of medication errors.*[3,4,5]
- Confirm in which ear you must administer the medication.[3,4,5]
- If your facility uses a bar code scanning system, scan your identification badge, the patient's identification bracelet, and the medication bar code.
- Provide privacy and explain the procedure to the patient.
- Put on gloves as needed *to comply with standard precautions.*[12,13]
- Have the patient sit or lie with his head turned to the unaffected side.
- Straighten the patient's ear canal. Pull the auricle (pinna) of the ear up and back. (See *Positioning the patient for eardrop instillation.*)
- Using a light source, examine the ear canal for drainage. If you find any, clean the canal with a tissue or cotton-tipped applicator *because drainage can reduce the medication's effectiveness.*
- *To avoid damaging the ear canal with the dropper,* gently support the hand holding the dropper against the patient's head. Straighten the patient's ear canal once again and instill the ordered number of drops. *To avoid patient discomfort,* position the dropper so that the drops fall against the sides of the ear canal, not on the eardrum. Hold the ear canal in position until you see the medication disappear down the canal. Then release the ear.
- Massage the tragus (the fleshy part in front of the ear canal) with your finger. *Doing so facilitates entry of the medication into the ear canal.*
- Instruct the patient to remain with his head to the side for 5 to 10 minutes *to allow the medication to run down into the ear canal.*
- If ordered, tuck a cotton ball loosely into the opening of the ear canal *to prevent the medication from leaking out.* Be careful not to insert it too deeply into the canal *because this would prevent drainage of secretions and increase pressure on the eardrum.*
- Clean and dry the outer ear with a tissue.
- If ordered, repeat the procedure in the other ear after 5 to 10 minutes.
- Assist the patient into a comfortable position.
- Remove and discard your gloves, if worn.[12,13]
- Perform hand hygiene.[6,7,8,9,10]
- Document the procedure.[14,15,16]

Special considerations

- Remember that some conditions make a normally tender ear canal even more sensitive, so be especially gentle when performing this procedure.
- *To prevent injury to the eardrum,* never insert a cotton-tipped applicator into the ear canal past the point where you can see the tip. After instilling eardrops to soften cerumen, irrigate the ear as ordered *to facilitate cerumen removal.*
- If the patient has vertigo, keep the side rails of his bed up and assist him during the procedure, as necessary. Also, move slowly *to avoid exacerbating his vertigo.*

Patient teaching

Teach the patient to instill the eardrops correctly so that he can continue treatment at home, if necessary. Review the procedure and let the patient try it himself while you observe.

Special considerations

When the ear canal is obstructed, performing ear cleaning, placing an ear wick, or both can enhance the delivery of topical preparations.[17]

Complications

Complications may include local reactions, such as redness and swelling of the ear canal, or systemic reactions. The patient may complain of dizziness, nausea, or discomfort if the medication is given while it's cold.

Documentation

Record the medication, the ear treated or whether you treated both ears, and the date, time, and number of eardrops instilled. Also note any adverse reactions that arise during the procedure, such as drainage, redness, vertigo, nausea, and pain. Document any patient teaching and the patient's comprehension of the teaching.

REFERENCES

1 Westbrook, J., et al. (2010). Association of interruptions with an increased risk and severity of medication administration errors. *Archives of Internal Medicine, 170,* 683–690. (Level IV)

2 Institute for Safe Medication Practices. (2013). Side tracks on the safety express: Interruptions lead to errors and unfinished...Wait, what was I doing? *Nurse Advise-ERR,* 11(2), 1–4. Accessed March 2015 via the Web at https://www.ismp.org/Newsletters/acutecare/showarticle.aspx?id=37 (Level VII)

3 The Joint Commission. (2015). Standard MM.06.01.01. *Comprehensive accreditation manual for hospitals: The official handbook.* Oakbrook Terrace, IL: The Joint Commission. (Level VII)
4 Centers for Medicare & Medicaid Services, Department of Health and Human Services. (2014). Condition of participation: Nursing services. 42 C.F.R. § 482.23(c).
5 American Osteopathic Association. (2014). Standard 16.01.03. *Healthcare Facilities Accreditation Program: Accreditation requirements for acute care hospitals.* Chicago, IL: American Osteopathic Association. (Level VII)
6 The Joint Commission. (2015). Standard NPSG.07.01.01. *Comprehensive accreditation manual for hospitals: The official handbook.* Oakbrook Terrace, IL: The Joint Commission. (Level VII)
7 Centers for Disease Control and Prevention. (2002). Guideline for hand hygiene in health-care settings: Recommendations of the Healthcare Infection Control Practices Advisory Committee and the HICPAC/SHEA/APIC/IDSA Hand Hygiene Task Force. *MMWR Recommendations and Reports, 51*(RR-16), 1–45. Accessed March 2015 via the Web at http://www.cdc.gov/mmwr/pdf/rr/rr5116.pdf (Level II)
8 World Health Organization. (2009). "WHO guidelines on hand hygiene in health care: First global patient safety challenge, clean care is safer care" [Online]. Accessed March 2015 via the Web at http://whqlibdoc.who.int/publications/2009/9789241597906_eng.pdf (Level IV)
9 Centers for Medicare & Medicaid Services, Department of Health and Human Services. (2014). Condition of participation: Infection control. 42 C.F.R. § 482.42.
10 American Osteopathic Association. (2014). Standard 07.01.21. *Healthcare Facilities Accreditation Program: Accreditation requirements for acute care hospitals.* Chicago, IL: American Osteopathic Association. (Level VII)
11 The Joint Commission. (2015). Standard NPSG.01.01.01. *Comprehensive accreditation manual for hospitals: The official handbook.* Oakbrook Terrace, IL: The Joint Commission. (Level VII)
12 Siegel, J. D., et al. (2007). "2007 guideline for isolation precautions: Preventing transmission of infectious agents in healthcare settings" [Online]. Accessed March 2015 via the Web at http://www.cdc.gov/hicpac/pdf/isolation/Isolation2007.pdf (Level II)
13 American Osteopathic Association. (2014). Standard 07.01.10. *Healthcare Facilities Accreditation Program: Accreditation requirements for acute care hospitals.* Chicago, IL: American Osteopathic Association.
14 The Joint Commission. (2015). Standard RC.01.03.01. *Comprehensive accreditation manual for hospitals: The official handbook.* Oakbrook Terrace, IL: The Joint Commission. (Level VII)
15 American Osteopathic Association. (2014). Standard 10.00.03. *Healthcare Facilities Accreditation Program: Accreditation requirements for acute care hospitals.* Chicago, IL: American Osteopathic Association. (Level VII)
16 Centers for Medicare & Medicaid Services, Department of Health and Human Services. (2014). Condition of participation: Medical record services. 42 C.F.R. § 482.24(b).
17 Rosenfeld, R. M., et al. (2006, reaffirmed 2011). Clinical practice guideline: Acute otitis externa. *Otolaryngology, Head and Neck Surgery, 134*(Suppl. 4), S4–S23. Accessed March 2015 via the Web at http://oto.sagepub.com/content/134/4_suppl/S4.full.pdf (Level VII)

ADDITIONAL REFERENCE

Taylor, C., et al. (2011). *Fundamentals of nursing: The art and science of nursing care* (7th ed.). Philadelphia, PA: Lippincott Williams & Wilkins.

EAR IRRIGATION

Irrigating the ear involves washing the external auditory canal with a stream of solution to clean the canal of discharge, soften and remove impacted cerumen, or dislodge a foreign body. Sometimes, irrigation aims to relieve localized inflammation and discomfort. The procedure must be performed carefully so that it doesn't cause the patient discomfort or vertigo and to avoid increasing the risk of otitis externa. Because irrigation may contaminate the middle ear if the tympanic membrane is ruptured, an otoscopic examination always precedes ear irrigation.

NURSING ALERT *This procedure is contraindicated when a vegetable (such as a pea) obstructs the auditory canal.* This type of foreign body attracts and absorbs moisture. In contact with an irrigant or other solution, it swells, causing intense pain and complicating removal of the object by irrigation. *Ear irrigation is also contraindicated if the patient has a cold, a fever, an ear infection, or an injured or ruptured tympanic membrane. The presence of a battery (or a battery part) in the ear contraindicates irrigation* because battery acid could leak, and irrigation would spread caustic material throughout the canal. *Procedural modifications may be indicated for patients with structural abnormalities, diabetes, or an immunocompromised state or those taking anticoagulant therapy.*

Equipment

Ear irrigation syringe (rubber bulb) or irrigation system ■ otoscope with ear speculum ■ prescribed irrigant (such as normal saline solution) ■ large basin filled with hot water ■ emesis basin ■ gloves ■ fluid-impermeable pad ■ bath towel ■ washcloth ■ 4″ × 4″ (10-cm × 10-cm) gauze pad ■ Optional: adjustable light, cotton pledget, goggles, face shield.

Preparation of equipment

Select the appropriate syringe, and obtain the prescribed irrigant. Put the container of irrigant into the large basin filled with hot water *to warm the solution to body temperature: 98.6°F (37°C).* Avoid extreme temperature changes *because they can affect inner ear fluids, causing nausea and dizziness.*

Test the temperature of the solution by sprinkling a few drops on your inner wrist. Inspect equipment for breaks or cracks.

Implementation

- Verify the practitioner's order for irrigation.
- Perform hand hygiene.[1,2,3,4,5]
- Confirm the patient's identity using at least two patient identifiers.[6]
- Review the history of the patient's conditions, including signs and symptoms, diseases involving the ear, and the condition of the tympanic membrane.
- Provide privacy and explain the procedure to the patient.[7]
- Make sure you have adequate lighting.
- Put on gloves and follow standard precautions.[8,9]
- *To avoid getting foreign matter into the ear canal,* clean the auricle and the meatus of the auditory canal with a washcloth moistened with normal saline solution or other prescribed irrigating solution.
- If you haven't already done so, use the otoscope with ear speculum to inspect the auditory canal to be irrigated.

NURSING ALERT *The ear canal is very sensitive, and instrumentation can be painful. Use caution when examining the ear. The patient must remain still while you examine his ear and insert any instruments into the ear* to avoid ear canal damage.

- Help the patient to a sitting position. *To prevent the solution from running down his neck,* tilt his head slightly forward and toward the affected side. If he can't sit, have him lie on his back and tilt his head slightly forward and toward the affected ear.
- If the patient is sitting, place the fluid-impermeable pad (covered with the bath towel) on his shoulder and upper arm, under the affected ear. If he's lying down, cover his pillow and the area under the affected ear.
- Put on goggles or a face shield before irrigation, if necessary.[8,9]
- Draw the irrigant into the syringe and expel any air.
- Gently pull the pinna up and back *to straighten the ear canal.*[10] Have the patient hold an emesis basin beneath the ear (as shown on next page, top left) *to catch returning irritant.*

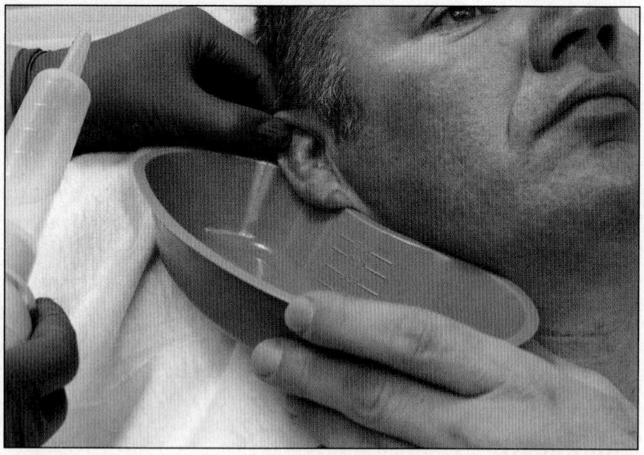

■ Position the tip of the irrigating syringe at the meatus of the auditory canal (as shown below). Don't block the meatus *because doing so will impede backflow and raise pressure in the canal.*

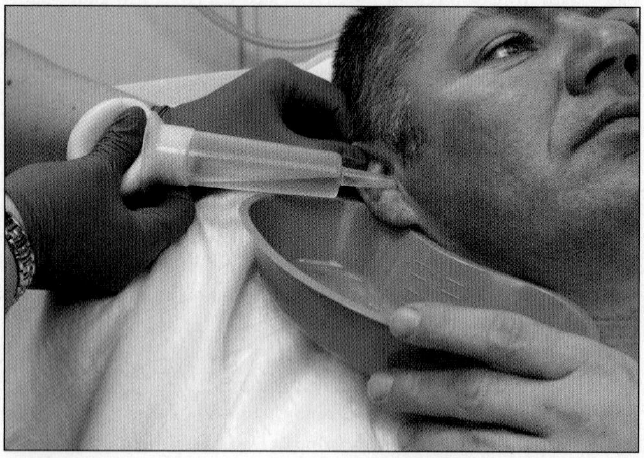

■ With the patient's head tilted toward the affected ear, point the syringe tip upward and toward the posterior ear canal. *This angle prevents damage to the tympanic membrane and guards against pushing debris farther into the ear canal.* Direct a steady stream of irrigant against the upper wall of the ear canal (as shown below).

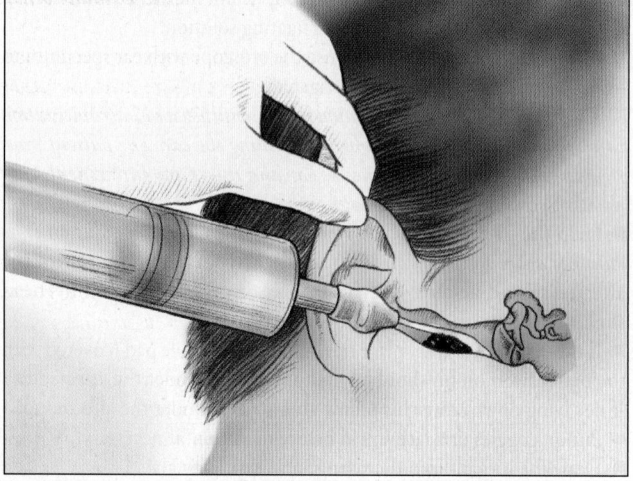

■ Throughout the irrigation, check the return flow and monitor the patient's tolerance of the procedure.

NURSING ALERT *During irrigation, observe the patient for signs of pain or dizziness. If he reports either, stop the procedure, recheck the temperature of the irrigant, inspect the patient's ear with the otoscope, and resume irrigation, as indicated.*

■ Remove the syringe when it's empty and inspect the return flow for cloudiness, cerumen, blood, or foreign matter. Then, refill the syringe, and continue the irrigation *until the return flow is clear.* Never use more than 500 mL of irrigant during this procedure.

■ Remove the syringe, and inspect the ear canal for cleanliness with the otoscope.

■ Dry the patient's auricle and neck.

■ Remove the bath towel and fluid-impermeable pad. Help the seated patient lie on his affected side with the 4″ × 4″ (10-cm × 10-cm) gauze pad under his ear *to promote drainage of residual debris and solution.*

■ Discard used supplies in the appropriate receptacles.[8]

■ Remove and discard your gloves and goggles or face shield, if worn.[8]

■ Perform hand hygiene.[1,2,3,4,5]

■ Document the procedure.[11,12,13]

Special considerations

■ Avoid dropping or squirting irrigant on the tympanic membrane, *which may startle the patient and cause discomfort.*

■ If the practitioner directs you to place a cotton pledget in the ear canal *to retain some of the solution,* pack the cotton loosely. Instruct the patient not to remove it.

■ If irrigation doesn't dislodge impacted cerumen, the practitioner may order you to instill several drops of glycerin, docusate, 2% acetic acid, 10% sodium bicarbonate, carbamide peroxide, or a similar preparation two to three times daily for 2 to 3 days, and then to irrigate the ear again.[14]

■ If you're performing the procedure on a patient with a hearing aid, remove the hearing aid and then inspect the ear canal with a handheld otoscope. If the patient has bilateral hearing aids, examine the second ear after replacing the first hearing aid *to facilitate communication.* Keep in mind that cerumen impaction may change hearing aid performance.[14]

Patient teaching

Discourage the patient from using manual methods to remove cerumen, such as inserting a cotton-tipped applicator. Suggest alternative measures to reduce cerumen impaction, such as instilling a prophylactic topical preparation, irrigating the ear canal, or having his practitioner routinely clean the ear canal every 6 to 12 months, as indicated. If the patient wears hearing aids, teach the patient and his caregiver how to care for and clean the hearing aids to decrease the risk of impaction.

NURSING ALERT *The Food and Drug Administration has concluded that no validated scientific evidence supports the efficacy of ear candles and warns against their use.*[14]

Complications

Possible complications include pain, vertigo, nausea, otitis externa, and otitis media (if the patient has a perforated or ruptured tympanic membrane). *Forceful instillation of irrigant can rupture the tympanic membrane.* Instilling cerumenolytic agents can also result in transient hearing loss and local irritation.

Documentation

Record the date and time of irrigation. Note which ear you irrigated or whether you treated both ears. Also note the volume and the solution used, the appearance of the canal before and after irrigation, the appearance of the return flow, the patient's tolerance of the procedure, and any comments he made about his condition, especially related to his hearing acuity.

REFERENCES

1 The Joint Commission. (2015). Standard NPSG.07.01.01. *Comprehensive accreditation manual for hospitals: The official handbook.* Oakbrook Terrace, IL: The Joint Commission. (Level VII)

2 Centers for Disease Control and Prevention. (2002). Guideline for hand hygiene in health-care settings: Recommendations of the Healthcare Infection Control Practices Advisory Committee and the HICPAC/SHEA/APIC/IDSA Hand Hygiene Task Force. *MMWR Recommendations and Reports, 51*(RR-16), 1–45. Accessed March 2015 via the Web at http://www.cdc.gov/mmwr/pdf/rr/rr5116.pdf (Level II)

3 World Health Organization. (2009). "WHO guidelines on hand hygiene in health care: First global patient safety challenge. Clean care is safer care" [Online]. Accessed March 2015 via the Web at http://whqlibdoc.who.int/publications/2009/9789241597906_eng.pdf (Level IV)

4 Centers for Medicare & Medicaid Services, Department of Health and Human Services. (2014). Condition of participation: Infection control. 42 C.F.R. § 482.42.

5 American Osteopathic Association. (2014). Standard 07.01.21. *Healthcare Facilities Accreditation Program: Accreditation requirements for acute care hospitals.* Chicago, IL: American Osteopathic Association. (Level VII)

6 The Joint Commission. (2015). Standard NPSG.01.01.01. *Comprehensive accreditation manual for hospitals: The official handbook.* Oakbrook Terrace, IL: The Joint Commission. (Level VII)

7 American Osteopathic Association. (2014). Standard 15.01.16. *Healthcare Facilities Accreditation Program: Accreditation requirements for acute care hospitals.* Chicago, IL: American Osteopathic Association. (Level VII)

8 Siegel, J. D., et al. (2007). "2007 guideline for isolation precautions: Preventing transmission of infectious agents in healthcare settings" [Online]. Accessed March 2015 via the Web at http://www.cdc.gov/hicpac/pdf/isolation/Isolation2007.pdf (Level II)

9 American Osteopathic Association. (2014). Standard 07.01.10. *Healthcare Facilities Accreditation Program: Accreditation requirements for acute care hospitals.* Chicago, IL: American Osteopathic Association. (Level VII)

10 Emergency Nurses Association. (2010). *Sheehy's emergency nursing principles and practice* (6th ed.). Philadelphia, PA: Lippincott Williams & Wilkins.

11 The Joint Commission. (2015). Standard RC.01.03.01. *Comprehensive accreditation manual for hospitals: The official handbook.* Oakbrook Terrace, IL: The Joint Commission. (Level VII)

12 Centers for Medicare & Medicaid Services, Department of Health and Human Services. (2014). Condition of participation: Medical record services. 42 C.F.R. § 482.24(b).

13 American Osteopathic Association. (2014). Standard 10.00.03. *Healthcare Facilities Accreditation Program: Accreditation requirements for acute care hospitals.* Chicago, IL: American Osteopathic Association. (Level VII)

14 Roland, P. S., et al. (2008). Clinical practice guideline: Cerumen impaction. *Otolaryngology: Head and Neck Surgery, 139,* S1–S21. Accessed March 2015 via the Web at http://www.entnet.org/Practice/upload/FINAL-CerumenImpaction-Journal-2008.pdf (Level I)

ADDITIONAL REFERENCES

Nettina, S. M. (2014). *Lippincott manual of nursing practice* (10th ed.). Philadelphia, PA: Wolters Kluwer.

Taylor, C., et al. (2011). *Fundamentals of nursing: The art and science of nursing care* (7th ed.). Philadelphia, PA: Lippincott Williams & Wilkins.

ELASTIC BANDAGE APPLICATION

Elastic bandages exert gentle, even pressure on a body part. By supporting blood vessels, these rolled bandages promote venous return. They can prevent pooling of blood in the legs and are sometimes used to replace antiembolism stockings to prevent venous thromboembolism, such as deep vein thrombosis and pulmonary embolism in postoperative or bedridden patients who can't stimulate venous return through muscle activity. Elastic bandages may also be used as compression wraps in patients with lower extremity edema and venous insuffucuency.[1,2]

Elastic bandages also have musculoskeletal indications. They can be used to minimize joint swelling after trauma to the musculoskeletal system and, when used with a splint, they can immobilize a fracture during healing. They can provide hemostatic pressure and anchor dressings over a fresh wound or after surgical procedures such as vein stripping.

Equipment

Elastic bandage of appropriate width and length ■ tape or self-closures ■ gauze pads or absorbent cotton ■ skin cleaner or mild soap and normal saline solution ■ Optional: gloves, skin barrier cream.[1]

Bandages usually come in 2″ to 6″ (5- to 15-cm) widths and 4′ and 6′ (1.2- and 1.8-M) lengths. The 3″ (7.6-cm) width is adaptable to most applications. An elastic bandage with self-closures is also available.

Preparation of equipment

Select a bandage that wraps the affected body part completely but isn't excessively long. Generally, use a narrower bandage for wrapping the foot, lower leg, hand, or arm and a wider bandage for the thigh or trunk. The bandage should be clean and rolled before application.

Implementation

- Verify the practitioner's order.
- Gather the appropriate equipment.
- Perform hand hygiene.[3,4,5,6,7]
- Put on gloves as needed *to comply with standard precautions.*[8,9,10]
- Confirm the patient's identity using at least two patient identifiers.[11]
- Provide privacy.[12]
- Explain the procedure to the patient *to allay anxiety and promote cooperation.*
- Position the patient comfortably, with the body part to be bandaged in normal functioning position *to promote circulation and prevent deformity and discomfort.*
- Inspect the area to be wrapped for the presence of lesions and skin breakdown.[1] If either condition is present, consult the practitioner before applying the elastic bandage.
- Clean and dry the skin surface of the area to be wrapped; apply a skin barrier cream, as indicated.[1]
- If the patient requires a compression wrap because of significant lower extremity edema, *the risk of impaired circulation is increased;* consult with a wound care nurse or another practitioner competent in the application of compression wraps *to ensure proper application,* as needed.[1]
- Before applying a bandage to an extremity with significant dependent edema, elevate the extremity for 15 to 30 minutes *to facilitate venous return.*[1]
- Don't let two skin surfaces touch when applying a bandage. Place gauze pads or absorbent cotton as needed between skin surfaces, such as between toes and fingers and under breasts and arms, *to prevent skin irritation.*
- Hold the bandage with the roll facing upward in one hand and the free end of the bandage in the other hand. Hold the bandage roll close to the part being bandaged *to ensure even tension and pressure.*
- Unroll the bandage as you wrap the body part using a spiral or spiral-reverse method. Never unroll the entire bandage before wrapping *because doing so could produce uneven pressure, which interferes with blood circulation and cell nourishment.*
- Overlap each layer of bandage by one-half to two-thirds the width of the strip. (See *Bandaging techniques,* page 262.)
- Wrap firmly, but not too tightly. As you wrap, ask the patient to tell you if the bandage feels comfortable. If he complains of tingling, itching, numbness, or pain, loosen the bandage.
- When wrapping an extremity, begin wrapping at the most distal part and work proximally *to promote venous return. Anchor the bandage initially* by circling the body part twice. *To prevent the bandage from slipping out*

Bandaging techniques

Circular
Each turn encircles the previous one, covering it completely. Use this technique to anchor a bandage.

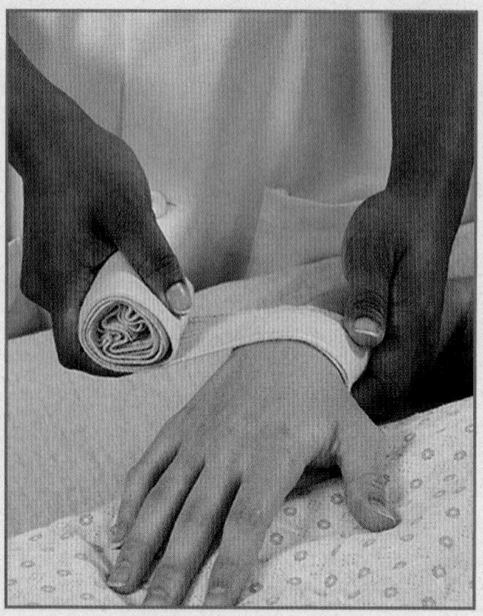

Spiral
Each turn partially overlaps the previous one. Use this technique to wrap a long, straight body part or one of increasing circumference.

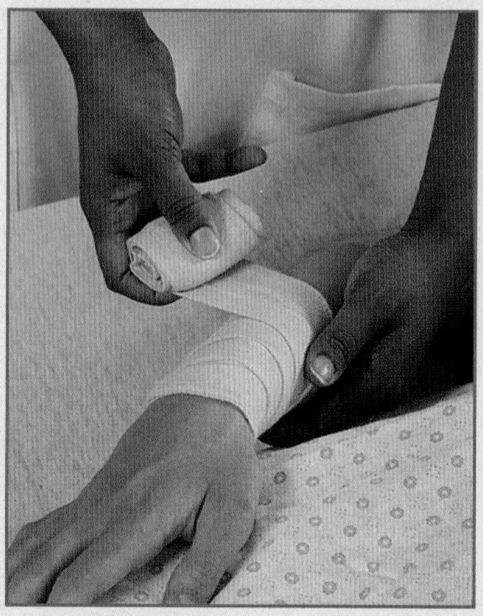

Spiral-reverse
Anchor the bandage and then reverse direction halfway through each spiral turn. Use this technique to accommodate the increasing circumference of a body part.

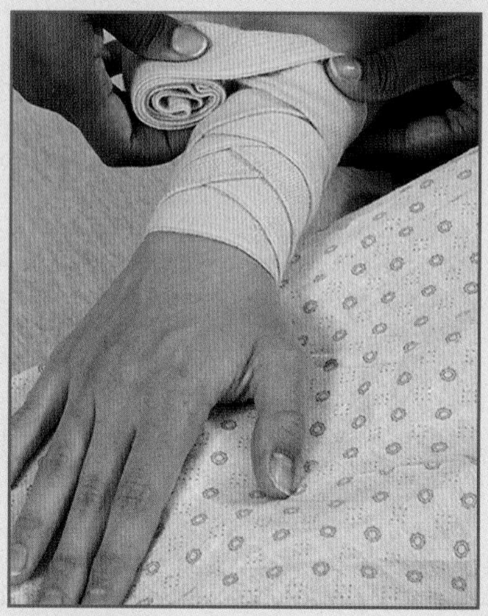

Figure eight
Anchor below the joint, and then use alternating ascending and descending turns to form a figure eight. Use this technique around joints.

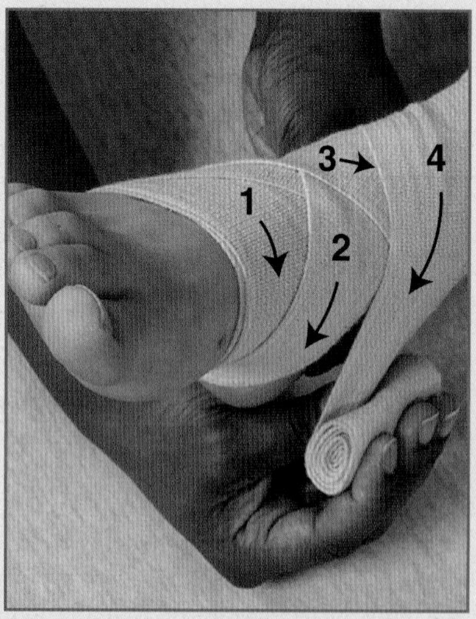

Recurrent
This technique includes a combination of recurrent and circular turns. Hold the bandage as you make each recurrent turn and then use the circular turns as a final anchor. Use this technique for a stump, a hand, or the scalp.

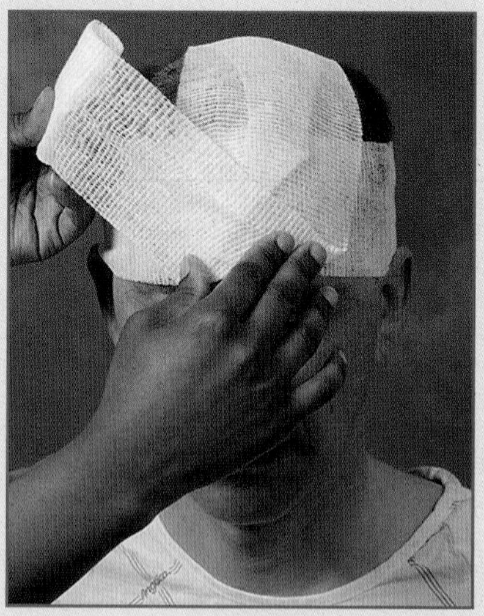

of place on the foot, wrap it in a figure eight around the foot, the ankle, and then the foot again before continuing. The same technique works on any joint, such as the knee, wrist, or elbow. Include the heel when wrapping the foot, but never wrap the toes (or fingers) unless absolutely necessary *because the distal extremities are used to detect impaired circulation.*

■ When you're finished wrapping, secure the end of the bandage with tape or self-closures. Be careful not to scratch or pinch the patient. Avoid using metal clips *because they typically come loose when the patient moves and can get lost in the bed linens and injure the patient.*

■ Assess distal circulation after the bandage is in place *because the elastic may tighten as you wrap* and every 4 hours thereafter *because an elastic bandage that's too tight can result in neurovascular damage.* Lift the distal end of the bandage and assess the skin underneath for color, temperature, and integrity.

■ If the wrapped body part is an extremity, elevate it for 15 to 30 minutes after wrapping *to facilitate venous return.*

- Remove the bandage every 8 hours or whenever it's loose and wrinkled. Roll it up as you unwrap *to ready it for reuse.* Observe the area and provide skin care before rewrapping the bandage.
- Change the bandage at least once daily. Bathe the skin, dry it thoroughly, and observe for irritation and breakdown before applying a fresh bandage.
- Remove and discard gloves if worn.[8]
- Perform hand hygiene.[3,4,5,6,7]
- Document the procedure.[13,14,15]

Special considerations

- If a patient has weeping lower-extremity edema, change elastic bandages frequently. Ensure that the bandage doesn't shift or crease, *which could cause constriction,* particularly around the heel and ankle.[1]
- Avoid leaving gaps in bandage layers, resulting in exposed skin surfaces between layers, *because doing so may result in uneven pressure on the body part.*
- Observe the patient for an allergic reaction *because some patients can't tolerate the sizing in a new bandage.* Laundering a new bandage before use reduces this risk.
- Launder the bandage daily or whenever it becomes limp *to restore the bandage's elasticity.* Always keep two bandages handy *so one can be applied while the other bandage is being laundered.*
- When using an elastic bandage after a surgical procedure on an extremity (such as vein stripping) or with a splint to immobilize a fracture, remove it only as ordered rather than every 8 hours.

Patient teaching

If the patient will be using an elastic bandage at home, teach him or a family member how to apply it correctly and how to assess for impaired circulation. Tell the patient to keep two bandages available *so he'll have one available while the other is being laundered.*

If the patient or a family member must apply the elastic bandage at home, demonstrate the procedure and observe a return demonstration before the patient's discharge. Make sure the patient has the information needed to obtain additional supplies.

Complications

Arterial obstruction—characterized by a decreased or absent distal pulse, blanching or bluish discoloration of the skin, dusky nail beds, numbness and tingling or pain and cramping, and cold skin—can result from elastic bandage application. Edema can occur from obstruction of venous return. Less serious complications include allergic reaction and skin irritation.

Documentation

Record the date and time of bandage application and removal, the application site, the bandage size, skin condition before application, skin care provided after removal, any complications, the patient's tolerance of the treatment, any patient teaching, and the patient's understanding of the teaching.

References

1 Cooper, K. L. (2011). Care of the lower extremities in patients with acute decompensated heart failure. *Critical Care Nurse, 31*(4), 21–29. Accessed March 2015 via the Web at http://ccn.aacnjournals.org/content/31/4/21.full.pdf

2 O'Meara, S., et al. (2012). Compression for venous leg ulcers. *Cochrane Database of Systematic Reviews, 2012*(11), CD000265. (Level I)

3 The Joint Commission. (2015). Standard NPSG.07.01.01. *Comprehensive accreditation manual for hospitals: The official handbook.* Oakbrook Terrace, IL: The Joint Commission. (Level VII)

4 Centers for Disease Control and Prevention. (2002). Guideline for hand hygiene in health-care settings: Recommendations of the Healthcare Infection Control Practices Advisory Committee and the HICPAC/SHEA/APIC/IDSA Hand Hygiene Task Force. *MMWR Recommendations and Reports, 51*(RR-16), 1–45. Accessed March 2015 via the Web at http://www.cdc.gov/mmwr/pdf/rr/rr5116.pdf (Level II)

5 World Health Organization. (2009). "WHO guidelines on hand hygiene in health care: First global patient safety challenge, clean care is safer care" [Online]. Accessed March 2015 via the Web at http://whqlibdoc.who.int/publications/2009/9789241597906_eng.pdf (Level IV)

6 Centers for Medicare & Medicaid Services, Department of Health and Human Services. (2014). Condition of participation: Infection control. 42 C.F.R. § 482.42.

7 American Osteopathic Association. (2014). Standard 07.01.21. *Healthcare Facilities Accreditation Program: Accreditation requirements for acute care hospitals.* Chicago, IL: American Osteopathic Association. (Level VII)

8 Occupational Safety and Health Administration. (n.d.). "Bloodborne pathogens, standard number 1910.1030" [Online]. Accessed March 2015 via the Web at http://www.osha.gov/pls/oshaweb/owadisp.show_document?p_table=STANDARDS&p_id=10051 (Level VII)

9 Siegel, J. D., et al. (2007). "2007 guideline for isolation precautions: Preventing transmission of infectious agents in healthcare settings" [Online]. Accessed March 2015 via the Web at http://www.cdc.gov/hicpac/pdf/isolation/Isolation2007.pdf (Level II)

10 American Osteopathic Association. (2014). Standard 07.01.10. *Healthcare Facilities Accreditation Program: Accreditation requirements for acute care hospitals.* Chicago, IL: American Osteopathic Association. (Level VII)

11 The Joint Commission. (2015). Standard NPSG.01.01.01. *Comprehensive accreditation manual for hospitals: The official handbook.* Oakbrook Terrace, IL: The Joint Commission. (Level VII)

12 American Osteopathic Association. (2014). Standard 15.01.16. *Healthcare Facilities Accreditation Program: Accreditation requirements for acute care hospitals.* Chicago, IL: American Osteopathic Association. (Level VII)

13 The Joint Commission. (2015). Standard RC.01.03.01. *Comprehensive accreditation manual for hospitals: The official handbook.* Oakbrook Terrace, IL: The Joint Commission. (Level VII)

14 Centers for Medicare & Medicaid Services, Department of Health and Human Services. (2014). Condition of participation: Medical record services. 42 C.F.R. § 482.24(b).

15 American Osteopathic Association. (2014). Standard 10.00.03. *Healthcare Facilities Accreditation Program: Accreditation requirements for acute care hospitals.* Chicago, IL: American Osteopathic Association. (Level VII)

Additional reference

Taylor, C., et al. (2011). *Fundamentals of nursing: The art and science of nursing care* (7th ed.). Philadelphia, PA: Lippincott Williams & Wilkins.

ELECTRICAL BONE GROWTH STIMULATION

Approximately 10% of patients in the United States who suffer bone fractures develop delayed bone healing.[1] By imitating the body's natural electrical forces, electrical bone growth stimulation initiates or accelerates the healing process in a fractured bone that fails to heal. This procedure is also used to help bones grow together after such procedures as spinal fusion.

Three basic electrical bone stimulation techniques are available: fully implantable (invasive) direct-current stimulation, semi-invasive percutaneous stimulation, and noninvasive electromagnetic coil stimulation. (See *Methods of electrical bone growth stimulation,* page 264.) The choice of technique depends on the fracture type and location, the practitioner's preference, and the patient's ability and willingness to comply with instructions. With invasive direct-current stimulation, implantation is performed under general anesthesia. After the bone fragments join together, the generator and leadwire are removed under local anesthesia. The device requires no patient involvement. With the other two methods, however, the patient must manage his own treatment schedule and maintain the equipment. Treatment time averages 3 to 6 months.

Methods of electrical bone growth stimulation

Electrical bone growth stimulation may be invasive or noninvasive.

Invasive system

An invasive system involves placing a spiral cathode inside the bone at the fracture site. A wire leads from the cathode to a battery-powered generator, also implanted in local tissues. The patient's body completes the circuit.

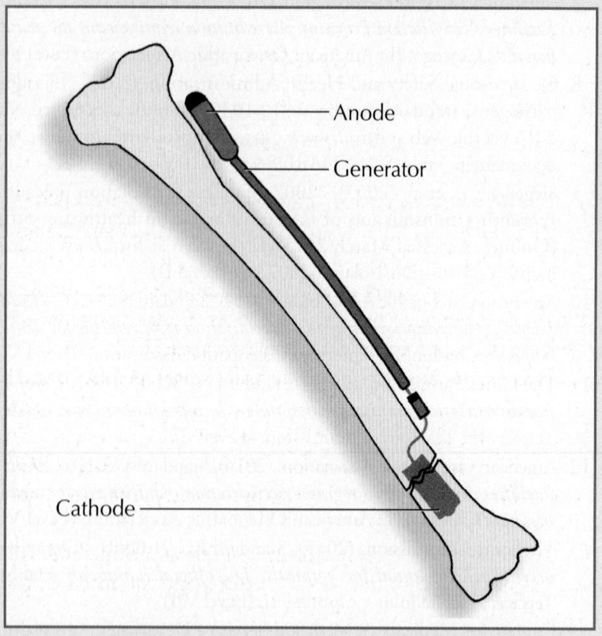

Noninvasive system

A noninvasive system may include a cuff-like transducer or fitted ring that wraps around the patient's limb at the level of the injury. Electrical current penetrates the limb.

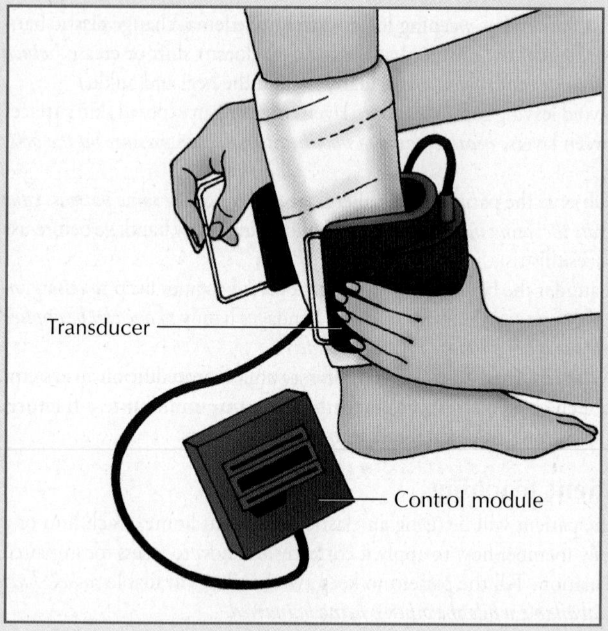

Equipment

Clippers ▪ ordered stimulation set.

For percutaneous stimulation

The stimulation set consists of an external anode skin pad with a lead-wire, lithium battery pack, and one to four Teflon-coated stainless steel cathode wires that are surgically implanted in the skin.

For electromagnetic stimulation

The stimulation set consists of a generator that plugs into a standard 110-volt outlet and two strong electromagnetic coils placed on either side of the injured area. The coils can be incorporated into a cast, cuff, or orthotic device.

Preparation of equipment

All equipment comes in sets with instructions provided by the manufacturer. Follow the instructions carefully and make sure that the equipment is operational.

Implementation

- Verify the practitioner's order.
- Ask the patient whether he's sensitive to nickel or chromium *because both are present in the electrical bone stimulation system.* If he is, notify the practitioner.
- Gather and prepare the equipment.
- Perform hand hygiene.[2,3,4]
- Confirm the patient's identity using at least two patient identifiers.[5]
- Explain the procedure to the patient.

Performing percutaneous stimulation

- Remove excessive body hair from the injured site using clippers.
- Apply the anode pad, making sure to avoid stressing or pulling on the anode wire.
- Instruct the patient to change the anode pad every 48 hours. Tell him to report local pain to his practitioner and not to bear weight on the injury site for the duration of the treatment.

Performing electromagnetic stimulation

- Show the patient where to place the coils.
- Tell the patient to apply the coils for 3 to 10 hours each day, as ordered by his practitioner. Many patients find it most convenient to perform the procedure at night.
- Urge the patient not to interrupt the treatments for more than 10 minutes at a time.
- Teach the patient how to use and care for the generator.
- Relay the practitioner's instructions for weight bearing. Usually, the practitioner will advise against bearing weight until evidence of bone healing appears on X-rays.

Completing the procedure

- Perform hand hygiene.[2,3,4]
- Document the procedure.[6,7]

Special considerations

- A patient undergoing direct-current electrical bone stimulation shouldn't undergo electrocauterization, diathermy, or magnetic resonance imaging (MRI). *Electrocautery may short-circuit the system; diathermy may potentiate the electrical current, possibly causing tissue damage; and MRI will interfere with or stop the current.*

- Percutaneous electrical bone stimulation is contraindicated if the patient has any kind of inflammatory process.
- Electromagnetic coils are contraindicated in patients who are pregnant, have a tumor, or have an arm fracture and a pacemaker.

Patient teaching

Teach the patient how to care for his cast or external fixation devices. Also tell him how to care for the electrical generator. Urge him to follow treatment instructions faithfully. If applicable, encourage the patient to stop smoking, provide smoking-cessation materials, and refer him to outpatient smoking-cessation counseling *because smoking delays wound healing.*[8,9]

Complications

Complications associated with any surgical procedure, including infection, can occur during insertion of direct-current electrical bone growth stimulation equipment. Local irritation or skin ulceration can occur around cathode pin sites with percutaneous devices. No complications are associated with use of electromagnetic coils or percutaneous simulation.

Documentation

Record the type of electrical bone stimulation equipment provided, including the date, time, and location, as appropriate. Note the patient's skin condition and tolerance of the procedure. Also record instructions given to the patient and family, as well as their ability to understand and act on those instructions.

REFERENCES

1 Galkowski, V., et al. (2009). Bone stimulation for fracture healing: What's all the fuss? *Indian Journal of Orthopaedics, 43,* 117–120.

2 Centers for Disease Control and Prevention. (2002). Guideline for hand hygiene in health-care settings: Recommendations of the Healthcare Infection Control Practices Advisory Committee and the HICPAC/SHEA/APIC/IDSA Hand Hygiene Task Force. *MMWR Recommendations and Reports, 51*(RR-16), 1–45. Accessed March 2015 via the Web at http://www.cdc.gov/mmwr/pdf/rr/rr5116.pdf (Level II)

3 World Health Organization. (2009). "WHO guidelines on hand hygiene in health care: First global patient safety challenge, clean care is safer care" [Online]. Accessed March 2015 via the Web at http://whqlibdoc.who.int/publications/2009/9789241597906_eng.pdf (Level IV)

4 The Joint Commission. (2015). Standard NPSG.07.01.01. *Comprehensive accreditation manual for hospitals: The official handbook.* Oakbrook Terrace, IL: The Joint Commission. (Level VII)

5 The Joint Commission. (2015). Standard NPSG.01.01.01. *Comprehensive accreditation manual for hospitals: The official handbook.* Oakbrook Terrace, IL: The Joint Commission. (Level VII)

6 The Joint Commission. (2015). Standard RC.01.03.01. *Comprehensive accreditation manual for hospitals: The official handbook.* Oakbrook Terrace, IL: The Joint Commission. (Level VII)

7 Centers for Medicare & Medicaid Services, Department of Health and Human Services. (2014). Condition of participation: Medical record services. 42 C.F.R. § 482.24(b).

8 National Association of Orthopaedic Nurses. (2013). *Core curriculum for orthopaedic nursing* (7th ed.). Boston, MA: Pearson Custom Publishing.

9 Centers for Medicare & Medicaid Services & The Joint Commission. (2014). "The specifications manual for national hospital inpatient quality measures (version 4.3)" [Online]. Accessed March 2015 via the Web at http://www.qualitynet.org/dcs/ContentServer?pagename=QnetPublic%2FPage%2FQnetTier2&cid=1141662756099

ADDITIONAL REFERENCE

Behrens, S. B., et al. (2013). A review of bone growth stimulation for fracture treatment. *Current Orthopaedic Practice, 24,* 84–91. (Level I)

ELECTROCARDIOGRAM, 12-LEAD

One of the most valuable and frequently used diagnostic tools, an electrocardiogram (ECG) can display the heart's electrical activity as waveforms. Impulses moving through the heart's conduction system create electrical currents that can be monitored on the body's surface. Electrodes attached to the skin can detect these electrical currents and transmit them to an instrument that produces a record of cardiac activity—the ECG. An ECG can be used to identify myocardial ischemia and infarction, rhythm and conduction disturbances, chamber enlargement, electrolyte imbalances, and drug toxicity.[1,2]

A standard 12-lead ECG uses a series of electrodes placed on the extremities and the chest wall to assess the heart from 12 different views (leads). The 12 leads consist of 3 standard bipolar limb leads (designated I, II, III), 3 unipolar augmented leads (aV_R, aV_L, aV_F), and 6 unipolar precordial leads (V_1 to V_6), which show the heart from the horizontal plane.

The ECG device measures and averages the differences between the electrical potential of the electrode sites for each lead and graphs them over time. This creates the standard ECG complex, made up of *P-QRS-T.* The P wave represents atrial depolarization; the QRS complex, ventricular depolarization; and the T wave, ventricular repolarization. (See *Reviewing ECG waveforms and components,* page 266.)

Variations of the standard ECG include the exercise ECG (stress ECG) and ambulatory ECG (Holter monitoring). The exercise ECG monitors heart rate, blood pressure, and ECG waveforms as the patient walks on a treadmill or pedals a stationary bicycle. For the ambulatory ECG, the patient wears a portable Holter monitor to record heart activity continually over 24 hours.

The ECG is accomplished using a multichannel method. All electrodes are attached to the patient at once, and the machine prints a simultaneous view of all leads.

Equipment

ECG machine with recording paper ▪ disposable pregelled electrodes ▪ 4″ × 4″ (10-cm × 10-cm) gauze pads or washcloth ▪ soap and water or cleaning pads ▪ bath blanket or sheet ▪ alcohol pads ▪ Optional: clippers, indelible marking pen, gloves.

Preparation of equipment

Place the ECG machine close to the patient's bed; check the cable and wires for fraying or breakage, and replace them or obtain another machine if necessary. Plug the cord into the wall outlet or, ensure functioning if the machine is battery operated. Turn on the machine and input the required patient information. If the patient is already connected to a cardiac monitor, move the electrodes *to accommodate the precordial leads and minimize electrical interference on the ECG tracing.* Keep the patient away from electrical fixtures and power cords. Make sure the centers of the pregelled electrodes are moist *to promote impulse transmission.*[3]

Implementation

- Verify the practitioner's order.
- Gather and prepare the appropriate equipment.
- Perform hand hygiene and put on gloves if needed *to follow standard precautions.*[4,5,6,7,8,9,10]
- Confirm the patient's identity using at least two patient identifiers.[11]
- Explain the procedure to the patient. Tell him that the test records the heart's electrical activity and that it may be repeated at certain intervals. Emphasize that no electrical current will enter his body. Also, tell him that the test typically takes just a few minutes.
- Provide privacy.[12,13]

Reviewing ECG waveforms and components

An electrocardiogram (ECG) waveform has three basic components: the P wave, QRS complex, and T wave. These elements can be further divided into the PR interval, J point, ST segment, U wave, and QT interval.

P wave and PR interval

The P wave represents atrial depolarization. The PR interval represents the time it takes an impulse to travel from the atria through the AV nodes and bundle of His. The PR interval measures from the beginning of the P wave to the beginning of the QRS complex.

QRS complex

The QRS complex represents ventricular depolarization (the time it takes for the impulse to travel through the bundle branches to the Purkinje fibers).

The Q wave, when present, appears as the first negative deflection in the QRS complex; the R wave, as the first positive deflection. The S wave appears as the second negative deflection or the first negative deflection after the R wave.

J point and ST segment

Marking the end of the QRS complex, the J point also indicates the beginning of the ST segment. The ST segment represents part of ventricular repolarization.

T wave and U wave

Usually following the same deflection pattern as the P wave, the T wave represents ventricular repolarization. The U wave follows the T wave, but isn't always seen.

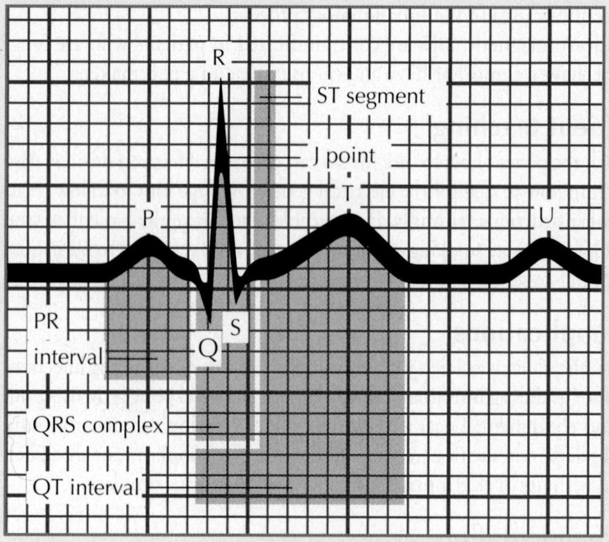

QT interval

The QT interval represents ventricular depolarization and repolarization. It extends from the beginning of the QRS complex to the end of the T wave.

■ Have the patient lie in the supine position in the center of the bed with his arms at his sides.[1,2] Raise the head of the bed if he desires *to promote comfort.*

■ Expose the patient's arms, legs, and chest, and then cover him appropriately with a bath blanket or sheet. His arms and legs should remain relaxed *to minimize trembling, which can cause electrical interference.*[2]

■ Select the electrode sites. Select flat, fleshy areas to place the limb lead electrodes. Avoid muscular and bony areas. If the patient has an amputated limb, choose a site on the stump. Mark the sites with an indelible marker if serial ECGs are likely.[3]

■ If an area is excessively hairy, clip the hair using clippers.

■ Clean the skin at each electrode site with a soap and water or cleaning pads and then dry it thoroughly *to enhance electrode contact.* Then clean any oils from the skin with an alcohol pad and allow the skin to dry.[3]

■ Rub the skin with a gauze pad or washcloth *to remove dead skin cells and promote impulse transmission.*[3]

■ Apply disposable pregelled electrodes to the patient's wrists and to the medial aspects of his ankles. Apply the pregelled electrodes directly to the prepared sites as recommended by the manufacturer's instructions. *To guarantee the best connection to the leadwire,* position electrodes on the patient's legs with the lead connections pointing superiorly.

■ Apply a pregelled electrode at each electrode position on the patient's chest. Place the chest electrodes below the breast tissue. If the patient is a woman, be sure to place the chest electrodes below the breast tissue. In a large-breasted woman, you may need to displace the breast tissue laterally. (See *Positioning chest electrodes.*)

■ Connect the leadwires to the electrodes. Note that the tip of each leadwire is lettered and color-coded *for easy identification.* The white or RA leadwire goes to the right arm; the green or RL leadwire, to the right leg; the red or LL leadwire, to the left leg; the black or LA leadwire, to the left arm; and the brown or V_1 to V_6 leadwires, to the chest electrodes.

■ Check to see that the paper speed selector is set to the standard 25 mm/second and that the machine is set to full voltage. The machine will record a normal standardization mark—a square that's the height of 2 large squares or 10 small squares on the recording paper.

■ If any part of the waveform height extends beyond the paper when you record the ECG, adjust the normal standardization to half-standardization. Note this adjustment on the ECG strip *because this will need to be considered in interpreting the results.*[2]

■ Ask the patient to relax and breathe normally. Tell him to lie still and not to talk when you record the ECG.

■ Press the AUTO or START button (as shown below). Observe the tracing quality. The machine will record all 12 leads automatically, recording 3 consecutive leads simultaneously. Some machines have a display screen so you can preview waveforms before the machine records them on paper.

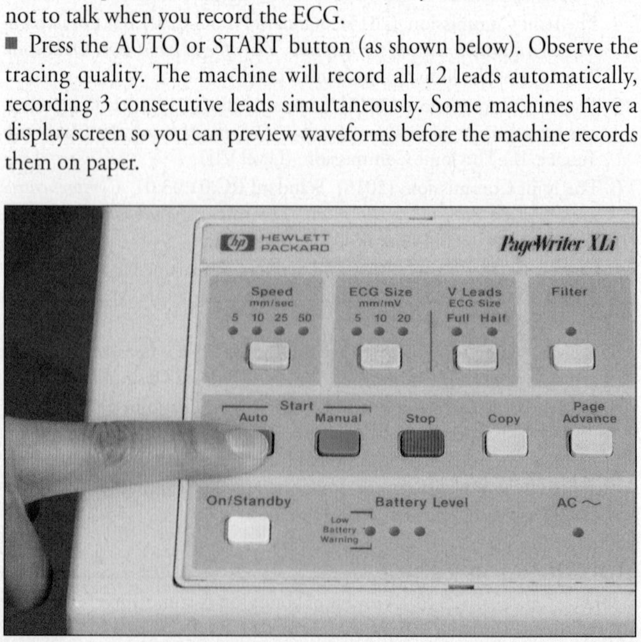

- When the machine finishes recording the 12-lead ECG, turn off the machine, remove the electrodes, and clean the patient's skin. After disconnecting the leadwires from the electrodes, dispose of the electrodes, as indicated.
- Remove and discard your gloves, if worn.
- Perform hand hygiene.[4,5,6,7,8,9]
- Document the procedure.[14,15,16]

Special considerations

- During the procedure, ask the patient to breathe normally. If his respirations distort the recording, ask him to hold his breath briefly *to reduce baseline wander in the tracing.*
- If the patient has a pacemaker, you can perform an ECG with or without a magnet, according to the practitioner's orders. Be sure to note the presence of a pacemaker and the use of the magnet on the ECG strip.

Documentation

Document the date and time the ECG was obtained and significant responses by the patient in the patient's medical record. Verify the date, time, patient's name, and assigned identification number on the ECG itself. Note any appropriate clinical information on the ECG.

Positioning chest electrodes

To ensure accurate test results, position chest electrodes as follows:

V_1: Fourth intercostal space at right border of sternum
V_2: Fourth intercostal space at left border of sternum
V_3: Halfway between V_2 and V_4
V_4: Fifth intercostal space at midclavicular line
V_5: Fifth intercostal space at anterior axillary line (halfway between V_4 and V_6)
V_6: Fifth intercostal space at midaxillary line, level with V_4

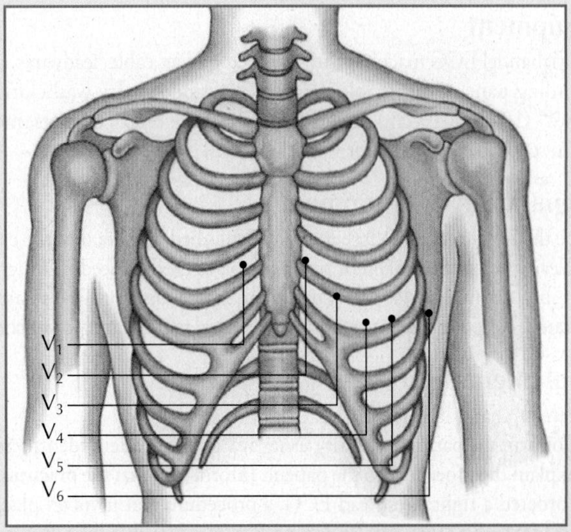

REFERENCES

1 Kligfield, P., et al. (2007). Recommendations for the standardization and interpretation of the electrocardiogram: Part I: The electrocardiogram and its technology: A scientific statement from the American Heart Association Electrocardiography and Arrhythmias Committee, Council on Clinical Cardiology; the American College of Cardiology Foundation; and the Heart Rhythm Society: Endorsed by the International Society for Computerized Electrocardiology. *Circulation, 115,* 1306–1324. (Level I)

2 Kadish, A. H., et al. (2001). ACC/AHA clinical competence statement on electrocardiography and ambulatory electrocardiography: A report of the ACC/AHA/ACP-ASIM Task Force on Clinical Competence (ACC/AHA Committee to Develop a Clinical Competence Statement on Electrocardiography and Ambulatory Electrocardiography).Endorsed by the International Society for Holter and Noninvasive Electrocardiology. *Circulation, 104,* 3169–3178. (Level I)

3 Lynn-McHale Wiegand, D. (Ed.). (2011). *AACN procedure manual for critical care* (6th ed.). St. Louis, MO: Saunders.

4 The Joint Commission. (2015). Standard NPSG.07.01.01. *Comprehensive accreditation manual for hospitals: The official handbook.* Oakbrook Terrace, IL: The Joint Commission. (Level VII)

5 Centers for Disease Control and Prevention. (2002). Guideline for hand hygiene in health-care settings: Recommendations of the Healthcare Infection Control Practices Advisory Committee and the HICPAC/SHEA/APIC/IDSA Hand Hygiene Task Force. *MMWR Recommendations and Reports, 51*(RR-16), 1–45. Accessed March 2015 via the Web at http://www.cdc.gov/mmwr/pdf/rr/rr5116.pdf (Level II)

6 World Health Organization. (2009). "WHO guidelines on hand hygiene in health care: First global patient safety challenge, clean care is safer care" [Online]. Accessed March 2015 via the Web at http://whqlibdoc.who.int/publications/2009/9789241597906_eng.pdf (Level IV)

7 Siegel, J. D., et al. (2007). "2007 guideline for isolation precautions: Preventing transmission of infectious agents in healthcare settings" [Online]. Accessed March 2015 via the Web at http://www.cdc.gov/hicpac/pdf/isolation/Isolation2007.pdf (Level II)

8 Centers for Medicare & Medicaid Services, Department of Health and Human Services. (2014). Condition of participation: Infection control. 42 C.F.R. § 482.42.

9 American Osteopathic Association. (2014). Standard 07.01.21. *Healthcare Facilities Accreditation Program: Accreditation requirements for acute care hospitals.* Chicago, IL: American Osteopathic Association. (Level VII)

10 American Osteopathic Association. (2014). Standard 07.01.10. *Healthcare Facilities Accreditation Program: Accreditation requirements for acute care hospitals.* Chicago, IL: American Osteopathic Association.

11 The Joint Commission. (2015). Standard NPSG.01.01.01. *Comprehensive accreditation manual for hospitals: The official handbook.* Oakbrook Terrace, IL: The Joint Commission. (Level VII)

12 American Osteopathic Association. (2014). Standard 15.01.16. *Healthcare Facilities Accreditation Program: Accreditation requirements for acute care hospitals.* Chicago, IL: American Osteopathic Association.

13 Centers for Medicare & Medicaid Services, Department of Health and Human Services. (2014). Condition of participation: Patient's rights. 42 C.F.R. § 482.13(c)(1).

14 The Joint Commission. (2015). Standard RC.01.03.01. *Comprehensive accreditation manual for hospitals: The official handbook.* Oakbrook Terrace, IL: The Joint Commission. (Level VII)

15 Centers for Medicare & Medicaid Services, Department of Health and Human Services. (2014). Condition of participation: Medical record services. 42 C.F.R. § 482.24.

16 American Osteopathic Association. (2014). Standard 10.00.03. *Healthcare Facilities Accreditation Program: Accreditation requirements for acute care hospitals.* Chicago, IL: American Osteopathic Association. (Level VII)

ADDITIONAL REFERENCES

American Heart Association. (2010). 2010 American Heart Association guidelines for cardiopulmonary resuscitation and emergency cardiovascular care. *Circulation, 122*(Suppl. 3), S640– S656.

Nettina, S. M. (2014). *Lippincott manual of nursing practice* (10th ed.). Philadelphia, PA: Wolters Kluwer.

ELECTROCARDIOGRAM, RIGHT CHEST LEAD

An electrocardiogram (ECG) measures the electrical activity of the heart. Unlike a standard 12-lead ECG, used primarily to evaluate left ventricular function, a right chest lead ECG reflects right ventricular function and provides clues to damage or dysfunction in this chamber. You might need to perform a right chest lead ECG for a patient with an inferior wall myocardial infarction (MI) and suspected right ventricular involvement. Between 25% and 50% of patients with this type of MI have right ventricular involvement.

Early identification of a right ventricular MI is essential because its treatment differs from treatment for other MIs. For instance, in left ventricular MI, treatment involves administering IV fluids judiciously to prevent heart failure. Conversely, in right ventricular MI, treatment typically requires administration of IV fluids to maintain adequate filling pressures on the right side of the heart. This helps the right ventricle eject an adequate volume of blood at an adequate pressure.

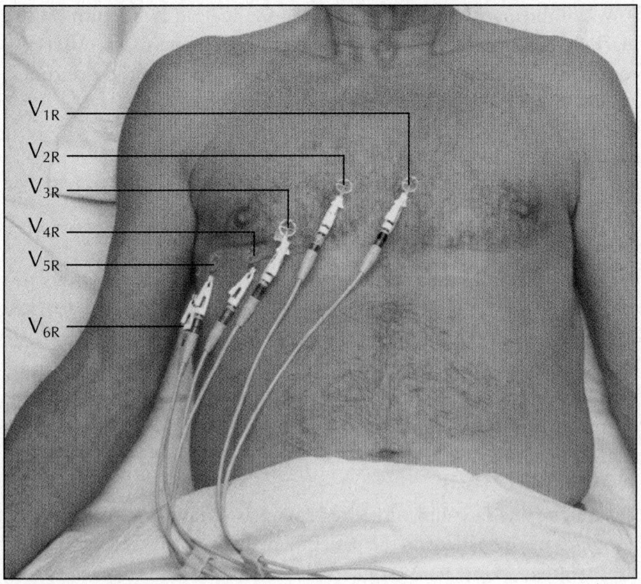

Equipment

Multichannel ECG machine with attached patient cable, leadwires, and recording paper ▪ disposable pregelled electrodes ▪ dry washcloth or 4″ × 4″ (10-cm × 10-cm) gauze pads ▪ Optional: drape, clippers, moist cloth, soap, towel, alcohol pad, marking pen, gloves.

Preparation of equipment

Place the ECG machine close to the patient's bed. Ensure that the cable and leadwires aren't broken or fraying; replace them if needed. Plug the cord into the wall outlet or, ensure the machine functions if it's battery operated. Keep the patient away from electrical fixtures and power cords.

Implementation

- Perform hand hygiene.[1,2,3,4,5]
- Confirm the patient's identity using at least two patient identifiers.[6]
- Explain the procedure to the patient. Inform him that the practitioner has ordered a right chest lead ECG, a procedure that involves placing electrodes on his arms, legs, and chest. Reassure him that the test is painless and takes only a few minutes, during which he'll need to lie quietly on his back.
- Have the patient lie in the supine position or, if he has difficulty lying flat, in the semi-Fowler position.[7]
- Provide privacy and expose his arms, chest, and legs. (Cover a female patient's chest with a drape until you apply the chest leads.)
- Put on gloves if needed *to comply with standard precautions.*[8]
- Select flat, fleshy areas to place the limb lead electrodes. Avoid muscular and bony areas. If the patient has an amputated limb, choose a site on the stump.
- *To enhance limb lead electrode contact,* prepare the application sites by washing them with soap and water and drying them thoroughly. If the patient is diaphoretic or if the skin is oily or has lotion on it, you may use an alcohol pad to remove the substance. If the area is excessively hairy, clip it.[9]
- Rub the electrode sites briskly with a dry washcloth or gauze pad *to remove dead skin cells and promote impulse transmission.*[9,10]
- For the limb leads, apply disposable pregelled electrodes to the patient's arms and legs, distal to the shoulders and hips.[9] Position them in approximately the same location on each limb. Apply each electrode directly to the prepared site, as recommended by the manufacturer's instructions. *To guarantee the best connection to the leadwire,* position disposable pregelled electrodes on the legs with the lead connection pointing superiorly
- Connect the leadwires to the electrodes. The leadwires are color-coded and lettered. Place the white or right arm (RA) wire on the right arm, the black or left arm (LA) wire on the left arm, the green or right leg (RL) wire on the right leg, and the red or left leg (LL) wire on the left leg.
- Examine the patient's chest *to locate the correct sites for chest lead placement* (as shown on top right). If the patient is female, place the electrodes under the breast tissue. Prepare the electrode application sites as done for the limb leads.
- Use your fingers to feel between the patient's ribs (the intercostal spaces). Start at the second intercostal space on the left (the notch felt at the top of the sternum, where the manubrium joins the body of the sternum). Count down two spaces to the fourth intercostal space at the left sternal border. Then apply a disposable pregelled electrode to the site and attach leadwire V_{1R} to that electrode.
- Move your fingers across the sternum to the fourth intercostal space at the right sternal border. Apply a disposable pregelled electrode to that site and attach lead V_{2R}.
- Move your finger down to the fifth intercostal space and over to the midclavicular line. Place a disposable pregelled electrode here and attach lead V_{4R}. Apply a disposable pregelled electrode midway on this line from V_{2R} and attach lead V_{3R}.
- Move your finger horizontally from V_{4R} to the right midaxillary line. Apply an electrode to this site and attach lead V_{6R}.
- Move your fingers along the same horizontal line to the midpoint between V_{4R} and V_{6R}. This is the right anterior midaxillary line. Apply a disposable pregelled electrode to this site and attach lead V_{5R}.
- Turn on the ECG machine and input the required patient information if necessary.
- Ask the patient to breathe normally and to refrain from talking during the recording *so that muscle movement won't distort the tracing.*
- Make sure that the paper speed is set at 25 mm/second and the amplitude at 1 mV/10 mm.[10,11]
- Press the AUTO or START key. The ECG machine will record all 12 leads automatically. Check your facility's policy for the number of readings to obtain. (Some facilities require at least two ECGs *so that one copy can be sent out for interpretation while the other remains at the bedside.*)
- Observe the tracing quality. If any part of the waveform height extends beyond the paper when you record the ECG, adjust the normal standardization to half-standardization. Note this adjustment on the ECG strip *because this will need to be considered in interpreting the results.*[11]
- When you're finished recording the ECG, turn off the machine. Make sure that the ECG is clearly labeled with the patient's name, identification number, date, and time. Also label the tracing as "RIGHT CHEST ECG" *to distinguish it from a standard 12-lead ECG.* Make sure that the tracings are correctly labeled V_{1R} through V_{6R}.
- If you think you may need more than one right chest lead ECG, use a marking pen to mark the electrode sites on the patient's skin. *This permits accurate comparisons for future tracings.*
- Remove the electrodes and discard them in the appropriate receptacle.[8]
- Ensure that the ECG machine is in working order and ready for the next use.

- Remove and discard your gloves, if worn.[8]
- Perform hand hygiene.[1,2,3,4,5]
- Place the tracing in the patient's medical record.
- Document the procedure.[12,13,14]

Special considerations

- For best results, place the electrodes symmetrically on the limbs. If the patient's wrist or ankle is covered by a dressing or if the patient is an amputee, choose an area that's available on both sides.
- If your facility has the capability of transmitting the patient's ECG from the ECG machine to the patient's medical record, verify that the ECG transmission was completed successful.

Complications

Prolonged application of the adhesive on the electrodes may cause skin irritation or tissue breakdown. Failure to identify the tracing as a right chest ECG could lead to misdiagnosis.

Documentation

Document the date and time the procedure was performed and the patient's tolerance to the procedure. Place a copy of the tracing in the patient's medical record.

REFERENCES

1 The Joint Commission. (2015). Standard NPSG.07.01.01. *Comprehensive accreditation manual for hospitals: The official handbook.* Oakbrook Terrace, IL: The Joint Commission. (Level VII)

2 Centers for Disease Control and Prevention. (2002). Guideline for hand hygiene in health care settings: Recommendations of the Healthcare Infection Control Practices Advisory Committee and the HICPAC/SHEA/APIC/IDSA Hand Hygiene Task Force. *MMWR Recommendations and Reports, 51*(RR-16), 1–45. Accessed March 2015 via the Web at http://www.cdc.gov/mmwr/pdf/rr/rr5116.pdf (Level II)

3 World Health Organization. (2009). "WHO guidelines on hand hygiene in health care: First global patient safety challenge, clean care is safer care" [Online]. Accessed March 2015 via the Web at http://whqlibdoc.who.int/publications/2009/9789241597906_eng.pdf (Level IV)

4 Centers for Medicare & Medicaid Services, Department of Health and Human Services. (2014). Condition of participation: Infection control. 42 C.F.R. § 482.42.

5 American Osteopathic Association. (2014). Standard 07.01.21. *Healthcare Facilities Accreditation Program: Accreditation requirements for acute care hospitals.* Chicago, IL: American Osteopathic Association. (Level VII)

6 The Joint Commission. (2015). Standard NPSG.01.01.01. *Comprehensive accreditation manual for hospitals: The official handbook.* Oakbrook Terrace, IL: The Joint Commission. (Level VII)

7 Feldman, T., et al. (1985). Relation of electrocardiographic R-wave amplitude to changes in left ventricular chamber size and position in normal subjects. *American Journal of Cardiology, 55,* 1168–1174. (Level VI)

8 Siegel, J. D., et al. (2007). "2007 guideline for isolation precautions: Preventing transmission of infectious agents in healthcare settings" [Online]. Accessed March 2015 via the Web at http://www.cdc.gov/hicpac/pdf/isolation/Isolation2007.pdf (Level II)

9 Kligfield, P., et al. (2007). Recommendations for the standardization and interpretation of the electrocardiogram: Part I: The electrocardiogram and its technology: A scientific statement from the American Heart Association Electrocardiography and Arrhythmias Committee, Council on Clinical Cardiology; the American College of Cardiology Foundation; and the Heart Rhythm Society: Endorsed by the International Society for Computerized Electrocardiology. *Circulation, 115,* 1306–1324. (Level VII)

10 Lynn-McHale Wiegand, D. (Ed.). (2011). *AACN procedure manual for critical care* (6th ed.). Philadelphia, PA: Saunders.

11 American College of Cardiology/American Heart Association. (2001). ACC/AHA clinical competence statement on electrocardiography and ambulatory electrocardiography. *Circulation, 104,* 3169–3178. (Level VII)

12 The Joint Commission. (2015). Standard RC.01.03.01. *Comprehensive accreditation manual for hospitals: The official handbook.* Oakbrook Terrace, IL: The Joint Commission. (Level VII)

13 Centers for Medicare & Medicaid Services, Department of Health and Human Services. (2014). Condition of participation: Medical record services. 42 C.F.R. § 482.24(b).

14 American Osteopathic Association. (2014). Standard 10.00.03. *Healthcare Facilities Accreditation Program: Accreditation requirements for acute care hospitals.* Chicago, IL: American Osteopathic Association. (Level VII)

ADDITIONAL REFERENCE

Nettina, S. M. (2014). *Lippincott manual of nursing practice* (10th ed.). Philadelphia, PA: Wolters Kluwer.

ELECTROCARDIOGRAM, POSTERIOR CHEST LEAD

An electrocardiogram (ECG) is a recording of the electrical activity of the heart. The 12-lead ECG is an essential diagnostic tool in the management and treatment of ischemic heart disease, but because of the location of the heart's posterior surface, changes associated with myocardial damage may not be apparent on a standard 12-lead ECG. To help identify posterior involvement, some practitioners recommend using posterior chest leads in addition to the limb leads of the 12-lead ECG. Despite lung and muscle barriers, posterior leads may provide clues to posterior wall infarction. Because patients with coexisting posterior infarction are at greater risk for complications, acute therapy, including thrombolysis and angioplasty, shouldn't be delayed.[1]

Equipment

Multichannel ECG machine with attached patient cables, leadwires, and recording paper ▪ disposable pregelled electrodes ▪ dry washcloth or 4″ × 4″ (10-cm × 10-cm) gauze pads ▪ Optional: gloves, clippers, moist cloth, soap, alcohol pad, marking pen.

Preparation of equipment

Place the ECG machine close to the patient's bed. Verify that cables and leadwires aren't frayed or broken; replace them if necessary. Plug the cord into the wall outlet, or ensure that the machine functions if it's battery operated. Keep the patient away from electrical fixtures and power cords.

Implementation

- Perform hand hygiene.[2,3,4,5,6]
- Confirm the patient's identity using at least two patient identifiers.[7]
- Provide privacy. As you set up the machine to record a posterior chest ECG, explain the procedure to the patient. Tell him that the test records the heart's electrical activity and that it may be repeated at certain intervals. Emphasize that no electrical current will enter his body. Also, tell him that the test typically takes about 5 minutes.
- Have the patient lie in the supine position in the center of the bed with his arms at his sides.[8] You may raise the head of the bed *to promote comfort.* Expose the patient's arms and legs, and cover him appropriately. His arms and legs should be relaxed *to minimize muscle trembling, which can cause electrical interference.*[9]
- Put on gloves, if necessary, *to comply with standard precautions.*[10]
- Select fleshy areas to place the limb lead electrodes. Avoid muscular and bony areas. If the patient has an amputated limb, choose a site on the stump.
- *To enhance limb lead electrode contact,* prepare the application sites by washing them with soap and water and drying them thoroughly. If the patient is diaphoretic or if the skin is oily or has lotion on it, you may use an alcohol pad to remove oils or lotion from the skin. If an area is extremely hairy, clip it.[11]
- Rub the electrode sites briskly with a dry washcloth or gauze pad *to remove dead skin cells and promote impulse transmission.*[11,12]

Placing electrodes for posterior ECG

To ensure an accurate electrocardiogram (ECG) reading, make sure that the posterior leads V_7, V_8, and V_9 are placed at the same level horizontally as the V_6 lead at the fifth intercostal space. Place V_6 at the midaxillary line. Place lead V_7 at the posterior axillary line, lead V_9 at the left paraspinal line, and lead V_8 halfway between leads V_7 and V_9.

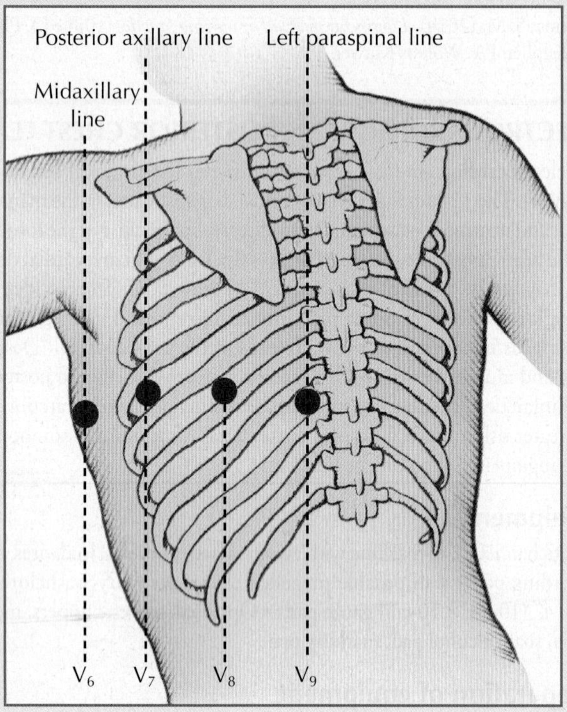

- For the limb leads, apply disposable pregelled electrodes to the patient's arms and legs, distal to the shoulders and hips. Position them in approximately the same location on each limb. Apply each electrode directly to the prepared site, as recommended by the manufacturer's instructions. *To guarantee the best connection to the leadwire,* position disposable pregelled electrodes on the legs with the lead connection pointing superiorly.
- Help the patient turn onto his right side and expose the left side of his back.
- Prepare the posterior electrode application sites as described for the limb leads.
- Attach a disposable pregelled electrode to the V_7 position on the left posterior axillary line, fifth intercostal space, at the same level as V_6. Then attach the V_4 leadwire to the V_7 electrode.
- Attach a disposable pregelled electrode to the patient's back at the V_9 position, just left of his spinal column at the left paraspinal line, at the same level as V_6 and V_7. Then, attach the V_6 leadwire to the V_9 electrode.
- Attach a disposable pregelled electrode to the patient's back at the V_8 position, halfway between leads V_7 and V_9, at the same level as V_6 and V_7, and attach the V_5 leadwire to this electrode. (See *Placing electrodes for posterior ECG.*)
- Turn on the machine and input the required patient information, if necessary.
- Ask the patient to breathe normally and to refrain from talking during the recording *so that muscle movement won't distort the tracing.*
- Make sure that the paper speed is set for 25 mm/second. If necessary, standardize the machine. Press AUTO or START.
- Observe the tracing quality. If any part of the waveform height extends beyond the paper when you record the ECG, adjust the normal standardization to half-standardization. Note this adjustment on the ECG strip *because this adjustment will need to be considered in interpreting the results.*
- When using a multichannel ECG machine, the unattached leads will print out as straight lines. Make sure that the leads are correctly labeled V_4, V_5, and V_6 to leads V_7, V_8, and V_9, respectively.
- When the ECG is complete, turn off the machine.
- Label the tracing with the patient's name and the date and time. Note whether the tracing is a right- or left-posterior chest lead ECG. Make sure the leads are correctly labeled V_7 through V_9.
- Remove the electrodes and discard them in the appropriate receptacle.[10]
- Clean the patient's skin with a gauze pad or a moist cloth. If you think you may need more than one posterior lead ECG, use a marking pen to mark the electrode sites on the patient's skin *to permit accurate comparison for future tracings.*
- Ensure that the ECG machine, cable, and leads are in working order and ready for the next use.
- Remove and discard your gloves, if worn.[10]
- Perform hand hygiene.[2,3,4,5,6]
- Place the ECG in the patient's medical record.
- Document the procedure.[13,14,15]

Special considerations

For best results, place the electrodes symmetrically on the limbs. If the patient's wrist or ankle is covered by a dressing or if the patient is an amputee, choose an area that's available on both sides. If your facility has the capability of transmitting the patient's ECG from the ECG machine to the patient's electronic medical record, verify that the ECG transmission was completed successfully.

Complications

Prolonged application of the adhesive on the electrodes may cause skin irritation or tissue breakdown. Failure to correctly label the ECG leads could lead to misdiagnosis.

Documentation

Document in your notes the test's date and time and significant responses by the patient. Verify the date, time, patient's name, and assigned identification number on the ECG itself. Note any appropriate clinical information on the ECG.

REFERENCES

1 van Gorselen, E. O. F., et al. (2007). "Posterior myocardial infarction: The dark side of the moon" [Online]. Accessed March 2015 via the Web at http://www.ncbi.nlm.nih.gov/pmc/articles/PMC1847720/ (Level V)

2 The Joint Commission. (2015). Standard NPSG.07.01.01. *Comprehensive accreditation manual for hospitals: The official handbook.* Oakbrook Terrace, IL: The Joint Commission. (Level VII)

3 Centers for Disease Control and Prevention. (2002). Guideline for hand hygiene in health-care settings: Recommendations of the Healthcare Infection Control Practices Advisory Committee and the HICPAC/SHEA/APIC/IDSA Hand Hygiene Task Force. *MMWR Recommendations and Reports, 51*(RR-16), 1–45. Accessed March 2015 via the Web at http://www.cdc.gov/mmwr/pdf/rr/rr5116.pdf (Level II)

4 World Health Organization. (2009). "WHO guidelines on hand hygiene in health care: First global patient safety challenge, clean care is safer care" [Online]. Accessed March 2015 via the Web at http://whqlibdoc.who.int/publications/2009/9789241597906_eng.pdf (Level IV)

5 Centers for Medicare & Medicaid Services, Department of Health and Human Services. (2014). Condition of participation: Infection control. 42 C.F.R. § 482.42.

6 American Osteopathic Association. (2014). Standard 07.01.21. *Healthcare Facilities Accreditation Program: Accreditation requirements for acute care hospitals.* Chicago, IL: American Osteopathic Association. (Level VII)

7 The Joint Commission. (2015). Standard NPSG.01.01.01. *Comprehensive accreditation manual for hospitals: The official handbook.* Oakbrook Terrace, IL: The Joint Commission. (Level VII)

8 Feldman, T., et al. (1985). Relation of electrocardiographic R-wave amplitude to changes in left ventricular chamber size and position in normal subjects. *American Journal of Cardiology, 55,* 1168–1174. (Level VI)

9 American College of Cardiology/American Heart Association. (2001). ACC/AHA clinical competence statement on electrocardiography and ambulatory electrocardiography. *Circulation, 104,* 3169–3178. (Level VII)

10 Siegel, J. D., et al. (2007). "2007 guideline for isolation precautions: Preventing transmission of infectious agents in healthcare settings" [Online]. Accessed March 2015 via the Web at http://www.cdc.gov/hicpac/pdf/isolation/Isolation2007.pdf (Level II)

11 American Heart Association, American College of Cardiology Foundation, Heart Rhythm Society. (2007). Recommendations for the standardization and interpretation of the electrocardiogram: Part I: The electrocardiogram and its technology: A scientific statement from the American Heart Association Electrocardiography and Arrhythmias Committee, Council on Clinical Cardiology; the American College of Cardiology Foundation; and the Heart Rhythm Society: Endorsed by the International Society for Computerized Electrocardiology. *Circulation, 115,* 1306–1324 (Level VII)

12 Lynn-McHale Wiegand, D. (Ed.). (2011). *AACN procedure manual for critical care* (6th ed.). Philadelphia, PA: Saunders.

13 The Joint Commission. (2015). Standard RC.01.03.01. *Comprehensive accreditation manual for hospitals: The official handbook.* Oakbrook Terrace, IL: The Joint Commission. (Level VII)

14 Centers for Medicare & Medicaid Services, Department of Health and Human Services. (2014). Condition of participation: Medical record services. 42 C.F.R. § 482.24(b).

15 American Osteopathic Association. (2014). Standard 10.00.03. *Healthcare Facilities Accreditation Program: Accreditation requirements for acute care hospitals.* Chicago, IL: American Osteopathic Association. (Level VII)

ADDITIONAL REFERENCES

Katoh, T., et al. (2011). Clinical significance of synthesized posterior/right-sided chest lead electrocardiograms in patients with acute chest pain. *Journal of Nippon Medical School, 78,* 22–29. (Level VI)

Khan, J. N., et al. (2012). Posterior myocardial infarction: Are we failing to diagnose this? *Emergency Medicine Journal, 29,* 15–18. Accessed March 2015 via the Web at http://emj.bmj.com/content/29/1/15.full.pdf+html (Level VI)

Nettina, S. M. (2014). *Lippincott manual of nursing practice* (10th ed.). Philadelphia, PA: Wolters Kluwer.

ELECTROCARDIOGRAM, SIGNAL-AVERAGED

An electrocardiogram (ECG) measures the electrical activity of the heart. A signal-averaged ECG is a more detailed type of ECG and helps to identify patients at risk for sustained ventricular tachycardia. Because this cardiac arrhythmia can be a precursor of sudden death after a myocardial infarction (MI), the results of a signal-averaged ECG can allow appropriate preventive measures.[1]

Using a computer-based ECG, signal averaging detects low-amplitude signals or late electrical potentials, which reflect slow conduction or disorganized ventricular activity through abnormal or infarcted regions of the ventricles. The signal-averaged ECG is developed by recording the noise-free surface ECG in three specialized leads for several hundred beats. (See *Placing electrodes for signal-averaged ECG.*) Signal averaging enhances signals that would otherwise be missed because of increased amplitude and sensitivity to ventricular activity. For instance, on the standard 12-lead ECG, "noise" created by muscle tissue, electronic artifacts, and electrodes masks late potentials, which have a low amplitude.

Placing electrodes for signal-averaged ECG

To prepare your patient for a signal-averaged electrocardiogram (ECG), place the electrodes in the X, Y, and Z orthogonal positions, as shown below. These positions bisect one another to provide a three-dimensional, composite view of ventricular activation.

Anterior chest

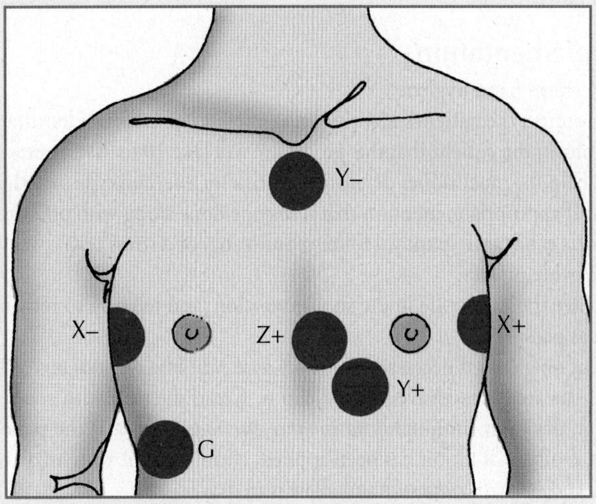

Posterior chest

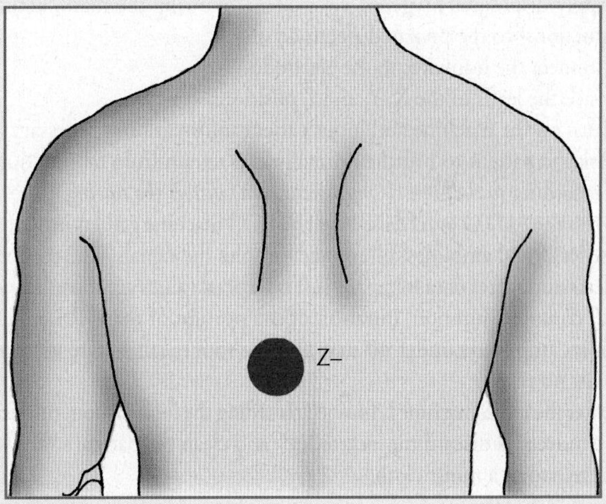

KEY

X+ Fourth intercostal space, midaxillary line, left side
X– Fourth intercostal space, midaxillary line, right side
Y+ Standard V_3 position (or proximal left leg)
Y– Superior aspect of manubrium
Z+ Standard V_2 position
Z– V_2 position, posterior
G Ground; eighth rib on right side

This procedure identifies the risk of sustained ventricular tachycardia in patients with malignant ventricular tachycardia, a history of MI, unexplained syncope, nonischemic congestive cardiomyopathy, or nonsustained ventricular tachycardia.

Equipment

Signal-averaged ECG machine with attached patient cable, leadwires, and recording paper ■ signal-averaged computer ■ record of patient's surface ECG for 200 to 300 QRS complexes ▪ three bipolar disposable pregelled electrodes ▪ Optional: moist cloth, soap, towel, alcohol pads, clippers, gloves.

Preparation of equipment

Place the ECG machine close to the patient's bed. Ensure that the cable and leadwires aren't broken or fraying; replace them if needed. Plug the machine's cord into the wall outlet, or ensure the machine functions if it's battery operated. Keep the patient away from the electrical fixtures and power cords.

Implementation

- Perform hand hygiene.[2,3,4,5,6]
- Confirm the patient's identity using at least two patient identifiers.[7]
- Inform the patient that this procedure will take 10 to 30 minutes and will help the practitioner determine his risk for a certain type of arrhythmia. If appropriate, mention that it may be done along with other tests, such as echocardiography, Holter monitoring, or a stress test.
- Provide privacy.[8]
- Have the patient lie in the supine position, and tell him to remain as still as possible.[9]
- Put on gloves if necessary *to comply with standard precautions.*[10,11]
- If the area is excessively hairy, clip it. Clean the skin with soap and water, drying it thoroughly *to enhance electrode contact.* If the patient's skin is oily or if lotion has been applied, clean the skin with an alcohol pad *to remove the substance* and allow it to dry.
- Rub the electrode sites briskly with a dry washcloth or gauze pad *to remove dry skin cells and promote impulse transmission.*[12]
- Apply disposable pregelled electrodes (following the manufacturer's instructions) to the prepared electrode sites.
- Connect the leadwires to the electrodes.
- Place the leads in the X, Y, and Z positions.
- Turn on the machine and input patient information if necessary.
- Ask the patient to breathe normally and refrain from talking during the recording *so that muscle movement won't distort the tracing.*
- Press the AUTO or START key. The ECG machine gathers input from these leads and amplifies, filters, and samples the signals. The computer collects and stores data for analysis. The crucial values are those showing QRS complex duration, duration of the portion of the QRS complex with an amplitude under 40 mV, and the root mean square voltage of the last 40 msec.
- After the ECG machine is finished recording the information, turn it off.
- Remove and discard the electrodes[10] and clean the patient's skin with a gauze pad or a moist cloth.
- Ensure that the machine is in working order and prepared for the next use.
- Remove and discard gloves your gloves, if worn.[10]
- Perform hand hygiene.[2,3,4,5,6]
- Place the ECG tracing in the patient's medical record for the practitioner to interpret.
- Document the procedure.[13,14,15]

Special considerations

- *Because muscle movements may cause a false-positive result,* patients who are restless or in respiratory distress are poor candidates for signal-averaged ECG. Proper electrode placement and skin preparation are essential to this procedure.
- Results indicating low-amplitude signals include a QRS complex duration greater than 110 msec, a duration of more than 40 msec for the amplitude portion under 40 mV, and a root mean square voltage of less than 25 mV during the last 40 msec of the QRS complex. However, all three factors don't need to be present to consider the result positive or negative. The final interpretation hinges on individualized patient factors.
- Results of signal-averaged ECG help the practitioner determine whether the patient is a candidate for invasive procedures, such as electrophysiologic testing or angiography.
- Keep in mind that the significance of signal-averaged ECG results in patients with bundle-branch heart block is unknown *because myocardial activation doesn't follow the usual sequence in these patients.*

Complications

Prolonged application of adhesive on the electrode may cause skin irritation or tissue breakdown at the application site.

Documentation

Document the time of the procedure, why the procedure was done, and how the patient tolerated it. Record any patient teaching and the patient's comprehension of your teaching.

REFERENCES

1 American College of Cardiology /American Heart Association. (2001). ACC/AHA clinical competence statement on electrocardiography and ambulatory electrocardiography. *Circulation, 104,* 3169–3178. (Level VII)

2 The Joint Commission. (2015). Standard NPSG.07.01.01. *Comprehensive accreditation manual for hospitals: The official handbook.* Oakbrook Terrace, IL: The Joint Commission. (Level VII)

3 Centers for Disease Control and Prevention. (2002). Guidelines for hand hygiene in health care settings: Recommendations of the Healthcare Infection Control Practices Advisory Committee and the HICPAC/SHEA/APIC/IDSA Hand Hygiene Task Force. *MMWR Recommendations and Reports, 51*(RR-16), 1–45. Accessed March 2015 via the Web at http://www.cdc.gov/mmwr/pdf/rr/rr5116.pdf (Level II)

4 World Health Organization. (2009). "WHO guidelines on hand hygiene in health care: First global patient safety challenge, clean care is safer care" [Online]. Accessed March 2015 via the Web at http://whqlibdoc.who.int/publications/2009/9789241597906_eng.pdf (Level IV)

5 Centers for Medicare & Medicaid Services, Department of Health and Human Services. (2014). Condition of participation: Infection control. 42 C.F.R. § 482.42.

6 American Osteopathic Association. (2014). Standard 07.01.21. *Healthcare Facilities Accreditation Program: Accreditation requirements for acute care hospitals.* Chicago, IL: American Osteopathic Association. (Level VII)

7 The Joint Commission. (2015). Standard NPSG.01.01.01. *Comprehensive accreditation manual for hospitals: The official handbook.* Oakbrook Terrace, IL: The Joint Commission. (Level VII)

8 American Osteopathic Association. (2014). Standard 15.01.16. *Healthcare Facilities Accreditation Program: Accreditation requirements for acute care hospitals.* Chicago, IL: American Osteopathic Association. (Level VII)

9 Feldman, T., et al. (1985). Relation of electrocardiographic R-wave amplitude to changes in left ventricular chamber size and position in normal subjects. *American College of Cardiology, 55,* 1168–1174. (Level VI)

10 Siegel, J. D., et al. (2007). "2007 guideline for isolation precautions: Preventing transmission of infectious agents in healthcare settings" [Online]. Accessed March 2015 via the Web at http://www.cdc.gov/hicpac/pdf/isolation/Isolation2007.pdf (Level II)

11 American Osteopathic Association. (2014). Standard 07.01.10. *Healthcare Facilities Accreditation Program: Accreditation requirements for acute care hospitals.* Chicago, IL: American Osteopathic Association. (Level VII)

12 Lynn-McHale Wiegand, D. (Ed.). (2011). *AACN procedure manual for critical care* (6th ed.). St. Louis, MO: Saunders.

13 The Joint Commission. (2015). Standard RC.01.03.01. *Comprehensive accreditation manual for hospitals: The official handbook.* Oakbrook Terrace, IL: The Joint Commission. (Level VII)

14 Centers for Medicare & Medicaid Services, Department of Health and Human Services. (2014). Condition of participation: Medical record services. 42 C.F.R. § 482.24(b).

15 American Osteopathic Association. (2014). Standard 10.00.03. *Healthcare Facilities Accreditation Program: Accreditation requirements for acute care hospitals.* Chicago, IL: American Osteopathic Association. (Level VII)

ADDITIONAL REFERENCE

Nettina, S. M. (2014). *Lippincott manual of nursing practice* (10th ed.). Philadelphia, PA: Wolters Kluwer.

ENDOSCOPIC THERAPY, ASSISTING

Endoscopic therapy allows visualization of the upper GI tract to help diagnose, control, or prevent bleeding and evacuate blood and clots.

During this procedure, the practitioner advances a fiber-optic endoscope through the patient's esophagus and into the stomach and duodenum to help look for a bleeding site. After locating the bleeding site, he may inject a sclerosing agent through an injector needle, which is inserted through a port in the endoscope. The practitioner injects the sclerosing agent into the bleeding vessel or tissue surrounding the vessel; he may also use laser or thermal therapy or apply a band to stop bleeding.

Equipment

Prescribed medications (anesthetics, sedatives, analgesics, sclerosing agent) ■ oral airway or bite block ■ water-soluble lubricant ■ oxygen administration equipment ■ suction apparatus ■ sterile normal saline solution or sterile water for irrigation ■ endoscope (rigid or flexible) ■ endoscopic injector needle (23G to 26G, 2- to 5-mm needle) ■ three 10-mL syringes filled with prescribed sclerosing agent ■ tonsil-tip suction device ■ gloves, gowns, masks, and goggles or face shields ■ two 30- to 60-mL syringes ■ cardiac monitor ■ pulse oximeter ■ capnometer ■ automatic blood pressure cuff ■ prescribed IV fluid ■ enzymatic detergent ■ lint-free cloth or sponge ■ Optional: endoscopic laser or thermal equipment, esophageal bands, specimen containers, laboratory biohazard transport bag, laboratory request form, nasogastric tube, IV catheter insertion equipment.

Preparation of equipment

Set up the suction apparatus and make sure it's functioning properly.[1] Prepare and label sedatives for administration, as ordered. Gather the emergency equipment and ensure proper function.

Label all medications, medication containers, and other solutions on and off the sterile field; on the label, include the medication name, dosage, strength, quantity, diluent and volume (if appropriate), and expiration date and time.[2,3]

Implementation

■ Verify the practitioner's orders.

■ Confirm that written informed consent was obtained and that the consent is in the patient's medical record.[4,5,6]

■ Conduct a preprocedure verification *to make sure that all relevant documentation, related information, and equipment are available and correctly identified to the patient's identifiers.*[7,8]

■ Verify that the laboratory and imaging studies have been completed as ordered and that the results are in the patient's medical record. Notify the practitioner of any unexpected results. If applicable, check the patient's medical record for pregnancy test results.[9]

■ Verify all medication or solution labels verbally and visually. *Verification is done by two individuals qualified to participate in the procedure whenever the person preparing the medication or solution isn't the person who'll be administering it.*[2,3]

■ Review baseline coagulation studies *because abnormal results increase the potential for bleeding.*[1] Review baseline hematocrit and hemoglobin levels.

■ Perform hand hygiene.[10,11,12,13,14]

■ Put personal protective equipment, as needed, *to comply with standard precautions.*[15,16,17]

■ Confirm the patient's identity using at least two patient identifiers.[18]

■ Reinforce the practitioner's explanation of the procedure, and answer the patient's questions *to evaluate his understanding of the information provided.*

■ Confirm the patient's nothing-by-mouth status before the procedure; minimum fasting recommendations include 2 hours for clear liquids, 6 or more hours for a light meal, and 8 hours or more for fried or fatty foods or meat.[1,19]

■ Assess the patient for conditions that may make ventilation difficult, such as significant obesity, a history of snoring or sleep apnea, facial hair, missing teeth, or the presence of stridor.[9]

■ Remove the patient's dentures, if appropriate, *because they can interfere with safe passage of the endoscope.*

■ Verify that the patient has an adequate-sized, patent IV catheter (an 18G catheter is preferred) *to administer sedation and any emergency medications or IV fluid, if necessary.* If an adequate catheter isn't in place, insert one. (See the "IV catheter insertion and removal" procedure, page 446.) Begin an IV infusion, as prescribed.

■ Provide goggles or a waterproof covering for the patient's eyes *to protect him against accidental exposure to blood or the sclerosing agent.*[15,16,17]

■ Attach the patient to the cardiac monitor, pulse oximeter, and automatic blood pressure cuff *for continuous monitoring during the procedure.*[1] Set the alarm limits appropriately for the patient's current condition and make sure that the alarms are turned on, functioning, and audible to staff.[20,21,22,23]

■ Attach the patient to a capnometer *to continuously monitor exhaled carbon dioxide during the procedure.* Make sure the alarm limits are set properly for the patient's current condition and alarms are turned on, functioning properly, and audible to staff.[20,21,22,23,24]

■ Obtain baseline vital signs and assess the patient's neurologic, cardiac, and respiratory status *to serve as a baseline for comparison during and after the procedure.*[1,25,26,27]

■ Determine the patient's sedation score based on vital signs, level of consciousness (LOC), and respiratory status using a facility-approved scoring system.[26,28]

■ Position the patient in the left lateral position. *This position is the position of choice to prevent aspiration and allow predictable views of the stomach as the scope is advanced; it allows secretions to collect in the dependent areas of the mouth for ease of suctioning.*[1]

■ Administer analgesia, sedation, or both as ordered, following safe medication administration practices, before endoscope insertion *to facilitate the insertion process.*[1]

NURSING ALERT *Moderate sedation agents are considered high-alert medications* because they can cause significant patient harm when used in error. *If required by your facility, before beginning the medication, have another nurse perform an independent double-check* to ensure safe medication administration.[30,31] (*See* **Double-checking high-alert medications**, page 274.)

■ After comparing results of the independent double-check with the other nurse (if required), administer the medication if there are no discrepancies. If discrepancies exist, rectify them before administering the medication.

■ Administer each medication separately in incremental doses, and titrate it to the desired effect *to decrease the risk of overdose and respiratory and circulatory depression.*[9]

■ Continuously monitor the patient's heart rate and function, oxygenation, and respiratory rate and adequacy of ventilation.[24,32,33]

■ Determine and evaluate the patient's blood pressure and heart rate at least every 5 minutes.[24,33]

■ Monitor the patient's LOC (by checking response to verbal commands when practical), comfort level, and skin condition at regular intervals.[9]

Double-checking high-alert medications[31]

When administering high-alert medications such as moderate sedation agents, if required by your facility, another nurse must perform an independent double-check of your preparation of the drug *to ensure safe administration.* The second nurse should do the following:

- Verify the patient's identity.
- Make sure that the correct medication is being given and in the prescribed concentration.
- Make sure that the medication's indication corresponds with the patient's diagnosis.
- Verify that the dosage calculations are correct and the dosing formula used to derive the final dose is correct.
- Verify that the route of administration is safe and appropriate for the patient.
- Ensure that pump settings are correct and that the infusion line is attached to the correct port, if appropriate.

- Administer supplemental oxygen if hypoxia occurs.[33] Determine the method and rate of flow by the patient's optimal oxygen saturation level according to pulse oximetry.[9]
- Assist the practitioner as indicated during the procedure.[13] If you're monitoring the patient, you can assist with minor, interruptible tasks when the patient's condition is stable. However, another trained staff member should assist with more complicated procedures.[32,34]
- The practitioner will anesthetize the posterior pharynx with a topical anesthetic agent. He'll insert an oral airway *to prevent the patient from biting down on the endoscope.*[1]
- The practitioner will lubricate the distal end of the endoscope with a water-soluble lubricant *to facilitate passage of the endoscope.*[1] Instruct the patient to swallow while the endoscope is being advanced *to help facilitate passage into the esophagus.*[1]
- Suction the oropharynx, as needed, using a tonsil-tip suction catheter *to prevent aspiration of secretions.*[1]
- Prepare the equipment for thermal or laser coagulation therapy, as needed, *which will be used to control bleeding.*[1]
- Assist with irrigation using sterile normal saline solution or sterile water through the endoscope *to improve visualization.*[1]
- If the site requires sclerosing, assist with the sclerosing needle and inject the sclerosing agent, as requested.[1]
- Provide the practitioner with endoscopic bands as requested if endoscopic variceal ligation (the treatment of choice for controlling variceal hemorrhage) is necessary.[35]
- If the practitioner obtains a specimen for testing, place it in the proper specimen container, label the container in the presence of the patient *to prevent mislabeling,* and place the container in a laboratory transport bag.[17,18]
- The practitioner will then carefully remove the endoscope.
- Insert a nasogastric tube, if ordered, *to assess for recurrent bleeding.* (See the "Nasogastric tube insertion and removal" procedure, page 531.)[1]
- Assess the patient for gag, swallow, and cough reflexes. Maintain the patient in the left lateral position until his gag, swallow, and cough reflexes return. After these reflexes return, reposition the patient *to promote comfort.*
- Remove your personal protective equipment and place it in the appropriate receptacle.[15,17]
- Perform hand hygiene.[10,11,12,13,14]
- After the procedure, continue to monitor the patient's using the same monitoring parameters used during the procedure; monitor him until discharge criteria are met. The patient should remain awake for at least 20 minutes without stimulation before he's considered ready for discharge. The duration and frequency of monitoring should be individualized depending on the level of sedation achieved, the patient's overall condition, and the nature of the procedure for which sedation was administered. If a reversal agent was given, monitor the patient for a sufficient time (for example, 2 hours) after the last administration of an antagonist *to make sure that the patient doesn't become resedated after the reversal effects have worn off.*[9,33,36]
- Immediately after use, preclean the endoscope before sending it for reprocessing: Wipe the insertion end of the endoscope with a wet sponge or lint-free cloth soaked in freshly prepared enzymatic detergent solution. Insert the distal portion of the endoscope into the solution container and use the suction device to suction the solution through the air, water, and biopsy channels. Alternate between suctioning the solution and air until the return solution is visibly clean. Flush or blow air through the channels according to the endoscope manufacturer's instructions. Detach the endoscope from the light source and suction setup. If you're using a videoendoscope, attach the protective video cap to the device. Place the endoscope in a container for transport to the reprocessing area.[37,38,39,40]
- Send specimens to the laboratory in the laboratory transport bag along with a completed laboratory request form.
- Perform hand hygiene.[10,11,12,13,14]
- Document the procedure.[41,42,43]

Special considerations

- Endoscope insertion and advancement may stimulate a vagal response in the patient, causing bradycardia. Closely monitor the patient.[1]
- Keep in mind that sedatives and topical anesthetics interfere with the patient's gag reflex, placing the patient at risk for aspiration. Moderate sedation may also put the patient at risk for respiratory depression.[1]
- The Joint Commission issued a sentinel event alert concerning medical device alarm safety *because alarm-related events have been associated with permanent loss of function or death.* Among the major contributing factors were improper alarm settings, alarm settings inappropriately turned off, and alarm signals not audible to staff. Make sure alarm limits are set appropriately, and that alarms are turned on, functioning properly, and audible to staff. Follow facility guidelines for preventing alarm fatigue.[21]

Complications

Complications include respiratory depression, hypotension, bradycardia, anaphylactic reaction to the sclerosing agent and premedications, aspiration, bleeding, temporary dysphagia, esophageal perforation, and decreased LOC.

Documentation

Record the patient's vital signs, pulse oximetry, and other assessment findings before, during and after the procedure. Document the date and time of the procedure, sclerosing agent administered, if applicable; any other therapies used during the procedure; and the patient's tolerance of the procedure. If any unexpected complications occurred, document the necessary interventions and the patient's response to such interventions. Also document any patient and family teaching and their understanding of the teaching.

REFERENCES

1 Lynn-McHale Wiegand, D. (Ed.). (2011). *AACN procedure manual for critical care* (6th ed.). St. Louis, MO: Saunders.

2 The Joint Commission. (2015). Standard NPSG.03.04.01. *Comprehensive accreditation manual for hospitals: The official handbook.* Oakbrook Terrace, IL: The Joint Commission. (Level VII)

3 American Osteopathic Association. (2014). Standard 25.01.27. *Healthcare Facilities Accreditation Program: Accreditation requirements for acute care hospitals.* Chicago, IL: American Osteopathic Association. (Level VII)
4 The Joint Commission. (2015). Standard RI.01.03.01. *Comprehensive accreditation manual for hospitals: The official handbook.* Oakbrook Terrace, IL: The Joint Commission. (Level VII)
5 Centers for Medicare & Medicaid Services, Department of Health and Human Services. (2014). Condition of participation: Patient's rights. 42 C.F.R. § 482.13(c)(1).
6 American Osteopathic Association. (2014). Standard 30.01.11. *Healthcare Facilities Accreditation Program: Accreditation requirements for acute care hospitals.* Chicago, IL: American Osteopathic Association. (Level VII)
7 The Joint Commission. (2015). Standard UP.01.01.01. *Comprehensive accreditation manual for hospitals: The official handbook.* Oakbrook Terrace, IL: The Joint Commission. (Level VII)
8 American Osteopathic Association. (2014). Standard 30.00.14. *Healthcare Facilities Accreditation Program: Accreditation requirements for acute care hospitals.* Chicago, IL: American Osteopathic Association. (Level VII)
9 Recommended practices for managing the patient receiving moderate sedation/analgesia. (2014). In R. Conner, et al. (Eds.), *Perioperative standards and recommended practices 2014.* Denver, CO: AORN, Inc.
10 Centers for Disease Control and Prevention. (2002). Guideline for hand hygiene in health care settings: Recommendations of the Healthcare Infection Control Practices Advisory Committee and the HICPAC/SHEA/APIC/IDSA Hand Hygiene Task Force. *MMWR Recommendations and Reports, 51*(RR-16), 1–45. Accessed March 2015 via the Web at http://www.cdc.gov/mmwr/pdf/rr/rr5116.pdf (Level II)
11 The Joint Commission. (2015). Standard NPSG.07.01.01. *Comprehensive accreditation manual for hospitals: The official handbook.* Oakbrook Terrace, IL: The Joint Commission. (Level VII)
12 World Health Organization. (2009). "WHO guidelines on hand hygiene in health care: First global patient safety challenge, clean care is safer care" [Online]. Accessed March 2015 via the Web at http://whqlibdoc.who.int/publications/2009/9789241597906_eng.pdf (Level IV)
13 American Osteopathic Association. (2014). Standard 07.01.21. *Healthcare Facilities Accreditation Program: Accreditation requirements for acute care hospitals.* Chicago, IL: American Osteopathic Association. (Level VII)
14 Centers for Medicare & Medicaid Services, Department of Health and Human Services. (2014). Condition of participation: Infection control. 42 C.F.R. § 482.42.
15 Siegel, J.D., et al. (2007). "2007 guideline for isolation precautions: Preventing transmission of infectious agents in healthcare settings" [Online]. Accessed March 2015 via the Web at http://www.cdc.gov/hicpac/pdf/isolation/Isolation2007.pdf (Level II)
16 American Osteopathic Association. (2014). Standard 07.01.10. *Healthcare Facilities Accreditation Program: Accreditation requirements for acute care hospitals.* Chicago, IL: American Osteopathic Association. (Level VII)
17 Occupational Safety and Health Administration. (n.d.). "Bloodborne pathogens, standard number 1910.1030" [Online]. Accessed March 2015 via the Web at http://www.osha.gov/pls/oshaweb/owadisp.show_document?p_table=STANDARDS&p_id=10051 (Level VII)
18 The Joint Commission. (2015). Standard NPSG.01.01.01. *Comprehensive accreditation manual for hospitals: The official handbook.* Oakbrook Terrace, IL: The Joint Commission. (Level VII)
19 American Society of Anesthesiologists. (2011). "Practice guidelines for preoperative fasting and the use of pharmacologic agents to reduce the risk of pulmonary aspiration: Application to healthy patients undergoing elective procedures" [Online]. Accessed March 2015 via the Web at http://journals.lww.com/anesthesiology/Fulltext/2011/03000/Practice_Guidelines_for_Preoperative_Fasting_and.13.aspx (Level VII)
20 The Joint Commission. (2015). Standard NPSG.06.01.01. *Comprehensive accreditation manual for hospitals: The official handbook.* Oakbrook Terrace, IL: The Joint Commission. (Level VII)
21 The Joint Commission. (2013). "Sentinel event alert: Medical device alarm safety in hospitals" [Online]. Accessed March 2015 via the Web at http://www.jointcommission.org/assets/1/18/SEA_50_alarms_4_5_13_FINAL1.PDF (Level VII)
22 Graham, K. C., & Cvach, M. (2010). Monitor alarm fatigue: Standardizing use of physiological monitors and decreasing nuisance alarms. *American Journal of Critical Care, 19,* 28–37.
23 American Association of Critical-Care Nurses. (2013). "AACN practice alert: Alarm management" [Online]. Accessed March 2015 via the Web at http://www.aacn.org/wd/practice/docs/practicealerts/alarm-management-practice-alert.pdf (Level VII)
24 American Society of Anesthesiologists. (2011). "Standards for basic anesthetic monitoring" [Online]. Accessed March 2015 via the Web at http://www.asahq.org/For-Members/Standards-Guidelines-and-Statements.aspx
25 The Joint Commission. (2015). Standard PC.03.01.03. *Comprehensive accreditation manual for hospitals: The official handbook.* Oakbrook Terrace, IL: The Joint Commission. (Level VII)
26 Centers for Medicare & Medicaid Services, Department of Health and Human Services. (2014). Condition of participation: Surgical services. 42 C.F.R. § 482.51.
27 American Osteopathic Association (2014). Standard 30.01.04. *Healthcare Facilities Accreditation Program: Accreditation requirements for acute care hospitals.* Chicago, IL: American Osteopathic Association. (Level VII)
28 The Joint Commission. (2015). Standard PC.03.01.03. *Comprehensive accreditation manual for hospitals: The official handbook.* Oakbrook Terrace, IL: The Joint Commission. (Level VII)
29 The Joint Commission. (2015). Standard UP.01.03.01. *Comprehensive accreditation manual for hospitals: The official handbook.* Oakbrook Terrace, IL: The Joint Commission. (Level VII)
30 Institute for Safe Medication Practices. (2012). "ISMP's list of high-alert medications" [Online]. Accessed March 2015 via the Web at http://www.ismp.org/tools/highalertmedications.pdf (Level VII)
31 Institute for Safe Medication Practices. (2008). Conducting an independent double-check. *ISMP Medication Safety Alert! Nurse Advise-ERR, 6*(12), 1. Accessed March 2015 via the Web at http://www.ismp.org/newsletters/nursing/Issues/NurseAdviseERR200812.pdf (Level VII)
32 Society of Gastroenterology Nurses and Associates, Inc. (2010). "Position statement: Statement on the use of sedation and analgesia in the gastrointestinal endoscopy setting" [Online]. Accessed March 2015 via the Web at http://www.sgna.org/Portals/0/Education/Position%20Statements/SedationFINAL.pdf
33 American Society of Anesthesiologists. (2002). Practice guidelines for sedation and analgesia by non-anesthesiologists. *Anesthesiology, 96,* 1004–1017.
34 Society of Gastroenterological Nurses and Associates, Inc. (2009). "Position statement: Manipulation of endoscopes during endoscopic procedures" [Online]. Accessed March 2015 via the Web at http://www.sgna.org/Portals/0/Education/Position%20Statements/ManipulationofEndoscopesPositionStatements.pdf
35 Qureshi, W., et al. (2002, updated 2005). ASGE guideline: The role of endoscopy in the management of variceal hemorrhage, updated July 2005. *Gastrointestinal Endoscopy, 62,* 651–655. Accessed March 2015 via the Web at http://www.asge.org/assets/0/71542/71544/e3123745d4604279a85d65f2cedc025d.pdf (Level VII)
36 Meyers, J. L., & Chaudhuri, S. (2011). Procedural sedation and analgesia: A practical review for non-anesthesiologists. *Journal of Surgical Radiology, 2,* 344–356.
37 Rutala, W. A., et al. (2008). "Guideline for disinfection and sterilization in healthcare facilities, 2008" [Online]. Accessed March 2015 via the Web at http://www.cdc.gov/hicpac/pdf/guidelines/Disinfection_Nov_2008.pdf (Level I)
38 Society of Gastroenterology Nurses Practice Committee. (2010). Reprocessing of endoscopic accessories and valves. *Gastroenterology Nursing, 33,* 139–140. (Level VII)
39 American Society for Gastrointestinal Endoscopy. (2011). "Multisociety guideline on reprocessing flexible gastrointestinal endoscopes: 2011" [Online]. Accessed March 2015 via the Web at http://www.asge.org/uploadedFiles/Publications_and_Products/Practice_Guidelines/Multisociety%20guideline%20on%20reprocessing%20flexible%20gastrointestinal.pdf (Level VII)

Administering endotracheal drugs

In an emergency, some drugs can be given through an endotracheal (ET) tube if IV or intraosseous access isn't available. They may be given using the syringe method or the adapter method. Before injecting any drug, check for proper placement of the ET tube using an end-tidal carbon dioxide detector, an esophageal detection device, or continuous waveform capnography. Make sure the patient is in the supine position with the head level with or slightly higher than the body.

Syringe method

Remove the needle before injecting medication into the ET tube. Insert the tip of the syringe into the ET tube, and inject the drug deep into the tube (as shown below).

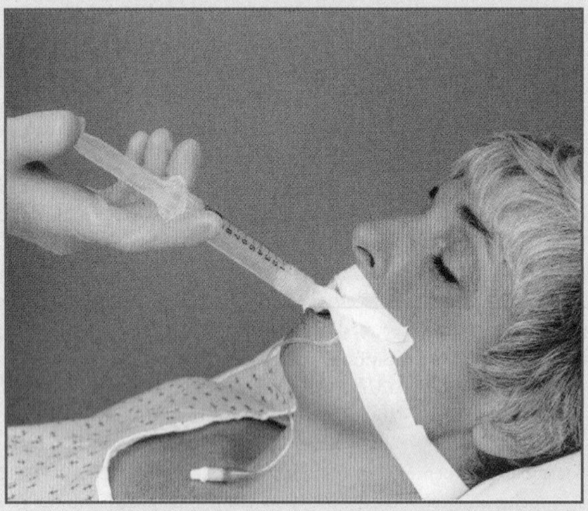

Adapter method

An adapter device for ET drug administration provides a more closed system of drug delivery than the syringe method. A special adapter placed on the end of the ET tube (as shown below) allows drug delivery through the closed stopcock.

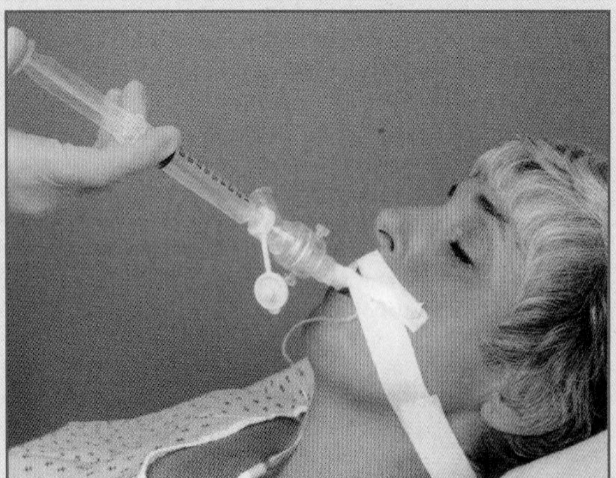

40 American Osteopathic Association. (2014). Standard 07.02.03. *Healthcare Facilities Accreditation Program: Accreditation requirements for acute care hospitals.* Chicago, IL: American Osteopathic Association. (Level VII)

41 The Joint Commission. (2015). Standard RC.01.03.01. *Comprehensive accreditation manual for hospitals: The official handbook.* Oakbrook Terrace, IL: The Joint Commission. (Level VII)

42 Centers for Medicare & Medicaid Services, Department of Health and Human Services. (2014). Condition of participation: Medical record services. 42 C.F.R. § 482.24(b).

43 American Osteopathic Association. (2014). Standard 10.00.03. *Healthcare Facilities Accreditation Program: Accreditation requirements for acute care hospitals.* Chicago, IL: American Osteopathic Association. (Level VII)

ENDOTRACHEAL DRUG ADMINISTRATION

When IV or intraosseous (IO) access isn't readily available, certain drugs can be administered into the respiratory system through an endotracheal (ET) tube. This route allows uninterrupted resuscitation efforts and avoids such complications as coronary artery laceration, cardiac tamponade, and pneumothorax, which can occur when emergency drugs are administered through an intrathoracic route.

Drugs given through an ET tube usually produce lower blood levels of the drug than the same dose given IV. According to the 2010 American Heart Association guidelines for cardiopulmonary resuscitation (CPR) and emergency cardiovascular care, studies show that these lower blood levels may actually be detrimental to the patient. For example, when epinephrine is administered through an ET tube, it can produce transient beta-adrenergic effects, causing vasodilation and subsequent hypotension and reducing the chance of patient survival. Because of this, although it's possible to administer some resuscitation drugs through an ET tube, IV or IO administration is preferred because these routes provide more predictable drug delivery and pharmacologic effect.[1]

When IV or IO access can't be established, epinephrine, vasopressin, and lidocaine may be administered through an ET tube during cardiac arrest. Typically, the dose given by the ET route is 2 to 2½ times the recommended IV dose. The drug should be diluted in 5 to 10 mL of sterile water or normal saline solution and then injected directly into the ET tube; better absorption may occur when epinephrine and lidocaine are diluted in sterile water rather than normal saline solution. Naloxone and atropine also can be administered through an ET tube.[1]

Drugs given endotracheally are typically administered in an emergency situation by a practitioner, an emergency medical technician, or a critical care nurse. Although guidelines may vary depending on state regulations, the basic administration method is the same.

Drugs may be given endotracheally using the syringe method or the adapter method. A swivel adapter can be placed on the end of the ET tube and, while ventilation continues through a bag-valve device, the drug can be delivered through the closed stopcock. (See *Administering endotracheal drugs.*)

Equipment

ET tube ▪ gloves ▪ end-tidal carbon dioxide (CO_2) detector, esophageal detection device, or continuous waveform capnography device ▪ handheld resuscitation bag ▪ prescribed medication ▪ syringe ▪ sterile water or normal saline solution ▪ stethoscope ▪ disinfectant pad ▪ Optional: swivel adapter, other personal protective equipment.

Implementation

- Avoid distractions and interruptions when preparing and administering the medication *to prevent medication errors.*[2,3]
- Verify the order on the patient's medication administration record by checking it against the practitioner's order.[4,5,6,7]
- Gather the prescribed medication and equipment.
- Compare the medication label with the order in the patient's medical record.[5,6,7]
- Check the patient's medical record for an allergy or a contraindication to the prescribed medication. If an allergy or a contraindication exists, don't administer the medication; instead, notify the practitioner.[5,6,7]

■ Check the expiration date on the medication. If the medication is expired, return it to the pharmacy and obtain new medication.[5,6,7]
■ Visually inspect the medication for particles, discoloration, and other signs of loss of integrity; don't administer the medication if its integrity is compromised.[5,6,7]
■ Discuss any unresolved concerns about the medication with the patient's practitioner.[5,6,7]
■ Perform hand hygiene.[8,9,10,11,12]
■ Put on gloves and other personal protective equipment as needed.[13,14]
■ Calculate the drug dose. Keep in mind that adult advanced cardiac life support guidelines recommend that drugs given endotracheally be administered at 2 to 2½ times the recommended IV dose.[1,7]
■ Draw up the correct amount of medication into the syringe. Dilute it in 5 to 10 mL of sterile water or normal saline solution. *Dilution increases drug volume and contact with the lung tissue.*
■ Label the syringe with the name and the dose of the medication.[15]
■ Confirm the patient's identity using at least two patient identifiers.[16]
■ Check ET tube placement by assessing chest expansion bilaterally and listening over the epigastrium (you shouldn't hear breath sounds) and by assessing the lung fields bilaterally (breath sounds should be equal and adequate). Also check placement by using a device such as an end-tidal CO_2 detector, esophageal detection device, or waveform capnography.[1]

NURSING ALERT ***Be aware that continuous waveform capnography combined with clinical assessment is recommended as the most reliable method of confirming correct ET tube placement.***[1]

■ If CPR is in progress, interrupt chest compressions briefly to administer the medication.[1,17]
■ Discontinue manual ventilation momentarily, remove the needle from the syringe, insert the tip of the syringe directly into the ET tube or into the swivel adapter, and inject the drug into the tube.
■ After injecting the drug, reattach the resuscitation bag and ventilate the patient briskly *to clear the ET tube of the drug and to disperse the drug into the airways.*
■ Discard the syringe and needle in a puncture-resistant sharps container.[13]
■ Remove and discard your gloves and any other personal protective equipment worn.[13]
■ Perform hand hygiene.[8,9,10,11,12]
■ Clean and disinfect your stethoscope with a disinfectant pad.[18,19]
■ Perform hand hygiene.[8,9,10,11,12]
■ Document the procedure.[20,21,22]

Special considerations

■ Keep in mind that, during cardiac arrest, drug administration should only briefly interrupt chest compressions.[1]

Complications

Potential complications of ET drug administration are related to the metabolism of the drug in the respiratory tract, which results in slow, erratic absorption and an unpredictable, reduced systemic effect.

Documentation

Document that ET tube placement was verified, and record the methods used for verification. Record the date and time of medication administration, the medication administered, the type and volume of diluent used, and the patient's response to the medication. Document any adverse effects, the practitioner notified, any prescribed interventions, and the patient's response to those interventions.

REFERENCES

1 American Heart Association. (2010). 2010 American Heart Association guidelines for cardiopulmonary resuscitation and emergency cardiovascular care. *Circulation, 122,* S729–S767. (Level II)

2 Institute for Safe Medication Practices. (2012). Side tracks on the safety express: Interruptions lead to errors and unfinished...Wait, what was I doing? *Nurse Advise-ERR,* 11(2), 1–4. Accessed March 2015 via the Web at https://www.ismp.org/Newsletters/acutecare/showarticle.aspx?id=37 (Level VII)

3 Westbrook, J., et al. (2010). Association of interruptions with an increased risk and severity of medication administration errors. *Archives of Internal Medicine, 170,* 683–690. (Level IV)

4 The Joint Commission. (2015). Standard MM.04.01.01. *Comprehensive accreditation manual for hospitals: The official handbook.* Oakbrook Terrace, IL: The Joint Commission. (Level VII)

5 The Joint Commission. (2015). Standard MM.06.01.01. *Comprehensive accreditation manual for hospitals: The official handbook.* Oakbrook Terrace, IL: The Joint Commission. (Level VII)

6 American Osteopathic Association. (2014). Standard 16.01.03. *Healthcare Facilities Accreditation Program: Accreditation requirements for acute care hospitals.* Chicago, IL: American Osteopathic Association. (Level VII)

7 Centers for Medicare & Medicaid Services, Department of Health and Human Services. (2014). Condition of participation: Nursing services. 42 C.F.R. § 482.23(c).

8 The Joint Commission. (2015). Standard NPSG.07.01.01. *Comprehensive accreditation manual for hospitals: The official handbook.* Oakbrook Terrace, IL: The Joint Commission. (Level VII)

9 World Health Organization. (2009). "WHO guidelines on hand hygiene in health care: First global patient safety challenge, clean care is safer care" [Online]. Accessed March 2015 via the Web at http://whqlibdoc.who.int/publications/2009/9789241597906_eng.pdf (Level IV)

10 Centers for Disease Control and Prevention. (2002). Guideline for hand hygiene in health-care settings: Recommendations of the Healthcare Infection Control Practices Advisory Committee and the HICPAC/SHEA/APIC/IDSA Hand Hygiene Task Force. *MMWR Recommendations and Reports, 51*(RR-16), 1–45. Accessed March 2015 via the Web at http://www.cdc.gov/mmwr/pdf/rr/rr5116.pdf (Level II)

11 American Osteopathic Association. (2014). Standard 07.01.21. *Healthcare Facilities Accreditation Program: Accreditation requirements for acute care hospitals.* Chicago, IL: American Osteopathic Association. (Level VII)

12 Centers for Medicare & Medicaid Services, Department of Health and Human Services. (2014). Condition of participation: Infection control. 42 C.F.R. § 482.42.

13 Siegel, J. D., et al. (2007). "2007 guideline for isolation precautions: Preventing transmission of infectious agents in healthcare settings" [Online]. Accessed March 2015 via the Web at http://www.cdc.gov/hicpac/pdf/isolation/Isolation2007.pdf (Level II)

14 American Osteopathic Association. (2014). Standard 07.01.10. *Healthcare Facilities Accreditation Program: Accreditation requirements for acute care hospitals.* Chicago, IL: American Osteopathic Association. (Level VII)

15 American Osteopathic Association. (2014). Standard 25.01.18. *Healthcare Facilities Accreditation Program: Accreditation requirements for acute care hospitals.* Chicago, IL: American Osteopathic Association. (Level VII)

16 The Joint Commission. (2015). Standard NPSG.01.01.01. *Comprehensive accreditation manual for hospitals: The official handbook.* Oakbrook Terrace, IL: The Joint Commission. (Level VII)

17 Meaney, P. A. et al. (2013). Cardiopulmonary resuscitation quality: Improving cardiac resuscitation outcomes both inside and outside the hospital: A consensus statement from the American Heart Association. *Circulation, 128,* 417–435. (Level VII)

18 American Osteopathic Association. (2014). Standard 07.02.03. *Healthcare Facilities Accreditation Program: Accreditation requirements for acute care hospitals.* Chicago, IL: American Osteopathic Association. (Level VII)

19 Rutala, W. A., et al. (2008). "Guideline for disinfection and sterilization in healthcare facilities, 2008" [Online]. Accessed March 2015 via the Web at http://www.cdc.gov/hicpac/pdf/guidelines/Disinfection_Nov_2008.pdf (Level I)

20 The Joint Commission. (2015). Standard RC.01.03.01. *Comprehensive accreditation manual for hospitals: The official handbook.* Oakbrook Terrace, IL: The Joint Commission. (Level VII)

21 Centers for Medicare & Medicaid Services, Department of Health and Human Services. (2014). Condition of participation: Medical record services. 42 C.F.R. § 482.24(b).

22 American Osteopathic Association. (2014). Standard 10.00.03. *Healthcare Facilities Accreditation Program: Accreditation requirements for acute care hospitals.* Chicago, IL: American Osteopathic Association. (Level VII)

Additional reference

Nettina, S. M. (2014). *Lippincott manual of nursing practice* (10th ed.). Philadelphia, PA: Wolters Kluwer.

Endotracheal intubation

Endotracheal (ET) intubation involves the oral or nasal insertion of a flexible tube through the larynx into the trachea for the purposes of controlling the airway and mechanically ventilating the patient. Performed by a practitioner, anesthetist, respiratory therapist, or nurse educated in the procedure, ET intubation typically occurs in emergencies such as cardiopulmonary arrest or in diseases such as epiglottitis. However, intubation may also occur under more controlled circumstances, such as just before surgery or in patients who can't clear their secretions effectively. In such situations, ET intubation requires patient teaching and preparation.

Advantages of the procedure are that it establishes and maintains a patent airway, protects against aspiration by sealing off the trachea from the digestive tract, permits removal of tracheobronchial secretions in patients who can't cough effectively, and provides a route for mechanical ventilation. Disadvantages are that it bypasses normal respiratory defenses against infection, reduces cough effectiveness, and prevents verbal communication.

ET intubation by the nasotracheal route (blind nasotracheal intubation) is more comfortable than oral intubation, but it's also more difficult to perform. Because the tube passes blindly through the nasal cavity, the procedure causes greater tissue trauma, increases the risk of infection by nasal bacteria introduced into the trachea, and risks pressure necrosis of the nasal mucosa. However, exact tube placement is easier, and the risk of dislodgment is lower. The cuff on the ET tube maintains a closed system that permits positive pressure ventilation and protects the airway from aspiration of secretions and gastric contents.

Oral ET intubation (direct visualization intubation) is preferred over the nasotracheal route because intubation by the nasotracheal route increases the risk of sinusitis, which may increase the risk of ventilator-associated pneumonia.[1] Nasotracheal intubation is contraindicated in patients with facial fractures or suspected basilar skull fractures and after cranial surgery such as transsphenoidal hypophysectomy.[2]

Equipment

Two ET tubes (one spare) of the appropriate size (normal female size is 7 to 8 mm; normal male size is 8 to 9 mm) with in-line or subglottic suctioning if available ■ 10-mL syringe ■ stethoscope ■ prescribed sedative ■ local anesthetic spray ■ overbed or other table ■ water-soluble lubricant ■ adhesive or other strong tape or commercial ET tube holder ■ skin preparation product ■ gloves ■ goggles and mask or face shield and other personal protective equipment ■ oral airway or bite block ■ suction equipment ■ handheld resuscitation bag with sterile swivel adapter ■ humidified oxygen source ■ carbon dioxide detector or waveform capnography equipment ■ oral care equipment ■ cuff pressure manometer ■ Optional: transparent semipermeable dressing.

For direct visualization intubation

Lighted laryngoscope with a handle and blades of various sizes, both curved and straight ■ Optional: prepackaged intubation tray, stylet.

For blind nasotracheal intubation

Mucosal vasoconstricting agent.

Preparation of equipment

Before direct visualization intubation, you may use a stylet to stiffen the tube. The entire stylet may be lubricated. Insert the stylet into the tube so that its distal tip lies about ½″ (1.3 cm) inside the distal end of the tube. Make sure the stylet doesn't protrude from the tube *to avoid vocal cord trauma.* Also, check the light in the laryngoscope by snapping the appropriate-sized blade into place; if the bulb doesn't light, replace the batteries or the laryngoscope (whichever will be quicker).

Prepare the humidified oxygen source and the suction equipment for immediate use. If the patient is in bed, remove the headboard to provide easier access.

Implementation

■ Verify the practitioner's order for intubation, if not an emergency situation.

■ Review the patient's medical record for a history of medical, surgical, and anesthetic factors that may increase the risk of difficult intubation.[1]

■ Conduct a preprocedure verification *to make sure all relevant documentation, related information, and equipment are available and correctly identified to the patient's identifiers.*[3,4]

■ Assess the patient's immediate history to see whether he has a suspected spinal cord injury or has undergone cranial surgery *to make sure that the proper intubation method is chosen.*[2]

■ Gather and prepare the necessary supplies.

■ Perform hand hygiene, and then put on gloves.[5,6,7,8,9,10,11]

■ Confirm the patient's identity using at least two patient identifiers, if possible.[12]

■ Using sterile technique, open the package containing the ET tube and, if desired, open the other supplies on an overbed table.

■ Attach the syringe to the port on the tube's exterior pilot cuff. Slowly inflate the cuff, observing for uniform inflation. Then use the syringe to deflate the cuff.

■ Lubricate the first 1″ (2.5 cm) of the distal end of the ET tube with water-soluble lubricant using sterile technique. Use only water-soluble lubricant *because it can be absorbed by the mucous membranes.*

■ If possible, assign a staff person *to provide information to the patient and his family and support them throughout the procedure;* offer family members the option of staying at the bedside *to allay the patient's and family's fears and to decrease anxiety.*[13]

■ Assess the patient's oral cavity for dentures or loose teeth; remove them if possible *because they might obstruct the airway.*[4] Inspect the patient's oral cavity, airway, head, and neck for factors that might increase the risk of difficult intubation.[1]

■ Determine when the patient last had something to eat *because recent food consumption increases the risk of aspiration;* handheld resuscitation bag use may also increase abdominal distention, further increasing the risk of aspiration.[2,14]

■ Assess the patient's level of consciousness, level of anxiety, and respiratory status *to determine whether he needs sedation, a paralytic agent, or both.*[2]

■ Insert an IV catheter if the patient doesn't already have a functioning catheter in place *to administer sedation and other emergency medications, if needed.*[2] (See the "IV catheter insertion and removal" procedure, page 446.)

■ Administer a sedative, or a sedative and paralytic agent, as ordered, *to decrease respiratory secretions, induce amnesia or analgesia, and help calm and relax a conscious patient.*[15,16]

NURSING ALERT *Sedatives and paralytic medications are considered high-alert medications* because they can cause significant harm when used in error. *If required in your facility, before administering these medications, have another nurse perform an independent double-check* to verify the patient's identity and make sure that the correct medication is being administered in the prescribed concentration, the medication's indication corresponds with the patient's diagnosis, the dosage calculations are correct and the dosing formula used to derive the final dose is correct, the route of administration is safe and proper for the patient, and, if the medication is administered through an infusion pump, the pump settings are correct and the infusion line is attached to the correct port.[17,18]

■ Compare the results of the independent double-check with another nurse (if required) and, if no discrepancies exist, administer the medication. If discrepancies exist, rectify them before administering the medication.[17]

■ Conduct a time-out immediately before starting the *procedure to perform a final assessment that the correct patient, site, position, and procedure are identified and, as applicable, that all relevant information and necessary equipment are available.*[3,19]

■ Remove and discard your gloves.

■ Perform hand hygiene.[5,6,7]

■ Put on goggles and a mask (or a mask with face shield), a gown, and gloves *because secretions may splash during intubation.*[8,11]

■ Preoxygenate the patient with 100% oxygen using a handheld resuscitation bag for at least 3 minutes; continue until the tube is inserted *to prevent hypoxia.*[2]

For direct visualization intubation

■ Place the patient in the supine, "sniffing" position so that his mouth, pharynx, and trachea are extended. If cervical spine injury is suspected, have an assistant maintain the patient's head in a neutral position with the spine immobilized.[2]

■ Spray a local anesthetic (such as lidocaine) deep into the posterior pharynx, if indicated, *to diminish the gag reflex and reduce patient discomfort.*

■ If necessary, suction the patient's pharynx just before tube insertion *to improve visualization of the patient's pharynx and vocal cords and to prevent aspiration of secretions.*

■ Be prepared to time each intubation attempt, limiting each attempt to less than 30 seconds *to prevent hypoxia.*[2,20] Ideally, each attempt should be limited to 10 seconds during cardiopulmonary resuscitation (CPR).[14] Hyperoxygenate the patient between attempts, if necessary.

■ Stand at the head of the patient's bed. Use the fingers of your right hand to open the patient's mouth *to provide access to the oral cavity.*[2]

■ Grasp the laryngoscope handle in your left hand, and gently slide the blade into the right side of the patient's mouth using the blade to push the tongue to the left *to visualize the glottis opening.*[2]

■ Advance the blade *to expose the epiglottis.* When using a straight blade, insert the tip under the epiglottis; when using a curved blade, insert the tip between the base of the tongue and the epiglottis.

■ Lift the laryngoscope handle upward and away from your body at a 45-degree angle *to reveal the vocal cords.* Avoid pivoting the laryngoscope against the patient's teeth *to avoid damaging them.*

■ Insert the ET tube into the right side of the patient's mouth.

■ Guide the tube into the vertical openings of the larynx between the vocal cords, being careful not to mistake the horizontal opening of the esophagus for the larynx. If the vocal cords are closed because of a spasm, wait a few seconds for them to relax; then gently guide the tube past them *to avoid traumatic injury.*

■ Advance the tube until the cuff disappears beyond the vocal cords. Avoid advancing the tube farther *to avoid occluding a major bronchus and precipitating lung collapse.*[2]

■ When the ET tube is placed properly, continue to hold it securely in place at the patient's lips while withdrawing the laryngoscope blade and then the stylet, if present.[2]

For blind nasotracheal intubation

■ Place the patient with his head and neck in a neutral position.

■ Spray a local anesthetic and a mucosal vasoconstrictor into the nasal passages *to anesthetize the nasal turbinates and reduce the chance of bleeding.*[2]

■ Be prepared to time each intubation attempt, limiting each attempt to less than 30 seconds to prevent hypoxia.[14] Ideally, each attempt should be limited to 10 seconds during CPR.[14] Hyperoxygenate the patient between attempts if necessary.[14]

■ Listen and feel for air movement through the tube as it's advanced *to ensure that the tube is properly placed in the airway.*

■ Insert the lubricated ET tube along the floor of the nasal cavity. Advance the tube between the vocal cords when the patient inhales *because the vocal cords separate on inhalation.*

■ Listen for the breath sounds to become louder when the tube is past the vocal cords. If breath sounds disappear at any time during tube advancement, withdraw the tube until they reappear.

After intubation

■ Inflate the tube's cuff with 5 to 10 mL of air according to the manufacturer's instructions. When the patient is mechanically ventilated, you'll use the minimal-leak technique or the minimal occlusive volume technique *to establish correct inflation of the cuff.* (For instructions, see the "Tracheal cuff-pressure measurement" procedure.) A cuff pressure between 20 and 25 cm H_2O is recommended *to provide an adequate seal and reduce the risk of complications.*[2,21]

■ *Confirm ET tube placement* using physical and nonphysical examination techniques. Physical examination techniques include auscultating for bilateral breath sounds, observing for bilateral chest expansion, and listening over the epigastrium (where breath sounds shouldn't be heard). The preferred nonphysical examination technique to confirm and monitor placement is continuous quantitative waveform capnography.[14]

NURSING ALERT *If ET tube insertion is occurring during emergency care, avoid interrupting chest compressions when confirming tube placement.*

NURSING ALERT *Intubation performed during cardiac arrest shouldn't delay initial CPR and defibrillation for ventricular fibrillation.*[14]

■ If any signs of esophageal intubation are present (stomach distention, belching, or a gurgling sound), immediately deflate the cuff and remove the tube. After reoxygenating the patient *to prevent hypoxia,* repeat insertion using a sterile tube *to prevent contamination of the trachea.* Auscultate bilaterally *to exclude the possibility of endobronchial intubation.* If you fail to hear breath sounds on both sides of the chest, you may have inserted the tube into one of the mainstem bronchi (usually the right one because of its wider angle at the bifurcation); such insertion occludes the other bronchus and lung and results in atelectasis on the obstructed side. It's also possible that the tube is resting on the carina, resulting in dry secretions that obstruct both bronchi. (The patient's coughing and fighting the ventilator will alert you to the problem.) To correct these situations, deflate the cuff, withdraw the tube 1 to 2 cm, auscultate for bilateral breath sounds, and then reinflate the cuff.

■ Once you have confirmed correct ET tube placement, administer oxygen or initiate mechanical ventilation and suction, if indicated. During CPR, deliver ventilations using a handheld resuscitation bag at a rate of one breath every 6 to 8 seconds.[14]

■ Insert a bite block or other oropharyngeal airway along the ET tube, if needed, *to prevent the patient from biting down on the tube.* Secure the bite block separately from the ET tube *to prevent ET tube dislodgement.*[2]

■ Measure the distance from the edge of the lip to the end of the tube and document the distance on the flow sheet or emergency sheet. If the tube has measurement markings on it, record the measurement where the tube exits at the lips. *By periodically monitoring this mark, you can detect tube displacement.*

■ Secure the ET tube using a commercial ET tube holder or tape *to prevent inadvertent extubation.*[2] (See *Methods to secure an ET tube,* page 280.)

■ Obtain a chest X-ray *to verify tube position.*[14]

Methods to secure an ET tube

An endotracheal (ET) tube should be secured with a commercial ET tube holder as recommended by The American Heart Association and American Pediatric Association. Alternatively, the tube may be taped in place *to prevent dislodgment.*

To secure the tube, use one of the following methods.

Method 1

Made of hard plastic or of softer materials, commercial ET tube holders are a convenient way to secure an ET tube in place. They're available in adult and pediatric sizes, and some models come with bite blocks attached. The strap is placed around the patient's neck and secured around the tube with Velcro fasteners. *Because each model is different,* check with the manufacturer's guidelines for correct placement and care.

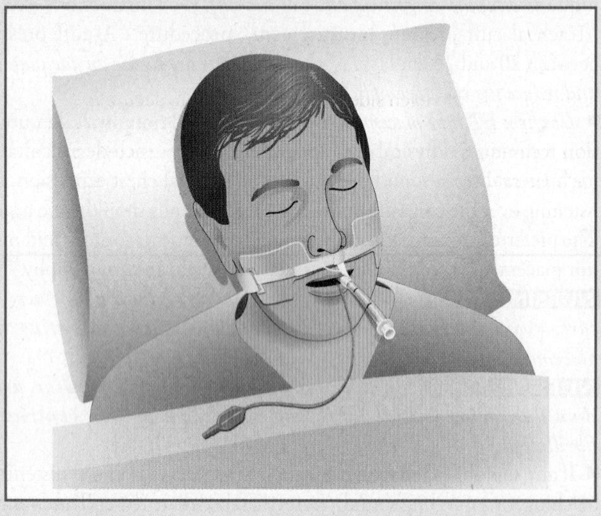

Method 2

Cut two 2″ (5-cm) strips and two 15″ (38-cm) strips of 1″ (2.5-cm) cloth adhesive tape. Then cut a 13″ (33-cm) slit in one end of each 15″ (38-cm) strip (as shown below). (Some facilities require the tape to encircle the patient's head.)

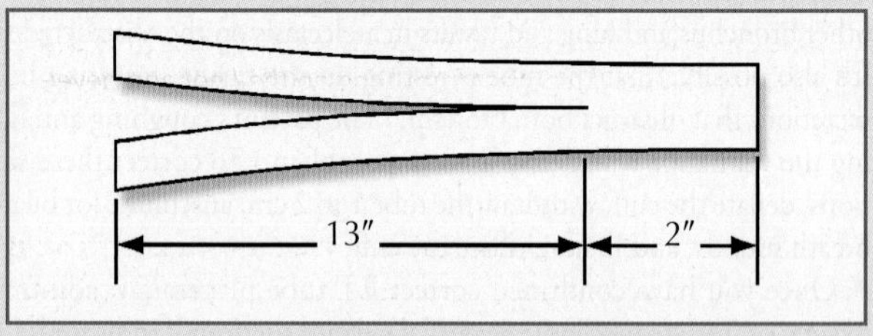

Apply skin preparation product to the patient's cheeks. Place the 2″ (5-cm) strips on his cheeks, creating a new surface on which to anchor the tape securing the tube. *When frequent retaping is necessary, this step helps preserve the patient's skin integrity.* If the patient's skin is excoriated or at risk, you can use a transparent semipermeable dressing to protect the skin.

Apply a skin preparation product to the part of the tube where you'll be applying the tape. On the side of the mouth where the tube will be anchored, place the unslit end of the long tape on top of the tape on the patient's cheek.

Wrap the top half of the tape around the tube twice, pulling the tape tightly around the tube. Then, directing the tape over the patient's upper lip, place the end of the tape on his other cheek. Cut off any excess tape. Use the lower half of the tape to secure an oral airway, if necessary (as shown below).

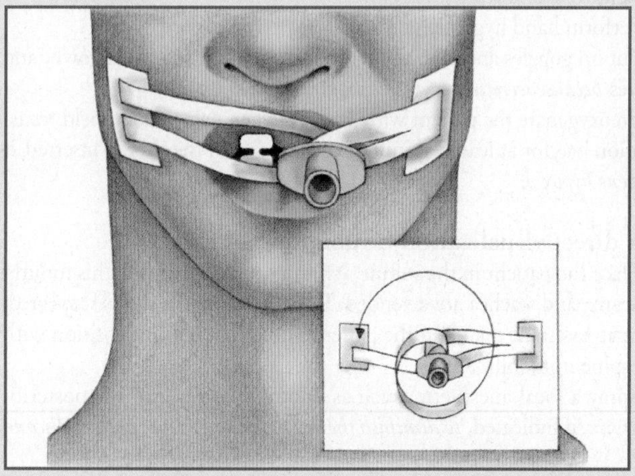

Alternatively, twist the lower half of the tape around the tube twice, and attach it to the original cheek. *Taping in opposite directions places equal traction on the tube.*

If an oral airway is taped in the mouth or you're concerned about the tube's stability, apply the other 15″ (38-cm) strip of tape in the same manner, starting on the other side of the patient's face (as shown below). If the tape around the tube is too bulky, use only the upper part of the tape and cut off the lower part. If the patient has copious oral secretions, seal the tape by cutting a 1″ (2.5-cm) piece of paper tape, coating it with a skin preparation product, and placing the paper tape over the adhesive tape.

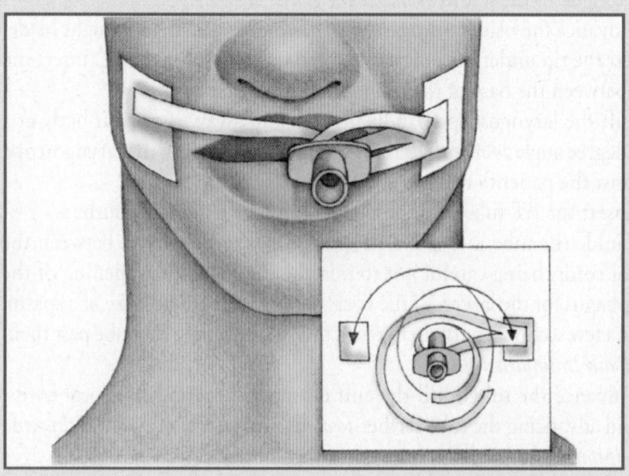

- If ordered, obtain an arterial blood sample for arterial blood gas analysis *to evaluate gas exchange.*
- Place a swivel adapter between the tube and the humidified oxygen *source to allow for intermittent suctioning and to reduce tube tension.*
- Position the patient with his head elevated 30 to 45 degrees *to reduce the risk of ventilator-associated pneumonia (VAP).*[21,22,23]
- Provide frequent oral care (use a chlorhexidine-based oral care solution daily, as prescribed),[21] and reposition the ET tube daily *to prevent formation of pressure ulcers and avoid excessive pressure on the sides of the mouth.*
- Suction secretions through the ET tube as the patient's condition indicates *to clear secretions and prevent mucus plugs from obstructing the tube.*

Methods to secure an ET tube *(continued)*

Method 3

Cut one piece of 1″ (2.5-cm) cloth adhesive tape long enough to wrap around the patient's head and overlap in front. Then cut an 8″ (20-cm) piece of tape and center it on the longer piece, sticky sides together. Next, cut a 5″ (13-cm) slit in each end of the longer tape (as shown below).

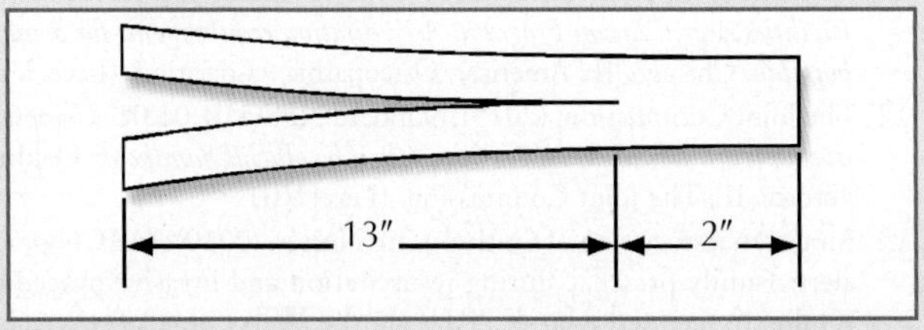

Apply a skin preparation product to the patient's cheeks, under his nose, and under his lower lip.

Place the top half of one end of the tape under the patient's nose, and wrap the lower half around the ET tube. Place the lower half of the other end of the tape along his lower lip, and wrap the top half around the tube (as shown below).

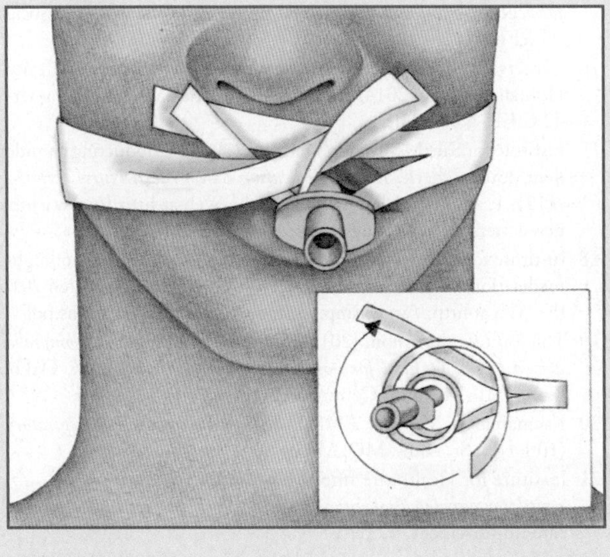

Method 4

Cut a tracheostomy tie in two pieces, one a few inches longer than the other, and cut two 6″ (15-cm) pieces of 1″ (2.5-cm) cloth adhesive tape. Then cut a 2″ (5-cm) slit in one end of both pieces of tape. Fold back the other end of the tape ½″ (1.3 cm) so that the sticky sides are together, and cut a small hole in it (as shown below).

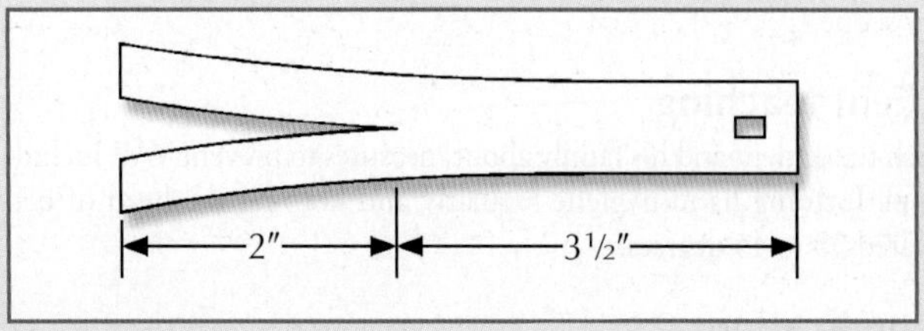

Apply a skin preparation product to the part of the ET tube that will be taped. Wrap the split ends of each piece of tape around the tube, one piece on each side. Overlap the tape *to secure it.*

Apply the free ends of the tape to both sides of the patient's face. Then insert tracheostomy ties through the holes in the tape and knot the ties (as shown below).

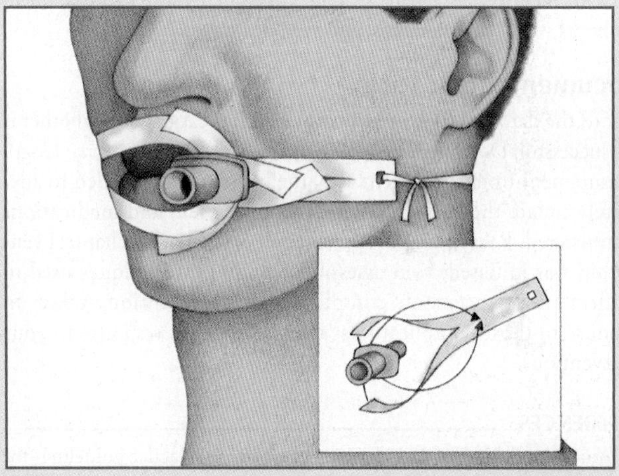

Bring the longer tie behind the patient's neck. *Knotting the ties on the side prevents the patient from lying on the knot and developing a pressure ulcer.*

- Remove and discard your gloves and other personal protective equipment.
- Perform hand hygiene.[5,6,7,9,10,11]
- Document the procedure.[24,25,26]

Special considerations

- Orotracheal intubation is preferred in emergencies *because insertion is easier and faster than it is with nasotracheal intubation.* However, maintaining exact tube placement is more difficult, and the tube must be well secured *to avoid kinking and to prevent bronchial obstruction or accidental extubation.*
- The routine use of cricoid pressure is no longer recommended except to help visualize the vocal cords in tracheal intubation.[14]
- Although low-pressure cuffs have significantly reduced the incidence of tracheal erosion and necrosis caused by cuff pressure on the tracheal wall, overinflation of a low-pressure cuff can negate the benefit. Use the minimal-leak technique to avoid these complications. Inflating the cuff a bit more to make a complete seal with the least amount of air is the next most desirable method. A gradual increase in cuff volume indicates tracheal dilatation or erosion. A sudden increase in volume indicates rupture of the cuff and requires immediate reintubation if the patient is being ventilated or if he requires continuous cuff inflation to maintain a high concentration of delivered oxygen. When the cuff has been inflated, measure its pressure at least every 8 hours *to avoid overinflation.* A minimal pressure of 20 cm H_2O is recommended *to prevent aspiration and VAP.*[27]
- Always record the volume of air needed to inflate the cuff. Cuff pressure should be monitored at least every 8 hours *to avoid overinflation and underinflation.*[27]
- If the patient requires mechanical ventilation, using a multidisciplinary approach, interrupt the patient's sedation daily and assess the patient's readiness to wean. *Doing so reduces the amount of time the patient spends on a ventilator and reduces the risk of VAP.*[21]

- If the patient requires mechanical ventilation, make sure he receives deep venous thrombosis prophylaxis (unless contraindicated), as prescribed, as well as peptic ulcer disease prophylaxis. *When combined with head-of-bed elevation, oral care, daily sedation interruption, and assessment of the readiness to wean, these measures reduce the incidence of VAP.*[21]
- Other techniques for managing a difficult airway include fiber-optic intubation, use of an intubating stylet or a tube changer, insertion of a supraglottic airway as an intubating conduit, use of laryngoscope blades of varying design and size, and use of a light wand or videolaryngoscope.[1]

Patient teaching

Teach the patient and his family about measures to prevent VAP, including performing hand hygiene regularly and keeping the head of bed elevated 30 to 45 degrees.

Complications

ET intubation can result in apnea caused by reflex breath holding or interruption of oxygen delivery; bronchospasm; aspiration of blood, secretions, or gastric contents; tooth damage or loss; and injury to the lips, mouth, pharynx, or vocal cords. It can also result in laryngeal edema and erosion and in tracheal stenosis, erosion, and necrosis. Nasotracheal intubation can result in nasal bleeding, laceration, sinusitis, otitis media, and VAP. Incorrect placement of an ET tube can result in hypoxia, pneumothorax, vocal cord paralysis, and even death.

Documentation

Record the date and time of intubation, its indication, and whether it was successful. Document the type and size of ET tube, external length measurement from the patient's lip, the volume of air needed to adequately inflate the cuff, inflation technique used, and medications administered. Record when supplemental oxygen or mechanical ventilation was initiated, your assessment findings, techniques used to confirm tube placement, complications, interventions taken in response to those complications, and the patient's response to your interventions.

References

1 American Society of Anesthesiologists. (2013). Practice guidelines for management of the difficult airway: An updated report by the American Society of Anesthesiologists Task Force on Management of the Difficult Airway. *Anesthesiology, 118,* 251–270. (Level VII)

2 Lynn-McHale Wiegand, D. (Ed.). (2011). *AACN procedure manual for critical care* (6th ed.). St. Louis, MO: Saunders.

3 American Osteopathic Association. (2014). Standard 30.00.14. *Healthcare Facilities Accreditation Program: Accreditation requirements for acute care hospitals.* Chicago, IL: American Osteopathic Association. (Level VII)

4 The Joint Commission. (2015). Standard UP.01.01.01. *Comprehensive accreditation manual for hospitals: The official handbook.* Oakbrook Terrace, IL: The Joint Commission. (Level VII)

5 The Joint Commission. (2015). Standard NPSG.07.01.01. *Comprehensive accreditation manual for hospitals: The official handbook.* Oakbrook Terrace, IL: The Joint Commission. (Level VII)

6 Centers for Disease Control and Prevention. (2002). Guideline for hand hygiene in health-care settings: Recommendations of the Healthcare Infection Control Practices Advisory Committee and the HICPAC/SHEA/APIC/IDSA Hand Hygiene Task Force. *MMWR Recommendations and Reports, 51*(RR-16), 1–45. Accessed March 2015 via the Web at http://www.cdc.gov/mmwr/pdf/rr/rr5116.pdf (Level II)

7 World Health Organization. (2009). "WHO guidelines on hand hygiene in health care: First global patient safety challenge, clean care is safer care" [Online]. Accessed March 2015 via the Web at http://whqlibdoc.who.int/publications/2009/9789241597906_eng.pdf (Level IV)

8 Siegel, J. D., et al. (2007). "2007 guideline for isolation precautions: Preventing transmission of infectious agents in healthcare settings" [Online]. Accessed March 2015 via the Web at http://www.cdc.gov/hicpac/pdf/isolation/Isolation2007.pdf (Level II)

9 American Osteopathic Association. (2014). Standard 07.01.21. *Healthcare Facilities Accreditation Program: Accreditation requirements for acute care hospitals.* Chicago, IL: American Osteopathic Association. (Level VII)

10 Centers for Medicare & Medicaid Services, Department of Health and Human Services. (2014). Condition of participation: Infection control. 42 C.F.R. § 482.42.

11 American Osteopathic Association. (2014). Standard 07.01.10. *Healthcare Facilities Accreditation Program: Accreditation requirements for acute care hospitals.* Chicago, IL: American Osteopathic Association. (Level VII)

12 The Joint Commission. (2015). Standard NPSG.01.01.01. *Comprehensive accreditation manual for hospitals: The official handbook.* Oakbrook Terrace, IL: The Joint Commission. (Level VII)

13 American Association of Critical-Care Nurses. (2010). "AACN practice alert: Family presence during resuscitation and invasive procedures" [Online]. Accessed March 2015 via the Web at http://www.aacn.org/wd/practice/docs/practicealerts/family%20presence%2004-2010%20final.pdf (Level VII)

14 American Heart Association. (2010). 2010 American Heart Association guidelines for cardiopulmonary resuscitation and emergency cardiovascular care. Circulation, 122, S729–S767. (Level II)

15 American Osteopathic Association. (2014). Standard 16.01.03. Healthcare Facilities Accred*itation Program: Accreditation requirements for acute care hospitals.* Chicago, IL: American Osteopathic Association. (Level VII)

16 Centers for Medicare & Medicaid Services, Department of Health and Human Services. (2014). Condition of participation: Nursing services. 42 C.F.R. § 482.23(c).

17 Institute for Safe Medication Practices. (2008). Conducting an independent double-check. *ISMP Medication Safety Alert! Nurse Advise-ERR, 6*(12), 1. Accessed March 2015 via the Web at http://www.ismp.org/newsletters/nursing/Issues/NurseAdviseERR200812.pdf

18 Institute for Safe Medication Practices. (2014). "ISMP list of high-alert medications in acute care settings" [Online]. Accessed March 2015 via the Web at http://www.ismp.org/tools/highalertmedications.pdf

19 The Joint Commission. (2015). Standard UP.01.03.01. *Comprehensive accreditation manual for hospitals: The official handbook.* Oakbrook Terrace, IL: The Joint Commission. (Level VII)

20 Kacmarek, R. M., et al. (2013). *Egan's fundamentals of respiratory care* (10th ed.). St. Louis, MO: Mosby.

21 Institute for Healthcare Improvement. (2012). *How-to guide: Prevent ventilator-associated pneumonia.* Cambridge, MA: Institute for Healthcare Improvement. (Level V)

22 American Association of Critical-Care Nurses. (2008). "AACN practice alert: Ventilator associated pneumonia" [Online]. Accessed March 2015 via the Web at http://www.aacn.org/WD/Practice/Docs/PracticeAlerts/Ventilator%20Associated%20Pneumonia%201-2008.pdf

23 Klompas, M., et al. (2014). Strategies to prevent ventilator-associated pneumonia in acute care hospitals: 2014 update. *Infection Control and Hospital Epidemiology, 35,* 915–936. Accessed March 2015 via the Web at http://www.jstor.org/stable/10.1086/677144 (Level I)

24 The Joint Commission. (2015). Standard RC.01.03.01. *Comprehensive accreditation manual for hospitals: The official handbook.* Oakbrook Terrace, IL: The Joint Commission. (Level VII)

25 American Osteopathic Association. (2014). Standard 10.00.03. *Healthcare Facilities Accreditation Program: Accreditation requirements for acute care hospitals.* Chicago, IL: American Osteopathic Association. (Level VII)

26 Centers for Medicare & Medicaid Services, Department of Health and Human Services. (2014). Condition of participation: Medical record services. 42 C.F.R. § 482.24(b).

27 Sole, M. L., et al. (2011). Evaluation of an intervention to maintain endotracheal tube cuff pressure within therapeutic range. *American Journal of Critical Care, 20,* 109–117. Accessed March 2015 via the Web at http://www.aacn.org/WD/CETests/Media/A1120023.pdf

ADDITIONAL REFERENCES

Nettina, S. M. (2014). *Lippincott manual of nursing practice* (10th ed.). Philadelphia, PA: Wolters Kluwer.

Thomas, A. N., et al. (2014). "Capnography guidelines" [Online]. Accessed March 2015 via the Web at http://www.guideline.gov/content.aspx?id=44354

Walls, R. M., & Murphy, M. F. (2012). *Manual of emergency airway management* (4th ed.). Philadelphia, PA: Lippincott Williams and Wilkins.

ENDOTRACHEAL TUBE CARE

An intubated patient requires meticulous care to ensure airway patency and prevent complications until the patient can maintain spontaneous ventilation. Care sometimes includes repositioning the endotracheal (ET) tube if it becomes partially dislodged or a chest X-ray shows improper placement.

Equipment

10-mL syringe ■ suction equipment ■ gloves ■ handheld resuscitation bag with mask ■ hospital-grade disinfectant ■ Optional: gown, mask, goggles, mask with face shield.

For repositioning an ET tube

Skin adhesive preparation product ■ stethoscope ■ adhesive or hypoallergenic tape or commercial tube holder ■ oxygen source ■ ET tube cuff pressure manometer ■ continuous waveform capnography equipment or end-tidal carbon dioxide monitoring equipment.

For removing an ET tube

Supplemental oxygen equipment ■ pulse oximeter ■ equipment for reintubation ■ equipment for obtaining vital signs.

Preparation of equipment

Gather all equipment at the patient's bedside. Set up the suction equipment. If appropriate, set up supplemental oxygen equipment. Have a handheld resuscitation bag with a mask available.

Implementation

■ Perform hand hygiene.[1,2,3,4,5]

■ Confirm the patient's identify using at least two patient identifiers.[6]

■ Explain the procedure to the patient *to decrease her anxiety and enhance cooperation.*[7]

■ Provide privacy.[8,9]

■ Put on gloves and personal protective equipment as needed *to comply with standard precautions.*[10,11]

For repositioning an ET tube

■ Obtain assistance from a respiratory therapist or another nurse *to prevent accidental extubation during the procedure if the patient coughs.*

■ Hyperoxygenate the patient for 30 to 60 seconds *to prevent suction-related hypoxemia.*[12]

■ Suction the patient's trachea through the ET tube *to remove any secretions, which can cause the patient to cough during the procedure. Coughing increases the risk of trauma and tube dislodgment.* Then suction the patient's pharynx *to remove any secretions that may have accumulated above the tube cuff, which helps to prevent aspiration of secretions during cuff deflation.*[7,13,14,15,16] *Aspiration increases the risk of ventilator-associated pneumonia.*[17,18]

■ *To prevent traumatic manipulation of the tube,* instruct the assisting nurse or respiratory therapist to hold the tube as you carefully untape the tube or unfasten the commercial tube holder (as shown on top right). When freeing the tube, locate the centimeter marking on the tube or measure the length from the patient's mouth to the top of the tube *so that you have a reference point when moving the tube.*[13]

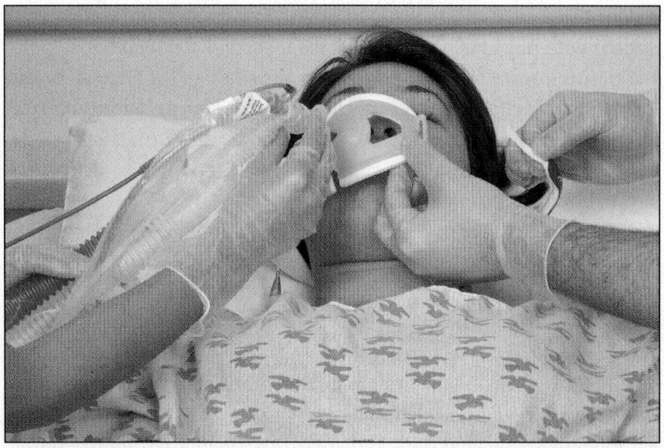

■ Next, deflate the cuff by attaching a 10-mL syringe to the pilot balloon port and aspirating air until you meet resistance and the pilot balloon deflates. Deflate the cuff before moving the tube (as shown below) *because the cuff forms a seal within the trachea and movement of an inflated cuff can damage the tracheal wall and vocal cords.*

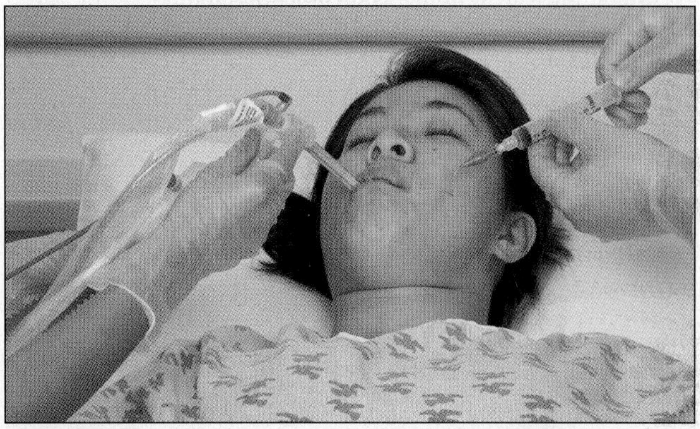

■ Reposition the tube, as necessary, noting new landmarks or measuring the length.

■ Reinflate the cuff immediately. To do this, instruct the patient to inhale, if able, and inflate the cuff slowly using the 10-mL syringe attached to the tube's pilot balloon port. As you do this, use your stethoscope to auscultate the patient's neck *to determine the presence of an air leak.* When air leakage ceases, stop cuff inflation and, while still auscultating the patient's neck, aspirate a small amount of air until you detect a slight leak (as shown below). *This maneuver creates a minimal air leak, which indicates that the cuff is inflated at the lowest pressure possible to create an adequate seal.* If the patient is being ventilated mechanically, aspirate to create a minimal air leak during the inspiratory phase of respiration *because the positive pressure of the ventilator during inspiration will create a larger leak around the cuff.*[13] Note the number of cubic centimeters of air required to achieve a minimal air leak.

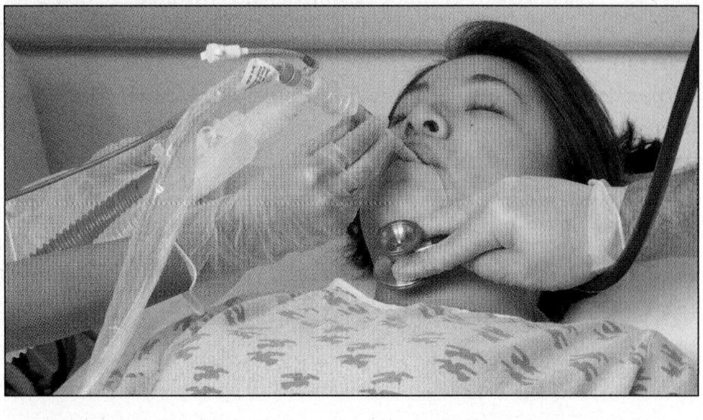

■ Measure the ET cuff pressure by using a manometer, and compare the reading with previous pressure readings *to prevent overinflation.*[16]
■ Confirm proper ET tube position by auscultating for bilateral breath sounds, looking for symmetrical chest wall movement, and using continuous waveform capnography. If continuous waveform capnography equipment isn't available, use clinical assessment and end-tidal carbon dioxide monitoring equipment.[19,20]
■ *Secure the ET tube in place* by applying a skin adhesive preparation product and adhesive or hypoallergenic tape or by refastening the commercial tube holder.

For removing an ET tube

■ Verify the practitioner's order or follow your facility's protocol (if present) for weaning and extubation.
■ Obtain baseline vital signs and assess the patient's respiratory status, including oxygen saturation level, *to identify that intubation is no longer necessary.*[7]
■ When you're authorized to remove the ET tube, obtain assistance from a respiratory therapist or another nurse *to prevent traumatic manipulation of the tube when it's untaped or unfastened.*
■ Position the patient in the semi-Fowler position (as shown below) *because respiratory muscles are more effective in an upright position than in a prone position.*[7]

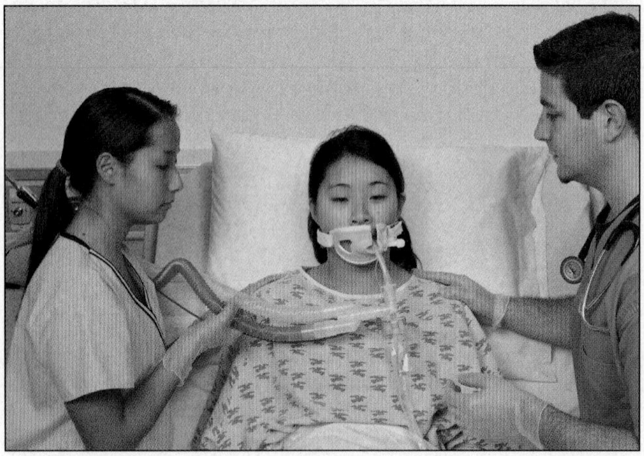

■ Hyperoxygenate the patient for 30 to 60 seconds *to prevent suctioning-related hypoxemia.*[7,14]
Suction the ET tube and the patient's oropharynx *to remove any accumulated secretions and to help prevent aspiration of secretions when the cuff is deflated.*[7,13,14]
■ Hyperoxygenate the patient for at least for at least 1 minute after suctioning *to allow oxygen saturation levels to recover after suctioning.*[7,14]
■ Untape or unfasten the ET tube while the assistant stabilizes the tube.
■ Attach a 10-mL syringe to the pilot balloon port, and aspirate air until you meet resistance and the pilot balloon deflates. If you fail to detect an air leak around the deflated cuff, notify the practitioner immediately and don't proceed with extubation. *Absence of an air leak may indicate marked tracheal edema, which can result in total airway obstruction if the ET tube is removed.*[14]
■ Instruct the patient to be calm and take a deep breath. At the peak of inspiration, *because vocal cords are maximally abducted,* remove the ET tube following the natural curve of the patient's mouth (as shown on top right).[7]

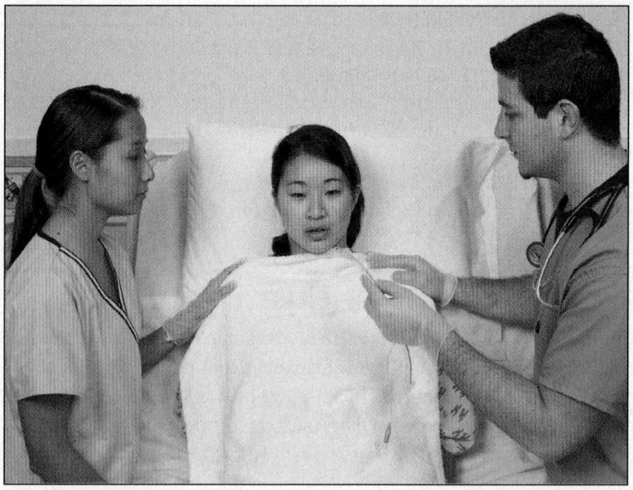

■ Administer supplemental humidified oxygen *to promote oxygenation and help decrease airway irritation, patient discomfort, and laryngeal edema.*
■ Suction the oropharynx, if needed, and encourage the patient to cough and deep-breathe. Remind her that a sore throat and hoarseness are to be expected and will gradually subside.
■ Closely monitor the patient's vital signs and respiratory status *to evaluate her tolerance of extubation and to watch for signs of respiratory distress.* Be alert for stridor or other evidence of upper airway obstruction. Obtain a sample for arterial sample for blood gas analysis, if ordered.

Completing the procedure

■ Remove and discard your gloves and any other personal protective equipment worn.[10,11]
■ Perform hand hygiene.[1,2,3,4,5]
■ Clean and disinfect reusable equipment properly using a hospital-grade disinfectant,[21,22] or dispose of equipment appropriately.
■ Perform hand hygiene.[1,2,3,4,5]
■ Document the procedure.[23,24,25]

Special considerations

■ When repositioning an ET tube, be especially careful in patients with highly sensitive airways. Sedation may be indicated in such patients.
■ If you inadvertently cut the pilot balloon on the cuff, immediately call the person in your facility who's responsible for *intubation so that the damaged tube can be replaced with one that's intact.* Don't remove the tube *because a tube with an air leak is better than no airway.*
■ The 2010 American Heart Association guidelines for cardiopulmonary resuscitation and emergency cardiovascular care recommend the use of end-tidal carbon dioxide monitoring in combination with clinical assessment to confirm initial ET tube placement in a patient in cardiac arrest when continuous waveform capnography isn't available.[19]
■ Measure ET tube cuff pressure at least every 8 hours *to avoid overinflation.*[16] (See the "Tracheal cuff-pressure measurement" procedure, page 750.)
■ Never extubate a patient unless someone skilled at intubation is readily available.
■ An ET tube should be removed as soon as it's no longer needed to reduce the risk of ventilator-associated events such as ventilator-associated pneumonia (VAP), sepsis, acute respiratory distress syndrome, pulmonary embolism, barotrauma, and pulmonary edema.[26,27]
■ Removal should occur when the patient is hemodynamically stable, can clear secretions without assistance, and the condition that required mechanical ventilation is reversed or improved to the point where mechanical ventilation is no longer needed.[7]

Complications

Traumatic injury to the larynx or trachea may result from tube manipulation, accidental extubation, or tube slippage into the right bronchus. Ventilatory failure and airway obstruction due to laryngospasm or marked tracheal edema are the gravest possible complications of extubation.

Documentation

After tube repositioning, record the date and time of the procedure, reason for repositioning (for example, malpositioning shown by chest X-ray), new tube position, total amount of air in the cuff after the procedure, complications and nursing actions taken, and the patient's tolerance of the procedure. Document any patient teaching and the patient's understanding of your teaching.

After extubation, record the date and time of extubation, vital signs, and assessment findings, including the presence or absence of stridor or other signs of upper airway edema. Document the type of supplemental oxygen administered, complications and required subsequent therapy, and the patient's tolerance of the procedure. Also document any patient teaching and the patient's understanding of your teaching.

References

1 The Joint Commission. (2015). Standard NPSG.07.01.01. *Comprehensive accreditation manual for hospitals: The official handbook.* Oakbrook Terrace, IL: The Joint Commission. (Level VII)

2 Centers for Disease Control and Prevention. (2002). Guideline for hand hygiene in health-care settings: Recommendations of the Healthcare Infection Control Practices Advisory Committee and the HICPAC/SHEA/APIC/IDSA Hand Hygiene Task Force. *MMWR Recommendations and Reports, 51*(RR-16), 1–45. Accessed March 2015 via the Web at http://www.cdc.gov/mmwr/pdf/rr/rr5116.pdf (Level II)

3 World Health Organization. (2009). "WHO guidelines on hand hygiene in health care: First global patient safety challenge, clean care is safer care" [Online]. Accessed March 2015 via the Web at http://whqlibdoc.who.int/publications/2009/9789241597906_eng.pdf (Level IV)

4 American Osteopathic Association. (2014). Standard 07.01.21. *Healthcare Facilities Accreditation Program: Accreditation requirements for acute care hospitals.* Chicago, IL: American Osteopathic Association. (Level VII)

5 Centers for Medicare & Medicaid Services, Department of Health and Human Services. (2014). Condition of participation: Infection control. 42 C.F.R. § 482.42.

6 The Joint Commission. (2015). Standard NPSG.01.01.01. *Comprehensive accreditation manual for hospitals: The official handbook.* Oakbrook Terrace, IL: The Joint Commission. (Level VII)

7 Lynn-McHale Wiegand, D. (Ed.). (2011). *AACN procedure manual for critical care* (6th ed.). St. Louis, MO: Saunders.

8 American Osteopathic Association. (2014). Standard 15.01.16. *Healthcare Facilities Accreditation Program: Accreditation requirements for acute care hospitals.* Chicago, IL: American Osteopathic Association. (Level VII)

9 Centers for Medicare & Medicaid Services, Department of Health and Human Services. (2014). Condition of participation: Patient's rights. 42 C.F.R. § 482.13(c)(1).

10 Siegel, J. D., et al. (2007). "2007 guideline for isolation precautions: Preventing transmission of infectious agents in healthcare settings" [Online]. Accessed March 2015 via the Web at http://www.cdc.gov/hicpac/pdf/isolation/Isolation2007.pdf (Level II)

11 American Osteopathic Association. (2014). Standard 07.01.10. *Healthcare Facilities Accreditation Program: Accreditation requirements for acute care hospitals.* Chicago, IL: American Osteopathic Association. (Level VII)

12 American Association for Respiratory Care (AARC). (2010). AARC clinical practice guidelines: Endotracheal suctioning of mechanically ventilated patients with artificial airways 2010. *Respiratory Care, 55,* 758–764. Accessed March 2015 via the Web at http://www.rcjournal.com/cpgs/pdf/06.10.0758.pdf (Level I)

13 American Association for Respiratory Care (AARC). (2007). AARC clinical practice guideline: Removal of the endotracheal tube—2007 revision & update. *Respiratory Care, 52,* 81–93. Accessed March 2015 via the Web at http://www.rcjournal.com/cpgs/pdf/removal_of_endotracheal_tube.pdf (Level VII)

14 American Association of Critical-Care Nurses. (2008). "AACN practice alert: Ventilator associated pneumonia" [Online]. Accessed March 2015 via the Web at http://www.aacn.org/WD/Practice/Docs/PracticeAlerts/Ventilator_Associated_Pneumonia_1-2008.pdf (Level VII)

15 Centers for Disease Control and Prevention. (2004). Guidelines for preventing health-care-associated pneumonia, 2003: Recommendations of CDC and the Healthcare Infection Control Practices Advisory Committee. *MMWR Recommendations and Reports, 53*(RR-3), 1–32. Accessed March 2015 via the Web at http://www.cdc.gov/mmwr/pdf/rr/rr5303.pdf (Level II)

16 Vyas, D., et al. (2002). Measurement of tracheal tube cuff pressure in critical care. *Anaesthesia, 57,* 275–277. (Level VI)

17 Association of Professionals in Infection Control and Epidemiology (APIC). (2009). "An APIC guide 2009: Guide to the elimination of ventilator-associated pneumonia" [Online]. Accessed March 2015 via the Web at http://www.apic.org/Resource_/EliminationGuideForm/18e326ad-b484-471c-9c35-6822a53ee4a2/File/VAP_09.pdf (Level IV)

18 Klompas, M., et al. (2014). Strategies to prevent ventilator-associated pneumonia in acute care hospitals: 2014 update. *Infection Control and Hospital Epidemiology, 35,* 915–936. Accessed March 2015 via the Web at http://www.jstor.org/stable/10.1086/677144 (Level I)

19 American Heart Association. (2010). 2010 American Heart Association guidelines for cardiopulmonary resuscitation and emergency cardiovascular care. *Circulation, 122,* S729–S767. (Level II)

20 Walsh, B. K., et al. (2011). AARC clinical practice guideline: Capnography/capnometry during mechanical ventilation: 2011. *Respiratory Care, 56,* 503–509. (Level VII)

21 Rutala, W. A., et al. (2008). "Guideline for disinfection and sterilization in healthcare facilities, 2008" [Online]. Accessed March 2015 via the Web at http://www.cdc.gov/hicpac/pdf/guidelines/Disinfection_Nov_2008.pdf (Level I)

22 American Osteopathic Association. (2014). Standard 07.02.03. *Healthcare Facilities Accreditation Program: Accreditation requirements for acute care hospitals.* Chicago, IL: American Osteopathic Association. (Level VII)

23 The Joint Commission. (2015). Standard RC.01.03.01. *Comprehensive accreditation manual for hospitals: The official handbook.* Oakbrook Terrace, IL: The Joint Commission. (Level VII)

24 American Osteopathic Association. (2014). Standard 10.00.03. *Healthcare Facilities Accreditation Program: Accreditation requirements for acute care hospitals.* Chicago, IL: American Osteopathic Association. (Level VII)

25 Centers for Medicare & Medicaid Services, Department of Health and Human Services. (2014). Condition of participation: Medical record services. 42 C.F.R. § 482.24(b).

26 Magill, S. S., et al. (2013). Developing a new national approach to surveillance for ventilator-associated events. *American Journal of Critical Care, 22,* 469–473.

27 Centers for Disease Control and Prevention. (2014). "Ventilator-associated event" [Online]. Accessed March 2015 via the Web at http://www.cdc.gov/nhsn/PDFs/pscManual/10-VAE_FINAL.pdf

Additional reference

Nettina, S. M. (2014). *Lippincott manual of nursing practice* (10th ed.). Philadelphia, PA: Wolters Kluwer.

End-tidal carbon dioxide monitoring

End-tidal carbon dioxide ($ETCO_2$) determines the carbon dioxide (CO_2) concentration in exhaled gas to provide information about a patient's pulmonary, cardiac, and metabolic status. Such information aids patient management and helps prevent clinical compromise.

In $ETCO_2$ monitoring, a photodetector measures the amount of infrared light absorbed by airway gas during inspiration and expiration. (Light absorption increases along with the CO_2 concentration.) A monitor converts these data to a CO_2 value and a corresponding waveform, or capnogram, if capnography is used. (See *How $ETCO_2$ monitoring works,* page 286.)

How ETCO$_2$ monitoring works

The optical portion of an end-tidal carbon dioxide (ETCO$_2$) monitor contains an infrared light source, a sample chamber, a special carbon dioxide (CO_2) filter, and a photodetector. The infrared light passes through the sample chamber and is absorbed in varying amounts, depending on the amount of CO_2 the patient has just exhaled. The photodetector measures CO_2 content and relays this information to the microprocessor in the monitor, which displays the CO_2 value and waveform.

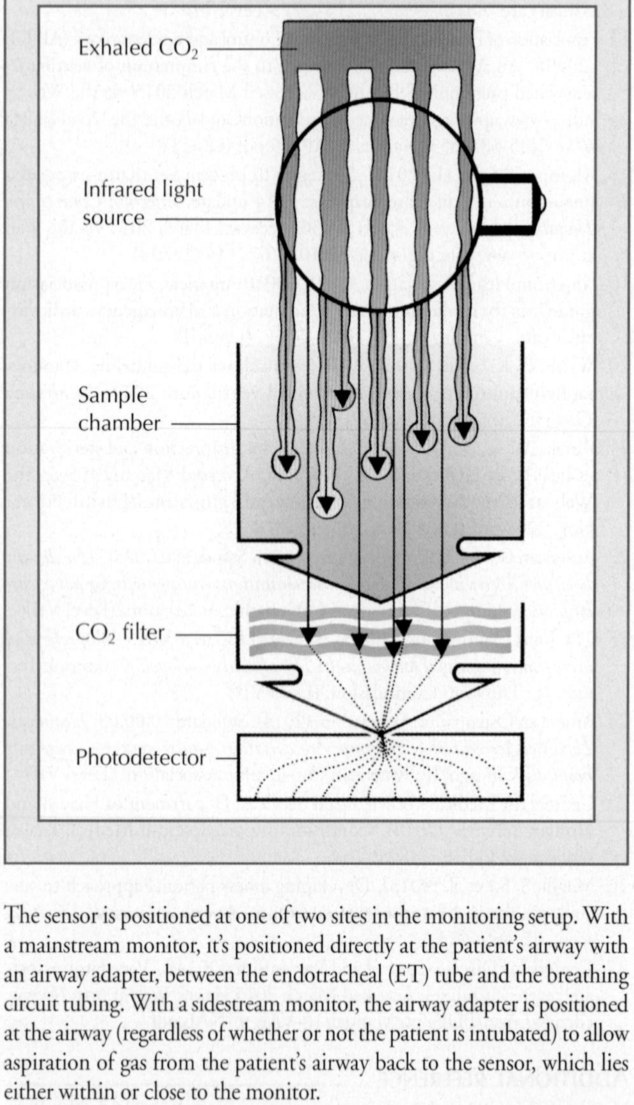

The sensor is positioned at one of two sites in the monitoring setup. With a mainstream monitor, it's positioned directly at the patient's airway with an airway adapter, between the endotracheal (ET) tube and the breathing circuit tubing. With a sidestream monitor, the airway adapter is positioned at the airway (regardless of whether or not the patient is intubated) to allow aspiration of gas from the patient's airway back to the sensor, which lies either within or close to the monitor.

Some CO_2 detection devices provide semiquantitative indications of CO_2 concentrations, supplying an approximate range rather than a specific value for ETCO$_2$. Other devices simply indicate whether CO_2 is present during exhalation. (See *Analyzing CO_2 levels.*)

The 2010 American Heart Association guidelines for cardiopulmonary resuscitation and emergency cardiovascular care recommend ETCO$_2$ monitoring in combination with clinical assessment to confirm initial ET tube placement in the patient in cardiac arrest when continuous quantitative waveform capnography isn't available.[1,2] Continuous quantitative waveform capnography can help monitor cardiopulmonary resuscitation quality in intubated patients and help detect fatigue in the person performing chest compressions.

ETCO$_2$ monitoring is recommended to guide ventilator management[1] and has become standard during anesthesia administration, such as in patients who are undergoing moderate sedation. It may also be used in those receiving epidural or patient-controlled analgesia. The ETCO$_2$ measurements can alert you to hypoventilation from oversedation.[3]

Detection of ETCO$_2$ during cardiac arrest is a good indicator that the ET tube is placed properly in the trachea. However, such conditions as pulmonary embolus, pulmonary edema, status asthmaticus, and gastric content contamination of the ETCO$_2$ detector can produce false results, so if you don't detect CO_2, use a second method to confirm ET tube placement, such as auscultation of breath sounds,[4] direct visualization, or use of an esophageal detector device.[2]

Equipment

Gloves ▪ mainstream or sidestream ETCO$_2$ monitor ▪ CO_2 sensor ▪ airway adapter, as recommended by the manufacturer (a neonatal adapter may have a much smaller dead space, making it appropriate for a smaller patient) ▪ ETCO$_2$ sensor ▪ hospital-grade disinfectant ▪ Optional: gown, mask, goggles, mask with face shield.

Preparation of equipment

If the monitor you're using isn't self-calibrating, calibrate it as the manufacturer directs *because failure to calibrate the device can lead to false readings.* If you're using a sidestream ETCO$_2$ monitor, replace the water trap between patients, if directed. *The trap allows humidity from exhaled gases to be condensed into an attached container.* Newer sidestream models don't require water traps.

Implementation

- Gather and prepare the equipment.
- Perform hand hygiene.[5,6,7,8,9]
- Confirm the patient's identity using at least two patient identifiers.[10]
- If the patient requires ET intubation, you'll typically apply an ETCO$_2$ detector or monitor immediately after the tube insertion. If he doesn't require intubation or is already intubated and alert, explain the purpose and expected duration of monitoring. Tell the patient that the monitor will painlessly measure the amount of CO_2 he exhales and track his CO_2 concentration *to make sure he's breathing is effectively.*
- Put on gloves and other personal protective equipment, as needed.[11,12]
- After turning on the monitor, position the airway adapter and sensor as directed by the manufacturer. For an intubated patient, position the adapter directly on the ET tube. For a nonintubated patient, place the adapter at or near the patient's airway.
- Set the alarm limits according to the patient's current condition. These alarms alert staff to potential life-threatening occurrences. Make sure the alarms are turned on, functioning properly, and audible to staff.[13,14,15]
- Remove and discard your gloves and any other personal protective equipment worn.[11,12]
- Perform hand hygiene.[5,6,7,8,9]
- Clean and disinfect reusable equipment after use.[1,16,17]
- Perform hand hygiene.[5,6,7,8,9]
- Document the procedure.[18,19,20]

Special considerations

- Note that The Joint Commission issued a sentinel event alert concerning medical device alarm safety *because alarm-related events have been associated with permanent loss of function and death.* Among the major contributing factors were improper alarm settings, inappropriately turned off alarms, and alarm signals that were not audible to staff. Make sure that alarm limits are appropriately set and that alarms are turned on and audible to staff. Follow facility guidelines for preventing alarm fatigue.[15]
- Make sure the adapter is changed with every breathing circuit and ET tube change.

EQUIPMENT

Analyzing CO_2 levels

Depending on which end-tidal carbon dioxide ($ETCO_2$) detector you use, the meaning of color changes within the detector dome may differ from the analysis for the Easy Cap detector described below. Follow the manufacturer's instructions for the specific detector you're using.

- The rim of the Easy Cap is divided into four segments (clockwise from the top): CHECK, A, B, and C. The CHECK segment is solid purple, signifying the absence of carbon dioxide (CO_2).
- The numbers in the other sections range from 0.03 to 5 and indicate the percentage of exhaled CO_2. The color should fluctuate during ventilation from purple (in section A) during inspiration to yellow (in section C) at the end of expiration. This indicates that the $ETCO_2$ levels are adequate, above 2%.
- An end-expiratory color change from the C range to the B range may be the first sign of hemodynamic instability.
- During cardiopulmonary resuscitation (CPR), an end-expiratory color change from the A or B range to the C range may mean the return of spontaneous ventilation.
- During prolonged cardiac arrest, inadequate pulmonary perfusion leads to inadequate gas exchange. The patient exhales little or no CO_2, so the color stays in the purple range even with proper intubation. Ineffective CPR also leads to inadequate pulmonary perfusion.
- Devices are available in adult and pediatric sizes.

Color indications on end-expiration

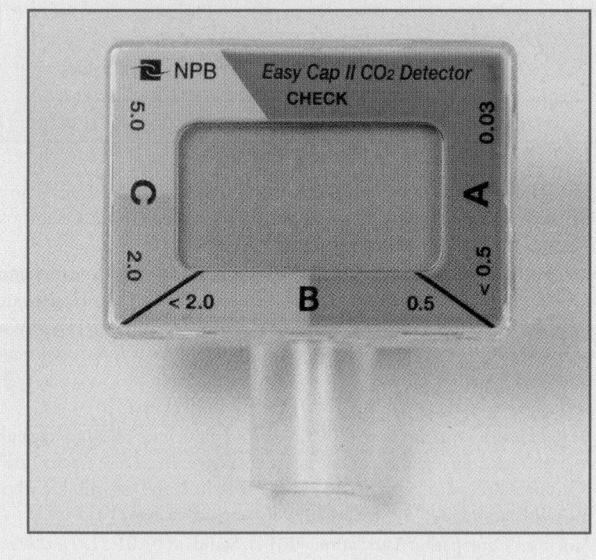

- Place the adapter on the ET tube *to avoid contaminating exhaled gases with fresh gas flow from the ventilator.* If you're using a heat and moisture exchanger, you may be able to position the airway adapter between the exchanger and breathing circuit.
- If the patient's $ETCO_2$ values differ from his partial pressure of arterial carbon dioxide, assess him for factors that can influence $ETCO_2$—especially when the differential between arterial and $ETCO_2$ values (the arterial absolute difference of carbon dioxide [$a\text{-}ADCO_2$]) is above normal.
- The $a\text{-}ADCO_2$ value, if correctly interpreted, provides useful information about the patient's status. For example, an increased $a\text{-}ADCO_2$ may mean that the patient has worsening dead space, especially if his tidal volume remains constant.
- Remember that $ETCO_2$ monitoring doesn't replace arterial blood gas (ABG) measurements *because it doesn't assess oxygenation or blood pH.*

Using a disposable $ETCO_2$ detector

When using a disposable end-tidal carbon dioxide ($ETCO_2$) detector, check the instructions and ensure ideal working conditions for the device. Here are some additional guidelines.

Avoiding high humidity, moisture, and heat

- Watch for changes indicating that the $ETCO_2$ detector's life span is decreasing—for example, sluggish color changes from breath to breath. A detector may be used for about 2 hours. However, using it with a ventilator that delivers high-humidity ventilation may shorten its usefulness to no more than 15 minutes.
- Don't use the detector with a heated humidifier or a nebulizer.
- Keep the detector protected from secretions, which render the device useless. If secretions enter the dome, remove and discard the detector.
- Use a heat and moisture exchanger to protect the detector. In some detectors, this filter fits between the endotracheal (ET) tube and the detector.
- If you're using a heat and moisture exchanger, remember that it may increase the patient's breathing effort. Be alert for increased resistance and breathing difficulties, and remove the exchanger if necessary.

Taking additional precautions

- Instilling epinephrine through the ET tube can damage the detector's indicator (the color may stay yellow). If this happens, discard the device.
- Frequently spot-check the $ETCO_2$ detector you're using for effectiveness.
- If you must transport the patient to another area for testing or treatment, use another method to verify the tube's placement.
- Never reuse a disposable $ETCO_2$ detector. It's intended for one-time, one-patient use only.

Supplementing $ETCO_2$ monitoring with pulse oximetry may provide more complete information.

- If the CO_2 waveform is available, assess it for height, frequency, rhythm, baseline, and shape *to help evaluate gas exchange.* Make sure you know how to recognize a normal waveform and can identify any abnormal waveforms in the patient's medical record. (See *CO_2 waveform,* page 288.)
- In a nonintubated patient, use $ETCO_2$ values to establish trends. Be aware that in such a patient, exhaled gas is more likely to mix with ambient air, and exhaled CO_2 may be diluted by fresh gas flow from the nasal cannula.
- $ETCO_2$ monitoring commonly is discontinued when the patient has been weaned effectively from mechanical ventilation or when he's no longer at risk for respiratory compromise. Carefully assess the patient's tolerance for weaning. After extubation, continuous $ETCO_2$ monitoring may detect the need for reintubation.
- Disposable $ETCO_2$ detectors are available. When using a disposable $ETCO_2$ detector, always check its color under fluorescent or natural light *because the dome looks pink under incandescent light.* (See *Using a disposable $ETCO_2$ detector.*)

Complications

Inaccurate measurements, such as from poor sampling technique, calibration drift, contamination of optics with moisture or secretions, or equipment malfunction, can lead to misdiagnosis and improper treatment.

The effects of manual resuscitation or ingestion of alcohol or carbonated beverages can alter the detector's findings. Color changes detected after fewer than six ventilations can be misleading.[2]

CO_2 waveform

The carbon dioxide (CO_2) waveform, or capnogram, produced in end-tidal carbon dioxide ($ETCO_2$) monitoring reflects the course of CO_2 elimination during exhalation. A normal capnogram (shown below) consists of several segments, which reflect the various stages of exhalation and inhalation.

Normally, any gas eliminated from the airway during early exhalation is dead-space gas, which hasn't undergone exchange at the alveolocapillary membrane. Measurements taken during this period contain no CO_2.

As exhalation continues, CO_2 concentration rises sharply and rapidly. The sensor now detects gas that has undergone exchange, producing measurable quantities of CO_2.

The final stages of alveolar emptying occur during late exhalation. During the alveolar plateau phase, CO_2 concentration rises more gradually *because alveolar emptying is more constant.*

The point at which the $ETCO_2$ value is derived is the end of exhalation, when CO_2 concentration peaks. Unless an alveolar plateau is present, this value doesn't accurately estimate alveolar CO_2. During inhalation, the CO_2 concentration declines sharply to zero.

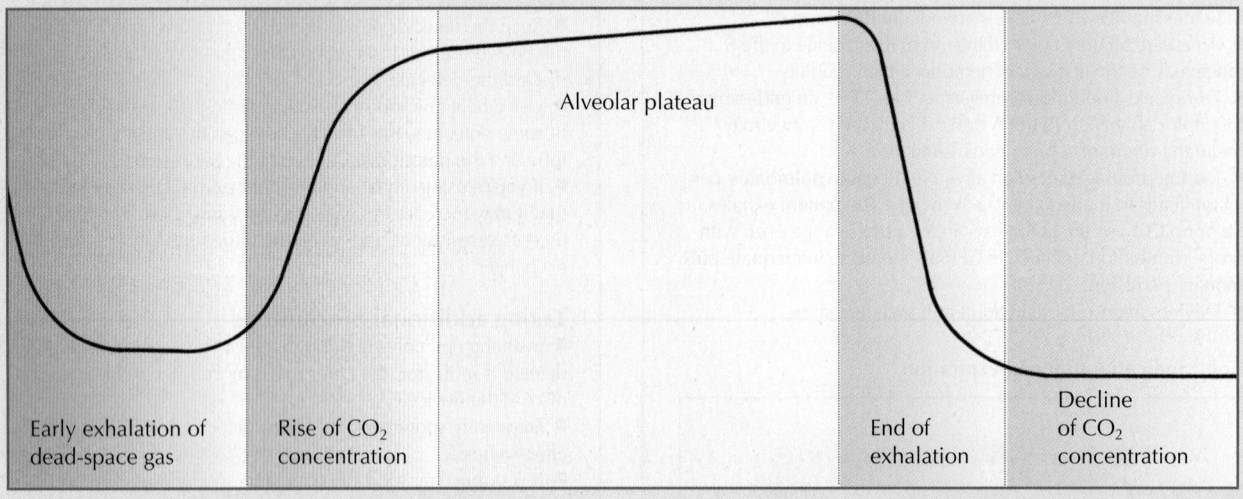

Documentation

Document the initial $ETCO_2$ value and all ventilator settings. Describe the waveform if one appears on the monitor. If the monitor has a printer, you may want to print out a sample waveform and include it in the patient's medical record.

Document $ETCO_2$ values at least as often as vital signs, whenever significant changes in waveform or patient status occur, and before and after weaning, respiratory procedures, and other interventions. Periodically obtain samples for ABG analysis as the patient's condition dictates, and document the corresponding $ETCO_2$ values.

REFERENCES

1 Walsh, B. K., et al. (2011). AARC clinical practice guideline: Capnography/capnometry during mechanical ventilation: 2011. *Respiratory Care, 56,* 503–509. Accessed March 2015 via the Web at http://rc.rcjournal.com/content/56/4/503.full.pdf (Level VII)

2 American Heart Association. (2010). 2010 American Heart Association guidelines for cardiopulmonary resuscitation and emergency cardiovascular care. *Circulation, 122,* S729–S767. (Level I)

3 Deitch, K., et al. (2010). Does end tidal CO2 monitoring during emergency department procedural sedation and analgesia with propofol decrease the incidence of hypoxic events? A randomized, controlled trial. *Annals of Emergency Medicine, 55,* 258–264. (Level II)

4 American College of Physicians. (2009). "AECP policy statement: Verification of endotracheal tube placement" [Online]. Accessed March 2015 via the Web at https://www.acep.org/Clinical—Practice-Management/Verification-of-Endotracheal-Tube-Placement/ (Level VII)

5 The Joint Commission. (2015). Standard NPSG.07.01.01. *Comprehensive accreditation manual for hospitals: The official handbook.* Oakbrook Terrace, IL: The Joint Commission. (Level VII)

6 Centers for Disease Control and Prevention. (2002). Guideline for hand hygiene in health-care settings: Recommendations of the Healthcare Infection Control Practices Advisory Committee and the HICPAC/SHEA/APIC/IDSA Hand Hygiene Task Force. *MMWR Recommendations and Reports, 51*(RR-16), 1–45. Accessed March 2015 via the Web at http://www.cdc.gov/mmwr/pdf/rr/rr5116.pdf (Level II)

7 World Health Organization. (2009). "WHO guidelines on hand hygiene in health care: First global patient safety challenge, clean care is safer care" [Online]. Accessed March 2015 via the Web at http://whqlibdoc.who.int/publications/2009/9789241597906_eng.pdf (Level IV)

8 American Osteopathic Association. (2014). Standard 07.01.21. *Healthcare Facilities Accreditation Program: Accreditation requirements for acute care hospitals.* Chicago, IL: American Osteopathic Association. (Level VII)

9 Centers for Medicare & Medicaid Services, Department of Health and Human Services. (2014). Condition of participation: Infection control. 42 C.F.R. § 482.42.

10 The Joint Commission. (2015). Standard NPSG.01.01.01. *Comprehensive accreditation manual for hospitals: The official handbook.* Oakbrook Terrace, IL: The Joint Commission. (Level VII)

11 Siegel, J. D., et al. (2007). "2007 guideline for isolation precautions: Preventing transmission of infectious agents in healthcare settings" [Online]. Accessed March 2015 via the Web at http://www.cdc.gov/hicpac/pdf/isolation/Isolation2007.pdf (Level II)

12 American Osteopathic Association. (2014). Standard 07.01.10. *Healthcare Facilities Accreditation Program: Accreditation requirements for acute care hospitals.* Chicago, IL: American Osteopathic Association. (Level VII)

13 American Association of Critical-Care Nurses. (2013). "AACN practice alert: Alarm management" [Online]. Accessed March 2015 via the Web

at http://www.aacn.org/wd/practice/docs/practicealerts/alarm-management-practice-alert.pdf (Level VII)

14 Graham, K. C., & Cvach, M. (2010). Monitor alarm fatigue: Standardizing use of physiological monitors and decreasing nuisance alarms. *American Journal of Critical Care, 19,* 28–37.

15 The Joint Commission. (2013). "Sentinel event alert: Medical device alarm safety in hospitals" [Online]. Accessed March 2015 via the Web http://www.jointcommission.org/assets/1/18/SEA_50_alarms_4_5_13_FINAL1.PDF (Level VII)

16 Rutala, W. A., et al. (2008). "Guideline for disinfection and sterilization in healthcare facilities, 2008" [Online]. Accessed March 2015 via the Web at http://www.cdc.gov/hicpac/pdf/guidelines/Disinfection_Nov_2008.pdf (Level I)

17 American Osteopathic Association. (2014). Standard 07.02.03. *Healthcare Facilities Accreditation Program: Accreditation requirements for acute care hospitals.* Chicago, IL: American Osteopathic Association. (Level VII)

18 The Joint Commission. (2015). Standard RC.01.03.01. *Comprehensive accreditation manual for hospitals: The official handbook.* Oakbrook Terrace, IL: The Joint Commission. (Level VII)

19 American Osteopathic Association. (2014). Standard 10.00.03. *Healthcare Facilities Accreditation Program: Accreditation requirements for acute care hospitals.* Chicago, IL: American Osteopathic Association. (Level VII)

20 Centers for Medicare & Medicaid Services, Department of Health and Human Services. (2014). Condition of participation: Medical record services. 42 C.F.R. § 482.24(b).

ADDITIONAL REFERENCE

Lynn-McHale Wiegand, D. (Ed.). (2011). *AACN procedure manual for critical care* (6th ed.). Philadelphia, PA: Saunders.

ENEMA ADMINISTRATION

Enema administration involves instilling a solution into the rectum and colon. In a retention enema, the patient holds the solution within the rectum or colon for 30 minutes to 1 hour. With a cleansing enema, the patient expels the solution almost completely within 15 minutes. Both types of enema stimulate peristalsis by mechanically distending the colon and stimulating rectal wall nerves.

Enemas are used to clean the lower bowel in preparation for diagnostic or surgical procedures, relieve distention and promote expulsion of flatus, lubricate the rectum and colon, and soften hardened stool for removal. Return-flow enemas are occasionally prescribed to expel flatus. In addition, a retention enema may be used to administer medications such as sodium polystyrene sulfonate for treatment of hyperkalemia, lactulose for treatment of hepatic encephalopathy, and vancomycin for the treatment of severe, complicated *Clostridium difficile* infection.[1,2]

Enemas are contraindicated in patients after recent colon or rectal surgery or myocardial infarction and in patients with acute abdominal conditions of unknown origin such as suspected appendicitis. They should be administered cautiously to patients with arrhythmia.

Equipment

Prescribed solution ▪ enema administration set or enema contained in a squeeze bottle ▪ gloves ▪ fluid-impermeable pads ▪ bath blanket ▪ bedpans or bedside commode ▪ toilet tissue ▪ hospital-grade disinfectant ▪ stethoscope ▪ disinfectant pad ▪ Optional: IV pole, additional personal protective equipment, water-soluble lubricant.

Prepackaged disposable enema kits are available, as are small-volume enema solutions in irrigating and retention types and in pediatric sizes.

Preparation of equipment

If you're using a concentrated enema solution, dilute the solution according to the manufacturer's instructions.[3] *Because some ingredients may be mucosal irritants,* make sure the proportions are correct and the agents are mixed thoroughly *to avoid local irritation.* Warm the solution until it's lukewarm *to reduce patient discomfort.* Clamp the tubing and fill the enema bag with the prescribed solution. Unclamp the tubing, flush the solution through the tubing, and then reclamp it. *Flushing detects leaks and removes air that could cause discomfort if introduced into the colon.* Hang the solution container on the IV pole and take all supplies to the patient's room.

If you're using an enema contained within a disposable squeeze bottle, no preparation is needed.

Implementation

- Avoid distractions and interruptions when preparing and administering medication *to prevent medication errors.*[4,5]
- Verify the order on the patient's medication record by checking it against the practitioner's order.[6,7,8]
- Gather the medication and the appropriate equipment.
- Compare the solution or medication label with the order in the patient's medical record.[6,7,8]
- Check the patient's medical record for an allergy or a contraindication to the prescribed solution. If an allergy or a contraindication exists, don't administer the solution; instead, notify the practitioner.[6,8,7]
- Check the expiration date on the medication. If the medication is expired, return it to the pharmacy and obtain new medication.[6,7,8]
- Visually inspect the solution for particles or discoloration or other loss of integrity; don't administer the solution if its integrity is compromised.[6,7,8]
- Discuss any unresolved concerns about the medication with the patient's practitioner.[6,7,8]
- Prepare the enema, as needed.
- Perform hand hygiene.[9,10,11,12,13]
- Confirm the patient's identity using at least two patient identifiers.[14]
- Provide privacy.[15]
- Explain the procedure to the patient *to allay his anxiety.* Ask the patient whether he's ever received an enema before. If so, ask whether he had difficulty retaining the enema *to determine your equipment needs.*
- If the patient is receiving the medication for the first time, teach him about potential adverse reactions and discuss any other concerns related to the medication.[6,7,8]
- Verify that the medication is being administered at the proper time, in the prescribed dose, and by the correct route *to reduce the risk of medication errors.*[6,7,8]
- Encourage the patient to empty his bladder *because fluid entering the rectum may cause discomfort if the patient has a full bladder.*[16]
- Place a bedpan or commode nearby for the patient to use. If the patient can use the bathroom, make sure that it will be available when the patient needs it. Have toilet tissue within the patient's reach.
- If your facility uses a bar code scanning system, scan your identification badge, the patient's identification bracelet, and the medication's bar code.
- Put on gloves and other personal protective equipment, as needed, *to comply with standard precautions.*[17,18]
- Remove any clothing below the patient's waist and cover him with a blanket.[16]
- Assess the patient's GI status for bowel sounds and abdominal distention *to serve as a baseline for comparison.*
- Position the patient on his left side with his knees bent or in the knee-to-chest position *to expose the anus and ease insertion of the enema.*[3,16]
- Place fluid-impermeable pads under the patient's buttocks *to prevent soiling the linens.*
- Remove the cap from the enema administration set and lubricate the distal tip of the administration tubing with water-soluble lubricant *to facilitate rectal insertion and reduce irritation.*[3] Alternatively, if you're using an administration set with a prelubricated tip or an enema contained in

a disposable squeeze bottle, remove the protective covering *to expose the prelubricated tip*. Expel excess air from the enema squeeze bottle *because air in the colon may cause discomfort.*[19]

- Gently insert the lubricated tip into the rectum, advancing it 2″ to 3″ (5 to 7.6 cm) with the tip pointing toward the umbilicus (as shown below). Don't force the tip into the rectum *because doing so can cause injury.* During insertion, instruct the patient to bear down as if having a bowel movement if able; this helps relax the muscles around the anus, easing insertion.[19]

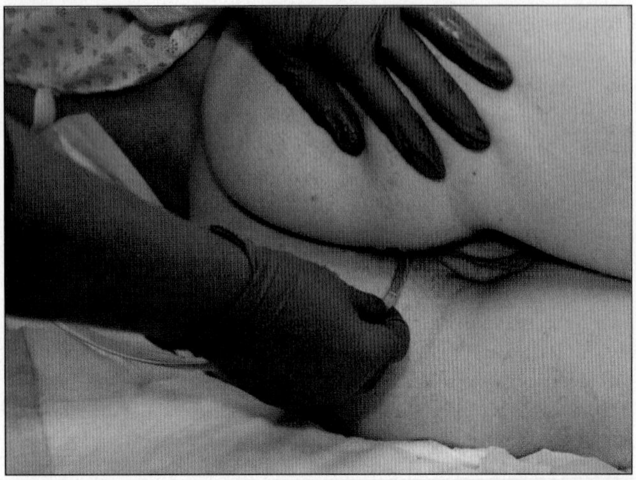

- Unclamp the enema administration set and allow the solution to flow into the rectum slowly. Advise the patient to tell you if he experiences discomfort, in which case you should slow the flow rate *because the flow is probably too fast.*[3] Alternatively, if you're using a squeeze bottle, squeeze the bottle until nearly all of the solution is gone (as shown below).

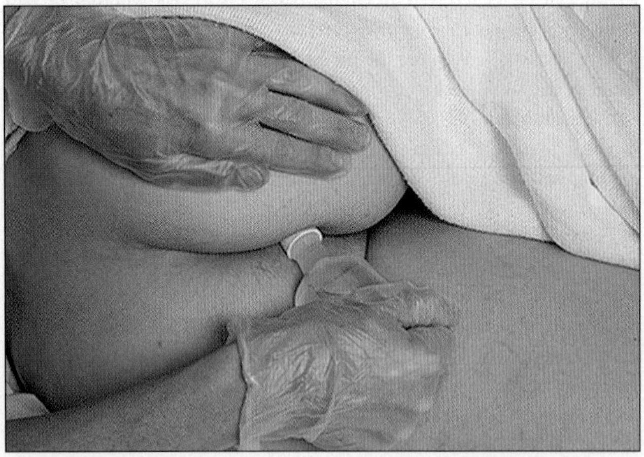

- Slowly withdraw the tip of the enema administration set tubing or squeeze bottle *to prevent a reflex emptying of the bowel.*[16]
- Instruct the patient to retain the enema, as prescribed. Explain that it's often easier to retain the enema while lying down.[16]
- Make sure the patient has access to a call light and a bedpan, commode, or bathroom.[16]
- Properly dispose of the enema equipment.[18] If additional enemas are scheduled, clean and disinfect reusable equipment with a hospital-grade disinfectant solution[20,21] and store it appropriately.
- Remove and discard your gloves and any other personal protective equipment worn.
- Perform hand hygiene.[9,10,11,12,13]
- Clean and disinfect your stethoscope with a disinfectant pad.[20,21]
- Perform hand hygiene.[9,10,11,12,13]
- Document the procedure.[22,23,24]

Special considerations

- *Because patients with salt-retention disorders, such as heart failure, may absorb sodium from the saline enema solution,* administer the solution to such patients cautiously and monitor electrolyte status.
- Double-bag all enema equipment and label it as isolation equipment if the patient is on enteric precautions.[18]

Patient teaching

Describe the procedure to the patient and his family. Emphasize that administering an enema to a person in a sitting position or on the toilet could injure the rectal wall. Tell the patient how to prepare and care for the equipment. Discuss relaxation techniques, and review measures for preventing constipation, including regular exercise, dietary modifications, and adequate fluid intake.

Complications

Enemas may produce dizziness or faintness, excessive irritation of the colonic mucosa resulting from repeated administration or from sensitivity to the enema ingredients, hyponatremia or hypokalemia from repeated administration of hypotonic solutions, and cardiac arrhythmias resulting from vasovagal reflex stimulation after insertion of the rectal catheter. Colonic water absorption may result from prolonged retention of hypotonic solutions, which may, in turn, cause hypervolemia or water intoxication.

Documentation

Record the date and time of enema administration; special equipment used; the type and amount of solution; retention time; the approximate amount returned; the color, consistency, and amount of the return; abnormalities within the return; any complications that occurred; and the patient's tolerance of the treatment.

REFERENCES

1 Lee, W. M., et al. (2011). "AASLD position paper: The management of acute liver failure: Update 2011" [Online]. Accessed March 2015 via the Web at http://www.aasld.org/practiceguidelines/Documents/AcuteLiverFailureUpdate2011.pdf (Level VII)

2 Cohen, S. H., et al. (2010). Clinical practice guidelines for Clostridium difficile infection in adults: 2010 update by the Society for Healthcare Epidemiology of America (SHEA) and the Infectious Diseases Society of America (IDSA). *Infection Control and Hospital Epidemiology, 31,* 431–455. (Level V)

3 Institute for Safe Medication Practices. (2013). "Administration of rectal suppositories and enemas" [Online]. Accessed March 2015 via the Web at http://www.consumermedsafety.org/component/k2/item/462-administration-of-rectal-suppositories-or-enemas

4 Westbrook, J., et al. (2010). Association of interruptions with an increased risk and severity of medication administration errors. *Archives of Internal Medicine, 170,* 683–690. (Level IV)

5 Institute for Safe Medication Practices. (2013). Side tracks on the safety express: Interruptions lead to errors and unfinished . . . Wait, what was I doing? *Nurse Advise-ERR, 11*(2), 1–4. Accessed March 2015 via the Web at https://www.ismp.org/Newsletters/acutecare/showarticle.aspx?id=37 (Level VII)

6 The Joint Commission. (2015). Standard MM.06.01.01. *Comprehensive accreditation manual for hospitals: The official handbook.* Oakbrook Terrace, IL: The Joint Commission. (Level VII)

7 American Osteopathic Association. (2014). Standard 16.01.03. *Healthcare Facilities Accreditation Program: Accreditation requirements for acute care hospitals.* Chicago, IL: American Osteopathic Association. (Level VII)

8 Centers for Medicare & Medicaid Services, Department of Health and Human Services. (2014). Condition of participation: Nursing services. 42 C.F.R. § 482.23(c).

9 Centers for Medicare & Medicaid Services, Department of Health and Human Services. (2014). Condition of participation: Infection control. 42 C.F.R. § 482.42.
10 American Osteopathic Association. (2014). Standard 07.01.21. *Healthcare Facilities Accreditation Program: Accreditation requirements for acute care hospitals.* Chicago, IL: American Osteopathic Association. (Level VII)
11 The Joint Commission. (2015). Standard NPSG.07.01.01. *Comprehensive accreditation manual for hospitals: The official handbook.* Oakbrook Terrace, IL: The Joint Commission. (Level VII)
12 World Health Organization. (2009). "WHO guidelines on hand hygiene in health care: First global patient safety challenge, clean care is safer care" [Online]. Accessed March 2015 via the Web at http://whqlibdoc.who.int/publications/2009/9789241597906_eng.pdf (Level IV)
13 Centers for Disease Control and Prevention. (2002). Guideline for hand hygiene in health-care settings: Recommendations of the Healthcare Infection Control Practices Advisory Committee and the HICPAC/SHEA/APIC/IDSA Hand Hygiene Task Force. *MMWR Recommendations and Reports, 51*(RR-16), 1–45. Accessed March 2015 via the Web at http://www.cdc.gov/mmwr/pdf/rr/rr5116.pdf (Level II)
14 The Joint Commission. (2015). Standard NPSG.01.01.01. *Comprehensive accreditation manual for hospitals: The official handbook.* Oakbrook Terrace, IL: The Joint Commission. (Level VII)
15 American Osteopathic Association. (2014). Standard 15.01.16. *Healthcare Facilities Accreditation Program: Accreditation requirements for acute care hospitals.* Chicago, IL: American Osteopathic Association. (Level VII)
16 Kyle, G. (2007). Bowel care: Administering an enema. *Nursing Times, 103*(45), 26–27.
17 American Osteopathic Association. (2014). Standard 07.01.10. *Healthcare Facilities Accreditation Program: Accreditation requirements for acute care hospitals.* Chicago, IL: American Osteopathic Association (Level VII)
18 Siegel, J. D., et al. (2007). "2007 guideline for isolation precautions: Preventing transmission of infectious agents in healthcare settings" [Online]. Accessed March 2015 via the Web at http://www.cdc.gov/hicpac/pdf/isolation/Isolation2007.pdf (Level II)
19 Fleet Laboratories. (2010). "Fleet enema saline laxative directions for use" [Online]. Accessed March 2015 via the Web at http://www.fleetlabs.com/directions/ICS4_5903Z03_OL.pdf
20 American Osteopathic Association. (2014). Standard 07.02.03. *Healthcare Facilities Accreditation Program: Accreditation requirements for acute care hospitals.* Chicago, IL: American Osteopathic Association. (Level VII)
21 Rutala, W. A., et al. (2008). "Guideline for disinfection and sterilization in healthcare facilities, 2008" [Online]. Accessed March 2015 via the Web at http://www.cdc.gov/hicpac/pdf/guidelines/Disinfection_Nov_2008.pdf (Level I)
22 American Osteopathic Association. (2014). Standard 10.00.03. *Healthcare Facilities Accreditation Program: Accreditation requirements for acute care hospitals.* Chicago, IL: American Osteopathic Association. (Level VII)
23 Centers for Medicare & Medicaid Services, Department of Health and Human Services. (2014). Condition of participation: Medical record services. 42 C.F.R. § 482.24(b).
24 The Joint Commission. (2015). Standard RC.01.03.01. *Comprehensive accreditation manual for hospitals: The official handbook.* Oakbrook Terrace, IL: The Joint Commission. (Level VII)

ADDITIONAL REFERENCE

Nettina, S. M. (2014). *Lippincott manual of nursing practice* (10th ed.). Philadelphia, PA: Wolters Kluwer.

EPICARDIAL PACING AND CARE

Epicardial pacing wires are commonly positioned on the epicardial (outer) surface of the heart after cardiac surgery to manage surgery-related arrhythmias. Depending on the patient's need, the surgeon may place positive and negative electrodes on the right atrium, right ventricle, or both. He'll loosely suture these electrodes to the epicardial surface and bring them out through the chest wall through small incisions.

If the patient requires pacing, you or the practitioner will connect epicardial pacing wires to the pulse generator of a temporary pacemaker. When the patient becomes hemodynamically stable and no longer requires pacing, the surgeon or a specially trained nurse removes the wires.

Equipment

For insertion and care

Pacemaker generator with new battery ▪ extra batteries ▪ connecting cable ▪ atrial epicardial wires ▪ ventricular epicardial wires ▪ sterile rubber finger cot, glove, or plastic cap ▪ sterile dressing materials ▪ gloves ▪ tape ▪ cardiac monitoring equipment (see the "Cardiac monitoring," procedure, page 117) ▪ automatic blood pressure monitoring equipment ▪ Optional: protective plastic cover, soft physical wrist restraints, prescribed pain medications.

For removal

Two pairs of gloves ▪ personal protective equipment (gown, goggles and mask or face shield with a mask) ▪ prescribed analgesic ▪ sterile gauze ▪ antiseptic solution (chlorhexidine-based) ▪ tape ▪ suture removal kit ▪ cardiac monitoring equipment ▪ thermometer ▪ blood pressure cuff and manometer ▪ stethoscope ▪ disinfectant pad ▪ emergency equipment (crash cart with cardiac medications, defibrillator, handheld resuscitation bag with mask, intubation equipment) ▪ temporary transcutaneous or transvenous pacing equipment ▪ Optional: IV catheter and catheter insertion equipment.

Preparation of equipment

For insertion

Insert a new battery into the pulse generator and make sure it's functioning properly. Make sure extra batteries are available.

For removal

Check that the emergency equipment and temporary transcutaneous or transvenous pacing equipment are readily available.

Implementation

For insertion and care

- Verify the practitioner's order.
- Gather and prepare the appropriate equipment.
- Confirm that a written informed consent has been obtained and is in the patient's medical record.[1,2,3,4]
- Perform a preprocedure verification *to make sure that all relevant documentation, related information, and equipment are available and correctly identified to the patient's identifiers.*[5,6]
- Verify that the laboratory and imaging studies have been completed as ordered and that the results are in the patient's medical record. Notify the practitioner of any unexpected results.
- Perform hand hygiene.[7,8,9,10,11]
- Confirm the patient's identity using at least two patient identifiers.[12]
- Reinforce the practitioner's explanation of the procedure to the patient and his family *to decrease anxiety.*
- The surgical team will conduct a time-out immediately before starting the procedure *to perform a final assessment that the correct patient, site, positioning, and procedure are identified and all relevant information and necessary equipment are available.*[13]
- The surgeon will hook epicardial wires into the epicardium just before the end of surgery. Depending on the patient's condition, the surgeon may insert atrial wires, ventricular wires, or both.
- Put on gloves *to prevent microshock.*[14]
- After insertion, attach the patient to the bedside cardiac monitor *to monitor the patient's heart rhythm and evaluate pacemaker function.*[14]

Sensitivity and stimulation threshold testing[14]

Sensitivity and stimulation threshold testing help determine the appropriate pacemaker rate and the amount of electrical current needed to initiate depolarization of the myocardium. Testing should occur on both chambers, as appropriate. Sensitivity threshold testing isn't necessary if the patient has no intrinsic rhythm. In some facilities, critical care nurses are permitted to perform sensitivity and stimulation threshold testing; in other facilities, the practitioner must perform the testing. Frequency of testing also varies by facility. Commonly, testing occurs at least every 24 hours *to make sure that the pacemaker is functioning properly and that it isn't delivering high levels of energy to the myocardium.*

Performing sensitivity threshold testing

- Slowly turn the sensitivity dial counterclockwise to a higher setting until the sensing indicator light stops flashing, which will occur when the device no longer senses the patient's intrinsic rhythm.
- Gradually turn the sensitivity dial clockwise to a lower setting until the sensing light begins flashing with each complex and the pacing light stops flashing; this setting is the sensing threshold.
- Set the sensitivity dial to the setting that's one-half the value of the sensing threshold.

Performing stimulation threshold testing

- Set the pacing rate about 10 beats/minute above the patient's intrinsic rate.
- Beginning at 20 milliamperes, slowly decrease the output until capture is lost.
- Gradually increase the milliamperes until you see a 1:1 capture and the pacing light flashes; this is the stimulation threshold.
- Set the milliamperes at least two times higher than the stimulation threshold.

- Attach the connecting cable to the pulse generator by connecting the positive pole on the cable to the positive pole on the pulse generator and the negative pole on the cable to the negative pole on the pulse generator.[14]
- Expose the epicardial pacing wires and identify the atrial and ventricular wires if both are present. *Epicardial wires that exit the chest to the right of the sternum originate in the atrium; wires that exit to the left of the sternum originate in the ventricle.*[14]
- Using the connecting cable, connect the epicardial wires to the pulse generator. Connect the positive electrode to the positive terminal on the pulse generator through the connecting cable; connect the negative electrode to the negative terminal.[14]
- Set the pacing mode, rate, and energy level (output or milliamperes) according to the practitioner's order, or as determined by sensitivity (the level at which intrinsic cardiac activity is sensed by electrodes) and stimulation threshold testing (the minimum amount of voltage necessary to initiate depolarization).[14] (See *Sensitivity and stimulation threshold testing.*)
- After adjusting the pacemaker settings, place the protective plastic cover over the pacemaker controls or lock the controls.[14]
- Apply a sterile occlusive dressing over the insertion site[14] and label it with the date, the time, and your initials *to prevent infection at the insertion site.*
- Secure the pulse generator *to prevent it from falling or becoming inadvertently detached.*[14]
- Insulate exposed wires using a plastic cap, glove, or finger cot.[14]
- Assess the patient's vital signs, skin color, level of consciousness, and peripheral pulses *to determine the effectiveness of the paced rhythm.* Perform a 12-lead electrocardiogram (ECG) *to serve as a baseline,* and then perform additional ECGs daily or with clinical changes. Also, if possible, obtain a rhythm strip before, during, and after pacemaker placement; after any adjustment in pacemaker settings; and whenever the patient receives treatment because of a pacemaker complication.
- Assess the patient for pain using techniques appropriate for the patient's age, condition, and ability to understand. Respond to the patient's pain appropriately.[15]

For removal

- Verify the practitioner's order in the patient's medical record for epicardial wire removal.
- Check laboratory data for coagulation and electrolyte results to make sure they're within normal limits *to reduce the risk of bleeding and cardiac arrhythmias.* Notify the practitioner of abnormal values.[14,16]
- Check the medication record to ensure that the patient isn't receiving anticoagulants *to reduce the risk of hemorrhage following the procedure.*[14]
- Gather and prepare the equipment and bring it to the patient's bedside.
- Perform hand hygiene.[7,8,9,10,11]
- Confirm the patient's identity using two patient identifiers.[12]
- Explain the procedure to the patient *to reduce anxiety and enhance cooperation* and tell him that he may feel a slightly painful pulling sensation.[17]
- Make sure the patient is attached to a cardiac monitor. Make sure the alarm limits are set appropriately for the patient's current condition and that the alarms are turned on, functioning properly, and audible to staff.[18,19,20,21]
- Perform a comprehensive pain assessment using techniques appropriate for the patient's age, condition, and ability to understand.[15]
- Administer an analgesic following safe medication administration practices 20 to 30 minutes before the procedure *to promote patient comfort.*[14,22,23]
- Obtain vital signs and an ECG rhythm strip, and assess the patient's cardiovascular status *to ensure the patient is stable before removing pacing wires and to provide a baseline for comparison.*[14]
- Confirm that the patient has patent IV access *in case emergency fluids or medications are required.*[14] Insert an IV catheter if patent access isn't available. (See the "IV catheter insertion and removal" procedure, page 446.)
- Perform hand hygiene[7,8,9,10,11] and put on personal protective equipment.[24,25]
- Place the patient in the supine position *so that the wires are readily accessible and the patient is properly positioned if emergency measures become necessary.*[14]
- Using sterile technique, open the suture removal kit and gauze packages and place them within reach.
- Carefully remove and discard the dressing[16] covering the exit site.
- Remove and discard your gloves,[16] perform hand hygiene,[7,8,9,10,11] and put on a new pair of gloves.[16,25]
- Clean the exit sites with antiseptic solution; clean at least a 3″ (7.6-cm) area around the exit sites.[14]
- Cut the sutures at the appropriate place and remove them. (See the "Suture removal" procedure, page 731.)[14]
- Grasp a wire and slowly and gently pull *to uncoil it from the epicardium.*[14] If you feel resistance, stop and notify the practitioner.
- While pulling each wire, observe the cardiac monitor for arrhythmias *because arrhythmias are common during epicardial pacing wire removal.*
- Inspect the pacing wire for a small piece of tissue at the tip, which indicates that you've removed the entire wire intact.[14]

- If you note bleeding at the exit site, apply pressure until hemostasis is achieved.[14]
- Observe the site, noting drainage, redness, or skin breakdown.
- Place sterile gauze pads over the exit sites and secure them with tape.[14]
- Dispose of soiled supplies appropriately *to reduce the risk of transmission of microorganism.*[24,26]
- Monitor vital signs and cardiac rhythm, and assess for signs of cardiac tamponade every 15 minutes for the first hour, every 30 minutes for the next 2 hours, and then hourly for 2 hours *to assess hemodynamic stability.*[14]
- Reassess the patient for pain and respond appropriately if the patient continues to have pain despite receiving the prescribed medication.[15]

Completing the procedure

- Discard supplies, remove and discard your gloves,[16] and perform hand hygiene.[7,8,9,10,11]
- Clean and disinfect your stethoscope using a disinfectant pad.[27,28]
- Perform hand hygiene.[7,8,9,10,11]
- Document the procedure.[17,18,19]

Special considerations

- Take care to prevent microshock, including warning the patient not to use any electrical equipment that isn't grounded, such as telephones, electric shavers, televisions, and lamps.
- If the patient is disoriented or uncooperative, use restraints if less restrictive measures aren't effective *to prevent accidental removal of the pacemaker wires.*
- If the patient needs emergency defibrillation, make sure the pacemaker can withstand the procedure. If you're unsure, disconnect the pulse generator *to avoid damage.*
- Continuously monitor the ECG reading, noting capture, sensing, rate, intrinsic beats, and competition of paced and intrinsic rhythms. If the pacemaker is sensing correctly, the sense indicator on the pulse generator should flash with each beat. (See *Handling pacemaker malfunction,* page 294.)
- Change the dressing at a frequency determined by your facility and the type of dressing used.[14] Clean the insertion site with an antiseptic solution, change the dressing, and label it with the date, the time, and your initials. Inspect the site for signs of infection.
- Assess and document sensitivity and stimulation thresholds (commonly every 24 hours) as required by your facility *to make sure the pacemaker is functioning properly.*[14]
- Monitor the pulse generator's battery light indicator and change the battery when necessary; battery life varies according to the pacing energy needed.[14]
- If the pulse generator is no longer needed, disconnect it from the pacing wires and insulate the wires using a plastic cap, glove, or finger cot *to prevent microshocks.*

Complications

Complications associated with pacemaker therapy include microshock, equipment failure, and competitive or fatal arrhythmias. Epicardial pacemakers carry a risk of infection, cardiac arrest, and diaphragmatic stimulation.

Complications following epicardial pacing wire removal occur more commonly in patients with a history of heart failure, repeat heart surgery, or anticoagulant therapy. Monitor for signs and symptoms of life-threatening cardiac tamponade, such as the Beck triad (hypotension, muffled heart tones, and jugular vein distention), tachycardia, decreased peripheral pulses, and dyspnea. Cardiac tamponade may not be immediately evident if the bleeding is slow, so you may need to monitor the patient closely for up to 2 hours. Other complications include infection, hemorrhage, hematoma, arrhythmias, hemodynamic instability, myocardial ischemia, and graft site trauma.

Documentation

Record the reason for pacing, the time it started, the locations of the electrodes, and the pacemaker settings. Note the patient's response to the procedure, along with any complications and interventions taken. If possible, obtain rhythm strips before, during, and after pacemaker placement and whenever pacemaker settings are changed or when the patient receives treatment for a complication caused by the pacemaker. As you monitor the patient, record his response to temporary pacing and note any changes in his condition. Document patient teaching and the patient's understanding of your teaching.

Record the date, time, and name of the person removing the wires. If an analgesic was administered, record the name, dose, route, and time it was given and the patient's rating of his pain level (on a 0 to 10 scale).

Describe the condition of the insertion sites, the ease with which you removed the wires, and whether you noted tissue at the end of the wires. Include vital signs, ECG strip, and patient assessment before, during, and after the procedure. Record how you dressed the site. Note the patient's tolerance of the procedure.

If any adverse effects occurred, note the time, name of the practitioner notified, orders given, nursing interventions, and the patient's response. Document frequent assessments on a frequent vital sign assessment sheet or in the electronic medical record. Include patient and family teaching provided and their understanding of your teaching.

REFERENCES

1 The Joint Commission. (2015). Standard RI.01.03.01. *Comprehensive accreditation manual for hospitals: The official handbook.* Oakbrook Terrace, IL: The Joint Commission. (Level VII)

2 American Osteopathic Association. (2014). Standard 30.01.11. *Healthcare Facilities Accreditation Program: Accreditation requirements for acute care hospitals.* Chicago, IL: American Osteopathic Association. (Level VII)

3 Centers for Medicare & Medicaid Services, Department of Health and Human Services. (2014). Condition of participation: Patient's rights. 42 C.F.R. § 482.13(b)(2).

4 Centers for Medicare & Medicaid Services, Department of Health and Human Services. (2012). Condition of participation: Surgical services. 42 C.F.R. § 482.51.

5 The Joint Commission. (2015). Standard UP.01.01.01. *Comprehensive accreditation manual for hospitals: The official handbook.* Oakbrook Terrace, IL: The Joint Commission. (Level VII)

6 American Osteopathic Association. (2014). Standard 30.00.14. *Healthcare Facilities Accreditation Program: Accreditation requirements for acute care hospitals.* Chicago, IL: American Osteopathic Association. (Level VII)

7 The Joint Commission. (2015). Standard NPSG.07.01.01. *Comprehensive accreditation manual for hospitals: The official handbook.* Oakbrook Terrace, IL: The Joint Commission. (Level VII)

8 World Health Organization. (2009). "WHO guidelines on hand hygiene in health care: First global patient safety challenge, clean care is safer care" [Online]. Accessed March 2015 via the Web at http://whqlibdoc.who.int/publications/2009/9789241597906_eng.pdf (Level IV)

9 Centers for Disease Control and Prevention. (2002). Guideline for hand hygiene in health-care settings: Recommendations of the Healthcare Infection Control Practices Advisory Committee and the HICPAC/SHEA/APIC/IDSA Hand Hygiene Task Force. *MMWR Recommendations and Reports, 51*(RR-16), 1–45. Accessed March 2015 via the Web at http://www.cdc.gov/mmwr/pdf/rr/rr5116.pdf (Level II)

10 Centers for Medicare & Medicaid Services, Department of Health and Human Services. (2014). Condition of participation: Infection control. 42 C.F.R. § 482.42.

11 American Osteopathic Association. (2014). Standard 07.01.21. *Healthcare Facilities Accreditation Program: Accreditation requirements for acute care hospitals.* Chicago, IL: American Osteopathic Association. (Level VII)

12 The Joint Commission. (2015). Standard NPSG.01.01.01. *Comprehensive accreditation manual for hospitals: The official handbook.* Oakbrook Terrace, IL: The Joint Commission. (Level VII)

TROUBLESHOOTING

Handling pacemaker malfunction

Occasionally, a temporary pacemaker may fail to function appropriately. When this occurs, you need to take immediate action *to correct the problem*. Follow these steps when your patient's pacemaker fails to pace, capture, or sense intrinsic beats.

Failure to pace

This problem happens when the pacemaker either doesn't fire or fires too often. The pulse generator may not be working properly, or it may not be conducting the impulse to the patient.

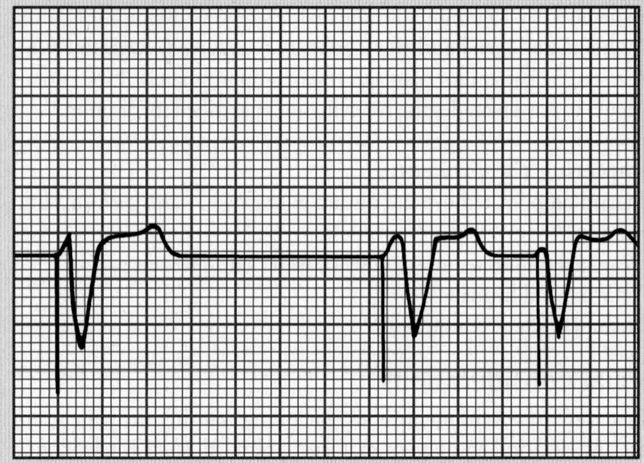

Nursing interventions

- If the pacing or sensing indicator flashes, check the patient, all connections, and the battery. Check the position of the pacing electrode in the patient by X-ray if ordered.
- If the pulse generator is turned on but the indicators still aren't flashing, change the battery. If that doesn't help, use a different pulse generator.
- Check the settings if the pacemaker is firing too rapidly. If the rate is correct or if increasing the sensitivity (according to the practitioner's order) doesn't help, change the pulse generator.
- Have a transcutaneous pacemaker on standby in case the pacemaker continues to malfunction and the patient becomes symptomatic. Notify the practitioner.

Failure to capture

In failure to capture, you can see the pacemaker spikes but the heart isn't responding. This malfunction may be caused by changes in the pacing threshold from ischemia, swelling at the insertion site, an electrolyte imbalance (high or low potassium or magnesium levels), acidosis, an adverse reaction to a medication, a perforated ventricle, fibrosis, or the electrode position.

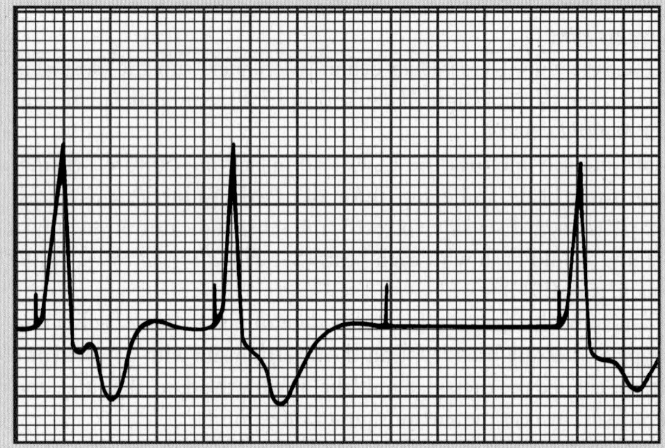

Nursing interventions

- Verify that the settings are correct, according to the practitioner's order.
- If the heart isn't responding, carefully check all connections, increase the milliamperes slowly as determined by your facility, and then notify the practitioner of the failure to capture.
- Have a transcutaneous pacemaker on standby in case the pacemaker continues to malfunction and the patient becomes symptomatic. Notify the practitioner.

Failure to sense intrinsic beats

Failure to sense intrinsic beats could cause ventricular tachycardia or ventricular fibrillation if the pacemaker fires on the vulnerable T wave. Possible causes include the pacemaker sensing an external stimulus as a QRS complex, which could lead to asystole, or the pacemaker not being sensitive enough, which means it could fire anywhere within the cardiac cycle.

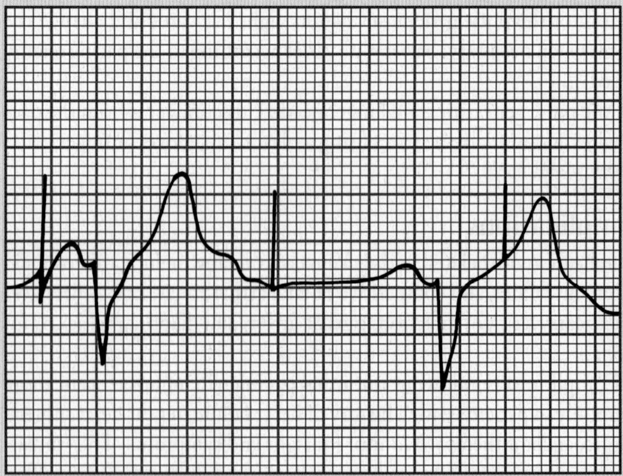

Nursing interventions

- If the pacing is undersensing, increase the sensitivity by turning down the voltage, usually to 2 to 5 millivolts (mV). If it's oversensing, decrease the sensitivity by turning up the voltage to 5 mV or higher.
- Change the battery and then the pulse generator.
- Remove items in the room causing electromechanical interference (such as razors, radios, and cautery devices). Check the ground wires on the bed and other equipment for obvious damage. Unplug each piece and see if the interference stops. When you locate the cause, notify the staff engineer and ask him to check it.
- If the pacemaker is still firing on the T wave and all else has failed to correct it, attach the patient to a transcutaneous pacemaker, turn off the epicardial pacemaker, and notify the practitioner.

13 The Joint Commission. (2015). Standard UP.01.03.01. *Comprehensive accreditation manual for hospitals: The official handbook.* Oakbrook Terrace, IL: The Joint Commission. (Level VII)

14 Lynn-McHale Wiegand, D. (Ed.). (2011). *AACN procedure manual for critical care* (6th ed.). St. Louis, MO: Saunders.

15 The Joint Commission. (2015). Standard PC.01.02.07. *Comprehensive accreditation manual for hospitals: The official handbook.* Oakbrook Terrace, IL: The Joint Commission. (Level VII)

16 The Joint Commission. (2015). Standard NPSG.02.03.01. *Comprehensive accreditation manual for hospitals: The official handbook.* Oakbrook Terrace, IL: The Joint Commission. (Level VII)

17 Mullin, M. H., et al. (2009). Sensations during removal of epicardial pacing wires after coronary artery bypass graft surgery. *Heart & Lung, 38,* 377–381. (Level VI)

18 Graham, K. C., & Cvach, M. (2010). Monitor alarm fatigue: Standardizing use of physiological monitors and decreasing nuisance alarms. *American Journal of Critical Care, 19,* 28–37.

19 American Association of Critical-Care Nurses. (2013). "AACN practice alert: Alarm management" [Online]. Accessed March 2015 via the Web at http://www.aacn.org/wd/practice/docs/practicealerts/alarm-management-practice-alert.pdf (Level VII)

20 The Joint Commission. (2015). Standard NPSG.06.01.01. *Comprehensive accreditation manual for hospitals: The official handbook.* Oakbrook Terrace, IL: The Joint Commission. (Level VII)

21 The Joint Commission. (2013). "Sentinel event alert: Medical device alarm safety in hospitals" [Online]. Accessed March 2015 via the Web at http://www.jointcommission.org/assets/1/18/SEA_50_alarms_4_5_13_FINAL1.PDF (Level VII)

22 Centers for Medicare & Medicaid Services, Department of Health and Human Services. (2014). Condition of participation: Nursing services. 42 C.F.R. § 482.23(c).

23 American Osteopathic Association. (2014). Standard 16.01.03. *Healthcare Facilities Accreditation Program: Accreditation requirements for acute care hospitals.* Chicago, IL: American Osteopathic Association. (Level VII)

24 Siegel, J. D., et al. (2007). "2007 guideline for isolation precautions: Preventing transmission of infectious agents in healthcare settings" [Online]. Accessed March 2015 via the Web at http://www.cdc.gov/hicpac/pdf/isolation/Isolation2007.pdf (Level II)

25 American Osteopathic Association. (2014). Standard 07.01.10. *Healthcare Facilities Accreditation Program: Accreditation requirements for acute care hospitals.* Chicago, IL: American Osteopathic Association. (Level VII)

26 Occupational Safety and Health Administration. (n.d.). "Bloodborne pathogens, standard number 1910.1030" [Online]. Accessed March 2015 via the Web at http://www.osha.gov/pls/oshaweb/owadisp.show_document?p_table=STANDARDS&p_id=10051 (Level VII)

27 Rutala, W. A., et al. (2008). "Guideline for disinfection and sterilization in healthcare facilities, 2008" [Online]. Accessed March 2015 via the Web at http://www.cdc.gov/hicpac/pdf/guidelines/Disinfection_Nov_2008.pdf (Level I)

28 American Osteopathic Association. (2014). Standard 07.02.03. *Healthcare Facilities Accreditation Program: Accreditation requirements for acute care hospitals.* Chicago, IL: American Osteopathic Association. (Level VII)

EPIDURAL ANALGESIC ADMINISTRATION

In epidural analgesic administration, the practitioner or specially trained nurse injects or infuses medication into the epidural space, which lies just outside the subarachnoid space where cerebrospinal fluid (CSF) flows. The drug diffuses slowly into the subarachnoid space of the spinal canal and then into the CSF, which carries it directly into the spinal area, bypassing the blood-brain barrier. In some cases, medication is injected directly into the subarachnoid space. (See *Understanding intrathecal injections.*)

Epidural analgesia helps manage acute or chronic pain, including moderate to severe postoperative pain. It's especially useful in patients with cancer or degenerative joint disease. This procedure works well because opioid receptors are located along the entire spinal cord. Opioid drugs act directly on the receptors of the dorsal horn to produce localized analgesia without motor blockage. Such opioids as preservative-free morphine, fentanyl, and hydromorphone are administered as a bolus dose or by continuous infusion, either alone or in combination with a local anesthetic. Infusion through an epidural catheter is preferred because it allows a smaller drug dosage to be given continuously. The epidural catheter, inserted into the epidural space, eliminates the risks of multiple IM injections, minimizes adverse cerebral and systemic effects, and eliminates the analgesic peaks and valleys that usually occur with intermittent IM injections. The American Society of Anesthesiologists recommends the use of epidural opioids ordered on an "as needed" basis. However, the risks and benefits should be carefully considered. (See *Placement of an epidural catheter,* page 296.)[1,2]

Typically, epidural catheter insertion is performed by an anesthesia practitioner using sterile technique. Once the catheter has been inserted, the nurse is responsible for monitoring the infusion and assessing the patient.[2]

Epidural analgesia is contraindicated in patients who have local or systemic infection, neurologic disease, coagulopathy, spinal arthritis or deformity, hypotension, marked hypertension, or an allergy to the prescribed drug as well as in those who are undergoing anticoagulant therapy.

Understanding intrathecal injections

An intrathecal injection allows the practitioner to inject medication into the subarachnoid space of the spinal canal. Certain drugs, such as anti-infectives or antineoplastics used to treat meningeal leukemia, are administered by this route *because they can't readily penetrate the blood-brain barrier through the bloodstream.* Intrathecal injection may also be used to deliver anesthetics such as lidocaine hydrochloride, to achieve regional anesthesia (as in spinal anesthesia), and for pain-management with such medications as preservative-free morphine.

An invasive procedure performed by a practitioner under sterile conditions with a nurse assisting, intrathecal injection requires informed consent. The injection site is usually between the third and fourth (or fourth and fifth) lumbar vertebrae, well below the spinal cord, *to avoid the risk of paralysis.* This procedure may be preceded by aspiration of spinal fluid for laboratory analysis.

Contraindications to intrathecal injection include inflammation or infection at the puncture site, septicemia, and spinal deformities (especially when considered as an anesthesia route).

Equipment

Epidural infusion pump with anti–free-flow protection ▪ epidural infusion tubing containing a 0.2 micron, surfactant-free, particulate-retentive filter[3] ▪ prescribed epidural solutions (preservative-free)[2,3] ▪ sterile transparent semipermeable dressing ▪ sterile tape measure ▪ sterile tape ▪ epidural tray ▪ label ▪ EPIDURAL INFUSION labels ▪ povidone-iodine solution ▪ tape ▪ sterile gloves ▪ gloves ▪ mask ▪ monitoring equipment for blood pressure, pulse, and temperature ▪ disinfectant pad ▪ emergency equipment (oxygen, intubation equipment, handheld resuscitation bag with mask, 0.4 mg of IV naloxone) ▪ Optional: chlorhexidine-impregnated sponge dressing, capnography monitor.

Preparation of equipment

Prepare the infusion device according to the manufacturer's instructions. Obtain an epidural tray. Make sure the pharmacy has been notified ahead of time about the medication order *because epidural solutions require special preparation.* Make sure that emergency equipment and drugs are readily available.

EQUIPMENT

Placement of an epidural catheter

An epidural catheter is implanted beneath the patient's skin and inserted near the spinal cord at the first lumbar (L1) interspace.

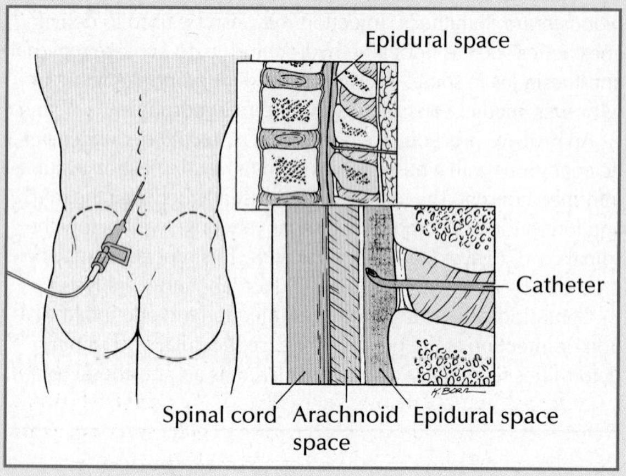

Implementation

- Avoid distractions and interruptions when preparing and administering the medication *to prevent medication errors.*[4,5]
- Verify the order on the patient's medical record by checking it against the practitioner's order.[6,7,8]
- Make sure that a consent form has been signed and is in the patient's medical record.[9,10,11]
- Conduct a preprocedure *verification to make sure that all relevant documentation, related information, and equipment are available and correctly identified to the patient's identifiers.*[12,13]
- Gather and prepare the medication and the appropriate equipment.
- Compare the medication label with the order in the patient's medical record.[6,7,8]
- Check the patient's medical record for an allergy or a contraindication to the prescribed medication. If an allergy or a contraindication exists, don't administer the medication; instead, notify the practitioner.[6,7,8]
- Check the expiration date on the medication. If the medication is expired, return it to the pharmacy and obtain new medication.[6,7,8]
- Visually inspect the solution for particulates, discoloration, and other signs of loss of integrity; don't administer the medication if its integrity is compromised.[6,7,8]
- Discuss any unresolved concerns about the medication with the patient's practitioner.[6,7,8]
- Perform hand hygiene.[14,15,16,17,18,19]
- Confirm the patient's identity using at least two patient identifiers.[20]
- If the patient is receiving the medication for the first time, teach him about potential adverse reactions and discuss any other concerns related to the medication.[6,7,8]
- Perform a comprehensive pain assessment using techniques appropriate for the patient's age, condition, and ability to understand.[21]
- Reinforce the practitioner's explanation of the procedure and its possible complications. Tell the patient that he'll feel some pain as the catheter is inserted. Answer any questions he has.
- Put on gloves and a mask.[22,23,24]
- Position the patient on his side in the knee-chest position, or have him sit on the edge of the bed and lean over a bedside table while the catheter is being inserted *to facilitate insertion.*[25]
- The anesthesia practitioner conducts a time-out immediately before starting the procedure *to perform a final assessment that the correct patient, site, position, and procedure are identified and, as applicable, that all relevant information and necessary equipment are available.*[26]
- After the catheter is in place, prime the infusion device with the prescribed epidural solution, confirm the appropriate medication and infusion rate, and then adjust the device for the correct rate.

NURSING ALERT ***Don't use preparations containing alcohol or acetone for preparing the site or disinfecting the catheter hub;* these agents can cause neurotoxic effects.**[3]

- If your facility uses a bar code scanning system, scan your identification badge, the patient's identification bracelet, and the medication's bar code.
- After the anesthesia practitioner aspirates the device to make sure that neither CSF nor blood is present, help to connect the infusion tubing to the epidural catheter. Trace the tubing from the patient to its point of origin *to make sure it's connected to the proper port* before beginning the infusion.[27] Then connect the tubing to the infusion pump.
- Bridge-tape all connection sites.
- Apply an EPIDURAL INFUSION label to the catheter, infusion tubing, and infusion pump *to prevent accidental infusion of other drugs.*[3]

NURSING ALERT ***Epidural medications are considered "high-alert" medications* because they can cause significant patient harm when used in error.**[28,29]

- If required by your facility, before beginning an epidural infusion, have another nurse perform an independent double-check to verify the patient's identity and to make sure that the correct medication is hanging in the prescribed concentration, the medication's indication corresponds with the patient's diagnosis, the dosage calculations are correct and the dosing formula used to derive the final dose is correct, the route of administration is safe and proper for the patient, the pump settings are correct, and the infusion line is attached to the correct port *to help prevent medication errors.*
- Compare the results of the independent double-check. If no discrepancies exist, move forward with medication administration. If discrepancies exist, rectify them before administering the medication.[29] Then start the infusion.
- Make sure the infusion pump alarm limits are set according to the patient's current condition and that the alarms are turned on, functioning properly, and audible to staff.[30,31,32]
- Lock the keypad on the pump *to prevent inadvertent infusion rate changes.*
- Remove and discard your gloves,[23,33] perform hand hygiene,[14,15,16,17,18,19] and put on sterile gloves.[23,34]
- Measure the external catheter length with a tape measure *to serve as a baseline for comparison to assess for catheter migration.*[34]
- Clean the insertion site with povidone-iodine solution, and then allow it to dry completely.[34]
- Place a chlorhexidine-impregnated sponge dressing around the insertion site if indicated *to reduce the risk of central nervous system infection.*[3,34]
- Secure the catheter to the skin with sterile tape, as needed.
- Place a transparent semipermeable dressing over the chlorhexidine-impregnated sponge dressing, if used; center the transparent dressing over the catheter insertion site.[34]
- Label the dressing with the date, the time, and your initials.[34]
- Discard all used supplies in the appropriate receptacles.[33]
- Remove and discard your mask and gloves.[23,33]
- Perform hand hygiene.[14,15,16,18,19]
- Tell the patient to report any pain immediately. Instruct him to use a pain scale from 0 to 10, with 0 denoting no pain and 10 denoting the worst pain imaginable. A response of 3 or less typically indicates tolerable pain. If the patient reports a higher pain score, the infusion rate may need to be increased. If the patient is unable to use a numerical pain scale, use

an assessment tool that's appropriate for the patient.[3,21] Call the practitioner or change the rate within prescribed limits.

■ Assess the following patient parameters hourly for the first 24 hours and then every 4 hours thereafter: vital signs, sedation level (if an opioid is being administered), pain status, adverse reactions (such as pruritus, nausea, urinary retention, orthostatic hypotension, and motor block), catheter and administration set connections, dressing intactness, signs and symptoms of infection (such as back pain, tenderness, erythema, swelling, drainage, fever, malaise, neck stiffness, progressive numbness, and motor block), sensory and motor function, changes that may indicate epidural hematoma (such as back or leg pain, bowel or bladder dysfunction, and motor block), analgesic use (including bolus doses needed), and accurate administration parameters.[3]

■ Notify the practitioner of inadequate pain relief and any adverse reactions.

■ Perform hand hygiene.[14,15,16,17,18,19]

■ Clean and disinfect your stethoscope with a disinfectant pad.[35,36]

■ Perform hand hygiene.[14,15,16,17,18,19]

■ Document the procedure.[37,38,39]

Special considerations

■ If ordered, monitor oxygen saturation levels with a pulse oximeter and carbon dioxide levels with a capnography monitor for the first 24 hours after beginning the infusion *because continuous infusions can cause drug accumulation that may produce adverse effects.*[1,3]

■ Routinely assess for catheter migration by measuring external catheter length; *catheter migration may cause inadequate pain control or an increase in adverse effects.*[1,3]

■ Note that routine dressing changes on short-term catheters aren't recommended *because of the risk of dislodgement and infection.* Semipermeable transparent dressings are commonly used for tunneled and implanted epidural catheters and should be changed every 7 days.[3]

■ Note that a change in sedation level (the patient becoming somnolent) is an early indicator of the respiratory depressant effects of an opioid. Respiratory depression usually occurs during the first 24 hours and is treated with IV naloxone. Nausea, vomiting, and pruritus may be treated with low-dose IV naloxone.

■ If sensorimotor loss occurs (numbness and leg weakness), large motor nerve fibers have been affected and dosage may need to be decreased. Notify the practitioner *because he may need to titrate the dosage to identify the dose that provides adequate pain control without causing excessive numbness and weakness.*

■ Keep in mind that drugs given epidurally diffuse slowly and may cause adverse effects, including excessive sedation, for up to 12 hours after epidural infusion has been discontinued.

ELDER ALERT ***Elderly patients may respond differently than younger patients to pain and analgesic medications* because of comorbidities.**[1]

■ Ensure that the patient always has a peripheral IV catheter (either continuous infusion or saline lock) *to allow immediate administration of emergency drugs.*[25]

■ Be aware that postdural puncture headache may result from accidental puncture of the dura mater during an attempted epidural insertion. The anesthesia practitioner will stop the procedure and may attempt the epidural again at a different lumbar interspace. If CSF leaks into the dura mater at the initial puncture site, the patient usually experiences a headache. This postanalgesia headache worsens with postural changes, such as standing or sitting. The headache can be treated with a blood patch, in which the patient's own blood (about 10 mL) is withdrawn from a peripheral vein and then injected into the epidural space. When the epidural needle is withdrawn, the patient is instructed to sit up. *Because the blood clots seal off the leaking area,* the blood patch should relieve the patient's headache immediately. The patient need not restrict his activity after this procedure.

■ Typically, the anesthesia practitioner orders analgesics and removes the catheter. However, your facility may allow a specially trained nurse to remove it.[3] If you feel resistance when removing the catheter, stop and call the practitioner for further orders. Be sure to save the catheter. *The practitioner will want to examine the catheter tip to rule out any damage during removal.*

■ Note that The Joint Commission has issued a sentinel event alert concerning medical device alarm safety *because alarm-related events have been associated with permanent loss of function and death.* Among the major contributing factors are improper alarm settings, inappropriately turned off alarms, and alarm signals that were not audible to staff. Make sure alarm limits are appropriately set and that alarms are turned on, functioning properly, and audible to staff. Follow facility guidelines for preventing alarm fatigue.[31]

■ Catheter migration occurs when the epidural catheter migrates out of the epidural space toward the skin. If migration occurs, the patient will have decreased pain relief and leakage at the catheter site. Notify the practitioner *because the infusion needs to be stopped and the catheter removed.* Contact the practitioner for further pain-management orders. The catheter can also migrate through the dura mater into the subarachnoid space; if the epidural dose is too high for the smaller subarachnoid space, the dose may eventually be toxic in high concentrations (the patient may show signs of increasing somnolence and, eventually, a decrease in respirations). Assess the patient and notify the practitioner immediately if these signs occur. The infusion needs to be stopped, the catheter must be removed, and the patient may need to be treated with IV naloxone and oxygen therapy.

Patient teaching

Home use of epidural analgesia is possible only if the patient or a family member is willing and able to learn the care needed. The patient also must be willing and able to abstain from alcohol and illegal drugs *because these substances potentiate opioid action.*

Complications

Potential complications of epidural analgesic administration include adverse reactions from opioids or local anesthetics and catheter-related problems, such as infection, epidural hematoma, and catheter migration. Postdural headache may occur if the practitioner accidently punctures the dura mater during catheter insertion.

Documentation

Document the infusion device type and gauge, the external catheter length, specific site preparation, infection prevention and safety precautions taken, the drug dose, and the rate of infusion. Record the patient's response to treatment, catheter patency, the condition of the dressing and insertion site, vital signs, and assessment results. Also document labeling of the epidural catheter, changing of the infusion bags, and the patient's response.

REFERENCES

1 American Society of Anesthesiologists Task Force on Acute Pain Management. (2012). Practice guidelines for acute pain management in the perioperative setting: An updated report by the American Society of Anesthesiologists Task Force on Acute Pain Management. *Anesthesiology, 116,* 248–273. (Level VII)

2 Pasero, C., et al. (2007). Registered nurse management and monitoring of analgesia by catheter techniques: Position statement. *Pain Management Nursing, 8,* 48–54. Accessed March 2015 via the Web at http://www.aspmn.org/Organization/documents/RegisteredNurseManagementandMonitoringofAnalgesiaByCatheterTechniquesPMNversion.pdf (Level VII)

3 Standard 58. Intraspinal access devices. Infusion nursing standards of practice. (2011). *Journal of Infusion Nursing, 34,* S81–S82. (Level VII)

4 Westbrook, J., et al. (2010). Association of interruptions with an increased risk and severity of medication administration errors. *Archives of Internal Medicine, 170,* 683–690. (Level IV)

5 Institute for Safe Medication Practices. (2013). Side tracks on the safety express: Interruptions lead to errors and unfinished... Wait, what was I doing? *Nurse Advise-ERR, 11*(2), 1–4. Accessed March 2015 via the Web at https://www.ismp.org/Newsletters/acutecare/showarticle.aspx?id=37 (Level VII)

6 The Joint Commission. (2015). Standard MM.06.01.01. *Comprehensive accreditation manual for hospitals: The official handbook.* Oakbrook Terrace, IL: The Joint Commission. (Level VII)

7 Centers for Medicare & Medicaid Services, Department of Health and Human Services. (2014). Condition of participation: Nursing services. 42 C.F.R. § 482.23(c).

8 American Osteopathic Association. (2014). Standard 16.01.03. *Healthcare Facilities Accreditation Program: Accreditation requirements for acute care hospitals.* Chicago, IL: American Osteopathic Association. (Level VII)

9 American Osteopathic Association. (2014). Standard 15.01.11. *Healthcare Facilities Accreditation Program: Accreditation requirements for acute care hospitals.* Chicago, IL: American Osteopathic Association. (Level VII)

10 The Joint Commission. (2015). Standard RI.01.03.01. *Comprehensive accreditation manual for hospitals: The official handbook.* Oakbrook Terrace, IL: The Joint Commission. (Level VII)

11 Centers for Medicare & Medicaid Services, Department of Health and Human Services. (2014). Condition of participation: Patient's rights. 42 C.F.R. § 482.13 (b)(2).

12 The Joint Commission. (2015). Standard UP.01.01.01. *Comprehensive accreditation manual for hospitals: The official handbook.* Oakbrook Terrace, IL: The Joint Commission. (Level VII)

13 American Osteopathic Association. (2014). Standard 30.00.14. *Healthcare Facilities Accreditation Program: Accreditation requirements for acute care hospitals.* Chicago, IL: American Osteopathic Association. (Level VII)

14 The Joint Commission. (2015). Standard NPSG.07.01.01. *Comprehensive accreditation manual for hospitals: The official handbook.* Oakbrook Terrace, IL: The Joint Commission. (Level VII)

15 Centers for Disease Control and Prevention. (2002). Guideline for hand hygiene in health-care settings: Recommendations of the Healthcare Infection Control Practices Advisory Committee and the HICPAC/SHEA/APIC/IDSA Hand Hygiene Task Force. *MMWR Recommendations and Reports, 51*(RR-16), 1–45. Accessed March 2015 via the Web at http://www.cdc.gov/mmwr/pdf/rr/rr5116.pdf (Level II)

16 World Health Organization. (2009). "WHO guidelines on hand hygiene in health care: First global patient safety challenge, clean care is safer care" [Online]. Accessed March 2015 via the Web at http://whqlibdoc.who.int/publications/2009/9789241597906_eng.pdf (Level IV)

17 Standard 19. Hand hygiene. Infusion nursing standards of practice. (2011). *Journal of Infusion Nursing, 34,* S26–S27. (Level VII)

18 American Osteopathic Association. (2014). Standard 07.01.21. *Healthcare Facilities Accreditation Program: Accreditation requirements for acute care hospitals.* Chicago, IL: American Osteopathic Association. (Level VII)

19 Centers for Medicare & Medicaid Services, Department of Health and Human Services. (2014). Condition of participation: Infection control. 42 C.F.R. § 482.42.

20 The Joint Commission. (2015). Standard NPSG.01.01.01. *Comprehensive accreditation manual for hospitals: The official handbook.* Oakbrook Terrace, IL: The Joint Commission. (Level VII)

21 The Joint Commission. (2015). Standard PC.01.02.07. *Comprehensive accreditation manual for hospitals: The official handbook.* Oakbrook Terrace, IL: The Joint Commission. (Level VII)

22 Siegel, J. D., et al. (2007). "2007 guideline for isolation precautions: Preventing transmission of infectious agents in healthcare settings" [Online]. Accessed March 2015 via the Web at http://www.cdc.gov/hicpac/pdf/isolation/Isolation2007.pdf (Level II)

23 Standard 18. Infection prevention. Infusion nursing standards of practice. (2011). *Journal of Infusion Nursing, 34,* S25–S26. (Level VII)

24 American Osteopathic Association. (2014). Standard 07.01.10. *Healthcare Facilities Accreditation Program: Accreditation requirements for acute care hospitals.* Chicago, IL: American Osteopathic Association. (Level VII)

25 Lynn-McHale Wiegand, D. (Ed.). (2011). *AACN procedure manual for critical care* (6th ed.). St. Louis, MO: Saunders.

26 The Joint Commission. (2015). Standard UP.01.03.01. *Comprehensive accreditation manual for hospitals: The official handbook.* Oakbrook Terrace, IL: The Joint Commission. (Level VII)

27 U.S. Food and Drug Administration. (n.d.). "Look. Check. Connect. Safe medical device connections save lives" [Online]. Accessed March 2015 via the Web at http://www.fda.gov/downloads/MedicalDevices/Safety/AlertsandNotices/UCM134873.pdf

28 Institute for Safe Medication Practices. (2012). "ISMP's list of high-alert medications" [Online]. Accessed March 2015 via the Web at http://www.ismp.org/tools/highalertmedications.pdf (Level VII)

29 Institute for Safe Medication Practices. (2008). Conducting an independent double-check. *ISMP Medication Safety Alert! Nurse Advise-ERR, 6*(12), 1. Accessed March 2015 via the Web at http://www.ismp.org/newsletters/nursing/Issues/NurseAdviseERR200812.pdf

30 Graham, K. C., & Cvach, M. (2010). Monitor alarm fatigue: Standardizing use of physiological monitors and decreasing nuisance alarms. *American Journal of Critical Care, 19,* 28–37.

31 The Joint Commission. (2013). "Sentinel event alert: Medical device alarm safety in hospitals" [Online]. Accessed March 2015 via the Web at http://www.jointcommission.org/assets/1/18/SEA_50_alarms_4_5_13_FINAL1.PDF (Level VII)

32 The Joint Commission. (2015). Standard NPSG.06.01.01. *Comprehensive accreditation manual for hospitals: The official handbook.* Oakbrook Terrace, IL: The Joint Commission. (Level VII)

33 Occupational Safety and Health Administration. (n.d.). "Bloodborne pathogens, standard number 1910.1030" [Online]. Accessed March 2015 via the Web at http://www.osha.gov/pls/oshaweb/owadisp.show_document?p_table=STANDARDS&p_id=10051 (Level VII)

34 Infusion Nurses Society. (2011). *Policies and procedures for infusion nursing* (4th ed.). Boston, MA: Infusion Nurses Society.

35 American Osteopathic Association. (2014). Standard 07.02.03. *Healthcare Facilities Accreditation Program: Accreditation requirements for acute care hospitals.* Chicago, IL: American Osteopathic Association. (Level VII)

36 Rutala, W. A., et al. (2008). "Guideline for disinfection and sterilization in healthcare facilities, 2008" [Online]. Accessed March 2015 via the Web at http://www.cdc.gov/hicpac/pdf/guidelines/Disinfection_Nov_2008.pdf (Level I)

37 The Joint Commission. (2015). Standard RC.01.03.01. *Comprehensive accreditation manual for hospitals: The official handbook.* Oakbrook Terrace, IL: The Joint Commission. (Level VII)

38 Centers for Medicare & Medicaid Services, Department of Health and Human Services. (2014). Condition of participation: Medical record services. 42 C.F.R. § 482.24(b).

39 American Osteopathic Association. (2014). Standard 10.00.03. *Healthcare Facilities Accreditation Program: Accreditation requirements for acute care hospitals.* Chicago, IL: American Osteopathic Association. (Level VII)

ADDITIONAL REFERENCES

Gramigni, E., et al. (2013). Epidural analgesia and postoperative orthostatic haemodynamic changes: Observational study. *European Journal of Anaesthesiology, 30,* 398–404. (Level VI)

Sawhney, M. (2012). Epidural analgesia: What nurses need to know. *Nursing, 42*(8), 36–41. Accessed May 2015 via the Web at http://www.nursingcenter.com/lnc/pdf?AID=1403661&an=00152193-201208000-00015&Journal_ID=54016&Issue_ID=1403510

Verduzco, L. A., et al. (2012). Subdural hematoma after an epidural blood patch. *International Journal of Obstetric Anesthesia, 21,* 189–192.

ESOPHAGOGASTRIC TAMPONADE TUBE CARE

Used to control hemorrhage from esophageal or gastric varices, an esophagogastric tamponade tube is inserted nasally or orally and advanced into the esophagus or stomach. (See *Types of esophagogastric tamponade tubes.*)

Although the practitioner inserts an esophagogastric tamponade tube, the nurse cares for the patient during and after intubation. Typically, the

EQUIPMENT

Types of esophagogastric tamponade tubes

When working with a patient who has an esophagogastric tamponade tube, remember the advantages of the most common types.

Blakemore-Sengstaken tube

A Blakemore-Sengstaken tube is a triple-lumen, double-balloon tube that has a gastric aspiration port, which allows you to obtain drainage from below the gastric balloon and also to instill medication.

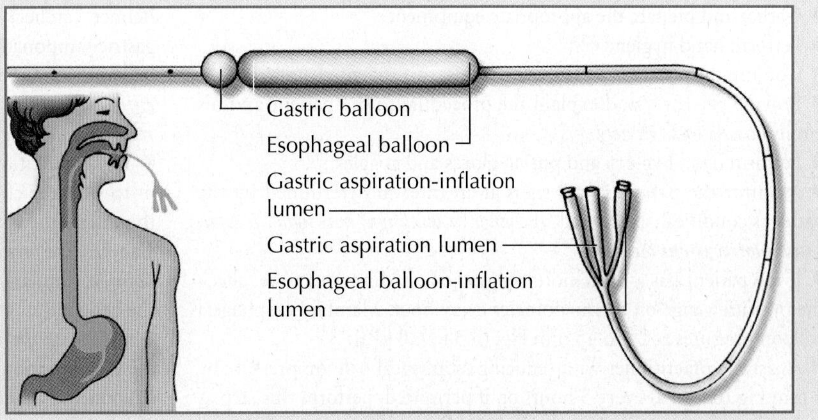

Linton tube

A Linton tube is a triple-lumen, single-balloon tube that has a port for gastric aspiration and one for esophageal aspiration. The Linton tube reduces the risk of esophageal necrosis *because it doesn't have an esophageal balloon.*

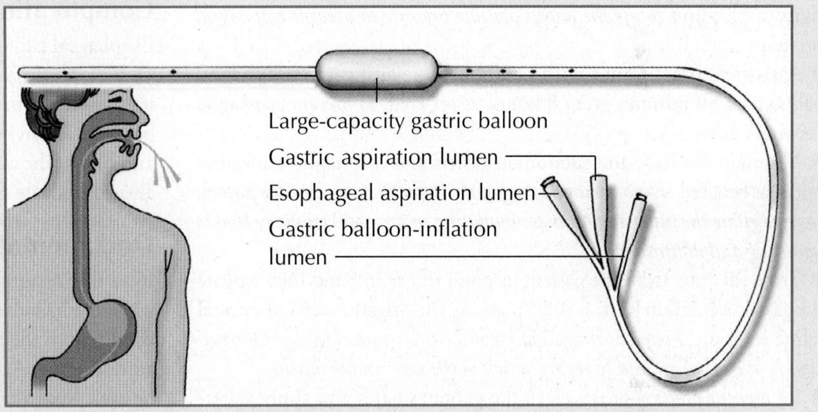

Minnesota esophagogastric tamponade tube

A Minnesota esophagogastric tamponade tube is an esophageal tube that has four lumens and two balloons. The device provides pressure-monitoring ports for both balloons without the need for Y-connectors. One port is used for gastric suction, the other for esophageal suction.

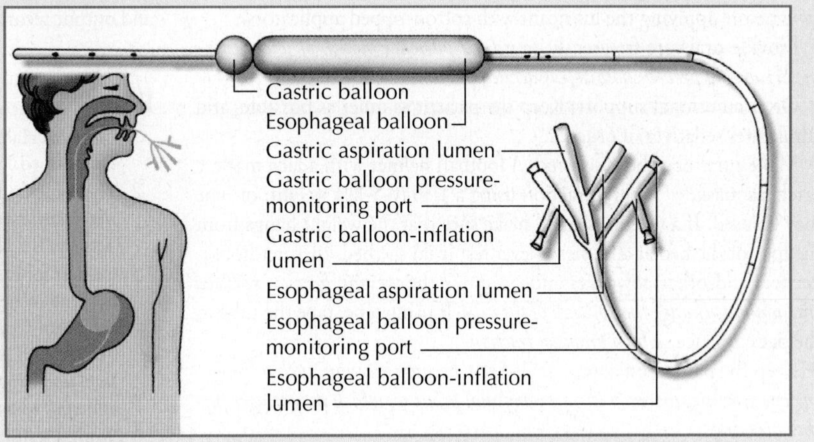

patient with an esophagogastric tamponade tube is on the intensive care unit for close observation and constant care. The patient may receive sedatives, but the dose should be individualized, especially for the patient with probable liver injury.[1] With the increasing use of endoscopic procedures to help control bleeding, the use of esophagogastric tamponade tubes is decreasing.

A patient who has an esophagogastric tamponade tube in place to control variceal bleeding (typically from portal hypertension) must be observed closely for possible esophageal rupture because varices weaken the esophagus. Possible traumatic injury from intubation or esophageal balloon inflation also increases the chance of rupture. Usually, emergency surgery is performed if a rupture occurs; the operation has a low success rate.

Equipment

Blood pressure monitoring equipment ▪ stethoscope ▪ disinfectant pad ▪ manometer ▪ normal saline solution ▪ irrigation set ▪ water-soluble lubricant ▪ several cotton-tipped applicators ▪ oral care equipment (see the "Oral care" procedure, page 560) ▪ suction equipment ▪ intake-and-output record ▪ gloves ▪ goggles ▪ traction weights, football helmet, catcher's mask, or tape ▪ scissors ▪ Optional: prescribed sedative.

Preparation of equipment

Make sure scissors and suction equipment are present at the patient's bedside; ensure that the suction equipment is functioning properly.

Implementation

- Verify the practitioner's order.
- Gather and prepare the appropriate equipment.
- Perform hand hygiene.[2,3,4,5,6]
- Confirm the patient's identity using at least two patient identifiers.[7]
- Provide privacy[8,9] and explain the procedure to the patient and his family *to ease their anxiety.*
- Perform hand hygiene and put on gloves and goggles.[10,11]
- Monitor the patient's vital signs at an interval determined by the patient's condition, as ordered. *A change in vital signs may signal complications or recurrent bleeding.*
- If the patient has a Blakemore-Sengstaken or Minnesota tube, check the pressure gauge on the manometer every hour. Maintain esophageal balloon pressures at 25 to 45 mm Hg. (3.3 to 6.0 kPa).[1]
- Assist the practitioner with reducing esophageal balloon pressure by 5 mm Hg (0.7 kPa) every 3 hours or, if permitted, perform this step as ordered until pressure is 25 mm Hg (3.3 kPa) and the patient shows no signs of bleeding *to use the lowest possible pressure to prevent esophageal necrosis.*[1]
- Assist the practitioner with completely deflating the esophageal balloon for 30 minutes every 8 hours, as ordered, *to prevent esophageal necrosis.*[1]
- Maintain drainage and suction on gastric and esophageal aspiration ports, as ordered. *Fluid accumulating in the stomach may cause the patient to regurgitate the tube, and fluid accumulating in the esophagus may lead to vomiting and aspiration.*
- Trace the tube from the patient its point of origin[12] and then irrigate the gastric aspiration port, as ordered, using the irrigation set and normal saline solution. *Frequent irrigation keeps the tube from clogging. Obstruction in the tube can lead to regurgitation of the tube and vomiting.*
- *To prevent pressure ulcers,* clean the patient's nares and apply water-soluble lubricant frequently. Use warm water *to loosen crusted nasal secretions* before applying the lubricant with cotton-tipped applicators.
- Provide oral care frequently *to rid the patient's mouth of foul-tasting matter and to prevent hospital-associated pneumonia.*[13]
- Offer emotional support. Keep the patient as quiet as possible, and administer sedatives, if ordered.
- Make sure the tube is secured. A football helmet with a face mask, a catcher's mask,[14,15] gentle traction using a 1-lb (0.5-kg) weight, or tape may be used. If a weight is used, make sure that the weight hangs from the foot of the bed at all times. Never rest it on the bed. Instruct housekeepers and other coworkers not to move the weight *because reduced traction may change the position of the tube.* If using tape, tape the tube to the patient's face, *which provides traction.*
- Keep the patient on complete bed rest *because exertion, such as coughing or straining, increases intra-abdominal pressure, which may trigger further bleeding.*
- Observe the patient carefully for esophageal rupture, indicated by signs and symptoms of shock, increased respiratory difficulties, and increased bleeding.
- Keep the head of the patient's bed elevated 30 to 45 degrees *to minimize aspiration and to prevent ventilator-associated pneumonia if the patient is intubated.*[1,16]
- Monitor intake and output, as ordered.
- Remove and discard your gloves and goggles.[10,11]
- Perform hand hygiene.[2,3,4]
- Clean and disinfect your stethoscope with a disinfectant pad.[17,18]
- Perform hand hygiene.[2,3,4]
- Document the procedure.[19,20,21]

Special considerations

- Keep scissors at the bedside *so you can cut the tube quickly to deflate the balloons if asphyxia develops.* When performing this emergency intervention, hold the tube firmly close to the nostril before cutting.[1]
- If you're using traction, be sure to release the tension before deflating any balloons. If a weight is being used, remove the weight. If a football helmet, catcher's mask, or tape supplies traction, untape the esophagogastric tamponade tube from the face guard or face before deflating the balloons. *Deflating the balloon under tension triggers a rapid release of the entire tube from the nose, which may injure mucous membranes, initiate recurrent bleeding, and obstruct the airway.*
- If the practitioner orders an X-ray study to check the tube's position or to view the chest, lift the patient in the direction of the pulley, and then place the X-ray film behind his back. Never roll him from side to side *because pressure exerted on the tube in this way may shift the tube's position.* Similarly, lift the patient to make the bed or to assist him with the bedpan.
- *To reduce the risk of necrosis and ulceration,* the maximum recommended duration for tamponade therapy is 36 hours for the esophageal balloon and 72 hours for the gastric balloon.[1]

Complications

Esophageal rupture, the most life-threatening complication associated with esophagogastric tamponade tube use, can occur at any time, but it's most likely to occur during intubation or inflation of the esophageal balloon. Asphyxia may result if the balloon moves up the esophagus and blocks the airway. Aspiration of pooled esophageal secretions may also complicate this procedure.

Documentation

Read the manometer hourly, and record the esophageal pressures. Note when the balloons are deflated and by whom. Document vital signs, the condition of the patient's nostrils, routine care provided, and any drugs administered. Also note the color, consistency, and amount of gastric returns. Record any signs and symptoms of complications and nursing actions taken. Document gastric port irrigations. Maintain accurate intake and output records.

REFERENCES

1 Lynn-McHale Wiegand, D. (Ed.). *AACN procedure manual for critical care* (6th ed.). Philadelphia, PA: Saunders.

2 The Joint Commission. (2015). Standard NPSG.07.01.01. *Comprehensive accreditation manual for hospitals: The official handbook.* Oakbrook Terrace, IL: The Joint Commission. (Level VII)

3 Centers for Disease Control and Prevention. (2002). Guideline for hand hygiene in health-care settings: Recommendations of the Healthcare Infection Control Practices Advisory Committee and the HICPAC/SHEA/APIC/IDSA Hand Hygiene Task Force. *MMWR Recommendations and Reports, 51*(RR-16), 1–45. Accessed March 2015 via the Web at http://www.cdc.gov/mmwr/pdf/rr/rr5116.pdf (Level II)

4 World Health Organization. (2009). "WHO guidelines on hand hygiene in health care: First global patient safety challenge, clean care is safer care" [Online]. Accessed March 2015 via the Web at http://whqlibdoc.who.int/publications/2009/9789241597906_eng.pdf (Level IV)

5 American Osteopathic Association. (2014). Standard 07.01.21. *Healthcare Facilities Accreditation Program: Accreditation requirements for acute care hospitals.* Chicago, IL: American Osteopathic Association. (Level VII)

6 Centers for Medicare & Medicaid Services, Department of Health and Human Services. (2014). Condition of participation: Infection control. 42 C.F.R. § 482.42.

7 The Joint Commission. (2015). Standard NPSG.01.01.01. *Comprehensive accreditation manual for hospitals: The official handbook.* Oakbrook Terrace, IL: The Joint Commission. (Level VII)

8 American Osteopathic Association. (2014). Standard 15.01.16. *Healthcare Facilities Accreditation Program: Accreditation requirements for acute care hospitals.* Chicago, IL: American Osteopathic Association. (Level VII) (Level VII)
9 Centers for Medicare & Medicaid Services, Department of Health and Human Services. (2014). Condition of participation: Patient's rights. 42 C.F.R. § 482.13(c)(1).
10 Siegel, J. D., et al. (2007). "2007 guideline for isolation precautions: Preventing transmission of infectious agents in healthcare settings" [Online]. Accessed March 2015 via the Web at http://www.cdc.gov/hicpac/pdf/isolation/Isolation2007.pdf (Level II)
11 American Osteopathic Association. (2014). Standard 07.01.10. *Healthcare Facilities Accreditation Program: Accreditation requirements for acute care hospitals.* Chicago, IL: American Osteopathic Association. (Level VII)
12 U.S. Food and Drug Administration. (n.d.). "Look. Check. Connect. Safe medical device connections save lives" [Online]. Accessed March 2015 via the Web at http://www.fda.gov/downloads/MedicalDevices/Safety/AlertsandNotices/UCM134873.pdf
13 American Association of Critical-Care Nurses. (2010). "AACN practice alert: Oral care for patients at risk for ventilator-associated pneumonia" [Online]. Accessed March 2015 via the Web at http://www.aacn.org/WD/Practice/Docs/PracticeAlerts/oral%20care%2004-2010%20final.pdf (Level VII)
14 Kashiwagi, H., et al. (1991). Technique for positioning the Sengstaken-Blakemore tube as comfortably as possible. *Surgery, Gynecology and Obstetrics, 172,* 63.
15 Irwin, R., et al. (2012). *Irwin & Rippe's procedures, techniques and minimally invasive monitoring in intensive care medicine* (5th ed). Philadelphia, PA: Lippincott Williams and Wilkins.
16 American Association of Critical-Care Nurses. (2008). "AACN practice alert: Ventilator-associated pneumonia" [Online]. Accessed March 2015 via the Web at http://www.aacn.org/WD/Practice/Docs/PracticeAlerts/Ventilator%20Associated%20Pneumonia%201-2008.pdf (Level VII)
17 Rutala, W. A., et al. (2008). "Guideline for disinfection and sterilization in healthcare facilities, 2008" [Online]. Accessed March 2015 via the Web at http://www.cdc.gov/hicpac/pdf/guidelines/Disinfection_Nov_2008.pdf (Level I)
18 American Osteopathic Association. (2014). Standard 07.02.03. *Healthcare Facilities Accreditation Program: Accreditation requirements for acute care hospitals.* Chicago, IL: American Osteopathic Association. (Level VII)
19 The Joint Commission. (2015). Standard RC.01.03.01. *Comprehensive accreditation manual for hospitals: The official handbook.* Oakbrook Terrace, IL: The Joint Commission. (Level VII)
20 American Osteopathic Association. (2014). Standard 10.00.03. *Healthcare Facilities Accreditation Program: Accreditation requirements for acute care hospitals.* Chicago, IL: American Osteopathic Association. (Level VII)
21 Centers for Medicare & Medicaid Services, Department of Health and Human Services. (2014). Condition of participation: Medical record services. 42 C.F.R. § 482.24(b).

ESOPHAGOGASTRIC TAMPONADE TUBE INSERTION AND REMOVAL

Used for the temporary control of hemorrhage from esophageal or gastric varices, an esophagogastric tamponade tube is inserted nasally or orally and advanced into the esophagus and stomach. Ordinarily, a practitioner inserts and removes the tube. However, in an emergency situation, a nurse may remove it. With the increase in endoscopy, the use of esophagogastric tamponade tubes is decreasing.

After the tube is inserted, a gastric balloon secured at the end of the tube can be inflated and drawn tightly against the cardia of the stomach. The inflated balloon secures the tube and exerts pressure on the cardia. The pressure, in turn, controls variceal bleeding.

Most tubes also contain an esophageal balloon to control esophageal bleeding. The esophageal balloon should be used to control bleeding for no longer than 36 hours; the gastric balloon, for no longer than 72 hours.[1] Pressure necrosis may develop and cause further hemorrhage or perforation.

Other procedures to control bleeding include irrigation with tepid or iced saline solution, drug therapy with a vasopressor, variceal banding, and transjugular intrahepatic portosystemic shunts. Used with the esophagogastric tamponade tube, these procedures provide effective, temporary control of acute variceal hemorrhage.

Equipment

For insertion

Esophagogastric tamponade tube ▪ two suction sources ▪ irrigation set ▪ normal saline solution ▪ two 60-mL catheter-tipped syringes ▪ water-soluble lubricant ▪ ½″ or 1″ (1.3- or 2.5-cm) adhesive tape ▪ stethoscope ▪ foam nose guard ▪ four rubber-shod clamps (two clamps and two plastic plugs for a Minnesota tube) ▪ traction equipment (football helmet, catcher's mask, or a basic frame with traction rope, pulleys, and a 1-lb [0.5-kg] weight) ▪ manometer ▪ basin of water ▪ scissors ▪ gloves ▪ gown ▪ goggles ▪ waterproof marking pen ▪ blood pressure monitoring equipment ▪ anesthetic spray ▪ Optional: Y-connector tube, nasogastric (NG) tube, cardiac monitor.

For removal

60-mL catheter-tipped syringe ▪ gloves ▪ gown ▪ goggles ▪ sphygmomanometer ▪ supplies for oral care. (See the "Oral care" procedure, page 560.)

Preparation of equipment

For insertion

Keep the traction helmet or mask at the bedside or attach traction equipment to the bed *so that traction is readily available after tube insertion.* Place the suction machines nearby and plug them in. Open the irrigation set and fill the container with normal saline solution. Place all equipment within reach. Place scissors at the bedside.

Test the balloons on the esophagogastric tamponade tube for air leaks by inflating them and submerging them in the basin of water. If no bubbles appear in the water, the balloons are intact. Remove them from the water and deflate them. Clamp the tube lumens *so that the balloons stay deflated during insertion.*

To prepare the Minnesota tube, connect the manometer to the gastric pressure monitoring port. Note the pressure when the balloon fills with 100, 200, 300, 400, and 500 mL of air.

Check the aspiration lumens for patency, and make sure they're labeled according to their purpose. If they aren't identified, label them carefully with the waterproof marking pen.

Implementation

- Verify the practitioner's order.
- Gather and prepare the necessary equipment.
- Perform hand hygiene.[2,3,4,5,6]
- Confirm the patient's identity using at least two patient identifiers.[7]
- Explain the procedure and its purpose to the patient, and provide privacy.[8,9]
- Attach the patient to a cardiac monitor (if not already attached) and assess the patient's cardiac rhythm.[1] (See the "Cardiac monitoring" procedure, page 117.) Set the upper and lower heart rate alarm limits according to the patient's current condition and make sure that alarms are turned on, functioning properly, and audible to staff.[10,11,12] Esophagogastric tamponade tube insertion can cause vagal stimulation and bradycardia.[1]
- Assess the patient's baseline respiratory status.[1]
- Put on gloves, a gown, and goggles to protect yourself from splashing blood.[13,14]
- Assist the patient into the semi-Fowler position. If the patient isn't alert, place him in the left lateral position. *These positions facilitate tube passage into the stomach and help prevent aspiration.*[1]

Securing an esophagogastric tamponade tube with a football helmet

If a basic frame isn't available, you can secure an esophagogastric tamponade tube to a football helmet or a catcher's mask *to reduce the risk of the gastric balloon's slipping down or away from the cardia of the stomach.* Tape the tube to the face guard, as shown below, and fasten the chin strap.

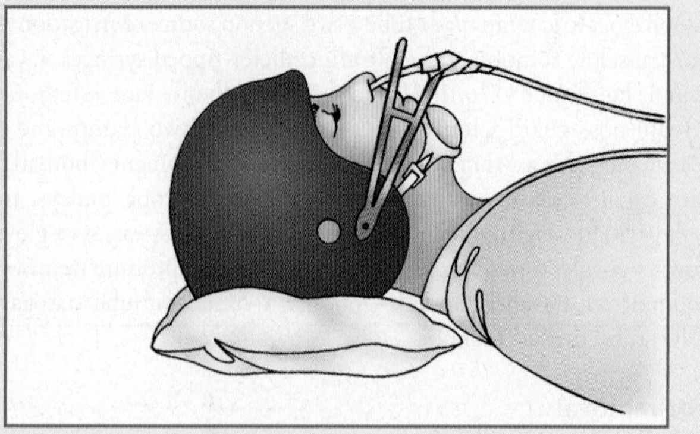

To remove the tube quickly, unfasten the chin strap and pull the helmet slightly forward. Cut the tape and the gastric balloon and esophageal balloon lumens. Be sure to hold onto the tube near the patient's nostril.

For insertion

■ Explain that the practitioner will inspect the patient's nostrils *for patency.*

■ *To determine the length of tubing needed,* hold the balloon at the patient's xiphoid process and then extend the tube to the patient's ear and forward to his nose. Using a waterproof pen, mark this point on the tubing.[1]

■ Inform the patient that the practitioner will spray his throat (posterior pharynx) and nostril with an anesthetic *to minimize discomfort and gagging during intubation.*

■ After lubricating the tip of the tube with water-soluble lubricant *to reduce friction and facilitate insertion,* the practitioner will pass the tube through the more patent nostril. As he does this, he'll direct the patient to tilt his chin toward his chest and to swallow when he senses the tip of the tube in the back of his throat. *Swallowing helps to advance the tube into the esophagus and prevents intubation of the trachea.* (If the practitioner introduces the tube orally, he'll direct the patient to swallow immediately.) As the patient swallows, the practitioner quickly advances the tube at least ½″ (1.3 cm) beyond the previously marked point on the tube.

■ *To confirm tube placement,* the practitioner will aspirate stomach contents through the gastric port. After partially inflating the gastric balloon with 50 to 100 mL of air, he'll order an X-ray of the abdomen *to confirm correct placement of the balloon.*[1] Before fully inflating the balloon, he'll use the 60-mL syringe to irrigate the stomach with normal saline solution and empty the stomach as completely as possible. *This irrigation helps the patient avoid regurgitating gastric contents when the balloon inflates.*

■ After confirming tube placement, the practitioner will fully inflate the gastric balloon (250 to 500 mL of air for a Blakemore-Sengstaken tube, and 700 to 800 mL of air for a Linton tube) and clamp the tube. If he's using a Minnesota tube, he'll connect the pressure-monitoring port for the gastric balloon lumen to the manometer and then inflate the balloon in 100-mL increments until it fills with up to 500 mL of air. As he introduces the air, he'll monitor the intragastric balloon pressure *to make sure the balloon stays inflated.* Then he'll clamp the ports. For the Blakemore-Sengstaken or Minnesota tube, the practitioner will gently pull on the tube until he feels resistance, *which indicates that the gastric balloon is inflated and exerting pressure on the cardia of the stomach.* When he senses that the balloon is engaged, he'll place the foam nose guard around the area where the tube emerges from the nostril.

■ Be ready to tape the nose guard in place around the tube *to help minimize pressure on the nostril from the traction and decrease the risk of necrosis.*[1]

■ With the nose guard secured, apply traction to the tube using the method preferred by the practitioner. Use a traction rope and a 1-lb weight, or pull the tube gently and tape it tightly to the face guard of a football helmet or catcher's mask. (See *Securing an esophagogastric tamponade tube.*) Alternatively, some facilities tape the tube to the side of the patient's face as a method of providing traction, *which helps eliminate any issues that may occur with weights or a helmet.*

■ Lavage the stomach through the gastric aspiration lumen with normal saline solution (iced or tepid) until the return fluid is clear. *The vasoconstriction from the lavage stops the hemorrhage; the lavage empties the stomach. Any blood detected later in the gastric aspirate indicates that bleeding remains uncontrolled.*

■ Attach one of the suction sources to the gastric aspiration lumen *to empty the stomach, help prevent nausea and possible vomiting, and allow continuous observation of the gastric contents for blood.*

■ If the practitioner inserted a Blakemore-Sengstaken or a Minnesota tube, he'll inflate the esophageal balloon as he inflates the gastric balloon *to compress the esophageal varices and control bleeding.*

■ With a Blakemore-Sengstaken tube, the Y-connector tube is attached to the esophageal lumen. Then a sphygmomanometer inflation bulb is attached to one end of the Y-connector and the manometer to the other end. The esophageal balloon is inflated until the pressure gauge ranges from 30 to 40 mm Hg (4.0 to 5.3 kPa) and the tube is clamped.

■ With a Minnesota tube, the manometer is attached directly to the esophageal pressure-monitoring outlet. Then, using the 60-mL syringe and pushing the air slowly into the esophageal balloon port, the balloon is inflated until the pressure gauge ranges from 35 to 45 mm Hg (4.7 to 6.0 kPa).

■ Set up esophageal suction *to prevent accumulation of secretions that may cause vomiting and pulmonary aspiration. This is important because swallowed secretions can't pass into the stomach if the patient has an inflated esophageal balloon in place.* If the patient has a Linton or a Minnesota tube, attach the suction source to the esophageal aspiration port. If the patient has a Blakemore-Sengstaken tube, advance an NG tube through the other nostril into the esophagus to the point where the esophageal balloon begins, and attach the suction source, as ordered.

■ Assess the patient for signs of airway obstruction.

■ Assess the patient's cardiac status.

For removal

■ The practitioner will deflate the esophageal balloon by aspirating the air with a syringe. (He may order the esophageal balloon to be deflated at 5-mm Hg [0.7-kPa] increments every 30 minutes for several hours.) Then, if bleeding doesn't recur, he'll remove the traction from the gastric tube and deflate the gastric balloon (also by aspiration). The gastric balloon is always deflated just before removing the tube *to prevent the balloon from riding up into the esophagus or pharynx and obstructing the airway or, possibly, causing asphyxia or rupture.*[12]

■ After disconnecting all suction tubes, the practitioner will gently remove the esophagogastric tamponade tube. If he feels resistance, he'll aspirate the balloons again. (To remove a Minnesota tube, he'll grasp it near the patient's nostril and cut across all four lumens approximately 3″ [7.5 cm] below that point *to ensure deflation of all balloons.*)

■ After the tube has been removed, assist the patient with oral care.

■ Discard equipment in the appropriate receptacles.

Completing the procedure

- Remove and discard your gloves and personal protective equipment.[13,14]
- Perform hand hygiene.[2,3,4,5,6]
- Document the procedure.[15,16,17]

Special considerations

- The Joint Commission issued a sentinel event alert concerning medical device alarm safety *because alarm-related events have been associated with permanent loss of function or death.* Among the major contributing factors were improper alarm settings, alarm settings inappropriately turned off, and alarm signals not audible to staff. Make sure that alarm limits are set appropriately and that alarms are turned on and audible. Follow facility guidelines for preventing alarm fatigue.[10]
- If the patient appears cyanotic or if other signs of airway obstruction develop during tube placement, remove the tube immediately *because it may have entered the trachea instead of the esophagus.*
- Many practitioners will intubate a patient before inserting an esophagogastric tamponade tube *to help eliminate the possibility of aspiration pneumonia during tube insertion and while the tube is in place.*
- After intubation, keep scissors at the bedside. If respiratory distress occurs, cut across all lumens while holding the tube at the nares, and remove the tube quickly.
- Unless contraindicated, the patient can sip water through a straw during intubation *to facilitate tube advancement.*
- Keep in mind that the intraesophageal balloon pressure varies with respirations and esophageal contractions. Baseline pressure is the important pressure to use when monitoring for complications.
- The balloon on the Linton tube should stay inflated no longer than 24 hours *because necrosis of the cardia may result.* Usually, the practitioner removes the tube only after a trial period (lasting at least 12 hours) with the esophageal balloon deflated or with the gastric balloon tension released from the cardia *to check for rebleeding.* In some facilities, the practitioner may deflate the esophageal balloon for 5 to 10 minutes every 6 hours *to temporarily relieve pressure on the esophageal mucosa.*

After removal, continue to monitor the patient for recurrence of bleeding.[1]

Complications

Aspiration is the most common complication of esophagogastric tamponade tube insertion. Erosion and perforation of the esophagus and gastric mucosa may result from the tension placed on these areas by the balloons during traction. Esophageal rupture may result if the gastric balloon accidentally inflates in the esophagus. Acute airway occlusion may result if the balloon dislodges and moves upward into the trachea. Other erosions, nasal tissue necrosis, and aspiration of oral secretions may complicate the patient's condition.

Documentation

Record the date and time of insertion and removal, the type of tube used, and the name of the practitioner who performed the procedure. Also document the intraesophageal balloon pressure (for the Blakemore-Sengstaken and Minnesota tubes), intragastric balloon pressure (for the Minnesota tube), or amount of air injected (for the Blakemore-Sengstaken and Linton tubes). Record the amount of fluid used for gastric irrigation and the color, consistency, and amount of gastric returns, both before and after lavage.

Record the date and time of removal and the name of the practitioner who performed the procedure. Document the patient's tolerance of the procedure, any complications, and, if complications occurred, the prescribed interventions and the patient's response to those interventions. Document patient and family teaching and their comprehension of your teaching.

REFERENCES

1 Lynn-McHale Wiegand, D. (Ed.). (2011). *AACN procedure manual for critical care* (6th ed.). St. Louis, MO: Saunders.

2 The Joint Commission. (2015). Standard NPSG.07.01.01. *Comprehensive accreditation manual for hospitals: The official handbook.* Oakbrook Terrace, IL: The Joint Commission. (Level VII)

3 Centers for Disease Control and Prevention. (2002). Guideline for hand hygiene in health-care settings: Recommendations of the Healthcare Infection Control Practices Advisory Committee and the HICPAC/SHEA/APIC/IDSA Hand Hygiene Task Force. *MMWR Recommendations and Reports, 51*(RR-16), 1–45. Accessed March 2015 via the Web at http://www.cdc.gov/mmwr/pdf/rr/rr5116.pdf (Level II)

4 World Health Organization. (2009). "WHO guidelines on hand hygiene in health care: First global patient safety challenge, clean care is safer care" [Online]. Accessed March 2015 via the Web at http://whqlibdoc.who.int/publications/2009/9789241597906_eng.pdf (Level IV)

5 American Osteopathic Association. (2014). Standard 07.01.21. *Healthcare Facilities Accreditation Program: Accreditation requirements for acute care hospitals.* Chicago, IL: American Osteopathic Association. (Level VII)

6 Centers for Medicare & Medicaid Services, Department of Health and Human Services. (2014). Condition of participation: Infection control. 42 C.F.R. § 482.42.

7 The Joint Commission. (2015). Standard NPSG.01.01.01. *Comprehensive accreditation manual for hospitals: The official handbook.* Oakbrook Terrace, IL: The Joint Commission. (Level VII)

8 American Osteopathic Association. (2014). Standard 15.01.16. *Healthcare Facilities Accreditation Program: Accreditation requirements for acute care hospitals.* Chicago, IL: American Osteopathic Association. (Level VII)

9 Centers for Medicare & Medicaid Services, Department of Health and Human Services. (2014). Condition of participation: Patient's rights. 42 C.F.R. § 482.13(c)(1).

10 The Joint Commission. (2012). "Sentinel events (SE)" [Online]. Accessed March 2015 via the Web at http://www.jointcommission.org/assets/1/6/CAMH_2012_Update2_24_SE.pdf (Level VII)

11 American Association of Critical-Care Nurses. (2013). "AACN practice alert: Alarm management" [Online]. Accessed March 2015 via the Web at http://www.aacn.org/wd/practice/docs/practicealerts/alarm-management-practice-alert.pdf (Level VII)

12 Graham, K. C., & Cvach, M. (2010). Monitor alarm fatigue: Standardizing use of physiological monitors and decreasing nuisance alarms. *American Journal of Critical Care, 19,* 28–37.

13 Siegel, J. D., et al. (2007). "2007 guideline for isolation precautions: Preventing transmission of infectious agents in healthcare settings" [Online]. Accessed March 2015 via the Web at http://www.cdc.gov/hicpac/pdf/isolation/Isolation2007.pdf (Level II)

14 American Osteopathic Association. (2014). Standard 07.01.10. *Healthcare Facilities Accreditation Program: Accreditation requirements for acute care hospitals.* Chicago, IL: American Osteopathic Association. (Level VII)

15 The Joint Commission. (2015). Standard RC.01.03.01. *Comprehensive accreditation manual for hospitals: The official handbook.* Oakbrook Terrace, IL: The Joint Commission. (Level VII)

16 American Osteopathic Association. (2014). Standard 10.00.03. *Healthcare Facilities Accreditation Program: Accreditation requirements for acute care hospitals.* Chicago, IL: American Osteopathic Association. (Level VII)

17 Centers for Medicare & Medicaid Services, Department of Health and Human Services. (2014). Condition of participation: Patient's rights. 42 C.F.R. § 482.24(b).

ADDITIONAL REFERENCE

Nettina, S. M. (2014). *Lippincott manual of nursing practice* (10th ed.). Philadelphia, PA: Wolters Kluwer.

EXTERNAL FIXATION MANAGEMENT

In external fixation, a practitioner inserts metal pins and wires through skin and muscle layers into the broken bones and affixes them to an adjustable external frame that maintains their proper alignment during

EQUIPMENT

Types of external fixation devices

The practitioner's selection of an external fixation device depends on the severity of the patient's fracture and on the type of bone alignment needed. Here are some examples of external fixation devices.

Universal day frame

The universal day frame is used to manage tibial fractures. This device allows the practitioner to readjust the position of bony fragments by angulation and rotation. The compression-distraction device allows compression and distraction of bony fragments.

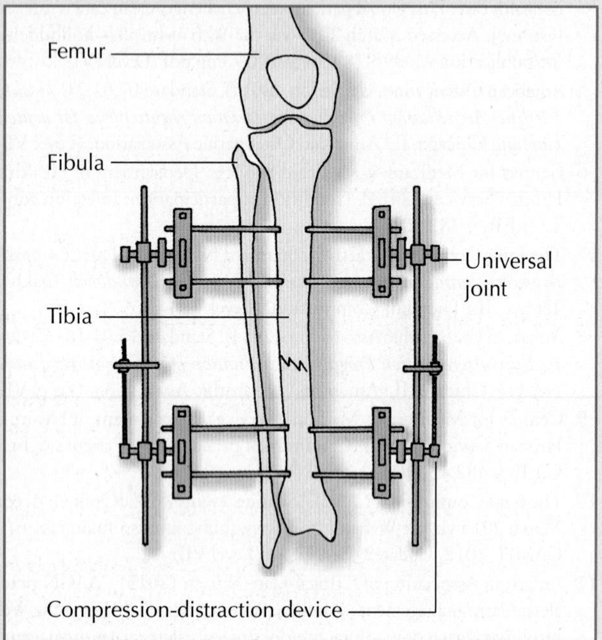

Portsmouth external fixation bar

The Portsmouth external fixation bar is a device used to manage complicated tibial fractures. The locking nut adjustment on the mobile carriage only allows bone compression, so the practitioner must accurately reduce bony fragments before applying the device.

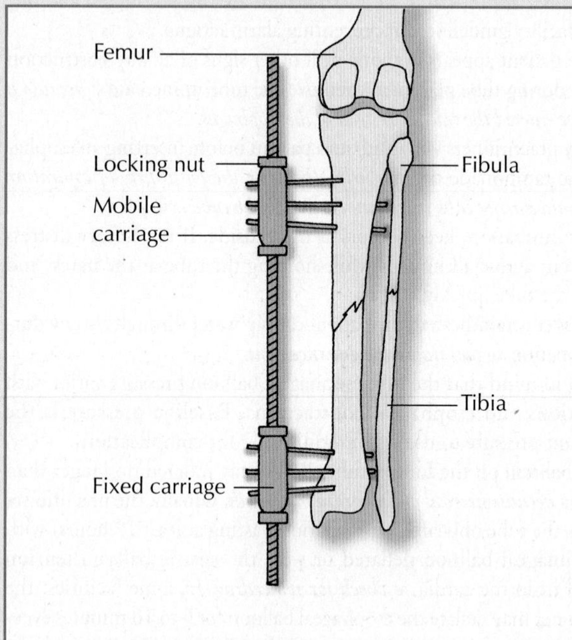

healing. (See *Types of external fixation devices.*) This procedure is used most commonly to treat open, unstable fractures with extensive soft-tissue damage, comminuted closed fractures, and septic, nonunion fractures and to facilitate surgical immobilization of a joint. Specialized types of external fixators may be used to lengthen leg bones or immobilize the cervical spine.

One advantage of external fixation over other immobilization techniques is that it stabilizes the fracture while allowing full visualization and access to open wounds. It also facilitates early ambulation, which reduces the risk of complications from immobilization.

The Ilizarov fixator is a special type of external fixation device. This device is a combination of rings and tensioned transosseous wires used primarily in limb lengthening, bone transport, and limb salvage. Highly complex, it provides gradual distraction that results in good-quality bone formation with a minimum of complications. It also provides enough stability to allow early unrestricted weight bearing.[1]

Equipment

External fixation set ▪ sterile gloves ▪ sterile container ▪ sterile cotton-tipped applicators ▪ prescribed antiseptic cleaning solution ▪ ice pack ▪ prescribed pain medication ▪ Optional: pillow, sterile dressing, sterile tape.

Equipment varies with the type of fixator and the type and location of the fracture. Typically, sets of pins, stabilizing rods, and clips are available from manufacturers.

Preparation of equipment

Make sure that the external fixation set includes all the equipment it's supposed to include and that the equipment has been sterilized.

Implementation

- Verify the practitioner's order.
- Gather and prepare the necessary equipment.
- Perform hand hygiene.[2,3,4,5,6]
- Confirm the patient's identity using at least two patient identifiers.[7]
- Provide privacy.[8,9]
- Explain the procedure to the patient *to reduce his anxiety.* Emphasize that he'll feel little pain after the fixation device is in place. Assure him that his feelings of anxiety are normal and that he'll be able to adjust to the apparatus.
- Tell the patient that he'll be able to move about with the apparatus in place, which may help him resume normal activities more quickly.
- Provide a comprehensive pain assessment using techniques appropriate for the patient's age, condition, and ability to understand. Provide medication, as ordered, using safe medication administration practices.[10,11,12] Perform a follow-up pain assessment and notify the practitioner if pain isn't adequately controlled.[13]
- After the fixation device is in place, perform neurovascular checks at an interval determined by your facility and the patient's condition *to assess for possible neurologic damage.* Assess color, warmth, motion, sensation, digital movement, edema, capillary refill, and pulses of the affected extremity. Compare with the unaffected side.

■ Apply an ice bag to the surgical site, as ordered, *to reduce swelling, relieve pain, and lessen bleeding.*
■ Perform a comprehensive pain assessment and administer pain medication, as ordered, 30 minutes to 1 hour before exercising or mobilizing the affected extremity *to promote comfort.*[10,11,12]
■ Monitor the patient for pain not relieved by analgesics and for burning, tingling, or numbness, *which may indicate nerve damage or circulatory impairment.*
■ Elevate the affected extremity, if appropriate, *to minimize edema.*
■ *To prevent* infection, perform pin site care, as ordered, following these guidelines: perform hand hygiene[2,3,4,5,6] and put on sterile gloves.[14,15] Using sterile technique, clean the pin site with a sterile cotton-tipped applicator dipped in the prescribed antiseptic solution.[16] If ordered, apply a loose sterile dressing.[16,17] Remove and discard your gloves[14,15] and perform hand hygiene.[2,3,4]
■ Perform pin site care, daily or weekly, after the first 48 to 72 hours, depending on the amount of drainage.[17,18]
■ Check for redness, tenting of the skin, prolonged or purulent drainage from the pin site, swelling, elevated body or pin site temperature, and any bowing or bending of pins, which may stress the skin.
■ Perform hand hygiene.[2,3,4,5,6]
■ Document the procedure.[19,20,21]

Special considerations

■ The National Association of Orthopaedic Nurses recommends using 2% chlorhexidine solution for pin site care.[22] Although studies have shown that chlorhexidine may be the most effective cleaning solution, continued research is needed to fully establish the most effective way to prevent infection.[23]
■ Because external fixation is commonly used in adolescents, pay special attention to the patient's psychosocial needs. Assess for depression, social issues, body image concerns, and sleep deprivation. Design a care plan with the patient and family to address these issues.
■ As appropriate, encourage the patient to stop smoking and provide smoking-cessation materials *because smoking delays bone healing.*[13]

For the patient with an Ilizarov fixator

■ When the device has been placed and preliminary calluses have begun to form at the insertion sites (in 5 to 7 days), gentle distraction is initiated by turning the appropriate screws one-quarter turn every 4 to 6 hours, as ordered.
■ Note that nonsteroidal anti-inflammatory drugs are usually contraindicated *because they may decrease the necessary inflammation caused by the distraction, resulting in delayed bone formation.*

Patient teaching

Before discharge, teach the patient and family members how to provide pin site care.[8] Although pin site care is a sterile procedure in the health care facility, the patient can use clean technique at home. Provide the patient and family with written instructions and have the patient demonstrate the procedure before leaving the health care facility.[8] Teach the patient to recognize signs and symptoms of pin site infection.[8] Tell him to keep the affected limb elevated when sitting or lying down.

For the patient with an Ilizarov fixator

Teach the patient that he must be consistent in turning the screws every 4 to 6 hours around the clock, or as ordered by the practitioner. Make sure he understands that he must be strongly committed to compliance with the protocol for the procedure to be successful. Because the treatment period may be prolonged (4 to 10 months), discuss with the patient and family members the psychological effects of long-term care.

Complications

Complications of external fixation include loosening of pins and loss of fracture stabilization, infection of the pin tract or wound, skin breakdown, nerve damage, and muscle impingement.

Ilizarov fixator pin sites are more prone to infection because of the extended treatment period and because of the pins' movement to accomplish distraction. The pins are also more likely to break because of their small diameter. Also, the large number of pins used increases the patient's risk of neurovascular compromise.

Documentation

Record the patient's response to the apparatus and to ambulation. Assess and document neurovascular status and the condition of the pin sites and surround skin. Document patient and family teaching performed and their understanding of that teaching. Also document the administration of any pain medication and its effectiveness.

References

1 Ramos, T., et al. (2013). Treatment of distal tibial fractures with the Ilizarov external fixator—A prospective observational study in 39 consecutive patients. *BMC Musculoskeletal Disorders, 14,* 30. Accessed March 2015 via the Web at http://www.ncbi.nlm.nih.gov/pmc/articles/PMC3626620/ (Level VI)

2 American Osteopathic Association. (2014). Standard 07.01.21. *Healthcare Facilities Accreditation Program: Accreditation requirements for acute care hospitals.* Chicago, IL: American Osteopathic Association. (Level VII)

3 Centers for Medicare & Medicaid Services, Department of Health and Human Services. (2014). Condition of participation: Infection control. 42 C.F.R. § 482.42.

4 The Joint Commission. (2015). Standard NPSG.07.01.01. *Comprehensive accreditation manual for hospitals: The official handbook.* Oakbrook Terrace, IL: The Joint Commission. (Level VII)

5 Centers for Disease Control and Prevention. (2002). Guideline for hand hygiene in health-care settings: Recommendations of the Healthcare Infection Control Practices Advisory Committee and the HICPAC/SHEA/APIC/IDSA Hand Hygiene Task Force. *MMWR Recommendations and Reports, 51*(RR-16), 1–45. Accessed March 2015 via the Web at http://www.cdc.gov/mmwr/pdf/rr/rr5116.pdf (Level II)

6 World Health Organization. (2009). "WHO guidelines on hand hygiene in health care: First global patient safety challenge, clean care is safer care" [Online]. Accessed March 2015 via the Web at http://whqlibdoc.who.int/publications/2009/9789241597906_eng.pdf (Level IV)

7 The Joint Commission. (2015). Standard NPSG.01.01.01. *Comprehensive accreditation manual for hospitals: The official handbook.* Oakbrook Terrace, IL: The Joint Commission. (Level VII)

8 Centers for Medicare & Medicaid Services, Department of Health and Human Services. (2014). Condition of participation: Patient's rights. 42 C.F.R. § 482.13(c)(1).

9 American Osteopathic Association. (2014). Standard 15.01.16. *Healthcare Facilities Accreditation Program: Accreditation requirements for acute care hospitals.* Chicago, IL: American Osteopathic Association. (Level VII)

10 The Joint Commission. (2015). Standard MM.06.01.01. *Comprehensive accreditation manual for hospitals: The official handbook.* Oakbrook Terrace, IL: The Joint Commission. (Level VII)

11 Centers for Medicare & Medicaid Services, Department of Health and Human Services. (2014). Condition of participation: Nursing services. 42 C.F.R. § 482.23(c).

12 American Osteopathic Association. (2014). Standard 16.01.03. *Healthcare Facilities Accreditation Program: Accreditation requirements for acute care hospitals.* Chicago, IL: American Osteopathic Association. (Level VII)

13 The Joint Commission. (2015). Standard PC.01.02.07. *Comprehensive accreditation manual for hospitals: The official handbook.* Oakbrook Terrace, IL: The Joint Commission. (Level VII)

14 Siegel, J. D., et al. (2007). "2007 guideline for isolation precautions: Preventing transmission of infectious agents in healthcare settings"

[Online]. Accessed March 2015 via the Web at http://www.cdc.gov/hicpac/pdf/isolation/Isolation2007.pdf (Level II)

15 American Osteopathic Association. (2014). Standard 07.01.10. *Healthcare Facilities Accreditation Program: Accreditation requirements for acute care hospitals.* Chicago, IL: American Osteopathic Association. (Level VII)

16 Holmes, S. B., & Brown, S. J. (2005). Skeletal pin site care: National Association of Orthopaedic Nurses guidelines for orthopaedic nursing. *Orthopaedic Nursing, 24,* 99–107. (Level VII)

17 Ferreira, N., & Marais, L. C. (2012). Prevention and management of external fixator pin track sepsis. *Strategies in Trauma and Limb Reconstruction, 7,* 67–72. Accessed January 2015 via the Web at http://www.ncbi.nlm.nih.gov/pmc/articles/PMC3535127/

18 Timms, A., et al. (2011). "Guidance on pin site care: Report and recommendations from the 2010 Consensus Project on Pin Site Care" [Online]. Accessed March 2015 via the Web at http://www.rcn.org.uk/__data/assets/pdf_file/0009/413982/004137.pdf

19 The Joint Commission. (2015). Standard RC.01.03.01. *Comprehensive accreditation manual for hospitals: The official handbook.* Oakbrook Terrace, IL: The Joint Commission. (Level VII)

20 Centers for Medicare & Medicaid Services, Department of Health and Human Services. (2014). Condition of participation: Medical record services. 42 C.F.R. § 482.24(b).

21 American Osteopathic Association. (2014). Standard 10.00.03. *Healthcare Facilities Accreditation Program: Accreditation requirements for acute care hospitals.* Chicago, IL: American Osteopathic Association. (Level VII)

22 National Association of Orthopaedic Nurses. (2013). *Core curriculum for orthopaedic nursing* (7th ed.). Boston, MA: Pearson.

23 Lethaby, A., et al. (2013). Pin site care for preventing infections associated with external bone fixators and pins. *Cochrane Database of Systematic Reviews, 2013*(12), CD004551. (Level I)

EYE CARE

Eye care is the practice of assessing, cleaning, or irrigating the eye or the instillation of prescribed ocular preparations. Eye care may be necessary to relieve pain and discomfort, prevent or treat infection or injury to the eye, detect disease at an early stage, detect drug-induced toxicity, prevent damage to the cornea in sedated or unconscious patients, maintain contact lenses, and care for false eye prostheses.[1]

Equipment

Towel ▪ sterile drape ▪ sterile basin ▪ powder-free gloves ▪ sterile gauze pads ▪ sterile normal saline solution ▪ Optional: prescribed eyedrops or eye ointment, eye patch or shield, hydrogel dressing, paper tape.

Implementation

- Gather the equipment at the patient's bedside and make sure the lighting is adequate.
- Perform hand hygiene.[2,3,4,5,6]
- Confirm the patient's identity using at least two patient identifiers.[7]
- Explain the procedure to the patient, even if he is comatose or appears unresponsive.
- Raise the head of the patient's bed to 30 degrees, unless contraindicated by the patient's condition.
- Make sure that the patient is in a comfortable position.
- Place a towel around the patient's neck.
- Create a sterile field using a sterile drape.
- Place the sterile basin and sterile gauze pads on the sterile field.
- Pour sterile normal saline solution into the sterile basin using sterile technique.
- Put on gloves.[8,9]
- Assess the patient's eyes and periorbital area for redness, drainage, bruising, presence of a foreign object, pupil size and reactivity, and subjective reports of pain, vision loss, itching, sensitivity to light, or sensation of something in the eye.
- Irrigate the eyes as needed and prescribed. (See the "Eye irrigation" procedure, page 308.)
- *To remove secretions or crusts adhering to the eyelids and eyelashes,* first soak a sterile gauze pad in sterile normal saline solution. Instruct the patient to close his eyes; then, without applying pressure, gently wipe the patient's eye with the moistened gauze pad, working from the inner canthus to the outer canthus *to prevent debris and fluid from entering the tear duct.*

NURSING ALERT *Don't use cotton swabs, tweezers, or anything else on the eye itself.*

- *To prevent cross-contamination,* use a new sterile gauze pad for each wipe until all discharge has been removed. *To prevent irritation,* avoid using soap for cleaning the eyes. Repeat the procedure for the other eye.
- *To keep the eyes moist after cleaning them,* instill eyedrops or apply eye ointment, as ordered, following safe medication administration practices. (See the "Eye medication administration" procedure, page 311.)
- Close the patient's eyelids gently using the back of your fingertip. Use an eye patch or shield or hydrogel dressing,[10] as indicated, *to promote eye closure in the patient with partial or incomplete eyelid closure.* Use paper tape *to secure the eye patch or shield.*[11]
- Dispose of the used supplies in the appropriate receptacle.[8]
- Remove and discard your gloves.[8]
- Perform hand hygiene.[2,3,4,5,6]
- Document the procedure.[12,13,14]

Special considerations

- Unconscious patients lose the protective corneal reflex of blinking, increasing the risk of corneal drying, abrasions, and eye injury. In these patients, keep the eyes *closed to maintain eye moisture and prevent injury.*[15]

Patient teaching

Teach the patient or caregiver about existing eye disorders, infections, or injuries, as appropriate, including proper hand hygiene to avoid contamination, safety measures to prevent eye injury, and current treatments for dry eye.

Documentation

Record the time and type of eye care in your notes. Document your assessment of the eyes and periorbital areas, noting redness, drainage, or bruising; the presence of any foreign object; pupil size and reactivity; and subjective reports of pain, vision loss, itching, sensitivity to light, or the sensation of something in the eye. If applicable, document any irrigation procedure performed or administration of eyedrops or ointment in the patient's medication record.

REFERENCES

1 NHS Wirral. (2014). "Procedures for eye care" [Online]. Accessed March 2015 via the Web at http://www.wirral.nhs.uk/document_uploads/Policies_and_Procedures_Nursing/NPENT02ProceduresEyeCare0510.pdf

2 The Joint Commission. (2015). Standard NPSG.07.01.01. *Comprehensive accreditation manual for hospitals: The official handbook.* Oakbrook Terrace, IL: The Joint Commission. (Level VII)

3 Centers for Disease Control and Prevention. (2002). Guideline for hand hygiene in health care settings: Recommendations of the Healthcare Infection Control Practices Advisory Committee and the HICPAC/SHEA/APIC/IDSA Hand Hygiene Task Force. *MMWR Recommendations and Reports, 51*(RR-16), 1–45. Accessed March 2015 via the Web at http://www.cdc.gov/mmwr/pdf/rr/rr5116.pdf (Level II)

4 World Health Organization. (2009). "WHO guidelines on hand hygiene in health care: First global patient safety challenge, clean care is safer care" [Online]. Accessed March 2015 via the Web at http://whqlibdoc.who.int/publications/2009/9789241597906_eng.pdf (Level IV)

5 Centers for Medicare & Medicaid Services, Department of Health and Human Services. (2014). Condition of participation: Infection control. 42 C.F.R. § 482.42.
6 American Osteopathic Association. (2014). Standard 07.01.21. *Healthcare Facilities Accreditation Program: Accreditation requirements for acute care hospitals.* Chicago, IL: American Osteopathic Association. (Level VII)
7 The Joint Commission. (2015). Standard NPSG.01.01.01. *Comprehensive accreditation manual for hospitals: The official handbook.* Oakbrook Terrace, IL: The Joint Commission. (Level VII)
8 Siegel, J. D., et al. (2007). "2007 guideline for isolation precautions: Preventing transmission of infectious agents in healthcare settings" [Online]. Accessed March 2015 via the Web at http://www.cdc.gov/hicpac/pdf/isolation/Isolation2007.pdf (Level II)
9 American Osteopathic Association. (2014). Standard 07.01.10. *Healthcare Facilities Accreditation Program: Accreditation requirements for acute care hospitals.* Chicago, IL: American Osteopathic Association. (Level VII)
10 Douglas, L., & Berry, S. (2011). Developing clinical guidelines in eye care for intensive care units. *Nursing Children and Young People, 23*(5), 14–20. (Level VII)
11 Perry, A., et al. (2013). *Clinical nursing skills and techniques* (8th ed.). St. Louis, MO: Mosby.
12 The Joint Commission. (2015). Standard RC.01.03.01. *Comprehensive accreditation manual for hospitals: The official handbook.* Oakbrook Terrace, IL: The Joint Commission. (Level VII)
13 Centers for Medicare & Medicaid Services, Department of Health and Human Services. (2014). Condition of participation: Medical record services. 42 C.F.R. § 482.24(b).
14 American Osteopathic Association. (2014). Standard 10.00.03. *Healthcare Facilities Accreditation Program: Accreditation requirements for acute care hospitals.* Chicago, IL: American Osteopathic Association. (Level VII)
15 Taylor, C., et al. (2011). *Fundamentals of nursing: The art and science of nursing care* (7th ed.). Philadelphia, PA: Lippincott Williams & Wilkins.

ADDITIONAL REFERENCE

Craven, R. F., & Hirnle, C. J. (2009). *Fundamentals of nursing: Human health and function* (6th ed.). Philadelphia, PA: Lippincott Williams & Wilkins.

EYE COMPRESS APPLICATION

Whether applied warm or cold, eye compresses are soothing and therapeutic. Because heat increases circulation, which enhances absorption and decreases inflammation, warm compresses may relieve discomfort and promote drainage of superficial infections.

The presence of ocular infection requires the use of sterile technique for this procedure.

Equipment

Prescribed solution (usually sterile water or normal saline solution) ▪ sterile basin ▪ sterile 4″ × 4″ (10-cm × 10-cm) gauze pads ▪ towel ▪ pillow ▪ Optional: gloves or sterile gloves, ophthalmic ointment or eyedrops, eye patch.

Additional equipment for a warm compress

Basin of warm water or access to hot tap water.

Additional equipment for a cold compress

Small plastic bag, ice pack, or latex-free glove ▪ ice chips ▪ ½″ (1.3-cm) hypoallergenic tape.

Preparation of equipment

If you're performing a sterile procedure, label all medications, medication containers, and solutions on and off the sterile field.[1]

For a warm compress

Place a capped bottle of sterile water or normal saline solution in a basin of hot water or under a stream of hot tap water. Allow the solution to become warm (no higher than 120°F [49°C]).[2] Pour the warm water or saline solution into a sterile basin, filling the basin about halfway. Place some of the sterile gauze pads in the basin.

For a cold compress

Place ice chips in a plastic bag, ice pack, or latex-free glove, if necessary. Keep the ice pack small *to avoid excessive pressure on the eye.* Remove excess air from the bag, pack, or glove, and then knot or close the open end. Cut a piece of hypoallergenic tape *to secure the ice pack.* Place all equipment on the bedside stand near the patient.

Implementation

- Verify the practitioner's order for solution, frequency, and duration of treatment.
- Gather and prepare the appropriate equipment.
- Perform hand hygiene and, as needed, put on gloves or sterile gloves.[3,4,5,6]
- Confirm the patient's identity using at least two patient identifiers.[7]
- Explain the procedure to the patient, make him comfortable, and provide privacy.
- Help the patient into the supine position, supporting his head with a pillow, and turning it slightly to the unaffected side. *This position will help hold the compress in place.*
- If the patient has an eye patch, remove and discard it.
- Remove and discard your gloves (if worn), perform hand hygiene, and put on new gloves.[3,4,5,6]
- Drape a towel around the patient's shoulders *to catch any spills.*

For a warm compress

- Remove two sterile gauze pads from the basin, and squeeze out the excess solution.
- Instruct the patient to close his eyes.
- Gently apply the pads—one on top of the other—to the affected eye. (If the patient complains that the compress feels too hot, remove it immediately.)
- Change the compress every few minutes during the prescribed length of time. After removing each compress, inspect the patient's skin for signs that the compress solution is too hot.

For a cold compress

- Moisten the middle of one of the sterile 4″ × 4″ (10-cm × 10-cm) gauze pads with the prescribed solution (sterile water, normal saline solution, or ophthalmic irrigating solution) *to help conduct the cold from the ice pack.* Keep the edges dry *so that they can absorb excess moisture.*
- Tell the patient to close his eyes.
- Place the moist gauze pad over the affected eye, place the ice pack on top of the gauze pad, and tape it in place.
- If the patient complains of pain, remove the ice pack. *Some patients may have an adverse reaction to cold.*
- Remove and discard your gloves, if worn.
- Perform hand hygiene.[3,4,5,6]
- After 15 to 20 minutes, or as ordered, perform hand hygiene and put on gloves, as needed.[3,4,5,6]
- Remove the tape, ice pack, and gauze pad and discard them.

For all compresses

- Use the remaining dry sterile gauze pads to clean and dry the patient's face.
- If ordered, apply ophthalmic ointment, instill drops, or apply an eye patch. (See the "Eye medication administration" procedure, page 311.)
- Discard used supplies.
- Remove and discard your gloves, if worn.
- Perform hand hygiene.[3,4,5,6]
- Document the procedure.[8,9]

Special considerations

- When applying warm compresses, change the compress as frequently as necessary *to maintain a constant temperature*—typically every 5 minutes—*to increase vasodilation and promote discharge.*[2,10]
- Don't use a microwave to warm the solution *because of the risk of overheating the solution.*
- Cold compresses are contraindicated in treating eye inflammation, such as keratitis and iritis, *because the capillary constriction inhibits delivery of nutrients to the cornea.*

Patient teaching

When teaching a patient to apply compresses at home, explain that he can substitute a clean basin and washcloth for the sterile equipment. If both eyes are infected, emphasize the importance of using separate equipment for each eye. Inform the patient that this approach will keep him from passing infection back and forth between the eyes. Teach him how to instill eyedrops or ophthalmic ointment correctly and without contaminating the medication container. Direct him to wash his hands thoroughly before and after treating each eye.

Documentation

Record the time and duration of the procedure. Describe the eye's appearance before and after treatment, any drainage, and the patient's comfort level. Note any ointments, eyedrops, or dressings applied to the eye. Record the patient's tolerance of the procedure. Document any patient teaching provided and the patient's understanding of the teaching.

References

1 The Joint Commission. (2015). Standard NPSG.03.04.01. *Comprehensive accreditation manual for hospitals: The official handbook.* Oakbrook Terrace, IL: The Joint Commission. (Level VII)

2 Blackie, C. A., et al. (2008). Inner eyelid surface temperature as a function of warm compress methodology. *Optometry and Vision Science, 85,* 675–683.

3 The Joint Commission. (2015). Standard NPSG.07.01.01. *Comprehensive accreditation manual for hospitals: The official handbook.* Oakbrook Terrace, IL: The Joint Commission. (Level VII)

4 World Health Organization. (2009). "WHO guidelines on hand hygiene in health care: First global patient safety challenge, clean care is safer care" [Online]. Accessed March 2015 via the Web at http://whqlibdoc.who.int/publications/2009/9789241597906_eng.pdf (Level IV)

5 Centers for Disease Control and Prevention. (2002). Guideline for hand hygiene in health-care settings: Recommendations of the Healthcare Infection Control Practices Advisory Committee and the HICPAC/SHEA/APIC/IDSA Hand Hygiene Task Force. *MMWR Recommendations and Reports, 51*(RR-16), 1–45. Accessed March 2015 via the Web at http://www.cdc.gov/mmwr/pdf/rr/rr5116.pdf (Level II)

6 Siegel, J. D., et al. (2007). "2007 guideline for isolation precautions: Preventing transmission of infectious agents in healthcare settings" [Online]. Accessed March 2015 via the Web at http://www.cdc.gov/hicpac/pdf/isolation/Isolation2007.pdf (Level II)

7 The Joint Commission. (2015). Standard NPSG.01.01.01. *Comprehensive accreditation manual for hospitals: The official handbook.* Oakbrook Terrace, IL: The Joint Commission. (Level VII)

8 The Joint Commission. (2015). Standard RC.01.03.01. *Comprehensive accreditation manual for hospitals: The official handbook.* Oakbrook Terrace, IL: The Joint Commission. (Level VII)

9 Centers for Medicare & Medicaid Services, Department of Health and Human Services. (2014). Condition of participation: Medical record services. 42 C.F.R. § 482.24(b).

10 American Optometric Association. (n.d.). "Blepharitis" [Online]. Accessed March 2015 via the Web at http://www.aoa.org/Blepharitis.xml

Additional reference

Hinkle, J. L., & Cheever, K. H. (2014). *Brunner & Suddarth's textbook of medical-surgical nursing* (13th ed.). Philadelphia, PA: Wolters Kluwer.

Eye irrigation

Used mainly to flush secretions, chemicals, and foreign bodies from the eye, eye irrigation also provides a way to administer medications for corneal and conjunctival disorders. In an emergency, tap water may serve as an irrigant.

The amount of solution needed to irrigate an eye depends on the contaminant. Secretions require a moderate volume; major chemical burns require a copious amount. Usually, an IV bottle or bag of normal saline solution (with IV tubing attached) supplies enough solution for continuous irrigation of a chemical burn. (See *Three devices for eye irrigation.*)

Equipment

Gloves ▪ fluid-impermeable pads ▪ emesis basin ▪ towel ▪ sterile gauze pads ▪ Optional: goggles, pH strips for eye testing, eyelid retractor, ophthalmic anesthetic drops, Morgan lens.

For moderate-volume irrigation

Prescribed sterile ophthalmic irrigant ▪ Optional: 60-mL sterile syringe, sterile squeeze bottle, sterile basin.

For copious irrigation

One or more 1,000-mL bottles or bags of normal saline solution or lactated Ringer solution ▪ standard IV infusion set ▪ IV pole.

Commercially prepared bottles of sterile ophthalmic irrigant are available.

Preparation of equipment

Read the label on the irrigant. Double-check its sterility, strength, and expiration date. All solutions should be warmed to 90°F to 100°F (32.2°C to 37.8°C), if possible, *to promote patient comfort.*[1,2]

For moderate-volume irrigation

Pour the sterile irrigant into the sterile basin. Fill the syringe or squeeze bottle with 30 to 60 mL of irrigant. If you're using a commercially prepared bottle of sterile irrigant, remove the cap from the irrigant container and place the container within easy reach. Be sure to keep the tip of the container sterile.

For copious irrigation

Use aseptic technique to set up the IV infusion set and the bag of normal saline or lactated Ringer solution. Hang the container on an IV pole, fill the IV tubing with the solution, and adjust the drip regulator valve *to ensure an adequate but not forceful flow.* Place all other equipment within easy reach.

Implementation

- Verify the practitioner's order.
- Gather and prepare the appropriate equipment.
- Perform hand hygiene and put on gloves and, if splashing is likely, goggles.[3,4,5,6]
- Confirm the patient's identity using at least two patient identifiers.[7]
- Explain the procedure to the patient and provide privacy. If the patient has a chemical burn, ease his anxiety by explaining that irrigation prevents further damage.
- If the patient is wearing contact lenses, remove and discard them immediately *to prevent further damage and to facilitate irrigation.*

NURSING ALERT ***If the patient has a history of acid or alkali exposure, irrigate the eye immediately and then perform a complete eye examination. The extent of the injury depends on the amount of exposure.*** **Irrigating immediately reduces damage.**[8]

Three devices for eye irrigation

Syringe or squeeze bottle
For moderate-volume irrigation—to remove eye secretions, for example—apply sterile ophthalmic irrigant to the eye directly from a 60-mL syringe or squeeze bottle (shown here) filled with ophthalmic irrigant. Direct the stream at the inner canthus, and position the patient so the stream washes across the cornea and exits at the outer canthus.

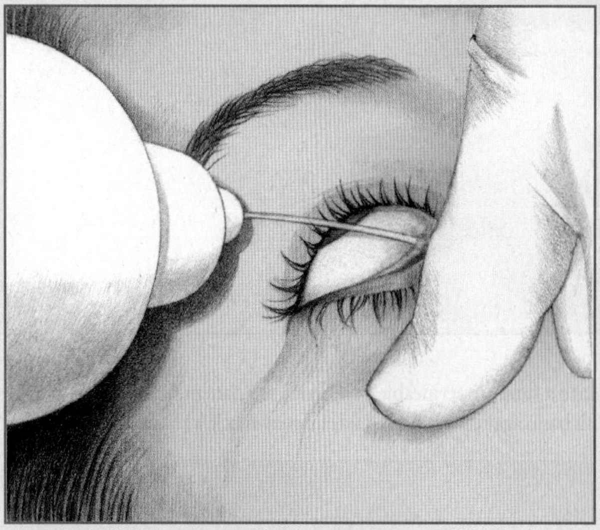

IV tube
For copious irrigation—to treat chemical burns, for example—set up an IV bag and tubing. Use the procedure described for moderate-volume irrigation to flush the eye for at least 15 minutes. Alkali burns may require irrigation for several hours.

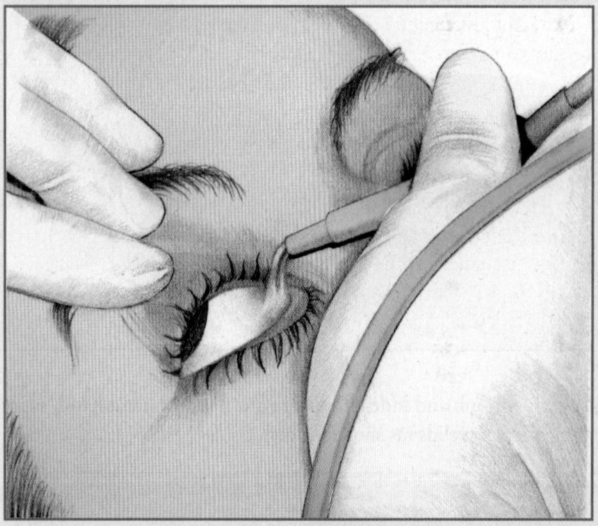

Morgan lens
Attached to IV tubing that's connected to a bag of IV fluid, a Morgan lens permits continuous lavage and also delivers medication to the eye. Begin the irrigation at the prescribed flow rate. To insert the device, ask the patient to look down as you insert the lens under the upper eyelid. Then have him look up as you retract and release the lower eyelid over the lens.

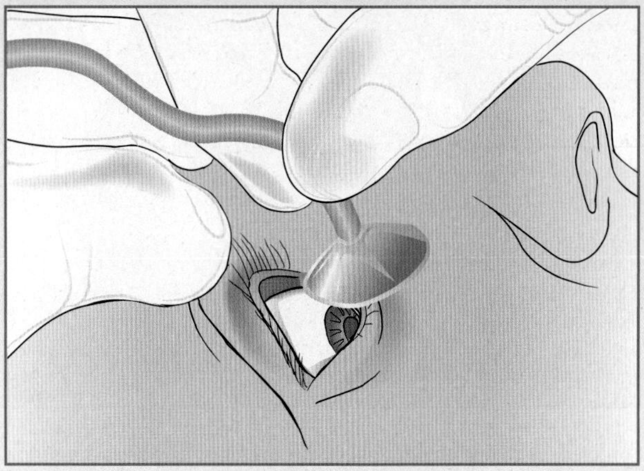

■ Help the patient into the supine position with the head of the bed elevated.
■ Gently remove visible external discharge or debris from the eye with sterile gauze pads. Wipe from the inner canthus to the outer canthus *to prevent debris from being washed back into the eye.* Use a new sterile gauze pad with each wipe *to prevent cross-contamination.*
■ Turn the patient's head slightly toward the affected side (as shown on next page, top left) *to prevent cross-contamination from the solution flowing over his nose and into the other eye.*

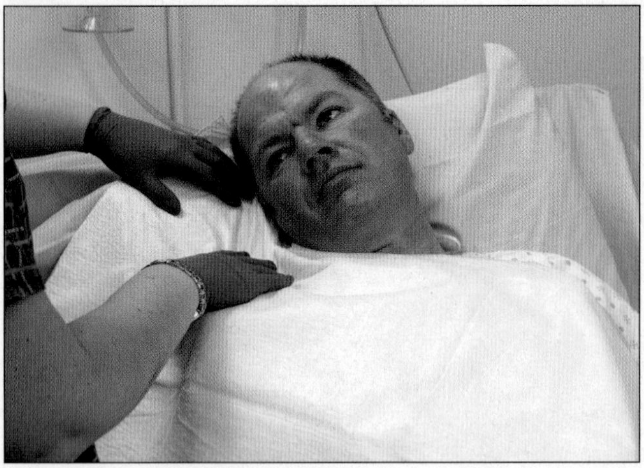

■ Place a fluid-impermeable pad under the patient's head, and hold the emesis basin against his affected side (as shown below) *to catch excess solution.*

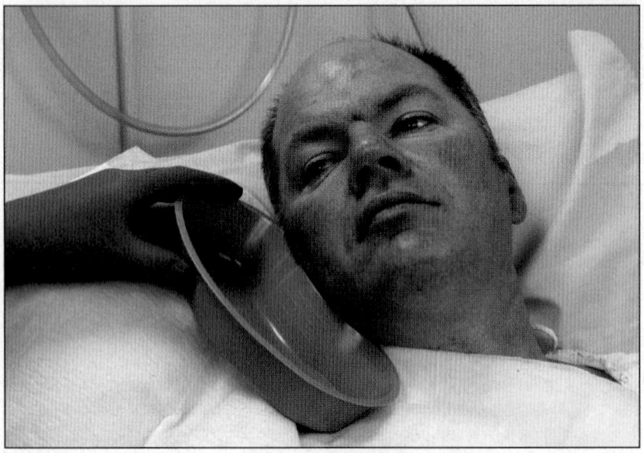

■ Using the thumb and index finger of your nondominant hand, separate the patient's eyelids (as shown below).

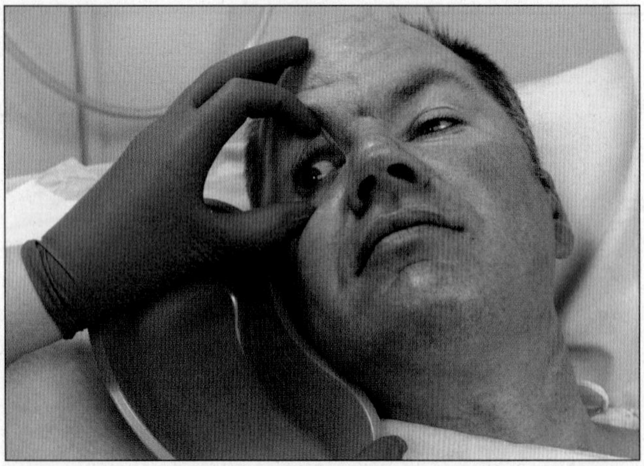

■ If ordered, instill ophthalmic anesthetic eyedrops *as a comfort measure.* Use them only once *because repeated use retards healing.*
■ *To irrigate the conjunctival cul-de-sac,* continue holding the eyelids apart with your thumb and index finger.
■ *To irrigate the upper eyelid (the superior fornix),* use an eyelid retractor. Steady the hand holding the retractor by resting it on the patient's forehead. *The retractor prevents the eyelid from closing involuntarily when solution touches the cornea and conjunctiva.*

Administering moderate-volume irrigation

■ Holding the syringe or squeeze bottle of sterile ophthalmic irrigant about 1″ (2.5 cm) from the eye, direct a constant, gentle stream at the inner canthus (as shown below) *so that the solution flows across the cornea to the outer canthus.*

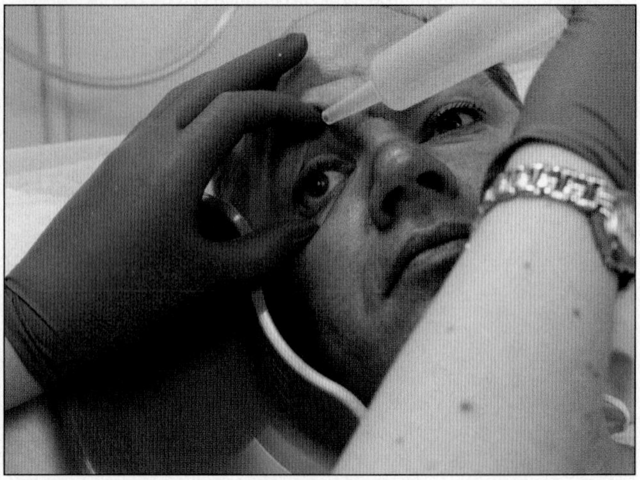

■ Use only enough force to gently remove secretions from the conjunctiva.
■ Make sure that you don't touch or press on the eyeball with the syringe or tip of the squeeze bottle while irrigating *to avoid causing discomfort and possible further injury to the patient.*
■ Evert the lower eyelid and then the upper eyelid *to inspect for retained foreign particles.*

Administering copious irrigation

■ Hold the control valve on the IV tubing about 1″ (2.5 cm) above the patient's eye, and direct a constant, gentle stream of normal saline or lactated Ringer solution at the inner canthus *so that the solution flows across the cornea to the outer canthus.*
■ Ask the patient to rotate his eye periodically while you continue the irrigation. *This action may dislodge foreign particles and ensures irrigation of the entire eye.*
■ Evert the lower eyelid and then the upper eyelid *to inspect for retained foreign particles.* (This inspection is especially important when the patient has caustic lime in his eye.)

Completing the procedure

■ Remove any foreign particles by gently touching the conjunctiva with a sterile gauze pad moistened with irrigant. Don't touch the cornea.
■ Resume irrigating the eye until all visible foreign particles have been removed.
■ Gently dry the patient's eyelids with a sterile gauze pad, wiping from the inner to the outer canthus. Use a new sterile gauze pad for each wipe. *This reduces the patient's need to rub his eye.*
■ Offer the patient a towel for drying his face and neck.
■ Discard waste and used supplies in the appropriate receptacle
■ Remove and discard your gloves, and remove your goggles, if worn.
■ Perform hand hygiene.[3,4,5]
■ Document the procedure.[9,10]

Special considerations

■ Arrange for follow-up care, when necessary.
■ When irrigating both eyes, have the patient tilt his head toward the side being irrigated *to avoid cross-contamination.*
■ For chemical burns, irrigate each eye for 15 to 30 minutes with normal saline or lactated Ringer solution *to dilute and wash out the harsh chemical.*[11]

After irrigation, close the patient's eye for about 5 minutes and then test the pH of the eye by touching the pH test strip to the area between the eyelid and globe. Continue irrigation until a neutral pH (7) is achieved and maintained for at least 30 minutes.[8]

■ After irrigating any chemical, note the time, date, and chemical for your own reference *in case you develop contact dermatitis.*[8]

■ For further information on chemicals, contact the American Association of Poison Control Centers at 1-800-222-1222 or access their Web site at http://www.aapcc.org.

■ Studies have shown that the most comfortable method of irrigation for patients is the use of the Morgan lens in combination with a lidocaine-saline solution.[12]

Patient teaching

If an ophthalmic anesthetic agent was used, instruct the patient to avoid touching his eye. *Touching the eye before the anesthetic has worn off may damage the cornea or conjunctiva.*[13]

Documentation

Note the duration of irrigation, the type and amount of solution used, and characteristics of the drainage. Record your assessment of the patient's eye before and after irrigation. Also note his response to the procedure.

REFERENCES

1 Ernst, A., et al. (1998). Warmed versus room temperature saline solution for ocular irrigation: A randomized clinical trial. *Annals of Emergency Medicine, 32,* 676–679. (Level II)

2 Agency for Healthcare Research and Quality. (2012). "Best evidence statement: Use of irrigation solution, warm versus room temperature, for irrigation procedures in the emergency department and urgent care" [Online]. Accessed March 2015 via the Web at http://www.guideline.gov/content.aspx?id=37635 (Level VII)

3 The Joint Commission. (2015). Standard NPSG.07.01.01. *Comprehensive accreditation manual for hospitals: The official handbook.* Oakbrook Terrace, IL: The Joint Commission. (Level VII)

4 World Health Organization. (2009). "WHO guidelines on hand hygiene in health care: First global patient safety challenge, clean care is safer care" [Online]. Accessed March 2015 via the Web at http://whqlibdoc.who.int/publications/2009/9789241597906_eng.pdf (Level IV)

5 Centers for Disease Control and Prevention. (2002). Guideline for hand hygiene in health-care settings: Recommendations of the Healthcare Infection Control Practices Advisory Committee and the HICPAC/SHEA/APIC/IDSA Hand Hygiene Task Force. *MMWR Recommendations and Reports, 51*(RR-16), 1–45. Accessed March 2015 via the Web at http://www.cdc.gov/mmwr/pdf/rr/rr5116.pdf (Level II)

6 Siegel, J. D., et al. (2007). "2007 guideline for isolation precautions: Preventing transmission of infectious agents in healthcare settings" [Online]. Accessed March 2015 via the Web at http://www.cdc.gov/hicpac/pdf/isolation/Isolation2007.pdf (Level II)

7 The Joint Commission. (2015). Standard NPSG.01.01.01. *Comprehensive accreditation manual for hospitals: The official handbook.* Oakbrook Terrace, IL: The Joint Commission. (Level VII)

8 Pokhrel, P. K., & Loftus, S. A. (2007). Ocular emergencies. *American Family Physician, 76,* 829–836. Accessed March 2015 via the Web at http://www.aafp.org/afp/2007/0915/p829.pdf

9 The Joint Commission. (2015). Standard RC.01.03.01. *Comprehensive accreditation manual for hospitals: The official handbook.* Oakbrook Terrace, IL: The Joint Commission. (Level VII)

10 Centers for Medicare & Medicaid Services, Department of Health and Human Services. (2014). Condition of participation: Medical record services. 42 C.F.R. § 482.24(b).

11 Rodrigues, Z. (2009). Irrigation of the eye after alkaline and acidic burns. *Emergency Nurse, 17*(8), 26–29.

12 O'Malley, G. F., et al. (2008). Eye irrigation is more comfortable with a lidocaine-containing irrigation solution compared with normal saline. *The Journal of Trauma: Injury, Infection, and Critical Care, 64,* 1360–1362.

13 Nettina, S. M. (2014). *Lippincott manual of nursing practice* (10th ed.). Philadelphia, PA: Wolters Kluwer.

ADDITIONAL REFERENCES

Khodabukus, R., & Tallouzi, M. (2009). Chemical eye injuries. 1: Presentation, clinical features, treatment and prognosis. *Nursing Times, 105*(22), 28–29.

Taylor, C., et al. (2011). *Fundamentals of nursing: The art and science of nursing care* (7th ed.). Philadelphia, PA: Lippincott Williams & Wilkins.

EYE MEDICATION ADMINISTRATION

During an eye examination, a practitioner can use eyedrops to anesthetize the eye, dilate the pupil to facilitate examination, and stain the cornea to identify corneal abrasions, scars, and other anomalies. Eye medications can also be used to lubricate the eye, treat certain eye conditions (such as glaucoma and infections), and lubricate the eye socket for insertion of a prosthetic eye.

Understanding the ocular effects of medications is important because certain drugs may cause eye disorders or have serious ocular effects. For example, anticholinergics, which are commonly used during eye examinations, can precipitate acute glaucoma in patients with a predisposition to the disorder.

Equipment

Prescribed eye medication ■ gloves ■ warm water or normal saline solution ■ sterile gauze pads ■ facial tissues ■ Optional: ocular dressing.

Preparation of equipment

Make sure the medication is labeled for ophthalmic use. Remember to date the container the first time you open it.[1,2] Follow your facility's guideline or the manufacturer's recommendations on when to discard an opened eye medication.

Implementation

■ Avoid distractions and interruptions when preparing and administering the medication *to prevent medication administration errors.*[3,4]

■ Verify the order on the patient's medication record by checking it against the practitioner's in the medical record.[5,6,7]

■ Gather and prepare the appropriate medication and equipment.

■ Compare the medication label with the practitioner's order *to verify the correct medication, indication, dose, route, and time of administration.*[5,6,7] Confirm which eye requires treatment.

NURSING ALERT ***Make sure you know which eye to treat* because the practitioner may order different medications and doses for each eye.**

■ Check the patient's medical record for an allergy or other contraindication to the prescribed medication. If an allergy or other contraindication is present, don't administer the medication; instead, notify the practitioner.[5,6,7]

■ Visually inspect the medication for discoloration or any other loss of integrity. Don't give the medication if its integrity is compromised.[5,6,7]

■ Discuss any unresolved concerns about the medication with the patient's practitioner.[5,6,7]

■ Warm the medication to room temperature, if needed.

■ Perform hand hygiene.[8,9,10,11,12]

■ Confirm the patient's identify using at least two patient identifiers.[7,13]

■ If the patient is receiving the medication for the first time, inform the patient or family about possible significant adverse reactions and discuss any other concerns related to the medication.[5,6,7]

Instilling eyedrops

To instill eyedrops, pull the lower lid down *to expose the conjunctival sac.* Have the patient look up and away, and then squeeze the prescribed number of drops into the sac. Release the patient's eyelid, and have him blink *to distribute the medication.*

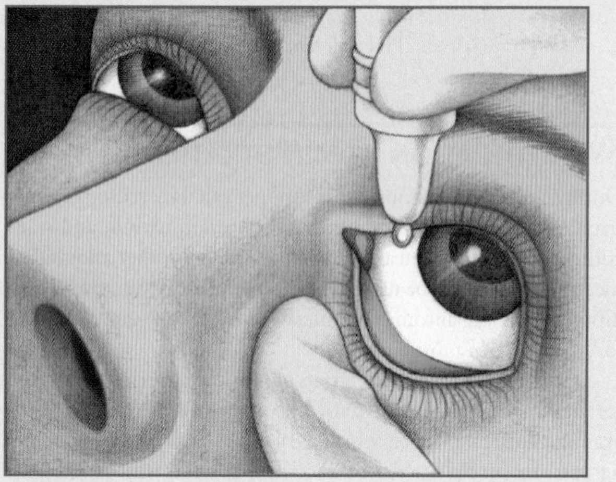

- If your facility uses a bar code scanning system, scan your identification badge, the patient's identification bracelet, and the medication's bar code.
- Explain the procedure to the patient and provide privacy.[14,15]
- Perform hand hygiene and then put on gloves.[8,9,10,11,12,16,17]
- If the patient is wearing an eye dressing, remove it by gently pulling it down and away from the patient's forehead. Take care not to contaminate your hands.
- Remove any discharge by cleaning around the eye with sterile gauze pads moistened with warm water or normal saline solution. With the patient's eye closed, clean from the inner to the outer canthus, using a fresh sterile gauze pad for each stroke.
- *To remove crusted secretions around the eye,* moisten a gauze pad with warm water or normal saline solution. Ask the patient to close the eye, and then place the gauze pad over it for 1 or 2 minutes. Remove the pad, and then repeat with new moist sterile gauze pads, as necessary, until the secretions are soft enough to be removed without traumatizing the mucosa.
- Remove and discard your gloves.
- Perform hand hygiene.[8,9,10,11,12]
- Put on new gloves.[16,17]
- Instruct the patient to tilt his head back and toward the side of the affected eye *so that excess medication can flow away from the tear duct, minimizing systemic absorption through the nasal mucosa.*

For eyedrops

- Remove the bottle top from the medication container, and place it on a clean, dry surface. Be careful to avoid contaminating the dropper tip or bottle top.
- Before instilling the eyedrops, instruct the patient to look up and away. *This position moves the cornea away from the lower lid and minimizes the risk of touching the cornea with the dropper if the patient blinks.*
- If necessary, steady the hand holding the dropper by resting it against the patient's forehead. With your other hand, gently pull down the lower lid of the affected eye and instill the drops in the conjunctival sac. Try to avoid placing the drops directly on the eyeball *to prevent the patient from experiencing discomfort.* (See *Instilling eyedrops.*)
- After instilling the eyedrops, instruct the patient to close both eyes gently, without squeezing the lids shut.
- *To prevent systemic absorption of medication,* gently press your thumb on the inner canthus for 2 to 3 minutes while the patient closes both eyes. *Doing so helps prevent medication from flowing into the tear ducts.*[18,19]
- Use a clean tissue to remove any excess solution leaking from the eye. Remember to use a fresh tissue for each eye *to prevent cross-contamination.*
- Replace the medication cap.
- Apply a new eye dressing, if necessary.
- Return the medication to the storage area. Make sure you store it according to the label's instructions.

For eye ointment

- Squeeze a small ribbon of medication on the edge of the conjunctival sac from the inner to the outer canthus. If necessary, steady the hand holding the medication tube by bracing it against the patient's forehead or cheek, taking care not to touch the tip of the tube to the eye or other surface. Cut off the ribbon by turning the tube.

For all eye medication

- Instruct the patient to close his eyes gently without squeezing the lids shut and to roll his eyes behind the closed lids *to help distribute the medication over the surface of the eyeball*
- Use a clean tissue *to remove any excess solution or ointment leaking from the eye.* Remember to use a fresh tissue for each eye *to prevent cross-contamination.*
- Replace the medication cap.
- Apply a new eye dressing, if necessary.
- Return the medication to the storage area. Make sure to store it according to the label's instructions.
- Remove and discard your gloves.
- Perform hand hygiene.[8,9,10,11,1]
- Document the procedure.[20,21,22]

Special considerations

- *To maintain the drug container's sterility,* never touch the tip of the bottle or dropper or the tip of the tube to the patient's eyeball, lids, or lashes. If the dropper tip becomes contaminated, discard the medication and obtain another sterile medication bottle.
- *To prevent cross-contamination,* never use a container of eye medication for more than one patient.
- If you're instilling more than one medication, wait at least 5 minutes between instillations. If the practitioner has ordered an eye ointment and eyedrops, administer the drops first *to enable the eyedrop medication to penetrate the eye without interference from the layer of ointment.*[19,23]
- Treat only the affected eye, unless otherwise ordered.

Complications

Instillation of some eye medications may cause transient burning, itching, and redness. Rarely, systemic effects may occur.

Patient teaching

If the practitioner has ordered eyedrops or ointment for home use, teach the patient the proper administration technique. Review the procedure and request a return demonstration. Ensure that the patient has refrigeration if needed to store the ointment or drops. Instruct the patient to contact the practitioner if the medication doesn't produce the desired effect within an indicated period or if eye irritation or changes in vision develop. Remind the patient that, to prevent cross-contamination, he must not share ophthalmic medications.

Documentation

Record the medication administered, eye or eyes treated, and date, time, and dose according to your facility's documentation format. Note the patient's response to the procedure and any adverse effects that occur. Document any patient teaching provided and the patient's understanding of that teaching.

REFERENCES

1 The Joint Commission. (2015). Standard MM.05.01.09. *Comprehensive accreditation manual for hospitals: The official handbook.* Oakbrook Terrace, IL: The Joint Commission. (Level VII)

2 American Osteopathic Association. (2014). Standard 25.01.18. *Healthcare Facilities Accreditation Program: Accreditation requirements for acute care hospitals.* Chicago, IL: American Osteopathic Association. (Level VII)

3 Westbrook, J., et al. (2010). Association of interruptions with an increased risk and severity of medication administration errors. *Archives of Internal Medicine, 170,* 683–690. (Level IV)

4 Institute for Safe Medication Practices. (2013). Side tracks on the safety express: Interruptions lead to errors and unfinished...Wait, what was I doing? *Nurse Advise-ERR, 11*(2), 1–4. Accessed March 2015 via the Web at https://www.ismp.org/Newsletters/acutecare/showarticle.aspx?id=37 (Level VII)

5 The Joint Commission. (2015). Standard MM.06.01.01. *Comprehensive accreditation manual for hospitals: The official handbook.* Oakbrook Terrace, IL: The Joint Commission. (Level VII)

6 Centers for Medicare & Medicaid Services, Department of Health and Human Services. (2014). Condition of participation: Nursing services. 42 C.F.R. § 482.23(c).

7 American Osteopathic Association. (2014). Standard 16.01.03. *Healthcare Facilities Accreditation Program: Accreditation requirements for acute care hospitals.* Chicago, IL: American Osteopathic Association. (Level VII)

8 The Joint Commission. (2015). Standard NPSG.07.01.01. *Comprehensive accreditation manual for hospitals: The official handbook.* Oakbrook Terrace, IL: The Joint Commission. (Level VII)

9 Centers for Disease Control and Prevention. (2002). Guideline for hand hygiene in health-care settings: Recommendations of the Healthcare Infection Control Practices Advisory Committee and the HICPAC/SHEA/APIC/IDSA Hand Hygiene Task Force. *MMWR Recommendations and Reports, 51*(RR-16), 1–45. Accessed March 2015 via the Web at http://www.cdc.gov/mmwr/pdf/rr/rr5116.pdf (Level II)

10 World Health Organization. (2009). "WHO guidelines on hand hygiene in health care: First global patient safety challenge, clean care is safer care" [Online]. Accessed March 2015 via the Web at http://whqlibdoc.who.int/publications/2009/9789241597906_eng.pdf (Level IV)

11 American Osteopathic Association. (2014). Standard 07.01.21. *Healthcare Facilities Accreditation Program: Accreditation requirements for acute care hospitals.* Chicago, IL: American Osteopathic Association. (Level VII)

12 Centers for Medicare & Medicaid Services, Department of Health and Human Services. (2014). Condition of participation: Infection control. 42 C.F.R. § 482.42.

13 The Joint Commission. (2015). Standard NPSG.01.01.01. *Comprehensive accreditation manual for hospitals: The official handbook.* Oakbrook Terrace, IL: The Joint Commission. (Level VII)

14 American Osteopathic Association. (2014). Standard 15.01.16. *Healthcare Facilities Accreditation Program: Accreditation requirements for acute care hospitals.* Chicago, IL: American Osteopathic Association. (Level VII)

15 Centers for Medicare & Medicaid Services, Department of Health and Human Services. (2014). Condition of participation: Patient's rights. 42 C.F.R. § 482.13(c)(1).

16 Siegel, J. D., et al. (2007). "2007 guideline for isolation precautions: Preventing transmission of infectious agents in healthcare settings" [Online]. Accessed March 2015 via the Web at http://www.cdc.gov/hicpac/pdf/isolation/Isolation2007.pdf (Level II)

17 American Osteopathic Association. (2014). Standard 07.01.10. *Healthcare Facilities Accreditation Program: Accreditation requirements for acute care hospitals.* Chicago, IL: American Osteopathic Association. (Level VII)

18 Taylor, C. R., et al. (2011). *Fundamentals of nursing: The art and science of nursing care* (7th ed.). Philadelphia, PA: Lippincott Williams & Wilkins.

19 Glaucoma Research Foundation. (2013). "Eye drop tips" [Online]. Accessed March 2015 via the Web at http://glaucoma.org/treatment/eyedrop-tips.php

20 The Joint Commission. (2015). Standard RC.01.03.01. *Comprehensive accreditation manual for hospitals: The official handbook.* Oakbrook Terrace, IL: The Joint Commission. (Level VII)

21 Centers for Medicare & Medicaid Services, Department of Health and Human Services. (2014). Condition of participation: Medical record services. 42 C.F.R. § 482.24(b).

22 American Osteopathic Association. (2014). Standard 10.00.03. *Healthcare Facilities Accreditation Program: Accreditation requirements for acute care hospitals.* Chicago, IL: American Osteopathic Association. (Level VII)

23 Callahan, D. (2014). "Using eye drops and ointment" [Online]. Accessed March 2015 via the Web at http://www.djo.harvard.edu/site.php?url=/patients/pi/413

ADDITIONAL REFERENCE

Nettina, S. M. (2014). *Lippincott manual of nursing practice* (10th ed.). Philadelphia, PA: Wolters Kluwer.

FALL PREVENTION AND MANAGEMENT

Falls are a major cause of injury and death among elderly people. Each year, one in three adults older than age 65 falls.[1] For hospitalized patients, falls are the most common safety incident, with rates of 1.7 to 25 falls per 1,000 patient stays.[2] One-third of these falls can be prevented.

Factors that contribute to falls among elderly patients include lengthy convalescent periods, incomplete recovery, medication use, increasing physical disability, and impaired vision, hearing, or mental status. For example, if an elderly person's equilibrium becomes impaired, it's likely to take longer to return to normal than it would for a younger adult—and, during that extended period of disequilibrium, the older adult is at an increased risk for falling. Falls not only cause physical injuries, but also trigger such psychological issues as a loss of self-confidence, which hastens dependence and a move to a long-term care facility or nursing home.

Extrinsic or environmental factors that increase the risk of falling include poor lighting, use of throw rugs, highly waxed floors, unfamiliar surroundings, or misuse of assistive devices. Intrinsic or physiologic factors include lower extremity weakness, vertigo, orthostatic hypotension, depression, failing eyesight, and functional or cognitive impairment.[3]

In a health care facility, an accidental fall can change a short stay for a minor problem into a prolonged stay for serious—and possibly life-threatening—problems. The risk of falling is highest during the first week of a stay in a health care or long-term care facility. (See *Who's at risk for a fall?*, page 314.)

Equipment

For fall management

Stethoscope ■ sphygmomanometer ■ thermometer ■ pillows ■ blankets ■ Optional: emergency equipment (crash cart with cardiac medications, defibrillator, hand-held resuscitation bag with mask, intubation equipment), electrocardiography (ECG) monitor, dressings, prescribed analgesics, cold and warm compresses.

Preparation of equipment

If you're helping a fallen patient, send an assistant to collect the assessment or resuscitation equipment you need.

Who's at risk for a fall?[3]

Preventing falls begins with identifying the patients at greatest risk. Consider a patient with one or more of the following characteristics to be at risk.

- Age 80 or older
- Lower extremity weakness
- Female gender
- A history of a recent fall
- Functional or cognitive impairment
- Dizziness
- Gait or balance impairment
- Depression
- Low body mass index
- Urinary incontinence
- Sensory deficits, particularly vision defects
- Orthostatic hypotension
- Use of more than four prescription medications
- Use of psychotropic medications
- Living in an environment that contains fall hazards

Implementation

- Perform hand hygiene.[4,5,6]
- Confirm the patient's identity using at least two patient identifiers.[7]

For fall prevention

- When the patient first enters the room, institute universal fall precautions *to make sure the environment is safe and the patient is comfortable.*[2] Orient the patient to the room and the call light *to help prevent falls related to an unfamiliar environment.* Have the patient perform a return demonstration on call light use.[8]
- Ask a patient who's age 65 or older or a patient who demonstrates unsteadiness or difficulty walking if he has fallen in the past 12 months. If he has, ask him about the frequency and circumstances of the fall, and evaluate him for gait and balance deficits.[3] Assess for proper use of assistive devices.
- Assess the patient's risk of falling, using either a standardized risk assessment form or one developed by your facility.[2] Assess such factors as the patient's history of falling, his mobility, what medications he takes, and his mental status. Note whether he's incontinent, has sensory deficits such as impaired vision, lives in an environment that contains fall hazards, or experiences orthostatic hypotension.[2] Perform a fall risk assessment after a change in the patient's condition, transfer from another unit, or a fall, or at a frequency determined by your facility. The optimal frequency for fall risk assessment hasn't yet been determined.[2]
- Make sure the patient is checked for potential dangers hourly during the daytime and evening and every 2 hours overnight *to comply with universal fall precautions.*[2] Correct potential dangers in the patient's room.
- Keep the call light positioned so it's within the patient's reach it at all times.[8]
- Provide adequate nighttime lighting.[8]
- Place the patient's personal belongings (such as a purse or wallet, books, and tissues) and assistive devices (such as a urinal or commode, cane, or walker) within easy reach.[8]
- Keep the bed in its lowest position *so the patient can easily reach the floor when he gets out of bed. This position also reduces the distance to the floor in case the patient falls.* Lock the bed's wheels.[8]
- Keep the patient's area uncluttered.[8]
- Keep floor surfaces clean and dry. Make sure spills are cleaned up immediately.[8]
- Instruct the patient to rise slowly from a supine position *to avoid possible dizziness and loss of balance.*[8]
- Advise the patient to wear well-fitting, nonskid footwear.[8]
- Respond promptly to the patient's call light *to help limit the number of times the patient gets out of bed without help.*
- Alert other caregivers to the patient's risk of falling and to the interventions you've implemented.[9]
- Assess the need for one-on-one patient monitoring, and arrange for it as needed.[8]
- Have a gait belt readily available at the patient's bedside, if needed, *for use during ambulation or transfer.*[8]
- Use a chair or bed alarm, if needed, *to alert staff members that the patient is attempting to get up without assistance.*[8]
- Encourage the patient to perform active range-of-motion (ROM) exercises *to improve flexibility and coordination.*
- Assist the patient with early and regular ambulation if his condition allows *because exercise reduces the risk of falling in older people.* Encourage the patient to use his regular assistive device for ambulation, such as a walker or cane or other equipment recommended by physical or occupational therapy.[8]
- If needed, regularly schedule assistance with toileting.[8]
- Review medications that may contribute to a fall.
- Perform hand hygiene.[4,5,6]
- Document the procedure.[10,11]

For fall management

- If you're with a patient as he falls, maintain your grip on the gait belt (if present) and place your elbow against the patient's waist or thigh *to prevent the patient from going down or to lessen the force of the fall.*[12] If you're with a bariatric patient, move any objects out of the way that could cause injury, and try to protect the patient's head from striking any objects or the floor *because there's very little you can do to prevent the fall.*[13]
- Remain calm and stay with the patient *to prevent any further injury.*
- Ask a coworker to collect any equipment you may need, such as a stethoscope, a sphygmomanometer, an ECG monitor, and (if necessary) dressings *to control bleeding.*
- Assess the patient's circulation, airway, and breathing *to be sure the fall wasn't caused by respiratory or cardiac arrest.* If the patient is unresponsive and his breathing is absent or abnormal (for example, if he's only gasping), call a code and have a coworker obtain a crash cart containing a defibrillator.
- Check for a pulse; if you don't feel a pulse within 10 seconds, immediately begin chest compressions. Compress the adult's chest at a rate of at least 100 compressions a minute, with a compression depth of at least 2″ (5 cm). After starting compressions, deliver rescue breaths (each over 1 second) using a compression ratio of 30 chest compressions to two ventilations. When the crash cart with the defibrillator arrives, check the patient's rhythm and defibrillate if the patient has a shockable rhythm; otherwise, continue cardiopulmonary resuscitation.[14]

NURSING ALERT *Don't move the patient until you fully evaluate his status* to prevent further injury if an injury has occurred as a result of the fall.[2]

- *To determine the extent of the patient's injuries,* look for lacerations, abrasions, and obvious deformities. Note any deviations from the patient's baseline condition and notify the practitioner of them. Determine whether the patient experienced a head trauma, *which requires further diagnostic evaluation to rule out subdural hematoma.*

NURSING ALERT *Patients taking anticoagulants or on aspirin therapy who experience head trauma are at increased risk for subdural hematoma.*

- Take steps to control bleeding (if indicated), and obtain an X-ray if you suspect a fracture. Provide first aid for minor injuries, as needed.

- If you weren't present during the fall, confirm the patient's identity using at least two patient identifiers.[7] Ask the patient or a witness what happened. Ask whether the patient experienced pain or a change in level of consciousness.
- Provide reassurance, as needed, and observe for such signs and symptoms as confusion, tremor, weakness, pain, and dizziness.
- Assess the patient's limb strength and motion. Don't perform ROM exercises if you suspect a fracture or if the patient complains of any odd sensations or limited movement. If you suspect an injury, don't move the patient until a practitioner examines him.
- While the patient lies on the floor until the practitioner arrives, offer pillows and blankets *for comfort.* However, if you suspect a spinal cord injury, don't place a pillow under the patient's head.
- If you don't detect any problems, return the patient to his bed with the help of another staff member. Never try to lift a patient alone *because you may injure yourself or the patient.*
- Even if the patient shows no signs of distress or has sustained only minor injuries, monitor his vital signs and assess his neurologic status frequently until his condition stabilizes. Notify the practitioner if you note any change from the baseline.
- Perform a comprehensive pain assessment using techniques appropriate for the patient's age, condition, and ability to understand.[15]
- Perform necessary measures *to relieve the patient's pain and discomfort.* Administer analgesics, as ordered, following safe medication administration practices. Apply cold compresses for the first 24 hours and warm compresses, as needed.
- Perform a postfall assessment *to determine the root cause of the fall.*[2] Gather assessment data from the patient, staff members, and any witnesses to the fall. Review the events that preceded the fall and any contributing factors. Discuss why it occurred and how it could have been prevented. Assess the patient's environment, looking for possible causes of the fall. Review medications, such as sedative and opioids, that may have contributed to the fall. (See *Medications associated with falls.*) Assess for gait disturbances or improper use of a cane, crutches, or a walker.[3]
- Monitor the patient's status for the next 48 hours or for a period determined by your facility and the patient's condition.[16]
- Perform hand hygiene.[4,5,6]
- Update the patient's risk profile.[2]
- Document the procedure.[10,11]

Special considerations

- If you don't already have a fall prevention program or interdisciplinary fall team in place in your facility, consider starting such a program.[2]

NURSING ALERT *Perform a risk assessment for falls on all admitted patients.*[3,9]

- Devise an alternative to physical restraints for high-risk patients *because physical restraints increase the risk of falling.* For example, consider using a pressure-pad alarm system in chairs and beds.[9] This system uses a pressure-sensor pad that's placed under a patient's bed linens or chair pad. When the patient gets out of bed or rises from the chair, the reduced pressure triggers an alarm that sounds at the nurses' station. A similar system consists of a control unit and a lightweight plastic pressure-sensor sheet that can be used on either a bed or a chair. Make sure you set it up according to the manufacturer's directions *to prevent false alarms.* An alternative alarm device consists of a sensor that the patient wears just above the knee; the sensor sounds an alarm when the patient moves his leg to a vertical position.
- *To promote patient safety,* add an appropriate notation (such as "Risk for falls") to the patient's medical record.[9]
- Provide emotional support. Let the elderly patient know that you recognize his limitations and acknowledge his fears. Point out measures that you'll take to provide a safe environment.

Medications associated with falls

This chart highlights some classes of drugs and the possible adverse effects of each that may increase a patient's risk of falling.

DRUG CLASS	ADVERSE EFFECTS
Diuretics	Hypovolemia, orthostatic hypotension, electrolyte imbalance, urinary incontinence
Antihypertensives	Hypotension, syncope
Beta-adrenergic blockers	Hypotension, syncope
Nitrates	Hypotension, syncope
Vasodilators	Hypotension, syncope
Tricyclic antidepressants	Orthostatic hypotension
Antipsychotics	Orthostatic hypotension, muscle rigidity, sedation
Benzodiazepines	Excessive sedation, confusion, paradoxical agitation, loss of balance
Antihistamines	Excessive sedation, confusion, paradoxical agitation, loss of balance
Opioids	Hypotension, sedation, motor incoordination, agitation
Hypnotics	Excessive sedation, ataxia, poor balance, confusion, paradoxical agitation
Antidiabetic drugs	Acute hypoglycemia
Alcohol	Intoxication, motor incoordination, agitation, sedation, confusion

- After a fall, review the patient's medical history *to determine whether he's at risk for other complications.* For example, if he hit his head, check his history to see whether he takes anticoagulants. If he does, he's at greater risk for intracranial bleeding, and you'll need to monitor him accordingly.

Patient teaching

Teach the patient how to fall safely. Show him how to protect his hands and face. If he uses a walker or a wheelchair, demonstrate how to cope with and recover from a fall. Instruct him to survey the room for a low, sturdy, supportive piece of furniture (such as a coffee table). Then review the proper procedure for lifting himself off the floor and either standing up with the walker or getting into the wheelchair. Also review with the patient how to call out for help if he can't get up.

Before discharge, teach the patient and his family how to prevent accidental falls at home by correcting common household hazards. Encourage them to take steps to ensure safety. (See *Promoting safety in the home,* page 316.)

PATIENT TEACHING

Promoting safety in the home

Before a patient leaves the health care facility, provide him and his family with a list of the following tips *to help ensure a safe home environment*:

- Secure all carpets and floor coverings around the edges, and tack down worn spots. Never use lightweight, loose mats or throw rugs on bare floors.
- Make sure potential hazards such as stairs are well lighted. Use white paint on either side of a staircase *to enhance visibility*.
- Install strong banisters along all indoor and outdoor steps.
- Use a bedside lamp or low-wattage night-light in the bedroom *to avoid the need to grope around in the dark when getting out of bed*.
- Fit secure handrails in convenient places in the shower and bathtub and around the toilet. Use nonskid mats inside and alongside every tub or shower.
- Minimize clutter. Store children's toys, especially those on wheels, when not in use.
- Walk carefully if you have a pet, such as a dog or a cat, *to avoid tripping*.
- Secure wires from electrical appliances to walls or moldings.
- Store frequently used clothing and other items in places where they can be reached without standing on a stool or chair.
- Sit on the edge of a bed or chair for a few minutes before rising, especially if you take a medication that can make you feel dizzy when you stand up.
- Use a walking stick, cane, or walker whenever you feel unsteady, but always inspect the condition of the assistive device before use.

As needed, refer the patient to the local visiting nurse association *so that nursing services can continue after discharge and during convalescence*.

Documentation

Document any measures taken to help prevent a fall, including patient and family teaching.

After a fall, complete a detailed incident report to help track frequent patient falls so that prevention measures can be used with high-risk patients. Used primarily for your facility's insurance carrier, this report isn't considered part of the patient's record. However, a copy will go to the facility's administrator, who will evaluate care given on the unit and propose new safety policies, as appropriate. It may also go to other patient care teams, such as fall prevention teams.

Make sure the incident report notes where and when the fall occurred, how the patient was found, and in what position. Include the events preceding the fall, the names of witnesses, the patient's reaction to the fall, and a detailed description of his condition based on assessment findings. Also include the patient's statement of the event. Note any interventions taken and the names of other staff members who helped care for the patient after the fall. Record the practitioner's name and the date and time that he was notified as well as the patient's health care power of attorney and the date and time he was notified. Include a copy of the practitioner's report. Also note whether the patient was sent for diagnostic tests or transferred to another unit.

Include all of the information about the fall in the patient's record. Also document his vital signs and whether you're monitoring the patient for a severe complication.

REFERENCES

1 Centers for Disease Control and Prevention, National Center for Injury Prevention and Control. (2012). "Falls among older adults: An overview" [Online]. Accessed March 2015 via the Web at http://www.cdc.gov/homeandrecreationalsafety/falls/adultfalls.html

2 Ganz, D. A., et al. (2013). Preventing falls in hospitals: A toolkit for improving quality of care (AHRQ Publication No. 13-0015-EF). Rockville, MD: Agency for Healthcare Research and Quality. (Level VII)

3 American Geriatrics Society & British Geriatrics Society. (2010). "Prevention of falls in older persons: AGS/BGS clinical practice guideline" [Online]. Accessed March 2015 via the Web at http://www.medcats.com/FALLS/frameset.htm (Level VI)

4 Centers for Disease Control and Prevention. (2002). Guideline for hand hygiene in health-care settings: Recommendations of the Healthcare Infection Control Practices Advisory Committee and the HICPAC/SHEA/APIC/IDSA Hand Hygiene Task Force. *MMWR Recommendations and Reports, 51*(RR-16), 1–45. Accessed March 2015 via the Web at http://www.cdc.gov/mmwr/pdf/rr/rr5116.pdf (Level II)

5 World Health Organization. (2009). "WHO guidelines on hand hygiene in health care: First global patient safety challenge, clean care is safer care" [Online]. Accessed March 2015 via the Web at http://whqlibdoc.who.int/publications/2009/9789241597906_eng.pdf (Level IV)

6 The Joint Commission. (2015). Standard NPSG.07.01.01. *Comprehensive accreditation manual for hospitals: The official handbook.* Oakbrook Terrace, IL: The Joint Commission. (Level VII)

7 The Joint Commission. (2015). Standard NPSG.01.01.01. *Comprehensive accreditation manual for hospitals: The official handbook.* Oakbrook Terrace, IL: The Joint Commission. (Level VII)

8 Institute for Clinical Systems Improvement. (2012). "Health care protocol: Prevention of falls (acute care) protocol (3rd ed.)" [Online] Accessed March 2015 via the Web at https://www.icsi.org/_asset/dcn15z/Falls-Interactive0412.pdf (Level VII)

9 The Joint Commission. (2015). Standard PC.01.02.08. *Comprehensive accreditation manual for hospitals: The official handbook.* Oakbrook Terrace, IL: The Joint Commission. (Level VII)

10 The Joint Commission. (2015). Standard RC.01.03.01. *Comprehensive accreditation manual for hospitals: The official handbook.* Oakbrook Terrace, IL: The Joint Commission (Level VII)

11 Centers for Medicare & Medicaid Services, Department of Health and Human Services. (2014). Condition of participation: Medical record services. 42 C.F.R. § 482.24(b).

12 Thompson Medical, Inc. (n.d.). "How to use a transfer/gait belt" [Online]. Accessed March 2015 via the Web at http://www.thompsonmedical.com/pdf/How%20to%20Use%20a%20Transfer.pdf

13 Waters, T. R., et al. (2009). "Safe patient handling training for schools of nursing (DHHS [NIOSH] Publication No. 2009-127)" [Online]. Accessed March 2015 via the Web at http://www.cdc.gov/niosh/docs/2009-127/pdfs/2009-127.pdf (Level VII)

14 American Heart Association. (2010). 2010 American Heart Association guidelines for cardiopulmonary resuscitation and emergency cardiovascular care. *Circulation, 122,* S676–S684. (Level II)

15 The Joint Commission. (2015). Standard PC.01.02.07. *Comprehensive accreditation manual for hospitals: The official handbook.* Oakbrook Terrace, IL: The Joint Commission. (Level VII)

16 Gray-Micelli, D., & Quigley, P. A. (2012). "Falls: Fall prevention: Assessment, diagnosis, and intervention strategies" [Online]. Accessed March 2015 via the Web at http://consultgerirn.org/topics/falls/want_to_know_more (Level VII)

ADDITIONAL REFERENCES

Boddice, S. D., & Kogan, P. (2009). Research on patient safety: Falls and medications. *Home Healthcare Nurse, 27*(9), 555–560.

Titler, M. G., et al. (2011). Factors associated with falls during hospitalization in an older adult population. *Research and Theory for Nursing Practice, 25,* 127–148.

FECAL IMPACTION REMOVAL, DIGITAL

Fecal impaction—a large, hard, dry mass of stool in the folds of the rectum and, at times, in the sigmoid colon—results from prolonged retention and accumulation of stool. Common causes include poor bowel habits, inactivity, dehydration, improper diet (especially inadequate fluid intake), constipation-inducing drugs, and incomplete bowel cleaning after a barium enema or barium swallow. Digital removal of fecal impaction is used when oil retention and cleansing enemas, suppositories, and laxatives fail to clear the impaction. It typically requires a practitioner's order.

Common manifestations of fecal impaction include abdominal cramping and bloating; leakage of liquid or sudden episodes of watery diarrhea in someone who has chronic constipation; rectal bleeding; small, semiformed stools; or straining when trying to pass stools. Other possible signs and symptoms include bladder pressure or loss of bladder control, lower back pain, or tachycardia or light-headedness from straining to pass stool.

This procedure is contraindicated during pregnancy; after rectal, genitourinary, abdominal, perineal, or gynecologic reconstructive surgery; in patients with myocardial infarction, coronary insufficiency, pulmonary embolus, heart failure, heart block, and Stokes-Adams syndrome (without pacemaker treatment); and in patients with GI or vaginal bleeding, hemorrhoids, rectal polyps, or blood dyscrasias.

Equipment

Equipment for measuring vital signs ■ gloves (two pairs) ■ fluid-impermeable pad ■ bedpan or bedside commode ■ toilet paper ■ disposal plastic bag ■ soap ■ water-filled basin ■ towel ■ water-soluble lubricant ■ washcloth ■ bath blanket ■ Optional: drawsheet.

Implementation

- Verify the practitioner's order.
- Gather the appropriate equipment.
- Perform hand hygiene.[1,2,3,4,5]
- Confirm the patient's identity using at least two patient identifiers.[6]
- Explain the procedure to the patient *to enhance cooperation.*
- Provide privacy.[7]
- Obtain baseline vital signs *because anal stimulation may cause a vagal response.*
- Position the patient on his left side and flex his knees *to allow easier access to the sigmoid colon and rectum.* (See *Side-lying position.*)
- Drape the patient with a bath blanket, and place a fluid-impermeable pad beneath the buttocks *to prevent soiling the bed linens.*
- Put on gloves.[8,9]
- Moisten an index finger with water-soluble lubricant *to reduce friction during insertion, avoiding injury to sensitive tissue.*
- Instruct the patient to breathe deeply *to promote relaxation.* Then gently insert your lubricated index finger beyond the anal sphincter until you touch the impaction. Rotate the finger gently around the stool *to dislodge and break it into small fragments.* Then work the fragments downward to the end of the rectum, and remove each one separately. Monitor the patient throughout the procedure.

NURSING ALERT *If the patient experiences pain, nausea, rectal bleeding, change in pulse rate or skin color, diaphoresis, or syncope, stop the procedure immediately and notify the practitioner.*

- Remove hardened fecal material gently from the rectum and dispose of it in the appropriate receptacle.[8]
- Gently stimulate the anal sphincter with a circular motion two or three times *to increase peristalsis and encourage evacuation before removing your finger.*
- Remove and discard your gloves.[8]
- Perform hand hygiene[1,2,3,4,5] and put on gloves.[8,9]
- Clean the anal area with a washcloth, soap, and water, and lightly pat it dry with a towel.

Side-lying position

Use a drawsheet or bath blanket to place the patient in a side-lying position.

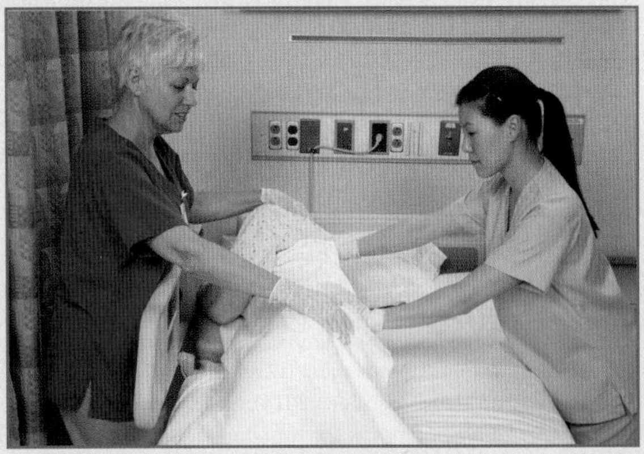

- Offer the patient the bedpan or commode and toilet tissue *because digital manipulation stimulates the urge to defecate.*
- Place the patient's call light within reach and instruct him to call for assistance as needed.
- Place disposable items in the disposable plastic bag, and discard properly.[8] If necessary, clean the bedpan and return it to the patient's bathroom.[10,11]
- Remove and discard your gloves.[8]
- Perform hand hygiene.[1,2,3,4,5]
- Document the procedure.[12,13,14]

Special considerations

- After the disimpaction is completed, you may need administer an enema or a suppository, as ordered, to complete stool removal. The most important aspect of care is preventing recurrence of elimination problems.

Patient teaching

Teach the patient about normal bowel physiology and function. Inform him that untreated fecal impaction can become a serious health problem, producing a chronically overdilated bowel, or megacolon, that can require surgical correction. In addition, rectal tissue can become damaged, ulcerated, or even necrotic. The most serious potential complication is complete obstruction of the lower bowel. Teach him strategies, such as diet and lifestyle changes, biofeedback, and bowel retraining, *to prevent a recurrence of fecal impaction.*

Complications

Digital removal of fecal impaction can stimulate the vagus nerve and may decrease heart rate and cause syncope. Potential damage to the mucous membrane lining of the bowel, which increases the risk of bleeding, inflammation, and infection, may also occur.

Documentation

Record the time and date of the procedure, the patient's response, and stool color, consistency, and odor.

REFERENCES

1 The Joint Commission. (2015). Standard NPSG.07.01.01. *Comprehensive accreditation manual for hospitals: The official handbook.* Oakbrook Terrace, IL: The Joint Commission. (Level VII)

2 Centers for Disease Control and Prevention. (2002). Guideline for hand hygiene in health-care settings: Recommendations of the Healthcare Infection Control Practices Advisory Committee and the HICPAC/SHEA/APIC/IDSA Hand Hygiene Task Force. *MMWR Recommendations and Reports, 51*(RR-16), 1–45. Accessed March 2015 via the Web at http://www.cdc.gov/mmwr/pdf/rr/rr5116.pdf (Level II)

3 World Health Organization. (2009). "WHO guidelines on hand hygiene in health care: First global patient safety challenge, clean care is safer care" [Online]. Accessed March 2015 via the Web at http://whqlibdoc.who.int/publications/2009/9789241597906_eng.pdf (Level IV)

4 Centers for Medicare & Medicaid Services, Department of Health and Human Services. (2014). Condition of participation: Infection control. 42 C.F.R. § 482.42.

5 American Osteopathic Association. (2014). Standard 07.01.21. *Healthcare Facilities Accreditation Program: Accreditation requirements for acute care hospitals.* Chicago, IL: American Osteopathic Association. (Level VII)

6 The Joint Commission. (2015). Standard NPSG.01.01.01. *Comprehensive accreditation manual for hospitals: The official handbook.* Oakbrook Terrace, IL: The Joint Commission. (Level VII)

7 American Osteopathic Association. (2014). Standard 15.01.16. *Healthcare Facilities Accreditation Program: Accreditation requirements for acute care hospitals.* Chicago, IL: American Osteopathic Association. (Level VII)

8 Siegel, J. D., et al. (2007). "2007 guideline for isolation precautions: Preventing transmission of infectious agents in healthcare settings" [Online]. Accessed March 2015 via the Web at http://www.cdc.gov/hicpac/pdf/isolation/Isolation2007.pdf (Level II)

9 American Osteopathic Association. (2014). Standard 07.01.10. *Healthcare Facilities Accreditation Program: Accreditation requirements for acute care hospitals.* Chicago, IL: American Osteopathic Association. (Level VII)

10 Rutala, W. A., et al. (2008). "Guideline for disinfection and sterilization in healthcare facilities, 2008" [Online]. Accessed March 2015 via the Web at http://www.cdc.gov/hicpac/pdf/guidelines/Disinfection_Nov_2008.pdf (Level I)

11 American Osteopathic Association. (2014). Standard 07.02.03. *Healthcare Facilities Accreditation Program: Accreditation requirements for acute care hospitals.* Chicago, IL: American Osteopathic Association. (Level VII)

12 The Joint Commission. (2015). Standard RC.01.03.01. *Comprehensive accreditation manual for hospitals: The official handbook.* Oakbrook Terrace, IL: The Joint Commission. (Level VII)

13 Centers for Medicare & Medicaid Services, Department of Health and Human Services. (2014). Condition of participation: Medical record services. 42 C.F.R. § 482.24(b).

14 American Osteopathic Association. (2014). Standard 10.00.03. *Healthcare Facilities Accreditation Program: Accreditation requirements for acute care hospitals.* Chicago, IL: American Osteopathic Association. (Level VII)

Additional references

Craven, R. F., & Hirnle, C. J. (2012). *Fundamentals of nursing: Human health and function* (7th ed.). Philadelphia, PA: Lippincott Williams & Wilkins.

Halawi, H. M., et al. (2012). Faecal impaction: In-hospital complications and their predictors in a retrospective study on 130 patients. *Colorectal Disease, 14,* 231–236. (Level IV)

Ness, W. (2013). Digital removal of faeces. *Nursing Times, 109*(17-18), 18–20.

Obokhare, I. (2012). Fecal impaction: A cause for concern? *Clinics in Colon and Rectal Surgery, 25,* 53–58. (Level V)

Fecal occult blood tests

Fecal occult blood tests are valuable for determining the presence of GI bleeding and for distinguishing between true melena and melena-like stools. (Certain medications, such as iron supplements and bismuth compounds, can darken stools so that they resemble melena.)

These tests are particularly important for early detection of colorectal cancer because 80% of patients with this disorder test positive. However, a single positive test result doesn't confirm GI bleeding or indicate colorectal cancer. To confirm a positive result, the test must be repeated at least three times while the patient follows a special diet, according to the manufacturer's recommendations for the particular occult blood test. Even then, a confirmed positive test doesn't necessarily indicate colorectal cancer; GI bleeding can also result from many causes other than cancer, such as ulcers, colon polyps, and diverticula. However, a positive result does indicate the need for further diagnostic studies.

Fecal occult blood tests are easily performed on collected specimens or smears from a digital rectal examination. The guaiac-based Hemoccult® tests, which include Hemoccult SENSA® and Hemoccult II®, are commonly used; of the two, Hemoccult SENSA® has greater sensitivity for cancer and advanced adenomas. Both tests produce a blue reaction in a fecal smear if occult blood loss exceeds 2 mL in 24 hours.

A newer test, the fecal immunochemical test (FIT), detects human globin, a protein that—along with heme—constitutes human hemoglobin; this makes the FIT more specific for human blood than such guaiac-based tests as the Hemoccult SENSA®. The FIT is also more specific for lower GI bleeding, which makes it more specific for detecting colorectal cancer. Some FITs also require fewer samples and less direct handling of stool.

Equipment

Gloves.

For a guaiac-based slide test

Guaiac test slide with quality-control monitors ■ guaiac developing solution ■ specimen applicator sticks.

For a FIT

FIT kit with long-handled brushes and test card ■ label ■ laboratory transport bag.

Preparation of equipment

Always check the condition and expiration dates of the slides and developing solution before use. Discard any damaged, discolored, or expired products. Hemoccult SENSA® test slides contain guaiac paper; keep the cover flap of the slide sealed until ready to use.

Implementation

- Verify the practitioner's order.
- Gather the appropriate equipment.
- Perform hand hygiene.[1,2,3,4,5]
- Confirm the patient's identity using at least two patient identifiers.[6]
- Explain the procedure to the patient.
- Check the patient's history for medications and conditions that may interfere with the test.
- Put on gloves.[7,8]
- Collect a stool specimen. (See the "Stool specimen collection" procedure, page 718.)

To perform a guaiac-based slide test

- Open the flap on the slide packet.[9]
- Use a specimen applicator stick to apply a thin smear of the stool specimen to the guaiac-impregnated filter paper exposed in box A. Alternatively, after performing a digital rectal examination, wipe the finger you used for the examination on a square of the filter paper.[9]
- Apply a second smear from another part of the specimen to the filter paper exposed in box B *because some parts of the specimen may not contain blood.*[9]
- Allow the specimen to dry for 3 to 5 minutes.[9]
- Open the flap on the reverse side of the slide package.[9]
- Place two drops of guaiac developing solution on the paper over each smear.[9]

■ Wait for a reaction; a blue reaction will appear in 30 to 60 seconds if the test is positive. Any trace of blue on or at the edge of the smear is positive for occult blood and can be recorded before the end of 60 seconds. Absence of blue at the end of 60 seconds is negative for occult blood. (Wait the full 60 seconds before recording a negative result.)[9]

NURSING ALERT *This test is visually read and requires color differentiation. You shouldn't interpret it if you have a blue color deficiency (color blindness).*[9]

■ *Perform a quality-control test* by applying 1 drop of developer between the positive and negative quality-control areas. Read the quality-control test results within 10 seconds. If the slide and developer are functioning properly, blue will appear in the positive area and no blue will appear in the negative area. If the quality-control test fails to react as expected after application of the developer, the patient's test results are invalid and shouldn't be documented. Repeat the procedure using new equipment.[9]
■ Record the results.
■ Discard the slide package in an appropriate receptacle.[7]
■ Remove and discard your gloves.[7]
■ Perform hand hygiene.[1,2,3,4,5]
■ Document the procedure.[10,11,12]

To perform a FIT

■ Open the flap of the test card.
■ Remove one of the long-handled brushes from the kit.
■ Gently brush the surface of the stool with the brush and then rinse the brush in the toilet water surrounding the stool.
■ Dab the brush onto the test card and then close the flap.
■ Label the specimen in the presence of the *patient to prevent mislabeling.*[6]
■ Place the test card in the laboratory biohazard transport bag and send it to the laboratory.[13]
■ Remove and discard your gloves.[7]
■ Perform hand hygiene.[1,2,3,4,5]
■ Document the procedure.[10,11,12]

Special considerations

■ Test stool specimens as soon as possible after collection, and make sure they aren't contaminated with urine, soap solution, iodine, or toilet tissue.
■ Test samples from several different portions of the same specimen *because occult blood from the upper GI tract isn't always evenly dispersed throughout the formed stool; likewise, blood from colorectal bleeding may occur mostly on the outer stool surface.*
■ Check the expiration date on Hemoccult® slides and developer, and protect unused slides from heat, moisture, light, and chemicals.
■ Don't exchange developers with different manufacturers or brands.
■ Make sure to develop the internal controls (performance monitors) after the patient's test has been developed; follow this practice with every test.
■ Don't collect specimens during or until 3 days after a female patient's menstrual period *to avoid a false-positive test resulting from contamination of the specimen.*
■ Be aware that ingestion of 2 to 5 mL of blood (such as from bleeding gums), active bleeding from hemorrhoids, or hematuria can produce false-positive results.
■ If repeated testing is necessary after a positive screening test, explain the test to the patient. Instruct him to maintain a high-fiber diet and to refrain from eating red meat, poultry, fish, turnips, and horseradish for 48 to 72 hours before the test as well as throughout the collection period *because these substances can alter test results.*
■ As ordered, have the patient discontinue the use of iron preparations, bromides, iodides, rauwolfia derivatives, indomethacin, colchicine, salicylates, potassium, bismuth compounds, steroids, and ascorbic acid for 48 to 72 hours before the test as well as during it *to ensure accurate test results and to avoid the possible bleeding that some of these compounds can cause.*
■ Guaiac slides and developer are ready for use as packaged but must be stored and used appropriately according to the manufacturer's instructions. Store products at a controlled room temperature of 59° to 86°F (15° to 30°C). Don't use them past the expiration date stamped on each slide and developer bottle. Protect them from heat, light, volatile chemicals, and refrigeration temperatures. Watch for signs of deterioration, including discoloration of the normally off-white guaiac paper and failure of the control system to react as expected (subsequent test results should be regarded as invalid).
■ Note that the developer is an irritant; avoid contact with the skin and eyes. If contact should occur, rinse promptly with water and consult a practitioner.

Patient teaching

If the patient will be using the Hemoccult® slide packet or the FIT at home, advise him to complete the label on the slide packet before specimen collection. If he'll be using a ColoCARE® test packet, inform him that this test is a preliminary screen for occult blood in his stool. Tell him he won't have to obtain a stool specimen to perform the test but that he should follow your instructions carefully. (See *Home tests for fecal occult blood.*)

Documentation

Record the time and date of the test, the name and title of the person interpreting the test, the test result, and any unusual characteristics of the stool tested. Report positive results to the practitioner. Document any patient teaching provided.

PATIENT TEACHING

Home tests for fecal occult blood

Although most fecal occult blood tests require the patient to collect a specimen of stool and to smear it on a slide, the ColoCARE test doesn't, making the procedure safer and simpler.

If the patient will be performing the ColoCARE test at home, tell him to avoid red meat and vitamin C supplements for 2 days beforehand. He should check with his practitioner about discontinuing any medications before the test. Drugs that may interfere with test results include aspirin, indomethacin, corticosteroids, reserpine, dietary supplements, anticancer drugs, and anticoagulants. The patient should also talk to the practitioner about his medical conditions *to determine the timing of the test.* For example, the patient shouldn't take the test if he has bleeding hemorrhoids, peptic ulcers, or gastritis. In addition, women who are at or near the time of menstruation shouldn't take the test.

To perform the test, tell the patient to follow these steps:
■ Flush the toilet twice just before performing the test *to remove any toilet-cleaning chemicals from the tank.*
■ Defecate into the toilet but don't throw toilet paper into the bowl.
■ Within 5 minutes, remove the test pad from its pouch and float it printed side up on the water.
■ Watch the pad for 15 to 30 seconds for any evidence of blue or green color changes
■ Record the result on the reply card.
■ Emphasize that the patient should perform this test with three consecutive bowel movements and then send the completed card to his practitioner. However, inform him that he should call his practitioner immediately if he notes a positive color change in the first test.

REFERENCES

1 The Joint Commission. (2015). Standard NPSG.07.01.01. *Comprehensive accreditation manual for hospitals: The official handbook.* Oakbrook Terrace, IL: The Joint Commission. (Level VII)

2 Centers for Disease Control and Prevention. (2002). Guideline for hand hygiene in health-care settings: Recommendations of the Healthcare Infection Control Practices Advisory Committee and the HICPAC/SHEA/APIC/IDSA Hand Hygiene Task Force. *MMWR Recommendations and Reports, 51*(RR-16), 1–45. Accessed March 2015 via the Web at http://www.cdc.gov/mmwr/pdf/rr/rr5116.pdf (Level II)

3 World Health Organization. (2009). "WHO guidelines on hand hygiene in health care: First global patient safety challenge, clean care is safer care" [Online]. Accessed March 2015 via the Web at http://whqlibdoc.who.int/publications/2009/9789241597906_eng.pdf (Level IV)

4 Centers for Medicare & Medicaid Services, Department of Health and Human Services. (2014). Condition of participation: Infection control. 42 C.F.R. § 482.42.

5 American Osteopathic Association. (2014). Standard 07.01.21. *Healthcare Facilities Accreditation Program: Accreditation requirements for acute care hospitals.* Chicago, IL: American Osteopathic Association. (Level VII)

6 The Joint Commission. (2015). Standard NPSG.01.01.01. *Comprehensive accreditation manual for hospitals: The official handbook.* Oakbrook Terrace, IL: The Joint Commission. (Level VII)

7 Siegel, J. D., et al. (2007). "2007 guideline for isolation precautions: Preventing transmission of infectious agents in healthcare settings" [Online]. Accessed March 2015 via the Web at http://www.cdc.gov/hicpac/pdf/isolation/Isolation2007.pdf (Level II)

8 American Osteopathic Association. (2014). Standard 07.01.10. *Healthcare Facilities Accreditation Program: Accreditation requirements for acute care hospitals.* Chicago, IL: American Osteopathic Association. (Level VII)

9 Beckman Coulter, Inc. (2009). "Hemoccult® Sensa®: Product instructions" [Online]. Accessed March 2015 via the Web at https://www.beckmancoulter.com/wsrportal/bibliography?docname=HOSEN%20-%20462489.EA.pdf

10 The Joint Commission. (2015). Standard RC.01.03.01. *Comprehensive accreditation manual for hospitals: The official handbook.* Oakbrook Terrace, IL: The Joint Commission. (Level VII)

11 Centers for Medicare & Medicaid Services, Department of Health and Human Services. (2014). Condition of Participation: Medical record services. 42 C.F.R. § 482.24(b).

12 American Osteopathic Association. (2014). Standard 10.00.03. *Healthcare Facilities Accreditation Program: Accreditation requirements for acute care hospitals.* Chicago, IL: American Osteopathic Association.

13 Occupational Safety and Health Administration. (n.d.). "Bloodborne pathogens, standard number 1910.1030" [Online]. Accessed March 2015 via the Web at http://www.osha.gov/pls/oshaweb/owadisp.show_document?p_table=STANDARDS&p_id=10051 (Level VII)

ADDITIONAL REFERENCES

Chubak, J., et al. (2013). Uptake and positive predictive value of fecal occult blood tests: A randomized controlled trial. *Preventive Medicine, 57,* 671–678. (Level II)

Fischbach, F., & Dunning, M. B. (2014). *A manual of laboratory and diagnostic tests* (9th ed.). Philadelphia, PA: Wolters Kluwer.

Hinkle, J. L. & Cheever, K. H. (2014). *Brunner & Suddarth's textbook of medical-surgical nursing* (13th ed.). Philadelphia, PA: Wolters Kluwer.

Nettina, S. M. (2014). *Lippincott manual of nursing practice* (10th ed.). Philadelphia, PA: Wolters Kluwer.

FEEDING

Various disabilities and conditions may prevent a patient from self-feeding, including cognitive deficits, neuromuscular disease, cancer, obstructive lung disease, and traumatic injury. A patient who can't self-feed is susceptible to malnutrition. The patient's condition or its associated treatment may also result in pain, nausea, depression, and anorexia. Meeting such a patient's nutritional needs requires determining food preferences; feeding the patient in a friendly, unhurried manner; encouraging self-feeding to promote independence and dignity; and documenting intake and output.

Equipment

Meal tray ▪ overbed table ▪ fluid-impermeable pad or towels ▪ flexible straws ▪ basin of water ▪ soap ▪ washcloth ▪ hand towel ▪ hospital-approved disinfectant ▪ spoon or feeding syringe ▪ Optional: assistive feeding devices, prescribed pain medication, clean linens.

Implementation

- Gather the appropriate equipment.
- Review the patient's medical record for conditions that may affect her ability to feed herself. Note any feeding problems and techniques that were recommended by the speech pathologist to remedy those problems. Review the patient's medications for adverse effects that might interfere with her appetite.[1]
- Collaborate with a speech pathologist, as indicated, *to assess the patient's swallowing and subsequent risk of aspiration.* Follow recommendations prescribed by the speech *pathologist to reduce the patient's risk of aspiration.*
- Perform hand hygiene.[2,3,4,5,6]
- Confirm the patient's identity using at least two patient identifiers.[7]
- Assess the patient's neurologic status, dentition, and functional *status to determine whether oral feeding is appropriate.*
- Collaborate with the patient and her family *to determine food preferences (including ethnic foods).* Ask about the normal consistency of her foods as well as the timing and frequency of her meal pattern.[1]
- Perform a comprehensive pain assessment using techniques appropriate for the patient's age, condition, and ability to understand.[8]
- Administer pain medication, as needed and prescribed, following safe medication administration practices.
- Explain the procedure to the patient.
- *Because many adults consider being fed demeaning,* allow the patient some control over mealtime, such as letting her set the pace of the meal or deciding the order in which she eats various foods.
- Position the patient with the head of the bed elevated 30 to 45 degrees (as shown below), unless contraindicated, *to ease swallowing and reduce the risk of aspiration.*[9]

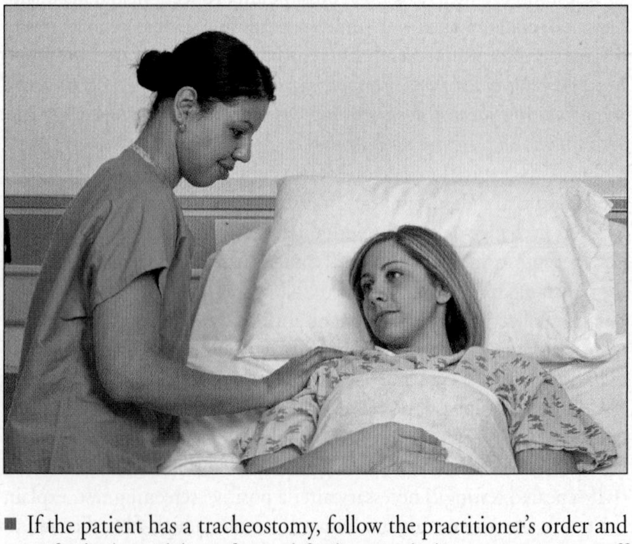

- If the patient has a tracheostomy, follow the practitioner's order and your facility's guidelines for oral feeding, including maintaining cuff pressure, applying a one-way valve, positioning the patient, and applying aspiration precautions.[10]

NURSING ALERT: *A tracheotomy may complicate feeding* because the tube interferes with normal swallowing. Between 20% and 70% of patients with a long-term tracheotomy experience at least one episode of aspiration every 48 hours. *In patients with prolonged critical illness or* *anticipated impaired swallowing, a fiber-optic evaluation of swallowing function is recommended before an oral feeding trial.*[10]

■ Before the meal tray arrives, give the patient soap, a basin of water or a wet washcloth, and a hand towel *to clean her hands.* If necessary, wash her hands for her (as shown below).

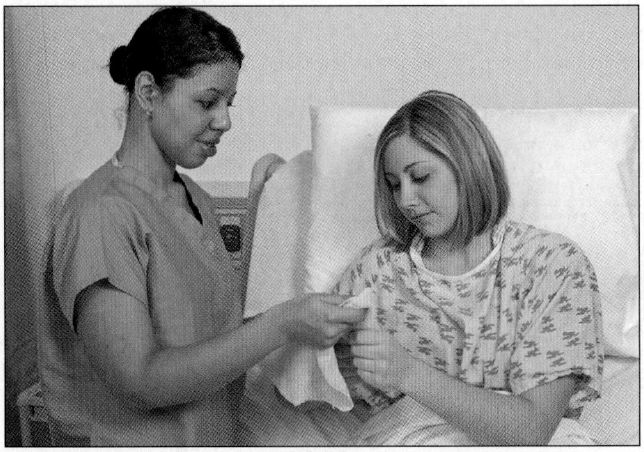

■ Wipe the overbed table with a hospital-approved disinfectant.[11]

■ Confirm that the correct tray has been delivered to the correct patient.

■ Check the tray to make sure it contains foods and fluids appropriate for the patient's condition.

■ Encourage the patient to feed herself if she can. If she's restricted to the prone or the supine position but can use her arms and hands, encourage her to try foods she can pick up, such as sandwiches. If she can assume the Fowler or semi-Fowler position but has limited use of her arms or hands, teach her how to use assistive feeding devices. (See *Using assistive feeding devices,* page 322.)

■ If necessary, tuck a napkin or towel under her chin *to protect her gown from spills* (as shown below). Use a fluid-impermeable pad or towel *to protect bed linens.*

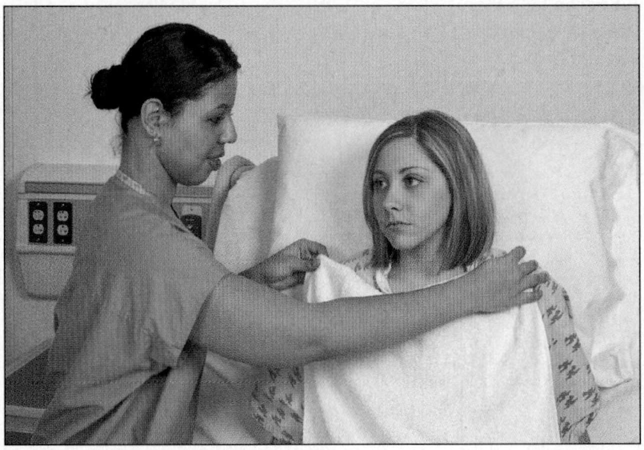

■ Position a chair next to the patient's bed *so you can sit comfortably if you need to feed her yourself.*

■ Face the patient during feeding, make eye contact, and use a gentle tone of voice.

■ Set up the patient's tray, remove the plate from the tray warmer, and discard all plastic wrappings. Then cut the food into bite-sized pieces (as shown on top right). Season food according to the patient's request, as appropriate.

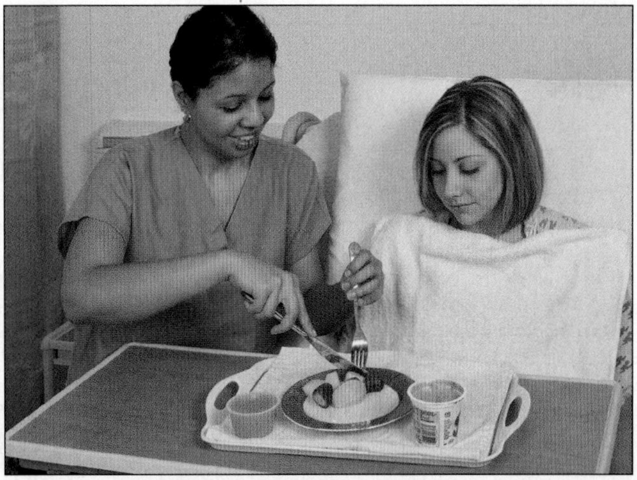

■ *To help a blind or visually impaired patient feed herself,* tell her that placement of various foods on her plate corresponds to the hours on a clock face. Maintain consistent placement for subsequent meals.

■ Ask the patient which food she prefers to eat first *to promote her sense of control over the meal. Some patients prefer to eat one food at a time; others prefer to alternate foods.*

■ Provide verbal encouragement to participate in eating by talking about the food's taste and smell and providing verbal prompts to chew and swallow.

■ Ask the patient to indicate when she's ready for another mouthful. Pause between courses and whenever the patient wants to rest. During the meal, wipe the patient's mouth and chin, as needed.

■ If the patient is at risk for aspiration, monitor her closely.

■ When the patient finishes eating, remove the tray. If necessary, clean up spills and change the bed linens.

■ Provide oral care. (See the "Oral care" procedure, page 560.)

■ Perform hand hygiene.[2,3,4,5,6]

■ Document oral intake, as ordered. (See *Recording fluid intake and output,* page 323.)

■ Document the procedure.[12,13,14]

Special considerations

■ A swallow evaluation is recommended before starting oral feeding in patients who require prolonged endotracheal intubation.[9]

■ If the patient is restricted to the supine position, provide foods that can be chewed easily, and feed her liquids carefully and only after she has swallowed any food in the mouth *to reduce the risk of aspiration.*

■ Establish a pattern for feeding the patient, and share this information with the other staff members *so the patient doesn't need to repeatedly instruct staff members about preferred feeding techniques.*

■ If the patient and family are willing, suggest that family members assist with feeding. *Such assistance will make the patient feel more comfortable at mealtimes and may ease discharge planning.*

Complications

Obstruction of the airway may lead to asphyxia, and aspiration of food can potentially cause hospital-acquired pneumonia. Undernutrition may occur in the patient with feeding dependence or if the patient denies feeding difficulties.

Documentation

Describe the feeding technique used in the nursing care plan to ensure continuity of care. Record the amount of food and fluid consumed; also note the fluids consumed on the intake and output record, if required. Note which foods the patient consistently fails to eat; then try to find the reason. Record the patient's level of independence. For a blind patient, record the pattern of feeding in the nursing care plan.

EQUIPMENT

Using assistive feeding devices

Various feeding devices can help the patient who has limited arm mobility, grasp, range of motion (ROM), or coordination. Before introducing the patient to an assistive feeding device, assess her ability to master it. Don't introduce a device she can't manage. If her condition is progressively disabling, encourage her to use the device only until her mastery of it falters.

Introduce the assistive device before mealtime, with the patient seated in a natural position. Explain its purpose, show the patient how to use it, and encourage her to practice. After meals, wash the device thoroughly and store it in the patient's bedside stand. Document the patient's progress and share it with staff and family members *to help reinforce the patient's independence*. Specific devices include the following:

Plate guard

This device blocks food from spilling off the plate. Attach the guard to the side of the plate opposite the hand the patient uses to feed herself. Guiding the patient's hand, show her how to push food against the guard *to secure it on the utensil*. Then have her try again with food of a different consistency. When the patient tires, feed her the rest of the meal. At subsequent meals, encourage the patient to feed herself for progressively longer periods until she can feed herself an entire meal.

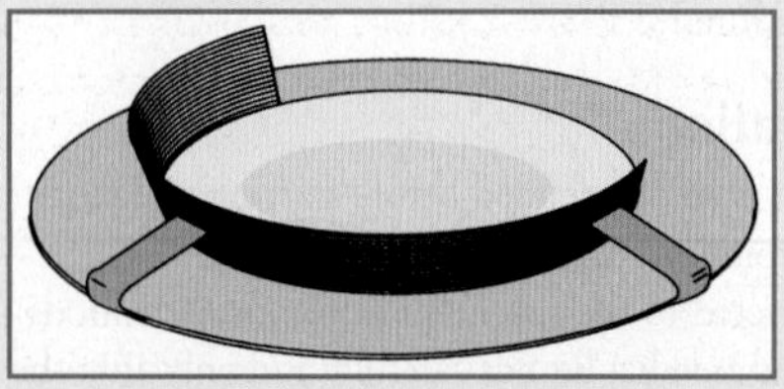

Swivel spoon

This utensil helps the patient with limited ROM in her forearm and will fit in universal cuffs.

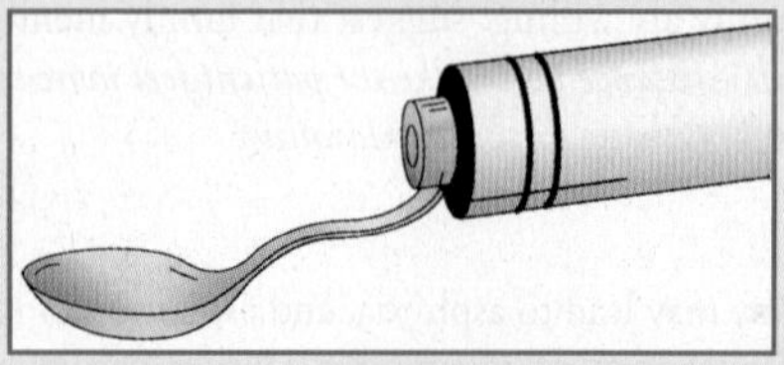

Universal cuffs

Universal cuffs are flexible bands that help the patient with flail hands or diminished grasp. Each cuff contains a slot that holds a fork or spoon. Attach the cuff to the hand the patient uses to feed herself. Then place the fork or spoon in the cuff slot. Bend the utensil *to facilitate feeding*.

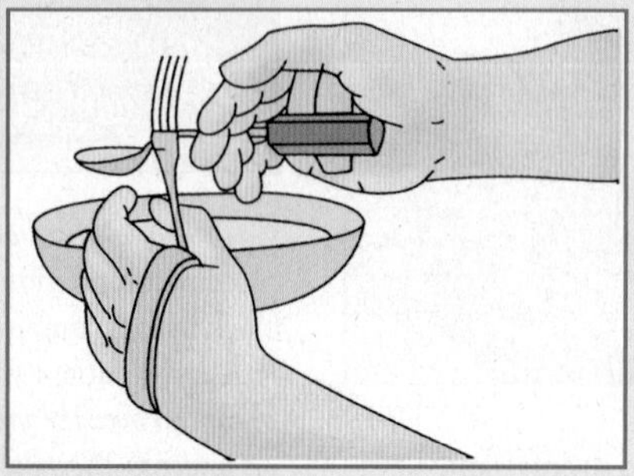

Long-handled utensils

These utensils have jointed stems to help the patient with limited ROM in her elbow and shoulder.

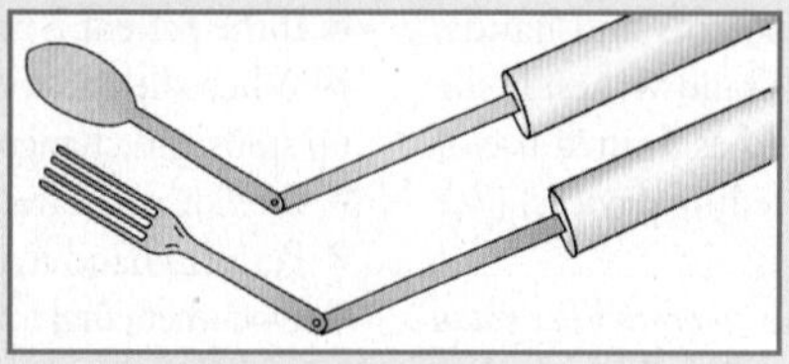

Utensils with built-up handles

Utensils with built up handles can help the patient with diminished grasp. They can be purchased or can be improvised by wrapping tape around the handles.

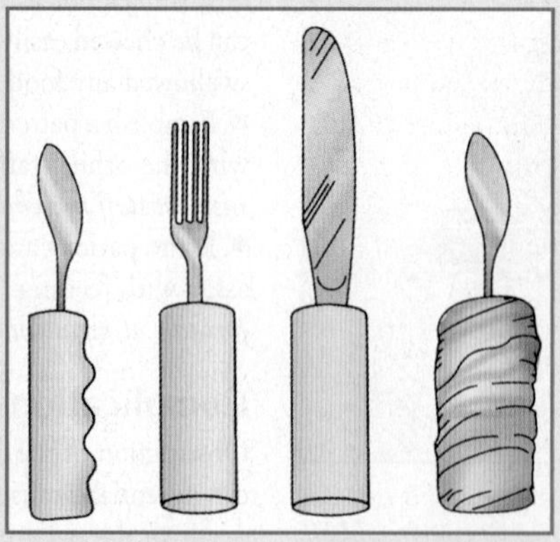

Spouted cups

Spouted cups have a spout that can be used *to prevent spills and burns* for patients experiencing tremors or who have unsteady arms and hands.

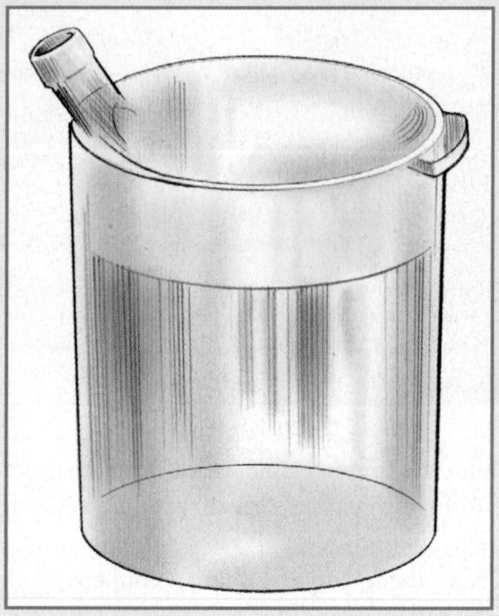

Slotted cups

Slotted (or nosey) cups have a cutout for the nose to allow the patient to drink without bending her neck or tilting her head. Some have handles on both sides *to ensure a firm grasp*.

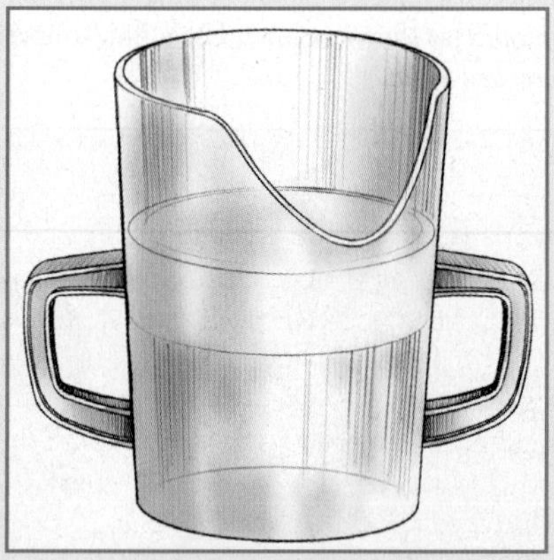

References

1 Vitale, C., et al. (2009). "Strategies for improving care for patients with advanced dementia and eating problems: Optimizing care through physician and speech pathologist collaboration" [Online]. Accessed March 2015 via the Web at http://www.annalsoflongtermcare.com/content/strategies-improving-care-patients-with-advanced-dementia-and-eating-problems-full-title-bel?page=0

2 The Joint Commission. (2015). Standard NPSG.07.01.01. *Comprehensive accreditation manual for hospitals: The official handbook.* Oakbrook Terrace, IL: The Joint Commission. (Level VII)

3 Centers for Disease Control and Prevention. (2002). Guideline for hand hygiene in health-care settings: Recommendations of the Healthcare Infection Control Practices Advisory Committee and the HICPAC/SHEA/APIC/IDSA Hand Hygiene Task Force. *MMWR Recommendations*

and Reports, 51(RR-16), 1–45. Accessed March 2015 via the Web at http://www.cdc.gov/mmwr/pdf/rr/rr5116.pdf (Level II)

4 World Health Organization. (2009). "WHO guidelines on hand hygiene in health care: First global patient safety challenge, clean care is safer care" [Online]. Accessed March 2015 via the Web at http://whqlibdoc.who.int/publications/2009/9789241597906_eng.pdf (Level IV)

5 Centers for Medicare & Medicaid Services, Department of Health and Human Services. (2014). Condition of participation: Infection control. 42 C.F.R. § 482.42.

6 American Osteopathic Association. (2014). Standard 07.01.21. *Healthcare Facilities Accreditation Program: Accreditation requirements for acute care hospitals.* Chicago, IL: American Osteopathic Association. (Level VII)

7 The Joint Commission. (2015). Standard NPSG.01.01.01. *Comprehensive accreditation manual for hospitals: The official handbook.* Oakbrook Terrace, IL: The Joint Commission. (Level VII)

8 The Joint Commission. (2015). Standard PC.01.02.07. *Comprehensive accreditation manual for hospitals: The official handbook.* Oakbrook Terrace, IL: The Joint Commission. (Level VII)

9 American Association of Critical Care Nurses (AACN). (2011). "Practice alert: Prevention of aspiration" [Online]. Accessed March 2015 via the Web at http://www.aacn.org/WD/practice/docs/practicealerts/aacn-aspiration-practice-alert.pdf (Level VII)

10 De Leyn, P., et al. (2007). Tracheotomy: A clinical review and guidelines. *European Journal of Cardiothoracic Surgery, 32,* 412–421. (Level VII)

11 Rutala, W. A., et al. (2008). "Guideline for disinfection and sterilization in healthcare facilities, 2008" [Online]. Accessed March 2015 via the Web at http://www.cdc.gov/hicpac/pdf/guidelines/Disinfection_Nov_2008.pdf (Level I)

12 The Joint Commission. (2015). Standard RC.01.03.01. *Comprehensive accreditation manual for hospitals: The official handbook.* Oakbrook Terrace, IL: The Joint Commission. (Level VII)

13 Centers for Medicare & Medicaid Services, Department of Health and Human Services. (2014). Condition of participation: Medical record services. 42 C.F.R. § 482.24(b).

14 American Osteopathic Association. (2014). Standard 10.00.03. *Healthcare Facilities Accreditation Program: Accreditation requirements for acute care hospitals.* Chicago, IL: American Osteopathic Association. (Level VII)

FEEDING TUBE INSERTION AND REMOVAL

Inserting an enteral feeding tube nasally or orally into the stomach or duodenum allows a patient to receive nourishment if he's unable to do so orally. The enteral feeding tube also permits supplemental feedings in a patient who has very high nutritional requirements, such as one with extensive burns. The preferred feeding tube insertion route is nasal, but the oral route may be used for patients with such conditions as a head injury, deviated septum, or other nose injury.

The practitioner may order duodenal feeding when the patient can't tolerate gastric feeding or when he expects gastric feeding to produce aspiration. Bowel sounds and other evidence of bowel function (passing flatus or stool) aren't necessary to begin enteral feeding. Contraindications to feeding tube use include bowel obstruction, ileus, severe upper GI bleeding, and intractable vomiting or diarrhea.

Enteral feeding tubes differ somewhat from standard nasogastric tubes. Made of silicone or polyurethane, feeding tubes have small diameters and great flexibility. These features reduce oropharyngeal irritation, necrosis from pressure on the tracheoesophageal wall, distal esophageal irritation, and discomfort when swallowing. To facilitate passage, some feeding tubes are weighted with tungsten, and some need a guide wire to keep them from curling in the back of the throat.

These small-bore tubes usually have radiopaque markings and a water-activated coating, which provides a lubricated surface.

Recording fluid intake and output

Accurate intake and output records help evaluate a patient's fluid and electrolyte balance, suggest various diagnoses, and influence the choice of fluid therapy. These records are mandatory for patients with burns, renal failure, electrolyte imbalance, recent surgical procedures, heart failure, or severe vomiting and diarrhea and for patients receiving diuretics or corticosteroids. Intake and output records are also significant in monitoring patients with nasogastric (NG) tubes or drainage collection devices and for those receiving IV therapy.

Fluid intake comprises all fluid entering the patient's body, including beverages, fluids contained in solid foods taken by mouth, and foods that aren't liquid at room temperature, such as flavored gelatin, custard, ice cream, and some beverages. Additional intake includes GI instillations, bladder irrigations, fluids ingested with medications, and IV fluids.

Fluid output consists of all fluid that leaves the patient's body, including urine, loose stools, vomitus, aspirated fluid loss, and drainage from surgical drains, NG tubes, and chest tubes.

When recording fluid intake and output, enlist the patient's help if possible. Record the amount in milliliters (mL). Measure; don't estimate. Monitor intake and output during each shift, and notify the practitioner if amounts differ significantly over a 24-hour period. Document your findings in the appropriate location; describe any fluid restrictions and the patient's compliance.

Equipment

For feeding tube insertion

Enteral feeding tube (#5 to #8 French, with or without a guide wire) ■ fluid-impermeable pad ■ gloves ■ hypoallergenic tape ■ water-soluble lubricant ■ cotton-tipped applicators ■ skin preparation product (such as compound benzoin tincture) ■ facial tissues ■ penlight ■ ice chips or a small cup of water with a straw ■ emesis basin ■ sterile water ■ permanent marker ■ Optional: commercial securement device, gown, mask with face shield, mask, goggles, capnography equipment, bedside glucose monitoring equipment, pH test strip, promotility agent, mouthwash or saline solution.

For feeding tube removal

Oral care supplies ■ fluid-impermeable pad ■ tube clamp ■ 60-mL syringe ■ gloves ■ Optional: equipment for nasal care, gown, mask with face shield, mask, goggles.

Preparation of equipment

For feeding tube insertion

Typically, the practitioner orders the smallest-bore tube that will allow free passage of the liquid feeding formula. Read the instructions on the tubing package carefully *because tube characteristics vary according to the manufacturer.* (For example, some tubes have marks at the appropriate lengths for gastric, duodenal, and jejunal insertion.) Examine the tube *to make sure it's free from defects, such as cracks or rough or sharp edges.* Run water through the tube *to check for patency, activate the coating, and facilitate removal of the guide wire.*

Implementation

- Verify the practitioner's order.
- Gather and prepare the necessary equipment.
- Perform hand hygiene.[1,2,3,4,5]
- Confirm the patient's identity using at least two patient identifiers.[6]
- Explain the procedure to the patient and show him the enteral feeding tube *to allay his fears.*

■ Provide privacy.[7,8]
■ Perform hand hygiene and put on gloves.[1,2,3]
■ Assess the patient for the risk of aspiration.[9]
■ Put on gloves and other personal protective equipment as needed.[10]
■ Assist the patient into the semi-Fowler or high Fowler position *to facilitate enteral feeding tube advancement into the esophagus.*[11]
■ Place a fluid-impermeable pad across on the patient's chest *to protect him from soiling.*

Inserting a feeding tube

■ *To determine the enteral tube length needed to reach the stomach,* first extend the distal end of the tube from the tip of the patient's nose to his earlobe. Coil this portion of the tube around your fingers *so the end stays curved until you insert it.* Then extend the uncoiled portion from the patient's earlobe to the bottom of the xiphoid process.[11] Use a small piece of hypoallergenic tape *to mark the total length of the two portions.*

Inserting the tube nasally

■ Using the penlight, assess nasal patency. Inspect nasal passages for a deviated septum, polyps, or other obstructions. Occlude one nostril, and then the other, *to determine which has the better airflow.* Assess the patient's history for nasal injury or surgery.[11]
■ Lubricate the curved tip of the tube and the feeding tube guide wire, if appropriate, with a small amount of water-soluble lubricant *to ease insertion and prevent tissue injury.*
■ Instruct the patient, if able, to hold an emesis basin and facial tissues in case he needs them.
■ *To advance the enteral feeding tube,* insert the curved, lubricated tip into the more patent nostril and direct it along the nasal passage.
■ When the enteral feeding tube passes the nasopharyngeal junction, you'll feel some resistance. Unless contraindicated, instruct the patient to lower his chin to his chest *to close the trachea.* Then give him a small cup of water with a straw or ice chips. Direct him to sip the water or suck on the ice and swallow frequently *to ease the tube's passage.* Advance the tube as he swallows.

Inserting the tube orally

■ Instruct the patient lower his chin (unless contraindicated) *to close his trachea,* and ask him to open his mouth.
■ Place the tip of the enteral feeding tube at the back of the patient's tongue, give him a small cup of water and a straw, and instruct him to sip the water and swallow frequently. Remind him to avoid clamping his teeth down on the tube. Advance the tube as he swallows.

Positioning the tube

■ Continue advancing the enteral feeding tube until the tape marking the appropriate length reaches the patient's nostril or lips. If you meet resistance, rotate the tube gently.
■ Use various bedside methods *to determine enteral feeding tube location during insertion.*[12] Watch for signs and symptoms of respiratory distress (such as coughing or dyspnea).[12] Use capnography equipment, if available, to detect carbon dioxide in the tube, *which indicates inadvertent tracheal insertion.*[9,12] Measure the pH of tube aspirate, if pH test strips are available and pH measurement is performed in your facility. *Fasting gastric pH is usually 5 or less, even in patients receiving gastric acid inhibitors;* however, this method may not be reliable, *because gastric pH sometimes has a high pH.*[9,12] Inspect the tube aspirate; *fasting gastric secretions commonly appear grass-green or clear and colorless.*[12]
■ *To advance the enteral feeding, especially a tungsten-weighted tube, to the duodenum,* position the patient on his right side *to use gravity to assist tube passage through the pylorus.* Move the tube forward 2″ to 3″ (5 to 7.5 cm) hourly. Observe for a change in aspirate as the tube progresses from the stomach to the duodenum; use these findings to determine the approximate time to confirm placement.[9] Tube placement must be confirmed by X-ray before feeding begins *because duodenal feeding can cause nausea and vomiting if accidentally delivered to the stomach.*[12]
■ Ensure that enteral feeding tube placement is confirmed by X-ray and documented before initial use; *a properly obtained and interpreted X-ray is recommended to confirm correct placement of any blindly inserted enteral tube before its initial use for feeding or medication.*[9,12,13]
■ After X-ray confirmation of placement has been confirmed, if the enteral feeding tube has a guide wire, remove the guide wire with one hand while holding the tube in place at the nostrils.[11]
■ Remove the tape marking the enteral feeding tube length, and mark the tube's exit point from the mouth or nostril with a permanent marker.
■ Apply a skin preparation product to the patient's nose or cheek *to help the enteral feeding tube adhere to the skin and prevent irritation.*[11]
■ Use a commercial securement device *to secure the enteral feeding tube,* or tape the tube securely to the patient's nose or cheek *to avoid excessive pressure on his nostrils or face.*[13]

Removing a feeding tube

■ Using a 60-mL syringe, flush the enteral feeding tube with air; then clamp or pinch the tube *to prevent fluid aspiration during withdrawal.*
■ Remove the tape or the commercial tube holder securing the enteral feeding tube.
■ Withdraw the tube gently but quickly.
■ Cover the enteral feeding tube promptly with the fluid-impermeable pad, and discard the used tube.
■ Perform oral care. (See the "Oral care" procedure, page 560.)
■ Perform nasal care if the enteral feeding tube was inserted through the naris.

Completing the procedure

■ Remove and discard your gloves and any other personal protective equipment worn.[10]
■ Perform hand hygiene.[1,2,3,4,5]
■ Document the procedure.[14]

Special considerations

■ Precise enteral feeding tube placement is important *because small-bore feeding tubes may slide into the trachea without causing immediate signs or symptoms of respiratory distress, such as coughing, choking, gasping, or cyanosis.* However, the patient usually coughs if the tube enters the larynx. *To make sure the tube clears the larynx,* ask the patient to speak. If he can't speak, the tube is in the larynx; withdraw the tube immediately, and reinsert it.
■ Check gastric residual contents before each feeding or every 4 hours during continuous feedings.[12,15] In a patients who isn't critically ill, measure gastric residual volume every 6 to 8 hours after the enteral feeding has been completed. If gastric residual volume is still greater than 250 mL after a second gastric residual volume check, consult with the practitioner about using a promotility agent. Withhold enteral feedings if gastric residual volume is greater than 500 mL, and reassess the patient's tolerance of enteral feedings by performing a GI assessment and evaluating his blood glucose levels. Minimize sedation and consider administering a promotility agent unless you've already done so.[9]
■ Flush the enteral feeding tube every 4 hours with 30 mL of warm water during continuous feeding, or before and after intermittent feedings[9] *to maintain tube patency.* If the tube is taped rather than secured with a commercial tube holder, retape the tube at least daily, or more frequently as needed. Alternate taping the tube toward the inner and outer side of the nose *to avoid constant pressure on the same nasal area.* Inspect the skin for redness and breakdown.

■ Provide nasal hygiene daily using cotton-tipped applicators and water-soluble lubricant *to remove crusted secretions.* Help the patient brush his teeth, gums, and tongue with mouthwash or saline solution at least twice daily.

■ Check enteral feeding tube placement every 4 hours after feedings have been started.[12] When aspirating gastric contents to check tube placement, pull gently on the syringe plunger *to prevent trauma to the stomach lining or bowel.* If you meet resistance during aspiration, stop the procedure *because the tube may be lying against the stomach wall.* If the tube coils above the stomach, you'll be unable to aspirate stomach contents. To rectify this, change the patient's position or withdraw the tube a few inches, advance it again, and try to aspirate again. If the tube was inserted with a guide wire, don't use the guide wire to reposition the tube. The practitioner may use the guide wire under fluoroscopic guidance.

■ Check the permanent marking on the tube regularly (at least every 4 hours)[16] *to determine whether the length of the external portion of the tube has changed, indicating that the tube has moved.* If you observe a significant increase in the external length, use other bedside tests *to determine if the tube has become dislodged;* if in doubt, obtain an X-ray, as ordered, *to determine tube location.*[9]

■ Keep the head of the patient's bed elevated at a 30- to 45-degree angle at all times during the enteral tube feeding administration[9,15,16] and for 30 to 60 minutes after the feeding has been completed or stopped for any reason.[17]

■ If the patient requires enteral feeding for at least 4 weeks, a long-term feeding device should be considered in place of the enteral feeding tube.[9] One such long-term feeding device is a feeding button, which has a high success rate and patency rate and a low complication rate, making it a safe choice for patients who need long-term supplemental feedings.[18]

Patient teaching

If the patient will use an enteral feeding tube at home, make appropriate home care nursing referrals and teach the patient and his caregiver how to use and care for a feeding tube. Teach them how to obtain equipment, insert and remove the tube, prepare and store enteral formula, and solve problems related to tube position and patency.

Complications

Prolonged intubation may lead to sinusitis, esophagitis, esophagotracheal fistula, gastric ulceration, skin erosion at the nostril, and pulmonary and oral infection. (See *Managing enteral tube feeding problems,* page 326.)

Documentation

For enteral feeding tube insertion, record the date and time, tube type and size, the insertion site, the area of placement, and confirmation of proper placement. Document the patient's tolerance of the procedure, any patient teaching provided, and the patient's understanding of your teaching.

For enteral feeding tube removal, record the date and time of removal and the patient's tolerance of the procedure. Document any patient teaching provided and the patient's understanding of your teaching.

REFERENCES

1 The Joint Commission. (2015). Standard NPSG.07.01.01. *Comprehensive accreditation manual for hospitals: The official handbook.* Oakbrook Terrace, IL: The Joint Commission. (Level VII)

2 Centers for Disease Control and Prevention. (2002). Guideline for hand hygiene in health-care settings: Recommendations of the Healthcare Infection Control Practices Advisory Committee and the HICPAC/SHEA/APIC/IDSA Hand Hygiene Task Force. *MMWR Recommendations and Reports, 51*(RR-16), 1–45. Accessed March 2015 via the Web at http://www.cdc.gov/mmwr/pdf/rr/rr5116.pdf (Level II)

3 World Health Organization. (2009). "WHO guidelines on hand hygiene in health care: First global patient safety challenge, clean care is safer care" [Online]. Accessed March 2015 via the Web at http://whqlibdoc.who.int/publications/2009/9789241597906_eng.pdf (Level IV)

4 American Osteopathic Association. (2014). Standard 07.01.21. *Healthcare Facilities Accreditation Program: Accreditation requirements for acute care hospitals.* Chicago, IL: American Osteopathic Association. (Level VII)

5 Centers for Medicare and Medicaid Services, Department of Health and Human Services. (2014). Condition of participation: Infection control. 42 C.F.R. § 482.42.

6 The Joint Commission. (2015). Standard NPSG.01.01.01. *Comprehensive accreditation manual for hospitals: The official handbook.* Oakbrook Terrace, IL: The Joint Commission. (Level VII)

7 Centers for Medicare and Medicaid Services, Department of Health and Human Services. (2014). Condition of participation: Patient's rights. 42 C.F.R. § 482.13(c)(1).

8 American Osteopathic Association. (2014). Standard 15.01.16. *Healthcare Facilities Accreditation Program: Accreditation requirements for acute care hospitals.* Chicago, IL: American Osteopathic Association. (Level VII)

9 Bankhead, R., et al. (2009). A.S.P.E.N. enteral nutrition practice recommendations. *Journal of Parenteral and Enteral Nutrition, 33,* 122–167. (Level IV)

10 Siegel, J. D., et al. (2007). "2007 guideline for isolation precautions: Preventing transmission of infectious agents in healthcare settings" [Online]. Accessed March 2015 via the Web at http://www.cdc.gov/hicpac/pdf/isolation.Isolation2007.pdf (Level II)

11 Lynn-McHale Wiegand, D. (Ed.). (2011). *AACN procedure manual for critical care* (6th ed.). St. Louis, MO: Saunders.

12 American Association of Critical-Care Nurses. (2009). "AACN practice alert: Verification of feeding tube placement (blindly inserted)" [Online]. Accessed March 2015 via the Web at http://www.aacn.org/WD/Practice/Docs/PracticeAlerts/Verification_of_Feeding_Tube_Placement_05-2005.pdf (Level VII)

13 Ukelja, A., et al. (2010). Standards for nutrition support: Adult hospitalized patients. *Nutrition in Clinical Practice, 25,* 403–414. (Level V)

14 The Joint Commission. (2015). Standard RC.01.03.01. *Comprehensive accreditation manual for hospitals: The official handbook.* Oakbrook Terrace, IL: The Joint Commission. (Level VII)

15 American Association of Critical-Care Nurses. (2011). "AACN practice alert: Prevention of aspiration" [Online]. Accessed March 2015 via the Web at http://www.aacn.org/WD/practice/docs/practicealerts/aacn-aspiration-practice-alert.pdf (Level VII)

16 Urden, L. D., et al. (2013). *Critical care nursing: Diagnosis and management* (7th ed.). St. Louis: Mosby.

17 Kenny, D. J., & Goodman, P. (2010). Care of the patient with enteral tube feeding: An evidence-based protocol. *Nursing Research, 59,* S22–S31.

18 Power, S., et al. (2013). Insertion of balloon retained gastrostomy buttons: A 5-year retrospective review of 260 patients. *CardioVascular and Interventional Radiology, 36,* 484–491.

FEMORAL COMPRESSION

After a procedure involving a femoral arterial access site (such as cardiac catheterization or angiography), femoral compression maintains hemostasis at the puncture site. A femoral compression device applies direct pressure to the arterial access site. Application involves placing a wide strap under the patient's buttocks and attaching it to the device with an inflatable plastic dome. After the dome is positioned over the puncture site, it's inflated to the set pressure. A practitioner or specially trained nurses may apply a femoral compression device.

Equipment

Femoral compression device strap ■ compression arch with dome and three-way stopcock ■ pressure inflation device ■ sterile transparent dressing ■ gloves ■ mask and goggles or mask with face shield ■ indelible marker ■ cardiac monitoring equipment ■ blood pressure monitoring

Managing enteral tube feeding problems

COMPLICATIONS	NURSING INTERVENTIONS
Aspiration of gastric secretions	■ Discontinue feeding immediately. ■ Perform tracheal suction of aspirated contents, if possible. ■ Notify the practitioner; prophylactic antibiotics and chest ■ *physiotherapy may be ordered.* ■ Check tube placement before feeding *to prevent complications.*
Tube obstruction	■ Flush the tube with warm water. ■ After ensuring proper tube placement, administer a pancreatic enzyme, as ordered, *to unclog the tube.* Ensuring proper tube placement is vital *because pancreatic enzymes, if instilled into the respiratory tract, may cause severe respiratory complications.* Juice, coffee, soda, or meat tenderizer shouldn't be used *because their effectiveness is unproven and these substances may be contraindicated by the patient's condition.*[17] ■ If necessary, replace the tube. ■ The best solution for a clogged tube is prevention. Flush the tube with 30 mL of water after each feeding *to remove excess sticky formula, which could occlude the tube.*[9] Flush the tube with sterile water (at least 5 mL) before and after medication administration, especially when multiple medications are administered.
Oral, nasal, or pharyngeal irritation or necrosis	■ Provide frequent oral hygiene using mouthwash or swabs. Use petroleum jelly on cracked lips. ■ Change the tube's position. If necessary, replace the tube.
Vomiting, bloating, diarrhea, or cramps	■ Reduce the flow rate. ■ Check tube placement. ■ Administer metoclopramide as prescribed *to increase GI motility.* ■ Warm the formula to prevent GI distress. ■ After feeding has been completed, position the patient on his right side with his head elevated for 30 minutes *to facilitate gastric emptying.* ■ Notify the practitioner; *the amount of formula may need to be reduced.*
Constipation	■ Provide additional fluids if the patient can tolerate them. ■ Have the patient participate in an exercise program, if appropriate. ■ Administer a bulk-forming laxative, as ordered. ■ Review the patient's medications that may cause constipation with the practitioner; discontinue medications, as ordered. ■ Increase the fiber or sugar content of the formula.
Electrolyte imbalance	■ Monitor serum electrolyte levels. ■ Notify the practitioner; *the formula content may need to be adjusted to correct the imbalance.*
Hyperglycemia	■ Monitor blood glucose levels, as ordered. ■ Notify the practitioner of elevated levels; *the sugar content of the formula may need to be adjusted.* ■ Administer insulin, if ordered.

equipment ■ emergency equipment (crash cart with cardiac medications, defibrillator, handheld resuscitation bag with mask, intubation equipment) ■ Optional: prescribed pain medication, Doppler ultrasound device, gown.

Preparation of equipment

Make sure the emergency equipment is readily available and functioning properly before the procedure.[1]

Implementation

Before the procedure

■ Confirm the practitioner's order regarding the femoral compression device, including the length of time the device should remain in place.

■ Gather and prepare the appropriate equipment.

■ Perform hand hygiene.[2,3,4,5,6]

■ Confirm the patient's identity using at least two patient identifiers.[7]

■ Explain the procedure to the patient.

■ Make sure the patient is positioned on the stretcher or bed with the affected leg straight and the head of the bed flat.[1]

■ Obtain the patient's vital signs and monitor his cardiac rhythm *to detect bradyarrhythmias that can occur with a vasovagal reaction.*[1]

■ Perform a comprehensive pain assessment using techniques appropriate for the patient's age, condition, and ability to understand. Administer pain medication, as needed and prescribed, following safe medication administration practices.[1,8,9,10,11]

Applying the femoral compression device

■ Put on gloves, a mask and goggles or a mask with face shield, and a gown, as needed.[1,12,13]

■ Assess the condition of the puncture site and the neurovascular status of the affected extremity. Mark the distal pulses with an indelible marker *to facilitate locating pulses during and after the procedure.*[1]

■ Place the device strap under the patient's hips before sheath removal (in cases that warrant the use of a sheath).

■ With the assistance of another nurse, position the compression arch over the arterial puncture site, not the skin puncture site. The arterial puncture site is ½″ to ¾″ (1.3 cm to 1.9 cm) above the skin puncture site *because the practitioner inserts the arterial sheath at a 45-degree angle to the artery.*[1]
■ Apply manual pressure over the dome area while the straps are secured to the arch.
■ After the dome is properly positioned over the arterial puncture site, connect the pressure inflation device to the stopcock that's attached to the device.
■ Before inflation, verify the amplitude and location of the pedal pulse.
■ Turn the stopcock to the open position and inflate the dome with the pressure inflation device to the ordered pressure.
■ Immediately after removal of the arterial sheath, inflate the device to the ordered pressure. (See the "Arterial and venous sheath removal" procedure page 29.)
■ After 2 to 3 minutes, reduce the pressure following the manufacturer's recommendations and the practitioner's specific orders for pressure changes.
■ Assess the site for proper placement of the device and for signs of bleeding or hematoma.
■ Assess the distal pulses of the affected extremity, and perform a neurovascular assessment. Use a Doppler ultrasound device, if necessary.

Maintaining the device

■ Reassess the patient's vital signs, device placement, the puncture site, and peripheral vascular and neurovascular status of the affected extremity every 15 minutes for an hour, then every 30 minutes over the next hour, and then hourly for the following 4 hours.[1] Afterward, continue to monitor at an interval determined by your facility and the patient's condition.
■ If the dome isn't in the proper position, perform hand hygiene and put on gloves, protective eyewear, and a gown, as needed,[2,3,4,5,6,12,13] and then reposition the compression arch and dome, as necessary. Using the pressure inflation device, reinflate the device to the ordered pressure.
■ Recheck the applied pressure against the pressure stated in the practitioner's order.
■ Continue to monitor the patient's cardiac rhythm *to detect bradyarrhythmias that might occur with a vasovagal reaction.*[1]
■ Confirm distal pulses after any adjustments of the device.

Removing the device

■ Put on gloves, a mask and goggles or a mask with face shield, and a gown, as needed.[12,13]
■ Remove the air from the dome.
■ Leave the dome in place at 0 mm Hg pressure for at least 10 minutes; then loosen the straps and remove the device by rolling it off.
■ Assess the puncture site for bleeding and hematoma.
■ Apply a sterile transparent dressing over the puncture site.
■ Frequently assess the puncture site and neurovascular status of the extremity. Watch for signs of bleeding, hematoma, and infection.
■ Dispose of the device in an appropriate receptacle.
■ Raise the head of the bed up 30 degree after hemostasis is achieved, as desires by the patient, *to minimize back discomfort.*[1]

Completing the procedure

■ Instruct the patient to keep the affected leg straight, to maintain the head of the bed in its prescribed position, and to splint his groin if he needs to cough or sneeze. Tell him to call for assistance with elimination when necessary.
■ Ensure that the patient's call light and personal belongings are within his reach.
■ Remove and discard your gloves, mask and goggles or mask and face shield, and gown, if worn.
■ Perform hand hygiene.[2,3,4,5,6]
■ Document the procedure.[14,151,6]

Special considerations

■ Note that the venous sheath is usually removed 5 to 10 minutes after removal of the arterial sheath *because pressure needs to be applied to the arterial sheath for a longer period to achieve hemostasis.*[1]
■ Maintain the patient on bed rest for 2 to 6 hours after arterial sheath removal and for a maximum of 4 hours after venous sheath removal.[1]
■ If you note external bleeding or signs of internal bleeding, remove the device, apply manual pressure, and notify the practitioner.
■ Change the sterile transparent dressing at the puncture site every 24 to 48 hours. (The sterile transparent dressing permits inspection of the site for bleeding, drainage, or hematoma.)
■ If the patient received antiplatelet and antithrombotic regimens in conjunction with percutaneous coronary intervention, exercise caution *because the patient is at increased risk for bleeding.*
■ The length of time it takes to achieve hemostasis varies with the patient's condition. Tissue damage may occur with pressure maintained for longer than 2 hours.[1]

Complications

Complications associated with femoral compression include bleeding, hematoma, retroperitoneal bleeding, and pseudoaneurysm. Other potential complications may include infection, arteriovenous fistula formation, ischemia of the extremity, thrombosis, and embolization. Tissue damage can also occur if prolonged pressure is maintained.

Documentation

Document the initial application of the device, sheath removal, and the patient's tolerance of the procedure. Record vital signs, puncture site assessments, distal pulses, neurovascular assessments, periodic deflation, repositioning of the device, the length of time the device was in place, and removal of the device. Document patient and family teaching, complications, and interventions.

REFERENCES

1 Lynn-McHale Wiegand, D. (Ed.). (2011). *AACN procedure manual for critical care* (6th ed.). St. Louis, MO: Saunders.

2 The Joint Commission. (2015). Standard NPSG.07.01.01. *Comprehensive accreditation manual for hospitals: The official handbook.* Oakbrook Terrace, IL: The Joint Commission. (Level VII)

3 Centers for Disease Control and Prevention. (2002). Guideline for hand hygiene in health-care settings: Recommendations of Healthcare Infection Control Practices Advisory Committee and the HICPAC/SHEA/APIC/IDSA Hand Hygiene Task Force. *MMWR Recommendations and Reports, 51*(RR-16), 1–45. Accessed March 2015 via the Web at http://www.cdc.gov/mmwr/pdf/rr/rr5116.pdf (Level II)

4 World Health Organization. (2009). "WHO guidelines on hand hygiene in health care: First global patient safety challenge, clean care is safer care" [Online]. Accessed March 2015 via the Web at http://whqlibdoc.who.int/publications/2009/9789241597906_eng.pdf (Level IV)

5 American Osteopathic Association. (2014). Standard 07.01.21. *Healthcare Facilities Accreditation Program: Accreditation requirements for acute care hospitals.* Chicago, IL: American Osteopathic Association. (Level VII)

6 Centers for Medicare and Medicaid Services, Department of Health and Human Services. (2014). Condition of participation: Infection control. 42 C.F.R. § 482.42.

7 The Joint Commission. (2015). Standard NPSG.01.01.01. *Comprehensive accreditation manual for hospitals: The official handbook.* Oakbrook Terrace, IL: The Joint Commission. (Level VII)

8 The Joint Commission. (2015). Standard PC.01.02.07. *Comprehensive accreditation manual for hospitals: The official handbook.* Oakbrook Terrace, IL: The Joint Commission. (Level VII)

9 American Osteopathic Association. (2014). Standard 16.01.03. *Healthcare Facilities Accreditation Program: Accreditation requirements for acute care hospitals.* Chicago, IL: American Osteopathic Association. (Level VII)

Foot care for patients with diabetes

Because diabetes mellitus can reduce blood supply to the feet, normally minor foot injuries can lead to dangerous infection. When caring for a patient with diabetes, keep these foot care guidelines in mind:

- Advise the patient to exercise his feet daily *to help improve circulation.* Teach him to sit on the edge of the bed and point his toes upward, then downward, 10 times. He should then make a circle with each foot 10 times.
- Explain that shoes must fit properly. Instruct the patient to break in new shoes gradually by increasing wearing time by 30 minutes each day.[1] Also tell him to check his old shoes frequently *for rough spots in the lining.*
- Tell the patient to wear clean socks daily and to avoid socks with holes, darned spots, or rough, irritating seams.
- Advise the patient to see a practitioner if he has corns or calluses.[1]
- Tell the patient to wear warm socks or slippers and to use extra blankets *to avoid cold feet.*
- Advise the patient to avoid heating pads or hot-water bottles *because these items may cause burns.*
- Teach the patient to regularly inspect the skin on his feet for cuts, cracks, blisters, or red, swollen areas and to use a mirror to check the soles as needed. Inform him that even slight cuts on the feet should receive a practitioner's attention. As a first-aid measure, tell him to wash the cut thoroughly and apply a mild antiseptic. Urge him to avoid harsh antiseptics, such as iodine, *because they can damage tissue.*
- Advise the patient to avoid tight-fitting garments and activities that can decrease circulation, especially wearing elastic garters, sitting with his knees crossed, picking at sores or rough spots on his feet, walking barefoot, or applying adhesive tape to the skin on his feet.

10 The Joint Commission. (2015). Standard MM.06.01.01. *Comprehensive accreditation manual for hospitals: The official handbook.* Oakbrook Terrace, IL: The Joint Commission. (Level VII)

11 Centers for Medicare and Medicaid Services, Department of Health and Human Services. (2014). Condition of participation: Nursing services. 42 C.F.R. § 482.23(c).

12 Siegel, J. D., et al. (2007). "2007 guideline for isolation precautions: Preventing transmission of infectious agents in healthcare settings" [Online]. Accessed March 2015 via the Web at http://www.cdc.gov/hicpac/pdf/isolation/Isolation2007.pdf (Level II)

13 American Osteopathic Association. (2014). Standard 07.01.10. *Healthcare Facilities Accreditation Program: Accreditation requirements for acute care hospitals.* Chicago, IL: American Osteopathic Association. (Level VII)

14 The Joint Commission. (2015). Standard RC.01.03.01. *Comprehensive accreditation manual for hospitals: The official handbook.* Oakbrook Terrace, IL: The Joint Commission. (Level VII)

15 American Osteopathic Association. (2014). Standard 10.00.03. *Healthcare Facilities Accreditation Program: Accreditation requirements for acute care hospitals.* Chicago, IL: American Osteopathic Association. (Level VII)

16 Centers for Medicare and Medicaid Services, Department of Health and Human Services. (2014). Condition of participation: Medical record services. 42 C.F.R. § 482.24(b).

ADDITIONAL REFERENCES

Das, R., et al. (2011). Arterial closure devices versus manual compression for femoral haemostasis in interventional radiological procedures: A systematic review and meta-analysis. *Cardiovascular and Interventional Radiology, 34,* 723–738. (Level I)

Deuling, J. H., et al. (2008). Closure of the femoral artery after cardiac catheterization: A comparison of Angio-Seal, StarClose, and manual compression. *Catheterization and Cardiovascular Interventions, 71,* 518–523.

Hamel, W. J. (2009). Femoral artery closure after cardiac catheterization. *Critical Care Nurse, 29*(1), 39–46. Accessed March 2015 via the Web at http://ccn.aacnjournals.org/content/29/1/39.full

Khaldi, A., et al. (2011). Delayed complication from a percutaneous vascular closure device following a neuro-interventional procedure. *Interventional Neuroradiology, 17,* 495–500.

Schwartz, B. G., et al. (2010). Review of vascular closure devices. *Journal of Invasive Cardiology, 22,* 599–607.

Schwarz, T., et al. (2009). Mechanical compression versus haemostatic wound dressing after femoral artery sheath removal: A prospective, randomized study. *Vasa, 38,* 53–59. (Level II)

Sulzbach-Hoke, L. M., et al. (2010). Predictors of complications following sheath removal with percutaneous coronary intervention. *Journal of Cardiovascular Nursing, 25*(3), E1–E8.

Tavris, D. R., et al. (2012). Bleeding and vascular complications at the femoral access site following percutaneous coronary intervention (PCI): An evaluation of hemostasis strategies. *Journal of Invasive Cardiology, 24,* 328–334. (Level VI)

FOOT CARE

Daily bathing of feet and regular trimming of toenails promotes cleanliness, prevents infection, stimulates peripheral circulation, and controls odor by removing debris from between toes and under toenails. It's particularly important for bedridden patients and those especially vulnerable to foot infection. Increased susceptibility may be caused by peripheral vascular disease, diabetes mellitus, poor nutritional status, arthritis, or any condition that impairs peripheral circulation. In at-risk patients, proper foot care should include meticulous cleanliness and regular observation for signs of skin breakdown.

When you perform a foot examination, inspect the patient's foot, assess foot pulses, and test for loss of protective sensation. Ask the patient about any history of previous foot ulceration or amputation, neuropathic or peripheral vascular signs and symptoms, impaired vision, tobacco use, and foot care practices.[1] (See *Foot care for patients with diabetes.*) Teach the at-risk patient proper foot care on at least a yearly basis.[1]

Toenail trimming is contraindicated in patients with toe infections, diabetes mellitus, neurologic disorders, renal failure, or peripheral vascular disease, unless performed by a practitioner. Some facilities prohibit nurses from trimming toenails. Check to see whether you're permitted by your facility before trimming the patient's toenails.

Equipment

Bath blanket ■ large basin ■ soap ■ water ■ towel ■ fluid-impermeable pad ■ pillow ■ washcloth ■ disposable, single-use toenail clippers ■ emery board ■ cotton-tipped applicators ■ cotton ■ lotion ■ water-absorbent powder ■ bath thermometer ■ hospital-grade disinfectant ■ puncture-proof sharps container ■ Optional: gloves, heel protectors, protective boots, 2″ × 2″ (5-cm × 5-cm) gauze pads.

Preparation of equipment

Fill the basin halfway with warm water. Test water temperature with a bath thermometer *because patients with diminished peripheral sensation could burn their feet in excessively hot water (over 105°F [40.6°C]) without feeling any warning pain.*

Implementation

- Gather the equipment at the patient's bedside.
- Perform hand hygiene.[2,3,4,5,6]
- Put on gloves if needed *to comply with standard precautions.*[7,8]
- Confirm the patient's identity using at least two patient identifiers.[9]
- Explain to the patient that you're going to wash his feet and provide foot and toenail care.

■ Cover the patient with a bath blanket. Fanfold the top linen to the foot of the bed.
■ Place a fluid-impermeable pad and a towel under the patient's feet *to keep the bottom linen dry.* Then position the basin on the pad.
■ Insert a pillow beneath the patient's knee *to provide support,* and cushion the rim of the basin with the edge of the towel *to prevent pressure on the patient's leg.*
■ Immerse one foot in the basin. Allow it to soak for about 10 minutes and then wash it thoroughly with soap and water. *Soaking softens the skin and toenails, loosens debris under toenails, and comforts and refreshes the patient.*
■ After washing the foot, rinse it with a washcloth, remove it from the basin, and place it on the towel.
■ Gently and thoroughly dry the patient's foot; *don't rub, especially between the toes, because doing so can cause skin breakdown.*
■ Empty the basin, and refill it with warm water at the appropriate temperature
■ Soak the other foot.
■ While the second foot is soaking, give the first one a pedicure. Using a cotton-tipped applicator, carefully clean the patient's toenails. Use an emery board to smooth the nails as indicated *to prevent self-inflicted skin tears.*[10]
■ Consult a podiatrist (if required by your facility) if the patient's nails need trimming.
■ Clean and rinse the foot that has been soaking, dry it thoroughly, and give it a pedicure.
■ Apply lotion *to moisten dry skin,* or lightly dust water-absorbent powder between the toes *to absorb moisture.* Don't apply lotion between the toes *because lotion can cause skin maceration.*[11]
■ Remove and clean[12] or dispose[7] of all equipment appropriately.
■ Remove and discard your gloves, if worn.[7]
■ Perform hand hygiene.[2,3,4,5,6]
■ Document the procedure.[13,14,15]

Special considerations

■ While providing foot care, observe the color, shape, and texture of the toenails. If you see redness, drying, cracking, blisters, discoloration, or other signs of traumatic injury, especially in a patient with impaired peripheral circulation, notify the practitioner. *Because such a patient is vulnerable to infection and gangrene,* the patient needs prompt treatment.[1]
■ If a patient's toenail grows inward at the corners, tuck a wisp of cotton under it *to relieve pressure on the toe.*
■ When providing foot care for a bedridden patient, perform range-of-motion exercises, unless contraindicated, *to stimulate circulation and prevent foot contractures and muscle atrophy.* Tuck folded 2″ × 2″ (5-cm × 5-cm) gauze pads between overlapping toes *to protect the skin from the toenails.* Apply heel protectors or protective boots *to prevent skin breakdown.*

Patient teaching

Instruct the patient to notify his practitioner right away if he observes discoloration (any part of the leg or foot turns blue or black); notes reduced sensation to pain or temperature; develops an injury that doesn't heal or becomes infected; experiences unusual numbness, tingling, cold, cramping, or pain in the feet; or develops pain while walking that's relieved by rest.

If a patient can't perform proper foot care and inspection because of visual difficulties, physical constraints that prevent movement, or cognitive problems that impair his ability to assess the condition of his foot and to institute appropriate responses, teach family members or another caregiver to assist in his care.[1]

Complications

Injury to the subungual skin may occur.

Documentation

Record the date and time of foot care in your notes. Record and report any abnormal findings and any nursing actions you take. If toenail trimming was necessary, specify the name of the person who performed the trimming.

REFERENCES

1 American Diabetes Association. (2011). "Standards of medical care in diabetes—2011" [Online]. Accessed March 2015 via the Web at http://care.diabetesjournals.org/content/34/Supplement_1/S11.full#sec-64 (Level VII)

2 Centers for Disease Control and Prevention. (2002). Guideline for hand hygiene in health-care settings: Recommendations of the Healthcare Infection Control Practices Advisory Committee and the HICPAC/SHEA/APIC/IDSA Hand Hygiene Task Force. *MMWR Recommendations and Reports, 51*(RR-16), 1–45. Accessed March 2015 via the Web at http://www.cdc.gov/mmwr/pdf/rr/rr5116.pdf (Level II)

3 World Health Organization. (2009). "WHO guidelines on hand hygiene in health care: First global patient safety challenge, clean care is safer care" [Online]. Accessed March 2015 via the Web at http://whqlibdoc.who.int/publications/2009/9789241597906_eng.pdf (Level IV)

4 The Joint Commission. (2015). Standard NPSG.07.01.01. *Comprehensive accreditation manual for hospitals: The official handbook.* Oakbrook Terrace, IL: The Joint Commission. (Level VII)

5 Centers for Medicare & Medicaid Services, Department of Health and Human Services. (2014). Condition of participation: Infection control. 42 C.F.R. § 482.42.

6 American Osteopathic Association. (2014). Standard 07.01.21. *Healthcare Facilities Accreditation Program: Accreditation requirements for acute care hospitals.* Chicago, IL: American Osteopathic Association. (Level VII)

7 Siegel, J. D., et al. (2007). "2007 guideline for isolation precautions: Preventing transmission of infectious agents in healthcare settings" [Online]. Accessed March 2015 via the Web at http://www.cdc.gov/hicpac/pdf/isolation/Isolation2007.pdf (Level II)

8 American Osteopathic Association. (2014). Standard 07.01.10. *Healthcare Facilities Accreditation Program: Accreditation requirements for acute care hospitals.* Chicago, IL: American Osteopathic Association.

9 The Joint Commission. (2015). Standard NPSG.01.01.01. *Comprehensive accreditation manual for hospitals: The official handbook.* Oakbrook Terrace, IL: The Joint Commission. (Level VII)

10 LeBlanc, K., et al. (2013). International skin tear advisory panel: A tool kit to aid in the prevention, assessment, and treatment of skin tears using a simplified classification system. *Advances in Skin & Wound Care, 26,* 459–476.

11 Heitzman, J. (2010). Foot care for patients with diabetes. *Topics in Geriatric Rehabilitation, 26,* 250–263.

12 Rutala, W. A., et al. (2008). "Guideline for disinfection and sterilization in healthcare facilities, 2008" [Online]. Accessed March 2015 via the Web at http://www.cdc.gov/hicpac/pdf/guidelines/Disinfection_Nov_2008.pdf (Level I)

13 The Joint Commission. (2015). Standard RC.01.03.01. *Comprehensive accreditation manual for hospitals: The official handbook.* Oakbrook Terrace, IL: The Joint Commission. (Level VII)

14 Centers for Medicare & Medicaid Services, Department of Health and Human Services. (2014). Condition of participation: Medical record services. 42 C.F.R. § 482.24(b).

15 American Osteopathic Association. (2014). Standard 10.00.03. *Healthcare Facilities Accreditation Program: Accreditation requirements for acute care hospitals.* Chicago, IL: American Osteopathic Association. (Level VII)

FOREIGN-BODY AIRWAY OBSTRUCTION AND MANAGEMENT

Most cases of foreign-body airway obstruction in adults occur while they're eating. Foreign bodies can cause mild or severe airway obstruction. In a child, foreign-body airway obstruction occurs most often when they're eating or playing and typically involves such items as balloons and small objects, or such foods as hot dogs, rounded candies, nuts, or grapes. In infants, airway obstruction typically results from a liquid.

Foreign bodies can cause mild or severe airway obstruction. If the obstruction is mild and the patient is coughing forcefully, there's no reason to intervene; spontaneous coughing and breathing typically relieve the obstruction.[1]

If severe obstruction develops, you must intervene quickly to relieve the obstruction;[1] anoxia resulting from the obstruction may cause brain damage and death in 4 to 6 minutes. Intervene by administering abdominal thrusts, also called the *Heimlich maneuver,* which uses a subdiaphragmatic abdominal thrust to create diaphragmatic pressure in the static lung below the foreign body sufficient to expel the obstruction. Abdominal thrusts are used in conscious adult patients who can't speak, cough, or breathe.

If abdominal thrusts are ineffective, you may consider administering chest thrusts; this maneuver forces air out of the lungs, creating an artificial cough. Also use chest thrusts for an obese patient, if you're unable to encircle the patient's abdomen, and for a patient who's in the late stages of pregnancy.[1]

For infants, deliver repeated cycles of five back blows followed by five chest compressions until the foreign body is expelled or the infant becomes unresponsive. Abdominal thrusts aren't recommended for infants because they may damage the infant's liver.

If a patient is unconscious or becomes unconscious despite your efforts, start cardiopulmonary resuscitation (CPR) immediately.

Equipment

No special equipment is required.

Implementation

■ Determine whether the patient is choking by asking, "Are you choking?" If the victim indicates "yes" by nodding her head without speaking, she has a severe airway obstruction.[1]

■ Activate the emergency response system quickly if the patient is having difficulty breathing. If another person is present, have him activate the system.[1]

■ *To calm the patient,* talk to the patient and explain what you're doing. Tell the patient that you'll try to dislodge the foreign body.

For a conscious adult or child

■ Standing behind the patient, wrap your arms around the waist. Make a fist with one hand, and place the thumb side against the abdomen, slightly above the umbilicus and well below the xiphoid process. Then grasp your fist with the other hand (as shown below).

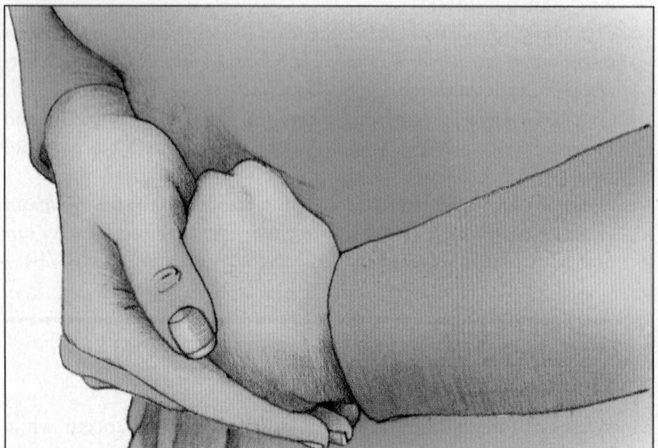

■ Squeeze the patient's abdomen using quick inward and upward thrusts. Each thrust should be a separate and distinct movement; each should be forceful enough to create an artificial cough that will dislodge an obstruction. Continue the abdominal thrust in rapid sequence until the obstruction is relieved or the patient becomes unresponsive.

■ Make sure you have a firm grasp on the patient *because the patient may lose consciousness and need to be lowered to the floor.*[1] Support the head and neck *to prevent injury.* If the patient becomes unconscious, start CPR and follow the steps for an unconscious adult or child.

■ Examine the patient for injuries, such as ruptured or lacerated abdominal or thoracic viscera, resulting from the procedure.

For an obese or pregnant adult

■ If the patient is conscious, stand behind her and place your arms under her armpits and around her chest.

■ Place the thumb side of your clenched fist against the middle of the sternum, avoiding the margins of the ribs and the xiphoid process (as shown below).

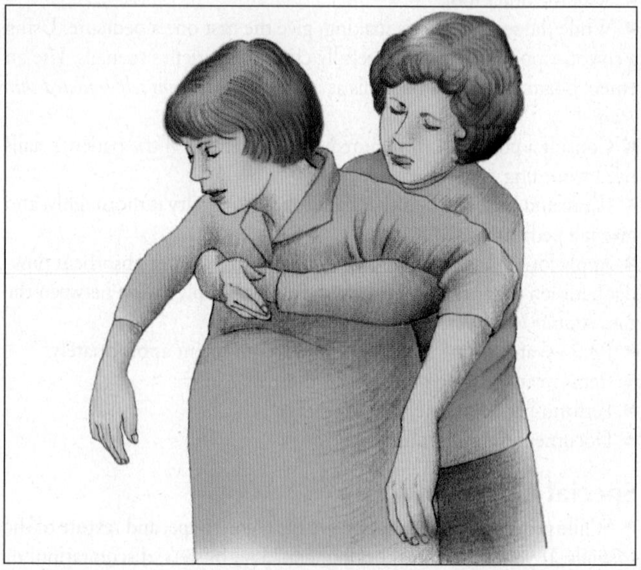

■ Grasp your fist with your other hand and perform a chest thrust with enough force to expel the foreign body. Continue until the patient expels the obstruction or loses consciousness. If the patient loses consciousness, carefully lower her to the floor and follow the steps outlined below for an unconscious adult or child.

■ Examine the patient for injuries, such as ruptured or lacerated abdominal or thoracic viscera, resulting from the procedure.

■ Notify the practitioner of the patient's status, especially with loss of consciousness.

For an unconscious adult or child

■ For a patient who has become unresponsive while you are trying to remove a foreign object, carefully lower the patient to the ground and call for help or activate the emergency response system.[1]

■ If you come upon an unconscious patient, establish unresponsiveness by tapping the patient and shouting, "Are you alright?" Check to see if the patient is apneic or only gasping. If the patient is unresponsive and apneic or only gasping, call for help or activate the emergency response system.[1]

■ Begin CPR immediately, starting with chest compressions; use a ratio of 30 chest compression to two ventilations.[1] (See the "Cardiopulmonary resuscitation, adult" and "Cardiopulmonary resuscitation, child" procedures, pages 124, 131.)

■ Each time the airway is opened using a head-tilt, chin-lift maneuver, look for an object in the patient's mouth.[1]

■ Remove the object, if seen.[1]

NURSING ALERT *Never perform a blind finger-sweep to retrieve an object from a patient's airway. Remove visible objects.*[1]

■ Attempt to ventilate the patient and follow with 30 chest compressions; continue CPR until the object is expelled.[1]

■ Examine the patient for injuries, such as ruptured or lacerated abdominal or thoracic viscera, resulting from the procedure.

For an infant

■ Determine whether the infant has a severe foreign body object obstruction. *If it's severe, the infant won't be able to cough or make a sound.*[1]

■ If severe obstruction exists, place the infant face down so that he's straddling your arm with his head lower than his trunk.[1]

■ Rest your forearm on your thigh and deliver five back blows with the heel of your hand between the infant's shoulder blades (as shown below).[1]

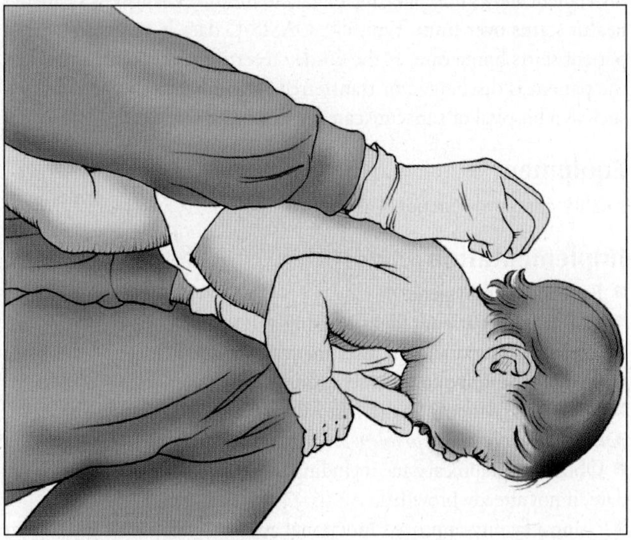

■ If the back blows don't remove the obstruction, place your free hand on the infant's back.

■ Supporting his neck, jaw, and chest with your other hand, turn him over onto your thigh keeping his head lower than his trunk.

■ Imagine a line between the infant's nipples and place the index finger of your free hand on his sternum, just below this imaginary line. Then place your middle and ring fingers next to your index finger and lift the index finger off his chest (as shown below).[1]

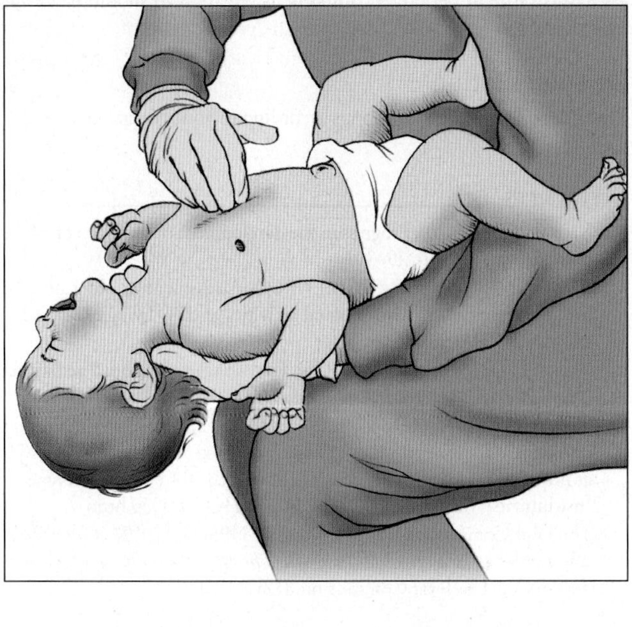

■ Deliver five chest thrusts as you would for chest compression, but at a slower rate.[1]

■ Repeat the above steps until you've relieved the obstruction or the infant becomes unconscious.

■ If the infant becomes unconscious, call for help, and start to perform CPR beginning with chest compressions.[1] (See the "Cardiopulmonary resuscitation, infant" procedure, page 134.)

■ After 30 chest compressions, open the airway.[1]

■ Before performing rescue breaths, look in the infant's mouth for the foreign body. If you see the object, remove it. Never perform a blind finger-sweep on an infant *because it may push the foreign body further back into the pharynx and damage the oropharynx.*[1]

■ Attempt ventilation and follow with chest compressions at a rate of 30 chest compressions to two ventilations until the object is removed.[1]

■ Activate the emergency response system after 2 minutes if no one else has done so.[1] Continue with CPR until the emergency response or code team arrives.

Completing the procedure

■ Perform hand hygiene.[2,3,4,5,6]

■ Document the procedure.[7,8,9]

Special considerations

■ If the patient vomits during abdominal thrusts, quickly wipe out his mouth with your fingers and resume the maneuver, as necessary.

■ Even if your efforts to clear the airway don't seem to be effective, keep trying. *As oxygen deprivation increases, smooth and skeletal muscles relax, making your maneuvers more likely to succeed.*

■ Never perform a blind finger-sweep to retrieve an object from a patient's airway. *You could end up pushing the object further into the airway rather than removing the object.*

Complications

Nausea, regurgitation, bruising, and achiness may develop after the patient can breathe independently. He may also be injured, possibly from incorrect placement of the rescuer's hands or because of osteoporosis or metastatic lesions that increase the risk of fracture.

Documentation

Record the date and time of the procedure, the patient's actions before the obstruction, the approximate length of time it took to clear the airway, and the type and size of the object removed. Also, note the patient's vital signs after the procedure, any complications that occurred and nursing actions taken, and the patient's tolerance of the procedure.

REFERENCES

1 American Heart Association. (2010). Adult basic life support: 2010 American Heart Association guidelines for cardiopulmonary resuscitation and emergency cardiovascular care. *Circulation, 122,* S685–S705. Accessed March 2015 via the Web at http://circ.ahajournals.org/content/122/18_suppl_3/S685.full (Level I)

2 The Joint Commission. (2015). Standard NPSG.07.01.01. *Comprehensive accreditation manual for hospitals: The official handbook.* Oakbrook Terrace, IL: The Joint Commission. (Level VII)

3 Centers for Disease Control and Prevention. (2002). Guideline for hand hygiene in health-care settings: Recommendations of the Healthcare Infection Control Practices Advisory Committee and the HICPAC/SHEA/APIC/IDSA Hand Hygiene Task Force. *MMWR Recommendations and Reports, 51*(RR-16), 1–45. Accessed March 2015 via the Web at http://www.cdc.gov/mmwr/pdf/rr/rr5116.pdf (Level II)

4 World Health Organization. (2009). "WHO guidelines on hand hygiene in health care: First global patient safety challenge, clean care is safer care" [Online]. Accessed March 2015 via the Web at http://whqlibdoc.who.int/publications/2009/9789241597906_eng.pdf (Level IV)

5 Centers for Medicare & Medicaid Services, Department of Health and Human Services. (2014). Conditions of participation: Infection control. 42 C.F.R. § 482.42.
6 American Osteopathic Association. (2014). Standard 07.01.10. *Healthcare Facilities Accreditation Program: Accreditation requirements for acute care hospitals.* Chicago, IL: American Osteopathic Association. (Level VII)
7 The Joint Commission. (2015). Standard RC.01.03.01. *Comprehensive accreditation manual for hospitals: The official handbook.* Oakbrook Terrace, IL: The Joint Commission. (Level VII)
8 Centers for Medicare & Medicaid Services, Department of Health and Human Services. (2014). Condition of participation: Medical records services. 42 C.F.R. § 482.24(b).
9 American Osteopathic Association. (2014). Standard 10.00.03. *Healthcare Facilities Accreditation Program: Accreditation requirements for acute care hospitals.* Chicago, IL: American Osteopathic Association. (Level VII)

Additional references

Kenth, J., & Ng, C. (2013). Foreign body airway obstruction causing a ball valve effect. *Journal of the Royal Society of Medicine, 4*(6), 1–4. Accessed March 2015 via the Web at http://shr.sagepub.com/content/4/6/2042533313482458.full.pdf+html
Nettina, S.M. (2014). *Lippincott manual of nursing practice* (10th ed.). Philadelphia, PA: Wolters Kluwer.

Functional assessment

A functional assessment is used to evaluate the older adult's overall well-being and self-care abilities. It helps identify individual needs and care deficits, provide a basis for developing a care plan that enhances the abilities of the older adult with coexisting disease and chronic illness, and provide feedback about treatment and rehabilitation. The goal of a functional assessment is to help an older adult maintain his independence by matching his needs with such services as housekeeping, home health care, and day care. Several tools are available to help perform a methodical functional assessment. Become familiar with the functional assessment tool used in your facility.

The *Katz Index of Independence in Activities of Daily Living* is a widely used tool for evaluating a person's ability to perform six daily personal care activities: bathing, dressing, toileting, transferring, continence, and feeding. It describes functional level at a specific point in time and objectively assigns a total score based on points accrued for dependence or independence in each of the six functional areas.[1]

Another widely used tool, the *Lawton Instrumental Activities of Daily Living Scale* evaluates a person's ability to perform more complex personal care activities. It addresses the activities needed to support independent living, such as the ability to use a telephone, shop, prepare food, perform housekeeping tasks, do laundry, use transportation, handle medications, and manage finances. Each of the activities is rated on a three-point scale, ranging from independence to complete disability.[2] (See *Lawton Instrumental Activities of Daily Living Scale.*) When using the Lawton scale, make sure you evaluate the patient in terms of safety. For example, a person may be able to cook a small meal but may leave the stove burner on after cooking.

The *Barthel Index* is commonly used in rehabilitation settings to assess the person's need for assistance with activities of daily living and to document improvement in the patient's abilities. The Barthel Index ranks functional status of the following 10 self-care functions: feeding, moving from wheelchair to bed and returning, performing personal toileting, getting on and off the toilet, bathing, walking on a level surface or propelling a wheelchair, ascending and descending stairs, dressing and undressing, maintaining bowel continence, and controlling the bladder. The Barthel Index ranks functional status as either independent or dependent, and each item is scored according to the degree of assistance needed; over time, results reveal improvement or decline.[3] A similar scale, called the *Barthel Self-Care Rating Scale,* is a more detailed evaluation of function. Both tools provide information to help you determine the type of assistance needed.

A standardized assessment tool called the *Minimum Data Set* (MDS) was developed by the Centers for Medicare & Medicaid Services Nursing Quality Initiative to make patient assessments more consistent and reliable throughout the country. The MDS includes assessment information that can be used to identify potential nutritional problems, risk factors, and potential for improved function. The use of this tool is required in all extended-care facilities that receive federal funding. MDS 3.0, the latest version of the MDS, replaced MDS 2.0 in 2012. It has improved the tool's reliability and accuracy and includes the patient in the assessment process.[4]

The *Outcome and Assessment Information Set-C,* now known as *OASIS-C,* is a standardized form required by the Health Care Financing Administration for Medicare-certified agencies. This form is a comprehensive assessment of home care patients. The OASIS-C was developed specifically to measure outcomes for adults who receive home care. This instrument allows the collection of data to measure changes in a patient's health status over time. Typically, OASIS-C data is collected when a patient starts home care, at the 60-day recertification point, and when the patient is discharged or transferred to another health care facility, such as a hospital or subacute care facility.

Equipment

Facility-approved functional assessment tool.

Implementation

- Perform hand hygiene.[5,6,7]
- Confirm the patient's identity using at least two patient identifiers.[8]
- Explain to the patient the assessment as well as where it will take place (the patient's room or a treatment room).
- Review the patient's health history *to obtain subjective data about the patient and insight into problem areas and subtle physical changes.*
- Obtain biographical data, including the patient's name, age, and birth date, if not already provided.
- Using a facility-approved functional assessment tool, ask the patient to answer the questions. If the patient is unable to answer, have his caregiver do so.
- Perform hand hygiene.[5,6,7]
- Document the procedure.[9,10]

Special considerations

- In a long-term care facility, the physical assessment and care plan should be completed by a licensed nurse within 24 hours of a patient's admission. Functional assessment should be completed after a 7- to 14-day assessment period. A comprehensive care plan should be developed within 21 days.

Documentation

Document all assessment findings according to your facility's assessment scale.

References

1 Katz, S., et al. (1970). Progress in the development of the index of ADL. *The Gerontologist, 10,* 20–30.
2 Lawton, M. P., & Brody, E. M. (1969). Assessment of older people: Self-maintaining and instrumental activities of daily living. *The Gerontologist, 9,* 179–186.
3 Mahoney, F. I. & Barthel, D. (1965). Functional evaluation: The Barthel Index. *Maryland State Medical Journal, 14,* 56–61.
4 Centers for Medicare & Medicaid Services. (2012). "MDS 3.0 for nursing homes and swing bed providers" [Online]. Accessed March 2015 via the Web at http://www.cms.gov/Medicare/Quality-Initiatives-Patient-Assessment-Instruments/NursingHomeQualityInits/NHQIMDS30.html
5 The Joint Commission. (2015). Standard NPSG.07.01.01. *Comprehensive accreditation manual for hospitals: The official handbook.* Oakbrook Terrace, IL: The Joint Commission. (Level VII)

Lawton Instrumental Activities of Daily Living Scale

The Lawton scale evaluates more sophisticated functions than those evaluated by the Katz index. Patients or their caregivers can complete the form in a few minutes. The first answer in each case—except for 8a—indicates independence; the second indicates capability with assistance; and the third indicates dependence. In this version, the maximum score is 29, although scores have meaning only for a particular patient (for example, declining scores over time reveal deterioration). Questions 4 to 7 tend to be gender specific; modify them as necessary.

Name: ______________________________

Rated by: ______________________________ Date: ______________

1. Can you use the telephone?	
without help	3
with some help	2
completely unable	1
2. Can you go shopping for groceries?	
without help	3
with some help	2
not without special arrangements	1
3. Can you prepare your own meals?	
without help	3
with some help	2
completely unable	1
4. Can you do your own housework?	
without help	3
with some help	2
completely unable	1
5. Can you do your own handyman work?	
without help	3
with some help	2
completely unable	1
6. Can you do your own laundry?	
without help	3
with some help	2
completely unable	1
7. Can you get to places beyond walking distance?	
without help	3
with some help	2
completely unable	1
8a. Do you take medicines or use any medications?	
Yes (If yes, answer Question 8b.)	1
No (If no, answer Question 8c.)	2
8b. Do you take your own medicine?	
without help (in the right doses at the right times)	3
with some help (if someone prepares it for you and/or reminds you to take it)	2
completely unable	1
8c. If you had to take medicine, could you do it?	
without help (in the right doses at the right time)	3
with some help (if someone prepared it for you and reminded you to take it)	2
completely unable	1
9. Can you manage your own money?	
without help	3
with some help	2
completely unable	1

Adapted with permission from Lawton, M. P., & Brody, E. M. (1969). Assessment of older people: Self-maintaining and instrumental activities of daily living. *The Gerontologist, 9*(3), 179–186.

6 World Health Organization. (2009). "WHO guidelines on hand hygiene in health care: First global patient safety challenge, clean care is safer care" [Online]. Accessed March 2015 via the Web at http://whqlibdoc.who.int/publications/2009/9789241597906_eng.pdf (Level IV)

7 Centers for Disease Control and Prevention. (2002). Guideline for hand hygiene in health-care settings: Recommendations of the Healthcare Infection Control Practices Advisory Committee and the HICPAC/SHEA/APIC/IDSA Hand Hygiene Task Force. *MMWR Recommendations and Reports, 51*(RR-16), 1–45. Accessed March 2015 via the Web at http://www.cdc.gov/mmwr/pdf/rr/rr5116.pdf (Level II)

8 The Joint Commission. (2015). Standard NPSG.01.01.01. *Comprehensive accreditation manual for hospitals: The official handbook.* Oakbrook Terrace, IL: The Joint Commission. (Level VII)

9 The Joint Commission. (2015). Standard RC.01.03.01. *Comprehensive accreditation manual for hospitals: The official handbook.* Oakbrook Terrace, IL: The Joint Commission. (Level VII)

10 Centers for Medicare & Medicaid Services, Department of Health and Human Services. (2014). Condition of participation: Medical record services. 42 C.F.R. § 482.24(b).

Additional reference

Hinkle, J. L., & Cheever, K. H. (2014). *Brunner & Suddarth's textbook of medical-surgical nursing* (13th ed.). Philadelphia, PA: Wolters Kluwer.

G

Gait belt use

A gait belt is a safety device made of cloth or plastic that buckles securely around a patient's waist. The device provides a secure grasping surface to aid with patient transfer and ambulation.[1,2] Commonly used for patients who are at risk for falling, a gait belt can help safely lower a patient to the ground if the patient begins to fall or loses balance during transfer or ambulation. When combined with proper body mechanics, a gait belt also improves caregiver safety by preventing back injury.

Before gait belt use, assess the patient for contraindications, including recent abdominal, back, or chest surgery; hernia; severe cardiac or respiratory conditions; abdominal aneurysm; or the presence of a gastrostomy tube or other equipment that might be compromised by gait belt use.

Equipment

Shoes or slippers with nonskid soles ▪ robe ▪ gait belt ▪ blood pressure equipment ▪ stethoscope ▪ disinfectant pad ▪ Optional: assistive devices (walker, cane, crutches), prescribed pain medication.

Preparation of equipment

Inspect the gait belt before use. Check the belt for broken stitches and torn or frayed material. Don't use the device if the buckle is cracked or broken or it doesn't fasten securely.[3] Check for proper buckle closure and test the buckle to make sure that it doesn't slip when you pull on it. Make sure that the bed and wheelchair, if used, are in a locked position.

Implementation

- Perform hand hygiene.[4,5,6,7,8]
- Confirm the patient's identity using at least two patient identifiers.[9]
- Explain the reason for gait belt use to the patient and family.
- Assess the patient's risk of falling and tolerance of recent activities. Check for any conditions that would contraindicate gait belt use.[10,11]
- Obtain vital signs to *serve as baselines for comparison.*
- Perform a comprehensive pain assessment using techniques appropriate for the patient's age, condition, and ability to understand. Administer pain medication, as needed and prescribed, following safe medication administration practices.[12,13,14]
- Assist the patient to a comfortable sitting position; then allow for a brief *rest to help the patient adjust to postural changes.*
- Help the patient put on a robe and appropriate footwear, such as nonskid socks or slippers, *to maintain dignity and reduce the risk of falling.*[1]
- Wrap the belt around the patient's waist and over any clothing, with the buckle facing front.
- Adjust the belt so that it fits snugly around the patient's waist (as shown below). Slide your open hand between the belt and the patient *to make sure that the device fits snugly but isn't too tight.*[3]

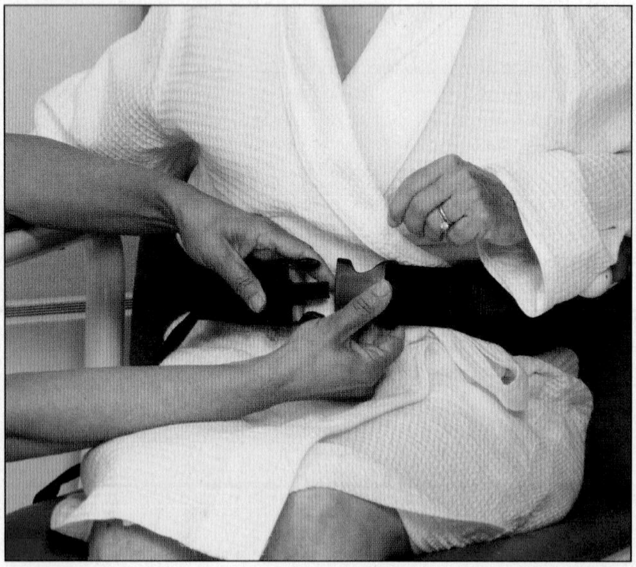

- Keep clothing as wrinkle-free as possible under the gait belt *to prevent skin breakdown.*

Transferring the patient

- If the patient has one-sided weakness, position the destination surface (wheelchair, commode, or chair) on the patient's unaffected side.
- Position yourself close to the patient so that you're facing each other.
- Grasp both sides of the gait belt using an underhand grip.
- While firmly gripping the gait belt, keep your back straight, bend your knees slightly, position your feet in a wide stance *to maintain proper body mechanics* (as shown on top right), and begin rocking back and forth *to overcome forces resisting transfer.* Instruct the patient, on a count of three, to push off of the surface he's sitting on *to encourage independence.*

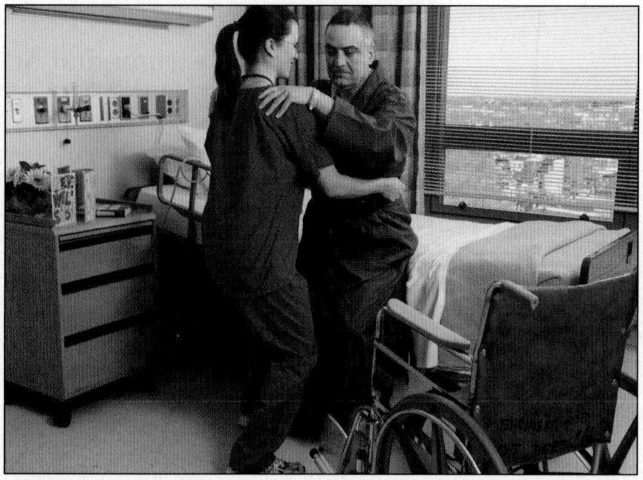

- Allow the patient to stand for a moment *to ensure balance.*
- Instruct the patient to pivot and to bear as much weight as possible on the unaffected side. Support the affected side *because the patient will tend to lean to this side.*
- Pivot on your back foot, guiding the patient to the destination surface. Maintain contact between the destination surface and the patient's legs *because doing so helps ensure proper positioning before the patient sits.*
- Flex your knees and hips while assisting the patient onto the destination surface. *Using good body mechanics prevents back injury by supporting weight with large muscle groups.*
- When you reach the destination surface, keep a firm grip on the gait belt and gently lower the patient onto the surface. Tell the patient to reach and grasp the armrests (as shown below), using them to bear some weight, if possible.

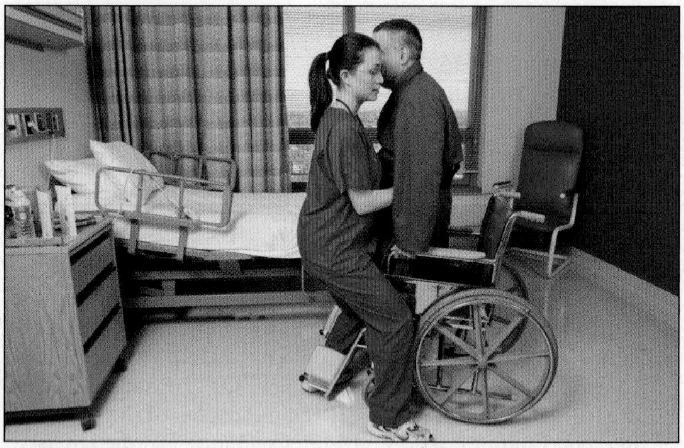

Ambulating the patient

- Position yourself close to the patient so that you're facing each other.
- Grasp both sides of the gait belt using an underhand grip.
- While firmly gripping the gait belt, keep your back straight, bend your knees slightly, position your feet in a wide stance *to maintain proper body mechanics,* and begin rocking back and forth *to overcome forces resisting transfer.* Instruct the patient to push off of the mattress on a count of three *to encourage independence.*
- Allow the patient to stand for a moment *to ensure balance.*
- Place one hand under the gait belt in back of the patient. If the patient is weaker on one side, make sure to walk on that side when ambulating (as shown on next page, top left), *because the patient will tend to lean to this side.* Encourage the patient to use a handrail if available.

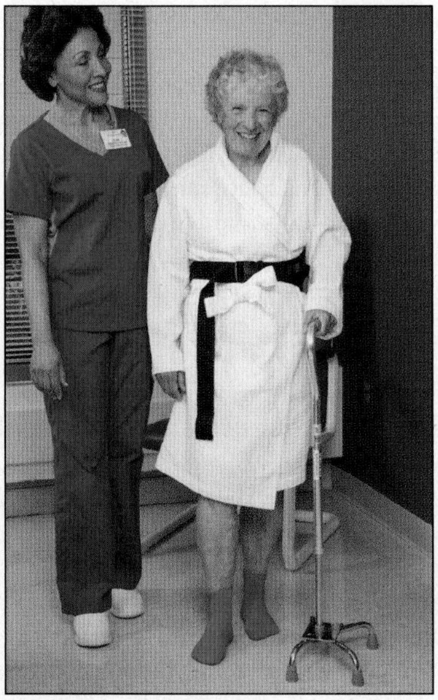

- Walk closely behind and slightly to the side of the patient, keeping the same pattern and pace as the patient.
- Allow for rest periods as needed.

Completing the procedure

- Remove the gait belt after use *to prevent patient harm.*
- Store the gait belt at the patient's bedside for immediate use.[1]
- Perform hand hygiene.[4,5,6,7,8]
- Clean and disinfect your stethoscope using a disinfectant pad.[15,16]
- Perform hand hygiene.[4,5,6,7,8]
- Document the procedure.[17,18,19]

Special considerations

- Don't leave a gait belt applied to a patient who's unattended in a chair or bed. *The gait belt could become displaced and result in strangulation or other patient injury.*
- If the patient is morbidly obese or can't bear weight, consider using lift equipment to transfer the patient instead of a gait belt *to ensure patient safety and prevent caregiver injury.*
- If the patient loses weight-bearing ability during ambulation or transfer, maintain your grip on the gait belt, pull the patient as close to your body as possible, and gently slide him to the floor using the large muscles in your upper leg. Call for assistance, and place the patient back into the chair or bed or in another sitting position.
- Before ambulation, decide with the patient the distance the patient can walk and your destination. *Planning helps ensure safety.*

Patient teaching

If the patient's family members or other caregivers will be using a gait belt at home, teach them how to use it and have them perform a return demonstration *so that you can evaluate their technique.* Instruct the family members or other caregivers to remove throw rugs and small pieces of furniture *to reduce tripping hazards.* Advise the patient to always wear shoes with nonskid soles.

Documentation

Document the patient's tolerance of the procedure; the distance that the patient ambulated, if applicable; and any associated complications. If complications occurred, record the date, time, and name of the practitioner notified; the prescribed interventions; and the patient's response to those interventions. Document teaching provided to the patient and family and their comprehension of that teaching.

References

1 Degelau, J., et al. (2012). "Institute for Clinical Systems Improvement: Health care protocol: Prevention of falls (acute care) (3rd ed.)" [Online]. Accessed March 2015 via the Web at https://www.icsi.org/_asset/dcn15z/Falls-Interactive0412.pdf (Level VII)

2 U.S. Department of Labor, Occupational Safety and Health Administration. (2009). "Guidelines for nursing homes: Ergonomics for the prevention of musculoskeletal disorders" [Online]. Accessed March 2015 via the Web at http://www.osha.gov/ergonomics/guidelines/nursinghome/final_nh_guidelines.html (Level I)

3 Posey Company. (2010). "Posey EZ clean gait belts" [Online]. Accessed March 2015 via the Web at http://www.posey.com/files/M6022-Posey®-EZ-Clean-Gait-Belts.pdf

4 Centers for Disease Control and Prevention. (2002). Guideline for hand hygiene in health-care settings: Recommendations of the Healthcare Infection Control Practices Advisory Committee and the HICPAC/SHEA/APIC/IDSA Hand Hygiene Task Force. *MMWR Recommendations and Reports, 51*(RR-16), 1–45. Accessed March 2015 via the Web at http://www.cdc.gov/mmwr/pdf/rr/rr5116.pdf (Level II)

5 World Health Organization. (2009). "WHO guidelines on hand hygiene in health care: First global patient safety challenge, clean care is safer care" [Online]. Accessed March 2015 via the Web at http://whqlibdoc.who.int/publications/2009/9789241597906_eng.pdf (Level IV)

6 The Joint Commission. (2015). Standard NPSG.07.01.01. *Comprehensive accreditation manual for hospitals: The official handbook.* Oakbrook Terrace, IL: The Joint Commission. (Level VII)

7 Centers for Medicare and Medicaid Services, Department of Health and Human Services. (2014). Condition of participation: Infection control. 42 C.F.R. § 482.42.

8 American Osteopathic Association. (2014). Standard 07.01.21. *Healthcare Facilities Accreditation Program: Accreditation requirements for acute care hospitals.* Chicago, IL: American Osteopathic Association. (Level VII)

9 The Joint Commission. (2015). Standard NPSG.01.01.01. *Comprehensive accreditation manual for hospitals: The official handbook.* Oakbrook Terrace, IL: The Joint Commission. (Level VII)

10 The Joint Commission. (2015). Standard PC.01.02.08. *Comprehensive accreditation manual for hospitals: The official handbook.* Oakbrook Terrace, IL: The Joint Commission. (Level VII)

11 American Osteopathic Association. (2014). Standard 16.02.02. *Healthcare Facilities Accreditation Program: Accreditation requirements for acute care hospitals.* Chicago, IL: American Osteopathic Association. (Level VII)

12 The Joint Commission. (2015). Standard PC.01.02.07. *Comprehensive accreditation manual for hospitals: The official handbook.* Oakbrook Terrace, IL: The Joint Commission. (Level VII)

13 American Osteopathic Association. (2014). Standard 16.01.03. *Healthcare Facilities Accreditation Program: Accreditation requirements for acute care hospitals.* Chicago, IL: American Osteopathic Association. (Level VII)

14 Centers for Medicare and Medicaid Services, Department of Health and Human Services. (2014). Condition of participation: Nursing services. 42 C.F.R. § 482.23(c).

15 Rutala, W. A., et al. (2008). "Guideline for disinfection and sterilization in healthcare facilities, 2008" [Online]. Accessed March 2015 via the Web at http://www.cdc.gov/hicpac/pdf/guidelines/Disinfection_Nov_2008.pdf (Level I)

16 American Osteopathic Association. (2014). Standard 07.02.03. *Healthcare Facilities Accreditation Program: Accreditation requirements for acute care hospitals.* Chicago, IL: American Osteopathic Association. (Level VII)

17 The Joint Commission. (2015). Standard RC.01.03.01. *Comprehensive accreditation manual for hospitals: The official handbook.* Oakbrook Terrace, IL: The Joint Commission. (Level VII)

18 American Osteopathic Association. (2014). Standard 10.00.03. *Healthcare Facilities Accreditation Program: Accreditation requirements for acute care hospitals.* Chicago, IL: American Osteopathic Association. (Level VII)

19 Centers for Medicare and Medicaid Services, Department of Health and Human Services. (2014). Condition of participation: Medical record services. 42 C.F.R. § 482.24(b).

ADDITIONAL REFERENCES

Craven, R. F., & Hirnle, C. J. (2012). *Fundamentals of nursing: Human health and function* (7th ed.). Philadelphia, PA: Lippincott Williams & Wilkins.

Rendon, A. A., et al. (2012). The effect of virtual reality gaming on dynamic balance in older adults. *Age and Ageing, 41*, 549–552. (Level II)

GASTRIC LAVAGE

Gastric lavage flushes the stomach and removes ingested substances through a gastric lavage tube. The procedure may be used to empty the stomach in preparation for endoscopic examination or after poisoning or a drug overdose, especially in patients who have central nervous system depression or an inadequate gag reflex. However, the American Academy of Clinical Toxicology doesn't recommend routinely using gastric lavage to manage instances of poisoning because its benefits are unfounded, it may delay treatment with activated charcoal and other therapies, and it may be associated with serious complications.[1]

Gastric lavage should be performed in the emergency department or on the intensive care unit by a practitioner, gastroenterologist, or nurse who has received proper training.[1] A large-bore lavage tube may be inserted by a gastroenterologist.

This procedure is contraindicated after ingestion of a corrosive substance (such as lye, petroleum distillates, ammonia, alkalis, or mineral acids) because the lavage tube may perforate the already compromised esophagus.[1] It's also contraindicated for patients with an unprotected airway, when lavage increases the risk and severity of aspiration, for a patient at risk for hemorrhage or GI perforation because of pathology or recent surgery, and for a patient who resists or refuses to cooperate.[1] Gastric lavage used to manage upper GI hemorrhage is controversial.[1] Studies show that it allows endoscopy to be performed more quickly, but it doesn't affect clinical outcomes.[3]

Correct lavage tube placement is essential for patient safety because accidental misplacement (in the lungs, for example) followed by lavage can be fatal.

Equipment

2 to 3 L of normal saline solution, tap water, or appropriate antidote, as ordered ▪ graduated container ▪ Ewald tube or any large-lumen gastric tube, typically #36 to #40 French (see *Using wide-bore gastric tubes*) ▪ connection tubing ▪ intermittent suction setup ▪ water-soluble lubricant or anesthetic ointment ▪ emesis basin ▪ ½″ (1.3 cm) hypoallergenic tape ▪ 60-mL bulb or catheter-tip syringe or prepackaged syringe irrigation kit ▪ gloves ▪ face shield ▪ gown ▪ fluid-impermeable pad or towel ▪ Yankauer or tonsil-tip suction device attached to suction ▪ cardiac monitor ▪ pulse oximeter and probe ▪ automated blood pressure cuff ▪ emergency equipment (crash cart with cardiac medications, defibrillator, handheld resuscitation bag with mask, intubation equipment) ▪ Optional: charcoal tablets or solution, endotracheal tube.

Preparation of equipment

Make sure emergency equipment is readily available and functioning properly. Set up the lavage and suction equipment. Lubricate the end of the lavage tube with the water-soluble lubricant or anesthetic ointment. Set up the Yankauer or tonsil-tip catheter for oropharyngeal suctioning.

Implementation

- Verify the practitioner's order.
- Gather and prepare the appropriate equipment.
- Perform hand hygiene.[4,5,6,7,8]
- Confirm the patient's identity using at least two patient identifiers.[9]
- Provide privacy.[10,11]
- Explain the procedure to the patient.
- Attach the patient to a cardiac monitor, automated blood pressure cuff, and pulse oximeter *for monitoring during the procedure.*[12] Make sure the upper and lower alarm limits are set according to the patient's current condition and that the alarms are turned on, functioning properly, and audible to staff.[13,14,15]
- Put on a gown, gloves, and a face shield.[16,17]
- Drape a towel or fluid-impermeable pad over the patient's chest *to protect him from soiling.*[12]
- Place the bed in the semi-Fowler position, ensuring the head of the bed is elevated 10 to 20 degrees, creating a slight reverse-Trendelenburg position.[12]
- Place the patient in the left lateral decubitus position.
- The practitioner or nurse inserts the lavage tube nasally or orally and advances it slowly and gently *because forceful insertion may injure tissues.* The tube's placement is checked by aspirating stomach contents with a 60-mL syringe and obtaining X-ray confirmation.[12]
- *Because the patient may vomit when the lavage tube reaches the posterior pharynx during insertion,* be prepared to suction the airway immediately with either a Yankauer or a tonsil-tip suction device.[1]
- After placement is confirmed, secure the lavage tube nasally or orally with tape.
- Trace the tubing from the patient to its point of origin *to make sure that it's attached to the proper port.*[18]
- Aspirate stomach contents using a 60-mL syringe.
- Begin gastric lavage by slowly instilling 200 to 300 mL of fluid (for adults) using the 60-mL syringe.[12]
- Aspirate the irrigant with the syringe and empty it into a graduated container or connect the lavage tube to the intermittent suction.[12]
- Measure the outflow amount to make sure that it equals at least the amount of irrigant you instilled *to prevent accidental stomach distention and vomiting.* If the drainage amount falls significantly short of the instilled amount, reposition the tube until sufficient solution flows out.
- Repeat the procedure as indicated.
- If the procedure is being performed for hemorrhage, repeat lavage intermittently until returned fluids appear clear, *signaling that bleeding has stopped.*
- If the procedure is being performed for an overdose, repeat lavage intermittently until the aspirated fluid is clear of toxic substances.
- Assess the patient's vital signs, cardiac rhythm, oxygen saturation level, and level of consciousness (LOC) during and after the procedure.[12] Notify the practitioner of any changes.
- If ordered, remove the lavage tube by clamping the tube and then pulling it out slowly and steadily.
- Dispose of soiled items in the appropriate receptacles.[16]
- Remove your gloves, gown, and face shield.[16,17]
- Perform hand hygiene.[4,5,6,7,8]
- Document the procedure.[19,20,21]

Special considerations

NURSING ALERT *Never leave a patient alone during gastric lavage.*

- Watch closely for airway obstruction caused by vomiting or excess oral secretions. As needed, suction the oral cavity frequently throughout gastric lavage *to ensure an open airway and prevent aspiration.* Be aware that, for the same reasons, and if the patient doesn't exhibit an adequate gag reflex or is comatose, the patient may require an endotracheal tube before the procedure.[1]
- If ordered, after lavage to remove poisons or drugs, mix charcoal tablets or solution with the irrigant (water or normal saline solution) and administer the mixture through the nasogastric (NG) tube. *The charcoal will absorb any remaining toxic substances.* Note that the tube may be clamped temporarily, allowed to drain via gravity, attached to intermittent suction, or removed.

EQUIPMENT

Using wide-bore gastric tubes

If you need to deliver a large volume of fluid rapidly through a gastric tube (for example, when irrigating the stomach of a patient with profuse gastric bleeding or poisoning), a wide-bore gastric tube usually serves best. Typically inserted orally, these tubes remain in place only long enough to complete the lavage and evacuate stomach contents.

Ewald tube

In an emergency, using an Ewald tube (a single-lumen tube with several openings at the distal end) allows you to aspirate large amounts of gastric contents quickly.

Levacuator tube

The Levacuator tube has two lumens. Use the larger lumen for evacuating gastric contents; use the smaller one for instilling an irrigant.

Edlich tube

The single-lumen Edlich tube has four openings near the closed distal tip. A funnel or syringe can be connected at the proximal end. Like the Ewald tube, the Edlich tube lets you withdraw large quantities of gastric contents quickly.

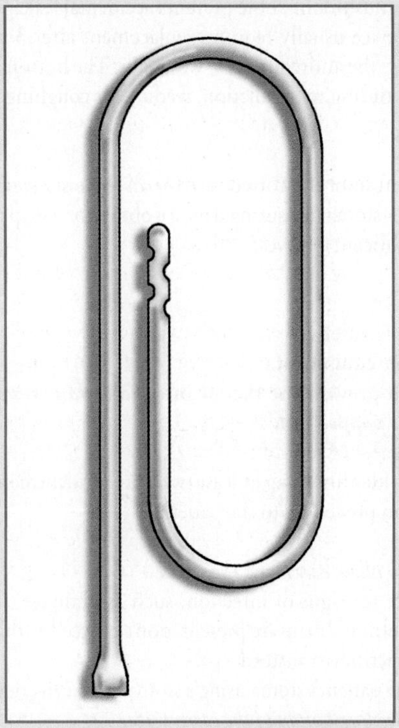

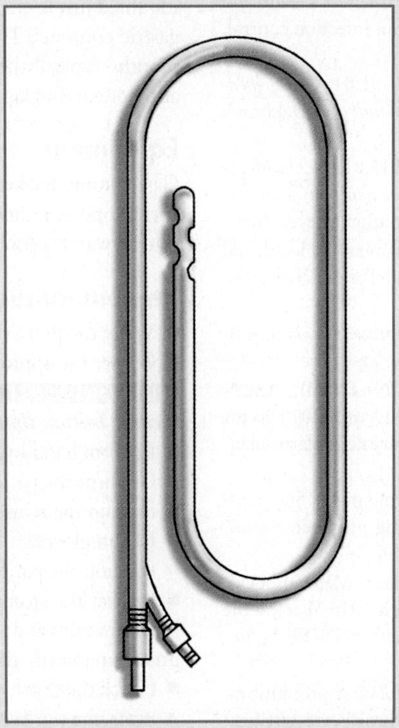

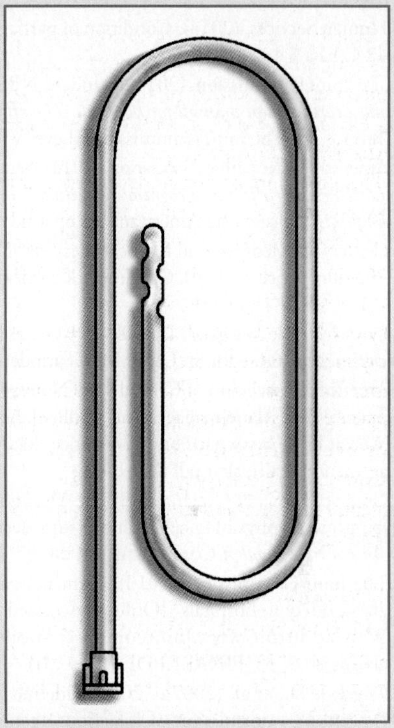

- When performing gastric lavage to stop bleeding, keep precise intake and output records *to determine the amount of bleeding.*
- Be aware that you may need to measure serum electrolyte and arterial blood gas levels during or after lavage when large volumes of fluid are instilled and withdrawn.
- Note that The Joint Commission issued a sentinel event alert concerning medical device alarm safety *because alarm-related events have been associated with permanent loss of function and death.* Among the major contributing factors were improper alarm settings, inappropriately turned off alarms, and alarm signals that were not audible to staff. Make sure that alarm limits are appropriately set and that alarms are turned on, functioning properly, and audible to staff. Follow facility guidelines for preventing alarm fatigue.[15]

Complications

Aspiration pneumonia, laryngospasm, arrhythmias, esophageal and stomach perforation, fluid and electrolyte imbalances, respiratory distress, and small conjunctival hemorrhages are complications of gastric lavage.[1]

Documentation

Record the date and time of lavage, size and type of gastric tube used, volume and type of irrigant, and amount of drained gastric contents. Record this information on the intake-and-output record sheet, and include your observations, including the color and consistency of drainage. Also keep precise records of the patient's vital signs, cardiac rhythm, oxygen saturation level, and LOC; any drugs instilled through the tube; the time the tube was removed; and the patient's tolerance of the procedure. Document patient and family teaching performed and their understanding of that teaching.

REFERENCES

1 Benson, B. E., et al. (2013). Position paper update: Gastric lavage for gastrointestinal decontamination. *Clinical Toxicology, 51,* 140–146. (Level VII)

2 Saltzman, J. R. Approach to acute upper gastrointestinal bleeding in adults. (2014). In: *UpToDate,* Feldman, M., & Travis, A. C. (Eds.). Accessed March 2015 via the Web at http://www.uptodate.com/contents/search

3 Huang, E. S., et al. (2011). Impact of nasogastric lavage on outcomes in acute GI bleeding. *Gastrointestinal Endoscopy, 74,* 971–980. (Level VI)

4 Centers for Disease Control and Prevention. (2002). Guideline for hand hygiene in health-care settings: Recommendations of the Healthcare Infection Control Practices Advisory Committee and the HICPAC/SHEA/APIC/IDSA Hand Hygiene Task Force. *MMWR Recommendations and Reports, 51*(RR-16), 1–45. Accessed March 2015 via the Web at http://www.cdc.gov/mmwr/pdf/rr/rr5303.pdf (Level II)

5 World Health Organization. (2009). "WHO guidelines on hand hygiene in health care: First global patient safety challenge, clean care is safer care" [Online]. Accessed March 2015 via the Web at http://whqlibdoc.who.int/publications/2009/9789241597906_eng.pdf (Level IV)

6 The Joint Commission. (2015). Standard NPSG.07.01.01. *Comprehensive accreditation manual for hospitals: The official handbook.* Oakbrook Terrace, IL: The Joint Commission. (Level VII)

7 American Osteopathic Association. (2014). Standard 07.01.21. *Healthcare Facilities Accreditation Program: Accreditation requirements for acute care hospitals.* Chicago, IL: American Osteopathic Association. (Level VII)

8 Centers for Medicare and Medicaid Services, Department of Health and Human Services. (2014). Condition of participation: Infection control. 42 C.F.R. § 482.42.

9 The Joint Commission. (2015). Standard NPSG.01.01.01. *Comprehensive accreditation manual for hospitals: The official handbook.* Oakbrook Terrace, IL: The Joint Commission. (Level VII)

10 American Osteopathic Association. (2014). Standard 15.01.16. *Healthcare Facilities Accreditation Program: Accreditation requirements for acute care hospitals.* Chicago, IL: American Osteopathic Association. (Level VII)

11 Centers for Medicare and Medicaid Services, Department of Health and Human Services. (2014). Condition of participation: Patient's rights. 42 C.F.R. § 482.13(c)(1).

12 Lynn-McHale Wiegand, D. (Ed.). (2011). *AACN procedure manual for critical care* (6th ed.). St. Louis, MO: Saunders.

13 American Association of Critical-Care Nurses (AACN). (2013). "AACN practice alert: Alarm management" [Online]. Accessed March 2015 via the Web at http://www.aacn.org/wd/practice/docs/practicealerts/alarm-management-practice-alert.pdf (Level VII)

14 Graham, K. C., & Cvach, M. (2010). Monitor alarm fatigue: Standardizing use of physiological monitors and decreasing nuisance alarms. *American Journal of Critical Care, 19,* 28–37.

15 The Joint Commission. (2013). "Sentinel event alert: Medical device alarm safety in hospitals" [Online]. Accessed March 2015 Year via the Web at http://www.jointcommission.org/assets/1/18/SEA_50_alarms_4_5_13_FINAL1.PDF (Level VII)

16 Siegel, J. D., et al. (2007). "2007 guideline for isolation precautions: Preventing transmission of infectious agents in healthcare settings" [Online]. Accessed March 2015 via the Web at http://www.cdc.gov/hicpac/pdf/isolation/Isolation2007.pdf (Level II)

17 American Osteopathic Association. (2014). Standard 07.01.10. *Healthcare Facilities Accreditation Program: Accreditation requirements for acute care hospitals.* Chicago, IL: American Osteopathic Association. (Level VII)

18 U.S. Food and Drug Administration. (n.d.). "Look. Check. Connect. Safe medical device connections save lives" [Online]. Accessed March 2015 via the Web at http://www.fda.gov/downloads/MedicalDevices/Safety/AlertsandNotices/UCM134873.pdf

19 The Joint Commission. (2015). Standard RC.01.03.01. *Comprehensive accreditation manual for hospitals: The official handbook.* Oakbrook Terrace, IL: The Joint Commission. (Level VII)

20 American Osteopathic Association. (2014). Standard 10.00.03. *Healthcare Facilities Accreditation Program: Accreditation requirements for acute care hospitals.* Chicago, IL: American Osteopathic Association. (Level VII)

21 Centers for Medicare and Medicaid Services, Department of Health and Human Services. (2014). Condition of participation: Medical record services. 42 C.F.R. § 482.24(b).

ADDITIONAL REFERENCE

Pitera, A., & Sarko, J. (2010). Just say no: Gastric aspiration and lavage rarely provide benefit. *Annals of Emergency Medicine, 55*(4), 365–366.

GASTROSTOMY FEEDING BUTTON REINSERTION

A gastrostomy feeding button serves as an alternative to a standard gastrostomy tube. The low-profile feeding device is generally used for an ambulatory patient or a pediatric patient who's receiving long-term enteral feedings. Gastrostomy feeding buttons are approved by the U.S. Food and Drug Administration for 6-month implantation.

The button has a mushroom dome at one end and two wing tabs and a flexible safety plug at the other. When inserted into an established stoma, the button lies almost flush with the skin, with only the tabs and the top of the safety plug visible.

The button usually can be inserted into a stoma in less than 15 minutes. Besides its cosmetic appeal, the device is easily maintained, reduces skin irritation and breakdown, and is less likely to become dislodged or migrate than an ordinary feeding tube. A one-way, antireflux valve mounted just inside the mushroom dome prevents accidental leakage of gastric contents. The device usually requires replacement after 3 to 4 months, typically because the antireflux valve wears out. The button can also potentially pop out during manipulation, feeding, or coughing.

Equipment

Gastrostomy feeding button of the correct size (or all three sizes, if the correct one isn't known) ■ stoma measuring device ■ obturator ■ soap and water ■ water-soluble lubricant ■ gloves.

Implementation

- Verify the practitioner's order.
- Gather the appropriate equipment.

NURSING ALERT **To prevent the risk of infection, *don't reuse a feeding button that has popped out.***[1]

- Perform hand hygiene.[2,3,4,5,6]
- Confirm the patient's identify using at least two patient identifiers.[7]
- Explain the reinsertion procedure to the patient.
- Put on gloves.[8,9]
- Position the patient *to allow easy access the stoma.*
- Inspect the stoma site for signs of infection, such as drainage, pus, inflammation, and tenderness. If any are present, don't proceed with the procedure; notify the practitioner instead.
- Check the depth of the patient's stoma using a stoma measuring device *to make sure you have a feeding button of the correct size.*[1]
- Clean around the stoma with mild soap and water.
- Lubricate the obturator with a water-soluble lubricant, and distend the button several times *to ensure patency and function of the antireflux valve within the button.*
- Lubricate the mushroom dome and the stoma.
- Gently push the button through the stoma into the stomach (as shown below).

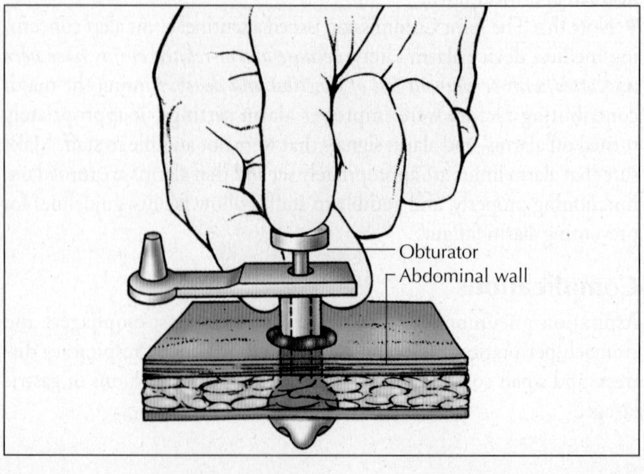

■ Remove the obturator by gently rotating it as you withdraw it *to keep the antireflux valve from adhering to it.*
■ After removing the obturator, confirm placement by rotating the button and gently pushing it into the stoma. If you feel no resistance, the device is properly placed.[1]
■ Close the flexible safety plug (as shown below), which should be relatively flush with the skin surface. The button is now ready for administration of enteral feedings.

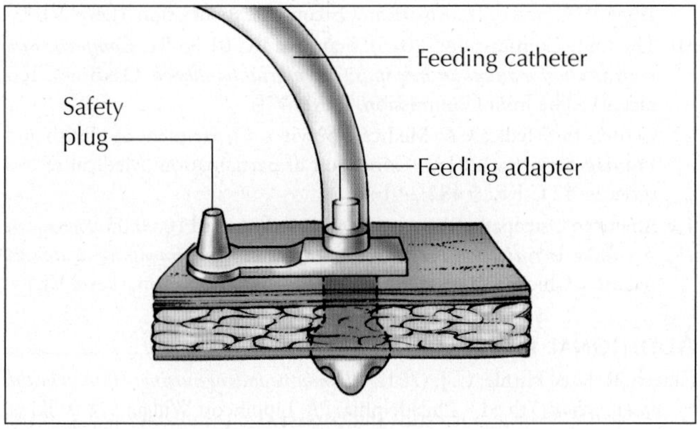

■ Discard used disposable equipment in the appropriate receptacle.
■ Remove and discard your gloves.
■ Perform hand hygiene.[2,3,4,5,6]
■ Document the procedure.[10,11,12]

Special considerations

■ Once daily, clean the peristomal skin with mild soap and water and let the skin air-dry for 20 minutes *to avoid skin irritation.* Also clean the site whenever spillage from the feeding bag occurs.

Patient teaching

Before discharge, make sure the patient can insert and care for the gastrostomy feeding button. If possible, teach him or a family member how to reinsert the button by first practicing on a model. Offer written instructions and answer questions on obtaining replacement supplies.

Complications

Complications from gastrostomy button reinsertion are rare and include irritation of the surrounding skin from leakage of gastric contents.

Documentation

Record the reason for reinsertion, the size of the button used, and the patient's tolerance of the procedure. Document any complications and nursing actions taken. Note the appearance of the stoma and surrounding skin. Also document any patient teaching provided to the patient and family and their understanding of that teaching.

REFERENCES

1 Bard Access Systems, Inc. (2012). "BARD button replacement gastrostomy device:m Information for use" [Online]. Accessed March 2015 via the Web at http://www.bardaccess.com/assets/pdfs/ifus/0732755_CE_Button_Replace_Gastro_IFU_web.pdf
2 The Joint Commission. (2015). Standard NPSG.07.01.01. *Comprehensive accreditation manual for hospitals: The official handbook.* Oakbrook Terrace, IL: The Joint Commission. (Level VII)
3 Centers for Disease Control and Prevention. (2002). Guideline for hand hygiene in health-care settings: Recommendations of the Healthcare Infection Control Practices Advisory Committee and the HICPAC/SHEA/APIC/IDSA Hand Hygiene Task Force. *MMWR Recommendations and Reports, 51*(RR-16), 1–45. Accessed March 2015 via the Web at http://www.cdc.gov/mmwr/pdf/rr/rr5116.pdf (Level II)
4 World Health Organization. (2009). "WHO guidelines on hand hygiene in health care: First global patient safety challenge, clean care is safer care" [Online]. Accessed March 2015 via the Web at http://whqlibdoc.who.int/publications/2009/9789241597906_eng.pdf (Level IV)
5 American Osteopathic Association. (2014). Standard 07.01.21. *Healthcare Facilities Accreditation Program: Accreditation requirements for acute care hospitals.* Chicago, IL: American Osteopathic Association. (Level VII)
6 Centers for Medicare & Medicaid Services, Department of Health and Human Services. (2014). Condition of participation: Infection control. 42 C.F.R. § 482.42.
7 The Joint Commission. (2015). Standard NPSG.01.01.01. *Comprehensive accreditation manual for hospitals: The official handbook.* Oakbrook Terrace, IL: The Joint Commission. (Level VII)
8 Siegel, J. D., et al. (2007). "2007 guideline for isolation precautions: Preventing transmission of infectious agents in healthcare settings" [Online]. Accessed March 2015 via the Web at http://www.cdc.gov/hicpac/pdf/isolation/Isolation2007.pdf (Level II)
9 American Osteopathic Association. (2014). Standard 07.01.10. *Healthcare Facilities Accreditation Program: Accreditation requirements for acute care hospitals.* Chicago, IL: American Osteopathic Association. (Level VII)
10 The Joint Commission. (2015). Standard RC.01.03.01. *Comprehensive accreditation manual for hospitals: The official handbook.* Oakbrook Terrace, IL: The Joint Commission. (Level VII)
11 Centers for Medicare & Medicaid Services, Department of Health and Human Services. (2014). Condition of participation: Medical record services. 42 C.F.R. § 482.24(b).
12 American Osteopathic Association. (2014). Standard 10.00.03. *Healthcare Facilities Accreditation Program: Accreditation requirements for acute care hospitals.* Chicago, IL: American Osteopathic Association. (Level VII)

ADDITIONAL REFERENCES

Hinkle, J. L., & Cheever, K. H. (2014). *Brunner & Suddarth's textbook of medical-surgical nursing* (13th ed.). Philadelphia, PA: Wolters Kluwer.
Nettina, S. M. (2014). *Lippincott manual of nursing practice* (10th ed.). Philadelphia, PA: Wolters Kluwer.
Taylor, C., et al. (2011). *Fundamentals of nursing: The art and science of nursing care* (7th ed.). Philadelphia, PA: Lippincott Williams & Wilkins.

H

HAIR CARE

Combing and brushing a patient's hair stimulates scalp circulation, removes dead cells and debris, and distributes hair oils to produce a healthy sheen. The frequency of hair care depends on the length and texture of the patient's hair, the duration of hospitalization, and the patient's condition. Usually, hair should be combed and brushed daily.

Equipment

Comb ■ brush ■ bath towel ■ Optional: gloves, alcohol or oil, hair ties, hair pins.

Preparation of equipment

The comb and brush should be clean. If necessary, wash them in hot, soapy water. The comb should have dull, even teeth *to prevent scratching the scalp.* The brush should have stiff bristles *to enhance vigorous brushing and stimulation of circulation.*

Implementation

■ Gather the equipment on the patient's bedside stand.
■ Perform hand hygiene.[1,2,3,4,5]
■ Confirm the patient's identity using at least two patient identifiers.[6]

■ Tell the patient you're going to comb and brush his hair. If possible, encourage him to do this himself, assisting him as necessary.
■ Adjust the bed to a comfortable working height *to prevent back strain.* If the patient's condition allows, help him to a sitting position by raising the head of the bed.
■ Provide privacy.[7]
■ Drape a bath towel over the patient's pillow and shoulders *to catch loose hair and dirt.*
■ Put on gloves if the patient has open scalp lesions.[8,9]
■ For short hair, comb and brush one side at a time. For long or curly hair, turn the patient's head away from you, and then part his hair down the middle from front to back. Comb and brush the hair on the side facing you. Then turn the patient's head and comb and brush the opposite side. Part hair into small sections *for easier handling.* Comb one section at a time, working from the ends toward the scalp *to remove tangles.* Anchor each section of hair above the area being combed *to avoid hurting the patient.*
■ If the hair is tangled, rub alcohol or oil on the hair strands *to loosen them.* Then, comb and brush the hair, making sure to get all the tangles out.
■ Style the hair as the patient prefers. Braiding long or curly hair helps prevent snarling. To braid, part hair down the middle of the scalp and begin braiding near the face. Don't braid too tightly *to avoid patient discomfort.* Fasten the ends of the braids with hair ties. Pin the braids across the top of the patient's head or let them hang, as the patient desires, *so the finished braids don't press against the patient's scalp.*
■ After styling the hair, carefully remove the towel by folding it inward. *This technique prevents loose hairs and debris from falling onto the pillow or into the patient's bed.*
■ Remove and discard your gloves, if worn.[8]
■ Perform hand hygiene.[1,2,3,4,5]
■ Document the procedure.[10,11,12]

Special considerations

■ When providing hair care, check the patient's scalp carefully for signs of scalp disorders or skin breakdown, particularly if the patient is bedridden.
■ Make sure each patient has his own comb and brush *to avoid cross-contamination.*

Documentation

Describe any scalp abnormalities in your notes.

References

1 The Joint Commission. (2015). Standard NPSG.07.01.01. *Comprehensive accreditation manual for hospitals: The official handbook.* Oakbrook Terrace, IL: The Joint Commission. (Level VII)
2 Centers for Disease Control and Prevention. (2002). Guideline for hand hygiene in health-care settings: Recommendations of the Healthcare Infection Control Practices Advisory Committee and the HICPAC/SHEA/APIC/IDSA Hand Hygiene Task Force. *MMWR Recommendations and Reports, 51*(RR-16), 1–45. Accessed March 2015 via the Web at http://www.cdc.gov/mmwr/pdf/rr/rr5116.pdf (Level II)
3 World Health Organization. (2009). "WHO guidelines on hand hygiene in health care: First global patient safety challenge, clean care is safer care" [Online]. Accessed March 2015 via the Web at http://whqlibdoc.who.int/publications/2009/9789241597906_eng.pdf (Level IV)
4 Centers for Medicare & Medicaid Services, Department of Health and Human Services. (2014). Condition of participation: Infection control. 42 C.F.R. § 482.42.
5 American Osteopathic Association. (2014). Standard 07.01.21. *Healthcare Facilities Accreditation Program: Accreditation requirements for acute care hospitals.* Chicago, IL: American Osteopathic Association. (Level VII)
6 The Joint Commission. (2015). Standard NPSG.01.01.01. *Comprehensive accreditation manual for hospitals: The official handbook.* Oakbrook Terrace, IL: The Joint Commission. (Level VII)
7 American Osteopathic Association. (2014). Standard 15.01.16. *Healthcare Facilities Accreditation Program: Accreditation requirements for acute care hospitals.* Chicago, IL: American Osteopathic Association. (Level VII)
8 Siegel, J. D., et al. (2007). "2007 guideline for isolation precautions: Preventing transmission of infectious agents in healthcare settings" [Online]. Accessed March 2015 via the Web at http://www.cdc.gov/hicpac/pdf/isolation/Isolation2007.pdf (Level II)
9 American Osteopathic Association. (2014). Standard 07.01.10. *Healthcare Facilities Accreditation Program: Accreditation requirements for acute care hospitals.* Chicago, IL: American Osteopathic Association. (Level VII)
10 The Joint Commission. (2015). Standard RC.01.03.01. *Comprehensive accreditation manual for hospitals: The official handbook.* Oakbrook Terrace, IL: The Joint Commission. (Level VII)
11 Centers for Medicare & Medicaid Services, Department of Health and Human Services. (2014). Condition of participation: Medical record services. 42 C.F.R. § 482.24(b).
12 American Osteopathic Association. (2014). Standard 10.00.03. *Healthcare Facilities Accreditation Program: Accreditation requirements for acute care hospitals.* Chicago, IL: American Osteopathic Association. (Level VII)

Additional reference

Craven, R. F., & Hirnle, C. J. (2012). *Fundamentals of nursing: Human health and function* (7th ed.). Philadelphia, PA: Lippincott Williams & Wilkins.

Halo-vest traction management

Halo-vest traction is a nonsurgical treatment used to immobilize the head and neck and protect the cervical spine after traumatic cervical vertebrae injury as well as to prevent further injury to the spinal cord. When surgical intervention is indicated, halo-vest traction may be used preoperatively to reduce spinal misalignment and postoperatively to allow bone healing.[1] An orthopedic surgeon or a neurosurgeon applies halo-vest traction, with nursing assistance, in an emergency department, in a specially equipped room, on the intensive care unit, or in the operating room after surgical reduction of vertebral injuries.

Components of a halo-vest traction device include a metal ring that fits over the patient's skull pins, anterior and posterior portions of a vest, a vest lining, four upright bars, and two transverse bars that distribute the weight of the entire apparatus around the chest. Halo-vest traction allows a patient greater mobility than other forms of cervical traction.

The halo-vest unit is a single-use item. Application of halo-vest traction requires sterile technique and signed informed consent. Duration of treatment varies, but traction is commonly needed for up to 12 weeks.[1]

Halo-vest traction offers several advantages; it immobilizes cervical spine fractures while allowing patient mobility, facilitates surgery of the cervical spine, permits flexion and extension, and allows airway intubation without losing skeletal traction. Adjustments at the junction of the threaded support rods and horizontal frame also allows for necessary alignment. Halo-vest traction can't be used for a patient with an unstable skull fracture or an open chest wound.

Equipment

Halo-vest kit (vest, liners, head ring, skull pins with plastic cap covers, suprastructure, wrenches, and lock nuts) ■ cap ■ gown ■ mask ■ positioning device ■ tape measure ■ clippers ■ 4″ × 4″ (10-cm × 10-cm) sterile gauze pads ■ antiseptic solution or antiseptic swabs ■ sterile and clean gloves ■ anesthetic agent ■ alcohol pads ■ syringe ■ 25G needles ■ torque screwdrivers ■ Optional: prescribed analgesic, prescribed sedative, cervical collar, crescent wrench, sheepskin vest liner, normal saline solution, wash cloth and towel, large plastic bag, shampoo, cotton-tipped applicators, chlorhexidine or another facility-approved antiseptic solution.

Preparation of equipment

The practitioner measures the patient's head at the greatest circumference of the skull (about 1 cm above the ears); depending on the device type, he may also measure the mediolateral and anterior-posterior diameter of the head *to determine proper ring size. To determine the proper vest size,* the practitioner measures the patient's chest circumference at the xiphoid process. If the patient has a pendulous abdomen, the practitioner measures the widest portion of the costal margin. *To determine anterior vest size,* the practitioner measures the patient's sternal length.[2,3]

Check the expiration date of the prepackaged kit, and check the outside covering for damage *to ensure the sterility of the contents.*

Implementation

- Verify the practitioner's order.[4]
- Gather the necessary equipment.
- Confirm that the practitioner has obtained written informed consent and that the consent form is in the patient's medical record.[5,6,7]
- Conduct a preprocedure verification *to make sure that all relevant documentation, related information, and equipment are available and correctly identified to the patient's identifiers.*[8,9]
- Verify that the laboratory and imaging studies have been completed as ordered and that the results are in the patient's medical record. Notify the practitioner of any unexpected results.
- Perform hand hygiene.[10,11,12,13,14]
- Confirm the patient's identity using at least two patient identifiers.[15]
- Provide privacy.[16,17]
- Explain the procedure to the patient *to allay his anxiety and to promote cooperation with the procedure.*
- Obtain baseline vital signs, and assess the patient's neurologic and respiratory status.
- Perform a comprehensive pain assessment using techniques appropriate for the patient's age, condition, and ability to understand.[18]
- Administer an analgesic, as needed and ordered, following safe medication administration practices *to help manage the patient's pain.*[1,19,20]
- Administer a sedative, as ordered, following safe medication administration practices *to help the patient relax during the procedure.*[3,19,20]

Assisting with halo application

- Have a coworker assist with the procedure *to maintain proper cervical spine precautions and prevent patient injury.*
- Elevate the bed to a comfortable working height and remove the headboard from the bed.
- Maintain the patient in the supine position.[2,3]
- Maintain cervical spine alignment by supporting the patient's head using the positioning device.
- The practitioner selects four pin sites: ½″ (1.3 cm) above the lateral one-third of each eyebrow and ½″ (1.3 cm) above the top of each ear in the occipital area. He also takes into account the degree and type of correction needed to provide proper cervical alignment.
- Trim the hair at the intended pin sites with clippers *to facilitate subsequent care and to help prevent infection.*[2,3]
- Perform hand hygiene.[10,11,12,13,14]
- Put on gloves and other personal protective equipment as needed *to comply with standard precautions.*[2,3,21,22]
- Use an antiseptic swab or 4″ × 4″ (10-cm × 10-cm) sterile gauze pads soaked in antiseptic solution to prepare the pin site areas for pin application. Allow the solution to dry following the manufacturer's instructions.[2,3]
- Open the halo-vest unit using sterile technique *to avoid contamination.* (See the "Sterile technique, basic" procedure, page 715.)
- The practitioner puts on a cap, a gown, a mask, and sterile gloves and then removes the halo and Allen wrench.
- Conduct a time-out immediately before starting the procedure *to perform a final assessment that the correct patient, site, positioning, and procedure are identified and, as applicable, that all relevant information and necessary equipment are available.*[9,23]
- The practitioner positions the ring on the patient's head using the positioning pins; the positioning pins should accommodate access to the selected skull pin sites.
- Assist the practitioner with preparing the anesthetic agent, if necessary.
- Clean and disinfect the injection port of the anesthetic with an alcohol pad, and allow it to dry.
- Invert the vial so that the practitioner can insert a 25G needle attached to a syringe and withdraw the anesthetic.
- The practitioner injects the anesthetic at each of the four pin sites;[2,3] note that an anesthetic without epinephrine is preferred *to prevent necrosis around the injection site.*[2] Change the needle on the syringe after each injection.
- Using sterile technique, the practitioner threads each skull pin through its halo ring hole until it touches the skin. He then tightens the pins by hand using one of two methods, according to the manufacturer's instructions. For an opposing pair, he simultaneously tightens the pins opposite each other; for a posterior-anterior pair, he tightens the two posterior pins first and then the two anterior pins.[2,3]
- The practitioner visually checks the pins' positioning and then tightens them in incremental steps using the torque screwdrivers and following the manufacturer's instructions; the pins are commonly tightened 6 to 8 inch-pounds (0.68 to 0.90 newton meters).[2,3]
- The practitioner removes the positioning pins and then applies and tightens the lock nuts to the pins by hand *to secure the pins in place.*[2,3] He applies plastic caps over the free ends of the pins *to prevent them from snagging on linens and clothing.*[3]

Applying the vest

- Separate the anterior and posterior portions of the vest, if necessary.[3]
- If not already in place, position the liners inside the anterior and posterior portions of the vest *to make it more comfortable to wear and to help prevent pressure ulcers.*
- With assistance from a coworker, raise the patient from the waist, maintaining proper cervical spine precautions; properly position the posterior portion of the vest according to the manufacturer's instructions.[2,3]
- Carefully return the patient to the supine position, and then check the position of the posterior portion of the vest.[2,3]
- The practitioner then positions the anterior portion of the vest on the patient's chest and secures it in place with the posterior portion using the waist stabilizers and straps and shoulder straps.[2,3]
- As you continue to maintain cervical spine precautions, the practitioner aligns and attaches the superstructure to the halo ring and tightens the screws or bolts.[2,3]
- After application is complete, help the practitioner bring the patient to a sitting position *so that the practitioner can check that the head is in alignment with the body and that the halo superstructure is symmetrical.*[3]
- When halo-vest traction is in place, arrange for an X-ray, as ordered, *to make sure that the desired alignment has been achieved.*[3]

Caring for the patient

- Gather the necessary equipment at the patient's bedside.
- Perform hand hygiene.[10,11,12,13,14]
- Confirm the patient's identity using at least two patient identifiers.[15]
- Explain the procedure to the patient and his family.
- Assess the patient's vital signs and neurologic status, as ordered.

NURSING ALERT *Notify the practitioner immediately if you observe any loss of motor function or any decreased sensation from baseline* because these changes could indicate spinal cord trauma.

■ *Because the vest limits chest expansion,* routinely assess the patient's pulmonary status, especially in a patient with pulmonary disease.

ELDER ALERT *Respiratory complications from halo fixation are more common in older patients.*[24]

■ Perform hand hygiene and put on gloves.[10,11,12,13,14]

■ Using cotton-tipped applicators, gently clean the pin sites with chlorhexidine or another facility-approved antiseptic solution (povidone-iodine shouldn't be used *because it interferes with tissue* healing) every 8 hours or as indicated.[25]

■ Use a clean cotton-tipped applicator for each individual site, and rinse each site afterward with normal saline solution to remove any excess cleaning solution.[13] *Meticulous pin-site care prevents infection and removes debris that might block drainage and lead to abscess formation.*

■ If crusting is present, wrap the pin site with gauze soaked in normal saline solution for 15 to 20 minutes and then remove the gauze. Using a gentle rolling motion, remove the crust with a cotton-tipped applicator that has been soaked in normal saline solution.[26]

■ Observe for loose pins and signs and symptoms of infection—including swelling, redness, purulent drainage, tracking (an open area where skin has pulled away from the pin), and pain at the site—and notify the practitioner if any develop.[26]

■ The practitioner retightens the skull pins with the torque screwdriver 24 and 48 hours after the halo is applied.

■ If the patient complains of a headache after the pins are tightened, obtain an order for an analgesic. If pain occurs with jaw movement or if any movement of the head or neck occurs, notify the practitioner immediately *because this symptom may indicate that pins have slipped.*

■ Examine the halo-vest unit every shift *to make sure that the unit is secure and that the patient's head is centered within the halo.* If the vest fits correctly, you should be able to insert one or two fingers under the jacket at the shoulder and chest when the patient is in the supine position.

■ Wash the patient's chest and back daily; be careful not to put any stress on the apparatus, *which could knock it out of alignment and lead to subluxation of the cervical spine.* Place the patient on his back. Loosen the bottom Velcro straps *so you can get to the chest and back.* Turn the patient on his side (less than 45 degrees) to wash his back. Reaching under the vest, wash and dry the skin. Check for tender, reddened areas, or pressure spots that may develop into ulcers. If itching occurs, check to see whether the patient is allergic to sheepskin and whether any drug he's taking might cause a skin rash. Change the vest lining, as needed. Close the vest.

NURSING ALERT *Don't use lotions or powders underneath the vest. A cotton pillowcase or undershirt can be worn or placed under the vest* for comfort and perspiration absorption; *change this item regularly.*[26]

■ Shampoo the patient's hair regularly. Place the patient in the supine position in bed with a towel or large plastic bag along the back and shoulders of the halo-vest *to protect the lining from getting wet.* The halo crown, pins, and bars can all safely get wet.[1]

Completing the procedure

■ Discard used supplies in the appropriate receptacles.[26]

■ Remove and discard your gloves and any other personal protective equipment worn.[21]

■ Perform hand hygiene.[10,11,12,13,14]

■ Document the procedure.[27,28,29]

Special considerations

NURSING ALERT *Keep two wrenches available at all time. A wrench should accompany the patient when he's away from the unit for testing. In the event of cardiac arrest, know the type of vest that the patient is wearing. Some vests have a hinged front to raise the breastplate for cardiopulmonary resuscitation (CPR). If the patient doesn't have one of these vests, you will need to use a wrench* to remove the distal anterior bolts. *Pull the two upright bars outward, unfasten the Velcro straps, and remove the front of the vest. Use the sturdy back of the vest as a board for CPR.* To prevent subluxating the cervical injury, *perform a jaw thrust to open the airway, which avoids hyperextension of the neck. Pull the patient's mandible forward while maintaining proper head and neck alignment.* This positioning pulls the tongue forward to open the airway.

■ Be aware that there are many different types of halo and vest components. Make sure that you're familiar with the equipment used by your facility. Confirm that the device is compatible with magnetic resonance imaging, as indicated.

■ Ensure that the practitioner examines the patient about 24 hours after halo-vest application *to assess pin tightness and to check for complications.*[2,3]

■ Note that some devices require the skull pins to be removed at least once every 14 days to be cleaned and retorqued; follow the manufacturer's instructions.[3]

■ If countertraction will be applied, position the patient with the head of the bed flat and on shock blocks or in the reverse Trendelenburg position.[26]

■ Never lift up a patient by the vertical bars of a halo-vest traction device. *Doing so could strain or tear the skin at the pin sites or misalign the traction.*

■ *To prevent falls in an ambulatory patient,* walk with him. Remember that the patient will have trouble seeing objects at or near his feet and that the weight of the halo-vest unit (about 10 lb [4.5 kg]) may throw him off balance. If the patient is in a wheelchair, lower the leg rests *to prevent the chair from tipping backward.*

■ *Because the vest limits chest expansion,* routinely assess pulmonary function, especially in a patient with pulmonary disease.

Patient teaching

If the patient is to be discharged home with halo-vest traction, teach him and his family how to care for the halo-vest apparatus and the pins, stress the importance of vigilant skin care, and explain how to perform such activities of daily living as bathing, dressing, sleeping, and ambulating. Stress the importance avoiding bending, heavy lifting, and driving, and explain that the patient may need to alter clothing as necessary while in the halo-vest. Have the patient and a family member teach back the information to confirm their understanding. A physical therapist may teach the patient how to use assistive devices. Instruct the patient and his family not to adjust the pins.

Provide information about follow-up appointments. Tell the patient to notify the practitioner if he develops signs and symptoms of infection, any loosening or dislodgment at the pin site, skin breakdown, swallowing problems, headache, malaise, or visual changes or if he experiences a fall or other trauma.[1]

Complications

Manipulating the patient's neck during application of halo-vest traction can cause subluxation of the spinal cord or could push a bone fragment into the spinal cord, possibly compressing the cord and causing paralysis below the break.

Inaccurate positioning of the skull pins can lead to a puncture of the dura mater, causing a loss of cerebrospinal fluid and a serious central nervous system infection. Multiple retorquing of the pins increases the potential for a dural puncture.

Nonsterile technique during application of the halo or inadequate pin-site care can lead to infection at the pin sites and other complications, including pin-site loosening or dislodgement, swallowing problems, and ring migration.

Pressure ulcers can develop if the vest fits poorly or chafes the skin.

Documentation

Record the date and time that the halo-vest traction was applied. Also note the length of the procedure and the patient's response. Record the patient's vital signs and neurologic, pain, and pulmonary assessment findings. Document that a preprocedure verification and time-out were performed. Document the appearance of pin insertion sites, analgesics provided, and patient education performed.

When providing care to the patient with halo-vest traction, record routine vital signs as well as pain, pulmonary, and neurologic assessments. Document pin-site care. Note any signs or symptoms of infection or loose pins. Document patient teaching and the patient's comprehension of that teaching.

REFERENCES

1 Sarro, A., et al. (2010). Developing a standard of care for halo-vest and pin site care including patient and family education: A collaborative approach among three greater Toronto area teaching hospitals. *Journal of Neuroscience Nursing, 42,* 169–173.

2 Ossur, H. F. (2009). "Practitioner primer: Ossur halo systems" [Online]. Accessed March 2015 via the Web at http://www.ossur.com/lisalib/getfile.aspx?itemid=18100

3 Friddle's Orthopedic Appliances. (n.d.). "The Friddle MRI halo system: Model D: Application manual" [Online]. Accessed March 2015 via the Web at http://store.friddles.com/graphics/Halo%20Application%20Manual.pdf

4 The Joint Commission. (2015). Standard MM.04.01.01. *Comprehensive accreditation manual for hospitals: The official handbook.* Oakbrook Terrace, IL: The Joint Commission. (Level VII)

5 The Joint Commission. (2015). Standard RI.01.03.01. *Comprehensive accreditation manual for hospitals: The official handbook.* Oakbrook Terrace, IL: The Joint Commission. (Level VII)

6 Centers for Medicare & Medicaid Services, Department of Health and Human Services. (2014). Condition of participation: Patient's rights. 42 C.F.R. § 482.13.

7 American Osteopathic Association. (2014). Standard 30.01.11. *Healthcare Facilities Accreditation Program: Accreditation requirements for acute care hospitals.* Chicago, IL: American Osteopathic Association. (Level VII)

8 The Joint Commission. (2015). Standard UP.01.01.01. *Comprehensive accreditation manual for hospitals: The official handbook.* Oakbrook Terrace, IL: The Joint Commission. (Level VII)

9 American Osteopathic Association. (2014). Standard 30.00.14. *Healthcare Facilities Accreditation Program: Accreditation requirements for acute care hospitals.* Chicago, IL: American Osteopathic Association. (Level VII)

10 The Joint Commission. (2015). Standard NPSG.07.01.01. *Comprehensive accreditation manual for hospitals: The official handbook.* Oakbrook Terrace, IL: The Joint Commission. (Level VII)

11 Centers for Disease Control and Prevention. (2002). Guideline for hand hygiene in health-care settings: Recommendations of the Healthcare Infection Control Practices Advisory Committee and the HICPAC/SHEA/APIC/IDSA Hand Hygiene Task Force. *MMWR Recommendations and Reports, 51*(RR-16), 1–45. Accessed March 2015 via the Web at http://www.cdc.gov/mmwr/pdf/rr/rr5116.pdf (Level II)

12 World Health Organization. (2009). "WHO guidelines on hand hygiene in health care: First global patient safety challenge, clean care is safer care" [Online]. Accessed March 2015 via the Web at http://whqlibdoc.who.int/publications/2009/9789241597906_eng.pdf (Level IV)

13 American Osteopathic Association. (2014). Standard 07.01.21. *Healthcare Facilities Accreditation Program: Accreditation requirements for acute care hospitals.* Chicago, IL: American Osteopathic Association. (Level VII)

14 Centers for Medicare & Medicaid Services, Department of Health and Human Services. (2014). Condition of participation: Infection control. 42 C.F.R. § 482.42.

15 The Joint Commission. (2015). Standard NPSG.01.01.01. *Comprehensive accreditation manual for hospitals: The official handbook.* Oakbrook Terrace, IL: The Joint Commission. (Level VII)

16 American Osteopathic Association. (2014). Standard 15.01.16. *Healthcare Facilities Accreditation Program: Accreditation requirements for acute care hospitals.* Chicago, IL: American Osteopathic Association. (Level VII)

17 Centers for Medicare & Medicaid Services, Department of Health and Human Services. (2014). Condition of participation: Patient's rights. 42 C.F.R. § 482.13(c)(1).

18 The Joint Commission. (2015). Standard PC.01.02.07. *Comprehensive accreditation manual for hospitals: The official handbook.* Oakbrook Terrace, IL: The Joint Commission. (Level VII)

19 American Osteopathic Association. (2014). Standard 16.01.03. *Healthcare Facilities Accreditation Program: Accreditation requirements for acute care hospitals.* Chicago, IL: American Osteopathic Association. (Level VII)

20 Centers for Medicare & Medicaid Services, Department of Health and Human Services. (2014). Condition of participation: Nursing services. 42 C.F.R. § 482.23(c).

21 American Osteopathic Association. (2014). Standard 07.01.10. *Healthcare Facilities Accreditation Program: Accreditation requirements for acute care hospitals.* Chicago, IL: American Osteopathic Association. (Level VII)

22 Siegel, J. D., et al. (2007). "2007 guideline for isolation precautions: Preventing transmission of infectious agents in healthcare settings" [Online]. Accessed March 2015 via the Web at http://www.cdc.gov/hicpac/pdf/isolation/Isolation2007.pdf (Level II)

23 The Joint Commission. (2015). Standard UP.01.03.01. *Comprehensive accreditation manual for hospitals: The official handbook.* Oakbrook Terrace, IL: The Joint Commission. (Level VII)

24 Benzel, E. C. (2012). *The cervical spine* (5th ed.). Philadelphia, PA: Lippincott Williams & Wilkins.

25 Lagerquist, D., et al. (2012). Care of external fixator pin sites. *American Journal of Critical Care, 21,* 288–295.

26 Lynn-McHale Wiegand, D. (Ed.). (2011). *AACN procedure manual for critical care* (6th ed.). St. Louis, MO: Saunders.

27 American Osteopathic Association. (2014). Standard 10.00.03. *Healthcare Facilities Accreditation Program: Accreditation requirements for acute care hospitals.* Chicago, IL: American Osteopathic Association. (Level VII)

28 Centers for Medicare & Medicaid Services, Department of Health and Human Services. (2014). Condition of participation: Medical record services. 42 C.F.R. § 482.24(b).

29 The Joint Commission. (2015). Standard RC.01.03.01. *Comprehensive accreditation manual for hospitals: The official handbook.* Oakbrook Terrace, IL: The Joint Commission. (Level VII)

ADDITIONAL REFERENCES

Holmes, S. B., & Brown, S. J. (2005). Skeletal pin site care: National Association of Orthopaedic Nurses guidelines for orthopaedic nursing. *Orthopaedic Nursing, 24*(2), 99–107.

Ivanic, P.C., et al. (2009). Effect of halo-vest components on stabilizing the injured cervical spine. *Spine, 34*(2), 167–175.

Lauweryns, P. (2010). Role of conservative treatment of cervical spine injury. *European Spine Journal, 19*(Suppl.), S23–S26.

Van Middendorp, J. J., et al. (2009). Incidence of and risk factors for complications associated with halo-vest immobilization: A prospective, descriptive cohort study of 239 patients. *Journal of Bone and Joint Surgery, 91*(1), 71–79.

HAND HYGIENE

"Hand hygiene" is a general term used by the Centers for Disease Control and Prevention (CDC) and the World Health Organization (WHO) to refer to hand washing, antiseptic hand washing, antiseptic hand rubbing, or surgical hand asepsis.[1,2,3]

The hands are the conduits for almost every transfer of potential pathogens from one patient to another, from a contaminated object to the patient, or from a staff member to the patient. Because of this, hand hygiene is the single most important procedure in preventing infection.[1,4] To protect patients from health care–associated infections, hand hygiene must be performed routinely and thoroughly.[5] In effect, clean and healthy hands with intact skin, short fingernails, and no rings minimizes the risk of contamination. Artificial nails may serve as a reservoir for microorganisms[6] as may rough or chapped hands.[1]

Your 5 moments for hand hygiene

According to the World Health Organization (WHO), there are 5 key moments during patient care when health care workers should perform hand hygiene.

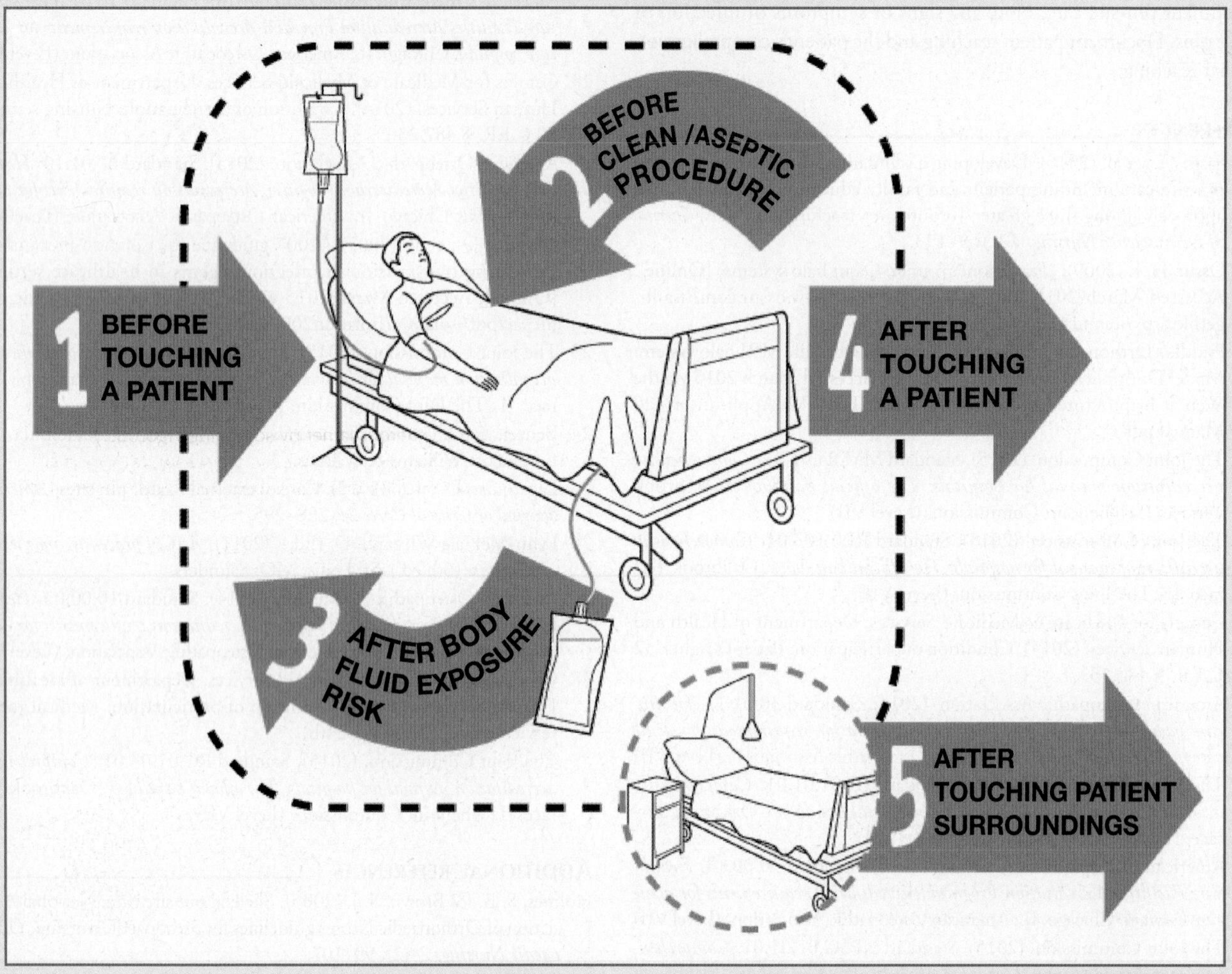

Based on "My 5 Moments for Hand Hygiene" URL: http://www.who.int/gpsc/5may/background/5moments/en/index.html

Washing with soap and water is appropriate when hands are visibly soiled or contaminated with blood or other body fluids, when exposure to potential spore-forming pathogens (such as *Clostridium difficile* or *Bacillus anthracis*) is strongly suspected or proven, and after using the restroom. Using an alcohol-based hand sanitizer is appropriate for decontaminating the hands before direct patient contact; before putting on gloves; before inserting an invasive device; after contact with the patient; when moving from a contaminated-body site to a clean-body site during patient care; after contact with body fluids, excretions, mucous membranes, nonintact skin, or wound dressings (if hands aren't visibly soiled); after removing gloves; and after contact with inanimate objects in the patient's environment.[1,2,7] (See *Your 5 moments for hand hygiene.*)

The CDC recommends performing hand hygiene with soap and water before eating;[1] the WHO recommends using either an alcohol-based hand rub or washing with soap and water before preparing food or handling medication.[2]

Equipment

Hand washing

Soap ▪ warm running water ▪ paper towels ▪ Optional: emollient hand cream or lotion.

Hand sanitizing

▪ Alcohol-based hand rub ▪ Optional: emollient hand cream or lotion.

Implementation

Hand washing

▪ Remove rings according to your facility's policy *because they harbor dirt and skin microorganisms.* Remove your watch and bracelets or wear them well above the wrist. If you wear nail polish, it must be kept in good repair *to minimize its potential to harbor microorganisms*; refer to your facility's guidelines regarding nail polish. Natural nails should be short (less than ¼″ [0.6 cm]).[1,6,8]

▪ Wet your hands and wrists with warm (not hot) water,[1,2] and apply soap from a dispenser.[1] Don't use bar soap *because it allows cross-contamination.*[1]

Hold your hands below elbow level *to prevent water from running up your arms and back down, contaminating clean areas.* (See *Proper hand-washing technique.*)

■ Work up a generous lather by rubbing your hands together vigorously for about 20 seconds.[1] *Soap and warm water reduce surface tension, which, aided by friction, loosens surface microorganisms, which wash away in the lather.*

■ Pay special attention to the area under your fingernails and around your cuticles and to your thumbs, knuckles, and the sides of your fingers and hands *because microorganisms thrive in these protected or overlooked areas.* If you don't remove your rings, move them up and down your finger *to clean beneath them.*[1]

■ Avoid splashing water on yourself or the floor *because microorganisms spread more easily on wet surfaces and because slippery floors are dangerous.* Avoid touching the sink or faucets *because they're considered contaminated.*

■ Rinse your hands and wrists well *because running water flushes away suds, soil, and microorganisms.*

■ Pat your hands and wrists dry with a paper towel. Avoid rubbing, *which can cause abrasion and chapping.*

■ If the sink isn't equipped with knee or foot controls, turn off the faucets by gripping them with a dry paper towel *to avoid recontaminating your hands.*

Hand sanitizing

■ Apply alcohol-based hand rub to the palm of one hand and then rub your hands together to cover all surfaces of the hands.[1,2]

■ Continue rubbing your hands together until all of the product has dried (usually about 30 seconds).[1,2]

Special considerations

■ Bundling supplies and clustering tasks reduces the number of times health care workers need to be in patients' rooms, resulting in fewer instances in which workers need to perform hand hygiene, which likely increases compliance.[9]

■ Before participating in any sterile procedure or whenever your hands are grossly contaminated, also wash your forearms, and clean under your fingernails and in and around your cuticles. Don't use brushes, metal files, or other hard objects *because they can injure your skin and, if reused, may be a source of contamination.*

■ The CDC hand hygiene guideline recommends that artificial nails or extenders not be worn by health care workers who have direct contact with patients at high risk for acquiring infections, such as patients on intensive care or transplant units.[1] Similarly, the WHO's guidelines on hand hygiene in health care recommend that artificial nails or extenders not be worn when having direct contact with all patients.[2]

■ If your hands aren't visibly soiled, you can use an alcohol-based hand rub for routine decontamination.[1]

■ If you're providing care in the patient's home, bring your own supply of soap and disposable paper towels. If running water isn't available, disinfect your hands with an alcohol-based hand rub.

■ Keep in mind that glove use doesn't eliminate the need for hand hygiene. (See *Getting to the root of hand hygiene failure,* page 346.)

■ Teach patients and their families about the importance of hand hygiene in preventing the spread of infection, and encourage them to remind health care workers to perform hand hygiene when necessary.[1,2]

■ *To prevent your hands from becoming dry or chapped,* apply an emollient hand cream after performing hand hygiene, or switch to a different cleaning agent. Make sure that the hand cream or lotion you use won't cause the material in your gloves to deteriorate. If you develop dermatitis, you may need to be evaluated by your employee health care provider to determine whether you should continue to work until the condition resolves.

Proper hand-washing technique

To minimize the spread of infection, follow these basic hand-washing instructions.

With your hands angled downward under the faucet, adjust the water temperature until it's comfortably warm.

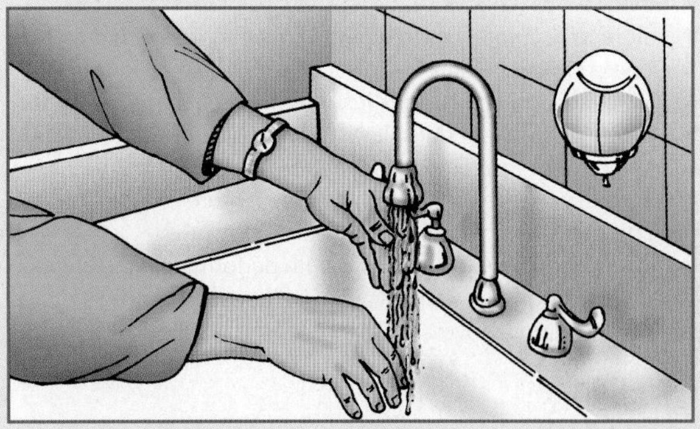

Work up a generous lather by scrubbing vigorously for at least 20 seconds.[1] Be sure to clean beneath your fingernails, around your knuckles, and along the sides of your fingers and hands.

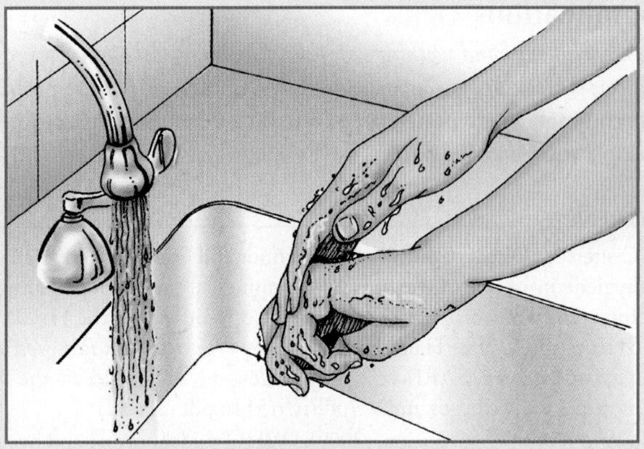

Rinse your hands completely *to wash away suds and microorganisms.* Pat dry with a paper towel. *To prevent recontaminating your hands on the faucet handles,* cover each one with a dry paper towel when turning off the water.[1]

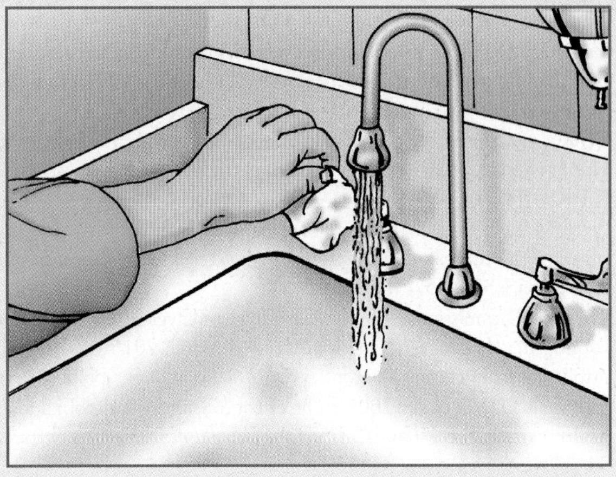

Getting to the root of hand hygiene failure[9]

Through observation of health care workers at eight participating hospitals, The Joint Commission's Hand Hygiene Project has identified the following 10 root causes of hand hygiene failure:

- ineffective placement of dispensers or sinks
- failure to accurately or frequently collect or report hand hygiene compliance data
- lack of accountability and "just-in-time" coaching
- a safety culture that doesn't stress hand hygiene at all levels
- ineffective or insufficient education
- hands that are frequently full, making it more difficult to perform hand hygiene
- glove wearing, which interferes with performing hand hygiene
- the perception that hand hygiene isn't needed if a health care worker is wearing gloves
- forgetfulness
- distractions.

Hands with dermatitis are more susceptible to becoming colonized with transient bacteria.

Complications

Because frequent hand washing strips the skin of natural oils, it can result in dryness, cracking, and irritation. However, these effects are probably more common after repeated use of antiseptic cleaning agents, especially in people with sensitive skin.

References

1 Centers for Disease Control and Prevention. (2002). Guideline for hand hygiene in health-care settings: Recommendations of the Healthcare Infection Control Practices Advisory Committee and the HICPAC/SHEA/APIC/IDSA Hand Hygiene Task Force. *MMWR Recommendations and Reports, 51*(RR-16), 1–45. Accessed March 2015 via the Web at http://www.cdc.gov/mmwr/pdf/rr/rr5116.pdf (Level I)

2 World Health Organization. (2009). "WHO guidelines on hand hygiene in health care: First global patient safety challenge, clean care is safer care" [Online]. Accessed March 2015 via the Web at http://whqlibdoc.who.int/publications/2009/9789241597906_eng.pdf (Level I)

3 The Joint Commission. (2015). Standard NPSG.07.01.01. *Comprehensive accreditation manual for hospitals: The official handbook.* Oakbrook Terrace, IL: The Joint Commission. (Level I)

4 Larson, E. (1988). A causal link between handwashing and risk of infection? Examination of the evidence. *Infection Control and Hospital Epidemiology, 9,* 28–36. (Level V)

5 Centers for Medicare & Medicaid Services, Department of Health and Human Services. (2014). Condition of participation: Patient's rights. 42 C.F.R. § 482.42.

6 Parry, M. F., et al. (2001). Candida osteomyelitis and diskitis after spinal surgery: An outbreak that implicates artificial nail use. *Clinical Infectious Diseases, 32,* 352–357. (Level IV)

7 The Joint Commission. (2009). "Measuring hand hygiene adherence: Overcoming the challenges" [Online]. Accessed March 2015 via the Web at http://www.jointcommission.org/assets/1/18/hh_monograph.pdf (Level I)

8 Salisbury, D. M., et al. (2001). The effect of rings on microbial load of health care workers' hands. *American Journal of Infection Control, 25,* 24–27. (Level VI)

9 Health Research & Educational Trust. (2010). Hand Hygiene Project: Best practices from hospitals participating in The Joint Commission Center for Transforming Healthcare Project. Chicago, IL: Health Research & Educational Trust. Accessed March 2015 via the Web at http://www.hpoe.org/Reports-HPOE/hand_hygiene_project.pdf (Level VII)

Additional references

Chow, A., et al. (2012). Alcohol handrubbing and chlorhexidine hand washing protocols for routine hospital practice: A randomized clinical trial of protocol efficacy. *American Journal of Infection Control, 40,* 800–805. (Level II)

Cohen, B., et al. (2011). Relationship between systems-level factors and hand hygiene adherence. *Journal of Nursing Care Quality, 26,* 30–38. Accessed March 2015 via the Web at http://www.ncbi.nlm.nih.gov/pmc/articles/PMC2927786/ (Level VI)

Nevo, I., et al. (2010). The efficacy of visual cues to improve hand hygiene compliance. *Simulation in Healthcare, 5,* 325–331. (Level II)

Siegel, J. D., et al. (2007). "2007 guideline for isolation precautions: Preventing transmission of infectious agents in healthcare settings" [Online]. Accessed March 2015 via the Web at http://www.cdc.gov/hicpac/pdf/isolation/Isolation2007.pdf (Level II)

Hearing aid care

Hearing is an anatomic function in which the external ear collects sounds and sends them to the eardrum, or tympanic membrane, which separates the outer ear from the inner ear. Sounds are then interpreted by the brain, which processes the appropriate response. The three primary bones involved in sound transmission are the malleus (hammer), incus (anvil), and stapes (stirrup).

Causes of hearing loss include chronic ear infections, trauma (pressure changes), age changes (presbycusis), long-term exposure to loud noises, and neuromas on the acoustic nerve. Additionally, certain drugs can contribute to hearing loss or degradation, including aspirin, naproxen, and ketorolac. Accumulation of cerumen can also affect hearing ability, leading to conductive hearing loss.

Hearing aids can help some patients regain some of their lost hearing. Several types of hearing aids are available in digital and analog form. Analog hearing aids simply amplify speech and sound; digital hearing aids provide amplification that can be individualized for the patient's type of hearing loss. All hearing aids have a microphone, a speaker, and an amplifier. Several types of hearing aids are available:[1]

- An *open-behind-the-ear aid* is a slim tube inserted into the external ear canal. This aid leaves the ear canal open, so it's best for mild to moderate high-frequency hearing loss in which low-frequency hearing is still normal or near normal.
- A *full-shell aid* is custom-made and fills most of the bowl-shaped area of the outer ear. It's used for mild to severe hearing loss.
- A *half-shell aid* is custom-made and fills the lower portion of the bowl-shaped area of the outer ear. It provides optimum performance and maximum comfort. They're used for mild to severe hearing loss.
- A *canal aid* fits partially inside the external ear canal and is used for mild to moderately severe hearing loss.
- A *mini-canal aid* fits almost completely inside the external ear canal and is appropriate for mild to moderately severe hearing loss.
- A *completely-in-the-canal aid* fits deeply within the external ear canal. This type decreases wind noise, has less feedback, and provides a more natural sound. Those with mild to moderately severe hearing loss can benefit from this type of aid.

Patients generally wear hearing aids only during the day. At night and at times of rest, most patients remove their hearing aids. Because of the fragile nature of the hearing aid, the device must be cleaned properly and carefully to avoid damage.

Equipment

Hearing aid ■ facial tissue ■ towel ■ cleaning tools as recommended by the manufacturer ■ storage case ■ washcloth ■ warm water ■ soap ■ Optional: spare battery, dryer for hearing aids, gloves.

Implementation

- Gather the appropriate equipment.
- Perform hand hygiene.[2,3,4,5,6]
- Confirm the patient's identity using at least two patient identifiers.[7]

Removing and cleaning the hearing aid

- Inspect the patient's ear. If drainage is present, put on gloves.[8,9]
- Gently turn the hearing aid off *to prevent feedback, in the form of whistling or squealing, during removal.*
- Grasp the hearing aid and remove it, following the contour of the patient's ear.
- Wipe the outside of the hearing aid with a tissue.
- Carefully inspect the hearing aid and look for accumulated cerumen (earwax). *Cerumen can block sound and the pressure equalizer channel and create a feeling of ear pressure.*
- Inspect the hearing aid for any rough areas that may irritate the ear canal.
- Open the battery compartment of the hearing aid *to conserve battery life and allow internal components exposure to air to dry.*
- Place the hearing aid and battery in a storage case labeled with the patient's name, room number, and identification number.
- Assess the patient's ear for drainage, redness, and irritation.
- Place a towel under the patient's ear and gently clean the ear and ear canal using a washcloth, soap, and warm water.

NURSING ALERT *Don't use alcohol or other solvents on the hearing aid because they may cause breakdown of the material.*

Inserting the hearing aid

- Gently remove the hearing aid from the storage case.
- Close the battery compartment door.
- Cupping your hand over the hearing aid, test the battery by slowing turning the volume to high. You should hear feedback; when you do, decrease the volume.
- Insert the hearing aid into the appropriate ear by holding it with the thumb and index finger of your dominant hand and placing it in the ear, following the contour of the patient's ear. Note that some hearing aids are color-coded red for right and blue for left.
- Turn the volume up slowly until it reaches a comfortable level for the patient.
- If you or the patient hears feedback after insertion, decrease the volume, reposition the device, and check the ear canal.

Completing the procedure

- Remove and discard your gloves, if worn.[8]
- Perform hand hygiene.[2,3,4,5,6]
- Document the procedure.[10,11,12]

Special considerations

- Many individuals with severe hearing loss have learned to read lips. Although this skill improves reception of the words, it doesn't improve the ability to hear. Face the patient when you speak to him and speak slowly.
- Keep background noise to a minimum if possible. *White noise can cause distractions, especially at higher frequencies.*
- Keep in mind that higher voices may be more difficult to hear, especially if the hearing loss is in the higher frequency, as occurs in elderly patients. Patients with hearing loss may also have difficulty hearing such consonants and sounds as "p," "k," "f," "th," and "s."
- Avoid placing the hearing aid in direct sunlight or direct heat.

Patient teaching

Teach the patient how to properly remove, clean, and insert the hearing aid.

ELDER ALERT *Some elderly patients may have difficulty manipulating hearing aids, making it difficult to correctly insert and clean them. In such a case, refer the patient to an audiologist, who can recommend a hearing aid that will better fit the patient's lifestyle.*

Tell the patient to keep the hearing aid in the storage case when not in use *to avoid damage.* Also, tell the patient to keep the hearing aid out of reach of children and animals. *Dogs are attracted to the smell of hearing aids and may damage them if they can reach them.* Tell the patient to keep the hearing aid dry and to remove it before showering, swimming, or participating in an activity with water. The patient should also avoid getting hairspray or cologne on the hearing aid.

Refer the patient for counseling and rehabilitative training, as needed, *to help him cope with hearing impairment and to learn ways to modify his environment to accommodate hearing loss.*[13]

Complications

Dropping the hearing aid may damage it. If moisture enters the hearing aid, either during wear or during cleaning, the device might stop transmitting sound.

Documentation

Document the proper functioning, insertion, removal, and cleaning of each hearing aid. Also document skin integrity and the presence of redness, drainage, or excessive cerumen. Note the locations where the hearing aid was stored. If you conducted patient teaching, record the teaching performed and the patient's response to the teaching.

REFERENCES

1 The Mayo Clinic. (2011). "Hearing aids: How to choose the right one" [Online]. Accessed March 2015 via the Web at http://www.mayoclinic.com/health/hearing-aids/HQ00812

2 The Joint Commission. (2015). Standard NPSG.07.01.01. *Comprehensive accreditation manual for hospitals: The official handbook.* Oakbrook Terrace, IL: The Joint Commission. (Level VII)

3 Centers for Disease Control and Prevention. (2002). Guideline for hand hygiene in health-care settings: Recommendations of the Healthcare Infection Control Practices Advisory Committee and the HICPAC/SHEA/APIC/IDSA Hand Hygiene Task Force. *MMWR Recommendations and Reports, 51*(RR-16), 1–45. Accessed March 2015 via the Web at http://www.cdc.gov/mmwr/pdf/rr/rr5116.pdf (Level II)

4 World Health Organization. (2009). "WHO guidelines on hand hygiene in health care: First global patient safety challenge, clean care is safer care" [Online]. Accessed March 2015 via the Web at http://whqlibdoc.who.int/publications/2009/9789241597906_eng.pdf (Level IV)

5 American Osteopathic Association. (2014). Standard 07.01.21. *Healthcare Facilities Accreditation Program: Accreditation requirements for acute care hospitals.* Chicago, IL: American Osteopathic Association. (Level VII)

6 Centers for Medicare & Medicaid Services, Department of Health and Human Services. (2014). Condition of participation: Infection control. 42 C.F.R. § 482.42.

7 The Joint Commission. (2015). Standard NPSG.01.01.01. *Comprehensive accreditation manual for hospitals: The official handbook.* Oakbrook Terrace, IL: The Joint Commission. (Level VII)

8 Siegel, J. D., et al. (2007). "2007 guideline for isolation precautions: Preventing transmission of infectious agents in healthcare settings" [Online]. Accessed March 2015 via the Web at http://www.cdc.gov/hicpac/pdf/isolation/Isolation2007.pdf (Level II)

9 American Osteopathic Association. (2014). Standard 07.01.10. *Healthcare Facilities Accreditation Program: Accreditation requirements for acute care hospitals.* Chicago, IL: American Osteopathic Association. (Level VII)

10 The Joint Commission. (2015). Standard RC.01.03.01. *Comprehensive accreditation manual for hospitals: The official handbook.* Oakbrook Terrace, IL: The Joint Commission. (Level VII)

11 American Osteopathic Association. (2014). Standard 10.00.03. *Healthcare Facilities Accreditation Program: Accreditation requirements for acute care hospitals.* Chicago, IL: American Osteopathic Association. (Level VII)

12 Centers for Medicare & Medicaid Services, Department of Health and Human Services. (2014). Condition of participation: Medical records services. 42 C.F.R. § 482.24(b).

13 Lin, F. R. (2012). Hearing loss in older adults: Who's listening? *JAMA, 307,* 1147–1148.

ADDITIONAL REFERENCES

National Institute on Deafness and Other Communication Disorders. (2007). "Hearing aids" [Online]. Accessed March 2015 via the Web at http://www.nidcd.nih.gov/health/hearing/pages/hearingaid.aspx#hearingaid_09

Perez, E., & Edmonds, B. A. (2012). A systematic review of studies measuring and reporting hearing aid usage in older adults since 1999: A descriptive summary of measurement tools. *PLoS One, 7*(3), e31831. (Level V)

Perry, A. G., & Potter, P. A. (2013). *Clinical nursing skills and techniques* (8th ed.). St. Louis, MO: Mosby.

Saunders, G. H., & Forsline, A. (2012). Hearing-aid counseling: Comparison of single-session informational counseling with single-session performance-perceptual counseling. *International Journal of Audiology, 51,* 754–764. (Level VI)

HEAT APPLICATION

Heat applied directly to the patient's body raises tissue temperature and enhances the inflammatory process by causing vasodilation and increasing local circulation, which promotes leukocytosis, suppuration, drainage, and healing. Heat also increases tissue metabolism; reduces pain caused by muscle spasm, muscle strains, or minor aches and stiffness; and decreases congestion in deep visceral organs.

Direct heat may be dry or moist. Dry heat can be delivered at a higher temperature and for a longer time than moist heat. Devices for applying dry heat include the hot-water bottle, electric heating pad, K pad, and chemical hot pack.

Moist heat softens crusts and exudates, penetrates deeper than dry heat, is less drying to the skin, produces less perspiration, and is usually more comfortable for the patient. Devices for applying moist heat include warm compresses for small body areas and warm packs for large areas.

Direct heat treatment can't be used on a patient at risk for hemorrhage. It also is contraindicated if the patient has a sprained limb in the acute stage (because vasodilation would increase pain and swelling) or if he has a condition associated with acute inflammation such as appendicitis. Direct heat should be applied cautiously to pediatric and elderly patients and to patients with impaired kidney, cardiac, or respiratory function; arteriosclerosis or atherosclerosis; impaired sensation; diabetes; or spinal cord injury. It should be applied with extreme caution to heat-sensitive areas, such as scar tissue and stomas. Don't apply heat to an open wound after trauma; to inflamed or edematous areas, a localized malignant tumor, the testes, or the abdomen of a pregnant woman; or over metallic implants.[1]

NURSING ALERT *Don't apply heat over a fentanyl transdermal system or its surrounding area* because an increase in temperature increases fentanyl release from the system, which may result in overdose and death.[2]

Equipment

For all methods

Thermometer ▪ adhesive tape or roller gauze ▪ absorbent, protective cloth covering ▪ dressing materials ▪ Optional: gloves.

For a hot-water bottle

Hot-water bottle ▪ hot tap water ▪ pitcher ▪ bath (utility) thermometer.

For an electric heating pad

Electric heating pad.

For a K pad

K pad ▪ distilled water ▪ temperature-adjustment key.

For a chemical hot pack (disposable)

Chemical hot pack.

For a warm compress or pack (sterile or nonsterile)

Warm compress or pack ▪ basin of hot tap water ▪ container of sterile water, normal saline solution, or other prescribed solution ▪ clean or sterile bowl or basin ▪ fluid-impermeable pad ▪ clean or sterile bath (utility) thermometer ▪ clean or sterile waterproof covering ▪ hot-water bottle, K pad, or chemical hot pack ▪ Optional: sterile forceps, clean container, clean or sterile towel, bedside sterilizer.

Preparation of equipment

Hot-water bottle

Fill the bottle with hot tap water *to detect leaks and warm the bottle;* then empty it. Run hot tap water into a pitcher and measure the water temperature with the bath thermometer. Adjust the temperature as ordered, usually to 115° to 125°F (46.1° to 51.7°C) for adults.

PEDIATRIC ALERT *Adjust water temperature to between 105° and 115°F (40.6° to 46.1°C) for children younger than age 2.*

ELDER ALERT *Adjust water temperature to between 105° and 115°F (40.6° to 46.1°C) for elderly patients.*

Next, pour hot water into the bottle, filling it one-half to two-thirds full. *Partially filling the bottle keeps it lightweight and flexible to mold to the treatment area.* Squeeze the bottle until the water reaches the neck *to expel any air that would make the bottle inflexible and reduce heat conduction.* Fasten the top and check the bag for leaks. Place the bag in an absorbent cloth covering, and secure the cover with tape or roller gauze.

Electric heating pad

Check the cord for frayed or damaged insulation. Then plug in the pad and adjust the control switch to the desired setting. Wrap the pad in a protective cloth covering, and secure the cover with tape or roller gauze. If the pad comes with its own cover, inspect the cover and fasteners *to ensure that all are intact.*

K pad

Check the cord for frayed or damaged insulation, and fill the control unit two-thirds full with distilled water according to the manufacturer's directions. Don't use tap water *because it leaves mineral deposits in the unit.* Check for leaks, and then tilt the unit in several directions *to clear the pad's tubing of air.* Tighten the cap, and then loosen it a quarter turn *to allow heat expansion within the unit.* After making sure the hoses between the control unit and the pad are free of tangles, place the unit on the bedside table, slightly above the patient *so that gravity can assist water flow.* Use the temperature-adjustment key provided to set the temperature on the control unit. The usual temperature is 105°F (40.6°C). Then place the pad in a protective cloth covering and secure the cover with tape or roller gauze. Plug in the unit, turn it on, and allow the pad to warm for 2 minutes.

Chemical hot pack

Select a pack of the correct size. Then follow the manufacturer's directions (strike, squeeze, or knead) *to activate the heat-producing chemicals.* Place the pack in a protective cloth covering and secure the cover with tape or roller gauze.

Sterile warm compress or pack

Warm the container of sterile water or solution by setting it in a sink or basin of hot water. Measure its temperature with a sterile bath thermometer. Adjust the temperature by adding hot or cold water to the sink or basin until the solution reaches 120°F (A48.9°C) for adults.[3]

PEDIATRIC ALERT *Adjust the water temperature to 100°F (37.8°C) for children.*[3]

ELDER ALERT *Adjust the water temperature to 100°F (37.8°C) for elderly patients.*[3]

NURSING ALERT *Adjust the water temperature to 100°F (37.8°C) for an eye compress.*[3]

Pour the heated solution into a sterile bowl or basin. Then, using the sterile forceps and sterile technique, soak the compress or pack in the heated solution and wring out excess solution while maintaining sterility. If necessary, prepare a hot-water bottle, K pad, or chemical hot pack *to keep the compress or pack warm.*

Nonsterile warm compress or pack

Fill a bowl or basin with hot tap water or other solution, and measure the temperature of the fluid with a bath thermometer. Adjust the temperature as ordered, usually to 120°F (48.9°C) for adults.[3]

PEDIATRIC ALERT *Adjust the water temperature to 100°F (37.8°C) for children.*[3]

ELDER ALERT *Adjust the water temperature to 100°F (37.8°C) for elderly patient.*[3]

NURSING ALERT *Adjust the water temperature to 100°F (37.8°C) for an eye compress.*[3]

Soak the compress or pack in the hot liquid and wring out excess liquid. If necessary, prepare a hot-water bottle, K pad, or chemical hot pack *to keep the compress or pack warm.*

Implementation

- Verify the practitioner's order if needed.
- Gather and prepare the equipment.
- Perform hand hygiene.[4,5,6,7,8]
- Confirm the patient's identity using at least two patient identifiers.[9]
- Explain the procedure to the patient, and tell him not to lean or lie directly on the heating device *because direct contact reduces air space and increases the risk of burns.* Warn him against adjusting the temperature of the heating device or adding hot water to a hot-water bottle. Advise him to report pain immediately and to remove the device if necessary.
- Provide privacy and make sure the room is warm and free of drafts.
- Obtain the patient's temperature, pulse, and respirations *to serve as a baseline.* If heat treatment is being applied to raise the patient's body temperature, monitor the patient's temperature, pulse, and respirations throughout the application.
- Put on gloves or sterile gloves as needed *to comply with standard precautions.*[10,11]
- Expose only the treatment area *because vasodilation will make the patient feel chilly.*
- Assess the treatment area for open lesions, edema, bleeding, and evidence of altered circulation *because the risk of damage to tissue is increased if the area is already traumatized.*[1]

Applying a hot-water bottle, an electric heating pad, a K pad, or a chemical hot pack

- Before applying the heating device, press it against your inner forearm *to test its temperature and heat distribution.* If it heats unevenly, obtain a new device.
- Apply the device to the treatment area and, if necessary, secure it with tape or roller gauze. Begin timing the application.
- Assess the patient's skin condition frequently; remove the device if you observe increased swelling or excessive redness, blistering, maceration, or pallor, or if the patient reports discomfort. Refill the hot-water bottle as necessary *to maintain the correct temperature.*
- Remove the device after 20 to 30 minutes, or as ordered.

Applying a warm compress or pack

- Place a fluid-impermeable pad under the site.
- Remove the warm compress or pack from the bowl or basin. (Use sterile forceps throughout the procedure if needed.)
- Wring excess solution from the compress or pack. *Excess moisture increases the risk of burns.*
- Apply the compress or pack gently to the affected site. After a few seconds, lift the device and check the skin for excessive redness, maceration, or blistering. When you're sure the compress or pack isn't causing a burn, mold it firmly to the skin *to keep air out, which reduces the temperature and effectiveness of the compress or pack.* Work quickly *so the compress or pack retains its heat.*
- Apply a waterproof covering (sterile, if necessary) to the device. Secure it with tape or roller gauze *to prevent it from slipping.*
- Place a hot-water bottle, K pad, or chemical hot pack and waterproof covering over the compress or pack *to maintain the correct temperature.* Begin timing the application.
- Assess the patient's skin at regular intervals. Remove the device if the skin shows excessive redness, maceration, or blistering or if the patient experiences pain or discomfort. Change the compress or pack as needed *to maintain the correct temperature.*
- After 15 or 20 minutes or as ordered, remove the device. Discard it into a waterproof trash bag.

Completing the procedure

- As necessary, dry the patient's skin with a towel (sterile, if necessary). Note the condition of the skin and re-dress the area, if necessary. Obtain the patient's temperature, pulse, and respirations *to compare with the baseline.* Then make sure the patient is comfortable.
- Remove and discard your gloves, if worn, and perform hand hygiene.[4,5,6,7,8]
- If the treatment is to be repeated, store the equipment in the patient's room, out of his reach; otherwise, return it for proper cleaning and disinfection.
- Document the procedure.[12,13,14]

Special considerations

- Make sure that closure devices aren't in direct contact with the skin *because closure devices can cause burns.*
- If the patient is unconscious, anesthetized, cognitively or neurologically impaired, or insensitive to heat, stay with him throughout the treatment.
- When direct heat is ordered to decrease congestion within internal organs, the application must cover a large enough area *to increase blood volume at the skin's surface.* For relief of pelvic organ congestion, for example, apply heat over the patient's lower abdomen, hips, and thighs. *To achieve local relief,* you may concentrate heat only over the specified area. (See *Using moist heat to relieve muscle spasm,* page 350.)
- As an alternative method to apply a sterile moist compress, use a bedside sterilizer *to sterilize the compress.* Saturate the compress with tap water or another solution and wring it dry. Then place it in the bedside sterilizer at 275°F (135°C) for 15 minutes. Remove the compress with sterile forceps or sterile gloves, and wring out the excess solution. Then place the compress in a sterile bowl, measure its temperature with a sterile thermometer, and allow it to cool to 120°F (48.9°C).[3]
- Follow the manufacturer's instructions for heating compresses, and avoid overheating.

PATIENT TEACHING

Using moist heat to relieve muscle spasm

Tell patients to choose moist heat rather than dry heat when attempting to ease muscle tension or spasm. *Moist heat is less drying to the skin, less apt to cause burns, less likely to cause excessive fluid and salt loss through sweating, and more likely to penetrate deeper tissues.* Instruct the patient to apply heat for 20 to 30 minutes, as follows:

- Place a moist towel over the painful area.
- Cover the towel with a hot-water bottle properly filled and at the correct temperature.
- Remove the hot-water bottle and towel after 20 to 30 minutes. Don't continue the application for longer than 30 minutes *because therapeutic value decreases after that time.*

Patient teaching

If the patient is to continue heat application at home, teach him how to use the equipment and to make sure the equipment is safe. Also teach him to check his skin at regular intervals for signs and symptoms of excessive exposure to heat.

Complications

Because tissue damage may result from direct heat application, monitor the temperature of the compress carefully. Frequently assess the condition of the patient's skin under the heat application device.

Documentation

Record the time and date of heat application; the type, temperature or heat setting, duration, and site of application; the patient's temperature, pulse, respirations, and skin condition before, during, and after treatment; signs of complications; and the patient's tolerance of the treatment. Document any patient teaching and the patient's understanding of your teaching.

REFERENCES

1 Taylor, C., et al. (2011). *Fundamentals of nursing: The art and science of nursing care* (7th ed.). Philadelphia, PA: Lippincott Williams & Wilkins.
2 Janssen Pharmaceuticals, Inc. (2012). "Duragesic (fentanyl transdermal system) prescribing information" [Online]. Accessed March 2015 via the Web at http://www.duragesic.com/sites/default/files/pdf/duragesic_0.pdf
3 Burn Foundation. (n.d.). "Safety facts on scald burns" [Online]. Accessed March 2015 via the Web at http://www.burnfoundation.org/programs/resource.cfm?c=1&a=3
4 American Osteopathic Association. (2014). Standard 07.01.21. *Healthcare Facilities Accreditation Program: Accreditation requirements for acute care hospitals.* Chicago, IL: American Osteopathic Association. (Level VII)
5 Centers for Medicare & Medicaid Services, Department of Health and Human Services. (2014). Condition of participation: Infection control. 42 C.F.R. § 482.42.
6 The Joint Commission. (2015). Standard NPSG 07.01.01. *Comprehensive accreditation manual for hospitals: The official handbook.* Oakbrook Terrace, IL: The Joint Commission. (Level VII)
7 Centers for Disease Control and Prevention. (2002). Guideline for hand hygiene in health-care settings: Recommendations of the Healthcare Infection Control Practices Advisory Committee and the HICPAC/SHEA/APIC/IDSA Hand Hygiene Task Force. *MMWR Recommendations and Reports, 51*(RR-16), 1–45. Accessed March 2015 via the Web at http://www.cdc.gov/mmwr/pdf/rr/rr5116.pdf (Level II)
8 World Health Organization. (2009). "WHO guidelines on hand hygiene in health care: First global patient safety challenge, clean care is safer care" [Online]. Accessed March 2015 via the Web at http://whqlibdoc.who.int/publications/2009/9789241597906_eng.pdf (Level IV)
9 The Joint Commission. (2015). Standard NPSG.01.01.01. *Comprehensive accreditation manual for hospitals: The official handbook.* Oakbrook Terrace, IL: The Joint Commission. (Level VII)
10 American Osteopathic Association. (2014). Standard 07.01.10. *Healthcare Facilities Accreditation Program: Accreditation requirements for acute care hospitals.* Chicago, IL: American Osteopathic Association. (Level VII)
11 Siegel, J. D., et al. (2007). "2007 guideline for isolation precautions: Preventing transmission of infectious agents in healthcare settings" [Online]. Accessed March 2015 via the Web at http://www.cdc.gov/hicpac/pdf/isolation/Isolation2007.pdf (Level II)
12 The Joint Commission. (2015). Standard RC 01.03.01. *Comprehensive accreditation manual for hospitals: The official handbook.* Oakbrook Terrace, IL: The Joint Commission. (Level VII)
13 Centers for Medicare & Medicaid Services, Department of Health and Human Services. (2014). Condition of participation: Medical records services. 42 C.F.R. § 482.24(b).
14 American Osteopathic Association. (2014). Standard 10.00.03. *Healthcare Facilities Accreditation Program: Accreditation requirements for acute care hospitals.* Chicago, IL: American Osteopathic Association. (Level VII)

ADDITIONAL REFERENCE

Craven, R. F., & Hirnle, C. J. (2012). *Fundamentals of nursing: Human health and function* (7th ed.). Philadelphia, PA: Lippincott Williams & Wilkins.

HEIGHT AND WEIGHT MEASUREMENT

Height and weight are routinely measured during admission to a health care facility. An accurate record of the patient's height and weight is essential for calculating dosages of drugs, anesthetics, and contrast agents; assessing nutritional status and bone health; and determining the height-weight ratio, body surface area, and body mass index (BMI).[1] And because body weight provides the best overall picture of fluid status, monitoring weight daily proves important for patients receiving sodium-retaining or diuretic medications. Rapid weight gain may signal fluid retention; rapid weight loss, diuresis.

Accurate weight measurement, rather than estimation, is important because errors in estimation have been reported to be as high as 42%; errors occur even when patients estimate their own weight.[2,3,4] Weight can be measured with a standing scale, chair scale, portable bed scale, or built-in bed scale. (See *Types of scales.*)

The Institute for Safe Medication Practices recommends that weight be measured in metric units only (kilograms for adults, adolescents, children, and infants, and grams for neonates) because official product labeling for medications provides weight-based dosing using only the metric system. Significant medication errors have occurred when a patient's weight was documented in nonmetric units of measure and confused with kilograms or grams. Numerous errors have been reported when health care workers convert weights from one measurement system to another, or weigh a patient in pounds but accidently record the value as kilograms in the patient's medical record, resulting in a greater than twofold dosing error.[5]

Equipment

Standing scale with measurement bar or chair or bed scale ▪ drawsheet (for bed scale) ▪ paper towel ▪ gloves ▪ hospital-grade disinfectant ▪ Optional: tape measure and ruler (if scale doesn't have measuring bar), wheelchair, pillow, transfer device.

Preparation of equipment

Select the appropriate scale, usually a standing scale for an ambulatory patient or a chair or bed scale for an acutely ill or debilitated patient.

EQUIPMENT

Types of scales

Scale selection varies and is influenced by the status of the patient.

For ambulatory patients

Standing scale

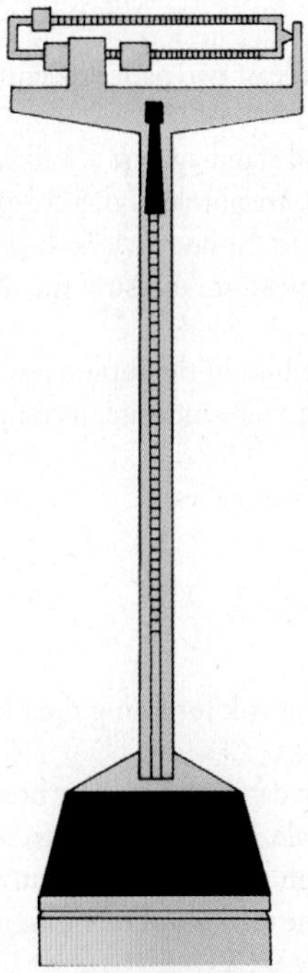

For acutely ill or debilitated patients

Chair scale

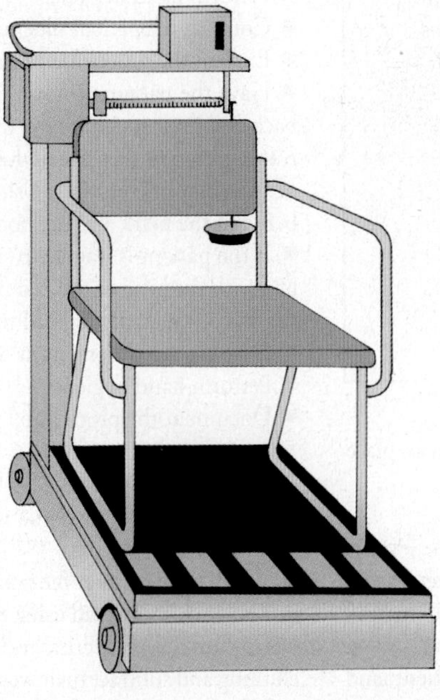

Bed scale

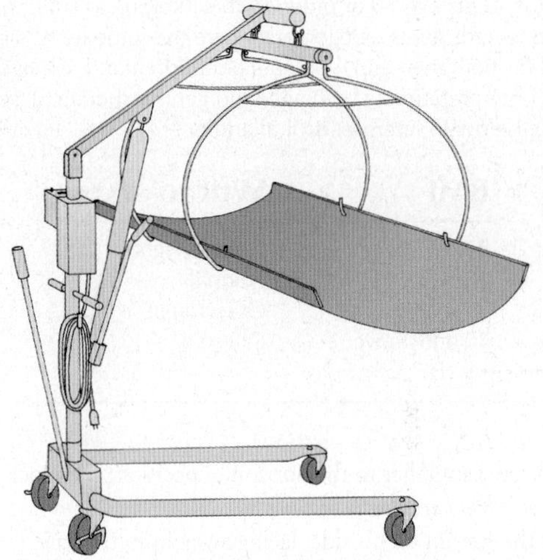

Then check to make sure the scale is balanced. *Standing scales and, to a lesser extent, bed scales may become unbalanced when transported.*

Implementation

- Perform hand hygiene.[6,7,8,9,10]
- Confirm the patient's identity using at least two patient identifiers.[11]
- Explain the procedure to the patient.

Using a standing scale

- Place a paper towel on the scale's platform.
- Check that the scale reads 0 *to ensure accurate measurement.* If the scale has wheels, lock them before the patient steps on *to prevent it from accidently moving.*
- Tell the patient to remove his robe and slippers or shoes.
- Assist the patient onto the scale and remain close to him *to prevent falls.*
- If you're using an upright balance (gravity) scale, slide the lower rider to the groove representing the largest increment below the patient's estimated weight. Then slide the small upper rider until the beam balances. Add the upper and lower rider figures *to determine the patient's weight.* Return the weight holder to its proper place.
- If the scale is digital, read the display with the patient standing as still as possible.
- While the patient is still on the scale, tell the patient to stand erect. Then raise the measuring bar beyond the top of the patient's head, extend the horizontal bar, and lower the bar until it touches the top of the patient's head. Read the patient's height.
- Help the patient off the scale
- Give the patient his robe and slippers or shoes.

Using a chair scale

- Transport the patient to the weighing area or the scale to the patient's bedside.
- Lock the scale in place *to prevent it from moving accidentally.*
- If you're using a scale with a swing-away chair arm, unlock the arm. *When unlocked, the arm swings back 180 degrees to permit easy access.*
- Position the scale beside the patient's bed or wheelchair with the chair arm open.
- Transfer the patient onto the scale.
- Swing the chair arm to the front of the scale, and lock the arm in place.
- If the chair scale is digital, make sure the display reads 0 before use *to ensure accurate measurement.*
- Press the button and record the patient's weight. If using a multiple-weight scale, follow the same process used with a standing scale to determine the weight.
- Transfer the patient from the chair scale to the bed or wheelchair.
- Lock the main beam *to avoid damaging the scale during transport* and unlock the wheels; remove the scale from the patient's room, if applicable.

Using a portable digital bed scale

- Provide privacy, and tell the patient that you're going to weigh him on a bed scale. Demonstrate its operation if appropriate.[12]
- Before using a bed scale, cover its stretcher with a drawsheet.
- Zero the scale with the drawsheet in place *to ensure accurate weighing.*

Calculating and interpreting BMI[20]

Body mass index (BMI) is a number calculated from a person's weight and height to determine if he's overweight or obese. BMI allows you to compare the patient's weight status with the general population. To calculate the patient's BMI, use the following formula: BMI = weight (kg) ÷ [height (M)]^2. For example, for a patient weighing 68 kg and measuring 1.65 m the calculation is 68 kg ÷ (1.65 M)^2 = BMI of 25.

For adults age 20 or older, BMI is interpreted using standard weight status categories that are the same for all ages and for both men and women. For children and teenagers, BMI interpretation is both age- and gender-specific. Use the table below to interpret BMI in adults.

BMI	WEIGHT STATUS
Below 18.5	Underweight
18.5 to 24.9	Normal
25 to 29.9	Overweight
30 and above	Obese

■ Release the stretcher to the horizontal position; then lock it in place *to prevent it from accidently moving.*
■ Turn the patient on his side, facing away from the scale.
■ Roll the base of the scale under the patient's bed. Adjust the lever *to widen the base of the scale, providing stability.* Then lock the scale's wheels.
■ Center the stretcher above the bed, lower it onto the mattress, and roll the patient onto the stretcher.
■ Position the circular weighing arms of the scale over the patient, and attach them securely to the stretcher bars.
■ Pump the handle with long, slow strokes *to raise the patient a few inches off the bed.* Ensure that the patient doesn't lean on or touch the headboard, side rails, or other bed equipment *because this will affect weight measurement.*
■ Press the OPERATE button.
■ Read the patient's weight on the digital display panel.
■ Press on the scale's handle *to lower the patient.*
■ Detach the circular weighing arms from the stretcher bars, roll the patient off the stretcher and remove the stretcher.
■ Position the patient comfortably in bed.
■ Release the wheel lock and withdraw the scale from under the bed. Return the stretcher to its vertical position.

Using a built-in bed scale

■ Before placing the patient in a bed with a built-in scale, prepare the bed. If required by the manufacturer, place the bed in the weighing position, typically with the head of bed elevated less than 40 degrees. Make sure the bed isn't touching anything, such as the wall or medical devices, *to prevent an inaccurate reading.* Prepare the sleep surface with pillows, sheets, and any other items that don't vary in weight that the patient will be using. Place a list of these items by the patient's bedside, if needed, *to make sure the patient is weighed with these items consistently;* some facilities have a protocol that designates the specific items that should be on the bed consistently. Zero the bed scale with the items in place, making sure that no one is touching the bed during this time.
■ With the assistance of coworkers and a transfer device, place the patient on the bed, making sure that he's centered in the bed and lying still.
■ If the scale doesn't function automatically, begin obtaining the patient's weight following the manufacturer's instructions.

Completing the procedure

■ Perform hand hygiene.[6,7,8,9,10]
■ Calculate the patient's BMI if necessary *to determine whether the patient is at a healthy weight.* (See *Calculating and interpreting BMI.*)
■ Put on gloves and clean and disinfect the scale using a hospital-grade disinfectant.[13,14,15]
■ Remove and discard your gloves and perform hand hygiene.[6,7,8,9,10]
■ Document the procedure.[16,17,18,19]

Measuring height without a scale

■ Perform hand hygiene.[6,7,8,9,10]
■ Confirm the patient's identity using at least two patient identifiers.[11]
■ Explain the procedure to the patient.
■ Have the patient remove his shoes and stand against a wall with his back and heels touching the wall. Place a straight, level object (such as a ruler) on top of the patient' head parallel to the floor. Mark the location of the ruler on the wall. Using a tape measure, measure the distance between the mark and the floor.
■ If the patient is unable to stand, place him in the supine position in bed with the head of the bed flat.[12] Using a tape measure, measure from the top of the patient's head to his heels.
■ Note the measurement in centimeters (or inches).
■ Perform hand hygiene.[6,7,8,9,10]
■ Document the procedure.[16,17,18,19]

Special considerations

■ Reassure and steady patients who are at risk for losing their balance on a scale.
■ Weigh the patient at the same time each day (usually before breakfast), in similar clothing, and using the same scale. If the patient uses crutches, weigh him with the crutches. Then weigh the crutches and any heavy clothing and subtract their weight from the total *to determine the patient's weight.*
■ When rolling the patient onto the stretcher, be careful not to dislodge IV catheters, indwelling catheters, and other supportive equipment.
■ Report any change in weight of more than 1 kg (2.2 lb) per day.
■ Measuring height can be difficult for bedbound patients, patients with structural anomalies, and patients with contractures. Alternative methods for estimating height in such patients include measuring recumbent length, knee height, forearm length, and demispan.[21]

Complications

Inaccurate measurement can lead to errors in medication administration and other treatments.

Documentation

Record the patient's weight using metric measurements.[5] Record the date and time of measurement and the type of scale used.[22] If the patient was weighed using a bed scale, note the items that were in place when the scale was reset to 0 before use.[22]

REFERENCES

1 Tipton, P. H., et al. (2012). Patient safety: Consider the accuracy of height and weight measurements. *Nursing, 42*(5), 50–52. (Level V)
2 Breuer, L., et al. (2010). Weight approximation in stroke before thrombolysis: The WAIST-Study: A prospective observational "dose-finding" study. *Stroke, 41,* 2867–2871. (Level VI)
3 Maskin, L. P., et al. (2010). Accuracy of weight and height estimation in an intensive care unit. *Anaesthesia Intensive Care, 38,* 930–934.
4 Sanchez, L. D., et al. (2005). Accuracy of weight estimation by ED personnel. *American Journal of Emergency Medicine, 23,* 915–916.
5 Institute for Safe Medication Practices. (2014). "2014-15 targeted medication safety best practices for hospitals" [Online]. Accessed March 2015

via the Web at http://www.ismp.org/tools/bestpractices/TMSBP-for-Hospitals.pdf (Level VII)

6 Centers for Disease Control and Prevention. (2002). Guideline for hand hygiene in health-care settings: Recommendations of the Healthcare Infection Control Practices Advisory Committee and the HICPAC/SHEA/APIC/IDSA Hand Hygiene Task Force. *MMWR Recommendations and Reports,* 51(RR-16), 1–45. Accessed March 2015 via the Web at http://www.cdc.gov/mmwr/pdf/rr/rr5116.pdf (Level II)

7 World Health Organization. (2009). "WHO guidelines on hand hygiene in health care: First global patient safety challenge, clean care is safer care" [Online]. Accessed March 2015 via the Web at http://whqlibdoc.who.int/publications/2009/9789241597906_eng.pdf (Level IV)

8 The Joint Commission. (2015). Standard NPSG.07.01.01. *Comprehensive accreditation manual for hospitals: The official handbook.* Oakbrook Terrace, IL: The Joint Commission. (Level VII)

9 American Osteopathic Association. (2014). Standard 07.01.21. *Healthcare Facilities Accreditation Program: Accreditation requirements for acute care hospitals.* Chicago, IL: American Osteopathic Association. (Level VII)

10 Centers for Medicare & Medicaid Services, Department of Health and Human Services. (2014). Condition of participation: Infection control. 42 C.F.R. § 482.42.

11 The Joint Commission. (2015). Standard NPSG.01.01.01. *Comprehensive accreditation manual for hospitals: The official handbook.* Oakbrook Terrace, IL: The Joint Commission. (Level VII)

12 Freitag, E., et al. (2010). Determination of body weight and height measurement for critically ill patients admitted to the intensive care unit: A quality improvement project. *Australian Critical Care, 23,* 197–207.

13 American Osteopathic Association. (2014). Standard 15.01.16. *Healthcare Facilities Accreditation Program: Accreditation requirements for acute care hospitals.* Chicago, IL: American Osteopathic Association. (Level VII)

14 American Osteopathic Association. (2014). Standard 07.02.03. *Healthcare Facilities Accreditation Program: Accreditation requirements for acute care hospitals.* Chicago, IL: American Osteopathic Association.

15 Rutala, W. A., et al. (2008). "Guideline for disinfection and sterilization in healthcare facilities, 2008" [Online]. Accessed March 2015 via the Web at http://www.cdc.gov/hicpac/pdf/guidelines/Disinfection_Nov_2008.pdf (Level I)

16 The Joint Commission. (2015). Standard RC.01.03.01. *Comprehensive accreditation manual for hospitals: The official handbook.* Oakbrook Terrace, IL: The Joint Commission. (Level VII)

17 Centers for Medicare & Medicaid Services, Department of Health and Human Services. (2014). Condition of participation: Patient's rights. 42 C.F.R. § 482.24.

18 American Osteopathic Association. (2014). Standard 10.00.03. *Healthcare Facilities Accreditation Program: Accreditation requirements for acute care hospitals.* Chicago, IL: American Osteopathic Association. (Level VII)

19 Centers for Medicare & Medicaid Services, Department of Health and Human Services. (2014). Condition of participation: Medical record services. 42 C.F.R. § 482.24(b).

20 Centers for Disease Control and Prevention. (2011). "Healthy weight—it's not a diet, it's a lifestyle!: About BMI for adults" [Online]. Accessed March 2015 via the Web at http://www.cdc.gov/healthyweight/assessing/bmi/adult_bmi/index.html

21 Froehlich-Grobe, K., et al. (2011). Measuring height without a stadiometer. *American Journal of Physical Medicine and Rehabilitation, 90,* 658–666. Accessed March 2015 via the Web at http://www.ncbi.nlm.nih.gov/pmc/articles/PMC3148840/

22 Byrd, J., et al. (2011). Scale consistency study: How accurate are in-patient hospital scales? *Nursing, 41*(11), 21–24. Accessed March 2015 via the Web at http://www.nursingcenter.com/_PDF_.aspx?an=00152193-201111000-00008

ADDITIONAL REFERENCE

Craven, R. F., & Hirnle, C. J. (2012). *Fundamentals of nursing: Human health and function* (7th ed.). Philadelphia, PA: Lippincott Williams & Wilkins.

HEMODIALYSIS

Hemodialysis is a potentially lifesaving procedure that removes blood from the body, circulates it through an artificial kidney known as a *dialyzer,* and then returns it to the body. Various access sites can be used for this procedure. (See *Hemodialysis access,* page 354.) The access can be temporary or long-term, depending on the patient's condition and needs. Catheters are used for short-term access; arteriovenous (AV) fistulas and AV grafts provide more long-term access for hemodialysis.

AV fistulas are preferred for long-term access because research shows they result in the longest survival, fewer access-related procedures, fewer hospitalizations because of infection, and lower overall costs of care. The Centers for Medicare & Medicaid Services and the Institute for Healthcare Improvement developed the Fistula First Breakthrough Initiative, a national campaign to increase the use of AV fistulas over catheters in patients who require hemodialysis. One challenge to using an AV fistula first is that planning is required so that the fistula can be created and can mature before a patient with stage 4 chronic kidney disease transitions to chronic kidney failure.[1]

The underlying mechanism in hemodialysis is differential diffusion across a semipermeable membrane, which extracts the by-products of protein metabolism (urea) as well as creatinine and excess water. The membrane doesn't permit diffusion of large molecules, such as blood cells and plasma proteins. This process restores or maintains the balance of the body's buffer system and electrolytes. Hemodialysis promotes a rapid return to normal serum values and helps prevent complications associated with uremia. (See *How hemodialysis works,* page 355.)

Hemodialysis provides temporary support for patients with acute kidney injury. It's also used for the regular long-term treatment of patients with chronic end-stage kidney disease. Hemodialysis may also be needed to remove toxic substances from the blood in patients suffering from various acute poisoning or barbiturate or analgesia overdose. The patient's condition, along with such variables as the rate of creatinine accumulation and weight gain, determines the number and duration of hemodialysis treatments. To determine the patient's ultrafiltration requirements, his present weight is compared with his weight after his last dialysis treatment and his target weight. Blood pressure and hemodynamic status are also considered.

Hemodialysis is typically performed on a hemodialysis unit by specially trained personnel. However, if the patient is acutely ill and unstable, it can be performed at the bedside on an intensive care unit. With increasing frequency, hemodialysis is even performed at home by the patient and his family.

Equipment

For initiating hemodialysis with AV access

Scale ▪ hemodialysis machine with appropriate dialyzer and dialysate ▪ stethoscope ▪ sphygmomanometer ▪ gloves, gown, and face shield ▪ sterile drape ▪ two 15G or 16G winged fistula needles ▪ two 10-mL syringes ▪ prescribed flush solution ▪ fluid-impermeable pad ▪ antiseptic swabs (chlorhexidine, povidone-iodine, or 70% alcohol)[5] ▪ antiseptic solution or antibacterial soap and water ▪ sterile 4″ × 4″ (10-cm × 10-cm) gauze pads ▪ adhesive tape ▪ medications, as ordered ▪ supplies for blood sampling, as indicated ▪ Optional: tourniquet; topical anesthetic, as ordered; heparin.[6]

For initiating hemodialysis with a double-lumen catheter

Scale ▪ hemodialysis machine with appropriate dialyzer and dialysate ▪ clean and sterile gloves ▪ gown and face shield ▪ sterile barrier ▪ sterile drape ▪ sterile 4″ × 4″ (10-cm × 10-cm) and 2″ × 2″ (5-cm × 5-cm) gauze pads ▪ antiseptic swabs and solution ▪ fluid-impermeable pad ▪ stethoscope ▪ sphygmomanometer ▪ two 3-mL syringes ▪ two 10-mL

Hemodialysis access

Hemodialysis requires vascular access. The site and type of access may vary, depending on the expected duration of dialysis, the practitioner's preference, and the patient's condition.

Subclavian vein catheterization

Typically, double-lumen catheters are placed in the internal jugular vein; use of the subclavian vein for catheter placement isn't recommended for patients who require permanent arteriovenous (AV) fistulas *because the risk of thrombosis can compromise AV fistula creation.*[2]

Using the Seldinger technique, the practitioner inserts an introducer needle into the subclavian vein. He then inserts a guide wire through the introducer needle and removes the needle. Using the guide wire, he then threads a 5″ to 12″ (13- to 30-cm) plastic or Teflon catheter (with a Y hub) into the patient's vein.

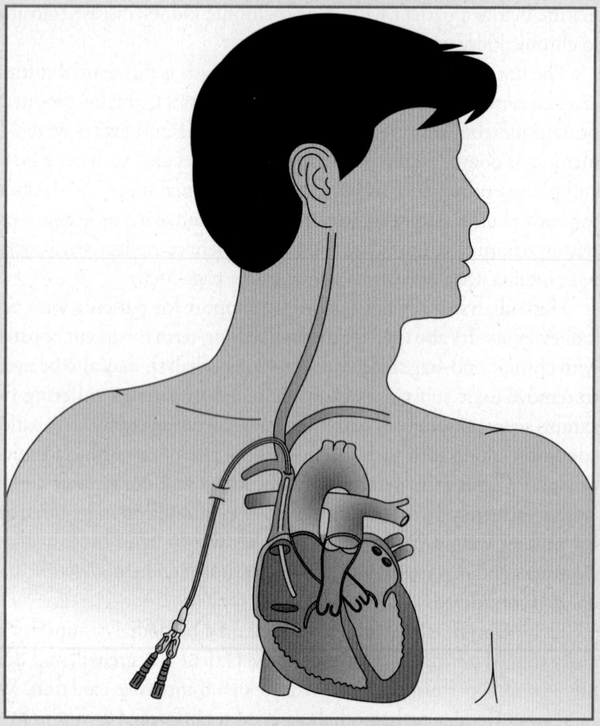

Several types of double-lumen catheters can be used for dialysis access, depending on the patient's condition, the practitioner's preference, and the anticipated length of time that the catheter will be needed. The internal diameter of each lumen is approximately 12G to allow for high flow rates. The catheters have two ports—one red and one blue. The red port is used for withdrawing the patient's blood and sending it to the dialyzer, and the blue port is used for returning dialyzed blood to the patient.

Most double-lumen catheters are considered temporary dialysis accesses. However, a double-lumen tunneled catheter with a Dacron cuff may be used for months.[3] This catheter is tunneled from the skin insertion site to the selected vein, and the Dacron cuff on the catheter under the skin acts as a barrier to infection.

Femoral vein catheterization

Using the Seldinger technique, the practitioner inserts an introducer needle into the left or right femoral vein. He then inserts a guide wire through the introducer needle and removes the needle.

Using the guide wire, the practitioner then threads a 5″ to 12″ (13- to 30-cm) plastic or Teflon catheter with a Y hub or two catheters, one for inflow and another placed about ½″ (1 cm) distal to the first for outflow. This site should be used only when no other access site is available *because it's associated with an increased risk of infection and deep vein thrombosis.*[4]

AV fistula

To create an AV fistula, a surgeon makes an incision into the patient's wrist or lower forearm and then makes two additional small incisions, one in the side of an artery and another in the side of a vein. He sutures the edges of the incisions together to make a common opening 0.12″ to 0.3″ (3 to 8 mm) long. Because an AV fistula requires a 4- to 6-week maturing time before it can be used as a dialysis access site, creation of a fistula is recommended before hemodialysis is needed *so that the fistula is matured and ready for use when needed.*

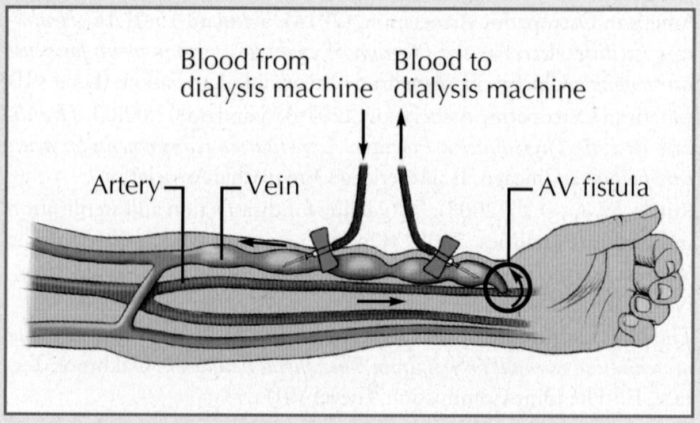

AV graft

To create an AV graft, the practitioner makes an incision in the patient's forearm, upper arm, or thigh. He then tunnels a natural or synthetic graft under the skin and sutures the distal end to an artery and the proximal end to a vein.

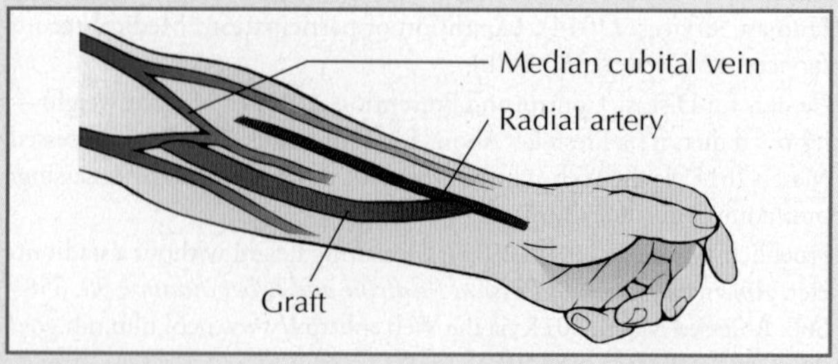

syringes with saline flush solution ▪ prescribed medications ▪ supplies for blood sampling ▪ Optional: prescribed anticoagulant.

For discontinuing hemodialysis with AV access

Gloves ▪ sterile 4″ × 4″ (10-cm × 10-cm) gauze pads ▪ dry sterile dressing ▪ scale.

For discontinuing hemodialysis with a double-lumen catheter

Clean and sterile gloves ▪ gown and face shield ▪ sterile barrier ▪ two 10-mL syringes with preservative-free normal saline solution ▪ two 5-mL syringes with prescribed anticoagulant flush solution ▪ two sterile luer-lock caps ▪ stethoscope ▪ sphygmomanometer ▪ antiseptic swabs and

EQUIPMENT

How hemodialysis works

In hemodialysis, blood flows from the patient to an external dialyzer (or artificial kidney) through an access site. Inside the dialyzer, blood and dialysate flow countercurrently, divided by a semipermeable membrane. The composition of the dialysate resembles normal extracellular fluid. The blood contains an excess of specific solutes (metabolic waste products and some electrolytes), and the dialysate contains electrolytes that may be at abnormal levels in the patient's bloodstream. The dialysate's electrolyte composition can be modified to raise or lower electrolyte levels, depending on need.

Excretory function and electrolyte homeostasis are achieved by *diffusion,* the movement of a molecule across the dialyzer's semipermeable membrane from an area of higher solute concentration to an area of lower concentration. Water (solvent) crosses the membrane from the blood into the dialysate by *ultrafiltration.* This process removes excess water, waste products, and other metabolites through *osmotic pressure* and *hydrostatic pressure.* Osmotic pressure is the movement of water across the semipermeable membrane from an area of lesser solute concentration to one of greater solute concentration. Hydrostatic pressure forces water from the blood compartment into the dialysate compartment. Cleaned of impurities and excess water, the blood returns to the body through a venous site.

Dialyzer

The hollow-fiber dialyzer contains fine capillaries, with a semipermeable membrane enclosed in a plastic cylinder. Blood flows through these capillaries as the system pumps dialysate in the opposite direction on the outside of the capillaries.

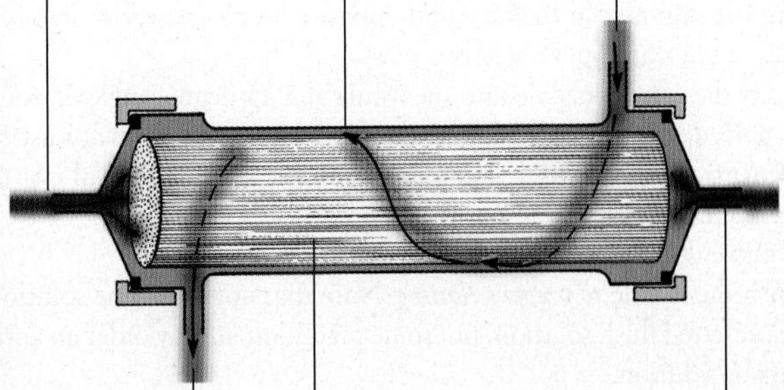

Dialysate delivery systems

Three system types can be used to deliver dialysate. The *batch system* uses a reservoir for recirculating dialysate. The *regenerative system* uses sorbents to purify and regenerate recirculating dialysate. The *proportioning system* (the most common) mixes concentrate with water to form dialysate, which then circulates through the dialyzer and goes down a drain after a single pass, followed by fresh dialysate.

solution ■ sterile drape ■ sterile 4″ × 4″ (10-cm × 10-cm) gauze pads ■ two 5-mL syringes with prescribed anticoagulant flush ■ scale ■ central venous access catheter dressing change kit ■ Optional: sterile specimen container, povidone-iodine ointment or polymyxin B, bacitracin zinc, and gramicidin ointment.

Preparation of equipment

NURSING ALERT **To avoid a pyrogenic reaction and bacteremia with septicemia resulting from contamination, *use strict sterile technique during preparation of the machine. Discard equipment that has been disconnected and exposed to the air.*[2]**

Prepare the hemodialysis equipment following the manufacturer's instructions. *To maintain catheter patency,* carefully follow the manufacturer's instructions for specific catheter care and flushing procedures. Maintain strict sterile technique *to prevent introducing pathogens into the patient's bloodstream during dialysis.* Test the dialyzer and dialysis machine for residual disinfectant after rinsing; this may require a double-check by a second nurse or technician.[5] Make sure the dialysis machine alarms limits are set appropriately and that the alarms are turned on, functioning properly, and audible to staff.[7]

Implementation

Initiating hemodialysis

- Verify the practitioner's order.[8]
- Gather and prepare the necessary equipment.
- Perform hand hygiene.[9,10,11,12,13,14]
- Confirm the patient's identity using at least two patient identifiers.[15]
- Explain the procedure to the patient.
- Weigh the patient. Estimate his dry weight and compare it with his predialysis and most recent postdialysis weight.[16]
- Record the patient's baseline vital signs, including blood pressure measurements, with the patient sitting and standing.
- Auscultate the heart for rate, rhythm, and abnormalities.
- Assess respiratory rate, rhythm, and quality. Auscultate breath sounds for crackles, *an indication of possible fluid overload,* and check for edema.
- Assess the patient's mental status.
- Evaluate previous laboratory data.
- Determine whether the patient had any problems with his last dialysis treatment.
- Help the patient into a comfortable position (supine or sitting in a recliner chair with the feet elevated). Make sure the access site is well supported and resting on a fluid-impermeable pad.
- Apply a topical anesthetic to the AV puncture site, as ordered, approximately 45 to 60 minutes before cannulation.[6]
- Perform hand hygiene.[9,10,11,12,13,14]
- Put on gloves, a gown, and a mask with face shield and follow standard precautions.[10,17,18]

Initiating hemodialysis with AV access

- Assess the AV access for patency. Check for the quality of the thrill and auscultate the bruit. Check for the presence of swelling, edema, erythema, or drainage.
- Draw up the prescribed flush solution into each 10-mL syringe, and prime and clamp the tubing and needle just before cannulation.[2]
- Wash the patient's access site using an antiseptic solution or antibacterial soap and water.[19]
- Remove the fluid-impermeable pad and place the patient's access limb on a sterile barrier.[20]
- Clean the skin over the AV access with antiseptic swabs according to the manufacturer's instructions.[5] To apply chlorhexidine, use a back-and-forth friction scrub for 30 seconds and then allow it to dry. To apply alcohol, use a rubbing motion for 1 minute immediately before accessing the fistula. To apply povidone-iodine, apply the solution and allow it to dry for 2 to 3 minutes.[19]

■ Remove and discard your gloves.[18]
■ Perform hand hygiene.[9,10,11,12]
■ Put on another pair of gloves.[10,18]
■ Apply a tourniquet to the upper portion of the arm containing the fistula.[19]
■ Remove the needle guard from the first fistula needle (arterial), and then squeeze the wings together.
■ Pull the skin taut in the direction opposite needle insertion; stabilize the vessel but don't apply excessive pressure.[2]
■ Insert the arterial needle into the fistula at a 25-degree angle or, for a graft, a 45-degree angle. Make sure the needle insertion site is at least 1″ (2.5 cm) from the arterial-venous anastomotic site. Be careful not to puncture the posterior wall of the access.
■ Remove the tourniquet.[19]
■ Flush the needle *to prevent clotting.* Note that normal saline solution is the preferred flush solution, but some practitioners may order an anticoagulant solution.
■ Clamp the arterial needle tubing and secure the wing tips of the needle to the skin with adhesive tape *to prevent accidental needle dislodgement.*
■ Perform the second access (venous) puncture with the other fistula needle, a few inches beyond the arterial needle (farther from the arterial-venous anastomosis). Be careful not to puncture the posterior wall of the access.
■ Flush the needle with the appropriate solution.
■ Clamp the venous needle tubing, and secure the wing tips of the venous needle to the patient's skin with adhesive tape. Use caution when taping needles, and don't lift up on the needle after it's in the vein. *Lifting up on the needle or improper taping can cause infiltration.*[19]
■ Remove the syringe from the end of the arterial needle tubing, uncap the arterial dialyzer tubing, and connect the two lines. Tape the connection securely *to prevent accidental separation of the tubing.*[16]
■ Remove the syringe from the end of the venous needle tubing, uncap the venous dialyzer tubing, and connect the two lines. Tape the connection securely *to prevent accidental separation of the tubing.*
■ Unclamp the tubing, and begin the hemodialysis treatment. Check for complications over the first 1 to 2 minutes.[16]
■ Keep the access and connections visible at all times.[16]
■ Monitor the patient's condition and vital signs at an interval determined by your facility and the patient's condition.
■ Administer medications and obtain clotting times, as ordered.

Initiating hemodialysis with a double-lumen catheter

■ Have the patient put on a mask.[16]
■ Clamp the catheter tubing *to prevent air from entering either lumen of the catheter.*
■ Prepare a sterile field.
■ Place sterile drapes and sterile 4″ × 4″ (10-cm × 10-cm) sterile gauze pads on the sterile field.
■ Identify the red (arterial) and the blue (venous) ports, and place them near the sterile field. Also place the dialyzer arterial and venous blood lines near the field. (A dual-lumen venous catheter is used for this procedure. The line that pulls blood from the catheter is referred to as the arterial line, and the line that returns the blood to the patient is referred to as the venous line.)
■ Open the sterile syringes and place them on the sterile field.
■ Prepare the normal saline flush solution in the 10-mL syringes, as indicated.
■ Remove the dressing from the catheter exit site, making sure you don't dislodge the catheter.
■ Discard the soiled dressing in the appropriate receptacle, and remove and discard your gloves.[17,18]
■ Perform hand hygiene and put on sterile gloves.[9,10,11,12]
■ Place a sterile drape beneath the catheter.
■ Saturate 4″ × 4″ (10-cm × 10-cm) sterile gauze pads with antiseptic solution.
■ Use a saturated gauze pad to scrub the red port for 1 minute. Wrap a saturated gauze pad around the red port and leave it in place for 3 to 5 minutes. Remove the gauze pad and discard it in the appropriate receptacle. Repeat these steps for the blue port.[20]
■ Remove and discard the luer-lock cap on the red port and replace it with a 3-mL syringe.
■ Unclamp the red port, aspirate and discard 1.5 to 3 mL of blood, and then reclamp the port.
■ Soak 2″ × 2″ (5-cm × 5-cm) sterile gauze pads in antiseptic solution and then clean the connection site with them.[20]
■ Connect one of the 10-mL syringes with saline flush solution to the red port, unclamp the port, aspirate 1.5 to 3 mL of blood, gently instill the solution, and then reclamp the red port.
■ Remove and discard the luer-lock cap on the blue port, and replace it with a 3-ml syringe.
■ Gently aspirate 1.5 to 3 mL of blood, discard it, and then reclamp the port.
■ Connect the other 10-mL syringe (with saline flush solution) to the blue port, unclamp the port, aspirate and discard 1.5 to 3 mL of blood, gently instill the solution, and then reclamp the blue port.
■ Remove the syringe from the red port, and attach the red port to the line leading to the arterial port of the dialyzer.
■ Administer the prescribed anticoagulant *to prevent clotting in the extracorporeal circuit.*
■ Remove the syringe from the blue port, and then attach the blue port to the line leading to the venous port of the dialyzer.
■ Trace the tubing from the patient to its point of origin *to prevent misconnections.*
■ Secure the tubing to the patient *to reduce tension on the connections and prevent trauma to the catheter insertion site.*
■ Open the clamps to the arterial and venous dialyzer tubing.
■ Remove the patient's mask.
■ Begin the hemodialysis treatment. Check for complications over the first 1 to 2 minutes.[16]
■ Keep the access and connection lines visible at all times.[16]
■ Monitor the patient's condition and vital signs at an interval determined by your facility and the patient's condition.
■ Administer medications, and obtain clotting times during hemodialysis, as ordered.

Discontinuing hemodialysis with AV access

■ Perform hand hygiene.[9,10,11,12,13]
■ Put on gloves.[10,18]
■ Turn the blood pump on the hemodialysis machine to 50 to 100 mL/minute.
■ Remove the tape from the connection site of the arterial lines.
■ Clamp the needle tubing and disconnect the lines. The blood in the arterial line will continue to flow toward the dialyzer, followed by normal saline solution. Clamp the blood line just before the blood reaches the point where the saline solution enters the line.
■ Unclamp the saline solution to allow a small amount of saline to flow through the line.
■ Unclamp the dialyzer line and allow all the blood to flow into the dialyzer, where it passes through the filter and back to the patient through the venous line.
■ After the blood is retransfused, clamp the venous needle tubing and the dialyzer's venous line and turn off the blood pump.
■ Remove the tape from the connection site of the venous lines and disconnect the lines.
■ Apply a folded 4″ × 4″ (10-cm × 10-cm) sterile gauze pad over the needle site, but don't apply pressure.

■ Carefully remove the needle at approximately the same angle as it was inserted *to prevent dragging the needle across the patient's skin and to avoid puncturing the vein wall.*[19]
■ Apply pressure to the site with the folded 4″ × 4″ (10-cm × 10-cm) sterile gauze pad using two fingers until the bleeding stops. *If inadequate pressure is used, a hematoma may develop; if excessive pressure is used, the access may thrombose.* Bleeding usually stops within 10 minutes.
■ Cover the site with a dry sterile dressing.[3,5] Avoid circumferential taping of the dressing.
■ Repeat the procedure on the arterial needle and site.
■ When dialysis is complete, weigh the patient, obtain vital signs (including blood pressure while the patient is sitting and standing), and assess mental status. Compare these findings with the predialysis assessment data.
■ Remove and discard your gloves.[18]
■ Perform hand hygiene.[9,11,12,13,14]
■ Put on a new pair of gloves.[18]
■ Rinse and disinfect the delivery system according to the manufacturer's instructions.[21]
■ Dispose of used equipment in appropriate receptacles.[17]

Discontinuing hemodialysis with a double-lumen catheter

■ Perform hand hygiene.[9,10,11,12,13]
■ Put on a gown, clean gloves, and a face shield, and follow standard precautions.[10,18]
■ Prepare a sterile field using a sterile barrier.
■ Open the syringes, luer-lock caps, and gauze pads, and place them on the sterile field.
■ Fill the two 5-mL syringes with the prescribed amount of anticoagulant flush solution.
■ Fill the two 10-mL syringes with preservative-free normal saline solution for injection, as indicated.
■ Clamp the tubing to the red and the blue catheter ports and the blood lines to the dialyzer.
■ Place a sterile drape beneath the ports.
■ Clean the connection points on the catheter, the clamps, and the blood lines with antiseptic solution.
■ Place a sterile drape under the catheter, and then place two sterile 4″ × 4″ (10-cm × 10-cm) sterile gauze pads beneath the catheter ports.[20]
■ Soak the 4″ × 4″ (10-cm × 10-cm) gauze pads with antiseptic solution.
■ Remove and discard your gloves.[18]
■ Perform hand hygiene. [9,10,11,12,13]
■ Put on sterile gloves.[4,5,6,7,16]
■ Grasping the red port connection with a gauze pad, disconnect it from the arterial dialyzer tubing. The line that pulls blood from the catheter is referred to as the arterial line, and the line that returns the blood to the patient is referred to as the venous line.
■ Attach a 10-mL syringe (with normal saline solution) to the red port on the catheter, and then slowly flush the tubing.
■ Replace the 10-mL syringe on the red port with the 5-mL syringe filled with the prescribed anticoagulant flush solution and instill it.
■ Remove the syringe, and then cap the port with a sterile luer-lock cap.
■ Grasping the blue port connection with a gauze pad, disconnect it from the venous dialyzer tubing
■ Attach a 10-mL syringe (with normal saline solution) to the blue catheter port, and slowly flush the tubing.
■ Replace the 10-mL syringe on the blue port with the 5-mL syringe filled with the prescribed anticoagulant flush solution and instill it.
■ Remove the syringe, and cap the port with a sterile luer-lock cap.
■ Clamp both ports.
■ Place the patient in the supine position with his head facing away from the catheter.
■ Perform catheter insertion site care, and obtain a drainage specimen for culture, if necessary. (See the "Central venous access catheter" procedure, page 145.) If compatible with the hemodialysis catheter material, apply povidone-iodine ointment or polymyxin B, bacitracin zinc, and gramicidin ointment (as prescribed) to the catheter insertion site *to reduce the risk of central line–associated bloodstream infection.*[4]
■ Obtain the patient's postdialysis weight, vital signs, and neurologic, respiratory, and hemodynamic parameters, and compare them with his predialysis baseline.
■ Remove and discard your gloves and other personal protective equipment.[18]
■ Perform hand hygiene.[9,11,12,13,14]
■ Put on a new pair of gloves.[18]
■ Rinse and disinfect the delivery system.[21]
■ Dispose of used equipment in the appropriate receptacles.[17]

Completing the procedure

■ Remove and discard your gloves.
■ Perform hand hygiene.[9,11,12,13,14]
■ Document the procedure.[22,23,24]

Special considerations

■ The Joint Commission issued a sentinel event alert concerning medical device alarm safety *because alarm-related events have been associated with permanent loss of function and death.* Among the major contributing factors were improper alarm settings, inappropriately turned off alarms, and alarm signals not audible to staff. Make sure that alarm limits are appropriately set and that alarms are turned on and audible to staff. Follow facility guidelines for preventing alarm fatigue.[7]
■ Immediately report any suspected machine malfunction or equipment defect.

NURSING ALERT ***Make sure you complete each step in the hemodialysis procedure correctly.*** **Overlooking a single step or performing it incorrectly can cause unnecessary blood loss or inefficient treatment from poor clearances or inadequate fluid removal. *For example, when preparing the equipment, never allow a normal saline solution bag to run dry while priming and soaking the dialyzer* because that could cause air to enter the patient portion of the dialysate system. *Failure to perform accurate hemodialysis therapy can lead to patient injury or death.***

■ If the patient receives meals during dialysis, make sure they're light.
■ Continue necessary drug administration during the hemodialysis treatment unless the drug would be removed in the dialysate; if so, administer the medication after dialysis.
■ If you meet resistance while instilling the anticoagulant flush solution into either port of a dual-lumen catheter, stop flushing immediately. Clamp the port, replace the sterile luer-lock cap, and notify the practitioner. Place a "Do not use" message on the port until its patency is verified.

Patient teaching

After surgery to create an AV access site

In the postoperative period, teach the patient to care for his AV access site. Teach him to keep the incision clean and dry to prevent infection and to clean it daily until it heals completely and the sutures are removed (usually 10 to 14 days after surgery). Teach him how to use a stethoscope to auscultate for his access bruit and how to palpate a thrill. He should check the access several times a day. He should notify the practitioner of pain, swelling, redness, drainage, and any decrease in the access thrill or bruit.

Explain that after the access site heals, he may use the arm freely. Exercise is beneficial because it stimulates vein enlargement. He may start by squeezing a small rubber ball or other soft object for 15 minutes as advised by his practitioner.

Teach the patient to avoid putting excessive pressure on the arm. He shouldn't sleep on it, wear constricting clothing, or lift heavy objects with it. Also teach the patient that he shouldn't allow anyone to take his blood pressure or draw blood from his access arm.

If the patient will be performing hemodialysis at home, thoroughly review all aspects of the procedure with the patient and family. Give them the phone number of the dialysis center. Emphasize that training for home hemodialysis is a complex process requiring 2 to 3 months to ensure that the patient or family member performs it safely and competently. Keep in mind that this procedure is stressful.

After hemodialysis

Teach the patient to keep the dressings on the access site for several hours after his treatment. Teach him not to loosen the scabs on the needle insertion sites because they may bleed or become infected. If bleeding should occur, teach the patient to apply pressure to the needle sites with a clean towel or gauze for 10 to 15 minutes without lifting the pressure. Prematurely releasing the pressure may disturb the clot formation. Tell him to use enough pressure to stop the bleeding but not enough to occlude the pulse in his access. Instruct the patient to tape the dressing in place when the bleeding stops. Instruct him never to wrap the tape all the way around his arm. Tell him to go to the emergency department if he can't stop the bleeding.

Complications

Bacterial endotoxins in the dialysate may cause fever. Improper access care and needle site asepsis can introduce bacteria into the bloodstream and cause sepsis. Rapid fluid removal and electrolyte changes during dialysis can cause early dialysis disequilibrium syndrome. Signs and symptoms include headache, nausea, vomiting, restlessness, hypertension, muscle cramps, backache, and seizures.

Excessive removal of fluid during ultrafiltration can cause hypovolemia and hypotension. Diffusion of the sugar and sodium content of the dialysate solution into the blood can cause hyperglycemia and hypernatremia and subsequent hyperosmolarity.

Cardiac arrhythmias can occur as the result of electrolyte and pH changes in the blood. They can also develop if the patient is taking antiarrhythmics because the drugs may be removed during the treatment. Angina can develop in patients with anemia and in those with preexisting arteriosclerotic disease. Patients with reduced oxygen levels resulting from extracorporeal blood flow or membrane sensitivity may require oxygen administration during hemodialysis.

Some complications of hemodialysis can be fatal. An air embolus can result from tubing disconnection, if the dialyzer contains air, or from an empty saline solution container. Signs and symptoms include dyspnea, chest pain, coughing, and cyanosis.

Hemolysis of the blood cells can result from obstructed flow of the dialysate concentrate or from incorrect setting of the conductivity alarm limits. Signs and symptoms include cherry red blood, chest pain, dyspnea, arrhythmias, hyperkalemia, and an abrupt decrease in hematocrit.

Hyperthermia, which can result from overheating of the dialysate, is potentially fatal.

Exsanguination can result if the connections on the blood lines become separated or ruptured or the dialyzer membrane ruptures.

Improper access site cannulation or needle site care can cause hematoma, pseudoaneurysm formation, and even rupture of the graft, which is accompanied by excessive bleeding.

Documentation

Record the time the treatment began, along with the patient's predialysis assessment data and vital signs. Note any complications and nursing actions taken. Note any blood samples sent and the laboratory results obtained.

Record the time the treatment was completed and the patient's response to it. Record the condition of the AV access site or catheter insertion site with the date and time of the dressing change, the time hemostasis was obtained, and any culture specimens obtained.

REFERENCES

1 Vassalotti, J. A., et al. (2012). Fistula First Breakthrough Initiative: Targeting catheter last in fistula first. *Seminars in Dialysis, 25*(3), 303–310. Accessed March 2015 via the Web at http://fistulafirst.org/LinkClick.aspx?fileticket=GN8QYytKHFo%3d&tabid=39

2 National Kidney Foundation. (2006). "2006 updates: Clinical practice guidelines and clinical practice recommendations: November adequacy" [Online]. Accessed March 2015 via the Web at http://www.kidney.org/professionals/kdoqi/guideline_uphd_pd_va/va_guide3.htm (Level I)

3 Centers for Disease Control and Prevention. (2011). "Guidelines for the prevention of intravascular catheter-related infections" [Online]. Accessed March 2015 via the Web at http://www.cdc.gov/hicpac/pdf/guidelines/bsi-guidelines-2011.pdf (Level I)

4 Marschall, J., et al. (2014). SHEA/IDSA practice recommendation: Strategies to prevent central line-associated bloodstream infections in acute care hospitals. *Infection Control and Hospital Epidemiology, 35,* 753–771. Accessed March 2015 via the Web at http://www.jstor.org/stable/10.1086/676533 (Level I)

5 Centers for Disease Control and Prevention. (2012). "Dialysis safety: Dialysis bloodstream infection (BSI) prevention collaborative" [Online]. Accessed March 2015 via the Web at http://www.cdc.gov/dialysis/collaborative/

6 Çelik, G., et al. (2011). Vapocoolant spray vs lidocaine/prilocaine cream for reducing the pain of venipuncture in November patients: A randomized, placebo-controlled, crossover study. *International Journal of Medical Science, 8,* 623–627. Accessed March 2015 via the Web at http://www.medsci.org/v08p0623.pdf (Level II)

7 The Joint Commission. (2013). "Sentinel event alert: Medical device alarm safety in hospitals" [Online]. Accessed March 2015 via the Web at http://www.jointcommission.org/assets/1/18/SEA_50_alarms_4_5_13_FINAL1.PDF (Level VII)

8 The Joint Commission. (2015). Standard MM.04.01.01. *Comprehensive accreditation manual for hospitals: The official handbook.* Oakbrook Terrace, IL: The Joint Commission. (Level VII)

9 The Joint Commission. (2015). Standard NPSG.07.01.01. *Comprehensive accreditation manual for hospitals: The official handbook.* Oakbrook Terrace, IL: The Joint Commission. (Level VII)

10 Centers for Disease Control and Prevention. (2001). Recommendations for preventing transmission of infections among chronic November patients. *MMWR Recommendations and Reports, 50*(RR-5), 1–43. (Level II)

11 Centers for Disease Control and Prevention. (2002). Guideline for hand hygiene in health-care settings: Recommendations of the Healthcare Infection Control Practices Advisory Committee and the HICPAC/SHEA/APIC/IDSA Hand Hygiene Task Force. *MMWR Recommendations and Reports, 51*(RR-16), 1–45. Accessed March 2015 via the Web at http://www.cdc.gov/mmwr/pdf/rr/rr5116.pdf (Level II)

12 World Health Organization. (2009). "WHO guidelines on hand hygiene in health care: First global patient safety challenge, clean care is safer care" [Online]. Accessed March 2015 via the Web at http://whqlibdoc.who.int/publications/2009/9789241597906_eng.pdf (Level IV)

13 American Osteopathic Association. (2014). Standard 07.01.21. *Healthcare Facilities Accreditation Program: Accreditation requirements for acute care hospitals.* Chicago, IL: American Osteopathic Association. (Level VII)

14 Centers for Medicare & Medicaid Services, Department of Health and Human Services. (2014). Condition of participation: Infection control. 42 C.F.R. § 482.42.

15 The Joint Commission. (2015). Standard NPSG.01.01.01. *Comprehensive accreditation manual for hospitals: The official handbook.* Oakbrook Terrace, IL: The Joint Commission. (Level VII)

16 American Nephrology Nurses' Association. (2011). *Nephrology nursing: Scope and standards of practice* (7th ed.). Pitman, NJ: American Nephrology Nurses' Association.

17 Occupational Safety and Health Administration. (n.d.). "Bloodborne pathogens, standard number 1910.1030" [Online]. Accessed March 2015 via the Web at http://www.osha.gov/pls/oshaweb/owadisp.show_document?p_table=STANDARDS&p_id=10051 (Level VII)
18 American Osteopathic Association. (2014). Standard 07.01.10. *Healthcare Facilities Accreditation Program: Accreditation requirements for acute care hospitals.* Chicago, IL: American Osteopathic Association. (Level VII)
19 National Kidney Foundation. (2006). "2006 updates: Clinical practice guidelines and clinical practice recommendations: Vascular access" [Online]. Accessed March 2015 via the Web at http://www.kidney.org/professionals/kdoqi/pdf/12-50-0210_JAG_DCP_Guidelines-VA_Oct06_SectionC_ofC.pdf
20 Lynn-McHale Wiegand, D. (Ed.). (2011). *AACN procedure manual for critical care* (6th ed.). St. Louis, MO: Saunders.
21 American Osteopathic Association. (2014). Standard 07.02.03. *Healthcare Facilities Accreditation Program: Accreditation requirements for acute care hospitals.* Chicago, IL: American Osteopathic Association. (Level VII)
22 The Joint Commission. (2015). Standard RC.01.03.01. *Comprehensive accreditation manual for hospitals: The official handbook.* Oakbrook Terrace, IL: The Joint Commission. (Level VII)
23 American Osteopathic Association. (2014). Standard 10.00.03. *Healthcare Facilities Accreditation Program: Accreditation requirements for acute care hospitals.* Chicago, IL: American Osteopathic Association. (Level VII)
24 Centers for Medicare & Medicaid Services, Department of Health and Human Services. (2014). Condition of participation: Medical record services. 42 C.F.R. § 482.24(b).

ADDITIONAL REFERENCES

Hinkle, J. L., & Cheever, K. H. (2014). *Brunner & Suddarth's textbook of medical-surgical nursing* (13th ed.). Philadelphia, PA: Wolters Kluwer.
Nettina, S. M. (2014). *Lippincott manual of nursing practice* (10th ed.). Philadelphia, PA: Wolters Kluwer.

HEMOGLOBIN TESTING, BEDSIDE

Hemoglobin level can be measured at the patient's bedside using a portable device. This method involves obtaining a fingerstick specimen and placing it in the device, which immediately determines the hemoglobin level and allows for prompt intervention, if necessary. In contrast, the traditional method involves obtaining a blood specimen using venipuncture (or a vascular access device) and then sending the sample to the laboratory for interpretation.

Several portable testing systems are available for bedside hemoglobin monitoring. These systems are also convenient for the patient's home use.

Normal hemoglobin values for adults range from 12.5 to 15 mg/dL (125 to 150 mmol/L). Normal hemoglobin ranges by vary age in children. A below-normal hemoglobin value may indicate anemia, recent hemorrhage, or fluid retention, all of which result in hemodilution. An elevated hemoglobin value suggests hemoconcentration from polycythemia or dehydration.

Equipment

Portable photometer ■ single-use, auto-disabling lancet ■ microcuvette ■ photometer ■ two pairs of gloves ■ alcohol pads ■ gauze pads ■ disinfectant pads.

Preparation of equipment

Note the expiration date on the microcuvette vial. If opening the vial for the first time, label the vial with the date and time it was opened. *Microcuvettes can be stored for up to 2 years; however, after the vial is opened, the shelf life of the microcuvettes is 90 days.* Turn on the photometer. If the photometer hasn't been used recently, insert the control microcuvette *to make sure that the photometer is working properly.*

Implementation

- Verify the practitioner's order.
- Gather and prepare the appropriate equipment.
- Perform hand hygiene and put on gloves.[1,2,3,4,5,6,7]
- Confirm the patient's identity using at least two patient identifiers.[8]
- Explain the procedure to the patient or to the parents or guardian, if applicable.
- Tell the patient that he'll feel a pinprick in his finger during blood sampling.
- Select an appropriate puncture site. In most cases, use the fingertip for an adult or child, and the heel or the great toe for an infant. For an adult, the middle and fourth fingers are the best choices *because the second finger is usually the most sensitive, and the thumb may have thickened skin or calluses. Blood should circulate freely in the finger from which you're drawing blood,* so avoid using a ring-bearing finger. *To ensure an adequate blood sample,* don't use a cold, cyanotic, or swollen area as the puncture site.
- If necessary, dilate the capillaries by applying warm, moist compresses to the area for about 10 minutes.
- Clean the intended puncture site with an alcohol pad, and allow it to dry completely *because any remaining alcohol may interfere with the test results.*[9]
- To collect the sample from the fingertip, use a single-use, auto-disabling lancet. Position the lancet on the side of the patient's fingertip, perpendicular to the lines of the fingerprints.[9] Puncture the skin with a quick, continuous, and deliberate stroke *to achieve a good flow of blood and to prevent the need to repeat the puncture.*[9]
- If required by your facility, wipe away the first drop of blood using a gauze pad *because it may be contaminated with tissue, fluid, or debris.*[9]
- Apply the microcuvette, which automatically collects a precise amount of blood (approximately 5 mL). Don't squeeze the patient's finger too tightly *because doing so may dilute the specimen with plasma.*[9]
- Insert the microcuvette into the photometer. Hemoglobin test results appear on the photometer screen in 40 seconds to 4 minutes.
- Place a gauze pad over the puncture site and apply firm pressure *to stop bleeding.*
- Dispose of the lancet and microcuvette in appropriate containers.[10]
- Remove and discard your gloves and perform hand hygiene.[1,2,3,5,6]
- Put on a pair of new gloves and clean and disinfect the photometer using a disinfectant pad *so that it's ready to use for another patient.*[7,11,12]
- Remove and discard your gloves and perform hand hygiene.[1,2,3,5,6]
- Notify the practitioner if the test result is outside the expected parameters.[13]
- Document the procedure.[14,15,16]

Special considerations

- Bedside hemoglobin testing is considered a waived test, meaning the test system was approved for waiver under the Clinical Laboratory Improvement Amendments of 1988 by the U.S. Food and Drug Administration. To qualify for waived test status, the test must be simple to perform and have low risk for erroneous test results. However, keep in mind that errors can occur anywhere in the testing process; make sure you follow the manufacturer's instructions for use *to prevent testing errors that could result in treatment errors.*[17]

Documentation

Document the values obtained from the photometer as well as the date and time of the test. Record the date and time the practitioner was notified of abnormal results, any interventions performed, and the patient's response to these interventions.

REFERENCES

1 The Joint Commission. (2015). Standard NPSG.07.01.01. *Comprehensive accreditation manual for hospitals: The official handbook.* Oakbrook Terrace, IL: The Joint Commission. (Level VII)

2 Centers for Disease Control and Prevention. (2002). Guideline for hand hygiene in health-care settings: Recommendations of the Healthcare Infection Control Practices Advisory Committee and the HICPAC/SHEA/APIC/IDSA Hand Hygiene Task Force. *MMWR Recommendations and Reports, 51*(RR-16), 1–45. Accessed March 2015 via the Web at http://www.cdc.gov/mmwr/pdf/rr/rr5116.pdf (Level II)

3 World Health Organization. (2009). "WHO guidelines on hand hygiene in health care: First global patient safety challenge, clean care is safer care" [Online]. Accessed March 2015 via the Web at http://whqlibdoc.who.int/publications/2009/9789241597906_eng.pdf (Level IV)

4 Siegel, J. D., et al. (2007). "2007 guideline for isolation precautions: Preventing transmission of infectious agents in healthcare settings" [Online]. Accessed March 2015 via the Web at http://www.cdc.gov/hicpac/pdf/isolation/Isolation2007.pdf (Level II)

5 Centers for Medicare & Medicaid Services, Department of Health and Human Services. (2014). Condition of participation: Infection control. 42 C.F.R. § 482.42.

6 American Osteopathic Association. (2014). Standard 07.01.21. *Healthcare Facilities Accreditation Program: Accreditation requirements for acute care hospitals.* Chicago, IL: American Osteopathic Association. (Level VII)

7 American Osteopathic Association. (2014). Standard 07.01.10. *Healthcare Facilities Accreditation Program: Accreditation requirements for acute care hospitals.* Chicago, IL: American Osteopathic Association. (Level VII)

8 The Joint Commission. (2015). Standard NPSG.01.01.01. *Comprehensive accreditation manual for hospitals: The official handbook.* Oakbrook Terrace, IL: The Joint Commission. (Level VII)

9 World Health Organization. (2010). "WHO guidelines on drawing blood: Best practices in phlebotomy" [Online]. Accessed March 2015 via the Web at http://www.who.int/injection_safety/phleb_final_screen_ready.pdf (Level IV)

10 Occupational Safety and Health Administration. (n.d.). "Bloodborne pathogens, standard number 1910.1030" [Online]. Accessed March 2015 via the Web at http://www.osha.gov/pls/oshaweb/owadisp.show_document?p_table=STANDARDS&p_id=10051 (Level VII)

11 Rutala, W. A., et al. (2008). "Guideline for disinfection and sterilization in healthcare facilities, 2008" [Online]. Accessed March 2015 via the Web at http://www.cdc.gov/hicpac/pdf/guidelines/Disinfection_Nov_2008.pdf (Level I)

12 American Osteopathic Association. (2014). Standard 07.02.03. *Healthcare Facilities Accreditation Program: Accreditation requirements for acute care hospitals.* Chicago, IL: American Osteopathic Association. (Level VII)

13 The Joint Commission. (2015). Standard NPSG.02.03.01. *Comprehensive accreditation manual for hospitals: The official handbook.* Oakbrook Terrace, IL: The Joint Commission. (Level VII)

14 The Joint Commission. (2015). Standard RC.01.03.01. *Comprehensive accreditation manual for hospitals: The official handbook.* Oakbrook Terrace, IL: The Joint Commission. (Level VII)

15 Centers for Medicare & Medicaid Services, Department of Health and Human Services. (2014). Condition of participation: Medical record services. 42 C.F.R. § 482.24.

16 American Osteopathic Association. (2014). Standard 10.00.03. *Healthcare Facilities Accreditation Program: Accreditation requirements for acute care hospitals.* Chicago, IL: American Osteopathic Association. (Level VII)

17 Centers for Disease Control and Prevention (2013). "Clinical Laboratory Improvement Amendments: Waived tests" [Online]. Accessed March 2015 via the Web at http://wwwn.cdc.gov/CLIA/Resources/WaivedTests/default.aspx

ADDITIONAL REFERENCES

Sanchis-Gomar, F., et al. (2013). Hemoglobin point-of-care testing: The HemoCue System. *Journal of Laboratory Automation, 18,* 198–205. Accessed March 2015 via the Web at http://jla.sagepub.com/content/early/2012/09/04/2211068212457560.full.pdf

Skelton, V. A., et al. (2013). Evaluation of point-of-care haemoglobin measuring devices: A comparison of Radical-7™ pulse co-oximetry, HemoCue(®) and laboratory haemoglobin measurements in obstetric patients. *Anaesthesia, 68,* 40–45.

HIP ARTHROPLASTY CARE

Hip arthroplasty involves surgical replacement of the hip joint. It may be total (replacing the femoral head and acetabulum) or partial (replacing only one joint component). (See *Total hip replacement.*)

Hip arthroplasty is performed to decrease or eliminate pain and improve functional status. It's most commonly used to treat osteoarthritis. Other indications include rheumatoid arthritis, avascular necrosis, traumatic arthritis, hip fractures, benign and malignant bone tumors, ankylosing spondylitis, and juvenile rheumatoid arthritis.

Arthroplasty postprocedure care includes providing routine postoperative care, maintaining alignment of the affected joint, and assisting with exercises. Nursing responsibility includes teaching, safe mobility, home care, and exercises that may continue for several years.

Equipment

Incentive spirometer ▪ antiembolism stocking or sequential compression device ▪ ice bag ▪ skin lotion ▪ warm water ▪ crutches or walker ▪ closed-wound drainage system ▪ pillow ▪ marker ▪ over-the-bed trapeze bar ▪ prescribed anticoagulants ▪ prescribed pain medications ▪ blood pressure monitoring device ▪ stethoscope ▪ disinfectant pad ▪ Optional: gloves, programmable IV infusion pump, sterile dressings, hypoallergenic tape, prescribed beta-adrenergic agent.

Implementation

- Verify the practitioner's orders.
- Perform hand hygiene and put on gloves, if necessary, *to comply with standard precautions.*[1,2,3,4]
- Confirm the patient's identity using at least two patient identifiers.[5]
- Explain all procedures to the patient.
- Monitor vital signs at an interval determined by your facility and the patient's condition; *no evidence-based research is available to dictate the best practice for the frequency of vital signs monitoring.*[6] Report changes in vital signs *because these changes may indicate the presence of infection, hemorrhage, and other postoperative complications.*
- Perform a comprehensive pain assessment using techniques appropriate for the patient's age, condition, and ability to understand. Administer pain medications, as ordered, following safe medication administration practices. Perform a follow-up assessment, and notify the practitioner if pain isn't adequately controlled.[7]
- Assess the patient for postoperative nausea and vomiting, and intervene if needed.[6]
- Perform bilateral neurovascular assessments regularly as needed[6] *to monitor for signs and symptoms of complications.* Assess the affected leg for color, temperature, toe movement, sensation, edema, capillary filling, and pedal pulse. Investigate complaints of pain, burning, numbness, and tingling.
- Assess and address the patient's safety needs to reduce the risk of patient harm.[6]
- Direct the patient to perform deep-breathing and coughing exercises and incentive spirometry *to prevent postprocedure atelectasis.*[8]
- Apply an antiembolism stocking or sequential compression device, as ordered, *to promote venous return and prevent venous thromboembolism (VTE).* (See the "Sequential compression therapy" and "Antiembolism stocking application" procedures, pages 687, 21.) Note that the Centers for Medicare & Medicaid Services considers deep vein thrombosis and pulmonary embolism in hip and total knee replacement surgery a hospital-acquired conditions.[9]
- Make sure baseline coagulation studies have been obtained and are documented in the patient's medical record. (International Normalized Ratio [INR] should be monitored if the patient is receiving warfarin.) If a continuous infusion of heparin is prescribed, administer it using a

programmable pump (preferably a smart pump with dose-range alerts) *to provide consistent and accurate dosing.*[10]

- Administer anticoagulant therapy, as ordered, *to minimize the risk of VTE.*[11]
- Observe for signs and symptoms of phlebitis, such as warmth, swelling, tenderness, and redness.
- Monitor laboratory results, such as complete blood count, prothrombin time, partial thromboplastin time, and INR.
- Inspect the dressings for excessive bleeding. Circle any drainage on the dressing and mark it with your initials, the date, and the time.
- Observe the closed-wound drainage system for discharge color. (See the "Closed-wound drain management" procedure, page 190.) *Proper drainage prevents hematoma. Purulent discharge and fever may indicate infection.* Empty and measure drainage, as ordered, using clean technique *to prevent infection.*
- Monitor fluid intake and output daily; include wound drainage in the output measurement.
- If an indwelling urinary catheter was inserted for surgery, remove the catheter on postoperative day 1 or 2 (with the day of surgery considered day 0), or as soon as it's no longer needed *to reduce the risk of catheter-associated urinary tract infection.*[11,12,13] (See the "Indwelling urinary catheter care and removal" procedure, page 391.)
- Make sure prophylactic antibiotics are discontinued within 24 hours after surgery.[12,14]
- Apply an ice bag, as ordered, to the affected site for the first 48 hours *to reduce swelling, relieve pain, and control bleeding.*
- Help the patient use the trapeze bar for repositioning every 2 hours.[15] *Position changes enhance comfort, prevent pressure ulcers, and help prevent respiratory complications.*
- Provide skin care for the back and buttocks, as indicated.
- Position the patient according to the surgical approach used and the surgeon's preference. Depending on the surgical approach, an abduction splint may be necessary *to keep the hip in a neutral position.*
- Encourage the patient to begin plantar flexion and dorsiflexion exercises of the ankles and feet *to prevent VTE.*
- Collaborate with physical therapy professionals, as appropriate, *to formulate an individualized exercise plan for the patient.*
- Before ambulation, assess the patient's pain and give pain medication, as ordered, *because movement is very painful.* Encourage the patient during exercise.
- Help the patient with progressive ambulation, using assistive devices when needed.
- If the patient was receiving a beta-adrenergic blocker before surgery, collaborate with the patient's practitioner to make sure he receives it during the perioperative period, as appropriate.[11]
- Remove and discard your gloves, if worn.
- Perform hand hygiene.[1,2,3]
- Disinfect your stethoscope using a disinfectant pad.[16]
- Perform hand hygiene.[1,2,3]
- Document the procedure.[17,18]

Special considerations

- Note that progressive ambulation protocols vary. Most patients are permitted to begin transfer and progressive ambulation with assistive devices on the first day. Collaborate with physical therapy professionals, as appropriate.
- Educate the patient and family about measures to prevent surgical site infection.[19]

Complications

Immobility after arthroplasty may result in such complications as shock, pulmonary embolism, pneumonia, phlebitis, paralytic ileus, urine retention, and bowel impaction. A deep wound or infection at the prosthesis site is a serious complication that may force removal of the prosthesis. Although these are the most common complications, their incidence has been significantly reduced because of the use of prophylactic antibiotics and anticoagulants and early mobilization. Dislocation of a total hip prosthesis may occur after violent hip flexion or adduction or during internal rotation. Signs of dislocation include inability to rotate the hip or bear weight, shortening of the leg, and increased pain.

Fat embolism, a potentially fatal complication resulting from release of fat molecules in response to increased intramedullary canal pressure from the prosthesis, may develop within 72 hours after surgery. Watch for such signs and symptoms as apprehension, diaphoresis, fever, dyspnea, hypoxia, pulmonary effusion, tachycardia, cyanosis, seizures, decreased level of consciousness, and a petechial rash on the chest and shoulders; hypoxia is an early sign that may occur hours before the onset of respiratory complaints.[20]

Total hip replacement

To form a totally artificial hip, the surgeon cements a femoral head prosthesis in place to articulate with a cup, which is then cemented into the deepened acetabulum. The surgeon may avoid using cement by implanting a prosthesis with a porous coating that promotes bony ingrowth.

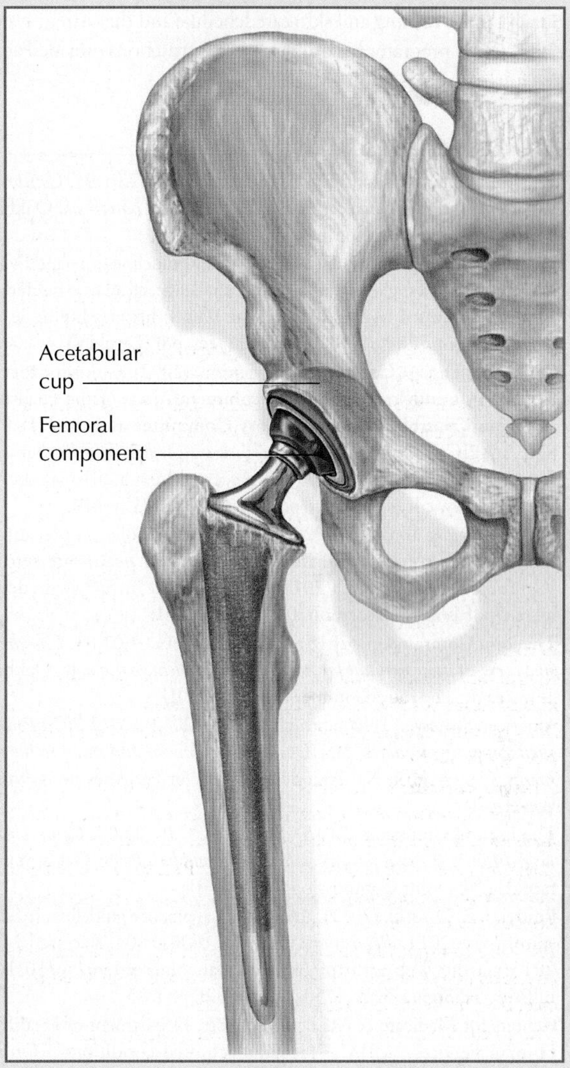

Documentation

Document signs and symptoms of infection. Record the patient's neurovascular status. Document the patient's pain and response to pain medication. Describe the patient's position (especially the position of the affected leg), skin care and condition, respiratory care and condition, and the use of antiembolism stockings. Document all exercises performed and their effect; also record ambulatory efforts, the type of support used, and the amount of traction weight.

On the appropriate flowchart, record vital signs and fluid intake and output. Note the turning and skin care schedule and the current exercise and ambulation program. Record discharge instructions provided as well as the patient's understanding of them.

References

1 The Joint Commission. (2015). Standard NPSG.07.01.01. *Comprehensive accreditation manual for hospitals: The official handbook.* Oakbrook Terrace, IL: The Joint Commission. (Level VII)

2 World Health Organization. (2009). "WHO guidelines on hand hygiene in health care: First global patient safety challenge, clean care is safer care" [Online]. Accessed March 2015 via the Web at http://whqlibdoc.who.int/publications/2009/9789241597906_eng.pdf (Level IV)

3 Centers for Disease Control and Prevention. (2002). Guideline for hand hygiene in health-care settings: Recommendations of the Healthcare Infection Control Practices Advisory Committee and the HICPAC/SHEA/APIC/IDSA Hand Hygiene Task Force. *MMWR Recommendations and Reports, 51*(RR-16), 1–45. Accessed March 2015 via the Web at http://www.cdc.gov/mmwr/pdf/rr/rr5116.pdf (Level II)

4 Siegel, J. D., et al. (2007). "2007 guideline for isolation precautions: Preventing transmission of infectious agents in healthcare settings" [Online]. Accessed March 2015 via the Web at http://www.cdc.gov/hicpac/pdf/isolation/Isolation2007.pdf (Level II)

5 The Joint Commission. (2015). Standard NPSG.01.01.01. *Comprehensive accreditation manual for hospitals: The official handbook.* Oakbrook Terrace, IL: The Joint Commission. (Level VII)

6 American Society of PeriAnesthesia Nurses. (2012). *2012-2014 Perianesthesia nursing standards, practice recommendations and interpretive statements.* Cherry Hill, NJ: American Society of PeriAnesthesia Nurses. (Level VII)

7 The Joint Commission. (2015). Standard PC.01.02.07. *Comprehensive accreditation manual for hospitals: The official handbook.* Oakbrook Terrace, IL: The Joint Commission. (Level VII)

8 Restrepo, R. D., et al. (2011). AARC clinical practice guideline: Incentive spirometry: 2011. *Respiratory Care, 56,* 1600–1604. Accessed March 2015 via the Web at http://rc.rcjournal.com/content/56/10/1600.full?sid=5a58b341-5f24-4d50-8d0a-3862f23b4e85

9 Centers for Medicare & Medicaid Services, Department of Health and Human Services. (2014). "Hospital-acquired conditions" [Online]. Accessed March 2015 via the Web at http://www.cms.gov/Medicare/Medicare-Fee-for-Service-Payment/HospitalAcqCond/Hospital-Acquired_Conditions.html

10 The Joint Commission. (2015). Standard NPSG.03.05.01. *Comprehensive accreditation manual for hospitals: The official handbook.* Oakbrook Terrace, IL: The Joint Commission. (Level VII)

11 Centers for Medicare & Medicaid Services & The Joint Commission. (2014). "The specifications manual for national hospital inpatient quality measures" [Online]. Accessed March 2015 via the Web at http://www.qualitynet.org/dcs/ContentServer?pagename=QnetPublic%2FPage%2FQnetTier2&cid=1141662756099 (Level VII)

12 The Joint Commission. (2015). Standard NPSG.07.06.01. *Comprehensive accreditation manual for hospitals: The official handbook.* Oakbrook Terrace, IL: The Joint Commission. (Level VII)

13 Healthcare Infection Control Practices Advisory Committee. (2010). "Guideline for prevention of catheter-associated urinary tract infections, 2009" [Online]. Accessed March 2015 via the Web at http://www.cdc.gov/hicpac/pdf/CAUTI/CAUTIguideline2009final.pdf (Level I)

14 Anderson, D. J., et al. (2014). SHEA/IDSA practice recommendation: Strategies to prevent surgical site infections in acute care hospitals: 2014 update. *Infection Control and Hospital Epidemiology, 35,* 605–627. Accessed March 2015 via the Web at http://www.jstor.org/stable/10.1086/676022 (Level IV)

15 Institute for Clinical Systems Improvement. (2012). "Health care protocol: Pressure ulcer prevention and treatment protocol (3rd ed.)" [Online]. Accessed March 2015 via the Web at https://www.icsi.org/_asset/6t7kxy/

16 Rutala, W. A., et al. (2008). "Guideline for disinfection and sterilization in healthcare facilities, 2008" [Online]. Accessed March 2015 via the Web at http://www.cdc.gov/hicpac/pdf/guidelines/Disinfection_Nov_2008.pdf (Level I)

17 The Joint Commission. (2015). Standard RC.01.03.01. *Comprehensive accreditation manual for hospitals: The official handbook.* Oakbrook Terrace, IL: The Joint Commission. (Level VII)

18 Centers for Medicare & Medicaid Services, Department of Health and Human Services. (2014). Condition of participation: Medical record services. 42 C.F.R. § 482.24(b).

19 The Joint Commission. (2015). Standard NPSG.07.05.01. *Comprehensive accreditation manual for hospitals: The official handbook.* Oakbrook Terrace, IL: The Joint Commission. (Level VII)

20 Shaikh, N. (2009). Emergency management of fat embolism syndrome. *Journal of Emergencies, Trauma, and Shock, 2*(1), 29–33. Accessed March 2015 via the Web at http://www.onlinejets.org/article.asp?issn=0974-2700%3Byear=2009%3Bvolume=2%3Bissue=1%3Bspage=29%3Bepage=33%3Baulast=Shaikh

Hour-of-sleep care

Hour-of-sleep care meets the patient's physical and psychological needs in preparation for sleep. It includes providing for the patient's hygiene, making the bed clean and comfortable, and ensuring safety. For example, raising the bed's side rails can prevent the drowsy or sedated patient from falling out. This type of care also provides an opportunity to answer the patient's questions about the next day's tests and procedures and to discuss his worries and concerns.

Effective hour-of-sleep care prepares the patient for a good night's sleep. Ineffective care may contribute to sleeplessness, which can intensify patient anxiety and interfere with treatment and recuperation. Promoting the patient's sleep on the challenging environment of a nursing unit dictates not only that you be sensitive to the patient's needs and attuned to the environment but also that you have the tools and resources necessary to implement effective strategies.

Equipment

Basin ▪ skin cleaner ▪ towel ▪ washcloth ▪ toothbrush and toothpaste ▪ lotion ▪ blankets ▪ facial tissues ▪ Optional: gloves, bedpan or urinal, earplugs, eye mask, clean linens, patient gown, denture cup, commercial denture cleaner, dressing materials, prescribed medications.

Preparation of equipment

Gather the equipment at the patient's bedside. For an ambulatory patient who's capable of self-care, gather skin cleaner, a washcloth, a towel, and oral hygiene items at the sink.

Implementation

- Perform hand hygiene[1,2,3,4,5] and put on gloves, if necessary.[6,7]
- Confirm the patient's identity using at least two patient identifiers.[8]
- Tell the patient you will help him prepare for sleep, and provide privacy.
- Offer a bedpan or urinal to a patient on bed rest. Alternatively, assist the ambulatory patient to the bathroom or commode.
- Fill the basin with warm water and bring it to the patient's bedside. Offer the skin cleaner and encourage the patient to wash himself, if possible,

to promote independence. Otherwise, wash the patient's face and hands and dry them thoroughly.

■ Provide toothpaste or a properly labeled denture cup and commercial denture cleaner. Assist the patient with oral hygiene, as necessary. (See the "Oral care" procedure, page 560.) If the patient prefers to wear dentures until bedtime, leave denture care items within easy reach.

■ After providing oral care, turn the patient on his side or stomach. Wash, rinse, and dry the patient's back and buttocks. Massage the back with lotion *to help him relax.* (See the "Back care" procedure, page 50.)

■ While providing back care, observe the skin for redness, cracking, or other signs of breakdown. If the patient's gown is soiled or damp, provide a clean one and help him put it on, if necessary.

■ Check dressings, binders, antiembolism stockings, or other aids, changing or readjusting them as needed.

■ Refill the water container, and place it and a box of facial tissues within the patient's easy reach *to prevent falls if the patient needs to reach for these items.*

■ Straighten or change bed linens, as necessary, and fluff the patient's pillow. Clean linens are only needed if the linen is soiled. Cover the patient with a blanket or place one within easy reach *to prevent chills during the night.* Then position him comfortably.

■ Offer the patient ear plugs, if appropriate, *to help block noise from the unit.*[9]

■ If the patient appears distressed, restless, or in pain, administer medications as needed and ordered following safe medication administration practices.

■ After making the patient comfortable, evaluate his mental and physical condition.

■ Place the bed in a low position and, if appropriate, raise the side rails *to promote safety.*

■ Place the call light within the patient's easy reach, and instruct him to use it whenever necessary.

■ Move all breakables from the overbed table out of the patient's reach, and remove any equipment and supplies that could cause him to fall if he gets up during the night.

■ Turn off the lights.[10]

NURSING ALERT ***Monitor alarms should be on, set appropriately, and audible to staff; volumes should never be decreased if contraindicated by the patient's clinical status.***[11]

■ Remove and discard your gloves, if worn.[6]

■ Perform hand hygiene.[1,2,3,4,5]

■ Close the patient's door if not contraindicated.

■ Document the procedure.[12,13,14]

Special considerations

■ Ask the patient about his sleep routine at home and, whenever possible, let him follow it while taking into consideration his social and cultural background *because sleep, while biological, can also be shaped by societal and cultural values and beliefs.*

■ Try to observe certain rituals, such as a bedtime snack, *which can aid sleep.* A back massage, a tub bath, or a shower can also help relax the patient and promote a restful night. If the patient normally bathes or showers before bedtime, let him do so if his condition and practitioner's orders permit it.

■ Because of the nature of the intensive care unit, periods of quiet time that coincide with circadian rhythms should be provided. *Efforts to reduce controllable noise and light at particular times throughout the day have been shown to contribute to patient sleep, even during day-shift hours.*[15]

Documentation

Record the time and type of hour-of-sleep care in your notes. Include use of any special procedures such as relaxation techniques.

REFERENCES

1 The Joint Commission. (2015). Standard NPSG.07.01.01. *Comprehensive accreditation manual for hospitals: The official handbook.* Oakbrook Terrace, IL: The Joint Commission. (Level I)

2 Centers for Disease Control and Prevention. (2002). Guideline for hand hygiene in health-care settings: Recommendations of the Healthcare Infection Control Practices Advisory Committee and the HICPAC/SHEA/APIC/IDSA Hand Hygiene Task Force. *MMWR Recommendations and Reports, 51*(RR-16), 1–45. Accessed March 2015 via the Web at http://www.cdc.gov/mmwr/pdf/rr/rr5116.pdf (Level I)

3 World Health Organization. (2009). "WHO guidelines on hand hygiene in health care: First global patient safety challenge, clean care is safer care" [Online]. Accessed March 2015 via the Web at http://whqlibdoc.who.int/publications/2009/9789241597906_eng.pdf (Level I)

4 American Osteopathic Association. (2014). Standard 07.01.21. *Healthcare Facilities Accreditation Program: Accreditation requirements for acute care hospitals.* Chicago, IL: American Osteopathic Association. (Level VII)

5 Centers for Medicare & Medicaid Services, Department of Health and Human Services. (2014). Condition of participation: Infection control. 42 C.F.R. § 482.42.

6 Siegel, J. D., et al. (2007). "2007 guideline for isolation precautions: Preventing transmission of infectious agents in healthcare settings" [Online]. Accessed March 2015 via the Web at http://www.cdc.gov/hicpac/pdf/isolation/Isolation2007.pdf (Level II)

7 American Osteopathic Association. (2014). Standard 07.01.10. *Healthcare Facilities Accreditation Program: Accreditation requirements for acute care hospitals.* Chicago, IL: American Osteopathic Association. (Level VII)

8 The Joint Commission. (2015). Standard NPSG.01.01.01. *Comprehensive accreditation manual for hospitals: The official handbook.* Oakbrook Terrace, IL: The Joint Commission. (Level I)

9 Jones, C., & Dawson, D. (2012). Eye masks and earplugs improve patient's perception of sleep. *Nursing in Critical Care, 17,* 247–254. (Level VI)

10. Thomas, K. P., et al. (2012). Sleep rounds: A multidisciplinary approach to optimize sleep quality and satisfaction in hospitalized patients. *Journal of Hospital Medicine, 7,* 508–512. (Level VI)

11 The Joint Commission. (2015). Standard NPSG 06.01.01. *Comprehensive accreditation manual for hospitals: The official handbook.* Oakbrook Terrace, IL: The Joint Commission. (Level I)

12 The Joint Commission. (2015). Standard RC.01.03.01. *Comprehensive accreditation manual for hospitals: The official handbook.* Oakbrook Terrace, IL: The Joint Commission. (Level I)

13 American Osteopathic Association. (2014). Standard 10.00.03. *Healthcare Facilities Accreditation Program: Accreditation requirements for acute care hospitals.* Chicago, IL: American Osteopathic Association. (Level VII)

14 Centers for Medicare & Medicaid Services, Department of Health and Human Services. (2014). Condition of participation: Medical records services. 42 C.F.R. § 482.24(b).

15 Dennis, C. M., et al. (2010). Benefits of quiet time for neuro-intensive care patients. *Journal of Neuroscience Nursing, 42,* 217–224. (Level VI)

ADDITIONAL REFERENCE

Craven, R. F., & Hirnle, C. J. (2012). *Fundamentals of nursing: Human health and function* (7th ed.). Philadelphia, PA: Lippincott Williams & Wilkins.

HUMIDIFIER THERAPY

Humidifiers, which deliver a maximum amount of water vapor without producing particulate water, are used to prevent drying and irritation of the upper airway. They're used in the treatment of such conditions as croup, in which the upper airway is inflamed, and when secretions are particularly thick and tenacious.

Several types of humidifiers are available. (See *Types of humidifiers,* page 364.) *Diffusion head humidifiers* (also known as *in-line humidifiers*) humidify only the air being delivered to the patient by an oxygen delivery system. One type of diffusion head humidifier—the *cascade bubble*

EQUIPMENT

Types of humidifiers

	Description and uses	Advantages	Disadvantages
Bedside humidifier	■ Spinning disk splashes water against a baffle, creating small drops and increasing evaporation. A motor disperses mist to directly humidify room air.	■ Can be used with all oxygen masks and nasal cannulas ■ Easy to operate ■ Inexpensive	■ Produces humidity inefficiently ■ Can't be used for a patient with a bypassed upper airway ■ Can harbor bacteria and mold
Cascade bubble diffusion humidifier	■ Gas is forced through a plastic grid in a reservoir of warmed water to create fine bubbles. It's commonly used in patients receiving mechanical ventilation or continuous positive airway pressure therapy.	■ Delivers 100% humidity at body temperature ■ Most effective of all evaporative humidifiers	■ If correct water level isn't maintained, can irritate the mucosa
Diffusion head humidifier	■ Depending on the design, a diffusion head humidifier can deliver low- or high-flow oxygen. Gas flows through the porous diffuser in the reservoir to increase gas-liquid interface, providing humidification to patients using a nasal cannula, oxygen mask (except the Venturi mask), or tracheostomy collar.	■ Easy to operate ■ Inexpensive	■ Possibility of microorganisms growing in standing water and then being dispersed by the device ■ Can't be used for a patient with a bypassed upper airway unless the patient has a tracheostomy collar
Heated vaporizer	■ Water heated in the reservoir directly humidifies room air.	■ May be used with all oxygen masks and nasal cannulas ■ Easy to operate ■ Inexpensive	■ Can't deliver a precise amount of humidification ■ Can harbor bacteria and mold ■ Can result in scald or burn injuries

diffusion humidifier—heats water vapor, which raises the moisture-carrying capacity of gas and increases the amount of humidity delivered to the patient. A diffusion head humidifier can be added to a low-flow oxygen delivery system to humidify the air being delivered to the patient, but it doesn't heat the water vapor. *Bedside humidifiers* and *heated vaporizers* sit at the patient's bedside and are plugged into an electrical outlet. A heated vaporizer heats water vapor to raise the moisture-carrying capacity of gas, adding humidity to an entire room.

Equipment

Appropriate humidifier ■ sterile, distilled water (for all types) or tap water (if the unit has a demineralizing capability) ■ container for waste water.

Bedside humidifier and heated vaporizer

Hospital-grade disinfectant.

Diffusion head humidifier (including cascade bubble diffusion humidifier)

Flowmeter ■ oxygen source ■ oxygen delivery device ■ Optional: drainage bag, commercially prepared disposable unit ■ Optional: gloves.

Preparation of equipment

For a bedside humidifier

Open the reservoir and add sterile, distilled water to the fill line; then close the reservoir. Keep all room windows and doors closed tightly *to maintain adequate humidification.*

For a cascade bubble diffusion humidifier

Install the cascade bubble diffuser into the ventilator circuit according to the manufacturer's instructions. Unscrew the cascade reservoir and add sterile, distilled water to the fill line. Then screw the top back onto the reservoir. For routine use on an intubated patient, plug in the heater unit and set the temperature to between 93.2°F (34°C) and 105.8°F (41°C) at the circuit Y-connector.[1] Use an audible temperature alarm, as recommended; set the high-temperature alarm no higher than 105.8°F (41°C), with a 109.4°F (43°C) over-temperature limit, and the low-temperature alarm no lower than 3.6°F (2°C) below the desired temperature at the circuit Y-connector. Test the device and alarm periodically *for proper functioning.*[1]

For a diffusion head humidifier

Unscrew the humidifier reservoir and add sterile, distilled water to the appropriate level. (If you're using a disposable unit, screw the cap with the extension onto the top of the unit.) Then screw the reservoir back onto the humidifier, and attach the flowmeter to the oxygen source.

Screw the humidifier onto the flowmeter until the seal is tight. Then set the flowmeter at a rate of 2 L/minute and check for gentle bubbling, *indicating that the flowmeter is working properly.* Next, check the positive-pressure release valve by occluding the end valve on the humidifier. The pressure should back up into the humidifier, signaled by a high-pitched whistle. If this whistle doesn't occur, tighten all connections and try again. Make sure the device is set up and functioning properly.

For a heated vaporizer

Remove the top of the vaporizer and fill the reservoir to the fill line with sterile, distilled water (or tap water if permitted). Replace the top securely. Make sure the vaporizer has been properly prepared.

Implementation

- Verify the practitioner's order.
- Gather and prepare the necessary equipment.
- Perform hand hygiene.[2,3,4,5,6]

■ Confirm the patient's identity using at least two patient identifiers.[7]
■ Explain the procedure to the patient *to reduce anxiety.*

Bedside humidifier

■ Plug the unit into an electrical outlet and then turn on the unit. Make sure the device is functioning properly.
■ Check for a fine mist emission from the nozzle, *which indicates proper operation.*
■ Direct the humidifier unit's nozzle toward the patient but away from the patient's face for effective treatment.
■ Check the unit every 4 hours for proper operation and water level.
■ Clean and refill the unit as needed *to reduce the risk of bacterial growth.* Unplug the unit. Discard the old water. Clean and disinfect the unit with a hospital-grade disinfectant.[8,9] Rinse the reservoir container. Refill the container with water.

Cascade bubble diffusion humidifier

■ Assess the temperature of the inspired gas near the patient's airway, every 2 hours or as determined by your facility. If the cascade becomes too hot, check the heater unit and reset or replace the unit, as necessary *because overheated water vapor can cause respiratory tract burns.*
■ Check the reservoir's water level every 2 to 4 hours, and fill it as necessary. *If the water level falls below the minimum water level mark, humidity will decrease to that of room air.*
■ Frequently check for condensation buildup in the tubing, *which can result from the high humidification produced by the cascade.*
■ Empty the condensate as necessary *so it can't drain into the patient's respiratory tract, encourage growth of microorganisms, or obstruct dependent sections of tubing.* Follow the manufacturer's recommendations for removing condensation from the patient unit. *Condensate is infectious waste and shouldn't be drained back into the humidifier.*[1]
■ Assess the quantity and consistency of the patient's secretions *to evaluate the effectiveness of treatment.*[1]

Diffusion head humidifier

■ Attach the oxygen delivery device to the humidifier and then to the patient. Adjust the flowmeter to the appropriate oxygen flow rate and look for a gentle bubbling.
■ If appropriate, add a drainage bag to the low point of the tubing *to prevent condensate from accumulating in the tubing.*
■ Check the reservoir every 4 hours. If the water level drops too low, empty the remaining water, rinse the jar, and refill it with sterile, distilled water. Alternately, replace a commercially prepared disposable unit at its low water mark. *As the reservoir water level decreases, the evaporation of water in the gas decreases, reducing humidification of the delivered gas.*
■ Assess the patient's sputum periodically; *sputum that's too thick can hinder mobilization and expectoration.* If thick sputum occurs, the patient requires a device that can provide higher humidity.

Heated vaporizer

■ Place the vaporizer about 4′ (1.2 m) from the patient so that the steam will be directed toward, but not directly onto, the patient. Place the unit in a spot where it can't be overturned *to avoid hot-water burns.* This step is especially important if children will be in the room.
■ Plug the unit into an electrical outlet. Steam should soon rise from the unit into the air. Close all windows and doors *to maintain adequate humidification.*

NURSING ALERT *Position the cord out of the way* to prevent a fall hazard.

■ Every 4 hours, check the water level and check the unit for proper functioning. To refill, unplug the unit, discard any old water, clean and disinfect with a hospital-grade disinfectant, rinse the reservoir, and refill the unit with sterile, distilled water.[8,9] If the steam production seems insufficient, consider refilling with half sterile, distilled water and half tap water.

Completing the procedure

■ Perform hand hygiene.[2,3,4,5,6]
■ Document the procedure.[10,11,12]

Special considerations

■ Replace a bedside humidifier unit every 7 days or as determined by your facility, and send used units for proper decontamination.
■ Assess the patient regularly *to determine the effectiveness of therapy because a bedside humidifier or vaporizer doesn't deliver a precise amount of humidification.* Ask the patient whether he has noticed any improvement, and evaluate his sputum.
■ The Joint Commission has issued a sentinel event alert concerning medical device alarm safety *because alarm-related events have been associated with permanent loss of function or death.* Among the major contributing factors were improper alarm settings, alarm settings inappropriately turned off, and alarm signals not audible to staff members. Make sure that alarm limits are set appropriately and that alarms are turned on and audible. Follow facility guidelines for preventing alarm fatigue.[13]
■ Change the ventilator circuit when it's not functioning properly or is visibly soiled, unless otherwise specified by the manufacturer.[1]
■ Change the cascade at an interval specified by your facility.
■ *Because the diffusion head humidifier creates a level of humidity comparable to that of ambient air,* the diffusion head humidifier is use only for oxygen flow rates greater than 4 L/minute.
■ For patients receiving oxygen by tracheostomy or a transtracheal device in which the device bypasses the upper airway, humidification of inspired gas is necessary even at low flow rates.[14]
■ Keep in mind that a humidifier that's not kept clean can cause or aggravate respiratory problems, especially for people allergic to molds.[9,15]
■ If humidifier therapy is prescribed for a child, use cool mist instead of warm *mist to reduce the risk of scalding and burns.*[16]

Patient teaching

Make sure the patient and his family understand the reason for using a humidifier and know how to use the equipment. Give them specific written guidelines concerning all aspects of home care.

Instruct a patient using a bedside humidifier at home to fill it with plain tap water but to periodically use sterile, distilled water *to prevent mineral buildup* or to follow the manufacturer's instructions for use. Also tell the patient to run white vinegar through it *to help clean it, prevent bacterial buildup, and dissolve deposits.*

Complications

If contaminated, humidifiers can cause infection. Improper cleaning can lead to mold growth, which may exacerbate certain respiratory conditions such as asthma.

Cascade bubble diffusion humidifiers can cause aspiration of tubal condensation, pulmonary burns if the air is heated, and infection if contaminated. Improper humidifier temperature settings may also lead to hyperthermia.[1]

Documentation

Record the date and time when humidification began and was discontinued, the type of humidifier used, the patient's response to humidification, and any patient teaching provided.[6]

REFERENCES

1 Restrepo, R. D., & Walsh, B. K. (2012). AARC clinical practice guideline: Humidification during mechanical ventilation: 2012. *Respiratory Care,*

57, 782–788. Accessed March 2015 via the Web at http://rc.rcjournal.com/content/57/5/782.full.pdf
2 The Joint Commission. (2015). Standard NPSG.07.01.01. *Comprehensive accreditation manual for hospitals: The official handbook.* Oakbrook Terrace, IL: The Joint Commission. (Level VII)
3 Centers for Disease Control and Prevention. (2002). Guideline for hand hygiene in health-care settings: Recommendations of the Healthcare Infection Control Practices Advisory Committee and the HICPAC/SHEA/APIC/IDSA Hand Hygiene Task Force. *MMWR Recommendations and Reports, 51*(RR-16), 1–45. Accessed March 2015 via the Web at http://www.cdc.gov/mmwr/pdf/rr/rr5116.pdf (Level II)
4 World Health Organization. (2009). "WHO guidelines on hand hygiene in health care: First global patient safety challenge, clean care is safer care" [Online]. Accessed March 2015 via the Web at http://whqlibdoc.who.int/publications/2009/9789241597906_eng.pdf (Level IV)
5 American Osteopathic Association. (2014). Standard 07.01.21. *Healthcare Facilities Accreditation Program: Accreditation requirements for acute care hospitals.* Chicago, IL: American Osteopathic Association (Level VII)
6 Centers for Medicare & Medicaid Services, Department of Health and Human Services. (2014). Condition of participation: Infection control. 42 C.F.R. § 482.42.
7 The Joint Commission. (2015). Standard NPSG.01.01.01. *Comprehensive accreditation manual for hospitals: The official handbook.* Oakbrook Terrace, IL: The Joint Commission. (Level VII)
8 Rutala, W. A., et al. (2008). "Guideline for disinfection and sterilization in healthcare facilities, 2008" [Online]. Accessed March 2015 via the Web at http://www.cdc.gov/hicpac/pdf/guidelines/Disinfection_Nov_2008.pdf (Level I)
9 American Osteopathic Association. (2014). Standard 07.02.03. *Healthcare Facilities Accreditation Program: Accreditation requirements for acute care hospitals.* Chicago, IL: American Osteopathic Association. (Level VII)
10 The Joint Commission. (2015). Standard RC.01.03.01. *Comprehensive accreditation manual for hospitals: The official handbook.* Oakbrook Terrace, IL: The Joint Commission. (Level VII)
11 American Osteopathic Association. (2014). Standard 10.00.03. *Healthcare Facilities Accreditation Program: Accreditation requirements for acute care hospitals.* Chicago, IL: American Osteopathic Association. (Level VII)
12 Centers for Medicare & Medicaid Services, Department of Health and Human Services. (2014). Condition of participation: Medical record services. 42 C.F.R. § 482.24(b).
13 The Joint Commission. (2013). "Sentinel event alert: Medical device alarm safety in hospitals" [Online]. Accessed March 2015 via the Web at http://www.jointcommission.org/assets/1/18/SEA_50_alarms_4_5_13_FINAL1.PDF (Level VII)
14 American Thoracic Society. (2014). "Oxygen sources and delivery devices" [Online]. Accessed March 2015 via the Web at http://www.thoracic.org/clinical/copd-guidelines/for-health-professionals/management-of-stable-copd/long-term-oxygen-therapy/oxygen-sources-and-delivery-devices.php
15 Bailey, W. Patient information: Trigger avoidance in asthma (beyond the basics). (2013). In: *UpToDate,* Feldweg, A. M. (Ed). Accessed March 2015 via the Web at http://www.uptodate.com/contents/search
16 Defendi, G. L. (2014). "Croup treatment & management" [Online]. Accessed March 2015 via the Web at http://emedicine.medscape.com/article/962972-treatment

Additional reference

Craven, R. F., & Hirnle, C. J. (2012). *Fundamentals of nursing: Human health and function* (7th ed.). Philadelphia, PA: Lippincott Williams & Wilkins.

Hyperthermia-hypothermia blanket use

A blanket-sized aquathermia K pad, the hyperthermia-hypothermia blanket raises, lowers, or maintains body temperature through conductive heat or cold transfer between the blanket and the patient. It can be operated manually or automatically.

In manual operation, a nurse or the practitioner sets the temperature on the unit. The blanket reaches and maintains this temperature regardless of the patient's temperature. The temperature setting must be adjusted manually to reach a different setting. The patient's body temperature is monitored with a conventional thermometer or with a bladder thermometer (if the patient has an indwelling urinary catheter with a temperature transducer).

In automatic operation, the unit directly and continually monitors the patient's temperature by means of a thermistor probe (rectal, skin, or esophageal) and alternates heating and cooling cycles as necessary to achieve and maintain the desired body temperature. The thermistor probe also may be used in conjunction with manual operation but isn't essential. The unit is equipped with an alarm to warn of abnormal temperature fluctuations and a circuit breaker that protects against current overload.

The blanket is used most commonly to reduce high fever when more conservative measures—such as baths, ice packs, and antipyretics—are unsuccessful. Its other uses include maintaining normal temperature during surgery or shock; inducing hypothermia during surgery to decrease metabolic activity, which reduces oxygen requirements; reducing intracranial pressure; controlling bleeding and intractable pain in patients with amputations, burns, or cancer; and providing warmth in cases of mild to moderate hypothermia.

Equipment

Hyperthermia-hypothermia control unit ▪ sterile, distilled water ▪ thermistor probe (rectal, skin, or esophageal) ▪ patient thermometer ▪ one or two hyperthermia-hypothermia blankets ▪ one or two disposable blanket covers (or one or two sheets or bath blankets) ▪ adhesive tape ▪ towel ▪ sphygmomanometer ▪ stethoscope ▪ disinfectant pads ▪ pillow ▪ Optional: gloves, hospital gown with cloth ties, protective wraps for the patient's hands and feet.

Disposable hyperthermia-hypothermia blankets are available for single-patient use.

Preparation of equipment

First, read the operation manual. Inspect the control unit and each blanket for leaks and the plugs and connecting wires for broken prongs, kinks, and fraying. If you detect or suspect malfunction, don't use the equipment.

Prepare one or two blankets by covering them with disposable covers (or use a sheet or bath blanket when positioning the blanket on the patient). *The cover absorbs perspiration and condensation, which could cause tissue breakdown if left on the skin.* Connect the blanket to the control unit, and set the controls for manual or automatic operation and for the desired blanket or body temperature. Make sure the machine is properly grounded before plugging it in. Turn on the machine and add sterile, distilled water to the unit reservoir, if necessary, as the sterile, distilled water fills the blanket. Allow the blanket to preheat or precool *so that the patient receives immediate thermal benefit.*

Implementation

- Verify the practitioner's order.
- Gather and prepare the equipment.
- If required by your facility, make sure that the patient or a responsible family member has signed a consent form.[1,2,3]
- Perform hand hygiene.[4,5,6,7,8]
- Confirm the patient's identity using at least two patient identifiers.[9]
- If the patient isn't already wearing a hospital gown, ask him to put one on. Use a gown with cloth ties rather than metal snaps or pins *to prevent heat or cold injury.*
- Assess the patient's condition and explain the procedure to him.
- Provide privacy and make sure the room is warm and free from drafts.

■ Obtain the patient's temperature, pulse, respirations, and blood pressure *to serve as a baseline,* and assess his level of consciousness, pupil reaction, limb strength, and skin condition.

■ Keeping the bottom sheet in place and the patient recumbent, roll the patient to one side and slide the blanket halfway underneath him so that its top edge aligns with his neck. Then roll the patient back, and pull and flatten the blanket across the bed. Place a pillow under the patient's head. Make sure the patient's head doesn't lie directly on the blanket *because the blanket's rigid surface may be uncomfortable and the heat or cold may lead to tissue breakdown.* Use a disposable cover, sheet, or bath blanket as insulation between the patient and the blanket. (See *Using a cooling system.*)

■ If you're using an automatic operation, perform hand hygiene and put on gloves.[4,5,6,7,8,10,11] Insert the thermistor probe in the patient's rectum and tape it in place *to prevent accidental dislodgment.* If rectal insertion is contraindicated, tuck a skin probe deep into the axilla, and secure it with tape. If the patient is comatose or anesthetized, you may want to insert an esophageal probe.

■ Remove and discard your gloves, perform hand hygiene,[4,5,6,7,8] and plug the other end of the probe into the correct jack on the unit's control panel.

■ Place a sheet or, if ordered, the second hyperthermia-hypothermia blanket over the patient *to increase the thermal benefit by trapping cooled or heated air.*

■ Wrap the patient's hands and feet if he wishes *to minimize chilling and promote comfort.*

■ Monitor the patient's vital signs and neurologic status at regular intervals, as indicated by the patient's condition.

■ Assess fluid intake and output hourly or as ordered. Observe the patient regularly for color changes in skin, lips, and nail beds, and for edema, induration, inflammation, pain, or sensory impairment. If these complications occur, discontinue the procedure and notify the practitioner.

■ Reposition the patient every 30 minutes to 1 hour, unless contraindicated, *to prevent skin breakdown.* Keep the patient's skin, bedclothes, and blanket cover free of perspiration and condensation.

Discontinuing hyperthermia-hypothermia blanket use

■ After turning off the machine, follow the manufacturer's directions. *Some units must remain plugged in for at least 30 minutes to allow the condenser fan to remove water vapor from the mechanism.* Continue to monitor the patient's temperature until it stabilizes *because body temperature can fall as much as 5°F (2.8°C) after this procedure.*

■ Remove all equipment from the bed. Dry the patient and make him comfortable. Supply a fresh hospital gown, if necessary. Cover him lightly.

■ Continue to monitor the patient's vital signs and condition regularly, as indicated by the patient's conditions.

■ Return the equipment to the central supply department for cleaning, disinfecting, servicing, and storage.

Completing the procedure

■ Perform hand hygiene.[4,5,6,7,8]

■ Clean and disinfect your stethoscope with a disinfectant pad.[12,13]

■ Perform hand hygiene.[4,5,6,7,8]

■ Document the procedure.[14,15,16]

Special considerations

■ If the patient shivers excessively during hypothermia treatment, discontinue the procedure and notify the practitioner immediately. *By increasing metabolism, shivering elevates body temperature and increases oxygen consumption.*

EQUIPMENT

Using a cooling system

A hypothermia or cooling blanket is used to lower a patient's body temperature. The pad contains coils that circulate a chilled solution. While the blanket is in use, you must monitor the patient's temperature. The blanket's temperature can be adjusted to help keep the patient's temperature in the ordered range.

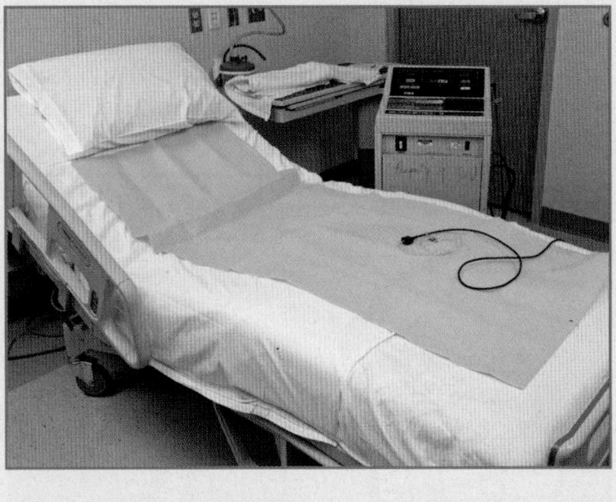

■ Avoid lowering the temperature more than 1°F (0.6°C) every 15 minutes *to prevent premature ventricular contractions.*

■ Don't use pins to secure catheters, tubes, or blanket covers *because an accidental puncture can result in fluid leakage and burns.*

■ With hyperthermia or hypothermia therapy, the patient may experience a secondary defense reaction (vasoconstriction or vasodilation, respectively) that causes body temperature to rebound, defeating the treatment's purpose.

■ If the patient requires isolation, place the blanket, blanket cover, and probe in a plastic bag clearly marked with the type of isolation *so that the central supply department can give it special handling.* If the blanket is disposable, discard it, using appropriate precautions.

■ *To avoid bacterial growth in the reservoir or blankets,* always use sterile, distilled water and change it monthly. Check to see if facility policy calls for adding a bacteriostatic agent to the water. Avoid using deionized water *because it may corrode the system.*

■ *To gradually increase body temperature, especially in postoperative patients,* the practitioner may order a disposable blanket warming system. (See *Using a warming system,* page 368.)

Complications

Use of a hyperthermia-hypothermia blanket can cause shivering, marked changes in vital signs, increased intracranial pressure, respiratory distress or arrest, cardiac arrest, oliguria, and anuria.

Documentation

Document the patient's vital signs, fluid intake and output, skin condition, and position changes. Record neurologic assessment findings. Also document the type of hyperthermia-hypothermia unit used; control settings (manual or automatic and temperature settings); date, time, duration, and patient's tolerance of treatment; and signs of complications. Document any patient teaching and the patient's understanding of your teaching.

EQUIPMENT

Using a warming system

Shivering, the compensatory response to falling body temperature, may use more oxygen than the body can supply—especially in a surgical patient. In the past, you would cover the patient with blankets to warm his body. Now, health care facilities may supply a warming system, such as the Bair Hugger patient-warming system.[17]

The Bair Hugger patient-warming system helps to gradually increase body temperature. Like a large hair dryer, the warming unit draws air through a filter, warms the air to the desired temperature, and circulates it through a hose to a warming blanket placed over the patient.

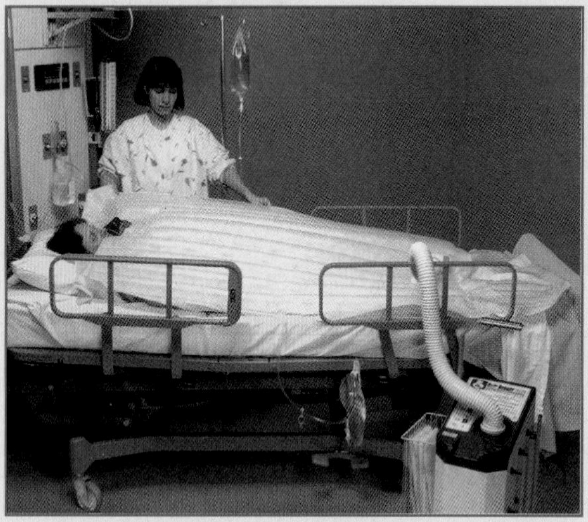

When using the warming system, be sure to take the following steps:

- Use a bath blanket in a single layer over the warming blanket *to minimize heat loss.*
- Place the warming blanket directly over the patient with the paper side facing down and the clear tubular side facing up.
- Make sure the connection hose is at the foot of the bed.
- Monitor the patient's temperature at regular intervals, according to the patient's condition, while the warming blanket is in use.
- Obtain guidelines from the patient's practitioner for discontinuing use of the warming blanket.

REFERENCES

1 Centers for Medicare & Medicaid Services, Department of Health and Human Services. (2014). Condition of participation: Patient's rights. 42 C.F.R. § 482.13(b)(2).

2 The Joint Commission. (2015). Standard RI.01.03.01. *Comprehensive accreditation manual for hospitals: The official handbook.* Oakbrook Terrace, IL: The Joint Commission. (Level VII)

3 American Osteopathic Association. (2014). Standard 15.01.11. *Healthcare Facilities Accreditation Program: Accreditation requirements for acute care hospitals.* Chicago, IL: American Osteopathic Association. (Level VII)

4 The Joint Commission. (2015). Standard NPSG 07.01.01. *Comprehensive accreditation manual for hospitals: The official handbook.* Oakbrook Terrace, IL: The Joint Commission. (Level VII)

5 Centers for Disease Control and Prevention. (2002). Guideline for hand hygiene in health-care settings: Recommendations of the Healthcare Infection Control Practices Advisory Committee and the HICPAC/SHEA/APIC/IDSA Hand Hygiene Task Force. *MMWR Recommendations and Reports, 51*(RR-16), 1–45. Accessed March 2015 via the Web at http://www.cdc.gov/mmwr/pdf/rr/rr5116.pdf (Level II)

6 World Health Organization. (2009). "WHO guidelines on hand hygiene in health care: First global patient safety challenge, clean care is safer care" [Online]. Accessed March 2015 via the Web at http://whqlibdoc.who.int/publications/2009/9789241597906_eng.pdf (Level IV)

7 American Osteopathic Association. (2014). Standard 07.01.21. *Healthcare Facilities Accreditation Program: Accreditation requirements for acute care hospitals.* Chicago, IL: American Osteopathic Association. (Level VII)

8 Centers for Medicare & Medicaid Services, Department of Health and Human Services. (2014). Condition of participation: Infection control. 42 C.F.R. § 482.42.

9 The Joint Commission. (2015). Standard NPSG.01.01.01. *Comprehensive accreditation manual for hospitals: The official handbook.* Oakbrook Terrace, IL: The Joint Commission. (Level VII)

10 Siegel, J. D., et al. (2007). "2007 guideline for isolation precautions: Preventing transmission of infectious agents in healthcare settings" [Online]. Accessed March 2015 via the Web at http://www.cdc.gov/hicpac/pdf/isolation/Isolation2007.pdf (Level II)

11 American Osteopathic Association. (2014). Standard 07.01.10. *Healthcare Facilities Accreditation Program: Accreditation requirements for acute care hospitals.* Chicago, IL: American Osteopathic Association. (Level VII)

12 Rutala, W. A., et al. (2008). "Guideline for disinfection and sterilization in healthcare facilities, 2008" [Online]. Accessed March 2015 via the Web at http://www.cdc.gov/hicpac/pdf/guidelines/Disinfection_Nov_2008.pdf (Level I)

13 American Osteopathic Association. (2014). Standard 07.02.03. *Healthcare Facilities Accreditation Program: Accreditation requirements for acute care hospitals.* Chicago, IL: American Osteopathic Association. (Level VII)

14 The Joint Commission. (2015). Standard RC 01.03.01. *Comprehensive accreditation manual for hospitals: The official handbook.* Oakbrook Terrace, IL: The Joint Commission. (Level VII)

15 Centers for Medicare & Medicaid Services, Department of Health and Human Services. (2014). Condition of participation: Medical record services. 42 C.F.R. § 482.24(b).

16 American Osteopathic Association. (2014). Standard 10.00.03. *Healthcare Facilities Accreditation Program: Accreditation requirements for acute care hospitals.* Chicago, IL: American Osteopathic Association. (Level VII)

17 3M. (n.d.). "3M infection prevention patient warming product brochure, warm every patient" [Online]. Accessed March 2015 via the Web at http://multimedia.3m.com/mws/mediawebserver?mwsId=66666UgxGCuNyXTt5XT_MxftEVtQEcuZgVs6EVs6E666666–&fn=B_8.1_Bair%2520Hugger%2520Product%2520Catalo

ADDITIONAL REFERENCE

Recommended practices for the prevention of unplanned perioperative hypothermia. (2014). In R. Conner, et al. (Eds.), *Perioperative standards and recommended practices 2014.* Denver, CO: AORN, Inc. (Level VII)

I

IM INJECTION

IM injections deposit medication deep into muscle tissue. This route of administration provides rapid systemic action and absorption of relatively large doses (up to 5 mL in appropriate sites).[1] IM injections are recommended for patients who can't take medication orally, when IV administration is inappropriate or inaccessible, and for drugs that are altered by digestive juices. Because muscle tissue has few sensory nerves, IM injections allow less painful administration of irritating drugs.

The site for an IM injection must be chosen carefully, taking into account the patient's general physical status and the purpose of the injection. IM injections shouldn't be administered at inflamed, edematous, or irritated sites or at sites that contain moles, birthmarks, scar tissue, or other lesions. IM injections may also be contraindicated in patients with

Selecting the appropriate syringe and needle

For an IM injection, the size of the syringe and the gauge and length of the needle are determined by several factors, including the amount and viscosity of the medication, the injection site chosen, and the patient's weight and amount of adipose tissue. Needles used for IM injections are longer than subcutaneous needles *because they must reach deep into the muscl.*

The volume of medication administered IM is usually 1 to 4 mL, so a 3- or 5-mL syringe is usually appropriate. The appropriate gauge of the needle is determined by the medication being administered. Biological agents and medications in aqueous solutions should be administered with a 20G to 25G needle. Medications in oil-based solutions should be administered with an 18G to 25G needle.

Needle length depends on the injection site, the patient's size, and the amount of subcutaneous fat covering the muscle. Patients who are obese may require a longer needle (1½" [3.8 cm] or longer)[3] and thin or emaciated patients may require a shorter needle (½" to 1" [1.25 cm to 2.5 cm]). When choosing the needle size and injection site, take into consideration muscle size, thickness of adipose tissue at the injection site, volume of the material to be administered, injection technique, and depth below the muscle surface into which you'll inject the medication:[4]

- Vastus lateralis: ½" to 1" (1.25 cm to 2.5 cm)
- Deltoid: ½" to 1½" (1.25 cm to 3.8 cm)
- Ventrogluteal: ½" to 1½" (1.25 cm to 3.8 cm)

impaired coagulation mechanisms, occlusive peripheral vascular disease, edema, and shock; after thrombolytic therapy; and during an acute myocardial infarction (MI) because these conditions impair peripheral absorption. IM injections require sterile technique to maintain the integrity of muscle tissue.

The Z-track method is preferred for administering IM injections. By leaving a zigzag path that seals the needle track, this technique prevents drug leakage into the subcutaneous tissue, helps seal the drug in the muscle, and minimizes irritation.[1]

Equipment

Patient's medication administration record ■ prescribed medication ■ single-use sterile syringe and needle of appropriate size and gauge (a self-sheathing needle is recommended)[2] ■ alcohol pads ■ gauze pads ■ Optional: gloves, 1" (2.5-cm) tape, ice, filter needle.

The prescribed medication must be sterile. The needle may be packaged separately or already attached to the syringe. (See *Selecting the appropriate syringe and needle.*)

Implementation

■ Avoid distractions and interruptions when preparing and administering medications *to prevent medication errors.*[5,6]

■ Verify the order in the patient's medication record by checking it against the practitioner's order.[7,8,9]

■ Choose equipment appropriate to the prescribed medication and injection site, and make sure it works properly. The needle should be straight, smooth, and free from burrs.

■ Compare the medication label with the order in the patient's medical record.[7,8,9]

■ Check the patient's medical record for an allergy or a contraindication to the prescribed medication. If an allergy or contraindications exist, don't administer the medication; instead, notify the practitioner.[7,8,9]

■ Check the expiration date on the medication. If the medication is expired, return it to the pharmacy and obtain new medication.[7,8,9]

■ Visually inspect the solution for particles, discoloration, or other loss of integrity; don't administer the medication if its integrity is compromised.[7,8,9] Remember that for some drugs (such as suspensions), the presence of drug particles is normal. If in doubt, check with the pharmacist and the manufacturer's instructions.

■ Discuss any unresolved concerns about the medication with the patient's practitioner.[7,8,9]

■ Perform hand hygiene.[10,11,12,13,14]

■ Carefully calculate the dose. If it's a high-alert medication that can cause significant patient harm when used in error, perform an independent double-check with another nurse if required by your facility.[15,16]

■ Read the medication label again as you draw up the medication for injection if needed. (See *Drawing up medication for injection,* page 370.)

■ Perform hand hygiene.[10,11,12,13,14]

■ Confirm the patient's identity using at least two patient identifiers.[18]

■ If the patient is receiving the medication for the first time, teach him about potential adverse reactions and discuss any other concerns related to the medication.[7,8,9]

■ Verify that the medication is being administered at the proper time, in the prescribed dose, and by the correct route *to reduce the risk of medication errors.*[7,8,9]

■ If your facility uses a bar code scanning system, scan your identification badge, the patient's identification bracelet, and the medication's bar code.

■ Provide privacy and explain the procedure to the patient.[19,20]

■ Put on gloves if contact with blood or body fluids is likely or if your skin or the patient's skin isn't intact; *gloves aren't required for routine IM injection because they don't protect against needle-stick injury.*[2,21]

■ Select an appropriate injection site. The ventrogluteal site is used most commonly for healthy adults, although the deltoid muscle may be used for a small-volume injection (2 mL or less). (See *Locating IM injection sites,* page 371.) Remember to always rotate injection sites for patients who require repeated injections.

NURSING ALERT *If using the ventrogluteal site, take care to correctly identify anatomic landmarks before administration.* Use of the dorsogluteal site isn't recommended because of the potential for nerve damage.[1,22,23]

■ Position and drape the patient appropriately using his bed linens, making sure the site is well exposed and that lighting is adequate (as shown below).

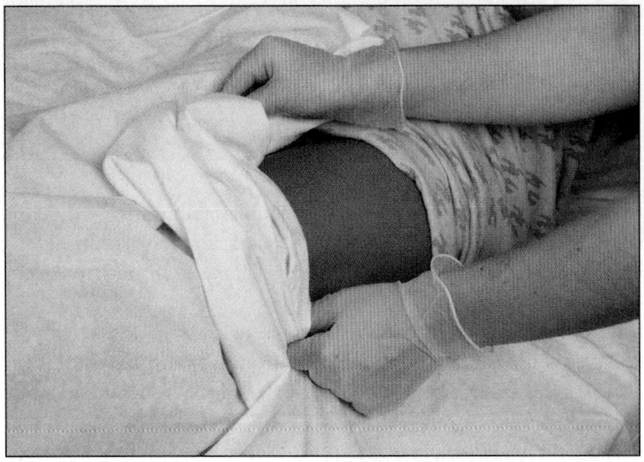

■ After selecting the injection site, clean the skin with an alcohol pad. Move the pad outward in a circular motion to a circumference of about 2" (5 cm) from the injection site and allow the skin to dry (as shown on next page, left middle).[21]

Drawing up medication for injection

Your technique for drawing up the medication will vary according to the type of container in which the medication is manufactured.

For single-dose ampules: Wrap an alcohol pad around the ampule's neck and snap off the top, directing the force away from your body. Attach a filter needle to the syringe and withdraw the medication, keeping the needle's bevel tip below the level of the solution. Tap the syringe *to clear air from it*. Cover the needle with the needle sheath. Before discarding the ampule, check the medication label against the patient's medication record.[7,8,9] Discard the filter needle and the ampule in the appropriate receptacle. Attach the appropriate needle to the syringe.

For single-dose or multidose vials: Whenever possible, use a single-dose vial instead of a multidose vial, especially when medications will be administered to multiple patients.[17] Reconstitute powdered drugs according to instructions. Make sure all crystals have dissolved in the solution. Warm the vial by rolling it between your palms *to help the drug dissolve faster.* Wipe the stopper of the medication vial with an alcohol pad, and then draw up the prescribed amount of medication. Read the medication label as you select the medication, as you draw it up, and after you have drawn it up *to verify the correct medication and dosage.*

Don't use an air bubble in the syringe. *Modern, disposable syringes are calibrated to give the correct dose without an air bubble.* Change the needle if it has become damaged or contaminated; cover the needle with the needle sheath.[2] Store all multidose vials according to the manufacturer's guidelines.

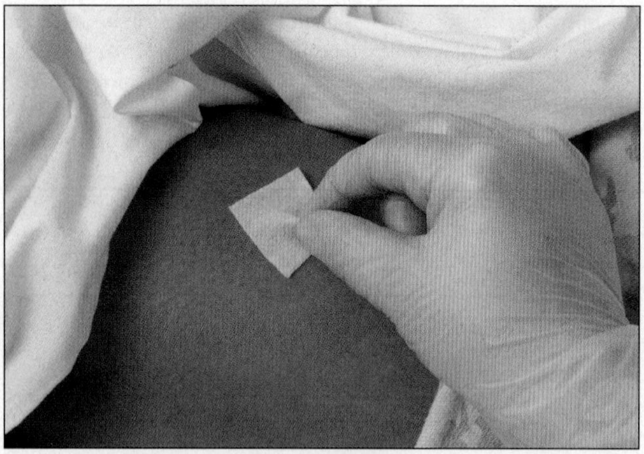

■ With the thumb and index finger of your nondominant hand, gently displace the skin and subcutaneous tissue of the injection site by pulling the skin laterally for the Z-track technique.[1] (See the "Z-track injection" procedure, page 842.)

■ Position the syringe at a 90-degree angle to the skin surface, with the needle a couple of inches (about 5 cm) from the skin. Tell the patient that he'll feel a prick as you insert the needle. Then quickly and smoothly insert the needle through the skin and subcutaneous tissue, deep into the muscle at a 90-degree angle.

■ Support the syringe with your nondominant hand if desired. Pull back slightly on the plunger with your dominant hand to aspirate for blood if appropriate. Aspiration of blood isn't recommended for administration of immunizations and vaccines.[4] If no blood appears, slowly inject the medication into the muscle. A slow, steady injection rate allows the muscle to distend gradually and accept the medication under minimal pressure. You should feel little or no resistance against the force of the injection.

NURSING ALERT *If blood appears in the syringe on aspiration, the needle is in a blood vessel. If this occurs, stop the injection, withdraw the needle, prepare another injection with new equipment, and inject another site. Don't inject the bloody solution.*

■ After the injection, wait 10 seconds to allow the medication to begin to diffuse into the surrounding muscle tissue; then withdraw the needle slowly at a 90-degree angle.[1,24,25] If present, activate the needle's safety mechanism *to prevent accidental needle-stick injury.*[2,26]

■ Release the displaced skin and subcutaneous tissue *to seal the needle track.*

■ Cover the injection site immediately with a gauze pad (as shown below), and apply gentle pressure.

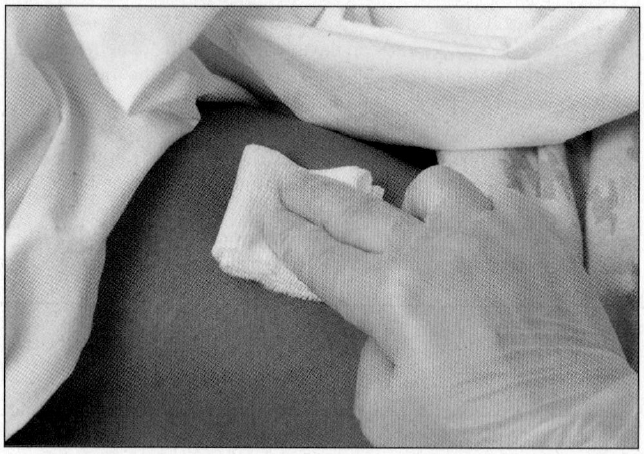

■ Remove the gauze pad, and inspect the injection site for signs of active bleeding or bruising. If bleeding continues, apply pressure to the site; if bruising occurs, you may apply ice.

■ Monitor for adverse reactions at the site for 10 to 30 minutes after the injection.[27]

ELDER ALERT *An elderly patient may bleed or ooze from the site after the injection* because of decreased tissue elasticity. *Applying a small pressure bandage may be helpful.*

■ Discard all equipment appropriately. Don't recap needles; dispose of them in an appropriate sharps container *to avoid needle-stick injuries.*[2,21]

■ Remove and discard your gloves if worn and perform hand hygiene.[10,11,12,13,14]

■ Document the procedure.[28,29,30]

Special considerations

■ *To slow their absorption,* some drugs for IM administration are dissolved in oil or other special solutions. Mix these preparations well before drawing them into the syringe.

■ Never inject into sensitive muscles, especially those that twitch or tremble when you assess site landmarks and tissue depth. *Injections into these trigger areas may cause sharp or referred pain, such as the pain caused by nerve trauma.*

■ Keep a rotation record that lists all available injection sites, divided into various body areas, for patients who require repeated injections. Rotate from a site in the first area to a site in each of the other areas. Then return to a site in the first area that's at least 1″ (2.5 cm) away from the previous injection site in that area.

■ If the patient has experienced pain or emotional trauma from repeated injections, consider numbing the area before cleaning it by holding ice on it for several seconds. If you must inject more than 4 mL of solution, divide the solution and inject it at two separate sites.

Locating IM injection sites

Deltoid

Have the patient sit or stand. Find the lower edge of the acromial process and the point on the lateral arm in line with the axilla. Insert the needle 1″ to 2″ (2.5 to 5 cm) below the acromial process, usually two or three fingerbreadths, at a 90-degree angle or angled slightly toward the process. Typical injection: 0.5 mL (range: 0.5 to 2.0 mL).[1]

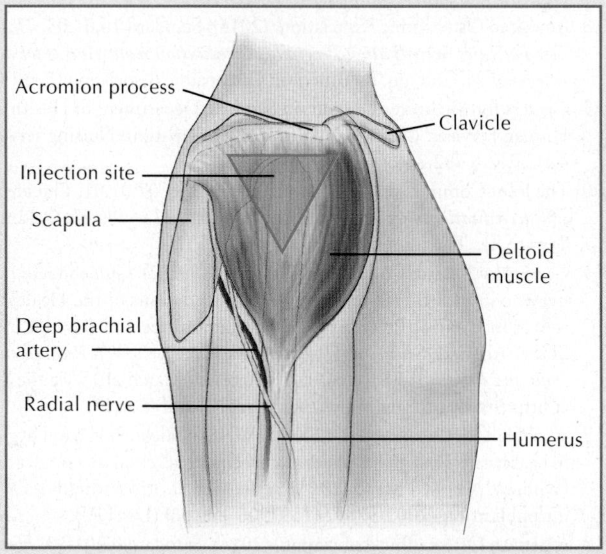

Ventrogluteal

Have the patient sit, stand, lie laterally, or lie supine. Locate the greater trochanter of the femur with the heel of your hand. Then spread your index and middle fingers from the anterior superior iliac spine to as far along the iliac crest as you can reach. Insert the needle between the two fingers at a 90-degree angle to the muscle. (Remove your fingers before inserting the needle.) Typical injection: 2.5 to 5 mL (range: 1 to 5 mL).[1]

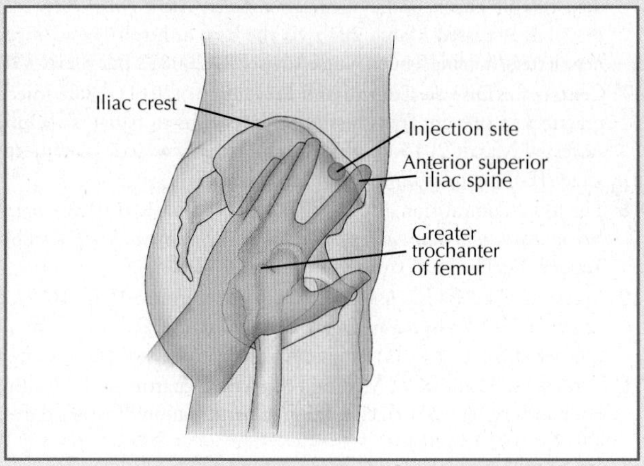

Vastus lateralis

Have the patient sit or lie supine. The knee may be slightly flexed and the foot may be externally rotated *to help relax the muscle.* Use the lateral muscle of the quadriceps group, from a handbreadth below the greater trochanter to a handbreadth above the knee. Insert the needle into the middle third of the muscle parallel to the surface on which the patient is lying. Typical injection: 5 mL (range: 1 to 5 mL).[1]

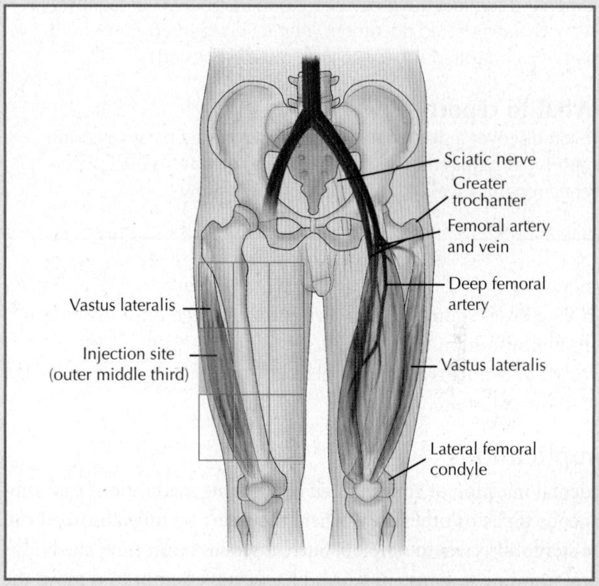

- Always encourage the patient to relax the muscle you'll be injecting *because injections into tense muscles are typically more painful and may bleed more readily.*
- IM injections can damage local muscle cells, causing elevations in serum enzyme levels (creatine kinase [CK]) that can be confused with elevations resulting from damage to cardiac muscle, as in MI. *To distinguish between skeletal and cardiac muscle damage,* diagnostic tests for suspected MI must identify the isoenzyme of CK specific to cardiac muscle (CK-MB) and include tests to determine lactate dehydrogenase and aspartate aminotransferase levels. If it's important to measure these enzyme levels, suggest that the practitioner switch to IV administration and adjust dosages accordingly.
- If the medication isn't going to be administered immediately, clearly label the medication syringe *to prevent a medication error.* An immediately administered medication is one that's prepared, taken directly to the patient, and administered without any break in the process.[31,32,33]

Documenting administration of controlled substances

Some facilities use a computerized system that confirms the opioid count for each drug as it's used or removed from the system via a secure identification code. This system eliminates the need for opioid counts during the day.

Before administering a controlled substance, regardless of the system being used, always verify the amount of drug in the container and sign out the medication as required by your facility. A second nurse should document your activity and observe you if part of a controlled substance dose must be wasted.

What to report

If you discover a discrepancy in the controlled substance count, report it as required by your facility. You'll need to file an occurrence report as well. An investigation will follow.

- Vaccine doses shouldn't be drawn into a syringe until immediately before administration.[4]
- Dosage adjustments are usually necessary when changing from the IM route to the oral route.

Complications

Accidental injection of concentrated or irritating medications into subcutaneous tissue or other areas where they can't be fully absorbed can cause sterile abscesses to develop. Such abscesses result from the body's natural immune response in which phagocytes attempt to remove the foreign matter.

Failure to rotate sites in patients who require repeated injections can lead to deposits of unabsorbed medications. Such deposits can reduce the desired pharmacologic effect and may lead to abscess formation or tissue fibrosis. Improper technique can also result in injury to bone, blood vessels, and peripheral nerves.[1]

ELDER ALERT Because elderly patients typically have decreased muscle mass, *IM medications can be absorbed more quickly than expected.*

Documentation

Document the drug administered, dose, date, time, route of administration, and injection site according to your facility's documentation format. Also, note the patient's tolerance of the injection and the injection's effects, including any adverse effects. (See *Documenting administration of controlled substances.*)

References

1 Hopkins, H., & Arias, C. Y. (2013). Large-volume IM injections: A review of best practices. *Oncology Nurse Advisor, 2013,* 32–37. Accessed March 2015 via the Web at http://media.oncologynurseadvisor.com/documents/44/ona_feature0213_injections_10767.pdf

2 Occupational Safety and Health Administration. (n.d.). "Bloodborne pathogens, standard number 1910.1030" [Online]. Accessed March 2015 via the Web at http://www.osha.gov/pls/oshaweb/owadisp.show_document?p_table=STANDARDS&p_id=10051 (Level VII)

3 Tanioka, T., et al. (2013) Optimal needle insertion length for intramuscular injection of risperidone long-acting injectable (RLAI). *Health, 5,* 1939–1945.

4 Centers for Disease Control and Prevention. (2011). General recommendations on immunization: Recommendations of the Advisory Committee on Immunization Practices (ACIP). *MMWR Recommendations and Reports, 60*(RR-02), 1–60. Accessed March 2015 via the Web at http://www.cdc.gov/mmwr/pdf/rr/rr6002.pdf (Level II)

5 Westbrook, J., et al. (2010). Association of interruptions with an increased risk and severity of medication administration errors. *Archives of Internal Medicine, 170,* 683–690. (Level IV)

6 Institute for Safe Medication Practices. (2013). Side tracks on the safety express: Interruptions lead to errors and unfinished . . . Wait, what was I doing? *Nurse Advise-ERR,* 11(2), 1–4. Accessed March 2015 via the Web at https://www.ismp.org/Newsletters/acutecare/showarticle.aspx?id=37 (Level VII)

7 The Joint Commission. (2015). Standard MM.06.01.01. *Comprehensive accreditation manual for hospitals: The official handbook.* Oakbrook Terrace, IL: The Joint Commission. (Level VII)

8 American Osteopathic Association. (2014). Standard 16.01.03. *Healthcare Facilities Accreditation Program: Accreditation requirements for acute care hospitals.* Chicago, IL: American Osteopathic Association (Level VII)

9 Centers for Medicare & Medicaid Services, Department of Health and Human Services. (2014). Condition of participation: Nursing services. 42 C.F.R. § 482.23(c).

10 The Joint Commission. (2015). Standard NPSG.07.01.01. *Comprehensive accreditation manual for hospitals: The official handbook.* Oakbrook Terrace, IL: The Joint Commission. (Level VII)

11 Centers for Disease Control and Prevention. (2002). Guideline for hand hygiene in health-care settings: Recommendations of the Healthcare Infection Control Practices Advisory Committee and the HICPAC/SHEA/APIC/IDSA Hand Hygiene Task Force. *MMWR Recommendations and Reports, 51*(RR-16), 1–45. Accessed March 2015 via the Web at http://www.cdc.gov/mmwr/pdf/rr/rr5116.pdf (Level II)

12 World Health Organization. (2009). "WHO guidelines on hand hygiene in health care: First global patient safety challenge, clean care is safer care" [Online]. Accessed March 2015 via the Web at http://whqlibdoc.who.int/publications/2009/9789241597906_eng.pdf (Level IV)

13 American Osteopathic Association. (2014). Standard 07.01.10. *Healthcare Facilities Accreditation Program: Accreditation requirements for acute care hospitals.* Chicago, IL: American Osteopathic Association (Level VII)

14 Centers for Medicare & Medicaid Services, Department of Health and Human Services. (2014). Condition of participation: Infection control. 42 C.F.R. § 482.42.

15 Institute for Safe Medication Practices. (2012). "ISMP's list of high-alert medications" [Online]. Accessed March 2015 via the Web at http://www.ismp.org/tools/highalertmedications.pdf (Level VII)

16 Institute for Safe Medication Practices. (2008). Conducting an independent double-check. *ISMP Medication Safety Alert! Nurse Advise-ERR, 6*(12), 1. Accessed March 2015 via the Web at http://www.ismp.org/newsletters/nursing/Issues/NurseAdviseERR200812.pdf (Level VII)

17 Centers for Disease Control and Prevention. (2011). "Safe injection practices to prevent transmission of infections to patients" [Online]. Accessed March 2015 via the Web at http://www.cdc.gov/injectionsafety/IP07_standardPrecaution.html (Level II)

18 The Joint Commission. (2015). Standard NPSG.01.01.01. *Comprehensive accreditation manual for hospitals: The official handbook.* Oakbrook Terrace, IL: The Joint Commission. (Level VII)

19 American Osteopathic Association. (2014). Standard 15.01.16. *Healthcare Facilities Accreditation Program: Accreditation requirements for acute care hospitals.* Chicago, IL: American Osteopathic Association (Level VII)

20 Centers for Medicare & Medicaid Services, Department of Health and Human Services. (2014). Condition of participation: Patient's rights. 42 C.F.R. § 482.13(c)(1).

21 World Health Organization. (2010). "WHO best practices for injections and related procedures toolkit" [Online]. Accessed March 2015 via the Web at http://whqlibdoc.who.int/publications/2010/9789241599252_eng.pdf (Level IV)

22 Mishra, P., & Stringer, M. D. (2010). Sciatic nerve injury from intramuscular injection: A persistent and global problem. *International Journal of Political Practice, 64,* 1573–1579. (Level V)

23 Cocoman, A., & Murray, J. (2010). Recognizing the evidence and changing practice on injection sites. *British Journal of Nursing, 19,* 1170–1174. (Level V)

24 Nicoll, L. H. & Hesby, A. (2002). Intramuscular injection: An integrative research review and guideline for evidence-based practice. *Applied Nursing Research, 15,* 149–162. (Level V)

25 Taylor, C., et al. (2011). *Fundamentals of nursing: The art and science of nursing care* (7th ed.). Philadelphia, PA: Lippincott Williams & Wilkins.

26 Occupational Safety and Health Administration. (n.d.). "Safety and health topics: Bloodborne pathogens and needlestick prevention" [Online]. Accessed March 2015 via the Web at http://www.osha.gov/SLTC/bloodbornepathogens (Level VII)

27 The Joint Commission. (2015). Standard MM.07.01.03. *Comprehensive accreditation manual for hospitals: The official handbook.* Oakbrook Terrace, IL: The Joint Commission. (Level VII)

28 The Joint Commission. (2015). Standard RC.01.03.01. *Comprehensive accreditation manual for hospitals: The official handbook.* Oakbrook Terrace, IL: The Joint Commission. (Level VII)

29 American Osteopathic Association. (2014). Standard 10.00.03. *Healthcare Facilities Accreditation Program: Accreditation requirements for acute care hospitals.* Chicago, IL: American Osteopathic Association (Level VII)

30 Centers for Medicare & Medicaid Services, Department of Health and Human Services. (2014). Condition of participation: Medical record services. 42 C.F.R. § 482.24(b).

31 The Joint Commission. (2015). Standard MM.05.01.09. *Comprehensive accreditation manual for hospitals: The official handbook.* Oakbrook Terrace, IL: The Joint Commission. (Level VII)

32 American Osteopathic Association. (2014). Standard 25.01.18. *Healthcare Facilities Accreditation Program: Accreditation requirements for acute care hospitals.* Chicago, IL: American Osteopathic Association. (Level VII)

33 The Joint Commission. (2015). Standard NPSG.03.04.01. *Comprehensive accreditation manual for hospitals: The official handbook.* Oakbrook Terrace, IL: The Joint Commission. (Level VII)

ADDITIONAL REFERENCES

Craven, R. F., & Hirnle, C. J. (2012). *Fundamentals of nursing: Human health and function* (7th ed.). Philadelphia, PA: Lippincott Williams & Wilkins.

Davidson, K. M., & Rourke, L. (2013). Teaching best evidence: Deltoid intramuscular injection technique. *Journal of Nursing Education and Practice, 3*(7), 120–128. Accessed March 2015 via the Web at http://www.sciedu.ca/journal/index.php/jnep/article/viewFile/1888/1291

Nettina, S. M. (2014). *Lippincott manual of nursing practice* (10th ed.). Philadelphia, PA: Wolters Kluwer.

IMPAIRED SWALLOWING AND ASPIRATION PRECAUTIONS

Patients may experience impaired swallowing as a result of several specific problems. The first of these—oropharyngeal dysphagia—is impaired swallowing associated with deficits in oral and pharyngeal structure or function. These patients are at especially high risk for aspiration, and many of them have silent aspiration (aspiration without visible signs of swallowing difficulty such as coughing or gagging before, during, or after swallowing).[1,2] Patients at risk for oropharyngeal dysphagia include those with nervous system damage, such as stroke, head injury, or spinal cord injury; neuromuscular diseases, such as muscular dystrophy or cerebral palsy; progressive neurologic diseases, such as Parkinson's disease, multiple sclerosis, amyotrophic lateral sclerosis, and dementia; facial, oral, or neck surgery or trauma; or head and neck cancer as well as those who have been intubated for longer than 3 days.

The second impaired swallowing problem is associated with esophageal dysphagia and aspiration due to gastroesophageal reflux disease, esophageal dysmotility or structural abnormality, delayed gastric emptying, or nasogastric intubation.

Finally, impaired swallowing can be associated with tracheostomies or ventilation support that results in decreased sensation of the oral and pharyngeal cavities, decreased sensation of food or fluids penetrating the laryngeal vestibule and aspirating (dropping below the level of the vocal cords), decreased ability to cough aspirated material off the vocal cords, and decreased laryngeal elevation and airway closure.

Equipment

Meal tray ▪ call light ▪ wall suction or portable suction apparatus ▪ suction kit ▪ gloves ▪ oral care supplies ▪ protective eyewear ▪ pulse oximeter ▪ scale ▪ Optional: denture care supplies, irrigation tray with 60-mL syringe, pH test strips, adaptive feeding devices, tape measure.

Implementation

- Gather the appropriate equipment.
- Perform hand hygiene.[3,4,5,6,7]
- Confirm the patient's identity using at least two patient identifiers.[8]
- Explain the procedure to the patient and his family.
- Maintain the head of the bed at 30 to 60 degrees unless contraindicated by the patient's conditions.[9]
- Put on gloves and protective eyewear, if indicated, before suctioning the patient or providing oral care.[10]
- Request a referral for and assist with a bedside swallow evaluation (usually conducted by a speech-language pathologist), as indicated.[2,9,11] *A swallowing evaluation can determine if the patient is at risk for aspiration.*

Managing impaired swallowing due to oropharyngeal dysphagia

- After the swallowing evaluation is completed, develop a multidisciplinary management plan that includes common swallowing strategies and takes into consideration the patient's nutritional status and required supervision.[2,12]

Using common swallowing strategies

- Have suction equipment available at the bedside.
- Verify the patient's diet modifications, as ordered.[12]
- Position the patient at a 90-degree angle during meals *to decrease the risk of aspiration.*[13]
- Implement additional strategies of body positioning and posture, as recommended, *to alter the speed and flow direction of a food or liquid bolus,* commonly with the intent of protecting the airway *to facilitate a safe swallow.*[12,13,14]
- Have the patient to sit up for 30 minutes, as recommended, after meals.[14]
- Assist with or perform oral care before and after meals, and check for food residue.[13]
- If applicable, ensure that dentures are in place, free from debris, and fit well.
- Make sure the patient uses any recommended adaptive devices and provide assistance, as needed.[12]
- Crush medications, as appropriate, and mix in applesauce, if appropriate.
- Avoid mixed consistencies.
- If applicable, ensure that the temperature, consistency, and amount of foods and liquids are appropriate.[2] Chill water; avoid tepid liquids or food.
- Minimize distractions when the patient is eating and drinking.[13]
- Encourage small sips with liquids and slow intake with adequate chewing.
- If one side of the patient's face is paralyzed, place food on the unaffected side. Check the affected side of the mouth for food that may lodge in the cheek during and after meals. If appropriate, teach the patient to perform a finger-sweep.
- Employ swallowing maneuvers, as recommended, *to improve the safety or efficiency of swallow function.*[12,14]
- If fatigue impairs swallowing, provide rest periods before and during meals as needed.[13]

■ Assess swallowing between bites by feeling the rise and fall of the larynx (Adam's apple).
■ Be alert for patient feedback during meals and modify the presentation and pace of feeding, as needed.[12,13]
■ Avoid medications that dry up secretions, *which may make swallowing more difficult for the patient.*[13]
■ Post swallowing precautions and feeding instructions in the patient's room.

Monitoring nutritional status
■ Ask the dietitian to conduct a nutrition evaluation.
■ Monitor the patient's hydration and nutrition. *Poor compliance with modified diets may lead to reduced food and fluid intake and an increased risk of malnutrition and dehydration.*[12]
■ Implement calorie counts as ordered.
■ Weigh the patient daily or as ordered.
■ Consult with the patient and family regarding food and fluid preferences.
■ Provide small, frequent meals and supplements.
■ Praise the patient and family for achieving nutritional goals.

Using one-on-one supervision
■ Ensure that someone remains with the patient throughout every meal.
■ Provide feeding assistance or cueing for feeding and swallowing strategies during the entire meal, or ensure that a family member does so.[2,12]
■ Encourage the patient to take 30 to 45 minutes to eat. *(Patients with dysphagia typically need to eat slowly.)*
■ Monitor the patient for signs of aspiration, such as coughing or gagging.

Using close supervision
■ Check on the patient frequently during the meal; spend 3 to 5 minutes each time by recueing and reminding the patient to use swallowing strategies.[2]
■ Monitor the patient for signs of aspiration, such as coughing or gagging.
■ Encourage the patient to increase intake, if needed, and provide other options *to maximize safety and nutritional intake.*
■ Keep the call light within reach.

Using distant supervision
■ Provide initial cueing *to initiate swallowing strategies.*[2]
■ Check on the patient by walking past his room frequently.
■ Monitor the patient for signs of aspiration, such as coughing or gagging.
■ Assess the patient's progress at least two to three times during meals.
■ Keep the call light within reach.

Completing the procedure
■ Remove and discard gloves and protective eyewear if used.[10]
■ Perform hand hygiene.[3,4,5,6,7]
■ Document the procedure.[15,16,17]

Managing impaired swallowing due to esophageal dysphagia
■ Monitor for reflux and aspiration risks related to esophageal dysphagia.
■ Consult with a speech-language pathologist and registered dietitian *to determine the need for alternative nutrition.*
■ Monitor respiratory rate and depth; monitor breath sounds for crackles or wheezes, *which may indicate aspiration and airway obstruction.* Monitor for dyspnea and cyanosis.
■ Monitor bowel sounds and assess for abdominal distention. *Absence of bowel sounds and increasing abdominal distention may indicate an ileus or bowel obstruction with resulting vomiting and risk for aspiration.*
■ Monitor the patient's intake and output and daily weight. *Weight loss may indicate an esophageal problem.*
■ Implement strategies for oral intake.
■ Position the patient at a 90-degree angle during oral feeding and maintain the position for 2 hours after the meal *to decrease the risk of reflux, regurgitation, and aspiration.*[14]
■ Offer thickened liquids and pureed and moist foods that may be easier to swallow if esophageal dysmotility exists.[2]
■ Feed the patient slowly; allow adequate time for esophageal emptying.
■ If the patient feels full quickly, offer small, frequent meals of high-calorie foods.
■ Alternate liquids and solids during feedings *to improve esophageal emptying of solids.*
■ Avoid spicy and acidic foods, and decrease caffeine intake *to decrease reflux.*
■ Tell the patient to avoid eating before bed, and keep the head of his bed elevated at a 30- to 40-degree angle at night, unless contraindicated.[9]
■ Remove and discard gloves and protective eyewear if used.[10]
■ Perform hand hygiene.[3,4,5,6,7]
■ Document the procedure.[15,16,17]

Managing a patient with a feeding tube
■ Initiate a dietary consult.
■ Provide oral care for the patient who is on nothing-by-mouth status *to decrease colonization of bacteria in the mouth because he is at risk for secretion aspiration.*
■ After feeding tube insertion, confirm tube placement by X-ray. *X-ray confirmation of placement, especially of small-bore feeding tubes, is the gold standard for safe placement.*[18]
■ Trace the tubing from the patient to its point of origin before administering the feeding through the feeding tube *to make sure the feeding is administered through the proper port.*[19]
■ Assess placement of the feeding tube before feeding and every 4 hours for a patient with a continuous feeding using the following methods, as appropriate: Measure the external portion of the catheter *to detect a change in the external length, indicating tube migration.* Aspirate contents from the tube and observe for changes in volume, appearance, and color. If pH test strips are available, test the pH of the aspirate; *fasting gastric pH is usually 5 or less.* Review routine chest and abdominal X-rays *for placement.* If tube placement is in doubt, obtain an X-ray *to confirm placement,* as ordered.[9,18,20]
■ If the assessment indicates the possibility of feeding solution in mucus coughed or suctioned from the trachea, test the mucus for glucose. *A positive result may indicate tube displacement and aspiration of feeding solution.*
■ Monitor the patient receiving feedings through a gastric tube for tolerance of feedings by assessing for abdominal distention; noting complaints of abdominal pain, nausea, and vomiting; observing for passage of flatus and stool; and monitoring gastric residual volumes.[9,13] If vomiting is present, stop the feeding and notify the practitioner.
■ Check gastric residuals every 4 hours during the first 48 hours of gastric feedings; after the enteral feeding goal rate is achieved, monitor residual volume every 6 to 8 hours in patients who aren't critically ill. For critically ill patients, monitor gastric residual volume every 4 hours.[9] Return residual to the stomach. Flush the feeding tube with 30 mL of water after measuring residual volume.
■ If residual volume is 250 mL or more, after a second residual check, a medication to improve gastric motility may be needed.[13] Hold the feedings for a residual volume greater than 500 mL (or as required by your facility) and assesses GI status.[21]
■ Maintain the patient in the semi-Fowler position (30 to 45 degrees) during feedings and for 30 to 45 minutes after each feeding *to promote movement of feeding solution through the stomach and into the small intestine, decreasing the risk of regurgitation and aspiration.*[9,13]
■ Remove and discard gloves and protective eyewear if used.[10]

- Perform hand hygiene.[3,4,5,6,7]
- Document the procedure.[15,16,17]

Managing impaired swallowing due to tracheostomies or endotracheal tubes

- Maintain the head of the bed at an angle of 30 to 45 degrees, unless contraindicated.[9,13]
- Use sedatives as sparingly as feasible *because sedation causes reduced cough and gag reflexes, may interfere with the patient's ability to handle secretions and refluxed gastric contents, and may slow gastric emptying.*[9,13]
- Maintain tracheal cuff pressures, as indicated. Suction secretions from above the cuff before deflating the cuff *to prevent aspiration of secretions and subsequent health care–associated pneumonia.*[9]
- Suction the patient as needed *to maintain a patent airway.*
- Obtain a practitioner's order for speaking valve trials, as appropriate.
- Discard used supplies in the appropriate receptacles.[10]

Managing impaired swallowing due to speaking valve trials

- Have the speech-language pathologist assess the patient's tolerance for the speaking valve. *The speaking valve permits hands-free speech and can return oropharyngeal sensation and taste.*
- Deflate the cuff before placing the valve. Monitor oxygen saturation at baseline, with the valve in place, and with valve removal.
- Follow speaking valve recommendations for cleaning and wearing schedules.
- Ensure the speaking valve is in place during meals (according to the speech-language pathologist's recommendations) *because it's usually safer to eat with the valve in place. The patient's ability to cough material off the vocal cords is increased.*

Completing the procedure

- Remove and discard gloves and protective eyewear if used.[10]
- Perform hand hygiene.[3,4,5,6,7]
- Document the procedure.[15,16,17]

Special considerations

- Patients with ischemic or hemorrhagic stroke should undergo dysphagia screening with an evidence-based, facility-approved bedside testing protocol before being given food, fluids, or medication by mouth.[22]
- Monitor the patient for signs and symptoms of swallowing problems and aspiration. These include coughing before, during, or after eating; wet or "gurgling" voice; increased chest congestion after eating; multiple swallows on one mouthful or washing down food with liquids; complaints of food getting "stuck" or painful swallowing; unexplained changes in the amount or rate of eating; drooling or spitting food out of the mouth; difficulty breathing during meals; weight loss and poor oral intake; recurrent pneumonias; low-grade temperatures shortly after meals; increased white blood cell counts; and leakage from the tracheostomy site. Currently, videofluoroscopic and videoendoscopic evaluations are the most accurate methods for diagnosing aspiration.[4]
- Small-bowel feedings are recommended when patients are intolerant of gastric feedings or have documented aspiration.[9]
- Angiotensin-converting enzyme inhibitors may improve the swallowing reflex in older patients with aspiration pneumonia.

Patient teaching

A patient with dysphagia may need to learn exercises to improve oral control or the overall strength, coordination, and initiation of oropharyngeal swallowing; how to use adaptive feeding devices; and overall strategies to reduce the risk of aspiration.

Train and supervise the family to feed the patient as needed. Teach family members how to perform the abdominal thrust and how to use suction equipment as needed.

Complications

Patients with impaired swallowing are more prone to airway obstruction and aspiration during meals. Aspiration may result in pneumonitis or pneumonia. Difficulty swallowing may result in decreased oral intake and eventually lead to dehydration and malnutrition.

Documentation

Record the amount of intake, daily weight measurements, the patient's food preferences, progress with meals, and any techniques effective in helping the swallowing process. Document patient tolerance to tube feedings, volume of gastric residual volume, and pH values, as indicated. Document the effectiveness of patient and family teaching, complications that arose, and interventions taken to remedy the problem. Document any aspiration precautions taken.

REFERENCES

1 Eisenstadt, E. S. (2010). Dysphagia and aspiration pneumonia in older adults. *Journal of the American Academy of Nurse Practitioners, 22,* 17–22. (Level V)

2 Smith Hammond, C. A., & Goldstein, L. B. (2006). Cough and aspiration of food and liquids due to oral-pharyngeal dysphagia: ACCP evidence-based clinical practice guidelines. *Chest, 129,* 154S–168S. Accessed March 2015 via the Web at http://journal.publications.chestnet.org/data/Journals/CHEST/22039/154S.pdf (Level I)

3 The Joint Commission. (2015). Standard NPSG.07.01.01. *Comprehensive accreditation manual for hospitals: The official handbook.* Oakbrook Terrace, IL: The Joint Commission. (Level VII)

4 Centers for Disease Control and Prevention. (2002). Guideline for hand hygiene in health-care settings: Recommendations of the Healthcare Infection Control Practices Advisory Committee and the HICPAC/SHEA/APIC/IDSA Hand Hygiene Task Force. *MMWR Recommendations and Reports, 51*(RR-16), 1–45. Accessed March 2015 via the Web at http://www.cdc.gov/mmwr/pdf/rr/rr5116.pdf (Level II)

5 World Health Organization. (2009). "WHO guidelines on hand hygiene in health care: First global patient safety challenge, clean care is safer care" [Online]. Accessed March 2015 via the Web at http://whqlibdoc.who.int/publications/2009/9789241597906_eng.pdf (Level IV)

6 American Osteopathic Association. (2014). Standard 07.01.21. *Healthcare Facilities Accreditation Program: Accreditation requirements for acute care hospitals.* Chicago, IL: American Osteopathic Association. (Level VII)

7 Centers for Medicare & Medicaid Services, Department of Health and Human Services. (2014). Condition of participation: Infection control. 42 C.F.R. § 482.42.

8 The Joint Commission. (2015). Standard NPSG.01.01.01. *Comprehensive accreditation manual for hospitals: The official handbook.* Oakbrook Terrace, IL: The Joint Commission. (Level VII)

9 American Association of Critical-Care Nurses. (2011). "AACN practice alert: Prevention of aspiration" [Online]. Accessed March 2015 via the Web at http://www.aacn.org/WD/practice/docs/practicealerts/aacn-aspiration-practice-alert.pdf (Level VII)

10 Siegel, J. D., et al. (2007). "2007 guideline for isolation and precautions: Preventing transmission of infectious agents in healthcare settings" [Online]. Accessed March 2015 via the Web at http://www.cdc.gov/hicpac/pdf/isolation/Isolation2007.pdf (Level II)

11 Scottish Intercollegiate Guidelines Network. (2010). *Management of patients with stroke: Identification and management of dysphagia—A national clinical guideline.* Edinburgh, UK: Scottish Intercollegiate Guidelines Network. (Level VII)

12 Sura, L., et al. (2012). Dysphagia in the elderly: Management and nutritional considerations. *Clinical Interventions in Aging, 2012,* 287–298. Accessed March 2015 via the Web at http://www.ncbi.nlm.nih.gov/pmc/articles/PMC3426263/

13 Metheny, N. A. (2012). "Preventing aspiration in older adults with dysphagia" [Online]. Accessed March 2015 via the Web at http://consultgerirn.org/uploads/File/trythis/try_this_20.pdf

14 Hitoshi, K., et al. (2011). Body positions and functional training to reduce aspiration in patients with dysphagia. *Japan Medical Association Journal, 54,* 35–38. Accessed March 2015 via the Web at http://www.med.or.jp/english/journal/pdf/2011_01/035_038.pdf

15 The Joint Commission. (2015). Standard RC.01.03.01. *Comprehensive accreditation manual for hospitals: The official handbook.* Oakbrook Terrace, IL: The Joint Commission. (Level VII)

16 Centers for Medicare & Medicaid Services, Department of Health and Human Services. (2014). Condition of participation: Medical record services. 42 C.F.R. § 482.24(b).

17 American Osteopathic Association. (2014). Standard 10.00.03. *Healthcare Facilities Accreditation Program: Accreditation requirements for acute care hospitals.* Chicago, IL: American Osteopathic Association. (Level VII)

18 American Association of Critical-Care Nurses. (2009). "AACN practice alerts: Verification of feeding tube placement" [Online]. Accessed March 2015 via the Web at http://www.aacn.org/WD/Practice/Docs/PracticeAlerts/Verification_of_Feeding_Tube_Placement_05-2005.pdf (Level VII)

19 U.S. Food and Drug Administration. (n.d.). "Look. Check. Connect. Safe medical device connections save lives" [Online]. Accessed March 2015 via the Web at http://www.fda.gov/downloads/MedicalDevices/Safety/AlertsandNotices/UCM134873.pdf

20 Simons, S. R., et al. (2012). Bedside assessment of enteral tube placement: Aligning practice with evidence. *American Journal of Nursing, 112*(2), 40–46. (Level V)

21 Bankhead, R., et al. (2009). ASPEN enteral nutrition practice recommendations. *Journal of Parenteral and Enteral Nutrition, 33,* 122–167. Accessed March 2015 via the Web at http://www.ismp.org/tools/articles/ASPEN.pdf (Level VII)

22 The Joint Commission. (2008). "Disease-specific care certification program: Stroke performance measurement implementation guide (2nd ed.)" [Online]. Accessed March 2015 via the Web at http://www.jointcommission.org/assets/1/18/stroke_pm_implementation_guide_ver_2a.pdf

Additional references

Gomes, C. A., Jr, et al. (2012). Percutaneous endoscopic gastrostomy versus nasogastric tube feeding for adults with swallowing disturbances. *Cochrane Database of Systematic Reviews, 2012*(3), CD008096.

Shem, K. L., et al. (2012). Diagnostic accuracy of bedside swallow evaluation versus videofluoroscopy to assess dysphagia in individuals with tetraplegia. *PM&R: The Journal of Injury, Function and Rehabilitation, 4,* 283–289.

Implanted port use

Surgically implanted by a surgeon or interventional radiologist using local anesthesia, an implanted port, also known as a *vascular access device* or a *vascular access port,* is a type of central venous access device. It consists of a Silastic® or polyurethane catheter attached to a reservoir, which is covered with a self-sealing silicone septum. The practitioner places the catheter in the central venous system and typically implants the reservoir in a subcutaneous pocket in the upper arm, abdomen, side, or back.

Use of an implanted port is most common when some type of long-term IV therapy is required and an external central venous device isn't appropriate or desirable. Depending on patient needs, the type of port selected may have one or two lumens. A port can be used immediately after placement, although some edema and tenderness may persist for about 72 hours, making the device initially difficult to palpate and slightly uncomfortable for the patient. (See *Understanding implanted ports.*)

For a patient who requires repeated computerized axial tomography scans with contrast, the practitioner may implant a port specially developed to withstand the high pressures of power injectors. Use of a power injector requires a specialized access needle and tubing approved for power injection to ensure that the tubing and connections won't rupture or separate.[1]

Equipment

Assisting with insertion

Noncoring needles of appropriate type and gauge ▪ implanted port and guide wire ▪ sterile gloves ▪ sterile gown ▪ mask ▪ cap ▪ sterile drapes ▪ antiseptic pads (chlorhexidine-based, alcohol, or tincture of iodine) ▪ chlorhexidine sponges ▪ local anesthetic (lidocaine without epinephrine) ▪ prefilled syringes of heparin flush solution ▪ prefilled syringes of preservative-free normal saline flush solution ▪ sterile dressings (gauze or transparent semipermeable membrane) ▪ needleless connector ▪ skin closure devices: suture material, surgical glue, or adhesive skin closures ▪ insertion checklist ▪ Optional: prescribed IV solution, other surgical equipment, prescribed prophylactic antibiotics, extension tubing.

Accessing a top-entry port

Gloves ▪ mask ▪ sterile gloves ▪ sterile drape ▪ noncoring needle with extension set tubing ▪ antiseptic swabs (chlorhexidine is preferred) ▪ 10-mL syringes prefilled with preservative-free normal saline solution ▪ sterile transparent semipermeable dressing ▪ sterile needleless connector ▪ catheter securement device, sterile tape, or sterile adhesive strips ▪ Optional: antiseptic soap, water, local anesthetic, ice pack, syringe prefilled with heparinized saline flush solution (100 units/mL or 10 units/mL, as prescribed), ordered IV fluid, IV administration set, sterile 2″ × 2″ (5-cm × 5-cm) gauze dressing, chlorhexidine-impregnated sponge dressing.

Some facilities use an implantable port access kit.

Obtaining a blood sample

Gloves ▪ antiseptic pads (alcohol, tincture of iodine, or chlorhexidine-based) ▪ 10-mL syringes prefilled with preservative-free normal saline solution ▪ blood collection tubes ▪ laboratory request forms and labels ▪ laboratory biohazard transport bag ▪ Optional: protective eyewear or mask with face shield, sterile injection cap, 10-mL syringe prefilled with locking solution (such as heparin lock).

For needleless blood collection tube holder method

Needleless blood collection tube holder with needleless adapter.

For syringe method

Blood transfer device ▪ sterile 10-mL syringe for discard blood.

Administering a bolus injection

Patient's medication administration record ▪ prescribed medication in a syringe ▪ gloves ▪ watch with second hand ▪ 10-mL syringes filled with preservative-free normal saline solution ▪ antiseptic pads (alcohol, tincture of iodine, or chlorhexidine-based) ▪ Optional: port access equipment, bar code scanner, 10-mL syringe, sterile needleless connector, 5-micron filter needle, appropriate diluent as indicated, 10-mL syringe prefilled with locking solution (such as heparin lock, 100 unit/mL).

Administering a continuous infusion

Prescribed IV solution ▪ IV administration set ▪ gloves ▪ antiseptic pads (alcohol, tincture of iodine, or chlorhexidine-based) ▪ 10-mL syringe prefilled with preservative-free normal saline solution ▪ Optional: infusion pump, filter.

Preparation of equipment

Assisting with insertion

Confirm with the practitioner the size and type of the device and the insertion site. Attach the tubing to the solution container and prime the tubing with the prescribed solution. Prime the noncoring needle with the extension set. Use strict sterile technique for all priming, and ensure all tubing is free of air.[2] After you've primed the tubing, recheck all connections for tightness. Make sure that sealed caps cover all open end.

Administering a bolus injection

If needed, access the port using the appropriate noncoring needle. Review the medication monograph so that you know the actions, adverse effects, and administration rate of the medication you'll be injecting.[29,30]

If needed, draw up the prescribed medication in the syringe and dilute it, if necessary. Whenever possible, administer pharmacy-prepared or commercially available products. Many medications come in unit-dose syringes.

Administering a continuous infusion

Review the patient's medical record *to determine the location of the implanted port and whether it's currently accessed with a noncoring needle.* If needed, access the port using the appropriate noncoring needle.

Implementation

Assisting with insertion

- Conduct a preprocedure verification *to make sure that all relevant documentation, related information, and equipment are available and correctly identified to the patient's identifiers.*[4]
- Check the patient's history for hypersensitivity to local anesthetics or chlorhexidine.
- Make sure the practitioner has obtained informed consent and that the consent is in the patient's medical record.[5,6,7,8]
- Use an insertion checklist to adhere to infection prevention and safety practices during insertion.[2,9,10,11] Stop the procedure immediately if you observe any breaks in sterile technique.[9]
- Perform hand hygiene *to prevent spreading microorganisms.*[2,10,11,12,13,14,15,16,17]
- Confirm the patient's identity using at least two patient identifiers.[18]
- Reinforce to the patient the practitioner's explanation of the procedure, its benefit and risks, and what's expected of the patient during and after implantation.
- Answer questions about movement restrictions, cosmetic concerns, and management regimens *to allay the patient's fears.*
- Administer an antibiotic, as prescribed, following safe medication administration practices. *To reduce the risk of vascular catheter–related infections in patients who are immunocompromised,* routine use isn't recommended.[19,20]
- Put on the mask, cap, sterile gloves, and sterile gown.[2,9,11,21,22]
- The practitioner, who will surgically implant the port, will most likely use a local anesthetic. Occasionally, however, he may use a general anesthetic.
- Prepare the insertion site using chlorhexidine-based antiseptic sponges and allow it to dry.[2,9,10]

Before beginning the procedure, the practitioner will drape the patient from head to toe *to comply with maximal barrier precautions.*[2,9,10,11] When the practitioner begins the procedure, you may be responsible for handing equipment and supplies to him.

- Conduct a time-out immediately before starting the procedure *to determine that the correct patient, site, positioning, and procedure are identified, and to confirm, as applicable, that relevant information and necessary equipment are available.*[23]
- The practitioner makes a small incision and introduces the guide wire and catheter, which he'll typically advance into the subclavian vein, terminating in the superior vena cava. After fluoroscopy verifies correct placement of the catheter tip, the practitioner creates a subcutaneous pocket over a bony prominence in the chest wall. He then tunnels the catheter to the pocket. Next, he connects the catheter to the reservoir, places the reservoir in the pocket, and flushes it with heparin flush solution. Lastly, he sutures the reservoir to the underlying fascia and closes the incision with the preferred skin closure device.
- Access the implanted port with a noncoring needle and attach the primed extension set and needleless injection cap, as ordered. (See "Accessing a top-entry port.")

EQUIPMENT

Understanding implanted ports

Typically, an implanted port is used to deliver intermittent infusions of medication, parenteral nutrition, chemotherapy, and blood products.[2,3] The patient's skin covers the device completely, *reducing the risk of extrinsic contamination.* Patients may prefer this type of central line *because it doesn't alter body image, requires less routine catheter care, only minimally restricts patient activity, and carries a decreased risk of infection compared with other central venous access devices.* The implanted port consists of a catheter connected to a small reservoir. A septum designed to withstand multiple punctures seals the reservoir. To access the port, a special noncoring needle is inserted perpendicular to the reservoir.

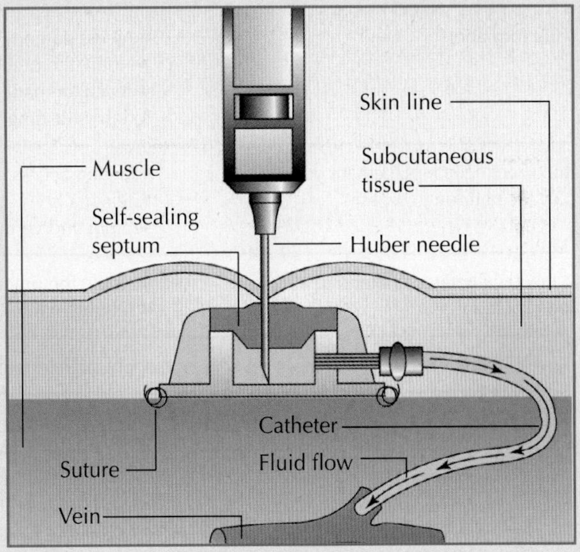

- Apply a sterile occlusive dressing.[1,24]
- Dispose of used equipment and discard of waste in the appropriate receptacle.[21]
- Remove and discard your personal protective equipment[21] and perform hand hygiene.[2,10,12,13,14,15,17]
- Document the procedure.[25,26,27,28]

Accessing a top-entry port

- Review the patient's medical record *to determine the type (such as a power-injectable device) and location of the implanted port, whether it has been previously accessed, and the patient's response to the procedure.*
- Ensure that placement of the catheter tip has been confirmed.
- Verify the practitioner's order for the size and length of the noncoring needle to use.
- Determine whether the patient has a history of allergies or contraindications to the antiseptic, anesthetic, or prescribed solution.
- Gather the necessary supplies.
- Perform hand hygiene.[2,10,11,12,13,14,15,16,17]
- Confirm the patient's identity using at least two patient identifiers.[18]
- Explain the procedure to the patient and answer any questions *to decrease his anxiety and promote his cooperation.*
- Assess the patient's pain tolerance and discuss his preferences for using a local anesthetic before accessing the port.[29,30]
- Administer a topical anesthetic, as needed and prescribed.[29,30,31]
- Perform hand hygiene.[2,10,11,12,13,14,15,16,17]
- Put on gloves.[2,9,11,21,22]

TROUBLESHOOTING

Managing implanted port problems

This chart outlines common problems with implanted ports along with possible causes and nursing interventions.

PROBLEMS AND POSSIBLE CAUSES	NURSING INTERVENTIONS
INABILITY TO FLUSH THE DEVICE OR DRAW BLOOD	
Catheter lodged against the vessel wall	■ Reposition the patient. ■ Raise the arm that's on the same side as the catheter. ■ Roll the patient to his opposite side. ■ Have the patient cough, sit up, or take a deep breath. ■ Regain access to the implanted port using a new needle. ■ Teach the patient to change his position to free the catheter from the vessel wall.
Clot formation	■ Assess patency by trying to flush the port while the patient changes position. ■ Notify the practitioner; obtain an order for fibrinolytic agent instillation. ■ Teach the patient to recognize clot formation; notify the practitioner if it occurs and avoid forcibly flushing the implanted port.
Incorrect needle placement or needle not advanced through septum	■ Regain access to the device. ■ Teach a home care patient to push down firmly on the noncoring needle device in the septum and verify needle placement by aspirating for blood return.
Kinked catheter, catheter migration, or port rotation	■ Notify the practitioner immediately. ■ Tell the patient to notify the practitioner if he has trouble using the implanted port.
Kinked tubing or closed clamp	■ Check the tubing or clamp.
INABILITY TO PALPATE THE DEVICE	
Deeply implanted port	■ Note the portal chamber scar. ■ Use a deep palpation technique. ■ Ask another nurse to try locating the port. ■ Use a 1½″ or 2″ (3.8-cm to 5-cm) noncoring needle to access the implanted port.

■ Position the patient for comfort with his head turned away from the implanted port.[29,30]
■ Palpate and locate the septum; assess the for device rotation.[29,30]
■ Remove and discard your gloves.[21]
■ Perform hand hygiene.[2,10,11,12,13,14,15,16,17]
■ Put on a mask.[29,30]
■ Open the supplies, and prepare a sterile field using a sterile drape. Using sterile technique, place the supplies on the sterile field.[29,30]
■ Put on sterile gloves.[29,30]
■ Clean the implanted port access site with antiseptic swabs following the manufacturer's instructions: For chlorhexidine, apply using a back-and-forth scrubbing motion for at least 30 seconds, and allow the area to dry.[29,30] For povidone-iodine solution, apply in a concentric circle; begin at the intended insertion site, moving outward. Allow the solution to remain on the skin for 2 minutes or longer if needed to dry completely.[29,30]
■ Attach a needleless connector to the extension set, which is connected to the noncoring needle.[29,30]
■ Thoroughly disinfect the needleless connector with a antiseptic pad using friction, and allow it to dry.[29,30]
■ Maintaining sterility of the syringe tip, attach a syringe containing preservative-free normal saline solution to the needleless connector and prime the extension set and noncoring needle.[29,30]
■ With your nondominant hand, palpate and stabilize the implanted port.[29,30]
■ Grasp the noncoring needle with your dominant hand, and insert the noncoring needle perpendicular to the skin through the septum of the port until the needle tip comes in contact with the back of the port.[29,30]
■ Aspirate for blood return *to confirm device patency* and then flush the port with preservative-free normal saline solution; the flushing volume varies with the diameter and type of catheter and fluid volume status of the patient.[29,30,32]

NURSING ALERT ***If you can't aspirate blood return*** **to confirm needle placement,** ***have the patient change positions, raise his arms, cough, or perform the Valsalva maneuver*** **to increase thoracic pressure and increase yield for blood return.** ***If you still can't obtain blood return or confirm needle placement, clamp the tubing and notify the practitioner before proceeding.***[30] (See *Managing implanted port problems.*)

■ Secure the noncoring needle with sterile tape. Support the wings of the noncoring needle (if present) with sterile gauze; make sure the gauze doesn't prevent visualization of the needle insertion site.[29,30]
■ If applicable, place a chlorhexidine-impregnated sponge dressing beneath the needle. The edges of the radial slit of the sponge dressing must touch *to maximize antimicrobial action.* Always follow the manufacturer's directions.[2,9,24]
■ Apply a sterile transparent semipermeable dressing over the insertion site, noncoring needle, and upper portion of the extension *tubing to maintain sterility of the system and enable visualization of the needle and insertion site.*[29,30]

■ Thoroughly disinfect the needleless connector device with an antiseptic pad using friction, and allow it to dry.[29,30]
■ Attach the primed IV administration set to the needleless connector and begin infusion therapy, as ordered. (See "Administering a continuous infusion," page 380.) Trace the tubing from the patient to its point of origin *to make sure that you are attaching the tubing to the correct port before beginning the infusion.*[33,34] Alternatively, lock the device with heparin lock solution.
■ Dispose of equipment and waste in an appropriate receptacle.[29,30]
■ Remove and discard your gloves[21] and mask and perform hand hygiene.[2,10,11,12,13,14,15,16,17]
■ Document the procedure.[25,26,27,28]

Obtaining a blood sample

■ Verify the practitioner's order for blood sampling.[35]
■ Perform hand hygiene.[2,10,11,12,13,14,15,16,17]
■ Confirm the patient's identity using at least two patient identifiers.[18]
■ Ensure that placement of the catheter tip has been confirmed.
■ If fasting is required before testing, verify that the patient has fasted. If any other preparations (such as administering or holding medication) are required before testing, make sure that they were completed.[35]
■ Place the patient in the supine position with his head slightly elevated *to allow for optimal access.*
■ Label the discard blood collection tube *to prevent confusing it with the actual specimen.* If it isn't already clearly marked, label the preservative-free normal saline flush syringe.
■ Perform hand hygiene.[2,10,11,12,13,14,15,16,17]
■ Put on gloves; also put on protective eyewear or a mask with face shield if splashing is likely.[29,30]
■ Locate the noncoring needle extension tubing.[1]
■ Stop infusions that are infusing through the port for at least 1 minute before drawing the blood sample *to prevent inaccurate blood test results.*[36] Trace the tubing from the patient to its point of origin *to make sure you've stopped the proper infusion.*[33] Close the clamp on the extension tubing, and clamp and disconnect the IV tubing, maintaining sterility. Cover the IV tubing end with a sterile cap.[3,35]
■ Assess the skin overlying the port, the tissue surrounding the port, and the site of needle entry. Observe for signs of infection, thrombosis, device rotation, and skin erosion. Hold the procedure and call the practitioner if you observe any complications.[37]
■ Close the clamp on the extension tubing.
■ Thoroughly disinfect the needleless connector with an antiseptic pad using friction and then allow it to dry.[3,30,38]
■ Maintaining the sterility of the syringe tip, attach a prefilled 10-mL syringe containing preservative-free normal saline solution and then open the clamp.
■ Aspirate for blood return and then instill the normal saline solution *to check the patency of the catheter.* The minimum volume of normal saline solution instilled should be twice the internal volume of the catheter system.
■ Reclamp the tubing and remove the syringe.[3,32]
■ Thoroughly disinfect the needleless connector with an antiseptic pad using friction, and then allow it to dry.[3,30,38]

Needleless blood collection tube holder method

■ Attach the needleless adapter to the needleless connector,[39] release the clamp, and engage the labeled discard blood collection tube *to aspirate the discard volume to clear the catheter's dead space volume and remove blood diluted by flush solution.* Limit the discard amount to 1.5 to 2 times the fill volume of the catheter.[30,36]
■ Clamp the extension tubing and remove the labeled discard blood collection tube from the needleless blood collection tube holder.
■ Insert another blood collection tube, unclamp the catheter, and obtain a sample following the correct order of draw. Repeat as necessary until you've obtained all blood samples. Draw only the volume of blood needed for accurate testing *to prevent complications associated with blood loss.*[35]
■ Clamp the extension tubing and remove the needleless blood collection tube holder and needleless adapter from the needleless connector.
■ Thoroughly disinfect the needleless connector with an antiseptic pad using friction, and then allow it to dry.[3,30,38]
■ Maintaining the sterility of the syringe tip, connect a syringe containing preservative-free normal saline solution to the needleless connector.
■ Open the clamp, inject the normal saline solution, and then close the clamp.[36]
■ Thoroughly disinfect the needleless connector with an antiseptic pad using friction, and then allow it to dry.[3,30,38]
■ Lock the device with the prescribed locking solution if the patient doesn't have a continuous infusion prescribed. Clamp the device according to the type of needleless connector used *to avoid reflux of blood into the catheter tip.*[30,32,36]
■ Clamp the noncoring needle extension tubing.[3]
■ If needed, apply a new, primed needleless connector using strict sterile technique.[3,38] *The needleless connector should be changed if it contains blood or debris or becomes contaminated and as directed by the manufacturer or by your facility.*[39]

Syringe method

■ Connect an empty labeled discard syringe to the catheter, release the clamp, and aspirate the discard volume. Limit the discard volume to 1.5 to 2 times the full volume of the catheter *to ensure that a minimal amount of blood is taken from the patient as waste.*[3,36]
■ Clamp the catheter and remove the labeled discard blood syringe and dispose of it appropriately.[40]
■ Thoroughly disinfect the needleless connector with an antiseptic pad using friction, and then allow it to dry.[3,30,38]
■ Connect an empty syringe to the catheter, release the clamp, and slowly withdraw the blood sample. If necessary, obtain multiple syringes of samples; draw only the volume of blood needed for accurate testing *to prevent complications associated with blood loss.*[35]
■ Clamp the extension tubing and remove the syringe.
■ Thoroughly disinfect the needleless connector with an antiseptic pad using friction, and then allow it to dry.[3,30,38]
■ Maintaining the sterility of the syringe tip, connect a syringe containing preservative-free normal saline solution to the needleless connector.
■ Open the clamp, slowly inject the preservative-free normal saline flush, and then close the clamp.
■ Thoroughly disinfect the needleless connector with an antiseptic pad using friction, and then allow it to dry.[3,30,38]
■ If the patient doesn't have a continuous infusion prescribed, lock the device with the prescribed locking solution.
■ If needed, apply a new primed needleless connector using strict sterile technique.[26] *The needleless connector should be changed if it contains blood or debris or becomes contaminated and as directed by the manufacturer or your facility.*[39]
■ Place the collected blood in the appropriate tubes for the ordered tests: Attach the blood transfer device to the collection syringes and designated specimen tubes. If you must draw blood with a syringe, you must use engineered sharps injury protection and safe work practices and you must implement needleless blood transfer devices.[40] Allow the blood to transfer from the syringe to the tube using the tube's vacuum. Don't depress the plunger of the syringe. When the appropriate number of tubes are filled, dispose of the syringe and blood transfer device as one unit in an appropriate receptacle.[21,40]

Completing the procedure

■ Label the samples in the presence of the patient *to prevent mislabeling.*[18,35]
■ Place all blood collection tubes in a laboratory biohazard transport bag and send them to the laboratory with a completed laboratory request form.[40]
■ Dispose of the equipment in the appropriate receptacle.[21]
■ Remove and discard your gloves and protective eyewear or mask with face shield, if worn.[21]
■ Perform hand hygiene.[2,10,11,12,13,14,15,16,17]
■ Document the procedure.[25,26,27,28]

Administering a bolus injection

■ Review the patient's medical record *to determine the location of the implanted port, whether it's currently accessed with a noncoring needle, and the patient's response to previous procedures.*
■ Ensure that the placement of the catheter tip has been confirmed.
■ Compare the medication label with the order in the patient's medical record.[20,29,30]
■ Check the patient's medical record for an allergy or contraindication to the prescribed medication. If an allergy or contraindication exists, don't administer the medication; instead, notify the practitioner.[19,20,29,30]
■ Check the expiration date on the medication. If the medication is expired, return it to the pharmacy and obtain new medication.[19,20,29,30]
■ Visually inspect the solution for particles, discoloration, or other loss of integrity; don't administer the medication if its integrity is compromised.[19,20,29,30]
■ Discuss any unresolved concerns about the medication with the patient's practitioner.[20]
■ Verify that the medication is being administered at the proper time, in the prescribed dose, and by the correct route *to reduce the risk of medication errors.*[20,34]
■ Review the patient's baseline vital signs and observe for changes that may indicate a local or systemic infection.
■ Perform hand hygiene.[2,10,12,13,14,15,16,17]
■ Confirm the patient's identity using at least two patient identifiers.[18]
■ Explain the procedure to the patient. If the patient is receiving the medication for the first time, teach him about potential adverse reactions and discuss any other concerns related to the medication.[20]
■ If your facility uses a bar code scanning system, scan your identification badge, the patient's identification bracelet, and the medication's bar code.
■ Perform hand hygiene.[2,10,12,13,14,15,16,17]
■ Put on gloves.[2,9,11,21,22]
■ Thoroughly disinfect the needleless connector of the access tubing with an antiseptic pad using friction, and then allow it to dry.[3,30,38]
■ Maintaining the sterility of the syringe tip, connect a syringe containing preservative-free normal saline solution to the needleless connector.[32]
■ Release the clamp and aspirate slowly *to verify blood return.*[32] If you can't aspirate blood return, troubleshoot the device; notify the practitioner if you're unsuccessful.
■ Slowly flush the tubing with preservative-free normal saline solution *to clear the blood from the catheter.*[29,30,32]
■ Examine the skin surrounding the needle for signs of infiltration, such as swelling and tenderness. If you note these signs, stop the injection and intervene appropriately.
■ Remove and discard the saline syringe.
■ Thoroughly disinfect the needleless connector of the access tubing with an antiseptic pad using friction, and then allow it to dry.[3,30,38]
■ Maintaining the sterility of the syringe tip, connect the syringe with the medication for the IV bolus injection into the injection port of the needleless connector.
■ Inject the medication at the rate indicated on the label; consult with the pharmacist before injection if a rate isn't present.[29,30]
■ Remove the syringe from the needleless connector.
■ Thoroughly disinfect the needleless connector of the access tubing with an antiseptic pad using friction, and then allow it to dry.[3,30,38]
■ Maintaining the sterility of the syringe tip, connect a syringe filled with preservative-free normal saline solution to the needleless connector and slowly inject the solution *to flush the tubing.*[29,36] (Remember to flush with preservative-free normal saline solution between infusions of incompatible drugs or fluids.) Remove and discard the syringe.[29,32]
■ Proceed with locking the device if necessary. Thoroughly disinfect the needleless connector of the access tubing with an antiseptic pad using friction, and then allow it to dry.[3,30,38]
■ Maintaining the sterility of the syringe tip, connect a syringe containing locking solution (such as heparin lock solution) to the needleless connector.[29,30]
■ Slowly inject the locking solution.
■ Close the clamp on the access tubing according to the type of needleless connector used *to reduce blood reflux.* For a positive-pressure needleless connector, clamp the catheter after disconnecting the syringe.[29,30] For a negative-pressure needleless connector, maintain pressure on the syringe while clamping the catheter.[29,30] For a neutral needleless connector, clamp the catheter before or after disconnecting the syringe.[29,30]
■ Dispose of equipment and waste in an appropriate receptacle.[29,30]
■ Remove and discard your gloves[21] and perform hand hygiene.[2,10,11,12,13,14,15,16,17]
■ Document the procedure.[25,26,27,28]

Administering a continuous infusion

■ Make sure that confirmation of the placement of the catheter tip has been obtained.
■ Verify the practitioner's order for the type of infusion to be administered.
■ Review the patient's baseline vital signs and observe for changes that may indicate a local or systemic infection.
■ Gather the necessary equipment.
Compare the IV solution label with the order in the patient's medical record.[34]
■ Visually inspect the IV solution for particulates, discoloration, or other loss of integrity, and check the expiration date. Replace the solution if the integrity is compromised or it's expired.[19,34]
■ Determine whether the patient has a history of allergies.[19]
■ Perform hand hygiene.[2,10,12,13,14,15,16,17]
■ Confirm the patient's identity using at least two patient identifiers.[18]
■ Explain the procedure to the patient.
■ Locate the noncoring needle extension tubing under the patient's gown.
■ Assess the skin overlying the port, the tissue surrounding the port, and the site of needle entry. Observe for signs of infection, thrombosis, device rotation, and skin erosion. Hold the procedure and notify the practitioner if you observe any complications.
■ If your facility uses a bar code scanning system, scan your identification badge, the patient's identification bracelet, and the solution's bar code.[19]
■ Put on gloves.[2,9,11,21,22]
■ Close the clamp on the IV administration set tubing, remove the protective cover from the administration set's spike and the IV infusion container, insert the spike into the solution container, and hang the container on an IV pole.[29,30]
■ Prime the administration set tubing of the IV administration set *to purge the tubing of air.* (See the "IV therapy preparation" procedure, page 468.) If using an infusion pump, set the correct infusion parameters

according to the practitioner's orders and the manufacturer's instructions.[29,30,41] (See the "IV pump use" procedure, page 462.)

- Thoroughly disinfect the needleless connector on the extension tubing with an antiseptic pad using friction, and then allow it to dry.[3,30,38]
- Maintaining the sterility of the syringe tip, connect a syringe containing preservative-free normal saline solution to the needleless connector.[29,30]
- Release the clamp on the extension tubing.
- Slowly aspirate until you obtain brisk blood return.[34] If you can't aspirate blood return, have the patient change positions, raise his arms over his head, take a deep breath and hold it, or cough *to increase intrathoracic pressure and increase yield for blood return.*[29] If you're still unable to obtain blood return or confirm noncoring needle placement, notify the practitioner.
- Slowly inject preservative-free normal saline solution into the implanted port. Don't inject against resistance. If you meet resistance, further evaluate the port.[29,30,31]
- Clamp the extension set and remove the saline solution syringe.[29,30]
- Thoroughly disinfect the needleless connector on the extension tubing with an antiseptic pad using friction, and then allow it to dry.[3,30,38]
- Connect and secure the administration set tubing of the prescribed IV solution to the needleless connector of the extension tubing. Trace the tubing from the patient to its point of origin *to make sure it's connected to the proper port before beginning the infusion.*[29,30,33]
- Slowly open the clamp of the administration set to begin the infusion, or start the electronic infusion device.[29,30]
- Monitor the drops per minute or observe the electronic infusion device for 1 to 2 minutes *to ensure the proper administration rate.*[29,30]
- Examine the skin surrounding the needle for signs of extravasation or infiltration, such as swelling and tenderness. If you note these signs or if the patient complains of stinging, burning, or pain at the site, stop the infusion and intervene appropriately.
- Label the IV solution container with the date and time it was started and your initials.[34]
- Label the IV tubing with the date and time of its first use and your initials. *Doing so helps identify proper change times.*[34]
- Dispose of equipment and waste in an appropriate receptacle.[29,30]
- Remove and discard your gloves[21] and perform hand hygiene.[2,10,11,12,13,14,15,16,17]
- Document the procedure.[25,26,27,28]

Special considerations

- *Assess the implantation site for infection* by visually monitoring and palpating the site through an intact dressing. If the patient has a fever without an obvious source, tenderness at the insertion site, or other signs or symptoms suggesting local or bloodstream infection, remove the dressing and inspect the site thoroughly.[9]
- Always use the smallest noncoring size needle necessary to accommodate the infusion *to prolong the life of the port and lessen the amount of pain experienced by the patient.*[1]
- Change the transparent semipermeable dressing at least every 7 days; change it sooner if its integrity is compromised.[2,42]
- Change add-on devices with each administration set replacement, or as defined by your facility, and whenever device integrity is compromised or if contamination is suspected.[29,30,38]
- Change the needleless connector if the connector is removed for any reason, if there's blood or debris visible within the connection, upon contamination, before drawing a blood culture through the catheter, and routinely as established by your facility.[29,30,39]
- As long as the gauze used to support the wings of the needle doesn't obscure or cover the catheter insertion site, it isn't considered a gauze dressing and doesn't require routine changing.[42]
- Alternative pain management strategies, such as distraction or relaxation techniques, may be helpful.
- Assess for catheter function before each use, observing for such clinical signs and symptoms as lack of blood return, difficulty or inability to flush, edema, the patient's reports of hearing gurgling, flow stream sounds with flushing, paresthesia, and neurologic effects. Also assess the implantation site for signs of infection, device rotation, and skin erosion.[2,13,43]
- Assess the implantation site for infection by visually monitoring and palpating the site through an intact dressing. If the patient has a fever without an obvious source, tenderness at the insertion site, or other signs or symptoms suggestive of local or bloodstream infection, remove the dressing and inspect the site thoroughly.[9]
- Assess for and identify signs of central venous access device occlusion, including sluggish flow and the inability to withdraw blood, flush, or infuse through the device. If clotting threatens to occlude the implanted port, the practitioner may order a fibrinolytic agent *to clear the catheter.*[44] *Because such agents increase the risk of bleeding,* this intervention may be contraindicated in patients who have had surgery within the past 10 days, who have active internal bleeding such as GI bleeding, or who have experienced central nervous system damage, such as infarction, hemorrhage, traumatic injury, surgery, or primary or metastatic disease within the past 2 months.
- When the implanted port isn't being used, flush it every 4 weeks with the prescribed locking solution.
- Besides performing routine care measures, you must be prepared to handle several common problems that may arise during an infusion with an implanted port, such as an inability to flush the port, withdraw blood from it, or palpate it.
- Change the tubing and solution as you would for a long-term central venous infusion.
- When obtaining a blood sample, use the minimal amount of discard blood *to help prevent anemia.*
- If total parenteral nutrition is infusing in the lumen from which blood is to be drawn, flush the line with 20 mL of normal saline solution before drawing blood.[36]
- Blood drawn from an implanted port isn't recommended for blood cultures, unless the port is suspected to be the source of infection. If you must draw blood cultures from the port, replace the needleless connector with a new one before obtaining the blood cultures or draw the blood cultures directly from the port.[36]
- When drawing blood for therapeutic drug levels, draw blood from a lumen other than the lumen being used for the drug infusion when possible. Use caution in interpreting results when therapeutic drug levels are drawn from the same lumen being used to administer the medication.[36]
- Aim to consolidate all daily tests into one sampling *to reduce the risk for central line–associated bloodstream infections.*[35]
- *Because there are different types of injection and access caps or needleless connectors,* always follow the manufacturer's guidelines for flush technique and when to clamp.[38,39]
- If you're having difficulty aspirating blood, have the patient change position, cough, move his arms above his head, or take a deep breath and hold it.[30]
- If using a heparin flush, be aware of any effects it may have on specimens and flush the catheter before drawing a discard sample, if necessary.
- When preparing to administer a bolus injection, always check drug compatibilities *because a drug may be incompatible with normal saline solution or heparin.*
- Assess the implantation site for signs of infection, device rotation, and skin erosion.
- While the patient is hospitalized, a needleless injection or access cap may be attached to the end of the extension set *to provide ready access for intermittent infusions. A cap reduces the discomfort of accessing the port and*

prolongs the life of the port septum by decreasing the number of needle punctures.

■ With a continuous infusion, when the solution container is almost empty, obtain a new IV solution container, as ordered, and prepare it for administration.

■ Change the transparent dressing and needle every 7 days with a continuous infusion. Change gauze dressings every 48 hours. However, any dressing should be changed immediately if its integrity is compromised. If gauze is used to support the wings of an access needle and it doesn't obscure the insertion site under the transparent semipermeable dressing, it can be changed every 7 days.[1]

■ Change the continuous infusion tubing no more frequently than every 96 hours; however, change it immediately upon suspected contamination or when the integrity of the product or system has been compromised.

Patient teaching

If the patient is going home, he'll need thorough teaching about procedures as well as follow-up visits from a home care nurse *to ensure safety and successful treatment.* Tell the patient what type of port that he has in place and explain the importance of carrying a port identification card.

If the patient will be accessing the port himself, explain that the most uncomfortable part of the procedure is the actual insertion of the needle into the skin. Once the needle has penetrated the skin, the patient will feel mostly pressure. Eventually, the skin over the port will become desensitized from frequent needle punctures. Until then, the patient may want to use a topical anesthetic.

Stress the importance of pushing the needle into the port until the patient feels the needle bevel touch the back of the port. *Many patients tend to stop short of the back of the port, leaving the needle bevel in the rubber septum.* Also stress the importance of monthly flushes when no more infusions are scheduled.

If possible, instruct a family member in all aspects of care as well.

If the patient is receiving an infusion at home, teach the patient and a family member about checking the dressing daily. Also teach the patient how to dress and undress to avoid pulling at the needle site; how to protect the site during bathing; to immediately report pain, burning, stinging, or soreness at the site; and to stop the infusion and report immediately any wetness, leaking, or swelling at the site.[1]

Complications

A patient who has an implanted port faces risks similar to those associated with central venous access devices, including infection, thrombus formation, catheter malposition, and occlusion.

Documentation

Document the site of the implanted port; site preparation; infection prevention; safety measures taken; the type, length, and gauge of the catheter; the manufacturer and lot number of the catheter; the number and location of insertion attempts; and the date and time of insertion. Record medications given, any complications that occurred, and how the patient tolerated the procedure. Also document patient teaching provided.[26]

Document your assessment findings, including the location and appearance of the site. Record the needle gauge and length used to access the site, the appearance of blood return, and any unexpected outcomes and your interventions. If you initiated an infusion, include the type, amount, and rate of the infusion.

Also keep a record of all needle and dressing changes for continuous infusions; blood samples obtained, including the type and amount; and patient-teaching topics covered.

Note the amount of blood withdrawn for discard and the amount withdrawn for testing. When obtaining a blood sample, document the time and type of sample drawn, the volume of blood withdrawn, the amount and types of flushes used, the patency of the catheter, and the patient's tolerance of the procedure. When administering a bolus injection, document the drug, route, dose, time, and rate of administration; the type and amount of flush solution used; the presence of blood return; and the condition of the site. When administering a continuous infusion, include the type, amount, rate, and duration of the infusion; the appearance of the site; and any adverse reactions. Record the date and time you notified the practitioner as well as the practitioner's name and any orders received from him. Note the type and amount of flush solution used, the presence or absence of blood return, any resistance to flushing and, if you encountered resistance, what interventions you took.

Also keep a record of all needle and dressing changes for continuous infusions; blood samples obtained, including the type and amount; and patient-teaching topics covered. Finally, document the removal of the infusion needle, status of the site, use of heparin flush, and any problems you found and resolved.

References

1 Standard 39. Implanted vascular access ports. Infusion nursing standards of practice. (2011). *Journal of Infusion Nursing, 34,* S50–S51. (Level VII)

2 Centers for Disease Control and Prevention. (2011). "Guidelines for the prevention of intravascular catheter-related infections" [Online]. Accessed March 2015 via the Web at http://www.cdc.gov/hicpac/pdf/guidelines/bsi-guidelines-2011.pdf (Level I)

3 Lynn-McHale Wiegand, D. (Ed.). (2011). *AACN procedure manual for critical care* (6th ed.). St. Louis, MO: Saunders.

4 The Joint Commission. (2015). Standard UP.01.01.01. *Comprehensive accreditation manual for hospitals: The official handbook.* Oakbrook Terrace, IL: The Joint Commission. (Level VII)

5 Standard 12. Informed consent. Infusion nursing standards of practice. (2011). *Journal of Infusion Nursing, 34,* S17–S19. (Level VII)

6 The Joint Commission. (2015). Standard RI.01.03.01. *Comprehensive accreditation manual for hospitals: The official handbook.* Oakbrook Terrace, IL: The Joint Commission. (Level VII)

7 Centers for Medicare & Medicaid Services, Department of Health and Human Services. (2014). Condition of participation: Patient's rights. 42 C.F.R. § 482.13(b).

8 American Osteopathic Association. (2014). Standard 15.01.11. *Healthcare Facilities Accreditation Program: Accreditation requirements for acute care hospitals.* Chicago, IL: American Osteopathic Association. (Level VII)

9 The Joint Commission. (2012). *Preventing central line-associated bloodstream infections: A global challenge, a global perspective.* Oakbrook Terrace, IL: Joint Commission Resources. Accessed March 2015 via the Web at http://www.jointcommission.org/assets/1/18/CLABSI_Monograph.pdf (Level VII)

10 The Joint Commission. (2015). Standard NPSG.07.04.01. *Comprehensive accreditation manual for hospitals: The official handbook.* Oakbrook Terrace, IL: The Joint Commission. (Level VII)

11 Centers for Medicare & Medicaid Services & The Joint Commission. (2014). "The specifications manual for national hospital inpatient quality measures (version 4.3)" [Online]. Accessed March 2015 via the Web at http://www.qualitynet.org/dcs/ContentServer?pagename=QnetPublic%2FPage%2FQnetTier2&cid=1141662756099

12 Centers for Disease Control and Prevention. (2002). Guideline for hand hygiene in health-care settings: Recommendations of the Healthcare Infection Control Practices Advisory Committee and the HICPAC/SHEA/APIC/IDSA Hand Hygiene Task Force. *MMWR Recommendations and Reports, 51*(RR-16), 1–45. Accessed March 2015 via the Web at http://www.cdc.gov/mmwr/pdf/rr/rr5116.pdf (Level II)

13 The Joint Commission. (2015). Standard NPSG.07.01.01. *Comprehensive accreditation manual for hospitals: The official handbook.* Oakbrook Terrace, IL: The Joint Commission. (Level VII)

14 Standard 19. Hand hygiene. Infusion nursing standards of practice. (2011). *Journal of Infusion Nursing, 34,* S26–S27. (Level VII)

15 World Health Organization. (2009). "WHO guidelines on hand hygiene in health care: First global patient safety challenge, clean care is safer care" [Online]. Accessed March 2015 via the Web at http://whqlibdoc.who.int/publications/2009/9789241597906_eng.pdf (Level IV)
16 Centers for Medicare & Medicaid Services, Department of Health and Human Services. (2014). Condition of participation: Infection control. 42 C.F.R. § 482.42.
17 American Osteopathic Association. (2014). Standard 07.01.21. *Healthcare Facilities Accreditation Program: Accreditation requirements for acute care hospitals.* Chicago, IL: American Osteopathic Association. (Level VII)
18 The Joint Commission. (2015). Standard NPSG.01.01.01. *Comprehensive accreditation manual for hospitals: The official handbook.* Oakbrook Terrace, IL: The Joint Commission. (Level VII)
19 Centers for Medicare & Medicaid Services, Department of Health and Human Services. (2014). Condition of participation: Nursing services. 42 C.F.R. § 482.23(c).
20 The Joint Commission. (2015). Standard MM.06.01.01. *Comprehensive accreditation manual for hospitals: The official handbook.* Oakbrook Terrace, IL: The Joint Commission. (Level VII)
21 Siegel, J. D., et al. (2007). "2007 guideline for isolation precautions: Preventing transmission of infectious agents in healthcare settings" [Online]. Accessed March 2015 via the Web at http://www.cdc.gov/hicpac/pdf/isolation/Isolation2007.pdf (Level II)
22 American Osteopathic Association. (2014). Standard 07.01.10. *Healthcare Facilities Accreditation Program: Accreditation requirements for acute care hospitals.* Chicago, IL: American Osteopathic Association. (Level VII)
23 The Joint Commission. (2015). Standard UP.01.03.01. *Comprehensive accreditation manual for hospitals: The official handbook.* Oakbrook Terrace, IL: The Joint Commission. (Level VII)
24 American Society of Anesthesiologists. (2012). Practice guidelines for central venous access. *Anesthesiology, 116,* 539–573. Accessed March 2015 via the Web at http://www.guideline.gov/content.aspx?id=36196 (Level IV)
25 The Joint Commission. (2015). Standard RC.01.03.01. *Comprehensive accreditation manual for hospitals: The official handbook.* Oakbrook Terrace, IL: The Joint Commission. (Level VII)
26 Standard 14. Documentation. Infusion nursing standards of practice. (2011). *Journal of Infusion Nursing, 34,* S20–S21. (Level VII)
27 Centers for Medicare & Medicaid Services, Department of Health and Human Services. (2014). Condition of participation: Medical record services. 42 C.F.R. § 482.24.
28 American Osteopathic Association. (2014). Standard 10.00.03. *Healthcare Facilities Accreditation Program: Accreditation requirements for acute care hospitals.* Chicago, IL: American Osteopathic Association. (Level VII)
29 Infusion Nurses Society. (2010). *Infusion nursing: An evidence-based approach* (3rd ed.). St. Louis, MO: Saunders.
30 Infusion Nurses Society. (2013). *Policies and procedures for infusion nursing of the older adult* (2nd ed.). Boston, MA: Infusion Nurses Society.
31 Standard 34. Local anesthesia. Infusion nursing standards of practice. (2011). *Journal of Infusion Nursing, 34,* S43–S44. (Level VII)
32 Standard 45. Flushing and locking. Infusion nursing standards of practice. (2011). *Journal of Infusion Nursing, 34,* S59–S63. (Level VII)
33 U.S. Food and Drug Administration. (n.d.). "Look. Check. Connect. Safe medical device connections save lives" [Online]. Accessed March 2015 via the Web at http://www.fda.gov/downloads/MedicalDevices/Safety/AlertsandNotices/UCM134873.pdf
34 Standard 61. Parenteral medication and solution administration. Infusion nursing standards of practice. (2011). *Journal of Infusion Nursing, 34,* S86–S87. (Level VII)
35 Standard 57. Phlebotomy. Infusion nursing standards of practice. (2011). *Journal of Infusion Nursing, 34,* S77–S80. (Level VII)
36 The Nebraska Medical Center. (2012). *Standardizing central venous catheter care: Hospital to home.* (2nd ed.). Omaha, NE: The Nebraska Medical Center. Accessed March 2015 via the Web at http://www.nebraskamed.com/App_Files/pdf/careers/education-programs/asp/SCORCH-guidelines.pdf
37 Standard 18. Infection prevention. Infusion nursing standards of practice. (2011). *Journal of Infusion Nursing, 34,* S25–S26. (Level VII)
38 Standard 26. Add-on devices. Infusion nursing standards of practice. (2011). *Journal of Infusion Nursing, 34,* S31–S33. (Level VII)
39 Standard 27. Needleless connectors. Infusion nursing standards of practice. (2011). *Journal of Infusion Nursing, 34,* S32–S33. (Level VII)
40 Occupational Safety and Health Administration. (n.d.). "Bloodborne pathogens, standard number 1910.1030" [Online]. Accessed March 2015 via the Web at http://www.osha.gov/pls/oshaweb/owadisp.show_document?p_table=STANDARDS&p_id=10051 (Level VII)
41 Standard 29. Flow-control devices. Infusion nursing standards of practice. (2011). *Journal of Infusion Nursing, 34,* S34–S35. (Level VII)
42 Standard 46. Vascular access device site care and dressing change. Infusion nursing standards of practice. (2011). *Journal of Infusion Nursing, 34,* S63–S64. (Level VII)
43 Standard 53. CVAD malposition. Infusion nursing standards of practice. (2011). *Journal of Infusion Nursing, 34,* S72–S74. (Level VII)
44 Standard 56. Catheter clearance: Occluded central vascular access devices. Infusion nursing standards of practice. (2011). *Journal of Infusion Nursing, 34,* S76–S77. (Level VII)

INCENTIVE SPIROMETRY

Incentive spirometry involves using a device to help the patient achieve maximal ventilation by providing feedback on respiratory effort. The device measures respiratory flow or respiratory volume and induces the patient to take a deep breath and hold it for several seconds. This deep breath increases lung volume, boosts alveolar inflation, and promotes venous return. Incentive spirometry is designed to replicate the natural mechanisms of sighing or yawning, preventing and reversing the alveolar collapse that causes atelectasis and pneumonitis.

Devices used for incentive spirometry provide an immediate visual incentive to breathe deeply. Some are activated when the patient inhales a certain volume of air; the device then estimates the amount of air inhaled. Others contain plastic floats, which rise according to the amount of air the patient pulls through the device during inhalation. Any device used for incentive spirometry should be volume-oriented.[1]

Incentive spirometry is used in conjunction with deep breathing, directed coughing, early mobilization, and optimal analgesia to prevent postoperative complications.[1] It's contraindicated in patients who are unable to cooperate, who can't receive instruction on or supervision of the proper use of the device, and who can't generate adequate inspiration because of pain, diaphragmatic dysfunction, or opiate analgesic use.[1]

Direct supervision of incentive spirometry use isn't necessary after the patient is able to demonstrate proper technique. However, periodic reassessment is necessary to make sure the patient complies with proper technique.[1,2]

Equipment

Flow or volume incentive spirometer, as indicated, with disposable tube and mouthpiece ▪ plastic storage bag ▪ stethoscope ▪ gloves ▪ watch ▪ pencil and paper ▪ hospital-grade disinfectant pad or wipe ▪ Optional: pillow, prescription pain medication.

Preparation of equipment

Read the manufacturer's instructions for spirometer setup and operation. Remove the flow tube and mouthpiece from the package, and attach them to the device according to the manufacturer's instructions. Set the flow rate or volume goal as determined by the practitioner or respiratory therapist and based on the patient's preoperative performance. Turn on the machine, if applicable.

Implementation

- Gather and prepare the appropriate equipment.
- Perform hand hygiene and follow standard precautions.[3,4,5,6,7,8,9]
- Confirm the patient's identity using at least two patient identifiers.[10]
- Assess the patient's condition.
- Perform a comprehensive pain assessment using techniques appropriate for the patient's age, condition, and ability to understand. Administer pain medication as needed and prescribed.[11]
- Explain the procedure to the patient, making sure she understands the importance of performing this exercise regularly *to maintain alveolar inflation.* Advise her to avoid this exercise at mealtimes *to prevent nausea.*
- Help the patient sit comfortably or assume the semi-Fowler position *to promote optimal lung expansion.* If the patient is using a flow incentive spirometer and can't assume or maintain the sitting or semi-Fowler position, she can perform the procedure in any position as long as the device remains upright. *Tilting a flow incentive spirometer decreases the required patient effort and reduces the exercise's effectiveness.*
- Auscultate the patient's breath sounds *to provide a baseline for comparison with posttreatment auscultation.*
- If the patient has an incision, have her splint the incision with a pillow.
- Instruct the patient to exhale normally, insert the mouthpiece, close her lips tightly around the mouthpiece *because a weak seal can alter flow and volume readings,* and then inhale as slowly and as deeply as possible (as shown below). If the patient has difficulty with this step, tell her to suck as she would through a straw but more slowly. Ask the patient to retain the entire volume of air she inhaled for at least 5 seconds or, if you're using a device with a light indicator, until the light turns off. This deep breath creates sustained transpulmonary pressure near the end of inspiration and is sometimes called a *sustained maximal inspiration.*[1]

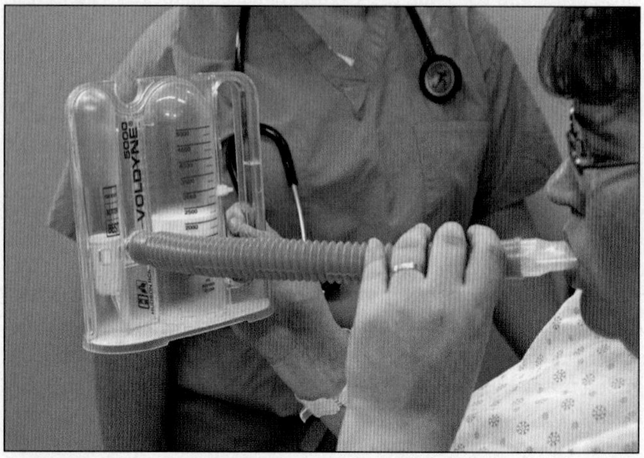

- Tell the patient to remove the mouthpiece and exhale normally. Allow her to relax and take several normal breaths before attempting another breath with the spirometer. Note tidal volumes.
- After proper instruction and return demonstration, encourage the patient to use the incentive spirometer independently.[1] *Because of a lack of evidence for specific frequency of use,* the patient may take 10 breaths every 1 to 2 hours while awake; 10 breaths five times per day; or 15 breaths every 4 hours.[1]
- Evaluate the patient's ability to cough effectively, and encourage her to cough during and after each exercise session *because deep lung inflation can loosen secretions, facilitating their removal.*
- Inspect any expectorated secretions.
- Auscultate the patient's breath sounds. Compare the findings with baseline auscultation findings.
- Put on gloves.[6,9]
- Wash the mouthpiece in warm water and dry it.[12,13] Avoid immersing the spirometer itself in water *because water enhances bacterial growth and impairs the internal filter's effectiveness in preventing inhalation of extraneous material.*
- Place the mouthpiece in a plastic storage bag between exercises, and label it and the spirometer, if applicable, with the patient's name *to avoid inadvertent use by another patient.*[1] Keep the incentive spirometer within the patient's reach.
- Remove and discard your gloves.
- Perform hand hygiene.[3,4,5,8,9]
- Disinfect your stethoscope using a disinfectant pad or wipe.[12,13]
- Perform hand hygiene.[3,4,5,8,9]
- Document the procedure.[14,15,16]

Special considerations

- If the patient is scheduled for surgery, make a preoperative assessment of her respiratory pattern and capability *to ensure the development of appropriate postoperative goals.* Teach the patient how to use the spirometer before surgery *so that she can concentrate on your instructions and practice the exercise.*
- Some research suggests that routine use of incentive spirometry to prevent atelectasis isn't beneficial to patients who have undergone upper abdominal or coronary artery bypass graft surgery. However, it's not clear whether the lack of benefit is related to noncompliance or to an inherent ineffectiveness of the procedure.[1,2]
- Provide paper and a pencil *so the patient can note exercise times.*
- Premedicate for pain as needed, following safe medication administration practices *to improve comfort and effort.*
- Note that some spirometers can be adapted for use by patients who have a tracheal stoma.
- If applicable, remove the patient's dentures *to create a better seal.*

Patient teaching

If the patient is learning the skill preoperatively and taking the instrument home, provide oral and written instructions for use, including cleaning and storage, frequency of sessions, and volumes desired. Demonstrate the procedure and observe return demonstrations.

Instruct the patient to contact the practitioner if shortness of breath, dizziness, extreme exacerbation of coughing, or extreme fatigue or pain associated with use of the incentive spirometer occur.

Complications

Complications of incentive spirometry include hyperventilation, which could lead to respiratory alkalosis; hypoxemia secondary to interruption of prescribed oxygen; fatigue; and pain.[1] Incentive spirometry can be ineffective if not performed as instructed.[1]

Documentation

Record any teaching you provided and the patient's ability to perform a return demonstration. Document the flow or volume levels, date and time of the procedure, type of spirometer, and number of breaths taken. Also record the patient's condition before and after the procedure, tolerance of the procedure, and the results of preprocedure and postprocedure auscultation. (See *Documenting flow and volume levels.*)

REFERENCES

1 Restrepo, R. D., et al. (2011). AARC clinical practice guideline: Incentive spirometry: 2011. *Respiratory Care, 56,* 1600–1604. Accessed March 2015 via the Web at http://rc.rcjournal.com/content/56/10/1600.full.pdf (Level I)

2 Hassanzadeh, H., et al. (2012). Postoperative incentive spirometry use. *Orthopedics, 35,* e927–e931. Accessed March 2015 via the Web at http://www.healio.com/orthopedics/journals/ortho/%7Bea909f29-0520-4b14-b047-223489e3ee6b%7D/postoperative-incentive-spirometry-use

3 The Joint Commission. (2015). Standard NPSG.07.01.01. *Comprehensive accreditation manual for hospitals: The official handbook.* Oakbrook Terrace, IL: The Joint Commission. (Level VII)

4 Centers for Disease Control and Prevention. (2002). Guideline for hand hygiene in health-care settings: Recommendations of the Healthcare Infection Control Practices Advisory Committee and the HICPAC/SHEA/APIC/IDSA Hand Hygiene Task Force. *MMWR Recommendations and Reports, 51*(RR-16), 1–45. Accessed March 2015 via the Web at http://www.cdc.gov/mmwr/pdf/rr/rr5116.pdf (Level II)

5 World Health Organization. (2009). "WHO guidelines on hand hygiene in health care: First global patient safety challenge, clean care is safer care" [Online]. Accessed March 2015 via the Web at http://whqlibdoc.who.int/publications/2009/9789241597906_eng.pdf (Level IV)

6 Siegel, J. D., et al. (2007). "2007 guideline for isolation precautions: Preventing transmission of infectious agents in healthcare settings" [Online]. Accessed March 2015 via the Web at http://www.cdc.gov/hicpac/pdf/isolation/Isolation2007.pdf (Level II)

7 American Osteopathic Association. (2014). Standard 07.01.21. *Healthcare Facilities Accreditation Program: Accreditation requirements for acute care hospitals.* Chicago, IL: American Osteopathic Association. (Level VII)

8 Centers for Medicare & Medicaid Services, Department of Health and Human Services. (2014). Condition of participation: Infection control. 42 C.F.R. § 482.42.

9 American Osteopathic Association. (2014). Standard 07.01.10. *Healthcare Facilities Accreditation Program: Accreditation requirements for acute care hospitals.* Chicago, IL: American Osteopathic Association. (Level VII)

10 The Joint Commission. (2015). Standard NPSG.01.01.01. *Comprehensive accreditation manual for hospitals: The official handbook.* Oakbrook Terrace, IL: The Joint Commission. (Level VII)

11 The Joint Commission. (2015). Standard PC.01.02.07. *Comprehensive accreditation manual for hospitals: The official handbook.* Oakbrook Terrace, IL: The Joint Commission. (Level VII)

12 Rutala, W. A., et al. (2008). "Guideline for disinfection and sterilization in healthcare facilities, 2008" [Online]. Accessed March 2015 via the Web at http://www.cdc.gov/hicpac/pdf/guidelines/Disinfection_Nov_2008.pdf (Level I)

13 American Osteopathic Association. (2014). Standard 07.02.03. *Healthcare Facilities Accreditation Program: Accreditation requirements for acute care hospitals.* Chicago, IL: American Osteopathic Association. (Level VII)

14 The Joint Commission. (2015). Standard RC.01.03.01. *Comprehensive accreditation manual for hospitals: The official handbook.* Oakbrook Terrace, IL: The Joint Commission. (Level VII)

15 Centers for Medicare & Medicaid Services, Department of Health and Human Services. (2014). Condition of participation: Medical record services. 42 C.F.R. § 482.24(b).

16 American Osteopathic Association. (2014). Standard 10.00.03. *Healthcare Facilities Accreditation Program: Accreditation requirements for acute care hospitals.* Chicago, IL: American Osteopathic Association. (Level VII)

ADDITIONAL REFERENCES

Nettina, S. M. (2014). *Lippincott manual of nursing practice* (10th ed.). Philadelphia, PA: Wolters Kluwer.

Taylor, C., et al. (2015). *Fundamentals of nursing: The art and science of nursing care* (8th ed.). Philadelphia, PA: Wolters Kluwer.

Documenting flow and volume levels

If you've used a flow incentive spirometer, compute the volume by multiplying the setting by the duration that the patient kept the ball (or balls) suspended. For example, if the patient suspended the ball for 3 seconds at a setting of 500 mL during each of 10 breaths, multiply 500 mL by 3 seconds and then record this total (1,500 mL) and the number of breaths, as follows: 1,500 mL × 10 breaths.

If the patient is using a volume incentive spirometer, take the volume reading directly from the spirometer. For example, record 1,000 mL × 5 breaths.

INCONTINENCE DEVICE APPLICATION, MALE

Many patients don't require an indwelling urinary catheter to manage their incontinence. An external catheter, also known as a *condom catheter or penile sheath,* is an alternative to an indwelling urinary catheter for cooperative male patients who don't have urinary retention or bladder outlet obstruction.[1] This male incontinence device reduces the risk of urinary tract infection from catheterization, promotes bladder retraining when possible, helps prevent skin breakdown, and improves the patient's self-image. The device consists of a condom catheter secured to the shaft of the penis and connected to a leg bag or drainage bag.

Contraindications to placement include latex or adhesive allergy, skin irritation or open lesions on the glans penis or penile shaft, phimosis or paraphimosis, catheter-induced hypospadias and, if the patient is highly agitated or confused, a high risk of trauma related to improper catheter removal.[2]

Equipment

Condom catheter of appropriate size and type[2] ■ drainage bag ■ extension tubing ■ gloves ■ basin ■ soap ■ washcloth ■ towel ■ Optional: electric clippers, commercial adhesive strip, skin protectant, scissors.

Preparation of equipment

Fill the basin with lukewarm water. Then bring the basin and the remaining equipment to the patient's bedside.

Follow the manufacturer's instructions for condom sizing.[2]

Implementation

Applying the device

- Review the patient's medical record for an allergy to latex or adhesive.[2]
- Perform hand hygiene.[1,3,4,5,6,7]
- Confirm the patient's identity using at least two patient identifiers.[8]
- Provide privacy and explain the procedure to the patient.[9]
- Put on gloves.[10,11]
- If the patient is circumcised, wash the penis with soap and water, rinse well, and pat dry with a towel. If the patient is uncircumcised, gently retract the foreskin and clean beneath it. Rinse well but don't dry *because moisture provides lubrication and prevents friction during foreskin replacement.* Replace the foreskin *to avoid penile constriction.* Then, if necessary, clip hair from the base and shaft of the penis *to prevent the adhesive strip or skin-bond cement from pulling pubic hair.*
- Apply a skin protectant, as indicated, and allow it to dry completely.[2]
- If you're using a precut commercial adhesive strip for a nonadhesive-coated condom catheter, insert the glans penis through its opening, and position the strip 1″ (2.5 cm) from the scrotal area. If you're using uncut adhesive for a nonadhesive-coated condom catheter, cut a strip to fit around the shaft of the penis. Remove the protective covering from one side of the adhesive strip and press this side firmly to the penis *to enhance adhesion.* Then remove the covering from the other side of the strip.
- If you're using an adhesive-coated condom catheter, there's no need for additional adhesive strips or securing devices.
- Position the rolled condom catheter at the tip of the penis, leaving ½″ (1.3 cm) between the condom end and the tip of the penis, with the drainage opening at the urinary meatus.
- Unroll the catheter upward, past the adhesive strip (if using a nonadhesive-coated condom catheter) on the shaft of the penis. Then gently press the sheath against the strip until it adheres. (See *How to apply a condom catheter,* page 386.)
- Using extension tubing, connect the condom catheter to the leg bag or drainage bag.

How to apply a condom catheter

Apply an adhesive strip to the shaft of the penis about 1″ (2.5 cm) from the scrotal area.

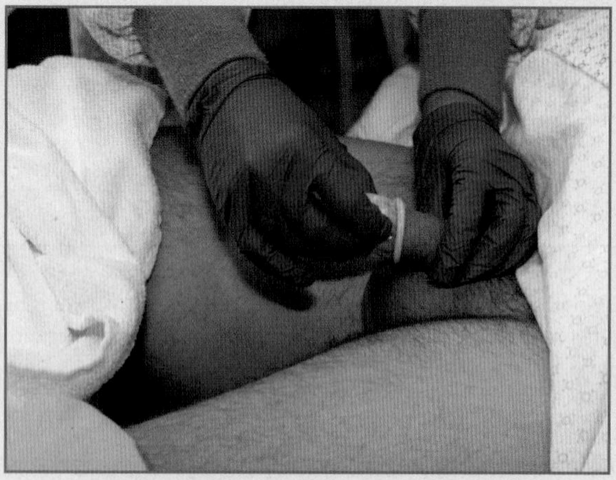

Then roll the condom catheter onto the penis past the adhesive strip. Leave about ½″ (1.3 cm) clearance at the end.

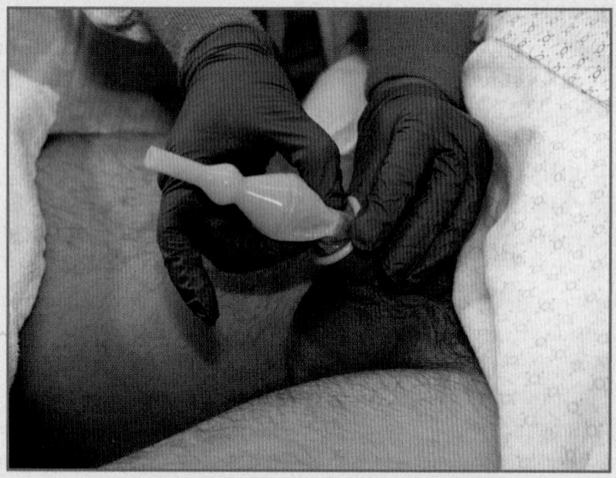

Press the sheath gently against the strip until it adheres.

■ Regularly inspect the catheter and extension tubing for kinks or twists, which could obstruct urine flow and cause the catheter to balloon, eventually dislodging it.
■ Regularly assess the penile skin for signs of irritation or breakdown.[2]
■ Remove and discard your gloves.
■ Perform hand hygiene.[1,3,4,5,6,7]
■ Document the procedure.[12,13,14]

Removing the device
■ Perform hand hygiene.[1,3,4,5,6,7]
■ Confirm the patient's identity using at least two patient identifiers.[8]
■ Provide privacy and explain the procedure to the patient.
■ Put on gloves.[10,11]
■ *To facilitate removal,* soak the penis with warm water and a washcloth for 30 seconds.[2]
■ Simultaneously roll the condom catheter and adhesive strip off the penis and discard them.
■ Clean the penis with lukewarm water, rinse thoroughly, and dry. Check for swelling or signs of skin breakdown.
■ Remove the leg bag by closing the drain clamp, unlatching the leg straps, and disconnecting the extension tubing at the top of the bag.
■ Remove and discard your gloves.
■ Perform hand hygiene.[1,3,4,5,6,7]
■ Document the procedure.[12,13,14]

Special considerations
■ When fitting an uncircumcised male, allow adequate space within the catheter to prevent the foreskin from being drawn into the outlet during voiding.[2]
■ If the penis retracts with position changes, a shorter catheter or different type of product may be necessary.[2]
■ When using an external catheter to collect a clean-catch urinary specimen, collect the urine in an unused and newly applied catheter and drainage bag.[2]

Patient teaching
If being discharged with a catheter, instruct the patient and caregiver in routine catheter care; signs and symptoms of occlusion, skin irritation, and infection; and when to report problems to a practitioner.[2]

Documentation
Record the date and time of application and removal of the incontinence device. Also note skin condition and the patient's response to the device, including voiding pattern, to assist with bladder retraining.

REFERENCES

1 Healthcare Infection Control Practices Advisory Committee. (2010). "Guideline for prevention of catheter-associated urinary tract infections, 2009" [Online]. Accessed March 2015 via the Web at http://www.cdc.gov/hicpac/pdf/CAUTI/CAUTIguideline2009final.pdf (Level I)
2 Wound, Ostomy and Continence Nurses Society. (2008). "External catheter fact sheet" [Online]. Accessed March 2015 via the Web at http://c.ymcdn.com/sites/www.wocn.org/resource/collection/6D79B935-1AA0-4791-886F-E361D29F152D/External_Catheter_-_FS_(2008).pdf
3 The Joint Commission. (2015). Standard NPSG.07.01.01. *Comprehensive accreditation manual for hospitals: The official handbook.* Oakbrook Terrace, IL: The Joint Commission. (Level VII)
4 Centers for Disease Control and Prevention. (2002). Guideline for hand hygiene in health-care settings: Recommendations of the Healthcare Infection Control Practices Advisory Committee and the HICPAC/SHEA/APIC/IDSA Hand Hygiene Task Force. *MMWR Recommendations and Reports, 51*(RR-16), 1–45. Accessed March 2015 via the Web at http://www.cdc.gov/mmwr/pdf/rr/rr5116.pdf (Level VII)
5 World Health Organization. (2009). "WHO guidelines on hand hygiene in health care: First global patient safety challenge, clean care is safer care" [Online]. Accessed March 2015 via the Web at http://whqlibdoc.who.int/publications/2009/9789241597906_eng.pdf (Level IV)
6 Centers for Medicare & Medicaid Services, Department of Health and Human Services. (2014). Condition of participation: Infection control. 42 C.F.R. § 482.42.
7 American Osteopathic Association. (2014). Standard 07.01.21. *Healthcare Facilities Accreditation Program: Accreditation requirements for acute care hospitals.* Chicago, IL: American Osteopathic Association. (Level VII)
8 The Joint Commission. (2015). Standard NPSG.01.01.01. *Comprehensive accreditation manual for hospitals: The official handbook.* Oakbrook Terrace, IL: The Joint Commission. (Level VII)
9 American Osteopathic Association. (2014). Standard 15.01.16. *Healthcare Facilities Accreditation Program: Accreditation requirements for acute care hospitals.* Chicago, IL: American Osteopathic Association. (Level VII)
10 American Osteopathic Association. (2014). Standard 07.01.10. *Healthcare Facilities Accreditation Program: Accreditation requirements for acute care hospitals.* Chicago, IL: American Osteopathic Association. (Level VII)

11 Siegel, J. D., et al. (2007). "2007 guideline for isolation precautions: Preventing transmission of infectious agents in healthcare settings" [Online]. Accessed March 2015 via the Web at http://www.cdc.gov/hicpac/pdf/isolation/Isolation2007.pdf (Level II)

12 The Joint Commission. (2015). Standard RC.01.03.01. *Comprehensive accreditation manual for hospitals: The official handbook.* Oakbrook Terrace, IL: The Joint Commission. (Level VII)

13 Centers for Medicare & Medicaid Services, Department of Health and Human Services. (2014). Condition of participation: Medical record services. 42 C.F.R. § 482.24(b).

14 American Osteopathic Association. (2014). Standard 10.00.03. *Healthcare Facilities Accreditation Program: Accreditation requirements for acute care hospitals.* Chicago, IL: American Osteopathic Association. (Level VII)

15 Dwivedi, A. K., et al. (2013). Massive urethral diverticulum: A complication of condom catheter use. *British Journal of Nursing, 21,* S20–S22.

ADDITIONAL REFERENCES

Gray, M., et al. (2010). Reducing catheter-associated urinary tract infection in the critical care unit. *AACN Advanced Critical Care, 21,* 247–257.

Kyle, G. (2011). The use of urinary sheaths in male incontinence. *British Journal of Nursing, 20,* 338.

Sauter, J. (2012). Preventing catheter-associated UTIs. *Nursing Critical Care,* 7(1), 17–21.

INCONTINENCE MANAGEMENT, FECAL

Fecal incontinence is the involuntary passage of feces, which may occur gradually (as in dementia) or suddenly (as in spinal cord injury). It usually results from fecal stasis and impaction secondary to reduced activity, inappropriate diet, or untreated painful anal conditions. It can also result from chronic laxative use; reduced fluid intake; neurologic deficit; pelvic, prostatic, or rectal surgery; and the use of certain medications, including antihistamines, psychotropics, and iron preparations.

In elderly patients, fecal incontinence commonly follows any loss or impairment of anal sphincter control. The incontinence may be transient or permanent and affects up to 10% of patients in assisted living or extended care facilities. Not usually a sign of serious illness, fecal incontinence can seriously impair an elderly patient's physical and psychological well-being. Patients with fecal or urinary incontinence are at risk for incontinence-associated dermatitis, which can result in the development of pressure ulcers and secondary skin infection.[1]

Successful management of these patients depends on identifying and treating the underlying cause or causes. Most can be treated; some can even be cured. Treatment aims to control the condition through bowel retraining or other behavioral management techniques, diet modification, drug therapy, pessaries and, possibly, surgery. Despite appropriate management, some patients may remain incontinent because of dementia, immobility, or comorbid issues. In such cases, management aims to prevent associated complications.[2]

Equipment

Gloves ■ stethoscope ■ skin barrier or skin protectant ■ appropriate skin cleaners ■ incontinence pads ■ bedside commode or bedpan ■ specimen container label ■ laboratory request form ■ Optional: skin moisturizer, stool collection kit, fecal incontinence collector or fecal management system, absorbent adult brief.

Implementation

- Perform hand hygiene.[3,4,5]
- Confirm the patient's identity using at least two patient identifiers.[6]
- Ask the patient to identify his fecal incontinence onset, duration, severity, and pattern (for instance, determine whether it occurs at night or with diarrhea). Focus the history on GI, neurologic, and psychological disorders. Asses for chronic constipation or laxative abuse.[7]
- Assess the patient's medication regimen. Check for drugs that affect bowel activity, such as antibiotics, aspirin, some anticholinergic antiparkinsonian agents, aluminum hydroxide, calcium carbonate antacids, diuretics, iron preparations, opiates, sedatives, tricyclic antidepressants, and phenothiazines.
- Review the patient's diet. Note whether the patient receives enteral nutrition, and include the type, volume, and frequency of administration *because osmotic diarrhea-induced incontinence should be considered.*[2]
- Note the frequency, consistency, and volume of stools passed in the past 24 hours.
- Put on gloves.
- Protect the patient's bed with an incontinence pad.

NURSING ALERT *Use superabsorbent adult disposable briefs designed to absorb and wick moisture from incontinence away from the skin when the patient is ambulating. Using an incontinence pad when the patient is in bed and a brief when he's out of bed is generally recommended.*[1,8]

- Inspect the abdomen for distention, and auscultate for bowel sounds. If not contraindicated, check for fecal impaction (a factor in overflow incontinence), as ordered
- Obtain a stool specimen, if ordered. (See the "Stool specimen collection" procedure, page 718.)
- Provide ongoing assessment of the perineal skin, observing its general condition and looking for signs of skin breakdown, such as visible areas of skin redness and erosion.[8,9]
- Maintain effective hygienic care *to increase the patient's comfort and prevent skin breakdown and infection.*[9,10] Clean the perineal area frequently with an appropriate skin cleaner; if possible, use a no-rinse skin cleaner with a pH range similar to that or normal skin instead of soap and water *to help prevent incontinence-associated dermatitis.* If a moisturizer isn't already incorporated into the skin cleaner, apply a moisturizer daily, as needed. Apply a skin barrier or protectant after every incontinence episode. Use measures to control odor.

NURSING ALERT *Clean the skin gently, using care to avoid rigorous scrubbing or friction* to minimize the risk of compromising the skin barrier function. *In situations of dried or difficult-to-remove feces, gently apply a moistened cloth on the area and softly pat it around, if needed.*[8]

- Provide bowel retraining for a neurologically capable patient with chronic incontinence. Offer the patient the commode or bedpan every 1 to 2 hours as appropriate.[1]
- If the patient has intact perineal skin, apply a fecal incontinence collector or fecal management system, as indicated and ordered.[1]
- Replace soiled linens promptly, as needed. Check the patient's incontinence pad (if applicable) at least every 2 hours *to ensure that it's dry. Because the skin lying on an underpad is commonly moist,* expose this area to air when turning the patient *to allow moisture to evaporate and the skin to dry.* Regularly and promptly remove soil and irritants from the skin, and prevent or minimize exposure of the skin to damaging irritants.[8]
- Remove and discard your gloves, and perform hand hygiene.[3,4,5]
- Document the procedure.[11,12]

Special considerations

- Schedule extra time to provide encouragement and support for the patient, who may feel shame, embarrassment, and powerlessness from loss of control.
- Minimize the use of incontinence pads. If used, ensure that pads aren't layered and have no wrinkles *to reduce pressure risk and subsequent skin damage.* Avoid the regular use of containment devices such as adult briefs, *which trap heat and moisture and progress skin damage.*[9]
- Antifungal products, steroidal-based topical anti-inflammatory products, and topical antibiotics to treat incontinence-associated dermatitis are recommended only in specific situations.[9,10]

Complications

Skin breakdown and infection may result from incontinence. Psychological problems resulting from incontinence include social isolation, loss of independence, lowered self-esteem, and depression.

Documentation

Record all bladder and bowel retraining efforts, noting scheduled bathroom times, food and fluid intake, and elimination amounts, as appropriate. Document the duration of continent periods. Note any complications, including emotional problems and signs of skin breakdown and infection as well as the treatments given for them.

References

1 Davis-Zeek, D., et al. (2010). "Changing our methods of adult incontinence management to decrease skin breakdown and improve patient satisfaction" [Online]. Accessed March 2015 via the Web at http://www.northshorecare.com/pdf/WOCN_2page_Study_Results_Handout_5.27.10.pdf

2 Leung, F. W., & Rao, S. S. (2011). Approach to fecal incontinence and constipation in older hospitalized patients. *Hospital Practice, 39,* 97–104.

3 Centers for Disease Control and Prevention. (2002). Guideline for hand hygiene in health-care settings: Recommendations of the Healthcare Infection Control Practices Advisory Committee and the HICPAC/SHEA/APIC/IDSA Hand Hygiene Task Force. *MMWR Recommendations and Reports, 51*(RR-16), 1–45. Accessed March 2015 via the Web at http://www.cdc.gov/mmwr/pdf/rr/rr5116.pdf (Level II)

4 World Health Organization. (2009). "WHO guidelines on hand hygiene in health care: First global patient safety challenge, clean care is safer care" [Online]. Accessed March 2015 via the Web at http://whqlibdoc.who.int/publications/2009/9789241597906_eng.pdf (Level IV)

5 The Joint Commission. (2015). Standard NPSG.07.01.01. *Comprehensive accreditation manual for hospitals: The official handbook.* Oakbrook Terrace, IL: The Joint Commission. (Level VII)

6 The Joint Commission. (2015). Standard NPSG.01.01.01. *Comprehensive accreditation manual for hospitals: The official handbook.* Oakbrook Terrace, IL: The Joint Commission. (Level VII)

7 Whitehead, W. E., et al. (2009). Fecal incontinence in US adults: Epidemiology and risk factors. *Gastroenterology, 137,* 512–517.

8 Langemo, D., et al. (2011). Incontinence and incontinence-associated dermatitis. *Advances in Skin and Wound Care, 24,* 126–140.

9 Chatham, N., & Carls, C. (2012). How to manage incontinence-associated dermatitis: Prevention and prompt action are keys to managing this painful and costly complication. *Wound Care Advisor, 1*(1), 7–10. Accessed March 2015 via the Web at http://woundcareadvisor.com/wp-content/uploads/2012/05/WCA_M-J-2012_Dermatitis.pdf

10 Beeckman, D., et al. (2012). Incontinence-associated dermatitis: A comprehensive review and update. *Journal of Wound, Ostomy and Continence Nursing, 39,* 61–74.

11 The Joint Commission. (2015). Standard RC.01.03.01. *Comprehensive accreditation manual for hospitals: The official handbook.* Oakbrook Terrace, IL: The Joint Commission. (Level VII)

12 Centers for Medicare & Medicaid Services, Department of Health and Human Services. (2014). Condition of participation: Medical record services. 42 C.F.R. § 482.24(b).

Additional reference

Hardin, S. (2012). Engaging families to participate in care of older critical care patients. *Critical Care Nurse, 32*(3), 35–40.

Incontinence Management, Urinary

In elderly patients, urinary incontinence commonly follows any loss or impairment of urinary sphincter control. The incontinence may be transient or permanent. About 10 million adults experience some form of urinary incontinence; this includes about 50% of the 1.5 million people in extended-care facilities.

Contrary to popular opinion, urinary incontinence is neither a disease nor a part of normal aging. It isn't inevitable and can be avoided or reversed with support and interventions. Incontinence may be caused by childbirth, confusion, dehydration, fecal impaction, or restricted mobility. It's also a sign of various disorders, such as prostatic hyperplasia, bladder calculus, bladder cancer, urinary tract infection (UTI), stroke, diabetic neuropathy, Guillain-Barré syndrome, multiple sclerosis, prostatic cancer, prostatitis, spinal cord injury, and urethral stricture. It may also result from urethral sphincter damage after prostatectomy. In addition, certain drugs, including diuretics, hypnotics, sedatives, anticholinergics, antihypertensives, and alpha antagonists, may trigger urinary incontinence.

Urinary incontinence is classified as acute or chronic. Acute urinary incontinence results from disorders that are potentially reversible, such as delirium, dehydration, urine retention, restricted mobility, fecal impaction, infection or inflammation, drug reactions, and polyuria. Chronic urinary incontinence occurs in several types and includes stress, overflow, urge, mixed, reflex, and functional (total) incontinence.

In *stress incontinence,* leakage results from a sudden physical strain, such as a sneeze, cough, or quick movement. In *overflow incontinence,* urine retention causes dribbling because the distended bladder can't contract strongly enough to force a urine stream. In *urge incontinence,* the patient can't control the impulse to urinate. In *mixed incontinence,* the patient has symptoms of both stress incontinence and urge incontinence (overactive bladder syndrome with incontinence). In *reflex incontinence,* the bladder muscle contracts and urine leaks without any warning or urge.[1,2] In *functional incontinence,* urine leaks despite a normally functioning bladder and urethra and is usually related to cognitive or mobility factors.

Patients with urinary incontinence should be carefully assessed for underlying disorders. Most can be treated; some can even be cured. Treatment aims to control the condition through bladder retraining or other behavioral management techniques, diet modification, drug therapy, pessaries and, possibly, surgery. Corrective surgery for urinary incontinence includes transurethral resection of the prostate in males, urethral collagen injections for males or females, repair of the anterior vaginal wall or retropelvic suspension of the bladder in females, urethral sling, and bladder augmentation. (See *Artificial urinary sphincter implant.*)

Equipment

Bladder retraining record sheet ▪ gloves ▪ appropriate skin cleaner ▪ skin protectant or skin barrier product ▪ incontinence pads ▪ bedside commode, bedpan, or urinal ▪ specimen container ▪ label ▪ laboratory request form ▪ Optional: skin moisturizer, absorbent adult brief, male external catheter.

Implementation

- Perform hand hygiene.[3,4,5]
- Confirm the patient's identity using at least two patient identifiers.[6]
- Obtain an incontinence history as needed. Ask when the patient first noticed urine leakage and whether it began suddenly or gradually. Have him describe his typical urinary pattern: Does he usually experience incontinence during the day or at night? Does he get the urge to go again immediately after emptying the bladder? Does he get strong urges to go? Ask him to rate his urinary control: Does he have moderate control, or is he completely incontinent? If he sometimes urinates with control, ask him to identify when and how much he usually urinates.
- Assess for related problems, such as urinary hesitancy, frequency, urgency, nocturia, and decreased force or interruption of the urine stream. Ask the patient to describe any previous treatment received for incontinence or measures the patient has performed. Ask about medications, including nonprescription drugs.[7]

■ Assess the patient's environment. Is a toilet or commode readily available, and how long does the patient take to reach it? After the patient is in the bathroom, assess his manual dexterity; for example, how easily does he manipulate his clothes?
■ Evaluate the patient's mental status and cognitive function.
■ Quantify the patient's normal daily fluid intake.
■ Review the patient's medication and diet history for drugs and foods that affect digestion and elimination.
■ Review or obtain the patient's medical history, noting especially any incidence of UTI, diabetes, spinal injury or tumor, stroke, and bladder or pelvic surgery. For a female patient, also note the number and route of births and whether she's had a hysterectomy; for a male, note any prostate surgery. Assess for such disorders as delirium, dehydration, urine retention, restricted mobility, fecal impaction, infection, inflammation, and polyuria.[7]
■ Perform hand hygiene and put on gloves.[3,4,5]
■ Protect the patient's bed with an incontinence pad.

NURSING ALERT *Use superabsorbent adult disposable briefs designed to absorb and wick moisture from incontinence away from the skin when the patient is ambulating. Using an incontinence pad in bed and a brief when out of bed is generally recommended.*[8,9]

■ Inspect the urethral meatus for obvious inflammation or anatomic defects. Have a female patient bear down while you note any urine leakage.
■ Gently palpate the abdomen for bladder distention, which signals urine retention.
■ Assess for costovertebral angle tenderness. If possible, have the patient examined by a urologist.
■ Obtain specimens for appropriate laboratory tests, as ordered. (See the "Urine specimen collection" procedure, page 817.)
■ Begin incontinence management by implementing an appropriate bladder retraining program. (See *Correcting urinary incontinence with bladder retraining,* page 390.)

NURSING ALERT *Obtain a 3- to 7-day bladder diary before implementing bladder retraining.*[7]

■ *To manage stress incontinence,* begin an exercise program to help strengthen the pelvic floor muscles. (See *Strengthening pelvic floor muscles,* page 391.)
■ *To manage functional incontinence,* frequently assess the patient's mental and functional status. Regularly remind him to void. Respond to his calls promptly, and help him get to the bathroom quickly.
■ Provide positive reinforcement.
■ Assess the patient's perineal area, observing its general condition and looking for signs of breakdown, such as visible areas of skin redness and erosion.[9,10]
■ Check the patient's incontinence pad at least every 2 hours *to ensure that it's dry.* Replace soiled linens promptly, as needed. When turning the patient, expose the area that comes in contact with the incontinence pad to air *to promote drying of the skin surface.*[9]
■ Maintain effective hygienic care *to increase the patient's comfort and prevent skin breakdown and infection.*[10,11] Clean the perineal area frequently with an appropriate skin cleaner, preferably a no-rinse skin cleaner with a pH range similar to that of normal skin instead of soap and water *to help prevent incontinence-associated dermatitis.* If a moisturizer isn't already incorporated into the skin cleaner, apply a moisturizer daily, as needed. Apply a skin barrier or skin protectant product after every incontinence episode. Use measures to control odors.

NURSING ALERT *Clean the skin gently, using care to avoid rigorous scrubbing or friction* to minimize the risk of compromising the skin barrier function.[9]

■ Remove and discard your gloves and perform hand hygiene.[3,4,5]
■ Document the procedure.[12]

EQUIPMENT

Artificial urinary sphincter implant

An artificial urinary sphincter implant can help restore continence to a patient with a neurogenic bladder. Criteria for inserting an implant include:
■ incontinence associated with a weak urinary sphincter
■ incoordination between the detrusor muscle and the urinary sphincter (if drug therapy fails)
■ inadequate bladder storage (if intermittent catheterization and drug therapy are unsuccessful).

Configuration and placement

An implant consists of a control pump, an occlusive cuff, and a pressure-regulating cuff. The cuff is placed around the bladder neck, and the balloon is placed under the rectus muscle in the abdomen. The balloon holds fluid that inflates the cuff. In males, the practitioner places the control pump in the scrotum (as shown below); in females, the practitioner places the pump in the labium.

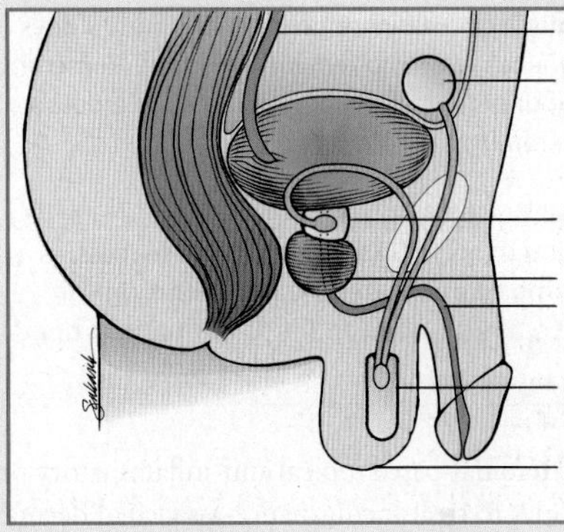

Using the implant

To void, the patient squeezes the bulb to deflate the cuff, which opens the urethra by returning fluid to the balloon. After voiding, the cuff reinflates automatically, sealing the urethra until the patient needs to void again.

Complications and care

If complications develop, the implant may need to be repaired or removed. Possible complications include cuff leakage (uncommon), trapped blood or other fluid contaminants (which can cause control pump problems), skin erosion around the bulb or erosion in the bladder neck or the urethra, infection, inadequate occlusion pressures, and kinked tubing. If the bladder holds residual urine, intermittent self-catheterization may be needed.

Care includes avoiding strenuous activity for about 6 months after surgery and having regular checkups.

Special considerations

■ External male catheters may be indicated to prevent wetness that results from temporary or chronic urinary incontinence in males who have little or no postvoid residual. External catheters may be preferred over indwelling catheters *because external devices are less invasive and carry less risk of urinary complications associated with instrumentation of the urethra.* External catheters can be used in conjunction with clean intermittent catheterization.[8,13]
■ Minimize the use of incontinent pads. If used, ensure that pads aren't layered and have no wrinkles *to reduce pressure risk and subsequent skin damage.* Avoid the regular use of certain containment devices such as adult briefs, *which trap heat and moisture and progress skin damage.*[10]

PATIENT TEACHING

Correcting urinary incontinence with bladder retraining

An incontinent patient typically feels frustrated, embarrassed, and hopeless. Fortunately, his problem can usually be corrected by bladder retraining—a program that aims to establish a regular voiding pattern. Follow these guidelines.

Assess elimination patterns

First, assess the patient's intake and voiding patterns and reason for each accidental voiding (such as a coughing spell). Use an incontinence monitoring record.

Establish a voiding schedule

Encourage the patient to void regularly, for example, every 2 hours. When he can stay dry for 2 hours, increase the interval by 30 minutes every day until he achieves a 3- to 4-hour voiding schedule. Teach the patient to practice relaxation techniques such as deep breathing, which help decrease the sense of urgency.

Record results and remain positive

Keep a record of continence and incontinence for about 5 days *to help reinforce the patient's efforts to remain continent.* Remember, both your own and your patient's positive attitudes are crucial to his successful bladder retraining.

Take steps for success

Here are some additional tips to boost the patient's success:

- Be sure to locate the patient's bed near a bathroom or portable toilet. Leave a light on at night. If the patient needs assistance getting out of bed or a chair, promptly answer the call for help.
- Teach the patient measures to prevent urinary tract infections, such as adequate fluid intake (at least 2,000 mL/day unless contraindicated), drinking cranberry juice *to help acidify urine,* wearing cotton underpants, and bathing with nonirritating soaps. If the patient has urge incontinence, cranberry juice is contraindicated.
- Encourage the patient to empty his bladder completely before and after meals and at bedtime.
- Advise him to urinate whenever the urge arises and never to ignore it.
- Instruct the patient to take prescribed diuretics upon rising in the morning.
- Advise him to limit the use of sleeping aids, sedatives, and alcohol; *they decrease the urge to urinate and can increase incontinence, especially at night.*
- If the patient is overweight, encourage weight loss.
- Suggest exercises to strengthen pelvic muscles.
- Instruct the patient to increase dietary fiber *to decrease constipation and incontinence.*
- Monitor the patient for signs of anxiety and depression.
- Reassure the patient that periodic incontinent episodes don't mean that the program has failed. Encourage persistence, tolerance, and a positive attitude.

- Antifungal products, steroidal-based topical anti-inflammatory products, and topical antibiotics to treat incontinence-associated dermatitis are recommended only in specific situations.[10,11]
- *To ensure healthful hydration and to prevent UTI,* encourage the patient to maintain an adequate daily intake of fluid (six to eight 8-oz glasses [about 1.5 to 2 L]). Restrict oral fluid intake after 6 p.m., as appropriate.
- Schedule extra time to provide encouragement and support for the patient, who may feel shame, embarrassment, and powerlessness from loss of control.

Patient teaching

Teach the patient and family member or other caregiver about normal lower urinary tract function, what's known about the patient's particular type of incontinence, and the benefits as well as the risks and burdens of available treatment options. Explain that, to achieve symptom control, the patient may need to try several therapeutic options.[14]

Complications

Skin breakdown and infection may result from incontinence. Psychological problems resulting from incontinence include social isolation, loss of independence, lowered self-esteem, and depression.

Documentation

Record all bladder retraining efforts, noting scheduled bathroom times, food and fluid intake, and elimination amounts, as appropriate. Document the duration of continent periods. Note any complications, including emotional problems and signs of skin breakdown and infection as well as the treatments given for them.

REFERENCES

1 Harvard Health Publications. (2011). *Urinary incontinence: Better bladder and bowel control.* Palm Coast, FL: Harvard Health Publications.

2 Dannecker, C., et al. (2010). "Urinary incontinence in women: Part 1 of a series of articles on incontinence" [Online]. Accessed March 2015 via the Web at http://www.ncbi.nlm.nih.gov/pmc/articles/PMC2896999/

3 Centers for Disease Control and Prevention. (2002). Guideline for hand hygiene in health-care settings: Recommendations of the Healthcare Infection Control Practices Advisory Committee and the HICPAC/SHEA/APIC/IDSA Hand Hygiene Task Force. *MMWR Recommendations and Reports, 51*(RR-16), 1–45. Accessed March 2015 via the Web at http://www.cdc.gov/mmwr/pdf/rr/rr5116.pdf (Level II)

4 World Health Organization. (2009). "WHO guidelines on hand hygiene in health care: First global patient safety challenge, clean care is safer care" [Online]. Accessed March 2015 via the Web at http://whqlibdoc.who.int/publications/2009/9789241597906_eng.pdf (Level IV)

5 The Joint Commission. (2015). Standard NPSG.07.01.01. *Comprehensive accreditation manual for hospitals: The official handbook.* Oakbrook Terrace, IL: The Joint Commission. (Level VII)

6 The Joint Commission. (2015). Standard NPSG.01.01.01. *Comprehensive accreditation manual for hospitals: The official handbook.* Oakbrook Terrace, IL: The Joint Commission. (Level VII)

7 Ghoniem, G., et al. (2008). Evaluation and outcome measures in the treatment of female urinary stress incontinence: International Urogynecological Association (IUGA) guidelines for research and clinical practice. *International Urogynecology Journal and Pelvic Floor Dysfunction, 19,* 5–33. (Level VII)

8 Davis-Zeek, D., et al. (2010). "Changing our methods of adult incontinence management to decrease skin breakdown and improve patient satisfaction" [Online]. Accessed March 2015 via the Web at http://www.northshorecare.com/pdf/WOCN_2page_Study_Results_Handout_5.27.10.pdf

9 Langemo, D., et al. (2011). Incontinence and incontinence-associated dermatitis. *Advances in Skin and Wound Care, 24,* 126–140.

10 Chatham, N., & Carls, C. (2012). How to manage incontinence-associated dermatitis: Prevention and prompt action are keys to managing this painful and costly complication. *Wound Care Advisor, 1*(1), 7–10.

PATIENT TEACHING

Strengthening pelvic floor muscles

Stress incontinence, the most common kind of urinary incontinence in females, usually results from weakening of the urethral sphincter. In males, it may sometimes occur after a radical prostatectomy.

You can help male and female patients prevent or minimize stress incontinence by teaching pelvic floor (Kegel) exercises to strengthen the pubococcygeal muscles.[7]

Learning Kegel exercises

First, explain how to locate the muscles of the pelvic floor. Instruct the patient to tense the muscles around the anus, as if to retain stools.

To identify this area initially, teach the patient to tighten the muscles of the pelvic floor to stop the flow of urine while urinating and then to release the muscles to restart the flow. Once learned, these exercises can be done anywhere. Although Kegel exercises shouldn't be done while urinating, they can be done at any other time.

Establishing a regimen

Explain to the patient that contraction and relaxation exercises are essential to muscle retraining. Suggest that the patient start out by contracting the pelvic floor muscles for 5 seconds, relaxing for 5 seconds, and then repeating the procedure as often as needed. Typically, the patient starts with 10 contractions in the morning and 10 at night, gradually increasing the relaxation and contraction time.

Advise the patient not to use stomach, leg, or buttock muscles. Also discourage leg crossing or breath holding during these exercises.

Accessed March 2015 via the Web at http://woundcareadvisor.com/wp-content/uploads/2012/05/WCA_M-J-2012_Dermatitis.pdf

11 Beeckman, D., et al. (2012). Incontinence-associated dermatitis: A comprehensive review and update. *Journal of Wound, Ostomy and Continence Nursing, 39,* 61–74.

12 The Joint Commission. (2015). Standard RC.01.03.01. *Comprehensive accreditation manual for hospitals: The official handbook.* Oakbrook Terrace, IL: The Joint Commission. (Level VII)

13 Wound, Ostomy and Continence Nurses Society. (2008). "External catheter fact sheet" [Online]. Accessed March 2015 via the Web at http://c.ymcdn.com/sites/www.wocn.org/resource/resmgr/c_extcat.pdf

14 Gormely, E. A., et al. (2012). "American Urological Association (AUA) guideline: Diagnosis and treatment of overactive bladder (non-neurogenic) in adults" [Online]. Accessed March 2015 via the Web at http://www.auanet.org/content/media/OAB_guideline.pdf (Level VII)

INDWELLING URINARY CATHETER CARE AND REMOVAL

The Centers for Disease Control and Prevention estimates that 15% to 25% of hospitalized patients have an indwelling urinary catheter inserted at some time during their hospitalization. Catheters are often inserted for inappropriate indications.[1] Appropriate indications for catheter use include perioperative use for selected surgical procedures, such as urologic surgery or surgery on contiguous structures of the genitourinary tract, prolonged surgery, large-volume infusions or diuretic use during surgery, or when intraoperative urine output monitoring is needed; hourly urine output measurement in critically ill patients; acute urinary retention or urinary obstruction; open pressure ulcers or skin grafts for selected patients with urinary incontinence; and at the patient's request to improve comfort during end-of-life care.[2]

Catheter-associated urinary tract infection (CAUTI) is the most common type of health care–associated infection. Researchers estimate that as much as 70% of these infections are preventable by following a variety of evidence-based practices.[3]

An indwelling urinary catheter should be removed when bladder decompression is no longer necessary, when the patient can resume voiding, or when the catheter is obstructed.[1] Depending on the length of the catheterization, the practitioner may order bladder retraining before catheter removal. The need for the catheter should be reviewed daily, and it should be removed as soon as it's no longer needed *to prevent CAUTI.*[1,2,3,4]

HOSPITAL-ACQUIRED CONDITION ALERT *The Centers for Medicare & Medicaid Services has identified CAUTI as a hospital-acquired condition that has payment implications* because CAUTI can be reasonably prevented using a variety of best practices. *When caring for a patient with an indwelling urinary catheter, follow infection-prevention practices, such as performing hand hygiene; maintaining a sterile, closed drainage system; properly securing the catheter; keeping the collection bag below the level of the bladder; maintaining unobstructed urine flow; emptying the collection bag regularly; performing routine hygiene during daily bathing; and removing the catheter as soon as it's no longer needed* to reduce the risk of CAUTI.[2,4,5,6,7,8,9]

Equipment

Gloves ■ washcloth ■ soap and water ■ catheter securement device ■ Optional: tape, specimen container, disinfectant pad, gown, goggles, mask, mask with face shield, perineal cleaner, leg bag.

For catheter removal

Fluid-impermeable pad ■ gloves ■ 10-mL syringe with a luer lock ■ bedpan ■ perineal care supplies ■ Optional: gown.

Implementation

Catheter care

■ Gather the equipment and supplies at the patient's bedside.

■ Perform hand hygiene.[7,10,11,12,13,14]

■ Confirm the patient's identity using at least two patient identifiers.[15]

■ Provide privacy.[16,17]

■ Explain the procedure and its purpose to the patient. Discuss the risks associated with indwelling urinary catheter use and the necessary measures *to reduce the risk of CAUTI.*[9] Advise the patient to remind staff members to perform hand hygiene before and after handling the catheter if they fail to do so.[9]

■ Make sure the lighting is adequate *so that you can clearly see the perineum and catheter tubing.*

■ Perform hand hygiene.[7,10,11,12,13,14]

■ Put on gloves and other personal protective equipment, as needed, *to comply with standard precautions.*[18,19]

■ Review the necessity of continued catheter use; remove the catheter (as ordered or according to protocol) as soon as it's no longer clinically indicated *to reduce the risk of CAUTI.*[2,5,6,7,8,9]

■ Inspect the catheter system for disconnections and leakage *because a sterile, continuously closed system is required to reduce the risk of CAUTI.* Replace the catheter and drainage system using sterile technique when breaks in sterile technique, disconnection, or leakage occurs.[2,5,6,7,8,9]

■ Provide routine hygiene for meatal care; note that cleaning the meatal area with antiseptic solutions isn't necessary.[2,5,6,7,8,9] *To avoid contaminating the urinary tract,* always clean by wiping away from—never toward—the urinary meatus. Use soap and water or a perineal cleaner to clean the periurethral area after each bowel movement; avoid frequent and vigorous cleaning of the area. Gently retract the foreskin of an uncircumcised male and clean the area, and then return the foreskin to its normal position.[20]

NURSING ALERT *When cleaning the periurethral area, clean the area carefully* **to prevent catheter movement and urethral traction, which increase the risk of CAUTI.**[20]

- Inspect the periurethral area for signs of inflammation and infection.
- Make sure the catheter is properly secured.[2] Assess the securement device daily and change it when clinically indicated and as recommended by the manufacturer.[21] If a new securement device is needed, connect it to the catheter before applying the device to the skin. If a securement device isn't available, use a piece of adhesive tape to secure the catheter.[22] If using tape, retape the catheter on the side opposite from where it was previously *to prevent skin hypersensitivity and irritation.*

NURSING ALERT *Provide enough slack before securing the catheter* **to prevent tension on the tubing, which could injure the urethral lumen and bladder wall.**[7]

- Monitor intake and output, as ordered. Monitor for changes in urine output, including volume and color.[2,3] Notify the practitioner of abnormal changes.
- Keep the catheter and drainage tubing free from kinks *to allow the free flow of urine,* and keep the drainage bag below the level of the patient's bladder *to prevent backflow of urine into the bladder, which increases the risk of CAUTI.*[2,6,7]
- Don't place the drainage bag on the floor *to reduce the risk of contamination and subsequent CAUTI.*[2,4,5,6]
- Dispose of all used supplies in appropriate waste receptacles.
- Remove and discard your gloves and any other personal protective equipment worn.[19]
- Perform hand hygiene.[10,11,12,13,14]
- Document the procedure.[23,24,25]

Catheter removal

- Gather the equipment and supplies at the patient's bedside.
- Perform hand hygiene.[7,10,11,12,13,14]
- Confirm the patient's identity using at least two patient identifiers.[15]
- Verify the practitioner's order.
- Explain the procedure and its purpose to the patient and tell him that he may feel slight discomfort.
- Provide the patient with the necessary equipment for self-cleaning, if possible.
- Provide privacy.
- Perform hand hygiene.[7,10,11,12,13,14]
- Put on gloves and a gown, if necessary, *to comply with standard precautions.*[18,19]
- Place the patient on a fluid-impermeable pad *to protect the bed linens.*
- Explain to the patient that you'll check him periodically during the first 6 to 24 hours after catheter removal *to make sure he resumes voiding.*
- Attach the syringe to the luer-lock mechanism on the catheter.
- Pull back on the plunger of the syringe *to deflate the balloon by aspirating the injected fluid.* The amount of fluid injected is usually indicated on the tip of the catheter's balloon lumen and in the patient's medical record.
- Ask the patient to take a deep breath in and then out *to help relax the pelvic floor muscles;* as the patient exhales, gently remove the catheter. Warn a male patients that he may feel discomfort as the deflated balloon passes through the prostatic urethra.[26]
- Offer the patient a bedpan and perineal care.[26]
- Measure and record the amount of urine in the collection bag before discarding it.
- If the patient's condition allows, encourage him to maintain an oral intake of 30 mL/kg/day *to flush the bladder of microorganisms that might be associated with indwelling urinary catheter use.*[26]
- Dispose of used equipment in the appropriate receptacles.
- Remove and discard your gloves and gown if worn.[19]
- Perform hand hygiene.[10,11,12,13,14]
- Document the procedure.[23,24,25]

Special considerations

- Empty the drainage bag regularly when it becomes one-half to two-thirds full *to prevent undue traction on the urethra from the weight of urine in the bag.* Use a separate collecting container for each patient to empty the drainage. During emptying, avoid splashing and don't allow the drainage spigot to come in contact with the nonsterile collecting container.[2,5,6,7,20]
- Unless obstruction is anticipated (for example, from bleeding after prostate or bladder surgery), bladder irrigation isn't recommended. If obstruction is anticipated, continuous irrigation is suggested *to prevent obstruction.*[20]
- If you need to collect a small urine specimen or culture, thoroughly disinfect the needleless sampling port with a disinfectant pad and then allow it to dry. Collect the sample by aspirating urine from the needleless sampling port with a sterile syringe or sterile urine collection tube system and a cannula adapter.[20] (See the "Urine specimen collection" procedure, page 817.)
- If a large volume of urine is needed for special analysis, obtain the sample from the drainage bag using sterile technique.[2]
- When possible, attach a leg bag *to allow the patient greater mobility.*
- Unless otherwise clinically indicated, consider using the smallest bore catheter possible, consistent with good drainage *to minimize bladder neck and urethral trauma.*[2,20]
- After catheter removal, assess the patient for incontinence (or dribbling), urgency, persistent dysuria or bladder spasms, fever, chills, or palpable bladder distention. Report these conditions to the practitioner.

Patient teaching

If the patient will be discharged with an indwelling catheter, teach him how to use a leg bag. (See *Teaching about leg bags.*) Instruct the patient to wash the urinary meatus and perineal area with soap and water twice daily and the anal area after each bowel movement. Provide the patient and family with information regarding additional methods of infection control as well as the signs and symptoms of urinary tract infection and obstruction.[27] Also review with the patient reasons to notify the practitioner.

Inform the patient that he may experience transient incontinence, urgency, frequency, dysuria, discomfort, and urinary retention after indwelling urinary catheter removal. Advise him to notify his practitioner if signs and symptoms persist for more than 48 hours.[26]

Complications

Complications associated with indwelling urinary catheter use include CAUTI, genitourinary trauma, epididymitis (in males), retained balloon fragments, bladder fistula (with prolonged use), bladder stone formation, and incontinence.[28,29]

Indwelling urinary catheter balloon rupture may occur with indwelling urinary catheter removal. If balloon rupture occurs, cystoscopy may be performed to remove balloon fragments.

Documentation

Document the reason for continued catheter use,[9] maintenance care given,[2] your assessment findings, and patient and family teaching performed and their understanding of that teaching. Record any specimens collected, including the collection method.

Document the date and time the indwelling urinary catheter was removed and the patient's tolerance of the procedure. Record the time and amount of the patient's first void after catheter removal, any signs

PATIENT TEACHING

Teaching about leg bags

A urine drainage bag attached to the leg provides the catheterized patient with greater mobility. *Because the bag is hidden under clothing,* it may also help him feel more comfortable about catheterization. Leg bags are usually worn during the day and are replaced at night with a standard drainage bag.

If the patient will be discharged with an indwelling urinary catheter, teach him how to attach and remove a leg bag. To demonstrate, you'll need a bag with a short drainage tube, two straps, an alcohol pad, adhesive tape, and a screw clamp or hemostat.

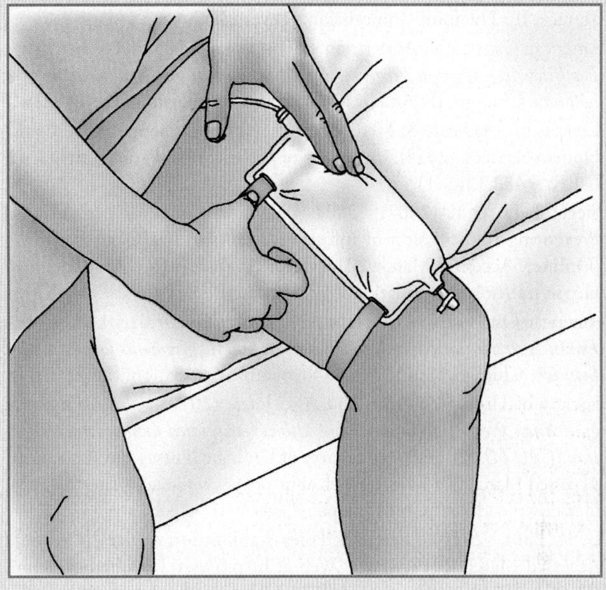

Attaching the leg bag

- Provide privacy, and explain the procedure. Describe the advantages of a leg bag, but caution the patient that a leg bag is smaller than a standard drainage bag and may have to be emptied more frequently.
- Remove the protective covering from the tip of the drainage tube. Then show the patient how to clean the tip with an alcohol pad, wiping away from the opening *to avoid contaminating the tube.*
- Show him how to attach the tube to the catheter.
- Place the drainage bag on the patient's calf or thigh. Have him fasten the straps securely (as shown right), and then show him how to tape the catheter to his leg. Emphasize that he must leave slack in the catheter *to minimize pressure on the bladder, urethra, and related structures. Excessive pressure or tension can lead to tissue breakdown.*

Avoiding complications

- Although most leg bags have a valve in the drainage tube that prevents urine reflux into the bladder, urge the patient to keep the drainage bag lower than his bladder at all times *because urine in the bag is a perfect growth medium for bacteria.* Caution him also not to go to bed or take long naps while wearing the leg bag.
- *To prevent a full leg bag from damaging the bladder wall and urethra,* encourage the patient to empty the bag when it's half full or every 3 to 6 hours.[22] He should also inspect the catheter and drainage tube periodically for compression or kinking, *which could obstruct urine flow and result in bladder distention.*
- Instruct the patient to avoid fastening the straps too tightly *because doing so may impede circulation.*
- Tell the patient to wash the leg bag with soap and water or a bacteriostatic solution before each use *to prevent infection.*

and symptoms associated with catheter removal, your interventions, and the patient's response to those interventions. Document patient teaching and the patient's comprehension of your teaching.

REFERENCES

1 Gould, C. (n.d.). "Catheter-associated urinary tract infection (CAUTI) toolkit" [Online]. Accessed March 2015 via the Web at http://www.cdc.gov/HAI/pdfs/toolkits/CAUTItoolkit_3_10.pdf

2 Lo, E., et al. (2014). SHEA/IDSA practice recommendation: Strategies to prevent catheter-associated urinary tract infections in acute care hospitals: 2014 update. *Infection Control and Hospital Epidemiology, 35,* 464–479. Accessed March 2015 via the Web at http://www.jstor.org/stable/10.1086/675718 (Level I)

3 Seckel, M. A. (2013). Maintaining urinary catheters: What does the evidence say? *Nursing, 43*(2), 63–65.

4 Jarrett, N., et al. (2013). "Evidence-based guidelines for selected and previously considered hospital-acquired conditions: Final report" [Online]. Accessed March 2015 via the Web at http://www.cms.gov/Medicare/Medicare-Fee-for-Service-Payment/HospitalAcqCond/Downloads/Evidence-Based-Guidelines.pdf

5 American Osteopathic Association. (2014). Standard 07.01.17. *Healthcare Facilities Accreditation Program: Accreditation requirements for acute care hospitals.* Chicago, IL: American Osteopathic Association. (Level VII)

6 The Joint Commission. (2015). Standard NPSG.07.06.01. *Comprehensive accreditation manual for hospitals: The official handbook.* Oakbrook Terrace, IL: The Joint Commission. (Level VII)

7 Healthcare Infection Control Practices Advisory Committee. (2010). "Guideline for prevention of catheter-associated urinary tract infections, 2009" [Online]. Accessed March 2015 via the Web at http://www.cdc.gov/hicpac/pdf/CAUTI/CAUTIguideline2009final.pdf (Level I)

8 Institute for Healthcare Improvement. (2012). *How-to guide: Prevent catheter-associated urinary tract infection.* Cambridge, MA: Institute for Healthcare Improvement. (Level VII)

9 Association of Professionals in Infection Control and Epidemiology (APIC). (2014). "APIC implementation guide: Guide to preventing catheter-associated urinary tract infections" [Online]. Accessed March 2015 via the Web at http://apic.org/Resource_/EliminationGuideForm/6473ab9b-e75c-457a-8d0f-d57d32bc242b/File/APIC_CAUTI_web_0603.pdf (Level IV)

10 Centers for Disease Control and Prevention. (2002). Guideline for hand hygiene in health-care settings: Recommendations of the Healthcare Infection Control Practices Advisory Committee and the HICPAC/SHEA/APIC/IDSA Hand Hygiene Task Force. *MMWR Recommendations and Reports, 51*(RR-16), 1–45. Accessed March 2015 via the Web at http://www.cdc.gov/mmwr/pdf/rr/rr5116.pdf (Level II)

11 The Joint Commission. (2015). Standard NPSG.07.01.01. *Comprehensive accreditation manual for hospitals: The official handbook.* Oakbrook Terrace, IL: The Joint Commission. (Level VII)

12 World Health Organization. (2009). "WHO guidelines on hand hygiene in health care: First global patient safety challenge, clean care is safer care" [Online]. Accessed March 2015 via the Web at http://whqlibdoc.who.int/publications/2009/9789241597906_eng.pdf (Level IV)

13 American Osteopathic Association. (2014). Standard 07.01.21. *Healthcare Facilities Accreditation Program: Accreditation requirements for acute care hospitals.* Chicago, IL: American Osteopathic Association. (Level VII)

14 Centers for Medicare & Medicaid Services, Department of Health and Human Services. (2014). Condition of participation: Infection control. 42 C.F.R. § 482.42.
15 The Joint Commission. (2015). Standard NPSG.01.01.01. *Comprehensive accreditation manual for hospitals: The official handbook.* Oakbrook Terrace, IL: The Joint Commission. (Level VII)
16 American Osteopathic Association. (2014). Standard 15.01.16. *Healthcare Facilities Accreditation Program: Accreditation requirements for acute care hospitals.* Chicago, IL: American Osteopathic Association. (Level VII)
17 Centers for Medicare & Medicaid Services, Department of Health and Human Services. (2014). Condition of participation: Patient's rights. 42 C.F.R. § 482.13(c)(1).
18 Siegel, J. D., et al. (2007). "2007 guideline for isolation precautions: Preventing transmission of infectious agents in healthcare settings" [Online]. Accessed March 2015 via the Web at http://www.cdc.gov/hicpac/pdf/isolation/Isolation2007.pdf (Level II)
19 American Osteopathic Association. (2014). Standard 07.01.10. *Healthcare Facilities Accreditation Program: Accreditation requirements for acute care hospitals.* Chicago, IL: American Osteopathic Association. (Level VII)
20 Society of Urologic Nurses and Associates. (2010). *Clinical practice guidelines: Prevention & control of catheter-associated urinary tract infection (CAUTI).* Pittman, NJ: Society of Urologic Nurses and Associates. Accessed March 2015 via the Web at http://www.suna.org/sites/default/files/download/cautiGuideline.pdf (Level VII)
21 C. R. Bard. (2010). "StatLock Foley stabilization device" [Online]. Accessed March 2015 via the Web at http://www.bardmedical.com/Resources/Products/Documents/Posters/Vascular/StatLock%20Foley%20Poster%20M1034.pdf
22 Society of Urologic Nurses and Associates Clinical Practice Guidelines Task Force. (2006). Care of the patient with an indwelling catheter. *Urologic Nursing, 26,* 80–81. (Level VII)
23 The Joint Commission. (2015). Standard RC.01.03.01. *Comprehensive accreditation manual for hospitals: The official handbook.* Oakbrook Terrace, IL: The Joint Commission. (Level VII)
24 American Osteopathic Association. (2014). Standard 10.00.03. *Healthcare Facilities Accreditation Program: Accreditation requirements for acute care hospitals.* Chicago, IL: American Osteopathic Association. (Level VII)
25 Centers for Medicare & Medicaid Services, Department of Health and Human Services. (2014). Condition of participation: Medical record services. 42 C.F.R. § 482.24(b).
26 European Association of Urology Nurses. (2012). "Evidence-based guidelines for best practice in urologic healthcare: Catheterisation of indwelling catheters in adults" [Online]. Accessed March 2015 via the Web at http://www.uroweb.org/fileadmin/EAUN/guidelines/EAUN_Paris_Guideline_2012_LR_online_file.pdf
27 Herter, R., & Kazer, M. W. (2010). Best practices in urinary catheter care. *Home Healthcare Nurse, 28,* 342–349.
28 Leuck, A. M., et al. (2012). Complications of Foley catheters—Is infection the greatest risk? *Journal of Urology, 187,* 1662–1666.
29 Schaeffer, A. J. Complications of urinary bladder catheters and preventive strategies. (2013). In: *UpToDate,* Richie, J. P. (Ed.). Accessed March 2015 via the Web at http://www.uptodate.com/contents/search

ADDITIONAL REFERENCE

Nettina, S. M. (2014). *Lippincott manual of nursing practice* (10th ed.). Philadelphia, PA: Wolters Kluwer.

INDWELLING URINARY CATHETER INSERTION

An indwelling urinary (Foley) catheter remains in the bladder to provide continuous urine drainage. A balloon inflated at the catheter's distal end prevents it from slipping out of the bladder after insertion.

An indwelling urinary catheter should be inserted only when absolutely necessary because its use is associated with an increased risk of developing a urinary tract infection, with the risk increasing with each day of use.[1,2] Catheter-associated urinary tract infection (CAUTI) is the most common type of health care–associated infection in the United States, accounting for 35% of all such infections.

HOSPITAL-ACQUIRED CONDITION ALERT *The Centers for Medicare & Medicaid Services has identified CAUTI as a hospital-acquired condition that has payment implications* because various best practices can reasonably prevent these infections. *Make sure to follow infection-prevention practices when inserting an indwelling urinary catheter.*[3,4,5,6,7]

To reduce the risk of CAUTI, consider alternatives to indwelling urinary catheterization, such as intermittent catheterization, when appropriate, for patients with spinal cord injury or bladder emptying dysfunction.[2] Ensure that you insert an indwelling urinary catheter only for an appropriate indication, including acute urinary retention or bladder outlet obstruction, the need for accurate urine output measurements in a critically ill patient, perioperative use for a patient undergoing urologic surgery or another procedure on structures of the genitourinary tract, prolonged surgery (with removal of catheters inserted for this purpose in the postanesthesia care unit), large-volume infusions or diuretic administration anticipated during surgery with the need for intraoperative monitoring of urinary output, assistance in the healing of open sacral or perineal wounds or skin grafts in certain incontinent patients,[4] prolonged immobilization (such as potentially unstable thoracic or lumbar spine and multiple traumatic injuries, including pelvic fractures), and improved comfort for end-of-life care if needed.[2]

Use sterile technique when inserting, manipulating, and maintaining the catheter. Maintain a sterile, continuously closed drainage system; don't disconnect the catheter from the drainage bag unless you can only irrigate the catheter manually or if you need to attach new tubing. Avoid irrigation unless necessary (such as in the case of catheter obstruction).[1] Make sure urinary flow is unobstructed and that the drainage bag remains below the patient's bladder to facilitate drainage. Empty the urine drainage bag at least once per shift using a container designated for that patient only. When the patient has an indwelling urinary catheter inserted for surgery, ensure its discontinuation within 24 hours of surgery unless another indication exists. Review the need for the indwelling urinary catheter daily and remove it as soon as it's no longer necessary.[1,2,4,5,6]

Equipment

Sterile indwelling catheter (latex or silicone #10 to #22 French [average adult sizes are #16 to #18 French]) ▪ syringe filled with 5 to 8 mL of sterile water ▪ fluid-impermeable pads ▪ gloves ▪ sterile gloves ▪ sterile drape ▪ sterile fenestrated drape ▪ antiseptic swabs ▪ urine receptacle ▪ single-use packet of sterile, water-soluble lubricant ▪ sterile drainage collection device ▪ intake and output record ▪ securement device or tape ▪ Optional: insertion checklist, antiseptic solution, sterile cotton-tipped applicators (or cotton balls and plastic forceps), topical anesthetic such as 2% lidocaine gel, urine specimen container, laboratory request form, gooseneck lamp or flashlight, bladder ultrasonography device, gown, mask with face shield or mask and goggles.

Prepackaged sterile disposable kits that usually contain all the necessary equipment are available. The syringes in these kits are prefilled with 10 mL of sterile water

Implementation

- Verify the practitioner's order.
- Check the patient's medical record for allergies, including to latex and iodine.[8]
- Gather the appropriate equipment. Use the smallest bore catheter possible that will support adequate urine drainage (unless otherwise clinically indicated) *to minimize bladder neck and urethral trauma.*[4,9,10]
- Obtain the assistance of a coworker to help with patient positioning; provide a light source, as needed; make sure that sterile technique is maintained during insertion.

■ Use an insertion checklist if available in your facility *to guide the insertion process.*[11]
■ Perform hand hygiene.[2,12,13,14,15,16,17]
■ Confirm the patient's identity using at least two patient identifiers.[18]
■ Provide privacy.[19,20]
■ Explain the procedure to the patient; explain the reason for catheterization and what to expect in the way of discomfort.[12] Discuss the risks associated with indwelling urinary catheter use and the necessary measures to reduce the risk of CAUTI. Advise the patient and family to remind staff members to perform hand hygiene before and after handling the catheter if they fail to do so.[11]
■ Put on personal protective equipment, as needed, *to comply with standard precautions.*[21,22]
■ Assess the patient to make sure that an indwelling urinary catheter is indicated; assess for alternatives to indwelling urinary catheter use.[23] If necessary, use bladder ultrasonography to measure the volume of urine in the patient's bladder *to avoid unnecessary catheterization.*[2]

For a female patient

■ Place the patient in the supine or lithotomy position with her knees bent and legs abducted *to allow visualization of the urinary meatus.*[12] Alternatively, position the patient on her side in a knee-chest position if she's unable to tolerate supine or lithotomy positioning.
■ Place a fluid-impermeable pad on the bed between the patient's legs and under her hips *to avoid soiling the linens.*
■ Wash the patient's genital area with warm water and soap. Rinse and dry thoroughly.
■ Remove and discard your gloves.
■ Perform hand hygiene.[12,13,14,15,16,17]
■ *To create the sterile field,* open the prepackaged kit or equipment tray and place it between the patient's legs. If the sterile gloves are the first item on the top of the tray, put them on.
■ Place a sterile fenestrated drape over the perineal area *to create a sterile field* (as shown below).[12] Take care not to contaminate your gloves if you have them on already.

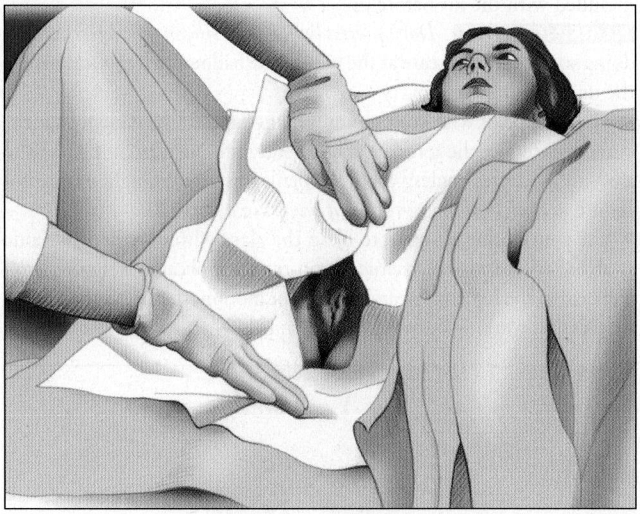

■ Open the rest of the insertion kit. Put on the sterile gloves if you haven't already done so.
■ Tear open the packet of antiseptic swabs or saturate the sterile cotton balls or applicators with antiseptic solution. Be careful not to spill the solution on the equipment.
■ Open the packet of water-soluble lubricant.[12]
■ If necessary, attach the drainage bag to the other end of the catheter. (If you're using a commercial kit, the drainage bag may already be attached.)
■ Attach the syringe filled with sterile water to the balloon inflation port. If required by the manufacturer, inflate the balloon, as directed, *to inspect for leaks.* Be aware that some manufacturers recommend not inflating the balloon before insertion *because of the risk of microtears that may cause infection;* before use, check the manufacturer's instructions included with the kit.
■ Separate the labia majora and labia minora as widely as possible with the thumb, middle, and index fingers of your nondominant hand *so you have a full view of the urinary meatus.* Keep the labia well separated throughout the procedure *so they don't obscure the urinary meatus or contaminate the area when it's cleaned.*
■ With your dominant hand, use a sterile, antiseptic swab or sterile, antiseptic-soaked, cotton-tipped applicator (or pick up a sterile cotton ball with the plastic forceps) to wipe from the meatus toward the anus in a downward stroke (as shown below). Repeat this procedure several times using a new swab or applicator with each wipe.[12]

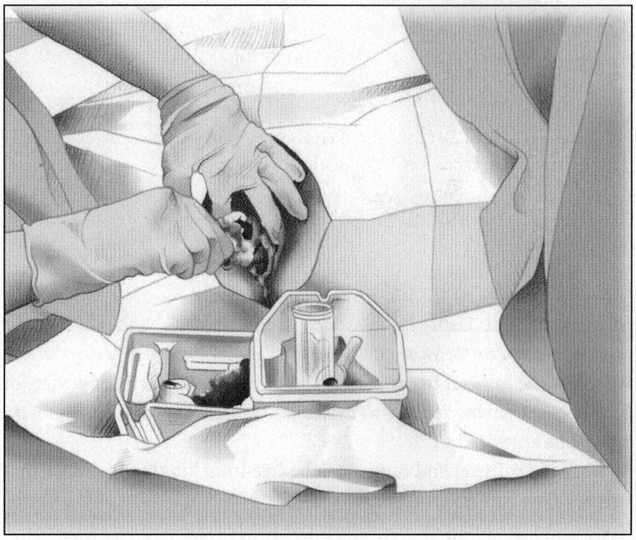

■ Maintaining sterile technique, pick up the catheter with your dominant hand and lubricate the catheter tip with the water-soluble lubricant.[12]
■ Hold the catheter 2″ to 3″ (5 to 7.5 cm) from the tip, (as shown below) and slowly insert the lubricated catheter tip into the urinary meatus; you'll typically be able to advance the catheter without meeting resistance.[12]

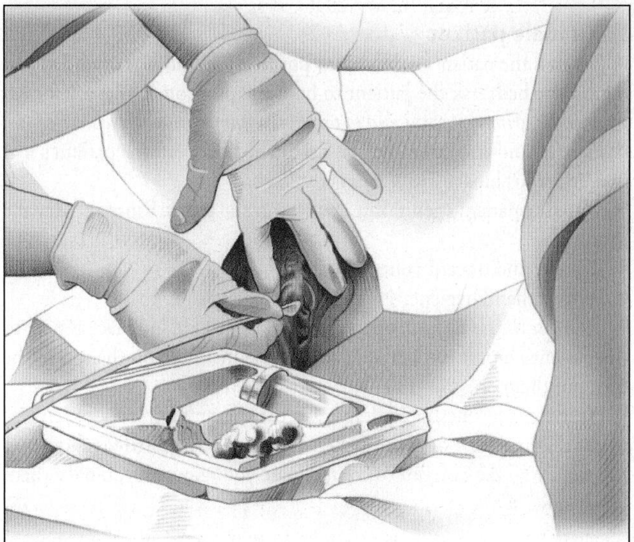

■ Continue to hold the labia apart until urine begins to flow, and advance the catheter about 2″ to 3″ (5 to 7.5 cm) further *to make sure the balloon is in the bladder and not in the urethra.*[12] If urine doesn't begin to flow, ask your coworker to apply gentle pressure to the suprapubic region, which may initiate urine flow.[24] If the catheter is inadvertently inserted into the vagina, leave it there as a landmark. Then begin the procedure over again using new supplies.

■ Inflate the balloon using the water-filled syringe (as shown below) *to secure the catheter inside the bladder.*[12]

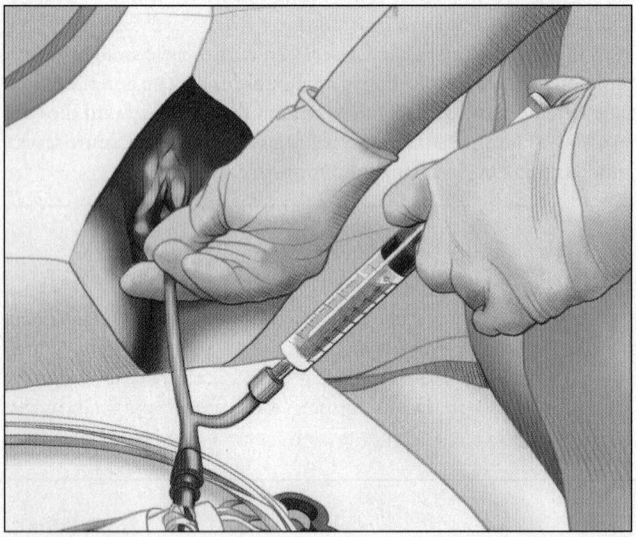

■ Secure the catheter to the patient's thigh using a securement device (or tape if a securement device isn't available) *to prevent possible tension on the urogenital trigone.*[2,12]

■ Keep the catheter and drainage tube free from kinking to ensure that urinary flow isn't obstructed.[1,2,4,6]

■ Position the drainage bag below the level of the patient's bladder *to facilitate drainage and prevent stasis of urine, which increases the risk of CAUTI.*[1,2] Don't place the drainage bag on the floor.[2]

■ Dispose of all used supplies in the appropriate receptacles.

■ Remove and discard your gloves and any other personal protective equipment worn.[22]

■ Perform hand hygiene.[2,12,13,14,15,16,17]

■ Document the procedure.[25,26,27]

For a male patient

■ Position the patient in the supine position with his legs extended and flat on the bed. Ask the patient to hold the position *to give you a clear view of the urinary meatus and to prevent contamination of the sterile field.*

■ Place a fluid-impermeable pad on the bed between the patient's legs and under his hips *to avoid soiling the linens.*

■ Wash the patient's genital area with soap and water. Rinse and dry the thoroughly.

■ Remove and discard your gloves.

■ Perform hand hygiene.[12,13,14,15,16,17]

■ *To create the sterile field,* open the prepackaged kit and place it next to the patient's hip. If the sterile gloves are the first item on the top of the tray, put them on.

■ Place a sterile fenestrated drape over the patient's lower abdomen and upper thighs so that only the genital area remains exposed (as shown on top right).[12] Take care not to contaminate your gloves if you have them on already.

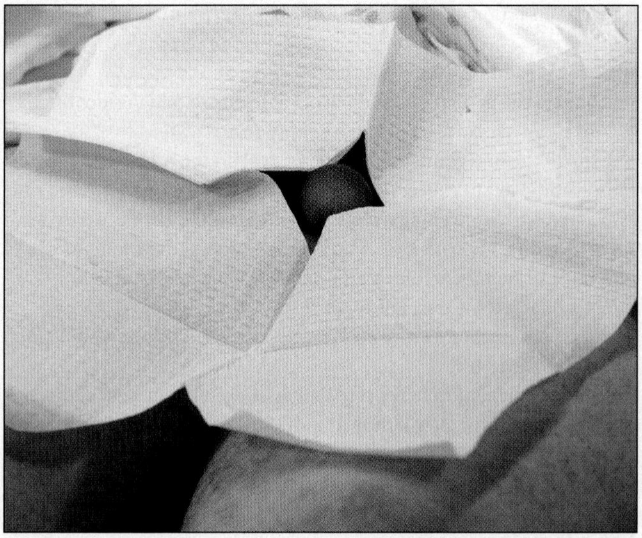

■ Open the rest of the kit or tray. Put on the sterile gloves if you haven't already done so.

■ Tear open the packet of antiseptic swabs or saturate the sterile cotton balls or cotton-tipped applicators with antiseptic solution. Be careful not to spill the solution on the equipment.

■ Open the packet of water-soluble lubricant.

■ If necessary, attach the drainage bag to the other end of the catheter, making sure that the tubing remains sterile. (If you're using a commercial kit, the drainage bag may already be connected.) Make sure the clamp at the emptying port of the drainage bag is closed *to prevent urine leakage.*

■ Attach the syringe filled with sterile water to the balloon inflation port. If required by the manufacturer, inflate the balloon, as directed, *to inspect it for leaks.* Be aware that some manufacturers recommend not inflating the balloon before insertion *because of the risk of microtears that may cause infection;* check the manufacturer's instructions included with the kit before use.

NURSING ALERT *Don't pretest balloons on silicone catheters* because doing so can cause a crease at the base of the balloon that can traumatize the urethra on insertion.

■ Hold the penis with your nondominant hand. If the patient is uncircumcised, retract the foreskin. Then gently lift and stretch the penis to a 60- to 90-degree angle.[12] Hold the penis this way throughout the procedure *to straighten the urethra and maintain a sterile field.*

■ Use your dominant hand to clean the glans with a sterile, antiseptic swab or antiseptic-soaked sterile cotton-tipped applicator or sterile cotton ball held in the forceps. Clean in a circular motion, starting at the urinary meatus and working outward (as shown below).[12]

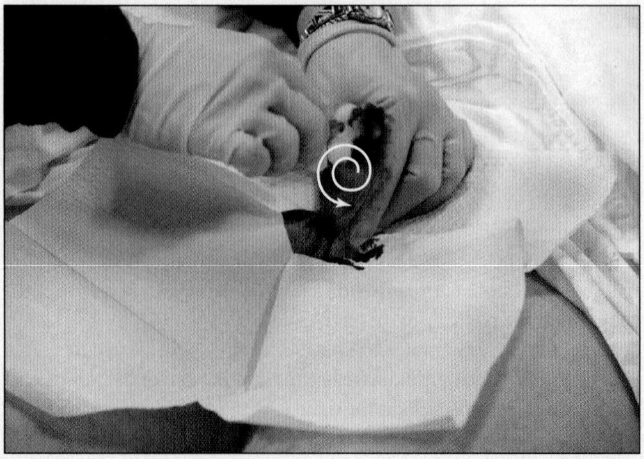

■ Repeat the procedure, using another swab, sterile applicator, or cotton ball, taking care not to contaminate your sterile glove.
■ Maintaining sterile technique, pick up the catheter with your dominant hand and lubricate the catheter tip with the water-soluble lubricant.[12]
■ Hold the catheter 2″ to 3″ (5 to 7.5 cm) from the tip, and prepare to insert the lubricated tip into the urinary meatus (as shown below). *To facilitate insertion by relaxing the sphincter,* ask the patient to cough as you insert the catheter. Tell him to breathe deeply and slowly *to further relax the sphincter and help prevent spasms.*[12]

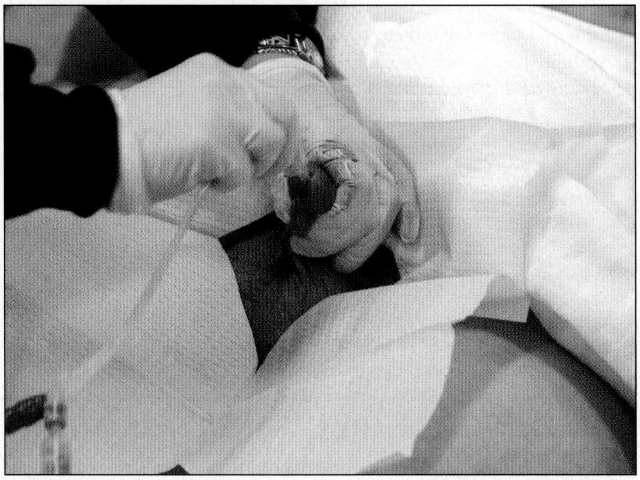

NURSING ALERT *Never force a catheter during insertion. Maneuver it gently as the patient bears down or coughs. If you still meet resistance, stop and notify the practitioner.*[12] Sphincter spasms, strictures, or an enlarged prostate can cause resistance.
■ Advance the catheter to the bifurcation and check for urine flow.[12] If urine fails to flow, ask a coworker to apply gently pressure to the suprapubic area. If the foreskin was retracted, replace it *to prevent compromised circulation and painful swelling.*
■ When urine stops flowing, inflate the balloon using the water-filled syringe attached to the inflation port *to keep the catheter in place in the bladder.*[12]
NURSING ALERT *Never inflate a balloon without first establishing urine flow,* which confirms that the catheter is in the bladder.
■ Hang the collection bag below the level of the patient's bladder *to prevent urine reflux into the bladder, which can cause CAUTI, and to facilitate gravity drainage of the bladder.*[1,2] Don't place the drainage bag on the floor.[2]
■ Secure the catheter using a catheter securement device. If a securement device isn't available, tape the catheter to the patient's abdomen or thigh *to prevent pressure on the urethra at the penoscrotal junction, which can lead to formation of urethrocutaneous fistulas.*[2,12] *Taping this way also prevents traction on the bladder and alteration in the normal direction of urine flow in males.*
■ Dispose of all used supplies in an appropriate receptacles.
■ Remove and discard your gloves and any other personal protective equipment worn.[22]
■ Perform hand hygiene.[2,12,13,14,15,16,17]
■ Document the procedure.[25,26,27]

Special considerations

■ Patients at high risk for latex hypersensitivity include those with spina bifida, spinal cord injury, atopy, certain food allergies, and occupational exposure. Provide these patients with a latex-free environment by avoiding all products containing latex proteins, including gloves, catheters, condoms, drains, and injection ports.[8]
■ In addition to hypersensitivity reactions, latex urethral catheters have been associated with an increased risk of cytotoxicity, urethritis, stricture, urinary tract infection, and encrustation. Selection of an alternative material, such as 100% silicone, reduces these risks, particularly when you anticipate long-term catheterization.[8]
■ Empty the drainage bag at least once per shift using a separate, clean collecting container for each patient; avoid splashing and prevent contact of the drainage spigot with the collecting container.[12]
■ If you need a small urine sample for laboratory examination (for culture or urinalysis), thoroughly disinfect the needleless sampling port with a disinfectant pad and allow it to dry and aspirate urine from the sampling port using a sterile adapter or syringe. If you need a large volume for special analysis (not culture), obtain the sample from the drainage bag using sterile technique.[28]
■ Monitor and record the patient's intake and output.[1]
■ Inspect the catheter and tubing periodically while they're in place *to detect compression or kinking that could obstruct urine flow.* Explain the basic principles of gravity drainage *so that the patient realizes the importance of keeping the drainage tubing and collection bag lower than the bladder at all times.*[4,6]

Patient teaching

If the patient will be discharged with a long-term indwelling catheter, teach the patient or family all aspects of daily catheter maintenance, including care of the skin and urinary meatus, signs and symptoms of urinary tract infection or obstruction, how to irrigate the catheter (if appropriate), and the importance of adequate fluid intake to maintain patency.[9]

Complications

Complications associated with indwelling urinary catheter use include CAUTI, genitourinary trauma, retained balloon fragments, bladder fistula (with prolonged use), bladder stone formation, and incontinence.[29,30]

Documentation

Document your assessment findings and the indication for catheter use. Record the date and time of insertion and the size and type of catheter used. Note the characteristics of the urine obtained. Record the patient's intake and output. Document any complications, the date and time the practitioner was notified, the prescribed interventions, and the patient's response to those interventions. Record patient teaching and the patient's comprehension of your teaching.

REFERENCES

1 Agency for Healthcare Research and Quality and U.S. Department of Health and Human Services. (2012). "On the CUSP: Stop CAUTI implementation guide" [Online]. Accessed March 2015 via the Web at http://www.onthecuspstophai.org/on-the-cuspstop-cauti/toolkits-and-resources/on-the-cusp-stop-cauti-implementation-guide/ (Level V)
2 Healthcare Infection Control Practices Advisory Committee. (2010). "Guideline for prevention of catheter-associated urinary tract infections, 2009" [Online]. Accessed March 2015 via the Web at http://www.cdc.gov/hicpac/pdf/CAUTI/CAUTIguideline2009final.pdf (Level I)
3 Jarrett, N., et al. (2013). "Evidence-based guidelines for selected and previously considered hospital-acquired conditions: Final report" [Online]. Accessed March 2015 via the Web at http://www.cms.gov/Medicare/Medicare-Fee-for-Service-Payment/HospitalAcqCond/Downloads/Evidence-Based-Guidelines.pdf
4 Lo, E., et al. (2014). SHEA/IDSA practice recommendation: Strategies to prevent catheter-associated urinary tract infections in acute care hospitals: 2014 update. *Infection Control and Hospital Epidemiology, 35,* 464–479. Accessed March 2015 via the Web at http://www.jstor.org/stable/10.1086/675718 (Level I)
5 Conway, L. J., & Larson, E. L. (2012). Guidelines to prevent catheter-associated urinary tract infection: 1980 to 2010. *Heart Lung, 41,* 271–283. Accessed March 2015 via the Web at http://www.ncbi.nlm.nih.gov/pmc/articles/PMC3362394/

6 The Joint Commission. (2015). Standard NPSG.07.06.01. *Comprehensive accreditation manual for hospitals: The official handbook.* Oakbrook Terrace, IL: The Joint Commission. (Level VII)

7 Association of Professionals in Infection Control and Epidemiology (APIC). (2014). "APIC implementation guide: Guide to preventing catheter-associated urinary tract infections" [Online]. Accessed March 2015 via the Web at http://apic.org/Resource_/EliminationGuideForm/6473ab9b-e75c-457a-8d0f-d57d32bc242b/File/APIC_CAUTI_web_0603.pdf

8 Achmetov, T., & Gray, M. (n.d.). Adverse reactions to latex in the clinical setting: A urologic perspective. *Infection Control Resource, 2*(2), 1–5. Accessed March 2015 via the Web at http://www.infectioncontrolresource.org/assets/ic6.pdf

9 Herter, R., & Kazer-Wallace, M. (2010). Best practices in urinary catheter care. *Home Healthcare Nurse, 28,* 342–349.

10 American Osteopathic Association. (2014). Standard 07.01.17. *Healthcare Facilities Accreditation Program: Accreditation requirements for acute care hospitals.* Chicago, IL: American Osteopathic Association. (Level VII)

11 Institute for Healthcare Improvement (2012). *How-to guide: Prevent catheter-associated urinary tract infections.* Cambridge, MA: Institute for Healthcare Improvement. (Level VII)

12 Society of Urologic Nurses and Associates Clinical Practice Guidelines Task Force. (2005). "Female urethral catheterization" [Online]. Accessed March 2015 via the Web at http://www.suna.org/sites/default/files/download/femaleCatheterization.pdf (Level V)

13 The Joint Commission. (2015). Standard NPSG.07.01.01. *Comprehensive accreditation manual for hospitals: The official handbook.* Oakbrook Terrace, IL: The Joint Commission. (Level VII)

14 Centers for Disease Control and Prevention. (2002). Guideline for hand hygiene in health-care settings: Recommendations of the Healthcare Infection Control Practices Advisory Committee and the HICPAC/SHEA/APIC/IDSA Hand Hygiene Task Force. *MMWR Recommendations and Reports, 51*(RR-16), 1–45. Accessed March 2015 via the Web at http://www.cdc.gov/mmwr/pdf/rr/rr5116.pdf (Level II)

15 World Health Organization. (2009). "WHO guidelines on hand hygiene in health care: First global patient safety challenge, clean care is safer care" [Online]. Accessed March 2015 via the Web at http://whqlibdoc.who.int/publications/2009/9789241597906_eng.pdf (Level IV)

16 American Osteopathic Association. (2014). Standard 07.01.21. *Healthcare Facilities Accreditation Program: Accreditation requirements for acute care hospitals.* Chicago, IL: American Osteopathic Association. (Level VII)

17 Centers for Medicare & Medicaid Services, Department of Health and Human Services. (2014). Condition of participation: Infection control. 42 C.F.R. § 482.42.

18 The Joint Commission. (2015). Standard NPSG.01.01.01. *Comprehensive accreditation manual for hospitals: The official handbook.* Oakbrook Terrace, IL: The Joint Commission. (Level VII)

19 American Osteopathic Association. (2014). Standard 15.01.16. *Healthcare Facilities Accreditation Program: Accreditation requirements for acute care hospitals.* Chicago, IL: American Osteopathic Association. (Level VII)

20 Centers for Medicare & Medicaid Services, Department of Health and Human Services. (2014). Condition of participation: Patient's rights. 42 C.F.R. § 482.13(c)(1).

21 Siegel, J. D., et al. (2007). "2007 guideline for isolation precautions: Preventing transmission of infectious agents in healthcare settings" [Online]. Accessed March 2015 via the Web at http://www.cdc.gov/hicpac/pdf/isolation/Isolation2007.pdf (Level II)

22 American Osteopathic Association. (2014). Standard 07.01.10. *Healthcare Facilities Accreditation Program: Accreditation requirements for acute care hospitals.* Chicago, IL: American Osteopathic Association. (Level VII)

23 American Association of Critical-Care Nurses. (2011). "AACN practice alert: Catheter-associated urinary tract infections" [Online]. Accessed March 2015 via the Web at http://www.aacn.org/WD/practice/docs/practicealerts/catheter-associated-uti-practice-alert.pdf (Level VII)

24 Schaeffer, A. Placement and management of urinary bladder catheters. (2014) In: *UpToDate,* Richie, J. P. (Ed.). Accessed March 2015 via the Web at http://www.uptodate.com/contents/search

25 The Joint Commission. (2015). Standard RC.01.03.01. *Comprehensive accreditation manual for hospitals: The official handbook.* Oakbrook Terrace, IL: The Joint Commission. (Level VII)

26 American Osteopathic Association. (2014). Standard 10.00.03. *Healthcare Facilities Accreditation Program: Accreditation requirements for acute care hospitals.* Chicago, IL: American Osteopathic Association. (Level VII)

27 Centers for Medicare & Medicaid Services, Department of Health and Human Services. (2014). Condition of participation: Medical record services. 42 C.F.R. § 482.24(b).

28 Society of Urologic Nurses and Associates Prevention of Catheter Associated Infection Task Force. (2010). "Clinical practice guidelines: Prevention and control of catheter-associated urinary tract infection (CAUTI)" [Online]. Accessed March 2015 via the Web at http://www.suna.org/sites/default/files/download/cautiGuideline.pdf

29 Leuck, A. M., et al. (2012). Complications of Foley catheters: Is infection the greatest risk? *Journal of Urology, 187,* 1662–1666.

30 Schaeffer, A. J. Complications of urinary bladder catheters and preventive strategies. (2014). In: *UpToDate,* Richie, J. P. (Ed.). Accessed March 2015 via the Web at http://www.uptodate.com/contents/search

ADDITIONAL REFERENCE

Nettina, S. M. (2014). *Lippincott manual of nursing practice* (10th ed.). Philadelphia, PA: Wolters Kluwer.

INDWELLING URINARY CATHETER IRRIGATION

Indwelling urinary catheter irrigation shouldn't be performed routinely. However, obstructions sometimes occur and require irrigation. To relieve an obstruction resulting from clots, mucus, or other causes, an intermittent method of irrigation may be used.[1] Whenever possible, the catheter should be irrigated through a closed system to decrease the risk for infection.[2,3] If an obstruction is anticipated, closed continuous irrigation may be used to prevent it. (See the "Continuous bladder irrigation" procedure, page 221.)

Signs and symptoms that a catheter might be obstructed include absence of urine flow from the catheter, urine flow bypassing the catheter, and suprapubic pain that becomes more pronounced as the bladder fills. If the obstruction remains unrelieved, vasovagal signs such as sweating, tachycardia, and hypotension can also occur.[4]

Before initiating catheter irrigation, a bladder scanner may be used to confirm whether a decrease in urine output results from a blockage or reduced urine in the bladder, decreasing the number of unnecessary irrigations and minimizing breaks in the closed drainage system.[5]

If an obstruction occurs and it's likely that the catheter material is contributing to obstruction, change the catheter.[2] To prevent catheter-associated urinary tract infection (CAUTI), review the need for the catheter daily, and remove the catheter as soon as it's no longer needed.[1,2,3,5,6,7]

HOSPITAL-ACQUIRED CONDITION ALERT *The Centers for Medicare & Medicaid Services has identified CAUTI as a hospital-acquired condition with payment implications* because it can be reasonably prevented using a variety of best practices. *When caring for a patient with an indwelling urinary catheter, follow CAUTI prevention practices. such as performing hand hygiene before and after any catheter manipulation; maintaining a sterile, continuously closed drainage system; maintaining unobstructed urine flow; emptying the collection bag regularly; replacing the catheter and collection system using sterile technique when breaks in sterile technique, disconnection, or leakage occur; and discontinuing the catheter as soon as it's no longer clinically indicated* to reduce the risk of CAUTI.[1,2,3,5,6,8]

Equipment

Prescribed irrigating solution (such as normal saline solution) ▪ sterile basin ▪ 30- to 60-mL syringes ▪ 18G blunt-end needle (if system isn't needleless) ▪ antiseptic pads ▪ gloves ▪ fluid-impermeable pad ▪ intake and output record ■ clamp ■ Optional: gown, mask, goggles, mask with face shield, graduated cylinder.

Commercially packaged kits containing sterile irrigating solution, a graduated receptacle, and a 50-mL catheter tip syringe may be available.

Preparation of equipment

Check the expiration date on the irrigating solution. *To prevent vesical spasms during instillation of solution,* warm it to room temperature. Never heat the solution on a burner or in a microwave oven; *hot irrigating solution can injure the patient's bladder.*

Implementation

- Verify the practitioner's order.
- Gather and prepare the appropriate equipment.
- Perform hand hygiene.[9,10,11,12,13]
- Confirm the patient's identity using at least two patient identifiers.[14]
- Explain the procedure to the patient, and provide privacy.[15,16]
- Perform hand hygiene.[2,3,9,10,11,12,13]
- Put on gloves and other protective equipment, as needed.[17]
- Empty the catheter drainage bag. Measure the amount of urine, noting the color and characteristics of the urine.
- Expose the catheter's aspiration port and place a fluid-impermeable pad under it *to protect the bed linens.*
- Clamp the catheter tubing below the aspiration port (as shown below).

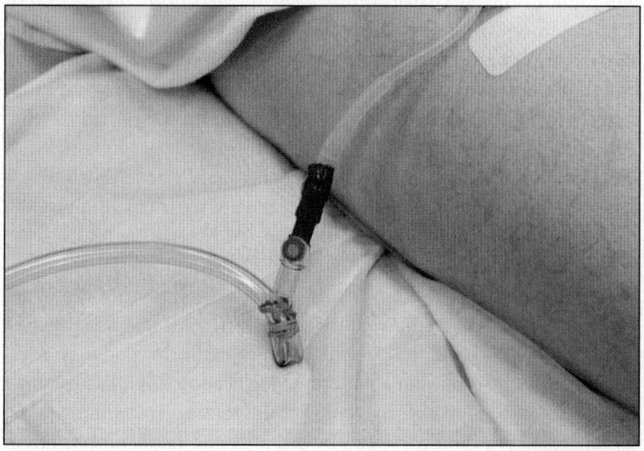

- Create a sterile field at the patient's bedside.
- Using sterile technique, pour the prescribed amount of solution into the basin.
- Place the tip of the syringe into the solution and fill the syringe with the appropriate amount (as shown below).

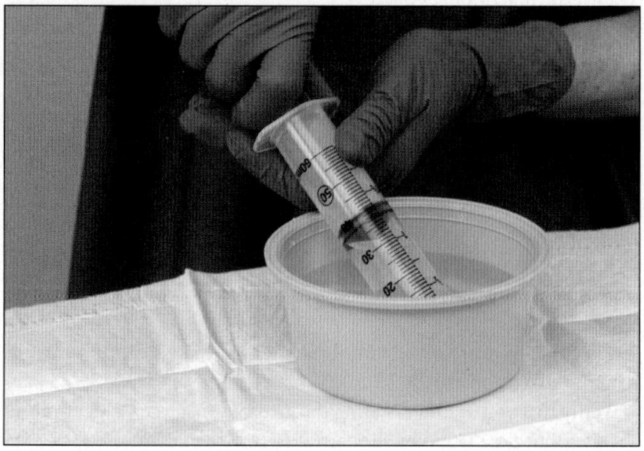

- Thoroughly disinfect the aspiration port with an antiseptic pad (as shown below) and then allow it to dry *to remove as many bacterial contaminants as possible.*

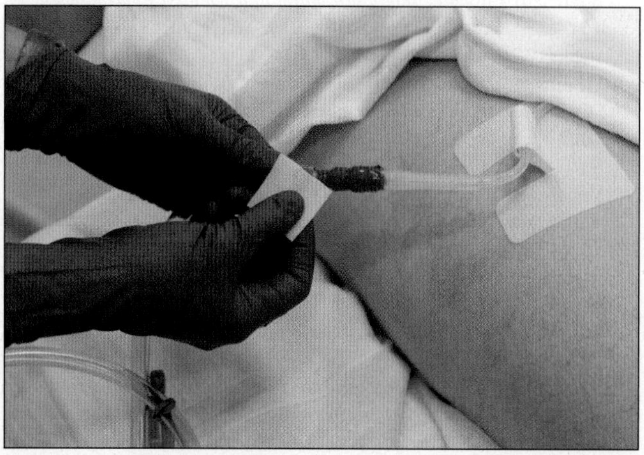

- Maintaining sterility of the syringe tip, attach the syringe to the aspiration port, or insert the blunt-tip needle into the port if a needleless system isn't in place.
- Instill the irrigating solution into the catheter. If necessary, refill the syringe and repeat this step until you've instilled the prescribed amount of irrigating solution.
- Remove the syringe and unclamp the drainage tube *to allow the irrigant and urine to flow into the drainage bags.*
- Make sure the catheter tubing is secured to the patient's leg and free from kinking and that the drainage bag is below the level of the bladder *to reduce the risk of CAUTI.*[2,3,6]
- Dispose of all used supplies in the appropriate receptacle.
- Remove your gloves and any other personal protective equipment worn.[2,17]
- Perform hand hygiene.[9,10,11,12,13]
- Document the procedure.[18,19,20]

Special considerations

- If you encounter any resistance during instillation of the irrigating solution, don't try to force the solution into the bladder. Instead, stop the procedure and notify the practitioner. If an indwelling catheter becomes totally obstructed, obtain an order to remove it and replace it with a new one *to prevent bladder distention, acute renal failure, urinary stasis, and subsequent infection.*
- Use caution if the patient has had open bladder surgery or renal transplantation *because increased pressure on the suture lines can result in suture line disruption and extravasation of urine.*[4]
- Encourage catheterized patients who aren't on restricted fluid intake to increase intake to 30 mL/kg/day *to help flush the urinary system and reduce sediment formation.*[3]

Complications

CAUTI is a complication associated with indwelling urinary catheter irrigation.

Documentation

Document the date and time the irrigation was performed as well as the type and volume of irrigant instilled. Note the amount, color, and consistency of return urine flow, and document the patient's tolerance of the procedure. Also note any resistance during instillation of the solution. If the return flow volume is less than the amount of solution instilled, note this on the intake and output record and in your notes.

References

1 Lo, E., et al. (2014). SHEA/IDSA practice recommendation: Strategies to prevent catheter-associated urinary tract infections in acute care hospitals: 2014 update. *Infection Control and Hospital Epidemiology, 35,* 464–479. Accessed March 2015 via the Web at http://www.jstor.org/stable/10.1086/675718 (Level I)

2 Healthcare Infection Control Practices Advisory Committee. (2010). "Guideline for prevention of catheter-associated urinary tract infections, 2009" [Online]. Accessed March 2015 via the Web at http://www.cdc.gov/hicpac/pdf/CAUTI/CAUTIguideline2009final.pdf (Level I)

3 Society of Urologic Nurses and Associates Clinical Practice Guidelines Task Force. (2006). Care of the patient with an indwelling catheter. *Urologic Nursing, 26,* 80–81. (Level I)

4 McLeod, P., & McDonald, C. (2008, revised 2012). "Bladder irrigation guidelines" [Online]. Accessed March 2015 via the Web at http://www.aci.health.nsw.gov.au/__data/assets/pdf_file/0007/165589/Bladder-Irrigation-Toolkit.pdf

5 Association of Professionals in Infection Control and Epidemiology. (2014). "APIC implementation guide: Guide to preventing catheter-associated urinary tract infections" [Online]. Accessed March 2015 via the Web at http://apic.org/Resource_/EliminationGuideForm/6473ab9b-e75c-457a-8d0f-d57d32bc242b/File/APIC_CAUTI_web_0603.pdf

6 The Joint Commission. (2015). Standard NPSG.07.06.01. *Comprehensive accreditation manual for hospitals: The official handbook.* Oakbrook Terrace, IL: The Joint Commission. (Level VII)

7 Herter, R., & Kazer, M. W. (2010). Best practices in urinary catheter care. *Home Healthcare Nurse, 28,* 342–349.

8 Jarrett, N., et al. (2013). "Evidence-based guidelines for selected and previously considered hospital-acquired conditions: Final report" [Online]. Accessed March 2015 via the Web at http://www.cms.gov/Medicare/Medicare-Fee-for-Service-Payment/HospitalAcqCond/Downloads/Evidence-Based-Guidelines.pdf

9 The Joint Commission. (2015). Standard NPSG.07.01.01. *Comprehensive accreditation manual for hospitals: The official handbook.* Oakbrook Terrace, IL: The Joint Commission. (Level VII)

10 Centers for Disease Control and Prevention. (2002). Guideline for hand hygiene in health-care settings: Recommendations of the Healthcare Infection Control Practices Advisory Committee and the HICPAC/SHEA/APIC/IDSA Hand Hygiene Task Force. *MMWR Recommendations and Reports, 51*(RR-16), 1–45. Accessed March 2015 via the Web at http://www.cdc.gov/mmwr/pdf/rr/rr5116.pdf (Level II)

11 World Health Organization. (2009). "WHO guidelines on hand hygiene in health care: First global patient safety challenge, clean care is safer care" [Online]. Accessed March 2015 via the Web at http://whqlibdoc.who.int/publications/2009/9789241597906_eng.pdf (Level IV)

12 American Osteopathic Association. (2014). Standard 07.01.21. *Healthcare Facilities Accreditation Program: Accreditation requirements for acute care hospitals.* Chicago, IL: American Osteopathic Association. (Level VII)

13 Centers for Medicare & Medicaid Services, Department of Health and Human Services. (2014). Condition of participation: Infection control. 42 C.F.R. § 482.42.

14 The Joint Commission. (2015). Standard NPSG.01.01.01. *Comprehensive accreditation manual for hospitals: The official handbook.* Oakbrook Terrace, IL: The Joint Commission. (Level VII)

15 American Osteopathic Association. (2014). Standard 15.01.16. *Healthcare Facilities Accreditation Program: Accreditation requirements for acute care hospitals.* Chicago, IL: American Osteopathic Association. (Level VII)

16 Centers for Medicare & Medicaid Services, Department of Health and Human Services. (2014). Condition of participation: Patient's rights. 42 C.F.R. § 482.13(c)(1).

17 American Osteopathic Association. (2014). Standard 07.01.10. *Healthcare Facilities Accreditation Program: Accreditation requirements for acute care hospitals.* Chicago, IL: American Osteopathic Association. (Level VII)

18 The Joint Commission. (2015). Standard RC.01.03.01. *Comprehensive accreditation manual for hospitals: The official handbook.* Oakbrook Terrace, IL: The Joint Commission. (Level VII)

19 American Osteopathic Association. (2014). Standard 10.00.03. *Healthcare Facilities Accreditation Program: Accreditation requirements for acute care hospitals.* Chicago, IL: American Osteopathic Association. (Level VII)

20 Centers for Medicare & Medicaid Services, Department of Health and Human Services. (2014). Condition of participation: Medical record services. 42 C.F.R. § 482.24(b).

Additional Reference

Nettina, S. M. (2014). *Lippincott manual of nursing practice* (10th ed.). Philadelphia, PA: Wolters Kluwer.

Intermittent Infusion Device Drug Administration

An intermittent infusion device, or *saline lock,* eliminates the need for multiple venipunctures or maintaining venous access with a continuous IV infusion. This device allows intermittent administration by infusion or by the IV bolus injection method.

When administering IV fluids to older adults, keep in mind that these patients commonly have compromised cardiac, hepatic, or renal systems, placing them at risk during IV fluid administration. Administering an infusion too rapidly or in a greater volume than appropriate may result in heart failure, shock, or cardiac arrest. Older patients in particular may be unable to articulate symptoms because of such underlying conditions as stroke, intubation, tracheostomy, dementia, or delirium; monitor these patients closely during all IV infusions. Speed shock may also result from rapid administration of a bolus medication or an infusion. Symptoms of speed shock, such as dizziness and headache, occur rapidly, which may make it difficult for the patient to articulate such symptoms. These early symptoms may progress to chest tightness, hypotension, irregular pulse, and anaphylactic shock. Close observation and careful control of medication or solutions administered parentally to older adults is crucial.[1]

Equipment

Patient's medication record ■ gloves ■ antiseptic pads (alcohol, tincture of iodine, or chlorhexidine) ■ 10-mL syringes prefilled with preservative-free normal saline solution ■ prescribed medication in an IV container (for IV infusion) or in a syringe (for IV bolus injection) ■ administration set ■ needleless connector ■ watch with a second hand ■ intermittent infusion device, 10-mL syringe prefilled with dextrose 5% in water.

Implementation

- Avoid distractions and interruptions when preparing and administering medications *to prevent medication errors.*[2,3]
- Verify the order in the patient's medication record by checking it against the practitioner's order.[1,4,5,6,7,8]
- Compare the medication label with the order in the patient's medical record.[5,6,8]
- Check the patient's medication record for an allergy or other contraindication to the prescribed medication. If an allergy or other contraindication exists, don't administer the medication; instead, notify the practitioner.[1,4,7,8,9]
- Check the expiration date on the medication. If it has expired, return the medication to the pharmacy and obtain a new medication.[5,7,8,9]
- Visually inspect the medication for particles, discoloration, or any other loss of integrity; don't administer the medication if its integrity is compromised.[1,4,5,7,8,9]
- Discuss any unresolved concerns about the medication with the patient's practitioner.[8]
- Verify that you're administering the medication at the proper time, in the prescribed dose, and by the correct route *to reduce the risk of medication errors.*[5,8,9]

- Perform hand hygiene.[10,11,12,13,14,15]
- Confirm the patient's identity using at least two patient identifiers.[16]
- Explain the procedure to the patient. If the patient is receiving the medication for the first time, teach him about potential adverse reactions and discuss any other concerns related to the medication.[8]
- Put on gloves.[17,18,19]
- Prepare the medication and administration set: For an IV infusion, remove the protective cover of the administration set's spike and the infusion container, insert the spike into the infusion container, attach a needleless connector to the opposite end of the administration set tubing, and then prime the tubing and needleless connector.[1,4] For an IV bolus injection, attach a needleless connector to the syringe containing the prescribed medication and prime the needleless connector.[1,4]
- Assess the IV site *to ensure that it's free from signs and symptoms of infection (tenderness, erythema, and induration within 2 cm of the insertion site, and purulence at the exit site), phlebitis (tenderness at the site, erythema, warmth, swelling, induration, purulent drainage, and palpable venous cord), and infiltration (blanching, bruising, or redness around the insertion site; edema in any direction from the insertion site; skin temperature changes; pain, burning, or stinging with injection or infusion; blisters; impaired mobility; numbness or tingling; slowed capillary refill; and fluid leaking from the insertion site).*[1,4,20]
- If your facility uses a bar code scanning system, scan your identification badge, the patient's identification bracelet, and the medication's bar code.
- Thoroughly disinfect the needleless connector of the intermittent infusion device with an antiseptic pad using friction, and allow it to dry.[1,4,21,22]
- Maintaining sterility of the syringe tip, attach a prefilled syringe containing preservative-free normal saline solution to the intermittent infusion device's needleless connector.[1,4,5,23]
- Open the intermittent infusion device clamp, if present.[1,4]
- Slowly aspirate for blood return *to verify the patency of the device.*[1,4]
- Slowly inject preservative-free normal saline solution into the intermittent infusion device, noting any resistance; stop the injection if you meet resistance, and assess the device. Insert a new intermittent infusion device at another location, if needed.[1,4]
- Remove and discard the syringe.[1,4]
- Thoroughly disinfect the needleless connector with an antiseptic pad using friction, and allow it to dry.[1,4,21,22]

Administering an IV bolus injection

- Attach the syringe containing the prescribed medication to the needleless connector of the intermittent infusion device.[1,4]
- Administer the medication at the rate indicated on the medication label; consult with the pharmacist if the rate isn't specified.[1,4]
- Remove and discard the syringe.[1,4]

Administering an IV drug infusion

- Remove the protective cover from the distal end of the administration set tubing.[1,4]
- Connect the administration set tubing to the intermittent infusion device's needleless connector.[1,4]
- Slowly open the clamp of the administration set tubing, and adjust the flow rate to begin the infusion. Alternatively, turn on the electronic infusion device and begin the infusion at the prescribed flow rate.[1,4]
- If using a gravity-flow administration set, monitor the drops per minute by counting the drops; if using an electronic infusion pump, watch the device display for 1 to 2 minutes *to ensure the proper administration rate.*[1,4]
- When the infusion is complete, clamp the administration set tubing and disconnect the tubing from the intermittent infusion device.

Completing the procedure

- Thoroughly disinfect the needleless connector with an antiseptic pad using friction, and allow it to dry.[1,4,21,22]
- Maintaining sterility of the syringe tip, attach a prefilled syringe containing preservative-free normal saline solution to the intermittent infusion device's needleless connector.[1,4,23,24]
- Slowly aspirate for blood return *to verify the patency of the device.*[1,4]
- Slowly inject preservative-free normal saline solution into the intermittent infusion device.[1,4]
- Follow a clamping sequence *to reduce blood reflux* based on the type of needleless connector: For a positive-pressure needleless connector, clamp the catheter after disconnecting the syringe;[1,4] for a negative-pressure needleless connector, maintain pressure on the syringe while clamping the catheter;[1,4] and for a neutral needleless connector, clamp the catheter before or after disconnecting the syringe.[1,4]
- Dispose of used equipment in the appropriate receptacle.[17,18,25]
- Remove and discard your gloves.[17,18,25]
- Perform hand hygiene.[10,11,12,13,14,15]
- Document the procedure.[26,27,28,29]

Special considerations

- Before administering an injectable drug, make sure you know the prescribed infusion rate and infusion time period.[5,8]
- You'll typically flush an intermittent infusion device with preservative-free normal saline solution. However, when the medication to be infused is incompatible with preservative-free normal saline solution, flush the device with dextrose 5% in water instead; after medication administration, flush with dextrose 5% in water and then follow by flushing with preservative-free normal saline solution.[23]

Patient teaching

Teach the patient about the medication, including its purpose and its potential adverse effects.

Complications

Infiltration, infection, phlebitis, and reactions specific to the infused medication are the most common complications.

Documentation

Document the type, concentration, dosage, and volume of drug administered and the times of administration. On the intake record, record the type and volume of all IV solutions used to dilute the medication and to flush the line.

References

1 Infusion Nurses Society. (2013). *Policies and procedures for infusion nursing of the older adult* (2nd ed.). Boston, MA: Infusion Nurses Society.

2 Westbrook, J., et al. (2010). Association of interruptions with an increased risk and severity of medication administration errors. *Archives of Internal Medicine, 170,* 683–690. (Level IV)

3 Institute for Safe Medication Practices. (2013). Side tracks on the safety express: Interruptions lead to errors and unfinished...Wait, what was I doing? *Nurse Advise-ERR,* 11(2), 1–4. Accessed March 2015 via the Web at https://www.ismp.org/Newsletters/acutecare/showarticle.aspx?id=37

4 Infusion Nurses Society. (2011). *Policies and procedures for infusion nursing* (4th ed.). Boston, MA: Infusion Nurses Society.

5 Standard 61. Parenteral medication and solution administration. Infusion nursing standards of practice. (2011). *Journal of Infusion Nursing, 34,* S86–S87. (Level VII)

6 Centers for Medicare & Medicaid Services, Department of Health and Human Services. (2014). Condition of participation: Pharmaceutical services. 42 C.F.R. § 482.25.

7 American Osteopathic Association. (2012). Standard 16.01.03. *Healthcare Facilities Accreditation Program: Accreditation standards for acute care hospitals.* Chicago, IL: American Osteopathic Association. (Level VII)
8 The Joint Commission. (2015). Standard MM.06.01.01. *Comprehensive accreditation manual for hospitals: The official handbook.* Oakbrook Terrace, IL: The Joint Commission. (Level VII)
9 Centers for Medicare & Medicaid Services, Department of Health and Human Services. (2013). Condition of participation: Nursing services. 42 C.F.R. § 482.23(c).
10 Centers for Disease Control and Prevention. (2002). Guideline for hand hygiene in health-care settings: Recommendations of the Healthcare Infection Control Practices Advisory Committee and the HICPAC/SHEA/APIC/IDSA Hand Hygiene Task Force. *MMWR Recommendations and Reports, 51*(RR-16), 1–45. Accessed March 2015 via the Web at http://www.cdc.gov/mmwr/pdf/rr/rr5116.pdf (Level II)
11 The Joint Commission. (2015). Standard NPSG.07.01.01. *Comprehensive accreditation manual for hospitals: The official handbook.* Oakbrook Terrace, IL: The Joint Commission. (Level VII)
12 Standard 19. Hand hygiene. Infusion nursing standards of practice. (2011). *Journal of Infusion Nursing, 34,* S26–S27. (Level VII)
13 World Health Organization. (2009). "WHO guidelines on hand hygiene in health care: First global patient safety challenge, clean care is safer care" [Online]. Accessed March 2015 via the Web at http://whqlibdoc.who.int/publications/2009/9789241597906_eng.pdf (Level IV)
14 Centers for Disease Control and Prevention. (2011). "Guidelines for the prevention of intravascular catheter-related infections" [Online]. Accessed March 2015 via the Web at http://www.cdc.gov/hicpac/pdf/guidelines/bsi-guidelines-2011.pdf (Level I)
15 American Osteopathic Association. (2012). Standard 07.01.21. *Healthcare Facilities Accreditation Program: Accreditation standards for acute care hospitals.* Chicago, IL: American Osteopathic Association. (Level VII)
16 The Joint Commission. (2015). Standard NPSG.01.01.01. *Comprehensive accreditation manual for hospitals: The official handbook.* Oakbrook Terrace, IL: The Joint Commission. (Level VII)
17 Occupational Safety and Health Administration. (n.d.). "Bloodborne pathogens, standard number 1910.1030" [Online]. Accessed March 2015 via the Web at http://www.osha.gov/pls/oshaweb/owadisp.show_document?p_table=STANDARDS&p_id=10051 (Level VII)
18 Siegel, J. D., et al. (2007). "2007 guideline for isolation precautions: Preventing transmission of infectious agents in healthcare settings" [Online]. Accessed March 2015 via the Web at http://www.cdc.gov/hicpac/pdf/isolation/Isolation2007.pdf (Level II)
19 American Osteopathic Association. (2012). Standard 07.01.10. *Healthcare Facilities Accreditation Program: Accreditation standards for acute care hospitals.* Chicago, IL: American Osteopathic Association. (Level VII)
20 Standard 48. Infiltration and extravasation. Infusion nursing standards of practice. (2011). *Journal of Infusion Nursing, 34,* S66–S68. (Level VII)
21 Standard 27. Needleless connectors. Infusion nursing standards of practice. (2011). *Journal of Infusion Nursing, 34,* S32–S33. (Level VII)
22 Infusion Nurses Society. (2010). *Infusion nursing: An evidence-based approach* (3rd ed.). St. Louis, MO: Saunders.
23 Standard 45. Flushing and locking. Infusion nursing standards of practice. (2011). *Journal of Infusion Nursing, 34,* S59–S63. (Level VII)
24 Hadaway, L. (2012). Needleless connectors for IV catheters: How to avoid complications associated with various models and practices. *American Journal of Nursing, 112*(11), 32–44. Accessed March 2015 via the Web at http://www.hadawayassociates.com/Needleless_Connectors_for_IV_Catheters_23.pdf
25 Standard 22. Safe handling and disposal of sharps, hazardous materials, and hazardous waste. Infusion nursing standards of practice. (2011). *Journal of Infusion Nursing, 34,* S28–S29. (Level VII)
26 The Joint Commission. (2015). Standard RC.01.03.01. *Comprehensive accreditation manual for hospitals: The official handbook.* Oakbrook Terrace, IL: The Joint Commission. (Level VII)
27 Standard 14. Documentation. Infusion nursing standards of practice. (2011). *Journal of Infusion Nursing, 34,* S20–S21. (Level VII)
28 Centers for Medicare & Medicaid Services, Department of Health and Human Services. (2014). Condition of participation: Medical record services. 42 C.F.R. § 482.24(b).
29 American Osteopathic Association. (2012). Standard 10.00.03. *Healthcare Facilities Accreditation Program: Accreditation standards for acute care hospitals.* Chicago, IL: American Osteopathic Association. (Level VII)

ADDITIONAL REFERENCES

Nettina, S. M. (2014). *Lippincott manual of nursing practice* (10th ed.). Philadelphia, PA: Wolters Kluwer.
Taylor, C., et al. (2011). *Fundamentals of nursing: The art and science of nursing care* (7th ed.). Philadelphia, PA: Lippincott Williams & Wilkins.

INTERMITTENT INFUSION DEVICE FLUSHING AND LOCKING

An intermittent infusion device consists of an IV cannula with an injection cap attached. These devices are used to maintain venous access in patients receiving IV medications intermittently as well as in those who might need medications if an emergency situation arises.

An intermittent infusion device should be flushed before each infusion, after each infusion (to prevent the mixing of incompatible medications and solutions), and after blood sampling. The volume of flush solution required for flushing depends on the type and size of the catheter and the type of infusion therapy prescribed. A volume equal to twice the internal volume of the catheter is recommended, but a larger volume may be required after blood sampling or transfusion.[1]

Needleless systems such as the intermittent infusion device also offer benefits to health care workers. By protecting workers from needle stick and other sharps-related injuries that can expose them to bloodborne pathogens, they help meet the Occupational Safety and Health Administration's recommendation for the use of safer medical devices.[2]

Equipment

Antiseptic pads (alcohol, tincture of iodine, or chlorhexidine-based) ■ syringe with preservative-free normal saline solution ■ gloves.

Implementation

■ Verify the practitioner's order and the patient's medication administration record for time intervals for flushing the IV cannula, *which improves the duration of catheter patency.*

■ Gather the necessary equipment.

■ Perform hand hygiene.[3,4,5,6,7,8,9]

■ Confirm the patient's identity using at least two patient identifiers.[10]

■ Explain the procedure to the patient and his family.

■ Put on gloves.[2,11,12,13,14]

■ Assess the IV site *to ensure that it's free from signs of infection, infiltration, and phlebitis.* (See *Complications of IV therapy.*)

■ Thoroughly disinfect the injection cap with an antiseptic pad using friction, and then allow it to dry.[15]

■ Maintaining the sterility of the syringe tip, attach the syringe containing preservative-free normal saline solution to the injection cap. Unclamp the clamp on the T-connector tubing, if necessary.[1]

■ *Verify catheter patency* by gently pulling back the syringe plunger and aspirating for blood return.[1]

■ Slowly inject the solution into the catheter while assessing for resistance, *which may mean that the catheter is blocked or otherwise not functioning properly.*[1]

NURSING ALERT *If resistance occurs, don't continue to inject the solution. Stop and evaluate the cause.*[1]

■ Close the clamp and remove the syringe according to the type of needleless injection cap used: For a positive-pressure needleless cap, clamp after the syringe is disconnected; for a negative-pressure needleless

Complications of IV therapy

This chart details common complications of IV therapy and associated interventions.

COMPLICATION	NURSING INTERVENTION
Bacteremia, or bacteria in the blood, may result in the IV system being contaminated.	■ Don't apply compresses to the IV site *because doing so may potentiate infection.* ■ Notify the practitioner and obtain an order for antibiotics.
Bleeding, typically mild, may occur at the IV insertion site for the first 24 hours after placement.	■ Apply a gauze dressing after initial IV placement, and change the first dressing in 24 hours. ■ Limit movement of the extremity, using an arm board as necessary. ■ If bleeding increases or persists after the first 24 hours, notify the practitioner.
Infiltration—the inadvertent accumulation of medication or solution in the tissue surrounding the IV site—may be indicated by an increase in the circumference of the extremity. Treatment depends on the properties of the infiltrated medication or solution, the manufacturer's guidelines for that agent, and the severity of the infiltration.	■ When assessing the IV site, assess along the path of the catheter. ■ Measure the circumference of the extremity above the IV site, and compare serial measurements. ■ If infiltration occurs, discontinue the infusion, disconnect the administration set, and aspirate fluid from the catheter using a small syringe. Estimate the volume of fluid that escaped into the tissues (based on the infusion rate and the time of your last assessment). Notify the practitioner of the infiltration, solution or medications infusing at the time of infiltration, and the site's appearance. ■ Obtain a practitioner's order for an agent to treat infiltration if the solution was a vesicant. ■ Immediately elevate the extremity *to promote venous return;* maintain elevation for 24 to 48 hours.
Hematoma formation indicates trauma to the vessel wall or extravasation of blood into the extravascular space.	■ Apply a warm compress to the extremity *to alleviate discomfort.* ■ If signs and symptoms increase, discontinue IV use at the site.
Mechanical issues include catheter migration, breaks in the catheter or connective tubing, or the accidental catheter dislodgement.	■ Evaluate for excessive patient movement, loose tape, or too much give in the IV tubing. ■ Encourage the patient to limit movement of the extremity. ■ Place the extremity on an arm board, and securely fasten the catheter and tubing.
Nerve damage may result from trauma to an adjacent nerve during IV insertion.	■ Remove the IV catheter. ■ Insert an IV catheter at another site.
Phlebitis, or vein inflammation, typically results from mechanical irritation from catheter trauma and is an early sign of infection.	■ Assess the severity of inflammation using a standardized scale. ■ Discontinue the infusion and remove the venous access device. ■ Determine the cause. ■ Apply a warm compress to the extremity *to ease discomfort.* ■ Notify the practitioner. ■ Replace the device in the opposite extremity.

cap, maintain pressure on the syringe plunger while closing the clamp; and for a neutral needleless cap, clamp before or after syringe disconnection.[11,12]

■ Assess the IV site after any manipulation of the catheter *to check for infiltration at the cannula insertion site.*[16]

■ Dispose of the syringe in an appropriate receptacle.[2,17]

■ Remove and discard your gloves.[2,13,14,17]

■ Perform hand hygiene.[3,4,5,6,7,8,9]

■ Document the procedure.[18,19,20,21]

Special considerations

■ If the patient reports a burning sensation during injection of the flush solution, stop the injection and check cannula placement. If the cannula is in the vein, inject the flush at a slower rate *to minimize irritation.*

■ Change needleless connectors no more frequently than every 72 hours or according to manufacturers' recommendations.[4]

Patient teaching

If the patient will be discharged with an intermittent infusion device and orders for intermittent IV infusions or medications, begin discharge planning with a home health nurse as early as possible. Communicate with the home health nurse about the type of catheter being used, including manufacturer and catheter size, if known; the date of insertion; dressing change and flush protocols taught at the facility; and any complications after placement.

Teach the patient and his family about hand hygiene techniques, dressing changes, device flushing, medication administration and syringe pump use (as applicable), disposal techniques for syringes, and any other relevant information about managing the intermittent infusion device.

Before discharge, demonstrate the procedure for the patient and his family, and have them perform a return demonstration. In addition, to ensure that the patient and family understand the information, have them repeat what they have learned about the most common complications of IV therapy (for example, sepsis and accidental removal), what signs to look for, and what to do if complications occur.[22]

Instruct the patient to contact the practitioner if the IV becomes dislodged, a fever develops, or the IV insertion site becomes red or swollen or oozes fluid or blood.

Complications

Complications associated with intermittent infusion device flushing and locking include mechanical issues, infiltration, extravasation, and infection.

Documentation

Record the date and time; concentration and amount of flush solution used; presence or absence of blood return and any resistance to flushing; appearance of the site (including the presence or absence of redness, swelling, drainage, tenderness, or streaking); and interventions for any complications that occurred. Also note the patient's tolerance of the procedure, any patient teaching, and patient's understanding of the teaching.

References

1 Standard 45. Flushing and locking. Infusion nursing standards of practice. (2011). *Journal of Infusion Nursing, 34,* S59–S63. (Level VII)
2 Occupational Safety and Health Administration. (n.d.). "Bloodborne pathogens, standard number 1910.1030" [Online]. Accessed March 2015 via the Web at https://www.osha.gov/pls/oshaweb/owadisp.show_document?p_id=10051&p_table=STANDARDS (Level VII)
3 The Joint Commission. (2015). Standard NPSG.07.01.01. *Comprehensive accreditation manual for hospitals: The official handbook.* Oakbrook Terrace, IL: The Joint Commission. (Level VII)
4 Centers for Disease Control and Prevention. (2011). "Guidelines for the prevention of intravascular catheter-related infections" [Online]. Accessed March 2015 via the Web at http://www.cdc.gov/hicpac/pdf/guidelines/bsi-guidelines-2011.pdf (Level I)
5 Centers for Disease Control and Prevention. (2002). Guideline for hand hygiene in health-care settings: Recommendations of the Healthcare Infection Control Practices Advisory Committee and the HICPAC/SHEA/APIC/IDSA Hand Hygiene Task Force. *MMWR Recommendations and Reports, 51*(RR-16), 1–45. Accessed March 2015 via the Web at http://www.cdc.gov/mmwr/pdf/rr/rr5116.pdf (Level II)
6 World Health Organization. (2009). "WHO guidelines on hand hygiene in health care: First global patient safety challenge, clean care is safer care" [Online]. Accessed March 2015 via the Web at http://whqlibdoc.who.int/publications/2009/9789241597906_eng.pdf (Level IV)
7 Standard 19. Hand hygiene. Infusion nursing standards of practice. (2011). *Journal of Infusion Nursing, 34,* S26–S27. (Level VII)
8 American Osteopathic Association. (2014). Standard 07.01.21. *Healthcare Facilities Accreditation Program: Accreditation requirements for acute care hospitals.* Chicago, IL: American Osteopathic Association. (Level VII)
9 Centers for Medicare & Medicaid Services, Department of Health and Human Services. (2014). Condition of participation: Infection control. 42 C.F.R. § 482.42.
10 The Joint Commission. (2015). Standard NPSG.01.01.01. *Comprehensive accreditation manual for hospitals: The official handbook.* Oakbrook Terrace, IL: The Joint Commission. (Level VII)
11 Infusion Nurses Society. (2013). *Policies and procedures for infusion nursing of the older adult* (2nd ed.). Boston, MA: Infusion Nurses Society.
12 Infusion Nurses Society. (2011). *Policies and procedures for infusion nursing* (4th ed.). Boston, MA: Infusion Nurses Society.
13 Siegel, J. D., et al. (2007). "2007 guideline for isolation precautions: Preventing transmission of infectious agents in healthcare settings" [Online]. Accessed March 2015 via the Web at http://www.cdc.gov/hicpac/pdf/isolation/Isolation2007.pdf (Level II)
14 American Osteopathic Association. (2014). Standard 07.01.10. *Healthcare Facilities Accreditation Program: Accreditation requirements for acute care hospitals.* Chicago, IL: American Osteopathic Association. (Level VII)
15 Standard 27. Needleless connectors. Infusion nursing standards of practice. (2011). *Journal of Infusion Nursing, 34,* S32–S33. (Level VII)
16 Standard 48. Infiltration and extravasation. Infusion nursing standards of practice. (2011). *Journal of Infusion Nursing, 34,* S66–S68. (Level VII)
17 Standard 22. Safe handling and disposal of sharps, hazardous materials, and hazardous waste. Infusion nursing standards of practice. (2011). *Journal of Infusion Nursing, 34,* S28–S29. (Level VII)
18 The Joint Commission. (2015). Standard RC.01.03.01. *Comprehensive accreditation manual for hospitals: The official handbook.* Oakbrook Terrace, IL: The Joint Commission. (Level VII)
19 Standard 14. Documentation. Infusion nursing standards of practice. (2011). *Journal of Infusion Nursing, 34,* S20–S21. (Level VII)
20 American Osteopathic Association. (2014). Standard 10.00.03. *Healthcare Facilities Accreditation Program: Accreditation requirements for acute care hospitals.* Chicago, IL: American Osteopathic Association. (Level VII)
21 Centers for Medicare & Medicaid Services, Department of Health and Human Services. (2014). Condition of participation: Medical record services. 42 C.F.R. § 482.24(b).
22 Standard 11. Patient education. Infusion nursing standards of practice. (2011). *Journal of Infusion Nursing, 34,* S16–S17. (Level VII)

INTERMITTENT INFUSION DEVICE INSERTION

Also called a *saline lock,* an intermittent infusion device consists of a catheter with a needleless connector attached. Filled with preservative-free normal saline solution to prevent blood clot formation, the device maintains venous access in patients who receive IV medication regularly or intermittently but who don't require continuous infusion.

An intermittent infusion device has several advantages over an IV catheter that's maintained at a moderately slow infusion rate. It minimizes the risk of fluid overload and electrolyte imbalance, cuts costs, reduces the risk of contamination by eliminating IV solution containers and administration sets, increases patient comfort and mobility, reduces patient anxiety and, if inserted in a large vein, allows collection of multiple blood samples without repeated venipuncture.

To insert an intermittent infusion device, choose a vein on the dorsal or ventral surface of the upper extremities, such as the metacarpal, cephalic, basilic, or median vein. When choosing a site, avoid areas of flexion; areas where there's pain on palpation; veins that are compromised by bruising, infiltration, phlebitis, sclerosis, or cord formation; and areas where procedures are planned. Also avoid the lateral surface of the wrist because of the risk of nerve damage. Don't use the ventral surface of the wrist because of the associated pain on insertion and the risk of nerve damage, and don't use veins on the lower extremities because of the increased risk of tissue damage, thrombophlebitis, and ulceration. You should also avoid using veins in an upper extremity on the side of the body where a patient has had lymphedema or who has undergone radiation therapy or breast surgery with axillary node dissection as well as veins in an extremity affected by stroke. If the patient has stage 4 or 5 chronic kidney disease, avoid using upper arm or forearms veins that could be used for dialysis access. Collaborate with the patient and practitioner to discuss the risks and benefits of using a vein in an affected extremity if no other options exist.[1]

Equipment

IV access device with safety shield[2] ▪ needleless connector ▪ prefilled syringe of preservative-free normal saline solution ▪ single-use tourniquet (preferably latex-free) ▪ antiseptic pads (chlorhexidine [preferred], alcohol, or tincture of iodine) ▪ antiseptic (chlorhexidine or, if a contraindication to chlorhexidine exists, tincture of iodine, povidone iodine, or alcohol) ▪ sterile gauze pad ▪ transparent semipermeable dressing ▪ catheter securement device, sterile hypoallergenic tape, or sterile surgical strips ▪ gloves ▪ Optional: warm packs, soap and water, scissors or electric clippers, prescribed local anesthetic, visualization technology, dressing label, marker, 1-mL syringe, swabs.

Implementation

■ Gather the appropriate equipment.
■ Perform hand hygiene.[3,4,5,6,7,8,9]
■ Confirm the patient's identity using at least two patient identifiers.[10]
■ Review the patient's medical records for allergies to antiseptic solutions or latex.
■ Explain the procedure to the patient *to enhance cooperation,* and describe the purpose of the intermittent infusion device. Provide the patient with information about the insertion process, expected duration of therapy, care and maintenance of the device, and signs and symptoms of complications and when to report them.[11,12]
■ Remove the intermittent infusion device from its packaging, thoroughly disinfect the injection port with an antiseptic pad using friction, and allow it to dry.[13,14]
■ Maintaining sterility of the syringe tip, attach the syringe containing preservative-free normal saline solution to the device's injection port and inject preservative-free normal saline solution to fill the tubing and needleless system device and purge the system of air *to prevent air embolism.*[15]
■ Select the insertion site. If you anticipate long-term therapy, start with a vein at the most distal site *so that you can move proximally as needed for subsequent IV insertion sites.*[11] For infusion of an irritating medication, choose a large vein distal to any nearby joint. Make sure the intended vein can accommodate the catheter.[1] If the patient is an older adult, select an area with more subcutaneous tissue and skeletal support *for better device stabilization;* keep in mind the need to conserve peripheral access for future therapy.[16]
■ Place the patient in a comfortable reclining position, leaving the arm in a dependent position *to increase venous fill of the lower arms and hands.* If the patient's skin is cold, cover his entire arm with warm packs for 5 to 10 minutes.[11]

Applying the tourniquet and dilating the vein

■ Apply a tourniquet about 4″ to 6″ (10 to 15 cm) above the intended puncture site *to dilate the vein.*
■ Check for a radial pulse. If it isn't present, release the tourniquet and reapply it with less tension *to prevent arterial occlusion.*[17]
■ Lightly palpate the vein with the index and middle fingers of your nondominant hand. Stretch the skin *to anchor the vein.* If the vein feels hard or ropelike, select another.
■ If the vein is easily palpable but not sufficiently dilated, place the extremity in a dependent position for several seconds or lightly stroke the vessel downward. If you have selected a vein in the arm or hand, tell the patient to open and close his fist several times.[16,18]
■ Release the tourniquet.[16,18]

Preparing the site

■ If the intended insertion site is visibly soiled, clean it with soap and water before applying the antiseptic solution.[11,16,18]
■ Remove excess hair, if necessary; clip the hair with scissors or electric clippers if needed.[3,11,16,18]
■ Perform hand hygiene[3,4,5,6,7] and put on gloves as needed.[11,19,21]
■ Administer a local anesthetic, if indicated and prescribed.[16,18] (See *Easing the pain of intermittent infusion device insertion.*)
■ Disinfect the site with a facility-approved antiseptic following the manufacturer's instructions: For chlorhexidine (which is preferred), apply it with an applicator using a back-and-forth scrubbing motion for at least 30 seconds and allow the area to dry.[3,11,16,18] For povidone-iodine, apply it in a concentric circle using a swab. Begin at the intended insertion site, moving outward. Allow the solution to remain on the skin for at least 2 minutes or longer if needed to dry completely.[16,18]
■ Reapply the tourniquet.
■ Use visualization technology *to locate the vein* if necessary.[11,16,18]

Easing the pain of intermittent infusion device insertion[16,18]

You can ease the pain of intermittent infusion device insertion by administering an anesthetic agent before insertion:

For anesthetic cream

■ Apply the recommended amount of anesthetic cream to the implanted port access site.
■ Cover the area with a transparent semipermeable dressing.
■ Note the time of application on the dressing with a marker.
■ After the recommended application time, remove the dressing, wipe off the cream, evaluate the
■ effectiveness of the anesthetic, and assess for any adverse reactions to the anesthetic.

For an anesthetic dermal patch

■ Apply the dermal patch to the intended access site.
■ Leave the patch on the skin for the recommended application time.
■ Remove the patch, evaluate the effectiveness of the anesthetic, and assess the site for any adverse reactions to the anesthetic patch.

For an intradermal anesthetic

■ Disinfect the skin of the intended access site with antiseptic pad and allow it to dry.
■ Withdraw 0.3 mL of injectable anesthetic into a 1-mL syringe.
■ With the needle bevel up, gently insert the needle intradermally above the intended access site.
■ Aspirate *to make sure that you didn't inadvertently insert the needle into a vessel.*
■ Inject 0.1 to 0.3 mL of the anesthetic, forming a wheal at the intended access site.
■ Remove the needle and discard the syringe in a puncture-resistant sharps container.
■ Evaluate the effectiveness of the anesthetic, and assess for any adverse reactions.

■ Using the thumb of your nondominant hand, stretch the skin taut below the puncture site *to stabilize the vein.*
■ Grasp the access cannula with your dominant hand, remove the cover, and examine the cannula tip.[11] If the edge isn't smooth, discard and replace the device.

Inserting the device

■ Tell the patient that you're about to insert the device.
■ Hold the needle bevel up and enter the skin directly over the vein at a 0- to 15-degree angle.
■ Aggressively push the needle directly through the skin and into the vein in one motion. Check the flashback chamber behind the hub for blood return, *which signifies that you've properly accessed the vein.* (You might not see a blood return in a small vein.)
■ Level the insertion device slightly by lifting the tip of the device up *to prevent puncturing the back wall of the vein with the access device.*
■ Advance the needle fully, if possible, and hold it in place.
■ Release the tourniquet and remove the stylet.
■ While stabilizing the vein with one hand, use the other to advance the catheter into the vein.
■ Attach a needleless connector and any other appropriate add-on devices primed with preservative-free normal saline solution.[16,18]

Converting an IV line to an intermittent infusion device

To convert an existing IV line into an intermittent infusion device, follow these steps:

- Prime the needleless connector with preservative-free normal saline solution.
- Clamp the IV catheter.
- Clamp the IV tubing, and then remove the administration set from the cannula hub.
- Thoroughly disinfect the catheter hub with a disinfectant pad using friction, and allow it to dry.
- Remove the protective cap from the needleless connector.
- Attach the needleless connector to the catheter hub. Rotate the device *to tighten it.*
- Thoroughly disinfect the needleless connector with an antiseptic pad using friction, and allow it to dry.
- Attach a syringe containing preservative-free normal saline solution, aspirate for a brisk blood return, and then slowly inject the normal saline solution.
- Clamp the catheter *to reduce blood reflux;* the clamping sequence depends on the type of needleless connector used: For a positive-pressure needleless port, clamp the catheter after removing the syringe; for a negative-pressure needleless port, maintain pressure on the syringe plunger while clamping the catheter; and for a neutral needleless port, clamp the device before or after disconnecting the syringe.

Needleless connectors

The photo below features three types of needleless connectors: positive-pressure (left), negative-pressure (center), and neutral (right).

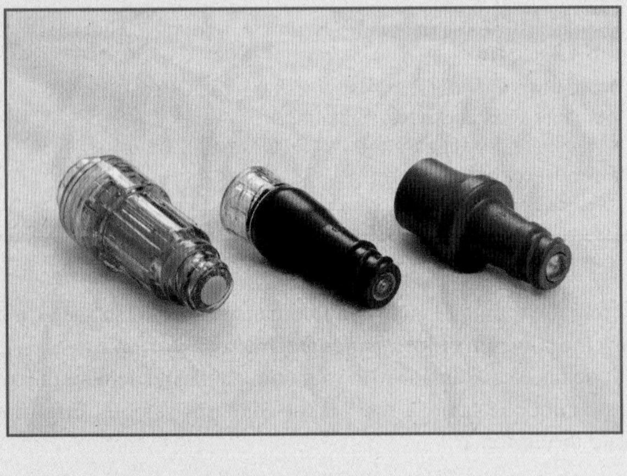

- Thoroughly disinfect the needleless connector with an antiseptic pad using friction, and then allow it to dry.[13,14]
- Attach the prefilled syringe of preservative-free normal saline solution to the needleless connector.[18,22]
- Slowly aspirate until you obtain a brisk blood return, and then slowly flush the catheter with the preservative-free normal saline solution.[18,22] Watch the site for signs of swelling or listen for patient complaints of discomfort or pain during injection; remove the device if such signs are present.
- Clamp the catheter *to reduce blood reflux*; the clamping sequence depends on the type of needleless connector used:[16,18] For a positive-pressure needleless port, clamp the catheter after removing the syringe; for a negative-pressure needleless port, maintain pressure on the syringe plunger while clamping the catheter; and for a neutral needleless port, clamp the device before or after disconnecting the syringe.
- Clean the skin surrounding the insertion site.[11]
- Secure the catheter using a catheter securement device, sterile hypoallergenic tape, or sterile surgical strips.[16,18,23]
- Apply a transparent semipermeable dressing.[3,24] If the patient has fragile skin, use a specially designed dressing *to prevent skin tearing or stripping.*[25]
- On a dressing label, write the time, the date, your initials, and the gauge and length of the catheter; place the label on the dressing.[24]
- Discard used supplies in the appropriate receptacle.[19,21,26]
- Remove and discard your gloves.[19,21,26]
- Perform hand hygiene.[3,4,5,6,7,8,9]
- Perform hand hygiene.[4,6,8,9]
- Document the procedure.[27,28,29,30]

Special considerations

- According to the Centers for Disease Control and Prevention, there's no need to replace a peripherally inserted intermittent infusion device more frequently than every 72 to 96 hours.[3,31]
- If the patient reports a burning sensation during the injection of the preservative-free normal saline solution, stop the injection and check catheter placement. If the catheter is in the vein, inject the preservative-free normal saline solution at a slower rate *to minimize irritation.* If the catheter isn't in the vein, remove and discard it; then select a new venipuncture site and, using fresh equipment, restart the procedure.[32]
- If the practitioner orders discontinuing an IV infusion and orders an intermittent infusion device in its place, convert the existing line by disconnecting the IV tubing and attach a needleless connector. (See *Converting an IV line to an intermittent infusion device.*)

Complications

Complications associated with intermittent infusion device insertion include intravascular catheter–related bloodstream infection, insertion site infection, phlebitis, infiltration, hematoma formation, and vasospasm.

Documentation

Record the date and time of insertion; the type, brand, and gauge and length of the intermittent infusion device; the local anesthetic, if used, the anatomic location of the insertion site; site preparation; whether an ultrasound device was used to guide insertion; the patient's tolerance of the procedure; the number and location of attempts; and the functionality of the device.

References

1 Standard 33. Site selection. Infusion nursing standards of practice. (2011). *Journal of Infusion Nursing, 34,* S40–S43. (Level VII)

2 Standard 32. Vascular access device selection. Infusion nursing standards of practice. (2011). *Journal of Infusion Nursing, 34,* S37–S40. (Level VII)

3 Centers for Disease Control and Prevention. (2011). "Guidelines for the prevention of intravascular catheter–related infections" [Online]. Accessed March 2015 via the Web at http://www.cdc.gov/hicpac/pdf/guidelines/bsi-guidelines-2011.pdf (Level I)

4 The Joint Commission. (2015). Standard NPSG.07.01.01. *Comprehensive accreditation manual for hospitals: The official handbook.* Oakbrook Terrace, IL: The Joint Commission. (Level VII)

5 Standard 19. Hand hygiene. Infusion nursing standards of practice. (2011). *Journal of Infusion Nursing, 34,* S26–S27. (Level VII)

6 Centers for Disease Control and Prevention. (2002). Guideline for hand hygiene in health-care settings: Recommendations of the Healthcare Infection Control Practices Advisory Committee and the HICPAC/SHEA/APIC/IDSA Hand Hygiene Task Force. *MMWR Recommendations and Reports, 51*(RR-16), 1–45. Accessed March 2015 via the Web at http://www.cdc.gov/mmwr/pdf/rr/rr5116.pdf (Level II)

7 World Health Organization. (2009). "WHO guidelines on hand hygiene in health care: First global patient safety challenge, clean care is safer care" [Online]. Accessed March 2015 via the Web at http://whqlibdoc.who.int/publications/2009/9789241597906_eng.pdf (Level IV)

8 American Osteopathic Association. (2014). Standard 07.01.21. *Healthcare Facilities Accreditation Program: Accreditation requirements for acute care hospitals.* Chicago, IL: American Osteopathic Association (Level VII)

9 Centers for Medicare & Medicaid Services, Department of Health and Human Services. (2014). Condition of participation: Infection control. 42 C.F.R. § 482.42.

10 The Joint Commission. (2015). Standard NPSG.01.01.01. *Comprehensive accreditation manual for hospitals: The official handbook.* Oakbrook Terrace, IL: The Joint Commission. (Level VII)

11 Standard 35. Vascular access site preparation and device placement. Infusion nursing standards of practice. (2011). *Journal of Infusion Nursing, 34,* S44–S46. (Level VII)

12 The Joint Commission. (2015). Standard RI.01.01.03. *Comprehensive accreditation manual for hospitals: The official handbook.* Oakbrook Terrace, IL: The Joint Commission. (Level VII)

13 Standard 27. Needleless connectors. Infusion nursing standards of practice. (2011). *Journal of Infusion Nursing, 34,* S32–S33. (Level VII)

14 Infusion Nurses Society. (2010). *Infusion nursing: An evidence-based approach* (3rd ed.). St. Louis, MO: Saunders.

14 Standard 50. Air embolism. Infusion nursing standards of practice. (2011). *Journal of Infusion Nursing, 34,* S69–S70. (Level VII)

16 Infusion Nurses Society. (2013). *Policies and procedures for infusion nursing of the older adult* (2nd ed.). Boston, MA: Infusion Nurses Society.

17 Standard 31. Tourniquets. Infusion nursing standards of practice. (2011). *Journal of Infusion Nursing, 34,* S36. (Level VII)

18 Infusion Nurses Society. (2011). *Policies and procedures for infusion nursing* (4th ed.). Boston, MA: Infusion Nurses Society.

19 Siegel, J. D., et al. (2007). "2007 guideline for isolation precautions: Preventing transmission of infectious agents in healthcare settings" [Online]. Accessed March 2015 via the Web at http://www.cdc.gov/hicpac/pdf/isolation/Isolation2007.pdf (Level II)

20 American Osteopathic Association. (2014). Standard 07.01.10. *Healthcare Facilities Accreditation Program: Accreditation requirements for acute care hospitals.* Chicago, IL: American Osteopathic Association. (Level VII)

21 Occupational Safety and Health Administration. (n.d.). "Bloodborne pathogens, standard number 1910.1030" [Online]. Accessed March 2015 via the Web at http://www.osha.gov/pls/oshaweb/owadisp.show_document?p_table=standards&p_id=10051 (Level VII)

22 Standard 45. Flushing and locking. Infusion nursing standards of practice. (2011). *Journal of Infusion Nursing, 34,* S59–S63. (Level VII)

23 Standard 36. Vascular access device stabilization. Infusion nursing standards of practice. (2011). *Journal of Infusion Nursing, 34,* S46–S47. (Level VII)

24 Standard 46. Vascular access device site care and dressing changes. Infusion nursing standards of practice. (2011). *Journal of Infusion Nursing, 34,* S63–S64. (Level VII)

25 LeBlanc, K., et al. (2013). International skin tear advisory panel: A tool kit to aid in the prevention, assessment, and treatment of skin tears using a simplified classification system. *Advances in Skin and Wound Care, 26,* 459–476. (Level IV)

26 Standard 22. Safe handling and disposal of sharps, hazardous materials, and hazardous waste. Infusion nursing standards of practice. (2011). *Journal of Infusion Nursing, 34,* S28–S29. (Level VII)

27 The Joint Commission. (2015). Standard RC.01.03.01. *Comprehensive accreditation manual for hospitals: The official handbook.* Oakbrook Terrace, IL: The Joint Commission. (Level VII)

28 Standard 14. Documentation. Infusion nursing standards of practice. (2011). *Journal of Infusion Nursing, 34,* S20–21. (Level VII)

29 American Osteopathic Association. (2014). Standard 10.00.03. *Healthcare Facilities Accreditation Program: Accreditation requirements for acute care hospitals.* Chicago, IL: American Osteopathic Association. (Level VII)

30 Centers for Medicare & Medicaid Services, Department of Health and Human Services. (2014). Condition of participation: Medical record services. 42 C.F.R. § 482.24(b).

31 Centers for Medicare & Medicaid Services, & The Joint Commission. (2014). "The specifications manual for national hospital inpatient quality measures (version 4.3)" [Online]. Accessed March 2015 via the Web at http://www.qualitynet.org/dcs/ContentServer?pagename=QnetPublic%2FPage%2FQnetTier2&cid=1141662756099

32 Standard 48. Infiltration and extravasation. Infusion nursing standards of practice. (2011). *Journal of Infusion Nursing, 34,* S66–S67. (Level VII)

ADDITIONAL REFERENCES

Nettina, S. M. (2014). *Lippincott manual of nursing practice* (10th ed.). Philadelphia, PA: Wolters Kluwer.

Taylor, C., et al. (2011). *Fundamentals of nursing: The art and science of nursing care* (7th ed.). Philadelphia, PA: Lippincott Williams & Wilkins.

INTERMITTENT POSITIVE-PRESSURE BREATHING

Intermittent positive-pressure breathing (IPPB) delivers room air or oxygen into the lungs at a pressure higher than atmospheric pressure. This delivery ceases when pressure in the mouth or in the breathing circuit tube increases to a predetermined airway pressure.

IPPB was formerly the mainstay of pulmonary therapy, with its proponents claiming that the device delivered aerosolized medications deeper into the lungs, decreased the work of breathing, and assisted in the mobilization of secretions. Studies now show that IPPB has no clinical benefit over handheld nebulizers. However, it continues to be used selectively to treat atelectasis and to promote airway clearance when patients aren't responsive to other procedures, such as incentive spirometry and chest physiotherapy.[1,2] It may also be used to augment tidal volume and reduce the work of breathing in patients who become easily fatigued and find airway clearance difficult.[2]

Equipment

IPPB machine with all necessary circuit tubing ■ mouthpiece or mask ■ source of pressurized gas at 50 psi ■ prescribed medication or normal saline solution ■ 3-mL syringe ■ sphygmomanometer ■ stethoscope ■ disinfectant pad ■ facial tissues and waste bag or specimen cup ■ warm, soapy water; sterile water; and clean plastic bag ■ Optional: suction equipment, oxygen, gloves, nose clip.

Preparation of equipment

Follow the manufacturer's instructions to set up the equipment properly. Label all medications, medication containers, and other solutions.

Implementation

- Verify the practitioner's orders.
- Gather and prepare the necessary equipment.
- Perform hand hygiene.[3,4,5,6,7]
- Put on gloves if needed *to comply with standard precautions.*[8,9]
- Confirm the patient's identity using at least two patient identifiers.[10]
- Explain the procedure to the patient *to decrease anxiety and ensure his cooperation.*
- Instruct the patient to sit erect in a chair, if possible, *to allow for optimal lung expansion.* If the patient can't sit, position him in the semi-Fowler or supine position.[2,11]
- Obtain baseline blood pressure and heart rate measurements, especially if a bronchodilator will be administered, and auscultate breath sounds *for posttreatment comparisons.*
- Instill the ordered medication or normal saline solution into the nebulizer cup.
- Turn on the IPPB machine at the appropriate settings as determined by the practitioner or respiratory therapist.
- Instruct the patient to insert the mouthpiece into his mouth and to make a tight seal with his lips.

- Instruct the patient to breathe deeply and slowly through his mouth as if sucking on a straw. Encourage the patient to let the machine do the work.
- During treatment, instruct the patient to hold his breath for a few seconds after full inspiration *to allow for greater distribution of gas and medication, if administered,* and then to exhale normally.
- During treatment, obtain the patient's blood pressure and heart rate. *IPPB treatment increases intrathoracic pressure and may temporarily decrease cardiac output and venous return, resulting in tachycardia, hypotension, and headache. Monitoring also detects reactions to the bronchodilator, if administered.* If you note a sudden change in blood pressure or increase in heart rate of 20 or more beats/minute, stop the treatment and notify the practitioner.
- If the patient is tolerating the treatment, continue until the medication or normal saline solution in the nebulizer is exhausted, usually about 10 minutes.
- After treatment and as needed, have the patient either expectorate into tissues and discard them in a waste bag or expectorate in a specimen cup; alternatively, you can suction him as necessary.
- Auscultate the patient's breath sounds, and compare the findings with the pretreatment assessment findings *to evaluate the effectiveness of therapy.*
- Shake excess moisture from the nebulizer and the mouthpiece or mask.
- After 24 hours of use, discard the equipment or clean it with warm, soapy water; rinse it with sterile water; and then air-dry it. When it's dry, store it in a clean plastic bag.[12]
- Remove and discard your gloves, if worn.[8]
- Perform hand hygiene.[3,4,5,6,7]
- Clean and disinfect your stethoscope with a disinfectant pad.
- Perform hand hygiene.[3,4,5,6,7]
- Document the procedure.[13,14,15]

Special considerations

- If possible, avoid administering IPPB treatment immediately before or after a meal *because the treatment may induce nausea and because a full stomach reduces lung expansion.*
- Never give IPPB treatment without medication or sterile saline in the nebulizer; *doing so could dry the patient's airway, making secretions more difficult to mobilize.*
- If the purpose of treatment is to mobilize secretions, ensure the patient expectorates into a specimen cup to measure the secretions obtained.
- If the patient wears dentures, leave them in place *to ensure a proper seal,* but remove them if they slide out of position.
- If the patient has an artificial airway, use a special adapter, such as mechanical ventilation tubing, to give IPPB treatments.
- When using a mask to administer treatments, allow the patient frequent rest periods, and observe for gastric distention *because this issue is more likely to occur with a mask.*
- If the patient's blood pressure is stable during the initial treatment, you may not need to check it during subsequent treatments unless he has a history of cardiovascular disease, hypotension, or sensitivity to any drug delivered in the treatment.

Patient teaching

If the patient will be using IPPB at home, provide appropriate patient teaching. Have him demonstrate the proper setup, use, and cleaning of the equipment before discharge. Tell him that he shouldn't change the pressure settings without checking with his practitioner. Suggest he avoid using IPPB immediately before or after a meal because of possible nausea and reduced lung expansion. Instruct him to discontinue treatment and call his practitioner if he experiences dizziness.

Complications

Gastric insufflation may result from swallowed air and occurs more commonly with a mask than with a mouthpiece. Dizziness can result from hyperventilation. The work of breathing can be increased, especially if the patient is uncomfortable with or frightened by the machine. Decreased blood pressure can result from decreased venous return, especially in a patient with hypovolemia or cardiovascular disease. Increased intracranial pressure can result from impeded venous return from the brain. Spontaneous pneumothorax may result from increased intrathoracic pressure; this complication is rare but is most likely to occur in patients with emphysematous blebs.

Documentation

Record the date, time, and duration of treatment; medication administered, if applicable; pressure used; vital signs; breath sounds before and after treatment; amount of sputum produced; any complications and nursing actions taken; the patient's tolerance of the procedure; and any patient teaching provided.

References

1 American Association for Respiratory Care. (1993, revised 2003). AARC clinical practice guideline: Intermittent positive pressure breathing—2003 revision & update. *Respiratory Care, 48,* 540–546. Accessed March 2015 via the Web at http://rc.rcjournal.com/content/48/5/540.full.pdf (Level VII)

2 Bott, J., et al. (2009). Guidelines for the physiotherapy management of the adult, medical, spontaneously breathing patient. *Thorax, 64,* i1–i51. Accessed March 2015 via the Web at http://thorax.bmj.com/content/64/Suppl_1/i1.full.pdf+html (Level I)

3 The Joint Commission. (2015). Standard NPSG.07.01.01. *Comprehensive accreditation manual for hospitals: The official handbook.* Oakbrook Terrace, IL: The Joint Commission. (Level VII)

4 Centers for Disease Control and Prevention. (2002). Guideline for hand hygiene in health-care settings: Recommendations of the Healthcare Infection Control Practices Advisory Committee and the HICPAC/SHEA/APIC/IDSA Hand Hygiene Task Force. *MMWR Recommendations and Reports,* 51(RR-16), 1–45. Accessed March 2015 via the Web at http://www.cdc.gov/mmwr/pdf/rr/rr5116.pdf (Level II)

5 World Health Organization. (2009). "WHO guidelines on hand hygiene in health care: First global patient safety challenge, clean care is safer care" [Online]. Accessed March 2015 via the Web at http://whqlibdoc.who.int/publications/2009/9789241597906_eng.pdf (Level IV)

6 American Osteopathic Association. (2014). Standard 07.01.21. *Healthcare Facilities Accreditation Program: Accreditation requirements for acute care hospitals.* Chicago, IL: American Osteopathic Association. (Level VII)

7 Centers for Medicare & Medicaid Services, Department of Health and Human Services. (2014). Condition of participation: Infection control. 42 C.F.R. § 482.42.

8 Siegel, J. D., et al. (2007). "2007 guideline for isolation precautions: Preventing transmission of infectious agents in healthcare settings" [Online]. Accessed March 2015 via the Web at http://www.cdc.gov/hicpac/pdf/isolation/Isolation2007.pdf (Level II)

9 American Osteopathic Association. (2014). Standard 07.01.10. *Healthcare Facilities Accreditation Program: Accreditation requirements for acute care hospitals.* Chicago, IL: American Osteopathic Association. (Level VII)

10 The Joint Commission. (2015). Standard NPSG.01.01.01. *Comprehensive accreditation manual for hospitals: The official handbook.* Oakbrook Terrace, IL: The Joint Commission. (Level VII)

11 Guérin, C., et al. (2010). The short-term effects of intermittent positive pressure breathing treatments on ventilation in patients with neuromuscular disease. *Respiratory Care, 55,* 866–872. Accessed March 2015 via the Web at http://rc.rcjournal.com/content/55/7/866.full.pdf

12 American Osteopathic Association. (2014). Standard 07.02.03. *Healthcare Facilities Accreditation Program: Accreditation requirements for acute care hospitals.* Chicago, IL: American Osteopathic Association. (Level VII)

13 The Joint Commission. (2015). Standard RC.01.03.01. *Comprehensive accreditation manual for hospitals: The official handbook.* Oakbrook Terrace, IL: The Joint Commission. (Level VII)
14 American Osteopathic Association. (2014). Standard 10.00.03. *Healthcare Facilities Accreditation Program: Accreditation requirements for acute care hospitals.* Chicago, IL: American Osteopathic Association. (Level VII)
15 Centers for Medicare & Medicaid Services, Department of Health and Human Services. (2014). Condition of participation: Medical record services. 42 C.F.R. § 482.24(b).

ADDITIONAL REFERENCES

Nettina, S. M. (2014). *Lippincott manual of nursing practice* (10th ed.). Philadelphia, PA: Wolters Kluwer.
Taylor, C., et al. (2015). *Fundamentals of nursing: The art and science of nursing care* (8th ed.). Philadelphia, PA: Wolters Kluwer.

INTERMITTENT URINARY CATHETERIZATION

Intermittent (straight) urinary catheter insertion involves inserting a temporary catheter into the bladder to drain urine. In contrast with an indwelling urinary catheter, an intermittent catheter is removed as soon as the urine is drained. It's a preferred alternative to indwelling urinary catheter insertion for managing patients with neurogenic bladder and urinary retention because it's associated with lower infection rates than indwelling urinary catheterization.[1,2,3,4]

Intermittent urinary catheterization has been used in patients with spinal cord injury, spinal tumors, diabetic neuropathy, multiple sclerosis, spina bifida, myelodysplasia, bladder outlet obstruction, and continent urinary diversion. It's also been used to manage incontinence and postoperative urinary retention as well as to collect urine samples for culture and sensitivity.

Intermittent urinary catheterization is used long-term or short-term, depending on the patient's condition. When used routinely, it should be performed at regular intervals throughout the day according to the patient's fluid intake to prevent bladder overdistention.[2]

In the health care facility, use sterile or clean technique for insertion, as required your facility. At home, the patient may use clean technique without increasing the risk for a urinary tract infection.[4]

Equipment

Sterile urethral catheter (#10 to #22 French) ▪ washcloth ▪ towel ▪ soap and water ▪ gloves ▪ two fluid-impermeable pads ▪ sterile gloves ▪ sterile drape ▪ sterile fenestrated drape ▪ antiseptic swabs ▪ urine drainage receptacle ▪ sterile water-soluble lubricant ▪ intake and output record ▪ Optional: antiseptic cleaning agent; sterile cotton-tipped applicators or cotton balls and plastic forceps; urine specimen container, laboratory request form, and biohazard transport bag; gooseneck lamp or flashlight; ultrasonography bladder scanner; catheter storage container; topical anesthetic.

Prepackaged sterile disposable kits that usually contain all the necessary equipment are available.

Implementation

- Verify the practitioner's order.
- Check the patient's medical record for a history of hypersensitivity to iodine or latex.[5]
- Gather the appropriate equipment. Use the smallest catheter possible *to minimize urethral damage.*[3]

NURSING ALERT *Large-size catheters (#18 French or larger) can increase erosion of the bladder neck and urethral mucosa, cause stricture formation, and impede drainage or periurethral gland secretions.*[6]

- Perform hand hygiene.[7,8,9,10,11]
- Put on gloves, as needed, *to comply with standard precautions.*[12,13]
- Confirm the patient's identity using at least two patient identifiers.[14]
- Provide privacy.[15,16]
- Explain the procedure to the patient *to allay anxiety and promote cooperation during the procedure.*
- Check the patient's intake and output record *to see the time and amount of the last recent void*; confirm the time with the patient.
- Percuss and palpate the patient's bladder *to establish baseline data.* Ask if the patient feels the urge to void. If possible, measure the volume of urine in the bladder using bladder ultrasonography; *ultrasonography helps prevent unnecessary catheterization.*[2]
- Have a coworker hold a flashlight or place a gooseneck lamp next to the patient's bed *so that you have sufficient light to see the urinary meatus.*

For a female patient

- Place the patient in the supine position, with her knees flexed and separated and her feet flat on the bed, about 2′ (61 cm) apart. If she finds this position uncomfortable, have her flex one knee and keep the other leg flat on the bed. Or have the patient lie on her side with her knees drawn up to her chest during the catheterization procedure (as shown below). *This position may be especially helpful for elderly or disabled patients, such as those with severe contractures.*

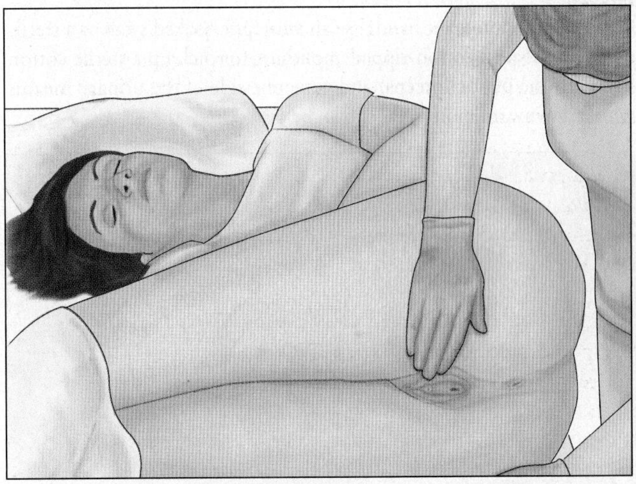

- You may need an assistant to help the patient stay in position. Ask the patient to hold her position *to give you a clear view of the urinary meatus and to prevent contamination of the sterile field.*
- Place fluid-impermeable pads on the bed between the patient's legs and under her hips *to prevent inadvertent soiling of the patient's bed linens.*
- Use warm, soapy water and a washcloth to clean the patient's genital area and perineum thoroughly. Dry the area with the towel.
- Remove and discard your gloves.[13]
- Perform hand hygiene.[7,8,9,10,11]
- *To create the sterile field,* open the prepackaged kit or equipment tray and place it at an area near the patient or between the patient's legs. If the sterile gloves are the first item on the top of the tray, put them on. Place the sterile drape under the patient's hips. Then drape the patient's lower abdomen with the sterile fenestrated drape so that only the genital area remains exposed (as shown on next page, top left). Make sure you don't contaminate your gloves if you have them on already.[3,8,17,18]
- Open the rest of the kit or tray. Put on the sterile gloves if you haven't already done so.
- Tear open the packet of antiseptic cleaning solution, and use it to saturate the sterile cotton balls or cotton-tipped applicators.
- Open the packet of water-soluble lubricant, and apply it to the catheter tip.[4]

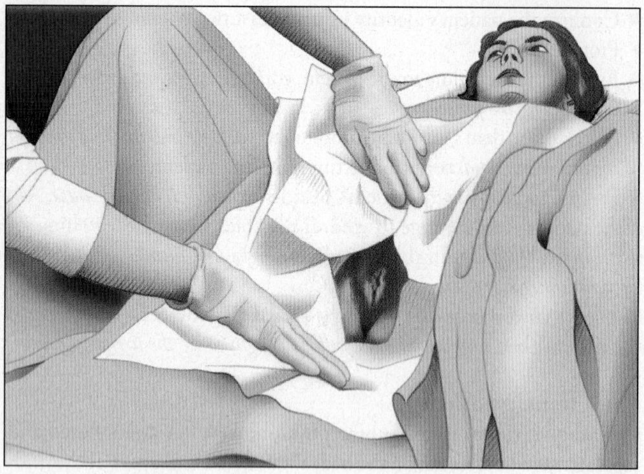

■ Separate the labia majora and labia minora as widely as possible with the thumb, middle, and index fingers of your nondominant hand *so you have a full view of the urinary meatus.* Keep the labia well separated throughout the procedure *so they don't obscure the urinary meatus or contaminate the area when it's cleaned.*

■ With your dominant hand, use an antiseptic-soaked swab or a sterile antiseptic-soaked cotton-tipped applicator (or pick up a sterile cotton ball with the plastic forceps) and wipe one side of the urinary meatus with a downward motion (as shown below).

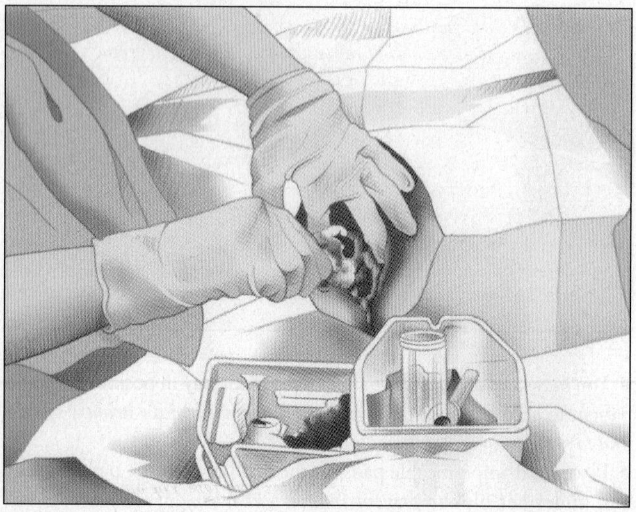

■ Wipe the other side with another sterile applicator or cotton ball using the same technique. Then wipe directly over the meatus with a third swab, sterile applicator, or cotton ball. Take care not to contaminate your sterile glove.

■ Pick up the straight catheter with your dominant hand, holding it about 2″ to 3″ (5 to 7.5 cm) from the tip, and prepare to insert the lubricated tip into the urinary meatus. *To facilitate insertion by relaxing the sphincter,* ask the patient to cough as you insert the catheter. Tell her to breathe deeply and slowly *to further relax the sphincter and reduce spasms.*[18]

NURSING ALERT ***Never force a catheter during insertion. Maneuver it gently as the patient bears down or coughs. If you still meet resistance, stop and notify the practitioner.* Sphincter spasms, strictures, or misplacement in the vagina may cause resistance.**

■ Slowly and gently advance the catheter 2″ to 4″ (5 to 10 cm) while continuing to hold the labia apart until urine begins to flow.[4] If the catheter is inadvertently inserted into the vagina, leave it there as a landmark. Then begin the procedure over again using new supplies.

■ Drain the urine into the urine receptacle.

■ Hold the catheter in place until the urine flow stops and the bladder is empty.

■ When flow has stopped, slowly remove the catheter, allowing urine to drain from the lower half of the bladder. Completely remove the catheter when there's no further urine flow.[4]

■ If the catheter is disposable, discard it in the appropriate receptacle. If it's reusable, clean the catheter with mild soap and water and store it in a clean, dry container.[4]

■ Discard all the used supplies in the appropriate receptacles.

■ Remove and discard your gloves.[12,13]

■ Perform hand hygiene.[7,8,9,10,11]

■ Document the procedure.[19,20,21]

For a male patient

■ Place the patient in the supine position with his legs extended and flat on the bed. Ask the patient to remain in that position *to give you a clear view of the urinary meatus and to prevent contamination of the sterile field.*

■ Place a fluid-impermeable pad on the bed between the patient's legs and under his hips *to prevent inadvertent soiling of bed linens.*

■ Use warm, soapy water and a washcloth to clean the patient's genital area and perineum thoroughly. Dry the area with the towel.

■ Place a new fluid-impermeable pad under the patient if the existing one is wet or soiled.

■ Remove and discard your gloves.[12,13]

■ Perform hand hygiene.[7,8,9,10,11]

■ *To create the sterile field,* open the prepackaged kit or equipment tray and place it next to the patient's hip. If the sterile gloves are the first item on the top of the tray, put them on. Place the sterile drape under the patient's hips. Then drape the patient's lower abdomen with the sterile fenestrated drape so that only the genital area remains exposed. Make sure you don't contaminate your gloves if you have them on already.[3,8,17,18]

■ Open the rest of the kit or tray.

■ Put on the sterile gloves if you haven't already done so.

■ Open a packet of antiseptic swabs or use an antiseptic cleaning agent *to saturate sterile cotton balls or cotton-tipped applicators.*

■ Open the packet of water-soluble lubricant and apply it to the catheter tip.[4]

■ Hold the penis with your nondominant hand. If the patient is uncircumcised, retract the foreskin. Then gently lift and stretch the penis to a 60- to 90-degree angle. Hold the penis this way throughout the procedure *to straighten the urethra and maintain a sterile field.*

■ Use your dominant hand to clean the glans with an antiseptic swab, antiseptic-soaked cotton-tipped applicator, or antiseptic-soaked sterile cotton ball held in the forceps. Clean in a circular motion, starting at the urinary meatus and working outward (as shown below).

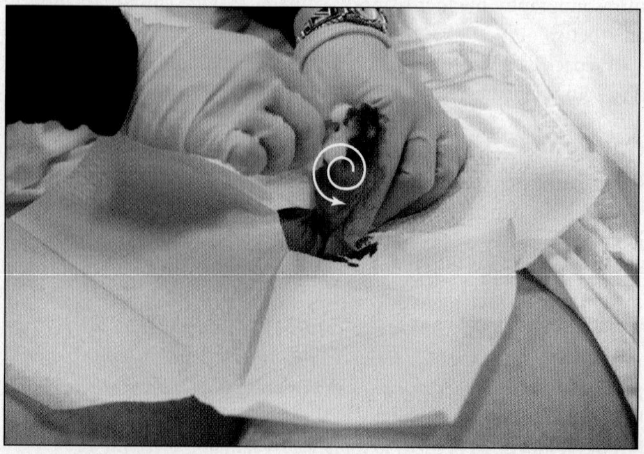

■ Repeat the procedure, using another swab or antiseptic-soaked applicator or cotton ball. Make sure that you don't contaminate your sterile glove.
■ Pick up the catheter with your dominant hand, holding it about 2″ to 3″ (5 to 7.5 cm) from the tip, and prepare to insert the lubricated tip into the urinary meatus. *To facilitate insertion by relaxing the sphincter,* ask the patient to cough as you insert the catheter. Tell him to breathe deeply and slowly *to further relax the sphincter and reduce spasms.*
■ Gently insert the catheter into the meatus, approximately 6″ to 8″ (15 to 20 cm) or until the urine begins to flow.[4]
■ As you reach the level of the prostate, you'll meet some resistance. Tell the patient to breathe deeply and slowly as you continue to advance the catheter.

NURSING ALERT *Never force a catheter during insertion. Maneuver it gently as the patient bears down or coughs. If you still meet resistance, stop and notify the practitioner.* **Sphincter spasms, strictures, or an enlarged prostate may cause resistance.**

■ If the foreskin was retracted, replace it *to prevent compromised circulation and painful swelling.*
■ Drain the urine into the urine receptacle.
■ Hold the catheter in place until the urine flow stops and the bladder is empty.
■ When urine flow has stopped, slowly remove the catheter, allowing urine to drain from the lower half of the bladder. Completely remove the catheter when there's no further urine flow.[4]
■ If the catheter is disposable, discard it in the appropriate receptacle. If it is reusable, clean the catheter with mild soap and water and store it in a clean, dry container.[4]
■ Discard all the used supplies in the appropriate receptacle.
■ Remove and discard your gloves.[12,13]
■ Perform hand hygiene.[7,8,9,10,11]
■ Document the procedure.[19,20,21]

Special considerations

■ Patients with spina bifida, spinal cord injury, atopy, certain food allergies, and occupational latex exposure are at increased risk for latex allergy. Provide these patients with a latex-free environment by avoiding all products containing latex proteins, including gloves, catheters, condoms, drains, and injection ports.[5]
■ If ordered, a topical anesthetic may be instilled directly into the urethra before catheter insertion *to prevent pain and trauma to the urethral lining.*[22]
■ Some practitioners use a syringe prefilled with water-soluble lubricant and instill the lubricant directly into the male urethra instead of on the catheter tip. A topical anesthetic gel may also be instilled into the urethra before catheter insertion. *These methods help prevent pain and trauma to the urethral lining as well as possible urinary tract infection.*[23]
■ If the practitioner orders a urine specimen for laboratory analysis, obtain it from the urine receptacle with a specimen collection container at the time of catheterization, label it in the presence of the patient *to prevent mislabeling,* and send it to the laboratory in a biohazard transport bag with the appropriate laboratory request form.

Patient teaching

Before discharge, teach the patient and caregiver about self-catheterization as needed. Review proper hand hygiene, catheterization technique, and daily care of the urinary meatus, as well as maintenance of catheter supplies. Instruct the patient to report signs and symptoms of urinary tract infection or obstruction.

Complications

Complications include urethral false passages, urethral strictures, bladder perforation, and deterioration of the upper urinary tracts.[4] Urinary tract infection can result from the introduction of bacteria into the bladder. Improper insertion can cause traumatic injury to the urethral and bladder mucosa. Bladder atony or spasms can result from rapid decompression of a severely distended bladder.

Documentation

Record the date, time, and size and type of catheter used. Also describe the amount, color, and other characteristics of urine emptied from the bladder. Your facility may require only the intake and output record for fluid-balance data. Describe the patient's tolerance of the procedure. Note whether a urine specimen was sent for laboratory analysis.

REFERENCES

1 Association of Professionals in Infection Control and Epidemiology. (2014). "APIC implementation guide: Guide to preventing catheter-associated urinary tract infections" [Online]. Accessed March 2015 via the Web at http://apic.org/Resource_/EliminationGuideForm/6473ab9b-e75c-457a-8d0f-d57d32bc242b/File/APIC_CAUTI_web_0603.pdf (Level IV)

2 Healthcare Infection Control Practices Advisory Committee. (2010). "Guideline for prevention of catheter-associated urinary tract infections, 2009" [Online]. Accessed March 2015 via the Web at http://www.cdc.gov/hicpac/pdf/CAUTI/CAUTI_GuidelineAppendices2009final.pdf (Level I)

3 Lo, E., et al. (2014). SHEA/IDSA practice recommendation: Strategies to prevent catheter-associated urinary tract infections in acute care hospitals: 2014 update. *Infection Control and Hospital Epidemiology, 35,* 464–479. Accessed March 2015 via the Web at http://www.jstor.org/stable/10.1086/675718 (Level I)

4 Society of Urologic Nurses and Associates. (2006). "Clinical practice guidelines: Adult clean intermittent catheterization" [Online]. Accessed March 2015 via the Web at http://www.suna.org/resources/adultCICGuide.pdf (Level VII)

5 Achmetov, T., & Gray, M. (n.d.). Adverse reactions to latex in the clinical setting: A urologic perspective. *Infection Control Resource, 2*(2), 1–5. Accessed March 2015 via the Web at http://www.covidien.com/imageServer.aspx?contentID=20455&contenttype=application/pdf

6 Herter, R., & Kazer-Wallace, M. (2010). Best practices in urinary catheter care. *Home Healthcare Nurse, 28,* 342–349.

7 Centers for Disease Control and Prevention. (2002). Guideline for hand hygiene in health-care settings: Recommendations of the Healthcare Infection Control Practices Advisory Committee and the HICPAC/SHEA/APIC/IDSA Hand Hygiene Task Force. *MMWR Recommendations and Reports, 51*(RR-16), 1–45. Accessed March 2015 via the Web at http://www.cdc.gov/mmwr/pdf/rr/rr5116.pdf (Level II)

8 The Joint Commission. (2015). Standard NPSG.07.01.01. *Comprehensive accreditation manual for hospitals: The official handbook.* Oakbrook Terrace, IL: The Joint Commission. (Level VII)

9 World Health Organization. (2009). "WHO guidelines on hand hygiene in health care: First global patient safety challenge, clean care is safer care" [Online]. Accessed March 2015 via the Web at http://whqlibdoc.who.int/publications/2009/9789241597906_eng.pdf (Level IV)

10 American Osteopathic Association. (2014). Standard 07.01.21. *Healthcare Facilities Accreditation Program: Accreditation requirements for acute care hospitals.* Chicago, IL: American Osteopathic Association. (Level VII)

11 Centers for Medicare & Medicaid Services, Department of Health and Human Services. (2014). Condition of participation: Infection control. 42 C.F.R. § 482.42.

12 Siegel, J. D., et al. (2007). "2007 guideline for isolation precautions: Preventing transmission of infectious agents in healthcare settings" [Online]. Accessed March 2015 via the Web at http://www.cdc.gov/hicpac/pdf/isolation/Isolation2007.pdf (Level I)

13 American Osteopathic Association. (2014). Standard 07.01.10. *Healthcare Facilities Accreditation Program: Accreditation requirements for acute care hospitals.* Chicago, IL: American Osteopathic Association. (Level VII)

14 The Joint Commission. (2015). Standard NPSG.01.01.01. *Comprehensive accreditation manual for hospitals: The official handbook.* Oakbrook Terrace, IL: The Joint Commission. (Level VII)

EQUIPMENT

Reviewing internal fixation devices

In trochanteric or subtrochanteric fractures, the surgeon may use a hip pin or nail, with or without a screw plate. A pin or plate with extra nails stabilizes the fracture by impacting the bone ends at the fracture site.

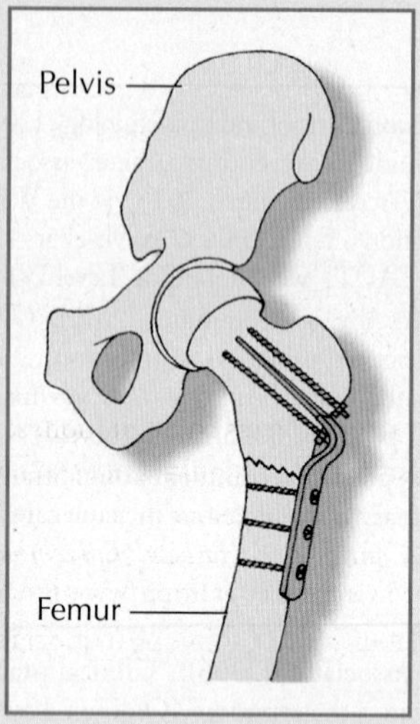

In an uncomplicated fracture of the femoral shaft, the surgeon may use an intramedullary rod. This device permits early ambulation with partial weight bearing.

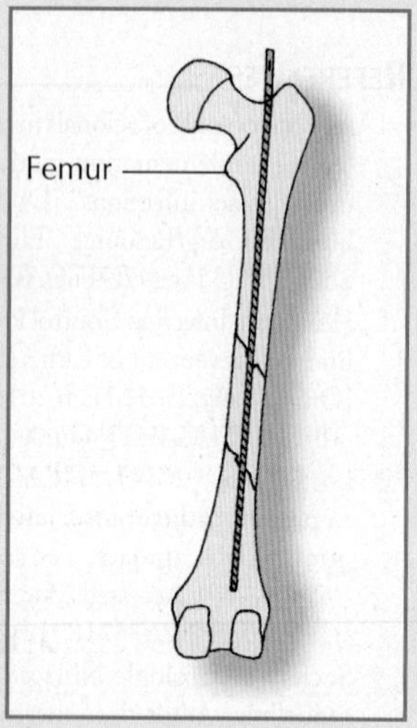

Another choice for fixation of a long-bone fracture is a screw plate, shown here on the tibia.

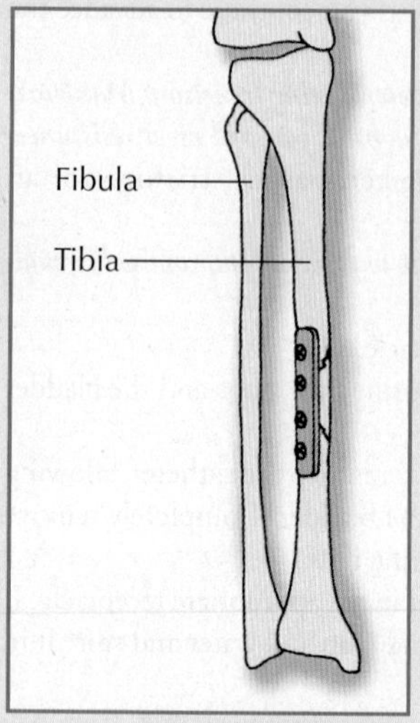

In an arm fracture, the surgeon may fix the involved bones with a plate, rod, or nail. Most radial and ulnar fractures may be fixed with plates, whereas humeral fractures are commonly fixed with rods.

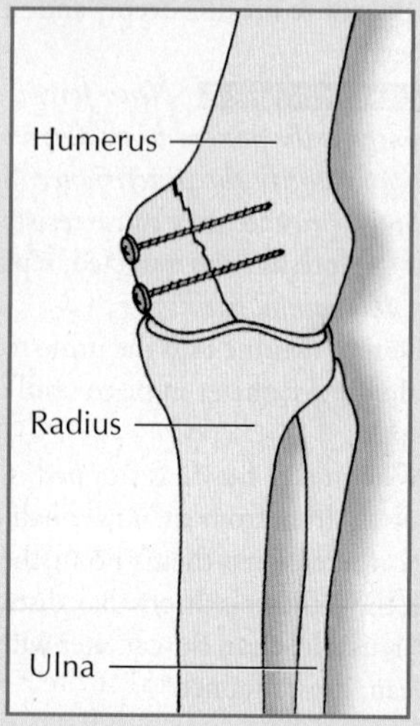

15 American Osteopathic Association. (2014). Standard 15.01.16. *Healthcare Facilities Accreditation Program: Accreditation requirements for acute care hospitals.* Chicago, IL: American Osteopathic Association. (Level VII)

16 Centers for Medicare & Medicaid Services, Department of Health and Human Services. (2014). Condition of participation: Patient's rights. 42 C.F.R. § 482.13(c)(1).

17 The Joint Commission. (2015). Standard NPSG.07.06.01. *Comprehensive accreditation manual for hospitals: The official handbook.* Oakbrook Terrace, IL: The Joint Commission. (Level VII)

18 Society of Urologic Nurses and Associates. (2005). "Clinical practice guidelines: Female urethral catheterization" [Online]. Accessed March 2015 via the Web at http://www.suna.org/resources/femaleCatheterization.pdf

19 The Joint Commission. (2015). Standard RC.01.03.01. *Comprehensive accreditation manual for hospitals: The official handbook.* Oakbrook Terrace, IL: The Joint Commission. (Level VII)

20 American Osteopathic Association. (2014). Standard 10.00.03. *Healthcare Facilities Accreditation Program: Accreditation requirements for acute care hospitals.* Chicago, IL: American Osteopathic Association. (Level VII)

21 Centers for Medicare & Medicaid Services, Department of Health and Human Services. (2014). Condition of participation: Medical record services. 42 C.F.R. § 482.24(b).

22 Shlamovitz, G. Z. (2012). "Urethral catheterization in women periprocedural care" [Online]. Accessed March 2015 via the Web at http://emedicine.medscape.com/article/80735-periprocedure

23 Villanueva, C., & Hemstreet, G. P. III. (2008). Difficult male urethral catheterization: A review of different approaches. *International Brazilian Journal of Urology, 34,* 401–412.

INTERNAL FIXATION MANAGEMENT

In internal fixation, also known as *surgical reduction* or *open reduction–internal fixation,* the practitioner implants fixation devices to stabilize the fracture. Internal fixation devices include nails, screws, pins, wires, and rods, all of which may be used in combination with metal plates. These devices remain in the body indefinitely unless the patient experiences adverse reactions after the healing process is complete. (See *Reviewing internal fixation devices.*)

Typically, internal fixation is used to treat fractures of the face and jaw, spine, and arms and legs as well as fractures involving a joint (most commonly, the hip). Internal fixation permits earlier mobilization and can shorten hospitalization, particularly in elderly patients with hip fractures.

Nursing management for a patient who undergoes internal fixation involves monitoring neurovascular status, administering medications, managing the patient's pain, preventing infection, and assisting with ambulation and exercises.

Equipment

Stethoscope ■ thermometer ■ blood pressure cuff ■ pulse oximeter ■ ice bag ■ pain medication ■ incentive spirometer ■ compression stockings ■ sequential compression device ■ prescribed IV fluid ■ preoperative checklist ■ Optional: IV insertion kit, prescribed medications, patient-controlled analgesia (PCA) pump.

For a patient with a leg fracture, you may also need an overhead frame with trapeze, pressure-relief mattress, crutches or walker, and pillow; hip fractures may require abductor pillows and a padded splint.[1]

Implementation

Preoperative care

■ Review the patient's medical record for relevant information, such past medical and surgical history (including postoperative nausea and vomiting), allergies, sensitivities, medication use, disabilities, substance use or abuse, physical and mental impairments, mobility limitations, external or implanted medical devices, home use of noninvasive positive-pressure ventilation, and sensory limitations.[2]

■ Verify that laboratory and imaging studies have been completed, as ordered, and that the results are in the patient's medical record. Notify the practitioner of unexpected results.[3,4]
■ Conduct a preprocedure verification *to make sure that all relevant documentation and related information or equipment are available and correctly identified to the patient's identifiers.*[3]
■ Verify the practitioner's orders.
■ Perform hand hygiene.[5,6,7]
■ Confirm the patient's identity using at least two patient identifiers.[8]
■ Obtain the patient's vital signs and oxygen saturation level *to serve as a baseline for comparison.*
■ Assess the patient's cardiac and respiratory status *to serve as a baseline for comparison.*
■ Assess the neurovascular status of the affected extremity, if appropriate, and compare your results with findings in the unaffected extremity *to promptly detect signs of neurovascular compromise.*[9]
■ Immobilize and elevate the affected extremity, if appropriate, *to reduce associated discomfort, promote venous return, and reduce swelling.* Support the extremity adequately when moving or elevating it.[9]
■ Apply ice to the affected site, if needed and prescribed, *to promote comfort and to reduce swelling.*[9]
■ Assess and address the patient's safety, emotional, and psychological needs.[2]
■ Begin a preoperative checklist.
■ Reinforce the practitioner's explanation of the procedure, and answer the patient's questions.
■ Ensure that the patient has signed a consent form and that the form is in the patient's medical record.[10]
■ Perform a comprehensive pain assessment using techniques appropriate for the patient's age, condition, and ability to understand.[2,11]
■ Administer pain medication, as needed and prescribed, following safe medication administration practices. Perform a follow-up pain assessment and notify the practitioner if pain isn't adequately controlled.[11]
■ Tell the patient what to expect during postoperative assessment, monitoring, and care.
■ Teach the patient how to cough, deep breathe, and use an incentive spirometer *to reduce the risk of postprocedure pneumonia.* (See the "Incentive spirometry" procedure, page 383.)[12,13]
■ Prepare the patient for proposed exercise and progressive ambulation regimens if necessary.
■ Encourage the patient to perform active range-of-motion (ROM) exercises of the uninvolved joints, unless contraindicated.[9]
■ Ensure that the patient has had nothing by mouth before the procedure (unless emergent) *to ensure gastric emptying and to reduce the risk of aspiration*; minimum fasting recommendations include 2 hours for clear liquids, 6 or more hours for a light meal or nonhuman milk, and 8 hours or more for fried or fatty foods or meat.[14]
■ Confirm that the patient has patent IV access *to administer prophylactic antibiotics*[4] *(commonly administered 1 hour before the incision, or 2 hours before if vancomycin or fluoroquinolones are prescribed), IV fluids, and blood products, as prescribed.* Insert an IV catheter if necessary. (See the "IV catheter insertion and removal" procedure, page 446.)[15]
■ Verify the surgical procedure and site with the patient and his family, if present.[9]
■ Verify that the prescribed surgical preparation, such as appropriate skin cleaning, has been completed, as indicated.
■ Provide hand-off communication for the person who'll be assuming care of the patient during the procedure; allow the opportunity for questions, as needed.
■ Perform hand hygiene.[5,6,7]
■ Document the procedure.[16]

Postoperative care

■ Receive hand-off communication from the person who assumed care of the patient on the postanesthesia care unit; ask questions as needed.[17]
■ Verify the practitioner's orders.
■ Perform hand hygiene.[4,5,6,7]
■ Confirm the patient's identity using at least two patient identifiers.[8]
■ Assess the patient's cardiac and neurologic status, sedation level, respiratory status, and oxygen saturation level.[2,18]

NURSING ALERT *Patients determined to have respiratory depression (defined as a rate of less than eight breaths/minute), poor respiratory quality or effort, oxygen desaturation, advancing sedation level, snoring, or other noisy respiration should be aroused immediately and instructed to take a deep breath.*

■ Monitor the patient's vital signs at an interval determined by your facility and the patient's condition *because there's no evidence-based research to indicate the best practice for frequency of vital sign assessments.*[2]
■ Assess the patency of the patient's IV catheter; insert a new one if necessary and administer IV fluids as prescribed.
■ Trace each tubing that the patient has in place from the patient to its point of origin *to detect misconnections.*[19]
■ Monitor fluid intake and output.
■ Assess the patient's neurovascular status.[2] Assess color, motion, sensation, digital movement, edema, capillary refill, and pulses of the affected area. Compare your findings with the unaffected side.
■ Apply an ice bag to the operative site, as ordered, *to reduce swelling, relieve pain, and lessen bleeding.*
■ Assess the patient's comfort level, including positioning, temperature, and postoperative nausea and vomiting.[2]
■ Perform a comprehensive pain assessment using techniques appropriate for the patient's age, condition, and ability to understand.[2,11]
■ Administer pain medication as needed and prescribed, following safe administration practices, *to promote comfort.* If the patient is using PCA, instruct him to administer a dose before exercising or moving.
■ Assess the patient's safety needs, including his risk of falling. Implement the appropriate measures *to ensure patient safety.*[2]
■ Reassess the patient's pain[2,11] and ask about the presence of burning, tingling, or numbness in the affected area, *which may indicate infection or impaired circulation.*
■ Elevate the affected limb on a pillow, if appropriate, *to minimize edema.*[9]
■ Assess the condition and color of the patient's skin.[2]
■ Monitor he patient's surgical dressings for excessive drainage or bleeding.[2]
■ Assist and encourage the patient to perform ROM and other muscle-strengthening exercises, as ordered, *to promote circulation, improve muscle tone, and maintain joint function.*
■ *To prevent postprocedure pneumonia,* have the patient cough, deep breathe, and use an incentive spirometer according to the practitioner's order.[12,13] (See the "Incentive spirometry" procedure, page 383.) Tell the patient that early ambulation and optimal pain management also reduce the risk of postoperative pulmonary complications.[13]
■ Apply compression stockings or a sequential compression device, as appropriate, *to prevent venous thromboembolism (VTE).*[20,21] The patient may also require a pressure-relief mattress *to prevent skin breakdown.* (See the "Sequential compression therapy" procedure, page 687.)
■ Teach the patient to perform early progressive ambulation and mobilization[12,20] using an overhead frame with a trapeze, crutches, or a walker and splint, as appropriate. (See the "Crutch use" procedure, page 237.)
■ Continue anticoagulation therapy as ordered by the practitioner *to prevent VTE.* Make sure baseline coagulation studies have been obtained and are documented in the patient's medical record. (Monitor the patient's International Normalized Ratio if he's receiving warfarin.)[20,21]
■ Make sure prophylactic antibiotics are discontinued within 24 hours after surgery.[21]

- Encourage the patient to consume fluids, as his condition allows, and administer a stool softener, as ordered, *to prevent constipation, because immobility and opioid use can slow colonic activity, causing constipation.*[1]
- If the patient has an indwelling urinary catheter that was inserted for surgery, remove the catheter on postoperative day 1 or 2 (with the day of surgery considered day 0), according to your facility's protocol or the practitioner's order, *to reduce the risk for catheter-associated urinary tract infection.*[21] (See the "Indwelling urinary catheter care and removal" procedure, page 391.)
- If the patient was receiving a beta-adrenergic blocker before surgery, collaborate with his practitioner to ensure that he receives it during the perioperative period.[21]
- Perform hand hygiene.[4,5,6,7]
- Document the procedure.[16]

Special considerations

- After the initial postoperative dressing is removed, begin assessing the incision site for signs and symptoms of infection, such as erythema, drainage, edema, and unusual pain.
- The use of capnography in the postoperative setting can be a useful indicator of respiratory depression in high-risk patients.[18]

Patient teaching

Before discharge, instruct the patient and family members how to care for the incisional site, including the importance of proper hygiene and how to recognize signs and symptoms of surgical site infection. Also, teach the patient and family members about administering pain medication, practicing an exercise regimen (if any), and using assistive ambulation devices (such as crutches or a walker), if appropriate. Teach the patient measures to prevent postoperative pneumonia. Teach the signs and symptoms of VTE and when and how to seek treatment. Also teach the patient about the prescribed anticoagulation regimen.[20,22]

Complications

Surgical site infection and, more critically, infection involving metal fixation devices may require reopening the incision, draining the suture line and, possibly, removing the fixation device. Any such infection would require wound dressings and antibiotic therapy. Other complications may include malunion, nonunion, fat or pulmonary embolism, neurovascular impairment, compartment syndrome,[1] and chronic pain.

Documentation

In the patient's medical record, document perioperative findings on cardiovascular, respiratory, and neurovascular status. Document pain medications administered, including the amount, the route, and the patient's tolerance. Describe wound appearance and alignment of the affected bone. Document the patient's response to teaching about appropriate exercise, care of the incision site, use of assistive devices (if appropriate), anticoagulant therapy, signs and symptoms that should be reported to the practitioner, and where and when to seek treatment.

REFERENCES

1 Horn, P. L., et al. (2011). Orthopedic trauma: Pilon fractures. *Orthopaedic Nursing, 30,* 293–300.

2 American Society of PeriAnesthesia Nurses. (2012). *Perianesthesia nursing standards, practice recommendations, and interpretive statements: 2012-2014.* Cherry Hill, NJ: American Society of PeriAnesthesia Nurses. (Level VII)

3 The Joint Commission. (2015). Standard UP.01.01.01. *Comprehensive accreditation manual for hospitals: The official handbook.* Oakbrook Terrace, IL: The Joint Commission. (Level VII)

4 World Health Organization. (2009). "WHO guidelines for safe surgery, 2009: Safe surgery saves lives" [Online]. Accessed March 2015 via the Web at http://whqlibdoc.who.int/publications/2009/9789241598552_eng.pdf (Level VI)

5 Centers for Disease Control and Prevention. (2002). Guideline for hand hygiene in health-care settings: Recommendations of the Healthcare Infection Control Practices Advisory Committee and the HICPAC/SHEA/APIC/IDSA Hand Hygiene Task Force. *MMWR Recommendations and Reports, 51*(RR-16), 1–45. Accessed March 2015 via the Web at http://www.cdc.gov/mmwr/pdf/rr/rr5116.pdf (Level II)

6 World Health Organization. (2009). "WHO guidelines on hand hygiene in health care: First global patient safety challenge, clean care is safer care" [Online]. Accessed March 2015 via the Web at http://whqlibdoc.who.int/publications/2009/9789241597906_eng.pdf (Level IV)

7 The Joint Commission. (2015). Standard NPSG.07.01.01. *Comprehensive accreditation manual for hospitals: The official handbook.* Oakbrook Terrace, IL: The Joint Commission. (Level VII)

8 The Joint Commission. (2015). Standard NPSG.01.01.01. *Comprehensive accreditation manual for hospitals: The official handbook.* Oakbrook Terrace, IL: The Joint Commission. (Level VII)

9 Hinkle, J. L., & Cheever, K. H. (2014). *Brunner & Suddarth's textbook of medical-surgical nursing* (13th ed.). Philadelphia, PA: Wolters Kluwer.

10 The Joint Commission. (2015). Standard RI.01.03.01. *Comprehensive accreditation manual for hospitals: The official handbook.* Oakbrook Terrace, IL: The Joint Commission. (Level VII)

11 The Joint Commission. (2015). Standard PC.01.02.07. *Comprehensive accreditation manual for hospitals: The official handbook.* Oakbrook Terrace, IL: The Joint Commission. (Level VII)

12 Centers for Disease Control and Prevention. (2003). "Guidelines for preventing health-care-associated pneumonia, 2003" [Online]. Accessed March 2015 via the Web at http://www.cdc.gov/mmwr/preview/mmwrhtml/rr5303a1.htm (Level II)

13 American Association for Respiratory Care. (2011). AARC clinical practice guideline, incentive spirometry: 2011. *Respiratory Care, 56,* 1600–1604. (Level VII)

14 American Society of Anesthesiologists. (2011). "Practice guidelines for preoperative fasting and the use of pharmacologic agents to reduce the risk of pulmonary aspiration: Application to healthy patients undergoing elective procedures" [Online]. Accessed March 2015 via the Web at http://journals.lww.com/anesthesiology/fulltext/2011/03000/practice_guidelines_for_preoperative_fasting_and.13.aspx (Level VII)

15 The Joint Commission. (2015). Standard NPSG.07.05.01. *Comprehensive accreditation manual for hospitals: The official handbook.* Oakbrook Terrace, IL: The Joint Commission. (Level VII)

16 The Joint Commission. (2015). Standard RC.01.03.01. *Comprehensive accreditation manual for hospitals: The official handbook.* Oakbrook Terrace, IL: The Joint Commission. (Level VII)

17 Recommended practices for transfer of patient care information. (20143). In Conner, R., et al. (Eds.), *Perioperative standards and recommended practices, 2014.* Denver, CO: AORN, Inc. (Level VII)

18 Jarzyna, D., et al. (2011). American Society for Pain Management: Nursing guidelines on monitoring for opioid-induced sedation and respiratory depression. *Pain Management Nursing, 12,* 118–145. Accessed March 2015 via the Web at http://www.aspmn.org/organization/documents/GuidelinesonMonitoringforOpioid-InducedSedationandRespiratoryDepression.pdf (Level VII)

19 U.S. Food and Drug Administration. (n.d.). "Look. Check. Connect. Safe medical device connections save lives" [Online]. Accessed March 2015 via the Web at http://www.fda.gov/downloads/MedicalDevices/Safety/AlertsandNotices/UCM134873.pdf

20 Institute for Clinical Systems Improvement. (2012). "Health care guideline: Venous thromboembolism prophylaxis (9th ed.)" [Online]. Accessed March 2015 via the Web at http://www.guideline.gov/content.aspx?id=39350 (Level IV)

21 Centers for Medicare & Medicaid Services, & The Joint Commission. (2014). "The specifications manual for national hospital inpatient quality measures (version 4.3)" [Online]. Accessed March 2015 via the Web at http://www.qualitynet.org/dcs/ContentServer?pagename=QnetPublic%2FPage%2FQnetTier2&cid=1141662756099

22 Anderson, D. J., et al. (2014). SHEA/IDSA practice recommendation: Strategies to prevent surgical site infections in acute care hospitals: 2014 update. *Infection Control and Hospital Epidemiology, 35,* 605–627. Accessed March 2015 via the Web at http://www.jstor.org/stable/10.1086/676022 (Level IV)

INTRA-ABDOMINAL PRESSURE MONITORING

Intra-abdominal pressure (IAP) monitoring measures the pressure in the abdominal compartment. It can be assessed indirectly with an indwelling urinary catheter by measuring the urinary bladder pressure with a pressure transducer, or by inserting an IV catheter into the sampling port of the urinary catheter. Pressure in the abdomen may result from such conditions as intraperitoneal bleeding, third-space fluid resuscitation, peritonitis, ascites, gaseous bowel distention, abdominal surgery, and trauma.

If pressure in the abdominal cavity becomes greater than the pressure in the capillaries that perfuse the abdominal organs, ischemia and infarction may result. Increased IAP can also lead to reduced cardiac output, increased systemic vascular resistance, increased peripheral vascular resistance, reduced venous return, and increased intrathoracic pressure, which limits expansion of the diaphragm, resulting in hypoventilation and hypoxia.[1] By measuring IAP, the nurse can detect a rise in pressure and initiate lifesaving measures.[2]

The urinary catheter should be removed as soon as it's no longer needed to prevent catheter-associated urinary tract infection (CAUTI).[3,4] **HOSPITAL-ACQUIRED CONDITION ALERT** *The Centers for Medicare & Medicaid Services has identified CAUTI as a hospital-acquired condition with payment implications* because it can be reasonably prevented using a variety of best practices. *When caring for the patient with an indwelling urinary catheter, follow CAUTI prevention practices, such as performing hand hygiene before and after catheter manipulation; maintaining a sterile, continuously closed drainage system; maintaining unobstructed urine flow; emptying the collection bag regularly; replacing the catheter and collection system using sterile technique when breaks in sterile technique, disconnection, or leakage occur; and discontinuing the catheter as soon as it's no longer clinically indicated,* to reduce the risk of CAUTI.[3,4,5]

Equipment

Indwelling urinary catheter with drainage collection bag ■ gloves ■ cardiac monitor with pressure transducer cable ■ 500-mL IV bag of normal saline solution ■ pressure bag ■ IV tubing ■ pressure tubing ■ pressure transducer with flush device ■ three-way stopcocks ■ 60-mL luer-lock syringe ■ dead-end caps ■ clamp ■ antiseptic pads ■ tape ■ IV pole.

Several commercially prepared kits are available. Examples include the Bard® Intra-abdominal Pressure Monitoring Device and the AbViser™ Intra-abdominal Pressure Monitoring System.

Preparation of equipment

Perform hand hygiene and put on appropriate personal protective equipment.[6,7,8,9,10] Maintain sterile technique throughout preparation. (For instructions on setting up and priming the monitoring system, see the "Transducer system setup" procedure.)

Assemble the equipment, taking care not to contaminate dead-end caps, stopcocks, and syringes. Connect the IV tubing to the transducer, the transducer to two successive stopcocks, and then the second stopcock to the pressure tubing and monitor cable. Attach a 60-mL syringe to the side port of the first stopcock. Place the transducer in the transducer holder attached to the IV pole. Hang the bag of normal saline solution from the IV pole, attach the IV tubing, and flush the air from the entire line. Use the pressure bag to pressurize the system to 300 mm Hg. Attach the cable from the transducer to the cardiac monitor, turn on the monitor, and select a 30-mm Hg scale for monitoring pressure.

Evaluating intra-abdominal pressure[2]

SEVERITY	INTRA-ABDOMINAL PRESSURE READING
Normal	5 to 7 mm Hg
Grade I	12 to 15 mm Hg
Grade II	16 to 20 mm Hg
Grade III	21 to 25 mm Hg
Grade IV	Greater than 25 mm Hg

Implementation

- Verify the practitioner's order.[11]
- Gather and prepare the necessary equipment.
- Perform hand hygiene.[6,7,8,9,10]
- Confirm the patient's identity using at least two patient identifiers.[12]
- Explain the procedure to the patient, including the purpose of IAP monitoring and anticipated duration of catheter placement, *to reduce anxiety and enhance cooperation.*
- Put on gloves *to comply with standard precautions.*[13,14]
- Insert an indwelling urinary catheter, if the patient doesn't already have one in place. (See the "Indwelling urinary catheter insertion" procedure, page 394.)
- Place the IV pole with the monitoring system next to the patient.
- With the patient in the supine position and the head of the bed flat, level and zero the transducer so that it's level with the iliac crest at the midaxillary line *to cancel out the effect of atmospheric pressure.*[2,15]
- If possible, keep the patient in the supine position with the head of the bed flat *to prevent the abdominal organs from exerting pressure on the bladder.* If the patient is at risk for ventilator-associated pneumonia, you may need to elevate the head of the bad at least 30 degrees. *Because pressure measurements may differ with varying positions,* use consistent positioning for each measurement *to ensure accuracy.*[15,16,17]
- Thoroughly disinfect the indwelling urinary catheter sampling port with an antiseptic pad using friction and allow it to air-dry *to reduce the risk of infection.*
- Attach the end of the pressure tubing to the sampling port.[3,4]
- Clamp the urinary catheter just distal to the connection of the catheter and drainage collection bag *to prevent normal saline solution from draining out of the bladder while filling the bladder.*
- Remove air from the clamp and the urinary catheter by opening the clamp, allowing the normal saline solution to flow past the clamp, and then reclamping the tubing.
- Open the stopcock from the flush line to the syringe and fill the syringe with 25 mL of normal saline solution.[1]
- Close the stopcock to the flush line and open it to the urinary catheter, and instill 25 mL of normal saline solution into the bladder. *This volume won't overdistend the bladder and produce a falsely high reading.*[1]
- Close the stopcock to the syringe, and open it to the pressure tubing and the transducer.
- Wait 10 to 30 seconds after instilling the saline solution,[2] and then obtain the IAP with the patient in the supine position.[2,15]
- Obtain the IAP reading at the end of the patient's expiration with the graphic scale on the monitor display and numeric display of the mean pressure.[1] (See *Evaluating intra-abdominal pressure.*)
- After obtaining the reading, turn the stopcock off to the pressure tubing and catheter, release the clamp, and allow the bladder to drain.
- Measure urine output, making sure to subtract the 25 mL of instilled normal saline solution *to maintain accurate intake and output.*[1]
- Remove the pressure tubing from the sampling port or leave it in place if subsequent monitoring is necessary. Tape the connections securely.
- Dispose of used supplies in appropriate receptacles.

- Remove and discard your gloves.[14]
- Perform hand hygiene.[6,7,8,9,10]
- Document the procedure.[18,19,20]

Special considerations

- Monitor IAP at least every 2 hours or as clinically indicated;[2] report an increasing IAP to the practitioner. *An IAP of 12 mm Hg or greater signals intra-abdominal hypertension; an IAP above 20 mm Hg indicates abdominal compartment syndrome, which may require decompression surgery.*[1]
- IAP typically displayed on the cardiac monitor is a mean pressure that reflects the pressure during both inspiration and expiration. If noticeable differences exist in the IAP reading during inspiration and expiration, consider obtaining a more precise end-expiration IAP reading by using a printed waveform strip or the graphic scale on the cardiac monitor.[1]
- Assess patients at risk for intra-abdominal hypertension for signs and symptoms of reduced organ perfusion, including decreased or absent urine output; hypotension; reduced cardiac output; increased serum creatinine levels, central venous and pulmonary artery pressures, intracranial pressure, serum lactate levels, and peak airway pressure; decreased tidal volume; hypoxemia; hypercapnia; and impaired peripheral circulation.
- IAP readings may not be accurate in a patient with intraperitoneal adhesions, pelvic hematomas, pelvic fractures, abdominal packs, or a neurogenic bladder *because accurate IAP measurement requires free movement of the bladder wall.* Chronically increased IAP due to morbid obesity, pregnancy, or ascites can also complicate accurate measurement.[17,21]
- Mechanical ventilation increases intrathoracic pressure, causing a direct influence on IAP as the increased pressure is transmitted across the patient's abdomen. Closely monitor IAP in critically ill patients on ventilator support, even if such patients have no other apparent risk factors for increased IAP.[22]
- When using the AbViser™ system, attach the AbViser™ valve to the pressure tubing and insert it into the hub of the urinary catheter using sterile technique. A special one-way valve in the AbViser™ allows for instillation of fluid, a dwell time of 1 minute to allow for pressure reading, and then automatic drainage into the drainage tubing of the urinary catheter. This valve maintains a closed system, *which reduces the risk of infection.*[23]

Complications

An IAP that exceeds 20 mm Hg is usually associated with irreversible organ damage, leading to abdominal compartment syndrome and multiple-organ-dysfunction syndrome. With increased pressure readings and signs of reduced organ perfusion, surgical intervention may be required to preserve organ function and decrease morbidity and mortality associated with intra-abdominal hypertension and abdominal compartment syndrome. The presence of an indwelling urinary catheter and entering the closed system for pressure monitoring increases the risk of CAUTI.

Documentation

Record the date and time and result of the IAP reading. (Frequent IAP readings may be recorded on a frequent parameter assessment sheet.) Document whether the system was leveled and zeroed and the patient's position during the reading. Record the amount of normal saline solution instilled. Document the practitioner who was notified of an abnormal reading, any orders given, interventions performed, and the patient's response to interventions.

Record any vital signs and assessments performed at the time of the IAP reading. Record urinary output, making sure to subtract the instilled normal saline solution. Document any urinary catheter care performed. If a printed waveform strip is available, label it "intra-abdominal pressure;" write the date, time, and patient's name on the strip; and place it in the patient's medical record.

Note the patient's tolerance of the procedure. Document any patient teaching provided and the patient's understanding of the teaching.

References

1 Lynn-McHale Wiegand, D. (Ed.). (2011). *AACN procedure manual for critical care* (6th ed.). St. Louis, MO: Saunders.

2 Malbrain, M. L., et al. (2006). Results from the International Conference of Experts on Intra-abdominal Hypertension and Abdominal Compartment Syndrome. I. Definitions. *Intensive Care Medicine, 32,* 1722–1732.

3 The Joint Commission. (2015). Standard NPSG.07.06.01. *Comprehensive accreditation manual for hospitals: The official handbook.* Oakbrook Terrace, IL: The Joint Commission. (Level VII)

4 Lo, E., et al. (2014). SHEA/IDSA practice recommendation: Strategies to prevent catheter-associated urinary tract infections in acute care hospitals: 2014 update. *Infection Control and Hospital Epidemiology, 35,* 464–479. Accessed March 2015 via the Web at http://www.jstor.org/stable/10.1086/675718 (Level I)

5 Jarrett, N., et al. (2013). "Evidence-based guidelines for selected and previously considered hospital-acquired conditions: Final report" [Online]. Accessed March 2015 via the Web at http://www.cms.gov/Medicare/Medicare-Fee-for-Service-Payment/HospitalAcqCond/Downloads/Evidence-Based-Guidelines.pdf

6 The Joint Commission. (2015). Standard NPSG.07.01.01. *Comprehensive accreditation manual for hospitals: The official handbook.* Oakbrook Terrace, IL: The Joint Commission. (Level VII)

7 Centers for Disease Control and Prevention. (2002). Guideline for hand hygiene in health-care settings: Recommendations of the Healthcare Infection Control Practices Advisory Committee and the HICPAC/SHEA/APIC/IDSA Hand Hygiene Task Force. *MMWR Recommendations and Reports, 51*(RR-16), 1–45. Accessed March 2015 via the Web at http://www.cdc.gov/mmwr/pdf/rr/rr5116.pdf (Level II)

8 World Health Organization. (2009). "WHO guidelines on hand hygiene in health care: First global patient safety challenge, clean care is safer care" [Online]. Accessed March 2015 via the Web at http://whqlibdoc.who.int/publications/2009/9789241597906_eng.pdf (Level IV)

9 American Osteopathic Association. (2014). Standard 07.01.21. *Healthcare Facilities Accreditation Program: Accreditation requirements for acute care hospitals.* Chicago, IL: American Osteopathic Association. (Level VII)

10 Centers for Medicare & Medicaid Services, Department of Health and Human Services. (2014). Condition of participation: Infection control. 42 C.F.R. § 482.42.

11 The Joint Commission. (2015). Standard MM.04.01.01. *Comprehensive accreditation manual for hospitals: The official handbook.* Oakbrook Terrace, IL: The Joint Commission. (Level VII)

12 The Joint Commission. (2015). Standard NPSG.01.01.01. *Comprehensive accreditation manual for hospitals: The official handbook.* Oakbrook Terrace, IL: The Joint Commission. (Level VII)

13 Siegel, J. D., et al. (2007). "2007 guideline for isolation precautions: Preventing transmission of infectious agents in healthcare settings" [Online]. Accessed March 2015 via the Web at http://www.cdc.gov/hicpac/pdf/isolation/Isolation2007.pdf (Level II)

14 American Osteopathic Association. (2014). Standard 07.01.10. *Healthcare Facilities Accreditation Program: Accreditation requirements for acute care hospitals.* Chicago, IL: American Osteopathic Association. (Level VII)

15 Soler Morejon, C., et al. (2012). Effects of zero reference position on bladder pressure measurements: An observational study. *Annals of Intensive Care, 2,* S13. Accessed March 2015 via the Web at http://www.ncbi.nlm.nih.gov/pmc/articles/PMC3390299/

16 Yi, M., et al. (2012). The evaluation of the effect of body positioning on intra-abdominal pressure measurement and the effect of intra-abdominal pressure at different body positioning on organ function and prognosis in critically ill patients. *Journal of Critical Care, 27*(2), e1–e6.

17 Gestring, M. Abdominal compartment syndrome. (2014). In: *UpToDate,* Sanfrey, H., & Franke., H. L. (Eds.). Accessed March 2015 via the Web at http://www.uptodate.com/contents/search

18 The Joint Commission. (2015). Standard RC.01.03.01. *Comprehensive accreditation manual for hospitals: The official handbook.* Oakbrook Terrace, IL: The Joint Commission. (Level VII)

19 American Osteopathic Association. (2014). Standard 10.00.03. *Healthcare Facilities Accreditation Program: Accreditation requirements for acute care hospitals.* Chicago, IL: American Osteopathic Association. (Level VII)

20 Centers for Medicare & Medicaid Services, Department of Health and Human Services. (2014). Condition of participation: Medical record services. 42 C.F.R. § 482.24(b).

21 Papavramidis, T. S. (2011). Abdominal compartment syndrome—intra-abdominal hypertension: Defining, diagnosing, and managing. *Journal of Emergency, Trauma, and Shock, 4,* 279–291. Accessed March 2015 via the Web at http://www.ncbi.nlm.nih.gov/pmc/articles/PMC3132369/

22 Soler Morejon, C., & Barbeito, T. (2012). Effect of mechanical ventilation on intra-abdominal pressure in critically ill patients without other risk factors for abdominal hypertension: An observational multicenter epidemiological study. *Annals of intensive Care, 2*(Suppl. 1), S22–S34. Accessed March 2015 via the Web at http://www.annalsofintensivecare.com/content/pdf/2110-5820-2-S1-S22.pdf

23 ConvaTec. (2012). "AbViser™: Intra-abdominal pressure monitor" [Online]. Accessed March 2015 at http://abviser.com/products/abviser-iap-monitoring-device/

ADDITIONAL REFERENCE

Kirkpatrick, A. W., et al. (2013). Intra-abdominal hypertension and the abdominal compartment syndrome: Updated consensus definitions and clinical practice guidelines from the World Society of the Abdominal Compartment Syndrome. *Intensive Care Medicine, 39,* 1190–1206. Accessed March 2015 via the Web at http://link.springer.com/article/10.1007/s00134-013-2906-z/fulltext.html

INTRA-AORTIC BALLOON COUNTERPULSATION

Providing temporary support for the heart's left ventricle, intra-aortic balloon counterpulsation (IABC) mechanically displaces blood within the aorta by means of an intra-aortic balloon attached to an external pump console, referred to as an *intra-aortic balloon pump* (IAPB). The balloon is usually inserted through the common femoral artery and positioned with its tip just distal to the left subclavian artery. It's made of polyethylene and is inflated with gas driven by the pump. Helium is commonly used because its low density facilitates rapid transfer of gas from the IABP to the balloon. It's also easily absorbed into the bloodstream if the balloon ruptures.[1]

When used correctly, IABC improves two key aspects of myocardial physiology: It increases the supply of oxygen-rich blood to the myocardium, and it decreases myocardial oxygen demand and consumption. Several physiologic and nonphysiologic factors can affect IABC efficacy, including the patient's cardiac function, hemodynamic conditions, the position and size of the balloon catheter used, and signal quality.[2]

IABC is indicated for patients with a wide range of low-cardiac-output disorders or cardiac instability. (See *Indications and contraindications for IABC*). Perioperatively, the technique is used to support and stabilize patients with a suspected high-grade lesion who are undergoing such procedures as angioplasty, thrombolytic therapy, cardiac surgery, and cardiac catheterization. Available evidence no longer supports routine use in patients with acute myocardial infarction complicated by cardiogenic shock who are receiving early revascularization.[3,4]

Indications and contraindications for IABC[2]

Various indications and contraindications exist for intra-aortic balloon counterpulsation (IABC). Indications include:

- acute myocardial infarction
- refractory left ventricular failure
- cardiogenic shock
- refractory ventricular arrhythmias
- acute mitral regurgitation and ventricular septal defect
- cardiomyopathies
- sepsis
- refractory unstable angina
- complex cardiac anomalies (in infants and children)
- cardiac surgery
- cardiac catheterization and angioplasty
- weaning from cardiopulmonary bypass.

Contraindications are categorized as absolute or relative. Absolute contraindications include:

- aortic regurgitation
- aortic dissection
- chronic end-stage cardiac disease
- chronic end-stage kidney disease
- aortic stents.

Relative contraindications include:

- uncontrolled sepsis
- abdominal aortic aneurysm
- tachyarrhythmias
- severe peripheral vascular disease
- major arterial reconstructive surgery.

Equipment

For assisting with insertion

IABP, cables, and appropriate-sized balloon catheters ▪ balloon insertion kit ▪ 30-mL luer-lock syringe ▪ 10-mL sterile syringes of prefilled flush solution ▪ helium gas source ▪ Dacron graft (for a surgically inserted balloon) ▪ electrocardiogram (ECG) monitor and electrodes ▪ pulse oximeter ▪ automated blood pressure cuff ▪ temperature probe ▪ clippers ▪ prescribed sedative or analgesic ▪ transducer system ▪ prepared bag of ordered flush solution ▪ 18G angiography needle ▪ antiseptic solution ▪ sterile drape ▪ sterile gloves ▪ sterile occlusive dressing ▪ sterile gowns ▪ caps ▪ masks ▪ sutures or other stabilization device ▪ suction equipment ▪ defibrillator and emergency medications ▪ temporary pacemaker equipment ▪ fluoroscope ▪ Optional: lead apron, backup helium supply, mechanical ventilator, supplemental oxygen, central line insertion kit, arterial catheter insertion equipment, pulmonary artery catheter insertion equipment, IV insertion and administration equipment, indwelling urinary catheter insertion equipment, arterial blood gas (ABG) kit, tubes for laboratory studies, heparin.

For maintaining IABC

IABP and balloon catheters ▪ ECG monitor and electrodes ▪ transducer system setup ▪ IV flush solution ▪ automated blood pressure cuff ▪ pulse oximeter ▪ thermometer ▪ stethoscope ▪ oxygen administration equipment ▪ emergency equipment and medications ▪ ABG kits ▪ equipment for obtaining samples (blood collection tubes, labels, laboratory request forms, laboratory biohazard transport bag, antiseptic pads) ▪ central venous catheter dressing change kit ▪ gloves ▪ vasoactive medications ▪ Optional: pain medications, as prescribed; mechanical ventilatory support equipment, as required; incentive spirometer, pressure-relief device, prescribed blood products.

For assisting with removal

Dressing materials ▪ gloves ▪ suture removal kit ▪ Optional: mechanical compression device.

Preparation of equipment

As determined by your facility, you or a perfusionist must zero and balance the pressure transducer in the IABP and calibrate the oscilloscope monitor *to ensure accuracy.* Refer to the manufacturer's instructions.

Plug the IABP into a nearby power outlet and then turn it on. Open the helium tank and verify that an adequate helium supply is available. Set up the IABP according to the manufacturer's instructions.

Make sure that the defibrillator, the suction setup, the temporary pacemaker setup, and emergency medications readily available *in case*

EQUIPMENT

How the intra-aortic balloon pump works

Made of polyurethane, the intra-aortic balloon is attached to an external pump console (called the *intra-aortic balloon pump*) by means of a large-lumen catheter. These illustrations show the direction of blood flow when the pump inflates and deflates the balloon.

Balloon inflation

The balloon inflates as the aortic valve closes and diastole begins. The balloon inflation displaces blood superiorly, which, in turn, augments coronary artery blood flow.

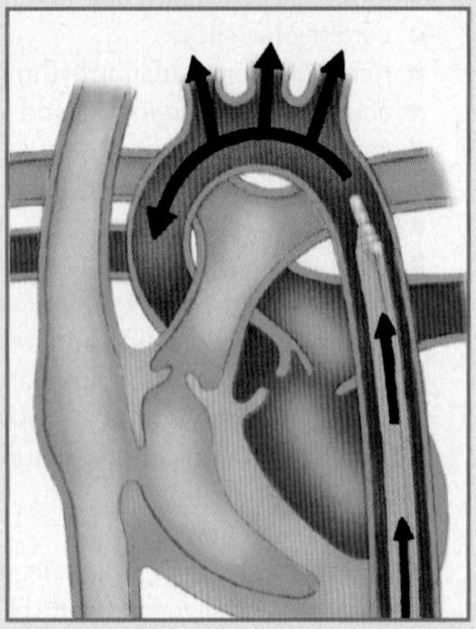

Balloon deflation

The balloon deflates before ventricular ejection, when the aortic valve opens. This deflation permits ejection of blood from the left ventricle against a lowered resistance. As a result, aortic end-diastolic pressure and afterload decrease and cardiac output rises.

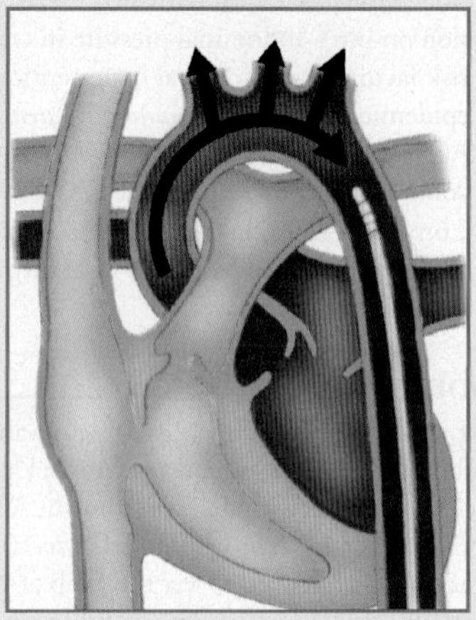

the patient develops a severe complication (such as an arrhythmia) during insertion.

Implementation

- Verify the practitioner's order.
- Gather and prepare the appropriate equipment.
- Confirm that written informed consent has been obtained and that the signed consent form is in the patient's medical record.[5,6,7]
- Conduct a preprocedure verification *to make sure that all relevant documentation, related information, and equipment are available and correctly identified to the patient's identifiers.*[8,9]
- Verify that a complete blood count, coagulation studies, and other ordered studies have been completed as ordered *to check for conditions that may increase the risk of bleeding.* Ensure that the results are in the patient's medical record.[10] Notify the practitioner of unexpected results.[11]
- Perform hand hygiene.[12,13,14,15,16]
- Confirm the patient's identity using at least two patient identifiers.[9,17]

For assisting with insertion

- Reinforce the practitioner's explanation of the procedure, explaining to the patient that the practitioner will place a special balloon catheter into the aorta *that increases oxygen supply to the heart, decreases the heart's workload, and increases cardiac output and perfusion of vital organs.* Briefly explain the insertion procedure, and mention that the catheter will be connected to a large console next to the bed. Tell the patient that the balloon will be removed after his heart can resume an adequate workload. (See *How the intra-aortic balloon pump works.*)
- Make sure the patient has an arterial line *for withdrawing blood samples, monitoring blood pressure, and assessing the timing and effectiveness of therapy;* a pulmonary artery catheter *to allow measurement of pulmonary artery pressure (PAP), aspiration of blood samples, and cardiac output studies (increased PAP indicates increased myocardial workload and ineffective balloon pumping)*; a peripheral IV catheter or central venous access device *for administering fluids and medications*; and an indwelling urinary catheter, if ordered, *to assess fluid balance and renal function.*
- Connect all monitoring equipment, including the ECG monitor, pulse oximeter, automated blood pressure cuff, temperature probe, and hemodynamic monitoring lines, as needed. Set alarm limits appropriately for the patient's current condition, and make sure alarms are turned on, functioning properly, and audible to staff.[18,19,20,21]
- Apply chest electrodes based on desired trigger mode. *A trigger is the signal the IABP uses to identify the beginning of the next cardiac cycle.* Select the desired ECG source from the waveform selector in the IABP controls. Obtain a baseline ECG.[22]
- Attach another set of ECG electrodes to the patient *unless the ECG pattern is being transmitted from the patient's bedside monitor to the IAPB through another cable.*
- Obtain the patient's baseline vital signs, including pulse oximetry.
- Administer supplemental oxygen as ordered and as necessary.
- *To reduce the risk of infection,* clip hair at the insertion site as needed.[23,24]
- Assess and record the patient's peripheral leg pulse and document sensation, movement, color, and temperature of the legs *to help determine the best insertion site.*
- Administer a sedative or an analgesic, as ordered, following safe medication administration practices.[25,26,27]
- Prepare the sterile field.[24,28]
- Place the catheter, insertion kit, and other supplies on the sterile field as indicated.[24]
- Make sure that all medications on and off the sterile field are labeled *to prevent medication administration errors.*[29,30]
- Perform hand hygiene.[12,13,14,15,16]
- Put on a cap, a mask, a sterile gown, and sterile gloves *to comply with maximal barrier precautions.*[24,28]
- Before the practitioner inserts the balloon, he puts on a cap, a mask, a sterile gown, and sterile gloves. He then cleans the site with antiseptic solution and drapes the patient using a sterile drape and observing maximal barrier precautions.[24,28]
- Conduct a time-out immediately before starting the procedure *to determine that the correct patient, site, positioning, and procedure are identified, and confirm, as applicable, that relevant information and necessary equipment are available.*[9,31]
- Administer a heparin bolus if prescribed following safe medication administration practices.[10,25,26,27]

NURSING ALERT ***Heparin is considered a high-alert medication because it can cause significant patient harm when used in error.***[32]

- If required by your facility, before administering heparin, have another nurse perform an independent double-check *to verify the patient's identity and to make sure that the correct medication is hanging in the prescribed concentration, the medication's indication corresponds with the patient's diagnosis, the dosage calculations are correct and the dosing formula used to derive the final dose is correct, the route of administration is safe and proper for the patient, the pump settings are correct, and the infusion line is attached to the correct port.*[33]

- Assist the practitioner with the procedure as needed.
- Attach the 30-mL syringe with one-way valve to the distal end of the balloon lumen.[22]
- Pull back on the syringe until all air is aspirated, and then disconnect the syringe while keeping the valve in place, creating a vacuum.[10,22]
- Lubricate the balloon catheter according to the manufacturer's instructions.[10]
- Flush the inner lumen of the balloon catheter before insertion according to the manufacturer's instructions.

Inserting the intra-aortic balloon percutaneously

- The practitioner may insert the balloon percutaneously through the femoral artery into the descending thoracic aorta using a modified Seldinger technique.
- First, the practitioner accesses the vessel with an 18G angiography needle and removes the inner stylet.
- Next, he passes the guide wire through the needle and removes the needle.
- After advancing a vessel dilator over the guide wire into the vessel, he removes the vessel dilator, leaving the guide wire in place.
- Next, the practitioner passes an introducer (dilator and sheath assembly) over the guide wire into the vessel until about 1″ (2.5 cm) remains above the insertion site. He then removes the inner dilator, leaving the introducer sheath and guide wire in place.
- After passing the balloon over the guide wire into the introducer sheath, the practitioner advances the catheter into position, ⅜″ to ¾″ (1 to 2 cm) distal to the left subclavian artery under fluoroscopic guidance.
- The practitioner secures the balloon catheter to the patient's leg at the entry site using sutures or another stabilization device, as indicated.[22]
- Apply an occlusive dressing *to cover the insertion site.*

Inserting the intra-aortic balloon surgically

- If the practitioner chooses not to insert the catheter percutaneously, he usually inserts it by femoral arteriotomy. (See *Surgical insertion sites for the intra-aortic balloon.*)
- After making an incision and isolating the femoral artery, the practitioner attaches a Dacron graft to a small opening in the arterial wall.
- The practitioner then passes the catheter through this graft. Using fluoroscopic guidance, as necessary, he advances the catheter up the descending thoracic aorta and places the catheter tip between the left subclavian artery and the renal arteries.
- The practitioner sews the balloon catheter to the patient's leg using sutures or a stabilization device, as indicated.[22]
- Apply an occlusive dressing *to cover the insertion site.*

Connecting the catheter to the IABP

- The practitioner removes the one-way valve from the balloon catheter and connects the balloon catheter to a catheter extender. The practitioner or nurse then connects the catheter extender to the pneumatic module of the IABP.
- Assist the practitioner or connect the previously prepared and zeroed transducer system to the aortic arterial line lumen (inner lumen) of the balloon catheter. Verify blood return, gently flush the lumen using the flush device, and then level the transducer with the patient's midaxillary line and zero it *to ensure accuracy.*

Surgical insertion sites for the intra-aortic balloon

If an intra-aortic balloon can't be inserted percutaneously, the practitioner will insert it surgically, using a femoral or transthoracic approach.

Femoral artery approach

Insertion through the femoral artery requires a cutdown and an arteriotomy. The practitioner passes the balloon through a Dacron graft that has been sewn to the artery.

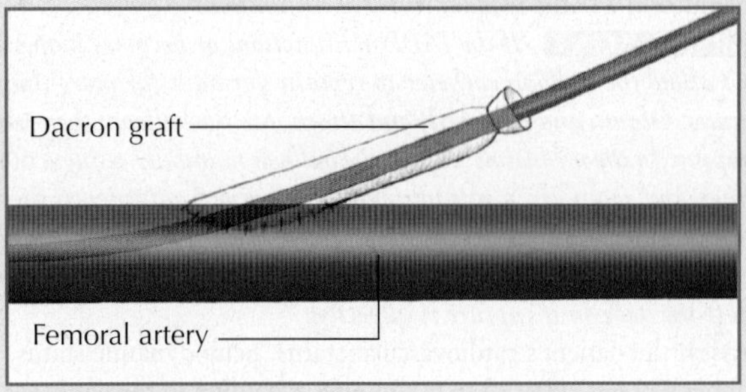

Subclavian artery approach

Although traditionally inserted in the femoral artery, the balloon can be inserted through the. subclavian artery, giving the patient more mobility than the femoral site.[40] For this approach, the practitioner inserts the balloon in an antegrade direction through the subclavian artery and then positions it in the descending thoracic aorta.

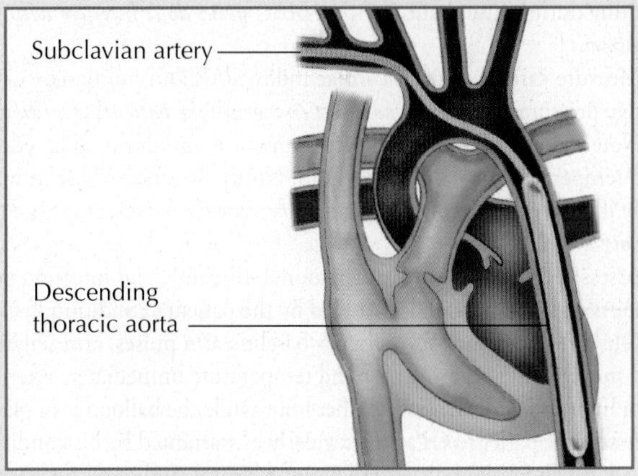

- Trace all connections from the patient to their point of origin *to make sure that they're connected to the proper ports and to make sure that all connections are tight and secure to prevent disconnections.*[34]
- Obtain a portable chest X-ray, as ordered, *to confirm balloon catheter placement.* Place the IABP on standby, as indicated, *for clearer visualization.*[10]
- Initiate counterpulsation therapy, as ordered, following the manufacturer's instructions.
- Monitor the patient's vital signs, hemodynamic parameters, and clinical status according to the patient's condition.[35]

Completing the procedure

- Discard used supplies appropriately.[36]
- Remove and discard your personal protective equipment.
- Perform hand hygiene.[12,13,14,15,16]
- Document the procedure.[37,38,39]

For maintaining IABC

■ Put on gloves, as needed, throughout the procedure *to follow standard precautions.*[9]
■ Verify that the pump settings coincide with the practitioner's order.
■ Ensure that alarm limits are set appropriately for the patient's current condition and that alarms are turned on, functioning properly, and audible to staff.[18,19,20,21]
■ Interpret waveforms and monitor balloon function. (See *Interpreting intra-aortic balloon waveforms.*)
■ Maintain accurate IABP timing according to waveform interpretation; *proper IABP inflation and deflation balance oxygen supply and demand, reducing the risk of further ischemia and compromised contractility.*[2]
■ Monitor the IABP *to make sure that it's functioning properly.*

NURSING ALERT *If the IABP malfunctions or becomes inoperable, don't allow the balloon catheter to remain dormant for more than 15 minutes. Obtain another IABP, and attach it to the balloon; then resume pumping. In the meantime, inflate the balloon manually, using a 60-mL syringe and room air, a minimum of once every 5 minutes* to prevent thrombus formation in the catheter. *The volume of inflation is equal to 10 mL less than the balloon size marked on the catheter. Never manually inflate the balloon if rupture is suspected.*

■ Assess the patient's cardiovascular status, hemodynamic status, and peripheral pulses every 15 to 60 minutes according to the patient's condition. Notify the practitioner immediately if you note changes.[10]
■ Monitor the patient's vital signs and level of consciousness at an interval determined by the patient's condition.
■ Monitor oxygen saturation and provide supplemental oxygen and noninvasive or invasive ventilatory support as required and ordered.[41]
■ Auscultate heart and breath sounds at an interval determined by the patient's condition. If the patient's condition permits, put the IABC on standby during auscultation *so that IABC noises don't interfere with your assessment.*[10]
■ Measure cardiac output, cardiac index, PAP, and pulmonary artery wedge pressure, as ordered, *to detect changes in the patient's condition.*
■ Note pulses, color, capillary refill, sensation, motor function, edema, and temperature in the affected limb. Notify the practitioner immediately if you detect circulatory changes *because the balloon may need to be removed.*[35]
■ Assess the insertion site for hematoma, bleeding, and infection every 2 hours or at an interval determined by the patient's condition.[10,28]
■ Observe and record the patient's baseline arm pulses, arm sensation and movement, and arm color and temperature immediately after balloon insertion and then every other hour while the balloon is in place.
■ Assess the patient's GI status regularly as warranted by his condition. Check for abdominal distention and tenderness, and assess for changes in elimination patterns.
■ Monitor the patient's urine output every hour.[10]
■ Perform a comprehensive pain assessment using techniques appropriate for the patient's age, condition, and ability to understand.[42,43] Administer pain medications as ordered using safe medication practices.[25,26,27]
■ Maintain the head of the bed at less than 45 degrees *to prevent kinking and migration of the catheter.*[10]
■ Assess skin integrity regularly. Logroll the patient as tolerated for assessment and care.
■ Consider the use of pressure-relief devices or a restraint, as ordered, *to maintain catheter position and function.*[44]
■ Perform range-of-motion exercises *to prevent venous stasis and muscle atrophy.*
■ As appropriate, encourage coughing and deep breathing and incentive spirometry use. Provide chest physiotherapy, as tolerated and ordered.[35]
■ Monitor the patient's hematologic status. Observe for bleeding gums, blood in the urine or stools, petechiae, and bleeding or hematoma at the insertion site. Monitor platelet count, hemoglobin level, and hematocrit daily. Expect to administer blood products to maintain hematocrit at 30%.
■ If platelet count drops, expect to administer platelets.
■ If heparin is used for arterial lumen patency, monitor partial thromboplastin time (PTT) every 6 hours while the heparin dose is adjusted to maintain PTT at 1½ to 2 times the normal value, and then every 12 to 24 hours while the balloon remains in place.
■ Obtain samples for ABG analysis, as ordered.
■ Monitor serum electrolyte levels, especially sodium and potassium, as ordered, *to assess the patient's fluid and electrolyte balance and help prevent arrhythmias.*

NURSING ALERT *Avoid sampling from the central lumen of the balloon* to avoid thrombus formation.[35]

■ Obtain an ECG, as ordered.
■ Obtain a chest X-ray, as ordered.
■ Watch for signs and symptoms of a dissecting aortic aneurysm, including a blood pressure differential between the left and right arms, elevated blood pressure, syncope, pallor, diaphoresis, dyspnea, a throbbing abdominal mass, a reduced red blood cell count with an elevated white blood cell count, and pain in the chest, abdomen, or back. Notify the practitioner immediately if you detect any of these signs and symptoms.
■ Administer vasoactive medications, as prescribed, following safe medication administration practices.[20,21,22]
■ Identify parameters that demonstrate clinical readiness to wean from IABC therapy.
■ Appropriately discard used supplies.[36]
■ Remove and discard your gloves.
■ Perform hand hygiene.[12,13,14,15,16]
■ Document the procedure.[37,38,39]

Weaning a patient from IABC

■ Verify the practitioner's order.
■ Perform hand hygiene.[12,13,14,15,16]
■ Confirm the patient's identity using at least two patient identifiers.[9,17]
■ To begin weaning, gradually decrease the frequency of balloon augmentation to 1:2, as ordered. Although each facility has its own weaning protocol, be aware that assist frequency is usually maintained for an hour or longer. If the patient's hemodynamic indices remain stable during this time, weaning may continue by decreasing the frequency of balloon augmentation to 1:3, and so on.
■ Avoid leaving the patient on a low augmentation volume for more than 2 hours *to prevent embolus formation.*
■ If augmentation volume is reduced for weaning, return the pump to full augmentation volume at a ratio of 1:1 for 5 minutes each hour *to decrease the risk of platelet aggregation.*
■ Assess the patient's tolerance of weaning by monitoring his vital signs, ECG, mental status, urine output, distal perfusion, cardiac output, and cardiac index.[35] Signs and symptoms of poor tolerance include hypotension, confusion, disorientation, urine output below 30 mL/hour, cold and clammy skin, chest pain, arrhythmias, ischemic ECG changes, and elevated pulmonary artery pressure. If the patient develops any of these problems, notify the practitioner immediately.
■ Perform hand hygiene.[12,13,14,15,16]
■ Document the procedure.[37,38,39]

For assisting with removal

■ Verify that coagulation studies are within normal limits before the balloon is removed *to prevent hemorrhage from the insertion site.*
■ Perform hand hygiene.[12,13,14,15,16]
■ Put on gloves.[24,28]
■ Confirm the patient's identity using at least two patient identifiers.[9,17]
■ Discontinue the heparin infusion at least 4 hours before removal, if ordered.[35]

Interpreting intra-aortic balloon waveforms

To function properly, the inflation-deflation cycle of an intra-aortic balloon pump (IABP) must be synchronized to appropriate events in the patient's cardiac cycle. During intra-aortic balloon counterpulsation (IABC), you can use electrocardiogram (ECG) and arterial pressure waveforms to determine whether the IABP is functioning properly. The central lumen of the double-lumen intra-aortic balloon catheter allows monitoring of the pressure in the descending aorta during the cardiac cycle. Timing of the IABP is always performed using the arterial waveform as a guide.[35]

Many IABP models automatically adjust timing setting to accommodate changes in the patient's heart rate.[2]

Normal inflation-deflation timing

Balloon inflation occurs after aortic valve closure; deflation, during isovolumetric contraction, just before the aortic valve opens. In a properly timed waveform, such as the one shown below, the inflation point lies at or slightly above the dicrotic notch. Both inflation and deflation cause a sharp V. Peak diastolic pressure exceeds peak systolic pressure; peak systolic pressure exceeds assisted peak systolic pressure.

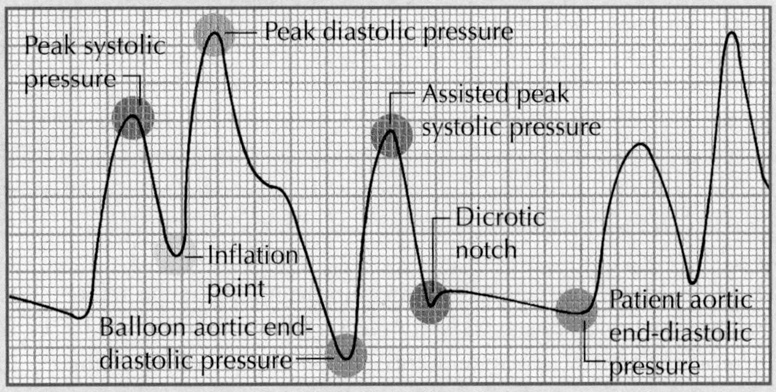

Early inflation

With *early inflation*, the inflation point lies before the dicrotic notch as shown right. Early inflation dangerously increases myocardial stress and decreases cardiac output.

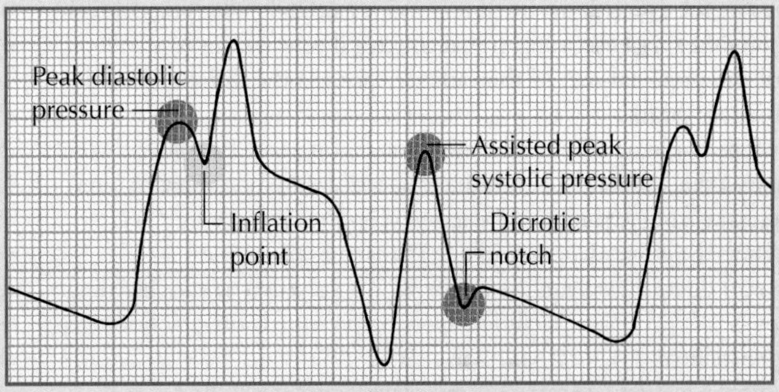

Early deflation

Early deflation results in a U shape on the arterial waveform, as shown right. Peak systolic pressure is less than or equal to assisted peak systolic pressure. Early deflation won't decrease afterload or myocardial oxygen consumption.

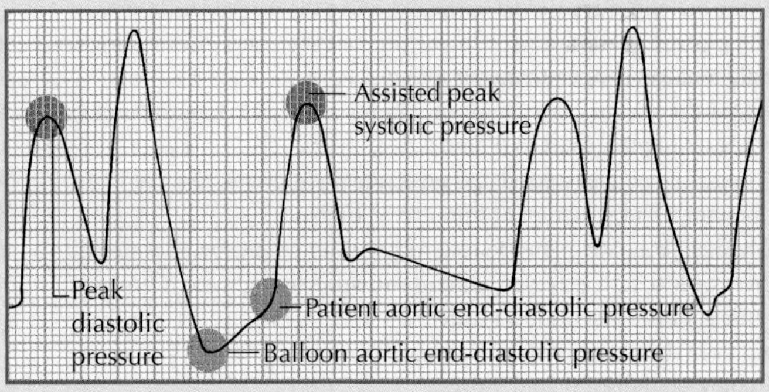

Late inflation

With *late inflation*, the dicrotic notch precedes the inflation point, and the notch and the inflation point create a W shape, as shown right. Late inflation can lead to a reduction in peak diastolic pressure, coronary and systemic perfusion augmentation time, and augmented coronary perfusion pressure.

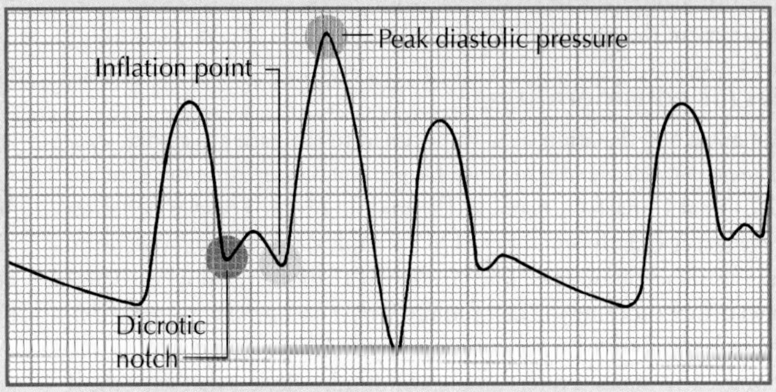

(continued)

Interpreting intra-aortic balloon waveforms *(continued)*

Late deflation

With *late deflation,* peak systolic pressure exceeds assisted peak systolic pressure. This event threatens the patient by increasing afterload, myocardial oxygen consumption, cardiac workload, and preload. It occurs when the balloon has been inflated for too long or fails to receive the input signal from the ECG, indicating the start of systole (QRS complex).

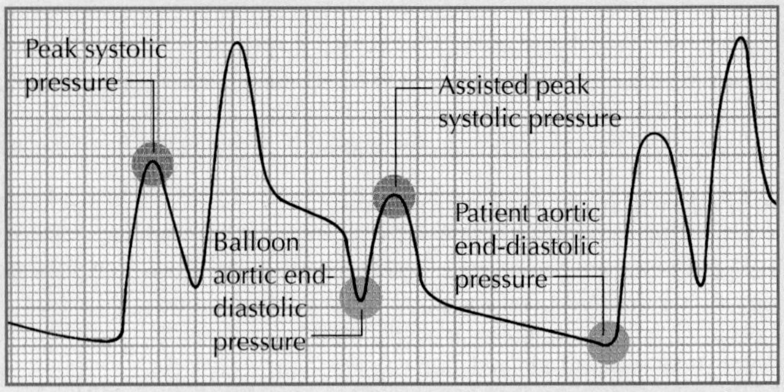

- Make sure that the patient's PTT is within the normal range before the balloon is removed *to prevent hemorrhage at the insertion site.*
- Turn off the control system and disconnect the connection tubing from the catheter *to ensure balloon deflation.*
- Assist the practitioner with removal, as needed. The practitioner removes the sutures securing the balloon and then withdraws the balloon until the proximal end of the catheter contacts the distal end of the introducer sheath.
- While applying pressure below the puncture site, the practitioner removes the balloon and introducer sheath as a unit, allowing a few seconds of free bleeding *to prevent thrombus formation.*
- Assess the integrity of the balloon after removal.
- Apply direct pressure to the site for 30 to 45 minutes or until bleeding stops.[10] (*Note:* In some facilities, applying pressure is the practitioner's responsibility.)
- Apply a mechanical compression device, as ordered.
- If the balloon was inserted surgically, assist the surgeon with closure of the Dacron graft and suturing of the insertion site. A cardiologist usually removes the percutaneous catheter.
- Assess the site for bleeding or hematoma. Apply a pressure dressing and keep it in place for 2 to 4 hours.[10]
- Record the patient's pedal and posterior tibial pulses, and the color, temperature, and sensation of the affected limb.
- Maintain the patient on bed rest, with the head of the bed elevated 30 degrees or less, and keep the affected extremity straight for 8 hours or according to the practitioner's order.[10]
- Appropriately discard used supplies.[36]
- Remove and discard your gloves.
- Perform hand hygiene.[12,13,14,15,16]
- Document the procedure.[37,38,39]

Special considerations

- Inflation and deflation need to be timed to the patient's cardiac *cycle to achieve optimal counterpulsation.* Determine timing using the patient's ECG signal (inflation occurs in the middle of the T wave; deflation occurs just before the end of the QRS complex), his arterial waveform, or the intrinsic pump rate. The goal of IABC therapy should be determined before choosing the best timing *method because inappropriate timing can be detrimental to left ventricular performance.*[2]
- Some IABP manufacturers produce autotiming devices that sense the R wave on the ECG tracing and use this as the trigger source.[2,10,45]
- The Joint Commission issued a sentinel event alert concerning medical device alarm safety *because alarm-related events have been associated with permanent loss of function or death.* Among the major contributing factors were improper alarm settings, alarm settings inappropriately turned off, and alarm signals not audible to staff. Make sure that alarm limits are set appropriately and that alarms are turned on, functioning properly, and audible to staff. Follow facility guidelines for preventing alarm fatigue.[10,19,20,21]
- Be aware that site care and frequency depend on the type of dressing used. Change a transparent semipermeable dressing at least every 7 days, and a gauze dressing every 2 days.[28] Change the dressing sooner if drainage, site tenderness, signs of infection, or compromised dressing integrity occur. Clean the catheter site junction with an antiseptic pad (chlorhexidine-based is preferred), allow it to dry, replace the securement device (if used), and then apply a sterile occlusive dressing.[46] If you use povidone-iodine solution, don't allow it to come in contact with the catheter.
- Watch for pump interruptions, which may result from loose ECG electrodes or leadwires, static or 60-cycle interference, catheter kinking, or improper body alignment.
- After removal, assess the patient's vital signs and hemodynamic parameters every 15 minutes for 1 hour, every 30 minutes for the next hour, and then hourly as the patient's condition warrants.[10] Notify the practitioner of any abnormalities.

Complications

IABC may cause numerous complications. The most common, arterial embolism, stems from clot formation on the balloon surface. Other potential complications include extension or rupture of an aortic aneurysm, femoral or iliac artery perforation, femoral artery occlusion, balloon rupture, sepsis, and limb ischemia. Bleeding at the insertion site may become aggravated by pump-induced thrombocytopenia caused by platelet aggregation around the balloon.

Removal of IABC can cause bleeding and hematoma formation at the insertion site. The risk of bleeding at the insertion site increases with the use of anticoagulants and the presence of thrombocytopenia, which may be caused by the balloon itself.

Documentation

Document all aspects of patient preparation and assessment, including any patient and family teaching provided. Also document the procedure, interventions, complications, and the patient's response.

When managing IABC, document all aspects of patient assessment and management, including the patient's response to therapy. If you're responsible for the IABC device, document all routine checks, problems, and troubleshooting measures. If a technician is responsible for the IABC device, record only when and why the technician was notified as well as the result of his actions on the patient, if any. Also document any teaching of the patient and family as well as their responses.

Document all aspects of patient assessment and management related to removal, including the condition of the insertion site after removal, wound care performed, and the patient's tolerance of the procedure. Document any patient teaching and the patient's understanding of your teaching.

REFERENCES

1 Krishna, M., & Zacharowski, K. (2009). Principles of intra-aortic balloon pump counterpulsation. *Continuing Education in Anaesthesia, Critical Care & Pain, 9,* 24–28. Accessed March 2015 via the Web at http://ceaccp.oxfordjournals.org/content/9/1/24.full

2 Hanlon-Pena, P. M., & Quaal, S. J. (2011). Intra-aortic balloon pump timing: Review of evidence supporting current practice. *American Journal of Critical Care, 20,* 323–334. Accessed March 2015 via the Web at http://ajcc.aacnjournals.org/content/20/4/323.full

3 Thiele, H., et al. (2012). Intraaortic balloon support for myocardial infarction with cardiogenic shock. *New England Journal of Medicine, 367,* 1287. (Level II)

4 Menon, V., & Hochman, J. S. Prognosis and treatment of cardiogenic shock complicating acute myocardial infarction. (2013). In: *UpToDate,* Gersh, B. J., et al. (Eds.). Accessed March 2015 via the Web at http://www.uptodate.com/contents/search

5 The Joint Commission. (2015). Standard RI.01.03.01. *Comprehensive accreditation manual for hospitals: The official handbook.* Oakbrook Terrace, IL: The Joint Commission. (Level VII)

6 Centers for Medicare & Medicaid Services, Department of Health and Human Services. (2014). Condition of Participation: Patient's rights. 42 C.F.R. § 482.13(b)(2).

7 American Osteopathic Association. (2014). Standard 30.01.11. *Healthcare Facilities Accreditation Program: Accreditation requirements for acute care hospitals.* Chicago, IL: American Osteopathic Association. (Level VII)

8 The Joint Commission. (2015). Standard UP.01.01.01. *Comprehensive accreditation manual for hospitals: The official handbook.* Oakbrook Terrace, IL: The Joint Commission. (Level VII)

9 American Osteopathic Association. (2014). Standard 30.00.14. *Healthcare Facilities Accreditation Program: Accreditation requirements for acute care hospitals.* Chicago, IL: American Osteopathic Association. (Level VII)

10 Lynn-McHale Wiegand, D. (Ed.). (2011). *AACN procedure manual for critical care* (6th ed.). St. Louis, MO: Saunders.

11 The Joint Commission. (2015). Standard NPSG.02.03.01. *Comprehensive accreditation manual for hospitals: The official handbook.* Oakbrook Terrace, IL: The Joint Commission. (Level VII)

12 The Joint Commission. (2015). Standard NPSG.07.01.01. *Comprehensive accreditation manual for hospitals: The official handbook.* Oakbrook Terrace, IL: The Joint Commission. (Level VII)

13 Centers for Disease Control and Prevention. (2002). Guideline for hand hygiene in health-care settings: Recommendations of the Healthcare Infection Control Practices Advisory Committee and the HICPAC/SHEA/APIC/IDSA Hand Hygiene Task Force. *MMWR Recommendations and Reports, 51*(RR-16), 1–45. Accessed March 2015 via the Web at http://www.cdc.gov/mmwr/pdf/rr/rr5116.pdf (Level II)

14 World Health Organization. (2009). "WHO guidelines on hand hygiene in health care: First global patient safety challenge, clean care is safer care" [Online]. Accessed March 2015 via the Web at http://whqlibdoc.who.int/publications/2009/9789241597906_eng.pdf (Level IV)

15 Centers for Medicare & Medicaid Services, Department of Health and Human Services. (2014). Condition of participation: Infection control. 42 C.F.R. § 482.42.

16 American Osteopathic Association. (2014). Standard 07.01.10. *Healthcare Facilities Accreditation Program: Accreditation requirements for acute care hospitals.* Chicago, IL: American Osteopathic Association. (Level VII)

17 The Joint Commission. (2015). Standard NPSG.01.01.01. *Comprehensive accreditation manual for hospitals: The official handbook.* Oakbrook Terrace, IL: The Joint Commission. (Level VII)

18 The Joint Commission. (2015). Standard NPSG.06.01.01. *Comprehensive accreditation manual for hospitals: The official handbook.* Oakbrook Terrace, IL: The Joint Commission. (Level VII)

19 The Joint Commission. (2013). "Sentinel event alert: Medical device alarm safety in hospitals" [Online]. Accessed March 2015 via the Web at http://www.jointcommission.org/assets/1/18/SEA_50_alarms_4_5_13_FINAL1.PDF (Level VII)

20 American Association of Critical-Care Nurses (AACN). (2013). "AACN practice alert: Alarm management" [Online]. Accessed March 2015 via the Web at http://www.aacn.org/wd/practice/docs/practicealerts/alarm-management-practice-alert.pdf (Level VII)

21 Graham, K. C., & Cvach, M. (2010). Monitor alarm fatigue: Standardizing use of physiological monitors and decreasing nuisance alarms. *American Journal of Critical Care, 19,* 28–37.

22 Maquet Getinge Group. (2012). "Quick reference guide: IAB insertion/Cardiosave™ IABP operation" [Online]. Accessed March 2015 via the Web at http://ca.maquet.com/file_assets/educational-materials/en/Quick-Reference-Guide-IAB-Insertion-CARDIOSAVE-IABP-Operation.pdf

23 Standard 35. Vascular access site preparation and device management. Infusion nursing standards of practice. (2011). *Journal of Infusion Nursing, 34,* S44–S45. (Level VII)

24 The Joint Commission. (2015). Standard NPSG.07.04.01. *Comprehensive accreditation manual for hospitals: The official handbook.* Oakbrook Terrace, IL: The Joint Commission. (Level VII)

25 Centers for Medicare & Medicaid Services, Department of Health and Human Services. (2014). Condition of participation: Preparation and administration of drugs. 42 C.F.R. § 482.23(c).

26 American Osteopathic Association. (2014). Standard 16.01.03. *Healthcare Facilities Accreditation Program: Accreditation requirements for acute care hospitals.* Chicago, IL: American Osteopathic Association. (Level VII)

27 The Joint Commission. (2015). Standard MM.06.01.01. *Comprehensive accreditation manual for hospitals: The official handbook.* Oakbrook Terrace, IL: The Joint Commission. (Level VII)

28 Centers for Disease Control and Prevention. (2011). "Guidelines for the prevention of intravascular catheter-related infections" [Online]. Accessed March 2015 via the Web at http://www.cdc.gov/hicpac/pdf/guidelines/bsi-guidelines-2011.pdf (Level I)

29 The Joint Commission. (2015). Standard NPSG.03.04.01. *Comprehensive accreditation manual for hospitals: The official handbook.* Oakbrook Terrace, IL: The Joint Commission. (Level VII)

30 American Osteopathic Association. (2014). Standard 25.01.27. *Healthcare Facilities Accreditation Program: Accreditation requirements for acute care hospitals.* Chicago, IL: American Osteopathic Association. (Level VII)

31 The Joint Commission. (2015). Standard UP.01.03.01. *Comprehensive accreditation manual for hospitals: The official handbook.* Oakbrook Terrace, IL: The Joint Commission. (Level VII)

32 Institute for Safe Medication Practices. (2012)."ISMP's list of high-alert medications" [Online]. Accessed March 2015 via the Web at http://www.ismp.org/tools/highalertmedications.pdf (Level VII)

33 Institute for Safe Medication Practices. (2008). Conducting an independent double-check. *ISMP Medication Safety Alert! Nurse Advise-ERR, 6*(12), 1. Accessed March 2015 via the Web at http://www.ismp.org/newsletters/nursing/Issues/NurseAdviseERR200812.pdf (Level VII)

34 U.S. Food and Drug Administration. (n.d.). "Look. Check. Connect. Safe medical device connections save lives" [Online]. Accessed March 2015 via the Web at http://www.fda.gov/downloads/MedicalDevices/Safety/AlertsandNotices/UCM134873.pdf

35 Goldich, G. (2011). Getting in sync with intra-aortic balloon pump therapy. *Nursing Critical Care, 6*(3), 10–13. Accessed March 2015 via the Web at http://www.nursingcenter.com/lnc/pdfjournal?AID=1254563&an=00152193-201110001-00003&Journal_ID=&Issue_ID=

36 Occupational Safety and Health Administration. (n.d.). "Bloodborne pathogens, standard number 1910.1030" [Online]. Accessed March 2015 via the Web at http://www.osha.gov/pls/oshaweb/owadisp.show_document?p_table=STANDARDS&p_id=10051 (Level VII)

37 The Joint Commission. (2015). Standard RC.01.03.01. *Comprehensive accreditation manual for hospitals: The official handbook.* Oakbrook Terrace, IL: The Joint Commission. (Level VII)

38 Centers for Medicare & Medicaid Services, Department of Health and Human Services. (2014). Condition of participation: Medical record services. 42 C.F.R. § 482.24(b).

EQUIPMENT

Understanding ICP monitoring

Intracranial pressure (ICP) can be monitored using one of four systems.

Intraventricular catheter monitoring

For intraventricular catheter monitoring, which provides direct monitoring of ICP, the practitioner inserts a small catheter into the lateral ventricle through a burr hole. Although this method provides the most accurate measure of ICP and is the only type of ICP monitoring that allows evaluation of brain compliance and drainage of significant amounts of cerebrospinal fluid (CSF), it carries the greatest risk of infection. Contraindications usually include stenotic cerebral ventricles, cerebral aneurysms in the path of catheter placement, and suspected vascular lesions.

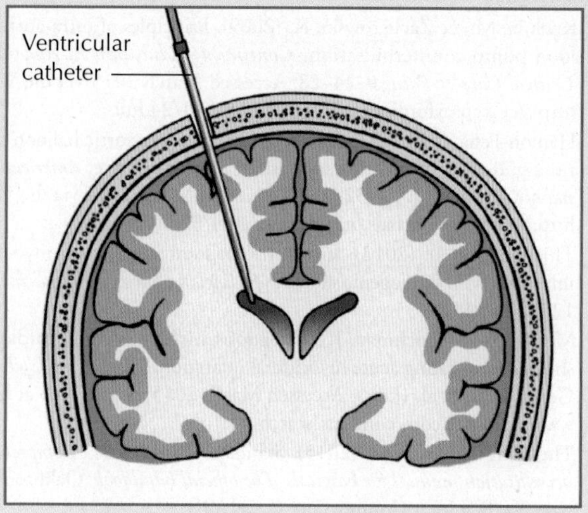

Subarachnoid bolt monitoring

Subarachnoid bolt monitoring involves insertion of a special bolt into the subarachnoid space through a twist-drill burr hole that's positioned in the front of the skull behind the hairline. Placing the bolt is easier than placing an intraventricular catheter, especially if a computed tomography scan reveals that the cerebrum has shifted or the ventricles have collapsed. This type of ICP monitoring also carries less risk of infection and parenchymal damage *because the bolt doesn't penetrate the cerebrum.*

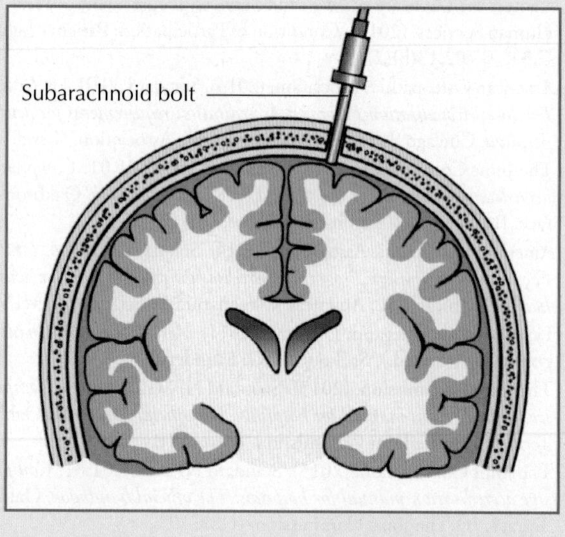

39 American Osteopathic Association. (2014). Standard 10.00.03. *Healthcare Facilities Accreditation Program: Accreditation requirements for acute care hospitals.* Chicago, IL: American Osteopathic Association. (Level VII)

40 Raman, J., et al. (2010). Subclavian artery access for ambulatory balloon pump insertion. *Annals of Thoracic Surgery, 90,* 1032–1034.

41 McMurray, J. J. V., et al. (2012). ESC guidelines for the diagnosis and treatment of acute and chronic heart failure 2012. *European Heart Journal, 33,* 1787–1847. Accessed March 2015 via the Web at http://eurheartj.oxfordjournals.org/content/33/14/1787.full.pdf (Level VII)

42 The Joint Commission. (2015). Standard PC.01.02.07. *Comprehensive accreditation manual for hospitals: The official handbook.* Oakbrook Terrace, IL: The Joint Commission. (Level VII)

43 American Osteopathic Association. (2014). Standard 16.02.01. *Healthcare Facilities Accreditation Program: Accreditation requirements for acute care hospitals.* Chicago, IL: American Osteopathic Association. (Level VII)

44 American Osteopathic Association. (2014). Standard 16.02.02. *Healthcare Facilities Accreditation Program: Accreditation requirements for acute care hospitals.* Chicago, IL: American Osteopathic Association. (Level VII)

45 Yarham, G., et al. (2013). Fiber-optic intra-aortic balloon therapy and its role within cardiac surgery.

46 Standard 46. Vascular access device site care and dressing changes. Infusion nursing standards of practice. (2011). *Journal of Infusion Nursing, 34,* S63–S64. (Level VII)

INTRACRANIAL PRESSURE MONITORING

Intracranial pressure (ICP) monitoring measures pressure exerted by the brain, blood, and cerebrospinal fluid (CSF) against the inside of the skull. Indications for monitoring ICP include head trauma with bleeding or edema, overproduction or insufficient absorption of CSF, cerebral hemorrhage, and space-occupying brain lesions. ICP monitoring can detect elevated ICP early, before clinical danger signs develop.[1] Prompt intervention can then help avert or diminish neurologic damage caused by cerebral hypoxia and shifts of brain mass.

The four basic ICP monitoring systems are intraventricular catheter, subarachnoid bolt, epidural or subdural sensor, and intraparenchymal

EQUIPMENT

Understanding ICP monitoring *(continued)*

Epidural or subdural sensor monitoring

ICP can also be monitored from the epidural or subdural space. For epidural monitoring, the practitioner inserts a fiber-optic sensor into the epidural space through a burr hole. This system's main drawback is its questionable accuracy *because it doesn't measure ICP directly from a CSF-filled space.*

For subdural monitoring, the practitioner tunnels a fiber-optic transducer-tipped catheter through a burr hole, placing its tip on brain tissue under the dura mater. The main drawback to this method is its inability to drain CSF.

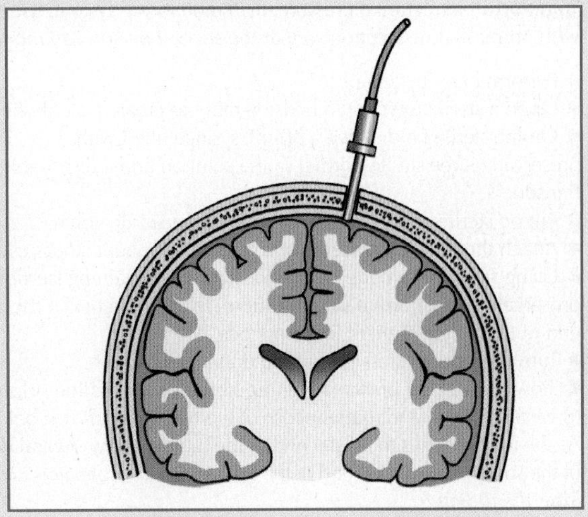

Intraparenchymal pressure monitoring

For intraparenchymal monitoring, the practitioner inserts a catheter through a small subarachnoid bolt and, after puncturing the dura mater, advances the catheter a few centimeters into the brain's white matter. One advantage of this method is that the equipment doesn't need to be balanced or calibrated the after insertion. Although this method doesn't provide direct access to CSF, measurements are accurate *because brain tissue pressures correlate well with ventricular pressures.*

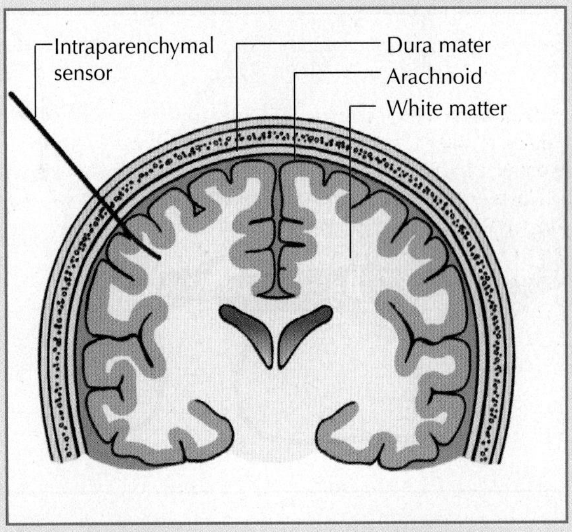

pressure monitoring. Intraventricular catheters are considered the gold standard for measuring ICP because they're inserted directly into the ventricle through a burr hole, which permits ICP monitoring and therapeutic CSF drainage to control ICP.[1] (See *Understanding ICP monitoring.*) Regardless of which system is used, the procedure is typically performed by a neurosurgeon in the operating room or emergency department or on the intensive care unit. Insertion of an ICP monitoring device requires sterile technique to reduce the risk of central nervous system (CNS) infection. Setting up equipment for the monitoring systems also requires strict sterile technique.[1]

Equipment

Intracranial access kit ■ catheter ■ flushless transducer ■ pressure cable and module ■ sterile 4″ × 4″ (10-cm × 10-cm) gauze pads ■ fluid-impermeable pads ■ electric or disposable clippers ■ sterile drapes or towels ■ antiseptic solution or sterile prep kit ■ sterile gown ■ sterile gloves ■ mask ■ caps ■ sterile marker ■ sterile labels ■ preservative-free normal saline solution ■ 30-mL or 40-mL syringe ■ lidocaine local anesthetic ■ leveling device ■ dead-end caps ■ monitoring equipment ■ Optional: tape; prescribed sedation, pain medication, and osmotic diuretic; prescribed IV fluid; IV pole; external ventricular drainage system.

You may need to gather other equipment as instructed by the practitioner, such as the drill and bits, a scalp retractor, and a scalp staple.

Preparation of equipment

Various types of preassembled ICP monitoring units are available, each with its own setup protocols. These units are designed to reduce the risk of infection by eliminating the need for multiple stopcocks, manometers, and transducer dome assemblies. When preparing the equipment, label all medications, medication containers, and other solutions on and off the sterile field.[2] Prepare and set up the monitoring system according to the manufacturer's instructions. (See *Setting up an ICP monitoring system,* page 426.)

- Lower the flow chamber to zero, and turn the stopcock off to the dead-end cap.
- Remove and discard your personal protective equipment.[9]
- Perform hand hygiene.[3,4,5,6,7]

Implementation

For catheter insertion

- Verify the practitioner's order.
- Gather and prepare the equipment, personnel, and supplies needed for device insertion.

EQUIPMENT

Setting up an ICP monitoring system

To set up an intracranial pressure (ICP) monitoring system, use strict sterile technique. Use the two-person method when priming the tubing with normal saline solution *so that the second person can monitor the sterile technique and assist as needed.*[1] Follow these steps:

- Perform hand hygiene.[3,4,5,6,7]
- Open a sterile towel on a bedside table to create a sterile field.
- On the sterile field, place a 30-mL syringe filled with preservative-free sterile normal saline solution and a disposable transducer.
- Put on sterile gloves, a cap, a mask, and a sterile gown.[8,9]
- Attach the flushless transducer to the panel mount stopcock.[1]
- Using sterile technique, attach the syringe containing sterile preservative-free normal saline solution to the stopcock at the distal end of the tubing (patient line stopcock).[1]
- Turn the stopcock off toward the drainage device.[1]
- Slowly inject the preservative-free sterile normal saline solution toward the distal end (patient end) of the tubing (as shown below). As the fluid reaches the distal end of the tubing, allow several drops of the solution to exit the end of the tubing *to make sure air is cleared from the tubing.*[1]

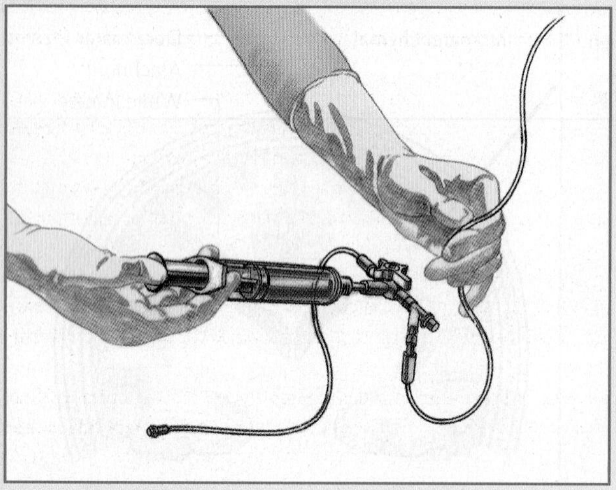

- Turn the stopcock off to the distal end of the tubing, keeping the syringe in place. Make sure that the panel mount stopcock is open to the flushless transducer. Prime through the vented caps in the flushless transducer. Replace the vented caps with dead-end caps.[1]
- With the syringe remaining in place, turn the stopcock off to the transducer and prime fluid into the drip chamber.[1]
- After priming the system, keep the stopcock on the distal end (patient end) of the tubing *off to make sure that no normal saline solution leaks from the system before connection.*[1]
- Connect the transducer to the bedside monitor with a pressure cable that's plugged into the designated pressure module.[1]
- Align the zero point with the center line of the patient's head, level with the middle of the ear.
- The key to accurate ICP measurement is to use the same landmark each time you check the zero reference level.[1]
- Lower the flow chamber to zero, and turn the stopcock off to the dead-end cap.
- With a clean hand, balance the system according to the manufacturer's guidelines.
- Remove and discard your gloves.
- Perform hand hygiene.[3,4,5,6,7]
- Turn the stopcock off to the distal end of the tubing, keeping the syringe in place. Make sure that the panel mount stopcock is open to the flushless transducer. Prime through the vented caps in the flushless transducer. Replace the vented caps with dead-end caps.[1]
- With the syringe remaining in place, turn the stopcock off to the transducer and prime fluid into the drip chamber.[1]
- After priming the system, keep the stopcock on the distal end (patient end) of the tubing off to make sure that no normal saline solution leaks from the system prior to connection.[1]
- Connect the transducer to the bedside monitor with a pressure cable that's plugged into the designated pressure module.[1]
- Align the zero point with the center line of the patient's head, level with the middle of the ear; the key to accurate ICP measurement is to use the same landmark each time you check the zero reference level.[1]

- Confirm that written informed consent has been obtained and that the consent form is in the patient's medical record.[10,11,12]
- Conduct a preprocedure verification *to make sure that all relevant documentation, related information, and equipment are available and correctly identified to the patient's identifiers.*[13,14]
- Verify that ordered laboratory and imaging studies have been completed and that the results are in the patient's medical record. Notify the practitioner of any unexpected results.
- Check the patient's history for an allergy or a hypersensitivity to iodine, latex, or the ordered local anesthetic.
- Perform hand hygiene.[3,4,5,6,7]
- Confirm the patient's identity using at least two patient identifiers.[15]
- Explain the procedure to the patient or his family.
- Make sure the patient is attached to a cardiac monitor and pulse oximeter.[1] Assist with arterial catheter insertion, if ordered, *because vigilant monitoring of mean arterial blood pressure is necessary to avoid decreased cerebral perfusion pressure (CPP).*[1] Make sure the alarm limits are set appropriately for the patient's current condition and that the alarms are turned on, functioning properly, and audible to staff.[16,17,18,19]
- If the monitoring device is to be inserted outside the operating room, make sure that conditions model the operating room; use maximum barrier precautions and close the doors to the room where the procedure is being performed. Make sure anyone in the room wears a mask and cap.[1]
- Obtain baseline routine and neurologic vital signs *to aid in prompt detection of decompensation during the procedure.*[1]
- Assess the patient's sedation and pain management needs in collaboration with the practitioner.
- Administer medications, as indicated and prescribed, *to ensure the patient's comfort during the procedure.*[1,20,21]
- Perform hand hygiene.[3,4,5,6,7]
- Put on gloves, a cap, and a mask.[1,8,9]
- Place the patient in the supine position with the head in a neutral position and the head of the bed elevated to 30 degrees (or as ordered).[1]
- Place fluid-impermeable pads under the patient's head.
- Verify that the insertion site has been identified before preparing the site *to minimize the risk of preparing the wrong area.*[22]
- Braid or clip hair at the insertion site. If the hair is clipped, use tape or some similar sticky product *to remove residual hair clippings.*[1]
- Immobilize the patient's head *to prevent patient movement and facilitate catheter insertion.*[1]
- Clean the incision site with an antiseptic solution using a circular motion. Note that 2% chlorhexidine preparation isn't recommended when contact with the meninges is possible.[1,23]

■ Drape the areas surrounding the insertion site with sterile drapes using maximal barrier precautions.[1]
■ The practitioner puts on a cap, a mask, a sterile gown, and sterile gloves.[19]
■ Conduct a time-out immediately before the practitioner begins the procedure *to identify the correct patient, site, positioning, and procedure and to ensure that all relevant information and necessary equipment are available.*[14,24]
■ The practitioner opens the interior wrap of the sterile supply tray, infiltrates the scalp with an anesthetic agent,[1] and proceeds with insertion of the ICP monitoring device. Assist with the procedure, as needed.
■ During insertion, continually monitor the patient's heart rate and rhythm, respiratory rate, and oxygen saturation level. Frequently monitor the patient's blood pressure. Assess neurologic status every 15 minutes *because serial assessments are necessary to immediately identify neurologic changes and ensure prompt treatment.*[1]
■ After insertion, assist the practitioner with connecting the catheter to the monitoring equipment while maintaining sterility and preventing contamination of the site, catheter, and sterile field.[1]
■ Trace the tubing from the patient to the point of origin *to make sure that it's connected to the proper port.*[25]
■ Clean around the insertion site with antiseptic solution, allow it to dry, and then apply a sterile occlusive dressing to the site.[1]
■ Clearly label the access port of an external ventricular drain *to indicate that it's an external ventricular drain, preventing accidental mix-up of the port with an IV line.*[1]
■ Maintain the patient in an upright position with the head of the bed elevated 30 degrees or as ordered *to promote venous return.* Make sure that the head is at the top of the bed in a midline position to the rest of the body *because flexion or rotation of the head or neck can obstruct venous return and thereby increase ICP.*[1]
■ Maintain the ICP transducer at the foramen of Monro. Anatomically, the reference point is equivalent to the level of the ear or the outer canthus of the eye. *Transducer placement at a point above or below the anatomically correct position will result in false readings.*
■ Zero and calibrate the device after insertion, if required by the type of device used. If the device requires recalibration after it's in use, rezero at least every 12 hours.[1]
■ If the patient has an external ventricular drain, maintain the drip chamber at the prescribed zero reference and pressure levels.[1]
■ Make sure that the monitor's alarm limits are set appropriately for the patient's current condition and that the alarms are turned on, functioning properly, and audible to staff.[16]
■ Begin ICP monitoring; obtain an ICP tracing and assess the waveform. Use this tracing as a baseline for comparison. (See *Interpreting ICP waveforms*, page 428.) If the patient has an external ventricular drain, turn the stopcock off to the drain and open to the transducer *to obtain an accurate ICP numeric value and waveform.*[1]
■ Observe ICP in relation to other hemodynamic parameters, such as mean arterial pressure.[1]
■ Dispose of insertion instruments and equipment appropriately *to prevent exposure to potentially infectious materials.*[1]
■ Remove and discard your personal protective equipment.[9]
■ Perform hand hygiene.[3,4,5,6,7]
■ Arrange for a computed tomography scan, if ordered, *to confirm catheter placement.*[1]
■ Document the procedure.[26,27,28]

ICP monitoring and care

■ Assess the patient's neurologic status hourly, or more frequently if the patient's condition warrants. Notify the practitioner immediately if the patient's ICP exceeds established parameters. If no parameters exist, notify the practitioner if ICP exceeds 20 mm Hg. Watch for signs and symptoms of increased ICP, such as decreased level of consciousness, nausea, vomiting, headache, lethargy, and agitation.[1] (See *Managing ICP*, page 429.)
■ If the bedside monitor doesn't calculate CPP, calculate CPP hourly by subtracting the patient's ICP from his mean arterial pressure (MAP) (CPP = MAP – ICP). If CPP isn't within the specified parameters, notify the practitioner.[1]
■ Assess CSF drainage hourly for color and clarity.[1]
■ Assess external ventricular drain patency as needed by lowering the entire system briefly to assess drip rate into the graduated burette.[1]
■ Check the patient's position hourly to ensure that the transducer is at the ordered reference level *to prevent overdrainage or underdrainage if an external ventricular drain is in place and to ensure accurate ICP readings.*[1]
■ Assess the catheter system at least every 4 hours to ensure the system is intact and has no leaks, kinks, or clots *to decrease the risk of increased ICP related to catheter flow and drainage and to ensure accurate pressure readings and waveforms consistent with neurologic assessment.*[1]
■ Record an ICP tracing each shift and as waveform changes occur; compare these tracings with previous tracings.[1]
■ If the patient has an external ventricular drain, inform him and his family that the bed position should only be changed with assistance *because raising the level of the bed with the external ventricular drain at fixed zero and reference levels can result in a large increase in CSF drainage.*[1]
■ Clamp an external ventricular drain any time there is a patient response (coughing, vomiting, or response to care) or procedure (suctioning, repositioning, and transport) that may cause CSF overdrainage.[1]
■ If an ICP waveform doesn't appear, troubleshoot the system. If the patient has an external ventricular drain, then air bubbles, clots, or debris within the drainage tubing or across the transducer may be the cause. Systematically assess the system for air and debris. Make sure the drain is leveled at the appropriate landmark and the system rezeroed. If a waveform still fails to appear, replace the pressure cable, module, or transducer; change only one at a time.[1]
■ Don't routinely change the drainage tubing; leave it in place for the duration of external ventricular drainage. If the drainage tubing becomes accidently disconnected, maintain the sterility of the ventricular catheter, and obtain and connect a new sterile drainage system.[1]
■ When accessing an external ventricular drainage system, perform hand hygiene, put on a mask, set up a sterile field, and put on sterile gloves. Scrub the access port for 3 minutes using povidone-iodine or use another facility-approved antiseptic and follow the manufacturer's instructions for use.[1]
■ Maintain the drainage bag in an upright position. If it must be laid down, drain the CSF to the lower collection bag *to decrease the transfer of bacteria in the collection chamber to the drainage bag.* Change the drainage bag when it's nearly full, wearing sterile gloves and a mask.[1]
■ Change the dressing every 48 hours, when soiled, or as directed by your facility.[1] Follow these steps when changing the dressing: put on sterile gloves and a mask and remove and discard the dressing. Clip any hair that has grown back at the site. Inspect the site for CSF leakage and signs of infection. Remove and discard your gloves and perform hand hygiene. Put on a new pair of sterile gloves and place a new sterile occlusive dressing over the site. Remove and discard your gloves.[1]
■ Perform hand hygiene.[3,4,5,6,7]
■ Document the procedure.[26,27,28]

Special considerations

■ The Joint Commission issued a sentinel event alert concerning medical device alarm safety *because alarm-related events have been associated with permanent loss of function and death.* Among the major contributing factors were improper alarm settings, alarms turned off inappropriately,

Interpreting ICP waveforms

Three waveforms—A, B, and C—are used to monitor intracranial pressure (ICP). A waves are an ominous sign of intracranial decompensation and poor compliance. B waves correlate with changes in respiration, and C waves correlate with changes in arterial pressure.

Normal waveform

A normal ICP waveform typically shows a steep upward systolic slope followed by a downward diastolic slope with a dicrotic notch. In most cases, this waveform occurs continuously and indicates an ICP between 0 and 15 mm Hg—normal pressure.

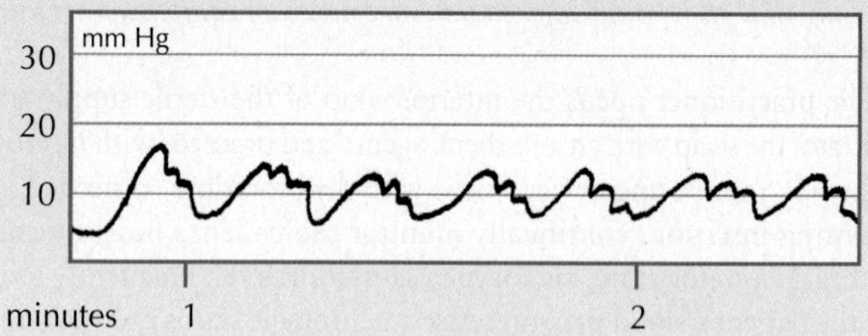

A waves

The most clinically significant ICP waveforms are A waves, which may reach elevations of 50 to 100 mm Hg, persist for 5 to 20 minutes, and then drop sharply—signaling exhaustion of the brain's compliance mechanisms. A waves may come and go, spiking from temporary rises in thoracic pressure or from any condition that increases ICP beyond the brain's compliance limits. Activities such as sustained coughing or straining during defecation can cause temporary elevations in thoracic pressure. *Because A waves are an ominous sign,* they require emergency treatment.

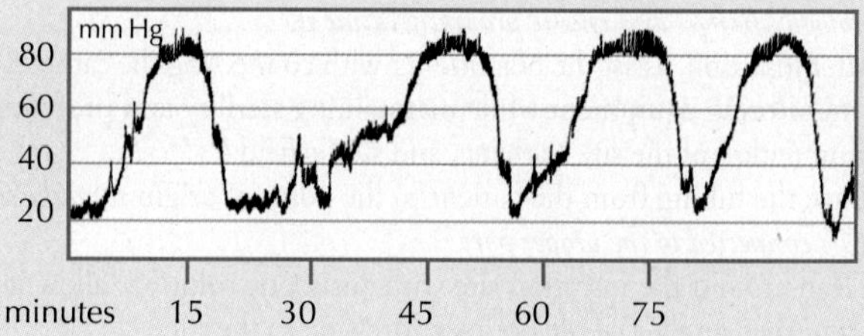

B waves

B waves, which appear sharp and rhythmic with a sawtooth pattern, occur every 1½ to 2 minutes and may reach elevations of 50 mm Hg. The clinical significance of B waves isn't clear, but the waves correlate with respiratory changes and may occur more frequently with decreasing compensation. *Because B waves sometimes precede A waves,* notify the practitioner if B waves occur frequently.

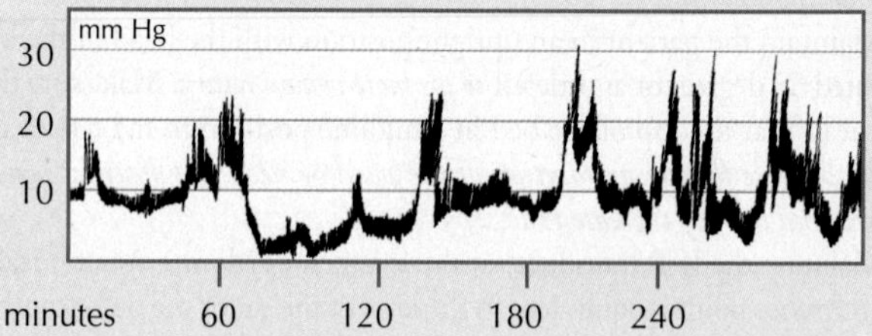

C waves

C waves are rapid and rhythmic, but not sharp, and last 1 to 2 minutes with an ICP of 20 to 50 mm Hg. Clinically insignificant, they may fluctuate with respirations or systemic blood pressure changes.

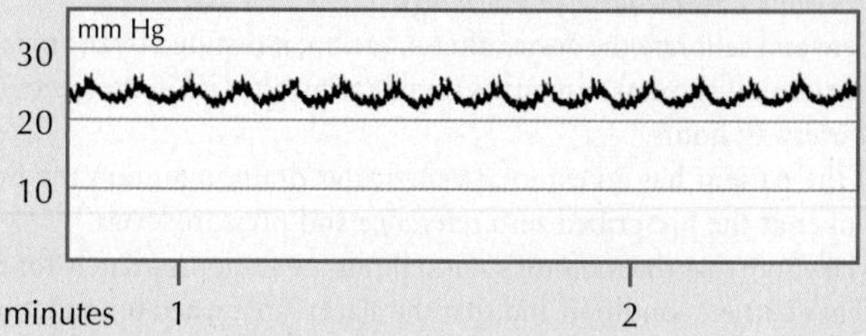

Waveform showing equipment problem

A waveform such as the one shown below signals a problem with the transducer or monitor. Check for line obstruction, and determine if the transducer needs rebalancing. If the patient has a low ICP reading, this waveform may be normal.

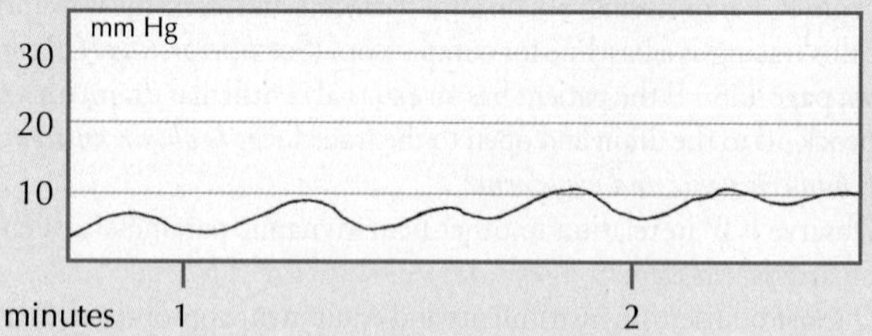

and alarm signals that were not audible to staff. Make sure that alarm limits are set appropriately and that alarms are turned on, functioning properly, and audible to staff. Follow facility guidelines for preventing alarm fatigue.[19]

- If the patient develops increased ICP, open the external ventricular drain to drain CSF, as ordered; administer hyperosmolar therapy with hypertonic saline solution or mannitol, if prescribed.[29]
- Be aware that induced hypothermia may reduce ICP initially but can cause cerebral edema during rewarming and isn't recommended for treatment of increased ICP.[29]

Complications

CNS infection, the most common hazard of ICP monitoring, can result from contamination of the equipment setup or of the insertion site.

NURSING ALERT *Excessive loss of CSF can result from faulty stopcock placement or a drip chamber that's positioned too low. Such loss can rapidly decompress the cranial contents and damage bridging cortical veins, leading to hematoma formation. Decompression can also lead to rupture of existing hematomas or aneurysms, causing hemorrhage.*

Managing ICP

By performing nursing care gently, slowly, and cautiously, you can best help manage—or even significantly reduce—increased intracranial pressure (ICP). If possible, urge the patient to participate in his own care. Here are some steps you can take to manage increased ICP.

- Plan your care to include rest periods between activities and minimize external stimulation *to allow the patient's ICP to return to baseline, thus avoiding lengthy and cumulative pressure elevations.*
- Speak to the patient before attempting any procedures, even if he appears comatose. Touch him on an arm or leg first before touching him in a more personal area, such as the face or chest. This is especially important if the patient doesn't know you or if he's confused or sedated.
- Suction the patient only when it's necessary to remove secretions and maintain airway patency.
- Hyperventilate the patient with 100% oxygen as ordered. *Hyperventilation with oxygen from a handheld resuscitation bag or ventilator helps rid the patient of excess carbon dioxide, thereby constricting cerebral vessels and reducing cerebral blood volume and ICP. However, only normal brain tissues respond because blood vessels in damaged areas have reduced vasoconstrictive ability.* Hyperventilation should only be used in an acute situation to decrease ICP until other measures can be instituted *because it can cause ischemia.*[1]
- *To promote venous drainage,* keep the patient's head in the midline position, even when he's positioned on his side.[1] Avoid flexing the neck or hip more than 90 degrees, and keep the head of the bed elevated 30 to 45 degrees. Keep endotracheal tube ties and rigid cervical collars secure but loose enough *to prevent compression of the jugular veins.*
- Avoid placing the patient in the prone position.
- *To avoid increasing intrathoracic pressure, which raises ICP,* discourage the Valsalva maneuver and isometric muscle contractions. *To avoid isometric contractions,* distract the patient when giving him painful injections (by asking him to wiggle his toes and by massaging the area before injection *to relax the muscle*) and have him concentrate on breathing through difficult procedures such as bed-to-stretcher transfers. *To keep the patient from holding his breath when moving around in bed,* tell him to relax as much as possible during position changes. If necessary, administer a stool softener *to help prevent constipation and unnecessary straining during defecation.*
- If the patient is heavily sedated, monitor his respiratory rate and blood gas levels. *Depressed respirations will compromise ventilations and oxygen exchange. Maintaining adequate respiratory rate and volume helps reduce ICP.*

Watch for signs of impending or overt decompensation: pupillary dilation (unilateral or bilateral); decreased pupillary response to light; decreasing level of consciousness; rising systolic blood pressure and widening pulse pressure; bradycardia; slowed, irregular respirations; and, in late decompensation, decerebrate posturing.

Documentation

Record the time and date of the insertion procedure and the patient's response. Note the insertion site and the type of monitoring system used. Record ICP digital readings and waveforms and CPP hourly in your notes or a flowchart, or directly on readout strips, depending on your facility's documentation format. Document any factors that may affect ICP (for example, drug therapy, stressful procedures, and sleep).

Record routine and neurologic vital signs hourly, and describe the patient's clinical status. Note the amount, character, and frequency of any CSF drainage (for example, "between 6 p.m. and 7 p.m., 15 mL of blood-tinged CSF"). Also record the ICP reading in response to drainage.

REFERENCES

1 American Association of Neuroscience Nurses (AANN). (2011). *Care of the patient undergoing intracranial pressure monitoring/external ventricular drainage or lumbar drainage: AANN clinical practice guideline series.* Glenview, IL: American Association of Neuroscience Nurses. Accessed March 2015 via the Web at http://www.aann.org/uploads/AANN11_ICPEVDnew.pdf (Level VII)

2 The Joint Commission. (2015). Standard NPSG.03.04.01. *Comprehensive accreditation manual for hospitals: The official handbook.* Oakbrook Terrace, IL: The Joint Commission. (Level VII)

3 The Joint Commission. (2015). Standard NPSG.07.01.01. *Comprehensive accreditation manual for hospitals: The official handbook.* Oakbrook Terrace, IL: The Joint Commission. (Level VII)

4 Centers for Disease Control and Prevention. (2002). Guideline for hand hygiene in health-care settings: Recommendations of the Healthcare Infection Control Practices Advisory Committee and the HICPAC/SHEA/APIC/IDSA Hand Hygiene Task Force. *MMWR Recommendations and Reports, 51*(RR-16), 1–45. Accessed March 2015 via the Web at http://www.cdc.gov/mmwr/pdf/rr/rr5116.pdf (Level II)

5 World Health Organization. (2009). "WHO guidelines on hand hygiene in health care: First global patient safety challenge, clean care is safer care" [Online]. Accessed March 2015 via the Web at http://whqlibdoc.who.int/publications/2009/9789241597906_eng.pdf (Level IV)

6 American Osteopathic Association. (2014). Standard 07.01.21. *Healthcare Facilities Accreditation Program: Accreditation requirements for acute care hospitals.* Chicago, IL: American Osteopathic Association. (Level VII)

7 Centers for Medicare & Medicaid Services, Department of Health and Human Services. (2014). Condition of participation: Infection control. 42 C.F.R. § 482.42.

8 Siegel, J. D., et al. (2007). "2007 guideline for isolation precautions: Preventing transmission of infectious agents in healthcare settings" [Online]. Accessed March 2015 via the Web at http://www.cdc.gov/hicpac/pdf/isolation/Isolation2007.pdf (Level II)

9 American Osteopathic Association. (2014). Standard 07.01.10. *Healthcare Facilities Accreditation Program: Accreditation requirements for acute care hospitals.* Chicago, IL: American Osteopathic Association. (Level VII)

10 The Joint Commission. (2015). Standard RI.01.03.01. *Comprehensive accreditation manual for hospitals: The official handbook.* Oakbrook Terrace, IL: The Joint Commission. (Level VII)

11 Centers for Medicare & Medicaid Services, Department of Health and Human Services. (2014). Condition of participation: Patient's rights. 42 C.F.R. § 482.13.

12 American Osteopathic Association. (2014). Standard 30.01.11. *Healthcare Facilities Accreditation Program: Accreditation requirements for acute care hospitals.* Chicago, IL: American Osteopathic Association. (Level VII)

13 The Joint Commission. (2015). Standard UP.01.01.01. *Comprehensive accreditation manual for hospitals: The official handbook.* Oakbrook Terrace, IL: The Joint Commission. (Level VII)

14 American Osteopathic Association. (2014). Standard 30.00.14. *Healthcare Facilities Accreditation Program: Accreditation requirements for acute care hospitals.* Chicago, IL: American Osteopathic Association. (Level VII)

15 The Joint Commission. (2015). Standard NPSG.01.01.01. *Comprehensive accreditation manual for hospitals: The official handbook.* Oakbrook Terrace, IL: The Joint Commission. (Level VII)

16 American Association of Critical-Care Nurses (AACN). (2013). "AACN practice alert: Alarm management" [Online]. Accessed March 2015 via

Intradermal injection sites

The most common intradermal injection site is the ventral forearm. Other sites (indicated by dotted areas) include the upper chest, upper arms, and shoulder blades. Skin in these areas is usually lightly pigmented, thinly keratinized, and relatively hairless, facilitating detection of adverse reactions.

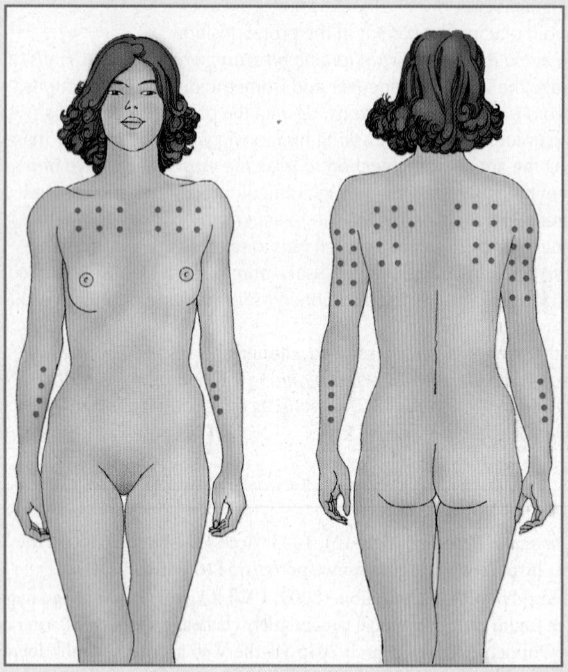

the Web at http://www.aacn.org/wd/practice/docs/practicealerts/alarm-management-practice-alert.pdf (Level VII)

17 Graham, K. C., & Cvach, M. (2010). Monitor alarm fatigue: Standardizing use of physiological monitors and decreasing nuisance alarms. *American Journal of Critical Care, 19,* 28–37.

18 The Joint Commission. (2015). Standard NPSG.06.01.01. *Comprehensive accreditation manual for hospitals: The official handbook.* Oakbrook Terrace, IL: The Joint Commission. (Level VII)

19 The Joint Commission. (2013). "Sentinel event alert: Medical device alarm safety in hospitals" [Online]. Accessed March 2015 via the Web at http://www.jointcommission.org/assets/1/18/SEA_50_alarms_4_5_13_FINAL1.PDF (Level VII)

20 American Osteopathic Association. (2014). Standard 16.01.03. *Healthcare Facilities Accreditation Program: Accreditation requirements for acute care hospitals.* Chicago, IL: American Osteopathic Association. (Level VII)

21 Centers for Medicare & Medicaid Services, Department of Health and Human Services. (2014). Condition of participation: Nursing services. 42 C.F.R. § 482.23(c).

22 The Joint Commission. (2015). Standard UP.01.02.01. *Comprehensive accreditation manual for hospitals: The official handbook.* Oakbrook Terrace, IL: The Joint Commission. (Level VII)

23 CareFusion. (n.d.). "ChloraPrep product label" [Online]. Accessed March 2015 via the Web at http://www.carefusion.com/medical-products/infection-prevention/skin-preparation/

24 The Joint Commission. (2015). Standard UP.01.03.01. *Comprehensive accreditation manual for hospitals: The official handbook.* Oakbrook Terrace, IL: The Joint Commission. (Level VII)

25 U.S. Food and Drug Administration. (n.d.). "Look. Check. Connect. Safe medical device connections save lives" [Online]. Accessed March 2015 via the Web at http://www.fda.gov/downloads/MedicalDevices/Safety/AlertsandNotices/UCM134873.pdf

26 The Joint Commission. (2015). Standard RC.01.03.01. *Comprehensive accreditation manual for hospitals: The official handbook.* Oakbrook Terrace, IL: The Joint Commission. (Level VII)

27 American Osteopathic Association. (2014). Standard 10.00.03. *Healthcare Facilities Accreditation Program: Accreditation requirements for acute care hospitals.* Chicago, IL: American Osteopathic Association. (Level VII)

28 Centers for Medicare & Medicaid Services, Department of Health and Human Services. (2014). Condition of participation: Medical record services. 42 C.F.R. § 482.24(b).

29 Ropper, A. H. (2012). Hyperosmolar therapy for raised intracranial pressure. *New England Journal of Medicine, 367,* 746–752.

ADDITIONAL REFERENCES

Hickey, J.V. (2014). *The clinical practice of neurological and neurosurgical nursing* (7th ed.). Philadelphia, PA: Wolters Kluwer.

Lynn-McHale Wiegand, D. (Ed.). (2011). *AACN procedure manual for critical care* (6th ed.). Philadelphia, PA: Saunders.

INTRADERMAL INJECTION

Because little systemic absorption of intradermally injected agents takes place, intradermal injections are used primarily to produce a local effect, as in allergy or tuberculin testing. Intradermal injections are administered in small volumes—usually 0.01 to 0.1 mL—into the outer layers of the skin.

The ventral forearm is the most commonly used site for intradermal injection because of its easy accessibility and lack of hair. In extensive allergy testing, the outer aspect of the upper arms may be used. (See *Intradermal injection sites.*)

Equipment

Patient's medication administration record ▪ single-use tuberculin or 1-mL syringe with a 26G or 27G ⅜″ to ½″ (1.0- to 1.3-cm) needle ▪ prescribed medication or antigen ▪ alcohol pads ▪ Optional: gloves, pen, emergency resuscitation equipment, epinephrine.

Preparation of equipment

Make sure emergency equipment is readily available and functioning properly.

Use single-dose vials for parenteral medications whenever possible. Don't administer medications from single-dose vials or ampules to multiple patients or combine leftover contents for later use. If multidose vials must be used, both the needle or cannula and syringe used to access the multidose vial must be sterile.[1]

Implementation

- Avoid distractions and interruptions when preparing and administering the medication *to prevent medication errors.*[2]
- Verify the order in the patient's medical record by checking it against the practitioner's order.[3,4,5]
- Gather the equipment and the medication and select the appropriate-sized needle.
- Compare the medication label with the order in the patient's medical record.[3,4,5,6]
- Review the patient's medical record for drug allergies or contraindications to the prescribed medication. If an allergy or a contraindication exists, don't administer the medication; instead, notify the practitioner.[3,4,5]
- Check the expiration date on the medication. If the medication is expired, return it to the pharmacy and obtain new medication.[3,4,5]
- Visually inspect the prescribed medication for particles, discoloration, or other loss of integrity; don't administer the medication if its integrity is compromised.[3,4,5]

NURSING ALERT *Never use medication that's cloudy or discolored or that contains a precipitate unless the manufacturer's instructions allow it. Remember that for some drugs (such as suspensions), the* *presence of drug particles is normal. When in doubt, check with the pharmacist.*

■ Discuss any unresolved concerns about the medication with the patient's practitioner.[3,4,5]

■ Carefully calculate the dosage and draw up the medication.

■ Perform hand hygiene.[7,8,9,10,11,12]

■ Confirm the patient's identity using at least two patient identifiers.[13]

■ If the patient is receiving the medication for the first time, teach about potential adverse reactions and discuss any other concerns related to the medication.[3,4,5]

■ Verify that the medication is being administered at the proper time, in the prescribed dose, and by the correct route *to reduce the risk of medication errors.*[3,4,5]

■ If your facility uses a bar code scanning system, scan your identification badge, the patient's identification band, and the medication's bar code.

■ Explain the procedure to the patient. Tell the patient where you'll be giving the injection.
Provide privacy.[14,15]

■ Put on gloves if contact with blood or other body fluids is likely or if your skin or the patient's skin isn't intact; *gloves aren't recommended for routine intradermal injection because they don't protect against needlestick injury.*[7]

■ Instruct the patient to sit up and to extend her arm and support it on a flat surface, with the ventral forearm exposed (as shown below).

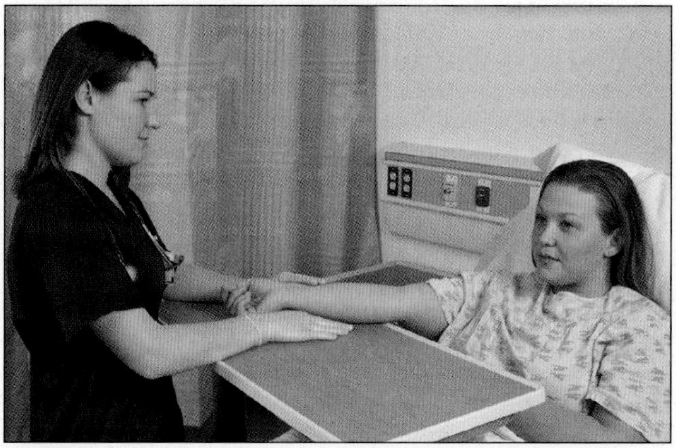

■ With an alcohol pad, clean the surface of the ventral forearm about two or three fingerbreadths distal to the antecubital space (as shown below). Wipe the area from the center of the injection site working outward.[7] Be sure the test site you have chosen is free of hair or blemishes. Allow the skin to dry completely before administering the injection.

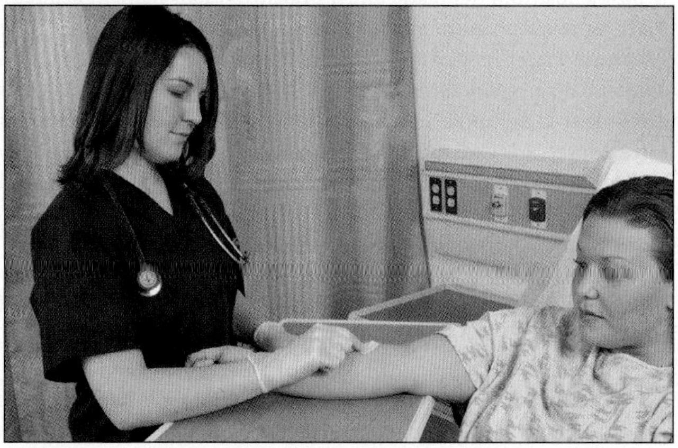

■ While holding the patient's forearm in your hand, stretch the skin taut with your thumb (as shown below).

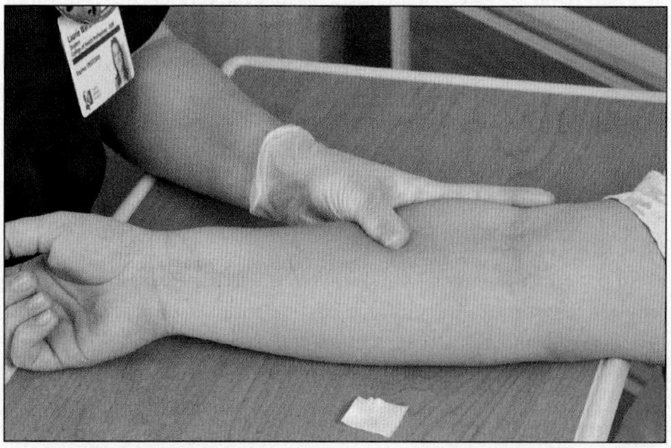

■ With your free hand, hold the needle at a 5- to 15-degree angle to the patient's arm, with its bevel up (as shown below).[16]

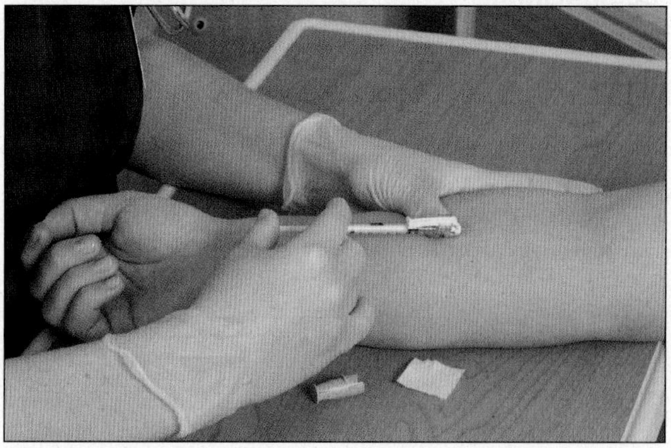

■ Insert the needle about ⅛″ (0.3 cm) below the epidermis. Stop when the needle's bevel tip is under the skin, and inject the antigen slowly. You should feel some resistance as you do this, and a wheal should form as you inject the antigen (as shown below). If no wheal forms, you have injected the antigen too deeply; withdraw the needle, and administer another test dose at least 2″ (5 cm) from the first site.

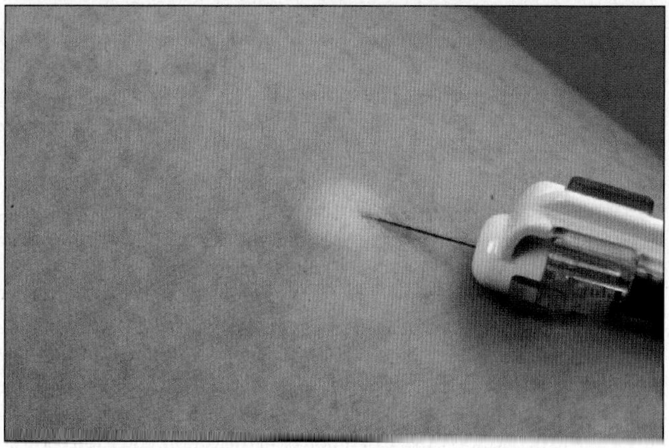

■ Withdraw the needle at the same angle you used to insert it. Don't rub the site. *Rubbing could irritate the underlying tissue, which may affect test results.*

■ If you're administering multiple antigens, inject them at sites at least 2″ (5 cm) apart. Circle each test site with a marking pen, and label each site according to the recall antigen given. Instruct the patient to refrain from washing off the circles until the test is completed.

■ Don't recap the needle. Dispose of needles and syringes in a leak-proof, puncture-resistance conainer.[7,17]

■ Remove and discard your gloves, if worn, and perform hand hygiene.[7,8,9,10,12,11]

■ Assess the patient's reaction; for tuberculin skin testing, assess the reaction in 48 to 72 hours.[18]

■ Document the procedure.[19,20,21]

Special considerations

■ In patients who are hypersensitive to the test antigens, a severe anaphylactic response can result. This reaction requires immediate epinephrine injection and other emergency resuscitation procedures. Be especially alert after giving a test dose of penicillin or tetanus antitoxin.

Patient teaching

Instruct the patient to return for follow-up testing or results interpretation as indicated.

Complications

An allergic reaction or pain may occur as a result of the medication injected.

Documentation

According to your facility's charting format, document the type and dosage of medication or antigen given, the lot number or expiration date as indicated, the time you gave it, and the injection site. Note skin reactions and other adverse reactions and any patient teaching provided.

References

1 Siegel, J. D., et al. (2007). "2007 guideline for isolation precautions: Preventing transmission of infectious agents in healthcare settings" [Online]. Accessed March 2015 via the Web at http://www.cdc.gov/hicpac/pdf/isolation/Isolation2007.pdf (Level I)

2 Westbrook, J., et al. (2010). Association of interruptions with an increased risk and severity of medication administration errors. *Archives of Internal Medicine, 170,* 683–690. (Level IV)

3 The Joint Commission. (2015). Standard MM.06.01.01. *Comprehensive accreditation manual for hospitals: The official handbook.* Oakbrook Terrace, IL: The Joint Commission. (Level VII)

4 American Osteopathic Association. (2014). Standard 16.01.03. *Healthcare Facilities Accreditation Program: Accreditation requirements for acute care hospitals.* Chicago, IL: American Osteopathic Association. (Level VII)

5 Centers for Medicare & Medicaid Services, Department of Health and Human Services. (2014). Condition of participation: Preparation and administration of drugs. 42 C.F.R. § 482.23(c).

6 The Joint Commission. (2015). Standard MM.04.01.01. *Comprehensive accreditation manual for hospitals: The official handbook.* Oakbrook Terrace, IL: The Joint Commission. (Level VII)

7 World Health Organization. (2010). "WHO best practices for injections and related procedures toolkit" [Online]. Accessed March 2015 via the Web at http://whqlibdoc.who.int/publications/2010/9789241599252_eng.pdf (Level IV)

8 American Osteopathic Association. (2014). Standard 07.01.10. *Healthcare Facilities Accreditation Program: Accreditation requirements for acute care hospitals.* Chicago, IL: American Osteopathic Association. (Level VII)

9 Centers for Medicare & Medicaid Services, Department of Health and Human Services. (2014). Condition of participation: Infection control. 42 C.F.R. § 482.42.

10 The Joint Commission. (2015). Standard NPSG.07.01.01. *Comprehensive accreditation manual for hospitals: The official handbook.* Oakbrook Terrace, IL: The Joint Commission. (Level VII)

11 World Health Organization. (2009). "WHO guidelines on hand hygiene in health care: First global patient safety challenge, clean care is safer care" [Online]. Accessed March 2015 via the Web at http://whqlibdoc.who.int/publications/2009/9789241597906_eng.pdf (Level IV)

12 Centers for Disease Control and Prevention. (2002). Guideline for hand hygiene in health-care settings: Recommendations of the Healthcare Infection Control Practices Advisory Committee and the HICPAC/SHEA/APIC/IDSA Hand Hygiene Task Force. *MMWR Recommendations and Reports, 51*(RR-16), 1–45. Accessed March 2015 via the Web at http://www.cdc.gov/mmwr/pdf/rr/rr5116.pdf (Level II)

13 The Joint Commission. (2015). Standard NPSG.01.01.01. *Comprehensive accreditation manual for hospitals: The official handbook.* Oakbrook Terrace, IL: The Joint Commission. (Level VII)

14 American Osteopathic Association (2014). Standard 15.01.16. *Healthcare Facilities Accreditation Program: Accreditation requirements for acute care hospitals.* Chicago, IL: American Osteopathic Association. (Level VII)

15. Centers for Medicare & Medicaid Services, Department of Health and Human Services. (2014). Condition of participation: Patient's rights. 42 C.F.R. § 482.13(c)(1).

16 Tarnow, K., & King, N. (2004). Intradermal injections: Traditional bevel up versus bevel down. *Applied Nursing Research, 17,* 275–282. (Level VI)

17 Occupational Safety and Health Administration. (n.d.). "Bloodborne pathogens, standard number 1910.1030" [Online]. Accessed March 2015 via the Web at http://www.osha.gov/pls/oshaweb/owadisp.show_document?p_table=standards&p_id=10051 (Level VII)

18 Centers for Disease Control and Prevention. (2012). "Fact sheet: Tuberculin skin testing" [Online]. Accessed March 2015 via the Web at http://www.cdc.gov/tb/publications/factsheets/testing/skintesting.html

19 The Joint Commission. (2015). Standard RC.01.03.01. *Comprehensive accreditation manual for hospitals: The official handbook.* Oakbrook Terrace, IL: The Joint Commission. (Level VII)

20 American Osteopathic Association. (2014). Standard 10.00.03. *Healthcare Facilities Accreditation Program: Accreditation requirements for acute care hospitals.* Chicago, IL: American Osteopathic Association (Level VII)

21 Centers for Medicare & Medicaid Services, Department of Health and Human Services. (2014). Condition of participation: Medical record services. 42 C.F.R. § 482.24(b).

Additional references

Craven, R. F., & Hirnle, C. J. (2012). *Fundamentals of nursing: Human health and function* (7th ed.). Philadelphia, PA: Lippincott Williams & Wilkins.

Nettina, S. M. (2014). *Lippincott manual of nursing practice* (10th ed.). Philadelphia, PA: Wolters Kluwer.

Taylor, C., et al. (2011). *Fundamentals of nursing: The art and science of nursing care* (7th ed.). Philadelphia, PA: Lippincott Williams & Wilkins.

Intraosseous infusion

When rapid venous access is difficult or impossible, intraosseous (IO) access allows short-term delivery of fluids, medications, or blood into the bone marrow. This technique is most common for infants and children in such emergencies as cardiopulmonary arrest or circulatory collapse, hypovolemia from traumatic injury or dehydration, status epilepticus, status asthmaticus, burns, near drowning, and overwhelming sepsis. The American Heart Association recommends inserting an IO device to administer emergency medications when you can't quickly insert another access device.[1] Advanced Trauma Life Support, Advanced Cardiovascular Life Support, and Pediatric Advanced Life Support guidelines currently recommend IO access as the immediate alternative route when peripheral IV access is unobtainable.[2] The onset of drug action and drug levels administered by this route are comparable to those of IV administration.[1]

An IO device can be placed manually or by using either an impact-driven or drill-powered device.[3,4,5] When used in adults, the preferred IO access site is the proximal tibia; however, the proximal humerus, distal femur, humeral head, radius, ulna, pelvis, clavicle, medial malleolus, and sternum are also possible sites.[4,5,6] Several studies show that an IO catheter can be placed more rapidly than a central venous catheter; however, unlike with other venous access devices, an IO device can only be left in place until conventional vascular access is obtained, and for no longer than 24 hours.[6,7]

Don't insert an IO access device in a site of previous IO access or attempted access, in a fracture at or above the site that required surgical repair of the bone, or in an area of known or suspected infection or local vascular compromise. IO access device insertion may be contraindicated in patients with osteogenesis imperfecta, osteopetrosis, or severe osteoporosis.[6] Only personnel trained in this procedure should perform it. Usually, a nurse assists; however, a qualified registered nurse may insert, maintain, and remove IO access devices.[8] (See *Understanding IO infusion.*)

Understanding IO infusion

During intraosseous (IO) infusion, the bone marrow serves as a noncollapsible vein; allowing fluid infused into the marrow cavity to rapidly enter the circulation by way of an extensive network of venous sinusoids. Here, the needle is shown positioned in the patient's tibia.

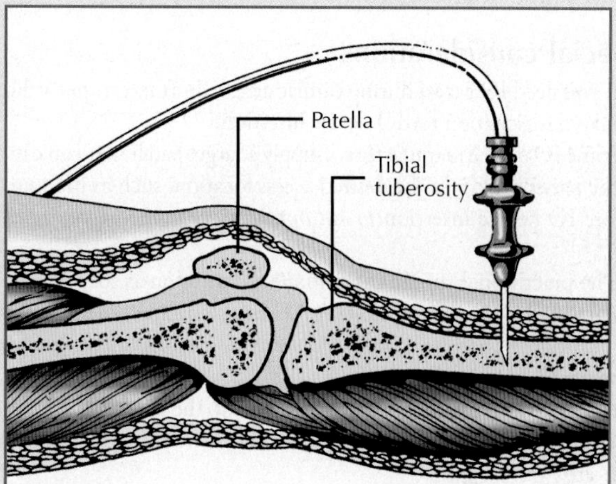

Equipment

Appropriate-sized IO infusion needle (bone marrow biopsy needle or specially designed IO infusion needle [cannula and obturator]), IO catheter insertion kit, or IO drill and drill needle ▪ antiseptic solution ▪ sterile gauze pads ▪ mask with face shield ▪ sterile gloves and gown ▪ sterile drape ▪ 10-mL syringes with preservative-free normal saline flush solution ▪ prescribed IV fluids or medications ▪ 1% lidocaine ▪ extension set or three-way stopcock ▪ administration set with needleless connector ▪ IV infusion pump or pressure bag ▪ tape ▪ sterile marker ▪ 3- to 5-mL syringes ▪ sterile labels ▪ Optional: IO alert armband, sedative, clippers, additional securement or protective device, antiseptic ointment.

Preparation of equipment

Prepare any prescribed IV fluids or medications, and prime the administration set and extension set or three-way stopcock. Using a sterile marker, label all medications, medication containers, and other solutions on and off the sterile field.[9,10]

Implementation

- Verify the practitioner's order.
- Gather and prepare the appropriate equipment.
- If time permits, confirm that written informed consent has been obtained and is in the patient's medical record.[11,12,13]
- Check the patient's history for hypersensitivity to the local anesthetic or contraindications to the procedure.
- If time permits, perform a preprocedure verification *to make sure that all relevant documentation, related information, and equipment are available and correctly identified to the patient's identifiers.*[14,15]
- Perform hand hygiene.[16,17,18,19,20]
- Confirm the patient's identity using at least two patient identifiers.[21]
- If the patient is conscious, explain the procedure *to allay his fears and promote his cooperation.* Tell the patient which bone site will receive the infusion. Inform him that he'll receive a local anesthetic but will feel pressure during needle insertion.
- Administer a sedative before the procedure, as ordered, following safe medication administration practices.[22,23,24]
- Position the patient appropriately for the selected puncture site.
- Remove excess hair from the site with clippers if necessary.[25]
- Perform hand hygiene.[16,17,18,19,20]
- Put on a mask with face shield, a sterile gown, and sterile gloves.[26]
- If time allows, conduct a time-out immediately before starting the procedure *to perform a final assessment that the correct patient, site, positioning, and procedure are identified and that all relevant information and necessary equipment are available.*[27]
- Using sterile technique, clean the puncture site with antiseptic solution, allow it to dry, and then cover the area with a sterile drape.
- Using sterile technique, hand the practitioner the 3- or 5-mL syringe with 1% lidocaine, as indicated, *so that he can anesthetize the insertion site.*[5,6,28]
- Assist the practitioner with the insertion, as needed.
- The practitioner inserts the IO device through the skin and into the bone. Alternatively, he may use an IO drill needle and handheld drill to place the needle.[29]
- The practitioner advances the device with a forward and backward rotary motion through the periosteum until the needle penetrates the marrow cavity. The device should "give" suddenly as it enters the marrow and should stand erect when released.
- The practitioner removes the stylet from the IO infusion device or the obturator from the needle and attaches a 5-mL syringe.
- The practitioner aspirates some bone marrow *to confirm needle placement.*
- The practitioner replaces the first syringe with a syringe containing preservative-free normal saline flush solution and then flushes the cannula *to confirm needle placement and to clear the cannula of clots and bone particles.*
- The practitioner may slowly inject lidocaine into the IO space after establishing access and before infusion *to prevent infusion-related pain.*[6,25,30]
- Connect the primed extension set or three-way stopcock to the IO hub according to the IO access device manufacturer's instructions *to facilitate infusion of medications and IV fluids.*
- Clean the infusion site with antiseptic solution and allow it to dry.
- Secure the device with tape and then cover the site with a sterile occlusive dressing and other protective or stabilization device, as required. *Certain IO device manufacturers provide a protective or stabilization device to cover and secure the IO access needle to prevent accidental dislodgment during patient transport and emergency procedures.*[5,6]
- Label the dressing with the date and time and your initials.[31]
- Attach the needleless connector from the IV administration set to the IO catheter extension set or three-way stopcock.
- Trace the IV tubing from the patient to the point of origin *to make sure that the tubing is connected to the correct cannula.*[32]
- Tape all connections *to prevent dangerous misconnections.*[32]
- Administer fluids and medications, as ordered.
- Place an IO alert armband on the patient *to notify staff members of IO device placement.*

- Monitor the patient's vital signs as warranted by the patient's condition.
- Check the infusion site for complications, such as bleeding and extravasation. Stop the infusion and notify the practitioner if complications occur.
- Assess perfusion in the extremity distal to the insertion site.
- Discard used equipment in appropriate receptacles.
- Remove and discard your personal protective equipment.[33]
- Perform hand hygiene.[16,17,18,19,20]
- Document the procedure.[34,35,36]

Special considerations

- If you need IO access during cardiac arrest, don't interrupt cardiopulmonary resuscitation for IO device insertion.
- Some IO device manufacturers supply a target patch that you can affix to the patient's skin in the desired access location, such as the sternum, before IO needle insertion *to aid in placement in the appropriate location.*[4,5,37]
- The practitioner should discontinue IO infusion as soon as conventional vascular access is possible. An IO infusion should remain in place for no longer than 24 hours *because prolonged infusion significantly increases the risk of infection.*[6,7]
- After needle removal, apply firm pressure to the site for 5 minutes and place antiseptic ointment and a sterile occlusive dressing over the injection site.
- Needle size and flow through the bone marrow determine IO flow rates. Fluids should flow freely if needle placement is correct; however, use of an IV pump or pressure bag is recommended.[5,38]
- If you're administering blood and blood products through the IO device, see the "Transfusion of blood and blood products" procedure, page 783.

Complications

Common complications include extravasation of fluid into subcutaneous tissue, resulting from incorrect needle placement; subperiosteal effusion, resulting from failure of fluid to enter the marrow space; and clotting in the needle from delayed infusion or failure to flush the needle after placement. Other complications include subcutaneous abscess, osteomyelitis, compartment syndrome, embolism of fat or bone fragment, necrosis, and epiphyseal injury.[25,39,40]

Documentation

Record the indications for insertion of the IO device, date and time of insertion, size, type, and location of the device, patient's tolerance of the procedure, and name of the person who placed the device. Also document assessment of the insertion site, including perfusion distal to the site. Record verification of IO catheter placement, the presence of any blood return, patency, and ease of flushing. Also document patient and family teaching performed as well as their understanding of that teaching. Document the type and volume of fluid infused and any medications given in the patient's medical record.

REFERENCES

1 American Heart Association. (2010). 2010 American Heart Association guidelines for cardiopulmonary resuscitation and emergency cardiovascular care. *Circulation, 122,* S729–S767. (Level II)

2 Lewis, G. C., et al. (2013). Critical skills and procedures in emergency medicine: Vascular access skills and procedures. *Emergency Medicine Clinics of North America, 31,* 59–86.

3 Consortium on Intraosseous Vascular Access in Healthcare Practice. (2010). Recommendations for the use of intraosseous vascular access for emergent and nonemergent situations in various health care settings: A consensus paper. *Critical Care Nurse, 30*(6), e1–e7. Accessed March 2015 via the Web at http://ccn.aacnjournals.org/content/30/6/e1.full.pdf+html (Level VII)

4 Day, M. W. (2011). Intraosseous devices for intravascular access in adult trauma patients. *Critical Care Nurse, 31*(2), 76–89. Accessed March 2015 via the Web at http://www.aacn.org/WD/CETests/Media/C1122.pdf

5 Luck, R. P., et al. (2010). Intraosseous access. *Journal of Emergency Medicine, 39,* 468–475. Accessed March 2015 via the Web at http://www.rigshospitalet.dk/NR/rdonlyres/8E0E2340-4B58-4F71-9F5C-44EDC23A4F86/0/HOC_ANOP_workshop_intraosseous_acces.pdf

6 Standard 59. Intraosseous access devices. Infusion nursing standards of practice. (2011). *Journal of Infusion Nursing, 34,* S82–S83. (Level VII)

7 Day, M. W. (2009). Boning up on intraosseous devices. *Nursing Critical Care, 4*(3), 22–26. Accessed March 2015 via the Web at http://www.nursingcenter.com/library/JournalArticle.asp?Article_ID=860674

8 Infusion Nurses Society. (2009). "INS position paper: The role of the registered nurse in the insertion of intraosseous (IO) access devices" [Online]. Accessed March 2015 via the Web at http://www.ins1.org/files/public/4_20_09_Position_paper_Intraosseous.pdf (Level VII)

9 The Joint Commission. (2015). Standard NPSG.03.04.01. *Comprehensive accreditation manual for hospitals: The official handbook.* Oakbrook Terrace, IL: The Joint Commission. (Level VII)

10 American Osteopathic Association. (2014). Standard 25.01.27. *Healthcare Facilities Accreditation Program: Accreditation requirements for acute care hospitals.* Chicago, IL: American Osteopathic Association. (Level VII)

11 The Joint Commission. (2015). Standard RI.01.03.01. *Comprehensive accreditation manual for hospitals: The official handbook.* Oakbrook Terrace, IL: The Joint Commission. (Level VII)

12 Centers for Medicare & Medicaid Services, Department of Health and Human Services. (2014). Condition of participation: Patient's rights. 42 C.F.R. § 482.13(b)(2).

13 American Osteopathic Association. (2014). Standard 15.01.11. *Healthcare Facilities Accreditation Program: Accreditation requirements for acute care hospitals.* Chicago, IL: American Osteopathic Association. (Level VII)

14 The Joint Commission. (2015). Standard UP.01.01.01. *Comprehensive accreditation manual for hospitals: The official handbook.* Oakbrook Terrace, IL: The Joint Commission. (Level VII)

15 American Osteopathic Association. (2014). Standard 30.00.14. *Healthcare Facilities Accreditation Program: Accreditation requirements for acute care hospitals.* Chicago, IL: American Osteopathic Association. (Level VII)

16 Centers for Disease Control and Prevention. (2002). Guideline for hand hygiene in health-care settings: Recommendations of the Healthcare Infection Control Practices Advisory Committee and the HICPAC/SHEA/APIC/IDSA Hand Hygiene Task Force. *MMWR Recommendations and Reports, 51*(RR-16), 1–45. Accessed March 2015 via the Web at http://www.cdc.gov/mmwr/pdf/rr/rr5116.pdf (Level II)

17 The Joint Commission. (2015). Standard NPSG.07.01.01. *Comprehensive accreditation manual for hospitals: The official handbook.* Oakbrook Terrace, IL: The Joint Commission. (Level VII)

18 World Health Organization. (2009). "WHO guidelines on hand hygiene in health care: First global patient safety challenge, clean care is safer care" [Online]. Accessed March 2015 via the Web at http://whqlibdoc.who.int/publications/2009/9789241597906_eng.pdf (Level IV)

19 Centers for Medicare & Medicaid Services, Department of Health and Human Services. (2014). Condition of participation: Infection control. 42 C.F.R. § 482.42.

20 American Osteopathic Association. (2014). Standard 07.01.10. *Healthcare Facilities Accreditation Program: Accreditation requirements for acute care hospitals.* Chicago, IL: American Osteopathic Association. (Level VII)

21 The Joint Commission. (2015). Standard NPSG.01.01.01. *Comprehensive accreditation manual for hospitals: The official handbook.* Oakbrook Terrace, IL: The Joint Commission. (Level VII)

22 The Joint Commission. (2015). Standard MM.06.01.01. *Comprehensive accreditation manual for hospitals: The official handbook.* Oakbrook Terrace, IL: The Joint Commission. (Level VII)

23 American Osteopathic Association. (2014). Standard 16.01.03. *Healthcare Facilities Accreditation Program: Accreditation requirements for acute care hospitals.* Chicago, IL: American Osteopathic Association. (Level VII)

24 Centers for Medicare & Medicaid Services, Department of Health and Human Services. (2014). Condition of participation: Nursing services. 42 C.F.R. § 482.23(c).

25 Infusion Nurses Society. (2011). *Policies and procedures for infusion nursing* (4th ed.). Boston, MA: Infusion Nurses Society.

26 Siegel, J. D., et al. (2007). "2007 guideline for isolation precautions: Preventing transmission of infectious agents in healthcare settings" [Online]. Accessed March 2015 via the Web at http://www.cdc.gov/hicpac/pdf/isolation/Isolation2007.pdf (Level II)

27 The Joint Commission. (2015). Standard UP.01.03.01. *Comprehensive accreditation manual for hospitals: The official handbook.* Oakbrook Terrace, IL: The Joint Commission. (Level VII)

28 Tobias, J. D., & Ross, A. K. (2010). Intraosseous infusions: A review for the anesthesiologist with a focus on pediatric use. *Anesthesia and Analgesia, 110*(2), 391–401. Accessed March 2015 via the Web at http://www.anesthesia-analgesia.org/content/110/2/391.full.pdf

29 Vidacare Corporation. (2008). "EZ-IO intraosseous infusion system: Directions for use" [Online]. Accessed March 2015 via the Web at http://www.fchn.org/docs/northstar/EZ-IO%20directions.pdf

30 Infusion Nurses Society. (2013). *Policies and procedures for infusion nursing of the older adult* (2nd ed.). Boston, MA: Infusion Nurses Society.

31 Standard 46. Vascular access device site care and dressing changes. Infusion nursing standards of practice. (2011). *Journal of Infusion Nursing, 34,* S63–S64. (Level VII)

32 U.S. Food and Drug Administration. (n.d.). "Look. Check. Connect. Safe medical device connections save lives" [Online]. Accessed March 2015 via the Web at http://www.fda.gov/downloads/MedicalDevices/Safety/AlertsandNotices/UCM134873.pdf

33 Occupational Safety and Health Administration. (n.d.). "Bloodborne pathogens, standard number 1910.1030" [Online]. Accessed March 2015 via the Web at http://www.osha.gov/pls/oshaweb/owadisp.show_document?p_table=STANDARDS&p_id=10051 (Level VII)

34 The Joint Commission. (2015). Standard RC.02.01.01. *Comprehensive accreditation manual for hospitals: The official handbook.* Oakbrook Terrace, IL: The Joint Commission. (Level VII)

35 Centers for Medicare & Medicaid Services, Department of Health and Human Services. (2014). Condition of participation: Medical record services. 42 C.F.R. § 482.24(b).

36 American Osteopathic Association. (2014). Standard 10.00.03. *Healthcare Facilities Accreditation Program: Accreditation requirements for acute care hospitals.* Chicago, IL: American Osteopathic Association. (Level VII)

37 Pyng Medical Corporation. (2011). "Fast1 intraosseous infusion system: Training device instructions" [Online]. Accessed March 2015 via the Web at http://www.pyng.com/wp/wp-content/uploads/2011/03/PM-097a%20FAST1%20Training%20Device%20Instructions.pdf

38 Emergency Nurses Association. (2013). "Clinical practice guideline: Difficult intravenous access" [Online]. Accessed March 2015 via the Web at http://www.ena.org/practice-research/research/CPG/Documents/DifficultIVAccessSynopsis.pdf

39 Lynn-McHale Wiegand, D. (Ed.). (2011). *AACN procedure manual for critical care* (6th ed.). St. Louis, MO: Saunders.

40 Te, E. T. (2013). "Intraosseous access" [Online]. Accessed March 2015 via the Web at http://reference.medscape.com/article/80431-overview#a01

ADDITIONAL REFERENCE

Nettina, S. M. (2014). *Lippincott manual of nursing practice* (10th ed.). Philadelphia, PA: Wolters Kluwer.

INTRAPLEURAL DRUG ADMINISTRATION

An intrapleural drug is injected through the chest wall into the pleural space or instilled through a chest tube placed intrapleurally for drainage. During intrapleural injection of a drug, the needle passes through the intercostal muscles and parietal pleura on its way to the pleural space. Intrapleurally administered drugs diffuse across the parietal pleura and innermost intercostal muscles to affect the intercostal nerves.

Practitioners use intrapleural administration to promote analgesia, treat spontaneous pneumothorax, resolve pleural effusion, and administer chemotherapy. Drugs commonly given by intrapleural injection include tetracycline, the combination of tissue plasminogen activator and deoxyribonuclease,[1] streptokinase, anesthetics, and chemotherapeutic agents (to treat malignant pleural effusion or lung adenocarcinoma).[2]

Contraindications for this route include pleural fibrosis or adhesions, which interfere with diffusion of the drug to the intended site; pleural inflammation; sepsis; and infection at the puncture site. Patients with bullous emphysema and those receiving respiratory therapy using positive end-expiratory pressure also shouldn't have intrapleural injections because the injections may exacerbate an already compromised pulmonary condition.

Equipment

An intrapleural drug is given through either a #16 to #20 or a #28 to #40 chest tube if the patient has emphysema, pleural effusion, or pneumothorax. Otherwise, it's given through a 16G to 18G blunt-tipped intrapleural (epidural) needle and catheter. Accessory equipment depends on the type of access device the practitioner uses. All equipment must be sterile.

For intrapleural catheter insertion

Sterile gloves ▪ cap ▪ mask ▪ sterile gown ▪ sterile gauze pads ▪ marker ▪ antiseptic solution ▪ sterile drape ▪ local anesthetic, such as 1% lidocaine ▪ 3- to 5-mL syringe with 22G 1″ (2.5-cm) and 25G ⅝″ (1.6-cm) needles ▪ 18G needle or scalpel ▪ saline-lubricated glass syringe ▪ sterile dressings ▪ sutures ▪ tape ▪ blunt-tipped intrapleural needle ▪ intrapleural catheter ▪ stethoscope ▪ vital signs monitoring equipment ▪ Optional: prescribed pain medications.

For chest tube insertion

Sterile drape ▪ sterile towels ▪ sterile gloves ▪ cap ▪ sterile mask ▪ sterile gown ▪ sterile gauze pads ▪ marker ▪ antiseptic solution ▪ 3- to 5-mL syringe ▪ local anesthetic, such as 1% lidocaine ▪ 18G needle or scalpel ▪ chest tube with or without trocar (#16 to #20 French catheter for air or serous fluid; #28 to #40 French catheter for blood, pus, or thick fluid) ▪ sutures ▪ petroleum dressing ▪ sterile drain dressings ▪ tape ▪ thoracic drainage system and tubing ▪ stethoscope ▪ vital signs monitoring equipment ▪ Optional: prescribed pain medications, two rubber-tipped clamps.

For drug administration

Gloves ▪ sterile gauze pads ▪ antiseptic solution ▪ prescribed medication ▪ appropriate-sized needles and syringes ▪ infusion pump ▪ dressings ▪ tape ▪ two rubber-tipped clamps ▪ Optional: 1% lidocaine.

For chemotherapy administration

Material safety data sheet for the prescribed chemotherapy drug ▪ nonlinting, nonabsorbent disposable gown ▪ powder-free chemotherapy gloves ▪ face shield ▪ National Institute for Occupational Safety and Health–approved respirator mask (if aerosolization is likely) ▪ antiseptic solution ▪ prescribed chemotherapeutic medication with the attached administration set ▪ vital signs monitoring equipment ▪ scale ▪ fluid-impermeable pad ▪ sterile gauze pads ▪ infusion pump with programmable dosing limits ▪ syringe with a luer-lock connector ▪ hazardous drug spill kit ▪ hazardous waste receptacle.

Preparation of equipment

Label all medications and solutions on and off the sterile filed *to prevent medication administration errors.*[3] When administering chemotherapy, make sure a spill kit is readily available *to clean up spills immediately should they occur.*

Inserting an intrapleural catheter

In intrapleural administration, the practitioner inserts a needle into the fourth to eighth intercostal space, 3″ to 4″ (7.5 to 10 cm) from the posterior midline. He then advances the needle medially over the superior edge of the patient's rib through the intercostal muscles until it tangentially penetrates the parietal pleura (as shown below). The practitioner advances the catheter into the pleural space through the needle, and then removes the needle. The nurse should assist the practitioner with insertion as necessary.

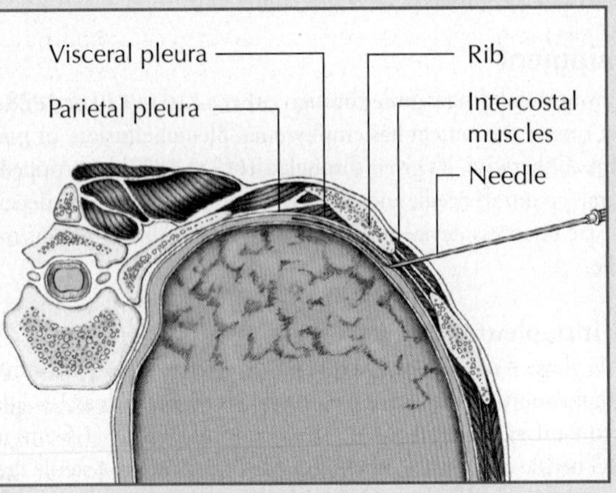

Implementation

■ Verify the practitioner's order.
■ Gather and prepare the appropriate equipment.
■ Confirm that written informed consent has been obtained and that the consent is in the patient's medical record.[4,5,6]
■ Conduct a preprocedure verification *to make sure that all relevant documentation, related information, and equipment are available and correctly identified to the patient's identifiers.*[7,8]
■ Perform hand hygiene.[9,10,11,12,13]
■ Confirm the patient's identity using at least two patient identifiers.[14]
■ Provide privacy.[15,16]
■ Explain the procedure to the patient *to allay his fears.* Encourage him to follow instructions.

Inserting an intrapleural catheter

■ Make sure that the insertion site is marked *to prevent inserting the catheter in the incorrect location.*[17]
■ Perform hand hygiene.[9,10,11,12,13]
■ Put on sterile gloves and other protective equipment as appropriate.[18]
■ The practitioner inserts the intrapleural catheter at the patient's bedside with the nurse assisting.
■ Position the patient on his side with the affected side up *to allow the practitioner access to the insertion site.* (See *Inserting an intrapleural catheter.*)
■ The practitioner puts on a cap, a mask, a sterile gown, and sterile gloves; cleans around the puncture site with an antiseptic-soaked gauze pad; allows it to dry; and then covers the area with a sterile drape.
■ Conduct a time-out immediately before starting the procedure *to perform a final assessment to ensure that the correct patient, site, positioning, and procedure are identified and, as applicable, that all relevant information and necessary equipment are available.*[8,19]
■ The practitioner fills a 3- to 5-mL syringe with local anesthetic and injects it into the skin and deep tissues.
■ The practitioner punctures the skin with the 18G needle or scalpel, which helps the blunt-tipped intrapleural needle penetrate the skin over the superior edge of the lower rib in the chosen interspace. Keeping the bevel tilted upward, he directs the needle medially at a 30- to 40-degree angle to the skin. When the needle tip punctures the posterior intercostal membrane, the practitioner removes the stylet and attaches a saline-lubricated glass syringe containing 2 to 4 mL of air to the needle hub.
■ The practitioner advances the needle slowly. When the needle punctures the parietal pleura, negative intrapleural pressure moves the plunger outward. He then removes the syringe from the needle and threads the intrapleural catheter through the needle until he has advanced it about 2″ (5 cm) into the pleural space. Without removing the catheter, he carefully withdraws the needle.
■ Tell the patient that he can breathe again (or reconnect mechanical ventilation).
■ The practitioner confirms placement by aspirating the catheter. *Resistance indicates placement in the pleural space; aspirated blood means that the catheter probably is misplaced in a blood vessel, and aspirated air means that it's probably in a lung.* The practitioner then orders a chest X-ray *to verify placement and to detect such complications as pneumothorax.*
■ Apply a sterile occlusive dressing over the insertion site *to prevent catheter dislodgment.* Label the dressing with the date, the time, and your initials.
■ Monitor the patient's vital signs after the procedure at an interval determined by your facility or by the patient's condition; *no evidence-based research is available to indicate best practice for frequency of vital signs.*[20]
■ Perform a comprehensive pain assessment using techniques appropriate for the patient's age, condition, and ability to understand. Respond appropriately to your findings.[21]

Inserting a chest tube

■ Make sure that the insertion site is marked *to prevent inserting the chest tube in the incorrect location.*[17]
■ Perform hand hygiene.[9,10,11,12,13]
■ Put on sterile gloves and other protective equipment as appropriate.[18]
■ The practitioner inserts the chest tube with the nurse assisting. (See the "Chest tube insertion, assisting" procedure, page 184.)
■ Position the patient with the affected side up, and drape him with sterile towels.
■ The practitioner puts on a cap, a mask, and a sterile gown and gloves; disinfects the appropriate site with an antiseptic-soaked gauze pad; allows the site to dry; and then applies a sterile drape.
■ Conduct a time-out immediately before starting the procedure to perform a final assessment to ensure that the correct patient, site, positioning, and procedure are identified and, as applicable, that all relevant information and necessary equipment are available.[8,19]
■ If the patient has a pneumothorax, the practitioner uses the second intercostal space as the access site *because air rises to the top of the pleural space.* If the patient has a hemothorax or pleural effusion, the practitioner uses the sixth to eighth intercostal space *because fluid settles to the bottom of the pleural space.*
■ The practitioner fills the syringe with a local anesthetic and injects it into the site.
■ The practitioner makes a small incision with the 18G needle or scalpel, inserts the appropriate-sized chest tube, and immediately connects it to the thoracic drainage system or clamps it close to the patient's chest. He then sutures the tube to the patient's skin.
■ Tape the chest tube to the patient's chest distal to the insertion site *to help prevent accidental dislodgment.* Also tape the junction of the chest tube and drainage tube *to prevent their separation.*

■ Apply a petroleum dressing at the junction between the skin and chest tube *to provide an airtight seal.*[22]
■ Apply sterile drain dressings, cover them with gauze, and tape them in place, creating an occlusive dressing. Label the dressing with the date, the time, and your initials.
■ After insertion, the practitioner uses X-rays *to verify tube placement and to monitor for complications.*[22]
■ Monitor the patient's vital signs at an interval determined by your facility or by the patient's condition.[20]
■ Perform a comprehensive pain assessment using techniques appropriate for the patient's age, condition, and ability to understand. Respond appropriately to the assessment findings.[21]
■ Auscultate the patient's breath sounds regularly according to your facility or based on the patient's condition *to assess air exchange in the affected lung. Diminished breath or absent breath sounds mean that the lung hasn't reexpanded.*

Administering medication

■ Assist the practitioner with medication preparation and administration, as required.
■ Avoid distractions and interruptions when preparing and administering medications *to prevent medication administration errors.*[23,24]
■ Verify the order in the patient's medication record by checking it against the practitioner's order.[25,26,27,28]
■ Perform hand hygiene.[9,10,11,12,13]
■ Compare the medication label with the order in the patient's medical record.[25,27,28]
■ Check the expiration date on the medication. If the medication is expired, return it to the pharmacy and obtain a new medication.[25,27,28]
■ Check the patient's medical record for an allergy or other contraindication to the prescribed medication. If an allergy or other contraindication exists, notify the practitioner.[25,27,28]
■ Visually inspect the medication for discoloration or other indication of loss of integrity. Don't prepare or administer the medication if its integrity is compromised.[25,27,28]
■ Confirm the patient's identity using at least two patient identifiers.[14]
■ Discuss any unresolved concerns about the medication with the patient's practitioner.[25,27,28]
■ If the patient is receiving the medication for the first time, teach him about potential adverse effects and discuss any other concerns related to the medication.[25,27,28]
■ Verify with the practitioner, as required, that the medication is administered at the proper time, in the prescribed dose, and by the correct route *to reduce the risk of medication errors.*[25,27,28,29]

NURSING ALERT ***Before administering a high-alert medication, if required by your facility, you and the practitioner may need to perform an independent double-check* to verify the patient's identity; ensure that the right medication is on hand; verify that the medication's indication corresponds with the patient's diagnosis; check that dosage calculations are correct; verify that the route of administration is safe and proper for the patient; and, if giving an infusion, ensure that the pump settings are correct and that the infusion line is attached to the correct port.**[29]

■ Perform hand hygiene[9,10,11,12,13] and put on gloves.
■ Position the patient with the affected side up *to gain access to the injection port.*
■ Assist the doctor with removing the dressing from the intrapleural catheter or chest tube and clamp the drainage tube, if present.
■ Discard the dressing in the appropriate receptacle.[30]
■ Remove and discard your gloves.
■ Perform hand hygiene.[9,10,11,12,13]
■ Put on a new pair of gloves.[18]
■ The practitioner disinfects the access port of the catheter or chest tube with an antiseptic-soaked gauze pad and allows it to dry.
■ Prepare the appropriate medication dose, as needed, and hand it to the practitioner.
■ The practitioner injects the medication. If it's an anesthetic, he gives a bolus or loading dose initially and then a continuous infusion. For another medication, he may also administer an anesthetic such as lidocaine *to alleviate pain during injection.*
■ Apply new dressings as needed.
■ Monitor the patient closely during and after drug administration *to gauge the effectiveness of drug therapy and to check for complications and adverse effects.*

Administering chemotherapy

■ Review the patient's medical record for verification of initial cancer diagnosis and staging or current cancer status; recent treatments, including surgery, radiation therapy, hormone therapy, cytotoxic therapy, and complementary therapy; medical, psychiatric, and surgical history; presence of allergic or hypersensitivity reactions; pregnancy and reproductive status, including the last menstrual period if applicable; and physical examination that includes assessment of height, weight, body surface area, and organ function appropriate for the planned treatment regimen.[2,31]
■ Verify the practitioner's order for the chemotherapeutic agent. Ensure that the order contains the patient's complete name and a second identifier, the date, the patient's diagnosis, any applicable allergies, the regimen name and number (if applicable), treatment criteria, the dosage calculation method, the patient's height and weight, and any other variables used to calculate the dose, dosage, route and rate of administration, administration schedule, duration of therapy, cumulative lifetime dose (if applicable), and sequence of drug administration (if applicable) as well as any supportive care treatments that are appropriate for the regimen.[5,25,27,28,31]
■ Verify that the patient has received written educational materials appropriate for his reading level and understanding, and include information about his diagnosis, his chemotherapy plan, possible long- and short-term adverse effects, risks associated with the regimen, signs and symptoms to report, monitoring, and follow-up care.[31]
■ Make sure that written informed consent has been obtained and that the form is in the patient's medical record.[5,31]
■ Verify that the prescribed medication dose is appropriate for the patient, diagnosis, and treatment plan. If you have concerns, consult with the prescribing practitioner or the pharmacist.[2,25,27,28,31]
■ Independently verify the chemotherapy order before medication preparation, confirming the two patient identifiers; medication name, dose, and volume; route of administration; calculation for dosing; and treatment cycle and where the patient is at in that cycle.[2,26,27,28,29,31]
■ Become familiar with the information in the material safety data sheet specific to the prescribed drug.[32,33]
■ Obtain the medication from the pharmacy.
■ Confirm the patient's identity using at least two patient identifiers.[14]
■ Review with the patient his current medications, including over-the-counter medications and complementary and alternative therapies; notify the practitioner of any changes.[31]
■ Assess the patient's clinical and performance status.[31]
■ Obtain the patient's vital signs and weight.[31]
■ Verify allergies, previous reactions, and treatment-related toxicities with the patient.[25,27,28,31]
■ Ask the patient about any psychosocial concerns or cultural or spiritual issues that may affect treatment, and take action as indicated.[31]
■ If premedication is prescribed before chemotherapy administration *to prevent adverse effects of the medication,* administer the medication before the procedure as ordered following safe medication administration practices.[25,27,28]
■ Wash your hands.[2,9,10,11,12,13]

- Put on personal protective equipment (two pairs of powder-free chemotherapy gloves; a nonlinting, nonabsorbent gown; a face shield; and a respirator if necessary). Make sure that your inner glove cuff is worn under the gown cuff and that the outer glove cuff extends over the gown cuff *to fully protect your skin.* Inspect your gloves *to make sure that they're physically intact.*[2,34]
- Position the patient in a sitting position and leaning forward on a sturdy surface *to gain access to the injection port.*[2]
- Assist the practitioner with removing the dressing from the intrapleural catheter or chest tube,
- Discard the dressing in the appropriate receptacle.[30] If pleural effusion is present, it must be completely drained from the pleural cavity before the medication is instilled.[2] Clamp the drainage tube, if present.
- Remove and discard your gloves.
- Wash your hands.[2,9,10,11,12,13]
- Confirm the treatment plan, drug route, and symptom management plan with the patient.[31]
- Verify the accuracy of the medication name, dose, and volume; route of administration; expiration date and time; and appearance and physical integrity of the medication. Document the verification process.[29,31]
- With the practitioner who is administering the chemotherapy, confirm the patient's identity using at least two patient identifiers.[9,29,31]

NURSING ALERT *Chemotherapy drugs are considered high-alert medications* because they can cause significant patient harm when used in error. *Perform an independent double-check with another practitioner who's qualified to prepare or administer chemotherapy before chemotherapy administration.*[31,35]

- Put on two new pairs of gloves.[2,34]
- Place a fluid-impermeable pad underneath the work area *to absorb droplets of the medication that may spill.*[31,33]
- Assist the practitioner with preparing the access port. The practitioner thoroughly disinfects the access port of the catheter or chest tube with an antiseptic-soaked gauze pad and then allows it to dry.
- The practitioner injects the medication or begins an infusion. Before the infusion begins, trace the tubing from the patient to its point of origin *to make sure the tubing is connected to the proper port.*[36]
- Apply new dressings, as needed. Label the dressings with the date, the time, and your initials.
- Discard the fluid-impermeable pad and other used equipment in the proper receptacles.[33]
- After instillation, clamp the tubing *so that all the chemotherapy agent remains in the intrapleural space for the prescribed dwell time.*[2]
- Monitor the patient closely for signs of respiratory distress, an allergic reaction, or other adverse reactions to the medication.
- If the medication was administered by infusion, remove the medication container with the tubing attached, and dispose of it in the proper receptacle; don't remove the spike from the container *to prevent exposure to the hazardous medication.*[2] If the medication container will be used to collect drainage after the prescribed dwell time, leave it hanging on an IV pole at the patient's bedside. After the prescribed dwell time, lower the bag to a dependent position, unclamp the tubing, and allow fluid to drain by gravity. After the prescribed volume drains, disconnect the tubing from the injection port and discard it, the fluid, and the container in the appropriate receptacle.

Completing the procedure

- Discard used supplies appropriately.[30]
- Remove your gloves and personal protective equipment and discard them in an appropriate receptacle.
- Perform hand hygiene.[9,10,11,12,13] If you administered chemotherapy, wash your hands with soap and water.[29,10,11,12,13]
- Document the procedure.[37,38,39]

Special considerations

- If the patient is receiving a continuous infusion, label the solution bag clearly. Cover all injection ports so that other drugs aren't injected into the pleural space accidentally.
- If the chest tube dislodges, cover the site at once with a sterile gauze pad and tape it in place. Stay with the patient, monitor his vital signs, and observe carefully for signs and symptoms of tension pneumothorax: hypotension, distended jugular veins, absent breath sounds, tracheal shift, hypoxemia, dyspnea, tachypnea, diaphoresis, chest pain, and a weak, rapid pulse. Have another nurse call the practitioner and gather the equipment for reinsertion.
- Keep rubber-tipped clamps at the bedside. If a commercial chest tube system cracks or a tube disconnects, use the clamps to clamp the chest tube close to the insertion site temporarily. Be sure to observe the patient closely for signs of tension pneumothorax *because no air can escape from the pleural space while the tube is clamped.*
- Each chemotherapy agent has unique adverse effects. Assess and monitor the patient for anticipated adverse effects for the agent administered. Evaluate, grade, and document treatment-related toxicities using standard definitions or criteria, as indicated.[31]
- When handling chemotherapy agents, change your gloves regularly (every 30 to 60 minutes), whenever your gloves become damaged, and when contact with the drug is known or suspected.[34]
- If some of the chemotherapy drug comes in contact with your skin, wash the involved area thoroughly with soap (not a germicidal agent) and water. If eye contact occurs, flood the eye with water or normal saline solution for at least 15 minutes while holding the eyelid open. Obtain a medical evaluation as soon as possible after accidental exposure.[2]
- If a chemotherapy spill occurs, use a chemotherapy spill kit to clean the area. Wear all personal protective equipment (double gloves, a gown, a face shield or goggles, booties, and a respirator if aerosolization is possible). Post a sign to warn others. Clean up the hazardous spill, as indicated. Report and document the spill appropriately.[3]

Patient teaching

Before a patient begins a chemotherapy regimen, he should receive written or electronic information regarding his diagnosis, goals of therapy, the planned schedule and duration of chemotherapy, the possible short- and long-term adverse effects, and regimen- or drug-specific symptoms that require medical attention.

Include emergency contact information for the practice or organization, signs and symptoms that should trigger a call, and who should be contacted. The patient should also receive a plan for monitoring and follow-up care. Ensure that the materials provided are appropriate for the patient's or caregiver's reading level and understanding.[31]

Complications

Pneumothorax or tension pneumothorax may occur if the practitioner accidentally injects air into the pleural cavity. These complications are more likely to occur in a patient who is on mechanical ventilation.

Accidental catheter placement in the lung can lead to respiratory distress; catheter placement within a vessel can increase the medication's effects; and laceration of intercostal vessels may cause bleeding. If the catheter fractures, lung puncture may occur.

Local anesthetic toxicity can lead to tinnitus, metallic taste, lightheadedness, somnolence, visual and auditory disturbances, restlessness, delirium, slurred speech, nystagmus, muscle tremor, seizures, arrhythmias, and cardiovascular collapse. A local anesthetic containing epinephrine can cause tachycardia and hypertension.

Intrapleural chemotherapeutic drugs can irritate the pleura chemically and cause such systemic effects as neutropenia and thrombocytopenia. Administering intrapleural tetracycline without an anesthetic can cause pain.

The insertion site can become infected. However, meticulous skin preparation, strict sterile technique, and sterile dressings usually prevent infection.

Documentation

Document the date and time of catheter insertion, the practitioner's name, the site of the catheter, and the patient's tolerance of the procedure. For drug administration, record the date, time, drug administered, drug dosage, patient's response to the treatment, and condition of the catheter insertion site. Document all preverification, including who was involved in the verification process. Also note any adverse reactions to the medication, the practitioner notified, the prescribed interventions, and the patient's response to the interventions.

REFERENCES

1 Ahmed, A. H., & Yacoub, T. E. (2010). Intrapleural therapy in management of complicated parapneumonic effusions and empyema. *Clinical Pharmacology, 2,* 213–221. Accessed March 2015 via the Web at http://www.ncbi.nlm.nih.gov/pmc/articles/PMC3262383/

2 Polovich, M., et al. (Eds.). (2014). *Chemotherapy and biotherapy guidelines and recommendations for practice* (4th ed.). Pittsburgh, PA: Oncology Nursing Society.

3 The Joint Commission. (2015). Standard NPSG.03.04.01. *Comprehensive accreditation manual for hospitals: The official handbook.* Oakbrook Terrace, IL: The Joint Commission. (Level VII)

4 The Joint Commission. (2015). Standard RI.01.03.01. *Comprehensive accreditation manual for hospitals: The official handbook.* Oakbrook Terrace, IL: The Joint Commission. (Level VII)

5 Centers for Medicare & Medicaid Services, Department of Health and Human Services. (2014). Condition of participation: Patient's rights. 42 C.F.R. § 482.13.

6 American Osteopathic Association. (2014). Standard 15.01.11. *Healthcare Facilities Accreditation Program: Accreditation requirements for acute care hospitals.* Chicago, IL: American Osteopathic Association. (Level VII)

7 The Joint Commission. (2015). Standard UP.01.01.01. *Comprehensive accreditation manual for hospitals: The official handbook.* Oakbrook Terrace, IL: The Joint Commission. (Level VII)

8 American Osteopathic Association. (2014). Standard 30.00.14. *Healthcare Facilities Accreditation Program: Accreditation requirements for acute care hospitals.* Chicago, IL: American Osteopathic Association. (Level VII)

9 The Joint Commission. (2015). Standard NPSG.07.01.01. *Comprehensive accreditation manual for hospitals: The official handbook.* Oakbrook Terrace, IL: The Joint Commission. (Level VII)

10 World Health Organization. (2009). "WHO guidelines on hand hygiene in health care: First global patient safety challenge, clean care is safer care" [Online]. Accessed March 2015 via the Web at http://whqlibdoc.who.int/publications/2009/9789241597906_eng.pdf (Level IV)

11 Centers for Disease Control and Prevention. (2002). Guideline for hand hygiene in health-care settings: Recommendations of the Healthcare Infection Control Practices Advisory Committee and the HICPAC/SHEA/APIC/IDSA Hand Hygiene Task Force. *MMWR Recommendations and Reports, 51*(RR-16), 1–45. Accessed March 2015 via the Web at http://www.cdc.gov/mmwr/pdf/rr/rr5116.pdf (Level II)

12 Centers for Medicare & Medicaid Services, Department of Health and Human Services. (2014). Condition of participation: Infection control. 42 C.F.R. § 482.42.

13 American Osteopathic Association. (2014). Standard 07.01.10. *Healthcare Facilities Accreditation Program: Accreditation requirements for acute care hospitals.* Chicago, IL: American Osteopathic Association. (Level VII)

14 The Joint Commission. (2015). Standard NPSG.01.01.01. *Comprehensive accreditation manual for hospitals: The official handbook.* Oakbrook Terrace, IL: The Joint Commission. (Level VII)

15 Centers for Medicare & Medicaid Services, Department of Health and Human Services. (2014). Condition of participation: Patient's rights. 42 C.F.R. § 482.13(c)(1).

16 American Osteopathic Association. (2014). Standard 15.01.16. *Healthcare Facilities Accreditation Program: Accreditation requirements for acute care hospitals.* Chicago, IL: American Osteopathic Association. (Level VII)

17 The Joint Commission. (2015). Standard UP.01.02.01. *Comprehensive accreditation manual for hospitals: The official handbook.* Oakbrook Terrace, IL: The Joint Commission. (Level VII)

18 Siegel, J. D., et al. (2007). "2007 guideline for isolation precautions: Preventing transmission of infectious agents in healthcare settings" [Online]. Accessed March 2015 via the Web at http://www.cdc.gov/hicpac/pdf/isolation/Isolation2007.pdf (Level II)

19 The Joint Commission. (2015). Standard UP.01.03.01. *Comprehensive accreditation manual for hospitals: The official handbook.* Oakbrook Terrace, IL: The Joint Commission. (Level VII)

20 American Society of PeriAnesthesia Nurses. (2012). *Perianesthesia nursing standards and practice recommendations: 2012-2014.* Cherry Hill, NJ: American Society of PeriAnesthesia Nurses.

21 The Joint Commission. (2015). Standard PC.01.02.07. *Comprehensive accreditation manual for hospitals: The official handbook.* Oakbrook Terrace, IL: The Joint Commission. (Level VII)

22 Lynn-McHale Wiegand, D. (Ed.). (2011). *AACN procedure manual for critical care* (6th ed.). St. Louis, MO: Saunders.

23 Westbrook, J., et al. (2010). Association of interruptions with an increased risk and severity of medication administration errors. *Archives of Internal Medicine, 170,* 683–690. (Level IV)

24 Institute for Safe Medication Practices. (2013). Side tracks on the safety express: Interruptions lead to errors and unfinished . . . Wait, what was I doing? *Nurse Advise-ERR,* 11(2), 1–4. Accessed March 2015 via the Web at https://www.ismp.org/Newsletters/acutecare/showarticle.aspx?id=37 (Level VII)

25 The Joint Commission. (2015). Standard MM.06.01.01. *Comprehensive accreditation manual for hospitals: The official handbook.* Oakbrook Terrace, IL: The Joint Commission. (Level VII)

26 The Joint Commission. (2015). Standard MM.04.01.01. *Comprehensive accreditation manual for hospitals: The official handbook.* Oakbrook Terrace, IL: The Joint Commission. (Level VII)

27 Centers for Medicare & Medicaid Services, Department of Health and Human Services. (2014). Condition of participation: Nursing services. 42 C.F.R. § 482.23(c).

28 American Osteopathic Association. (2014). Standard 16.01.03. *Healthcare Facilities Accreditation Program: Accreditation requirements for acute care hospitals.* Chicago, IL: American Osteopathic Association. (Level VII)

29 Institute for Safe Medication Practices. (2008). Conducting an independent double-check. *ISMP Medication Safety Alert! Nurse Advise-ERR, 6*(12), 1. Accessed March 2015 via the Web at http://www.ismp.org/newsletters/nursing/Issues/NurseAdviseERR200812.pdf (Level VII)

30 Occupational Safety and Health Administration. (n.d.). "Bloodborne pathogens, standard number 1910.1030" [Online]. Accessed March 2015 via the Web at http://www.osha.gov/pls/oshaweb/owadisp.show_document?p_table=STANDARDS&p_id=10051 (Level VII)

31 Neuss, M. N. et al. (2013). Updated American Society of Clinical Oncology/Oncology Nursing Society chemotherapy administration safety standards including standards for the safe administration and management of oral chemotherapy. *Journal of Oncology Practice, 9*(2S), 5–13. Accessed March 2015 via the Web at http://qopi.asco.org/Documents/2013updatedoralstandards.pdf (Level VII)

32 Department of Health and Human Services, Centers for Disease Control and Prevention, & the National Institute for Occupational Safety and Health. (2012). "NIOSH list of antineoplastic and other hazardous drugs in healthcare settings 2012" [Online]. Accessed March 2015 via the Web at http://www.cdc.gov/niosh/docs/2012-150/pdfs/2012-150.pdf (Level I)

33 Occupational Safety and Health Administration. (n.d.). "Toxic and hazardous substances, standard number 1910.1450, App A" [Online]. Accessed March 2015 via the Web at http://www.osha.gov/pls/oshaweb/owadisp.show_document?p_table=STANDARDS&p_id=10107

34 National Institute for Occupational Safety and Health. (2008). "Personal protective equipment for health care workers who work with hazardous drugs" [Online]. Accessed March 2015 via the Web at http://www.cdc.gov/niosh/docs/wp-solutions/2009-106/pdfs/2009-106.pdf

35 Institute for Safe Medication Practices. (2012). "ISMP's list of high-alert medications" [Online]. Accessed March 2015 via the Web at http://www.ismp.org/tools/highalertmedications.pdf (Level VII)
36 U.S. Food and Drug Administration. (n.d.). "Look. Check. Connect. Safe medical device connections save lives" [Online]. Accessed March 2015 via the Web at http://www.fda.gov/downloads/MedicalDevices/Safety/AlertsandNotices/UCM134873.pdf
37 The Joint Commission. (2015). Standard RC.02.01.01. *Comprehensive accreditation manual for 32. hospitals: The official handbook.* Oakbrook Terrace, IL: The Joint Commission. (Level VII)
38 Centers for Medicare & Medicaid Services, Department of Health and Human Services. (2014). Condition of participation: Medical record services. 42 C.F.R. § 482.24(b).
39 American Osteopathic Association. (2014). Standard 10.00.03. *Healthcare Facilities Accreditation Program: Accreditation requirements for acute care hospitals.* Chicago, IL: American Osteopathic Association. (Level VII)

Additional references

Demmy, T. L., et al. (2009). Chest tube-delivered bupivacaine improves pain and decreases opioid use after thoracoscopy. *Annals of Thoracic Surgery, 87*(4), 1040–1046; discussion 1046–1047.
Levinson, G. M., & Pennington, D. W. (2007). Intrapleural fibrinolytics combined with image-guided chest tube drainage for pleural infection. *Mayo Clinic Proceedings, 82*(4), 407–413.
Maskell, N., et al. (2006). Intrapleural streptokinase for pleural infection. *British Medical Journal, 332*(7540), 552.
Tokuda, Y., et al. (2006). Intrapleural fibrinolytic agents for empyema and complicated parapneumonic effusions: A meta-analysis. *Chest, 129*(3), 783–790.

Iontophoresis

Iontophoresis is a technique for delivering a dermal analgesia quickly with minimal discomfort and without distorting the tissue. One example is the Chattanooga Ionto™ Dual Channel Iontophoresis System.[1] This handheld device, which is powered by a 9-volt battery, has two electrodes that use a mild electric current to deliver charged ions of lidocaine 2% and epinephrine 1:100,000 solution into the skin.

Local anesthetic agents, such as those administered through iontophoresis, should be considered before vascular access device insertion.[2] Lidocaine iontophoresis has been found to be 80% to 100% effective in providing anesthetic action before such procedures as injections, abrasion treatment, and laser surgery and cautery.[3] Because iontophoresis act quickly, often within 10 minutes, it's an excellent choice for numbing IV insertion sites, especially in children.

Equipment

Dose-control device with battery and leadwires ■ drug-delivery electrode kit ■ lidocaine 2% with epinephrine 1:100,000 solution ■ mild soap and water ■ washcloths ■ syringe with needle ■ gloves ■ tongue blade ■ Optional: clippers, alcohol pads, disposable scissors.

Implementation

- Verify the practitioner's order.
- Perform hand hygiene.[4,5,6,7,8]
- Confirm the patient's identity using at least two patient identifiers.[9]
- Ask the patient or, if the patient is a child, ask the parents or guardian, about any allergies or sensitivity to medications or contraindications to treatment.

NURSING ALERT *Avoid iontophoresis in patients with electrically sensitive implanted devices such as pacemakers.*[1]

- Explain the procedure to the patient (or his parents or guardian), and tell him that he might feel tingling or warmth under the electrode pads while they're on the skin.
- Assess the patient for appropriate electrode placement. The medication-delivery electrode will be placed over the intended procedure site; the second electrode, which drives drug ions into the skin, must be applied over a muscle 4″ to 6″ (10 to 15 cm) from the first.
- Put on gloves.[10,11]
- Examine the patient's skin and select intact electrode placement sites, avoiding areas with pimples, unhealed wounds, or ingrown hairs.
- Prepare the skin by cleaning and drying it thoroughly; don't use alcohol to prepare the skin unless it's excessively oily.[1]
- If necessary, trim excess body hair at the application sites.
- Remove the paper flap from the back of the drug-delivery electrode.
- Draw up the lidocaine with epinephrine in a syringe as ordered, following safe medication administration practices.[12,13,14]
- Remove the needle from the syringe and saturate the medication pad with the amount of lidocaine and epinephrine solution indicated on the pad (as shown below). The amount of lidocaine and epinephrine solution required to saturate the pad varies with pad size: For a standard-sized pad, use about 1 mL; for a large pad, use about 2.5 mL.

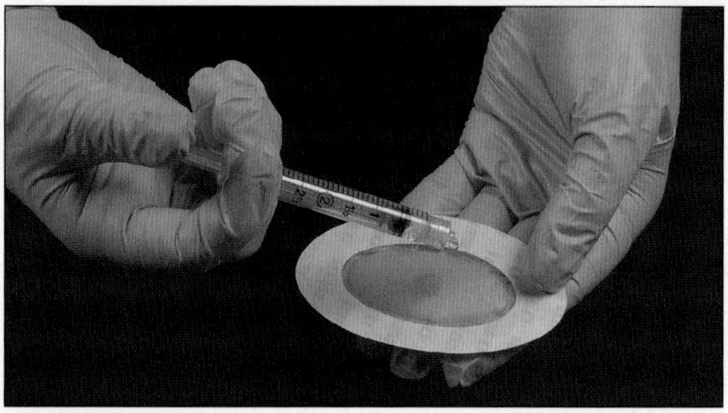

- Remove the remaining backing from the drug-delivery pad.
- Apply the pad to the selected site.
- Remove the backing from the grounding electrode, and then apply it to the second prepared site.
- Connect the lead clips to the electrodes according to the manufacturer's instructions.
- Make sure the device is turned off and then connect the leadwires to the device.
- Turn on the device (as shown below).

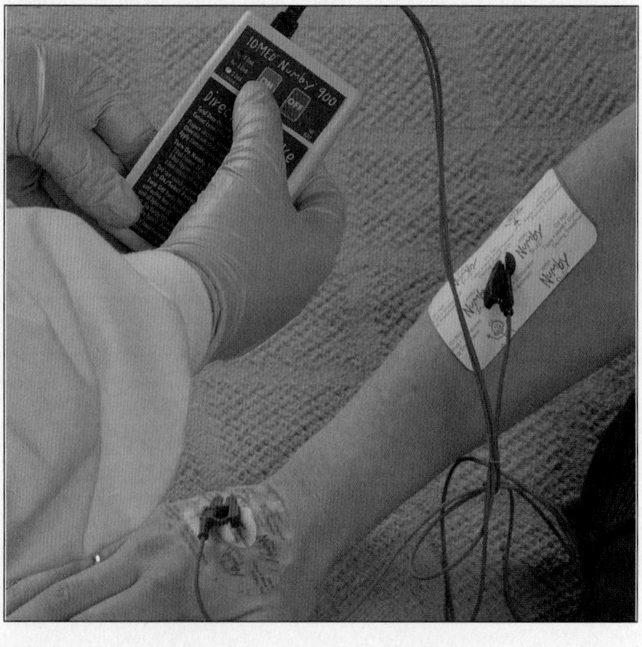

- Set the desired treatment dosage. The device is calibrated to deliver a dose of 40 milliamps (mA). Adjust the dosage by pressing the dosage arrow keys up or down until the correct dosage is displayed.
- Set the level of current. Adjust the device to the desired level of current using the current knobs. If you don't know the desired level, initiate treatment at a level lower than 2 mA and adjust in 0.1-mA increments; current is commonly set between 0.5 and 4 mA.[1]
- Initiate treatment by setting the treatment mode switch. Current will ramp up to the set intensity level in 30 seconds.
- Pause the treatment as needed *to assess for patient tolerance and comfort.*
- At the end of treatment, turn off the device.
- Disconnect the leadwires, and remove the electrodes.
- Assess the skin at the drug-delivery site *for numbness* by touching it with a blunt object, such as a tongue blade.
- Promptly prepare the site and perform the venipuncture or other procedure *because the numbness may last only a few minutes.*
- Remove and discard your gloves.
- Perform hand hygiene.[4,5,6,7,8]
- Document the procedure.[15,16,17]

Special considerations

- *To avoid interfering with energy emission,* don't tape or compress, or apply heat or cold to the electrode sites during treatment.
- If the device doesn't function, make sure that the battery is fresh and properly installed (check polarity markings) and that the battery contacts are clean. If a battery must be replaced during the treatment, record how much of the treatment was completed *because this information will be lost when the battery is replaced.*

Complications

Iontophoresis can cause transient erythema, inflammation, blanching, itching, burning, and a tingling sensation at the site, which usually disappears within 12 hours after treatment.[1] An allergic reaction may occur in patients sensitive to lidocaine or epinephrine.

Documentation

Document the treatment, sites used, and effectiveness in achieving analgesia. Also document any adverse reactions. Record any patient teaching and the patient's and, if applicable, parents' or guardian's understanding of the teaching.

References

1 The Chattanooga Group. (n.d.). "Chattanooga Ionto™ Dual Channel Iontophoresis System: Instruction for use manual" [Online]. Accessed March 2015 via the Web at https://content.pattersonmedical.com/PDF/spr/Product/257507.pdf

2 Standard 34. Local anesthesia for vascular access device placement and access. Infusion nursing standards of practice. (2011). *Journal of Infusion Nursing, 34,* S43–S44. (Level VII)

3 Tadicherla, S., & Berman, B. (2006). Percutaneous dermal drug delivery for local pain control. *Therapeutics and Clinical Risk Management, 2,* 99–113. Accessed March 2015 via the Web at http://www.ncbi.nlm.nih.gov/pmc/articles/PMC1661648/

4 Centers for Disease Control and Prevention. (2002). Guideline for hand hygiene in health-care settings: Recommendations of the Healthcare Infection Control Practices Advisory Committee and the HICPAC/SHEA/APIC/IDSA Hand Hygiene Task Force. *MMWR Recommendations and Reports, 51*(RR-16), 1–45. Accessed March 2015 via the Web at http://www.cdc.gov/mmwr/pdf/rr/rr5116.pdf (Level II)

5 World Health Organization. (2009). "WHO guidelines on hand hygiene in health care: First global patient safety challenge, clean care is safer care" [Online]. Accessed March 2015 via the Web at http://whqlibdoc.who.int/publications/2009/9789241597906_eng.pdf (Level IV)

6 The Joint Commission. (2015). Standard NPSG.07.01.01. *Comprehensive accreditation manual for hospitals: The official handbook.* Oakbrook Terrace, IL: The Joint Commission. (Level VII)

7 Centers for Medicare & Medicaid Services, Department of Health and Human Services. (2014). Condition of participation: Infection control. 42 C.F.R. § 482.42.

8 American Osteopathic Association. (2014). Standard 07.01.10. *Healthcare Facilities Accreditation Program: Accreditation requirements for acute care hospitals.* Chicago, IL: American Osteopathic Association. (Level VII)

9 The Joint Commission. (2015). Standard NPSG.01.01.01. *Comprehensive accreditation manual for hospitals: The official handbook.* Oakbrook Terrace, IL: The Joint Commission. (Level VII)

10 Siegel, J. D., et al. (2007). "2007 guideline for isolation precautions: Preventing transmission of infectious agents in healthcare settings" [Online]. Accessed March 2015 via the Web at http://www.cdc.gov/hicpac/pdf/isolation/Isolation2007.pdf (Level II)

11 American Osteopathic Association. (2014). Standard 07.01.10. *Healthcare Facilities Accreditation Program: Accreditation requirements for acute care hospitals.* Chicago, IL: American Osteopathic Association. (Level VII)

12 The Joint Commission. (2015). Standard MM.06.01.01. *Comprehensive accreditation manual for hospitals: The official handbook.* Oakbrook Terrace, IL: The Joint Commission. (Level VII)

13 Centers for Medicare & Medicaid Services, Department of Health and Human Services. (2014). Condition of participation: Nursing services. 42 C.F.R. § 482.23(c).

14 American Osteopathic Association. (2014). Standard 16.01.03. *Healthcare Facilities Accreditation Program: Accreditation requirements for acute care hospitals.* Chicago, IL: American Osteopathic Association. (Level VII)

15 The Joint Commission. (2015). Standard RC.01.03.01. *Comprehensive accreditation manual for hospitals: The official handbook.* Oakbrook Terrace, IL: The Joint Commission. (Level VII)

16 Centers for Medicare & Medicaid Services, Department of Health and Human Services. (2014). Condition of participation: Medical record services. 42 C.F.R. § 482.24(b).

17 American Osteopathic Association. (2014). Standard 10.00.03. *Healthcare Facilities Accreditation Program: Accreditation requirements for acute care hospitals.* Chicago, IL: American Osteopathic Association. (Level VII)

Additional reference

Taylor, M. B., et al. (2013). Successful short-term and long-term treatment of melasma and postinflammatory hyperpigmentation using vitamin C with a full-face iontophoresis mask and a mandelic/malic acid skin care regimen. *Journal of Drugs in Dermatology, 12,* 45–50.

Isolation garb use

Isolation precautions may be implemented to prevent the spread of infection from patient to patient, from patients to health care workers, or from health care workers to patients.[1,2,3,4] Central to the success of these precautions is the selection of the proper personal protective equipment and adequate training of those who use it.

Equipment

Materials required for isolation typically include personal protective equipment, an isolation cart or anteroom for storing equipment, and a door card or sign alerting staff members and others entering the room that isolation precautions are in effect.

Personal protective equipment

Fluid-resistant gown ▪ gloves ▪ goggles or face shield ▪ mask or respirator (each staff member must be trained in their proper use).

For removal

Trash container ▪ receptacles for gown and equipment.

Putting on a face mask

To avoid spreading airborne particles, wear a face mask. Position the mask to cover your nose and mouth, and secure it high enough *to ensure stability.* Tie the top strings at the back of your head above the ears. Then tie the bottom strings at the base of your neck (as shown below). Alternately, if the face mask has ear loops, secure them around your ears.[9]

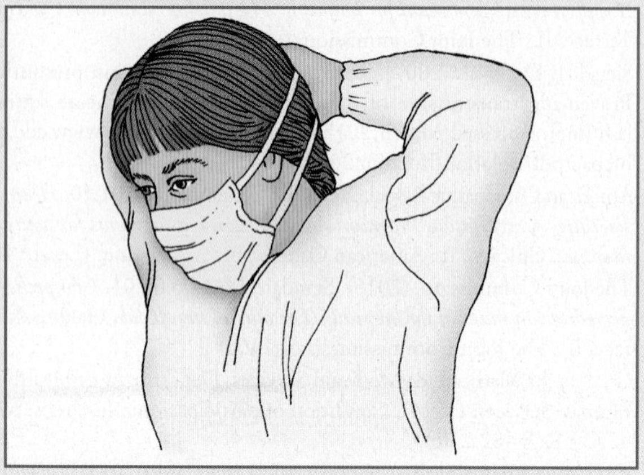

Adjust the metal nose strip if the mask has one (as shown below).[3,4]

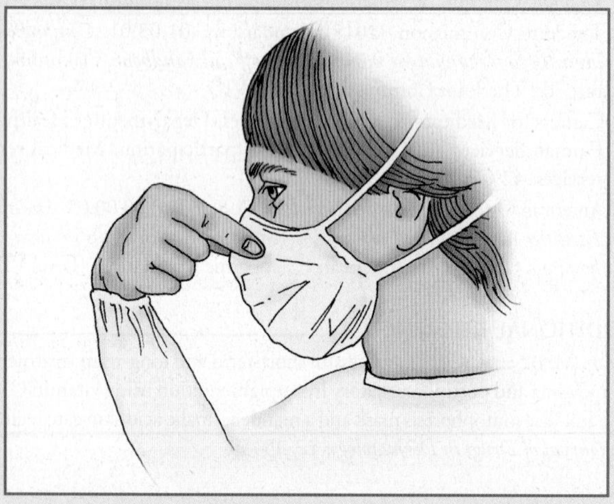

Preparation of equipment

Remove the cover from the isolation cart if necessary, and set up the work area. Check the cart or anteroom *to make sure enough of the proper isolation supplies are available for the designated isolation category.*

Implementation

Putting on isolation garb

- Remove your watch (or push it well up on your arm) and your rings if required by your facility. *These actions help prevent the spread of microorganisms hidden under your watch or rings.*
- Perform hand hygiene.[5,6,7,8,9]
- Pick up the gown and allow it to unfold in front of you without touching areas of your body that may be contaminated *to minimize the transmission of microorganisms.* Put on the gown and wrap it around the back of your uniform, making sure it overlaps and completely covers your uniform *to prevent contact with the patient or his environment.*[3,4] Tie the strings or fasten the snaps or pressure-sensitive tabs at the neck. Then tie the waist strings.
- Place the mask snugly over your nose and mouth. Secure the ear loops around your ears or tie the strings at the middle of the back of your head and neck *so that the mask won't slip off.* If the mask has a metal strip, squeeze it to fit your nose firmly but comfortably.[3,4] (See *Putting on a face mask.*) If you wear eyeglasses, tuck the upper edge of the mask under the lower edge of the glasses.
- Choose eye protection according to your risk of exposure. *Although goggles provide eye protection, they don't protect the rest of the face from splashing of potentially infectious substances.* Wear a face shield for any procedures that may involve spraying or splashing of respiratory secretions or other body fluids.[3,4]
- Select gloves according to your hand size *to make sure they fit securely.* Put on the gloves and pull them over the cuffs of your gown *to cover the edges of the gown's sleeves.*

Removing isolation garb

- After completing patient care, prepare to leave the room by collecting items that need to be removed.
- Remember that the outside surfaces of your goggles or face shield, mask or respirator, and barrier clothes (such as a gown) are contaminated.[3,4]
- Except for a respirator mask, remove all personal protective equipment at the patient's doorway or in the anteroom. Remove a respirator after leaving the patient's room and closing the door.[3,4,10]
- Remove your gloves using the appropriate technique. (See *Removing contaminated gloves.*) Don't touch any skin with the outside of either glove. Discard the gloves in the trash container,[4,5,11] and then perform hand hygiene.[5,6,7,8,9]
- To remove your goggles or face shield, grasp the ear pieces or headband and remove carefully. Place the equipment in the appropriate receptacle for reprocessing, or discard it in an appropriate receptacle.[3,4,10,11]
- To remove your gown, untie the neck straps and then the waist ties. Pull your gown away from your neck and shoulders, touching only the inside of the gown (as shown below). Turn the gown inside out as you remove it, folding it or rolling it into a bundle *to ensure containment of pathogens.* Discard the gown in the appropriate receptacle.[3,4,10,11]

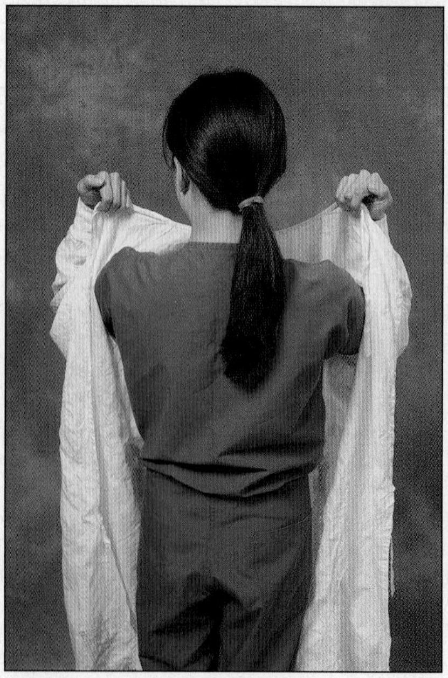

- To remove your mask or respirator, grasp the bottom tie or elastic and lift it over your head; then grasp the top tie or elastic, and carefully remove the mask or respirator. Don't touch the front of the mask *to*

Removing contaminated gloves[4]

Proper removal technique is essential for preventing the spread of pathogens from gloves to your skin surfaces. Follow these steps carefully to properly remove your contaminated gloves.

■ Grasp the outside of one glove with the opposite gloved hand and peel it off, turning the glove inside out as you pull it off (as shown below). Hold the removed glove in the remaining gloved hand

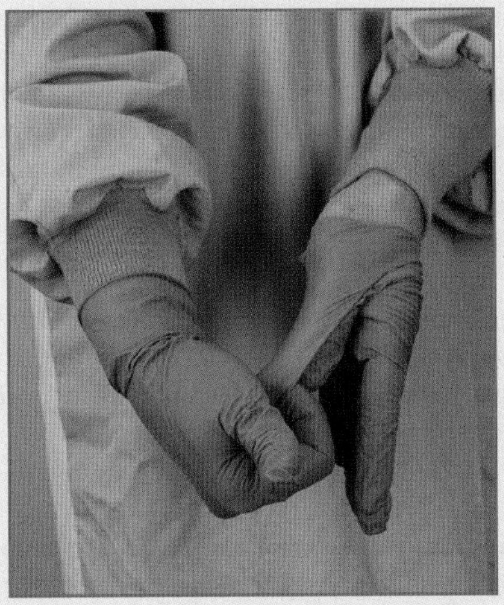

■ Slide the fingers of the ungloved hand under the remaining glove at the wrist, taking care not to touch the outer surface of the glove (as shown below).

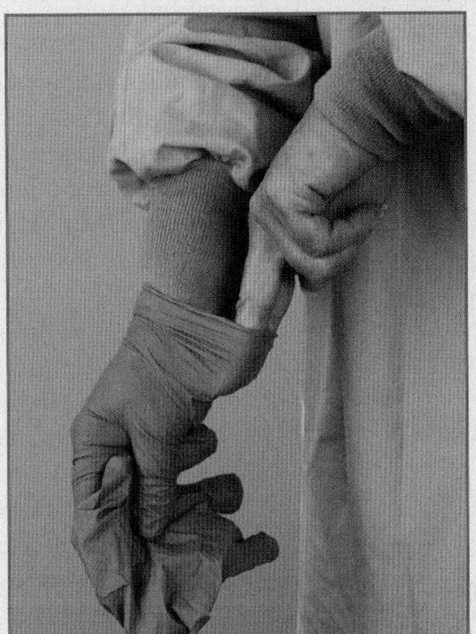

■ Peel off the glove over the first glove, containing the one glove inside the other (as shown below). Discard the gloves in an appropriate container,[3,4,6] and perform hand hygiene.[5,6,7,8,9]

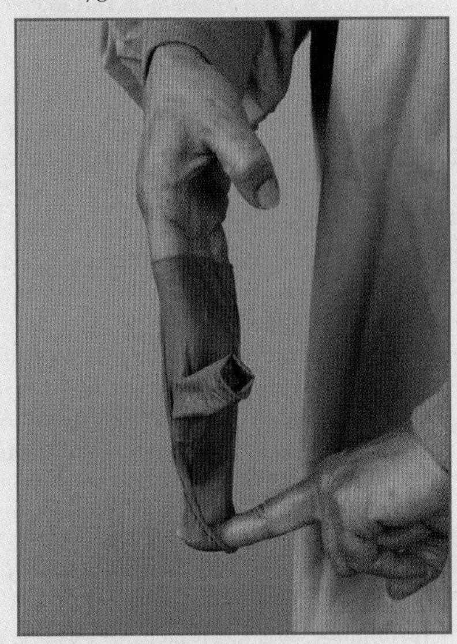

prevent contamination. Discard the mask in the appropriate receptacle.[3,4,10,11]

■ Perform hand hygiene immediately.[5,6,7,8,9]

Special considerations

■ If airborne precautions are required, wear an N95 or higher level particulate respirator approved by the Occupational Safety and Health Administration rather than a surgical mask.[3,4,10] (See the "Airborne precautions" procedure, page 10.) Employees who wear respirators must be properly fit-tested initially and then periodically thereafter according to federal, state, and local regulations.[11,12]

■ If your respirator is reusable, retain it for further use unless it's contaminated, damaged, or fails to form a good seal.[12] Store it according to your facility's policy. Reuse of respiratory protection may consist of removing and putting the device back on between patient encounters. *To avoid a transmission risk,* adhere to stringent hand hygiene before and after handling the respirator.[12,13]

■ Always perform hand hygiene before putting on gloves *to avoid contaminating the gloves with microorganisms from your hands.*[5,6,7,8,9]

■ Use gloves only once.[3,4] Be aware that isolation garb loses its effectiveness when wet *because moisture permits organisms to seep through the material.* Change masks and gowns as soon as moisture is noticeable or according to the manufacturer's recommendations or your facility's guidelines.[3,4,14]

■ Change masks and gowns as soon as moisture is noticeable or according to the manufacturer's recommendations or your facility's guidelines.[15]

■ Keep isolation supplies stocked *so that they're readily available for those who must enter the patient's room.*

Documentation

No documentation is needed for this procedure.

REFERENCES

1 The Joint Commission. (2015). Standard IC.02.01.01. *Comprehensive accreditation manual for hospitals: The official handbook.* Oakbrook Terrace, IL: The Joint Commission. (Level VII)

2 Centers for Medicare & Medicaid Services, Department of Health and Human Services. (2014). Condition of participation: Patient's rights. 42 C.F.R. § 482.13(b)(2).

3 American Osteopathic Association. (2014). Standard 07.01.10. *Healthcare Facilities Accreditation Program: Accreditation requirements for acute care hospitals.* Chicago, IL: American Osteopathic Association. (Level VII)

4 Siegel, J. D., et al. (2007). "2007 guideline for isolation precautions: Preventing transmission of infectious agents in healthcare settings" [Online]. Accessed March 2015 via the Web at http://www.cdc.gov/hicpac/pdf/isolation/Isolation2007.pdf (Level II)

5 The Joint Commission. (2015). Standard NPSG.07.01.01. *Comprehensive accreditation manual for hospitals: The official handbook.* Oakbrook Terrace, IL: The Joint Commission. (Level VII)

6 Centers for Disease Control and Prevention. (2002). Guideline for hand hygiene in health-care settings: Recommendations of the Healthcare Infection Control Practices Advisory Committee and the HICPAC/SHEA/APIC/IDSA Hand Hygiene Task Force. *MMWR Recommendations and Reports, 51*(RR-16), 1–45. Accessed March 2015 via the Web at http://www.cdc.gov/mmwr/pdf/rr/rr5116.pdf (Level II)

7 World Health Organization. (2009). "WHO guidelines on hand hygiene in health care: First global patient safety challenge, clean care is safer care" [Online]. Accessed March 2015 via the Web at http://whqlibdoc.who.int/publications/2009/9789241597906_eng.pdf (Level IV)

8 American Osteopathic Association. (2014). Standard 07.01.21. *Healthcare Facilities Accreditation Program: Accreditation requirements for acute care hospitals.* Chicago, IL: American Osteopathic Association. (Level VII)

9 Centers for Medicare & Medicaid Services, Department of Health and Human Services. (2014). Condition of participation: Infection control. 42 C.F.R. § 482.42.

EQUIPMENT

Using a ready injectable

A commercially premeasured medication packaged with a syringe and needle, the ready injectable enables rapid drug administration in an emergency. Preparing a ready injectable usually takes only 15 to 20 seconds. Other advantages include the reduced risk of breaking sterile technique during administration and the easy identification of medication and dose.

When using a ready injectable, be sure to give the precise dose prescribed. For example, if a 50-mg/mL cartridge is supplied but the patient's prescribed dose is 25 mg, you must administer only 0.5 mL, half of the volume contained in the cartridge. Be alert for potential medication errors whenever dispensing medications in premeasured dosage forms.

10 Centers for Disease Control and Prevention. (n.d.). "Sequence for donning and removing personal protective equipment" [Online]. Accessed March 2015 via the Web athttp://www.cdc.gov/HAI/pdfs/ppe/ppeposter1322.pdf

11 American Osteopathic Association. (2014). Standard 07.03.07. *Healthcare Facilities Accreditation Program: Accreditation requirements for acute care hospitals.* Chicago, IL: American Osteopathic Association. (Level VII)

12 Occupational Safety and Health Administration. (n.d.). "Respiratory protection, standard number 1910.134" [Online]. Accessed March 2015 via the Web at http://www.osha.gov/pls/oshaweb/owadisp.show_document?p_table=STANDARDS&p_id=12716 (Level VII)

13 Rebmann, T., et al. (2009). "APIC position paper: Extending the use and/or reusing respiratory protection in healthcare settings during disasters" [Online]. Accessed March 2015 via the Web at http://www.apic.org/Resource_/TinyMceFileManager/Advocacy-PDFs/APIC_Position_Ext_the_Use_and_or_Reus_Resp_Prot_in_Hlthcare_Settings1209l.pdf (Level VII)

14 Jensen, P., et al. (2005). Guidelines for preventing the transmission of *Mycobacterium tuberculosis* in health-care settings, 2005. *MMWR Recommendations and Reports, 54*(RR-17), 1–141. Accessed March 2015 via the Web at http://www.cdc.gov/mmwr/pdf/rr/rr5417.pdf (Level II)

15 Occupational Health and Safety Administration. (n.d.). "Bloodborne pathogens, standard number 1910.1030" [Online]. Accessed March 2015 via the Web at http://www.osha.gov/pls/oshaweb/owadisp.show_document?p_table=STANDARDS&p_id=10051 (Level VII)

IV BOLUS INJECTION

The IV bolus injection method allows rapid drug administration. It can be used in an emergency to provide an immediate drug effect. It can also be used to administer drugs that can't be given IM, to achieve peak drug levels in the bloodstream, and to deliver drugs that can't be diluted, such as diazepam, digoxin, and phenytoin. The term *bolus* usually refers to the concentration or amount of a drug.

Bolus doses of medication can be injected directly through an existing venous access device or through an implanted port. The medication administered by these methods usually takes effect rapidly, so the patient must be monitored for adverse reactions, such as cardiac arrhythmias and anaphylaxis. IV bolus injections are contraindicated when rapid drug administration could cause life-threatening complications. The safe rate of injection is specified by the drug's manufacturer.

Equipment

Patient's medication record ▪ gloves ▪ antiseptic pads (alcohol, tincture of iodine, or chlorhexidine-based) ▪ prescribed medication ▪ prefilled-syringe containing preservative-free normal saline solution (or other compatible flush solution if medication is incompatible with normal saline solution)[1] ▪ syringe and needleless adapter ▪ Optional: second syringe filled with preservative-free normal saline solution, diluent, dextrose 5% in water.

A useful dosage form is the ready injectable. (See *Using a ready injectable.*)

Implementation

- Avoid distractions and interruptions when preparing and administering medications *to prevent medication administration errors.*[2,3]
- Verify the practitioner's order.[4,5,6,7]
- Compare the medication label with the order in the patient's medical record.[5,8]
- Check the patient's medical record for an allergy or other contraindication to the prescribed medication. If an allergy or contraindications exist, don't administer the medication; instead, notify the practitioner.[5]
- Check the expiration date on the medication. If the medication is expired, return it to the pharmacy and obtain a new medication.[4,5]
- Visually inspect the medication for discoloration or any other loss of integrity; don't administer the medication if its integrity is compromised.[4,5,6,7]
- Review the drug monograph before administration (if necessary) *to ensure safe medication administration.*[6,7]
- Check the compatibility of the medication with the IV solution, other medicated infusions, and the flush solution.
- Discuss any unresolved concerns about the medication with the patient's practitioner.[5]
- If the patient is receiving the medication for the first time, teach about potential adverse reactions and discuss any other concerns related to the medication.[5]
- Verify that the medication is being administered at the proper time, in the prescribed dose, and by the correct route *to reduce the risk of medication errors.*[4,5]
- Perform hand hygiene.[6,7,9,10,11,12,13]
- Put on gloves.[14,15]
- If the medication isn't in a prefilled syringe, dilute it (if required) and draw it up in a syringe using sterile technique. Check the medication label three times while preparing it *to prevent medication administration errors.*
- In a perioperative or other procedural setting, if the medication or solution is transferred from the original packaging to another container or if it won't be administered immediately, label the container with the medication name, dosage, quantity, diluent and volume, and expiration date, as indicated.[16]
- Confirm the patient's identity using at least two patient identifiers.[6,7,17,18]
- Explain the procedure to the patient.[6,7]
- If your facility uses a bar code scanning system, scan your identification badge, the patient's identification bracelet, and the medication's bar code.
- If IV fluids are infusion, close the flow clamp of the IV administration tubing and pause the infusion pump, if used.[19]
- Thoroughly disinfect the lowest needleless injection port of the administration tubing,[19] if attached, or directly disinfect the needleless connector of the patient's venous access device (if used for intermittent infusion) with an antiseptic pad using friction, and then allow it to dry.[20]
- Assess the patient's IV site for pain, redness, or swelling.
- Attach a prefilled syringe containing preservative-free normal saline solution or other compatible solution[1] to the lowest injection port on the administration tubing or directly to the venous access device, as indicated; aspirate for blood return *to verify catheter patency* and then flush the catheter.[6,7,19,21]
- Attach the medication syringe to the injection port or venous access device and inject the medication, as prescribed and according to rate on

the medication label; consult with the pharmacist of a rate isn't specified.[6,7]

NURSING ALERT *Speed shock can result from rapid administration of a bolus medication. Carefully administer the medication at the proper rate and monitor the patient closely during administration. Symptoms of speed shock, such as dizziness and headache, can occur rapidity and progress to such signs and symptoms as chest tightness, hypotension, irregular pulse, and anaphylactic shock. Keep in mind that an older adult patient may not be able to articulate these symptoms* because of preexisting conditions, such as stroke, tracheotomy, endotracheal intubation, dementia, and delirium.[7]

- If the patient is receiving a continuous IV infusion and the bolus medication is compatible with the patient's prescribed IV solution, open the clamp on the administration tubing, adjust the flow rate, or restart the pump, as indicated; if the medication is incompatible, provide an additional flush of preservative-free normal saline solution into the injection port and then open the clamp, adjust the flow rate, or restart the pump, as indicated, *to rid the tubing and catheter of any dead-volume incompatible fluid.*[19,21] Alternately, flush and lock the patient's venous access device with preservative-free normal saline solution if the venous access device is used intermittently.[6,7]
- Discard used supplies in the appropriate receptacles.[14,15,22]
- Remove and discard your gloves[14,15,22] and perform hand hygiene.[9,10,11,12,13]
- Document the procedure.[23,24,25]

Special considerations

- If you're giving a medication that's incompatible with preservative-free normal saline solution, flush the device with dextrose 5% in water followed by preservative-free normal saline solution. Some medications, such as dantrolene, are incompatible with both normal saline and dextrose 5% in water. If unsure, consult your facility's pharmacist.[1,21]
- Use single-dose vials for parenteral medications whenever possible.[14,26]
- Never administer medications from the same syringe to more than one patient.[14,26]
- Don't enter a medication or fluid container with a used syringe.[14,26]
- Never use medications packaged as single-dose or single-use for more than one patient. This includes ampules, bags, and bottles of IV solutions.[14,26]
- Don't keep multidose vials in the immediate patient treatment area. Store them in accordance with the manufacturer's recommendations, and discard them if their sterility is compromised or questionable.[14,26]
- Always use sterile technique when preparing and administering injections.[14,26]
- Avoid using infusion pumps to deliver bolus doses *to prevent overinfusion of highly potent medications.*[19]

Patient teaching

Teach the patient about the medication and its potential adverse effects.

Complications

Because drugs administered by IV bolus injections are delivered directly into the circulatory system and can produce an immediate effect, an acute allergic reaction or anaphylaxis can develop rapidly. If signs of anaphylaxis (dyspnea, cyanosis, seizures, and increasing respiratory distress) occur, notify the practitioner immediately and begin emergency procedures, as necessary.

Excessively rapid drug administration may cause adverse effects, such as speed shock and other complications, depending on the medication administered.

Monitor for signs of local and systemic infections. Also watch for signs of extravasation, such as redness and swelling. If extravasation occurs, stop the injection, estimate the amount of infiltration, and notify the practitioner.

Documentation

Record the amount and type of drug administered, date and time of administration, route of administration, vascular access device used, appearance of the site, and patient's tolerance of the procedure.[6,7] Also note the medication's effect and any adverse reactions. Document patient teaching and the patient's understanding of your teaching.

References

1 Loubnan, V., & Nasser, S. C. (2010). A guide on intravenous drug compatibilities based on their pH. *Pharmacie Globale, 5*(1), 1–9.

2 Westbrook, J., et al. (2010). Association of interruptions with an increased risk and severity of medication administration errors. *Archives of Internal Medicine, 170,* 683–690. (Level IV)

3 Institute for Safe Medication Practices. (2013). Side tracks on the safety express: Interruptions lead to errors and unfinished . . . Wait, what was I doing? *Nurse Advise-ERR,* 11(2), 1–4. Accessed March 2015 via the Web at https://www.ismp.org/Newsletters/acutecare/showarticle.aspx?id=37

4 Centers for Medicare & Medicaid Services, Department of Health and Human Services. (2014). Condition of participation: Nursing services. 42 C.F.R. § 482.23 (c).

5 The Joint Commission. (2015). Standard MM.06.01.01. *Comprehensive accreditation manual for hospitals: The official handbook.* Oakbrook Terrace, IL: The Joint Commission. (Level VII)

6 Infusion Nurses Society. (2011). *Policies and procedures for infusion nursing* (4th ed.). Boston, MA: Infusion Nurses Society.

7 Infusion Nurses Society. (2013). *Policies and procedures for infusion nursing of the older adult* (2nd ed.). Boston, MA: Infusion Nurses Society.

8 Centers for Medicare & Medicaid Services, Department of Health and Human Services. (2014). Condition of participation: Pharmaceutical services. 42 C.F.R. § 482.25.

9 The Joint Commission. (2015). Standard NPSG.07.01.01. *Comprehensive accreditation manual for hospitals: The official handbook.* Oakbrook Terrace, IL: The Joint Commission. (Level VII)

10 Standard 19. Hand hygiene. Infusion nursing standards of practice. (2011). *Journal of Infusion Nursing, 34,* S26–S27. (Level VII)

11 Centers for Disease Control and Prevention. (2002). Guideline for hand hygiene in health-care settings: Recommendations of the Healthcare Infection Control Practices Advisory Committee and the HICPAC/SHEA/APIC/IDSA Hand Hygiene Task Force. *MMWR Recommendations and Reports, 51*(RR-16), 1–45. Accessed March 2015 via the Web at http://www.cdc.gov/mmwr/pdf/rr/rr5116.pdf (Level II)

12 World Health Organization. (2009). "WHO guidelines on hand hygiene in health care: First global patient safety challenge, clean care is safer care" [Online]. Accessed March 2015 via the Web at http://whqlibdoc.who.int/publications/2009/9789241597906_eng.pdf (Level IV)

13 Centers for Disease Control and Prevention. (2011). "Guidelines for the prevention of intravascular catheter-related infections" [Online]. Accessed March 2015 via the Web at http://www.cdc.gov/hicpac/pdf/guidelines/bsi-guidelines-2011.pdf

14 Siegel, J. D., et al. (2007). "2007 guideline for isolation precautions: Preventing transmission of infectious agents in healthcare settings" [Online]. Accessed March 2015 via the Web at http://www.cdc.gov/hicpac/pdf/isolation/Isolation2007.pdf (Level II)

15 Occupational Safety and Administration. (n.d.). "Bloodborne pathogens, standard number 1910.1030" [Online]. Accessed March 2015 via the Web at http://www.osha.gov/pls/oshaweb/owadisp.show_document?p_table=STANDARDS&p_id=10051 (Level VII)

16 The Joint Commission. (2015). Standard NPSG.03.04.01. *Comprehensive accreditation manual for hospitals: The official handbook.* Oakbrook Terrace, IL: The Joint Commission. (Level VII)

17 The Joint Commission. (2015). Standard NPSG.01.01.01. *Comprehensive accreditation manual for hospitals: The official handbook.* Oakbrook Terrace, IL: The Joint Commission. (Level VII)

18 Standard 61. Parenteral medication and solution administration. Infusion nursing standards of practice. (2011). *Journal of Infusion Nursing, 34,* S86–S87. (Level VII)
19 Health Technology Safety Research Team in Collaboration with ISMP Canada. (2012). "Mitigating the risks associated with multiple IV infusions: Recommendations based on a field study of twelve Ontario hospitals" [Online]. Accessed March 2015 via the Web at http://www.aami.org/htsi/infusion/wg/multiple/MultipleIVInfusions_Phase1bSummary_Recommendations%20and%20Rationale_June%202012.pdf (Level VII)
20 Standard 27. Needleless connectors. Infusion nursing standards of practice. (2011). *Journal of Infusion Nursing, 34,* S32–S33. (Level VII)
21 Standard 45. Flushing and locking. Infusion nursing standards of practice. (2011). *Journal of Infusion Nursing, 34,* S59–S63. (Level VII)
22 Standard 22. Safe handling and disposal of sharps, hazardous materials, and hazardous waste. Infusion nursing standards of practice. (2011). *Journal of Infusion Nursing, 34,* S28–S29. (Level VII)
23 The Joint Commission. (2015). Standard RC.01.03.01. *Comprehensive accreditation manual for hospitals: The official handbook.* Oakbrook Terrace, IL: The Joint Commission. (Level VII)
24 Standard 14. Documentation. Infusion nursing standards of practice. (2011). *Journal of Infusion Nursing, 34,* S20–S21. (Level VII)
25 Centers for Medicare & Medicaid Services, Department of Health and Human Services. (2014). Condition of participation: Medical record services. 42 C.F.R. § 482.24(b).
26 Centers for Disease Control and Prevention. (2011). "Safe injection practices to prevent transmission of infections to patients" [Online]. Accessed March 2015 via the Web at http://www.cdc.gov/injectionsafety/IP07_standardPrecaution.html (Level I)

ADDITIONAL REFERENCE

Jacobson, J. O., et al. (2012). Revisions to the 2009 American Society of Clinical Oncology/Oncology Nursing Society chemotherapy administration safety standards: Expanding the scope to include inpatient settings. *Journal of Oncology Practice, 8*(1), 2–6. Accessed March 2015 via the Web at http://intl-jop.ascopubs.org/content/8/1/2.full.pdf+html (Level VII)

IV CATHETER INSERTION AND REMOVAL

Peripheral IV catheter insertion involves selection of a venipuncture device and an insertion site, application of a tourniquet, site preparation, venipuncture, catheter securement, and dressing application. Selection of a venipuncture device and site depends on the type of solution to be used; frequency and duration of infusion; patency and location of accessible veins; the patient's age, size, and condition; and, when possible, the patient's preference.[1,2,3,4] For an older adult, choose an area with more subcutaneous tissue and skeletal support for better device stabilization, keeping in mind the need to conserve access for future therapy.[5]

A peripheral catheter allows administration of fluids, medication, blood, and blood components and maintains IV access to the patient. Peripheral catheters are recommended for use with infusates with a pH between 5 and 9, osmolality less than 600 mOsm/L, and a therapy regimen of short duration.[1,3]

Follow sterile technique when inserting an IV catheter to reduce the risk of vascular catheter–associated infection. According to the Centers for Disease Control and Prevention, a peripheral IV catheter should be replaced no more frequently than every 72 hours to reduce the risk of infection and phlebitis in adults.[1] If an IV catheter is inserted in an emergency, it should be removed as soon as possible, within a maximum of 48 hours, to reduce the risk of vascular catheter–associated infection.

HOSPITAL-ACQUIRED CONDITION ALERT *Keep in mind that a vascular catheter–associated infection is considered a hospital-acquired condition* because it can be reasonably prevented using best practices. *Follow infection prevention techniques (such as performing hand hygiene, preparing the site with an antiseptic, adhering to sterile technique during insertion and maintenance, and discontinuing the device when it's no longer needed)* to reduce the risk of vascular catheter–associated infection.[6,7]

Equipment

For insertion

Antiseptic solution (chlorhexidine [preferred];[8] tincture of iodine, povidone-iodine, or alcohol if a contraindication to chlorhexidine exists) ▪ gloves ▪ single-use tourniquet (preferably latex-free) ▪ peripheral catheters with passive and active safety mechanism[3] ▪ needleless connector ▪ IV solution with attached and primed administration set, as ordered ▪ 10-mL prefilled syringe containing preservative-free normal saline solution ▪ IV pole ▪ transparent semipermeable dressing ▪ catheter securement device, sterile hypoallergenic tape, or sterile surgical strips ▪ marker ▪ Optional: padded arm board, roller gauze, tube gauze, 2″ × 2″ (5-cm × 5-cm) sterile gauze pad, warm packs, scissors, clippers, visualization technology, local anesthetic, basin of water, soap, adhesive remover, culture swab and tube.

Commercial venipuncture kits come with or without an IV access device. (See *Comparing venous access devices.*) In many facilities, venipuncture equipment is kept on a tray or cart, allowing more choice of access devices and easy replacement of contaminated items.[9]

For removal

Gloves ▪ gauze pads ▪ tape ▪ Optional: culture swab and tube, single-patient-use tourniquet, warm compress, prescribed medications, adhesive remover, topical ointment, paper or silicone tape.

Preparation of equipment

Check the information on the label of the IV solution container, including the patient's name and identification number, the type of solution, the time and date of its preparation, the preparer's name, and the ordered infusion rate. Compare the practitioner's orders with the solution label *to verify that the solution is the correct one.*[10] Inspect the solution for discoloration and other signs of loss of integrity and make sure that it isn't expired.[10]

Select the catheter gauge that's appropriate for the patient's diagnosis, prescribed type and duration of therapy (therapy that's required for less than 1 week), available access sites, and your experience with insertion. Also take into consideration complications associated with the particular catheter type. If blood transfusion is necessary, a 14G to 24G catheter may be used in adults.[3]

If you're using a winged infusion set, connect the adapter to the administration set, and unclamp the line until fluid flows from the open end of the needle cover. Then close the clamp and place the needle on a sterile surface, such as the inside of its packaging. If you're using a catheter device, open its package *to allow easy access.*

Implementation

- Gather the appropriate equipment.
- Perform hand hygiene.[1,11,12,13,14,15,16]
- Place the IV pole in the proper slot in the patient's bed frame. If you're using a portable IV pole, position it close to the patient.
- Hang the IV solution with attached primed administration set on the IV pole.
- Confirm the patient's identity using at least two patient identifiers.[17]
- Explain the procedure to the patient *to ensure cooperation and reduce anxiety. Anxiety can cause a vasomotor response resulting in venous constriction.* Provide the patient with information about the insertion process, expected duration of therapy, care and maintenance of the IV catheter, and the signs and symptoms of complications and when to report them.[8,18]

Selecting the site

- Select the puncture site. Use the nondominant arm if possible. If long-term therapy is anticipated, start with a vein at the most distal site *so that*

EQUIPMENT

Comparing venous access devices

Most IV infusions are delivered through one of two basic types of venous access devices: an over-the-needle cannula or a winged infusion set. *To improve IV therapy and guard against accidental needle sticks,* you should use a needle-free system and shielded or retracting peripheral IV catheters. Steel-winged devices should be limited to single-dose or short-term administration.[3]

Over-the-needle cannula

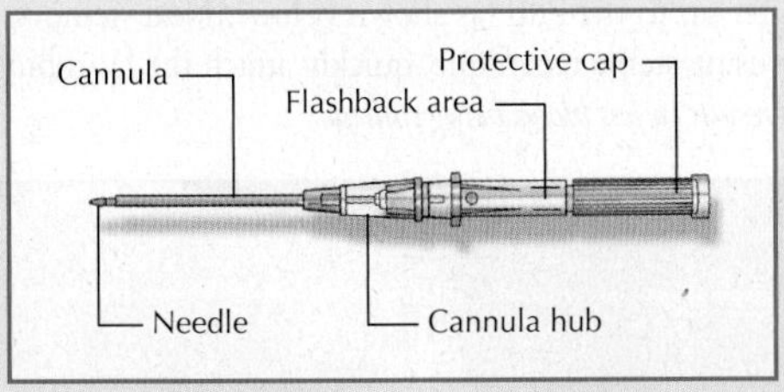

Purpose
Long-term therapy for an active or agitated patient

Advantages
More comfortable for the patient once it's in place; contains radiopaque thread for easy location; rarely requires an activity-restricting device, such as an arm board.

Disadvantage
More difficult to insert than other devices

Winged infusion set

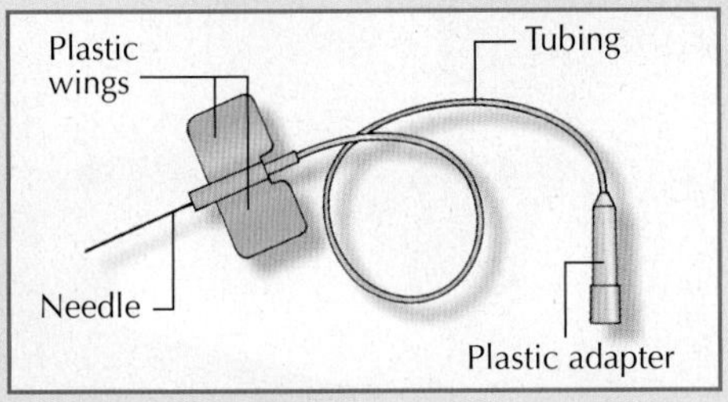

Purpose
Short-term therapy or single-dose administration.

Advantages
Less painful to insert; ideal for nonirritating IV push drugs.

Disadvantage
May easily cause infiltration

you can move proximally as needed for subsequent IV insertion sites.[2] For infusion of an irritating medication, choose a large vein distal to any nearby joint. Make sure the intended vein can accommodate the cannula.

■ Place the patient in a comfortable, reclining position. Position the extremity of the intended insertion site lower than the heart for several minutes *to promote vascular distention.*[8]

■ If the patient's skin is cold, consider using warm packs or dry warmth *to promote vascular dilation.*[8]

Applying the tourniquet

■ Apply a tourniquet at an appropriate location above the intended insertion site *to dilate the vein* (as shown below). Check for a pulse distal to the tourniquet location *because an arterial pulse should be easily palpable distal to the tourniquet location.*[4,19] If a pulse isn't present, release the tourniquet and reapply it with less tension *to prevent arterial occlusion.*

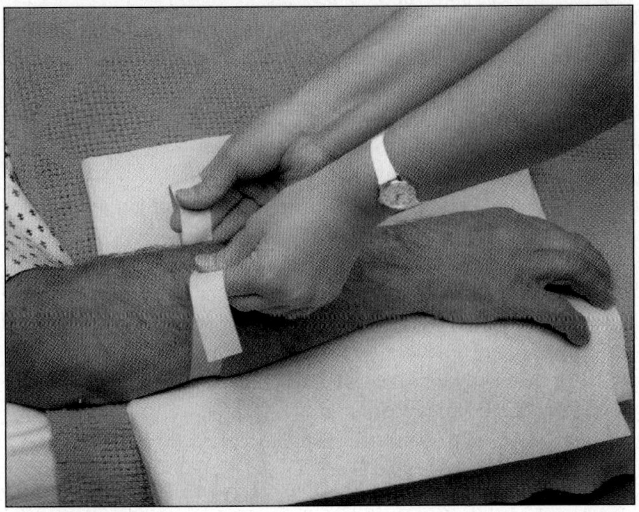

■ Lightly palpate the vein with the index and middle fingers of your nondominant hand *to assess vein condition.*[4]

■ If the vein is easily palpable but not sufficiently dilated, one or more of the following techniques may help raise the vein. Place the extremity in a dependent position for several seconds or lightly stroke the vessel downward. If you have selected a vein in the arm or hand, tell the patient to open and close his fist several times.[8]

■ Leave the tourniquet in place for no more than 3 minutes while you locate a suitable vein. Release the tourniquet for site preparation.

Preparing the site

■ If the intended insertion site is visibly soiled, clean it with soap and water before applying the antiseptic solution.[4,8]

■ Clip the hair around the insertion site, if needed, with scissors or electric clippers.[8]

■ Administer a local anesthetic if indicated and prescribed.[4,20,21] *Because there's less supportive underlying tissue in older adults,* take care not to nick or damage the vein when administering a local anesthetic; avoid inadvertently administering the anesthetic intravascularly.[5]

■ Perform hand hygiene.[1,11,12,13,14,15,16]

■ Put on gloves.[1,22,23,24]

■ Clean the site with chlorhexidine using a back-and-forth scrubbing motion for at least 30 seconds *to remove flora that would otherwise be introduced into the vascular system with the venipuncture.* Allow the antiseptic to dry.[4,8]

ELDER ALERT ***Be aware that, although antiseptic agents should be applied with friction, irritated skin may become more damaged, causing discomfort in older adults.*** **Antiseptics can cause stinging and irritation. Excessive amounts of alcohol may dry already compromised skin.**[5]

■ Reapply the tourniquet.

■ Use visualization technology (as shown on next page, top left) if necessary *to locate the vein.*

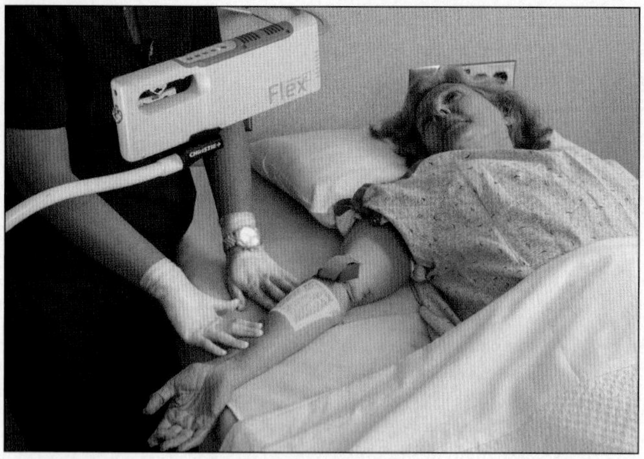

■ Using the thumb of your nondominant hand, stretch the skin taut below the puncture site *to stabilize the vein.*[4] If the patient is an older adult, anchor the vein distal to the intended insertion site; *the vein may be difficult to stabilize and penetrate because of the aging process.*[5]
■ Grasp the access cannula. If you're using a winged infusion set, hold the short edges of the wings (with the needle's bevel facing upward) between the thumb and forefinger of your dominant hand. Then squeeze the wings together. If you're using an over-the-needle cannula, grasp the plastic hub with your dominant hand, remove the cover, and examine the cannula tip. If the edge isn't smooth, discard and replace the device.

Inserting the device

■ Tell the patient that you are about to insert the device.
■ Hold the needle bevel up and enter the skin directly over the vein at a 0- to 15-degree angle.
■ Aggressively push the needle directly through the skin and into the vein in one motion. Check the flashback chamber behind the hub for blood return, *signifying that the vein has been properly accessed.* (You may not see a blood return in a small vein.)
■ Level the insertion device slightly by lifting the tip of the device up *to prevent puncturing the back wall of the vein with the access device.*
■ If you're using a winged infusion set, advance the needle fully, if possible, and hold it in place. Release the tourniquet, open the administration set clamp slightly, and check for free flow or infiltration.
■ If you're using an over-the-needle cannula, advance the device 2 to 3 mm *to ensure that the cannula itself, not just the introducer needle, has entered the vein.* Then release the tourniquet. Grasp the cannula hub to hold it in the vein, and withdraw the needle. As you withdraw it, press lightly on the catheter tip *to prevent bleeding* (as shown below).

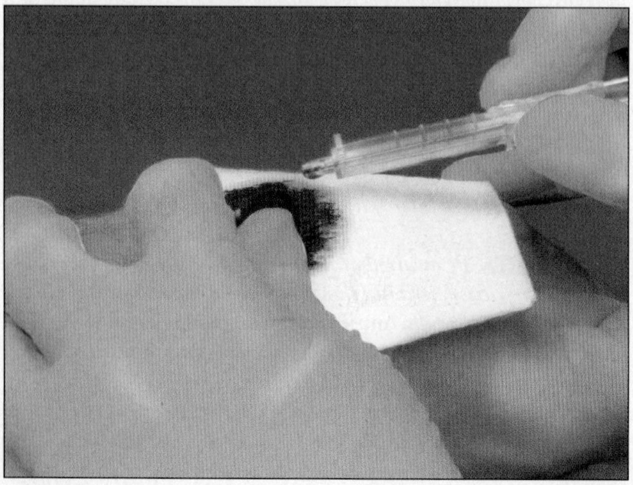

■ To advance the cannula while infusing IV solution, release the tourniquet and remove the inner needle. Using sterile technique, attach the IV tubing and begin the infusion. While stabilizing the vein with one hand, use the other to advance the catheter into the vein. When the catheter is advanced, decrease the IV flow rate. *This method reduces the risk of puncturing the vein's opposite wall because the catheter is advanced without the needle and because the rapid flow dilates the vein.*
■ To advance the cannula before starting the infusion, first release the tourniquet. While stabilizing the vein with one hand, use the other to advance the catheter up to the hub (as shown below). Next, remove the inner needle and, using sterile technique, quickly attach the IV tubing.[25] *This method often results in less blood being spilled.*

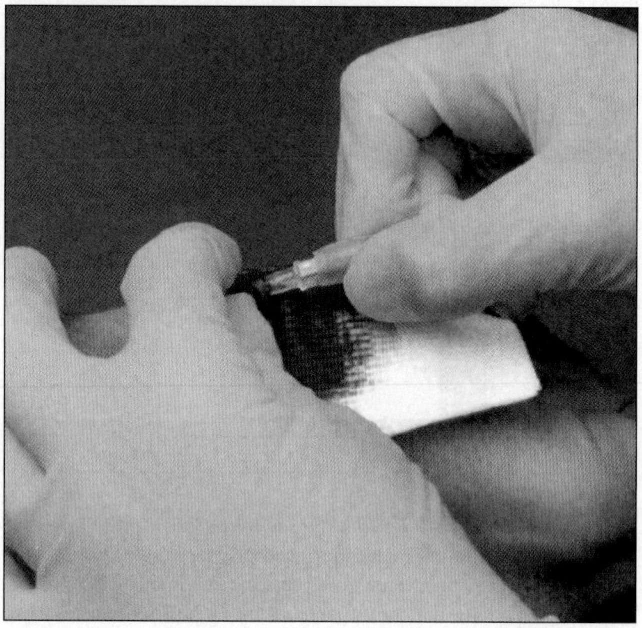

Dressing the site

■ After inserting the venous access device, clean the skin completely.
■ Apply a catheter securement device using a method that doesn't interfere with assessment and monitoring of the access site or impede vascular circulation or delivery of the prescribed therapy.[18] If a catheter securement device isn't available, use sterile 1″ (2.5-cm) hypoallergenic tape or sterile surgical strips *to secure the device.* (See *Methods of taping a venous access site.*)
■ Apply a transparent semipermeable dressing to the site.[18] (See *How to apply a transparent semipermeable dressing,* page 450.) If the patient has fragile skin, use a dressing specifically formulated for fragile skin *to prevent skin stripping or tearing with removal.*
■ Loop the IV tubing on the patient's limb, and secure the tubing with tape. *The loop allows some slack to prevent dislodgment of the cannula from tension on the line.*
■ Label the site with the type, gauge, and length of the catheter; the date and time of insertion; and your initials.[4,29]
■ Adjust the flow rate as ordered.
■ Trace the tubing from the patient to its point of origin *to make sure you've attached the tubing to the correct port.*[10,30]
■ If the puncture site is near a movable joint, place a padded arm board under the joint and secure it with roller gauze or tape *to provide stability because excessive movement can dislodge the venous access device and increase the risk of thrombophlebitis and infection.*[31]
■ Check frequently for impaired circulation distal to the infusion site anytime an arm board is used.[31]
■ Discard used supplies in an appropriate receptacle.[22,23,32]
■ Perform hand hygiene.[1,11,12,13,14]
■ Document the procedure.[33,34,35]

Methods of taping a venous access site

Securement devices are preferred for securing an IV catheter *because they're associated with fewer overall complications, fewer dislodgments, and a longer dwell time than securing with tape.*[26,27,28] If a securement device isn't available and you must use tape, make sure to use only sterile tape and avoid placing tape over the insertion site. When using tape to secure a venous access device, use one of the basic methods described below.

Chevron method

- Cut a long strip of ½″ (1.3-cm) tape and place it, sticky side up, under the cannula.
- Cross the ends of the tape over the cannula so that the tape sticks to the patient's skin (as shown below).
- Cut another piece of sterile tape and apply it across the two wings of the chevron; make sure that the tape is applied only to the chevron wings and cannula hub *so that the insertion site remains visible.*[27]
- Apply a sterile dressing and a label. On the label, write the date and time of insertion, length and gauge of the vascular access device, and your initials.[4,29]

U method

- Cut a 2″ (5-cm) strip of ½″ (1.3-cm) tape. With the sticky side up, place it under the hub of the cannula.
- Bring each side of the tape up, folding it over the wings of the cannula in a U shape (as shown below). Press it down parallel to the hub.
- Cut another piece of sterile tape and apply it across the U-shape tape and wings of the cannula; make sure that the cannula insertion site remains visible.[27]
- Apply a sterile dressing and a label. On the label, write the date and time of insertion, length and gauge of the vascular access device, and your initials.[4,29]

H method

- Cut three strips of 1″ (2.5-cm) tape.
- Place one strip of tape over each wing of the cannula, keeping the tape parallel to the cannula.
- Place the last strip of tape perpendicular to the first two, putting it on top of the wings (as shown below); make sure the cannula insertion site remains visible.
- Make sure the cannula is secure, and then apply a dressing and a label. On the label, write the date and time of insertion, length and gauge of the vascular access device, and your initials.[4,29]

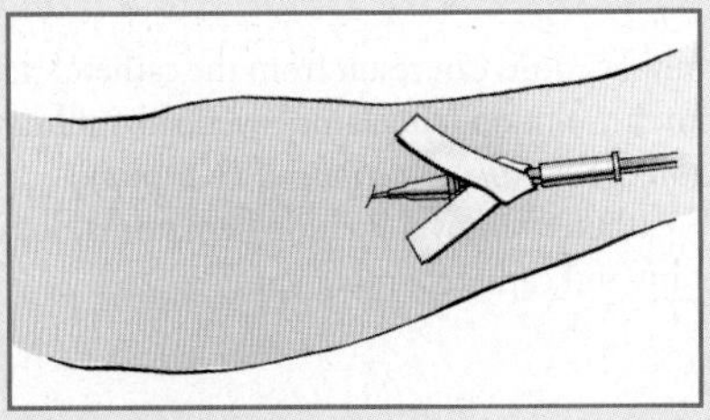

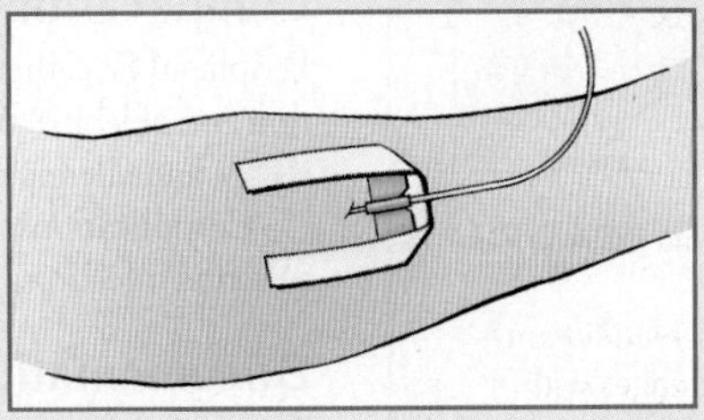

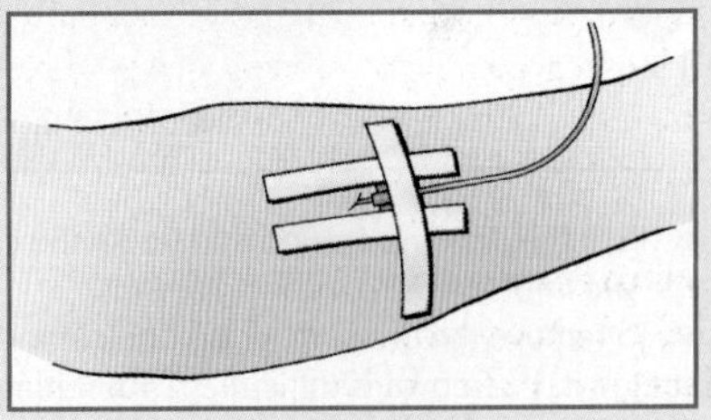

Removing an IV catheter

- Verify the order to remove the peripheral IV catheter.[36]
- Gather the appropriate equipment.
- Perform hand hygiene.[1,11,12,13,14]
- Confirm the patient's identity using at least two patient identifiers.[17]
- Open the gauze pads and place them within reach on a clean barrier.
- Put on gloves.[1,22,23,24]
- Clamp the IV tubing *to stop the flow of solution.*
- Gently remove the transparent dressing (and tape if present) by pulling the dressing edges back toward the insertion site (as shown below) *to avoid stripping or tearing the skin.* Use an adhesive remover if necessary.[5,42]

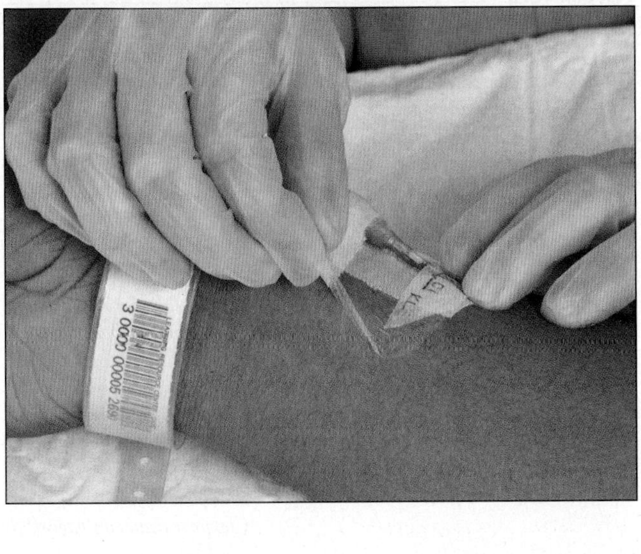

- Remove the catheter securement device.[4,5]
- Inspect the catheter-skin junction for signs of infection or phlebitis.[4,5,37,38,39]
- Hold the gauze pad over the puncture site with one hand, and use your other hand to withdraw the cannula slowly and smoothly, keeping it parallel to the skin (as shown below).

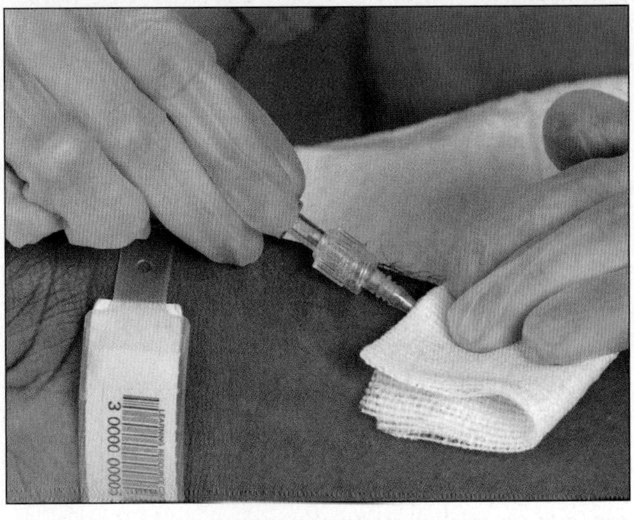

- Using the gauze pad, apply firm pressure over the puncture site until bleeding has stopped (for a minimum of 30 seconds).[4,5,36]
- Assess the integrity of the removed catheter. Compare the length of the catheter with the original insertion length *to make sure that the entire catheter has been removed.* If the catheter isn't intact and you

How to apply a transparent semipermeable dressing

To secure the IV insertion site, you can apply a transparent semipermeable dressing as follows:

- Make sure the insertion site is clean and dry.
- Remove the dressing from the package and, using sterile technique, remove the protective seal. Avoid touching the sterile surface.
- Place the dressing directly over the insertion site and the hub (as shown below). Don't cover the tubing. Also, don't stretch the dressing; *doing so may cause itching.*

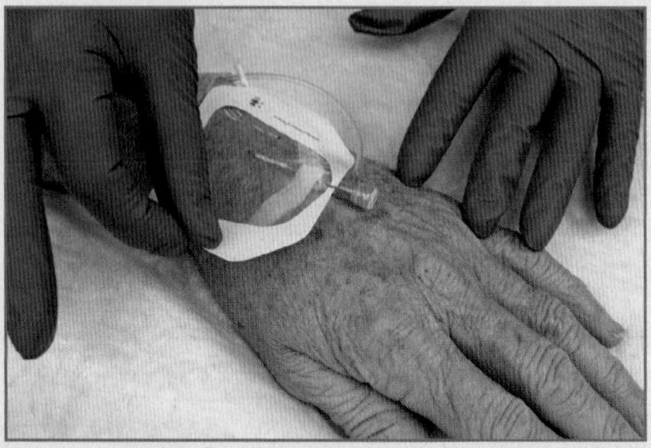

- Tuck the dressing around and under the cannula hub *to make the site impervious to microorganisms.*
- To remove the dressing, grasp one corner, and then lift and stretch it. If removal is difficult, try loosening the edges with alcohol or water.

suspect device embolism, place a tourniquet above the venipuncture site; check the patient's pulse frequently *to make sure that you aren't obstructing arterial flow,* and place the patient on bed rest. Notify the practitioner immediately, monitor the patient closely, and administer prescribed treatments.[4]

- If signs and symptoms of exit site infection are present (tenderness, erythema and induration within 2 cm [¾″] of the catheter-skin junction, and purulence at the exit site), notify the practitioner. Obtain a culture of the purulent exudate, and apply moist, warm compresses. Apply a topical ointment and initiate antibiotic therapy, as prescribed.[4]
- Apply a gauze pad and tape to the exit site.[4,36] If the patient has fragile skin, use nontraumatic paper or silicone tape *to avoid skin stripping or tearing.*[40]
- Discard used supplies in an appropriate receptacle.[22,23,32]
- Remove and discard your gloves.
- Perform hand hygiene.[1,11,12,13,14]
- Document the procedure.[33,34,35]

Special considerations

ELDER ALERT ***Apply the tourniquet carefully to avoid pinching the skin. If necessary, apply it over the patient's gown. Make sure skin preparation materials are at room temperature* to avoid vasoconstriction resulting from lower temperatures.**

- One nurse should make no more than two attempts at insertion *because unsuccessful attempts limit future attempts and cause the patient unnecessary pain.*[8]
- If you fail to see flashback after the needle enters the vein, pull back slightly and rotate the device. If you still fail to see flashback, remove the cannula and try again with a new cannula.
- According to the Centers for Disease Control and Prevention, peripheral IV catheters shouldn't be changed more frequently than every 72 hours *to reduce the risk of infection and phlebitis.*[1]
- Consider replacing IV catheters when clinically indicated based on the patient's condition, access site, skin and vein integrity, and length and type of therapy.[36]
- After removal, change the dressing every 24 hours until the exit site heals[5] and monitor the site for 48 hours *to detect postinfusion phlebitis.*[37]

Patient teaching

Teach the patient how to examine the site, and instruct him to notify the practitioner or home care nurse if redness, swelling, or discomfort develops or if the dressing becomes moist.

Teach the patient general strategies to prevent catheter complications. Also tell the patient to report any problems with the IV line, such as if the solution stops infusing or if an alarm goes off on an infusion pump. If the patient is using an intermittent infusion device, teach him how and when to flush it. Finally, teach the patient to document daily whether the IV site is free from pain, swelling, and redness.

Complications

Peripheral IV catheter complications can result from the catheter (infection and phlebitis) or from the solution (circulatory overload, infiltration, sepsis, and allergic reaction). (See *Risks of peripheral IV therapy.*)

Complications of IV catheter removal include hematoma, local or systemic infection, phlebitis and catheter embolism.

Documentation

Document the date and time of insertion; the type, gauge, and length of the vascular access device; the anatomic location of the insertion site; the number and location of attempts; and the functionality of the device.

Record the local anesthetic, if used, site preparation, and whether visualization technology was used to guide insertion.

Also document the type and flow rate of the IV solution, the name and dose of medication in the solution (if any), any adverse reactions and actions taken to correct them, patient teaching, and evidence of patient understanding.[8]

Record the date and time of catheter removal, the site from which the catheter was removed, the condition of the catheter site and catheter, the patient's tolerance of the procedure, and any patient teaching provided.

References

1 Centers for Disease Control and Prevention. (2011). "Guidelines for the prevention of intravascular catheter-related infections" [Online]. Accessed March 2015 via the Web at http://www.cdc.gov/hicpac/pdf/guidelines/bsi-guidelines-2011.pdf (Level I)

2 Standard 33. Site selection. Infusion nursing standards of practice. (2011). *Journal of Infusion Nursing, 34,* S40–S43. (Level VII)

3 Standard 32. Vascular access device selection. Infusion nursing standards of practice. (2011). *Journal of Infusion Nursing, 34,* S37–S40. (Level VII)

4 Infusion Nurses Society. (2011*). Policies and procedures for infusion nursing* (4th ed.). Boston, MA: Infusion Nurses Society.

5 Infusion Nurses Society. (2013). *Policies and procedures for infusion nursing of the older adult* (2nd ed.). Boston, MA: Infusion Nurses Society.

6 Jarrett, N., et al. (2013). "Evidence-based guidelines for selected and previously considered hospital-acquired conditions: Final report" [Online]. Accessed March 2015 via the Web at http://www.cms.gov/Medicare/Medicare-Fee-for-Service-Payment/HospitalAcqCond/Downloads/Evidence-Based-Guidelines.pdf

(*Text continues on page 455*)

Risks of peripheral IV therapy

COMPLICATIONS	SIGNS AND SYMPTOMS	POSSIBLE CAUSES	NURSING INTERVENTIONS
LOCAL COMPLICATIONS			
Phlebitis[37]	■ Tenderness at tip of and proximal to venous access device ■ Redness at tip of cannula and along vein ■ Warmth ■ Swelling and induration over vein ■ Palpable venous cord ■ Elevated temperature ■ Pain ■ Purulent drainage	■ Multiple manipulations of the infusion delivery system[4] ■ Large catheter gauge and catheter length[4] ■ Failure to stabilize the catheter adequately[4] ■ Catheter material and configuration[4] ■ Venous access device left in vein too long[4] ■ Inadequate skin asepsis, poor insertion technique, and inadequate catheter care and maintenance practices[4] ■ Drug or solution with high or low pH or high osmolarity[4]	■ Use a standardized scale *to assess the severity of phlebitis.*[37] ■ Discontinue the infusion and then remove the venous access device.[4,37] ■ Determine whether the cause was mechanical, chemical, or bacterial.[4] ■ Apply warm soaks for 20 minutes three to four times per day, as ordered.[4] ■ Notify the practitioner about the degree of phlebitis.[4] ■ Reassess the patient's vascular access needs. If a device is still needed, replace the device in the opposite extremity. Consult with the practitioner about central venous access device placement if the probable cause is irritating fluid.[4] ■ Document the patient's condition and your interventions.[33,34,37] ***Prevention*** ■ Use the smallest gauge and length of catheter needed to accommodate the prescribed therapy.[4] ■ Avoid inserting the device in an area of flexion.[4] ■ Thoroughly disinfect the patient's skin at the insertion site, and allow the antiseptic to dry completely before inserting the catheter.[4] ■ Secure the device *to prevent motion.*[4] ■ Follow sterile technique when accessing the catheter and administering IV fluids and medications.[4] ■ Use an infusate with a pH between 5 and 9, an osmolality of less than 600 mOsm/L, or a final dextrose concentration of less than 10%.[34]
Infiltration	■ Edema in any direction from the insertion site[4] ■ Changes in skin temperature, including coolness or warmth[4] ■ Changes in skin color, including blanching, bruising, or redness surrounding insertion site[4] ■ Pain, burning, or stinging with injection or infusion[4] ■ Fluid leakage from insertion site[4] ■ Blister development[4] ■ Impaired mobility of fingers, hand, or entire extremity[4] ■ Numbness, tingling, and other signs of paresthesia in extremity[4] ■ Slowed capillary refill time[4] ■ Loss of blood return during aspiration	■ Dislodgement of the venous access device from the vein or a perforated vein	■ Stop the infusion.[38] ■ Remove the catheter.[36,38] ■ Apply warm soaks *to aid absorption.* ■ Elevate the limb.[4] ■ Check for pulse and capillary refill periodically *to assess circulation.* ■ Restart the infusion in another limb. ■ Document the patient's condition and your interventions.[33,34,38] ■ Notify the practitioner that infiltration has occurred, if severe. Treatment depends on the severity and type of solution infiltrated. ***Prevention*** ■ Use the smallest gauge and length of catheter needed to accommodate the prescribed therapy.[4] ■ Avoid inserting the catheter in an area of flexion.[4] ■ Frequently check the IV site. ■ Don't rely on infusion pump alarms to detect infiltration.[4] ■ Aspirate for blood return *to ensure catheter patency before beginning the infusion.*[4,10,38] ■ Teach the patient to observe the IV site and report pain, burning, or swelling.[4] ■ Stabilize the catheter *to minimize movement at the insertion site.*[18,38] ■ Consider using a central venous access device for infusates with a pH of less than 5 or more than 9, an osmolarity of more than 600 mOsm/L, or a final dextrose concentration or more than 10%.[4]

(continued)

Risks of peripheral IV therapy *(continued)*

Complications	Signs and symptoms	Possible causes	Nursing interventions
Local complications *(continued)*			
			■ Infuse an irritating infusate into a large peripheral vein; avoid using a vein in the fingers or hand.[4] ■ If administering a vesicant, check device patency during vesicant administration, aspirating for blood return every 3 to 4 mL.[4] ■ Administer vesicants through the lowest injection port of free-flowing compatible solution.[4]
Cannula dislodgment	■ Cannula partly backed out of vein ■ Solution infiltrating	■ Loosened tape, or tubing snagged in bed linens, resulting in partial retraction of cannula ■ Removal by a confused patient	■ If no infiltration occurs, retape without pushing cannula back into vein. Never reinsert the cannula into the vein.[18] If pulled out, apply pressure to IV site with sterile dressing. ■ Document the patient's condition and your interventions.[33,34] ***Prevention*** ■ Secure the device on insertion.
Occlusion	■ Infusion doesn't flow ■ Infusion pump alarms "occlusion" ■ Discomfort at insertion site	■ IV flow interrupted ■ Saline lock not flushed ■ Blood backflow in line when patient walks ■ Line clamped too long ■ Hypercoagulable patient	■ Use mild flush injection; don't force it. ■ If unsuccessful, remove the IV catheter and insert a new one. ■ Document the patient's condition and your interventions.[33,34] ***Prevention*** ■ Maintain IV flow rate. ■ Flush promptly after intermittent piggyback administration. ■ Have the patient walk with his arm bent at the elbow *to reduce the risk of blood backflow.*
Vein irritation or pain at IV site	■ Pain during infusion ■ Possible blanching if vasospasm occurs ■ Red skin over vein during infusion ■ Rapidly developing signs of phlebitis	■ Solution with high or low pH or high osmolarity, such as phenytoin and some antibiotics (vancomycin and nafcillin)	■ Decrease the flow rate. ■ Try using an electronic flow device *to achieve a steady flow.* ■ Document the patient's condition and your interventions.[33,34] ***Prevention*** ■ Dilute solutions before administration. For example, give antibiotics in 250-mL solution rather than 100-mL solution. ■ If long-term therapy with an irritating drug is planned, ask the practitioner to use a central venous access device.
Severed cannula	■ Leakage from cannula shaft	■ Cannula inadvertently cut by scissors ■ Reinsertion of stylet into cannula	■ If a broken part is visible, attempt to retrieve it. If unsuccessful, notify the practitioner. ■ If a portion of the cannula enters the bloodstream, place a tourniquet above the IV site *to prevent progression of the broken part.* ■ Notify the practitioner and radiology department. ■ Document the patient's condition and your interventions.[33,34] ***Prevention*** ■ Don't use scissors around the IV site. ■ Never reinsert the stylet into the cannula.[8] ■ Remove an unsuccessfully inserted cannula and stylet together.

Risks of peripheral IV therapy *(continued)*

COMPLICATIONS	SIGNS AND SYMPTOMS	POSSIBLE CAUSES	NURSING INTERVENTIONS
LOCAL COMPLICATIONS *(continued)*			
Hematoma	■ Tenderness at venipuncture site ■ Bruised area around site ■ Inability to advance or flush IV catheter	■ Vein punctured through opposite wall at time of insertion ■ Leakage of blood from stylet displacement	■ Remove the venous access device.[36] ■ Apply direct pressure and elevate the extremity until bleeding has stopped. ■ Recheck for bleeding. ■ Document the patient's condition and your interventions.[33,34] ***Prevention*** ■ Choose a vein that can accommodate the size of the venous access device. ■ Release the tourniquet as soon as successful insertion is achieved.
Venous spasm	■ Pain along vein ■ Flow rate sluggish when clamp completely open ■ Blanched skin over vein	■ Severe vein irritation from irritating drugs or fluids ■ Administration of cold fluids or blood ■ Very rapid flow rate (with fluids at room temperature)	■ Apply warm soaks over the vein and surrounding area. ■ Decrease the flow rate. ■ Document the patient's condition and your interventions.[33,34] ***Prevention*** ■ Use a blood warmer for blood or packed red blood cells.
Thrombosis	■ Painful, reddened, and swollen vein ■ Sluggish or stopped IV flow	■ Injury to endothelial cells of vein wall, allowing platelets to adhere and thrombi to form	■ Remove the venous access device; restart the infusion in the opposite limb if possible. ■ Apply cold compresses. ■ Watch for IV therapy–related infection; *thrombi provide an excellent environment for bacterial growth.* ■ Document the patient's condition and your interventions.[33,34] ***Prevention*** ■ Use proper venipuncture technique *to reduce injury to the vein.* ■ Avoid starting an IV infusion in the lower extremities.[2]
Thrombophlebitis	■ Severe discomfort ■ Reddened, swollen, and hardened vein	■ Thrombosis and inflammation	■ Remove the venous access device; restart the infusion in the opposite limb if possible. ■ Apply cold compresses. ■ Watch for IV therapy–related infection; *thrombi provide an excellent environment for bacterial growth.* ■ Document the patient's condition and your interventions.[33,34] ***Prevention*** ■ Check the site frequently. Remove the venous access device at the first sign of redness and tenderness.
Nerve, tendon, or ligament damage	■ Extreme pain (similar to electrical shock when nerve is punctured) ■ Numbness and muscle contraction ■ Delayed effects, including paralysis, numbness, and deformity	■ Improper venipuncture technique, resulting in injury to surrounding nerves, tendons, or ligaments ■ Tight taping or improper splinting with arm board	■ Stop the procedure. ■ Remove the device. ■ Document the patient's condition and your interventions.[33,34] ***Prevention*** ■ Don't repeatedly penetrate tissues with a venous access device. ■ Don't apply excessive pressure when taping; don't encircle the limb with tape. ■ Pad arm boards and use tape to secure them if possible.

(continued)

Risks of peripheral IV therapy *(continued)*

Complications	Signs and symptoms	Possible causes	Nursing interventions
Local complications *(continued)*			
Vasovagal reaction	■ Sudden collapse of vein during venipuncture ■ Sudden pallor, sweating, faintness, dizziness, and nausea ■ Decreased blood pressure	■ Vasospasm from anxiety or pain	■ Lower the head of the bed. ■ Have the patient take deep breaths. ■ Check vital signs. ■ Document the patient's condition and your interventions.[33,34] ***Prevention*** ■ Prepare the patient for therapy *to relieve his anxiety.* ■ Use local anesthetic *to prevent pain.*
Systemic complications			
Circulatory overload	■ Discomfort ■ Neck vein engorgement ■ Respiratory distress ■ Increased blood pressure ■ Crackles ■ Increased difference between fluid intake and output	■ Roller clamp loosened to allow run-on infusion ■ Flow rate too rapid ■ Miscalculation of fluid requirements	■ Raise the head of the bed. ■ Slow the infusion rate, but don't remove the IV catheter. ■ Administer oxygen as needed. ■ Notify the practitioner. ■ Administer medications (probably furosemide) as prescribed. ■ Document the patient's condition and your interventions.[33,34] ***Prevention*** ■ Use a pump for elderly or compromised patients. ■ Recheck calculations of fluid requirements. ■ Monitor infusions frequently.
Systemic infection (septicemia or bacteremia)	■ Fever, chills, and malaise for no apparent reason ■ Contaminated IV site, usually with no visible signs of infection at site	■ Failure to maintain sterile technique during insertion or site care ■ Severe phlebitis, which can set up ideal conditions for organism growth ■ A poorly secured device that can move, which can introduce organisms into bloodstream ■ Prolonged indwelling time of device ■ Weak immune system	■ Notify the practitioner. ■ Administer medications as prescribed. ■ Culture the site and device.[39] ■ Monitor vital signs. ■ Document the patient's condition and your interventions.[33,34] ***Prevention*** ■ Use scrupulous sterile technique when handling solutions and tubing, inserting a venous access device, and discontinuing an infusion. ■ Secure all connections and use only luer-lock–designed devices.[30,41] ■ Change IV solutions, tubing, and venous access devices at recommended times.
Air embolism[42]	■ Sudden onset of dyspnea ■ Breathlessness ■ Tachyarrhythmias ■ Weak pulse ■ Increased central venous pressure ■ Hypotension ■ Loss of consciousness ■ Continued coughing ■ Chest pain ■ Jugular venous distention ■ Wheezing ■ Altered mental status ■ Altered speech ■ Numbness ■ Paralysis	■ Empty solution container (the solution container empties, and added container pushes air down the line if line not purged first) ■ Disconnected tubing from venous access device or IV bag	■ Clamp, fold, or close the existing catheter or occlude the insertion site.[42] ■ Place the patient in a left lateral decubitus position, if not contraindicated by other conditions.[42] ■ Administer oxygen. ■ Notify the practitioner. ■ Document the patient's condition and your interventions.[33,34] ***Prevention*** ■ Purge administration sets and add-on devices of air completely before starting an infusion.[4] ■ Use an air-detection device on the pump or an air-eliminating filter proximal to the IV site. ■ Secure connections.

Risks of peripheral IV therapy *(continued)*

Complications	Signs and symptoms	Possible causes	Nursing interventions
Systemic complications *(continued)*			
			■ Use luer-lock connections on catheter-administration set junctions.[4] ■ Place the patient in a position with the insertion site at or below heart level when changing administration sets or needleless connectors.[4] ■ Trace the tubing from the patient to its point of origin *to prevent misconnections.*[4,30] ■ Have the patient perform the Valsalva maneuver, if able, when you're changing administration tubing or the needleless connector if a clamp isn't present on the catheter's exterior. If it is present, clamp it.[4]
Allergic reaction	■ Itching ■ Watery eyes and nose ■ Bronchospasm ■ Wheezing ■ Urticarial rash ■ Edema at IV site ■ Anaphylactic reaction, which may occur within minutes or up to 1 hour after exposure (flushing, chills, anxiety, agitation, itching, palpitations, paresthesia, throbbing in ears, wheezing, coughing, seizures, cardiac arrest)	■ Allergens, such as medications	■ If a reaction occurs, stop the infusion immediately and infuse normal saline solution. ■ Maintain a patent airway. ■ Notify the practitioner. ■ Administer an antihistamine, a steroid, an anti-inflammatory, and antipyretic drugs, as prescribed. ■ Give epinephrine, as prescribed, for more severe reactions. Repeat as needed and prescribed. ■ Administer steroids if prescribed. ■ Document the patient's condition and your interventions.[33,34] ***Prevention*** ■ Obtain the patient's allergy history. Be aware of cross-allergies. ■ Assist with test dosing and document any new allergies. ■ Monitor the patient carefully during the first 15 minutes of administration of a new drug.

7 Standard 18. Infection prevention. Infusion nursing standards of practice. (2011). *Journal of Infusion Nursing, 34,* S25–S26. (Level VII)

8 Standard 35. Vascular access site preparation and device placement. Infusion nursing standards of practice. (2011). *Journal of Infusion Nursing, 34,* S44–S46. (Level VII)

9 Franklin, B. D., et al. (2012). The safe insertion of peripheral intravenous catheters: a mixed methods descriptive study of the availability of the equipment needed. *Antimicrobial Resistance and Infection Control, 1*(1), 15. Accessed March 2015 via the Web at http://www.aricjournal.com/content/pdf/2047-2994-1-15.pdf

10 Standard 61. Parenteral medication and solution administration. Infusion nursing standards of practice. (2011). *Journal of Infusion Nursing, 34,* S86–S87. (Level VII)

11 The Joint Commission. (2015). Standard NPSG.07.01.01. *Comprehensive accreditation manual for hospitals: The official handbook.* Oakbrook Terrace, IL: The Joint Commission. (Level VII)

12 Standard 19. Hand hygiene. Infusion nursing standards of practice. (2011). *Journal of Infusion Nursing, 34,* S26–S27. (Level VII)

13 Centers for Disease Control and Prevention. (2002). Guideline for hand hygiene in health-care settings: Recommendations of the Healthcare Infection Control Practices Advisory Committee and the HICPAC/SHEA/APIC/IDSA Hand Hygiene Task Force. *MMWR Recommendations and Reports, 51*(RR-16), 1–45. Accessed March 2015 via the Web at http://www.cdc.gov/mmwr/pdf/rr/rr5116.pdf (Level II)

14 World Health Organization. (2009). "WHO guidelines on hand hygiene in health care: First global patient safety challenge, clean care is safer care" [Online]. Accessed March 2015 via the Web at http://whqlibdoc.who.int/publications/2009/9789241597906_eng.pdf (Level IV)

15 American Osteopathic Association. (2014). Standard 07.01.21. *Healthcare Facilities Accreditation Program: Accreditation requirements for acute care hospitals.* Chicago, IL: American Osteopathic Association. (Level VII)

16 Centers for Medicare & Medicaid Services, Department of Health and Human Services. (2014). Condition of participation: Infection control. 42 C.F.R. § 482.42.

17 The Joint Commission. (2015). Standard NPSG.01.01.01. *Comprehensive accreditation manual for hospitals: The official handbook.* Oakbrook Terrace, IL: The Joint Commission. (Level VII)

18 Standard 36. Vascular access device stabilization. Infusion nursing standards of practice. (2011). *Journal of Infusion Nursing, 34,* S46–S47. (Level VII)

19 Standard 31. Tourniquets. Infusion nursing standards of practice. (2011). *Journal of Infusion Nursing, 34,* S36. (Level VII)

20 Standard 34. Local anesthesia for vascular access device placement and access. Infusion nursing standards of practice. (2011). *Journal of Infusion Nursing, 34,* S43–S44. (Level VII)

21 Page, D. E., & Taylor, D. M. (2010). Vapocoolant spray vs subcutaneous lidocaine injection for reducing the pain of intravenous cannulation: A randomized, controlled, clinical trial. *British Journal of Anaesthesia, 105,* 519–525. (Level II)

22 Occupational Safety and Health Administration. (n.d.). "Bloodborne pathogens, standard number 1910.1030" [Online]. Accessed March 2015 via the Web at http://www.osha.gov/pls/oshaweb/owadisp.show_document?p_table=STANDARDS&p_id=10051 (Level VII)
23 Siegel, J. D., et al. (2007). "2007 guideline for isolation precautions: Preventing transmission of infectious agents in healthcare settings" [Online]. Accessed March 2015 via the Web at http://www.cdc.gov/hicpac/pdf/isolation/Isolation2007.pdf (Level II)
24 American Osteopathic Association. (2014). Standard 07.01.10. *Healthcare Facilities Accreditation Program: Accreditation requirements for acute care hospitals.* Chicago, IL: American Osteopathic Association. (Level VII)
25 Standard 45. Flushing and locking. Infusion nursing standards of practice. (2011). *Journal of Infusion Nursing, 34,* S59–S63. (Level VII)
26 Gazda-Bausone, D., et al. (2010). A randomized controlled trial to compare the complications of 2 peripheral intravenous catheter-stabilization systems. *Journal of Infusion Nursing, 33,* 371–384. (Level II)
27 Infusion Nurses Society. (2010). *Infusion nursing: An evidence-based approach* (3rd ed.). St. Louis, MO: Saunders.
28 Gabriel, J. (2010). Vascular access devices: Securement and dressings. *Nursing Standard, 24*(52), 41–46.
29 Standard 46. Vascular access device site care and dressing changes. Infusion nursing standards of practice. (2011). *Journal of Infusion Nursing, 34,* S63–S64. (Level VII)
30 U.S. Food and Drug Administration. (n.d.). "Look. Check. Connect. Safe medical device connections save lives" [Online]. Accessed March 2015 via the Web at http://www.fda.gov/downloads/MedicalDevices/Safety/AlertsandNotices/UCM134873.pdf
31 Standard 37. Joint stabilization. Infusion nursing standards of practice. (2011). *Journal of Infusion Nursing, 34,* S47–S48. (Level VII)
32 Standard 22. Safe handling and disposal of sharps, hazardous materials, and hazardous waste. Infusion nursing standards of practice. (2011). *Journal of Infusion Nursing, 34,* S28–S29. (Level VII)
33 The Joint Commission. (2015). Standard RC.01.03.01. *Comprehensive accreditation manual for hospitals: The official handbook.* Oakbrook Terrace, IL: The Joint Commission. (Level VII)
34 Standard 14. Documentation. Infusion nursing standards of practice. (2011). *Journal of Infusion Nursing, 34,* S20–S21. (Level VII)
35 Centers for Medicare & Medicaid Services, Department of Health and Human Services. (2014). Condition of participation: Medical record services. 42 C.F.R. § 482.24(b).
36 Standard 44. Vascular access device removal. Infusion nursing standards of practice. (2011). *Journal of Infusion Nursing, 34,* S57–S59. (Level VII)
37 Standard 47. Phlebitis. Infusion nursing standards of practice. (2011). *Journal of Infusion Nursing, 34,* S65–S66. (Level VII)
38 Standard 48. Infiltration and extravasation. Infusion nursing standards of practice. (2011). *Journal of Infusion Nursing, 34,* S66–S68. (Level VII)
39 Standard 49. Infection. Infusion nursing standards of practice. (2011). *Journal of Infusion Nursing, 34,* S68–S69. (Level VII)
40 LeBlanc, K., et al. (2013). International skin tear advisory panel: A tool kit to aid in the prevention, assessment, and treatment of skin tears using a simplified classification system. *Advances in Skin & Wound Care, 26,* 459–476. (Level VII)
41 Standard 26. Add-on devices. Infusion nursing standards of practice. (2011). *Journal of Infusion Nursing, 34,* S31. (Level VII)
42 Standard 50. Air embolism. Infusion nursing standards of practice. (2011). *Journal of Infusion Nursing, 34,* S69–S70. (Level VII)

IV CATHETER MAINTENANCE

Routine maintenance of an IV site includes regular assessment of the site and periodic changes of the dressing, which help prevent complications, such as thrombophlebitis and infection. Routine site care and IV dressing changes aren't recommended for short peripheral IV catheters unless the dressing becomes soiled or damp or is no longer intact.[1,2] Dressings are also changed when the device is changed; the IV catheter should be changed when clinically indicated by the patient's condition, integrity of the vein and skin, length and type of prescribed therapy, integrity and patency of the existing catheter, and the patient's care location.[2,3] Peripheral IV catheters should be replaced no more frequently than every 72 hours to reduce the risk for infection and phlebitis in adults.[1] If an IV catheter is inserted during an emergency, it should be replaced as soon as possible, within a maximum of 48 hours to reduce the risk of vascular catheter–associated infection.[2]

HOSPITAL-ACQUIRED CONDITION ALERT *Keep in mind that vascular catheter–associated infection is considered a hospital-acquired condition* because it can be reasonably prevented using best practices. *Use infection-prevention techniques (such as performing hand hygiene, properly cleaning the insertion site with an antiseptic, and using sterile technique) when changing an IV dressing* to reduce the risk of vascular catheter–associated infection.[4]

Equipment

For a dressing change

Gloves ▪ antiseptic solution (chlorhexidine-based antiseptic is preferred; however, tincture of iodine, povidone-iodine, or alcohol may also be used)[2] ▪ transparent semipermeable dressing ▪ catheter securement device, sterile tape, or sterile surgical strips ▪ label ▪ marker ▪ Optional: sterile 2″ × 2″ (5-cm × 5-cm) gauze pads, adhesive bandage, dressing formulated for fragile skin, sterile needleless connector, extension set.

For a solution change

Solution container ▪ antiseptic pad (chlorhexidine-based, alcohol, or tincture of iodine) ▪ Optional: time tape.

For an IV tubing change

IV administration set ▪ new bag of prescribed IV fluids (as needed) ▪ gloves ▪ transparent semipermeable dressing ▪ sterile 2″ × 2″ (5-cm × 5-cm) gauze pads ▪ label.

For using a time tape

IV solution ▪ IV administration set with clamp ▪ 1″ (2.5-cm) paper or adhesive tape (or preprinted time tape) ▪ pen.

Preparation of equipment

If your facility keeps IV equipment and dressings in a tray or cart, have it nearby, if possible,[5] *because you may have to select a new venipuncture site, depending on the current site's condition.*

Implementation

- Gather the appropriate equipment.
- Perform hand hygiene *to prevent the spread of microorganisms.*[1,6,7,8,9,10]
- Confirm the patient's identity using at least two patient identifiers.[11]
- Explain the procedure to the patient *to allay his fears and ensure cooperation.*

Changing a dressing

- Open all supply using sterile technique.
- Put on gloves.[1,12,13,14]
- Remove the existing dressing (as shown on next page, top left). Begin at the catheter hub and gently pull the dressing perpendicular to the skin toward the insertion site *to prevent skin stripping or tearing and catheter dislodgment.*[15,16]

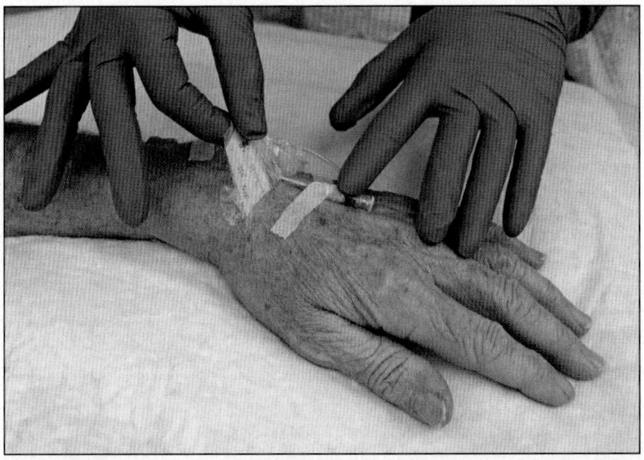

■ Remove the securement device; hold the cannula in place with your nondominant hand (as shown below) *to prevent accidental movement or dislodgment, which could puncture the vein and cause infiltration.*

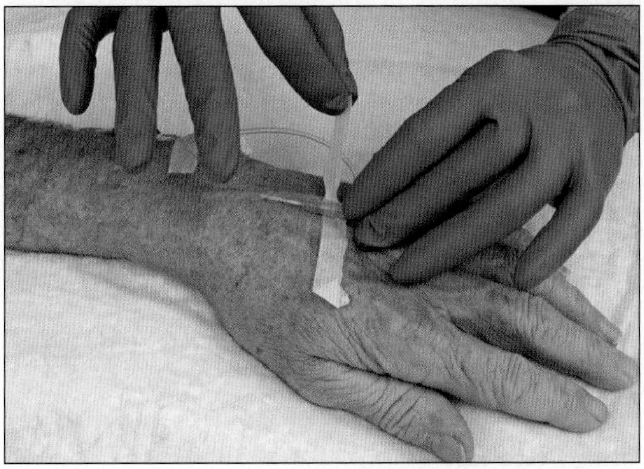

■ Assess the venipuncture site for signs and symptoms of infection (redness and pain at the puncture site), infiltration (coolness, blanching, and edema at the site), and thrombophlebitis (redness, firmness, tenderness, warmth, palpable venous cord, and edema).[1,2,15] If any such signs or symptoms are present, cover the area with a sterile 2″ × 2″ (5-cm × 5-cm) gauze pad and remove the catheter.[1] Apply pressure to the area until the bleeding stops, and apply an adhesive bandage. Then, using fresh equipment and solution, start the IV line in another appropriate site, preferably on the opposite extremity. (See the "IV catheter insertion and removal" procedure, page 446.)

■ If the venipuncture site is intact, stabilize the cannula and carefully clean around the puncture site with antiseptic solution (as shown on top right) *to decrease the risk of infection.* Cleaning methods vary with the type of antiseptic used. Apply chlorhexidine using a side-to-side motion for at least 30 seconds.[17] Allow the area to dry completely. If using povidone-iodine swabs, apply in a concentric circle beginning at the insertion site and moving outward. Allow the povidone-iodine solution to remain on the skin for at least 2 minutes until it dries completely *to ensure adequate antisepsis.*[15]

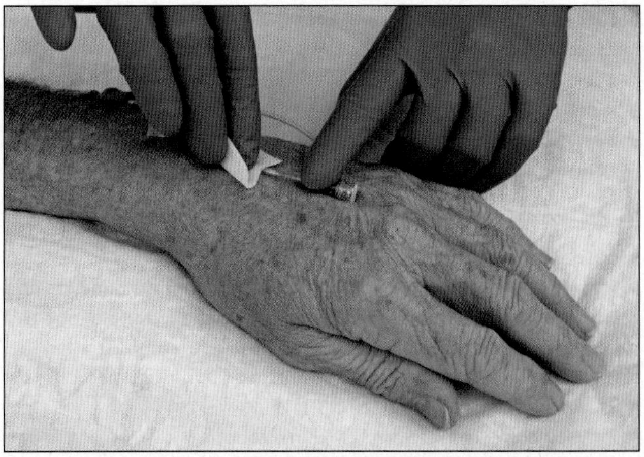

■ Secure the catheter with a catheter securement device, sterile tape, or sterile surgical strips. A catheter securement device is preferred over tape when feasible *because studies show overall reduction in complications and improved dwell time when a catheter securement device is used.*[1,2,18,19]

■ Place a transparent semipermeable dressing over the insertion site to halfway up the catheter (as shown below).[1,2] *The transparent dressing allows visualization of the insertion site and maintains sterility.* If the patient has fragile skin, use a dressing specifically formulated for fragile skin *to prevent tearing or stripping.*[16]

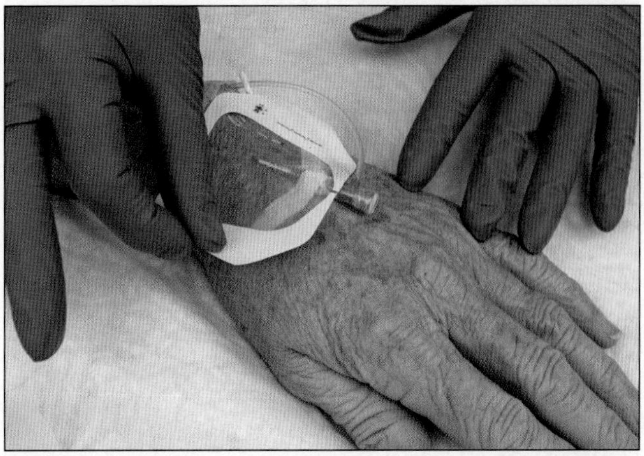

■ Label the dressing with the date and time of the procedure and your initials.[2]

■ Discard used supplies in appropriate receptacles.[12,13,20]

■ Remove and discard your gloves and perform hand hygiene.[1,6,7,8,9,10]

■ Document the procedure.[21,22,23,24]

Changing the solution

■ If your facility uses a bar code scanning system, scan your identification badge, the patient's identification band, and the IV fluid's bar code.

■ Inspect the new solution container for cracks, leaks, and other damage. Check the solution for discoloration, turbidity, and particulates. Note the date and time the solution was mixed and its expiration date.[25]

■ Clamp the tubing when inverting it *to prevent air from entering the tubing.* Keep the drip chamber half full. Put the IV pump on standby or pause.

■ If you're replacing a bag, remove the seal or tab from the new bag and remove the old bag from the pole. Remove the spike, insert it into the new bag, and adjust the flow rate or restart the pump.[17]

■ If you're replacing a bottle, remove the cap and seal from the new bottle and disinfect the rubber port with an antiseptic pad and allow it to dry. Clamp the line, pause the pump, remove the spike from the old bottle, and insert the spike into the new bottle. Then hang the new bottle and adjust the flow rate or restart the pump.

- Label the solution container with the date and time and place a time tape on the solution, if required by your facility.
- Discard used supplies in an appropriate receptacle.[12,13,20]
- Perform hand hygiene.[1,6,7,8,9,10]
- Document the procedure.[21,22,23,24]

Changing the tubing

- Hang the solution on an IV pole, squeeze the administration set's drip *chamber to fill it to the manufacturer's mark* (about one-third to one-half full), slowly open the clamp, and prime the new administration set, including add-on devices, if used. Clamp the administration set.[17]
- Put on gloves.[1,12,13,14]
- Assess the IV site for redness, swelling, or pain.[1]
- Remove the dressing over the IV catheter insertion site, if needed, *to access the catheter hub.*
- Stop or pause the electronic infusion pump, if indicated.
- Clamp the existing administration set.[15,17]
- Clamp the IV catheter *to prevent accidental exposure to blood and to reduce the risk of air embolism.*[15,17]
- Gently disconnect the existing tubing (as shown below), being careful not to dislodge the catheter.[15,17]

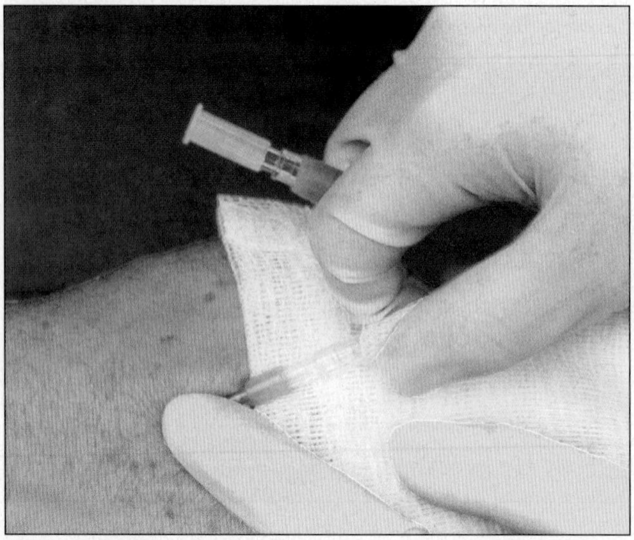

- Thoroughly disinfect the catheter hub with an antiseptic pad using friction and allow it to dry.[15,17]
- Remove the protective cap from the distal end of the new administration set, and attach it to the catheter hub.[15,17]
- Trace the tubing from the patient to its point of origin *to make sure you've connected the administration tubing to the proper port.*[26]
- Open the IV catheter clamp.
- Slowly open the clamp of the administration set *to begin the infusion* or place the administration set in the electronic infusion device and turn on the device.[15,17]
- Adjust the clamp (as shown on top right) *to maintain the appropriate flow rate*; manually count the drops per minute *to ensure the proper rate of infusion.* Alternatively, confirm that the right information is displayed on the electronic pump, unclamp the tubing, and begin the infusion. Watch the electronic infusion device for 1 to 2 minutes *to ensure the proper administration rate.*[15,17] (See the "IV pump use" procedure, page 462.)

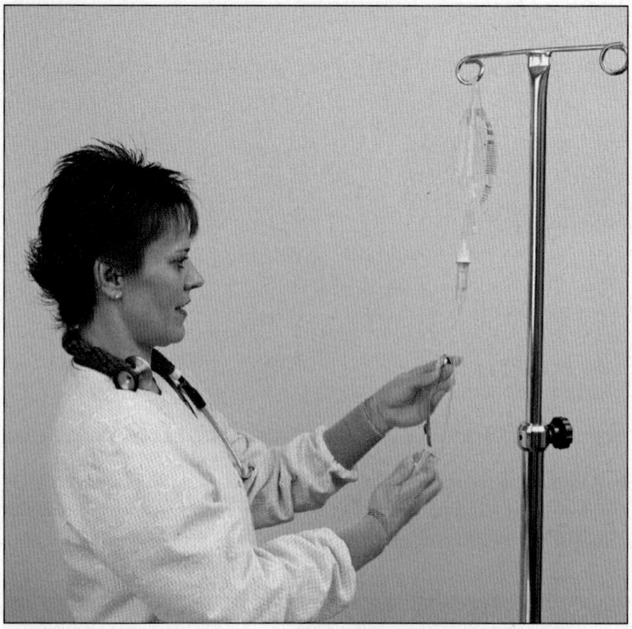

- Secure the catheter, as indicated, *to preserve the integrity of the access device, minimize catheter movement, and prevent catheter dislodgment.*[18]
- Perform insertion site care and apply a new transparent semipermeable dressing over the insertion site, if needed.[2]
- Check that all connections are secure *to prevent leaking, bleeding, contamination, and disconnections.*[27] Recheck the IV flow rate.
- Discard used supplies in an appropriate receptacle.[12,13,20]
- Remove and discard your gloves.[12,13,20]
- Perform hand hygiene.[1,6,7,8,9,10]
- Label the administration set and solution container with the date and time.[15,17,27]
- Document the procedure.[21,22,23,24]

Using a time tape

- Calculate the number of milliliters to be infused per hour.
- Place a piece of tape or preprinted time tape vertically on the container alongside the volume-increment markers.
- Starting at the current solution level, move down the number of milliliters to be infused in 1 hour, and mark the appropriate time and a horizontal line on the tape at this level. Then continue to mark 1-hour intervals until you reach the bottom of the container. Don't use a felt-tip pen to write directly on the plastic IV bag *because the ink may penetrate the container, contaminating the IV fluid.*[27]
- Check the flow rate every 15 minutes until stable, then hourly; adjust as needed.
- Compare the time with the appropriate infusion level on the tape and recheck the flow rate. Assess for deviations from recommended intake. (See *Managing IV flow rate deviations.*)
- With each check, inspect the IV site for complications, and assess the patient's response to therapy.[25]
- Perform hand hygiene.[1,6,7,8,9,10]
- Document the procedure.[21,22,23,24]

Patient teaching

Teach the patient about positioning and movement related to the IV site and tubing, and tell him to report any changes to the catheter site as well as any discomfort.

Special considerations

- If you crack the adapter or hub (or if you accidentally dislodge the cannula from the vein), remove the cannula. Apply pressure and an

TROUBLESHOOTING

Managing IV flow rate deviations

Problem	Possible causes	Nursing interventions
Flow rate too slow	■ Venous spasm after insertion	■ Apply warm soaks over the site.
	■ Venous obstruction from bending arm	■ Secure the arm with an arm board if necessary. ■ Change the IV site.
	■ Pressure change (decreasing fluid in bottle causes solution to run slower because of decreasing pressure)	■ Readjust the flow rate.
	■ Elevated blood pressure	■ Readjust the flow rate. Use an infusion *pump to ensure the correct flow rate.*
	■ Cold solution	■ Allow the solution to warm to room temperature before hanging.
	■ Change in solution viscosity from medication added	■ Readjust the flow rate.
	■ IV container too low or patient's arm too high	■ Hang the container higher or remind the patient to keep his arm below heart level.
	■ Bevel against vein wall (positional cannulation)	■ Withdraw the needle slightly, or place a folded 2″ × 2″ (5-cm × 5-cm) gauze pad over or under the catheter hub to change the angle.
	■ Excess tubing dangling below insertion site	■ Replace the tubing with a shorter piece, or tape excess tubing to the IV pole, below the flow clamp. (Make sure the tubing isn't kinked.)
	■ Catheter too small	■ Remove the catheter in use, and insert a larger-bore catheter, or use an infusion pump.
	■ Infiltration or clotted catheter	■ Remove the catheter in use, and insert a new catheter.
	■ Kinked tubing	■ Check the tubing over its entire length and unkink it. ■ Replace the tubing if it remains kinked.
	■ Clogged filter	■ Remove the filter and replace with it a new one.
	■ Tubing memory (tubing compressed at clamped area)	■ Massage or milk the tubing by pinching and wrapping it around a pencil four or five times. Quickly pull the pencil out of the coiled tubing. ■ Replace tubing if necessary.
Flow rate too fast	■ Clamp manipulated by patient or visitor	■ Instruct the patient not to touch the clamp. Place tape over it. Administer IV solution with infusion pump.
	■ Tubing disconnected from catheter	■ Restart IV with new a catheter with luer-lock connections.
	■ Change in patient position	■ Readjust the flow rate.
	■ Flow clamp drifted because of patient movement	■ Place tape below the clamp.

adhesive bandage *to stop any bleeding.* Perform a venipuncture at another site, and reinsert a new IV catheter.

■ The Centers for Disease Control and Prevention recommends replacing administration sets that are used continuously (including secondary sets and add-on devices) no more frequently than every 96 hours, but at least every 7 days for patients who aren't receiving blood, blood products, or fat emulsions. Tubing used to administer blood, blood products, or fat emulsions should be replaced within 24 hours of initiating the infusion.[1]

■ Replace the needleless connector with a new primed one if indicated. Change needleless connectors when removed for any reason, when blood or debris is present within the connector, before drawing a blood culture sample, or upon contamination.[25] Also, if an extension set is present and necessary, replace it with a new, primed one; however, keep in mind that the potential for contamination exists with all add-on devices, so their use should be limited.[28]

- Closely monitor the flow rate and correct as needed *because such factors as venous spasm, venous pressure changes, patient movement or manipulation of the clamp, and bent or kinked tubing can cause the rate to vary markedly.*
- If the infusion rate slows significantly, you may need to increase the flow rate slightly. If you must increase the rate by more than 30% to achieve the infusion volume goal, consult the practitioner. When infusing drugs, use an IV pump if possible *to avoid flow rate inaccuracies.* Always use a pump when infusing solutions through a central venous access device.
- Large-volume solution containers have about 10% more fluid than the amount indicated on the bag *to allow for tubing purges.* A 1,000-mL bag or bottle contains an additional 100 mL; similarly, a 500-mL container holds an extra 50 mL, and a 250-mL container holds an extra 25 mL.

Complications

Potential complications include catheter dislodgment and infection. An excessively slow flow rate may cause insufficient intake of fluids, drugs, and nutrients; an excessively rapid rate of fluid or drug infusion may cause circulatory overload, possibly leading to heart failure and pulmonary edema as well as adverse drug effects.

Documentation

For a dressing change, record the date and time of the dressing change and the appearance of the site, the dressing type, the type of stabilization device used, site care performed, and any patient reports of discomfort or pain. Document patient and family teaching and their understanding of the teaching.

For a solution change, record the time, date, and rate and type of solution (and any additives). Also record the appearance of the site.

For a tubing change, record the date and time of the tubing change, the appearance of the site, the type of dressing applied, and any patient teaching and the patient's understanding of your teaching. Document the patient's tolerance of the procedure as well as the type of IV fluid administered and the rate of infusion.

When using a time tape, record the original flow rate when beginning the infusion through the peripheral IV catheter. If you adjust the rate, record the change, the date and time, and your initials. Document any patient teaching provided and the patient's understanding of your teaching.

References

1 Centers for Disease Control and Prevention. (2011). "Guidelines for the prevention of intravascular catheter-related infections" [Online]. Accessed March 2015 via the Web at http://www.cdc.gov/hicpac/pdf/guidelines/bsi-guidelines-2011.pdf (Level I)

2 Standard 46. Vascular access device site care and dressing changes. Infusion nursing standards of practice. (2011). *Journal of Infusion Nursing, 34,* S63–S64. (Level VII)

3 Rickard, C. M., et al. (2012). Routine versus clinically indicated replacement of peripheral intravenous catheters: A randomised controlled equivalence trial. *Lancet, 380,* 1066–1074. (Level II)

4 Jarrett, N., et al. (2013). "Evidence-based guidelines for selected and previously considered hospital-acquired conditions: Final report" [Online]. Accessed March 2015 via the Web at http://www.cms.gov/Medicare/Medicare-Fee-for-Service-Payment/HospitalAcqCond/Downloads/Evidence-Based-Guidelines.pdf

5 Franklin, B. D., et al. (2012). The safe insertion of peripheral intravenous catheters: A mixed methods descriptive study of the availability of the equipment needed. *Antimicrobial Resistance and Infection Control, 1*(1), 15.

6 The Joint Commission. (2015). Standard NPSG.07.01.01. *Comprehensive accreditation manual for hospitals: The official handbook.* Oakbrook Terrace, IL: The Joint Commission. (Level VII)

7 Centers for Disease Control and Prevention. (2002). Guideline for hand hygiene in health-care settings: Recommendations of the Healthcare Infection Control Practices Advisory Committee and the HICPAC/SHEA/APIC/IDSA Hand Hygiene Task Force. *MMWR Recommendations and Reports, 51*(RR-16), 1–45. Accessed March 2015 via the Web at http://www.cdc.gov/mmwr/pdf/rr/rr5116.pdf (Level II)

8 World Health Organization. (2009). "WHO guidelines on hand hygiene in health care: First global patient safety challenge, clean care is safer care" [Online]. Accessed March 2015 via the Web at http://whqlibdoc.who.int/publications/2009/9789241597906_eng.pdf (Level IV)

9 Standard 19. Hand hygiene. Infusion nursing standards of practice. (2011). *Journal of Infusion Nursing, 34,* S26–S27. (Level VII)

10 American Osteopathic Association. (2014). Standard 07.01.21. *Healthcare Facilities Accreditation Program: Accreditation requirements for acute care hospitals.* Chicago, IL: American Osteopathic Association. (Level VII)

11 The Joint Commission. (2015). Standard NPSG.01.01.01. *Comprehensive accreditation manual for hospitals: The official handbook.* Oakbrook Terrace, IL: The Joint Commission. (Level VII)

12 Siegel, J. D., et al. (2007). "2007 guideline for isolation precautions: Preventing transmission of infectious agents in healthcare settings" [Online]. Accessed March 2015 via the Web at http://www.cdc.gov/hicpac/pdf/isolation/Isolation2007.pdf (Level II)

13 Occupational Safety and Health Administration. (n.d.). "Bloodborne pathogens, standard number 1910.1030" [Online]. Accessed March 2015 via the Web at http://www.osha.gov/pls/oshaweb/owadisp.show_document?p_table=STANDARDS&p_id=10051 (Level VII)

14 American Osteopathic Association. (2014). Standard 07.01.10. *Healthcare Facilities Accreditation Program: Accreditation requirements for acute care hospitals.* Chicago, IL: American Osteopathic Association. (Level VII)

15 Infusion Nurses Society. (2013). *Policies and procedures for infusion nursing of the older adult* (2nd ed.). Boston, MA: Infusion Nurses Society.

16 LeBlanc, K., et al. (2013). International skin tear advisory panel: A tool kit to aid in the prevention, assessment, and treatment of skin tears using a simplified classification system. *Advances in Skin & Wound Care, 26,* 459–476.

17 Infusion Nurses Society. (2011). *Policies and procedures for infusion nursing* (4th ed.). Boston, MA: Infusion Nurses Society.

18 Standard 36. Vascular access device stabilization. Infusion nursing standards of practice. (2011). *Journal of Infusion Nursing, 34,* S46–S47. (Level VII)

19 Gabriel, J. (2010). Vascular access devices: Securement and dressings. *Nursing Standard, 24*(52), 41–46.

20 Standard 22. Safe handling and disposal of sharps, hazardous materials, and hazardous waste. Infusion nursing standards of practice. (2011). *Journal of Infusion Nursing, 34,* S28–S29. (Level VII)

21 The Joint Commission. (2015). Standard RC.01.03.01. *Comprehensive accreditation manual for hospitals: The official handbook.* Oakbrook Terrace, IL: The Joint Commission. (Level VII)

22 Standard 14. Documentation. Infusion nursing standards of practice. (2011). *Journal of Infusion Nursing, 34,* S20–S21. (Level VII)

23 Centers for Medicare & Medicaid Services, Department of Health and Human Services. (2014). Condition of participation: Medical record services. 42 C.F.R. § 482.24(b).

24 American Osteopathic Association. (2014). Standard 10.00.03. *Healthcare Facilities Accreditation Program: Accreditation requirements for acute care hospitals.* Chicago, IL: American Osteopathic Association. (Level VII)

25 Standard 61. Parenteral medication and solution administration. Infusion nursing standards of practice. (2011). *Journal of Infusion Nursing, 34,* S86–S87. (Level VII)

26 U.S. Food and Drug Administration. (n.d.). "Look. Check. Connect. Safe medical device connections save lives" [Online]. Accessed March 2015 via the Web athttp://www.fda.gov/downloads/MedicalDevices/Safety/AlertsandNotices/UCM134873.pd

27 Smith, S., et al. (Eds.). (2012). *Clinical nursing skills: Basic to advanced skills* (8th ed.). Cranbury, NJ: Pearson.

28 Standard 26. Add-on devices. Infusion nursing standards of practice. (2011). *Journal of Infusion Nursing, 34,* S31. (Level VII)

29 Standard 48. Administration set change. Infusion nursing standards of practice. (2011). *Journal of Infusion Nursing, 34,* S55–S57. (Level VII)

IV INFUSION RATES AND MANUAL CONTROL

Calculated from a practitioner's order, flow rate is usually expressed as the total volume of IV solution infused over a prescribed interval or as the total volume given in milliliters per hour. Many devices can regulate the flow of IV solution, including clamps, flow regulators, and infusion pumps. (See *Using IV clamps.*)

When regulated by a clamp, flow rate is usually measured in drops per minute; by an infusion pump, in milliliters per hour. Flow regulators can be set to deliver the desired amount of solution, also in milliliters per hour. Less accurate than infusion pumps, flow regulators are most reliable when used with inactive adult patients. With any device, flow rate can easily be monitored by using a time tape, which indicates the prescribed solution level at hourly intervals. (See the "IV catheter maintenance" procedure, page 456.)

Equipment

IV solution ■ IV administration set with clamp ■ watch with second hand ■ Optional: drip rate chart.

Standard macrodrip sets deliver from 10 to 20 drops/mL, depending on the manufacturer; microdrip sets, 60 drops/mL; and blood transfusion sets, 10 drops/mL. A commercially available adapter can convert a macrodrip set to a microdrip system.

Implementation

- Verify the practitioner's order for the prescribed flow rate.
- Gather the appropriate equipment.
- Perform hand hygiene.[1,2,3,4,5,6,7]
- Confirm the patient's identity using at least two patient identifiers.[8]
- Attach the administration set to the IV solution and prime the tubing *to remove air.* (See the "IV therapy preparation" procedure, page 468.) Trace the tubing from the patient to its point of origin *to make sure you've connected it to the proper port before beginning the infusion.*[9,10]
- Determine the proper drip rate, or use your unit's drip rate chart. (See *Calculating infusion rates,* page 462.)
- After calculating the desired drip rate, remove your watch and hold it next to the drip chamber *so that you can observe the watch and drops simultaneously.*
- Release the clamp to the approximate drip rate. Then count drops for 1 minute *to account for flow irregularities.*
- Adjust the clamp as necessary, and count drops for 1 minute. Continue to adjust the clamp and count drops until the correct rate is achieved.
- Closely monitor the flow rate, inspect the IV site for complications, and assess the patient's response to therapy.
- Perform hand hygiene.[1,2,3,4,5,6,7]
- Document the procedure.[11,12,13,14]

Special considerations

- If the infusion rate slows significantly, a slight rate increase may be necessary. If the rate must be increased by more than 30% to achieve the infusion volume goal, consult the practitioner. When infusing drugs, use an IV pump, if possible, *to avoid flow rate inaccuracies.* Always use a pump when infusing solutions by way of a central venous access device.[15]
- Large-volume solution containers have about 10% more fluid than the amount indicated on the bag *to allow for tubing purges.* A 1,000-mL bag or bottle contains an additional 100 mL; similarly, a 500-mL container holds an extra 50 mL, and a 250-mL container holds an extra 25 mL.

Complications

An excessively slow flow rate may cause insufficient intake of fluids, drugs, and nutrients; an excessively rapid rate of fluid or drug infusion may cause circulatory overload—possibly leading to heart failure and pulmonary edema—as well as other adverse drug effects.

Using IV clamps

With a roller clamp, you can increase or decrease the flow through the IV line by turning a wheel.

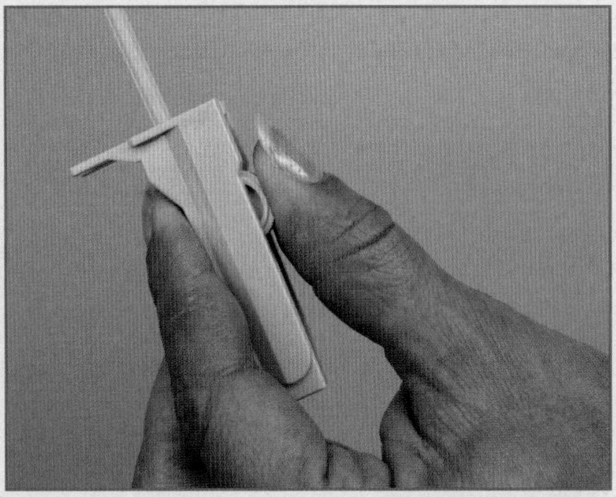

With a slide clamp, you can open or close the line by moving the clamp horizontally. However, you can't make fine adjustments to the flow rate.

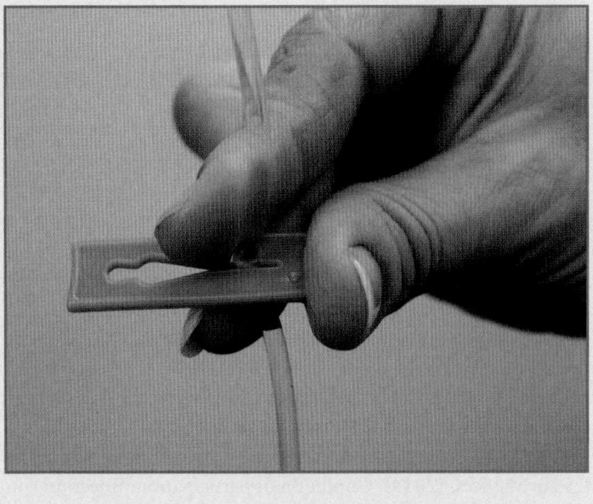

Documentation

Record the original flow rate when setting up a peripheral line. If you adjust the rate, record the change, the date and time, and your initials. Document the patient's response to therapy and any patient teaching provided.

References

1 The Joint Commission. (2015). Standard NPSG.07.01.01. *Comprehensive accreditation manual for hospitals: The official handbook.* Oakbrook Terrace, IL: The Joint Commission. (Level VII)

2 Centers for Disease Control and Prevention. (2002). Guideline for hand hygiene in health-care settings: Recommendations of the Healthcare Infection Control Practices Advisory Committee and the HICPAC/SHEA/APIC/IDSA Hand Hygiene Task Force. *MMWR Recommendations and Reports, 51*(RR-16), 1–45. Accessed March 2015 via the Web at http://www.cdc.gov/mmwr/pdf/rr/rr5116.pdf (Level II)

3 World Health Organization. (2009). "WHO guidelines on hand hygiene in health care: First global patient safety challenge, clean care is safer care"

Calculating infusion rates

When calculating the infusion rate of IV solutions, remember that the number of drops required to deliver 1 mL varies with the type and manufacturer of the administration set used. The first illustration shows a standard (macrodrip) set, which delivers from 10 to 20 drops/mL. The second illustration shows a pediatric (microdrip) set, which delivers about 60 drops/mL. The third illustration shows a blood transfusion set, which delivers about 10 drops/mL.

To calculate the infusion rate, you must know the calibration of the drip rate for each manufacturer's product. Use this formula to calculate specific drip rates:

$$\frac{\text{volume of infusion (in mL)}}{\text{time of infusion (in minutes)}} \times \text{drip factor (in drops/mL)} = \text{drops/minute}$$

Macrodrip set

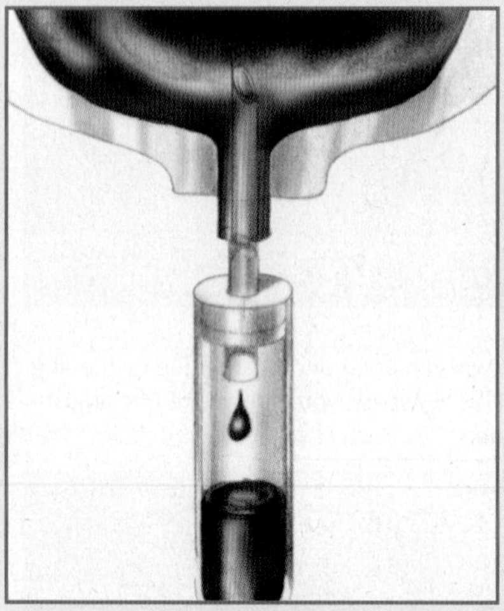

Microdrip set

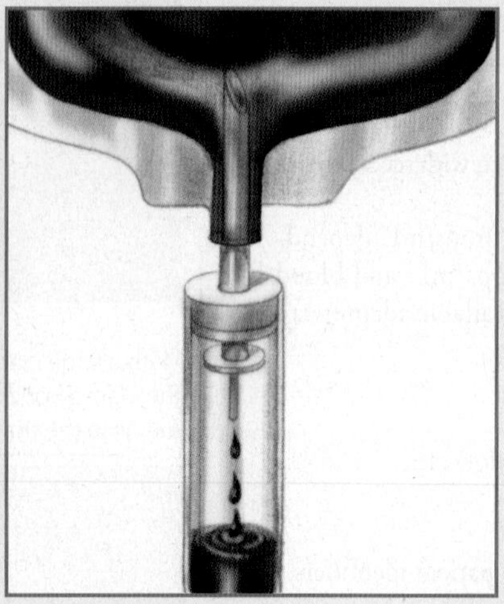

Blood transfusion set

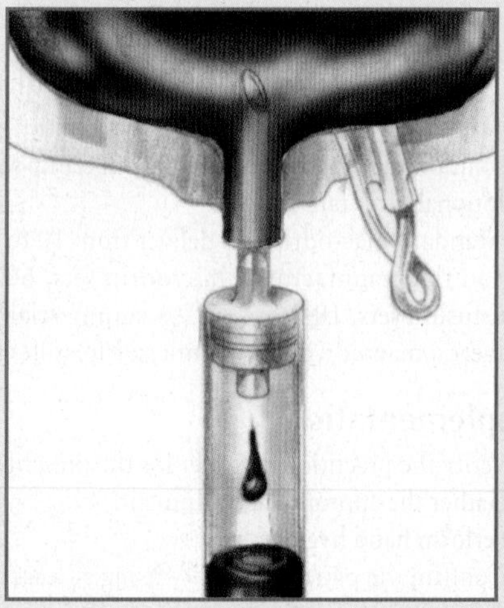

[Online]. Accessed March 2015 via the Web at http://whqlibdoc.who.int/publications/2009/9789241597906_eng.pdf (Level IV)

4 Standard 19. Hand hygiene. Infusion nursing standards of practice. (2011). *Journal of Infusion Nursing, 34,* S26–S27. (Level VII)

5 Centers for Disease Control and Prevention. (2011). "Guidelines for the prevention of intravascular catheter–related infections" [Online]. Accessed March 2015 via the Web at http://www.cdc.gov/hicpac/pdf/guidelines/bsi-guidelines-2011.pdf (Level I)

6 Centers for Medicare & Medicaid Services, Department of Health and Human Services. (2014). Condition of participation: Infection control. 42 C.F.R. § 482.42.

7 American Osteopathic Association. (2014). Standard 07.01.21. *Healthcare Facilities Accreditation Program: Accreditation requirements for acute care hospitals.* Chicago, IL: American Osteopathic Association. (Level VII)

8 The Joint Commission. (2015). Standard NPSG.01.01.01. *Comprehensive accreditation manual for hospitals: The official handbook.* Oakbrook Terrace, IL: The Joint Commission. (Level VII)

9 Standard 61. Parenteral medication and solution administration. Infusion nursing standards of practice. (2011). *Journal of Infusion Nursing, 34,* S86–S87. (Level VII)

10 U.S. Food and Drug Administration. (n.d.). "Look. Check. Connect. Safe medical device connections save lives" [Online]. Accessed March 2015 via the Web at http://www.fda.gov/downloads/MedicalDevices/Safety/AlertsandNotices/UCM134873.pdf

11 The Joint Commission. (2015). Standard RC.01.03.01. *Comprehensive accreditation manual for hospitals: The official handbook.* Oakbrook Terrace, IL: The Joint Commission. (Level VII)

12 Standard 14. Documentation. Infusion nursing standards of practice. (2011). *Journal of Infusion Nursing, 34,* S20–S21. (Level VII)

13 Centers for Medicare & Medicaid Services, Department of Health and Human Services. (2014). Condition of participation: Medical record services. 42 C.F.R. § 482.24(b).

14 American Osteopathic Association. (2014). Standard 10.00.03. *Healthcare Facilities Accreditation Program: Accreditation requirements for acute care hospitals.* Chicago, IL: American Osteopathic Association. (Level VII)

15 Standard 29. Flow-control devices. Infusion nursing standards of practice. (2011). *Journal of Infusion Nursing, 34,* S34–S35. (Level VII)

16 Infusion Nurses Society. (2011). *Policies and procedures for infusion nursing* (4th ed.). Boston, MA: Infusion Nurses Society.

IV PUMP USE

Various types of pumps electronically regulate the flow of IV solutions or drugs with great accuracy. Volumetric pumps, used for high-pressure infusion of drugs or for highly accurate delivery of fluids or drugs, have mechanisms to propel the solution at the desired rate under pressure. (Pressure is brought to bear only when gravity flow rates are insufficient to maintain preset infusion rates.) The peristaltic pump applies pressure to the IV tubing to force the solution through it. (Not all peristaltic pumps are volumetric; some count drops.) The piston-cylinder pump pushes the solution through special disposable cassettes. Most of these pumps operate at high pressures (up to 45 psi), delivering from 1 to 999 mL/hour with about 98% accuracy; some pumps operate at 10 to 25 psi. The portable syringe pump delivers very small amounts of fluid over a long period of time. It's used for administering fluids to infants and for delivering intra-arterial drugs.

Other specialized devices include bar code automated programming devices, smart pumps, the controlled-release infusion system, the secondary syringe converter, and patient-controlled analgesia. (See *Understanding smart pumps.*)

Pumps also have various detectors and alarms that automatically signal or respond to the completion of an infusion, air in the line, low battery power, and occlusion or inability to deliver at the set rate.

Understanding smart pumps

Conventional, general-purpose infusion pumps allow nurses to program an hourly infusion rate and volume. A smart pump has software that allows the pump to be programmed with a facility's guidelines for specific drugs and patients, making it a customized drug library. These pumps can help you intercept and correct potentially serious infusion mistakes before they happen.

Before smart pumps are used at the bedside, a facility programs the pumps with its own specific information. These profiles specify the infusion requirements for different types of patients, such as adults and children, and care areas, such as pediatric, maternal, oncology, intensive care, and postanesthesia care units. Each profile includes a drug library that contains facility-defined drug infusion parameters, such as acceptable concentrations, infusion rates, dosing units, and maximum and minimum loading and maintenance dose bolus limits. The maximum rate and pressure at which the infusion will run can also be programmed into the software. A team that typically consist of pharmacists, practitioners, and nurses within each facility sets up and manages these profiles based on the facility's own best-practice guidelines.

Smart pumps vary by manufacturer, with some pumps even incorporating bar code technology on each IV medication bag. The bar code automatically programs the pump according to a current drug order.

Programming the pump

When you turn on a typical smart pump, it asks you to designate the specific patient care area you're going to use it in. Then it automatically configures itself to provide you with the infusion parameters for that area. Because a pump may be used in different types of patient care units and departments throughout the facility, this feature adds an extra layer of safety.

You then program the pump by choosing the intended drug and concentration from the smart pump's list and entering the ordered dose and infusion rate. The pump checks this information against the drug library. If the parameters you've programmed match those in the pump's drug library for that patient care area, the pump allows the infusion to begin. However, if what you've programmed is outside of the specified limits, the pump alerts you with a visual and audible alarm and lets you know which parameter lies outside of the recommended range.

Depending on the pump's settings, it will sound a soft or hard alarm. If your facility permits it, you can override a soft alarm to allow the infusion to begin at the current settings. However, a hard alarm requires you to reprogram the pump with settings that lie within your facility's specified limits before allowing the infusion to run.

A smart pump also logs and tracks all alerts, recording the time, date, drug, concentration, and infusion rate, as well as your action—including whether you overrode the alert or reprogrammed the pump with different settings. This provides your facility with data it can use to shape current practice guidelines and identify process improvements.

Guidelines for safe administration

Health care facilities provide safer, more effective care when they follow these guidelines from the Institute for Healthcare Improvement before deploying smart pumps:

- Standardize concentrations within the health care facility; asking a health care worker to choose from several concentrations increases the risk of selection error.
- Standardize dosing units for a given drug; for instance, always use either mcg/minute or mcg/kg/minute for nitroglycerin, but not both.
- Standardize drug nomenclature; for example, agree to use the abbreviation KCl for potassium chloride consistently rather than allowing a variety of terms, such as K, pot chloride, or potassium chloride (spelled out).
- Make sure that all concentrations, dose units, and nomenclature used in the smart pump are consistent with those used in the medication administration record, pharmacy computer system, and electronic medical record.
- Meet with all relevant clinicians to agree on the proper upper and lower hard and soft dose limits.
- Monitor the frequency and type of alert overrides to determine if alert settings have been properly configured or if they need adjustment.
- Make sure the pump's smart feature is used in all parts of the facility; for instance, if the operating room sets up the pump volumetrically without the smart feature, but the intensive care unit uses the smart feature, an error may occur if the pump isn't reprogrammed properly.
- Make sure to establish upper and lower dose limits for bolus doses, when applicable.
- Have a biomedical technician identify previously unidentified risks for failure when the pumps are deployed.
- Establish procedures that allow staff members, when necessary, to administer drugs in nonstandard concentrations as well as to administer drugs that aren't in the drug library.
- Deploy one type of smart pump throughout the health care facility; doing so helps prevent errors that may occur when different types of pumps are used on different units.[1]

When administering IV fluids to older adults, keep in mind that these patients commonly have compromised cardiac, hepatic, or renal systems, which place them at risk during IV fluid administration. If infusions are too rapid or the volume is too great, the patient may develop heart failure, shock, or cardiac arrest. An older adult may be unable to articulate symptoms because of underlying conditions, such as stroke, intubation, tracheostomy, dementia, and delirium. Monitor the patient closely during all IV infusions. Rapid administration of a bolus medication or infusion may cause speed shock; symptoms associated with speed shock, such as dizziness and headache, occur rapidly, making it difficult for the patient to articulate such symptoms. Early symptoms of speed shock may progress to chest tightness, hypotension, irregular pulse, and anaphylactic shock. Carefully control any parenteral medication or solution and observe older adult patients closely.[2]

Equipment

IV pump ▪ IV pole ▪ prescribed IV solution ▪ sterile administration set ▪ antiseptic pads (alcohol, tincture of iodine, or chlorhexidine-based) ▪ prefilled syringe containing preservative-free normal saline ▪ gloves ▪ Optional: needleless connector.

Preparation of equipment

Gather the appropriate equipment. Attach the IV pump to the IV pole (as shown on next page, top left.)

Implementation

- Avoid distractions and interruptions when preparing and administering medications *to prevent medication errors*.[3,4,5]
- Verify the practitioner's order; make sure it contains the type and volume of fluid, medication and dosage (if a medicated infusion is prescribed), route of administration, frequency, and duration.[2,3,6,7,8]

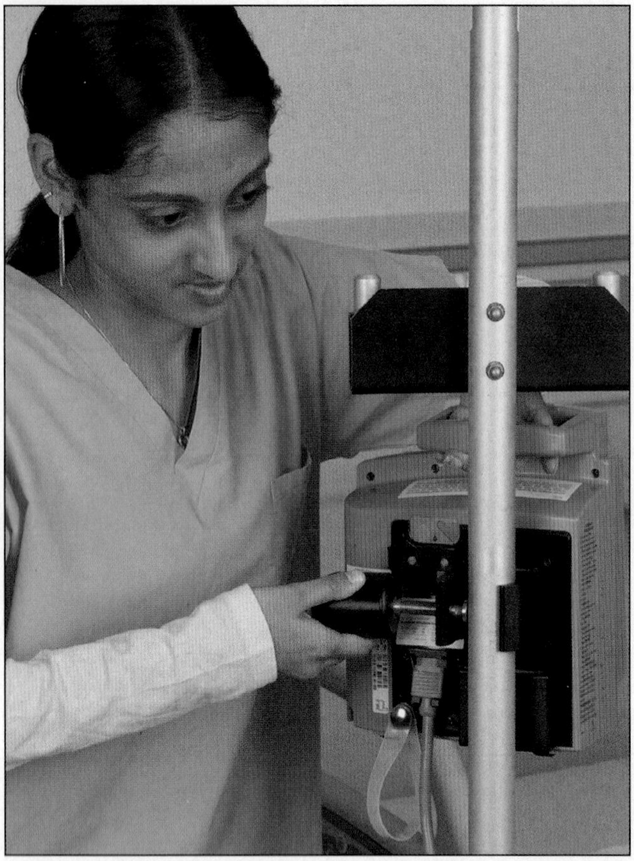

■ Check the patient's medical record for an allergy or contraindication to the prescribed medication. If an allergy or contraindication exists, don't administer the medication; instead, notify the practitioner.[7,8]
■ Inspect the IV solution for cracks, leaks, and contamination. Also verify that it has been labeled properly, contains the right solution in the right concentration, and hasn't expired.[2,3,6,7,8]
■ Discuss any unresolved concerns about the medication with the patient's practitioner.[7]
■ Verify that you're administering the medication at the proper time, in the prescribed dose, and by the correct route *to reduce the risk of medication errors.*[7,8]
■ Perform hand hygiene.[9,10,11,12,13,14]
■ Confirm the patient's identity using at least two patient identifiers.[15]
■ Explain the procedure to the patient *to ease his anxiety and ensure his cooperation.* If the patient is receiving the medication for the first time, teach him about potential adverse reactions and discuss any other concerns related to the medication.[7]
■ Access the port on the IV container and thoroughly disinfect it with an antiseptic pad using friction, if appropriate, and allow it to dry. (See the "IV therapy preparation" procedure, page 468.)
■ Insert the administration set spike, and fill the drip chamber to the manufacturer's mark (approximately one-third to one-half full) *to prevent air bubbles from entering the tubing.*[2,6]
■ Slowly open the clamp to prime the administration set tubing while holding the distal end of the administration set upright, permitting the filter to hang upside down. Prime the entire length of the administration set tubing, and then close the clamp.[2,6] Place the administration set tubing into the infusion pump following the manufacturer's instructions.
■ Alternatively, insert the administration set tubing into the infusion pump and use the pump's priming function to prime the administration set tubing.
■ If your facility uses a bar code automated pump, scan your identification badge, the patient's identification bracelet, and the bar code on the medication bag, or follow your facility's bar code system procedure.
■ Position the pump on the same side of the bed as the vascular access device or the anticipated insertion site *to avoid misconnections.*[16]
■ Plug in the electronic infusion pump.
■ Perform hand hygiene.[9,10,11,12,13,14]
■ Put on gloves.[10,17,18,19]
■ Assess the insertion site.[3]
■ Thoroughly disinfect the needleless connector with an antiseptic pad using friction, and allow it to dry.[2,6,20]
■ Maintaining sterility of the syringe tip, attach a syringe containing preservative-free normal saline solution to the needleless connector, and aspirate for a positive blood return from the vascular access device *to confirm patency.*[2,3,6]
■ Slowly flush the device with preservative-free normal saline solution *to assess catheter function.*[21]
■ If necessary, insert a new IV catheter or notify the practitioner if the patient has a central venous access catheter and you see signs of complications at the insertion site or catheter function is compromised. (See the "IV catheter insertion and removal" procedure, page 446.)[3]
■ Attach the IV tubing to the catheter hub using sterile technique.[2,6] If you're infusing an IV solution or medication via a secondary line, attach the secondary IV tubing to the injection port closest to the insertion site of the primary line with a needleless adapter. (See the "IV secondary line drug infusion" procedure, page 466.)
■ Trace the tubing from the patient to its point of origin *to make sure that you're connecting the tubing to the correct port before beginning the infusion.*[3,16]
■ Following specific pump operation, turn the pump on and enter the desired infusion rate and volume.
■ Confirm that the infusion pump's display screen is displaying the right information, open the tubing clamp, and then push the RUN or START button (as shown below).

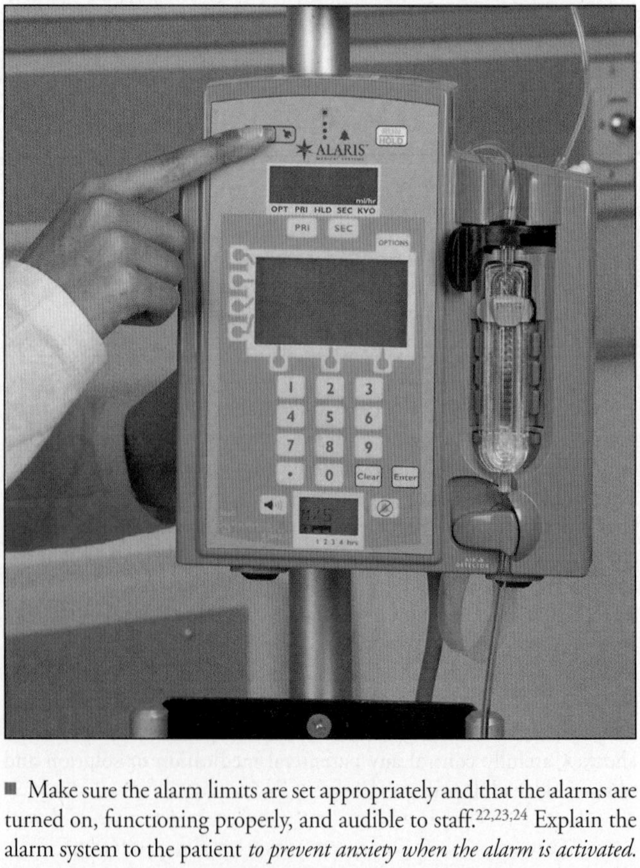

■ Make sure the alarm limits are set appropriately and that the alarms are turned on, functioning properly, and audible to staff.[22,23,24] Explain the alarm system to the patient *to prevent anxiety when the alarm is activated.*

- Recheck the patency of the IV catheter and watch for infiltration.[3,25]
- Check that all connections are secure *to prevent leaking, bleeding, contamination, and disconnections.*[16]
- Remove and discard your gloves.[17,18]
- Perform hand hygiene.[9,10,11,12,13,14]
- Document the procedure.[26,27,28,29]

Special considerations

- Monitor the pump and the patient frequently *to ensure the device's correct operation and flow rate and to detect complications, such as infiltration, infection and air embolism.*[25]
- Be aware that, if electrical power fails, the pumps automatically switch to battery power.
- Check the manufacturer's recommendations before administering opaque fluids, such as blood, *because some pumps fail to detect opaque fluids and others may cause hemolysis of infused blood.*
- Change the tubing and cassette no more frequently than every 96 hours and immediately upon suspected contamination or when the integrity of the product or system has been compromised.[10,30] Change a secondary infusion set that's detached from the primary administration set every 24 hours; change a secondary set that administers fluids other than lipids, blood, or blood products and remains attached to the primary administration set every 96 hours.[30]
- If you suspect a catheter-associated infection or see it documented in the patient's medical record, follow the practitioner's order regarding catheter changes.
- Remove IV solutions from the refrigerator 1 hour before infusing them *to help release small gas bubbles from the solution. Small bubbles in the solution can join to form larger bubbles, which can activate the pump's air-in-line alarm.* Aspirate large air bubbles from the tubing before they reach the cassette.
- If the alarm sounds, mute the alarm and check the pump for a problem message, such as INFUSION COMPLETE, OCCLUSION, AIR IN LINE, or LOW BATTERY. Address the problem, assess the IV and infusion components, restart the infusion, and reset the alarm.
- The Joint Commission issued a sentinel event alert concerning medical device alarm safety *because alarm-related events have been associated with permanent loss of function or death.* Among the major contributing factors were improper alarm settings, alarm settings inappropriately turned off, and alarm signals not audible to staff. Make sure alarm limits are set appropriately, and that alarms are turned on, functioning properly, and audible to staff. Follow facility guidelines for preventing alarm fatigue.[24]

Patient teaching

Make sure the patient and his family understand the purpose of using the pump. If necessary, demonstrate how the device works. Explain the signs and symptoms of IV infiltration to the patient; instruct him to call for assistance if they occur. Discuss potential adverse effects of IV medication administration, if appropriate, and what signs and symptoms to report. If the patient is ambulatory, discuss his ability to unplug the pump and wheel the IV pole with him. Discourage the patient from touching the controls on the infusion pump, and instruct him to call for assistance if the pump sounds an alarm.

Complications

Complications associated with IV solution and medication infusion via IV pumps can include circulatory overload and adverse effects from specific medication administration. General complications associated with IV infusion include infiltration, extravasation, phlebitis, infection, and air embolism. Keep in mind that infiltration can develop rapidly with infusion by a volumetric pump because the increased subcutaneous pressure won't slow the infusion rate until significant edema occurs. Never rely on infusion pump alarms to detect the presence of infiltration.

Documentation

In addition to routine documentation of the IV infusion, record the use of a pump. Also document any patient teaching provided and the patient's understanding of the teaching.

References

1 Institute for Safe Medication Practices. (2009). "Proceedings from the ISMP summit on the use of smart infusion pumps: Guidelines for safe implementation and use" [Online]. Accessed March 2015 via the Web at http://www.ismp.org/tools/guidelines/smartpumps/comments/printer-Version.pdf

2 Infusion Nurses Society. (2013). *Policies and procedures for infusion nursing of the older adult* (2nd ed.). Boston, MA: Infusion Nurses Society.

3 Standard 61. Parenteral medication and solution administration. Infusion nursing standards of practice. (2011). *Journal of Infusion Nursing, 34,* S86–S87. (Level VII)

4 Institute for Safe Medication Practices. (2013). Side tracks on the safety express: Interruptions lead to errors and unfinished . . . Wait, what was I doing? *Nurse Advise-ERR,* 11(2), 1–4. Accessed March 2015 via the Web at https://www.ismp.org/Newsletters/acutecare/showarticle.aspx?id=37

5 Westbrook, J., et al. (2010). Association of interruptions with an increased risk and severity of medication administration errors. *Archives of Internal Medicine, 170,* 683–690.

6 Infusion Nurses Society. (2011). *Policies and procedures for infusion nursing* (4th ed.). Boston, MA: Infusion Nurses Society.

7 The Joint Commission. (2015). Standard MM.06.01.01. *Comprehensive accreditation manual for hospitals: The official handbook.* Oakbrook Terrace, IL: The Joint Commission. (Level VII)

8 American Osteopathic Association. (2014). Standard 25.01.18. *Healthcare Facilities Accreditation Program: Accreditation requirements for acute care hospitals.* Chicago, IL: American Osteopathic Association.

9 Centers for Disease Control and Prevention. (2002). Guideline for hand hygiene in health-care settings: Recommendations of the Healthcare Infection Control Practices Advisory Committee and the HICPAC/SHEA/APIC/IDSA Hand Hygiene Task Force. *MMWR Recommendations and Reports, 51*(RR-16), 1–45. Accessed March 2015 via the Web at http://www.cdc.gov/mmwr/pdf/rr/rr5116.pdf (Level II)

10 Centers for Disease Control and Prevention. (2011). "Guidelines for the prevention of intravascular catheter-related infections" [Online]. Accessed March 2015 via the Web at http://www.cdc.gov/hicpac/pdf/guidelines/bsi-guidelines-2011.pdf (Level I)

11 Standard 19. Hand hygiene. Infusion nursing standards of practice. (2011). *Journal of Infusion Nursing, 34,* S26–S27. (Level VII)

12 The Joint Commission. (2015). Standard NPSG.07.01.01. *Comprehensive accreditation manual for hospitals: The official handbook.* Oakbrook Terrace, IL: The Joint Commission. (Level VII)

13 World Health Organization. (2009). "WHO guidelines on hand hygiene in health care: First global patient safety challenge, clean care is safer care" [Online]. Accessed March 2015 via the Web at http://whqlibdoc.who.int/publications/2009/9789241597906_eng.pdf (Level IV)

14 American Osteopathic Association. (2014). Standard 07.01.21. *Healthcare Facilities Accreditation Program: Accreditation requirements for acute care hospitals.* Chicago, IL: American Osteopathic Association. (Level VII)

15 The Joint Commission. (2015). Standard NPSG.01.01.01. *Comprehensive accreditation manual for hospitals: The official handbook.* Oakbrook Terrace, IL: The Joint Commission. (Level VII)

16 U.S. Food and Drug Administration. (n.d.). "Look. Check. Connect. Safe medical device connections save lives" [Online]. Accessed March 2015 via the Web at http://www.fda.gov/downloads/MedicalDevices/Safety/AlertsandNotices/UCM134873.pdf

17 Siegel, J. D., et al. (2007). "2007 guideline for isolation precautions: Preventing transmission of infectious agents in healthcare settings" [Online]. Accessed March 2015 via the Web at http://www.cdc.gov/hicpac/pdf/isolation/Isolation2007.pdf (Level II)

18 Occupational Safety and Health Administration. (n.d.). "Bloodborne pathogens, standard number 1910.1030" [Online]. Accessed March

2015 via the Web at http://www.osha.gov/pls/oshaweb/owadisp.show_document?p_table=STANDARDS&p_id=10051 (Level VII)

19 American Osteopathic Association. (2014). Standard 07.01.10. *Healthcare Facilities Accreditation Program: Accreditation requirements for acute care hospitals.* Chicago, IL: American Osteopathic Association. (Level VII)

20 Standard 27. Needleless connectors. Infusion nursing standards of practice. (2011). *Journal of Infusion Nursing, 34,* S32–S33. (Level VII)

21 Standard 45. Flushing and locking. Infusion nursing standards of practice. (2011). *Journal of Infusion Nursing, 34,* S59–S63. (Level VII)

22 The Joint Commission. (2015). Standard NPSG.06.01.01. *Comprehensive accreditation manual for hospitals: The official handbook.* Oakbrook Terrace, IL: The Joint Commission. (Level VII)

23 Graham, K. C., & Cvach, M. (2010). Monitor alarm fatigue: Standardizing use of physiological monitors and decreasing nuisance alarms. *American Journal of Critical Care, 19,* 28–37.

24 The Joint Commission. (2013). "Sentinel event alert: Medical device alarm safety in hospitals" [Online]. Accessed March 2015 via the Web at http://www.jointcommission.org/assets/1/18/SEA_50_alarms_4_5_13_FINAL1.PDF (Level VII)

25 Standard 29. Flow-control devices. Infusion nursing standards of practice. (2011). *Journal of Infusion Nursing, 34,* S34–S35. (Level VII)

26 The Joint Commission. (2015). Standard RC.01.03.01. *Comprehensive accreditation manual for hospitals: The official handbook.* Oakbrook Terrace, IL: The Joint Commission. (Level VII)

27 Standard 14. Documentation. Infusion nursing standards of practice. (2011). *Journal of Infusion Nursing, 34,* S20–S21. (Level VII)

28 Centers for Medicare & Medicaid Services, Department of Health and Human Services. (2014). Condition of participation: Medical record services. 42 C.F.R. § 482.24(b).

29 American Osteopathic Association. (2014). Standard 10.00.03. *Healthcare Facilities Accreditation Program: Accreditation requirements for acute care hospitals.* Chicago, IL: American Osteopathic Association. (Level VII)

30 Standard 43. Administration set change. Infusion nursing standards of practice. (2011). *Journal of Infusion Nursing, 34,* S55–S57. (Level VII)

IV SECONDARY LINE DRUG INFUSION

A secondary IV line is a complete IV set, container, tubing, and microdrip or macrodrip system connected to the lower Y port (secondary port) of a primary line instead of to the IV catheter. It can be used for continuous or intermittent drug infusion. When used continuously, a secondary IV line permits drug infusion and titration while the primary line maintains a constant total infusion rate.

A secondary IV line used for intermittent infusions is commonly called a *piggyback set.* In this case, the primary line maintains venous access between drug doses. Typically, a piggyback set includes a small IV container, short tubing, and a macrodrip system. This set connects to the primary line's upper Y port, also called a *piggyback port.* Antibiotics are most commonly administered by intermittent (piggyback) infusion. You should position the primary IV solution below the secondary solution to facilitate infusion. (The manufacturer provides an extension hook for that purpose.)

You should change a secondary administration set used to continuously administer fluids other than lipids, blood, or blood products at least every 7 days but no more frequently than every 96 hours, unless it becomes contaminated or otherwise compromised.[1,2] If the secondary administration set is detached from the primary administration set, it's considered a primary intermittent administration set and you should change it every 24 hours.[1]

Equipment

Patient's medical record ▪ patient's medication administration record ▪ gloves ▪ prescribed IV medication ▪ administration set with secondary injection port (luer-lock design recommended)[1] ▪ needleless adapter ▪ antiseptic pads (alcohol, tincture of iodine, or chlorhexidine-based) ▪ 1″ (2.5-cm) 10-mL prefilled syringe containing preservative-free normal saline solution ▪ time tape ▪ labels ▪ extension hook ▪ Optional: 10-mL prefilled syringe containing dextrose 5% in water if medication is incompatible with normal saline solution.

For intermittent infusion, the primary line typically has a piggyback port with a backcheck valve that stops the flow from the primary line during drug infusion and returns to the primary flow after infusion. You can also use a volume-control set with an intermittent infusion line.

Preparation of equipment

Gather the appropriate medication and equipment. Inspect the IV container for cracks, leaks, and contamination. Check drug compatibility with the primary solution. Confirm that the primary administration set contains a secondary port.

If necessary, add the drug to the secondary IV solution. (Whenever possible, administer pharmacy-prepared or commercially available products.) To do so, remove any seals from the secondary container, disinfect the main port with an antiseptic pad, and allow it to dry. Inject the prescribed medication using safe medication administration practices, and gently agitate the solution *to mix the medication thoroughly.* (See the "Safe medication administration practices, general" procedure, page 678.) Properly label the mixed IV solution as required by your facility. In a perioperative or procedural setting, the label should contain the medication name, strength, and quantity; diluent type and volume; and the expiration date.[3]

Insert the administration set spike and attach the needleless system. Open the flow clamp, prime the line, and then close the flow clamp. Initiate immediate-use medications within 1 hour of preparation or discard them.[4]

Implementation

- Avoid distractions and interruptions when preparing and administering medications *to prevent medication errors.*[5,6]
- Verify the practitioner's order.[7,8,9] Make sure it contains the type of fluid and volume, medication and dosage, route of administration, and frequency and duration of administration.[10,11]
- Compare the medication label with the order in the patient's medical record.[8,9,12]
- Check the patient's medical record for an allergy or a contraindication to the prescribed medication. If an allergy or contraindication exists, don't administer the medication; instead, notify the practitioner.[6,9,12]
- Check the expiration date on the medication. If the medication is expired, return it to the pharmacy, obtain new medication, and notify the practitioner.[6,9,12]
- Visually inspect the solution for particles, discoloration, or other loss of integrity; don't administer the medication if its integrity is compromised.[6,9,12]
- Discuss any unresolved concerns about the medication with the patient's practitioner.[6,9]
- Verify that you're administering the medication at the proper time, in the prescribed dose, and by the correct route *to reduce the risk of medication errors.*[6,9,12]
- Perform hand hygiene.[2,13,14,15,16,17]
- Confirm the patient's identity using at least two patient identifiers.[18]
- Explain the procedure to the patient. If the patient is receiving the medication for the first time, teach him about the potential adverse reactions and discuss any other concerns related to the medication.[9]
- If your facility uses a bar code scanning system, scan your identification badge, the patient's identification bracelet, and the medication's bar code.
- Put on gloves.[2,19,20,21]

■ If the prescribed drug is incompatible with the primary IV solution, replace the primary solution with a fluid that's compatible with both solutions, as ordered.[22,23]
■ Assess the patient's IV site for pain, redness, or swelling.[10,11,24]
■ Thoroughly disinfect the needleless connector with an antiseptic pad using friction, and allow it to dry.[10,11,25]
■ Maintaining sterility of the syringe tip, attach a syringe containing preservative-free normal saline solution to the needleless connector and aspirate for a positive blood return from the vascular access device *to confirm patency.*[10,11,24]
■ Slowly flush the device with preservative-free normal saline solution *to assess catheter function.*[10,11,22]
■ If necessary, insert a new IV catheter or notify the practitioner if the patient has a central venous access catheter and you see signs of complications at the insertion site or catheter function is compromised. (See the "IV catheter insertion and removal" procedure, page 446.)[24]
NURSING ALERT ***Don't administer continuous high-alert medications as a secondary infusion. Don't piggyback a secondary infusion into a primary infusion containing a high-alert drug* to avoid adverse drug events caused by infusion at indeterminate rates or pump programming errors.**[6,26,27]
■ Hang the secondary set's container.
■ With an antiseptic pad using friction, thoroughly disinfect the needleless connector of the primary line that's closest to the vascular access catheter, and allow it to dry.[10,11,25]
■ Trace the tubing from the patient to its point of origin *to make sure that you're connecting it to the proper port.*[24,26,28]
■ Insert the needleless adapter from the secondary line into the needleless connector, verify a proper connection, and secure it to the primary line, as needed.[28]
■ To run the secondary set's container by itself, lower the primary set's container with an extension hook. To run both containers simultaneously, place them at the same height. (See *Assembling a piggyback set.*)
■ Open the clamp and adjust the drip rate.
■ For continuous infusion, set the secondary solution to the desired drip rate; then adjust the primary solution *to achieve the desired total infusion rate.* Begin the secondary infusion
■ For intermittent infusion, perform a visual inspection of the drip chambers *to verify that the secondary infusion is active and that the primary infusion is not active.*[26] Adjust the primary drip rate, as required, on completion of the secondary solution. If you're reusing the secondary solution tubing, close the clamp on the tubing, remove the needleless adapter, and replace it with a new, sterile one.[1] Don't attach the exposed end of the administration set to a port on the same set.[1] If you won't reuse the tubing, discard it appropriately with the IV container.
■ Discard used supplies in appropriate receptacles.[19,20,29]
■ Remove and discard your gloves.[19,20,29]
■ Perform hand hygiene.[2,13,14,15,16,17]
■ Document the procedure.[30,31,32,33]

Special considerations

■ Use a pump for medication infusion *to maintain a constant infusion rate.* (See the "IV pump use" procedure, page 462.)
■ Unless you're piggybacking lipids, don't piggyback a secondary IV line to a total parenteral nutrition line *because of the risk of contamination.*

Patient teaching

Teach the patient about the medication and its potential adverse effects.

Complications

The patient may experience an adverse reaction to the infused drug. In addition, repeated punctures of the secondary injection port can damage the seal, possibly allowing leakage or contamination.

EQUIPMENT

Assembling a piggyback set

A piggyback set is useful for intermittent drug infusion. For the set to work properly, you must position the secondary set's container higher than the primary set's container.

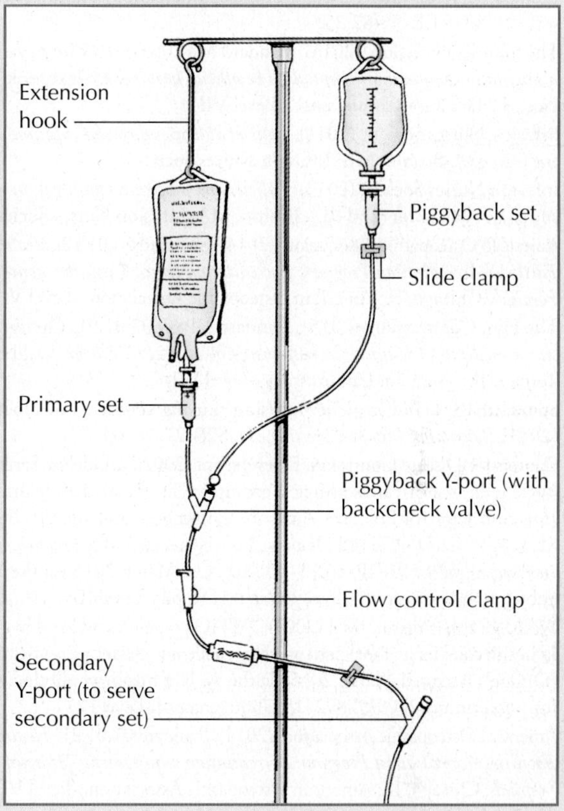

General complications of infusion therapy include phlebitis, infiltration, extravasation, air embolism, infection, and circulatory overload.

Documentation

Record the amount and type of drug administered and the amount of IV solution on the intake and output and medication records. Also note the date, duration and rate of infusion, and the patient's response, where applicable.

References

1 Standard 43. Administration set change. Infusion nursing standards of practice. (2011). *Journal of Infusion Nursing, 34,* S55–S56. (Level VII)
2 Centers for Disease Control and Prevention. (2011). "Guidelines for the prevention of intravascular catheter-related infections" [Online]. Accessed March 2015 via the Web at http://www.cdc.gov/hicpac/pdf/guidelines/bsi-guidelines-2011.pdf (Level I)
3 The Joint Commission. (2015). Standard NPSG.03.04.01. *Comprehensive accreditation manual for hospitals: The official handbook.* Oakbrook Terrace, IL: The Joint Commission. (Level VII)
4 Standard 20. Compounding of parenteral solutions and medications. Infusion nursing standards of practice. (2011). *Journal of Infusion Nursing, 34,* S27. (Level VII)
5 Westbrook, J., et al. (2010). Association of interruptions with an increased risk and severity of medication administration errors. *Archives of Internal Medicine, 170,* 683–690. (Level IV)

6 Centers for Medicare & Medicaid Services, Department of Health and Human Services. (2014). Condition of participation: Nursing services. 42 C.F.R. § 482.23(c).
7 The Joint Commission. (2015). Standard MM.04.01.01. *Comprehensive accreditation manual for hospitals: The official handbook.* Oakbrook Terrace, IL: The Joint Commission. (Level VII)
8 Centers for Medicare & Medicaid Services, Department of Health and Human Services. (2014). Condition of participation: Pharmaceutical services. 42 C.F.R. § 482.25.
9 The Joint Commission. (2015). Standard MM.06.01.01. *Comprehensive accreditation manual for hospitals: The official handbook.* Oakbrook Terrace, IL: The Joint Commission. (Level VII)
10 Infusion Nurses Society. (2011). *Policies and procedures for infusion nursing* (4th ed.). Boston, MA: Infusion Nurses Society.
11 Infusion Nurses Society. (2013). *Policies and procedures for infusion nursing of the older adult* (2nd ed.). Boston, MA: Infusion Nurses Society.
12 American Osteopathic Association. (2014). Standard 25.01.18. *Healthcare Facilities Accreditation Program: Accreditation requirements for acute care hospitals.* Chicago, IL: American Osteopathic Association. (Level VII)
13 The Joint Commission. (2015). Standard NPSG.07.01.01. *Comprehensive accreditation manual for hospitals: The official handbook.* Oakbrook Terrace, IL: The Joint Commission. (Level VII)
14 Standard 19. Hand hygiene. Infusion nursing standards of practice. (2011). *Journal of Infusion Nursing, 34,* S26–27. (Level VII)
15 Centers for Disease Control and Prevention. (2002). Guideline for hand hygiene in health-care settings: Recommendations of the Healthcare Infection Control Practices Advisory Committee and the HICPAC/SHEA/APIC/IDSA Hand Hygiene Task Force. *MMWR Recommendations and Reports, 51*(RR-16), 1–45. Accessed March 2015 via the Web at http://www.cdc.gov/mmwr/pdf/rr/rr5116.pdf (Level II)
16 World Health Organization. (2009). "WHO guidelines on hand hygiene in health care: First global patient safety challenge, clean care is safer care" [Online]. Accessed March 2015 via the Web at http://whqlibdoc.who.int/publications/2009/9789241597906_eng.pdf (Level IV)
17 American Osteopathic Association. (2014). Standard 07.01.21. *Healthcare Facilities Accreditation Program: Accreditation requirements for acute care hospitals.* Chicago, IL: American Osteopathic Association. (Level VII)
18 The Joint Commission. (2015). Standard NPSG.01.01.01. *Comprehensive accreditation manual for hospitals: The official handbook.* Oakbrook Terrace, IL: The Joint Commission. (Level VII)
19 Occupational Safety and Health Administration. (n.d.). "Bloodborne pathogens, standard number 1910.1030" [Online]. Accessed March 2015 via the Web at http://www.osha.gov/pls/oshaweb/owadisp.show_document?p_table=STANDARDS&p_id=10051 (Level VII)
20 Siegel, J. D., et al. (2007). "2007 guideline for isolation precautions: Preventing transmission of infectious agents in healthcare settings" [Online]. Accessed March 2015 via the Web at http://www.cdc.gov/hicpac/pdf/isolation/Isolation2007.pdf (Level II)
21 American Osteopathic Association. (2014). Standard 07.01.10. *Healthcare Facilities Accreditation Program: Accreditation requirements for acute care hospitals.* Chicago, IL: American Osteopathic Association.
22 Standard 45. Flushing and locking. Infusion nursing standards of practice. (2011). *Journal of Infusion Nursing, 34,* S59–S63. (Level VII)
23 Loubnan, V., & Nasser, S. C. (2010). A guide on intravenous drug compatibilities based on their pH. *Pharmacie Globale, 5*(1), 1–9.
24 Standard 61. Parenteral medication and solution administration. Infusion nursing standards of practice. (2011). *Journal of Infusion Nursing, 34,* S86–S87. (Level VII)
25 Standard 27. Needleless connectors. Infusion nursing standards of practice. (2011). *Journal of Infusion Nursing, 34,* S32–S33. (Level VII)
26 Health Technology Safety Research Team in Collaboration with ISMP Canada. (2012). "Mitigating the risks associated with multiple IV infusions: Recommendations based on a field study of twelve Ontario hospitals" [Online]. Accessed March 2015 via the Web at http://www.aami.org/htsi/infusion/wg/multiple/MultipleIVInfusions_Phase1bSummary_Recommendations%20and%20Rationale_June%202012.pdf (Level VII)
27 The Joint Commission. (2015). Standard MM.01.01.03. *Comprehensive accreditation manual for hospitals: The official handbook.* Oakbrook Terrace, IL: The Joint Commission. (Level VII)
28 U.S. Food and Drug Administration. (n.d.). "Look. Check. Connect. Safe medical device connections save lives" [Online]. Accessed March 2015 via the Web at http://www.fda.gov/downloads/MedicalDevices/Safety/AlertsandNotices/UCM134873.pdf
29 Standard 22. Safe handling and disposal of sharps, hazardous materials, and hazardous waste. Infusion nursing standards of practice. (2011). *Journal of Infusion Nursing, 34,* S28–S29. (Level VII)
30 The Joint Commission. (2015). Standard RC.01.03.01. *Comprehensive accreditation manual for hospitals: The official handbook.* Oakbrook Terrace, IL: The Joint Commission. (Level VII)
31 Standard 14. Documentation. Infusion nursing standards of practice. (2011). *Journal of Infusion Nursing, 34,* S20–S21. (Level VII)
32 Centers for Medicare & Medicaid Services, Department of Health and Human Services. (2014). Condition of participation: Medical record services. 42 C.F.R. § 482.24.
33 American Osteopathic Association. (2014). Standard 10.00.03. *Healthcare Facilities Accreditation Program: Accreditation requirements for acute care hospitals.* Chicago, IL: American Osteopathic Association. (Level VII)

ADDITIONAL REFERENCE

Nettina, S. M. (2014). *Lippincott manual of nursing practice* (10th ed.). Philadelphia, PA: Wolters Kluwer.

IV THERAPY PREPARATION

Selection and preparation of appropriate equipment are essential for accurate delivery of an IV solution. The type of IV administration set used depends on the rate and type of infusion desired and the type of IV solution container used. Two types of drip sets are available: the macrodrip and the microdrip. The macrodrip set can deliver a solution in large quantities at rapid rates because it delivers a larger amount with each drop. The microdrip set, used for pediatric patients and certain adult patients who require small or closely regulated amounts of IV solution, delivers a smaller quantity with each drop.

Although plastic bags are often used to hold IV fluids, there may be times when you'll use a bottle as a container. Glass bottles are usually used to hold medications that are unstable in a plastic bag, such as nitroglycerin. The bottle may be vented or nonvented.

Administration tubing with a secondary injection port permits separate or simultaneous infusion of two solutions; tubing with a piggyback port and a backcheck valve permits intermittent infusion of a secondary solution and, on its completion, a return to infusion of the primary solution. Assembly of IV equipment requires sterile technique to prevent contamination.[1]

Equipment

IV solution bag ▪ IV administration set ▪ IV pole ▪ label ▪ Optional: prescribed medication, antiseptic pads (chlorhexidine-based, alcohol, or tincture of iodine), marker, medication-added label.

Preparation of equipment

Verify the practitioner's order. Perform hand hygiene *to prevent introducing contaminants during preparation.*[2,3,4,5,6] Verify the type, volume, and expiration date of the IV solution. Discard outdated solution.[7,8] Squeeze the bag *to detect leaks.* Examine the IV solution for particles, abnormal discoloration, and cloudiness. If present, discard the solution and notify the pharmacy or dispensing department.[8,9] If ordered, add medication to the solution using sterile technique, and place a completed medication-added label on the bag.[10] However, whenever possible, administer pharmacy-prepared or commercially available products.[11] Remove the administration set from its box, and check for cracks, holes, and missing clamps.[9]

Implementation

Preparing the bag

■ Slide the flow clamp of the administration set tubing down to the drip chamber or injection port, and close the clamp.

■ Remove the protective cap or tear the tab from the tubing insertion port (as shown below).

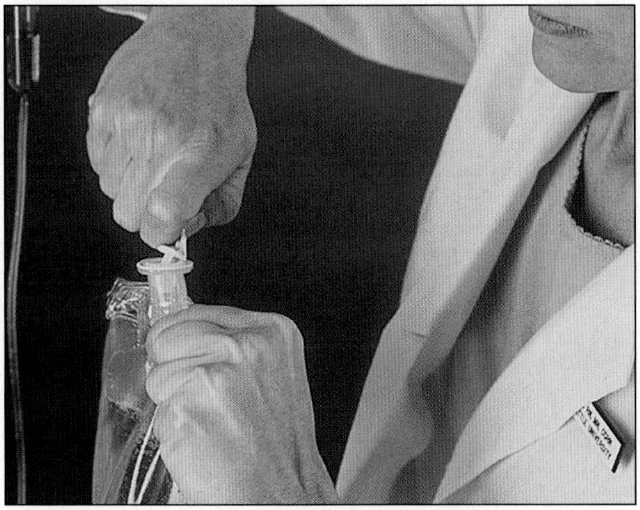

■ Remove the protective cap from the administration set spike.

■ Hold the port firmly with one hand, and insert the spike with your other hand (as shown below). Be careful not to contaminate the IV bag insertion port or the IV tubing spike.

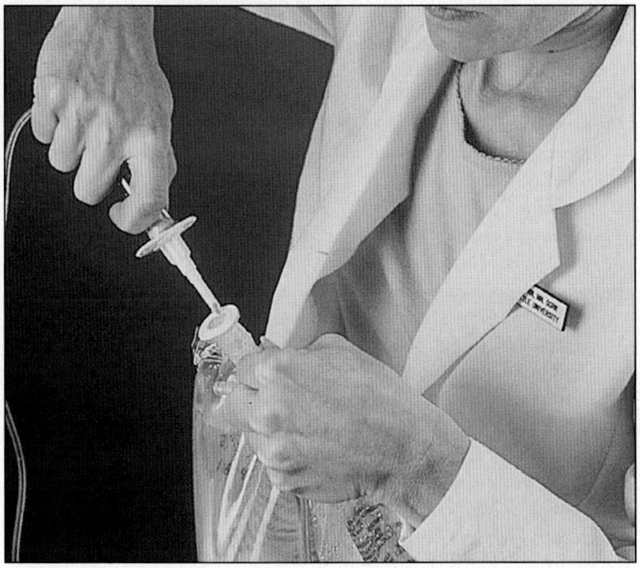

■ Hang the bag on the IV pole, if you haven't already, and squeeze the drip chamber until it's half full (as shown on top right).

■ Label the bag with the patient's name and identification number, date and time, the bag number, ordered rate and duration of infusion, and your initials.

■ Perform hand hygiene.[2,3,4,5,6]

■ Document the procedure.[12,13,14]

Preparing a bottle

■ Close the flow or roller clamp on the administration set tubing

■ For a nonvented bottle, remove the bottle's metal cap and inner disk, if present. For a vented bottle, remove the bottle's metal cap and latex

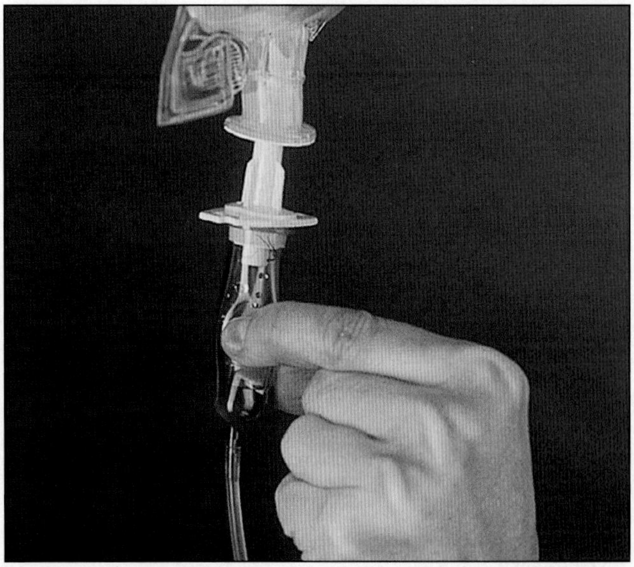

diaphragm *to release the vacuum.* If the vacuum isn't intact, discard the bottle and begin again.

■ Place the bottle on a stable surface and disinfect the rubber stopper with an antiseptic pad using friction and allow it to dry.

■ Remove the protective cap from the administration set spike, and push the spike through the center of the nonvented bottle's rubber stopper. Avoid twisting or angling the spike *to prevent pieces of the stopper from breaking off and falling into the solution.* If using a vented bottle, push the spike through the insertion port next to the air vent tube opening.

■ Invert the nonvented bottle. If its vacuum is intact, you'll hear a hissing sound and see air bubbles rise (this may not occur if you've already added medication). If the vacuum isn't intact, discard the bottle and begin again.

■ Hang the bottle on the IV pole.

■ Squeeze the drip chamber until it's half full.

■ Perform hand hygiene.[2,3,4,5,6]

■ Document the procedure.[12,13,14]

Priming the tubing

■ Hang the solution on the IV pole, if you haven't already, and squeeze the drip chamber until it's half full.

■ Leave the protective cover on the end of the tubing, hold the tubing above waist level, aim the distal end of the tubing over a wastebasket or sink, and slowly open the flow clamp.

■ If an in-line filter is necessary, purge the tubing before attaching it *to avoid forcing air into the filter and, possibly, clogging some filter channels.* Attach a filter to the end of the IV tubing, and follow the manufacturer's instructions for filling and priming it. Most filters are positioned with the distal end of the tubing facing upward *so that the solution will completely wet the filter membrane and all air bubbles will be eliminated from the line.*[15] (See *Indications for in-line filters,* page 470.)

■ Leave the clamp open until the IV solution flows through the entire length of tubing *to release trapped air bubbles and force out all the air.*

■ Invert all Y-ports and backcheck valves and tap them, if necessary, *to fill them with solution.*

■ Close the clamp. Then loop the tubing over the IV pole.

■ Label the IV container with the patient's name and room number, date and time, container number, ordered rate and duration of infusion, and your initials.

■ Perform hand hygiene.[2,3,4,5,6]

■ Document the procedure.[12,13,14]

Indications for in-line filters[15]

An in-line filter removes pathogens and particles from IV solutions, *which helps reduce the risk of infusion phlebitis. Because an in-line filter is expensive and its installation is awkward and time-consuming,* these filters aren't used routinely. Many health care facilities require that a filter be used only when administering an admixture. If you're not sure whether to use a filter, check your facility's policy and the manufacturer's specific recommendations. Use this list of do's and don'ts as a guide.

Do's

Do use an in-line filter:

- when administering solutions to an immunodeficient patient
- when administering total parenteral nutrition
- when using additives comprising many separate particles, such as antibiotics requiring reconstitution, or when administering several additives
- when using rubber injection ports or plastic diaphragms repeatedly
- when phlebitis is likely to occur.

Change the in-line filter according to the manufacturer's recommendations (and with administration set change). *If you don't, bacteria trapped in the filter releases endotoxin, a pyrogen small enough to pass through the filter into the bloodstream.*

Use an add-on filter of larger pore size (1.2 microns) when infusing lipid emulsions or total nutrient admixtures that require filtration.

If a positive-pressure electronic infusion device is used, consider the psi rating of the filter. If the psi from the infusion device exceeds that of the filter, the filter will crack or break under the pressure.

Don'ts

Don't use an in-line filter:

- when administering solutions with large particles, such as blood and its components, suspensions, lipid emulsions, and high-molecular-volume plasma expanders, *because the particle will clog the filter and stop IV flow*
- when administering a small-volume IV push medication *because the filter may absorb it.*

Special considerations

- Always use sterile technique when preparing IV solutions.[1] If you contaminate the administration set or container, replace it with a new one *to prevent introducing contaminants into the system.*
- Change the IV tubing no more frequently than 96 hours; however, change it immediately upon suspected contamination.[1,3] Change the filter according to the manufacturer's recommendations or sooner if it becomes clogged.
- Select flow-control devices on the basis of the patient's age and condition, prescribed infusion therapy, type of vascular access device, and care setting.[16]

Patient teaching

Before initiating IV therapy, teach the patient what to expect. Explain how to examine the site, and instruct the patient to notify the practitioner or home care nurse if redness, swelling, or discomfort develops or if the dressing becomes moist.

Teach the patient general strategies to prevent catheter complications. Also tell the patient to report problems with the IV line, such as the infusing stopping or an alarm going off on an infusion pump. If the patient must observe movement restrictions, make sure that he understands them. If the patient is using an intermittent infusion device, teach him how and when to flush it. Finally, teach the patient to document daily whether the IV site is free from pain, swelling, and redness.

Documentation

Document the type and amount of solution, the rate used, and any additives added to the solution.

References

1 Standard 43. Administration set change. Infusion nursing standards of practice. (2011). *Journal of Infusion Nursing, 34,* S55–S57. (Level VII)

2 The Joint Commission. (2015). Standard NPSG.07.01.01. *Comprehensive accreditation manual for hospitals: The official handbook.* Oakbrook Terrace, IL: The Joint Commission. (Level VII)

3 Centers for Disease Control and Prevention. (2011). "Guidelines for the prevention of intravascular catheter-related infections" [Online]. Accessed March 2015 via the Web at http://www.cdc.gov/hicpac/pdf/guidelines/bsi-guidelines-2011.pdf (Level I)

4 Standard 19. Hand hygiene. Infusion nursing standards of practice. (2011). *Journal of Infusion Nursing, 34,* S26–S27. (Level VII)

5 Centers for Disease Control and Prevention. (2002). Guideline for hand hygiene in health-care settings: Recommendations of the Healthcare Infection Control Practices Advisory Committee and the HICPAC/SHEA/APIC/IDSA Hand Hygiene Task Force. *MMWR Recommendations and Reports, 51*(RR-16), 1–45. Accessed March 2015 via the Web at http://www.cdc.gov/mmwr/pdf/rr/rr5116.pdf (Level II)

6 World Health Organization. (2009). "WHO guidelines on hand hygiene in health care: First global patient safety challenge, clean care is safer care" [Online]. Accessed March 2015 via the Web at http://whqlibdoc.who.int/publications/2009/9789241597906_eng.pdf (Level IV)

7 Standard 17. Verification of products and medications. Infusion nursing standards of practice. (2011). *Journal of Infusion Nursing, 34,* S24. (Level VII)

8 Standard 61. Parenteral medication and solution administration. Infusion nursing standards of practice. (2011). *Journal of Infusion Nursing, 34,* S86–S87. (Level VII)

9 Standard 16. Product evaluation, integrity, and defect reporting. Infusion nursing standards of practice. (2011). *Journal of Infusion Nursing, 34,* S22–S23. (Level VII)

10 The Joint Commission. (2015). Standard MM.05.01.09. *Comprehensive accreditation manual for hospitals: The official handbook.* Oakbrook Terrace, IL: The Joint Commission. (Level VII)

11 Standard 20. Compounding of parenteral solutions and medications. Infusion nursing standards of practice. (2011). *Journal of Infusion Nursing, 34,* S27. (Level VII)

12 The Joint Commission. (2015). Standard RC.01.03.01. *Comprehensive accreditation manual for hospitals: The official handbook.* Oakbrook Terrace, IL: The Joint Commission. (Level VII)

13 Standard 14. Documentation. Infusion nursing standards of practice. (2011). *Journal of Infusion Nursing, 34,* S20–S21. (Level VII)

14 Centers for Medicare & Medicaid Services, Department of Health and Human Services. (2013). Condition of participation: Medical record services. 42 C.F.R. § 482.24(b).

15 Standard 28. Filters. Infusion nursing standards of practice. (2011). *Journal of Infusion Nursing, 34,* S33. (Level VII)

16 Standard 29. Flow-control device. Infusion nursing standards of practice. (2011). *Journal of Infusion Nursing, 34,* S34. (Level VII)

Additional references

Infusion Nurses Society. (2011). *Policies and procedures for infusion nursing* (4th ed.). Boston, MA: Infusion Nurses Society.

Nettina, S. M. (2014). *Lippincott manual of nursing practice* (10th ed.). Philadelphia, PA: Wolters Kluwer.

Taylor, C., et al. (2011). *Fundamentals of nursing: The art and science of nursing care* (7th ed.). Philadelphia, PA: Lippincott Williams & Wilkins.

J

JUGULAR VENOUS OXYGEN SATURATION MONITORING

Jugular venous oxygen saturation ($SjvO_2$) monitoring measures the venous oxygenation saturation of blood as it leaves the brain, reflecting the oxygen saturation of blood after cerebral perfusion has taken place. Comparing $SjvO_2$ with the arterial venous oxygenation can help to determine whether blood flow to the brain matches the brain's metabolic demand.

The normal range for $SjvO_2$ is 55% to 70%. Values higher than 70% indicate hyperperfusion; values between 40% and 54% indicate relative hypoperfusion. Values lower than 40% indicate ischemia.

Data from monitoring can also be used to calculate:

- cerebral extraction of oxygen (CEO_2 = arterial oxygen saturation [SaO_2] – $SjvO_2$)
- cerebral arterial oxygen content (CaO_2 = 1.34 × hemoglobin [Hgb] × SaO_2 – 0.0031 × partial pressure of arterial oxygen [PaO_2])
- global cerebral oxygen extraction ratio (O_2ER = SaO_2 – $SjvO_2/SaO_2$) and jugular venous oxygen content saturation ($CjvO_2$ = 1.34 × Hgb × $SjvO_2$ + 0.0031 × jugular venous oxygen tension [$PjvO_2$])
- arteriovenous jugular oxygen content ($AVjDO_2$ = CaO_2 – $CjvO_2$).

These calculations help determine cerebral oxygen use, metabolic demand, and adequacy of oxygen delivery.

Monitoring of $SjvO_2$ allows the nurse to maximize the balance between cerebral perfusion, oxygenation, and metabolism. Indications for $SjvO_2$ monitoring include any neurologic injury in which ischemia is a threat, intraoperative monitoring, subarachnoid hemorrhage, and post-acute head injury with increased intracranial pressure (ICP).

Equipment

Sterile towels ▪ sterile drapes ▪ surgical caps ▪ gowns ▪ sterile gloves ▪ masks (with face shields or goggles, if needed) ▪ antiseptic solution (chlorhexidine is preferred) ▪ central venous catheter insertion kit ▪ 1% or 2% lidocaine without epinephrine ▪ 5- or 10-mL syringe with an 18G or 23G needle ▪ #5 French sterile percutaneous introducer ▪ #4 French fiber-optic $SjvO_2$ catheter ▪ oximetric monitor with cable ▪ 500 mL of normal saline solution (heparinized or nonheparinized) ▪ pressure tubing with continuous flush device ▪ pressure bag ▪ sterile occlusive dressing ▪ sterile labels ▪ Optional: supplies for venous blood sampling.

Implementation

- Gather the appropriate equipment.
- Confirm that the written informed consent has been obtained and that the signed consent form is in the patient's medical record.[1,2,3]
- Conduct a preprocedure verification *to make sure that all relevant documentation, related information, and equipment are available and correctly identified to the patient's identifiers.*[4,5]
- Verify that laboratory reports and imaging studies have been completed and that the results are in the patient's medical record. Notify the practitioner of any unexpected results.
- Perform hand hygiene.[6,7,8,9,10]
- Confirm the patient's identity using at least two patient identifiers.[11]
- Explain the procedure to the patient and provide privacy.

Inserting the catheter

- Prime the pressure tubing system, removing all air bubbles and maintaining sterility of the system for insertion.
- Apply a pressure bag a and inflate it to 300 mm Hg.[12]
- Follow the manufacturer's instructions for in vitro calibration of the catheter before insertion.
- Position the patient with his head elevated 30 to 45 degrees and his neck in a neutral position.[12]
- Document baseline ICP and cerebral perfusion pressure (CPP).[12]
- Turn the patient's head laterally, away from the site chosen for catheter insertion. Note and document any change in ICP and CPP.
- Perform hand hygiene.[6,7,8,9,10]
- Put on a cap, a mask (with face shield or goggles, if needed),[12] a gown, and sterile gloves.[13]
- Using sterile technique, open and prepare the central venous catheter insertion tray, and add a #5 French sterile percutaneous introducer and a #4 French fiber-optic $SjvO_2$ catheter.
- Label all medications, medication containers, and other solutions on and off the sterile field.[14,15]
- After the practitioner puts on a cap, a mask, a gown, and sterile gloves, he will scrub the insertion site with a chlorhexidine-based antiseptic solution for 30 seconds, using a vigorous side-to-side motion. He will then position the sterile drapes, using maximum barrier precautions and exposing only the insertion site.[16]
- Conduct a time-out *to make sure that the correct patient, site, and procedure are verified.*[17]
- Assist the practitioner during insertion, as needed, making sure sterile technique is maintained.
- Monitor the patient's neurologic status, vital signs, ICP, CPP, and pain during insertion and immediately after insertion.[12]

NURSING ALERT Because the catheter in the jugular bulb can inhibit venous outflow, *a sustained ICP of more than 5 mm Hg over preinsertion baseline may be an indication for catheter removal.*

- After the catheter is in place, carefully trace the pressure tubing from the point of origin *to make sure you are connecting the tubing to the correct line,* and then attach it to the line.[18]
- *Confirm the patency of both jugular catheter lumens* by aspirating and flushing them.
- Apply a sterile occlusive dressing.
- Make sure that the monitor alarm limits are set appropriately for the patient's current condition and that the alarms are turned on, functioning properly, and audible to staff.[19,20,21,22]
- Obtain a lateral cervical spine or lateral skull X-ray *to confirm catheter placement at the level of the jugular bulb.*
- Obtain an initial jugular venous blood gas sample and perform in vivo calibration according to the manufacturer's instructions. *In vivo calibration is necessary to ensure reliability of the data.*
- Discard used supplies in an appropriate receptacle.
- Remove and discard your gloves and other personal protective equipment.
- Perform hand hygiene.[6,7,8,9,10]
- Document the procedure.[23,24,25]

Performing ongoing monitoring

- Record baseline parameters for $SjvO_2$.
- Obtain blood samples for laboratory testing, as ordered; *hemoglobin and hematocrit values may be necessary to interpret $SjvO_2$ and to calculate other hemodynamic parameters.*[26]
- Calculate and record baseline $AVjDO_2$, CEO_2, and O_2ER values.
- Continuously monitor $SjvO_2$.
- Record $SjvO_2$ and ICP values and note trends. Assess ICP in relation to $SjvO_2$. Notify the practitioner of any deviation from the trend. *Increased ICP is a frequent cause of desaturation in patients with brain injury.*[27]
- Recalculate and record $AVjDO_2$, CEO_2, and O_2ER, as indicated.
- Identify $SjvO_2$ desaturations and notify the practitioner if any occur. (See *Common causes of desaturation,* page 472.)

TROUBLESHOOTING

Common causes of desaturation

During jugular venous oxygen saturation monitoring, you may encounter periods of desaturation and need to be prepared to take action. Below are common causes of desaturation and appropriate interventions.

CAUSE	NURSING INTERVENTIONS
■ Systemic hypoxemia (one of the most common causes of cerebral hypoxia)	■ If the oxygen saturation is less than 90%, increase the oxygen percentage or fraction of inspired oxygen and adjust the ventilator settings as ordered.
■ Anemia (hemoglobin less than 9 g/L)	■ Report abnormal results to the practitioner, and administer a blood transfusion if ordered.
■ Systemic hypotension (mean blood pressure less than 70 mm Hg)	■ Report abnormal results to the practitioner, and administer a fluid challenge or vasopressors, if ordered.
■ Increased intracranial pressure (greater than 20 mm Hg)	■ Elevate the head of the bed 30 degrees, decrease external stimuli, administer osmotic diuretics such as mannitol, and adjust the ventilator settings *to produce mild hyperventilation (partial pressure of arterial carbon dioxide of 30 to 35 mm Hg)*. Other measures may include drainage of cerebrospinal fluid and methods to reduce cerebral oxygen demand, such as sedation, neuromuscular blockade, or barbiturate coma.

NURSING ALERT *Repeated patterns of desaturation have been shown to be predictors of poor outcomes in patients with severe head injury. Desaturations are emergent events requiring immediate interventions* to restore cerebral blood flow and oxygen delivery.

■ Perform in vivo calibration with a jugular blood gas sample, as recommended by the monitor manufacturer (usually performed every 24 hours, with $SjvO_2$ desaturations, and when data reliability is in question).

NURSING ALERT *Significant changes in readings following sampling can signify errors related to aspiration of blood. Avoid errors by aspirating blood slowly (1 mL/minute) during sampling.*

■ Perform hand hygiene.[6,7,8,9,10]

■ Document the procedure.[23,24,25]

Special considerations

■ The Joint Commission issued a sentinel event alert concerning medical device alarm safety *because alarm-related events have been associated with permanent loss of function and death.* Among the major contributing factors were improper alarm settings, alarms turned off inappropriately, and alarm signals that were not audible to staff. Make sure that alarm limits are appropriately set and that alarms are turned on, functioning properly, and audible to staff. Follow facility guidelines for preventing alarm fatigue.[19]

■ Maintain a safe environment during monitoring *to prevent accidental dislodgement of the catheter.*

■ Use sedation or analgesia, as indicated, *to maintain, monitor, and enhance CPP.*

■ Change the dressing using sterile technique if it becomes soiled or loosened and at the interval determined by your facility for central venous access device redressing.

■ Change the IV solution and tubing for the catheter at the interval determined by your facility.

■ For an $SjvO_2$ catheter with low light intensity, check the fiber-optics *for obstruction, occlusion, and damage.* Aspirate the catheter until blood can be freely sampled and normal light intensity is displayed. If you can't aspirate a blood sample, the catheter needs to be replaced.

■ For an $SjvO_2$ catheter with high light intensity, adjust the patient's head *to ensure a neutral neck position. High light intensity indicates a vessel-wall artifact and is usually encountered during patient repositioning.*

■ *To prevent catheter coiling,* identify rhythmic fluctuations in $SjvO_2$ trends. Those unrelated to changes in ICP, CPP, or systemic blood pressure signify coiling of the catheter. Obtain a lateral cervical spine or lateral skull X-ray *to assess the position of the catheter in the external jugular vein* (compare it with the X-ray performed on insertion). If coiling is confirmed, consider replacing the catheter.

■ Assess line necessity daily, and make sure the line is removed when it's no longer needed *to reduce the risk of intravascular catheter–associated bloodstream infection.*

Complications

Complications associated with $SvjO_2$ monitoring are similar to complications that can occur with any central line, the most common being line sepsis. Other risks include pneumothorax, carotid artery puncture, internal jugular thrombosis, and excessive bleeding.

In rare instances, the catheter can also cause impaired cerebral venous drainage and increased ICP.

Documentation

Document difficulties encountered during insertion, depth (in centimeters) of the catheter, the patient's tolerance of the procedure, and ICP and CPP readings during insertion. Record the baseline $SjvO_2$ reading and initial CEO_2, $AVjDO_2$, and O_2ER calculations. Record $SjvO_2$ and ICP hourly. Record CEO_2, $AVjDO_2$, and O_2ER, when indicated. Document your assessment of the insertion site, expected and unexpected outcomes, nursing actions taken, and patient and education provided to the patient and his family.

REFERENCES

1 The Joint Commission. (2015). Standard RI.01.03.01. *Comprehensive accreditation manual for hospitals: The official handbook.* Oakbrook Terrace, IL: The Joint Commission. (Level VII)

2 American Osteopathic Association. (2014). Standard 30.01.11. *Healthcare Facilities Accreditation Program: Accreditation requirements for acute care hospitals.* Chicago, IL: American Osteopathic Association. (Level VII)

3 Centers for Medicare and Medicaid Services, Department of Health and Human Services. (2014). Condition of participation: Patient's rights. 42 C.F.R. § 482.13(b)(2).

4 The Joint Commission. (2015). Standard UP.01.01.01. *Comprehensive accreditation manual for hospitals: The official handbook.* Oakbrook Terrace, IL: The Joint Commission. (Level VII)

5 American Osteopathic Association. (2014). Standard 30.00.14. *Healthcare Facilities Accreditation Program: Accreditation requirements for acute care hospitals.* Chicago, IL: American Osteopathic Association. (Level VII)

6 The Joint Commission. (2015). Standard NPSG.07.01.01. *Comprehensive accreditation manual for hospitals: The official handbook.* Oakbrook Terrace, IL: The Joint Commission. (Level VII)

7 Centers for Disease Control and Prevention. (2002). Guideline for hand hygiene in health-care settings: Recommendations of the Healthcare Infection Control Practices Advisory Committee and the HICPAC/SHEA/APIC/IDSA Hand Hygiene Task Force. *MMWR Recommendations and Reports, 51*(RR-16), 1–45. Accessed March 2015 via the Web at http://www.cdc.gov/mmwr/pdf/rr/rr5116.pdf (Level II)

8 World Health Organization. (2009). "WHO guidelines on hand hygiene in health care: First global patient safety challenge, clean care is safer care" [Online]. Accessed March 2015 via the Web at http://whqlibdoc.who.int/publications/2009/9789241597906_eng.pdf (Level IV)

9 American Osteopathic Association. (2014). Standard 07.01.21. *Healthcare Facilities Accreditation Program: Accreditation requirements for acute care hospitals.* Chicago, IL: American Osteopathic Association. (Level VII)

10 Centers for Medicare and Medicaid Services, Department of Health and Human Services. (2014). Condition of participation: Infection control. 42 C.F.R. § 482.42.

11 The Joint Commission. (2015). Standard NPSG.01.01.01. *Comprehensive accreditation manual for hospitals: The official handbook.* Oakbrook Terrace, IL: The Joint Commission. (Level VII)

12 Lynn-McHale Wiegand, D. (Ed.). (2011). *AACN procedure manual for critical care* (6th ed.). St. Louis, MO: Saunders.

13 Siegel, J. D., et al. (2007). "2007 guideline for isolation precautions: Preventing transmission of infectious agents in healthcare settings" [Online]. Accessed March 2015 via the Web at http://www.cdc.gov/hicpac/pdf/isolation/Isolation2007.pdf (Level II)

14 The Joint Commission. (2015). Standard NPSG.03.04.01. *Comprehensive accreditation manual for hospitals: The official handbook.* Oakbrook Terrace, IL: The Joint Commission. (Level VII)

15 American Osteopathic Association. (2014). Standard 25.01.18. *Healthcare Facilities Accreditation Program: Accreditation requirements for acute care hospitals.* Chicago, IL: American Osteopathic Association. (Level VII)

16 Centers for Disease Control and Prevention. (2011). "Guidelines for the prevention of intravascular catheter-related infections" [Online]. Accessed March 2015 via the Web at http://www.cdc.gov/hicpac/pdf/guidelines/bsi-guidelines-2011.pdf (Level I)

17 The Joint Commission. (2014). Standard UP.01.03.01. *Comprehensive accreditation manual for hospitals: The official handbook.* Oakbrook Terrace, IL: The Joint Commission. (Level VII)

18 U.S. Food and Drug Administration. (n.d.). "Look. Check. Connect. Safe medical device connections save lives" [Online]. Accessed March 2015 via the Web at http://www.fda.gov/downloads/MedicalDevices/Safety/AlertsandNotices/UCM134873.pdf

19 The Joint Commission. (2013). "Sentinel event alert: Medical device alarm safety in hospitals" [Online]. Accessed March 2015 via the Web at http://www.jointcommission.org/assets/1/18/SEA_50_alarms_4_5_13_FINAL1.PDF (Level VII)

20 Graham, K. C., & Cvach, M. (2010). Monitor alarm fatigue: Standardizing use of physiological monitors and decreasing nuisance alarms. *American Journal of Critical Care, 19,* 28–37.

21 American Association of Critical-Care Nurses. (2013). "AACN practice alert: Alarm management" [Online]. Accessed March 2015 via the Web at http://www.aacn.org/wd/practice/docs/practicealerts/alarm-management-practice-alert.pdf (Level VII)

22 The Joint Commission. (2015). Standard NPSG.06.01.01. *Comprehensive accreditation manual for hospitals: The official handbook.* Oakbrook Terrace, IL: The Joint Commission. (Level VII)

23 The Joint Commission. (2015). Standard RC.01.03.01. *Comprehensive accreditation manual for hospitals: The official handbook.* Oakbrook Terrace, IL: The Joint Commission. (Level VII)

24 American Osteopathic Association. (2014). Standard 10.00.03. *Healthcare Facilities Accreditation Program: Accreditation requirements for acute care hospitals.* Chicago, IL: American Osteopathic Association. (Level VII)

25 Centers for Medicare and Medicaid Services, Department of Health and Human Services. (2014). Condition of participation: Medical record services. 42 C.F.R. § 482.24(b).

26 Cyrous, A., et al. (2012). New approaches to bedside monitoring in stroke. *Expert Review of Neurotherapeutics, 12,* 915–928.

27 Chiu, W., et al. (2012). "Application of brain tissue oxygen monitoring in traumatic brain injury" [Online]. Accessed March 2015 via the Web at http://www.internationalbrain.org/articles/application-of-brain-tissue-oxygen-monitoring-in-traumatic-brain-injury/

ADDITIONAL REFERENCES

Haddad, S. H., & Arabi, Y. M. (2012). Critical care management of severe traumatic brain injury in adults. *Scandinavian Journal of Trauma, Resuscitation & Emergency Medicine, 20,* 12–37. Accessed March 2015 via the Web at http://www.sjtrem.com/content/pdf/1757-7241-20-12.pdf

Meng, L., et al. (2012). Head-up tilt and hyperventilation produce similar changes in cerebral oxygenation and blood volume: An observational comparison study using frequency-domain near-infrared spectroscopy. *Canadian Journal of Anesthesiology, 59,* 357–365. Accessed March 2015 via the Web athttp://www.ics.uci.edu/~zhaoxia/publications/paper22_Yuzx_CanJAnesth2012.pdf

K

KNEE ARTHROPLASTY POSTPROCEDURE CARE

Knee arthroplasty involves surgical replacement of all or part of the knee joint. In partial knee replacement, either the medial or lateral compartment of the knee joint is replaced. Total knee replacement is commonly used to treat severe pain, joint contractures, and deterioration of joint surfaces, conditions that prohibit full extension or flexion.

Arthroplasty postprocedure care includes maintaining alignment of the affected joint, assisting with exercises, and providing routine postoperative care. Nursing responsibilities include teaching, safe mobility, home care, and exercises that may continue for several years.

Equipment

Incentive spirometer ■ continuous passive motion (CPM) machine ■ compression stockings or sequential compression device ■ gloves ■ ice bag ■ skin lotion ■ warm water ■ crutches or walker ■ pain medications ■ closed-wound drainage system ■ IV antibiotics ■ anticoagulants ■ stethoscope ■ thermometer ■ blood pressure cuff ■ pulse oximeter ■ pillow ■ Optional: infusion pump, sterile dressings, hypoallergenic tape, black marker or pen.

After total knee replacement, a knee immobilizer may be applied in the operating room, or the leg may be placed in CPM.

Implementation

- Verify the practitioner's orders.
- Perform hand hygiene.[1,2,3,4,5]
- Confirm the patient's identity using at least two patient identifiers.[6]
- Explain all the procedures.
- Obtain the patient's vital signs at an interval determined by your facility and the patient's condition. Report changes in vital signs *because they may indicate infection, hemorrhage, or postoperative complications.*
- Encourage the patient to perform deep-breathing and coughing exercises. Assist with incentive spirometry *to prevent healthcare-associated pneumonia.*[7]
- Perform a bilateral neurovascular assessment every 2 hours for the first 48 hours and then every 4 hours *for signs of complications.* Check the affected leg for color, temperature, toe movement, sensation, edema, capillary filling, and pedal pulse. Investigate any complaints of pain, burning, numbness, or tingling.[8]
- Apply the compression stockings or sequential compression device, as ordered, *to promote venous return and prevent venous thromboembolism.*[9] Remove the stockings or compression device regularly, inspect the patient's legs (especially the heels) for pressure ulcers, and reapply the stockings or device.

■ Perform a comprehensive pain assessment using techniques appropriate for the patient's age, condition, and ability to understand.[10] Administer pain medications, as ordered, following safe medication administration practices.[11]
■ If the patient was receiving a beta-adrenergic blocker before surgery, collaborate with the patient's practitioner *to make sure he receives it during the perioperative period, as appropriate.*[12]
■ Make sure prophylactic antibiotics are discontinued within 24 hours after surgery.[13,14]
■ Administer anticoagulant therapy, as ordered,[11,12,14] following safe medication administration practices[11] *to minimize the risk of venous thromboembolism.* If the practitioner prescribes a continuous infusion of heparin, administer it using a programmable pump (preferably a smart pump with dose-range alerts) *to provide consistent and accurate dosing.*[15]
■ Observe the patient for bleeding and for signs and symptoms of phlebitis, such as warmth, swelling, tenderness, and redness. Monitor laboratory results, such as complete blood count, prothrombin time, International Normalized Ratio, and partial thromboplastin time.[12]
■ Perform hand hygiene[1,2,3,4,5] and put on gloves as needed.
■ Inspect the patient's dressings for excessive bleeding. Circle any drainage on the dressing and mark it with your initials, the date, and the time. As needed, apply more sterile dressings, using hypoallergenic tape. Report excessive bleeding to the practitioner.

NURSING ALERT *During inspection, pay special attention to the incisional area. Monitor for bruising, and report redness, warmth, or swelling of the surgical site. Record drainage amounts, and report excess drainage immediately* because this could signal bleeding into the joint. *Be aware that many patients complain of slight numbness or tingling and mild swelling at the incision site.*[8]

■ Observe the closed-wound drainage system for discharge color. (See the "Closed-wound drain management" procedure, page 190.) *Proper drainage prevents hematoma. Purulent discharge and fever may indicate infection.* Empty and measure drainage, as ordered, using clean technique *to prevent infection.*
■ Monitor fluid intake and output daily; include wound drainage in the output measurement.
■ If the patient has an indwelling urinary catheter that was inserted for surgery, remove the catheter on postoperative day 1 or 2 (with the day of surgery considered day 0), according to your facility's protocol or the practitioner's order, *to reduce the risk of catheter-associated urinary tract infection.*[12] (See the "Indwelling urinary catheter care and removal" procedure, page 391.)
■ Apply an ice bag, as ordered, to the affected site for the first 48 hours *to reduce swelling, relieve pain, and control bleeding.*
■ Help the patient use the trapeze to reposition himself every 2 hours. *These position changes enhance comfort, prevent pressure ulcers, and help prevent respiratory complications.* Then provide skin care for the back and buttocks, using warm water and lotion, as indicated.
■ Instruct the patient to perform muscle-strengthening exercises for extremities, as ordered, *to help maintain muscle strength and range of motion and to help prevent phlebitis.* Collaborate with physical therapy professionals, as appropriate.
■ Instruct the patient to begin quadriceps exercises and straight-leg raises, when ordered (usually on the second postoperative day).
■ Encourage flexion-extension exercises, when ordered (usually after the first dressing change). Collaborate with physical therapy professionals, as appropriate.
■ Elevate the affected leg, as ordered, *to reduce swelling.*
■ If the practitioner orders use of the CPM machine, he will adjust the machine daily *to gradually increase the degree of flexion of the affected leg.* Typically, patients can dangle their feet on the first day after surgery and begin ambulation with partial weight-bearing (cemented knee) or toe-touch ambulation only (uncemented knee), as tolerated, by the second day. The patient may need to wear a knee immobilizer for support when walking; otherwise, he should be in CPM for most of the day and night or during waking hours only. (See the "Continuous passive motion device use" procedure, page 224.)
■ The degree of flexion, extension, and weight-bearing status depend on the practitioner's specific orders, the surgical approach used, and the surgeon's preference.
■ Before ambulation, ensure adequate pain management *because movement is very painful.* Encourage the patient during exercise.
■ Help the patient with progressive ambulation, using adjustable crutches or a walker when needed.[13,16]
■ Teach the patient and his family about measures to prevent surgical site infection.
■ Remove and discard your gloves and perform hand hygiene.[1,2,3,4,5]
■ Document the procedure.[18,19]

Special considerations

Fever within the first 48 hours after surgery is commonly due to atelectasis. Superficial wound infections commonly take 4 to 6 days for fever to develop.[20]

Patient teaching

During discharge teaching, teach the patient to[8] take prescribed medications, as ordered; have blood tests performed, as ordered (usually twice weekly), until discontinued by the practitioner; keep follow-up appointments with the practitioner; immediately report any signs or symptoms of deep vein thrombosis, such as increasing calf pain, tenderness, or swelling above or below the knee and increased swelling in the calf, ankle, or foot; immediately report warning signs and symptoms of a blood clot that has traveled to the lungs, including a sudden increase in shortness of breath, sudden chest pain, or localized chest pain with coughing; and promptly report signs and symptoms of possible infection, such as fever (a temperature above 101°F [38.3°C]), shaking chills, excessive incisional drainage, unusual warmth or swelling around the incision, and increasing knee pain.

Stress the importance of continuing with rehabilitation, not only to maintain physical function, but also to prevent complications. Caution the patient about the risk of falling, and teach him to avoid stairs until he's able to keep a strong and mobile balance. Urge the patient to wear strong, sturdy shoes, and emphasize that assistive devices are an important part of rehabilitation. Explain that he may need periodic X-rays to evaluate for loosening or wearing out of prosthesis components, as indicated.[8]

Complications

Immobility after arthroplasty may result in such complications as shock, pulmonary embolism, pneumonia, phlebitis, paralytic ileus, urine retention, and bowel impaction. A deep wound or infection at the prosthesis site is a serious complication that may force removal of the prosthesis.

Fat embolism, a potentially fatal complication resulting from release of fat molecules in response to increased intramedullary canal pressure from the prosthesis, may develop within 72 hours after surgery. Watch for such signs and symptoms as apprehension, diaphoresis, fever, dyspnea, pulmonary effusion, tachycardia, cyanosis, seizures, decreased level of consciousness, and a petechial rash on the chest and shoulders.

Documentation

Record the patient's neurovascular status and maintenance and settings of the CPM device. Describe the patient's position (especially the position of the affected leg), skin care and condition, respiratory care and condition, and the use of a sequential compression device. Document all exercises performed and their effect; also record ambulatory efforts, the type of support used, and the amount of traction weight.

On the appropriate flowchart, record vital signs and fluid intake and output. Note the turning and skin care schedule and the current exercise and ambulation program. Record discharge instructions and how well the patient seems to understand them.

REFERENCES

1 The Joint Commission. (2015). Standard NPSG.07.01.01. *Comprehensive accreditation manual for hospitals: The official handbook.* Oakbrook Terrace, IL: The Joint Commission. (Level VII)

2 Centers for Disease Control and Prevention. (2002). Guideline for hand hygiene in health-care settings: Recommendations of the Healthcare Infection Control Practices Advisory Committee and the HICPAC/SHEA/APIC/IDSA Hand Hygiene Task Force. *MMWR Recommendations and Reports, 51*(RR-16), 1–45. Accessed March 2015 via the Web at http://www.cdc.gov/mmwr/pdf/rr/rr5116.pdf (Level II)

3 World Health Organization. (2009). "WHO guidelines on hand hygiene in health care: First global patient safety challenge, clean care is safer care" [Online]. Accessed March 2015 via the Web at http://whqlibdoc.who.int/publications/2009/9789241597906_eng.pdf (Level IV)

4 American Osteopathic Association. (2014). Standard 07.01.21. *Healthcare Facilities Accreditation Program: Accreditation requirements for acute care hospitals.* Chicago, IL: American Osteopathic Association. (Level VII)

5 Centers for Medicare and Medicaid Services, Department of Health and Human Services. (2014). Condition of participation: Infection control. 42 C.F.R. § 482.42.

6 The Joint Commission. (2015). Standard NPSG.01.01.01. *Comprehensive accreditation manual for hospitals: The official handbook.* Oakbrook Terrace, IL: The Joint Commission. (Level VII)

7 Centers for Disease Control and Prevention. (2004). Guidelines for preventing health-care associated pneumonia, 2003: Recommendations for CDC and the Healthcare Infection Control Practices Advisory Committee. *MMWR Recommendations and Reports, 53*(RR-3), 1-32. Accessed March 2015 via the Web at http://www.cdc.gov/mmwr/pdf/rr/rr5303.pdf (Level III)

8 Loy-Turner, M. (2011). "Joint adventures: The path to total knee replacement" [Online]. Accessed March 2015 via the Web at http://www.americannursetoday.com/assets/0/434/436/440/7364/7542/7544/7566/9eeaff40-7aca-4eb2-a776-30b4dd7ce0b0.pdf

9 Centers for Medicare and Medicaid Services and The Joint Commission. (2014). "The specifications manual for national hospital inpatient quality measures (version 4.3)" [Online]. Accessed March 2015 via the Web at http://www.qualitynet.org/dcs/ContentServer?pagename=QnetPublic%2FPage%2FQnetTier2&cid=1141662756099

10 The Joint Commission. (2014). Standard PC.01.02.07. *Comprehensive accreditation manual for hospitals: The official handbook.* Oakbrook Terrace, IL: The Joint Commission. (Level VII)

11 Centers for Medicare and Medicaid Services, Department of Health and Human Services. (2014). Condition of participation: Nursing services. 42 C.F.R. § 482.23(c).

12 The Joint Commission. (2010). Surgical care improvement project national hospital inpatient quality measures. In *Specification manual for national hospital inpatient quality measures.* Oakbrook Terrace, IL: The Joint Commission.

13 Anderson, D. J., et al. (2014). SHEA/IDSA practice recommendation: Strategies to prevent surgical site infections in acute care hospitals: 2014 update. *Infection Control and Hospital Epidemiology, 35,* 605–627. Accessed March 2015 via the Web at http://www.jstor.org/stable/10.1086/676022 (Level IV)

14 American Academy of Orthopedic Surgeons. (2011). "Preventing venous thromboembolic disease in patients undergoing elective hip and knee arthroplasty: Evidence-based guideline and evidence report" [Online]. Accessed March 2015 via the Web at http://www.aaos.org/research/guidelines/VTE/VTE_full_guideline.pdf (Level IV)

15 The Joint Commission. (2015). Standard NPSG.03.05.01. *Comprehensive accreditation manual for hospitals: The official handbook.* Oakbrook Terrace, IL: The Joint Commission. (Level VII)

16 The Joint Commission. (2015). Standard NPSG.07.05.01. *Comprehensive accreditation manual for hospitals: The official handbook.* Oakbrook Terrace, IL: The Joint Commission. (Level VII)

17 The Joint Commission. (2015). Standard NPSG.07.01.01. *Comprehensive accreditation manual for hospitals: The official handbook.* Oakbrook Terrace, IL: The Joint Commission. (Level VII)

18 The Joint Commission. (2015). Standard RC.01.03.01. *Comprehensive accreditation manual for hospitals: The official handbook.* Oakbrook Terrace, IL: The Joint Commission. (Level VII)

19 Centers for Medicare & Medicaid Services, Department of Health and Human Services. (2014). Condition of participation: Medical record services. 42 C.F.R. § 482.24(b).

20 Hinkle, J. L., & Cheever, K. H. (2014). *Brunner & Suddarth's textbook of medical-surgical nursing* (13th ed.). Philadelphia, PA: Wolters Kluwer.

ADDITIONAL REFERENCES

Lee, R. M., et al. (2012). "Postoperative pain control for total knee arthroplasty: Continuous femoral nerve block versus intravenous patient controlled analgesia" [Online]. Accessed March 2015 via the Web at http://anesthpain.com/?page=article&article_id=3404

Selby, R., et al. (2012). Impact of thromboprophylaxis guidelines on clinical outcomes following total hip and total knee replacement. *Thrombosis Research, 130,* 166–172.

LARYNGEAL MASK AIRWAY INSERTION

The laryngeal mask airway (LMA) establishes and maintains a patent airway in the unconscious patient. Anesthesia personnel use it extensively in the operating room. It's also appropriate for emergency airway and ventilatory support when endotracheal (ET) intubation isn't immediately possible. Health care practitioners with special training in the use of the LMA may also use it in place of a face mask during adult, pediatric, and neonatal resuscitation.[1,2,3]

The LMA consists of a semirigid tube attached to a silicone mask. The mask is placed into the patient's mouth and advanced blindly until it rests above the larynx. The patient may then breathe spontaneously or be assisted with moderate positive-pressure ventilation. The LMA may not protect the patient from regurgitation and aspiration; however, when compared with the bag-mask device, regurgitation is less likely and aspiration uncommon.[1]

Because of the risks of regurgitation and aspiration, LMAs should be used in patients with full stomachs only in emergency situations in which intubation isn't possible, or if ventilation by face mask is ineffective. LMAs may be contraindicated for morbidly obese patients, patients more than 14 weeks pregnant, those with sustained multiple or massive injuries or acute adnominal or thoracic injuries, those with any condition that results in delayed gastric emptying, and those who have recently received opiate medication. Always follow the manufacturer's indications and instructions for use.[4]

Types of LMAs used outside of the operating room include the reusable LMA, which must be cleaned and sterilized between uses, and the disposable (single-patient use) LMA. In addition, an intubating LMA can be used to provide a patent airway before facilitating endotracheal intubation.

Occasionally, patients can't be adequately ventilated with the LMA after successful insertion. Supplies for ET intubation should be readily available if needed.[1]

Equipment

Appropriately sized LMA based on patient's weight (reusable, disposable, or intubating) (see *LMA specifications,* page 476) ▪ syringe of appropriate

LMA specifications

The following chart will help you choose the right size laryngeal mask airway (LMA) for your patient.

LMA SIZE	PATIENT SIZE	MAXIMAL CUFF INFLATION VOLUME	OVERINFLATION VOLUME FOR CUFF TEST
1	Up to 5 kg (11 lb)	4 mL	8 mL
1½	5–10 kg (11–22 lb)	7 mL	10 mL
2	10–20 kg (22–44 lb)	10 mL	15 mL
2½	20–30 kg (44–66 lb)	14 mL	21 mL
3	30–50 kg (66–110 lb)	20 mL	30 mL
4	50–70 kg (110–154 lb)	30 mL	45 mL
5	70–100 kg (154–220 lb)	40 mL	60 mL
6	Greater than 100 kg (220 lb)	50 mL	75 mL

size for inflating cuff ▪ water-soluble lubricant ▪ gloves and other personal protective equipment ▪ folded towel or blanket ▪ oxygen equipment ▪ tape or device to secure the tube ▪ handheld resuscitation bag with mask ▪ bite block ▪ stethoscope ▪ pulse oximeter and probe ▪ capnometer ▪ disinfectant pad ▪ Optional: prescribed anesthetic agent, cricothyroidotomy kit, suction equipment, intubation equipment, introducer.

Preparation of equipment

Remove the LMA from its package and visually inspect it for discoloration, cracks, or kinks in the tube; also make sure it's the right size. Inspect the airway opening and check that the aperture bars are intact. Manually tighten the connector, if needed.

Test the patency of the cuff by first withdrawing all air and then inflating it with air injected through the pilot balloon. While it's inflated, visually inspect the cuff for symmetry, and then deflate the cuff. Don't use the LMA if it's leaking air or if you note asymmetry of the cuff when you inflate it. Assemble suction equipment and check that it's working properly.

Implementation

- If this is a planned procedure, verify the order in the patient's medical record *to ensure that the right procedure is being performed on the right patient at the right time.*
- Gather and prepare the equipment.
- Perform hand hygiene.[5,6,7,8,9]
- Confirm the patient's identity using at least two patient identifiers.[10]
- Assess the patient's level of consciousness. The patient should be unconscious and unresponsive *because the LMA shouldn't be inserted into a patient who may resist insertion.*
- Teach the family about the procedure, as the patient's condition allows, *to provide them with information and reduce anxiety.*
- Put on gloves and personal protective equipment *to reduce the transmission of microorganisms and contact with body secretions.*[11]
- While the equipment is being prepared, ventilate and oxygenate the patient with a bag-valve mask device, if necessary.
- Lubricate the posterior surface of the LMA, using a water-soluble lubricant, *to ease insertion.*[12] Avoid getting the lubricant on the anterior surface of the cuff *because the lubricant may be aspirated.*
- Place the patient in the supine position with a folded towel or blanket under the head to flex the neck and extend the head (the "sniffing position") *to ease insertion of the LMA.*
- Stand behind the patient's head and place your nondominant hand under the patient's head, lifting the head slightly and keeping upward pressure.[12]
- Hold the LMA in your dominant hand like a pencil, with your index finger placed at the junction of the mask and the tube (as shown below). The lumen of the LMA should be facing up, with the lubricated posterior surface facing the floor.

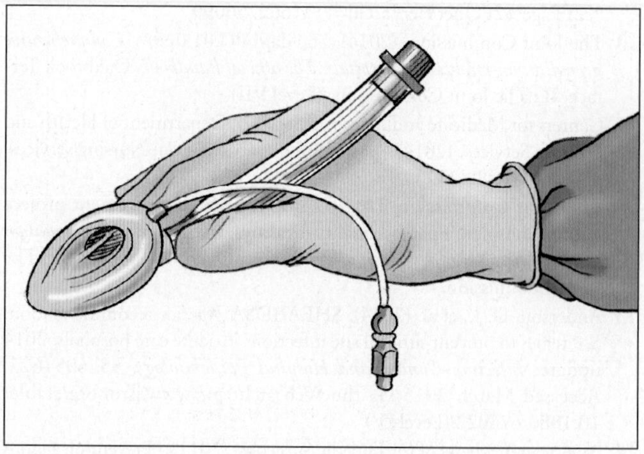

- Extend the patient's head while flexing the neck and flatten the LMA against the patient's hard palate.[4,12] Use your middle finger to gently press down on the patient's jaw.
- Flex your wrist fully so that the tip of the LMA points toward the patient's head and down, and use your index finger to insert the tip of the LMA into the patient's mouth (as shown on next page, top left).

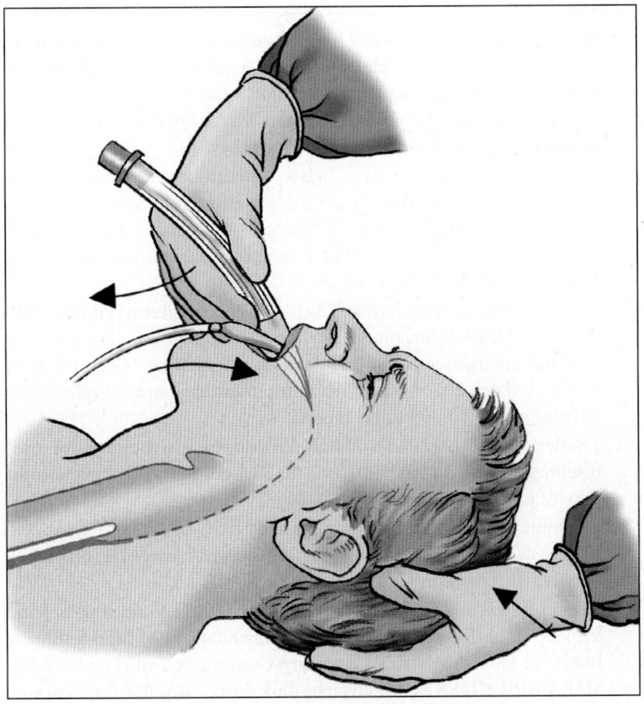

■ Press the posterior surface of the LMA against the hard palate and advance it into the oropharynx (as shown below).[4,12] *By applying pressure up against the hard palate, the LMA will advance to the proper position.*

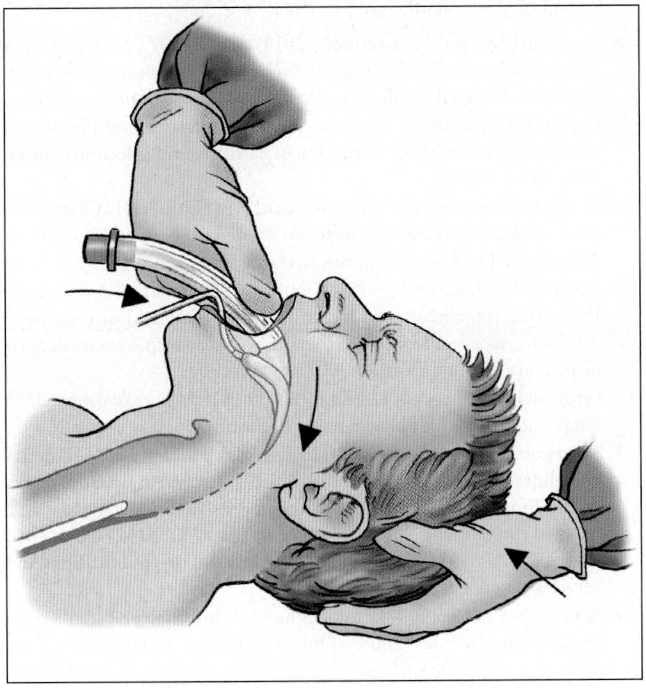

■ Use your middle finger to open the patient's jaw and check that the cuff is compressed against the hard palate. If the cuff isn't flattened against the hard palate, remove the LMA and insert it again.

■ While maintaining pressure on the LMA so that it stays pressed against the hard palate, extend your index finger fully while continuing to advance the LMA until you meet resistance at the hypopharynx (as shown on top right). The LMA should now be in the correct position.[4,12]

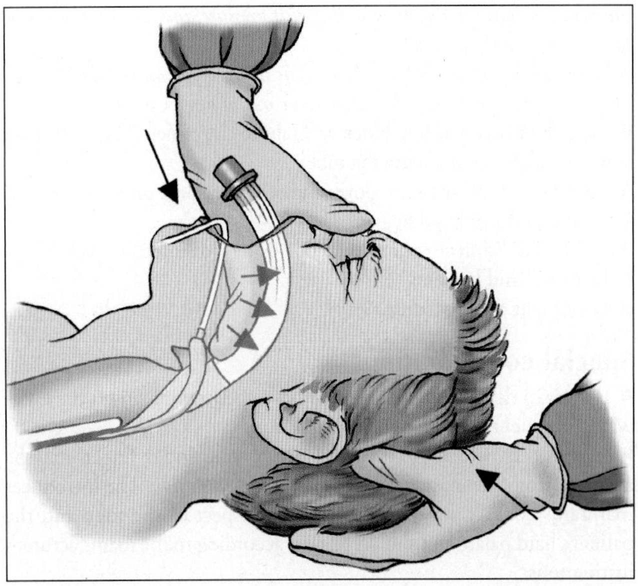

■ Remove your nondominant hand from under the patient's head, and use it to hold the LMA in place while removing your index finger (as shown below).[12]

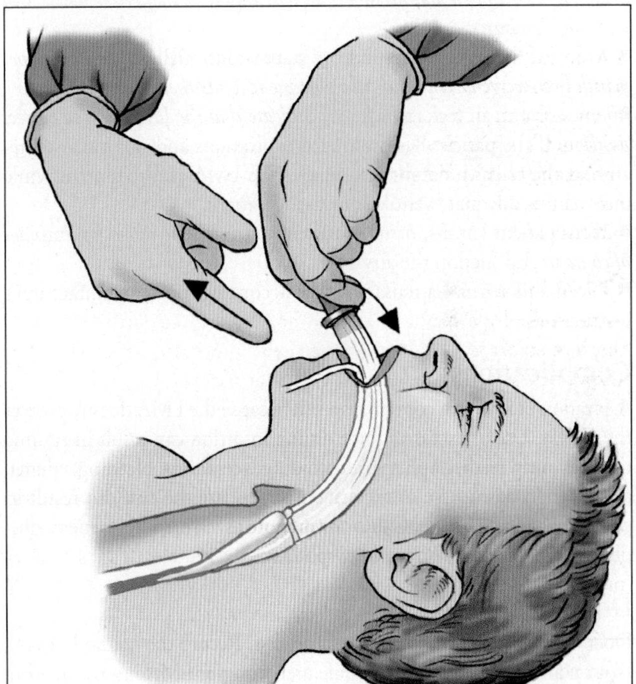

■ Without holding the LMA, use the syringe to inflate the cuff to an intracuff pressure of about 60 cm H_2O.[4,12] Only one-half the maximum inflation volume is required to make a seal. *Inflating the cuff without holding the tube allows it to settle itself into the correct position during cuff inflation.* Don't overinflate the cuff.

■ Check the patient's mouth to make sure the cuff isn't visible, and observe for minor outward movement of the tube and minor neck bulging in the area of the cricothyroid, *indicating proper tube placement and cuff inflation.*

■ Verify correct placement by auscultating for bilateral breath sounds with a stethoscope and by monitoring using pulse oximetry.[13]

■ Use a bag-valve device connected to an oxygen source, if indicated, to gently deliver ventilations using a peak airway pressure less than 20 cm H_2O and a tidal volume of 8 mL/kg of body weight or less. *Using low pressure ventilations avoids exceeding cuff pressure and reduces the risk of forcing air into the stomach.*

- Insert a bite block *to keep the patient from biting on the tube, which may cause it to become occluded or move out of proper position.*[4,12]
- Tape the LMA and bite block securely to the patient's face, or use a commercial device to secure the tube.
- Remove and discard your gloves and other personal protective equipment and perform hand hygiene.[5,6,7]
- Clean and disinfect your stethoscope using a disinfectant pad.[14,15]
- Perform hand hygiene.[5,6,7,8,9]
- Document the procedure.[16,17,18]

Special considerations

- If there's a risk that the patient may have neck trauma, insert the LMA with the patient's neck in a neutral position.
- Introducers, which are used in place of your index finger, may be available from the manufacturer *to assist with insertion.* The introducer maintains contact between the posterior aspect of the tube and the patient's hard palate and should be used according to the manufacturer's instructions.
- Never use extreme force when inserting a LMA.
- If there's any concern about the final placement of the LMA, remove and reposition the device.
- Avoid use of the LMA in patients who need high pressures for ventilation. *The LMA has a low-pressure seal, which may be ineffective when used with high pressures.*
- Monitor the patient's respiratory status continually *to ensure proper ventilation, oxygenation, and tube placement while the LMA is in place.*
- Assess for an air leak, *which may indicate that the LMA isn't in correct position.* If the patient has prolonged expirations and no oval swelling around the cricoid membrane, remove the LMA and reinsert it while maintaining adequate ventilations to the patient.
- If the patient vomits, turn the patient to the side *to allow for drainage of contents* and suction the airway.
- Clean and sterilize a reusable LMA according to the manufacturer's instructions.[4,15]

Complications

Aspiration of stomach contents is a risk because the LMA doesn't protect the airway. Use of excessive force during insertion can result in trauma to the mouth, teeth, or pharynx, including lacerations, bleeding, edema, and laryngospasm. Use of excessive air to inflate the cuff can result in edema or nerve damage. Other complications include hoarseness, dysphagia, stridor, dysarthria, and dysphonia.

Documentation

Document why LMA insertion was needed. Record the method of ventilation and oxygenation used while preparing for LMA insertion. Note that the cuff was tested for patency and that the device was visually inspected, with no irregularities observed. Record the date, time, and name of the person performing the procedure. Include the size of the LMA, volume of air used to inflate the cuff, and number of attempts to achieve proper placement. Record the methods used to determine proper tube placement. Include placement of the bite block and how the bite block and tube were secured. Document whether the patient was breathing spontaneously or receiving assisted or controlled ventilations. Include the amount of oxygen being delivered. Also document any evidence of trauma to the airway from insertion of the LMA. Record frequent assessments of tube placement and respiratory status on a frequent patient assessment record using the appropriate documentation format. Include any teaching and support given to the family.

References

1 American Heart Association. (2010). Adult advanced cardiovascular life support: 2010 American Heart Association guidelines for cardiopulmonary resuscitation and emergency cardiovascular care. *Circulation, 122,* 729–767. Accessed March 2015 via the Web at http://circ.ahajournals.org/content/122/18_suppl_3/S729.short (Level II)

2 American Heart Association. (2010). Pediatric advanced life support: 2010 American Heart Association guidelines for cardiopulmonary resuscitation and emergency cardiovascular care. *Circulation, 122,* 876–908. Accessed March 2015 via the Web at http://circ.ahajournals.org/content/122/18_suppl_3/S876.extract (Level II)

3 American Heart Association. (2010). Neonatal resuscitation: 2010 American Heart Association guidelines for cardiopulmonary resuscitation and emergency cardiovascular care. *Circulation, 122,* 909–919. Accessed March 2015 via the Web at http://circ.ahajournals.org/content/122/18_suppl_3/S909.full (Level II)

4 Teleflex Medical. (2013). "LMA Proseal™: Instructions for use" [Online]. Accessed March 2015 via the Web at http://www.lmana.com/viewifu.php?ifu=19

5 The Joint Commission. (2015). Standard NPSG.07.01.01. *Comprehensive accreditation manual for hospitals: The official handbook.* Oakbrook Terrace, IL: The Joint Commission. (Level VII)

6 Centers for Disease Control and Prevention. (2002). Guideline for hand hygiene in health-care settings: Recommendations of the Healthcare Infection Control Practices Advisory Committee and the HICPAC/SHEA/APIC/IDSA Hand Hygiene Task Force. *MMWR Recommendations and Reports, 51*(RR-16), 1–45. Accessed March 2015 via the Web at http://www.cdc.gov/mmwr/pdf/rr/rr5116.pdf (Level II)

7 World Health Organization. (2009). "WHO guidelines on hand hygiene in health care: First global patient safety challenge, clean care is safer care" [Online]. Accessed March 2015 via the Web at http://whqlibdoc.who.int/publications/2009/9789241597906_eng.pdf (Level IV)

8 American Osteopathic Association. (2014). Standard 07.01.10. *Healthcare Facilities Accreditation Program: Accreditation requirements for acute care hospitals.* Chicago, IL: American Osteopathic Association. (Level VII)

9 Centers for Medicare & Medicaid Services, Department of Health and Human Services. (2014). Condition of participation: Infection control. 42 C.F.R. § 482.42.

10 The Joint Commission. (2015). Standard NPSG.01.01.01. *Comprehensive accreditation manual for hospitals: The official handbook.* Oakbrook Terrace, IL: The Joint Commission. (Level VII)

11 Siegel, J. D., et al. (2007). "2007 guideline for isolation precautions: Preventing transmission of infectious agents in healthcare settings" [Online]. Accessed March 2015 via the Web at http://www.cdc.gov/hicpac/pdf/isolation/Isolation2007.pdf (Level II)

12 Lynn-McHale Wiegand, D. (Ed.). (2011). *AACN procedure manual for critical care* (6th ed.). Philadelphia, PA: Saunders.

13 American Society of Anesthesiologists Task Force. (2013). Practice guidelines for management of the difficult airway: An updated report by the American Society of Anesthesiologists Task Force on Management of the Difficult Airway. *Anesthesiology, 118,* 251–270. Accessed March 2015 via the Web at http://www.asahq.org/publicationsAndServices/practiceparam.htm (Level IV)

14 Rutala, W. A., et al. (2008). "Guideline for disinfection and sterilization in healthcare facilities, 2008" [Online]. Accessed March 2015 via the Web at http://www.cdc.gov/hicpac/pdf/guidelines/Disinfection_Nov_2008.pdf (Level I)

15 American Osteopathic Association. (2014). Standard 07.02.03. *Healthcare Facilities Accreditation Program: Accreditation requirements for acute care hospitals.* Chicago, IL: American Osteopathic Association. (Level VII)

16 The Joint Commission. (2015). Standard RC.01.03.01. *Comprehensive accreditation manual for hospitals: The official handbook.* Oakbrook Terrace, IL: The Joint Commission. (Level VII)

17 American Osteopathic Association. (2014). Standard 10.00.03. *Healthcare Facilities Accreditation Program: Accreditation requirements for acute care hospitals.* Chicago, IL: American Osteopathic Association. (Level VII)

18 Centers for Medicare & Medicaid Services, Department of Health and Human Services. (2014). Condition of participation: Medical record services. 42 C.F.R. § 482.24(b).

ADDITIONAL REFERENCE

Bosson, N. (2012). "Laryngeal mask airway" [Online]. Accessed March 2015 via the Web at http://emedicine.medscape.com/article/82527-overview#a30

LASER THERAPY, ASSISTING

Using the highly focused and intense energy of a laser beam, the surgeon can treat various skin lesions. Laser therapy has several advantages. As a surgical instrument, the laser offers precise control. It spares normal tissue, speeds healing, and deters infection by sterilizing the operative site. In addition, by sealing tiny blood vessels as it vaporizes tissue, the laser beam leaves a nearly bloodless operative field.

Laser therapy can be performed on an outpatient basis. The lasers used most commonly to treat skin lesions are vascular, pigment, and carbon dioxide (CO_2) lasers. (See *Understanding types of laser therapy.*)

In general, laser surgery is safe, although bleeding and scarring can result. One pronounced hazard, to the patient and treatment staff alike, is eye damage or other injury caused by unintended laser beam reflection. For this reason, anyone in the surgical suite, including the patient, must wear special goggles to filter laser light, and the surgeon must use special nonreflective instruments. Access to the room must be strictly controlled, and all windows must be covered.

Equipment

Laser ▪ filtration face masks ▪ protective eyewear (approved by the laser safety officer)[1] ▪ laser vacuum ▪ extra vacuum filters ▪ surgical drape ▪ prescribed cleaning solution ▪ skin preparation product ▪ sterile gauze ▪ wet towels ▪ normal saline solution ▪ nonadherent dressings ▪ surgical tape ▪ cotton-tipped applicators ▪ nonreflective surgical instruments ▪ gown ▪ cap ▪ sterile gloves ▪ prescribed local anesthetic ▪ laser-use warning signs.

Preparation of equipment

Perform hand hygiene[2,3,4] and gather the equipment. Prepare the tray, which should include a local anesthetic, as ordered, as well as both dry gauze and gauze saturated in normal saline solution. The gauze will be used *to control bleeding, protect healthy tissue, and abrade and remove any eschar,* which would otherwise inhibit laser absorption. Prepare nonreflective surgical instruments as needed.

Cover all the windows and door windows in the treatment room *to prevent the laser from being seen through the windows, creating a potential for exposure.*[1]

Fire is a significant hazard during laser use. No one should use a laser in an oxygen-rich environment. Use caution near flammable solutions as well as volatile or combustible chemicals or liquids.[5] Make sure that water, normal saline solution, and a fire extinguisher are readily available for use during the procedure.[1] Refer to the manufacturer's instructions for use and fire safety information.[5]

Implementation

- Make sure the practitioner has obtained informed consent and that it's documented in the patient's medical record.[6,7]
- Conduct a preprocedure verification *to make sure that all relevant documentation, related information, and equipment are available and correctly identified to the patient's identifiers.*[8]
- Perform hand hygiene.[2,3,4]
- Confirm the patient's identity using at least two patient identifiers.[9]

Understanding types of laser therapy

Laser therapy is now an essential tool for treating many types of skin lesions. The number of lasers used in dermatology continues to grow, with different types used for specific conditions.

The term *laser* is an acronym for Light Amplification by the Stimulated Emission of Radiation. When directed toward the skin, most of this light energy is absorbed by *chromophores,* substances that absorb specific wavelengths of light. This is the basis of selective photothermolysis, which has revolutionized cutaneous laser surgery. Melanin is the target chromophore in pigmented lesions, and oxyhemoglobin within microvessels is the target chromophore in vascular lesions.

Make sure you're familiar with the various types of lasers and the indications for each.

Lasers for vascular lesions

The laser most commonly used for vascular lesions is the pulsed dye laser (PDL). Other lasers used for vascular lesions include copper vapor, argon, argon-pumped tunable dye, potassium-titanyl-phosphate (KTP), krypton, and neodymium:yttrium-aluminum-garnet (Nd:YAG). Vascular lesions appropriate for laser therapy include port-wine stains, hemangiomas, venous lake, rosacea, telangiectasia, and Kaposi sarcoma.

Lasers for pigmented lesions

Lasers that are effective in treating tattoos and dermal and epidermal pigmented lesions include Q-switched ruby, Q-switched Nd:YAG, Q-switched alexandrite, and PDL. Pigmented lesions appropriate for laser treatment include tattoos, freckles, and birthmarks, including nevi of Ota, melasma, solar lentigo, café-au-lait spots, Becker nevi, and epidermal nevi.

Lasers for hair removal

Lasers used to eliminate unwanted hair include ruby, alexandrite, and Nd:YAG. Laser treatment is only effective in removing dark-colored hair; it doesn't effectively remove blonde, red, white, or gray hair.

- Explain to the patient how the laser works and name its benefits. Point out the equipment and outline the procedure *to help allay the patient's concerns.*
- Put on a cap, gown, and filtration face mask as well as protective eyewear.
- If appropriate, make sure that the surgical site is marked.[10]
- Position the patient comfortably, drape him, and place normal saline solution–saturated gauze, if needed, over exposed tissue around the operative site. *To avoid thermal injuries,* make sure that all surgical drapes at the site are moist.[1]
- Place protective eyewear on the patient: goggles or glasses designed for the type of laser, if the patient will remain awake during the procedure; wet eye pads, laser-specific eye shields, or as designated by the laser safety officer if the patient will undergo general anesthesia; or metal corneal eye shields if the patient will undergo laser surgery on or around the eyelids.[1]
- Confirm that everyone in the room, including the patient, is wearing protective eyewear *to filter the laser light.*[1]
- Keep the door to the surgical suite closed and post warning signs regarding the type of laser used at all entrances to the laser treatment area *to keep unprotected people from inadvertently entering the room.*[1]
- Make sure that the surgical team conducts a time-out immediately before the surgeon begins the procedure *to perform a final assessment that the correct patient, site, positioning, and procedure are identified and, as applicable, all relevant information and necessary equipment are available.*[11]

- Make sure that the skin preparation product and hand antiseptic agents are completely dry before the laser is turned on *to prevent surgical fires. Use of nonflammable preparation agents minimizes the risk.*[1]
- Keep sponges and drapes near the surgical site moist *to reduce the risk of fire.* Ensure that wet towels and normal saline solution are available on the sterile field *to extinguish a fire if one occurs.*[1]

NURSING ALERT *With high-enough energy and absorption, laser beams can ignite clothing, hair, or paper products. The risk increases in the presence of oxygen, methane, and alcohol. Take such precautions as removing or protecting hair and clothing within the treatment areas* to prevent this risk. *The high voltage required by lasers can also result in electric shock. Proper wiring during installation is critical.*[12]

- After the surgeon administers the anesthetic and it takes effect, activate the laser vacuum. The CO_2 laser has a vacuum hose attached to a separate apparatus. Use this apparatus *to clear the surgical site.* The vacuum has a filter that traps and collects most of the vaporized tissue. Change the filter whenever suction decreases, and follow facility guidelines for filter disposal.
- When the surgeon finishes the procedure, perform hand hygiene,[2,3,4] put on sterile gloves, and apply direct pressure with a sterile gauze pad to any bleeding wound *until hemostasis is achieved.* If a wound continues to bleed, notify the practitioner.
- When the bleeding is controlled, use sterile technique to clean the area with a cotton-tipped applicator dipped in the prescribed cleaning solution. Then size and cut a nonadherent dressing. Secure the dressing with surgical tape.
- Discard equipment and supplies.
- Remove and discard your gloves and other personal protective equipment and perform hand hygiene.[2,3,4]
- Document the procedure.[13]

Special considerations

- Vascular and pigment lasers won't result in a wound; only superficial skin changes will occur.
- Make sure you have thorough knowledge of how each laser operates and of laser safety considerations for both the patient and health care providers.[1]

Patient teaching

Before the procedure, tell the patient that the surgeon uses the laser beam much as he would a scalpel to excise the lesion. Explain that the laser causes a burnlike wound that can be deep. Inform the patient that the wound will appear charred. Also, tell the patient that some of the eschar will be removed during the initial postoperative cleaning and that more will gradually dislodge at home. Warn the patient to expect a burning odor and smoke during the procedure, and that a machine called a smoke evacuator, which sounds like a vacuum cleaner, will clear it away. Advise the patient that he may sense heat from the laser. Urge him to tell the surgeon at once if pain develops.

Teach the patient how to dress his wound or care for his skin daily as ordered by the surgeon. Tell him that he can take showers, but he shouldn't immerse the wound in water *to promote wound healing and prevent infection.* If the wound bleeds at home, demonstrate how to apply direct pressure on the site with clean gauze or a washcloth for 20 minutes. If pressure doesn't control the bleeding, tell the patient to call his practitioner.

If the patient's foot or leg was operated on, urge him to keep the extremity elevated and to use it as little as possible *because pressure can inhibit healing.* Warn the patient to protect the treated area from exposure to the sun *to avoid changes in pigmentation.* Tell him to call the practitioner if he develops a temperature of 100°F (37.8°C) or higher that persists longer than 1 day.

Complications

Pain, bruising, redness, and blistering may occur after laser surgery. Scarring, pigment changes, and infection are rare complications of laser surgery. Delayed wound healing and allergic reaction are also potential complications of certain types of laser therapies.[12]

Laser safety complications include ocular damage, burns, and electric shock. Depending on the laser and its indication, laser-tissue interaction may produce a smoke plume, tissue splatter, or both, potentially transmitting infectious microorganisms.[12]

Documentation

Most patients who have laser surgery for skin lesions are treated as outpatients. Note the patient's skin condition before and after the procedure. Also document any bleeding, the type of dressing applied, and any patient complaints of pain. Note whether the patient understands home care instructions.

REFERENCES

1 Recommended practices for laser safety. (2014). In Conner, R., et al. (Eds.), *Perioperative standards and recommended practices 2014.* Denver, CO: AORN. (Level VII)

2 Centers for Disease Control and Prevention. (2002). Guideline for hand hygiene in health-care settings: Recommendations of the Healthcare Infection Control Practices Advisory Committee and the HICPAC/SHEA/APIC/IDSA Hand Hygiene Task Force. *MMWR Recommendations and Reports, 51*(RR-16), 1–45. Accessed March 2015 via the Web at http://www.cdc.gov/mmwr/pdf/rr/rr5116.pdf (Level II)

3 World Health Organization. (2009). "WHO guidelines on hand hygiene in health care: First global patient safety challenge, clean care is safer care" [Online]. Accessed March 2015 via the Web at http://whqlibdoc.who.int/publications/2009/9789241597906_eng.pdf (Level IV)

4 The Joint Commission. (2015). Standard NPSG.07.01.01. *Comprehensive accreditation manual for hospitals: The official handbook.* Oakbrook Terrace, IL: The Joint Commission. (Level VII)

5 Safe environment of care. (2014). In Conner, R., et al. (Eds.), *Perioperative standards and recommended practices 2014.* Denver, CO: AORN. (Level VII)

6 The Joint Commission. (2015). Standard RI.01.03.01. *Comprehensive accreditation manual for hospitals: The official handbook.* Oakbrook Terrace, IL: The Joint Commission. (Level VII)

7 Centers for Medicare & Medicaid Services, Department of Health and Human Services. (2014). Condition of participation: Patient's rights. 42 C.F.R. § 482.13.

8 The Joint Commission. (2015). Standard UP.01.01.01. *Comprehensive accreditation manual for hospitals: The official handbook.* Oakbrook Terrace, IL: The Joint Commission. (Level VII)

9 The Joint Commission. (2015). Standard NPSG.01.01.01. *Comprehensive accreditation manual for hospitals: The official handbook.* Oakbrook Terrace, IL: The Joint Commission. (Level VII)

10 The Joint Commission. (2015). Standard UP.01.02.01. *Comprehensive accreditation manual for hospitals: The official handbook.* Oakbrook Terrace, IL: The Joint Commission. (Level VII)

11 The Joint Commission. (2015). Standard UP.01.03.01. *Comprehensive accreditation manual for hospitals: The official handbook.* Oakbrook Terrace, IL: The Joint Commission. (Level VII)

12 Brown, C. W. (2012). "Complications of dermatologic laser surgery" [Online]. Accessed March 2015 via the Web at http://emedicine.medscape.com/article/1120837-overview

13 The Joint Commission. (2015). Standard RC.01.03.01. *Comprehensive accreditation manual for hospitals: The official handbook.* Oakbrook Terrace, IL: The Joint Commission. (Level VII)

ADDITIONAL REFERENCE

Plauntz, L. (2013). Guidelines for staff administering laser therapy in an office setting. *Plastic Surgical Nursing, 33,* 29–35. (Level VII)

LATEX ALLERGY PROTOCOL

Latex—a natural product of the rubber tree—is used in many products in the health care field. With the increased use of latex in barrier protection and medical equipment, more nurses and patients are becoming hypersensitive to it. Certain groups of people are at increased risk for developing latex allergy. These groups include people who have had or will undergo multiple surgical procedures (such as those with a history of spina bifida), health care workers (especially those who work in emergency departments and operating rooms), workers who manufacture latex and latex-containing products, and people with a genetic predisposition to latex allergy. Some studies also suggest that pregnant patients are at a greater risk for latex allergy.[1]

People allergic to certain cross-reactive foods, including bananas, avocados, chestnuts, cherries, grapes, kiwis, passion fruit, tomatoes, and peaches, may also be allergic to latex. Exposure to latex elicits an allergic response similar to the one that occurs with these foods.

For people with latex allergy, latex becomes a hazard when the protein in latex comes in direct contact with mucous membranes or is inhaled, which happens with the use of powdered latex surgical gloves. People with asthma are at greater risk for developing worsening signs and symptoms from airborne latex.

The diagnosis of latex allergy is based on the patient's history and physical examination. The patient should undergo laboratory testing to confirm or eliminate the diagnosis. Laboratory tests include skin testing, such as the skin-prick or patch test; the radioallergosorbent test, which measures the serum level of latex-specific immunoglobulin E in the blood; and other serum blood tests, such as Pharmacia CAP, AlaSTAT, and HYTEC.

Latex allergy can produce a myriad signs and symptoms, including generalized itching (such as on the hands and arms); itchy, watery, or burning eyes; sneezing and coughing (hay fever–type signs and symptoms); rash; hives; bronchial asthma, scratchy throat, or difficulty breathing; edema of the face, hands, or neck; and anaphylaxis.

To help identify a patient at risk for latex allergy, ask latex allergy–specific questions during the health history. (See *Latex allergy screening.*) If the patient's history reveals a latex sensitivity, the practitioner assigns him to one of three categories based on the extent of his sensitization:

- Group 1 patients have a history of anaphylaxis or a systemic reaction when exposed to a natural latex product.
- Group 2 patients have a clear history of an allergic reaction of a nonsystemic type.
- Group 3 patients don't have a previous history of latex hypersensitivity but are considered high risk because of an associated medical condition, occupation, or crossover allergy.

If you determine that the patient has a sensitivity to latex, ensure that he doesn't come in contact with latex because such contact could result in a life-threatening hypersensitivity reaction. Creating a latex-safe environment is the only way to safeguard the patient. Many facilities now designate nonlatex equipment, which is usually kept on a cart that can be moved into the patient's room.

Equipment

Nonlatex equipment, including room contents ▪ nonlatex protective materials (such as cloth, transparent dressing material, and gauze) ▪ anaphylaxis kit ▪ Optional: latex allergy sign, face mask with cloth ties, gauze wrap, latex-allergy patient identification bracelet.

Preparation of equipment

After you've determined that the patient has a latex allergy or is sensitive to latex, arrange for him to be placed in a private room. If that isn't possible, make the room latex-safe, even if the roommate hasn't been designated as hypersensitive to latex. *This intervention prevents the spread of airborne particles from latex products used on other patients.*

Latex allergy screening

To determine if the patient has a latex sensitivity or allergy, ask him the following screening questions:

- What is your occupation?
- Have you experienced an allergic reaction, local sensitivity, or itching following exposure to any latex products, such as balloons, dishwashing gloves, or condoms?
- Have you experienced shortness of breath or wheezing after blowing up balloons or after a dental visit?

Have you experienced itching in or around your mouth after eating a banana?

If the patient answers yes to any of these questions, proceed with the following questions:

- Do you have a history of allergies, dermatitis, or asthma? If so, what type of reaction do you have?
- Do you have any congenital abnormalities? If yes, explain.
- Do you have any food allergies? If so, what specific allergies do you have? Describe your reaction.
- If you experience shortness of breath or wheezing when blowing up latex balloons, describe your reaction.
- Have you had any previous surgical procedures? Did you experience associated complications? If so, describe them.
- Have you had previous dental procedures? Did you experience associated complications? If so, describe them.
- Are you exposed to latex in your occupation, and have you ever had a reaction to these products? If so, describe your reaction.

Implementation

- Perform hand hygiene.[2,3,4,5,6]
- Confirm the patient's identify using at least two patient identifiers.[7]
- Assess for possible latex allergy in every patient admitted to a labor and delivery unit or short-procedure unit or scheduled for a surgical procedure.
- Explain the protocol to the patient.
- Gather the appropriate equipment.
- Document in the patient's medical record and in the facility database that the patient has a latex allergy or is at high-risk for latex allergy.
- If your facility requires the patient to wear a latex-allergy identification bracelet, place it on the patient.
- Post a LATEX ALLERGY sign in the patient's room.
- If the patient will be receiving anesthesia, make sure that "latex allergy" is clearly visible on the front of his medical record. Also notify the circulating nurse on the surgical unit, the nurses on the postanesthesia care unit, and any other team members that the patient has a latex allergy. (See *Anesthesia induction and latex allergy,* page 482.)
- Bring a cart with nonlatex supplies into the room.
- If the patient must be transported to another area of the health care facility, make certain that the nonlatex cart accompanies him and that all health care workers who come in contact with him are wearing nonlatex gloves. The patient may need to wear a mask with cloth ties when leaving his room *to protect him from inhaling airborne latex particles.*
- Check adhesives and tapes, including electrocardiogram (ECG), electrodes, and dressing supplies, for latex content.
- Notify central supply and the dietary and pharmacy departments about the patient's allergy.
- If the patient will have an IV line, ensure that all products used to establish IV access are nonlatex products. Post a LATEX ALLERGY sign on the IV tubing *to prevent access of the line using latex products.*

Anesthesia induction and latex allergy

Latex allergy can cause signs and symptoms in both conscious and anesthetized patients.

Causes of intraoperative reaction	Signs and symptoms in a conscious patient	Signs and symptoms in an anesthetized patient
■ Latex contact with mucous membrane ■ Latex contact with intraperitoneal serosal lining ■ Inhalation of airborne latex particles during anesthesia ■ Injection of antibiotics and anesthetic agents through latex ports	■ Abdominal cramping ■ Anxiety ■ Bronchoconstriction ■ Diarrhea ■ Feeling of faintness ■ Generalized pruritus ■ Itchy eyes ■ Nausea ■ Shortness of breath ■ Swelling of soft tissue (hands, face, tongue) ■ Vomiting ■ Wheezing	■ Bronchospasm ■ Cardiopulmonary arrest ■ Facial edema ■ Flushing ■ Hypotension ■ Laryngeal edema ■ Tachycardia ■ Urticaria ■ Wheezing

■ If you must use latex tubing, flush the tubing with 50 mL of IV solution *to rinse it out.*

■ Place a warning label on IV bags that reads "Do not use latex injection ports."

■ Use a nonlatex tourniquet if available. If not, use a latex tourniquet over clothing.

■ Remove the vial stopper to mix and draw up medications.

■ Use nonlatex oxygen administration equipment. Remove the elastic, and tie the equipment on with gauze.

■ Use nonlatex equipment if available. If not, wrap stethoscopes, blood pressure cuffs and tubing, and ECG wires with a nonlatex product *to protect the patient from latex contact.*

■ Apply a transparent dressing over the patient's finger before using pulse oximetry *to create a barrier.*

■ Use nonlatex syringes when administering medication through a syringe.

■ Make sure that an anaphylaxis kit is readily available *so that you can act immediately if the patient has an allergic reaction to latex.*

■ Have a special latex-free crash cart outside the patient's room at all times.

■ Document the procedure.[8,9,10]

Special considerations

■ Remember that signs and symptoms of latex allergy usually occur within 30 minutes of anesthesia induction. However, the time of onset can range from 10 minutes to several hours.

■ Keep in mind that, as a health care worker, you're susceptible to developing latex hypersensitivity. If you suspect that you're sensitive to latex, contact the employee health services department concerning facility protocol for latex-sensitive employees. Use nonlatex products as often as possible *to help reduce your exposure to latex.* If you must wear latex gloves, wear the powder-free variety when possible *because the natural rubber latex proteins in powdered gloves attach to the cornstarch powder particles and become airborne when putting on and removing gloves.*

■ Don't assume that if something doesn't look like rubber, it isn't latex. Latex is found in a variety of equipment, including ECG leads, oral and nasal airway tubing, tourniquets, nerve stimulation pads, temperature strips, and blood pressure cuffs.

Patient teaching

Teach the patient that the best way to prevent an allergic reaction is to avoid latex exposure. Encourage the patient to obtain and wear a medical identification bracelet and to carry nonlatex gloves.[11] Teach the patient with a severe group 1 allergy to latex about the benefits and use of a prescribed epinephrine self-injection pen.[11] Instruct the patient to tell all health care workers, including dentists, about his latex allergy. Instruct him to read labels on household rubber items for latex content.

Documentation

Document the results of latex allergy screening, the date and time of screening, and notification of staff members of the patient's status. Document placement of signs and warning labels and any patient teaching provided.

References

1 Draisci, G., et al. (2011). Latex sensitization: A special risk for the obstetric population? *Anesthesiology, 114,* 565–569.

2 The Joint Commission. (2015). Standard NPSG.07.01.01. *Comprehensive accreditation manual for hospitals: The official handbook.* Oakbrook Terrace, IL: The Joint Commission. (Level VII)

3 Centers for Disease Control and Prevention. (2002). Guideline for hand hygiene in health-care settings: Recommendations of the Healthcare Infection Control Practices Advisory Committee and the HICPAC/SHEA/APIC/IDSA Hand Hygiene Task Force. *MMWR Recommendations and Reports, 51*(RR-16), 1–45. Accessed March 2015 via the Web at http://www.cdc.gov/mmwr/pdf/rr/rr5116.pdf (Level II)

4 World Health Organization. (2009). "WHO guidelines on hand hygiene in health care: First global patient safety challenge, clean care is safer care" [Online]. Accessed March 2015 via the Web at http://whqlibdoc.who.int/publications/2009/9789241597906_eng.pdf (Level IV)

5 American Osteopathic Association. (2014). Standard 07.01.21. *Healthcare Facilities Accreditation Program: Accreditation requirements for acute care hospitals.* Chicago, IL: American Osteopathic Association. (Level VII)

6 Centers for Medicare & Medicaid Services, Department of Health and Human Services. (2014). Condition of participation: Infection control. 42 C.F.R. § 482.42.

7 The Joint Commission. (2015). Standard NPSG.01.01.01. *Comprehensive accreditation manual for hospitals: The official handbook.* Oakbrook Terrace, IL: The Joint Commission. (Level VII)

8 The Joint Commission. (2015). Standard RC.01.03.01. *Comprehensive accreditation manual for hospitals: The official handbook.* Oakbrook Terrace, IL: The Joint Commission. (Level VII)

9 American Osteopathic Association. (2014). Standard 10.00.03. *Healthcare Facilities Accreditation Program: Accreditation requirements for acute care hospitals.* Chicago, IL: American Osteopathic Association. (Level VII)

10 Centers for Medicare & Medicaid Services, Department of Health and Human Services. (2014). Condition of participation: Medical record services. 42 C.F.R. § 482.24(b).

11 Pollart, S. M., et al. (2009). Latex allergy. *American Family Physician, 80,* 1413–1418. Accessed March 2015 via the Web at http://www.aafp.org/afp/2009/1215/p1413.html

ADDITIONAL REFERENCES

AORN latex guideline. (2014). In R. Conner, et al. (Eds.), *Perioperative standards and recommended practices 2014.* Denver, CO: AORN, Inc. (Level VII)

Centers for Disease Control and Prevention & National Institute for Occupational Safety and Health. (1998). "Latex allergy: A prevention guide (NIH Publication No. 98-113)" [Online]. Accessed March 2015 via the Web at http://www.cdc.gov/niosh/docs/98-113/

LIPID EMULSION ADMINISTRATION

Given as a separate solution in conjunction with parenteral nutrition or as a component of a total nutrient admixture or three-in-one solution, lipid emulsions are a source of calories and essential fatty acids. A deficiency in essential fatty acids can hinder wound healing, adversely affect production of red blood cells, and impair prostaglandin synthesis.

Currently, all of the IV lipid emulsions available in the United States are soybean oil–based; however, other countries have used alternative oil-based lipid emulsions containing olive oil and fish oil. Studies show that these alternative lipid emulsions may have fewer proinflammatory effects, less immune suppression, and more antioxidant effects than the standard soybean oil products.[1,2] Further research is needed to develop specific guidelines for their use.[2]

When given alone, lipid emulsions can be administered through a peripheral or a central venous line. Central venous access is preferred when lipid emulsion administration accompanies hypertonic parenteral nutrition solution administration.[3]

Lipid emulsions are contraindicated in patients who have a condition that disrupts normal fat metabolism, such as pathologic hyperlipidemia, lipid nephrosis, or acute pancreatitis. They also can't be given to patients with severe egg allergies. They must be used cautiously in patients who have liver or pulmonary disease, anemia, or coagulation disorders as well as in those who are at risk for developing a fat embolism.

Equipment

Patient's medical record ▪ prescribed lipid emulsion ▪ diethylhexyl phthalate–free lipid administration set[4] ▪ appropriate-sized syringe of preservative-free normal saline solution ▪ needleless connector ▪ tape ▪ antiseptic pads (alcohol, tincture of iodine, or chlorhexidine) ▪ IV infusion pump ▪ gloves ▪ Optional: time tape.

If you're administering the lipid emulsion as part of a total nutrient admixture or a three-in-one solution, also obtain a filter that's 1.2 microns or greater *because lipids will clog a smaller filter.*[4,5,6]

Preparation of equipment

To prevent aggregation of fat globules, don't shake the lipid container excessively. Protect the emulsion from freezing, and never add anything to it.

PEDIATRIC ALERT *The U.S. Food and Drug Administration (FDA) specifically requires a black box warning on all lipid injectable emulsions approved for use in the United States, outlining the potential for significant morbidity and mortality* because of poor clearance of the IV fat emulsion. *Administration in premature and small-for-gestational-age infants shouldn't exceed 1 g/kg in 4 hours.* Infant deaths following infusion of IV fat emulsions have been reported, resulting in the FDA warning.[7,8]

Implementation

- Avoid distractions and interruptions when preparing and administering lipids *to prevent medication errors.*[9,10]
- Verify the order on the patient's medication record by checking it against the practitioner's order.[11]
- Gather the appropriate supplies and the lipid infusion.
- Compare the label on the lipid emulsion with the order in the patient's medical record. The label should contain the appropriate patient identifiers, the administration date and time, the patient's current weight, the route of administration, and the complete name and prescribed amount of lipid emulsion, including the total volume to be infused, the infusion rate in milliliters per hour, the duration of the infusion, and the expiration date.[6]
- Check the patient's medical record for an allergy or contraindication to the lipid emulsion. If an allergy or contraindication exists, don't administer it; instead, notify the practitioner.[12,13,14]
- Inspect the emulsion for opacity and consistency of color and texture. If the emulsion looks frothy or oily or contains particles, or if you think its stability or sterility is questionable, return the bottle to the pharmacy.[12,13,14]
- Discuss unresolved concerns about lipids with the patient's practitioner.[12,13,14]
- Perform hand hygiene.[15,16,17,18,19]
- Confirm the patient's identity using at least two patient identifiers.[20]
- If the patient is receiving lipids for the first time, teach him about potential adverse reactions or other concerns.[12,13,14]
- Verify that the lipid emulsion is being administered at the proper time, in the prescribed dose, and by the correct route *to reduce the risk of medication errors.*[12,13,14]
- If your facility uses a bar code scanning system, scan your identification badge, the patient's identification bracelet, and the lipid bar code.
- Explain the procedure to the patient *to promote cooperation.*
- Put on gloves.[21]
- Using aseptic technique, remove the protective cap from the lipid emulsion bottle, thoroughly disinfect the rubber stopper with an antiseptic pad, and allow the stopper to dry.
- Hold the bottle upright and, using strict aseptic technique, insert the vented spike through the inner circle of the rubber stopper.
- Invert the bottle, and squeeze the drip chamber until it fills to the level indicated in the tubing package instructions.
- Open the flow clamp and prime the tubing. Gently tap the tubing *to dislodge air bubbles trapped in the Y-ports.* If necessary, attach a time tape to the lipid emulsion container *to monitor fluid intake.*
- Label the tubing, noting the date and time the tubing was hung.[22]
- Thoroughly disinfect the needleless access port of the peripheral or central venous access device with an antiseptic pad using friction and allow it to dry.[23]
- Attach the needleless prefilled syringe to the needleless access port, unclamp the catheter, and slowly aspirate until you obtain a brisk blood return *to confirm the proper function and patency of the access device.*[22,24]
- Slowly inject the preservative-free normal saline flush solution and reclamp the catheter.
- Attach the primed lipid emulsion tubing to the needleless connector.
- Trace the tubing from the patient to its point of origin and then put the lipid emulsion tubing into the infusion pump.[25]
- Program the infusion pump following the manufacturer's instructions. For the patient's first lipid infusion, set the test dose at a rate of 1 mL/minute for 30 minutes or as ordered.

NURSING ALERT *A lipid infusion is considered a high-alert medication* because it can cause significant patient harm when used in error. *Another nurse must double-check certain procedure steps* to ensure safe medication administration.[26]

■ Before beginning a lipid infusion, if required by your facility, have another nurse perform an independent double-check *to verify the patient's identity and make sure that the correct medication is hanging in the prescribed concentration, the medication's indication corresponds with the patient's diagnosis, the dosage calculations are correct and the dosing formula used to derive the final dose is correct, the route of administration is safe and proper for the patient, the pump settings are correct, and the infusion line is attached to the correct port.*[27]
■ After comparing results of the independent double-check with another nurse (if required), begin infusing the medication if no discrepancies exist. If discrepancies exist, rectify them before beginning the infusion.
■ Unclamp the catheter and start the infusion pump.
■ Make sure that the infusion pump alarm limits are set appropriately and that the alarms are turned on, functioning properly, and audible to staff.[28,29,30]
■ Monitor the patient's vital signs, and watch for signs and symptoms of adverse reactions, such as fever; flushing, sweating, or chills; a pressure sensation over the eyes; nausea; vomiting; headache; chest and back pain; tachycardia; dyspnea; and cyanosis. An allergic reaction usually is due to either the source of lipids or to eggs, which occur in the emulsion as egg phospholipids, an emulsifying agent.
■ If the patient has no adverse reactions to the test dose, begin the infusion at the prescribed rate after an independent double-check with another nurse, if required.[27]
■ Dispose of supplies in appropriate receptacles.
■ Remove and discard your gloves.
■ Perform hand hygiene.[15,16,17,18,19]
■ Document the procedure.[31,32,33]

Special considerations

■ The Joint Commission issued a sentinel event alert concerning medical device alarm safety *because alarm-related events have been associated with permanent loss of function or death.* Among the major contributing factors were improper alarm settings, alarm settings inappropriately turned off, and alarm signals not audible to staff. Make sure alarm limits are set appropriately and that alarms are turned on and audible to staff. Follow facility guidelines for preventing alarm fatigue.[29]
■ Exercise caution when administering IV lipid emulsions to patients with severe liver damage, pulmonary disease, anemia, or blood coagulation disorders and when a danger of fat embolism is present.[7,8]
■ Be aware that IV lipid emulsions contain aluminum; levels can become toxic with prolonged use in patients with kidney impairment.[7,8]
■ Always maintain strict aseptic technique while preparing and handling equipment.[4,23]
■ If the lipid emulsion will be piggybacked into parenteral nutrition, connect it between the filter and the patient's access device; control flow rates of each infusion with separate pumps.[8]
■ If a multilumen catheter will be used to administer parenteral nutrition, one port should be designated exclusively for parenteral nutrition administration.[34]
■ Observe the patient's reaction to the lipid emulsion. Most patients report a feeling of satiety; some complain of an unpleasant metallic taste.
■ Change the administration set and the lipid emulsion container every 24 hours when given continuously.[4,6] If lipids are given intermittently, change the administration set with each new container. Change immediately upon suspected contamination, or when the integrity of the system has been compromised.[23]
■ Make sure a dietitian or clinician with expertise in nutrition performs a nutrition assessment and formulates a nutrition care plan that describes intervention and monitoring and reevaluation parameters.[34]
■ Monitor for lipid tolerance rate. Cloudy plasma in a centrifuged sample of citrated blood indicates that the lipids haven't been cleared from the patient's bloodstream.
■ Be aware that a lipid emulsion may clear from the blood at an accelerated rate in patients with full-thickness burns, multiple traumatic injuries, or a metabolic imbalance *because catecholamines, adrenocortical hormones, thyroxine, and growth hormone enhance lipolysis and embolization of fatty acids.*
■ Obtain weekly laboratory tests, as ordered. Usual tests include liver function studies, prothrombin time, platelet count, and serum triglyceride levels. Whenever possible, draw blood for triglyceride levels at least 6 hours after the completion of the lipid emulsion infusion *to avoid falsely elevated results.*
■ Never rehang a partially empty bottle of emulsion *because a lipid emulsion is an excellent medium for bacterial growth.*
■ Complete the infusion of lipid emulsions within 12 to 24 hours, as ordered.[4,34]

Complications

Immediate or early adverse reactions to lipid emulsion therapy, which occur in less than 1% of patients, include fever, dyspnea, cyanosis, nausea and vomiting, headache, flushing, diaphoresis, lethargy, syncope, chest and back pain, slight pressure over the eyes, irritation at the infusion site, hyperlipidemia, hypercoagulability, and thrombocytopenia.

PEDIATRIC ALERT *Thrombocytopenia has been reported in infants receiving a 20% IV lipid emulsion.*

Delayed but uncommon complications associated with prolonged administration of lipid emulsion include hepatomegaly, splenomegaly, jaundice secondary to central lobular cholestasis, and blood dyscrasias (such as thrombocytopenia, leukopenia, and transient increases in liver function studies). Dry or scaly skin, thinning hair, abnormal liver function studies, and thrombocytopenia may indicate a deficiency of essential fatty acids. For unknown reasons, some patients develop brown pigmentation in the reticuloendothelial system.

Documentation

Record the times of all dressing changes and solution changes, the condition of the catheter insertion site, your assessments of the patient's condition, and any complications and resulting interventions. Also document patient and family teaching and their understanding of the teaching.[35]

References

1 Barbosa, V. M., et al. (2010). Effects of a fish oil containing lipid emulsion on plasma phospholipid fatty acids, inflammatory markers, and clinical outcomes in septic patients: A randomized, controlled clinical trial. *Critical Care, 14*(1), R5. Accessed March 2015 via the Web at http://www.ncbi.nlm.nih.gov/pmc/articles/PMC2875515/ (Level I)
2 Vanek, V. W., et al. (2012). A.S.P.E.N. position paper: Clinical role for alternative intravenous fat emulsions. *Nutrition in Clinical Practice, 27,* 150–192.
3 Standard 32. Vascular access device selection. Infusion nursing standards of practice. (2011). *Journal of Infusion Nursing, 34,* S37–S40. (Level VII)
4 Standard 43. Administration set change. Infusion nursing standards of practice. (2011). *Journal of Infusion Nursing, 34,* S55–S57. (Level VII)
5 Standard 28. Filters. Infusion nursing standards of practice. (2011). *Journal of Infusion Nursing, 34,* S33–S34. (Level VII)
6 Ayers, P., et al. (2014). A.S.P.E.N. parenteral nutrition safety consensus recommendations. *Journal of Parenteral and Enteral Nutrition, 38,* 296–333. Accessed March 2015 via the Web at http://pen.sagepub.com/content/38/3/296.full.pdf+html (Level VII)
7 Hospira, Inc. (2005, revised 2009). "Liposyn III® intravenous fat emulsion" [Online]. Accessed March 2015 via the Web at http://www.drugs.com/pro/liposyn-iii.html
8 "Intralipid® 20%" [Online]. (2007). Accessed March 2015 via the Web at http://www.rxlist.com/intralipid-20-drug/indications-dosage.htm
9 Westbrook, J., et al. (2010). Association of interruptions with an increased risk and severity of medication administration errors. *Archives of Internal Medicine, 170,* 683–690. (Level IV)

10 Institute for Safe Medication Practices. (2013). Side tracks on the safety express: Interruptions lead to errors and unfinished . . . Wait, what was I doing? *Nurse Advise-Err, 11*(2), 1–4. Accessed March 2015 via the Web at https://www.ismp.org/Newsletters/acutecare/showarticle.aspx?id=37 (Level VII)

11 The Joint Commission. (2015). Standard MM.04.01.01. *Comprehensive accreditation manual for hospitals: The official handbook.* Oakbrook Terrace, IL: The Joint Commission. (Level VII)

12 The Joint Commission. (2015). Standard MM.06.01.01. *Comprehensive accreditation manual for hospitals: The official handbook.* Oakbrook Terrace, IL: The Joint Commission. (Level VII)

13 American Osteopathic Association. (2014). Standard 16.01.03. *Healthcare Facilities Accreditation Program: Accreditation requirements for acute care hospitals.* Chicago, IL: American Osteopathic Association. (Level VII)

14 Centers for Medicare & Medicaid Services, Department of Health and Human Services. (2014). Condition of participation: Nursing services. 42 C.F.R. § 482.23(c).

15 The Joint Commission. (2015). Standard NPSG.07.01.01. *Comprehensive accreditation manual for hospitals: The official handbook.* Oakbrook Terrace, IL: The Joint Commission. (Level VII)

16 Centers for Disease Control and Prevention. (2002). Guideline for hand hygiene in health-care settings: Recommendations of the Healthcare Infection Control Practices Advisory Committee and the HICPAC/SHEA/APIC/IDSA Hand Hygiene Task Force. *MMWR Recommendations and Reports, 51*(RR-16), 1–45. Accessed March 2015 via the Web at http://www.cdc.gov/mmwr/pdf/rr/rr5116.pdf (Level II)

17 World Health Organization. (2009). "WHO guidelines on hand hygiene in health care: First global patient safety challenge, clean care is safer care" [Online]. Accessed March 2015 via the Web at http://whqlibdoc.who.int/publications/2009/9789241597906_eng.pdf (Level IV)

18 American Osteopathic Association. (2014). Standard 07.01.10. *Healthcare Facilities Accreditation Program: Accreditation requirements for acute care hospitals.* Chicago, IL: American Osteopathic Association. (Level VII)

19 Centers for Medicare & Medicaid Services, Department of Health and Human Services. (2014). Condition of participation: Infection control. 42 C.F.R. § 482.42.

20 The Joint Commission. (2015). Standard NPSG.01.01.01. *Comprehensive accreditation manual for hospitals: The official handbook.* Oakbrook Terrace, IL: The Joint Commission. (Level VII)

21 Siegel, J. D., et al. (2007). "2007 guideline for isolation precautions: Preventing transmission of infectious agents in healthcare settings" [Online]. Accessed March 2015 via the Web at http://www.cdc.gov/hicpac/pdf/isolation/Isolation2007.pdf (Level II)

22 Infusion Nurses Society. (2011). *Policies and procedures for infusion nursing* (4th ed.). Boston, MA: Infusion Nurses Society.

23 Centers for Disease Control and Prevention. (2011). "Guidelines for the prevention of intravascular catheter-related infections" [Online]. Accessed March 2015 via the Web at http://www.cdc.gov/hicpac/pdf/guidelines/bsi-guidelines-2011.pdf (Level I)

24 Standard 45. Flushing and Locking. Infusion nursing standards of practice. (2011). *Journal of Infusion Nursing, 34,* S59–S63. (Level VII)

25 U.S. Food and Drug Administration. (n.d.). "Look. Check. Connect. Safe medical device connections save lives" [Online]. Accessed March 2015 via the Web at http://www.fda.gov/downloads/MedicalDevices/Safety/AlertsandNotices/UCM134873.pdf

26 Institute for Safe Medication Practices. (2012)."ISMP's list of high-alert medications" [Online]. Accessed March 2015 via the Web at http://www.ismp.org/tools/highalertmedications.pdf (Level VII)

27 Institute for Safe Medication Practices. (2008). Conducting an independent double-check. *ISMP Medication Safety Alert! Nurse Advise-ERR, 6*(12), 1. Accessed March 2015 via the Web at http://www.ismp.org/newsletters/nursing/Issues/NurseAdviseERR200812.pdf (Level VII)

28 The Joint Commission. (2015). Standard NPSG.06.01.01. *Comprehensive accreditation manual for hospitals: The official handbook.* Oakbrook Terrace, IL: The Joint Commission. (Level VII)

29 The Joint Commission. (2013). "Sentinel event alert: Medical device alarm safety in hospitals" [Online]. Accessed March 2015 via the Web at http://www.jointcommission.org/assets/1/18/SEA_50_alarms_4_5_13_FINAL1.PDF (Level VII)

30 Graham, K. C., & Cvach, M. (2010). Monitor alarm fatigue: Standardizing use of physiological monitors and decreasing nuisance alarms. *American Journal of Critical Care, 19,* 28–37.

31 The Joint Commission. (2015). Standard RC.01.03.01. *Comprehensive accreditation manual for hospitals: The official handbook.* Oakbrook Terrace, IL: The Joint Commission. (Level VII)

32 American Osteopathic Association. (2014). Standard 10.00.03. *Healthcare Facilities Accreditation Program: Accreditation requirements for acute care hospitals.* Chicago, IL: American Osteopathic Association. (Level VII)

33 Centers for Medicare & Medicaid Services, Department of Health and Human Services. (2014). Condition of participation: Medical record services. 42 C.F.R. § 482.24(b).

34 Ukleja, A., et al. (2010). Standards for nutrition support: Adult hospitalized patients. *Nutrition in Clinical Practice, 25,* 403–414.

35 Standard 14. Documentation. Infusion nursing standards of practice. (2011). *Journal of Infusion Nursing, 34,* S20–S21. (Level VII)

LOW-AIR-LOSS THERAPY BED USE

Low-air-loss therapy beds consist of segmented, air-filled cushions that provide surface area for pressure relief. Studies have shown that these beds are effective in preventing pressure ulcers in obese patients,[1] although recent research hasn't demonstrated that this type of support surface is superior in preventing and treating skin breakdown and minimizing pain than other support surfaces.[2] They're indicated for patients with skin grafts and surgical flaps, pressure ulcers, edema, and malnutrition as well as oncology, orthopedic, and transplant patients.

Low-air-loss therapy beds inflate to specific pressures based on the height and weight of the patient. The segmented air cushions, covered by a low-friction fabric, inflate and rest on a bed frame (similar to a standard bed frame), reducing pressure on skin surfaces and diminishing shearing forces when repositioning the patient. A maximum-inflate feature allows the entire surface to become firm for patient repositioning. The system is also capable of deflating quickly in emergencies. As with a standard bed frame, you can adjust the head and foot of the bed.

These beds also assist with microclimate management by circulating air, which helps to evaporate moisture and reduce temperature, reducing excess skin moisture and preventing maceration.[3] Some models are equipped with pulsation or rotational capability. Pulsation promotes circulation, which improves healing; lateral rotation capability raises one lung over the other, mobilizing secretions and preventing pulmonary complications.[4] Larger beds are available for bariatric patients, and some bed models allow pressure zone and lumbar support adjustment. (See *Low-air-loss therapy bed,* page 486.)

Keep in mind that, although pressure redistribution devices are helpful for preventing and managing pressure ulcers, they shouldn't replace repositioning protocols; instead, they should serve as adjunct therapy.[5] Low-air-loss therapy beds are contraindicated for patients with an unstable cervical, thoracic, or lumbar fracture. Patients with uncontrolled diarrhea, hemodynamic instability, severe agitation, or uncontrolled claustrophobia may not benefit from this bed.

Equipment

Low-air-loss therapy bed ■ turning sheet ■ Optional: assistive transfer device, pillows or foam wedges, gloves.

Preparation of equipment

Usually the manufacturer's representative or a trained staff member prepares the bed for use. The unit is plugged in and turned on to inflate the bed. Make sure the bed inflates properly and that the equipment is in working order. The settings (such as degrees of rotation) are adjusted as appropriate. Fully inflate the bed until the patient is moved onto it.

EQUIPMENT

Low-air-loss therapy bed

A low-air-loss therapy bed reduces pressure on skin surfaces and may be used for patients with such conditions as immobility, malnutrition, incontinence, contractures, fractures, or amputations. Some models come with special features, such as rotational or percussion options.

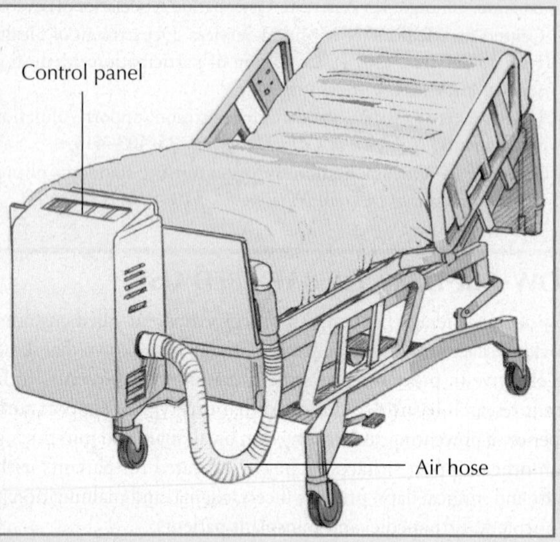

Implementation

- Perform hand hygiene and put on gloves, as necessary.[6,7,8,9,10,11,12]
- Confirm the patient's identity using at least two patient identifiers.[13]
- Explain and, if possible, demonstrate the operation of the low-air-loss therapy bed. Tell the patient the reason for its use. Explain the bed's special features, such as lumbar supports and rotation.
- With the help of four or more coworkers, transfer the patient to the bed using a lift sheet, or use a hydraulic lift.

NURSING ALERT *Use an assistive device, such as a hydraulic lift, for a one-person-dependent transfer to prevent injury. The device contains moveable and lockable wheels for positioning and moving, a base that can be widened to fit around chairs or toilets, and a hydraulic release valve that's tightened to close and lift and loosened to open and lower. Most are made up of a single seat sling made of canvas and nylon netting, chains, and hooks connected to a spreader bar.*[14,15]

- Start with the settings as set by the representative, monitor the patient for comfort, and ensure proper functioning of the bed.
- Adjust the inflation settings on the control panel according to the patient's comfort and therapeutic use.
- Remove and discard your gloves, if worn, and perform hand hygiene.[6,7,8,9,10]
- Document the procedure.[16,17,18]

Special considerations

- Encourage coughing and deep breathing every 2 hours.
- Turn the patient at least every 2 hours and reposition him using an approved turning sheet. Some beds come with special foam wedges that are used for repositioning.
- To turn and reposition the patient, use the maximum-inflate feature *to fully inflate the bed.* Use the turning sheet to position the patient and place the pillows or foam wedges. Then return the bed to the correct patient settings.
- If the bed is rotational, verify that invasive lines and tubes are secured at the correct angle *to minimize the risk for binding, disconnecting, or dislodging.*
- To position a bedpan, deflate the seat portion of the bed, roll the patient away from you, and place the bedpan on the turning sheet. Then reposition the patient. To remove the bedpan, hold it steady, roll the patient away from you, and remove the bedpan. Then reinflate the seat portion of the bed.
- Don't use pins or clamps to secure sheets or tubing *because they may puncture the bed and result in air loss.* Take care to avoid puncturing the bed when giving injections.
- Assess the patient's skin every 2 hours. Assess pressure ulcer risk on admission to your facility, at regular intervals, and with any signs of skin or wound deterioration.[5]
- Engage the emergency or cardiopulmonary resuscitation button during cardiac arrest *to help ensure adequate chest compressions.*

Documentation

Record the duration of therapy and the patient's response to it. Document the condition of the patient's skin, including the presence of pressure ulcers and other wounds. Document the patient's comfort level and tolerance of rotational angles, as applicable.

References

1 Pemberton, V., et al. (2009). The effect of using a low-air-loss surface on the skin integrity of obese patients: Results of a pilot study. *Ostomy/Wound Management, 55*(2), 44–48.

2 Somnath, S., et al. (2013). "Pressure ulcer treatment strategies: Comparative effectiveness review no. 90" [Online]. Accessed March 2015 via the Web at http://www.ncbi.nlm.nih.gov/books/NBK143657/pdf/TOC.pdf (Level I)

3 Krasner, D. L., et al. (2012). *Chronic wound care 5: A clinical source book for healthcare professionals.* Malvern, PA: HMP Communications, LLC.

4 Bryant, R. A., & Nix, D. P. (2012). *Acute and chronic wounds: Current management concepts* (4th ed.). St. Louis, MO: Mosby.

5 Wound, Ostomy and Continence Nurses Society (WOCN). (2003, revised 2010). "WOCN clinical practice guideline no. 2: Guideline for prevention and management of pressure ulcers" [Online]. Accessed March 2015 via the Web at http://guideline.gov/content.aspx?id=23868 (Level VII)

6 The Joint Commission. (2015). Standard NPSG.07.01.01. *Comprehensive accreditation manual for hospitals: The official handbook.* Oakbrook Terrace, IL: The Joint Commission. (Level VII)

7 Centers for Disease Control and Prevention. (2002). Guidelines for hand hygiene in health-care settings: Recommendations of the Healthcare Infection Control Practices Advisory Committee and the HICPAC/SHEA/APIC/IDSA Hand Hygiene Task Force. *MMWR Recommendations and Reports, 51*(RR-16), 1–45. Accessed March 2015 via the Web at http://www.cdc.gov/mmwr/pdf/rr/rr5116.pdf (Level II)

8 World Health Organization. (2009). "WHO guidelines on hand hygiene in health care: First global patient safety challenge, clean care is safer care" [Online]. Accessed March 2015 via the Web at http://whqlibdoc.who.int/publications/2009/9789241597906_eng.pdf (Level IV)

9 Centers for Medicare & Medicaid Services, Department of Health and Human Services. (2014). Condition of participation: Infection control. 42 C.F.R. § 482.42.

10 American Osteopathic Association. (2014). Standard 07.01.21. *Healthcare Facilities Accreditation Program: Accreditation requirements for acute care hospitals.* Chicago, IL: American Osteopathic Association. (Level VII)

11 Siegel, J. D., et al. (2007). "2007 guideline for isolation precautions: Preventing transmission of infectious agents in healthcare settings" [Online]. Accessed March 2015 via the Web at http://www.cdc.gov/hicpac/pdf/isolation/Isolation2007.pdf (Level II)

12 American Osteopathic Association. (2014). Standard 07.01.10. *Healthcare Facilities Accreditation Program: Accreditation requirements for acute care hospitals.* Chicago, IL: American Osteopathic Association. (Level VII)
13 The Joint Commission. (2015). Standard NPSG.01.01.01. *Comprehensive accreditation manual for hospitals: The official handbook.* Oakbrook Terrace, IL: The Joint Commission. (Level VII)
14 American Nurses Association. (2013). *Safe patient handling and mobility: Interprofessional national standards.* Silver Spring, MD: American Nurses Association.
15 Occupational Safety and Health Administration. (2009). "Guidelines for nursing homes: Ergonomics for the prevention of musculoskeletal disorders" [Online]. Accessed March 2015 via the Web at http://www.osha.gov/ergonomics/guidelines/nursinghome/final_nh_guidelines.html
16 The Joint Commission. (2015). Standard RC.01.03.01. *Comprehensive accreditation manual for hospitals: The official handbook.* Oakbrook Terrace, IL: The Joint Commission. (Level VII)
17 Centers for Medicare & Medicaid Services, Department of Health and Human Services. (2014). Condition of participation: Patient's rights. 42 C.F.R. § 482.13(b)(2).
18 American Osteopathic Association. (2014). Standard 10.00.03. *Healthcare Facilities Accreditation Program: Accreditation requirements for acute care hospitals.* Chicago, IL: American Osteopathic Association. (Level VII)

LUMBAR PUNCTURE, ASSISTING

Lumbar puncture involves the insertion of a sterile needle into the subarachnoid space of the spinal canal, usually between the third and fourth lumbar vertebrae. This procedure is used to determine the presence of blood in cerebrospinal fluid (CSF), obtain CSF specimens for laboratory analysis, inject dyes for contrast in radiologic studies, or administer drugs or anesthesia. The pressure of CSF, which flows freely between the brain and the spinal column, can also be measured during the procedure.

Performed by a practitioner with a nurse assisting, lumbar puncture requires sterile technique and careful patient positioning. This procedure is contraindicated in patients with increased intracranial pressure (ICP) with mass effect, a lumbar deformity, a platelet count of less than 50,000/mm, or an International Normalized Ratio greater than 1.5 as well as in those receiving anticoagulants[1] or who have an infection at the puncture site.

Equipment

Overbed or procedure table ■ sterile gloves ■ mask with face shield or mask and goggles ■ sterile gown ■ antiseptic solution ■ sterile gauze pads or antiseptic sponges ■ antiseptic pads ■ sterile fenestrated drape ■ 3-mL syringe ■ 25G ¾″ (1.9 cm) sterile needle ■ local anesthetic (usually 1% lidocaine without epinephrine) ■ 22G 3½″ (8.9 cm) spinal needle with stylet[2] ■ three-way stopcock ■ manometer ■ small adhesive bandage ■ three sterile collection tubes with caps ■ labels ■ light source ■ sterile marker ■ sterile labels ■ laboratory transport bag ■ Optional: patient-care reminder, prescribed analgesia or anxiolytic, prescribed contrast medium, laboratory request form.

Disposable lumbar puncture trays contain most of the needed sterile equipment.

Implementation

■ Verify the practitioner's order.
■ Gather the equipment and take it to the patient's bedside.
■ Confirm that the practitioner has obtained written informed consent and that the consent is in the patient's medical record.[3,4,5]
■ Perform a preprocedure verification *to make sure that all relevant documentation, related information, and equipment is available and is correctly identified to the patient's identifiers.*[6,7]
■ Verify that the laboratory and imaging studies are complete, as ordered, and that the results are in the patient's medical record. Notify the practitioner of any unexpected results.
■ Perform hand hygiene.[8,9,10,11,12]
■ Confirm the patient's identity using at least two patient identifiers.[13]
■ Provide privacy.[14,15]
■ Explain the procedure to the patient *to ease his anxiety and ensure his cooperation.*[3,4]
■ Inform the patient that he may experience a headache after lumbar puncture, but reassure him that his cooperation during the procedure will minimize such an effect.
■ Check the patient's history for hypersensitivity to local anesthetic, antiseptic solution, analgesia, or sedation.
■ Instruct the patient to void before the procedure.
■ If prescribed, give analgesia or anxiolytic medication using safe medication practices *to promote comfort and decrease anxiety so the patient can maintain his position during the procedure.*[16]
■ Perform hand hygiene.[8,9,10,17,18]
■ Open the equipment tray on an overbed or procedure table, being careful not to contaminate the sterile field when you open the wrapper.
■ Label all medications, medication containers, and other solutions on and off the sterile field.[19,20]
■ Provide adequate lighting at the puncture site, and adjust the height of the patient's bed *to allow the practitioner to perform the procedure comfortably.*
■ Position the patient and reemphasize the importance of remaining as still as possible *to minimize discomfort and trauma.* (See *Positioning for lumbar puncture,* page 488.)
■ Perform hand hygiene.[8,9,10,11,12]
■ Put on a cap, a mask with a face shield or a mask and goggles, a sterile gown, and sterile gloves.[1,16,21]
■ The practitioner cleans the puncture site with antiseptic solution and allows it to dry *to prevent contamination by the body's normal skin flora.* He then drapes the area with the sterile fenestrated drape *to provide a sterile field.* (If the practitioner uses antiseptic sponges instead of sterile gauze pads, he may remove his sterile gloves and put on another pair *to avoid introducing antiseptic solution into the subarachnoid space with the lumbar puncture needle.*)

NURSING ALERT *Studies suggest that chlorhexidine is neurotoxic; its use as an antiseptic agent for skin preparation before lumbar puncture is controversial.*[16,22,23]

■ Conduct a time-out before starting the procedure *to determine that the correct patient, site, positioning, and procedure are identified and confirmed as applicable.*[7,24]
■ If the equipment tray doesn't include an ampule of anesthetic, disinfect the injection port of a vial of anesthetic with an antiseptic pad. Then invert the vial 45 degrees *so that the practitioner can insert a 25G needle and syringe and withdraw the anesthetic for injection.*
■ Before the practitioner injects the anesthetic, tell the patient he'll experience a transient burning sensation and local pain. Ask him to report any other persistent pain or sensations *because they may indicate irritation or puncture of a nerve root, requiring repositioning of the needle.*
■ When the practitioner inserts the sterile spinal needle into the subarachnoid space between the third and fourth lumbar vertebrae, instruct the patient to remain still and breathe normally. If necessary, hold the patient firmly in position *to prevent sudden movement that may displace the needle.*
■ If the practitioner is performing lumbar puncture to administer contrast medium for radiologic studies or spinal anesthetic, he injects the dye or anesthetic at this time.
■ When the needle is in place, the practitioner attaches a manometer with a three-way stopcock to the needle hub *to read CSF pressure.* If

Positioning for lumbar puncture

Have the patient lie on his side at the edge of the bed, with his chin tucked to his chest and his knees drawn up to his abdomen. Make sure the patient's spine is curved and his back is at the edge of the bed (as shown below). *This position widens the spaces between the vertebrae, easing insertion of the needle.*

To help the patient maintain this position, place one of your hands behind his neck and the other hand behind his knees, and pull gently. Hold the patient firmly in this position throughout the procedure *to prevent accidental needle displacement.* Typically, the practitioner inserts the needle between the third and fourth lumbar vertebrae (as shown below).

Patient positioning

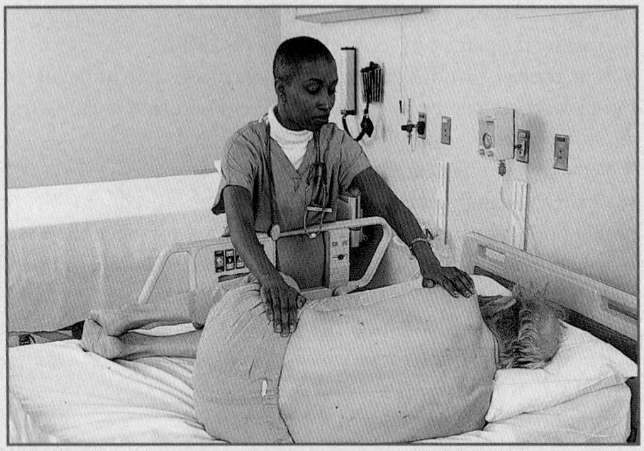

Needle insertion

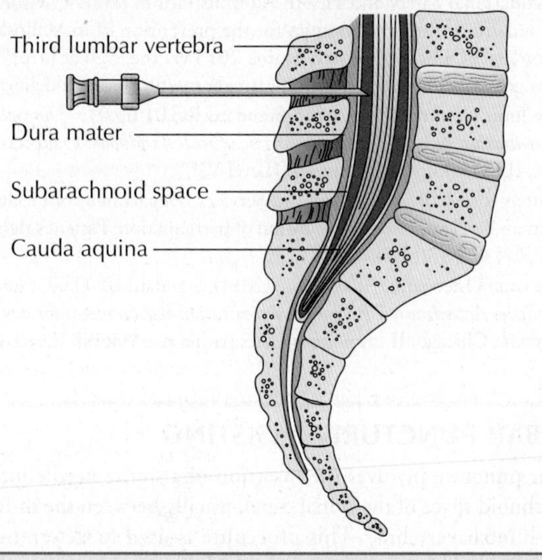

ordered, help the patient extend his legs *to provide a more accurate pressure reading.*

■ The practitioner then detaches the manometer and allows CSF to drain from the needle hub into the collection tubes. When he has collected 2 to 3 mL in each tube, mark the tubes in sequence and securely cap them. Label the specimens in the presence of the patient *to prevent mislabeling.*[13]

■ After the practitioner collects the specimens and removes the spinal needle, he applies a sterile occlusive dressing to the puncture site.[16]

■ Discard used supplies in the appropriate receptacle.[25]

■ Remove and discard your gloves and other personal protective equipment.[21]

■ Perform hand hygiene.[8,9,10,11,12]

■ Place the CSF specimens in a laboratory transport bag and send them to the laboratory immediately, with completed laboratory request forms if needed. Send collected CSF specimens to the laboratory immediately; they can't be refrigerated them for later transport *because refrigeration alters results.*[26]

■ Perform hand hygiene.[8,9,10,11,12]

■ Document the procedure.[27,28,29]

Special considerations

■ During lumbar puncture, watch closely for signs of an adverse reaction, including elevated pulse rate, pallor, and clammy skin. Alert the practitioner immediately of any significant changes.

■ Monitor CSF test results and report critical results to the practitioner within the time frame determined by your facility *to prevent treatment delays.*[30]

■ The practitioner may order the patient to remain flat or at a 30-degree angle for 30 minutes to several hours. Check the practitioner's orders for the specific position and duration.

■ Encourage the patient to drink fluids after the procedure *to restore spinal fluid volume and reduce the risk of headache.*

■ Check the puncture site for redness, swelling, and drainage every hour for the first 4 hours, and then every 4 hours for the next 24 hours.

■ If CSF pressure is elevated, assess the patient's neurologic status every 15 minutes for 4 hours. If he's stable, assess him every hour for 2 hours and then every 4 hours, or according to the pretest schedule.

■ For an obese patient, the practitioner may use an ultrasound *to help determine accurate needle placement.*[31]

Complications

Headache is the most common adverse effect of lumbar puncture. Others adverse effects may include a reaction to the anesthetic, meningitis, epidural or subdural abscess, bleeding into the spinal canal, CSF leakage through the dural defect remaining after needle withdrawal, local pain caused by nerve root irritation, edema or hematoma at the puncture site, transient difficulty voiding, and fever. The most serious complications of lumbar puncture, although rare, are tonsillar herniation and medullary compression.

Documentation

Record that you took a time-out before the procedure to verify the correct patient, correct site, and correct procedure.[24] Document the time that the procedure started and ended. Record the patient's response to the procedure, administration of drugs, number of specimen tubes collected, time of specimen transport to the laboratory, and color, consistency, and other characteristics of the collected specimens. Document patient teaching.

References

1 Siegel, J. D., et al. (2007). "2007 guideline for isolation precautions: Preventing transmission of infectious agents in healthcare settings" [Online]. Accessed March 2015 via the Web at http://www.cdc.gov/hicpac/pdf/isolation/Isolation2007.pdf (Level II)

2 Armon, C., et al. (2005, reaffirmed, 2008). Addendum to assessment: Prevention of post-lumbar puncture headaches. *Neurology, 65,* 510–512. Accessed March 2015 via the Web at http://www.neurology.org/content/65/4/510.abstract

3 The Joint Commission. (2015). Standard RI.01.03.01. *Comprehensive accreditation manual for hospitals: The official handbook.* Oakbrook Terrace, IL: The Joint Commission. (Level VII)
4 Centers for Medicare & Medicaid Services, Department of Health and Human Services. (2014). Condition of participation: Patient's rights. 42 C.F.R. § 482.13(b)(2).
5 American Osteopathic Association. (2014). Standard 15.01.11. *Healthcare Facilities Accreditation Program: Accreditation requirements for acute care hospitals.* Chicago, IL: American Osteopathic Association. (Level VII)
6 The Joint Commission. (2015). Standard UP.01.01.01. *Comprehensive accreditation manual for hospitals: The official handbook.* Oakbrook Terrace, IL: The Joint Commission. (Level VII)
7 American Osteopathic Association. (2014). Standard 30.00.14. *Healthcare Facilities Accreditation Program: Accreditation requirements for acute care hospitals.* Chicago, IL: American Osteopathic Association. (Level VII)
8 The Joint Commission. (2015). Standard NPSG.07.01.01. *Comprehensive accreditation manual for hospitals: The official handbook.* Oakbrook Terrace, IL: The Joint Commission. (Level VII)
9 Centers for Disease Control and Prevention. (2002). Guideline for hand hygiene in health-care settings: Recommendations of the Healthcare Infection Control Practices Advisory Committee and the HICPAC/SHEA/APIC/IDSA Hand Hygiene Task Force. *MMWR Recommendations and Reports, 51*(RR-16), 1–45. Accessed March 2015 via the Web at http://www.cdc.gov/mmwr/pdf/rr/rr5116.pdf (Level II)
10 World Health Organization. (2009). "WHO guidelines on hand hygiene in health care: First global patient safety challenge, clean care is safer care" [Online]. Accessed March 2015 via the Web at http://whqlibdoc.who.int/publications/2009/9789241597906_eng.pdf (Level IV)
11 American Osteopathic Association. (2014). Standard 07.01.21. *Healthcare Facilities Accreditation Program: Accreditation requirements for acute care hospitals.* Chicago, IL: American Osteopathic Association. (Level VII)
12 Centers for Medicare & Medicaid Services, Department of Health and Human Services. (2014). Condition of participation: Infection control. 42 C.F.R. § 482.42.
13 The Joint Commission. (2015). Standard NPSG.01.01.01. *Comprehensive accreditation manual for hospitals: The official handbook.* Oakbrook Terrace, IL: The Joint Commission. (Level VII)
14 American Osteopathic Association. (2014). Standard 15.01.16. *Healthcare Facilities Accreditation Program: Accreditation requirements for acute care hospitals.* Chicago, IL: American Osteopathic Association. (Level VII)
15 Centers for Medicare & Medicaid Services, Department of Health and Human Services. (2014). Condition of participation: Patient's rights. 42 C.F.R. § 482.13(c)(1).
16 Lynn-McHale Wiegand, D. (Ed.). (2011). *AACN procedure manual for critical care* (6th ed.). St. Louis, MO: Saunders.
17 Centers for Medicare & Medicaid Services, Department of Health and Human Services. (2014). Condition of participation: Nursing services. 42 C.F.R. § 482.23(c).
18 American Osteopathic Association. (2014). Standard 16.01.03. *Healthcare Facilities Accreditation Program: Accreditation requirements for acute care hospitals.* Chicago, IL: American Osteopathic Association. (Level VII)
19 The Joint Commission. (2015). Standard NPSG.03.04.01. *Comprehensive accreditation manual for hospitals: The official handbook.* Oakbrook Terrace, IL: The Joint Commission. (Level VII)
20 American Osteopathic Association. (2014). Standard 25.01.27. *Healthcare Facilities Accreditation Program: Accreditation requirements for acute care hospitals.* Chicago, IL: American Osteopathic Association. (Level VII)
21 American Osteopathic Association. (2014). Standard 07.01.10. *Healthcare Facilities Accreditation Program: Accreditation requirements for acute care hospitals.* Chicago, IL: American Osteopathic Association. (Level VII)
22 Daily, P. (2009). "Chlorhexidine or povidone-iodine: Do we follow the guidelines or the package insert?" [Online]. Accessed March 2015 via the Web at http://apicwv.org/docs/19.pdf
23 Recommended practices for preoperative patient skin antisepsis. (2014). In R. Connor, et al. (Eds.), *Perioperative standards and recommended practices 2014.* Denver, CO: AORN, Inc. (Level VII)
24 The Joint Commission. (2015). Standard UP.01.03.01. *Comprehensive accreditation manual for hospitals: The official handbook.* Oakbrook Terrace, IL: The Joint Commission. (Level VII)
25 Occupational Safety and Health Administration. (n.d.). "Bloodborne pathogens, standard number 1910.1030" [Online]. Accessed March 2015 via the Web at http://www.osha.gov/pls/oshaweb/owadisp.show_document?p_table STANDARDS&p_id 10051 (Level VII)
26 Fischbach, F., & Dunning, M. B. (2014). *A manual of laboratory and diagnostic tests* (8th ed.). Philadelphia, PA: Wolters Kluwer.
27 The Joint Commission. (2014). Standard RC.01.03.01. *Comprehensive accreditation manual for hospitals: The official handbook.* Oakbrook Terrace, IL: The Joint Commission. (Level VII)
28 American Osteopathic Association. (2014). Standard 10.00.03. *Healthcare Facilities Accreditation Program: Accreditation requirements for acute care hospitals.* Chicago, IL: American Osteopathic Association. (Level VII)
29 Centers for Medicare & Medicaid Services, Department of Health and Human Services. (2014). Condition of participation: Medical record services. 42 C.F.R. § 482.24(b).
30 The Joint Commission. (2015). Standard NPSG.02.03.01. *Comprehensive accreditation manual for hospitals: The official handbook.* Oakbrook Terrace, IL: The Joint Commission. (Level VII)
31 Strony, R. (2010). Ultrasound-assisted lumbar puncture in obese patients. *Critical Care Clinics, 26,* 661–664.

ADDITIONAL REFERENCE

Nettina, S. M. (2014). *Lippincott manual of nursing practice* (10th ed.). Philadelphia, PA: Wolters Kluwer.

MANUAL VENTILATION

A handheld resuscitation bag is an inflatable device that can be attached to a face mask or directly to an endotracheal (ET) or tracheostomy tube, allowing manual delivery of oxygen or room air to the lungs of a patient who can't breathe by himself. Typically used in emergencies, manual ventilation can also can be performed while a patient is temporarily disconnected from mechanical ventilation, such as during a tubing change, during transport, or before suctioning. In such instances, use of the handheld resuscitation bag maintains ventilation.

During cardiopulmonary resuscitation (CPR), however, using a handheld resuscitation bag to administer rescue breaths is less important than providing high-quality chest compressions. Lone rescuers should begin chest compressions first. After 30 compressions, the rescuer should then administer two breaths. When a second person arrives, that person can use a handheld resuscitation bag to administer two breaths after every 30 compressions.

Equipment

Handheld resuscitation bag with mask ▪ oxygen source ▪ oxygen tubing ▪ nipple adapter attached to oxygen flowmeter ▪ gloves ▪ oropharyngeal or nasopharyngeal airway ▪ suction apparatus ▪ suction tubing ▪ suction catheters ▪ Optional: personal protective equipment, oropharyngeal airway, oxygen accumulator (oxygen reservoir), emergency resuscitation equipment (crash cart with cardiac medications, defibrillator, and intubation equipment).

Preparation of equipment

Unless the patient is intubated or has a tracheostomy, select a mask that fits snugly over the mouth and nose. Attach the mask to the resuscitation bag.

If oxygen is readily available, connect the handheld resuscitation bag to the oxygen. Attach one end of the tubing to the bottom of the bag and the other end to the nipple adapter on the flowmeter of the oxygen source.

Turn on the oxygen and adjust the flow rate to 15 L/minute. If the patient has a low partial pressure of arterial oxygen, he'll need a higher fraction of inspired oxygen (FIO_2). *To increase the concentration of inspired oxygen,* you can add an oxygen accumulator (also called an oxygen reservoir). This device, which attaches to an adapter on the bottom of the bag, permits an FIO_2 of up to 100%. If time allows, set up suction equipment.

Implementation

■ Perform hand hygiene[1,2,3,4,5] and put on gloves and other personal protective equipment, as needed.[6,7]

■ Confirm the patient's identity using at least two patient identifiers.[8]

■ Explain the procedure to the patient.

■ Before using the handheld resuscitation bag, check the patient's upper airway for foreign objects. If present, remove them *because doing so may restore spontaneous respirations in some instances and because foreign matter or secretions can obstruct the airway and impede resuscitation efforts.*

■ Suction the patient *to remove any secretions that may obstruct the airway.* If necessary, insert an oropharyngeal or nasopharyngeal airway *to maintain airway patency.* If the patient has a tracheostomy or ET tube in place, suction the tube.

■ If appropriate, remove the bed's headboard and stand at the head of the bed *to help keep the patient's neck extended and to free space at the side of the bed for other activities such as CPR.*

■ Unless the patient has evidence of head or neck trauma, use the head-tilt, chin-lift maneuver to open the patient's airway *to move the tongue away from the base of the pharynx and prevent obstruction of the airway.*[9]

■ Apply the mask. (See *How to apply a handheld resuscitation bag and mask.*)

■ Keeping your nondominant hand on the patient's mask, exert downward pressure *to seal the mask against his face.* For the adult patient, use your dominant hand to compress the bag to deliver 600 mL of air over 1 second *to produce a rise in the patient's chest.*[9]

■ Deliver breaths with the patient's own inspiratory effort, if any is present. Don't attempt to deliver a breath as the patient exhales. During CPR, deliver two breaths (each over 1 second) during a brief pause (about 3 to 4 seconds) after 30 chest compressions.[9]

■ Observe the patient's chest *to ensure that it rises and falls with each compression.*[9] If ventilation fails to occur, check the fit of the mask and the patency of the patient's airway; if necessary, reposition his head and ensure patency with an oral airway.

■ Assist with ET intubation if necessary. (See the "Endotracheal intubation" procedure, page 278.)

■ Remove and discard your gloves and any other personal protective equipment worn, and perform hand hygiene.[1,2,3,4,5]

■ Document the procedure.[10,11,12]

Special considerations

■ Avoid neck hyperextension if the patient has a possible cervical injury; instead, use the jaw-thrust maneuver to open the airway. If you need both hands to keep the patient's mask in place with a good seal and maintain hyperextension, use the lower part of your arm to compress the bag against your side until another rescuer is available to assist.

■ Observe for vomiting through the clear part of the mask. If vomiting occurs, stop the procedure immediately, lift the mask, wipe and suction vomitus, and resume resuscitation.

■ An oropharyngeal airway should be inserted only in an unresponsive patient who has lost his gag reflex.

■ It isn't possible to deliver an accurate or exact tidal volume while using a handheld resuscitation bag and mask.[13]

■ If a second rescuer relieves you in performing chest compressions during CPR and you're using the handheld resuscitation bag and mask to deliver breaths, make sure the use of the bag doesn't interfere with the performance of chest compressions.[9]

Complications

Aspiration of vomitus may result in pneumonia, and gastric distention may result from air forced into the patient's stomach. In an emergency, hyperventilation of the patient may cause increased intrathoracic pressure with a subsequent decrease in coronary and cerebral perfusion pressures.

Documentation

In an emergency, record the date and time of the procedure, the reason for initiating the procedure, any complications and the nursing action taken, and the patient's response to treatment using your facility's documentation system or flow sheet for respiratory distress.

If it isn't an emergency, record the date and time of the procedure as well as the reason and length of time the patient was disconnected from mechanical ventilation and received manual ventilation. Note the patient's tolerance of the procedure, along with any complications and nursing actions taken. Document any patient and family teaching and their understanding of your teaching.

REFERENCES

1 The Joint Commission. (2015). Standard NPSG.07.01.01. *Comprehensive accreditation manual for hospitals: The official handbook.* Oakbrook Terrace, IL: The Joint Commission. (Level VII)

2 Centers for Disease Control and Prevention. (2002). Guideline for hand hygiene in health-care settings: Recommendations of the Healthcare Infection Control Practices Advisory Committee and the HICPAC/SHEA/APIC/IDSA Hand Hygiene Task Force. *MMWR Recommendations and Reports, 51*(RR-16), 1–45. Accessed May 2015 via the Web at http://www.cdc.gov/mmwr/pdf/rr/rr5116.pdf (Level II)

3 World Health Organization. (2009). "WHO guidelines on hand hygiene in health care: First global patient safety challenge, clean care is safer care" [Online]. Accessed May 2015 via the Web at http://whqlibdoc.who.int/publications/2009/9789241597906_eng.pdf (Level IV)

4 American Osteopathic Association. (2012). Standard 07.01.21. *Healthcare Facilities Accreditation Program: Accreditation requirements for acute care hospitals.* Chicago, IL: American Osteopathic Association. (Level VII)

5 Centers for Medicare & Medicaid Services, Department of Health and Human Services. (2014). Condition of participation: Infection control. 42 C.F.R. § 482.42.

6 Siegel, J. D., et al. (2007). "2007 guideline for isolation precautions: Preventing transmission of infectious agents in healthcare settings" [Online]. Accessed May 2015 via the Web at http://www.cdc.gov/hicpac/pdf/isolation/Isolation2007.pdf (Level II)

7 American Osteopathic Association. (2014). Standard 07.01.10. *Healthcare Facilities Accreditation Program: Accreditation requirements for acute care hospitals.* Chicago, IL: American Osteopathic Association. (Level VII)

8 The Joint Commission. (2015). Standard NPSG.01.01.01. *Comprehensive accreditation manual for hospitals: The official handbook.* Oakbrook Terrace, IL: The Joint Commission. (Level VII)

9 American Heart Association. (2010). 2010 American Heart Association guidelines for cardiopulmonary resuscitation and emergency cardiovascular care. *Circulation, 122,* S729–S767, S876–S908. (Level II)

10 The Joint Commission. (2015). Standard RC.02.01.01. *Comprehensive accreditation manual for hospitals: The official handbook.* Oakbrook Terrace, IL: The Joint Commission. (Level VII)

11 Centers for Medicare & Medicaid Services, Department of Health and Human Services. (2014). Condition of participation: Medical record services. 42 C.F.R. § 482.24(b).

12 American Osteopathic Association. (2014). Standard 10.00.03. *Healthcare Facilities Accreditation Program: Accreditation requirements for acute care hospitals.* Chicago, IL: American Osteopathic Association. (Level VII)

EQUIPMENT

How to apply a handheld resuscitation bag and mask

Place the mask over the patient's face so that the apex of the triangle covers the bridge of his nose and the base lies between his lower lip and chin *to create a tight seal*. Hold the mask in place (as shown below).

Using your nondominant hand, create a C shape with the thumb and index finger over the top of the mask and apply gentle downward pressure. Hook the remaining fingers around the mandible and lift it upward toward the mask, creating an E shape (as shown below). Make sure that the patient's mouth remains open underneath the mask. Attach the resuscitation bag to the mask and the tubing leading to the oxygen source.

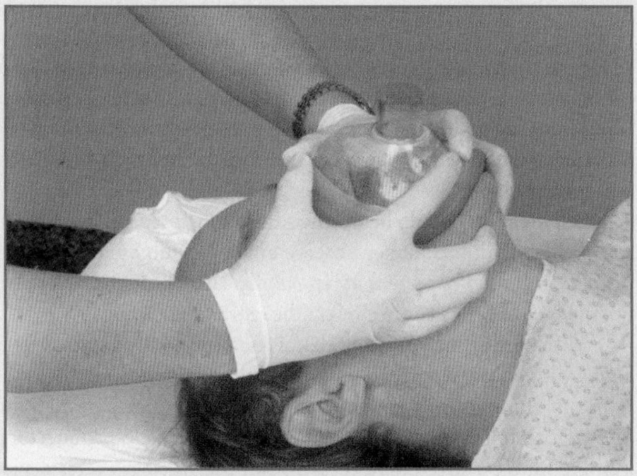

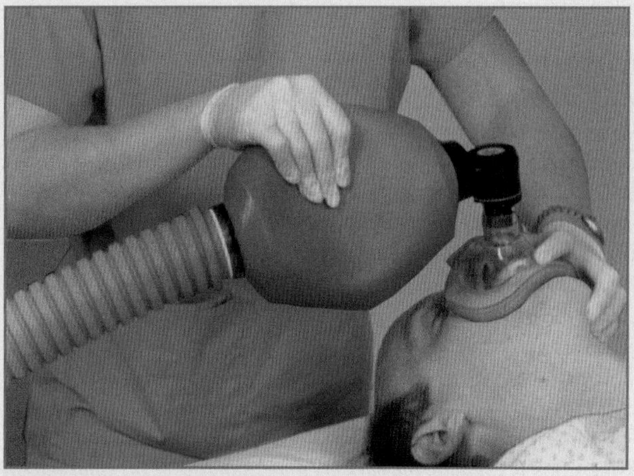

If the patient has a tracheostomy or endotracheal tube in place, remove the mask from the bag and attach the handheld resuscitation bag directly to the tube.

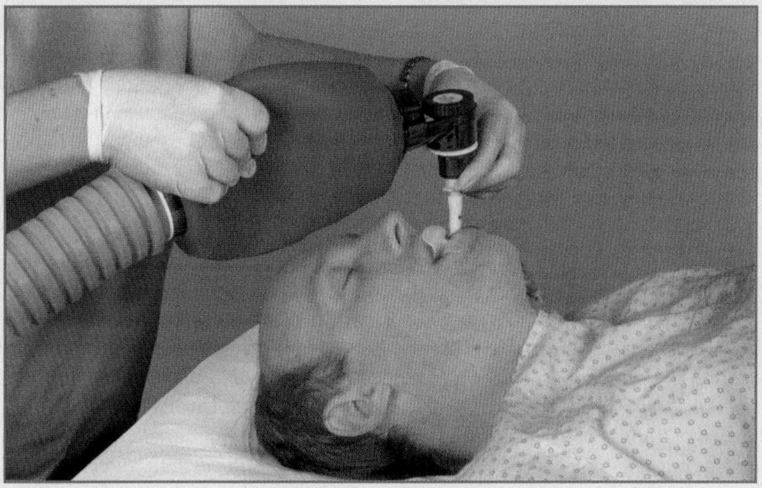

13 Lee, H. M., et al. (2008). Can you deliver accurate tidal volume by manual resuscitator? *Emergency Medicine Journal, 25,* 632–634. (Level VI)

ADDITIONAL REFERENCES

Lynn-McHale Wiegand, D. (Ed.). (2011). *AACN procedure manual for critical care* (6th ed.). Philadelphia, PA: Saunders.

Nettina, S. M. (2014). *Lippincott manual of nursing practice* (10th ed.). Philadelphia, PA: Wolters Kluwer.

MASSIVE INFUSION DEVICE USE

A massive infusion device is a mechanical device used in patients who need rapid fluid replacement with IV fluids or blood products. It can warm IV fluids or blood products to room temperature to prevent hypothermia and then administer the fluid rapidly at rates of up to 45,000 mL/hour.[1] The device requires specialized IV tubing that expands under pressure.[2] Patients with life-threatening conditions, such as severe trauma, GI or postoperative hemorrhage, septic shock, or burns, may need require the use of a rapid infusion device to receive large volumes of fluids within a short period.[2]

Equipment

Massive infusion device ▪ prescribed IV fluids or blood products ▪ 10-mL syringe containing preservative-free normal saline solution ▪ appropriate infusion set with warming device or heat exchanger[1,3] ▪ replacement filter or vent or large-capacity reservoir, as indicated[1,3] ▪ IV pole ▪ gloves ▪ gown ▪ mask with face shield ▪ antiseptic pads (chlorhexidine-based, alcohol, or tincture of iodine) ▪ needleless connector ▪

monitoring equipment ▪ blankets ▪ Optional: indwelling urinary catheter, IV catheter insertion equipment, supplies for blood gas sampling.

Preparation of equipment

Male sure that the equipment is safe for massive, rapid, or pressurized infusion.[4]

Set up and use a warming device or heat exchanger following the manufacturer's instructions for use. Make sure that systems are plugged into an outlet *to ensure that the infused fluid is heated properly.*[1,3] Make sure that the device alarm limits are set appropriately and that the alarms are turned on, functioning properly, and audible to staff.[4,5,6] Troubleshoot alarms according to the specific manufacturer's instructions for use.[1,3]

Implementation

▪ Verify the practitioner's orders, including whether you should warm the fluid or blood.[7,8,9]
▪ Confirm that the practitioner has obtained written informed consent and that the consent is in the patient's medical record.[10,11,12,13]
▪ Verify that baseline coagulation studies and hematocrit, electrolyte, and hemoglobin levels have been obtained *to serve as a comparison and help guide fluid replacement.*[2,14]
▪ Check the patient history for allergies, as indicated.
▪ Perform hand hygiene.[15,16,17,18,19,20,21,22]
▪ Confirm the patient's identity using at least two patient identifiers.[23]
▪ Reinforce the practitioner's explanation of the procedure and answer any questions *to evaluate the patient's understanding of the information provided and reduce anxiety.*
▪ If the patient doesn't already have one in place, insert an indwelling urinary catheter, as ordered, *to help monitor fluid resuscitation efforts.* (See the "Indwelling urinary catheter insertion" procedure, page 394.)
▪ Perform hand hygiene and put on gloves and other personal protective equipment as needed.[15,16,17,18,19,20,24]
▪ Make sure the patient has a large-bore, patent IV access.[8] If not, insert an IV catheter *to administer IV fluid and medications, as needed, until a central venous catheter can be inserted.* (See the "IV catheter insertion and removal" procedure, page 446.)
▪ Assist the practitioner with insertion of a central venous or pulmonary artery catheter *to facilitate administration of large fluid volumes and to help monitor the patient's fluid status.*[2]
▪ Assist the practitioner with arterial catheter insertion *for continuous blood pressure assessment.* (See the "Arterial pressure monitoring" procedure, page 31.)[2]
▪ Turn on the infusion device *to allow the system to warm up.*[2]
▪ If you're infusing blood products, perform a pretransfusion blood verification with another qualified health care provider *to prevent life-threatening blood incompatibility errors.*[8,23,25] (See the "Transfusion of blood and blood products" procedure, page 783.)

HOSPITAL-ACQUIRED CONDITION ALERT *Keep in mind that blood incompatibility errors are considered hospital-acquired conditions* because various best practices can reasonably prevent them. *Follow best practices, such as properly identifying the blood sample used for compatibility testing and the patient, before administering blood and blood products.*[26]

▪ Remove the appropriate administration set from its packaging. Inspect the administration sets for loose or missing luer and spike caps *to ensure sterility.*[1,3]

Using the Level 1 infuser

▪ Install the appropriate administration set into the infusion device according to the manufacturer's instructions.[3]
▪ Secure the heat exchanger and gas vent filter in their proper positions and turn them on, following the manufacturer's instructions.[2,3]
▪ Close all of the clamps on the Y-administration set.[3]
▪ Invert and spike the fluid or blood product bag. Squeeze the bag *to remove all air* and connect the ordered fluid or blood product to the Y-set. Then hang the bag on the hooks provided within the rapid infuser pressure chambers.[2] Close the pressure chamber door and secure the latch. Repeat for each fluid line you'll use.[3]
▪ Open the clamps above the drip chamber for each IV fluid bag you'll use.[3]
▪ Fill the drip chambers on the administration set halfway by squeezing them *to prevent air from entering the tubing.*[2] Repeat with each fluid line, as indicated.[3]
▪ Open the remaining clamps above the heat exchanger *so that fluid will flow into the gas vent filter assembly.*[3]
▪ Vigorously tap the gas vent filter assembly *to dislodge air bubbles from the filter screen,* according to the manufacturer's instructions. Inspect the tubing and filter when finished *to make sure there are no air bubbles.*[2]
▪ Remove the male luer cap from the distal end of the administration set tubing.[3]
▪ Open the pinch clamp below the gas vent filter assembly. Allow fluid to flow until you no longer observe air in the tubing and the line is primed with fluid *to prevent air embolism.* Then close the roller clamp. Put a new needleless connector on the end of the tubing.[3,27]
▪ Thoroughly disinfect the needleless connector of the patient's venous access with an antiseptic pad using friction, and allow it to dry.[21,27]
▪ Maintaining sterility of the syringe tip, attach a syringe containing preservative-free normal saline solution to the needleless connector and aspirate for a positive blood return from the vascular access device *to confirm patency.*[28,29]
▪ Slowly flush the device with preservative-free normal saline solution *to assess catheter function.*[28,29]
▪ Thoroughly disinfect the catheter hub or needleless connector with an antiseptic pad using friction, and allow it to dry.[28,29]
▪ Trace the tubing from the patient to its point of origin *to make sure that you're attaching the tubing to the proper port.*[30]
▪ Connect the distal end of the tubing to the patient's vascular access catheter.
▪ Complete functional testing of all audible and visual alarms according to the manufacturer's instructions. If any visual indicator doesn't illuminate or the audible signal doesn't sound, remove the device from service immediately.[3]
▪ After confirming proper infusion device operation, unclamp the tubing and begin the infusion, adjusting the infusion rate as needed.[2]

Using the Belmont infuser

▪ Install the appropriate administration set into the infusion device according to the manufacturer's instructions.[1]
▪ Confirm that the heat exchanger is secured properly.[1]
▪ As needed for infusion of larger volumes of fluid, replace the reservoir chamber with the larger-capacity reservoir. Using aseptic technique, remove the reservoir chamber from the administration set by disconnecting the luer connectors.[1]
▪ Attach the reservoir holder onto the IV pole and place the larger reservoir into the holder.[1]
▪ Attach the three fluid supply tails onto the top of the larger reservoir to be used.[1]
▪ Connect the larger reservoir to the administration set. Adjust the reservoir holder *to make sure that the connection leads underneath the reservoir aren't stretched or kinked.*[1]
▪ Hang the fluid bag on the IV pole.[1]
▪ Close the bag clamps, remove the bag spike cap, thoroughly disinfect the port with a disinfectant pad and allow it to dry, and then spike the fluid bag, piercing it fully *to ensure that fluids flow freely.*[1]
▪ Repeat with additional fluid lines that you'll use.[1]

■ Open the bag clamps.[1]
■ Prime the main system by pressing the PRIME button to recirculate 100 mL of fluid at 500 mL/minute *to remove air and replace the main system with fluid.*[1]
■ Prime the remainder of the administration tubing by opening the roller clamp and removing the male luer cap at the distal end of the tubing. Press the PT. LINE PRIME button once *to prime at 50 mL/minute* and press and hold the button *to prime at 200 mL/minute.* Press the STOP button after inspecting the tubing *to make sure there are no air bubbles.* Press the PT. LINE PRIME button again *to remove any remaining air.*[1]
■ Put a new needleless connector on the end of the tubing.[27]
■ Thoroughly disinfect the needleless connector of the patient's venous access device with an antiseptic pad using friction, and allow it to dry.[21,28,29,31]
■ Maintaining sterility of the syringe tip, attach a syringe containing preservative-free normal saline solution to the needleless connector and aspirate for a positive blood return from the vascular access device *to confirm patency.*[28,29]
■ Slowly flush the device with preservative-free normal saline solution *to assess catheter function.*
■ Thoroughly disinfect the catheter hub or needleless connector with an antiseptic pad using friction, and allow it to dry.[21,28,29]
■ Trace the tubing from the patient to its point of origin *to make sure that you're attaching the tubing to the proper port.*[30]
■ Connect the distal end of the tubing to the patient's vascular access catheter.[1]
■ Press INFUSE to start infusing and adjust the flow rate as needed.[1]

Completing the procedure

■ Monitor the patient's vital signs every 5 to 15 minutes, as indicated. As the patient's condition stabilizes, monitor vital signs less frequently (every 30 minutes until the patient's blood pressure is stable for longer than 2 hours).[2]
■ Monitor core temperature every 15 to 30 minutes and maintain a core temperature no lower than 96.8°F (36°C) *to prevent hypothermia-induced coagulopathies.*[2]
■ Assess the patient's hemodynamic parameters every 15 to 30 minutes and urine output every 30 to 60 minutes, as ordered, *to evaluate the patient's fluid volume status, which indicates the effectiveness of fluid resuscitation and can be used to guide therapy.*[2]
■ Inspect IV sites every 15 minutes *because rapid infusion increases the risk of infiltration.*[2]
■ If the patient is receiving blood products, monitor him closely for signs of a transfusion reaction, such as fever, chills, flushing, nausea, chest tightness, restlessness, apprehension, and back pain.[28]
■ Obtain an arterial blood gas sample, as ordered, *to monitor oxygenation and acid-base balance.* (See the "Arterial puncture for blood gas analysis" procedure, page 37.)
■ When the infusion is complete, change the IV fluid or blood bag according to the specific manufacturer's instructions.
■ Discard the empty infusion bag in the proper receptacle.[20,24] Note that some facilities require that empty blood transfusion bags be returned to the blood bank.
■ Obtain blood samples for hemoglobin, hematocrit, lactic acid, and electrolyte testing as well as coagulation studies, as ordered. (See the "Venipuncture" procedure, page 821.)
■ Report all critical test results to the practitioner within the time frame established by your facility *to prevent life-threatening treatment delays.*[32]
■ Cover the patient with blankets *to keep him warm and prevent hypothermia.*[2]
■ Dispose of used equipment in appropriate receptacles.[20,24]
■ Remove and discard your gloves and other personal protective equipment, as appropriate.[20,24]
■ Perform hand hygiene.[16,17,18,19]
■ Document the procedure.[33,34,35]

Special considerations

■ Rapid infusion devices are designed for use during rapid fluid infusion only; they aren't appropriate when a specific drip rate is required.
■ The rate of administration of resuscitation fluids should be adequate to support tissue perfusion.[14] Most devices increase the flow rate gradually *to prevent damage to the vein.* Adjust the roller clamp if the rate needs to be decreased.
■ Don't use these devices with pressure infusers; the system pump provides adequate pressure to infuse fluid.[1]
■ Replace gas vent filters and reservoirs according to the manufacturer's instructions.[1,3]
■ If you're administering blood products, prime the system with a compatible IV solution; don't prime with the blood product.[1,3]

Complications

Possible complications include electrolyte imbalances, fluid overload, acid-base imbalance, infiltration (extravasation), pulmonary edema, heart failure, interstitial edema, acute respiratory distress syndrome, and hypothermia.

Documentation

Document the transfusion of all blood products in the patient's record; include the product type, the date and time of the infusion, and the unique number or lot number for the blood products. Record the patient's core temperature before the start of a massive infusion and monitor it during and afterward. Include a meticulous account of the amounts of fluids, the types of fluids, and correlating vital signs. Incorporate documentation of massive fluid infusion into the existing required documentation protocol for resuscitation documentation.[33,34]

REFERENCES

1 Belmont Instrument Corporation. (n.d.). "The Belmont fluid management system FMS2000 operator's manual" [Online]. Accessed May 2015 via the Web at http://www.sh.lsuhsc.edu/policies/policy_manuals_via_ms_word/Nursing/Oper_Manuals/Belmont.pdf

2 Lynn-McHale Wiegand, D. (Ed.). (2011). *AACN procedure manual for critical care* (6th ed.). St. Louis, MO: Saunders.

3 Smiths Medical ASD, Inc. (2010). "Level 1® H-1200 fast flow fluid warmer: Operator's manual" [Online]. Accessed May 2015 via the Web at http://www.smiths-medical.com/upload/products/product_relateddocs/H-1200_Rev_0082.pdf

4 Gandhi, M. N., et al. (Eds.). (2011). *A practical approach to anesthesia for emergency surgery.* London, UK: Jaypee Brothers Medical Publishers.

5 Zoremba, N., et al. (2011). Air elimination capability in rapid infusion systems. *Anaesthesia, 66,* 1031–1034.

6 The Joint Commission. (2015). Standard NPSG.06.01.01. *Comprehensive accreditation manual for hospitals: The official handbook.* Oakbrook Terrace, IL: The Joint Commission. (Level VII)

7 Standard 10. Orders for the initiation and management of infusion therapy. Infusion nursing standards of practice. (2011). *Journal of Infusion Nursing, 34,* S15–S16. (Level VII)

8 Standard 66. Transfusion therapy. Infusion nursing standards of practice. (2011). *Journal of Infusion Nursing, 34,* S93–S95. (Level VII)

9 Standard 30. Blood and fluid warmers. Infusion nursing standards of practice. (2011). *Journal of Infusion Nursing, 34,* S35–S36. (Level VII)

10 The Joint Commission. (2015). Standard RI.01.03.01. *Comprehensive accreditation manual for hospitals: The official handbook.* Oakbrook Terrace, IL: The Joint Commission. (Level VII)

11 Standard 12. Informed consent. Infusion nursing standards of practice. (2011). *Journal of Infusion Nursing, 34,* S17–S18. (Level VII)

12 Centers for Medicare & Medicaid Services, Department of Health and Human Services. (2014). Condition of participation: Patient's rights. 42 C.F.R. § 482.13(b)(2).
13 American Osteopathic Association. (2014). Standard 15.01.11. *Healthcare Facilities Accreditation Program: Accreditation requirements for acute care hospitals.* Chicago, IL: American Osteopathic Association. (Level VII)
14 Kaur, P., et al. (2011). Transfusion protocol in trauma. *Journal of Emergency Trauma and Shock, 4,* 103–108. Accessed May 2015 via the Web at http://www.ncbi.nlm.nih.gov/pmc/articles/PMC3097557/
15 Centers for Disease Control and Prevention. (2002). Guideline for hand hygiene in health-care settings: Recommendations of the Healthcare Infection Control Practices Advisory Committee and the HICPAC/SHEA/APIC/IDSA Hand Hygiene Task Force. *MMWR Recommendations and Reports, 51*(RR-16), 1–45. Accessed May 2015 via the Web at http://www.cdc.gov/mmwr/pdf/rr/rr5116.pdf (Level II)
16 The Joint Commission. (2015). Standard NPSG.07.01.01. *Comprehensive accreditation manual for hospitals: The official handbook.* Oakbrook Terrace, IL: The Joint Commission. (Level VII)
17 Siegel, J. D., et al. (2007). "2007 guideline for isolation precautions: Preventing transmission of infectious agents in healthcare settings" [Online]. Accessed May 2015 via the Web at http://www.cdc.gov/hicpac/pdf/isolation/Isolation2007.pdf (Level II)
18 Standard 19. Hand hygiene. Infusion nursing standards of practice. (2011). *Journal of Infusion Nursing, 34,* S26–S27. (Level VII)
19 World Health Organization. (2009). "WHO guidelines on hand hygiene in health care: First global patient safety challenge, clean care is safer care" [Online]. Accessed May 2015 via the Web at http://whqlibdoc.who.int/publications/2009/9789241597906_eng.pdf (Level IV)
20 Occupational Safety and Health Administration. (n.d.). "Bloodborne pathogens, standard number 1910.1030" [Online]. Accessed May 2015 via the Web at http://www.osha.gov/pls/oshaweb/owadisp.show_document?p_table=Standards&p_id=10051 (Level VII)
21 Centers for Disease Control and Prevention. (2011). "Guidelines for the prevention of intravascular catheter–related infections" [Online]. Accessed May 2015 via the Web at http://www.cdc.gov/hicpac/pdf/guidelines/bsi-guidelines-2011.pdf
22 Centers for Medicare & Medicaid Services, Department of Health and Human Services. (2014). Condition of participation: Infection control. 42 C.F.R. § 482.42.
23 The Joint Commission. (2015). Standard NPSG.01.01.01. *Comprehensive accreditation manual for hospitals: The official handbook.* Oakbrook Terrace, IL: The Joint Commission. (Level VII)
24 Standard 22. Safe handling and disposal of sharps, hazardous materials, and hazardous waste. Infusion nursing standards of practice. (2011). *Journal of Infusion Nursing, 34,* S28–S29. (Level VII)
25 The Joint Commission. (2015). Standard NPSG.01.03.01. *Comprehensive accreditation manual for hospitals: The official handbook.* Oakbrook Terrace, IL: The Joint Commission. (Level VII)
26 Jarrett, N., et al. (2013). "Evidence-based guidelines for selected and previously considered hospital-acquired conditions: Final report" [Online]. Accessed May 2015 via the Web at http://www.cms.gov/Medicare/Medicare-Fee-for-Service-Payment/HospitalAcqCond/Downloads/Evidence-Based-Guidelines.pdf
27 Standard 27. Needleless connectors. Infusion nursing standards of practice. (2011). *Journal of Infusion Nursing, 34,* S32. (Level VII)
28 Infusion Nurses Society. (2013). *Policies and procedures for infusion nursing of the older adult* (2nd ed.). Boston, MA: Infusion Nurses Society.
29 Infusion Nurses Society. (2011). *Policies and procedures for infusion nursing* (4th ed.). Boston, MA: Infusion Nurses Society.
30 U.S. Food and Drug Administration. (n.d.). "Look. Check. Connect. Safe medical device connections save lives" [Online]. Accessed May 2015 via the Web at http://www.fda.gov/downloads/MedicalDevices/Safety/AlertsandNotices/UCM134873.pdf
31 Standard 27. Needleless connectors. Infusion nursing standards of practice. (2011). *Journal of Infusion Nursing, 34,* S32–S33. (Level VII)
32 The Joint Commission. (2015). Standard NPSG.02.03.01. *Comprehensive accreditation manual for hospitals: The official handbook.* Oakbrook Terrace, IL: The Joint Commission. (Level VII)
33 The Joint Commission. (2015). Standard RC.01.03.01. *Comprehensive accreditation manual for hospitals: The official handbook.* Oakbrook Terrace, IL: The Joint Commission. (Level VII)
34 Standard 14. Documentation. Infusion nursing standards of practice. (2011). *Journal of Infusion Nursing, 34,* S20–S21. (Level VII)
35 Centers for Medicare & Medicaid Services, Department of Health and Human Services. (2014). Condition of participation: Medical record services. 42 C.F.R. § 482.24(b).

ADDITIONAL REFERENCE

Kapoor, D., & Singh, M. (2011). Novel rapid infusion device for patients in emergency situations. *Scandinavian Journal of Trauma, Resuscitation and Emergency Medicine, 19,* 35. Accessed May 2015 via the Web at http://www.ncbi.nlm.nih.gov/pmc/articles/PMC3127777/

MECHANICAL TRACTION MANAGEMENT

Mechanical traction exerts a pulling force on a part of the body—usually the spine, pelvis, or long bones of the arms and legs. It can be used to reduce fractures, treat dislocations, correct or prevent deformities, improve or correct contractures, or decrease muscle spasms. Depending on the injury or condition, an orthopedist may order either skin or skeletal traction.

Applied directly to the skin and thus indirectly to the bone, skin traction is ordered when a light, temporary, or noncontinuous pulling force is required. Contraindications for skin traction include a severe injury with open wounds, an allergy to tape or other skin traction equipment, circulatory disturbances, dermatitis, and varicose veins.

With skeletal traction, an orthopedist inserts a pin or wire through the bone and attaches the traction equipment to the pin or wire to exert a direct, constant, longitudinal pulling force. Indications for skeletal traction include fractures of the tibia, femur, and humerus. Infections such as osteomyelitis contraindicate skeletal traction.

The IV-type basic frame is typically used for patients weighing up to 250 lb (113 kg).[1] The IV-type Balkan traction frame is generally used for special traction setups and for the increased weight-bearing of patients weighing between 250 lb and 450 lb (113 kg and 204 kg).[1] The claw-type basic frame is used on beds without IV sockets; this frame can hold patients weighing up to 200 lb (91 kg).[1]

After the patient is placed in the specific type of traction ordered by the orthopedist, the nurse is responsible for preventing complications from immobility; for routinely inspecting the equipment; for adding traction weights, as ordered; and, in patients with skeletal traction, for monitoring the pin insertion sites for signs of infection.[2]

Equipment

IV-type basic frame

102″ (259-cm) plain bar ▪ 27″ (69-cm) double-clamp bar ▪ 48″ (122-cm) swivel-clamp bar ▪ two 36″ (91-cm) plain bars ▪ four 4″ (10-cm) IV posts with clamps ▪ cross clamp ▪ trapeze with clamp ▪ wall bumper or roller.

IV-type Balkan traction frame

Two 102″ (259-cm) plain bars ▪ two 27″ (69-cm) double-clamp bars ▪ two 48″ (122-cm) swivel-clamp bars ▪ five 36″ (91-cm) plain bars ▪ four 4″ (10-cm) IV posts with clamps ▪ eight cross clamps ▪ trapeze with clamp ▪ wall bumper or roller.

Claw-type basic frame

102″ (259-cm) plain bar ▪ two 66″ (168-cm) swivel-clamp bars ▪ two upper-panel clamps ▪ two lower-panel clamps ▪ trapeze with clamp ▪ wall bumper or roller.

Preparation of equipment

Arrange with central supply or the appropriate department to have the traction equipment transported to the patient's room on a traction cart.

EQUIPMENT

IV-type basic traction frame

With an IV-type basic frame, IV posts, placed in IV holders, support the horizontal bars across the foot and head of the bed. These horizontal bars then support the two uprights.

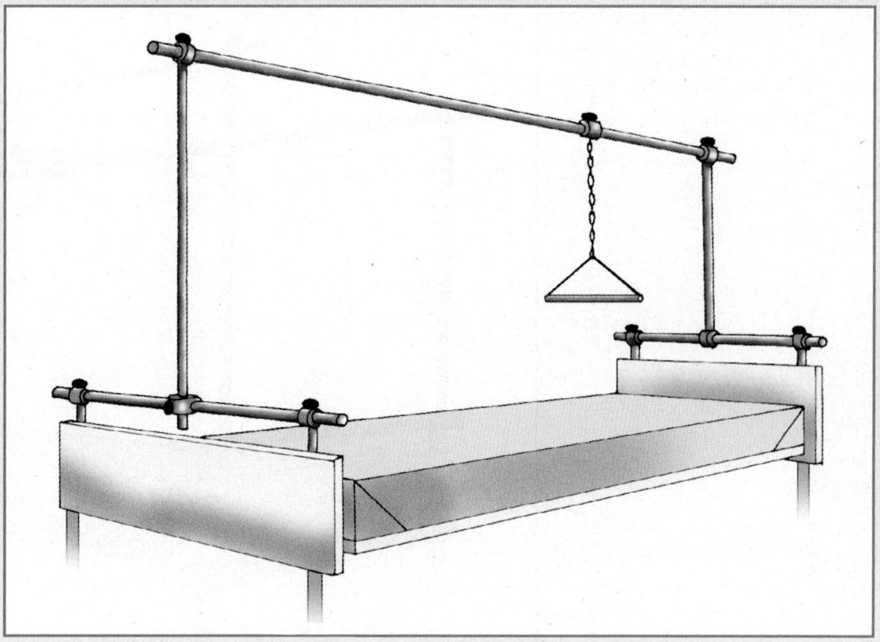

Implementation

- Verify the practitioner's order.
- Perform hand hygiene.[3,4,5]
- Confirm the patient's identity using at least two patient identifiers.[6]
- Explain the purpose of traction to the patient. Emphasize the importance of maintaining proper body alignment after the traction equipment is set up.

IV-type basic frame

- Attach one 4″ (10-cm) IV post with clamp to each end of both 36″ (91-cm) horizontal plain bars.
- Secure an IV post in each IV holder at the bed corners. Using a cross clamp, fasten the 48″ (122-cm) vertical swivel-clamp bar to the middle of the horizontal plain bar at the foot of the bed.
- Fasten the 27″ (69-cm) vertical double-clamp bar to the middle of the horizontal plain bar at the head of the bed.
- Attach the 102″ (259-cm) horizontal plain bar to the tops of the two vertical bars, making sure the clamp knobs point up.
- Using the appropriate clamp, attach the trapeze to the horizontal bar about 2′ (61 cm) from the head of the bed. (See *IV-type basic traction frame.*)
- Attach a wall bumper or roller to the vertical bar or bars at the head of the bed *to protect the walls from damage caused by the bed or equipment.*
- Perform hand hygiene.[3,4,5]
- Document the procedure.[7,8]

IV type Balkan traction frame

- Attach one 4″ (10-cm) IV post with clamp to each end of two 36″ (91-cm) horizontal plain bars.
- Secure an IV post in each IV holder at the bed corners.
- Attach a 48″ (122-cm) vertical swivel-clamp bar, using a cross clamp, to each IV post clamp on the horizontal plain bar at the foot of the bed.
- Fasten one 36″ (91-cm) horizontal plain bar across the midpoints of the two 48″ (122-cm) swivel-clamp bars, using two cross clamps.
- Attach a 27″ (69-cm) vertical double-clamp bar to each IV post clamp on the horizontal bar at the head of the bed.
- Using two cross clamps, fasten a 36″ (91-cm) horizontal plain bar across the midpoints of two 27″ double-clamp bars.
- Clamp a 102″ (259-cm) horizontal plain bar onto the vertical bars on each side of the bed; make sure the clamp knobs point up.
- Use two cross clamps to attach a 36″ (91-cm) horizontal plain bar across the two overhead bars, about 2′ (61 cm) from the head of the bed.
- Attach the trapeze to this 36″ (91-cm) horizontal bar. (See *IV-type Balkan traction frame,* page 496.)
- Attach a wall bumper or roller to the vertical bar or bars at the head of the bed *to protect the walls from damage caused by the bed or equipment.*
- Perform hand hygiene.[3,4,5]
- Document the procedure.[7,8]

Claw-type basic frame

- Attach one lower-panel and one upper-panel clamp to each 66″ (168-cm) swivel-clamp bar.
- Fasten one bar to the footboard and one to the headboard by turning the clamp knobs clockwise until they're tight and then pulling back on the upper clamp's rubberized bar until it's tight.
- Secure the 102″ (259-cm) horizontal plain bar atop the two vertical bars, making sure that the clamp knobs point up.
- Using the appropriate clamp, attach the trapeze to the horizontal bar about 2′ (61 cm) from the head of the bed. (See *Claw-type basic frame,* page 496.)
- Attach a wall bumper or roller to the vertical bar or bars at the head of the bed *to protect the walls from damage caused by the bed or equipment.*
- Perform hand hygiene.[3,4,5]
- Document the procedure.[7,8]

Special considerations

- Countertraction must always be provided by the patient's body weight, pull of weights in the opposite direction, or elevation of the bed.
- The line of pull should be maintained at all times.

EQUIPMENT

IV-type Balkan traction frame

The IV-type Balkan frame features IV posts and horizontal bars (secured in the same manner as those for the IV-type basic frame) that support four uprights.

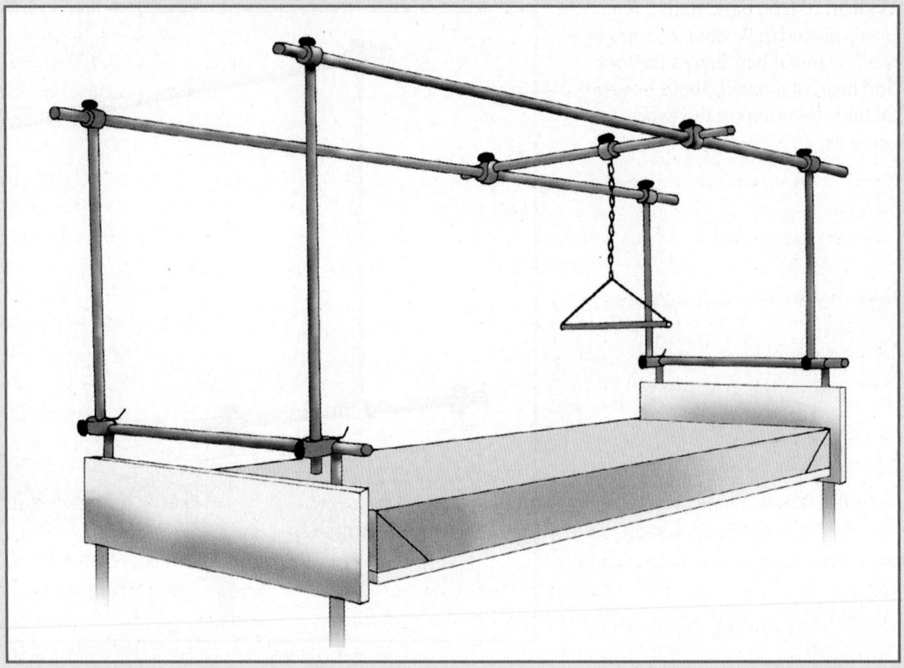

EQUIPMENT

Claw-type basic frame

With a claw-type basic frame, claw attachments secure the uprights to the footboard and headboard.

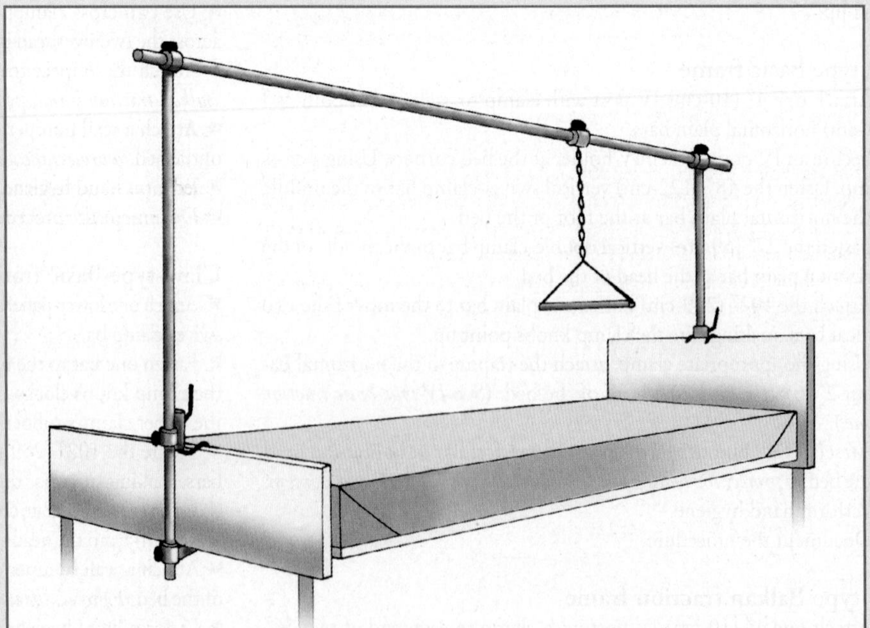

- The weights should hang freely at all times.
- Friction should be prevented on the traction apparatus.
- When using skin traction, apply ordered weights slowly and carefully *to avoid jerking the affected extremity.* Arrange the weights so that they don't hang over the patient *to avoid injury in case the ropes break.*

Patient teaching

Teach the patient to maintain proper body alignment.

Complications

Immobility during traction may result in pressure ulcers, osteoporosis, muscle atrophy, weakness, or contractures. Immobility can also cause GI disturbances such as constipation; urinary problems, including stasis and calculi; respiratory problems, such as stasis of secretions and hypostatic pneumonia; and circulatory disturbances, including stasis and thrombophlebitis.

Prolonged immobility, especially after traumatic injury, may promote depression or other emotional disturbances. Skeletal traction may cause osteomyelitis originating at the pin or wire sites.

Documentation

In the patient's record, document the time the traction was set up and the amount of traction weight used; note that the weight is hanging freely. Record the patient's tolerance of traction. Also document the patent's neurovascular integrity, skin condition, and respiratory status. Note whether any pain medications were administered and their effectiveness. Document any patient teaching and the patient's understanding of the teaching.

REFERENCES

1 Zimmer Orthopaedic Surgical Products, Inc. (2006). "Zimmer traction handbook: A complete reference guide to the basics of traction" [Online]. Accessed May 2015 via the Web at http://www.zimmer.com/content/pdf/en-US/zimmer_traction_handbook.pdf

2 Holmes, S. B., & Brown, S. J. (2005). National Association of Orthopaedic Nurses guidelines for orthopaedic nursing: Skeletal pin site care. *Orthopaedic Nursing, 24,* 99–107. (Level V)

3 Centers for Disease Control and Prevention. (2002). Guideline for hand hygiene in health-care settings: Recommendations of the Healthcare Infection Control Practices Advisory Committee and the HICPAC/SHEA/APIC/IDSA Hand Hygiene Task Force. *MMWR Recommendations and Reports, 51*(RR-16), 1–45. Accessed May 2015 via the Web at http://www.cdc.gov/mmwr/pdf/rr/rr5116.pdf (Level II)

4 World Health Organization. (2009). "WHO guidelines on hand hygiene in health care: First global patient safety challenge, clean care is safer care" [Online]. Accessed May 2015 via the Web at http://whqlibdoc.who.int/publications/2009/9789241597906_eng.pdf (Level IV)

5 The Joint Commission. (2015). Standard NPSG.07.01.01. *Comprehensive accreditation manual for hospitals: The official handbook.* Oakbrook Terrace, IL: The Joint Commission. (Level VII)

6 The Joint Commission. (2015). Standard NPSG.01.01.01. *Comprehensive accreditation manual for hospitals: The official handbook.* Oakbrook Terrace, IL: The Joint Commission. (Level VII)

7 The Joint Commission. (2015). Standard RC.01.03.01. *Comprehensive accreditation manual for hospitals: The official handbook.* Oakbrook Terrace, IL: The Joint Commission. (Level VII)

8 Centers for Medicare & Medicaid Services, Department of Health and Human Services. (2014). Condition of participation: Medical record services. 42 C.F.R. § 482.24(b).

MECHANICAL VENTILATION, POSITIVE PRESSURE

The purpose of positive-pressure mechanical ventilation is to promote gas exchange in the lungs by producing positive intrathoracic pressure and positive airway pressure. This positive-pressure mechanical ventilation may be delivered to the airway through an endotracheal (ET) or tracheostomy tube. The amount of gas exchange that takes place depends on the resistance and compliance of the lung itself.

Depending on how they provide ventilation, mechanical ventilators fall into three different categories. They can deliver a preset tidal volume (V_T), deliver a preset peak inspiratory pressure, or operate at a high frequency (60 to 3,000 oscillations per minute) with low V_T.

Positive-pressure ventilation is indicated for the patient with respiratory or ventilatory failure evidenced by hypoxemia, metabolic acidosis, respiratory acidosis, inadequate tissue oxygenation, and respiratory muscle fatigue. These signs and symptoms may result from acute or chronic lung injury; neurologic disorders; trauma; chemical or medical respiratory depressants, such as sedation, anesthesia, or pain killers; multiple-organ-dysfunction syndrome; or disease. The goals of positive-pressure ventilation include maintaining adequate alveolar ventilation, correcting hypoxemia, and decreasing the work of breathing while providing adequate respirations and rest for the patient.

Patients receiving ventilatory support may need sedation, pain medication, or a neuromuscular blocking agent intermittently or continuously to decrease the work of breathing and to allow the ventilator to work effectively.

A practitioner orders mechanical ventilation and, in collaboration with the respiratory therapist, sets ventilatory parameters to maintain appropriate pH, partial pressure of arterial carbon dioxide, partial pressure of arterial oxygen, and arterial oxygen saturation. The practitioner, respiratory therapist, and nurse must collaborate to manage the moment-to-moment ventilatory needs of the patient. The nurse must know how to assess, monitor, and care for patients on mechanical ventilation and understand basic ventilator mechanisms of action. (See *Mechanical ventilation terminology,* page 498.)

Equipment

Oxygen source ▪ air source that can supply 50 psi ▪ mechanical ventilator ▪ humidifier ▪ ventilator circuit tubing, connectors, and adapters ▪ condensation collection trap ▪ spirometer, respirometer, or electronic device to measure flow and volume ▪ in-line thermometer ▪ gloves ▪ handheld resuscitation bag with reservoir ▪ suction equipment ▪ sterile distilled water ▪ equipment for arterial blood gas (ABG) analysis ▪ vital signs monitoring equipment ▪ stethoscope ▪ disinfectant pad ▪ pulse oximeter ▪ capnography device ▪ oral care products ▪ emergency resuscitation equipment ▪ Optional: prescribed sedative, neuromuscular blocking agent, and other medications; chlorhexidine oral care product; replacement inserts or filters; other personal protective equipment.

Preparation of equipment

In most facilities, respiratory therapists assume responsibility for setting up a ventilator. If necessary, however, check the manufacturer's instructions for setting it up. In some cases, you'll need to add sterile distilled water to the humidifier and connect the ventilator to the appropriate gas source.

Plug the ventilator into an emergency electrical outlet (with generator backup) and turn it on. Adjust the settings on the ventilator, as ordered. Make sure the ventilator's alarms are set appropriately for the ventilator settings and the patient's current condition, and that the alarms are turned on, functioning properly, and audible to staff.[1,2] Make sure that the humidifier is filled with the sterile distilled water and that the heated humidifier is set to deliver an inspired gas temperature of 93.2°F to 105.8°F (34° to 41°C) at the circuit Y-piece and provide a minimum of 33 mg/L of water vapor.[3]

Attach a capnographic device to measure carbon dioxide levels *to confirm placement of the ET tube and detect any disconnection from the ventilator or other complications.*

Mechanical ventilation terminology

Make sure you're familiar with the following mechanical ventilation terminologies:

Assist-control mode: The ventilator delivers a preset tidal volume (V_T) at a preset rate; however, the patient can initiate additional breaths, which trigger the ventilator to deliver the preset V_T at positive pressure.

Continuous positive airway pressure (CPAP): This setting prompts the ventilator to deliver positive pressure to the airway throughout the respiratory cycle. It works only on patients who can breathe spontaneously.

Control mode: The ventilator delivers a preset V_T at a fixed rate, regardless of whether the patient is breathing spontaneously.

Fraction of inspired oxygen (F_{IO_2}): This is the percentage of oxygen delivered to the patient by the ventilator. The dial or digital display on the ventilator that sets this percentage is labeled OXYGEN CONCENTRATION or OXYGEN PERCENTAGE.

Inspiratory-expiratory (I:E) ratio: This ratio compares the duration of inspiration to the duration of expiration. The I:E ratio of normal, spontaneous breathing is 1:2, meaning that expiration is twice as long as inspiration.

Inspiratory flow rate (IFR): The IFR denotes the V_T delivered within a certain time. Its value can range from 20 to 120 L/minute.

Minute ventilation or minute volume (VE): This measurement results from the multiplication of respiratory rate and V_T.

Peak inspiratory pressure (PIP): Measured by the pressure manometer on the ventilator, PIP reflects the amount of pressure required to deliver a preset V_T.

Plateau pressure: Airway pressure measured after a 0.5 second pause at the end of inspiration, plateau pressure indicates the stiffness of the lungs.

Positive end-expiratory pressure (PEEP): In PEEP mode, the ventilator is triggered to apply positive pressure at the end of each expiration to increase the area for oxygen exchange by helping to inflate and keep open collapsed alveoli.

Pressure support: A ventilator adjunct, pressure support delivers positive pressure, supplementing the spontaneous breath of a patient on the ventilator. It's used to reduce the work of breathing associated with the artificial airway or increase the volume of the patient's spontaneous breath.

Respiratory rate: The number of breaths per minute delivered by the ventilator; also called *frequency*.

Sensitivity setting: A setting that determines the amount of effort the patient must exert to trigger the inspiratory cycle.

Sigh volume: A ventilator-delivered breath that's 1¼ times as large as the patient's V_T.

Synchronized intermittent mandatory ventilation (SIMV): The ventilator delivers a preset number of breaths at a specific V_T. The patient may supplement these mechanical ventilations with his own breaths, in which case the V_T and rate are determined by his own inspiratory ability.

Tidal volume (V_T): This refers to the volume of air delivered to the patient with each cycle, usually 8 to 10 mL/kg.

Implementation

- Verify the practitioner's order.
- If the patient isn't already intubated, prepare him for intubation. (See the "Endotracheal intubation" procedure, page 278.)
- Gather and prepare the necessary equipment.
- Perform hand hygiene.[4,5,6,7,8]
- Confirm the patient's identity using at least two patient identifiers.[9]
- When possible, explain the procedure to the patient and his family *to help reduce anxiety and fear.* Assure them that staff members are nearby to provide care.
- Make sure the patient is being adequately oxygenated.
- Put on gloves and other personal protective equipment as needed *to comply with standard precautions.*[10,11,12]
- As the patient's condition allows, perform a complete physical assessment, and obtain blood for ABG analysis *to establish baselines for comparison.*
- Assist with intubation (if necessary) and then connect the ET tube to the ventilator circuit.
- Observe for chest expansion, and auscultate for bilateral breath sounds *to verify that the patient is being ventilated.*[10]
- Monitor the patient's oxygen saturation level by pulse oximetry; make sure that the alarm limits are set appropriately for the patient's current condition and that the alarms are turned on, functioning properly, and audible to staff.[1,2,13,14]
- Use waveform capnography, an exhaled-carbon dioxide detector, or an esophageal detector device in addition to a chest X-ray *to confirm ET tube placement.*[15,16]
- Position the patient with the head of the bed elevated 30 to 45 degrees, unless contraindicated by the patient's condition, *to reduce the risk of aspiration and consequent ventilator-associated pneumonia (VAP).* If the patient can't bend at the waist, use a reverse Trendelenburg position.[17,18,19]
- Suction the patient's airway when necessary *to maintain airway patency by removing accumulated pulmonary secretions.*[16] Before performing suctioning, hyperoxygenate the patient, as needed, with 100% oxygen for 30 to 60 seconds. Suction the patient with a closed-suction catheter, limiting suctioning to 15 seconds. After suctioning, hyperoxygenate the patient for at least 1 minute using the same technique as you did before suctioning.[16,20]
- Monitor the patient's ABG values after the initial ventilator setup, after changes in ventilator settings, and as the patient's condition indicates, if ordered, *to determine whether the patient is being adequately ventilated and to avoid oxygen toxicity.* Be prepared to adjust ventilator settings based on ABG analysis.
- Check the ventilator tubing frequently for condensation, *which can cause resistance to airflow and which the patient may aspirate.* As needed, drain the condensate into a collection trap. Keep the circuit closed during condensate drainage *to prevent bacterial contamination.*[17] Don't drain the condensate into the humidifier *because the condensate may be contaminated with the patient's secretions.* Also avoid accidental drainage of condensation into the patient's airway when moving the tubing or the patient *because condensate is considered infectious waste.*[3,10]
- Inspect heat and moisture exchangers, and replace inserts or filters contaminated by secretions.
- Check the in-line thermometer *to make sure the temperature of the air delivered to the patient is close to body temperature.*
- If you're using a heated humidifier, monitor the inspired air temperature as close to the patient's airway as possible. The inspiratory gas shouldn't be warmer than 98.6°F (37°C) at the opening of the airway. Check that the high temperature alarm is set no higher than 105.8°F (41°C) and no lower than 3.6°F (2°C) below the desired temperature at the circuit Y-piece.[3]
- Monitor the patient's vital signs and respiratory status regularly. When monitoring the patient's vital signs, count spontaneous breaths as well as ventilator-delivered breaths.

■ Change, clean, or dispose of the ventilator tubing and equipment when it's visibly soiled or malfunctioning or at an interval determined by your facility *to reduce the risk of bacterial contamination.*[3,10,17,20]
■ Provide emotional support to the patient during all phases of mechanical ventilation *to reduce anxiety and promote successful treatment.* Even if the patient is unresponsive, continue to explain all procedures and treatments to him.
■ Confirm that the ventilator alarms are set appropriately for the patient's current condition. Make sure that the alarms are turned on, functioning, and audible to staff.[1,2,13,14]
■ Unless contraindicated, turn the patient from side to side every 1 to 2 hours *to facilitate lung expansion and removal of secretions* and perform active or passive range-of-motion exercises for all extremities *to reduce the hazards of immobility.*
■ Assess the patient's peripheral circulation, and monitor his intake and output *to assess for signs of decreased cardiac output.* Watch for signs and symptoms of fluid volume excess or dehydration.
■ Brush the patient's teeth, gums, and tongue at least twice a day using a soft pediatric or adult toothbrush *to prevent VAP.*[21,22]
■ Use a chlorhexidine rinse daily, as prescribed, *to reduce colonization of the oropharynx and prevent subsequent VAP.*[18,22,23] For a patient undergoing cardiac surgery, use the rinse twice a day during the perioperative period.[21]
■ Moisten the patient's lips and oral mucosa every 2 to 4 hours *to reduce oral inflammation and improve oral health.*[21,22]
■ Institute measures to prevent venous thromboembolism (VTE) and peptic ulcer disease (PUD), as prescribed, to reduce the risk of VAP.[17,18,22]
NURSING ALERT *Make sure that infection-prevention techniques (such as performing hand hygiene, providing oral care, positioning the patient with head of bed elevated 30 to 45 degrees, and instituting VTE and PUD prophylaxis) are followed when caring for the patient receiving mechanical ventilation* to reduce the risk of VAP.[10,17]
■ Place the call light within the patient's reach, and establish a method of communication, such as a communication board, *because intubation and mechanical ventilation impair the patient's ability to speak.* An artificial airway may help the patient to speak by allowing air to pass through his vocal cords.
■ Administer and titrate the patient's sedative and neuromuscular blocking agent as ordered following safe medication administration practices.[24,25] Maintain target sedation levels *to avoid oversedation.*[26] Remember that the patient receiving a neuromuscular blocking agent requires close observation *because of his inability to breathe or communicate.*
■ Take steps to ensure the patient's safety, such as raising the side rails of his bed while turning him and covering and lubricating his eyes.
■ Dispose of used supplies in the appropriate receptacle.[11]
■ Remove and discard your gloves and any other personal protective equipment worn.[11]
■ Perform hand hygiene.[4,5,6,7,8]
■ Clean and disinfect your stethoscope using a disinfectant pad.[27,28]
■ Perform hand hygiene.[4,5,6,7,8]
■ Document the procedure.[29,30,31]

Special considerations

■ The Joint Commission issued a sentinel event alert concerning medical device alarm safety *because alarm-related events have been associated with permanent loss of function and death.* Among the major contributing factors were improper alarm settings, alarms inappropriately turned off, and alarm signals not audible to staff. Make sure that alarm limits are set appropriately and that alarms are turned on, functioning properly, and audible to staff. Follow facility guidelines for preventing alarm fatigue.[2]
■ If an alarm sounds and you can't easily identify the problem, disconnect the patient from the ventilator and use a handheld resuscitation bag to ventilate him. (See *Responding to ventilator alarms,* page 500.)
■ If the patient is receiving a neuromuscular blocking agent, make sure that he also receives a sedative. *Neuromuscular blocking agents cause paralysis without altering the patient's level of consciousness (LOC).* Reassure the patient and his family that the paralysis is temporary. Also make sure emergency resuscitation equipment is readily available *in case the ventilator malfunctions or the patient is extubated accidentally.*
■ Discuss with the practitioner during multidisciplinary rounds a sedation vacation strategy *to assess for readiness for weaning.*[17,18]
■ Interrupt sedation daily, as ordered or according to your facility's protocol, and assess the patient's readiness to wean.[17,18]
■ If the patient is ready to wean, begin to wean him from the ventilator, as ordered. (See the "Weaning a patient from a ventilator" procedure, page 836.)
■ In a postoperative patient, perform a comprehensive pain assessment using techniques appropriate for the patient's age, condition, and ability to understand.[32] Administer analgesics, as needed and ordered, following safe medication administration practices.[24,25]
■ If the patient is receiving enteral feedings, avoid gastric overdistention *to reduce the risk of aspiration.*
■ Ensure that the patient gets adequate rest and sleep *because fatigue can delay weaning from the ventilator.* Provide subdued lighting, safely muffle equipment noises, and restrict staff access to the area *to promote quiet during rest periods.*
■ Teach the patient and family about measures to prevent VAP, including maintaining the head of the bed at 30 to 45 degrees. Encourage them to alert staff members when the bed doesn't appear to be positioned correctly.[18,19]

Patient teaching

If the patient will be discharged on a ventilator, evaluate the ability and motivation of the family or caregiver to provide care. Well before discharge, develop a teaching plan that addresses the patient's needs. For example, teaching should include information about ventilator care and settings, artificial airway care, suctioning, respiratory therapy, communication, nutrition, therapeutic exercise, signs and symptoms of infection, and ways to troubleshoot minor equipment malfunctions.

Also evaluate the patient's need for adaptive equipment, such as a hospital bed, wheelchair or walker with a ventilator tray, patient lift, and bedside commode. Determine whether the patient needs to travel; if so, select appropriate portable and backup equipment.

Before discharge, have the patient's caregiver demonstrate the ability to use the equipment. At discharge, contact a durable medical equipment vendor and a home health nurse to follow up with the patient. Also, refer the patient to community resources, if available.

Complications

Mechanical ventilation can cause tension pneumothorax, decreased cardiac output, oxygen toxicity, fluid volume excess caused by humidification, infection, and such GI complications as distention or bleeding from stress ulcers.

Documentation

Document the date and time mechanical ventilation was initiated. Name the type of ventilator used for the patient, and note its settings. Describe the patient's subjective and objective response to mechanical ventilation, including vital signs, breath sounds, neurologic status, readiness to wean, use of accessory muscles, intake and output, and weight. List any complications and nursing actions taken. Record all pertinent laboratory data, including ABG analysis results and oxygen saturation levels. Describe the patient's LOC, respiratory effort, arrhythmias, skin color, and need for suctioning. Document interventions, such as head of bed elevation, oral care, sedation interruption, and weaning, and the patient's response to these interventions. Also document any patient teaching provided.

If the patient was receiving pressure-support ventilation or using a T-piece or tracheostomy collar, note the duration of spontaneous breathing

TROUBLESHOOTING

Responding to ventilator alarms

SIGNAL	POSSIBLE CAUSE	NURSING INTERVENTIONS
Low-pressure alarm	■ Tube disconnected from ventilator	■ Reconnect the tube to the ventilator.
	■ Endotracheal (ET) tube displaced above vocal cords or tracheostomy tube extubated	■ Check tube placement and reposition if needed. If extubation or displacement has occu rred, ventilate the patient manually and call the practitioner immediately.
	■ Leaking tidal volume from low cuff pressure (from an underinflated or ruptured cuff or a leak in the cuff or one-way valve)	■ Listen for a whooshing sound around the tube, indicating an air leak. If you hear one, check cuff pressure. If you can't maintain pressure, call the practitioner; he may need to insert a new tube.
	■ Ventilator malfunction	■ Disconnect the patient from the ventilator and ventilate him manually if necessary. Obtain another ventilator.
	■ Leak in ventilator circuitry (from loose connection or hole in tubing, loss of temperature-sensitive device, or cracked humidification device)	■ Make sure all connections are intact. Check for holes or leaks in the tubing and replace if necessary. Check the humidification device and replace if cracked.
High-pressure alarm	■ Increased airway pressure or decreased lung compliance caused by worsening disease	■ Auscultate the lungs for evidence of increasing lung consolidation, barotrauma, or wheezing. Call the practitioner if indicated.
	■ Patient biting on oral ET tube	■ Insert a bite block if needed. ■ Consider pain medication or sedation if appropriate.
	■ Secretions in airway	■ Look for secretions in the airway; suction the patient's airway or have him cough to remove secretions as necessary.
	■ Condensate in large-bore tubing	■ Check tubing for condensate and drain the condensate from the tubing as necessary.
	■ Intubation of right mainstem bronchus	■ Auscultate for diminished or absent breath sounds in the left lung fields.
	■ Patient coughing, gagging, or attempting to talk	■ Check tube position. If it has become displaced, call the practitioner; he may need to reposition it.
	■ Chest wall resistance	■ If the patient's breathing is asynchronous with the ventilator, the practitioner may order a sedative or neuromuscular blocking agent and sedative.
	■ Failure of high-pressure relief valve	■ Reposition the patient to improve chest expansion. ■ Administer the prescribed analgesic if needed. ■ Replace faulty equipment.
	■ Bronchospasm	■ Assess the patient to try to determine the cause. Report your findings to the practitioner, and treat the patient as ordered.

and the patient's ability to maintain the weaning schedule. If using intermittent mandatory ventilation, with or without pressure-support ventilation, record the control breath rate, the time of each breath reduction, and the rate of spontaneous respirations. Document patient and family teaching.

REFERENCES

1 American Association of Critical-Care Nurses. (2013). "AACN practice alert: Alarm management" [Online]. Accessed May 2015 via the Web at http://www.aacn.org/wd/practice/docs/practicealerts/alarm-management-practice-alert.pdf (Level VII)

2 The Joint Commission. (2013). "Sentinel event alert: Medical device alarm safety in hospitals" [Online]. Accessed May 2015 via the Web at http://www.jointcommission.org/assets/1/18/SEA_50_alarms_4_5_13_FINAL1.PDF (Level VII)

3 Restrepo, R. D., & Walsh, B. K. (2012). AARC clinical practice guideline: Humidification during invasive and noninvasive mechanical ventilation: 2012. *Respiratory Care, 57,* 782–788. Accessed May 2015 via the Web at http://rc.rcjournal.com/content/57/5/782.full.pdf (Level VII)

4 The Joint Commission. (2015). Standard NPSG.07.01.01. *Comprehensive accreditation manual for hospitals: The official handbook.* Oakbrook Terrace, IL: The Joint Commission. (Level VII)

5 Centers for Disease Control and Prevention. (2002). Guideline for hand hygiene in health-care settings: Recommendations of the Healthcare Infection Control Practices Advisory Committee and the HICPAC/SHEA/APIC/IDSA Hand Hygiene Task Force. *MMWR Recommendations and Reports, 51*(RR-16), 1–45. Accessed May 2015 via the Web at http://www.cdc.gov/mmwr/pdf/rr/rr5116.pdf (Level II)

6 World Health Organization. (2009). "WHO guidelines on hand hygiene in health care: First global patient safety challenge, clean care is safer care" [Online]. Accessed May 2015 via the Web at http://whqlibdoc.who.int/publications/2009/9789241597906_eng.pdf (Level IV)

7 Centers for Medicare & Medicaid Services, Department of Health and Human Services. (2014). Condition of participation: Infection control. 42 C.F.R. § 482.42.

8 American Osteopathic Association. (2014). Standard 07.01.21. *Healthcare Facilities Accreditation Program: Accreditation requirements for acute care hospitals.* Chicago, IL: American Osteopathic Association. (Level VII)

9 The Joint Commission. (2015). Standard NPSG.01.01.01. *Comprehensive accreditation manual for hospitals: The official handbook.* Oakbrook Terrace, IL: The Joint Commission. (Level VII)

10 Centers for Disease Control and Prevention. (2004). Guidelines for preventing health-care-associated pneumonia, 2003: Recommendations of CDC and the Healthcare Infection Control Practices Advisory Committee. *MMWR Recommendations and Report, 53*(RR-3), 1–36. Accessed May 2015 via the Web at http://www.cdc.gov/mmwr/pdf/rr/rr5303.pdf (Level II)

11 Siegel, J. D., et al. (2007). "2007 guideline for isolation precautions: Preventing transmission of infectious agents in healthcare settings" [Online]. Accessed May 2015 via the Web at http://www.cdc.gov/hicpac/pdf/isolation/Isolation2007.pdf (Level II)

12 American Osteopathic Association. (2014). Standard 07.01.10. *Healthcare Facilities Accreditation Program: Accreditation requirements for acute care hospitals.* Chicago, IL: American Osteopathic Association. (Level VII)

13 The Joint Commission. (2015). Standard NPSG.06.01.01. *Comprehensive accreditation manual for hospitals: The official handbook.* Oakbrook Terrace, IL: The Joint Commission. (Level VII)

14 Graham, K. C., & Cvach, M. (2010). Monitor alarm fatigue: Standardizing use of physiological monitors and decreasing nuisance alarms. *American Journal of Critical Care, 19,* 28–37.

15 Walsh, B. K., et al. (2011). AARC clinical practice guideline: Capnography/capnometry during mechanical ventilation: 2011. *Respiratory Care, 56,* 503–509. Accessed May 2015 via the Web at http://rc.rcjournal.com/content/56/4/503.full.pdf (Level VII)

16 American Association for Respiratory Care (AARC). (2010). AARC clinical practice guidelines: Endotracheal suctioning of mechanically ventilated patients with artificial airways 2010. *Respiratory Care, 55,* 758–764. Accessed May 2015 via the Web at http://rc.rcjournal.com/content/55/6/758.full.pdf (Level VII)

17 Association of Professionals in Infection Control and Epidemiology (APIC). (2009). "An APIC guide 2009: Guide to the elimination of ventilator-associated pneumonia" [Online]. Accessed May 2015 via the Web at http://www.apic.org/Resource_/EliminationGuideForm/18e326ad-b484-471c-9c35-6822a53ee4a2/File/VAP_09.pdf (Level IV)

18 Institute for Healthcare Improvement. (2012). *How-to-guide: Prevent ventilator-associated pneumonia.* Cambridge, MA: Institute for Healthcare Improvement. (Level VII)

19 American Association of Critical-Care Nurses. (2008). "AACN practice alert: Ventilator associated pneumonia" [Online]. Accessed May 2015 via the Web at http://www.aacn.org/wd/practice/docs/practicealerts/vap.pdf?menu=aboutus (Level VII)

20 Hess, D. R., et al. (2003). AARC evidence-based clinical practice guideline: Care of the ventilator circuit and its relation to ventilator-associated pneumonia. *Respiratory Care, 48,* 869–879. Accessed May 2015 via the Web at http://rc.rcjournal.com/content/48/9/869.full.pdf (Level VII)

21 American Association of Critical-Care Nurses. (2010). "AACN practice alert: Oral care for patients at risk for ventilator-associated pneumonia" [Online]. Accessed May 2015 via the Web at http://www.aacn.org/WD/Practice/Docs/PracticeAlerts/oral%20care%2004-2010%20final.pdf (Level VII)

22 American Osteopathic Association. (2014). Standard 07.01.02. *Healthcare Facilities Accreditation Program: Accreditation requirements for acute care hospitals.* Chicago, IL: American Osteopathic Association. (Level VII)

23 Hillier, B., et al. (2013). Preventing ventilator-associated pneumonia through oral care, product selection, and application method. *AACN Advanced Critical Care, 24,* 38–58.

24 Centers for Medicare & Medicaid Services, Department of Health and Human Services. (2014). Condition of participation: Nursing services. 42 C.F.R. § 482.23(c).

25 American Osteopathic Association. (2014). Standard 16.01.03. *Healthcare Facilities Accreditation Program: Accreditation requirements for acute care hospitals.* Chicago, IL: American Osteopathic Association. (Level VII)

26 Grap, M. J., et al. (2012). Sedation in adults receiving mechanical ventilation: Physiological and comfort outcomes. *American Journal of Critical Care, 21,* e53–e64. Accessed May 2015 via the Web at http://www.aacn.org/wd/Cetests/media/A1221033.pdf (Level VI)

27 Rutala, W. A., et al. (2008). "Guideline for disinfection and sterilization in healthcare facilities, 2008" [Online]. Accessed May 2015 via the Web at http://www.cdc.gov/hicpac/pdf/guidelines/Disinfection_Nov_2008.pdf (Level I)

28 American Osteopathic Association. (2014). Standard 07.02.03. *Healthcare Facilities Accreditation Program: Accreditation requirements for acute care hospitals.* Chicago, IL: American Osteopathic Association. (Level VII)

29 The Joint Commission. (2015). Standard RC.01.03.01. *Comprehensive accreditation manual for hospitals: The official handbook.* Oakbrook Terrace, IL: The Joint Commission. (Level VII)

30 Centers for Medicare & Medicaid Services, Department of Health and Human Services. (2014). Condition of participation: Medical record services. 42 C.F.R. § 482.24(b).

31 American Osteopathic Association. (2014). Standard 10.00.03. *Healthcare Facilities Accreditation Program: Accreditation requirements for acute care hospitals.* Chicago, IL: American Osteopathic Association. (Level VII)

32 The Joint Commission. (2015). Standard PC.01.02.07. *Comprehensive accreditation manual for hospitals: The official handbook.* Oakbrook Terrace, IL: The Joint Commission. (Level VII)

ADDITIONAL REFERENCES

American Heart Association. (2010). 2010 American Heart Association guidelines for cardiopulmonary resuscitation and emergency cardiovascular care. *Circulation, 122,* S729–S767. (Level II)

Lynn-McHale Wiegand, D. (Ed.). (2011). *AACN procedure manual for critical care* (6th ed.). Philadelphia, PA: Saunders.

Nettina, S. M. (2014). *Lippincott manual of nursing practice* (10th ed.). Philadelphia, PA: Wolters Kluwer.

METERED-DOSE INHALER USE

A metered-dose inhaler (MDI) delivers topical medications to the respiratory tract, producing local and systemic effects. The mucosal lining of the respiratory tract absorbs the inhalant almost immediately. Examples of common inhalants include bronchodilators, which improve airway patency and facilitate mucous drainage; mucolytics, which attain a high local concentration to liquefy tenacious bronchial secretions; and corticosteroids, which decrease inflammation.

The use of MDIs may be contraindicated in patients who can't form an airtight seal around the device and in those who lack the coordination or clear vision to assemble the device. Some patients use a spacer to assist them with the airtight seal. Specific inhalants may also be contraindicated. For example, bronchodilators are contraindicated in patients with tachycardia or a history of cardiac arrhythmias associated with tachycardia.

Equipment

Patient's medication and medical records ■ prescribed MDI with mouthpiece ■ stethoscope ■ disinfectant pad ■ Optional: MDI spacer, water for gargling, emesis basin.

Implementation

- Avoid distractions and interruptions when preparing and administering medication *to prevent medication errors.*[1,2]
- Verify the practitioner's order.[3,4,5]
- Perform hand hygiene.[6,7,8,9,10]
- Compare the medication label with the order in the patient's medical record.[3,4,5]
- Check the patient's medical record for an allergy or other contraindication to the medication. If an allergy or a contraindication exists, don't administer the medication; notify the practitioner.[3,4,5]
- Check the expiration date on the medication. If the medication has expired, return it to the pharmacy and obtain new medication.[3,4,5]
- Inspect the prescribed MDI visually for loss of integrity; don't administer the medication if the MDI's integrity has been compromised.[3,4,5]
- Discuss any unresolved concerns about the medication with the practitioner.[3,4,5]
- Confirm the patient's identity using at least two patient identifiers.[11]
- Explain the procedure to the patient.
- If the patient is using the medication for the first time, teach him about potential adverse reactions and discuss any other concerns related to the medication.[3,4,5]
- Verify that the medication is being administered at the proper time, in the prescribed dose, and by the correct route *to reduce the risk of medication errors.*[3,4,5]
- If your facility uses a bar code scanning system, scan your identification badge, the patient's identification bracelet, and the medication's bar code.
- Assess the patient's breath sounds *to obtain a baseline for comparison.*
- Insert the metal stem of the prescribed MDI into the small hole on the flattened portion of the mouthpiece.
- Shake the prescribed MDI *to mix the medication and aerosol propellant.* Prime the MDI, as needed, according to the manufacturer's instructions; requirements for priming (spraying one or more puffs into the air before use) vary among devices and ensure that the inhaler is ready to use and will dispense the correct amount of medication.[12]
- Remove the mouthpiece cap. Attach the prescribed MDI to the spacer as indicated, making sure not to touch the mouthpiece. Keep in mind that some MDIs have a spacer built into the inhaler.
- Instruct the patient to exhale fully and then to hold the prescribed MDI, as instructed by the practitioner, 1″ to 2″ (2.5 cm to 5 cm) in front of his mouth (about the width of two fingers). The patient should then put the prescribed MDI into his mouth and close his lips around it, or place the end of the spacer into his mouth (as shown below).[13]

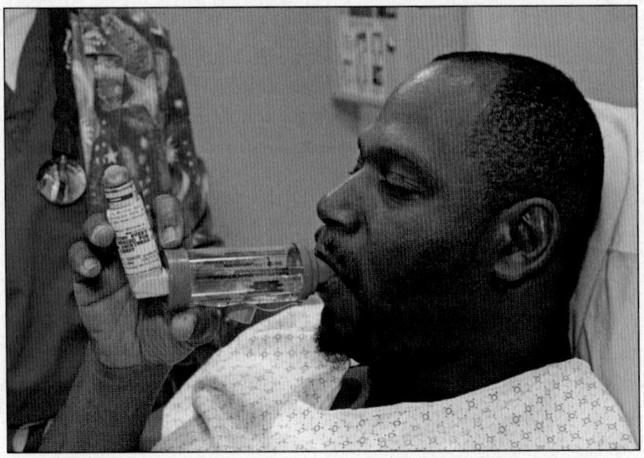

- Instruct the patient to press down on the prescribed MDI one time as he starts breathing in through his mouth slowly. (If a spacer is being used, instruct the patient to press down on the prescribed MDI first and then begin to breathe in slowly within 5 seconds.)
- Instruct the patient to continue breathing in slowly, as deeply as he can.[13] *This action draws the medication into his lungs.*
- Remove the mouthpiece from the patient's mouth, and instruct him to hold his breath as he slowly counts to 10, if possible,[13] *to allow the medication to reach the alveoli.* Then, instruct him to exhale slowly through pursed lips *to keep the distal bronchioles open, allowing increased absorption and diffusion of the drug and better gas exchange.* When inhaled quick-relief medications (beta$_2$-adrenergic agonists) are administered, the patient should wait about 15 to 30 seconds between inhalations. There's no need to wait between inhalations for other medications.[13]
- When inhaled corticosteroids (such as beclomethasone, budesonide, ciclesonide, flunisolide, fluticasone, and triamcinolone) are administered, instruct the patient to rinse and gargle with water and then to expectorate using an emesis basin, if necessary, after each dose *to help prevent an infection in the mouth.*[14,15]
- When all the ordered inhalations have been administered, remove the spacer (if used) from the MDI, and wash the spacer and mouthpiece according to the manufacturer's instructions.
- Put the cap back on the prescribed MDI after each use. Store the MDI and spacer, if used, with the patient's medication.
- Assess the patient's breath sounds after medication administration *to determine his response to the medication.*
- Allow the patient to gargle with water, if desired, *to remove the medication from his mouth and the back of his throat.*
- Perform hand hygiene.[6,7,8,9,10]
- Clean and disinfect your stethoscope using a disinfectant pad.[16,17]
- Perform hand hygiene.[6,7,8,9,10]
- Document the procedure.[18,19,20]

Special considerations

- MDIs with spacers may be recommended *to provide greater therapeutic benefit for children and for patients who have difficulty with coordination.* A spacer attachment is an extension to the inhaler's mouthpiece that provides more dead-air space for mixing the medication. Some MDIs have built-in spacers.
- If the patient is also using a steroid, instruct him to use the bronchodilator MDI first and then to wait 5 minutes before using the steroid MDI *because this process allows the bronchodilator to open the air passages for maximum effectiveness.*

Patient teaching

Teach the patient how to use the MDI *so that he can continue treatments himself after discharge.*. Explain that overdosage, which is common, can cause the medication to lose its effectiveness. Instruct the patient to record the date and time of each inhalation as well as his response *to prevent overdosage and to help the practitioner determine the drug's effectiveness.* If more than one inhalation is ordered, tell the patient if he should wait before repeating the procedure. During teaching, note whether the patient uses an unusual amount of medication (for instance, more than one cartridge every 3 weeks). Inform the patient of possible adverse reactions to the prescribed MDI.

Complications

Complications are related to the medication being administered by the MDI.

Documentation

Record the medication administered by the MDI as well as the dose and time. Document your respiratory assessment before MDI administration and the patient's response to treatment. Document any adverse reactions and interventions taken. Document any patient teaching and the patient's understanding of the teaching.

References

1 Westbrook, J., et al. (2010). Association of interruptions with an increased risk and severity of medication administration errors. *Archives of Internal Medicine, 170,* 683–690. (Level IV)

2 Institute for Safe Medication Practices. (2012). Side tracks on the safety express: Interruptions lead to errors and unfinished . . . Wait, what was I doing? *Nurse Advise-ERR, 11*(2), 1–4. Accessed May 2015 via the Web at https://www.ismp.org/Newsletters/acutecare/showarticle.aspx?id=37

3 The Joint Commission. (2015). Standard MM.06.01.01. *Comprehensive accreditation manual for hospitals: The official handbook.* Oakbrook Terrace, IL: The Joint Commission. (Level VII)

4 Centers for Medicare & Medicaid Services, Department of Health and Human Services. (2014). Condition of participation: Nursing services. 42 C.F.R. § 482.23(c).

5 American Osteopathic Association. (2014). Standard 16.01.03. *Healthcare Facilities Accreditation Program: Accreditation requirements for acute care hospitals.* Chicago, IL: American Osteopathic Association. (Level VII)

6 Centers for Disease Control and Prevention. (2002). Guideline for hand hygiene in health-care settings: Recommendations of the Healthcare Infection Control Practices Advisory Committee and the HICPAC/SHEA/APIC/IDSA Hand Hygiene Task Force. *MMWR Recommendations and Reports, 51*(RR-16), 1–45. Accessed May 2015 via the Web at http://www.cdc.gov/mmwr/pdf/rr/rr5116.pdf (Level II)

7 World Health Organization. (2009). "WHO guidelines on hand hygiene in health care: First global patient safety challenge, clean care is safer care" [Online]. Accessed May 2015 via the Web at http://whqlibdoc.who.int/publications/2009/9789241597906_eng.pdf (Level IV)

8 The Joint Commission. (2015). Standard NPSG.07.01.01. *Comprehensive accreditation manual for hospitals: The official handbook.* Oakbrook Terrace, IL: The Joint Commission. (Level VII)

9 Centers for Medicare & Medicaid Services, Department of Health and Human Services. (2014). Condition of participation: Infection control. 42 C.F.R. § 482.42.

10 American Osteopathic Association. (2014). Standard 07.01.21. *Healthcare Facilities Accreditation Program: Accreditation requirements for acute care hospitals.* Chicago, IL: American Osteopathic Association. (Level VII)

11 The Joint Commission. (2015). Standard NPSG.01.01.01. *Comprehensive accreditation manual for hospitals: The official handbook.* Oakbrook Terrace, IL: The Joint Commission. (Level VII)

12 American College of Chest Physicians. (2006). "Priming and cleaning your MDI: Patient education guide" [Online]. Accessed May 2015 via the Web at http://accpstorage.org/newOrganization/patients/inhaledDevices/patientEducation10LP.pdf

13 National Heart, Lung, and Blood Institute. National Asthma Education and Prevention Program. (2007). "Expert Panel Report 3: Guidelines for the diagnosis and management of asthma" [Online]. Accessed May 2015 at http://www.nhlbi.nih.gov/guidelines/asthma/asthgdln.pdf (Level VII)

14 American Academy of Allergy, Asthma & Immunology. (2013). "Inhaled asthma medications: Tips to remember" [Online]. Accessed May 2015 via the Web at http://www.aaaai.org/conditions-and-treatments/library/at-a-glance/inhaled-asthma-medications.aspx

15 National Asthma Education and Prevention Program. (2013). "How to use a metered-dose inhaler" [Online]. Accessed May 2015 via the Web at http://www.nhlbi.nih.gov/files/docs/public/lung/asthma_tipsheets.pdf

16 Rutala, W. A., et al. (2008). "Guideline for disinfection and sterilization in healthcare facilities, 2008" [Online]. Accessed May 2015 via the Web at http://www.cdc.gov/hicpac/pdf/guidelines/Disinfection_Nov_2008.pdf (Level I)

17 American Osteopathic Association. (2014). Standard 07.02.03. *Healthcare Facilities Accreditation Program: Accreditation requirements for acute care hospitals.* Chicago, IL: American Osteopathic Association. (Level VII)

18 The Joint Commission. (2015). Standard RC.01.03.01. *Comprehensive accreditation manual for hospitals: The official handbook.* Oakbrook Terrace, IL: The Joint Commission. (Level VII)

19 Centers for Medicare & Medicaid Services, Department of Health and Human Services. (2014). Condition of participation: Medical record services. 42 C.F.R. § 482.24(b).

20 American Osteopathic Association. (2014). Standard 10.00.03. *Healthcare Facilities Accreditation Program: Accreditation requirements for acute care hospitals.* Chicago, IL: American Osteopathic Association. (Level VII)

Additional references

Ari, A., & Restrepo, R. D. (2012). AARC clinical practice guideline: Aerosol delivery device selection for spontaneously breathing patients: 2012. *Respiratory Care, 57,* 613–626. Accessed May 2015 via the Web at http://rc.rcjournal.com/content/57/4/613.full.pdf (Level VII)

De Tratto, K., et al. (2014). Nurses' knowledge of inhaler technique in the inpatient hospital setting. *Clinical Nurse Specialist, 28,* 156–160. (Level IV)

Gardenhire, D. S., et al. (2013). "A guide to aerosol delivery devices for respiratory therapists (3rd ed.)" [Online]. Accessed May 2015 via the Web at https://www.aarc.org/resources/aerosol_resources/aerosol_guide_rt.pdf (Level VII)

Press, V. G., et al. (2012). Teaching the use of respiratory inhalers to hospitalized patients with asthma or COPD: A randomized trial. *Journal of General Internal Medicine, 27,* 1317–1325. (Level II)

Rennard, S., et al. (2014). Randomized study of the safety, pharmacokinetics, and bronchodilatory efficacy of a proprietary glycopyrronium metered-dose inhaler in study patients with chronic obstructive pulmonary disease. *BMC Pulmonary Medicine, 14,* 118. (Level II)

Mixed venous oxygen saturation monitoring

Mixed venous oxygen saturation (Svo_2) monitoring involves the use of a fiber-optic thermodilution pulmonary artery (PA) catheter to continuously monitor oxygen delivery to tissues and oxygen consumption by tissues. Monitoring of Svo_2 allows rapid detection of impaired oxygen delivery, such as from decreased cardiac output, hemoglobin level, or arterial oxygen saturation. It also helps evaluate a patient's response to drug therapy, endotracheal tube suctioning, ventilator setting changes, positive end-expiratory pressure (PEEP), and fraction of inspired oxygen. Svo_2 usually ranges from 60% to 80%.[1]

Equipment

Fiber-optic PA catheter ■ co-oximeter (monitor) ■ optical module and cable ■ gloves ■ mixed venous blood sampling equipment ■ laboratory biohazard bag.

Preparation of equipment

Review the manufacturer's instructions for assembly and use of the fiber-optic PA catheter. Connect the optical module and cable to the monitor. Next, peel back the wrapping covering the catheter just enough to uncover the fiber-optic connector. Attach the fiber-optic connector to the optical module while allowing the rest of the catheter to remain in its sterile wrapping. Calibrate the fiber-optic catheter by following the manufacturer's instructions. Enter the patient's most recent hemoglobin level during the calibration process.[2]

To prepare for the rest of the procedure, follow the instructions for pulmonary catheter insertion, as described in the "Pulmonary artery pressure and pulmonary artery wedge pressure monitoring" procedure. (See *Svo_2 monitoring equipment,* page 504.)

Implementation

- Verify the practitioner's order.
- Gather and prepare the necessary equipment.
- Confirm the patient's identity using at least two patient identifiers.[3]
- Perform hand hygiene.[4,5,6,7,8]
- Put on gloves *to comply with standard precautions.*[10,11,12]
- Explain the procedure to the patient and answer any questions *to allay his fears and promote cooperation.*
- Assist with the insertion of the fiber-optic catheter just as you would for a PA catheter insertion.

EQUIPMENT

SvO_2 monitoring equipment

A mixed venous oxygen saturation (SvO_2) monitoring system consists of a flow-directed pulmonary artery (PA) catheter with fiber-optic filaments, an optical module, and a co-oximeter. The co-oximeter displays a continuous digital SvO_2 value; the strip recorder prints a permanent record.

Catheter insertion follows the same technique as with any thermodilution flow-directed PA catheter. The distal lumen connects to an external PA pressure monitoring system, the proximal or central venous pressure lumen connects to another monitoring system or to a continuous flow administration unit, and the optical module connects to the co-oximeter unit.[9]

Normal SvO_2 waveform

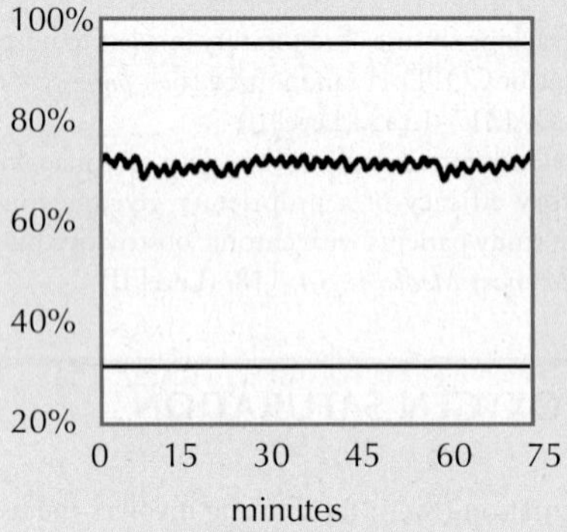

SvO_2 with patient activities

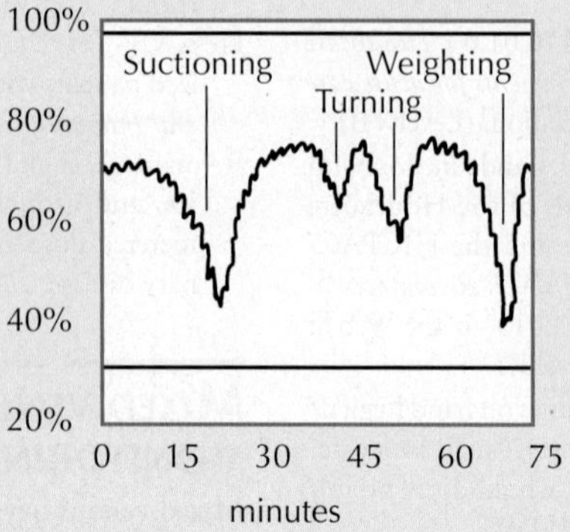

SvO_2 with positive end-expiratory pressure (PEEP) and fraction of inspired oxygen (FIO_2) changes

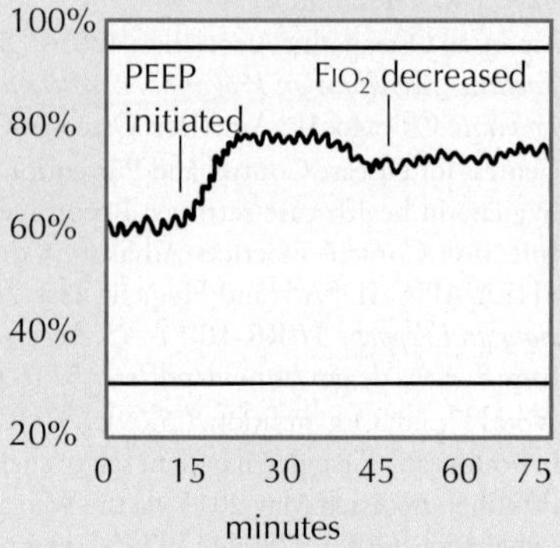

- After the catheter is inserted, confirm that the light intensity tracing on the graphic printout is within normal range *to ensure correct positioning and function of the catheter.*
- Observe the digital readout and record the SvO_2 on the graphic printout. Repeat readings at least once each hour *to monitor and document trends.*
- Make sure the machine alarms limits are set appropriately for the patient's current condition and that the alarms are turned on, functioning, and audible to staff.[13,14,15,16]

Recalibrating the monitor

- Draw a mixed venous blood sample from the distal port of the PA catheter. Label the sample in the presence of the patient *to prevent mislabeling.*[3] Send it to the laboratory for analysis in a laboratory biohazard transport bag[12] *to compare the laboratory's SvO_2 reading with that of the fiber-optic catheter.*
- If the catheter values and the laboratory values differ by more than 4%, follow the manufacturer's instructions to enter the SvO_2 value obtained by the laboratory into the co-oximeter.
- Recalibrate the monitor every 24 hours or whenever the catheter has been disconnected from the optical module.

Completing the procedure

- Remove and discard your gloves.[10]
- Perform hand hygiene.[4,5,6,7,8]
- Document the procedure.[17,18,19]

Special considerations

- The Joint Commission issued a sentinel event alert concerning medical device alarm safety *because alarm-related events have been associated with permanent loss of function and death.* Among the major contributing factors were improper alarm settings, alarms inappropriately turned off, and alarm signals not audible to staff. Make sure that alarm limits are set appropriately and that alarms are turned on, functioning properly, and audible to staff. Follow facility guidelines for preventing alarm fatigue.[14]
- If the patient's SvO_2 drops below 60% or varies by more than 10% for 3 minutes or longer, reassess the patient. If the SvO_2 doesn't return to the baseline value after nursing interventions, notify the practitioner. *A decreasing SvO_2, or a value less than 60%, indicates impaired oxygen delivery, which can occur in hemorrhage, hypoxia, shock, sepsis,*[20] *arrhythmias, or suctioning.* SvO_2 may also decrease as a result of increased oxygen demand from hyperthermia, shivering, or seizures.
- If the intensity of the tracing is low, ensure that all connections between the catheter and co-oximeter are secure and that the catheter is patent and not kinked.
- If the tracing is damped or erratic, try to aspirate blood from the catheter *to check for patency.* If you can't aspirate blood, notify the practitioner *so that he can replace the catheter.* Also check the PA waveform *to determine whether the catheter has wedged.* If the catheter has wedged, turn the patient from side to side and instruct him to cough. If the catheter remains wedged, notify the practitioner immediately.

Complications

Thrombosis can result from local irritation by the catheter; however, a heparinized flush helps prevent this complication. Thromboembolism also can occur if a thrombus breaks off and lodges in the circulatory system. Catheter insertion and maintenance may increase the risk of infection.

Documentation

Record the SvO_2 value, as ordered, and document a tracing. Note significant changes in the patient's status; the date, time, and name of the practitioner notified; prescribed interventions; and the results of any interventions. For comparison, note the SvO_2 as measured by the fiber-optic catheter whenever a blood sample is obtained for laboratory analysis of SvO_2. Document patient teaching and the patient's understanding of that teaching.

REFERENCES

1 Lynn-McHale Wiegand, D. (Ed.). (2011). *AACN procedure manual for critical care* (6th ed.). St. Louis, MO: Saunders.

2 Edwards Lifesciences. (2002). "Understanding continuous mixed venous oxygen saturation (SvO_2) monitoring with the Swan-Ganz oximetry TD system (2nd ed.)" [Online]. Accessed May 2015 via the Web at http://ht.edwards.com/resourcegallery/products/swanganz/pdfs/svo2edbook.pdf
3 The Joint Commission. (2015). Standard NPSG.01.01.01. *Comprehensive accreditation manual for hospitals: The official handbook.* Oakbrook Terrace, IL: The Joint Commission. (Level VII)
4 The Joint Commission. (2015). Standard NPSG.07.01.01. *Comprehensive accreditation manual for hospitals: The official handbook.* Oakbrook Terrace, IL: The Joint Commission. (Level VII)
5 Centers for Disease Control and Prevention. (2002). Guideline for hand hygiene in health-care settings: Recommendations of the Healthcare Infection Control Practices Advisory Committee and the HICPAC/SHEA/APIC/IDSA Hand Hygiene Task Force. *MMWR Recommendations and Reports, 51*(RR-16), 1–45. Accessed May 2015 via the Web at http://www.cdc.gov/mmwr/pdf/rr/rr5116.pdf (Level II)
6 World Health Organization. (2009). "WHO guidelines on hand hygiene in health care: First global patient safety challenge, clean care is safer care" [Online]. Accessed May 2015 via the Web at http://whqlibdoc.who.int/publications/2009/9789241597906_eng.pdf (Level IV)
7 Centers for Medicare & Medicaid Services, Department of Health and Human Services. (2014). Condition of participation: Infection control. 42 C.F.R. § 482.42.
8 American Osteopathic Association. (2014). Standard 07.01.21. *Healthcare Facilities Accreditation Program: Accreditation requirements for acute care hospitals.* Chicago, IL: American Osteopathic Association. (Level VII)
9 Edwards Lifesciences. (2004). "Advanced technology catheters" [Online]. Accessed May 2015 via the Web at http://ht.edwards.com/resourcegallery/products/swanganz/pdfs/advtechbroch.pdf
10 Siegel, J. D., et al. (2007). "2007 guideline for isolation precautions: Preventing transmission of infectious agents in healthcare settings" [Online]. Accessed May 2015 via the Web at http://www.cdc.gov/hicpac/pdf/isolation/Isolation2007.pdf (Level II)
11 American Osteopathic Association. (2014). Standard 07.01.10. *Healthcare Facilities Accreditation Program: Accreditation requirements for acute care hospitals.* Chicago, IL: American Osteopathic Association. (Level VII)
12 Occupational Safety and Health Administration. (n.d.). "Bloodborne pathogens, standard number 1910.1030" [Online]. Accessed May 2015 via the Web at http://www.osha.gov/pls/oshaweb/owadisp.show_document?p_table=STANDARDS&p_id=10051 (Level VII)
13 American Association of Critical-Care Nurses. (2013). "AACN practice alert: Alarm management" [Online]. Accessed May 2015 via the Web at http://www.aacn.org/wd/practice/docs/practicealerts/alarm-management-practice-alert.pdf (Level VII)
14 The Joint Commission. (2013). "Sentinel event alert: Medical device alarm safety in hospitals" [Online]. Accessed May 2015 via the Web at http://www.jointcommission.org/assets/1/18/SEA_50_alarms_4_5_13_FINAL1.PDF (Level VII)
15 The Joint Commission. (2015). Standard NPSG.06.01.01. *Comprehensive accreditation manual for hospitals: The official handbook.* Oakbrook Terrace, IL: The Joint Commission. (Level VII)
16 Graham, K. C., & Cvach, M. (2010). Monitor alarm fatigue: Standardizing use of physiological monitors and decreasing nuisance alarms. *American Journal of Critical Care, 19,* 28–37.
17 The Joint Commission. (2015). Standard RC.01.03.01. *Comprehensive accreditation manual for hospitals: The official handbook.* Oakbrook Terrace, IL: The Joint Commission. (Level VII)
18 Centers for Medicare & Medicaid Services, Department of Health and Human Services. (2014). Condition of participation: Medical record services. 42 C.F.R. § 482.24(b).
19 American Osteopathic Association. (2014). Standard 10.00.03. *Healthcare Facilities Accreditation Program: Accreditation requirements for acute care hospitals.* Chicago, IL; American Osteopathic Association. (Level VII)
20 Dellinger, R. P., et al. (2013). Surviving sepsis campaign: International guidelines for management of severe sepsis and septic shock: 2012. Critical Care Medicine, 41, 580–637. Accessed May 2015 via the Web at http://www.sccm.org/Documents/SSC-Guidelines.pdf (Level VII)

Levels of sedation[3]

Because a patient receiving sedation might not always respond as intended, make sure you can recognize the different levels of sedation. The American Society of Anesthesiologists describes levels of sedation as follows:

- *Minimal sedation (anxiolysis)* is a drug-induced state during which a patient responds normally to verbal commands. Cognitive function and physical coordination may be impaired, but airway reflexes and ventilatory and cardiovascular functions aren't affected.
- *Moderate sedation/analgesia (conscious sedation)* is a drug-induced depression of consciousness during which a patient responds purposefully to verbal commands, given either alone or accompanied by light tactile stimulation. (Reflex withdrawal from a painful stimulus isn't considered a purposeful response.) The patient doesn't require intervention to maintain a patent airway, has adequate spontaneous ventilation, and maintains cardiovascular function.
- *Deep sedation/analgesia* is a drug-induced depression of consciousness during which a patient can't be easily aroused but responds purposefully to repeated or painful stimulation. The patient's ability to independently maintain ventilatory function may be impaired. He may require assistance to maintain a patent airway and may not have adequate spontaneous ventilation, but typically maintains cardiovascular function.
- *General anesthesia* is a drug-induced loss of consciousness during which a patient can't be aroused, even by painful stimulation. The patient's ability to maintain ventilatory function independently is typically impaired. He's likely to require assistance to maintain a patent airway, and may need positive-pressure ventilation because of depressed spontaneous ventilation or drug-induced depression of neuromuscular function. Cardiovascular function may be impaired.

ADDITIONAL REFERENCES

Christensen, M. (2013). Mixed venous oxygen saturation monitoring revisited: Thoughts for critical care nursing practice. *Australian Critical Care, 25*(2), 78–90.
McGee, W. T., et al. (2014). "Quick guide to cardiopulmonary care (3rd ed.)" [Online]. Accessed May 2015 via the Web at http://ht.edwards.com/scin/edwards/sitecollectionimages/products/pressuremonitoring/ar11206-quickguide3rded.pdf

MODERATE SEDATION

Previously referred to as *conscious sedation,* moderate sedation is a drug-induced depression of consciousness in which the patient responds purposefully to verbal commands, either spontaneously or with light tactile stimulation. With moderate sedation, the patient is able to maintain a patent airway, protective reflexes (such as the ability to handle secretions without aspiration), adequate spontaneous ventilations, and cardiovascular function without interventions.[1]

Moderate sedation, or procedural sedation and analgesia,[2] is commonly administered so that patients can tolerate unpleasant procedures by relieving anxiety, discomfort, or pain; in children and uncooperative adults, it may be used to expedite procedures that aren't particularly uncomfortable but that require the patient to remain still.[1]

Because predicting a patient's response to sedation isn't always possible, health care providers must have an understanding of the different levels of sedation. (See *Levels of sedation.*)

In addition to the person administering moderate sedation, this procedure requires the presence of at least one other person capable of

ASA physical status classification system[4,8]

The American Society of Anesthesiologists (ASA) physical status classification system is widely used to estimate a patient's risk of developing complications. Patients classified as P1, P2, and medically stable P3 are commonly considered appropriate for registered nurse–administered moderate sedation.[4]

P1: normal, healthy patient
P2: patient with mild systemic disease
P3: patient with severe systemic disease
P4: patient with severe systemic disease that's a constant threat to life
P5: moribund patient who isn't expected to survive the procedure
P6: patient declared brain dead whose organs are being removed for donation

establishing a patent airway, administering positive-pressure ventilation to the patient, and summoning additional assistance if necessary. A person with advanced life support skills should be immediately available (within 1 to 5 minutes).[1,4]

A patient receiving moderate sedation requires sedation monitoring before the procedure, throughout the procedure, and during the recovery period. Health care workers permitted by their scope of practice to administer moderate sedation should receive special training.[1,4,5,6] Those administering the sedation who are responsible for the patient's care should understand the pharmacology of the agents as well as the role of reversal agents. Those monitoring the patient receiving moderate sedation should be able to recognize associated complications.[1] Health care workers responsible for monitoring a patient receiving moderate sedation/analgesia shouldn't have other responsibilities that would require leaving the patient unattended or that would compromise continuous monitoring during the procedure.[4]

Some patients who require a procedure may not be appropriate candidates for moderate sedation and may require anesthesia that's monitored by an anesthesia care provider. The American Society of Anesthesiologists (ASA) devised the ASA physical status classification system to provide a uniform guideline for evaluating the severity of systemic diseases, physiologic dysfunction, and anatomic abnormalities to determine a patient's risk of developing complications.[7] (See *ASA physical status classification system.*)

Moderate sedation is commonly administered for procedures that are performed in many settings outside the operating room, including GI procedure units, interventional radiology suites, bronchoscopy suites, emergency departments, interventional cardiology suites, and critical care units. Regardless of the location, adequately trained staff and appropriate monitoring equipment must be available to ensure the patient's safety.

Equipment

Sedation record ▪ positive-pressure oxygen delivery system ▪ supplemental oxygen administration equipment[1] ▪ suction apparatus ▪ suction catheter ▪ pulse oximeter ▪ blood pressure monitoring equipment ▪ capnometer ▪ stethoscope ▪ cardiac monitoring equipment ▪ thermometer ▪ disinfectant pad ▪ emergency cart that contains a defibrillator, IV access equipment, IV fluids, basic and advanced airway management equipment, and emergency medications[1,5] ▪ prescribed medications and reversal agents ▪ Optional: gloves, other personal protective equipment.

Preparation of equipment

Make sure the room where the patient will be receiving the sedation has all the necessary equipment, including emergency care supplies.[1,5] Test all monitoring equipment *to ensure that it's in proper working order* before attaching it to the patient.[1]

Implementation

▪ Avoid distractions and interruptions when preparing and administering medication *to prevent medication errors.*[9,10]

▪ Verify the practitioner's order for the prescribed medication.[11,12,13]

▪ Review the patient's medical record and verify documentation of preexisting medical conditions; a history of tobacco, alcohol, or substance use or abuse; previous anesthesia and sedation experiences; current medications; allergies; the last time the patient ate or had oral fluids; a recent height and weight measurement; and physical examination findings, including evaluation of the airway and a cardiac and respiratory assessment.[1,4,5,14,15,16]

NURSING ALERT *Contact the anesthesia care provider if the patient has any of the following conditions: a history of respiratory or hemodynamic instability; one or more significant comorbidities; pregnancy; sleep apnea; inability to communicate or cooperate; multiple drug allergies; multiple medications with potential for drug interactions with sedative analgesia; or current substance abuse.* **Extra precautions may need to be taken with these patients, including additional monitoring and medication management.**[4]

NURSING ALERT *Obese patients have special needs during moderate sedation* because they're at increased risk for complications due to altered physiology. *Consult with the anesthesia care provider.*[17]

▪ Check the patient's medical record for allergies and other contraindications to the prescribed medication. If either exists, don't administer the medication; notify the practitioner.[11,12,13]

▪ If applicable, check the patient's medical record for pregnancy test results.[4]

▪ Confirm that written informed consent has been obtained and is in the patient's medical record.[4,5,18,19,20,21]

▪ Conduct a preprocedure verification *to make sure that all relevant documentation, related information, and equipment are available and correctly identified to the patient's identifiers.*[22,23]

▪ Compare the medication label with the order in the patient's medical record.[11,12,13]

▪ Check the expiration date on the medication. If the medication is expired, return it to the pharmacy and obtain new medication.[11,12,13]

▪ Visually inspect the solution for particles or discoloration or other loss of integrity; don't administer the medication if its integrity is compromised.[11,12,13]

▪ Discuss any unresolved concerns about the medication with the patient's practitioner.[11,12,13]

▪ Perform hand hygiene.[24,25,26,27,28]

▪ Confirm the patient's identity using at least two patient identifiers.[29]

▪ Verify the scheduled invasive procedure and the correct site as stated by the patient, and compare it with the medical record.[22,30] Explain the sedation administration procedure to the patient and his family, and answer their questions *to reduce their anxiety.* Teach the patient and his family about potential adverse reactions and discuss any other concerns related to the medication.[11,12,13]

▪ If the patient is to be discharged less than 12 hours after receiving sedation, verify that arrangements have been made to transport the patient home and that an adult will be available in case complications arise.

▪ Confirm the patient's nothing-by-mouth status before the procedure; if not an emergency, minimum fasting recommendations include 2 hours for clear liquids, 6 or more hours for a light meal or nonhuman milk, and 8 or more hours for fried or fatty foods or meat. If the need for the procedure is an emergency, collaborate with the practitioner to compare the risks and benefits of the procedure, considering the amount and type of liquids or solids ingested.[31]

■ Assess the patient for conditions that might make ventilation difficult, such as significant obesity, history of snoring or sleep apnea, facial hair, missing teeth, and the presence of stridor.[4]
■ When the patient is in the room where sedation will be administered, perform hand hygiene and put on gloves and other personal protective equipment as needed *to comply with standard precautions.*[24,25,26,27,28,32,33]
■ Apply a pulse oximeter probe, turn on the machine, and record the patient's oxygen saturation level. Make sure that the alarm limits are set appropriately for the patient's current condition and that the alarms are turned on, functioning properly, and audible to staff.[4,34,35,36,37,38]
■ Attach the patient to a cardiac monitor *to monitor heart rate and function.*[4,34] Make sure that the alarm limits are set appropriately for the patient's current condition and that the alarms are turned on, functioning properly, and audible to staff.[1,35,36,37,38]
■ Attach the patient to a capnometer *to continuously monitor exhaled carbon dioxide during the procedure.* Make sure that the alarm limits are set appropriately for the patient's current condition and that alarms are turned on, functioning properly, and audible to staff.[34,35,36,37,38]
■ Record the patient's vital signs, level of consciousness (LOC), skin color, and respiratory status *to use as baselines.*[14,15]
■ Ensure that the patient has patent IV access. If a patent IV catheter isn't present, establish one.[1,18] (See the "IV catheter insertion and removal" procedure, page 446.)
■ Confirm that the procedure site has been marked appropriately, if indicated. Involve the patient in the process if possible.[7,23,39]
■ Confirm the medication dosage calculations based on the patient's weight or body surface area.
■ If your facility uses a bar code scanning system, scan your identification badge, the patient's identification bracelet, and the medication's bar code.
■ After the patient is prepped and draped for the procedure, conduct a time-out immediately before starting the procedure *to perform a final assessment that the correct patient, site, positioning, and procedure are identified and, as applicable, all relevant information and necessary equipment are available.*[7,30,40]

NURSING ALERT *Medications used for moderate sedation are considered high-alert medications* because they can cause significant patient harm when used in error.[41]

■ Before administering moderate sedation, have another nurse perform an independent double-check *to verify the patient's identity and to make sure that the correct medication is being administered in the prescribed concentration, the medication's indication corresponds with the patient's diagnosis, the dosage calculations are correct and the dosing formula used to derive the final dose is correct, and the route of administration is safe and proper for the patient.*[42]
■ Compare the results of the independent double-check with the other nurse and, if no discrepancies exist, begin administering the medication. If discrepancies exist, rectify them before administering the medication.[42]
■ Administer each medication separately in incremental doses and titrate it to the desired effect following safe medication administration practices *to decrease the risk of overdose and respiratory and circulatory depression.*[4,12,13]
■ Continuously monitor the patient's heart rate and function (using a cardiac monitor), oxygenation (using pulse oximetry), and respiratory rate and adequacy of ventilation (using continual observation of clinical status and capnography).[14]
■ Determine and evaluate the patient's blood pressure and heart rate at least every 5 minutes.[1,34]
■ Monitor the patient's LOC (by checking response to verbal commands when practical), comfort level, and skin condition at regular intervals.[4]
■ Administer supplemental oxygen if hypoxia occurs.[1] *The method and rate of flow should be determined by the patient's optimal oxygen saturation level according to pulse oximetry.*[4] *Hypoxemia may cause cardiopulmonary complications.*[4]

TROUBLESHOOTING

Responding to complications of sedation

This table reviews nursing interventions for various complications of sedation.

COMPLICATION	NURSING INTERVENTIONS
Airway obstruction or respiratory depression	■ Reposition the patient's head. ■ Suction the patient. ■ Insert an oral airway. ■ Tell the patient to take a deep breath. ■ Stimulate the patient by rubbing his arms or legs. ■ Administer oxygen. ■ Manually ventilate the patient with a handheld resuscitation bag.
Oversedation	■ Maintain circulation, airway, and breathing. ■ Have drugs to reverse sedation (such as naloxone for opiates or flumazenil for benzodiazepines) immediately available and administer, as ordered, if the patient is too deeply sedated. ■ Monitor respiratory status until stable.
Cardiac arrhythmias	■ Note baseline heart rate and rhythm. ■ Obtain an apical pulse for 1 minute. ■ Examine electrocardiogram patterns if indicated. ■ Ensure that the patient has a patent airway. ■ Monitor oxygen saturation levels. ■ Administer oxygen. ■ Administer fluids and antiarrhythmic drugs as ordered.
Hypotension	■ Investigate possible causes. ■ Support respiratory status. ■ Administer fluids and vasopressors as ordered.
Hypertension	■ Administer additional sedation or analgesia.

■ Monitor the patient's temperature when clinically significant changes in body temperature are intended, anticipated, or suspected.[34]
■ Monitor the patient for complications and intervene as indicated.[5] (See *Responding to complications of sedation.*)
■ When sedation administration is complete, use the same monitoring parameters used during the procedure and monitor the patient until discharge criteria are met. The patient should remain awake for at least 20 minutes without stimulation before he's considered ready for discharge. The duration and frequency of monitoring should be individualized, depending on the level of sedation achieved, the patient's overall condition, and the nature of the procedure for which sedation was administered. If a reversal agent was given, monitor the patient for a sufficient time interval (for example, 2 hours) after the last administration of an antagonist *to make sure that the patient doesn't become resedated after the reversal effects have worn off.*[1,2,4]

- Remove and discard your gloves and other personal protective equipment if worn.[32]
- Perform hand hygiene.[24,25,26,27,28]
- Clean and disinfect your stethoscope using a disinfectant pad.[43,44]
- Perform hand hygiene.[24,25,26,27,28]
- Document the procedure.[45,46,47,48]

Special considerations

- The Joint Commission issued a sentinel event alert concerning medical device alarm safety *because alarm-related events have been associated with permanent loss of function and death.* Among the major contributing factors were improper alarm settings, alarms inappropriately turned off, and alarm signals not audible to staff. Make sure that alarm limits are set appropriately and that alarms are turned on, functioning properly, and audible to staff. Follow facility guidelines for preventing alarm fatigue.[35]
- Before discharge, the patient should meet certain criteria, which may include a return to preprocedural baseline LOC and stable vital signs; a sufficient time interval (for example, 2 hours) since the last administration of an antagonist; the use of an objective patient assessment scoring system; absence of protracted nausea; intact protective reflexes (for example, gag or cough reflexes); adequate pain control; and return of sensory and motor control.[4] Use a recovery and discharge criteria scoring system, such as the Aldrete Post-Anesthesia Recovery Score and the Post-Anesthesia Discharge Scoring System, *to monitor the patient's status and to help determine when the patient is ready for discharge*; tailor use of the scoring system to the patient's specific needs.[2]

Patient teaching

After completion of the procedure, reinforce patient education with written instructions for the patient and his family. Teach the patient and his family about potential adverse reactions, and discuss other concerns related to the administered medications.[11] Explain when they should seek immediate emergency care, and provide the patient's escort with an emergency phone number.[2] Teach the patient and his family about pain management strategies. Reinforce the importance of having someone available to assist the patient with care for 24 hours after the procedure.

Complications

The patient can become oversedated during moderate sedation. Other complications of moderate sedation include aspiration of gastric contents, respiratory depression or failure, and adverse reactions to the medication. Observe the patient for airway obstruction, respiratory depression, hypotension, and drug-specific complications.

Advanced age and poor general health, such preexisting respiratory conditions as chronic obstructive pulmonary disease and asthma, and hepatic or renal dysfunction can increase the patient's risk of adverse reactions. In general, older adults, because of decreased renal and hepatic function and relative loss of muscle, are at greater risk. Drug interactions may occur; opioids when used in combination with sedatives may produce a synergistic effect.

Documentation

Document according to your facility's documentation system and include parameters your facility considers necessary. Such parameter include but aren't limited to preprocedure assessment findings, procedure and site verification, and time-out; the name, dose, route, time, and effects of all medications administered; the patient's LOC, ventilation, and oxygenation status; and the procedure start and end times. Documentation should also include vital signs at intervals determined by the type and quantity of medication administered and the patient's condition.[4]

References

1 American Society of Anesthesiologists. (2002). Practice guidelines for sedation and analgesia by non-anesthesiologists. *Anesthesiology, 96,* 1004–1017. Accessed May 2015 via the Web at http://journals.lww.com/anesthesiology/Fulltext/2002/04000/Practice_Guideline_for_Sedation_and_Analgesia_by.31.aspx(Level VII)

2 Meyers, J. L., & Chaudhuri, S. (2011). Procedural sedation and analgesia: A practical review for non-anesthesiologists. *Journal of Surgical Radiology, 2,* 344–356.

3 American Society of Anesthesiologists. (2009). "Continuum of depth of sedation: Definition of general anesthesia and levels of sedation/analgesia" [Online]. Accessed May 2015 via the Web at http://www.asahq.org/For-Members/Standards-Guidelines-and-Statements.aspx

4 Recommended practices for managing the patient receiving moderate sedation/analgesia. (2014). In R. Conner, et al. (Eds.), *Perioperative standards and recommended practices 2014.* Denver, CO: AORN, Inc. (Level VII)

5 American Society of PeriAnesthesia Nurses. (2015). *2015–2017 Perianesthesia nursing standards, practice recommendations and interpretive statements.* Cherry Hill, NJ: American Society of PeriAnesthesia Nurses. (Level VII)

6 American Osteopathic Association. (2014). Standard 30.01.04. *Healthcare Facilities Accreditation Program: Accreditation requirements for acute care hospitals.* Chicago, IL: American Osteopathic Association. (Level VII)

7 Rothrock, J. C. (2015). *Alexander's care of the patient in surgery* (15th ed.). St. Louis, MO: Mosby.

8 American Society of Anesthesiologists. (n.d.). "ASA physical status classification system" [Online]. Accessed May 2015 via the Web at http://www.asahq.org/Home/For-Members/Clinical-Information/ASA-Physical-Status-Classification-System

9 Westbrook, J., et al. (2010). Association of interruptions with an increased risk and severity of medication administration errors. *Archives of Internal Medicine, 170,* 683–690. (Level IV)

10 Institute for Safe Medication Practices. (2012). Side tracks on the safety express: Interruptions lead to errors and unfinished . . . Wait, what was I doing? *Nurse Advise-ERR, 11*(2), 1–4. Accessed May 2015 via the Web at https://www.ismp.org/Newsletters/acutecare/showarticle.aspx?id=37

11 The Joint Commission. (2015). Standard MM.06.01.01. *Comprehensive accreditation manual for hospitals: The official handbook.* Oakbrook Terrace, IL: The Joint Commission. (Level VII)

12 Centers for Medicare & Medicaid Services, Department of Health and Human Services. (2014). Condition of participation: Nursing services. 42 C.F.R. § 482.23(c).

13 American Osteopathic Association. (2014). Standard 16.01.03. *Healthcare Facilities Accreditation Program: Accreditation requirements for acute care hospitals.* Chicago, IL: American Osteopathic Association. (Level VII)

14 The Joint Commission. (2015). Standard PC.03.01.03. *Comprehensive accreditation manual for hospitals: The official handbook.* Oakbrook Terrace, IL: The Joint Commission. (Level VII)

15 Centers for Medicare & Medicaid Services, Department of Health and Human Services. (2014). Condition of participation: Surgical services. 42 C.F.R. § 482.51.

16 American Osteopathic Association. (2014). Standard 30.01.06. *Healthcare Facilities Accreditation Program: Accreditation requirements for acute care hospitals.* Chicago, IL: American Osteopathic Association. (Level VII)

17 Welliver, M., & Bednarzyk, M. (2009). Sedation considerations for the nonintubated obese patient in critical care. *Critical Care Nursing Clinics of North America, 21,* 341–352. (Level VII)

18 Standard 67. Moderate sedation/analgesia using intravenous infusion. Infusion nursing standards of practice. (2011). *Journal of Infusion Nursing, 34,* S95. (Level VII)

19 The Joint Commission. (2015). Standard RI.01.03.01. *Comprehensive accreditation manual for hospitals: The official handbook.* Oakbrook Terrace, IL: The Joint Commission. (Level VII)

20 Centers for Medicare & Medicaid Services, Department of Health and Human Services. (2014). Condition of participation: Patient's rights. 42 C.F.R. § 482.13(b)(2).

21 American Osteopathic Association. (2014). Standard 15.01.11. *Healthcare Facilities Accreditation Program: Accreditation requirements for acute care hospitals.* Chicago, IL: American Osteopathic Association. (Level VII)
22 The Joint Commission. (2015). Standard UP.01.01.01. *Comprehensive accreditation manual for hospitals: The official handbook.* Oakbrook Terrace, IL: The Joint Commission. (Level VII)
23 American Osteopathic Association. (2014). Standard 30.00.14. *Healthcare Facilities Accreditation Program: Accreditation requirements for acute care hospitals.* Chicago, IL: American Osteopathic Association. (Level VII)
24 The Joint Commission. (2015). Standard NPSG.07.01.01. *Comprehensive accreditation manual for hospitals: The official handbook.* Oakbrook Terrace, IL: The Joint Commission. (Level VII)
25 Centers for Disease Control and Prevention. (2002). Guideline for hand hygiene in health-care settings: Recommendations of the Healthcare Infection Control Practices Advisory Committee and the HICPAC/SHEA/APIC/IDSA Hand Hygiene Task Force. *MMWR Recommendations and Reports, 51*(RR-16), 1–45. Accessed May 2015 via the Web at http://www.cdc.gov/mmwr/pdf/rr/rr5116.pdf (Level II)
26 World Health Organization. (2009). "WHO guidelines on hand hygiene in health care: First global patient safety challenge, clean care is safer care" [Online]. Accessed May 2015 via the Web at http://whqlibdoc.who.int/publications/2009/9789241597906_eng.pdf (Level IV)
27 Centers for Medicare & Medicaid Services, Department of Health and Human Services. (2014). Condition of participation: Infection control. 42 C.F.R. § 482.42.
28 American Osteopathic Association. (2014). Standard 07.01.21. *Healthcare Facilities Accreditation Program: Accreditation requirements for acute care hospitals.* Chicago, IL: American Osteopathic Association. (Level VII)
29 The Joint Commission. (2015). Standard NPSG.01.01.01. *Comprehensive accreditation manual for hospitals: The official handbook.* Oakbrook Terrace, IL: The Joint Commission. (Level VII)
30 Policy and procedure template for use with recommended practices. (2014). In R. Conner, et al. (Eds.), *Perioperative standards and recommended practices 2014.* Denver, CO: AORN, Inc. (Level VII)
31 American Society of Anesthesiologists. (2011). Practice guidelines for preoperative fasting and the use of pharmacologic agents to reduce the risk of pulmonary aspiration: Application to healthy patients undergoing elective procedures: An updated report by the American Society of Anesthesiologists Committee on Standards and Practice Parameters. *Anesthesiology, 114,* 495–511. Accessed May 2015 via the Web at http://journals.lww.com/anesthesiology/Fulltext/2011/03000/Practice_Guidelines_for_Preoperative_Fasting_and.13.aspx (Level V)
32 Siegel, J. D., et al. (2007). "2007 guideline for isolation precautions: Preventing transmission of infectious agents in healthcare settings" [Online]. Accessed May 2015 via the Web at http://www.cdc.gov/hicpac/pdf/isolation/Isolation2007.pdf (Level II)
33 American Osteopathic Association. (2014). Standard 07.01.10. *Healthcare Facilities Accreditation Program: Accreditation requirements for acute care hospitals.* Chicago, IL: American Osteopathic Association. (Level VII)
34 American Society of Anesthesiologists. (2011). "Standards for basic anesthetic monitoring" [Online]. Accessed May 2015 via the Web at http://www.asahq.org/~/media/For%20Members/documents/Standards%20Guidelines%20Stmts/Basic%20Anesthetic%20Monitoring%202011.ashx (Level VII)
35 The Joint Commission. (2013). "Sentinel event alert: Medical device alarm safety in hospitals" [Online]. Accessed May 2015 via the Web at http://www.jointcommission.org/assets/1/18/SEA_50_alarms_4_5_13_FINAL1.PDF (Level VII)
36 Graham, K. C., & Cvach, M. (2010). Monitor alarm fatigue: Standardizing use of physiological monitors and decreasing nuisance alarms. *American Journal of Critical Care, 19,* 28–37.
37 The Joint Commission. (2014). Standard NPSG.06.01.01. *Comprehensive accreditation manual for hospitals: The official handbook.* Oakbrook Terrace, IL: The Joint Commission. (Level VII)
38 American Association of Critical-Care Nurses. (2013). "AACN practice alert: Alarm management" [Online]. Accessed May 2015 via the Web at http://www.aacn.org/wd/practice/docs/practicealerts/alarm-management-practice-alert.pdf (Level VII)
39 The Joint Commission. (2015). Standard UP.01.02.01. *Comprehensive accreditation manual for hospitals: The official handbook.* Oakbrook Terrace, IL: The Joint Commission. (Level VII)
40 The Joint Commission. (2015). Standard UP.01.03.01. *Comprehensive accreditation manual for hospitals: The official handbook.* Oakbrook Terrace, IL: The Joint Commission. (Level VII)
41 Institute for Safe Medication Practices. (2014). "ISMP list of high-alert medications in acute care settings" [Online]. Accessed May 2015 via the Web at http://www.ismp.org/tools/highalertmedications.pdf (Level VII)
42 Institute for Safe Medication Practices. (2008). Conducting an independent double-check. *ISMP Medication Safety Alert! Nurse Advise-ERR, 6*(12), 1. Accessed May 2015 via the Web at http://www.ismp.org/newsletters/nursing/Issues/NurseAdviseERR200812.pdf (Level VII)
43 Rutala, W. A., et al. (2008). "Guideline for disinfection and sterilization in healthcare facilities, 2008" [Online]. Accessed May 2015 via the Web at http://www.cdc.gov/hicpac/pdf/guidelines/Disinfection_Nov_2008.pdf (Level I)
44 American Osteopathic Association. (2014). Standard 07.02.03. *Healthcare Facilities Accreditation Program: Accreditation requirements for acute care hospitals.* Chicago, IL: American Osteopathic Association. (Level VII)
45 The Joint Commission. (2015). Standard RC.01.03.01. *Comprehensive accreditation manual for hospitals: The official handbook.* Oakbrook Terrace, IL: The Joint Commission. (Level VII)
46 The Joint Commission. (2015). Standard RC.02.01.03. *Comprehensive accreditation manual for hospitals: The official handbook.* Oakbrook Terrace, IL: The Joint Commission. (Level VII)
47 Centers for Medicare & Medicaid Services, Department of Health and Human Services. (2014). Condition of participation: Medical record services. 42 C.F.R. § 482.24(b).
48 American Osteopathic Association. (2014). Standard 10.00.03. *Healthcare Facilities Accreditation Program: Accreditation requirements for acute care hospitals.* Chicago, IL: American Osteopathic Association. (Level VII)

ADDITIONAL REFERENCES

Weaver, J. (2011). The latest ASA mandate: CO_2 monitoring for moderate and deep sedation. *Anesthesia Progress, 58,* 111–112. Accessed May 2015 via the Web at http://www.ncbi.nlm.nih.gov/pmc/articles/PMC3167153/
Weingart, S. D., & Bhagwan, S. D. (2010). Current guidelines for procedural sedation in the emergency department. *EM Practice Guidelines Update, 2*(3), 1–12. Accessed May 2015 via the Web at http://emcrit.org/wp-content/uploads/procedural-sedation-guidelines.pdf (Level VII)
Yang, K. S., et al. (2014). A prospective evaluation of adverse events in nurse-administered moderate sedation guided by sedation scores or bispectral index. *Anesthesia and Analgesia, 119,* 43–48. (Level IV)

MUCUS CLEARANCE DEVICE

Patients with chronic respiratory disorders, such as cystic fibrosis, bronchitis, or bronchiectasis, require therapy to mobilize and remove mucus secretions from the lungs. A handheld mucus clearance device can help such patients cough up secretions more easily. Two such devices on the market are the Flutter device and the Acapella device, both of which facilitate mucus removal with oscillatory positive expiratory pressure. Both devices have similar performance characteristics; however, Acapella's performance isn't gravity-dependent and may be easier for some patients to use, particularly at low expiratory flows.[1]

Both devices consist of a ball valve that vibrates as the patient exhales vigorously through it. The vibrations propagate throughout the airways during expiration, loosening mucus. As the patient repeats this process, the mucus progressively moves up the airway until the patient can easily cough it out. A licensed practitioner determines the frequency and duration of device use.

Use of a mucus clearance device in patients with chronic obstructive pulmonary disease has been shown to improve patient response to bronchodilators when a patient uses the device before bronchodilator therapy.[2]

Equipment

Disinfectant pad ▪ mucus clearance device ▪ emesis basin ▪ tissues ▪ trash bag ▪ stethoscope ▪ oral care supplies (see the "Oral care" procedure, page 560) ▪ Optional: gloves.

Implementation

- Verify the practitioner's order.
- Gather the appropriate equipment.
- Perform hand hygiene.[3,4,5,6,7]
- Confirm the patient's identity using at least two patient identifiers.[8]
- Put on gloves as needed *to comply with standard precautions.*[9,10]
- Provide privacy.[11,12]
- Explain the procedure to the patient. Tell him that this device will help move the mucus through his airways so that he can eventually expectorate it.
- Auscultate the patient's breath sounds *to obtain a baseline assessment for comparison.*
- Have the patient sit with his back straight and his head tilted backward slightly so that his throat and trachea are wide open. *This position allows exhaled air to flow smoothly from the lungs and out through the device.*
- If the patient prefers, he may place his elbows on a table at a height that prevents him from slouching, *which would interfere with smooth breathing.*
- For the Flutter device, tell the patient to hold the device so that the stem is parallel to the floor. *This position places the interior cone of the device at a 30-degree tilt, which allows the ball inside the device to bounce and roll freely in the cone.* For the Acapella device, tell the patient to hold the device parallel with the floor.
- Have the patient draw a deep breath and hold it for 2 to 3 seconds. This inhalation step is important *because it evenly distributes the inspired air throughout the lungs, especially in the small airways, where infection and airway damage can occur.*
- After 2 to 3 seconds, instruct the patient to place the device in his mouth and then exhale at a steady rate for as long as he can. *Explain that if he breathes out too quickly and forcefully, the vibration won't be effective, defeating the purpose of the device.*
- Tell the patient to keep his cheeks as flat and hard as possible while exhaling *to direct the air out through the device most effectively.* Suggest that he hold his cheeks lightly with his other hand *to help him learn the technique.*
- After the patient has completely exhaled, instruct him to remove the device from his mouth, take in another full breath, and cough.
- Tell the patient to expectorate the mucus into an emesis basin or tissue.
- Instruct the patient to repeat the entire procedure several times or as recommended by the practitioner.
- Assess the type, amount, color, and odor of expectorated secretions.
- Dispose of secretions appropriately.[9]
- Auscultate for breath sounds *to determine the effectiveness of coughing,* and compare your findings with the baseline assessment.
- Have the patient perform oral care.
- Remove and discard your gloves if worn.[9]
- Perform hand hygiene.[3,4,5,6,7]
- Clean and disinfect your stethoscope using a disinfectant pad.[13,14]
- Perform hand hygiene.[3,4,5,6,7]
- Document the procedure.[15,16,17]

Special considerations

- As an alternative to removing the device from his mouth after completely exhaling, the patient can leave the device in his mouth, draw another big breath through his nose, hold it for 2 to 3 seconds, and then exhale. He can breathe through the device up to five times before taking the final breath and coughing.
- *To help the patient achieve the best fluttering effect,* you may need to place one hand on his back and the other on his chest as he exhales through the device. If he's achieving the maximum effect, you'll feel the vibrations in his lungs as he exhales. If initial results are unsatisfactory, tell the patient to adjust the angle of the device until optimal fluttering occurs.
- Patients routinely perform multiple sets of 10 to 15 exhalations over 12 to 20 minutes. After each series of exhalations, the patient is instructed to "huff" (take repeated, controlled, short, rapid exhalations) and cough, *which aids expectoration.*[18,19]
- Observe the patient over several sets and evaluate his ability to self-administer the treatment.
- For the Flutter device, the oscillation frequency can be regulated by moving the device slightly up or down from its horizontal position.[18]
- All models of the Acapella device can be used with a mask or mouthpiece or in line with a nebulizer.[18]
- Patients with severe obstruction may not be able to generate sufficient airflow to cause the steel ball within the Flutter device to vibrate, limiting the device's effectiveness in such patients.[18]
- The Flutter and Acapella mucus clearance devices are recommended for single-patient use.

Patient teaching

Tell the patient to clean the device after each use *to remove mucus from the internal components.* Instruct him to clean it more thoroughly every 2 days, washing all parts in a solution of mild soap or detergent. Tell him not to use bleach or other chlorine-containing products. After thorough cleaning, tell the patient to rinse all parts under a stream of hot tap water, wipe them with a clean towel, and reassemble and store the device in a clean, dry place.

Documentation

Record patient teaching as well as the patient's tolerance of the procedure. Record the amount, color, and odor of any secretions that the patient expectorates. Document the patient's breath sounds before and after he's used the device and coughed. Also record the number of times the patient repeated the procedure and the success of his coughing efforts.

References

1 Volska, T. A., et al. (2003). Performance comparison of two oscillating positive expiratory pressure devices: Acapella versus Flutter. *Respiratory Care, 48,* 124–130. Accessed May 2015 via the Web at http://www.henleysmed.com/sites/default/files/acapella_vs_flutter.pdf (Level VI)

2 Wolkove, N., et al. (2004). A randomized trial to evaluate the sustained efficacy of a mucus clearance device in ambulatory patients with chronic obstructive pulmonary disease. *Canadian Respiratory Journal, 11,* 567–572. (Level II)

3 The Joint Commission. (2015). Standard NPSG.07.01.01. *Comprehensive accreditation manual for hospitals: The official handbook.* Oakbrook Terrace, IL: The Joint Commission. (Level VII)

4 Centers for Disease Control and Prevention. (2002). Guideline for hand hygiene in health-care settings: Recommendations of the Healthcare Infection Control Practices Advisory Committee and the HICPAC/SHEA/APIC/IDSA Hand Hygiene Task Force. *MMWR Recommendations and Reports, 51*(RR-16), 1–45. Accessed May 2015 via the Web at http://www.cdc.gov/mmwr/pdf/rr/rr5116.pdf (Level II)

5 World Health Organization. (2009). "WHO guidelines on hand hygiene in health care: First global patient safety challenge, clean care is safer care" [Online]. Accessed May 2015 via the Web at http://whqlibdoc.who.int/publications/2009/9789241597906_eng.pdf (Level IV)

6 Centers for Medicare & Medicaid Services, Department of Health and Human Services. (2014). Condition of participation: Infection control. 42 C.F.R. § 482.42.

7 American Osteopathic Association. (2014). Standard 07.01.21. *Healthcare Facilities Accreditation Program: Accreditation requirements for acute care hospitals.* Chicago, IL: American Osteopathic Association. (Level VII)
8 The Joint Commission. (2015). Standard NPSG.01.01.01. *Comprehensive accreditation manual for hospitals: The official handbook.* Oakbrook Terrace, IL: The Joint Commission. (Level VII)
9 Siegel, J. D., et al. (2007). "2007 guideline for isolation precautions: Preventing transmission of infectious agents in healthcare settings" [Online]. Accessed May 2015 via the Web at http://www.cdc.gov/hicpac/pdf/isolation/Isolation2007.pdf (Level II)
10 American Osteopathic Association. (2014). Standard 07.01.10. *Healthcare Facilities Accreditation Program: Accreditation requirements for acute care hospitals.* Chicago, IL: American Osteopathic Association. (Level VII)
11 Centers for Medicare & Medicaid Services, Department of Health and Human Services. (2014). Condition of participation: Patient's rights. 42 C.F.R. § 482.13(c)(1).
12 American Osteopathic Association. (2014). Standard 15.01.16. *Healthcare Facilities Accreditation Program: Accreditation requirements for acute care hospitals.* Chicago, IL: American Osteopathic Association. (Level VII)
13 Rutala, W. A., et al. (2008). "Guideline for disinfection and sterilization in healthcare facilities, 2008" [Online]. Accessed May 2015 via the Web at http://www.cdc.gov/hicpac/pdf/guidelines/Disinfection_Nov_2008.pdf (Level I)
14 American Osteopathic Association. (2014). Standard 07.02.03. *Healthcare Facilities Accreditation Program: Accreditation requirements for acute care hospitals.* Chicago, IL: American Osteopathic Association. (Level VII)
15 The Joint Commission. (2015). Standard RC.01.03.01. *Comprehensive accreditation manual for hospitals: The official handbook.* Oakbrook Terrace, IL: The Joint Commission. (Level VII)
16 Centers for Medicare & Medicaid Services, Department of Health and Human Services. (2014). Condition of participation: Medical record services. 42 C.F.R. § 482.24(b).
17 American Osteopathic Association. (2014). Standard 10.00.03. *Healthcare Facilities Accreditation Program: Accreditation requirements for acute care hospitals.* Chicago, IL: American Osteopathic Association. (Level VII)
18 Hristara-Papadopoulou, A., et al. (2008). Current devices of respiratory physiotherapy. *Hippokratia, 12,* 211–220. Accessed May 2015 via the Web at http://www.ncbi.nlm.nih.gov/pmc/articles/PMC2580042/ (Level V)
19 Lester, M. K., & Flume, P. A. (2009). Airway-clearance therapy guidelines and implementation. *Respiratory Care, 54,* 733–753. Accessed May 2015 via the Web at http://services.aarc.org/source/DownloadDocument/Downloaddocs/06.09.0733.pdf (Level VII)

ADDITIONAL REFERENCES

Aptalis Pharma U.S., Inc. (2013). "Flutter® mucus clearance device: Instructions for use" [Online]. Accessed May 2015 via the Web at http://www.aptalispharma.com/pdf/Flutter_PI.pdf
Kacmarek, R. M., et al. (2013). *Egan's fundamentals of respiratory care* (10th ed.). St. Louis, MO: Mosby.
Taylor, C. R., et al. (2015). *Fundamentals of nursing: The art and science of nursing care* (8th ed.). Philadelphia, PA: Lippincott Williams & Wilkins.
Wang, Q. X., et al. (2010). Effects of a flutter mucus-clearance device on pulmonary function test results in healthy people 85 years and older in China. *Respiratory Care, 55,* 1449–1452. Accessed May 2015 via the Web at http://www.rcjournal.com/contents/11.10/11.10.1449.pdf (Level II)

N

NASAL BRIDLE INSERTION AND REMOVAL

A nasal bridle is used to secure a nasally inserted gastric or enteral feeding tube to prevent the tube's inadvertent dislodgment or removal.[1]

Nasal bridle use is contraindicated in patients with nasal airway obstructions or abnormalities as well as in those with facial or cranial fractures. A nasal bridle shouldn't be used in a patient who may pull on the bridle hard enough to cause injury.[1] Before a nasal bridal is inserted, the practitioner should perform a nasal examination to ensure that the patient has adequate bone in the posterior septum to support the bridle system.[1]

A nasal bridle should be inserted only by those who have been specially trained in the insertion technique and have demonstrated competency to do so.

Equipment

Gloves ■ bridle catheter with attached umbilical tape and stylet ■ feeding tube retaining clip ■ retrieval probe ■ stylet guide ■ water-soluble lubricant ■ scissors ■ Optional: skin barrier, clip reopening tool, gown, mask and goggles or mask with face shield.

Implementation

■ Verify the practitioner's order.
■ Confirm that written informed consent has been obtained and is in the patient's medical record.[2,3,4]
■ Perform hand hygiene.[5,6,7,8,9]
■ Confirm the patient's identity using at least two patient identifiers.[10]
■ Put on gloves and other personal protective equipment as needed *to comply with standard precautions.*[11,12]

Inserting a nasal bridle

■ Lubricate the probe, catheter, and umbilical tape with water-soluble lubricant.
■ Place the patient in the supine position *to ease insertion.*[1]
■ Insert the retrieval (blue) probe into the patient's nostril; if the nasal enteral tube is already in place, insert the receiving probe in the nostril opposite the existing tube (as shown below) until the first rib is at the base of the nostril; make adjustments for a smaller patient.[1]

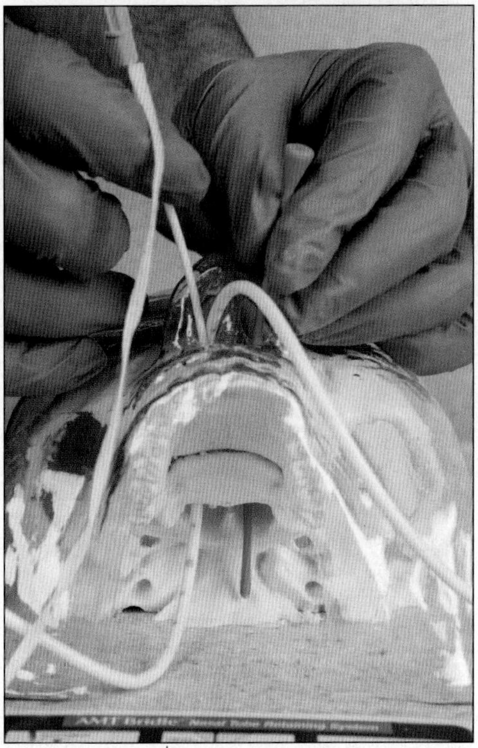

■ Insert the bridle (white) catheter into the opposite nostril to where the magnets would meet (as shown on next page, top left).

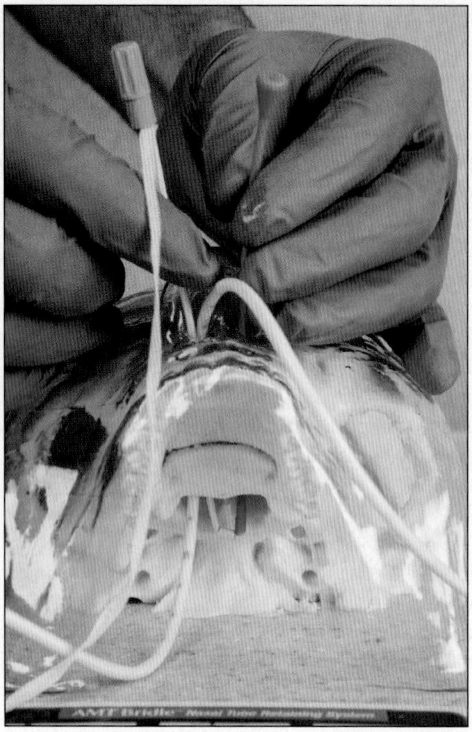

■ Pull back on the stylet about ½″ (1 cm) until the magnets connect; you should hear or feel the click of the magnets as they connect. If necessary, gently twist the probes from side to side or up and down *to encourage contact between the magnets.* If contact still doesn't occur, advance the probe and bridle catheter.[1]

■ Remove the stylet from the bridle catheter when the magnets connect (as shown below).[1]

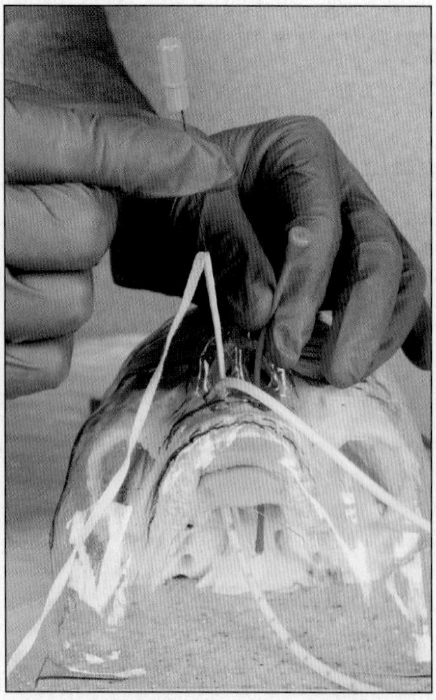

■ Slowly withdraw the probe (as shown on top right), and allow the catheter to advance through the nose; continue until the cloth umbilical tape is in the nose, creating a loop or bridle around the vomer bone. If the catheter and umbilical tape don't advance out of the opposite nostril, remove the catheter, replace the stylet, and repeat the procedure.[1]

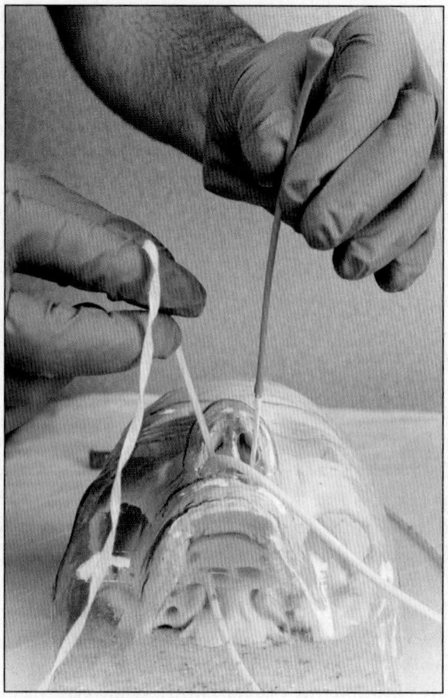

■ Using scissors, cut the catheter portion from the umbilical tape. Dispose of the catheter and probe.[1]

■ If the nasal enteral tube hasn't been inserted, insert it now.[1] (See the "Feeding tube insertion and removal" procedure, page 323.)

■ Place the nasal clip about ½″ (1 cm) or one finger width from the nostril (as shown below); make sure that the clip doesn't touch the nostril.[1]

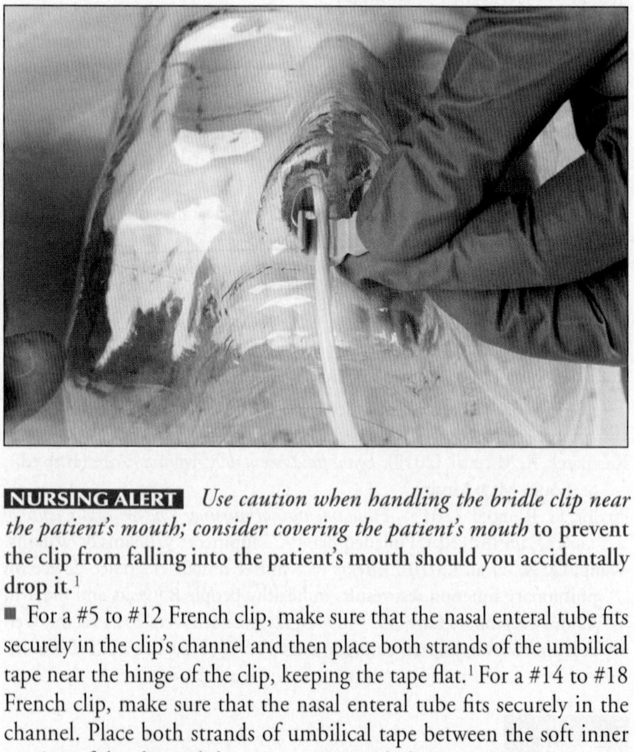

NURSING ALERT ***Use caution when handling the bridle clip near the patient's mouth; consider covering the patient's mouth*** **to prevent the clip from falling into the patient's mouth should you accidentally drop it.**[1]

■ For a #5 to #12 French clip, make sure that the nasal enteral tube fits securely in the clip's channel and then place both strands of the umbilical tape near the hinge of the clip, keeping the tape flat.[1] For a #14 to #18 French clip, make sure that the nasal enteral tube fits securely in the channel. Place both strands of umbilical tape between the soft inner portion of the clip and the outer, more rigid plastic section.[1]

■ Close the clip by folding over the plastic edge (as shown on next page, top left) and firmly snapping it shut; *the clip is difficult to reopen,* so make sure that the nasal enteral tube, umbilical tape, and clip are positioned properly before closing the clip. Don't use another object to open or close the clip *because the clip may become damaged, making it less secure.* If the clip becomes damaged, use a new one.[1]

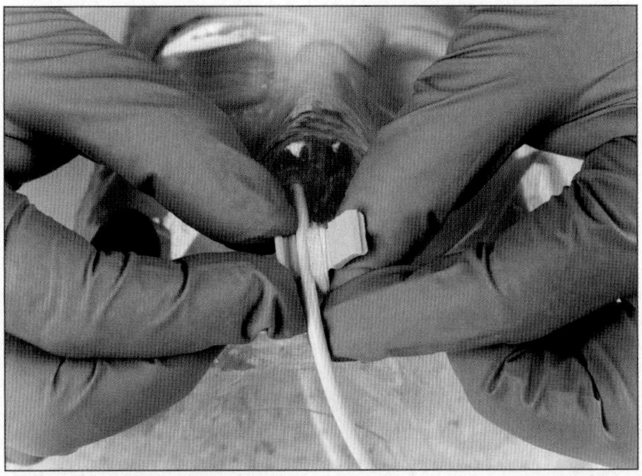

■ After closing the clip completely, tie the two umbilical tape ends together (excluding the tube) in a simple knot (as shown below). Knot the tape ends two to three times, and then cut the excess umbilical tape.

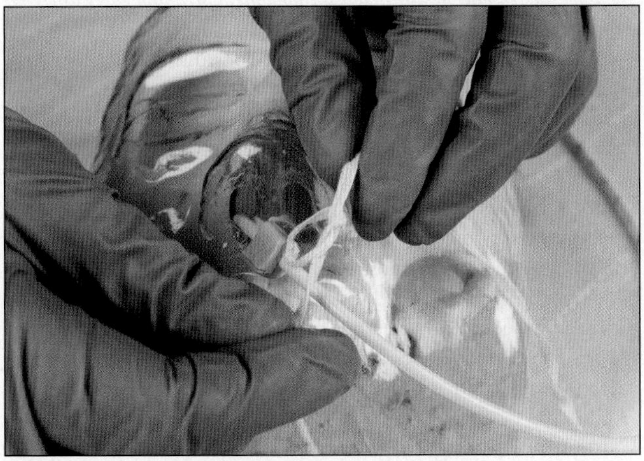

■ Make sure a thorough nasal examination is performed after nasal bridle insertion *to ensure that the umbilical tape loop has passed behind the nasal septum, not through a septal perforation.*[1]
■ Regularly monitor the position of the nasal enteral tube and clip for signs of enteral feeding tube migration.[1,13,14]
■ Monitor the insertion site for redness, swelling, drainage, and skin irritation. Use a skin barrier as necessary.[15]
■ Visually monitor the clip for signs of damage or loose attachment to the enteral tube; replace the clip if necessary.[1]
■ Assess the condition of the umbilical tape *because it can degrade over time, resulting in pieces being left in the patient's nose.*[1]

Removing a nasal bridle

To remove a nasal bridle and nasogastric or nasoenteral tube together

■ Using scissors, cut one strand of the umbilical tape.
■ Pull the nasal bridle and nasogastric or nasoenteral tube gently out of the patient's nose.[1]

To removal a nasal bridle alone

■ Leaving the clip in place, cut both ends of the umbilical tape near the clip.[1,13]
■ Secure the umbilical tape as you gently remove it *to avoid dislodging the nasogastric or nasoenteral tube during tape removal. Maintaining control of the tape also protects the patient from aspirating or swallowing pieces of the tape.*

Completing the procedure

■ Assess the patient's skin around the nostrils and upper lip for signs of bleeding, skin breakdown, or irritation.
■ Dispose of used supplies in the appropriate receptacle.
■ Remove and discard your gloves and any other personal protective equipment worn.[12]
■ Perform hand hygiene.[5,6,7,8,9]
■ Document the procedure.[16,17,18]

Special considerations

Use an alternative means of securing the enteral feeding tube if there's excessive traction on the nasal bridle *because excessive traction on the nasal bridle may cause tube displacement or nasal injury.*[1]

The bridle may remain in place for the entire time the nasal tube is in position; however, studies showed an increased risk of erosion of the nasal septum after more than 8 weeks when using a #5 French enteral tube to bridle the nasal tube as opposed to using a manufactured bridle setup.[19,20]

Complications

If the nasal bridle is secured too tightly, damage may occur to the internal and external tissues. The nasal enteral tube may become dislodged if the nasal bridle is secured too loosely.[13]

Documentation

Document that an assessment of the patient's nose was performed before the procedure. Record the patient's tolerance of the procedure, the size of the clip used, the position of the nasal enteral tube, and the condition of the patient's nose. Document patient and family teaching and their understanding of your teaching.

REFERENCES

1 Applied Medical Technology, Inc. (2011). "AMT Bridle™: Nasal retaining system" [Online]. Accessed May 2015 via the Web at http://www.amtinnovation.com/pdf/AMT_BridlePocketGuide.pdf
2 The Joint Commission. (2015). Standard RI.01.03.01. *Comprehensive accreditation manual for hospitals: The official handbook.* Oakbrook Terrace, IL: The Joint Commission. (Level VII)
3 Centers for Medicare & Medicaid Services, Department of Health and Human Services. (2014). Condition of participation: Patient's rights. 42 C.F.R. § 482.13(b)(2).
4 American Osteopathic Association. (2014). Standard 15.01.11. *Healthcare Facilities Accreditation Program: Accreditation requirements for acute care hospitals.* Chicago, IL: American Osteopathic Association. (Level VII)
5 The Joint Commission. (2015). Standard NPSG.07.01.01. *Comprehensive accreditation manual for hospitals: The official handbook.* Oakbrook Terrace, IL: The Joint Commission. (Level VII)
6 Centers for Disease Control and Prevention. (2002). Guideline for hand hygiene in health-care settings: Recommendations of the Healthcare Infection Control Practices Advisory Committee and the HICPAC/SHEA/APIC/IDSA Hand Hygiene Task Force. *MMWR Recommendations and Reports, 51*(RR-16), 1–45. Accessed May 2015 via the Web at http://www.cdc.gov/mmwr/pdf/rr/rr5116.pdf (Level II)
7 World Health Organization. (2009). "WHO guidelines on hand hygiene in health care: First global patient safety challenge, clean care is safer care" [Online]. Accessed May 2015 via the Web at http://whqlibdoc.who.int/publications/2009/9789241597906_eng.pdf (Level IV)
8 American Osteopathic Association. (2014). Standard 07.01.21. *Healthcare Facilities Accreditation Program: Accreditation requirements for acute care hospitals.* Chicago, IL: American Osteopathic Association. (Level VII)
9 Centers for Medicare & Medicaid Services, Department of Health and Human Services. (2014). Condition of participation: Infection control. 42 C.F.R. § 482.42.

10 The Joint Commission. (2015). Standard NPSG.01.01.01. *Comprehensive accreditation manual for hospitals: The official handbook.* Oakbrook Terrace, IL: The Joint Commission. (Level VII)
11 Siegel, J. D., et al. (2007). "2007 guideline for isolation precautions: Preventing transmission of infectious agents in healthcare settings" [Online]. Accessed May 2015 via the Web at http://www.cdc.gov/hicpac/pdf/isolation/Isolation2007.pdf (Level II)
12 American Osteopathic Association. (2014). Standard 07.01.10. *Healthcare Facilities Accreditation Program: Accreditation requirements for acute care hospitals.* Chicago, IL: American Osteopathic Association. (Level VII)
13 McGinnis, C. (2011). The feeding tube bridle: One inexpensive, safe, and effective method to prevent inadvertent feeding tube dislodgement. *Nutrition in Clinical Practice, 26,* 70–77.
14 Gunn, S. R., et al. (2009). Use of a nasal bridle prevents accidental nasoenteral feeding tube removal. *Journal of Parenteral and Enteral Nutrition, 33,* 50–54.
15 Lynn-McHale Wiegand, D. (Ed.). (2011). *AACN procedure manual for critical care* (6th ed.). St. Louis, MO: Saunders.
16 The Joint Commission. (2015). Standard RC.01.03.01. *Comprehensive accreditation manual for hospitals: The official handbook.* Oakbrook Terrace, IL: The Joint Commission. (Level VII)
17 Centers for Medicare & Medicaid Services, Department of Health and Human Services. (2014). Condition of participation: Medical record services. 42 C.F.R. § 482.24(b).
18 American Osteopathic Association. (2014). Standard 10.00.03. *Healthcare Facilities Accreditation Program: Accreditation requirements for acute care hospitals.* Chicago, IL: American Osteopathic Association. (Level VII)
19 Gurram, K. (2011). Nasal bridle: Married to your tube. *Practical Gastroenterology, 35*(1), 27–34. Accessed May 2015 via the Web at http://www.practicalgastro.com/pdf/January11/GurramArticle.pdf
20 Seder, C. W., et al. (2010). Nasal bridling decreases feeding tube dislodgment and may increase caloric intake in the surgical intensive care unit: A randomized, controlled trial. *Critical Care Medicine, 38,* 797–801. (Level II)

NASAL IRRIGATION

Irrigation of the nasal passages soothes irritated mucous membranes and washes away crusted mucus, secretions, and foreign matter. Left unattended, these deposits may impede sinus drainage and nasal airflow and cause headaches, infections, and unpleasant odors. Irrigation may be done with a bulb syringe or an electronic irrigating device.

Nasal irrigation benefits patients with acute or chronic nasal conditions, including sinusitis, rhinitis, Wegener granulomatosis, and Sjögren syndrome.[1] The procedure may also help people who regularly inhale toxins or allergens—paint fumes, sawdust, pesticides, or coal dust, for example.[2] Nasal irrigation is routinely recommended after some nasal surgeries to enhance healing by removing postoperative eschar and to aid remucosolization of the sinus cavities and ostia.[3]

Contraindications for nasal irrigation may include advanced destruction of the sinuses, frequent nosebleeds, and foreign bodies in the nasal passages (which could be driven farther into the passages by the irrigant). However, some patients with these conditions may benefit from irrigation.

Equipment

Bulb syringe or oral irrigating device ▪ rigid or flexible disposable nasal irrigation tips (for one-patient use) ▪ normal saline solution ▪ fluid-impermeable pad ▪ towels ▪ facial tissues ▪ bath basin ▪ gloves ▪ soap and water ▪ hospital-grade disinfectant.

Preparation of equipment

Attach the disposable nasal irrigation tip to the delivery device, as needed.

Warm the saline solution to about 105°F (40.6°C). If you'll be irrigating with a bulb syringe, draw some irrigant into the bulb and then expel it *to rinse any residual solution from the previous irrigation and to warm the bulb.*

If you're using an oral irrigating device, plug the instrument into an electrical outlet in an area near the patient. Then run about 1 cup (240 mL) of normal saline solution through the tubing *to rinse residual solution from the lines and to warm the tubing.* Next, fill the reservoir of the device with warm saline solution.

Implementation

- Gather and prepare the necessary equipment.
- Perform hand hygiene.[4,5,6,7,8]
- Confirm the patient's identity using at least two patient identifiers.[9]
- Explain the procedure to the patient.
- Put on gloves *to comply with standard precautions.*[12,13]
- Place a towel on the patient's upper body *to protect clothing from getting wet.* Place a fluid-impermeable pad on the bed if indicated.
- Have the patient sit comfortably near the equipment in a position that allows the bulb or catheter tip to enter the nose and the returning irrigant to flow into the bath basin or sink. (See *Positioning the patient for nasal irrigation.*)
- Remind the patient to keep the mouth open and to breathe rhythmically during irrigation. *This action causes the soft palate to seal the throat, allowing the irrigant to stream out the opposite nostril and carry discharge with it.*
- Instruct the patient not to speak or swallow during the irrigation *to avoid forcing infectious material into the sinuses or eustachian tubes.*
- *To avoid injuring the nasal mucosa,* remove the irrigating tip from the nostril if the patient reports the need to sneeze or cough.

Using a bulb syringe

- Fill the bulb syringe with saline solution and insert the tip about ½″ (1.3 cm) into the patient's nostril.
- Squeeze the bulb until a gentle stream of warm irrigant washes through the nose. Avoid forceful squeezing, *which may drive debris from the nasal passages into the sinuses or eustachian tubes and introduce infection.* Alternate the nostrils until the return irrigant runs clear.

Using an oral irrigating device

- Insert the irrigation tip into the nostril about ½″ to 1″ (1.3 to 2.5 cm).
- Turn on the irrigating device. Begin with a low pressure setting (increasing the pressure as needed) *to obtain a gentle stream of irrigant.* Be careful not to drive material from the nose into the sinuses or eustachian tubes. Irrigate both nostrils.

Completing the procedure

- Inspect the returning irrigant for purulence, *which may indicate infection, bleeding, or foreign bodies.* Report unexpected findings to the practitioner.
- After irrigation, have the patient wait a few minutes before blowing excess fluid from both nostrils at once. *Gentle blowing through both nostrils prevents fluid or pressure buildup in the sinuses. This action also helps to loosen and expel crusted secretions and mucus.*
- Clean the bulb syringe or irrigating device with soap and water and then disinfect it, as recommended. Rinse and dry the device. Clean the basin or sink with hospital-grade disinfectant.[14,15]
- Remove and discard your gloves.[12]
- Perform hand hygiene.[4,5,6,7,8]
- Document the procedure.[16,17,18]

Special considerations

- Expect fluid to drain from the patient's nose for a brief time after irrigation and before blowing the nose.
- Insert the irrigation tip far enough to ensure that the irrigant cleans the nasal membranes before draining out. A typical amount of irrigant ranges from 500 to 1,000 mL.

Patient teaching

■ To continue nasal irrigations at home, teach the patient how to prepare saline solution. Tell the patient to fill a clean 1-L plastic bottle (4 cups + 1 oz = 1L) with bottled or distilled water, add 1 tsp of salt, and shake the solution until the salt dissolves.

■ If the patient will use a commercial nasal rinsing device, teach the necessary steps, beginning with washing and drying the hands; checking that the device is clean and completely dry before use; using the appropriate irrigant as recommended by the device manufacturer (normal saline solution, sterile or distilled water, boiled and cooled tap water, or filtered tap water); following the manufacturer's directions for use; cleaning the device with distilled, sterile, or boiled and cooled tap water; and finally drying the inside with a paper towel or letting it air-dry between uses.[19]

■ Instruct the patient to notify the practitioner if signs and symptoms worsen or if headaches, nosebleeds, or fever develop.[19]

Complications

Use of nasal irrigation devices can lead to ear fullness, sinus discomfort, nosebleeds, and headaches. Infection is possible with improper use of the device.[19]

Documentation

Write down the time and duration of the procedure and the amount of irrigant used. Describe the appearance of the returned solution. Record your assessment of the patient's comfort level and breathing ease before and after the procedure. Document patient teaching and the patient's understanding of the teaching.

Positioning the patient for nasal irrigation

Whether you're teaching a patient to perform nasal irrigation with a bulb syringe or an oral irrigating device, the irrigation will progress more easily once the patient learns how to hold her head for optimal safety, comfort, and effectiveness.

Help the patient to sit upright with her head bent forward over the basin or sink and well-flexed on her chest. Her nose and ear should be on the same vertical plane.

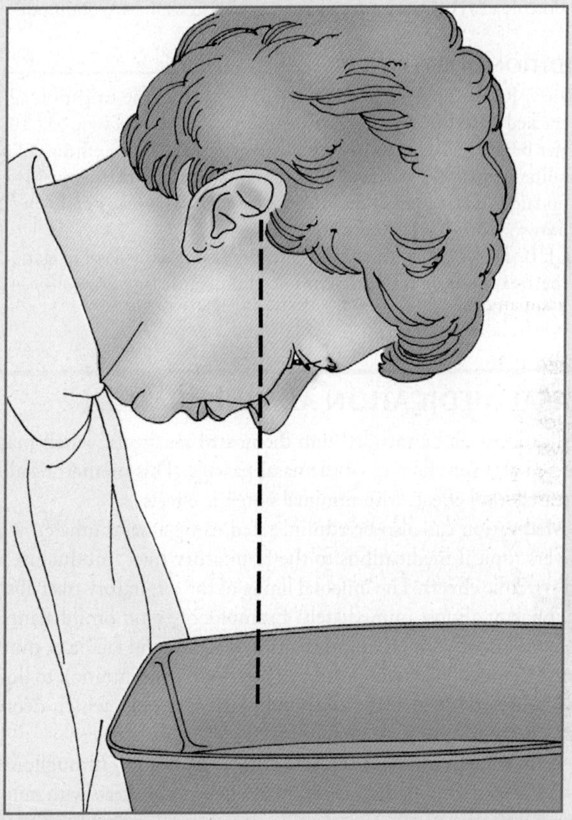

Explain that she's less likely to breathe in the irrigant when holding her head in this position. This position should also keep the irrigant from entering the eustachian tubes, which will now lie above the level of the irrigation stream.

REFERENCES

1 Rabago, D., & Zgierska, A. (2009). Saline nasal irrigation for upper respiratory conditions. *American Family Physician, 80,* 1117–1119.

2 Hermelingmeier, K. E., et al. (2012). Nasal irrigation as an adjunctive treatment in allergic rhinitis: A systematic review and meta-analysis. *American Journal of Rhinology and Allergy, 26,* e119–e125. (Level I)

3 Low, T. H., et al. (2014). A double-blind randomized controlled trial of normal saline, lactated Ringers, and hypertonic saline nasal irrigation solution after endoscopic sinus surgery. *American Journal of Rhinology and Allergy, 28,* 225–231. (Level II)

4 Centers for Disease Control and Prevention. (2002). Guideline for hand hygiene in health-care settings: Recommendations of the Healthcare Infection Control Practices Advisory Committee and the HICPAC/SHEA/APIC/IDSA Hand Hygiene Task Force. *MMWR Recommendations and Reports, 51*(RR-16), 1–45. Accessed May 2015 via the Web at http://www.cdc.gov/mmwr/pdf/rr/rr5116.pdf (Level II)

5 World Health Organization. (2009). "WHO guidelines on hand hygiene in health care: First global patient safety challenge, clean care is safer care" [Online]. Accessed May 2015 via the Web at http://whqlibdoc.who.int/publications/2009/9789241597906_eng.pdf (Level IV)

6 The Joint Commission. (2015). Standard NPSG.07.01.01. *Comprehensive accreditation manual for hospitals: The official handbook.* Oakbrook Terrace, IL: The Joint Commission. (Level VII)

7 Centers for Medicare & Medicaid Services, Department of Health and Human Services. (2014). Condition of participation: Infection control. 42 C.F.R. § 482.42.

8 American Osteopathic Association. (2014). Standard 07.01.21. *Healthcare Facilities Accreditation Program: Accreditation requirements for acute care hospitals.* Chicago, IL: American Osteopathic Association. (Level VII)

9 The Joint Commission. (2015). Standard NPSG.01.01.01. *Comprehensive accreditation manual for hospitals: The official handbook.* Oakbrook Terrace, IL: The Joint Commission. (Level VII)

10 Centers for Medicare & Medicaid Services, Department of Health and Human Services. (2014). Condition of participation: Patient's rights. 42 C.F.R. § 482.13(c)(1).

11 American Osteopathic Association. (2014). Standard 15.01.16. *Healthcare Facilities Accreditation Program: Accreditation requirements for acute care hospitals.* Chicago, IL: American Osteopathic Association. (Level VII)

12 Siegel, J. D., et al. (2007). "2007 guideline for isolation precautions: Preventing transmission of infectious agents in healthcare settings" [Online]. Accessed May 2015 via the Web at http://www.cdc.gov/hicpac/pdf/isolation/Isolation2007.pdf (Level II)

13 American Osteopathic Association. (2014). Standard 07.01.10. *Healthcare Facilities Accreditation Program: Accreditation requirements for acute care hospitals.* Chicago, IL: American Osteopathic Association. (Level VII)

14 Rutala, W. A., et al. (2008). "Guideline for disinfection and sterilization in healthcare facilities, 2008" [Online]. Accessed May 2015 via the Web at http://www.cdc.gov/hicpac/pdf/guidelines/Disinfection_Nov_2008.pdf (Level I)

15 American Osteopathic Association. (2014). Standard 07.02.03. *Healthcare Facilities Accreditation Program: Accreditation requirements for acute care hospitals.* Chicago, IL: American Osteopathic Association. (Level VII)

16 The Joint Commission. (2015). Standard RC.01.03.01. *Comprehensive accreditation manual for hospitals: The official handbook.* Oakbrook Terrace, IL: The Joint Commission. (Level VII)
17 Centers for Medicare & Medicaid Services, Department of Health and Human Services. (2014). Condition of participation: Medical record services. 42 C.F.R. § 482.24(b).
18 American Osteopathic Association. (2014). Standard 10.00.03. *Healthcare Facilities Accreditation Program: Accreditation requirements for acute care hospitals.* Chicago, IL: American Osteopathic Association. (Level VII)
19 U.S. Food and Drug Administration. (2012). "Is rinsing your sinuses safe?" [Online]. Accessed May 2015 via the Web at http://www.fda.gov/downloads/ForConsumers/ConsumerUpdates/UCM316649.pdf

ADDITIONAL REFERENCES

Khianey, R., & Oppenheimer, J. (2012). Is nasal saline irrigation all it is cracked up to be? *Annals of Asthma, Allergy, and Immunology, 109,* 20–28.
van der Berg, J. W., et al. (2014). Limited evidence: Higher efficacy of nasal saline irrigation over nasal saline spray in chronic rhinosinusitis—An update and reanalysis of the evidence base. *Otolaryngology Head and Neck Surgery, 150,* 16–21. (Level V)
Wei, J. L., et al. (2011). Safety and efficacy of once-daily nasal irrigation for the treatment of pediatric chronic rhinosinusitis. *Laryngoscope, 121,* 1989–2000.

NASAL MEDICATION ADMINISTRATION

Medications can be instilled into the nostril via drops, which may be directed at a specific area of the nasal passage. This method results in increased local effects with minimal systemic effects.

Medication can also be administered using a nasal inhaler, which delivers topical medications to the respiratory tract, producing local and systemic effects. The mucosal lining of the respiratory tract absorbs the inhalant almost immediately. Examples of common inhalants are bronchodilators, which improve airway patency and facilitate mucous drainage; mucolytics, which attain a high local concentration to liquefy tenacious bronchial secretions; and corticosteroids, which decrease inflammation.

A third method, nasal aerosols diffuse medication throughout the nasal passages. This method results in increased local effects with minimal systemic effects.

Most nasal medications such as phenylephrine are vasoconstrictors, which relieve nasal congestion by coating and shrinking swollen mucous membranes. However, because vasoconstrictors may be absorbed systemically, they're usually contraindicated in hypersensitive patients. Other types of nasal medications include serotonin-receptor agonists,[1] antiseptics, anesthetics, vaccines, and corticosteroids. Local anesthetics may be administered to promote patient comfort during rhinolaryngologic examination, laryngoscopy, bronchoscopy, and endotracheal intubation. Corticosteroids reduce inflammation in allergic or inflammatory conditions and nasal polyps.

Equipment

Prescribed medication ▪ patient's medication record ▪ emesis basin ▪ facial tissues ▪ Optional: pillow, appropriate-sized syringe, small piece of plastic tubing, atomization device, gloves, normal saline solution (or another appropriate solution) for gargling.

Implementation

- Avoid distractions and interruptions when preparing and administering medications *to prevent medication administration errors.*[2,3]
- Verify the order on the patient's medication record by checking it against the practitioner's order.[4,5,6]
- Gather the prescribed medication and appropriate equipment.
- Compare the medication label with the practitioner's order *to verify the correct medication, indication, dose, route, and time of administration.*[4,5,6] Verify the correct concentration of the medication. Phenylephrine, for example, is available in concentrations from 0.125% to 1%.
- Check the expiration date on the medication. If the medication is expired, return it to the pharmacy and obtain new medication.[4,5,6]
- Check the patient's medical record for an allergy or other contraindication to the prescribed medication. If an allergy or other contraindication exists, don't administer the medication; instead, notify the practitioner.[4,5,6]
- Visually inspect the medication for discoloration or other loss of integrity. Don't give the medication if its integrity is compromised.[4,5,6]
- Discuss any unresolved concerns about the medication with the patient's practitioner.[3,4,5]
- Perform hand hygiene.[7,8,9,10,11]
- Confirm the patient's identity using at least two patient identifiers.[12]
- If the patient is receiving the medication for the first time, inform the patient or family about significant adverse reactions and discuss any other concerns related to the medication.[4,5,6]
- Verify that the medication is being administered at the proper time, in the prescribed dose, and by the correct route *to reduce the risk of medication errors.*[4,5,6]
- If your facility uses a bar code scanning system, scan your identification badge, the patient's identification bracelet, and the medication's bar code.
- Explain the procedure, and provide privacy.[13,14]
- Put on gloves, if needed.[15]

For nose drop instillation

- When possible, position the patient so that the drops flow back into the nostrils, toward the affected area. (See *Positioning the patient for nose drop instillation.*)
- Draw the medication into the dropper or an appropriate-sized syringe.
- Push up the tip of the patient's nose slightly. Position the dropper just above the nostril, and direct its tip toward the midline of the nose *so that the drops flow toward the back of the nasal cavity rather than down the throat.*
- Insert the dropper about ⅜″ (1 cm) into the nostril. Don't let the dropper or syringe touch the sides of the nostril *because this would contaminate the dropper or could cause the patient to sneeze.*
- Instill the prescribed number of drops or milliliters, observing the patient carefully for signs of discomfort.
- *To prevent the drops from leaking out of the nostrils,* ask the patient to keep the head tilted back for at least 5 minutes and to breathe through the mouth. *This also allows sufficient time for the medication to constrict mucous membranes.*
- Keep an emesis basin handy *so that the patient can expectorate any medication that flows into the oropharynx and mouth.* Use a facial tissue to wipe any excess medication from the patient's nostrils and face.
- If used, clean the dropper by separating the plunger and pipette and flushing them with warm water. Allow them to air-dry.

For nasal inhaler

- Agitate the contents of the medication bottle for aqueous spray inhalers, as directed. Follow the manufacturer's instructions for loading and activating dry-powdered inhalers.[16]
- Remove the protective cap from the applicator tip.
- Have the patient tilt the head slightly forward.
- Tell the patient to keep the medication container upright and to place the applicator tip into one nostril, pointing it slightly away from the nasal septum, while occluding the other nostril with a finger.
- For aqueous spray inhalers, instruct the patient to place the thumb at the bottom of the bottle and the middle and index fingers on either side

Positioning the patient for nose drop instillation

To reach the ethmoid and sphenoid sinuses, have the patient lie on her back with her neck hyperextended and her head tilted back over the edge of the bed. Support her head with one hand *to prevent neck strain.*

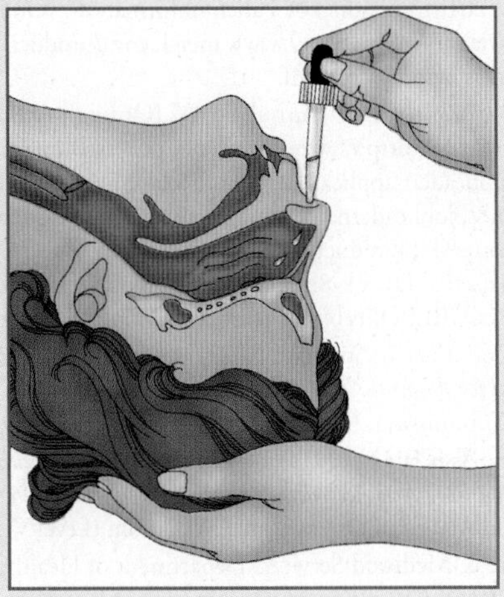

To reach the maxillary and frontal sinuses, have the patient lie on her back with her head toward the affected side and hanging slightly over the edge of the bed. Ask her to rotate her head laterally after hyperextension, and support her head with one hand *to prevent neck strain.*

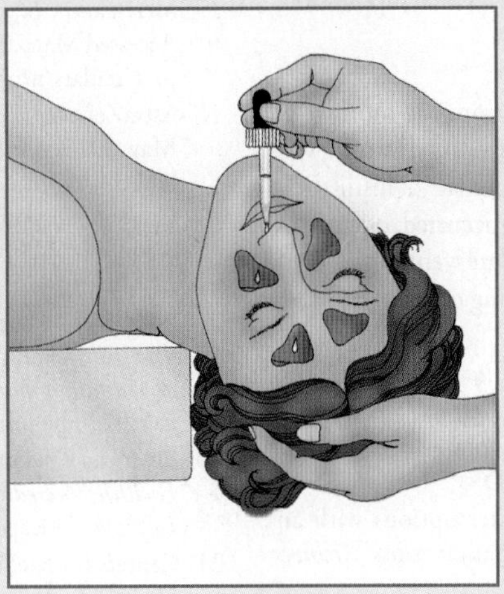

To administer drops for relief of ordinary nasal congestion, help the patient to a reclining or supine position with her head tilted slightly toward the affected side. Aim the dropper upward, toward the patient's eye, rather than downward, toward her ear.

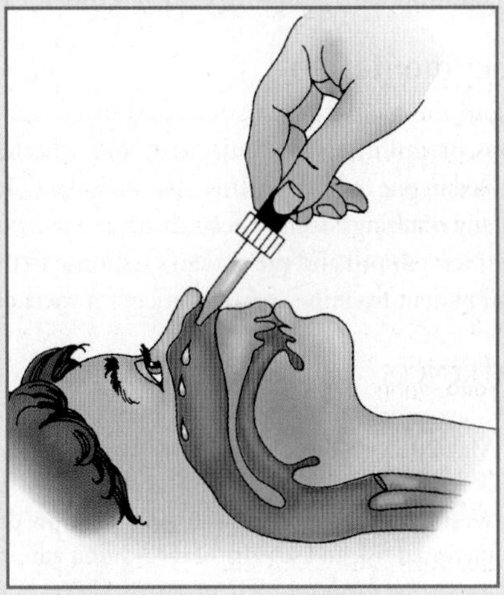

of the spray tip and then to press down firmly and quickly on the inhaler while inhaling deeply with the mouth closed.[17] For a dry-powder inhaler, instruct the patient to breathe in quickly and forcefully to release a premeasured, loaded dose of medication.[18]

- Tell the patient to remove the inhaler from the nostril and to hold his breath for a few seconds.
- Have the patient exhale through the mouth.
- Have the patient repeat the procedure in the other nostril, as directed.
- Have the patient tilt the head back for a few seconds and gargle with normal saline solution or water to remove the medication from the mouth and throat. Offer the patient an emesis basin, as needed.
- Clean the nasal applicator tip according to the manufacturer's instructions.

For nasal spray instillation

- Agitate the contents of the medication container according to the manufacturer's instructions.
- Remove the protective cap from the atomizer.
- *To prevent air from entering the nasal cavity and to allow the medication to flow properly,* occlude one of the patient's nostrils with your finger. Insert the atomizer tip into the open nostril.
- Instruct the patient to inhale with the mouth closed. As the patient inhales, squeeze the atomizer once, quickly and firmly. Use just enough force to coat the inside of the patient's nose with the medication. Then tell the patient to exhale through the mouth.
- If ordered, spray the nostril again. Then repeat the procedure in the other nostril.
- Instruct the patient to keep the head tilted back for several minutes and to breathe slowly through the nose so that the medication has time to work. Tell the patient to avoid nose blowing for several minutes.
- Keep an emesis basin handy so that the patient can expectorate any medication that flows into the oropharynx and mouth. Use a facial tissue to wipe any excess medication from the patient's nostrils and face.
- Rinse the tip of the nasal adapter in lukewarm water, and allow it to dry.

Completing the procedure

- Dispose of equipment in the appropriate receptacles.[19]
- Remove and discard your gloves, if worn.
- Perform hand hygiene.[7,8,9,10,11]
- Document the procedure.[20,21,22]

Special considerations

- Instruct the patient to avoid nose blowing for 15 minutes after the medication is given.

NURSING ALERT *To administer nasal medications more easily to a child or uncooperative patient, attach a small piece of tubing or an atomizer to a prefilled syringe of medication. Always follow the manufacturer's instructions for atomization device use.*[20]

- If using a metered-dose pump spray system, prime the delivery system with four sprays (or as directed by the manufacturer) or until a fine mist appears. Repeat the process to prime the system, as directed. Newer delivery system designs may reduce the need for priming and repriming and provide safety features *to enhance dosing control.* Always follow the manufacturer's instructions for use.[22]
- When using an aerosol, be careful not to puncture or incinerate the pressurized cartridge. Store it at temperatures below 120°F (49°C).
- *To prevent the spread of infection,* label the medication bottle so that it will be used only for that patient.[23]

Patient teaching

Teach the patient how to instill nasal medications correctly *so that the patient can continue treatment after discharge, if necessary.* Caution against using nasal medications longer than prescribed *because they may cause a rebound effect that worsens the condition.* A rebound effect occurs when the medication loses its effectiveness and relaxes the vessels in the nasal turbinates, producing a stuffiness that can be relieved only by discontinuing the medication. Teach good oral and nasal hygiene.

Explain that overdosage—which commonly occurs—can cause the medication to lose its effectiveness. Suggest recording the date and time of each inhalation or instillation as well as the patient's response *to prevent overdosage and to help the practitioner determine the drug's effectiveness.* Also, note whether the patient uses an unusual amount of medication. Inform the patient of possible adverse reactions.

Complications

Complications are related to the medication being administered. Use of nasal inhalers may also dry the nasal membranes and epistaxis.

Some nasal medications may cause restlessness, palpitations, nervousness, and other systemic effects. For example, excessive use of corticosteroid nose drops may cause hyperadrenocorticism and adrenal suppression.

Documentation

Record the medication instilled and its concentration, the number of drops or milliliters administered, and whether the medication was instilled in one or both nostrils. Also note the time and date of instillation and any resulting adverse effects. If adverse reactions occurred, document any interventions and the patient's response to the interventions. Document patient teaching and the patient's understanding of your teaching.

References

1 GlaxoSmithKline. (2013). "Imitrex® nasal spray" [Online]. Accessed May 2015 via the Web at https://www.gsksource.com/gskprm/htdocs/documents/IMITREX-NASAL-SPRAY-PI-PIL.PDF

2 Westbrook, J., et al. (2010). Association of interruptions with an increased risk and severity of medication administration errors. *Archives of Internal Medicine, 170,* 683–690. (Level IV)

3 Institute for Safe Medication Practices. (2013). Side tracks on the safety express: Interruptions lead to errors and unfinished... Wait, what was I doing? *Nurse Advise-ERR, 11*(2), 1–4. Accessed May 2015 via the Web at https://www.ismp.org/Newsletters/acutecare/showarticle.aspx?id=37

4 The Joint Commission. (2015). Standard MM.06.01.01. *Comprehensive accreditation manual for hospitals: The official handbook.* Oakbrook Terrace, IL: The Joint Commission. (Level VII)

5 American Osteopathic Association. (2014). Standard 16.01.03. *Healthcare Facilities Accreditation Program: Accreditation requirements for acute care hospitals.* Chicago, IL: American Osteopathic Association. (Level VII)

6 Centers for Medicare & Medicaid Services, Department of Health and Human Services. (2014). Condition of participation: Nursing services. 42 C.F.R. § 482.23(c).

7 The Joint Commission. (2015). Standard NPSG.07.01.01. *Comprehensive accreditation manual for hospitals: The official handbook.* Oakbrook Terrace, IL: The Joint Commission. (Level VII)

8 Centers for Disease Control and Prevention. (2002). Guideline for hand hygiene in health-care settings: Recommendations of the Healthcare Infection Control Practices Advisory Committee and the HICPAC/SHEA/APIC/IDSA Hand Hygiene Task Force. *MMWR Recommendations and Reports, 51*(RR-16), 1–45. Accessed May 2015 via the Web at http://www.cdc.gov/mmwr/pdf/rr/rr5116.pdf (Level II)

9 World Health Organization. (2009). "WHO guidelines on hand hygiene in health care: First global patient safety challenge, clean care is safer care" [Online]. Accessed May 2015 via the Web at http://whqlibdoc.who.int/publications/2009/9789241597906_eng.pdf (Level IV)

10 American Osteopathic Association. (2014). Standard 07.01.10. *Healthcare Facilities Accreditation Program: Accreditation requirements for acute care hospitals.* Chicago, IL: American Osteopathic Association. (Level VII)

11 Centers for Medicare & Medicaid Services, Department of Health and Human Services. (2014). Condition of participation: Infection control. 42 C.F.R. § 482.42.

12 The Joint Commission. (2015). Standard NPSG.01.01.01. *Comprehensive accreditation manual for hospitals: The official handbook.* Oakbrook Terrace, IL: The Joint Commission. (Level VII)

13 American Osteopathic Association. (2014). Standard 15.01.16. *Healthcare Facilities Accreditation Program: Accreditation requirements for acute care hospitals.* Chicago, IL: American Osteopathic Association. (Level VII)

14 Centers for Medicare & Medicaid Services, Department of Health and Human Services. (2014). Condition of participation: Patient's rights. 42 C.F.R. § 482.13(c)(1).

15 Siegel, J. D., et al. (2007). "2007 guideline for isolation precautions: Preventing transmission of infectious agents in healthcare settings" [Online]. Accessed May 2015 via the Web at http://www.cdc.gov/hicpac/pdf/isolation/Isolation2007.pdf (Level II)

16 Occupational Safety and Health Administration. (n.d.). "Bloodborne pathogens, standard number 1910.1030" [Online]. Accessed May 2015 via the Web at http://www.osha.gov/pls/oshaweb/owadisp.show_document?p_table=STANDARDS&p_id=10051 (Level VII)

17 Merck and Co., Inc. (2010). "Nasonex®: Patient information" [Online]. Accessed May 2015 via the Web at http://www.merck.com/product/usa/pi_circulars/n/nasonex/nasonex_ppi.pdf

18 AstraZeneca, (2013). "Rhinocort® Turbuhaler®" [Online]. Accessed May 2015 via the Web at http://www.astrazeneca.ca/cs/BlobServer?blobcol=pdffile&blobheader=application%2Fpdf&blobheadername1=Content-Disposition&blobheadername2=MDT-Type&blobheadervalue1=inline%3B+filename%3DProduct-Monograph.pdf&blobheadervalue2=abinary%3B+charset%3DUTF-8&blobkey=id&blobnocache=true&blobtable=AZ_FixedURLPDF&blobwhere=1285585477847&ssbin

19 The Joint Commission. (2015). Standard RC.01.03.01. *Comprehensive accreditation manual for hospitals: The official handbook.* Oakbrook Terrace, IL: The Joint Commission. (Level VII)

20 American Osteopathic Association. (2014). Standard 10.00.03. *Healthcare Facilities Accreditation Program: Accreditation requirements for acute care hospitals.* Chicago, IL: American Osteopathic Association. (Level VII)

21 Centers for Medicare & Medicaid Services, Department of Health and Human Services. (2014). Condition of participation: Medical record services. 42 C.F.R. § 482.24(b).

22 Djupesland, G. (2012). Nasal drug delivery devices: Characteristics and performance in a clinical perspective—a review. *Drug Delivery and Translational Research, 3,* 42–62. Accessed May 2015 via the Web at http://link.springer.com/content/pdf/10.1007%2Fs13346-012-0108-9.pdf (Level VII)

23 American Osteopathic Association. (2014). Standard 25.01.18. *Healthcare Facilities Accreditation Program: Accreditation requirements for acute care hospital.* Chicago, IL: American Osteopathic Association. (Level VII)

Additional references

Nettina, S. M. (2014). Lippincott manual of nursing practice (10th ed.). Philadelphia, PA: Wolters Kluwer.

Teva Respiratory, LLC. (2013). "Qnasl®: Patient information and instructions for use" [Online]. Accessed May 2015 via the Web at http://qnasl.com/Content/pdf/PIL.pdf

Nasal packing, assisting

In the highly vascular nasal mucosa, even seemingly minor injuries can cause major bleeding and blood loss. Initial treatment begins with ensuring a secure airway and hemodynamic stability. Most nasal bleeding originates at a plexus of arterioles and venules in the anteroinferior septum. About 90% of nosebleeds are anterior and can be controlled by pinching the anterior aspect of the nose.[1] Initially, direct pressure is applied for about 20 minutes. When direct pressure alone doesn't stop bleeding, topical vasoconstrictive drugs such as oxymetazoline or chemical cautery with silver nitrate sticks may be effective. Silver nitrate sticks are rolled over the area for 5 to 10 seconds until a gray eschar forms; then antibiotic ointment is applied to the area.[1]

If these steps are unsuccessful, nasal packing is typically the next step for persistent bleeding from epistaxis (nosebleed).[1,2] The patient may have to undergo nasal packing to stop anterior bleeding (which runs out of the nose) or posterior bleeding (which runs down the throat). If blood drains into the nasopharyngeal area or lacrimal ducts, the patient may also appear to bleed from the mouth and eyes.

The nurse typically assists a practitioner with anterior or posterior nasal packing. Commercially available balloons are relatively easy to insert and quite effective for anterior bleeding.[1] Whichever procedure the patient undergoes, he'll need ongoing encouragement and support to reduce his discomfort and anxiety as well as ongoing assessment to determine whether the procedure succeeded and to detect possible complications.

Equipment

Gowns ■ mask and goggles or mask with face shield ■ gloves ■ prescribed sedative ■ clamp ■ patient drape (towels or a gown) ■ emesis basin ■ nasal speculum and tongue blades (may be in preassembled head and neck examination kit) ■ light source (such as headlamp or fiber-optic nasal endoscope) ■ suction apparatus ■ sterile nasal aspirator tip ■ sterile bowl and sterile saline solution for flushing out suction apparatus ■ sterile tray or sterile towels ■ vial of 2% lidocaine ■ topical nasal vasoconstrictor decongestant (such as 0.5% phenylephrine) ■ sterile normal saline solution (1-g container and 60-mL syringe with luer-lock tip, or 5-mL bullets for moistening nasal tampons) ■ vital signs monitoring equipment ■ pulse oximeter ■ posterior packing materials[1] ■ commercially produced double-balloon tampon or indwelling urinary catheter, #10 to #14 French with a 30-mL (uninflated) balloon ■ Optional: cotton balls, cotton-tipped applicators, petroleum jelly, tape, epistaxis tray, supplemental humidified oxygen and face mask, arterial blood gas kit, supplies for blood sampling, flashlight, tongue blade, 20-mL syringe, hemostats, nasal dressing holder, prescribed medications, 10-mL syringe, Kelly clamp or bayonet forceps, antibiotic ointment, oral care supplies, 0-gauge silk suture material, two #14 or #16 French catheters (indwelling urinary catheter or some other type) with 30-mL (uninflated) balloon.

Preparation of equipment

Make sure the headlamp works. Plug in the suction apparatus if necessary or turn on the suction regulator. Connect the tubing from the collection container to the suction source. Test the suction equipment *to make sure it works properly.*

Implementation

- Gather all the equipment at the patient's bedside.
- Verify the practitioner's order.
- Perform hand hygiene.[3,4,5,6,7]
- Confirm the patient's identity using at least two patient identifiers.[8]
- Explain the procedure to the patient and offer reassurance *to reduce his anxiety and promote cooperation.*
- Obtain the patient's vital signs, and observe for hypotension with postural changes. *Hypotension and tachycardia suggest significant blood loss.* Obtain the patient's oxygen saturation level.
- Monitor airway patency and provide the patient with an emesis basin *because the patient will be at risk for aspirating or vomiting swallowed blood.*
- Perform a comprehensive pain assessment using techniques appropriate for the patient's age, condition, and ability to understand.[9]
- If ordered, administer a sedative, following safe medication administration practices, *to reduce the patient's anxiety and decrease sympathetic stimulation, which can exacerbate a nosebleed.*[1,10,11]
- Put on gloves, a gown, and a mask and goggles or a mask with face shield *to comply with standard precautions.*[12,13,14]
- Help the patient sit with his head tilted forward *to minimize blood drainage into the throat and prevent aspiration.*
- Drape the patient, as necessary.
- Make sure the suction regulator is turned on and attach the connecting tubing *so the practitioner can aspirate the nasal cavity to remove clots before locating the bleeding source.*
- At the bedside, create a sterile field. Using sterile technique, place all sterile equipment on the sterile field. Open the package containing the sterile nasal aspirating tip and place on the sterile field. Fill the sterile bowl with sterile normal saline solution *so that you can flush the suction tubing, as necessary.* Label all medications, medication containers, and solutions on and off the sterile field.[16] Thoroughly lubricate the posterior packing with antibiotic ointment.[1]

Inserting posterior nasal packing

Posterior packing consists of a gauze roll shaped and secured by three sutures (one suture at each end and one in the middle) or a balloon-type catheter. To insert the packing, the practitioner advances one or two soft catheters into the patient's nostrils (as shown below). When the catheter tips appear in the nasopharynx, the practitioner grasps them with a Kelly clamp or bayonet forceps and pulls them forward through the mouth. He secures the two end sutures to the catheter tip and draws the catheter back through the nostrils.

This step brings the packing into place with the end sutures hanging from the patient's nostril. (The middle suture emerges from the patient's mouth to free the packing, when needed.)

The practitioner may weigh the nose sutures with a clamp. Then he will pull the packing securely into place behind the soft palate and against the posterior end of the septum (nasal choana).

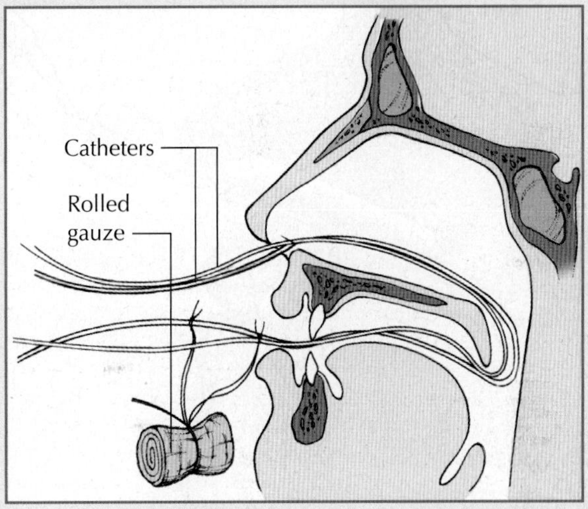

- *To inspect the nasal cavity,* the practitioner will use a nasal speculum and an external light source such as a headlamp or a fiber-optic nasal endoscope. *To remove collected blood and help visualize the bleeding vessel,* he may ask the patient to blow his nose or he may use suction.[1]
- Assist the practitioner with administering an anesthetic agent, if needed. He may administer a solution containing lidocaine, epinephrine, and tetracaine applied to cotton balls, which he'll then place in the nostrils for 10 minutes, or he may apply lidocaine spray.[2]
- Prepare to assist the practitioner with insertion of packing, as directed. (See *Inserting posterior nasal packing* and *Inserting anterior nasal packing,* pages 519, 520.)
- Lubricate the catheters *to ease insertion in the posterior nasal cavity.*
- Instruct the patient to breathe normally through his mouth during catheter insertion *to minimize gagging as the catheters pass through the nostril.*
- Help the practitioner with administering an anesthetic if needed. He may add 2% lidocaine to a topical nasal vasoconstricting agent and then have the patient inhale it.[2]
- Help the patient assume a comfortable position with his head elevated 45 to 90 degrees. Assess him for airway obstruction or any respiratory changes.

Inserting anterior nasal packing[1,15]

If bleeding persists despite chemical cautery, assist the practitioner with insertion of nasal packing to stop the bleeding. You may use a commercially available inflatable balloon or nasal tampon to pack the area.

Inflatable balloon device

One inflatable balloon device has a balloon that's coated with a carboxymethylcellulose hydrocolloid compound that acts as a platelet aggregator. The substance also creates a lubricant when it comes in contact with water *to ease insertion*. After soaking the device in sterile water, the practitioner inserts the device along the superior aspect of the hard palate until the fabric ring is well into the naris (as shown below). Then, using a 20-mL syringe, the practitioner inflates the balloon until the pilot cuff becomes rounded and feels firm when squeezed.

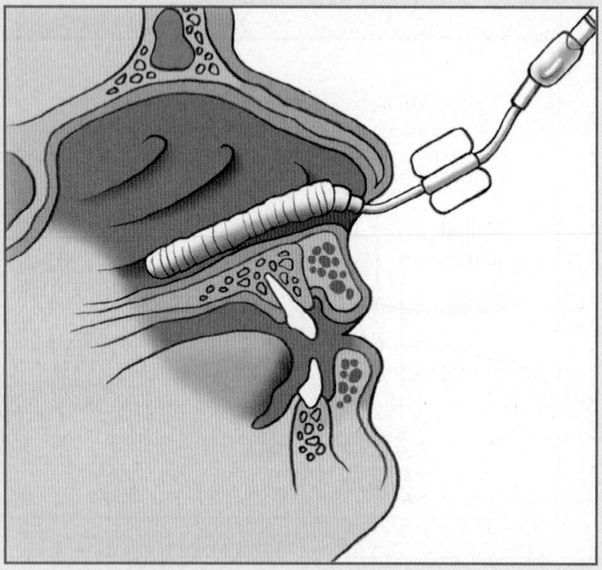

Reassess the device 15 to 20 minutes after insertion. If necessary, reinflate the cuff *to ensure proper pressure*. Tape the pilot balloon to the patient's cheek away from his upper lip. The device can remain in place for up to 72 hours, as needed.

Nasal tampon

Another alternative for anterior nasal packing is the nasal tampon. After coating the tampon with water-soluble lubricant (or antibiotic ointment, as prescribed), the practitioner grabs the string end with his gloved fingers or forceps. He inserts the tampon gently and quickly along the floor of the nasal cavity until the string reaches the naris (as shown below).

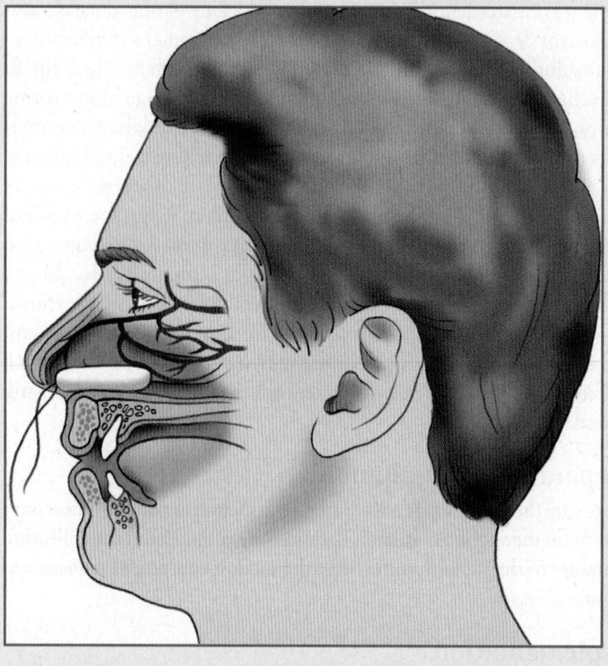

If the tampon doesn't expand within 30 seconds of insertion, the practitioner irrigates it with 10 mL of saline solution or water *so that the tampon expands*. Tape the string to the patient's nose *to secure the device in place* and trim the ends of the string, if necessary.

- Monitor the patient's vital signs *to detect changes that may indicate hypovolemia or hypoxemia.*
- Monitor the patient's respiratory status *to make sure his airway is patent*; monitor oxygen saturation level by pulse oximetry *to detect hypoxemia.* Make sure that the alarm limits are set appropriately for the patient's current condition and that the alarms are turned on, functioning properly, and audible to staff.[17,18,19,20]
- Administer supplemental humidified oxygen by face mask, if needed and ordered.
- Provide emotional support *because mouth breathing, which is necessary with the packing in place, may cause anxiety and hyperventilation.*
- If severe or recurrent bleeding or an underlying medical condition is present, obtain a blood sample for complete blood count and blood compatibility testing, as ordered. If the patient has renal or hepatic dysfunction or if he was taking an anticoagulant, obtain a specimen for coagulation studies, as ordered.[1] Notify the practitioner of critical test results within your facility's established timeframe *so the patient can receive prompt treatment.*[21]
- Check the posterior oropharynx frequently *to see whether there's bleeding into the back of the throat or whether the packing has slipped out of position.*
- Maintain the head of the bed at 30 degrees or higher.
- While the anterior packing is in place, use the cotton-tipped applicators to apply petroleum jelly to the patient's lips and nostrils *to prevent drying and cracking.*
- *Because a patient with nasal packing must breathe through his mouth,* provide frequent oral care. Artificial saliva, room humidification, and ample fluid intake also relieve dryness caused by mouth breathing.
- As ordered, administer an analgesic, antiemetic, decongestant, sedative, and prophylactic antibiotic following safe medication administration practices.[10,11] Avoid administration of aspirin and nonsteroidal anti-inflammatory agents for a few days *to reduce the risk of bleeding.*[1]
- Discard used supplies in the appropriate receptacle.[13]
- Remove and discard your gloves and other personal protective equipment.[12,13]
- Perform hand hygiene.[3,4,5,6,7]
- Reassess the patient's pain and respond appropriately.[9]
- Perform hand hygiene.[3,4,5,6,7]
- Clean and disinfect your stethoscope using a disinfectant pad.[22,23]
- Perform hand hygiene.[3,4,5,6,7]
- Document the procedure.[24,25,26]

Special considerations

■ Assist the practitioner, as required, in the balloon catheter method of posterior nasal packing insertion. If using a commercially produced double-balloon tampon, inflate the balloons according to the manufacturer's instructions.[15] If using an indwelling urinary catheter, inflate the balloon with up to 10 mL of sterile water. (Don't inflate the balloon to its full 30-mL capacity.)[2]

■ Patients with posterior packing are usually hospitalized for monitoring. If mucosal oozing persists, apply a moustache dressing by securing a folded gauze pad over the nasal vestibules with tape or a commercial nasal dressing holder. Change the pad when soiled.

■ Test the patient's call light *to make sure he can summon help if needed.* Also, keep emergency equipment (flashlight, tongue blade, syringe, and hemostats) at the patient's bedside *to speed packing removal if it becomes displaced and occludes the airway.*

■ After the packing is in place, compile assessment data carefully *to help detect the underlying cause of nosebleeds.* Mechanical factors include a deviated septum, injury, and a foreign body. Environmental factors include drying and erosion of the nasal mucosa. Other possible causes include upper respiratory tract infection, anticoagulant or salicylate therapy, blood dyscrasias, cardiovascular or hepatic disorders, tumors of the nasal cavity or paranasal sinuses, chronic nephritis, and familial hemorrhagic telangiectasia.

■ If significant blood loss occurs or if the underlying cause remains unknown, expect the practitioner to order a complete blood count and coagulation profile as soon as possible. Blood transfusion may be necessary.

■ The patient should remain on modified bed rest until removal of the pack.

■ The practitioner will usually remove nasal packing in 2 to 5 days.

■ The Joint Commission issued a sentinel event alert concerning medical device alarm safety *because alarm-related events have been associated with permanent loss of function or death.* Among the major contributing factors were improper alarm settings, alarms inappropriately turned off, and alarm signals not audible to staff. Make sure alarm limits are set appropriately, and that alarms are turned on, functioning properly, and audible to staff. Follow facility guidelines for preventing alarm fatigue.[17]

Patient teaching

Tell the patient to expect a reduced ability to detect smell and taste. Make sure he has a working smoke detector at home. Advise him to eat soft foods *because his eating and swallowing abilities will be impaired.* Instruct him to drink fluids often or to use artificial saliva to cope with dry mouth. Teach him measures to prevent nosebleeds, and instruct him to seek medical help if these measures fail to stop bleeding. (See *Preventing recurrent nosebleeds.*)

Complications

The pressure of a posterior pack on the soft palate may lead to hypoxemia. Patients with posterior packing are at special risk for aspiration of blood. Patients with underlying pulmonary conditions, such as chronic obstructive pulmonary disease and asthma, are at special risk for exacerbation of the condition or for hypoxemia while nasal packing is in place. You can detect hypoxemia with pulse oximetry. Signs and symptoms include tachycardia, confusion, cyanosis, and restlessness.

Airway obstruction may occur if a posterior pack slips backward. The patient may complain of difficulty swallowing, pain, or discomfort. In patients with posterior packs, otitis media may develop. Other possible complications include hematotympanum and pressure necrosis of nasal structures, especially the septum.

Sedation may cause hypotension in a patient with significant blood loss and may also increase the patient's risk of aspiration and hypoxemia.

PATIENT TEACHING

Preventing recurrent nosebleeds

Review these self-care guidelines with your patient *to reduce his risk of developing recurrent nosebleeds:*

■ *Because nosebleeds can result from dry mucous membranes,* suggest that the patient use a cool mist vaporizer or humidifier, as needed, especially in dry environments.

■ Teach the patient how to minimize pressure on nasal passages. Advise him, for instance, to avoid constipation and consequent straining during defecation. Recommend a fiber-rich diet and adequate fluid intake, and warn him to avoid extreme physical exertion for 24 hours after the nosebleed stops. Caution him to avoid aspirin, nonsteroidal anti-inflammatory drugs, alcoholic beverages, and tobacco for at least 5 days.

■ If the patient gets a nosebleed despite these precautions, tell him to keep his head higher than his heart and, using his thumb and forefinger, to press the soft portion of the nostrils together and against the facial bones. (Recommend against direct pressure if he has a facial injury or nasal fracture.) Tell him to maintain pressure for up to 10 minutes and then to reassess bleeding. If it's uncontrolled, he should reapply pressure for another 10 minutes with ice between the thumb and forefinger.

■ After a nosebleed or after nasal packing is removed, caution the patient to avoid rubbing or picking his nose, putting a handkerchief or tissue in his nose, or blowing his nose forcefully for at least 48 hours. After this time, he may blow his nose gently and use salt-water nasal spray to clear nasal clots.

Documentation

Record the type of pack used *to ensure its removal at the appropriate time.* On the intake-and-output record, document the estimated blood loss and all fluid administered. Note the patient's vital signs; his response to sedation, analgesics, or position changes; the results of any laboratory tests; and any drugs administered, including topical agents. Record any complications and interventions. Document patient teaching, discharge instructions, and clinical follow-up plans and the patient's understanding of them.

REFERENCES

1 Gilman, C. (2009). "Focus on: Treatment of epistaxis" [Online]. Accessed May 2015 via the Web at http://www.acep.org/Clinical—Practice-Management/Focus-On–Treatment-of-Epistaxis/

2 Goralnick, E. (2012). "Anterior epistaxis nasal pack" [Online]. Accessed May 2015 via the Web at http://emedicine.medscape.com/article/80526-overview

3 Centers for Disease Control and Prevention. (2002). Guideline for hand hygiene in health-care settings: Recommendations of the Healthcare Infection Control Practices Advisory Committee and the HICPAC/SHEA/APIC/IDSA Hand Hygiene Task Force. *MMWR Recommendations and Reports, 51*(RR-16), 1–45. Accessed May 2015 via the Web at http://www.cdc.gov/mmwr/pdf/rr/rr5116.pdf (Level II)

4 World Health Organization. (2009). "WHO guidelines on hand hygiene in health care: First global patient safety challenge, clean care is safer care" [Online]. Accessed May 2015 via the Web at http://whqlibdoc.who.int/publications/2009/9789241597906_eng.pdf (Level IV)

5 The Joint Commission. (2015). Standard NPSG.07.01.01. *Comprehensive accreditation manual for hospitals: The official handbook.* Oakbrook Terrace, IL: The Joint Commission. (Level VII)

6 Centers for Medicare & Medicaid Services, Department of Health and Human Services. (2014). Condition of participation: Infection control. 42 C.F.R. § 482.42.

7 American Osteopathic Association. (2014). Standard 07.01.21. *Healthcare Facilities Accreditation Program: Accreditation requirements for acute care hospitals.* Chicago, IL: American Osteopathic Association. (Level VII)

8 The Joint Commission. (2015). Standard NPSG.01.01.01. *Comprehensive accreditation manual for hospitals: The official handbook.* Oakbrook Terrace, IL: The Joint Commission. (Level VII)
9 The Joint Commission. (2015). Standard PC.01.02.07. *Comprehensive accreditation manual for hospitals: The official handbook.* Oakbrook Terrace, IL: The Joint Commission. (Level VII)
10 Centers for Medicare & Medicaid Services, Department of Health and Human Services. (2014). Condition of participation: Nursing services. 42 C.F.R. § 482.23(c).
11 American Osteopathic Association. (2014). Standard 16.01.03. *Healthcare Facilities Accreditation Program: Accreditation requirements for acute care hospitals.* Chicago, IL: American Osteopathic Association. (Level VII)
12 Siegel, J. D., et al. (2007). "2007 guideline for isolation precautions: Preventing transmission of infectious agents in healthcare settings" [Online]. Accessed May 2015 via the Web at http://www.cdc.gov/hicpac/pdf/isolation/Isolation2007.pdf (Level II)
13 Occupational Safety and Health Administration. (n.d.). "Bloodborne pathogens, standard number 1910.1030" [Online]. Accessed May 2015 via the web at http://www.osha.gov/pls/oshaweb/owadisp.show_document?p_table=STANDARDS&p_id=10051 (Level VII)
14 American Osteopathic Association. (2014). Standard 07.01.10. *Healthcare Facilities Accreditation Program: Accreditation requirements for acute care hospitals.* Chicago, IL: American Osteopathic Association. (Level VII)
15 ArthroCare ENT. (2013). "Rapid Rhino®: Epistaxis solutions" [Online]. Accessed May 2015 via the Web at http://www.arthrocareent.com/img/vfsroot/it_1298837673/Rapid%20Rhino%20Epistaxis%20Brochure%20-%20PN%20RR117_K.pdf
16 The Joint Commission. (2015). Standard NSPG.03.04.01. *Comprehensive accreditation manual for hospitals: The official handbook.* Oakbrook Terrace, IL: The Joint Commission. (Level VII)
17 The Joint Commission. (2013). "Sentinel event alert: Medical device alarm safety in hospitals" [Online]. Accessed May 2015 via the Web at http://www.jointcommission.org/assets/1/18/SEA_50_alarms_4_5_13_FINAL1.PDF (Level VII)
18 The Joint Commission. (2015). Standard NPSG.06.01.01. *Comprehensive accreditation manual for hospitals: The official handbook.* Oakbrook Terrace, IL: The Joint Commission. (Level VII)
19 Graham, K. C., & Cvach, M. (2010). Monitor alarm fatigue: Standardizing use of physiological monitors and decreasing nuisance alarms. *American Journal of Critical Care, 19,* 28–37. Accessed May 2015 via the Web at http://ajcc.aacnjournals.org/content/19/1/28.full.pdf
20 American Association of Critical-Care Nurses. (2013). "AACN practice alert: Alarm management" [Online]. Accessed May 2015 via the Web at http://www.aacn.org/wd/practice/docs/practicealerts/alarm-management-practice-alert.pdf (Level VII)
21 The Joint Commission. (2015). Standard NSPG.02.03.01. *Comprehensive accreditation manual for hospitals: The official handbook.* Oakbrook Terrace, IL: The Joint Commission. (Level VII)
22 Rutala, W. A., et al. (2008). "Guideline for disinfection and sterilization in healthcare facilities, 2008" [Online]. Accessed May 2015 via the Web at http://www.cdc.gov/hicpac/pdf/guidelines/Disinfection_Nov_2008.pdf (Level I)
23 American Osteopathic Association. (2014). Standard 07.02.03. *Healthcare Facilities Accreditation Program: Accreditation requirements for acute care hospitals.* Chicago, IL: American Osteopathic Association. (Level VII)
24 The Joint Commission. (2015). Standard RC.01.03.01. *Comprehensive accreditation manual for hospitals: The official handbook.* Oakbrook Terrace, IL: The Joint Commission. (Level VII)
25 Centers for Medicare & Medicaid Services, Department of Health and Human Services. (2014). Condition of participation: Medical record services. 42 C.F.R. § 482.24(b).
26 American Osteopathic Association. (2014). Standard 10.00.03. *Healthcare Facilities Accreditation Program: Accreditation requirements for acute care hospitals.* Chicago, IL: American Osteopathic Association. (Level VII)

NASOENTERIC-DECOMPRESSION TUBE CARE

A nasoenteric-decompression tube is used to aspirate intestinal contents for analysis and to treat intestinal obstruction. The tube may also help to prevent nausea, vomiting, and abdominal distention after GI surgery.

After initial tube insertion, the patient lies on his right side for about 2 hours to promote the tube's passage. When the tube advances past the pylorus, it can be advance 2″ to 3″ (5 to 7.5 cm) per hour until it reaches the desired position. The tube is then secure to the patient's gown or bed linens, taped to his face, and connected to a suction machine.

The patient with a nasoenteric-decompression tube needs special care, including precise intake-and-output records as well as continuous monitoring to ensure tube patency, maintain suction and bowel decompression, and detect such complications as fluid-electrolyte imbalances related to aspiration of intestinal contents. He'll also need frequent mouth and nose care to provide comfort and prevent skin breakdown, and encouragement and support during tube insertion and removal and while the tube is in place.

Equipment

Suction apparatus with intermittent suction capability ■ container of water ■ intake-and-output record sheets ■ mouthwash and water mixture ■ sponge swabs ■ petroleum jelly or water-soluble lubricant ■ cotton-tipped applicators ■ disposable irrigation set ■ normal saline solution ■ labels for tube lumens ■ Optional: gloves, gown, mask and goggles or mask with face shield, blood sampling supplies, mouthwash, gargles, viscous lidocaine, throat lozenges, ice collar, sour hard candy or gum.

Preparation of equipment

Assemble the suction apparatus and set up the suction unit. If indicated, test the unit by turning it on and placing the end of the suction tubing in a container of water. If the tubing draws in water, the unit works.

Implementation

- Gather the appropriate equipment.
- Perform hand hygiene.[1,2,3,4,5]
- Put on gloves and personal protective equipment as needed *to comply with standard precautions.*[6,7]
- Confirm the patient's identity using at least two patient identifiers.[8]
- Explain the purpose of the procedure to the patient and his family. Answer questions clearly and thoroughly *to ease anxiety and enhance cooperation.*
- Verify X-ray confirmation of tube placement.[9]
- Assess for tube migration by checking the external tube length and comparing it with the baseline measurement.[10]
- Check the suction machine at least every 2 hours *to confirm proper functioning and to ensure tube patency and bowel decompression. Excessive negative pressure may draw the mucosa into the tube openings, impair the suction's effectiveness, and injure the mucosa.* Using intermittent suction helps to avoid these problems. *To check functioning in an intermittent suction unit,* look for drainage in the connecting tube and dripping into the collecting container.
- Measure and record intake and output at least every 8 hours *to monitor fluid balance.*[11]
- Watch for signs and symptoms of pneumonia related to the patient's inability to clear his pharynx or cough effectively with a tube in place. Be alert for fever, chest pain, tachypnea or labored breathing, and diminished breath sounds over the affected area.
- Observe drainage characteristics, including color, amount, consistency, odor, and any unusual changes.
- Obtain blood samples for laboratory testing, as ordered, *to monitor fluids, electrolytes, and blood loss.*[12] (See the "Venipuncture" procedure, page 821.)

■ Provide oral care frequently (at least every 4 hours) *to increase patient comfort and promote a healthy oral cavity. If the tube remains in place for several days, mouth-breathing will leave the lips, tongue, and other tissues dry and cracked.* Encourage the patient to participate in oral care. (See the "Oral care" procedure, page 560.)
■ Lubricate the patient's lips with either sponge swabs or petroleum jelly applied with a cotton-tipped applicator.
■ At least every 4 hours, gently clean and lubricate the patient's external nostrils with either petroleum jelly or water-soluble lubricant on a cotton-tipped applicator *to prevent skin breakdown.*
■ Watch for peristalsis to resume, signaled by bowel sounds, passage of flatus, decreased abdominal distention and, possibly, a spontaneous bowel movement. *These signs may require tube removal.*
■ After decompression and before extubation, as ordered, provide a clear- to full-liquid diet *to assess bowel function.*
■ Remove and discard your gloves and any other personal protective equipment worn.[6,7]
■ Perform hand hygiene.[1,2,3,4,5]
■ Document the procedure.[13,14,15]

Special considerations

■ If no drainage is accumulating in the collection container, suspect an obstruction in the tube. As ordered, irrigate the tube with the irrigation set *to clear the obstruction.* (See *Clearing a nasoenteric-decompression tube obstruction.*) Record the amount of instilled irrigant as "intake." Typically, normal saline solution supersedes water as the preferred irrigant *because water, which is hypotonic, may increase electrolyte loss, especially if you must irrigate the tube often.*
■ If the patient is ambulatory and his tube connects to a portable suction unit, he may move short distances while connected to the unit. Alternatively, if feasible and ordered, you can disconnect the tube briefly while he moves about.
■ If the tubing irritates the patient's throat or makes him hoarse, offer relief with mouthwash, gargles, viscous lidocaine, throat lozenges, an ice collar, sour hard candy, or gum, as appropriate.
■ If the tip of the balloon falls below the ileocecal valve (confirmed by X-ray), you can't remove the tube nasally, but must advance it and remove it through the anus.
■ If the balloon at the end of the tube protrudes from the anus, notify the practitioner. Most likely, the practitioner can disconnect the tube from suction, sever the proximal end, and remove the remaining tube gradually through the anus manually or by peristalsis.

Complications

In addition to fluid-volume deficit, electrolyte imbalance, and pneumonia, potential complications include intussusception of the bowel (from the weight of the balloon).

Documentation

Record the frequency and type of oral and nasal care given. Describe the therapeutic effect, if any. Document in your notes the amount, color, consistency, and odor of the drainage obtained each time you empty the collection container.

Record the amount of drainage on the intake and output sheet. Always record the amount of any irrigant or other fluid introduced through the tube or taken orally by the patient.

If the suction machine malfunctions, note the length of time it wasn't functioning and nursing actions taken. Document the amount and character of any vomitus. Also note the patient's tolerance of the tube's insertion and removal. Document any patient teaching and the patient's understanding of that teaching.

TROUBLESHOOTING

Clearing a nasoenteric-decompression tube obstruction

If a patient's nasoenteric-decompression tube appears to be obstructed, notify the practitioner right away. He may order measures such as those listed below *to restore patency quickly and efficiently.*
■ Disconnect the tube from the suction source and irrigate with normal saline solution. Use gravity flow *to help clear the obstruction* unless ordered otherwise.
■ If irrigation doesn't reestablish patency, the tube may be obstructed by its position against the gastric mucosa. To rectify this problem, tug slightly on the tube *to move it away from the mucosa.*
■ If gentle tugging doesn't restore patency, the tube may be kinked and may need additional manipulation. Before proceeding, however, take these precautions:
– Never reposition or irrigate a nasoenteric-decompression tube (without a practitioner's order) in a patient who has had GI surgery.
– Avoid manipulating a tube in a patient who had the tube inserted during surgery. *Doing so may disturb new sutures.*
– Don't try to reposition a tube in a patient who was difficult to intubate (such as a patient with an esophageal stricture).

REFERENCES

1 The Joint Commission. (2015). Standard NPSG.07.01.01. *Comprehensive accreditation manual for hospitals: The official handbook.* Oakbrook Terrace, IL: The Joint Commission. (Level VII)

2 Centers for Disease Control and Prevention. (2002). Guideline for hand hygiene in health-care settings: Recommendations of the Healthcare Infection Control Practices Advisory Committee and the HICPAC/SHEA/APIC/IDSA Hand Hygiene Task Force. *MMWR Recommendations and Reports, 51*(RR-16), 1–45. Accessed May 2015 via the Web at http://www.cdc.gov/mmwr/pdf/rr/rr5116.pdf (Level II)

3 World Health Organization. (2009). "WHO guidelines on hand hygiene in health care: First global patient safety challenge, clean care is safer care" [Online]. Accessed May 2015 via the Web at http://whqlibdoc.who.int/publications/2009/9789241597906_eng.pdf (Level IV)

4 Centers for Medicare & Medicaid Services, Department of Health and Human Services. (2014). Condition of participation: Infection control. 42 C.F.R. § 482.42.

5 American Osteopathic Association. (2014). Standard 07.01.21. *Healthcare Facilities Accreditation Program: Accreditation requirements for acute care hospitals.* Chicago, IL: American Osteopathic Association. (Level VII)

6 Siegel, J. D., et al. (2007). "2007 guideline for isolation precautions: Preventing transmission of infectious agents in healthcare settings" [Online]. Accessed May 2015 via the Web at http://www.cdc.gov/hicpac/pdf/isolation/Isolation2007.pdf (Level II)

7 Occupational Safety and Health Administration. (n.d.). "Bloodborne pathogens, standard number 1910.1030" [Online]. Accessed May 2015 via the Web at http://www.osha.gov/pls/oshaweb/owadisp.show_document?p_table=STANDARDS&p_id=10051 (Level VII)

8 The Joint Commission. (2015). Standard NPSG.01.01.01. *Comprehensive accreditation manual for hospitals: The official handbook.* Oakbrook Terrace, IL: The Joint Commission. (Level VII)

9 American Association of Critical Care Nurses. (2009). "AACN practice alert: Verification of feeding tube placement (blindly inserted)" [Online]. Accessed May 2015 via the Web at http://www.aacn.org/WD/Practice/Docs/PracticeAlerts/Verification_of_Feeding_Tube_Placement_05-2005.pdf (Level VII)

10 Metheny, N. A., et al. (2012). Blind insertion of feeding tubes in intensive care units: A national survey. *American Journal of Critical Care, 21,*

EQUIPMENT

Common types of nasoenteric-decompression tubes

The type of nasoenteric-decompression tube chosen for the patient depends on the size of the patient and his nostrils, the estimated duration of intubation, and the reason for the procedure. For example, to remove viscous material from the patient's intestinal tract, the practitioner may select a tube with a wide bore and a single lumen.

Such tubes as the Andersen pre-weighted Miller-Abbot type intestinal tube (shown below), have a tungsten-weighted inflatable latex balloon tip designed for temporary management of mechanical obstruction in the small or large intestines.

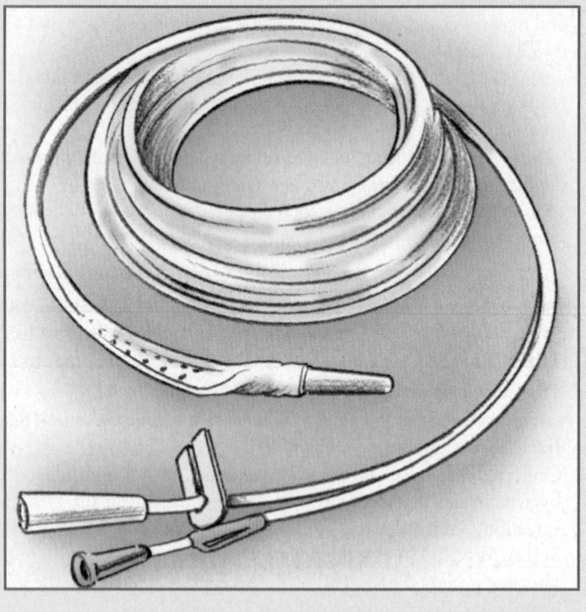

352–360. Accessed May 2015 via the Web at http://ajcc.aacnjournals.org/content/21/5/352.full.pdf+html (Level VI)

11 Hinkle, J. L., & Cheever, K. H. (2014). *Brunner and Suddarth's textbook of medical-surgical nursing* (13th ed.). Philadelphia, PA: Wolters Kluwer.

12 Jackson, P. G., & Raiji, M. (2011). Evaluation and management of intestinal obstruction. *American Family Physician, 83,* 159–165. Accessed May 2015 via the Web at http://www.aafp.org/afp/2011/0115/p159.html

13 The Joint Commission. (2015). Standard RC.01.03.01. *Comprehensive accreditation manual for hospitals: The official handbook.* Oakbrook Terrace, IL: The Joint Commission. (Level VII)

14 Centers for Medicare & Medicaid Services, Department of Health and Human Services. (2014). Condition of participation: Medical record services. 42 C.F.R. § 482.24(b).

15 American Osteopathic Association. (2014). Standard 10.00.03. *Healthcare Facilities Accreditation Program: Accreditation requirements for acute care hospitals.* Chicago, IL: American Osteopathic Association. (Level VII)

NASOENTERIC-DECOMPRESSION TUBE INSERTION AND REMOVAL

A nasoenteric-decompression tube, inserted nasally and advanced beyond the stomach into the intestinal tract, aspirates intestinal contents for analysis and to treat intestinal obstruction. The tube can also help to prevent nausea, vomiting, and abdominal distention after GI surgery. A practitioner usually inserts and removes a nasoenteric-decompression tube; however, a nurse may remove it in an emergency. An oroenteric-decompression tube is a good substitute if the patient has facial trauma, a nasal injury, or abnormal nasal anatomy.[1]

Some nasoenteric-decompression tubes have a pre-weighted tip and balloon at one end of the tube that holds air or water to stimulate peristalsis and facilitate the tube's passage through the pylorus and into the intestinal tract. (See *Common types of nasoenteric-decompression tubes.*)

Equipment

For insertion

Nasoenteric-decompression tube ▪ suction apparatus with intermittent suction capability ▪ gloves ▪ towel or fluid-impermeable pad ▪ water-soluble lubricant ▪ 4″ × 4″ (10-cm × 10-cm) gauze pad ▪ hypoallergenic tape or securement device ▪ bulb syringe or 60-mL catheter-tip syringe ▪ pH test paper ▪ waterproof pen ▪ glass of water with straw ▪ oral care supplies ▪ Optional: basin of ice or warm water, penlight, local anesthetic spray, liquid anesthetic, ice chips, gown, mask and goggles or mask with face shield, capnography monitor.

For removal

10-mL syringe ▪ gloves ▪ towel or fluid-impermeable pad ▪ clamp ▪ oral care supplies.

Preparation of equipment

Stiffen a flaccid tube by chilling it in a basin of ice *to facilitate insertion.* To make a stiff tube flexible, dip it into warm water.

Add air or water to the balloon either before or after insertion of the tube, depending on the type of tube used. Follow the manufacturer's recommendations.

Set up suction-decompression equipment, as ordered, and make sure it works properly.

Implementation

- Verify the practitioner's order.
- Gather the appropriate equipment.
- Perform hand hygiene.[2,3,4,5,6]
- Confirm the patient's identity using at least two patient identifiers.[7]
- Explain the procedure to the patient, including the fact that he might experience some discomfort.
- Provide privacy and adequate lighting.[8,9]

Inserting a nasoenteric-decompression tube

- Put on gloves and other personal protective equipment as needed *to comply with standard precautions.*[10,11,12]
- Position the patient as the practitioner specifies, usually in the semi-Fowler or high Fowler position. You might also need to help the patient hold his neck in a partially flexed position *to help facilitate proper insertion into the GI tract.*[13]
- Protect the patient's chest with a towel or fluid-impermeable pad.
- Agree with the patient on a signal that can be used to stop the insertion briefly if necessary.
- The practitioner assesses the patency of the patient's nostrils. *To evaluate which nostril has better airflow in a conscious patient,* he holds one nostril closed and then the other as the patient breathes. In an unconscious patient, he examines each nostril with a penlight *to check for polyps, a deviated septum, or other obstruction.*
- Apply a local anesthetic spray, if ordered, to the nostril or the back of the throat *to dull sensations and the gag reflex for intubation.* Letting the patient gargle with a liquid anesthetic or holding ice chips in his mouth for a few minutes serves the same purpose.
- *To decide how far the tube must be inserted to reach the stomach,* the practitioner places the tube's distal end at the tip of the patient's nose and then extends the tube to the earlobe and down to the xiphoid

process. He marks the tube with a waterproof pen or holds it at this point.

- The practitioner applies water-soluble lubricant to the first few inches of the tube *to reduce friction and tissue trauma and to facilitate insertion.*
- If the balloon already contains water, the practitioner holds it so the fluid runs to the bottom. Then he pinches the balloon closed *to retain the fluid as the insertion begins.*
- *To keep the tube out of the patient's eyes and help avoid undue skin irritation,* fold a 4″ × 4″ (10-cm × 10-cm) gauze pad in half and tape it to the patient's forehead with the fold directed toward the patient's nose. The practitioner can slide the tube through this sling, leaving enough slack for the tube to advance.
- Tell the patient to breathe through his mouth or to pant as the balloon enters his nostril. After the balloon begins its descent, the practitioner releases his grip on it, allowing the weight of the fluid or the pre-weighted tip to pull the tube into the nasopharynx. When the tube reaches the nasopharynx, the practitioner instructs the patient to lower his chin and to swallow. In some cases, the patient may sip water through a straw *to facilitate swallowing as the tube advances,* but not after the tube reaches the trachea (*to prevent injury from aspiration*). The practitioner continues to advance the tube slowly *to prevent it from curling or kinking in the stomach.*
- *To confirm the tube's passage into the stomach,* the practitioner may use various techniques to determine tube location during insertion, including watching for signs of respiratory distress (coughing and dyspnea); using capnography, if available, to detect carbon dioxide, which indicates inadvertent tracheal insertion; measuring pH aspirate from the tube if pH strips are available and pH measurement is performed in your facility (fasting gastric pH is usually 5 or less, even in patients receiving gastric acid inhibitors; however, this method isn't reliable enough to exclude the need for X-ray placement verification because gastric content occasionally has a high pH); and inspecting the visual characteristics of the tube aspirate (fasting gastric secretions commonly appear grassy-green or clear and colorless).[14,15]
- Position the patient as directed *to help advance the tube.* She'll typically lie on her right side until the tube clears the pylorus (about 2 hours).
- After the tube clears the pylorus, the practitioner may direct you to advance it 2″ to 3″ (5 to 7.5 cm) every hour and to reposition the patient until the premeasured mark reaches the patient's nostril. Gravity and peristalsis will help advance the tube. (Notify the practitioner if you can't advance the tube.) Keep the remaining premeasured length of tube well lubricated *to ease passage and prevent irritation.*
- After the tube progresses the necessary distance, the practitioner will order an X-ray; most tubes are impregnated with a radiopaque mark so that you can easily confirm placement by X-ray or other imaging technique.[14]
- When the tube is in place, secure the external tubing with hypoallergenic tape or a securement device *to help prevent further progression.*

NURSING ALERT *Don't secure the tube while it advances to the premeasured mark unless the practitioner asks you to do so.*

- Trace the tubing from the patient to its point of origin *to make sure that you're accessing the correct tube* and then attach the tube to intermittent suction.[16]

Removing a nasoenteric-decompression tube

- Put on gloves to comply with standard precautions.[10,11,12]
- Position the patient as the practitioner specifies, typically in the semi-Fowler or high Fowler position. You may also need to help the patient hold his neck in a hyperextended position.
- Protect the patient's chest with a fluid-impermeable pad or towel.
- Trace the tubing from the patient to its point of origin *to make sure you're accessing the correct tube.*[16]
- Clamp the tube and disconnect it from suction *to prevent the patient from aspirating gastric contents that leak from the tube during withdrawal.*
- If the patient has a tube with an inflated balloon tip, attach a 10-mL syringe to the balloon port and withdraw the air or water. Don't deflate the balloon until you're ready to remove the tube.
- Slowly withdraw 6″ to 8″ (15 to 20 cm) of the tube. Wait 10 minutes, withdraw another 6″ to 8″, and then wait another 10 minutes. Continue this procedure until the tube reaches the patient's esophagus (with 18″ [46 cm] of the tube remaining inside the patient). At this point, you can gently withdraw the tube completely.

NURSING ALERT *If the tube doesn't come out easily, don't force it. Notify the practitioner.*[17]

Completing the procedure

- Discard used equipment appropriately.
- Remove and discard your gloves.[10,11]
- Perform hand hygiene.[2,3,4,5,6]
- Document the procedure.[18,19,20]

Special considerations

- Blind insertion of a nasoenteric-decompression tube is commonly more successful when using an unweighted tube.[1]
- For a double- or triple-lumen tube, label which lumen accommodates balloon inflation and which accommodates drainage.
- Provide oral care regularly and check the patient's nostrils often for signs of irritation. (See the "Oral care" procedure, page 560.) If you see signs of irritation, resecure the tube *so that it doesn't cause tension* and then lubricate the nostril. Alternatively, check with the practitioner to see if the tube can be inserted through the other nostril.
- Provide oral care after removing the tube *to promote comfort and prevent oral colonization that may contribute to health care–associated pneumonia.*

Complications

Nasoenteric-decompression tubes may cause reflux esophagitis, nasal or oral inflammation, and nasal, laryngeal, or esophageal ulceration. Misplacement into the bronchial tree can result in pneumonitis, pneumonia, and pneumothorax if not recognized.[21,22]

Documentation

Record the date and time the nasoenteric-decompression tube was inserted and who performed it. Note the patient's tolerance of the procedure, the type of tube used, confirmation method of tube placement, suction type and amount, and color, amount, and consistency of drainage.

Record the date and time of tube removal, the name of the person removing the tube, and the patient's tolerance of the removal procedure. Record the color, consistency, and amount of drainage. Document any patient teaching and the patient's understanding of your teaching.

REFERENCES

1 Itkin, M., et al. (2011). Multidisciplinary practical guidelines for gastrointestinal access for enteral nutrition and decompression from the Society of Interventional Radiology and American Gastroenterological Association (AGA) Institute, with endorsement by Canadian Interventional Radiological Association (CIRA) and Cardiovascular and Interventional Radiological Society of Europe (CIRSE). *Journal of Vascular and Interventional Radiology, 22,* 1089–1106. Accessed May 2015 via the Web at http://www.sirweb.org/clinical/cpg/PIIS1051044311008505.pdf (Level VII)

2 The Joint Commission. (2015). Standard NPSG.07.01.01. *Comprehensive accreditation manual for hospitals: The official handbook.* Oakbrook Terrace, IL: The Joint Commission. (Level VII)

3 Centers for Disease Control and Prevention. (2002). Guideline for hand hygiene in health-care settings: Recommendations of the Healthcare Infection Control Practices Advisory Committee and the HICPAC/SHEA/APIC/IDSA Hand Hygiene Task Force. *MMWR Recommendations*

and Reports, 51(RR-16), 1–45. Accessed May 2015 via the Web at http://www.cdc.gov/mmwr/pdf/rr/rr5116.pdf (Level II)

4 World Health Organization. (2009). "WHO guidelines on hand hygiene in health care: First global patient safety challenge, clean care is safer care" [Online]. Accessed May 2015 via the Web at http://whqlibdoc.who.int/publications/2009/9789241597906_eng.pdf (Level IV)

5 Centers for Medicare & Medicaid Services, Department of Health and Human Services. (2014). Condition of participation: Infection control. 42 C.F.R. § 482.42.

6 American Osteopathic Association. (2014). Standard 07.01.21. *Healthcare Facilities Accreditation Program: Accreditation requirements for acute care hospitals.* Chicago, IL: American Osteopathic Association. (Level VII)

7 The Joint Commission. (2015). Standard NPSG.01.01.01. *Comprehensive accreditation manual for hospitals: The official handbook.* Oakbrook Terrace, IL: The Joint Commission. (Level VII)

8 Centers for Medicare & Medicaid Services, Department of Health and Human Services. (2014). Condition of participation: Patient's rights. 42 C.F.R. § 482.13(c)(1).

9 American Osteopathic Association. (2014). Standard 15.01.16. *Healthcare Facilities Accreditation Program: Accreditation requirements for acute care hospitals.* Chicago, IL: American Osteopathic Association. (Level VII)

10 Siegel, J. D., et al. (2007). "2007 guideline for isolation precautions: Preventing transmission of infectious agents in health care settings" [Online]. Accessed May 2015 via the Web at http://www.cdc.gov/hicpac/pdf/isolation/Isolation2007.pdf (Level II)

11 Occupational Safety and Health Administration. (n.d.). "Bloodborne pathogens, standard number 1910.1030" [Online]. Accessed May 2015 via the Web at http://www.osha.gov/pls/oshaweb/owadisp.show_document?p_table=STANDARDS&p_id=10051 (Level VII)

12 American Osteopathic Association. (2014). Standard 07.01.10. *Healthcare Facilities Accreditation Program: Accreditation requirements for acute care hospitals.* Chicago, IL: American Osteopathic Association. (Level VII)

13 Shlamovitz, G. V. (2013). "Nasogastric tube" [Online]. Accessed May 2015 via the Web at http://emedicine.medscape.com/article/80925-overview#a01

14 American Association of Critical-Care Nurses. (2009). "AACN practice alert: Verification of feeding tube placement (blindly inserted)" [Online]. Accessed May 2015 via the Web at http://www.aacn.org/WD/Practice/Docs/PracticeAlerts/Verification_of_Feeding_Tube_Placement_05-2005.pdf (Level VII)

15 Bankhead, R., et al. (2009). A.S.P.E.N. enteral nutrition practice recommendations. *Journal of Parenteral and Enteral Nutrition, 33,* 122–167. Accessed May 2015 via the Web at http://www.ismp.org/tools/articles/ASPEN.pdf (Level IV)

16 U.S. Food and Drug Administration. (n.d.). "Look. Check. Connect. Safe medical device connections save lives" [Online]. Accessed May 2015 via the Web at http://www.fda.gov/downloads/MedicalDevices/Safety/AlertsandNotices/UCM134873.pdf

17 Hinkle, J. L., & Cheever, K. H. (2014). *Brunner and Suddarth's textbook of medical-surgical nursing* (13th ed.). Philadelphia, PA: Wolters Kluwer.

18 The Joint Commission. (2015). Standard RC.01.03.01. *Comprehensive accreditation manual for hospitals: The official handbook.* Oakbrook Terrace, IL: The Joint Commission. (Level VII)

19 Centers for Medicare & Medicaid Services, Department of Health and Human Services. (2014). Condition of participation: Medical record services. 42 C.F.R. § 482.24(b).

20 American Osteopathic Association. (2014). Standard 10.00.03. *Healthcare Facilities Accreditation Program: Accreditation requirements for acute care hospitals.* Chicago, IL: American Osteopathic Association. (Level VII)

21 Stayner, J. L., et al. (2012). Feeding tube placement: Errors and complications. *Nutrition in Clinical Practice, 27,* 738–748. Accessed May 2015 via the Web at http://ncp.sagepub.com/content/27/6/738.full.pdf+html (Level V)

22 Sparks, D. A., et al. (2011). Pulmonary complications of 9931 narrow-bore nasoenteric tubes during blind placement: A critical review. *Journal of Parenteral and Enteral Nutrition, 35,* 625–629. Accessed May 2015 via the Web at http://pen.sagepub.com/content/35/5/625.full.pdf+html (Level I)

ADDITIONAL REFERENCE

Hodin, R. A., & Bordeianou, L. Nasogastric and nasoenteric tubes. (2014). In: *UpToDate,* Sanfey, H. (Ed.). Accessed May 2015 via the Web at http://www.uptodate.com/contents/search

NASOGASTRIC TUBE CARE

Providing effective nasogastric (NG) tube care requires meticulous monitoring of the patient and the equipment. Monitoring the patient involves checking drainage from the NG tube and assessing GI function. Monitoring the equipment involves verifying correct tube placement and function.

Equipment

Oral sponge swabs or toothbrush and toothpaste ▪ petroleum jelly ▪ cotton-tipped applicator ▪ ½″ (1.3-cm) or 1″ (2.5-cm) hypoallergenic tape or commercial securement device ▪ water-soluble lubricant ▪ stethoscope ▪ graduated container ▪ disinfectant pad ▪ gloves ▪ Optional: screening test for occult blood, skin preparation product, irrigation supplies, water, fluid-impermeable pad, emesis basin.

Preparation of equipment

Make sure suction that the equipment works properly. (See *Common gastric suction devices.*) When using a Salem sump tube with suction, connect the larger, primary lumen (for drainage and suction) to the suction equipment and select the appropriate setting, as ordered (usually low constant suction). If the practitioner doesn't specify the setting, follow the manufacturer's instructions. A Levin tube usually calls for intermittent low suction.

Implementation

- Gather the appropriate equipment.
- Perform hand hygiene.[1,2,3,4,5]
- Confirm the patient's identity using at least two patient identifiers.[6]
- Explain the procedure to the patient, and provide privacy.[7,8]
- Put on gloves *to comply with standard precautions.*[9,10,11]
- Provide oral care using oral sponge swabs to clean the patient's teeth, gums, and tongue, or assist him to brush his teeth with a toothbrush and toothpaste at least twice daily *to increase patient comfort and promote a healthy oral cavity.* (See the "Oral care" procedure, page 560.)[12] Encourage the patient to participate in oral care if possible.
- Lubricate the patient's lips with either sponge swabs or petroleum jelly applied with a cotton-tipped applicator. *If the tube remains in place for several days, mouth-breathing will leave the lips, tongue, and other tissues dry and cracked.*[12]
- Clean the skin and apply fresh tape (at least daily) or a new securement device, as needed. Use a skin preparation product as needed before application *to prevent irritation from the adhesive.*
- Regularly check the adherence of the hypoallergenic tape or other securement device *because sweat and nasal secretions may loosen the device.*
- Trace the tubing from the patient to its point of origin *to make sure that you're accessing the correct tube.*[13]
- Check the position of the NG tube regularly and before instilling any type of solution into the tube.[14,15,16] Use various techniques *to confirm placement,* including observing for a change in external tube length;[14] reviewing chest and abdominal X-ray reports *to look for notations about the tube's location;*[14] inspecting the visual characteristics of the tube aspirate (fasting gastric secretions commonly appear grassy-green or clean and colorless); measuring the pH of aspirate from the tube if pH strips are available and pH measurement is performed in your facility (fasting gastric pH is usually 5 or less, even in patients receiving gastric acid inhibitors);[14,15] and arranging for an X-ray, as ordered, if the tube's placement is uncertain.[14]

EQUIPMENT

Common gastric suction devices

A variety of wall-mounted suction devices are available for applying negative pressure to nasogastric (NG) and other drainage tubes. Two common types are shown here.

Portable suction machine

In a portable suction machine, a vacuum created intermittently by an electric pump draws gastric contents up the NG tube and into the collecting bottle. This type of suction is becoming less common because of the prevalence of stationary, or wall-mounted, units.

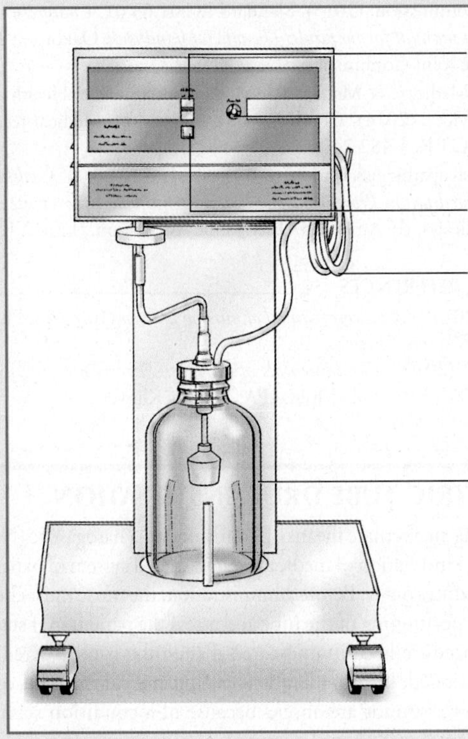

Stationary suction machine

A stationary wall-mounted unit can provide intermittent or continuous suction. Variable power settings let you set and adjust the suction force on either machine.

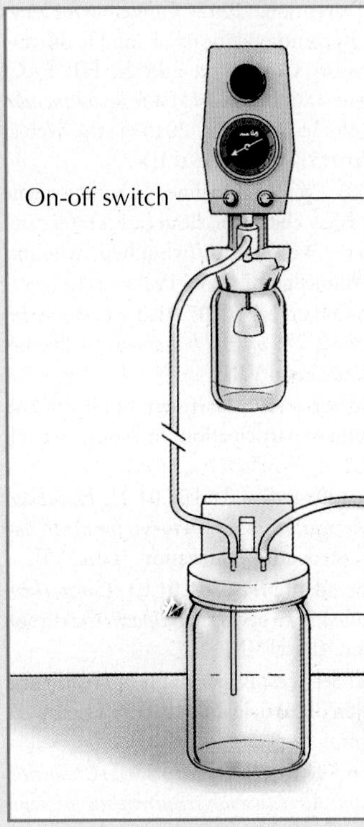

- Irrigate the tube, as ordered or necessary.[15]
- Assess bowel sounds every 4 to 8 hours *to verify GI function.*
- Measure the drainage amount and update the intake-and-output record every 8 hours. Be alert for electrolyte imbalances with excessive gastric output.
- Inspect gastric drainage and note its color, consistency, odor, and amount. Immediately report any drainage with a coffee-ground color, *which may indicate bleeding.* If you suspect that the drainage contains blood, use a screening test (such as Hematest) for occult blood.
- Remove and discard your gloves.[9,10]
- Perform hand hygiene.[1,2,3,4,5]
- Clean and disinfect your stethoscope using a disinfectant pad.[17,18]
- Perform hand hygiene.[1,2,3,4,5]
- Document the procedure.[19,20,21]

Special considerations

- NG tubes can become clogged or incorrectly positioned. Attempt to reposition the patient or rotate and reposition the tube. However, if the tube was inserted during surgery, avoid this maneuver *to ensure that the movement doesn't interfere with gastric or esophageal sutures.* Instead, notify the practitioner.
- If necessary, irrigate the NG tube and instill 30 mL of air into the vent tube *to maintain patency.* Don't attempt to stop reflux by clamping the vent tube. Unless contraindicated, elevate the patient's torso more than 30 degrees, and keep the vent tube above his midline *to prevent a siphoning effect.*
- If no drainage appears in the tube, check the suction equipment for proper function. Then, holding the NG tube over a fluid-impermeable pad or an emesis basin, separate the tube and the suction source. Check the suction equipment by placing the suction tubing in an irrigant container of water. If the apparatus draws water, check the NG tube for proper function. Note the amount of water drawn into the suction container on the intake-and-output record.
- If the patient is allowed to ambulate and you need to interrupt suction, disconnect the NG tube from the suction equipment. Clamp the tube *to prevent stomach contents from draining out of the tube.*

Complications

Epigastric or abdominal pain and vomiting may result from a clogged or improperly placed tube. Any NG tube—the Levin tube in particular—can move and aggravate esophagitis, ulcers, or esophageal varices, causing hemorrhage. Perforation may result from aggressive insertion technique. Dehydration and electrolyte imbalances can result from removing body fluids and electrolytes by suctioning. Pain, swelling, and salivary dysfunction may signal parotitis, which occurs in dehydrated, debilitated patients. Intubation can cause oral or nasal skin breakdown and discomfort and increased mucous secretions. Aspiration pneumonia may result from gastric reflux. Vigorous suction can damage the gastric mucosa and cause significant bleeding, possibly interfering with endoscopic assessment and diagnosis.

Documentation

Regularly confirm and record tube placement (usually every 4 to 8 hours). Keep a precise record of fluid intake and output. Describe drainage color, consistency, odor, and amount. Also note tape or securement device change times, oral care, and the condition of the nostrils.

References

1 Centers for Disease Control and Prevention. (2002). Guideline for hand hygiene in health-care settings: Recommendations of the Healthcare Infection Control Practices Advisory Committee and the HICPAC/SHEA/APIC/IDSA Hand Hygiene Task Force. *MMWR Recommendations and Reports, 51*(RR-16), 1–45. Accessed May 2015 via the Web at http://www.cdc.gov/mmwr/pdf/rr/rr5116.pdf (Level II)

2 World Health Organization. (2009). "WHO guidelines on hand hygiene in health care: First global patient safety challenge, clean care is safer care" [Online]. Accessed May 2015 via the Web at http://whqlibdoc.who.int/publications/2009/9789241597906_eng.pdf (Level IV)

3 The Joint Commission. (2015). Standard NPSG.07.01.01. *Comprehensive accreditation manual for hospitals: The official handbook.* Oakbrook Terrace, IL: The Joint Commission. (Level VII)

4 Centers for Medicare & Medicaid Services, Department of Health and Human Services. (2014). Condition of participation: Infection control. 42 C.F.R. § 482.42.

5 American Osteopathic Association. (2014). Standard 07.01.21. *Healthcare Facilities Accreditation Program: Accreditation requirements for acute care hospitals.* Chicago, IL: American Osteopathic Association. (Level VII)

6 The Joint Commission. (2015). Standard NPSG.01.01.01. *Comprehensive accreditation manual for hospitals: The official handbook.* Oakbrook Terrace, IL: The Joint Commission. (Level VII)

7 Centers for Medicare & Medicaid Services, Department of Health and Human Services. (2014). Condition of participation: Patient's rights. 42 C.F.R. § 482.13(c)(1).

8 American Osteopathic Association. (2014). Standard 15.01.16. *Healthcare Facilities Accreditation Program: Accreditation requirements for acute care hospitals.* Chicago, IL: American Osteopathic Association. (Level VII)

9 Siegel, J. D., et al. (2007). "2007 guideline for isolation precautions: Preventing transmission of infectious agents in healthcare settings" [Online]. Accessed May 2015 via the Web at http://www.cdc.gov/hicpac/pdf/isolation/Isolation2007.pdf (Level II)

10 Occupational Safety and Health Administration. (n.d.). "Bloodborne pathogens, standard number 1910.1030" [Online]. Accessed May 2015 via the Web at http://www.osha.gov/pls/oshaweb/owadisp.show_document?p_table=STANDARDS&p_id=10051 (Level VII)

11 American Osteopathic Association. (2014). Standard 07.01.10. *Healthcare Facilities Accreditation Program: Accreditation requirements for acute care hospitals.* Chicago, IL: American Osteopathic Association. (Level VII)

12 American Association of Critical-Care Nurses (AACN). (2010). "AACN practice alert: Oral care for patients at risk for ventilator-associated pneumonia" [Online]. Accessed May 2015 via the Web at http://www.aacn.org/WD/Practice/Docs/PracticeAlerts/oral%20care%2004-2010%20final.pdf (Level VII)

13 U.S. Food and Drug Administration. (n.d.). "Look. Check. Connect. Safe medical device connections save lives" [Online]. Accessed May 2015 via the Web at http://www.fda.gov/downloads/MedicalDevices/Safety/AlertsandNotices/UCM134873.pdf

14 American Association of Critical-Care Nurses (AACN). (2009). "AACN practice alert: Verification of feeding tube placement" [Online]. Accessed May 2015 via the Web at http://www.aacn.org/WD/Practice/Docs/PracticeAlerts/Verification_of_Feeding_Tube_Placement_05-2005.pdf (Level VII)

15 Bankhead, R., et al. (2009). A.S.P.E.N. enteral nutrition practice recommendations. *Journal of Parenteral and Enteral Nutrition, 33,* 122–167. Accessed May 2015 via the Web at http://www.ismp.org/tools/articles/ASPEN.pdf (Level IV)

16 Durai, R., et al. (2009). Nasogastric tubes. 1: Insertion technique and confirming the correct position. *Nursing Times, 105*(16), 12–13.

17 Rutala, W. A., et al. (2008). "Guideline for disinfection and sterilization in healthcare facilities, 2008" [Online]. Accessed May 2015 via the Web at http://www.cdc.gov/hicpac/pdf/guidelines/Disinfection_Nov_2008.pdf (Level I)

18 American Osteopathic Association. (2014). Standard 07.02.03. *Healthcare Facilities Accreditation Program: Accreditation requirements for acute care hospitals.* Chicago, IL: American Osteopathic Association. (Level VII)

19 The Joint Commission. (2015). Standard RC.01.03.01. *Comprehensive accreditation manual for hospitals: The official handbook.* Oakbrook Terrace, IL: The Joint Commission. (Level VII)

20 Centers for Medicare & Medicaid Services, Department of Health and Human Services. (2014). Condition of participation: Medical record services. 42 C.F.R. § 482.24(b).

21 American Osteopathic Association. (2014). Standard 10.00.03. *Healthcare Facilities Accreditation Program: Accreditation requirements for acute care hospitals.* Chicago, IL: American Osteopathic Association. (Level VII)

Additional references

Nettina, S. M. (2014). *Lippincott manual of nursing practice* (10th ed.). Philadelphia, PA: Wolters Kluwer.

Taylor, C., et al. (2015). *Fundamentals of nursing: The art and science of nursing care* (8th ed.). Philadelphia, PA: Wolters Kluwer.

Nasogastric tube drug instillation

Besides providing an alternate means of nourishment, a nasogastric (NG) tube allows direct instillation of medication into the GI system of patients who can't ingest drugs orally. Before administration, the nurse must check the patency and positioning of the tube and assess the patient's GI status because the procedure is contraindicated if the tube is obstructed or improperly positioned, if the patient is vomiting around the tube, or if the patient's bowel sounds are absent because of a condition such as mesenteric ischemia, small-bowel obstruction, or paralytic ileus.[1,2]

Administering medications enterally carries potential risks because most medications given via this route weren't originally formulated to be administered directly into the GI tract.[3] To address this issue, an increasing number of tablets and capsules have been designed as extended-, delayed-, or sustained-release preparations. Be aware that crushing or otherwise altering these types of medications to facilitate transport through the tube may result in reduced drug effects or increased drug toxicity.[2]

Equipment

Patient's medication administration and medical records ▪ prescribed medication ▪ towel or fluid-impermeable pad ▪ 30- or 60-mL piston-type catheter-tip syringe (make sure to use only syringes designed for oral or enteral use)[2] ▪ two 4″ × 4″ (10-cm × 10-cm) gauze pads ▪ pH test strip ▪ gloves ▪ sterile water[2] ▪ medicine cups ▪ spoon ▪ clamp ▪ Optional: mortar and pestle or other pill-crushing device, plastic bag (for crushing pills), needle and syringe (if administering medication in a soft gelatin capsule).[4]

Preparation of equipment

Gather equipment for use at the bedside. Make sure liquids are at room temperature. *Administering cold liquids through an NG tube can cause abdominal cramping.* Although this isn't a sterile procedure, make sure the cup, syringe, spoon, and gauze are clean.

If the patient is receiving a continuous tube feeding, turn off the pump at least 30 minutes before administering medications incompatible with the feeding, such as highly protein-bound medications (such as phenytoin and warfarin) and medications intended for administration on an empty stomach.

Implementation

■ Avoid distractions and interruptions when preparing and administering the medication *to prevent medication errors.*[5]

■ Verify the order on the patient's medication administration record by checking it against the practitioner's order.[5,6]

■ Compare the medication label with the order in the patient's medication record.[7,8,9]

■ Check the patient's medical record for an allergy to the prescribed medication. If an allergy or a contraindication exists, don't administer the medication; notify the practitioner.[7,8,9]

■ Check the expiration date on the medication. If the medication is expired, return it to the pharmacy and obtain a new medication.[7,8,9]

■ Visually inspect the medication for any loss of integrity; don't administer the medication if integrity is compromised.[7,8,9]

■ Discuss any unresolved concerns about the medication with the patient's practitioner.[7,8,9]

■ Consult with a pharmacist, as needed, for appropriateness of enteral medication administration, and request liquid forms of medications if available.[2] If the patient is concurrently receiving enteral nutrition or multiple medications, drug-formula and drug-drug incompatibilities may exist.[2,10] If liquid forms aren't available and the prescribed medication is an immediate-release tablet, crush the tablet individually into a fine powder in a cup or plastic bag designed for this purpose using a mortar and pestle or other pill-crushing device, unless contraindicated.

■ Review the patient's medical record for verification of the location of the distal tube tip before administering the medication *to ensure adequate administration and absorption of the drug.*[2,10,11,12]

■ Perform hand hygiene.[13,14,15,16,17]

■ Confirm the patient's identity using at least two patient identifiers.[18]

■ If the patient is receiving the medication for the first time, teach about potentially adverse reactions and discuss any other concerns related to the medication.[7,8,9]

■ Explain the procedure to the patient, if necessary, and provide privacy.[19,20]

■ Verify that the medication is being administered at the proper time, in the prescribed dose, and by the correct route *to reduce the risk of medication errors.*

■ If your facility uses a bar code scanning system, scan your identification badge, the patient's identification bracelet, and the medication's bar code.

■ Put on gloves *to comply with standard precautions.*[21,22]

■ *To avoid soiling the sheets during the procedure,* fold back the bed linens to the patient's waist and drape a towel or fluid-impermeable pad over the patient's chest.

■ Elevate the head of the bed so that the patient is in the Fowler position, as tolerated.

■ Trace the tubing from the patient to its point of origin *to make sure you're accessing the proper tube before beginning the medication administration.*[23]

■ Verify proper tube placement and patency before administering fluid or medication through the tube using various methods, including observing for a change in external length;[11] reviewing chest and abdominal X-ray reports to look for notations about the tube's location;[11] inspecting the visual characteristics of the tube aspirate (fasting gastric secretions commonly appear grassy-green or clear and colorless);[2,11] measuring the pH of aspirate from the tube if pH strips are available and pH measurement is performed in your facility (fasting gastric pH is usually 5 or less, even in patients receiving gastric acid inhibitors);[11] and arranging for an X-ray, as ordered, if there's a doubt about the tube's placement.[2,11]

■ If you meet resistance when aspirating, stop the procedure. *Resistance may indicate a nonpatent tube or improper tube placement.* (Keep in mind that some smaller NG tubes may collapse when aspiration is attempted.) If the tube seems to be in the stomach, resistance probably means the tube is lying against the stomach wall. *To relieve resistance,* withdraw the tube slightly or turn the patient.

■ After you have established that the tube is patent and in the correct position, flush the tube with at least 15 mL of sterile water.[2] Clamp the tube, detach the syringe, and lay the end of the tube on a 4″ × 4″ (10-cm × 10-cm) gauze pad.

■ If the prescribed medication is in a crushable form, crush the tablets with a mortar and pestle *to ready them for mixing in a cup with the diluting liquid.* Mix the crushed tablets with sterile water.[2] Make sure the particles are small enough to pass through the opening at the distal end of the NG tube.

■ If the medication is in capsule form, open the capsules and empty their contents into a medicine cup containing 5 to 10 mL of sterile water.[2] If the medication is in gelatin capsule form, puncture the capsule and express the contents into a medicine cup. Consult with a pharmacist, if necessary, *because expressing medication from a capsule may not deliver the intended dose.* Pour liquid medications directly into a medicine cup of 5 to 10 mL of sterile water.[2] Stir well with the spoon.

■ Reattach the syringe, without the piston, to the end of the tube and open the clamp.

■ Deliver the medication slowly and steadily. (See *Giving medications through an NG tube,* page 530.)

■ If the medication flows smoothly, slowly add more until you've administered the entire dose. If the medication doesn't flow properly, don't force it. Raise the syringe slightly. If you suspect that tube placement is inhibiting the flow, stop the procedure and reevaluate tube placement.

■ Flush the tube again with at least 15 mL of sterile water.[2]

NURSING ALERT *Take into account the patient's volume status when determining flush volumes.*[2,10]

■ Watch the patient's reaction throughout the instillation. If you observe any sign of discomfort, stop the procedure immediately.

■ Repeat with the next medication, as appropriate.[2]

■ As the last of the medication flows out of the syringe, start to irrigate the tube by adding at least 15 mL of sterile water. *Irrigation clears medication from the sides of the tube and from the distal end, reducing the risk of clogging.*

■ When the water stops flowing, quickly clamp the tube. Detach the syringe and discard it.

■ Remove the towel or fluid-impermeable pad and replace the bed linens.

■ Leave the patient in the Fowler position, or have the patient lie on the right side with the head of the bed partially elevated. Have the patient maintain this position for at least 30 minutes after the procedure *to facilitate the downward flow of medication into the stomach and prevent esophageal reflux.*

■ Discard used supplies in the appropriate receptacle.

■ Remove and discard your gloves.[21]

■ Perform hand hygiene.[13,14,15,16,17]

■ Document the procedure.[24,25,26]

Special considerations

■ *To prevent instillation of too much fluid* (more than 400 mL of liquid at one time for an adult), don't schedule the drug instillation with the patient's regular tube feeding if possible.

■ If you must schedule a tube feeding and medication instillation simultaneously, give the medication first *to ensure that the patient receives the prescribed drug therapy even if the patient can't tolerate an entire feeding.* Hold the feeding by 30 minutes or more *to avoid altering drug bioavailability.*[2]

■ If the NG tube is attached to suction, turn off the suction for 30 to 60 minutes after administering medication.

Giving medications through an NG tube

Holding the nasogastric (NG) tube at a level a little above the patient's nose, pour up to 30 mL of diluted medication into the syringe barrel. *To prevent air from entering the patient's stomach,* hold the tube at a slight angle and add more medication before the syringe empties. If necessary, raise the tube slightly higher *to increase the flow rate.*

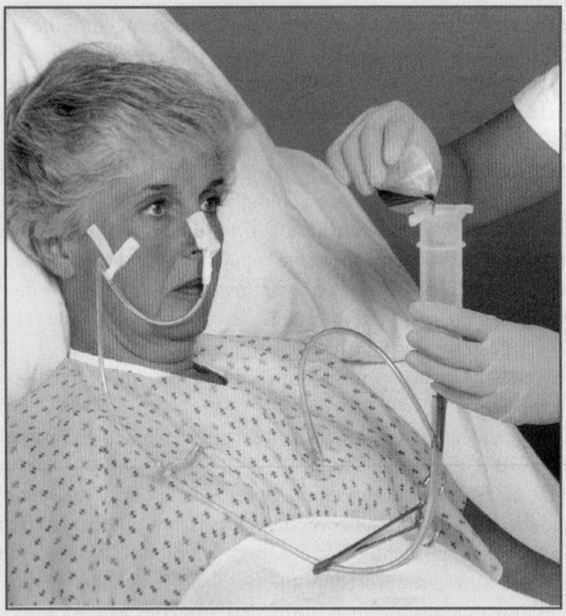

After you've delivered the entire dose, position the patient on her right side, head slightly elevated, *to minimize esophageal reflux.*

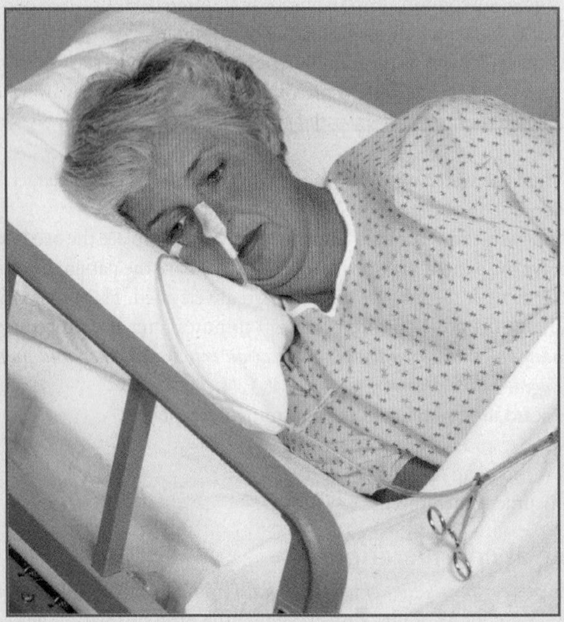

Patient teaching

If the patient will require an NG tube after discharge, give oral and written instructions for instilling medication through an NG tube to the patient and family, as appropriate. Make sure you're present when the patient performs the procedure for the first few times *so that you can provide assistance and answer any questions.* Offer encouragement, and correct any errors in technique, as necessary.

Complications

Aspiration can occur with improper tube placement. Administration of large volumes of liquid medications containing sorbitol (such as liquid acetaminophen) or those of high osmolality (such as electrolyte solutions) may cause cramping, abdominal discomfort, and diarrhea.[27]

Documentation

Record the instillation of medication, the date and time of instillation, the dose, and the patient's tolerance of the procedure. On the intake-and-output sheet, note the amount of fluid instilled. Document any patient teaching provided and whether the patient gave a return demonstration.

REFERENCES

1 Makic, M. B. F., et al. (2011). Evidence-based practice habits: Putting sacred cows out to pasture. *Critical Care Nurse, 31*(2), 38–62. Accessed May 2015 via the Web at http://ccn.aacnjournals.org/content/31/2/38.full.pdf+html

2 Bankhead, R., et al. (2009). A.S.P.E.N. enteral nutrition practice recommendations. *Journal of Parenteral and Enteral Nutrition, 33,* 122–167. Accessed May 2015 via the Web at http://www.ismp.org/tools/articles/ASPEN.pdf (Level IV)

3 White, R., & Bradnam, V. (2011). *Handbook of drug administration via enteral feeding tubes* (2nd ed.). London, UK: Pharmaceutical Press.

4 Boullata, J. I. (2009). Drug administration through an enteral feeding tube. *American Journal of Nursing, 109*(10), 34–42.

5 Westbrook, J., et al. (2010). Association of interruptions with an increased risk and severity of medication administration errors. *Archives of Internal Medicine, 170,* 683–690. (Level IV)

6 Institute for Safe Medication Practices. (2012). Side tracks on the safety express: Interruptions lead to errors and unfinished... Wait, what was I doing? *Nurse Advise-Err, 11*(2), 1–4. Accessed May 2015 via the Web at https://www.ismp.org/Newsletters/acutecare/showarticle.aspx?id=37

7 The Joint Commission. (2015). Standard MM.06.01.01. *Comprehensive accreditation manual for hospitals: The official handbook.* Oakbrook Terrace, IL: The Joint Commission. (Level VII)

8 Centers for Medicare & Medicaid Services, Department of Health and Human Services. (2014). Condition of participation: Nursing services. 42 C.F.R. § 482.23(c).

9 American Osteopathic Association. (2014). Standard 16.01.03. *Healthcare Facilities Accreditation Program: Accreditation requirements for acute care hospitals.* Chicago, IL: American Osteopathic Association. (Level VII)

10 Wilson, N., & Best, C. (2011). Administration of medicines via an enteral feeding tube. *Nursing Times, 107*(41), 18–20. Accessed May 2015 via the Web at http://www.nursingtimes.net/Journals/2011/10/17/l/d/v/Rev-nutrition.pdf

11 American Association of Critical-Care Nurses. (2009). "AACN practice alert: Verification of feeding tube placement" [Online]. Accessed May 2015 via the Web at http://www.aacn.org/WD/Practice/Docs/PracticeAlerts/Verification_of_Feeding_Tube_Placement_05-2005.pdf (Level VII)

12 Williams, N. T. (2008). Medication administration through enteral feeding tubes. *American Journal of Health-System Pharmacy, 65,* 2347–2357.

13 The Joint Commission. (2015). Standard NPSG.07.01.01. *Comprehensive accreditation manual for hospitals: The official handbook.* Oakbrook Terrace, IL: The Joint Commission. (Level VII)

14 Centers for Disease Control and Prevention. (2002). Guideline for hand hygiene in health-care settings: Recommendations of the Healthcare Infection Control Practices Advisory Committee and the HICPAC/SHEA/APIC/IDSA Hand Hygiene Task Force. *MMWR Recommendations and Reports, 51*(RR-16), 1–45. Accessed May 2015 via the Web at http://www.cdc.gov/mmwr/pdf/rr/rr5116.pdf (Level II)

15 World Health Organization. (2009). "WHO guidelines on hand hygiene in health care: First global patient safety challenge, clean care is safer care"

[Online]. Accessed May 2015 via the Web at http://whqlibdoc.who.int/publications/2009/9789241597906_eng.pdf (Level IV)

16 Centers for Medicare & Medicaid Services, Department of Health and Human Services. (2014). Condition of participation: Infection control. 42 C.F.R.§ 482.42.

17 American Osteopathic Association. (2014). Standard 07.01.21. *Healthcare Facilities Accreditation Program: Accreditation requirements for acute care hospitals.* Chicago, IL: American Osteopathic Association. (Level VII)

18 The Joint Commission. (2015). Standard NPSG.01.01.01. *Comprehensive accreditation manual for hospitals: The official handbook.* Oakbrook Terrace, IL: The Joint Commission. (Level VII)

19 Centers for Medicare & Medicaid Services, Department of Health and Human Services. (2014). Condition of participation: Patient's rights. 42 C.F.R. § 482.13(c)(1).

20 American Osteopathic Association. (2014). Standard 15.01.16. *Healthcare Facilities Accreditation Program: Accreditation requirements for acute care hospitals.* Chicago, IL: American Osteopathic Association. (Level VII)

21 Siegel, J. D., et al. (2007). "2007 guideline for isolation precautions: Preventing transmission of infectious agents in healthcare settings" [Online]. Accessed May 2015 via the Web at http://www.cdc.gov/hicpac/pdf/isolation/Isolation2007.pdf (Level II)

22 American Osteopathic Association. (2014). Standard 07.01.10. *Healthcare Facilities Accreditation Program: Accreditation requirements for acute care hospitals.* Chicago, IL: American Osteopathic Association. (Level VII)

23 U.S. Food and Drug Administration. (n.d.). "Look. Check. Connect. Safe medical device connections save lives" [Online]. Accessed May 2015 via the Web at http://www.fda.gov/downloads/MedicalDevices/Safety/AlertsandNotices/UCM134873.pdf

24 The Joint Commission. (2015). Standard RC.01.03.01. *Comprehensive accreditation manual for hospitals: The official handbook.* Oakbrook Terrace, IL: The Joint Commission. (Level VII)

25 Centers for Medicare & Medicaid Services, Department of Health and Human Services. (2014). Condition of participation: Medical record services. 42 C.F.R. § 482.24(b).

26 American Osteopathic Association. (2014). Standard 10.00.03. *Healthcare Facilities Accreditation Program: Accreditation requirements for acute care hospitals.* Chicago, IL: American Osteopathic Association. (Level VII)

27 Phillips, N. M., & Nay, R. (2008). A systematic review of nursing administration of medication via enteral tubes in adults. *Journal of Clinical Nursing, 17,* 2257–2265. (Level I)

ADDITIONAL REFERENCES

Nettina, S. M. (2014). *Lippincott manual of nursing practice* (10th ed.). Philadelphia, PA: Wolters Kluwer.

Taylor, C., et al. (2015). *Fundamentals of nursing: The art and science of nursing care* (7th ed.). Philadelphia, PA: Wolters Kluwer.

NASOGASTRIC TUBE INSERTION AND REMOVAL

Usually inserted to decompress the stomach, a nasogastric (NG) tube can prevent vomiting after major surgery. An NG tube is typically in place for 48 to 72 hours after surgery, by which time peristalsis usually resumes. It may remain in place for shorter or longer periods depending on its use.

An NG tube has other diagnostic and therapeutic applications, especially in assessing and treating upper GI bleeding, collecting gastric contents for analysis, performing gastric lavage, aspirating gastric secretions, and administering medications and nutrients.

Inserting an NG tube requires close observation of the patient and verification of proper placement. The tube must be inserted with extra care in pregnant patients and in those with an increased risk of complications. For example, the practitioner will order an NG tube for a patient with aortic aneurysm, myocardial infarction, gastric hemorrhage, or esophageal varices only if he believes that the benefits outweigh the risks of intubation.

Most NG tubes have a radiopaque marker or strip at the distal end so that the tube's position can be verified by X-ray. If the position can't be confirmed, the practitioner may order fluoroscopy to verify placement.

The most common NG tubes are the Levin tube, which has one lumen, and the Salem sump tube, which has two lumens—one for suction and drainage and a smaller one for ventilation. Air flows through the vent lumen continuously, which protects the delicate gastric mucosa by preventing a vacuum from forming should the tube adhere to the stomach lining. (See *Types of NG tubes,* page 532.)

Equipment

For insertion

Tube (usually #12, #14, #16, or #18 French for a normal adult) ▪ towel or fluid-impermeable pad ▪ facial tissues ▪ emesis basin ▪ penlight ▪ 1″ or 2″ (2.5- or 5-cm) hypoallergenic tape ▪ gloves ▪ water-soluble lubricant ▪ pH test strip or carbon dioxide detector ▪ tongue blade ▪ catheter-tip or bulb syringe, or irrigation set ▪ ordered suction equipment ▪ Optional: viscous lidocaine 2%, nebulized lidocaine, cup or glass of water with a straw, mask and goggles or mask with face shield, commercial securement device, basin of warm water or ice, tape formulated for fragile skin.

For removal

Stethoscope ▪ catheter-tip syringe ▪ normal saline solution ▪ towel or fluid-impermeable pad ▪ adhesive remover ▪ gloves ▪ disinfectant pad.

Preparation of equipment

Inspect the NG tube for defects, such as rough edges or partially closed lumens. Then check the tube's patency by flushing it with water. If you need to increase the tube's flexibility *to ease insertion,* coil it around your gloved fingers for a few seconds or dip it in warm water. If the tube is too flaccid, stiffen it by filling the tube with water and then freezing it[1] or dipping the tube in ice water.

Implementation

- Verify the practitioner's order for the type of tube to be inserted.
- Gather and prepare the equipment.
- Perform hand hygiene.[2,3,4,5,6]
- Confirm the patient's identity using at least two patient identifiers.[7]
- Explain the procedure to the patient *to ease anxiety and promote cooperation.*

Inserting an NG tube

- Inform the patient that she may experience some nasal discomfort, she may gag, and her eyes may water. Emphasize that swallowing will ease the tube advancement.
- Agree on a signal that the patient can use if she wants you to stop briefly during the procedure.
- Provide privacy and assist the patient into the high Fowler position unless contraindicated.[8,9]
- Stand at the patient's right side if you're right-handed or at her left side if you're left-handed *to ease insertion.*
- Drape the towel or fluid-impermeable pad over the patient's chest *to protect her gown and bed linens from spills.*
- Offer tissues, and have the patient gently blow her nose *to clear her nostrils.*
- Place the facial tissues and emesis basin well within the patient's reach.
- Help the patient face forward with her neck in a neutral position.
- Put on gloves *to comply with standard precautions* and other personal protective equipment, as needed, if splashing of body fluids is likely.[10,11,12]
- Determine the length of the tube to be inserted to reach the stomach: To do so, hold the end of the tube at the tip of the patient's nose (as shown on next page, middle left) and extend the tube to the patient's earlobe and then down to the xiphoid process.

EQUIPMENT

Types of NG tubes

The practitioner will choose the type and diameter of nasogastric (NG) tube that best suits the patient's needs, including lavage, aspiration, enteral therapy, and stomach decompression. Choices may include the Levin and Salem sump tubes.

Levin tube

The Levin tube is a rubber or plastic tube that has a single lumen, a length of 42″ to 50″ (107 to 127 cm), and holes at the tip and along the side.

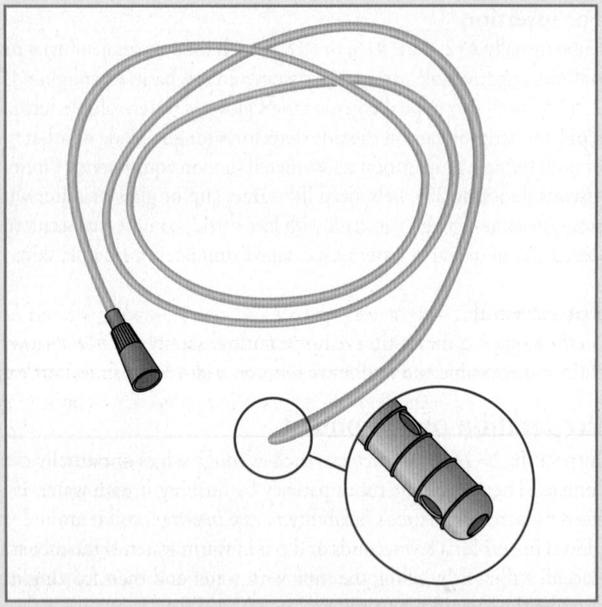

Salem sump tube

A Salem sump tube is a double-lumen tube that's made of clear plastic and has a blue sump port (pigtail) that allows atmospheric air to enter the patient's stomach. This air allows the tube to float freely and not adhere to or damage gastric mucosa. The larger port of this 48″ (122-cm) tube serves as the main suction conduit. The tube has openings at 45, 55, 65, and 75 cm as well as a radiopaque line *to verify placement.*

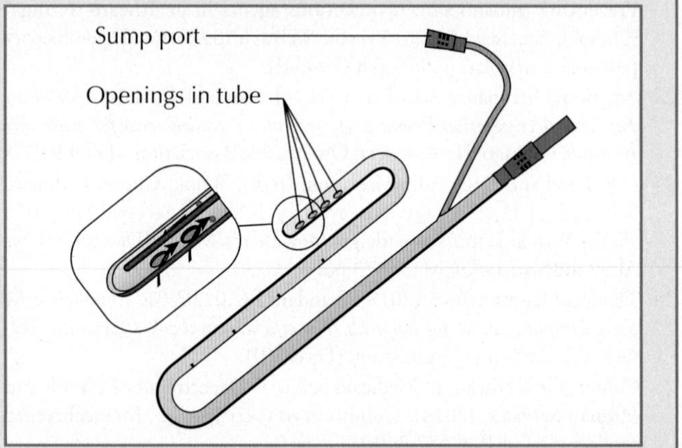

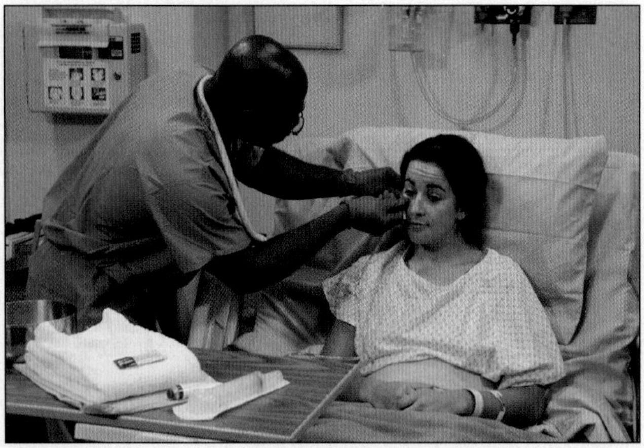

■ Mark this distance on the tubing with the tape. (Average measurements for an adult range from 22″ to 26″ [56 to 66 cm].) It may be necessary to add 2″ (5 cm) to this measurement in tall patients *to ensure entry into the stomach.*

■ Determine which nostril will allow easier access; use a penlight and inspect for a deviated septum or other abnormalities. Ask the patient if she ever had nasal surgery or a nasal injury. *Assess airflow in both nostrils* by occluding one nostril at a time while the patient breathes through her nose. Choose the nostril with the better airflow. If the patient can respond, ask whether she has previously undergone NG tube placement. If she has, then ask which nostril is better for insertion.

■ Administer viscous lidocaine 2% (for oral use) or nebulized lidocaine, as ordered, following safe medication administration practices. Ask the patient to sniff and swallow *to anesthetize the nasal and oropharyngeal mucosa.*[13,14,15,16,17]

■ *To minimize injury to the nasal passages,* lubricate the first 3″ (7.5 cm) of the tube with a water-soluble gel *to minimize injury to the nasal passages. Using a water-soluble lubricant prevents lipoid pneumonia, which may result from aspiration of an oil-based lubricant or from accidental slippage of the tube into the trachea.*

■ Instruct the patient to hold her head straight and upright.

■ Grasp the tube, curve it if necessary, and carefully insert it into the more patent nostril (as shown below).

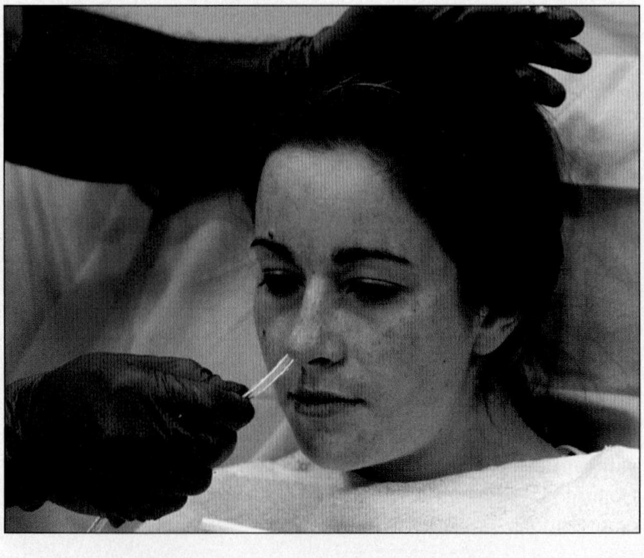

■ Aim the tube downward and toward the ear closer to the chosen nostril. Advance it slowly *to avoid pressure on the turbinates and resultant pain and bleeding.*

■ When the tube reaches the nasopharynx, you'll feel resistance. Instruct the patient to lower her head slightly *to close the trachea and open the esophagus.* Then rotate the tube 180 degrees toward the opposite nostril to redirect it *so that the tube won't enter the patient's mouth.*

■ Unless contraindicated, offer the patient a cup or glass of water with a straw. Direct her to sip and swallow as you slowly advance the tube *to help the tube pass to the esophagus* (as shown below). If you aren't using water, ask the patient to swallow.

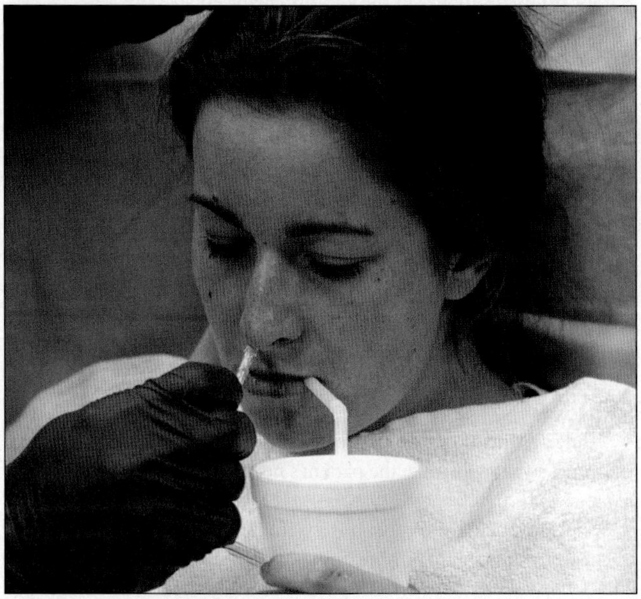

■ Use a tongue blade and penlight to examine the patient's mouth and throat for signs of a coiled section of tubing (especially in an unconscious patient). *Coiling may indicate an obstruction.*

■ Carefully advance the tube as the patient swallows and watch for signs of respiratory distress, *which may mean the tube is in the bronchus and must be removed immediately.*

■ Stop advancing the tube when the tape mark reaches the patient's nostril.

NURSING ALERT ***When confirming tube placement, never place the tube's end in a container of water*** **because accidental positioning of the tube in the trachea may cause the patient to aspirate water.** ***Water without bubbles doesn't confirm proper placement.***[18] ***Rather, it may indicate that the tube may be coiled in the trachea or the esophagus.***

■ Use various bedside *methods to determine tube location during insertion,* including watching for signs of respiratory distress, such as coughing and dyspnea; using capnography, if available, *to detect carbon dioxide, which indicates inadvertent tracheal insertion;*[19] measuring the pH of aspirate from the tube if pH strips are available and your facility allows pH measurement (fasting gastric pH is typically 5 or less, even in patients receiving gastric acid inhibitors; however, this method isn't reliable enough to exclude the need for X-ray placement verification *because gastric aspirate occasionally has a high pH*); and aspirating secretions with a catheter-tip or bulb syringe (as shown on top right) and inspecting the visual characteristics of the tube aspirate (fasting gastric secretions commonly appear grassy green or clear and colorless).[18,20]

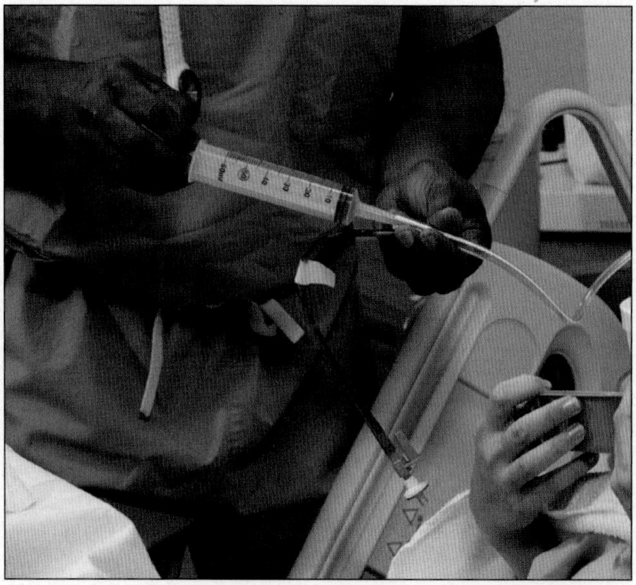

■ Anticipate an X-ray *to verify placement; a properly obtained and interpreted X-ray is recommended to confirm placement of any blindly inserted NG tube before its initial use for feedings or medication administration.*[18]

■ Mark the tube's exit site at the time of X-ray placement confirmation *to help monitor for tube dislocation.*[18]

NURSING ALERT ***If the patient has fragile skin and you're using tape to secure the tube, use tape specifically formulated for fragile skin*** **to prevent skin stripping and tearing during removal.**[21]

■ Secure the NG tube to the patient's nose using a commercial securement device or tape. If you're using a commercial securement device, follow the manufacturer's application instructions. If you're using tape, cut about a 4″ (10-cm) length of 1″ (2.5-cm) tape, split one end of the tape up the center about 1½″ (4 cm), make tabs on the split ends by folding the sticky sides together, stick the uncut tape end on the patient's nose so that the split in the tape starts about ½″ (1.3 cm) to 1½″ (4 cm) from the tip of her nose, crisscross the tabbed ends around the tube (as shown below), and then apply another piece of tape over the bridge of the nose *to secure the tube.*

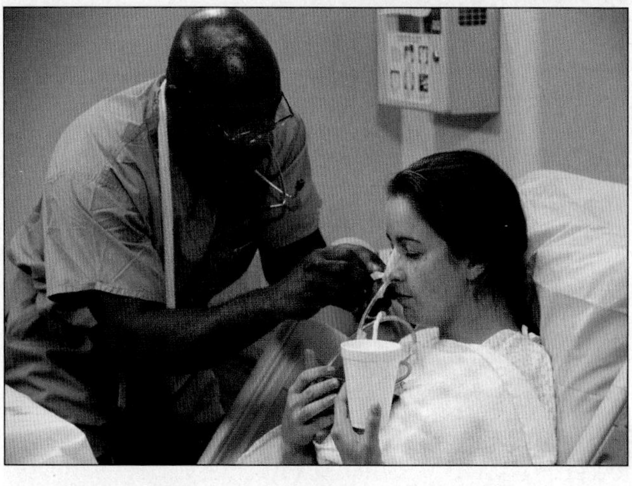

■ Trace the tubing from the patient to its point of origin *to make sure that you're connecting the correct tubing,* and then attach it to suction equipment, if ordered, and set the designated suction pressure.[22]

Removing an NG tube

■ Assess the patient's GI status; auscultate for peristalsis and ask the patient whether she's passing flatus *to evaluate bowel function.*

■ Help the patient into the semi-Fowler position. Then drape a towel or fluid-impermeable pad across her chest *to protect her gown and bed linens from spills* (as shown below).

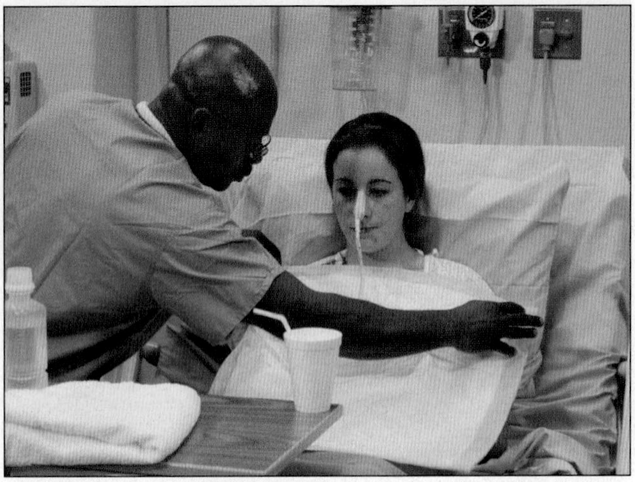

■ Put on gloves *to comply with standard precautions.*[10,11,12]
■ Trace the tubing from the patient to its point of origin *to make sure that you're accessing the correct tube.*[22] Check the placement of the tube and then use a catheter-tip syringe to flush the tube with 30 mL of air or normal saline solution *to ensure that the tube doesn't contain stomach contents that could irritate tissues during tube removal* (as shown below).

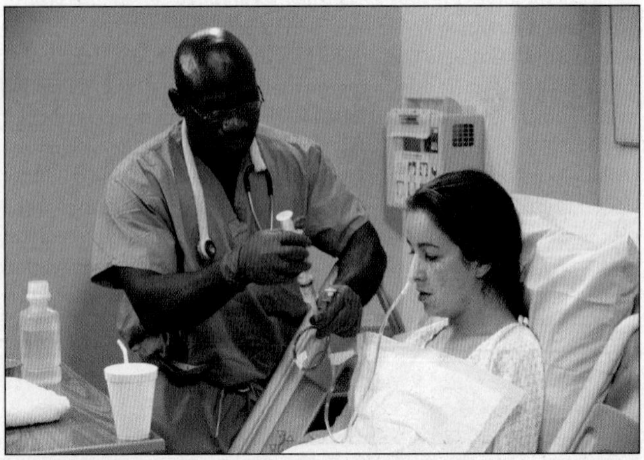

■ Carefully remove the tape from the patient's nose *to prevent skin stripping or tearing,*[21] or remove the securement device.
■ Clamp the tube by folding it in your hand (as shown below).

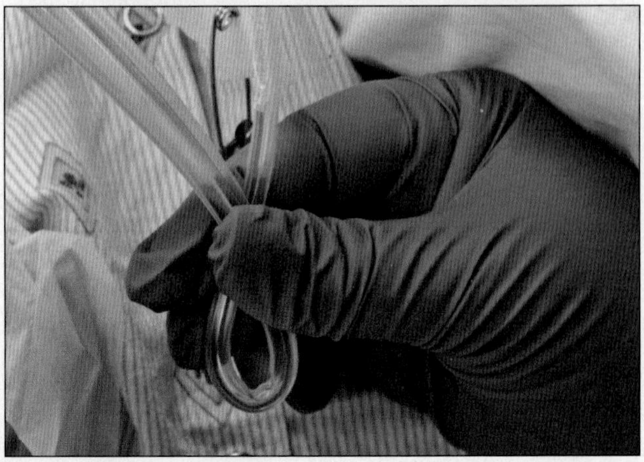

■ Ask the patient to hold her breath *to close the epiglottis.* Then withdraw the tube gently and steadily. (When the distal end of the tube reaches the nasopharynx, you can pull it quickly.)
■ When possible, immediately cover and remove the tube *because its sight and odor may nauseate the patient.*
■ Assist the patient with thorough oral care. (See the "Oral care" procedure, page 560.)
■ Clean the tape residue from the patient's nose with adhesive remover if necessary.

Completing the procedure

■ Discard used supplies in the appropriate receptacle.[10,11]
■ Remove and discard your gloves and any other personal protective equipment worn.[10,11]
■ Perform hand hygiene.[2,3,4,5,6]
■ Document the procedure.[23,24,25]

Special considerations

■ Provide frequent nasal and oral care while the NG tube is in place.
■ If the patient has a deviated septum or other nasal condition that prevents nasal insertion, pass the tube orally after removing dentures, if necessary. Sliding the tube over the tongue, proceed as you would for nasal insertion.
■ Tilt the unconscious patient's chin toward the chest *to close the trachea.* Then advance the tube between respirations *to ensure that it doesn't enter the trachea.*
■ While advancing the tube in an unconscious patient (or in a patient who can't swallow), stroke the patient's neck *to encourage the swallowing reflex and facilitate passage down the esophagus.*
■ While advancing the tube, observe for signs that it has entered the trachea, such as choking or breathing difficulties in a conscious patient and cyanosis in an unconscious patient or in a patient without a cough reflex. If these signs occur, remove the tube immediately. Allow the patient time to rest, and then try to reinsert the tube.
■ If vomiting occurs after tube placement, suspect tubal obstruction or incorrect position. Assess immediately *to determine the cause.*
■ For the next 48 hours after removal, monitor the patient for signs of GI dysfunction, including nausea, vomiting, abdominal distention, and food intolerance. *GI dysfunction may necessitate reinsertion of the NG tube.*

Patient teaching

A home care nurse, the patient, or a family member may insert an NG tube at home, deliver the feeding, and remove the tube. Indications for insertion include gastric decompression and short-term feeding. (See *Using an NG tube at home.*)

Complications

Potential complications of prolonged intubation with an NG tube include skin erosion at the nostril, sinusitis, esophagitis, esophagotracheal fistula, gastric ulceration, and pulmonary and oral infection. Complications that can result from suctioning include electrolyte imbalances and dehydration.

Documentation

Record the type and size of the NG tube as well as the date and time, the route of insertion, and the marked exit site. Include the method used to confirm tube placement. Also note the type and amount of suction, if used, and describe the drainage, including the amount, color, character, consistency, and odor. Note the patient's tolerance of the procedure. Include in your notes any signs and symptoms signaling complications, such as nausea, vomiting, and abdominal distention. Document subsequent irrigation procedures and continuing problems after irrigation. Document any patient and family teaching and their understanding of your teaching.

When you remove a nasogastric tube, record the date and time. Describe the color, consistency, and amount of gastric drainage. Note unusual events following NG tube removal, such as nausea, vomiting, abdominal distention, and food intolerance. Note the patient's tolerance of the procedure. Document any patient and the patient's understanding of your teaching.

REFERENCES

1 Chun, D. H., et al. (2009). A randomized, clinical trial of frozen versus standard nasogastric tube placement. *World Journal of Surgery, 33,* 1789–1792. (Level II)

2 The Joint Commission. (2015). Standard NPSG.07.01.01. *Comprehensive accreditation manual for hospitals: The official handbook.* Oakbrook Terrace, IL: The Joint Commission. (Level VII)

3 Centers for Disease Control and Prevention. (2002). Guideline for hand hygiene in health-care settings: Recommendations of the Healthcare Infection Control Practices Advisory Committee and the HICPAC/SHEA/APIC/IDSA Hand Hygiene Task Force. *MMWR Recommendations and Reports, 51*(RR-16), 1–45. Accessed May 2015 via the Web at http://www.cdc.gov/mmwr/pdf/rr/rr5116.pdf (Level II)

4 World Health Organization. (2009). "WHO guidelines on hand hygiene in health care: First global patient safety challenge, clean care is safer care" [Online]. Accessed May 2015 via the Web at http://whqlibdoc.who.int/publications/2009/9789241597906_eng.pdf (Level IV)

5 Centers for Medicare & Medicaid Services, Department of Health and Human Services. (2014). Condition of participation: Infection control. 42 C.F.R. § 482.42.

6 American Osteopathic Association. (2014). Standard 07.01.21. *Healthcare Facilities Accreditation Program: Accreditation requirements for acute care hospitals.* Chicago, IL: American Osteopathic Association. (Level VII)

7 The Joint Commission. (2015). Standard NPSG.01.01.01. *Comprehensive accreditation manual for hospitals: The official handbook.* Oakbrook Terrace, IL: The Joint Commission. (Level VII)

8 Centers for Medicare & Medicaid Services, Department of Health and Human Services. (2014). Condition of participation: Patient's rights. 42 C.F.R. § 482.13(c)(1).

9 American Osteopathic Association. (2014). Standard 15.01.16. *Healthcare Facilities Accreditation Program: Accreditation requirements for acute care hospitals.* Chicago, IL: American Osteopathic Association. (Level VII)

10 Siegel, J. D., et al. (2007). "2007 guideline for isolation precautions: Preventing transmission of infectious agents in healthcare settings" [Online]. Accessed May 2015 via the Web at http://www.cdc.gov/hicpac/pdf/isolation/Isolation2007.pdf (Level II)

11 Occupational Safety and Health Administration. (n.d.). "Bloodborne pathogens, standard number 1910.1030" [Online]. Accessed May 2015 via the Web at http://www.osha.gov/pls/oshaweb/owadisp.show_document?p_table=STANDARDS&p_id=10051 (Level VII)

12 American Osteopathic Association. (2014). Standard 07.01.10. *Healthcare Facilities Accreditation Program: Accreditation requirements for acute care hospitals.* Chicago, IL: American Osteopathic Association. (Level VII)

13 Uri, O., et al. (2011). Lidocaine gel as an anesthetic protocol for nasogastric tube insertion in the ED. *American Journal of Emergency Medicine, 29,* 386–390. (Level IV)

14 Kuo, Y. W., et al. (2010). Reducing the pain of nasogastric tube intubation with nebulized and atomized lidocaine: A systematic review and meta analysis. *Journal of Pain and Symptom Management, 40,* 613–620. (Level I)

15 Centers for Medicare & Medicaid services, Department of Health and Human Services. (2014). Condition of participation: Nursing services. 42 C.F.R. § 482.23(c).

16 American Osteopathic Association. (2014). Standard 16.01.03. *Healthcare Facilities Accreditation Program: Accreditation requirements for acute care hospitals.* Chicago, IL: American Osteopathic Association. (Level VII)

17 The Joint Commission. (2015). Standard MM.06.01.01. *Comprehensive accreditation manual for hospitals: The official handbook.* Oakbrook Terrace, IL: The Joint Commission. (Level VII)

PATIENT TEACHING

Using an NG tube at home

If the patient will need to have a nasogastric (NG) tube in place at home—for short-term feeding or gastric decompression, for example—find out who will insert the tube. If the patient will have a home care nurse, identify who it will be and, if possible, tell the patient when to expect her.

If the patient or a family member will perform the procedure, you'll need to provide additional instruction and supervision. Use this checklist to prepare such teaching topics as:

- obtaining equipment needed for home intubation
- inserting the tube
- verifying tube placement by aspirating stomach contents
- correcting tube misplacement
- preparing formula for tube feeding
- storing formula, if appropriate
- administering formula through the tube
- removing and disposing of a disposable NG tube, or cleaning and storing a reusable NG tube
- using the NG tube for gastric decompression, if appropriate
- setting up and operating suctioning equipment
- troubleshooting suctioning equipment
- performing mouth care and other hygienic procedures.

18 American Association of Critical-Care Nurses. (2009). "AACN practice alert: Verification of feeding tube placement (blindly inserted)" [Online]. Accessed May 2015 via the Web at http://www.aacn.org/WD/Practice/Docs/PracticeAlerts/Verification_of_Feeding_Tube_Placement_05-2005.pdf (Level VII)

19 Meyer, P., et al. (2009). Colorimetric capnography to ensure correct nasogastric tube position. *Journal of Critical Care, 24,* 231–235. (Level IV)

20 Bankhead, R., et al. (2009). A.S.P.E.N. enteral nutrition practice recommendations. *Journal of Parenteral and Enteral Nutrition, 33,* 122–167. Accessed May 2015 via the Web at http://www.ismp.org/tools/articles/ASPEN.pdf

21 LeBlanc, K., et al. (2013). International Skin Tear Advisory Panel: A tool kit to aid in the prevention, assessment, and treatment of skin tears using a simplified classification system. *Advances in Skin and Wound Care, 26,* 459–476. (Level VII)

22 U.S. Food and Drug Administration. (n.d.). "Look. Check. Connect. Safe medical device connections save lives" [Online]. Accessed May 2015 via the Web at http://www.fda.gov/downloads/MedicalDevices/Safety/AlertsandNotices/UCM134873.pdf

23 The Joint Commission. (2015). Standard RC.01.03.01. *Comprehensive accreditation manual for hospitals: The official handbook.* Oakbrook Terrace, IL: The Joint Commission. (Level VII)

24 Centers for Medicare & Medicaid Services, Department of Health and Human Services. (2014). Condition of participation: Medical record services. 42 C.F.R. § 482.24(b).

25 American Osteopathic Association. (2014). Standard 10.00.03. *Healthcare Facilities Accreditation Program: Accreditation requirements for acute care hospitals.* Chicago, IL: American Osteopathic Association. (Level VII)

ADDITIONAL REFERENCES

Craven, R. F., & Hirnle, C. J. (2012). *Fundamentals of nursing: Human health and function* (7th ed.). Philadelphia, PA: Lippincott Williams & Wilkins.

Nettina, S. M. (2014). *Lippincott manual of nursing practice* (10th ed.). Philadelphia, PA: Wolters Kluwer.

Taylor, C., et al. (2011). *Fundamentals of nursing: The art and science of nursing care* (7th ed.). Philadelphia, PA: Lippincott Williams & Wilkins.

Inserting a nasopharyngeal airway

First, hold the airway beside the patient's face *to make sure it's the proper size* (as shown below). It should be slightly smaller than the patient's nostril diameter and slightly longer than the distance from the tip of his nose to his earlobe.

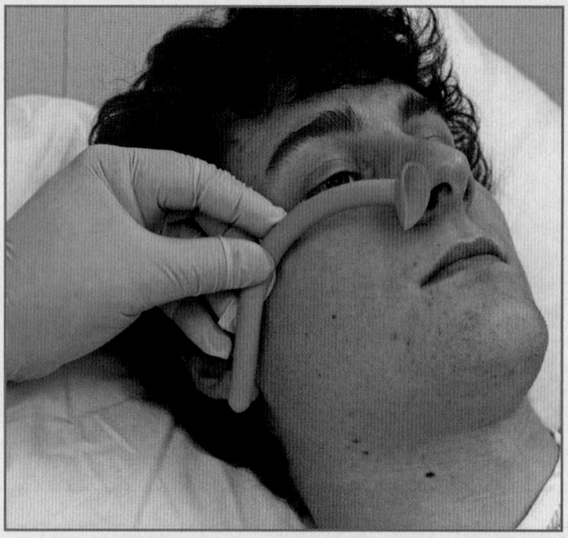

To insert the airway, hyperextend the patient's neck using a chin-lift or jaw-thrust technique *to anteriorly displace the patient's mandible* (unless contraindicated). Then push up the tip of his nose and pass the airway into his nostril (as shown below). Avoid pushing against any resistance *to prevent tissue trauma and airway kinking.*

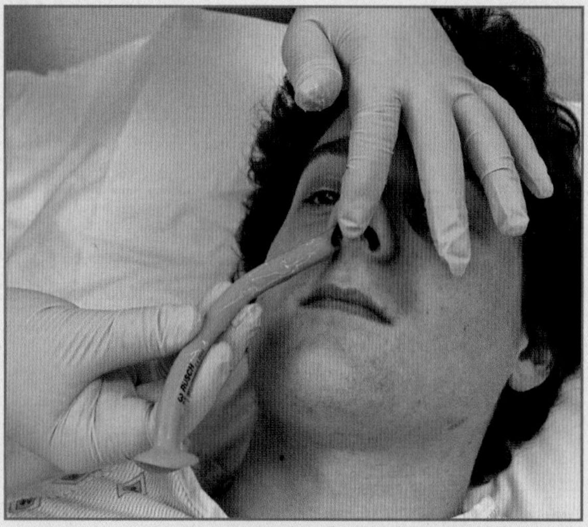

To check for correct airway placement, first close the patient's mouth. Then, place your finger over the tube's opening *to detect air exchange*. Also depress the patient's tongue with a tongue blade, and look for the airway tip behind the uvula.

NASOPHARYNGEAL AIRWAY INSERTION AND CARE

Insertion of a nasopharyngeal airway—a soft rubber or latex uncuffed catheter—establishes or maintains a patent airway. This airway is the typical choice for patients with airway obstruction or the risk of developing airway obstruction when conditions such as a clenched jaw or oral problems prevent placement of an oral airway.[1] It's also used to protect the nasal mucosa from injury when the patient needs frequent nasotracheal suctioning.

The airway follows the curvature of the nasopharynx, passing through the nose and extending from the nostril to the posterior pharynx. The bevel-shaped pharyngeal end of the airway facilitates insertion, and its funnel-shaped nasal end helps prevent slippage.

Insertion of a nasopharyngeal airway is preferred when an oropharyngeal airway is contraindicated or fails to maintain a patent airway. A nasopharyngeal airway is contraindicated for patients with pathologic nasopharyngeal deformities. An oropharyngeal airway is preferred for patients who have or are suspected of having traumatic brain injury, central facial fractures, basal skull fractures, or severe coagulopathy as well as for patients on anticoagulation therapy.[1,2,3]

Equipment

Nasopharyngeal airway of proper size ■ tongue blade ■ water-soluble lubricant ■ gloves ■ stethoscope ■ hospital-grade disinfectant ■ oral care supplies ■ Optional: suction equipment; flashlight; resuscitation mask, handheld resuscitation bag, or oxygen-powered breathing device.

Implementation

- Verify the practitioner's order.
- Gather the appropriate equipment.
- Perform hand hygiene.[4,5,6,7,8]
- Confirm the patient's identity using at least two patient identifiers.[9]
- In nonemergency situations, explain the procedure to the patient *to decrease anxiety and increase cooperation.*
- Measure the diameter of the patient's nostril and the distance from the tip of his nose to his earlobe. Select an airway whose diameter is slightly smaller than that of the nostril and whose length is about 1″ (2.5 cm) longer than from the nose tip to the earlobe. Airway sizes are labeled according to their internal diameter. The recommended airway size for a large adult is 8 to 9 mm; for a medium-sized adult, 7 to 8 mm; for a small adult, 6 to 7 mm. Lubricate the distal half of the airway's surface with a water-soluble lubricant *to prevent traumatic injury during insertion.*
- Place the patient in the supine or high Fowler position unless contraindicated *to provide easy access to the nostrils.*[2]
- Put on gloves *to comply with standard precautions.*[10,11]
- Properly insert the airway. (See *Inserting a nasopharyngeal airway.*)
- Immediately after insertion, auscultate the patient's respirations. If they're absent or inadequate, initiate artificial positive-pressure ventilation with a resuscitation mask, a handheld resuscitation bag, or an oxygen-powered breathing device.
- Suction the patient's airway as needed *to remove secretions.* (See the "Oronasopharyngeal suction" procedure, page 569.)
- Reassess the patient's respiratory status following suctioning and at an interval determined by the patient's condition and your facility.[2]
- Assess the patient's skin surrounding the nasopharyngeal airway regularly for redness, swelling, drainage, bleeding, or skin breakdown.[2]
- Check the airway regularly *to detect dislodgment or obstruction.*
- Provide oral moisturizing to the oral mucosa and lips every 2 to 4 hours and as needed. Brush the patient's teeth, gums, and tongue at least twice a day *to reduce the risk of pneumonia.* (See the "Oral care" procedure, page 560.)
- Remove and discard your gloves.[10]
- Perform hand hygiene.[4,5,6,7,8]
- Clean and disinfect your stethoscope using a disinfectant pad.[12,13]
- Perform hand hygiene.[4,5,6,7,8]
- Document the procedure.[14,15,16]

Special considerations

■ If the patient continues to cough or gag, the tube may be too long. If so, remove the airway and insert a shorter one.

■ Every 8 hours, remove and clean the airway *to check for skin breakdown.* Clean the airway according to the manufacturer's instructions. Reinsert the airway. Consider rotating to the other nostril *to prevent skin breakdown.*[2]

■ When the patient's natural airway is patent, remove the airway in one smooth motion. If the airway sticks, apply lubricant around the nasal end of the tube and around the nostril and then gently rotate the airway until it's free.

Complications

Sinus infection may result from obstruction of sinus drainage. Insertion of the airway may injure the nasal mucosa and cause bleeding and, possibly, aspiration of blood into the trachea. If the tube is too long, it may enter the esophagus and cause gastric distention and hypoventilation during artificial ventilation. Although semiconscious patients usually tolerate this type of airway better than conscious patients do, they may still experience laryngospasm and vomiting.

Documentation

Record the date and time of the airway's insertion, the size of the airway, removal and cleaning of the airway, shifts from one nostril to the other, the condition of the mucous membranes, suctioning, complications and nursing actions taken, and the patient's reaction to the procedure. Document patient teaching and the patient's understanding of your teaching.

REFERENCES

1 American Heart Association. (2010). 2010 American Heart Association guidelines for cardiopulmonary resuscitation and emergency cardiovascular care. *Circulation, 122,* S729–S767. (Level II)

2 Lynn-McHale Wiegand, D. (Ed.). (2011). *AACN procedure manual for critical care* (6th ed.). St. Louis, MO: Saunders.

3 Bullard, D., et al. (2012). Contraindications to nasopharyngeal airway insertion. *Nursing, 42*(10), 66–67. (Level V)

4 The Joint Commission. (2015). Standard NPSG.07.01.01. *Comprehensive accreditation manual for hospitals: The official handbook.* Oakbrook Terrace, IL: The Joint Commission. (Level VII)

5 Centers for Disease Control and Prevention. (2002). Guideline for hand hygiene in health-care settings: Recommendations of the Healthcare Infection Control Practices Advisory Committee and the HICPAC/SHEA/APIC/IDSA Hand Hygiene Task Force. *MMWR Recommendations and Reports, 51*(RR-16), 1–45. Accessed May 2015 via the Web at http://www.cdc.gov/mmwr/pdf/rr/rr5303.pdf (Level II)

6 World Health Organization. (2009). "WHO guidelines on hand hygiene in health care: First global patient safety challenge, clean care is safer care" [Online]. Accessed May 2015 via the Web at http://whqlibdoc.who.int/publications/2009/9789241597906_eng.pdf (Level IV)

7 Centers for Medicare & Medicaid Services, Department of Health and Human Services. (2014). Condition of participation: Infection control. 42 C.F.R. § 482.42.

8 American Osteopathic Association. (2014). Standard 07.01.21. *Healthcare Facilities Accreditation Program: Accreditation requirements for acute care hospitals.* Chicago, IL: American Osteopathic Association. (Level VII)

9 The Joint Commission. (2015). Standard NPSG.01.01.01. *Comprehensive accreditation manual for hospitals: The official handbook.* Oakbrook Terrace, IL: The Joint Commission. (Level VII)

10 Siegel, J. D., et al. (2007). "2007 guideline for isolation precautions: Preventing transmission of infectious agents in healthcare settings" [Online]. Accessed May 2015 via the Web at http://www.cdc.gov/hicpac/pdf/isolation/Isolation2007.pdf (Level II)

11 American Osteopathic Association. (2014). Standard 07.01.10. *Healthcare Facilities Accreditation Program: Accreditation requirements for acute care hospitals.* Chicago, IL: American Osteopathic Association. (Level VII)

12 Rutala, W. A., et al. (2008). "Guideline for disinfection and sterilization in healthcare facilities, 2008" [Online]. Accessed May 2015 via the Web at http://www.cdc.gov/hicpac/pdf/guidelines/Disinfection_Nov_2008.pdf (Level I)

13 American Osteopathic Association. (2014). Standard 07.02.03. *Healthcare Facilities Accreditation Program: Accreditation requirements for acute care hospitals.* Chicago, IL: American Osteopathic Association. (Level VII)

14 The Joint Commission. (2015). Standard RC.01.03.01. *Comprehensive accreditation manual for hospitals: The official handbook.* Oakbrook Terrace, IL: The Joint Commission. (Level VII)

15 Centers for Medicare & Medicaid Services, Department of Health and Human Services. (2014). Condition of participation: Medical record services. 42 C.F.R. § 482.24(b).

16 American Osteopathic Association. (2014). Standard 10.00.03. *Healthcare Facilities Accreditation Program: Accreditation requirements for acute care hospitals.* Chicago, IL: American Osteopathic Association. (Level VII)

ADDITIONAL REFERENCES

American Association of Critical-Care Nurses. (2010). "AACN practice alert: Oral care for patients at risk for ventilator-associated pneumonia" [Online]. Accessed May 2015 via the Web at http://www.aacn.org/WD/Practice/Docs/PracticeAlerts/oral%20care%2004-2010%20final.pdf (Level VII)

Taylor, C., et al. (2011). *Fundamentals of nursing: The art and science of nursing care* (7th ed.). Philadelphia, PA: Lippincott Williams & Wilkins.

NEBULIZER THERAPY

An established component of respiratory care, nebulizer therapy aids bronchial hygiene by restoring and maintaining mucous blanket continuity; hydrating dried, retained secretions; promoting expectoration of secretions; humidifying inspired oxygen; and delivering medications. Therapy may be administered through nebulizers that have a large or small volume, are connected to ventilator tubing, or are ultrasonic.

Large-volume nebulizers, such as the Venturi jet, are used to provide long-term 100% humidity for an artificial airway such as a tracheostomy or for certain pulmonary conditions such as cystic fibrosis. (See *Large-volume nebulizer,* page 538.) Cool aerosols can be used to treat upper airway disorders, such as croup, epiglottiditis, and postextubation edema.[1] Heated aerosols are used whenever the upper airway is bypassed, such as in patients who are intubated or have a tracheostomy, to prevent the dry gas from causing damage to the bronchial airways.[1] The aerosol mist can be delivered via mist tent, hood, mouthpiece, mask, T-piece, face tent, or tracheostomy collar. The amount of aerosol the nebulizer delivers varies depending on the design, gas flow, air entrainment port, and temperature.[1] Small-volume nebulizers are also used to deliver medications.

In-line nebulizers are used to deliver medications to patients who are being mechanically ventilated. In such cases, the nebulizer is placed in the inspiratory side of the ventilatory circuit.

Ultrasonic nebulizers are electrically driven and use high-frequency vibrations to break up surface water into particles. The resultant dense mist works to penetrate smaller airways and is useful for hydrating secretions, which induces a cough and sputum. The aerosol mist can be delivered to the patient via mist tent, hood, mouthpiece, mask, T-piece, face tent, or tracheostomy collar. Some ultrasonic nebulizers are also capable of aerosolizing medications, but this application hasn't been shown to be superior to a standard jet nebulizer.

Standard precautions for body fluid isolation should be used for all patients on nebulizer therapy. Airborne precautions should be implemented for patients with known or suspected tuberculosis, including enclosing and containing aerosol administration and filtering aerosols that bypass or are exhaled by the patient.

EQUIPMENT

Large-volume nebulizer

Connected to a flowmeter and pneumatically powered, an air entrainment port allows oxygen and air to mix to deliver a reliable oxygen concentration through a jet orifice. When connected to a liquid chamber, liquid is siphoned into the jet flow and creates an aerosol.[1]

Advantages
- Provides oxygen and aerosol therapy
- Can be used for long-term therapy

Disadvantages
- Increases the risk of bacterial growth (in reusable units)
- Results in condensate collection in large-bore tubing
- May cause mucosal irritation from breathing hot, dry air (if water level isn't maintained correctly in reservoir)
- Increases the risk of overhydration by mist (in infants)

Equipment

For large-volume nebulizer therapy
Stethoscope ■ pressurized gas source ■ flowmeter ■ patient interface device (such as a mask or collar) ■ large-bore oxygen tubing ■ nebulizer ■ sterile distilled water[1] ■ tissues and emesis basin or other container (for collection or disposal of expectorated sputum) ■ suction source and supplies ■ gloves ■ vital signs monitoring equipment ■ hospital-grade disinfectant ■ oral care supplies ■ Optional: oxygen blender (if a built-in adjustable oxygen controller isn't available), heater, in-line thermometer (if using a heater), gown, mask and goggles or mask with face shield.

For small-volume nebulizer therapy
Stethoscope ■ pressurized gas source ■ flowmeter ■ oxygen tubing ■ nebulizer cup ■ mouthpiece or mask ■ normal saline solution ■ prescribed medication ■ syringe and needle or needleless device ■ antiseptic pad ■ tissues and emesis basin or other container (for collection or disposal of expectorated sputum) ■ oral care supplies ■ gloves ■ hospital-grade disinfectant ■ Optional: spirometer or peak flow meter, suction source and supplies, sterile water, gown, mask and goggles or mask with face shield.

For in-line nebulizer therapy
Syringe or needleless device ■ disinfectant pad ■ pressurized gas source ■ flowmeter ■ in-line nebulizer cup ■ normal saline solution ■ prescribed medication ■ gloves ■ stethoscope ■ pulse oximeter ■ vital signs monitoring equipment ■ hospital-grade disinfectant ■ suction equipment ■ Optional: gown, mask and goggles or mask with face shield.

For ultrasonic nebulizer therapy
Stethoscope ■ ultrasonic gas-delivery device ■ large-bore oxygen tubing ■ patient interface device (such as a mask, mouthpiece, or collar[2]) ■ nebulizer couplet compartment ■ tissues and emesis basin or other container (for collection or disposal of expectorated sputum) ■ disinfectant pad ■ prescribed medication for inhalation ■ prescribed bronchodilator ■ oral care supplies ■ gloves ■ vital signs monitoring equipment ■ Optional: sterile distilled water, spirometer or peak flow meter, normal saline solution, suction source and supplies, gown, mask and goggles or mask with face shield; specimen container, laboratory transport bag, and labels.

Preparation of equipment
Assemble the ultrasonic nebulizer according to the manufacturer's instructions. *To ensure proper operation of the nebulizer,* check the connections with the AC adapter and electrical output or battery installation. Reconnect or reinstall, as needed.[2] Depending on the manufacturer, fill the reservoir of the device with sterile distilled water until it reaches exactly the level marked. This amount of water serves as a conductor for the ultrasonic waves and medication and will never be nebulized.[3]

Implementation
- For large-volume nebulizer therapy Verify the practitioner's order.
- Gather the appropriate equipment.
- Perform hand hygiene.[4,5,6,7,8]
- Confirm the patient's identity using at least two patient identifiers.[9]
- Explain the procedure to the patient.
- Put on gloves and other personal protective equipment as needed *to comply with standard precautions.*[10,11]
- Obtain the patient's vital signs, and perform a respiratory assessment *to establish a baseline.*
- If possible, place the patient in a sitting or high Fowler position *to encourage full lung expansion and promote aerosol dispersion.*
- Fill the water chamber to the indicated level with sterile distilled water.[1] Avoid using saline solution *to prevent corrosion.* Add a heating device, if ordered, and place an in-line thermometer between the outlet port and the patient, as close to the patient as possible, *to monitor the actual temperature of the inhaled gas and to avoid burning the patient.*
- If the nebulizer will supply oxygen to the patient, set the air entrainment port or adjust the external oxygen blender to the ordered oxygen concentration and analyze the flow at the patient's end of the tubing *to ensure delivery of the prescribed oxygen percentage.*
- Attach the delivery device to the patient.
- Encourage the patient to cough and expectorate sputum, and suction as needed.
- Check the water level in the nebulizer at frequent intervals and refill or replace, as indicated. When refilling a reusable container, discard the old water *to prevent infection from bacterial or fungal growth,* and refill the container to the indicator line with sterile distilled water.
- If the aerosol is heated, tell the patient to report warmth, discomfort, or hot tubing *because these may indicate a heater malfunction.* Use the in-line thermometer to monitor the temperature of the gas the patient is inhaling. If you turn off the flow for more than 5 minutes, unplug the heater *to avoid overheating the water and burning the patient when the aerosol is resumed.*
- Obtain the patient's vital signs and assess his respiratory status *to evaluate the effectiveness of therapy.*
- Change the nebulizer unit and tubing at an interval determined by your facility *to prevent bacterial contamination.*
- Assist the patient with oral care, as needed. (See the "Oral care" procedure, page 560.)
- Remove and discard your gloves and any other personal protective equipment worn.[10]
- Perform hand hygiene.[4,5,6,7,8]
- Clean and disinfect your stethoscope using a disinfectant pad.[12,13]
- Perform hand hygiene.[4,5,6,7,8]
- Document the procedure.[14,15,16]

For small-volume, in-line, or ultrasonic nebulizer therapy
- Avoid distractions and interruptions when preparing and administering medications *to prevent medication errors.*[17,18]
- Verify the practitioner's order.[19,20,21]
- Gather the necessary equipment.
- Compare the medication label with the order in the patient's medical record.[19,20,21]
- Check the patient's medical record for an allergy or a contraindication to the prescribed medication. If an allergy or a contraindications exists, don't administer the medication; notify the practitioner.[19,20,21]

- Check the expiration date on the medication. If the medication is expired, return it to the pharmacy and obtain new medication.[19,20,21]
- Visually inspect the medication for particles or discoloration or other signs of loss of integrity; don't administer the medication if its integrity is compromised.[19,20,21]
- Label all medications, medication containers, and other solutions and handle them using sterile technique.[22]
- Discuss any unresolved concerns about the medication with the patient's practitioner.[19,20,21]
- Perform hand hygiene.[4,5,6,7,8]
- Confirm the patient's identity using at least two patient identifiers.[9]
- Explain the procedure to the patient. If the patient is receiving the medication for the first time, teach him about potential adverse effects and discuss any other concerns related to the medication.[19,20,21]
- Put on gloves and other personal protective equipment as needed *to comply with standard precautions.*[10,11]
- Obtain the patient's vital signs, perform a respiratory assessment, and obtain a spirometry or peak flow reading, as ordered, *to establish a baseline.*
- If possible, place the patient in a sitting or high Fowler position *to encourage full lung expansion and promote aerosol dispersion.*
- Verify that the medication is being administered at the proper time, in the prescribed dose, and by the correct route *to reduce the risk of medication errors.*[19,20,21]
- If your facility uses a bar code scanning system, scan your identification badge, the patient's identification bracelet, and the medication's bar code.

Fos small-volume therapy

- Draw up the prescribed medication and inject it into the nebulizer cup. *To prevent contamination, don't touch the nebulizer.* Add normal saline solution or water to the prescribed dose volume according to the drug manufacturer's prescribing information.[1]
- After attaching the flowmeter to the gas source, attach the nebulizer to the flowmeter and then adjust the flow according to the manufacturer's recommendations, usually 6 to 10 L/minute (as shown below).[1]

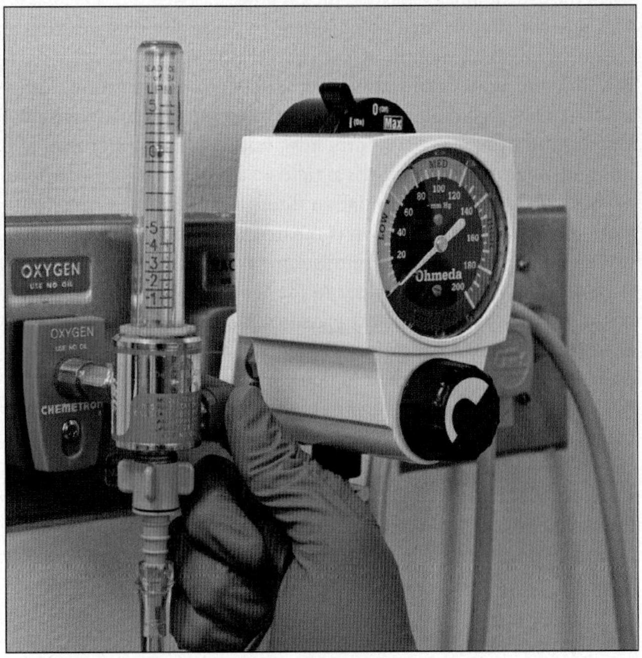

- Check the outflow port *to ensure adequate misting.*
- Assist the patient with the mouthpiece or mask, as needed, depending on the delivery system and patient-related factors such as age and physical and cognitive ability.[2] Instruct him to inhale slowly through his mouth at a normal tidal volume (as shown below).[1]

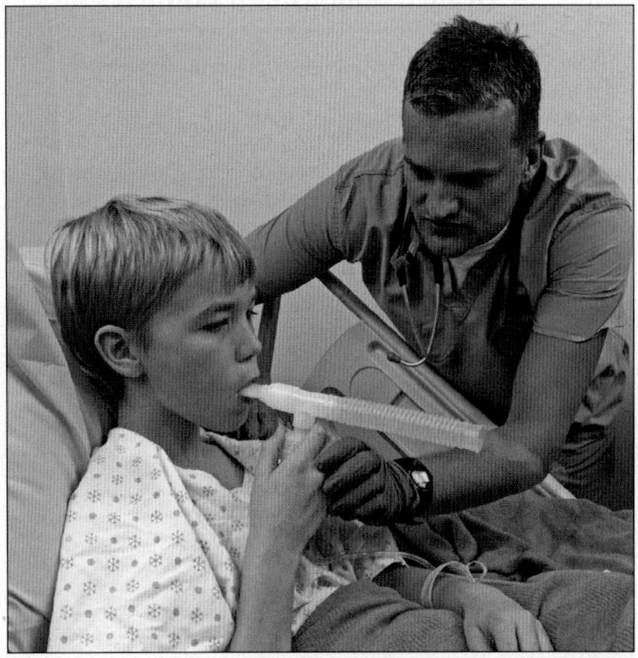

- Remain with the patient and continue the treatment until the nebulizer begins to sputter.[1] After treatment, obtain the patient's vital signs, assess his respiratory status, and obtain a spirometry or peak flow measurement, as indicated, *to detect any adverse reactions to the medication.*[23,24,25]
- Encourage the patient to cough and expectorate, or suction the patient's airway as needed.
- Auscultate the patient's lungs *to evaluate the effectiveness of therapy.*[1]
- Assist the patient with oral care. (See the "Oral care" procedure, page 560.)
- Rinse the nebulizer with sterile water and allow it to air-dry, or discard it after the treatment.[1]

For in-line nebulizer therapy

- Draw up the medication and diluent, open the nebulizer cup, inject the medication, and then replace the lid. Attach the cup to the gas source with the attached tubing.
- Insert the nebulizer cup adapter into the inspiratory limb of the ventilator circuit 6″ (15.2 cm) from the Y-connection *to create a reservoir of aerosolized medication in the inspiratory limb of the circuit and to reduce the amount of drug flushed into the expiratory limb.*[1]
- Remove the heat-moisture exchanger from the ventilator if it's attached.
- Initiate gas flow by using the nebulizer function on the ventilator if available. If this function isn't available, initiate gas flow from an external source *to create a mist.*[1]

NURSING ALERT *Adding an external gas flow to the ventilator can affect gas flow and volume delivery to the patient, causing alarms to trigger. Monitor the patient closely during a nebulizer treatment, and return ventilator settings to pretreatment levels as soon as possible after treatment.*[1]

- If the patient is being ventilated using a spontaneous pressure mode, encourage him to take slow, even breaths during the treatment.
- Remain with the patient during the treatment, which typically lasts 15 to 20 minutes, and monitor his vital signs, oxygen saturation level, and ventilator parameters *to detect any adverse reaction to the medication.*
- Discontinue treatment when medication administration is complete. Remove the nebulizer cup from the ventilatory circuit.

PATIENT TEACHING

Using a nebulizer at home

If the patient will be using a small-volume nebulizer at home, teach him the following steps:[2]

- Wash your hands with soap and warm water and dry thoroughly.
- Assemble the tubing, nebulizer cup, and mouthpiece or mask according to the manufacturer's directions.
- Put the prescribed medicine into the nebulizer cup.
- Sit in an upright position.
- Connect the nebulizer to a power source.
- Breathe normally, with occasional deep breaths, until sputtering occurs or until the end of nebulization.
- Make sure the nebulizer remains vertical during treatment.
- After treatment, rinse the nebulizer with sterile or distilled water and allow it to air-dry.
- Disinfect the nebulizer according to the manufacturer's instructions.

Teach the patient who will be using an ultrasonic nebulizer for home therapy the following steps:[2]

- Wash your hands with soap and warm water and dry them thoroughly.
- Assemble the nebulizer according to the manufacturer's directions.
- Following the manufacturer's instructions, perform a functionality test before the first use of a new nebulizer and after each disinfection *to verify proper operation.*
- Pour the prescribed medication or solution into the medication reservoir. Don't exceed the volume recommended by the manufacturer.
- Sit in an upright position.
- Turn on the power.
- Hold the nebulizer in the recommended position.
- Breathe normally, with occasional deep breaths.
- If you must interrupt treatment, turn off the unit *to avoid waste.*
- When you've completed the treatment, disassemble and clean the nebulizer as recommended by the manufacturer.
- Once or twice a week, disinfect the nebulizer following the manufacturer's instructions.

- Encourage the patient to cough, and suction excess secretions as needed.
- Clean and store the nebulizer cup according to the manufacturer's instructions.
- Perform a respiratory assessment *to evaluate the effectiveness of therapy.*[23,24,25]

For ultrasonic nebulizer therapy

- Fill the couplet compartment on the nebulizer with the prescribed medication or normal saline solution to the level indicated. If the dose to be inhaled is larger than the maximum capacity of the compartment, divide it into several separate inhalations.[3]
- Before beginning, administer an inhaled bronchodilator (metered-dose inhaler or small-volume nebulizer) *to prevent bronchospasm,* as ordered, following safe medication administration practices.[20,21]
- Turn on the nebulizer machine, and check the outflow port *to ensure proper misting.*
- Assist the patient with applying a mouthpiece, mask, or collar, as necessary, depending on the delivery system and patient-related factors such as age and physical and cognitive ability.[2]
- Encourage the patient to take slow, even breaths through his mouth.
- Check the patient frequently during the procedure *to observe for adverse reactions.* Watch for labored respirations *because ultrasonic nebulizer therapy may hydrate retained secretions and obstruct airways.* Observe for wheezing resulting from irritation of the airways.
- When medication delivery is complete, turn off the nebulizer.
- Clean and store the nebulizer and tubing appropriately to prevent bacterial contamination.
- Obtain the patient's vital signs, assess his respiratory status, and obtain a spirometry or peak flow measurement, as ordered, *to determine the efficacy of treatment.*[23,24,25]
- Encourage the patient to cough and expectorate, or suction his airway as needed.
- Dispose of sputum properly or send an ordered specimen to the laboratory immediately. (See the "Sputum collection" procedure, page 711.)
- Assist the patient with oral care. (See the "Oral care" procedure, page 560.)

Completing the procedure

- Dispose of used supplies in the appropriate receptacle.
- Remove and discard your gloves and any other personal protective equipment worn.[10]
- Perform hand hygiene.[4,5,6,7,8]
- Clean and disinfect your stethoscope using a disinfectant pad.[12,13]
- Perform hand hygiene.[4,5,6,7,8]
- Document the procedure.[14,15,16]

Special considerations

- When using large-volume nebulizer therapy in pediatric patients or patients with a delicate fluid balance, be alert for signs of overhydration (exhibited by unexplained weight gain occurring over several days after the initiation of therapy), pulmonary edema, crackles, and electrolyte imbalance.
- If a nebulizer device is for single-patient use, use it only for a single patient, label it with the proper patient identifiers, and discard it at the end of the patient's stay *to prevent cross-contamination.*[2]
- If oxygen is being delivered concomitantly, the fraction of inspired oxygen (FIO_2) may be diluted if the flow isn't adequate, so if the mist disappears when the patient inhales, increase the gas flow.
- A noseclip may be used if the patient has difficulty remembering to breathe through his mouth.
- Ventilator modes and settings can affect aerosol deposition. Lung-model studies suggest that low inspiratory flow rates, use of decelerating flow instead of square wave–form flow, tidal volume greater than 500 mL, and longer inspiratory times are all associated with improved aerosol deposition. Spontaneous inspiration through the ventilator circuit provides increased lung deposition compared with controlled, assist-controlled, and pressure-support ventilation.
- Adding gas from the nebulizer to the ventilator circuit may increase volumes, flows, and peak airway pressures, altering the intended pattern of ventilation. Reset ventilator settings at the end of treatment if you made changes to accommodate the additional gas flow during nebulization.
- Don't leave the nebulizer cup in the ventilator circuit between treatments *because doing so increases the risk of a pressure leak in the system.*

Patient teaching

If the patient needs to continue nebulizer therapy after discharge, teach him and his family how to use the equipment. (See *Using a nebulizer at home.*)

Complications

Nebulized particulates can irritate the mucosa and cause bronchospasm and dyspnea.[2] Other complications include airway burns (when a heating element is used), infection from contaminated equipment (rarely), overhydration, and adverse reactions to medications.

Documentation

Record the date, time, and duration of therapy; the type and amount of medication; FIO_2 or oxygen flow, if administered; vital signs, respiratory assessment, and peak flow or spirometry readings before and after treatment; the patient's response to treatment; and any patient teaching provided and the patient's understanding of the treatment.

REFERENCES

1 Kacmarek, R. M., et al. (2013). *Egan's fundamentals of respiratory care* (10th ed.). St. Louis, MO: Mosby.

2 Elliot, D., & Dunne, P. (2011). "Guide to aerosol delivery devices: For physicians, nurses, pharmacists, and other healthcare professionals" [Online]. Accessed May 2015 via the Web at http://www.aarc.org/resources/aerosol_nonrts.pdf (Level I)

3 GF Health Products, Inc. (2009). "Lumiscope® portable ultrasonic nebulizer model 6700 user manual" [Online]. Accessed May 2015 via the Web at http://www.grahamfield.com/nosync/productimagesV2/ProductAdditionalInfoItemOriginal2220.PDF

4 Centers for Disease Control and Prevention. (2002). Guideline for hand hygiene in health-care settings: Recommendations of the Healthcare Infection Control Practices Advisory Committee and the HICPAC/SHEA/APIC/IDSA Hand Hygiene Task Force. *MMWR Recommendations and Reports, 51*(RR-16), 1–45. Accessed May 2015 via the Web at http://www.cdc.gov/mmwr/pdf/rr/rr5116.pdf (Level II)

5 World Health Organization. (2009). "WHO guidelines on hand hygiene in health care: First global patient safety challenge, clean care is safer care" [Online]. Accessed May 2015 via the Web at http://whqlibdoc.who.int/publications/2009/9789241597906_eng.pdf (Level IV)

6 The Joint Commission. (2015). Standard NPSG.07.01.01. *Comprehensive accreditation manual for hospitals: The official handbook.* Oakbrook Terrace, IL: The Joint Commission. (Level VII)

7 Centers for Medicare & Medicaid Services, Department of Health and Human Services. (2014). Condition of participation: Infection control. 42 C.F.R. § 482.42.

8 American Osteopathic Association. (2014). Standard 07.01.21. *Healthcare Facilities Accreditation Program: Accreditation requirements for acute care hospitals.* Chicago, IL: American Osteopathic Association. (Level VII)

9 The Joint Commission. (2015). Standard NPSG.01.01.01. *Comprehensive accreditation manual for hospitals: The official handbook.* Oakbrook Terrace, IL: The Joint Commission. (Level VII)

10 Siegel, J. D., et al. (2007). "2007 guideline for isolation precautions: Preventing transmission of infectious agents in healthcare settings" [Online]. Accessed May 2015 via the Web at http://www.cdc.gov/hicpac/pdf/isolation/Isolation2007.pdf (Level II)

11 American Osteopathic Association. (2014). Standard 07.01.10. *Healthcare Facilities Accreditation Program: Accreditation requirements for acute care hospitals.* Chicago, IL: American Osteopathic Association. (Level VII)

12 Rutala, W. A., et al. (2008). "Guideline for disinfection and sterilization in healthcare facilities, 2008" [Online]. Accessed May 2015 via the Web at http://www.cdc.gov/hicpac/pdf/guidelines/Disinfection_Nov_2008.pdf (Level I)

13 American Osteopathic Association. (2014). Standard 07.02.03. *Healthcare Facilities Accreditation Program: Accreditation requirements for acute care hospitals.* Chicago, IL: American Osteopathic Association. (Level VII)

14 The Joint Commission. (2015). Standard RC.01.03.01. *Comprehensive accreditation manual for hospitals: The official handbook.* Oakbrook Terrace, IL: The Joint Commission. (Level VII)

15 Centers for Medicare & Medicaid Services, Department of Health and Human Services. (2014). Condition of participation: Medical record services. 42 C.F.R. § 482.24(b).

16 American Osteopathic Association. (2014). Standard 10.00.03. *Healthcare Facilities Accreditation Program: Accreditation requirements for acute care hospitals.* Chicago, IL: American Osteopathic Association. (Level VII)

17 Westbrook, J., et al. (2010). Association of interruptions with an increased risk and severity of medication administration errors. *Archives of Internal Medicine, 170,* 683–690. (Level IV)

18 Institute for Safe Medication Practices. (2013). Side tracks on the safety express: Interruptions lead to errors and unfinished . . . Wait, what was I doing? *Nurse Advise-ERR, 11*(2), 1–4. Accessed May 2015 via the Web at https://www.ismp.org/Newsletters/acutecare/showarticle.aspx?id=37

19 The Joint Commission. (2014). Standard MM.06.01.01. *Comprehensive accreditation manual for hospitals: The official handbook.* Oakbrook Terrace, IL: The Joint Commission. (Level VII)

20 Centers for Medicare & Medicaid Services, Department of Health and Human Services. (2014). Condition of participation: Nursing services. 42 C.F.R. § 482.23(c).

21 American Osteopathic Association. (2014). Standard 16.01.03. *Healthcare Facilities Accreditation Program: Accreditation requirements for acute care hospitals.* Chicago, IL: American Osteopathic Association. (Level VII)

22 The Joint Commission. (2015). Standard MM.05.01.09. *Comprehensive accreditation manual for hospitals: The official handbook.* Oakbrook Terrace, IL: The Joint Commission. (Level VII)

23 Brophy, C., et al. (2008). Quality of life measurements and bronchodilator responsiveness in prescribing nebulizer therapy in COPD. *Chronic Respiratory Disease, 5,* 13–18. (Level II)

24 Fanta, C. H. Treatment of acute exacerbations of asthma in adults. (2014). In: *UpToDate,* Bochner, B. S., & Hollingsworth, H. (Eds.). Accessed May 2015 via the Web at http://www.uptodate.com/contents/search

25 Global Initiative for Chronic Obstructive Lung Disease. (2013). "Global strategy for the diagnosis, management, and prevention of chronic obstructive pulmonary disease: Updated 2014" [Online]. Accessed May 2015 via the Web at http://www.goldcopd.org/uploads/users/files/GOLD_Report2014_Feb07.pdf (Level I)

NEGATIVE-PRESSURE WOUND THERAPY

Negative-pressure wound therapy encourages wound healing by applying localized negative pressure at the site of a wound.[1] Doing so removes excess wound fluids that can cause maceration and delay healing, reduces edema and bacterial colonization, and stimulates the formation of healthy granulation tissue. It also increases local blood flow and draws wound edges together. (See *Understanding negative-pressure wound therapy,* page 542.)

Negative-pressure wound therapy is indicated for acute and traumatic wounds, pressure ulcers, and chronic open wounds, such as diabetic ulcers, dehisced surgical wounds, partial-thickness burns, meshed grafts, and skin flaps.[2] It's contraindicated in patients with exposed vital organs, wounds that have been inadequately debrided; untreated coagulopathy, or an allergy to any component of the procedure.[3] This therapy should be used cautiously in patients with active bleeding, in those taking anticoagulants or platelet aggregate inhibitors, and when achieving wound hemostasis has been difficult.[4]

Equipment

Emesis basin ▪ sterile normal saline irrigating solution ▪ gloves ▪ sterile gloves ▪ fluid-impermeable pad ▪ irrigation kit with syringe ▪ suction tubing ▪ evacuation canister tubing ▪ skin protectant wipe ▪ evacuation canister ▪ negative-pressure wound therapy unit ▪ wound assessment tool and guide ▪ vital signs monitoring equipment ▪ Optional: gown, goggles, prescribed pain medication, scale, prescribed cleaning agent, additional skin barrier product.

For foam packing

Sterile scissors ▪ foam packing ▪ transparent dressing therapy drape ▪ transparent semipermeable dressing.

For gauze packing

Nonadherent gauze ▪ antimicrobial gauze packing moistened with sterile normal saline solution ▪ drain ▪ ostomy strip paste ▪ transparent dressings.

Understanding negative-pressure wound therapy

When a wound fails to heal in a timely manner, negative-pressure wound therapy may be an option. It involves placing a special dressing in a wound or over a graft or flap and using a vacuum-assisted closure device to create negative pressure within the wound bed, which enhances wound healing.

Depending on the type of wound, the selected manufacturer's equipment, and the practitioner's preference, gauze or foam packing will be ordered. Gauze is typically used in circumferential and tunneling wounds and explored fistulas. Gauze fits most wounds and tends to be more comfortable for the patient during application and removal. Foam packing is typically used in wounds with a lot of exudate. It's available in various sizes to fit a wide range of wound types and can be cut to accommodate any wound size.

Wound with gauze packing

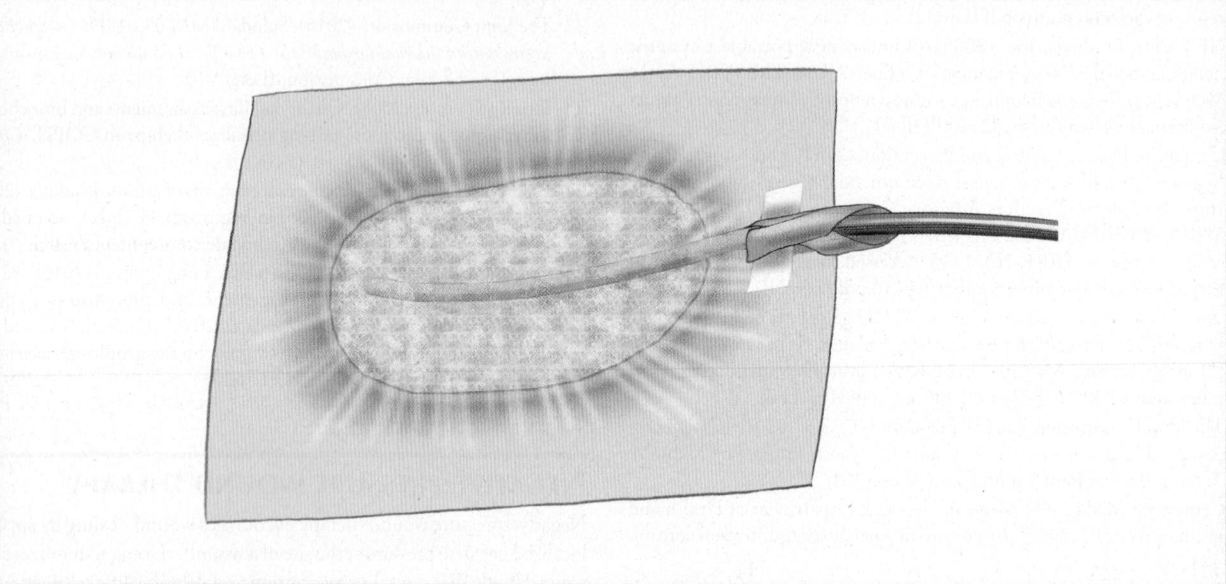

Wound with foam packing

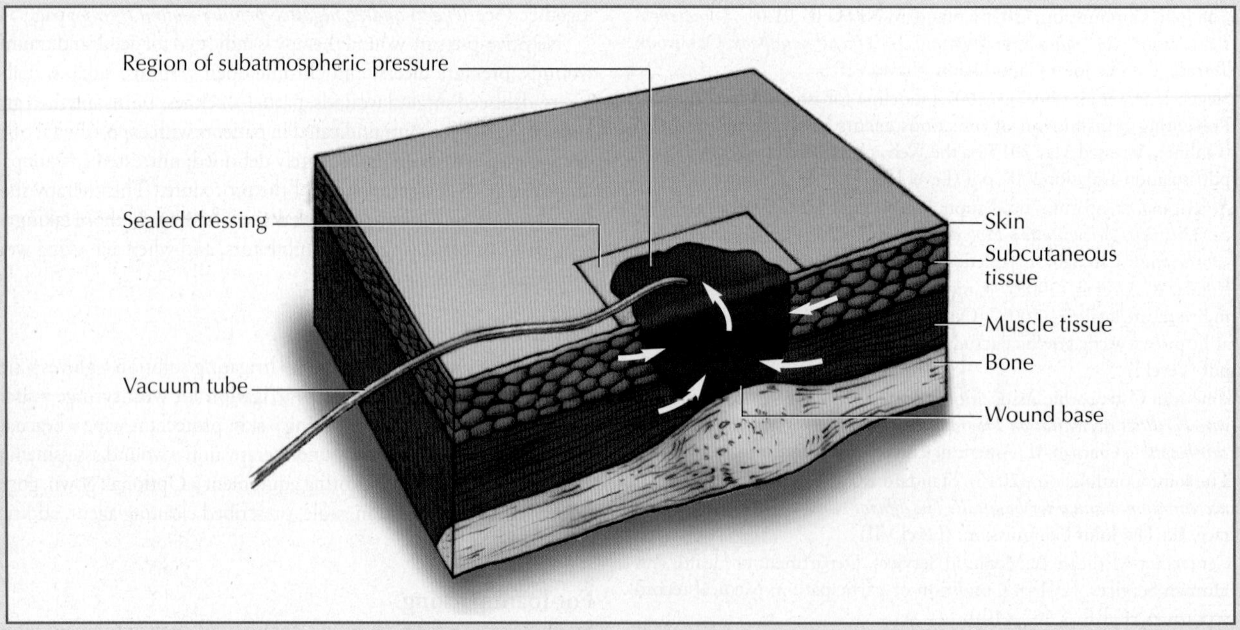

Preparation of equipment

Assemble the negative-pressure wound therapy unit at the bedside according to the manufacturer's instructions. Make sure the unit functions properly, dressings and supplies aren't expired and are intact and the tubing and canisters are appropriate for the unit and the patient's size, weight, condition, and wound characteristics. A large canister shouldn't be used for an elderly patient, a patient at high risk of bleeding, or a patient who can't tolerate large-volume fluid loss.[4,5] Set negative pressure according to the practitioner's order and the manufacturer's instructions (25 to 200 mm Hg). Prepare a place for the supplies that's within reach.

Warm the sterile irrigating solution to 90° to 95°F (32° to 35°C) *to reduce discomfort.* Pour irrigating solution into the container of the irrigation kit.

Implementation

■ Review the patient's medical record for allergies or contraindications to treatment. Also assess the patient's bleeding risk before initiation of therapy.[4,6]
■ Verify the practitioner's order for the appropriate wound cleaning agent, frequency of dressing change, type of negative pressure unit, type of wound packing, and settings for the negative-pressure unit.[6]
■ Confirm that written informed consent has been obtained and is in the patient's medical record, as required.[7,8,9,10]
■ Gather and prepare the equipment.
■ Perform hand hygiene.[11,12,13,14,15]
■ Confirm the patient's identity using at least two patient identifiers.[16]
■ Provide privacy and explain the procedure to the patient.[17,18,19]
■ Assess the patient's condition.
■ Perform a comprehensive pain assessment using techniques appropriate for the patient's age, condition, and ability to understand.[20]
■ Administer pain medication, as needed and prescribed, following safe medication administration practices.[21,22]
■ Put on gloves and, if necessary, a gown and goggles *to protect yourself from wound drainage and contamination.*[23]
■ Place a fluid-impermeable pad under the patient *to catch any spills and avoid linen changes.*
■ Position the patient *to allow maximum wound exposure.*
■ Place the emesis basin under the wound *to collect any drainage.*
■ Using sterile technique, prepare a sterile field and place all the supplies on the sterile field.
■ Remove the soiled dressing, weight it as ordered, and then discard it in an appropriate receptacle.[24]
■ Thoroughly inspect the wound *to ensure that all pieces of dressing components have been removed.* Verify that the number of removed pieces correlates with the number documented in the patient's medical record.[4,25,26]
■ Remove and discard your gloves, and perform hand hygiene.[11,12,13,14,15]
■ Replace your gown as needed, and put on a new pair of gloves.[23]
■ Irrigate the wound thoroughly using normal saline solution and an irrigation syringe. (See the "Wound irrigation" procedure, page 840.)
■ Clean the area around the wound with normal saline solution or ordered cleaning agent.[6]
■ Wipe the intact skin with a skin protectant wipe and allow it to dry *to prevent blistering when removing the dressing.* Apply addition skin barrier product, as indicated.[4,27]
■ Remove and discard your gloves and perform hand hygiene.[11,12,13,14,15]
■ Put on a new pair of sterile gloves.[23]
■ Assess the wound. Note the wound's precise location, any tunneling, tissue type and loss, size, color, odor, and the presence of warmth, edema, or drainage. Also assess the patient for increased pain, fever, and elevated white blood cell count.[27]

ELDER ALERT ***Closely monitor elderly patients, certain small adults, and those with large exudating wounds in relation to body size and weight for fluid loss and dehydration. When monitoring fluid output, consider the volume of fluid in both the tubing and canister and the weight of the dressing removed.***[4]

■ Measure the wound using your facility's assessment tool and guide. Obtain measurements at the baseline assessment, with the first dressing change, weekly, and when negative-pressure wound therapy is discontinued.
■ If your gloves are contaminated, remove them, perform hand hygiene, and put on a new pair of sterile gloves.[11,12,13,14,15,23]

Using foam packing

■ Using sterile scissors, cut the foam to the shape and measurement of the wound *to help maintain negative pressure to the entire wound.* More than one piece of foam may be necessary, depending on the size of the wound. Don't cut the foam directly over the wound *to prevent foam fragments from falling into the wound.* If a tunnel is present, cut the foam longer than the tunnel *to ensure the foam makes contact with the wound.*
■ Carefully place the foam in the wound, ensuring that the foam is in contact with the wound bed, margins, and any tunneled area or areas of undermining (if there's a groove in the foam, apply it with the groove side up). Don't pack the foam tightly into any areas of the wound *because doing so may delay healing.*
■ Apply the transparent therapy dressing drape over the foam leaving a 2″ (5-cm) margin of intact skin covered by the dressing around the wound *to ensure that the wound is covered completely and that the negative-pressure seal will be intact.*
■ Cut a small hole no bigger than 3/8″ (1 cm) in the center of the transparent therapy dressing drape (over the groove in the foam, if present). Don't cut a slit *because it could seal during therapy.*[4] The hole in the drape is the insertion point for the suction tubing. Depending on the equipment your facility uses, the tubing may be attached to an adhesive pad that you attach to this site.
■ If you're not using a preattached system, place the suction tubing into the center of the foam. The suction tubing embedded into the foam delivers negative pressure to the wound.
■ Apply a transparent semipermeable dressing over the insertion point of the suction tubing.

Using gauze packing

■ Using sterile scissors, trim a single layer of nonadherent gauze.
■ Lay the nonadherent gauze across the wound bed.
■ Apply saline-moistened antimicrobial gauze loosely into the wound, ensuring that the gauze is in contact with the nonadherent gauze, margins, and any tunneled area or areas of undermining. Don't overpack the wound *because doing so can delay healing.*
■ Position the drain tubing on top of the gauze. If a channel drain (a small, cylindrical drain) or round drain (a round, perforated drain) is used, wrap a layer of saline-moistened gauze around the drain.
■ Apply ostomy strip paste to a small portion of the wound edge at the location where the drain tubing exits the wound *to secure the tubing's position.* Position the drain tubing on top of the ostomy strip paste. Apply the ostomy strip paste over the top of the tubing and pinch it in place *to secure the tubing's position.*
■ Apply one or more transparent semipermeable dressing over the wound. Reinforce the seal by pinching the transparent occlusive film and ostomy strip paste together.

Completing the procedure

■ Connect the free end of the drain tubing to the canister tubing at the adapter.
■ Position the drain tubing on flat surfaces, away from the perineal area, bony prominences, or pressure areas *to prevent additional skin breakdown.*[4]
■ Anchor the drain tubing several inches away from the dressing *to prevent tension on the suction tubing.*
■ Dispose of soiled supplies appropriately.[24]
■ Remove and discard your gloves and any other personal protective equipment worn, and perform hand hygiene.[11,12,13,14]
■ Turn on the negative-pressure unit. Make sure the transparent dressing drape shrinks to the foam or gauze and the skin *to ensure a good seal.* This

seal is apparent by a raisin-like appearance of the dressing. Failure of the dressing drape to shrink to the foam or gauze under negative pressure indicates a break in the seal and will trigger the device's alarm; you might also hear a hissing sound if you auscultate with a stethoscope.

- Properly dispose of the drainage, solution, fluid-impermeable pad, and trash bag, and clean and dispose of soiled equipment and supplies.
- Make sure the device alarm limits are set appropriately and that the alarms are turned on, functioning properly, and audible to staff.[28,29,30]
- Make sure the patient is comfortable.
- Monitor the patient closely.
- Perform hand hygiene.[11,12,13,14]
- Document the procedure.[31,32,33]

Special considerations

- The Joint Commission issued a sentinel event alert concerning medical device alarm safety *because alarm-related events have been associated with permanent loss of function or death.* Among the major contributing factors were improper alarm settings, alarms inappropriately turned off, and alarm signals not audible to staff. Make sure alarm limits are set appropriately and that alarms are turned on and audible to staff. Follow facility guidelines for preventing alarm fatigue.[28]
- Many manufacturers have dressing kits that contain the necessary equipment. Make sure that you're using the correct kit for your patient's needs.
- Change the dressing according to the manufacturer's directions, usually 48 hours after the beginning of treatment and then two to three times per week.[27] More frequent dressing changes may be necessary if the wound has heavy drainage or drainage with sediment or if the wound is infected. Try to coordinate the dressing change with the practitioner's visit *so he can inspect the wound.*
- Measure and record the amount of drainage every shift.
- Be aware that audible and visual alarms alert you when the canister is full, the dressing has an air leak, the battery is low, or the tubing becomes blocked or dislodged.
- Change the canister once per week, when it's full, if it has any signs of damage.
- Never leave the dressing in place without suction. If the machine malfunctions, replace the dressing with a wet-to-damp dressing until the machine is repaired or replaced. Leaving the dressing in place without suction puts the patient at high risk for infection.
- If the patient requires defibrillation, disconnect the unit from the wound first. If the dressing interferes with defibrillation, remove the dressing.
- Be aware that many negative-pressure units aren't compatible with computed tomography or magnetic resonance imaging. Check the manufacturer's instructions before testing.
- Evaluate the effectiveness of negative-pressure wound therapy weekly using a comprehensive wound assessment tool and wound measurements. If the wound shows no steady improvement (10% decrease in wound size per week or 50% improvement in wound size over 4 weeks) or if the wound worsens, reevaluate the use of negative-pressure wound therapy.[34]
- If the wound is infected, notify the practitioner *so that treatment may begin with systemic antibiotics before the initiation of negative-pressure wound therapy.* Necrotic tissue should be debrided before the initiation of therapy.
- If the patient experiences pain from the negative-pressure wound therapy or dressing changes, consider premedicating the patient, decreasing the pressure settings, using continuous instead of intermittent suction, changing the type of filler dressing, applying a contact layer to the wound surface before inserting the foam, and instilling normal saline solution before removing the dressing.[35]
- For best results, ensure that the patient receives uninterrupted therapy for at least 22 hours daily.[34]

Patient teaching

If the patient will be using negative-pressure wound therapy at home, teach him and his family about the device, foam dressing changes using sterile technique, and possible complications with the machine or the wound. Tell them to remove the foam dressing and replace it with a wet-to-damp dressing if the machine malfunctions and to contact the practitioner as soon as possible if they observe signs of infection. Demonstrate dressing changes and observe return demonstrations. Answer all questions and provide guidance and encouragement as needed.

Complications

Local skin irritation may occur. The most serious complication is bleeding; carefully monitor the patient for indications of bleeding. Cleaning and care of wounds may temporarily increase the patient's pain and increase the risk of infection.[36]

Documentation

Document the frequency and duration of therapy; the amount of negative pressure applied; the size and condition of the wound, including the location, tissue type and loss, odor, drainage, and measurement; and the patient's response to treatment. Note the type of dressing applied as well as the verification of components removed and inserted.[4,25,26] Document any patient teaching and the patient's response to the teaching.

REFERENCES

1 Anesäter, E., et al. (2011). The influence of different sizes and types of wound fillers on wound contraction and tissue pressure during negative pressure wound therapy. *International Wound Journal, 8,* 336–342.

2 Andros, G., et al. (2006). "Consensus statement on negative pressure wound therapy (V.A.C. therapy) for the management of diabetic foot wounds" [Online]. Accessed May 2015 via the Web at http://www.o-wm.com/files/docs/071406_kci.pdf (Level I)

3 Agency for Healthcare Research and Quality. (2009). "Technology assessment on negative pressure wound therapy devices" [Online]. Accessed May 2015 via the Web at http://www.ahrq.gov/research/findings/ta/negative-pressure-wound-therapy/background.html

4 KCI®. (2012). "V.A.C.™ therapy clinical guidelines: A reference source for clinicians" [Online]. Accessed May 2015 via the Web at http://www.kci1.com/cs/Satellite?blobcol=urldata&blobheader=application%2Fpdf&blobkey=id&blobtable=MungoBlobs&blobwhere=1226689404554&ssbinary=true

5 Centers for Medicare & Medicaid Services. (2012). "Negative pressure wound therapy interpretive guidelines" [Online]. Accessed May 2015 via the Web at http://www.cms.gov/Medicare/Provider-Enrollment-and-Certification/MedicareProviderSupEnroll/Downloads/NPWTinterpretguidlines_finalcleared.pdf

6 Martindell, D. (2012). Safety monitor: The safe use of negative-pressure wound therapy. *American Journal of Nursing, 112*(6), 59–63. Accessed May 2015 via the Web at http://www.nursingcenter.com/lnc/pdfjournal?AID=1353037&an=00000446-201206000-00034&Journal_ID=&Issue_ID=

7 The Joint Commission. (2015). Standard RI.01.03.01. *Comprehensive accreditation manual for hospitals: The official handbook.* Oakbrook Terrace, IL: The Joint Commission. (Level VII)

8 Centers for Medicare & Medicaid Services, Department of Health and Human Services. (2014). Condition of participation: Patient's rights. 42 C.F.R. § 482.13.

9 Henderson, V., et al. (2010). NPWT in everyday practice made easy. *Wounds International, 1*(5), 1–6. Accessed May 2015 via the Web at http://www.woundsinternational.com/pdf/content_9720.pdf

10 American Osteopathic Association. (2012). Standard 15.01.11. *Healthcare Facilities Accreditation Program: Accreditation requirements for acute care hospitals.* Chicago, IL: American Osteopathic Association. (Level VII)

11 The Joint Commission. (2015). Standard NPSG.07.01.01. *Comprehensive accreditation manual for hospitals: The official handbook.* Oakbrook Terrace, IL: The Joint Commission. (Level VII)

12 Centers for Disease Control and Prevention. (2002). Guideline for hand hygiene in health-care settings: Recommendations of the Healthcare Infection Control Practices Advisory Committee and the HICPAC/SHEA/APIC/IDSA Hand Hygiene Task Force. *MMWR Recommendations and Reports, 51*(RR-16), 1–45. Accessed May 2015 via the Web at http://www.cdc.gov/mmwr/pdf/rr/rr5116.pdf (Level II)

13 World Health Organization. (2009). "WHO guidelines on hand hygiene in health care: First global patient safety challenge, clean care is safer care" [Online]. Accessed May 2015 via the Web at http://whqlibdoc.who.int/publications/2009/9789241597906_eng.pdf (Level IV)

14 American Osteopathic Association. (2014). Standard 07.01.10. *Healthcare Facilities Accreditation Program: Accreditation requirements for acute care hospitals.* Chicago, IL: American Osteopathic Association. (Level VII)

15 Centers for Medicare & Medicaid Services, Department of Health and Human Services. (2014). Condition of participation: Infection control. 42 C.F.R. § 482.42.

16 The Joint Commission. (2015). Standard NPSG.01.01.01. *Comprehensive accreditation manual for hospitals: The official handbook.* Oakbrook Terrace, IL: The Joint Commission. (Level VII)

17 American Osteopathic Association. (2014). Standard 30.00.14. *Healthcare Facilities Accreditation Program: Accreditation requirements for acute care hospitals.* Chicago, IL: American Osteopathic Association. (Level VII)

18 American Osteopathic Association. (2014). Standard 15.01.16. *Healthcare Facilities Accreditation Program: Accreditation requirements for acute care hospitals.* Chicago, IL: American Osteopathic Association. (Level VII)

19 Centers for Medicare & Medicaid Services, Department of Health and Human Services. (2014). Condition of participation: Patient's rights. 42 C.F.R. § 482.13(c)(1).

20 The Joint Commission. (2015). Standard PC.01.02.07. *Comprehensive accreditation manual for hospitals: The official handbook.* Oakbrook Terrace, IL: The Joint Commission. (Level VII)

21 American Osteopathic Association. (2014). Standard 16.01.03. *Healthcare Facilities Accreditation Program: Accreditation requirements for acute care hospitals.* Chicago, IL: American Osteopathic Association. (Level VII)

22 Centers for Medicare & Medicaid Services, Department of Health and Human Services. (2014). Condition of participation: Nursing services. 42 C.F.R. § 482.23(c).

23 Siegel, J. D., et al. (2007). "2007 guideline for isolation precautions: Preventing transmission of infectious agents in healthcare settings" [Online]. Accessed May 2015 via the Web at http://www.cdc.gov/hicpac/pdf/isolation/Isolation2007.pdf (Level II)

24 Occupational Safety and Health Administration. (n.d.). "Bloodborne pathogens, standard number 1910.1030" [Online]. Accessed May 2015 via the Web at http://www.osha.gov/pls/oshaweb/owadisp.show_document?p_table=standards&p_id=10051 (Level VII)

25 The Joint Commission. (2013). "Sentinel event alert: Preventing unintended retained foreign objects" [Online]. Accessed May 2015 via the Web at http://www.jointcommission.org/assets/1/6/SEA_51_URFOs_10_17_13_FINAL.pdf

26 National Quality Forum. (2011). "Serious reportable events in healthcare—2011 update: A consensus report" [Online]. Accessed May 2015 via the Web at http://www.nothingleftbehind.org/uploads/NQF_SRE_s_2011.pdf

27 Baranoski, S., & Ayello, E. A. (2012). *Wound care essentials: Practice principles* (3rd ed.). Philadelphia, PA: Lippincott Williams & Williams.

28 The Joint Commission. (2013). "Sentinel event alert: Medical device alarm safety in hospitals" [Online]. Accessed May 2015 via the Web at http://www.jointcommission.org/assets/1/18/SEA_50_alarms_4_5_13_FINAL1.PDF

29 The Joint Commission. (2015). Standard NPSG.06.01.01. *Comprehensive accreditation manual for hospitals: The official handbook.* Oakbrook Terrace, IL: The Joint Commission. (Level VII)

30 Graham, K .C., & Cvach, M. (2010). Monitor alarm fatigue: Standardizing use of physiological monitors and decreasing nuisance alarms. *American Journal of Critical Care, 19,* 28–37.

31 The Joint Commission. (2015). Standard RC.01.03.01. *Comprehensive accreditation manual for hospitals: The official handbook.* Oakbrook Terrace, IL: The Joint Commission. (Level VII)

32 American Osteopathic Association. (2014). Standard 10.00.03. *Healthcare Facilities Accreditation Program: Accreditation requirements for acute care hospitals.* Chicago, IL: American Osteopathic Association. (Level VII)

33 Centers for Medicare & Medicaid Services, Department of Health and Human Services. (2014). Condition of participation: Medical record services. 42 C.F.R. § 482.24(b).

34 Gupta, S. (Ed.). (2007). Differentiating negative pressure wound therapy devices: An illustrative case series. *Wounds, 19*(1), 1–9. Accessed May 2015 via the Web at http://www.woundsresearch.com/files/docs/LomaLinda.pdf

35 Netsch, D. (2012). Negative pressure wound therapy. In R. A. Bryant & D. P. Nix (Eds.). *Acute and chronic wounds current management concepts* (4th ed.). St. Louis, MO: Mosby.

36 U.S. Food and Drug Administration. (2009). "Negative pressure wound devices draw notice, advice" [Online]. Accessed May 2015 via the Web at http://www.fda.gov/downloads/ForConsumers/ConsumerUpdates/UCM193750.pdf (Level VII)

ADDITIONAL REFERENCES

Langer, V., et al. (2013). Negative pressure wound therapy as an adjunct in healing of chronic wounds. *International Wound Journal.* Advance online publication.

Schintler, M. V. (2012). Negative pressure therapy: Theory and practice. *Diabetes/Metabolism Research and Reviews, 28,* 72–77.

Sussman, C., & Bates-Jensen, B. (2012). *Wound care: A collaborative practice manual for health professionals* (4th ed.). Philadelphia, PA: Lippincott Williams & Wilkins.

NEPHROSTOMY AND CYSTOSTOMY TUBE DRESSING CHANGES

Two urinary diversion techniques—nephrostomy and cystostomy—ensure temporary or permanent drainage from the kidneys or bladder and help prevent urinary tract infection or kidney failure. (See *Urinary diversion techniques,* page 546.)

A nephrostomy tube drains urine directly from a kidney when a disorder inhibits the normal flow of urine. The practitioner usually places the tube percutaneously, although sometimes he'll insert it surgically through the renal cortex and medulla into the renal pelvis from a lateral flank incision. The practitioner will usually place the tube because of obstructive problems, such as ureteral or ureteropelvic junction calculi or tumors. Diverting urine with a nephrostomy tube also allows kidney tissue damaged from obstructive disease to heal.

A cystostomy tube drains urine from the bladder, diverting it from the urethra. The practitioner will use this type of tube after certain gynecologic procedures, bladder surgery, prostatectomy, severe urethral strictures, or traumatic injury. He inserts the tube into the bladder approximately 2″ (5 cm) above the pubic symphysis and may use it alone or in addition to an indwelling urethral catheter.

Equipment

Antiseptic swabs ▪ fluid-impermeable pad ▪ gloves ▪ sterile gloves ▪ sterile precut 4″ × 4″ (10 cm × 10-cm) drain dressings or transparent semipermeable dressing ▪ hypoallergenic adhesive tape or other securement device, tape formulated for fragile skin.

Implementation

- Verify the practitioner's order.
- Gather the appropriate equipment.

Urinary diversion techniques

A cystostomy or a nephrostomy can be used to create a permanent diversion to relieve obstruction from an inoperable tumor or provide an outlet for urine after cystectomy. A temporary diversion can relieve obstruction from a calculus or ureteral edema.

In a *cystostomy,* the practitioner inserts a catheter percutaneously through the suprapubic area into the bladder. In a *nephrostomy,* the practitioner inserts a catheter percutaneously through the flank into the renal pelvis.

Cystostomy

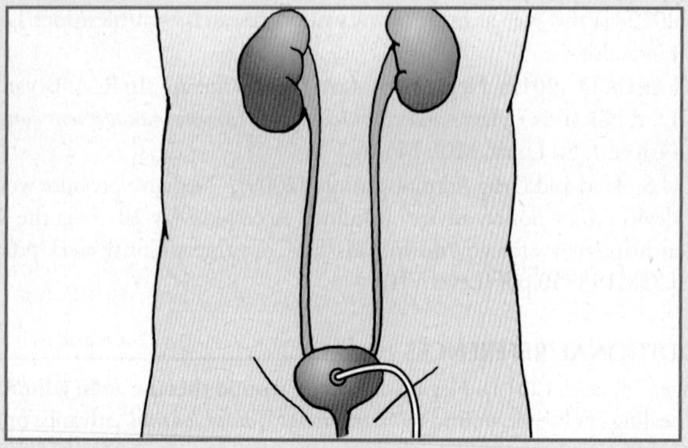

Nephrostomy

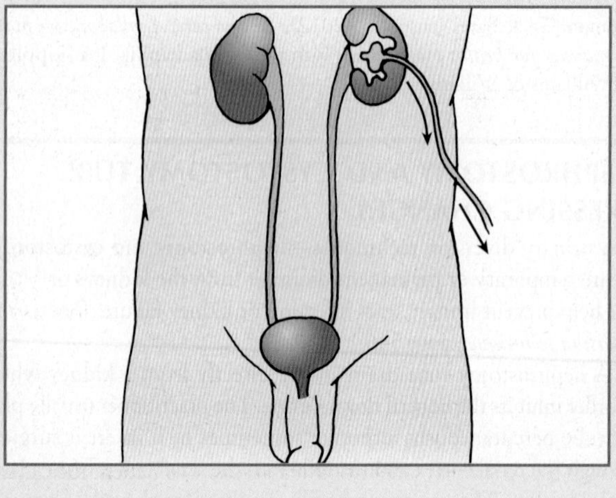

- Perform hand hygiene.[1,2,3,4,5]
- Confirm the patient's identity using at least two patient identifiers.[6]
- Provide privacy.[7,8]
- Explain the procedure to the patient *to enhance cooperation.*
- Open the antiseptic swabs, the sterile precut 4″ × 4″ (10-cm × 10-cm) drain dressings or transparent semipermeable dressing, and the sterile gloves using sterile technique.
- Position the patient *so you can clearly see the tube exit site.* If he has a nephrostomy tube, have him lie on his side opposite the tube. If the patient has a cystostomy tube, have him lie on his back.
- Place the fluid-impermeable pad under the patient *to absorb excess drainage and keep him dry.*
- Put on gloves *to comply with standard precautions.*[9,10]
- Carefully remove the tape around the tube, and remove the wet or soiled dressing.
- Note the markings on the tube at the insertion site *to check for accidental dislodgment.*
- Assess the tube exit site for redness, swelling, warmth, tenderness, or drainage *to note signs of infection and skin breakdown* and, if any are present, report them to the practitioner.
- Discard used supplies in the appropriate receptacle.[9]
- Remove and discard your gloves and perform hand hygiene.[1,2,3,4,5]
- Put on sterile gloves.[9]
- Use an antiseptic swab *to clean the skin,* wiping from the tube site outward.
- Discard the swab appropriately, being careful not to contaminate your gloves.[9]
- Repeat the skin cleaning procedure, if needed.
- Pick up a sterile precut 4″ × 4″ (10-cm × 10-cm) drain dressing and place it around the tube exit site. If necessary, overlap two drain dressings *for maximum absorption.* Alternatively, apply a transparent semipermeable dressing over the tube exit site *to enable observation of the site without removing the dressing.*
- Secure the dressing with hypoallergenic tape or another securement device.[11] Tape the tube to the patient's lateral abdomen *to prevent tension on the tube.*

NURSING ALERT ***If the patient has fragile skin, use dressings and tape specifically formulated for fragile skin*** **to prevent skin stripping and tearing during removal.**[12]

- Dispose of all equipment appropriately.
- Remove and discard your gloves.[9]
- Perform hand hygiene.[1,2,3,4,5]
- Help the patient to a comfortable position.
- Perform hand hygiene.[1,2,3,4,5]
- Document the procedure.[13,14,15]

Special considerations

- Change the dressings daily as needed.
- Check a nephrostomy tube frequently for kinks or obstructions. Kinks are likely to occur if the patient lies on the insertion site. Suspect an obstruction when the amount of urine in the drainage bag decreases or the amount of urine around the insertion site increases. Pressure created by urine backing up in the tube can damage nephrons. Gently curve a cystostomy tube *to prevent kinks.*
- Typically, cystostomy tubes for postoperative urologic patients should be checked hourly for 24 hours *to ensure adequate drainage and tube patency. To check tube patency,* note the amount of urine in the drainage bag and check the patient's bladder for distention.
- Keep the drainage bag below the level of the kidney at all times *to prevent urine reflux.*[11,16]
- If the tube becomes dislodged, cover the site with a sterile dressing and notify the practitioner immediately.
- The practitioner may order the nephrostomy tube to be clamped *to determine the patient's readiness for removal.* While the tube is clamped, assess the patient for flank pain and fever, and monitor his urine output.

Patient teaching

Teach the home care patient and caregiver how to clean the tube insertion site with soap and water, check for skin breakdown, and change the dressing daily. Teach them how to change the drainage bag or leg bag and perform irrigation, as indicated.[11] Explain that the patient can use a leg bag during the day and a larger drainage bag at night.

Tell the patient he can shower but not sit in a tub or go swimming. Stress the importance of reporting to his practitioner any signs of infection (red skin or white, yellow, or green drainage at the insertion site), oral temperature greater than 100.4°F (38°C), tube displacement (drainage that smells like urine), or severe flank pain.

Whether the patient uses a drainage bag or larger container, explain that he must wash it daily with a 1:3 vinegar-to-water solution and rinse and dry it thoroughly *to prevent crystalline buildup.* Encourage patients with unrestricted fluid intake to increase their daily intake to at least 3 qt (2.8 L) *to help flush the urinary system and reduce sediment formation.*

Complications

The patient has an increased risk of infection *because nephrostomy and cystostomy tubes provide a direct opening to the kidneys and bladder.*

Documentation

Describe the color and amount of drainage from the nephrostomy or cystostomy tube and record any color changes as they occur. Note the markings on the tube at the tube exit site and the presence of any signs of infection or skin breakdown. If the patient has more than one tube, describe the drainage (color, amount, and character) from each separate tube. Note any teaching performed and the patient's understanding of the teaching, as well as any complications and nursing actions taken.

REFERENCES

1 The Joint Commission. (2015). Standard NPSG.07.01.01. *Comprehensive accreditation manual for hospitals: The official handbook.* Oakbrook Terrace, IL: The Joint Commission. (Level VII)

2 Centers for Disease Control and Prevention. (2002). Guideline for hand hygiene in health-care settings: Recommendations of the Healthcare Infection Control Practices Advisory Committee and the HICPAC/SHEA/APIC/IDSA Hand Hygiene Task Force. *MMWR Recommendations and Reports, 51*(RR-16), 1–45. Accessed May 2015 via the Web at http://www.cdc.gov/mmwr/pdf/rr/rr5303.pdf (Level II)

3 World Health Organization. (2009). "WHO guidelines on hand hygiene in health care: First global patient safety challenge, clean care is safer care" [Online]. Accessed May 2015 via the Web at http://whqlibdoc.who.int/publications/2009/9789241597906_eng.pdf (Level IV)

4 Centers for Medicare & Medicaid Services, Department of Health and Human Services. (2014). Condition of participation: Infection control. 42 C.F.R. § 482.42.

5 American Osteopathic Association. (2014). Standard 07.01.21. *Healthcare Facilities Accreditation Program: Accreditation requirements for acute care hospitals.* Chicago, IL: American Osteopathic Association. (Level VII)

6 The Joint Commission. (2015). Standard NPSG.01.01.01. *Comprehensive accreditation manual for hospitals: The official handbook.* Oakbrook Terrace, IL: The Joint Commission. (Level VII)

7 Centers for Medicare & Medicaid Services, Department of Health and Human Services. (2014). Condition of participation: Patient's rights. 42 C.F.R. § 482.13(c)(1).

8 American Osteopathic Association. (2014). Standard 15.01.16. *Healthcare Facilities Accreditation Program: Accreditation requirements for acute care hospitals.* Chicago, IL: American Osteopathic Association. (Level VII)

9 Siegel, J. D., et al. (2007). "2007 guideline for isolation precautions: Preventing transmission of infectious agents in healthcare settings" [Online]. Accessed May 2015 via the Web at http://www.cdc.gov/hicpac/pdf/isolation/Isolation2007.pdf (Level II)

10 American Osteopathic Association. (2014). Standard 07.01.10. *Healthcare Facilities Accreditation Program: Accreditation requirements for acute care hospitals.* Chicago, IL: American Osteopathic Association. (Level VII)

11 National Institutes of Health. (2007). "Patient education: Caring for your percutaneous nephrostomy tube" [Online]. Accessed May 2015 via the Web at http://www.cc.nih.gov/ccc/patient_education/pepubs/percneph.pdf

12 LeBlanc, K., et al. (2013). International Skin Tear Advisory Panel: A tool kit to aid in the prevention, assessment, and treatment of skin tears using a simplified classification system. *Advances in Skin and Wound Care, 26,* 459–476. (Level IV)

13 The Joint Commission. (2015). Standard RC.01.03.01. *Comprehensive accreditation manual for hospitals: The official handbook.* Oakbrook Terrace, IL: The Joint Commission. (Level VII)

14 Centers for Medicare & Medicaid Services, Department of Health and Human Services. (2014). Condition of participation: Medical record services. 42 C.F.R. § 482.24(b).

15 American Osteopathic Association. (2014). Standard 10.00.03. *Healthcare Facilities Accreditation Program: Accreditation requirements for acute care hospitals.* Chicago, IL: American Osteopathic Association. (Level VII)

16 Agency for Clinical Innovation (ACI) Urology Network. (2013). "Management of patients with nephrostomy tubes: Clinical guideline and patient information" [Online]. Accessed May 2015 via the Web at http://www.aci.health.nsw.gov.au/__data/assets/pdf_file/0005/191066/ACI_Nephrostomy_Jan13.pdf#zoom=100 (Level VII)

ADDITIONAL REFERENCE

Doubleman, J. (2013). Ostomy 101: Colostomy, ileostomy, and urostomy: Understanding the types of ostomy surgeries can help you provide better patient care. *Wound Care Advisor, 2*(2), 31–36. Accessed May 2015 via the Web at http://woundcareadvisor.com/wp-content/uploads/2013/03/Ost_M-A13.pdf

NEUROLOGIC ASSESSMENT

Neurologic vital signs supplement the routine measurement of temperature, pulse rate, blood pressure, and respirations by evaluating the patient's level of consciousness (LOC), pupillary activity, and orientation to time, place, and person. They provide a simple, indispensable tool for checking the patient's neurologic status quickly.

A measure of environmental awareness and self-awareness, LOC reflects cortical function and usually provides the first sign of central nervous system deterioration. Changes in pupillary activity (pupil size, shape, equality, and response to light) may signal increased intracranial pressure (ICP) associated with a space-occupying lesion. Evaluating muscle strength and tone, reflexes, and posture also may help identify nervous system damage.

Changes in vital signs alone rarely indicate neurologic compromise, so any changes should be evaluated in light of a complete neurologic assessment. Because vital signs are controlled at the medullary level, changes in neurologic vital signs may signify ominous neurologic compromise.

Equipment

Low-pitched tuning fork ■ penlight ■ thermometer ■ sterile cotton ball or cotton-tipped applicator ■ stethoscope ■ sphygmomanometer ■ pupil size chart ■ pencil or pen ■ paperclip or key ■ safety pin ■ hospital-grade disinfectant.

Implementation

- Perform hand hygiene.[1,2,3,4,5]
- Confirm the patient's identity using at least two patient identifiers.[6]
- Explain the procedure to the patient, even if he's unresponsive.
- Provide privacy.[7,8]

Assessing LOC and orientation

- Assess the patient's LOC by evaluating his responses. Use standard methods such as the Glasgow Coma Scale (see *Using the Glasgow Coma Scale,* page 548) and the Rancho Los Amigos Cognitive Scale (see *Using the Rancho Los Amigos Cognitive Scale,* page 549). Begin by measuring the patient's response to verbal, light tactile (touch), or painful (nail bed pressure) stimuli. First, ask the patient his full name. If he responds appropriately, assess his orientation to time, place, and person. Ask him where he is and then what day, season, and year it is. (Expect disorientation to affect the sense of date first, then time, place, caregivers and, lastly, self.) When he responds verbally, assess the quality of his replies. For example, garbled words indicate difficulty with the motor nerves that govern speech muscles. Rambling responses indicate difficulty with thought processing and organization.

ELDER ALERT **Because of decreased hearing, vision, and tactile sensation with aging,** ***cues in the environment are an important feedback mechanism for older adults. When an older adult experiences a change***

Using the Glasgow Coma Scale

The Glasgow Coma Scale provides a standard reference for assessing or monitoring level of consciousness in a patient with a suspected or confirmed brain injury. This scale measures three responses to stimuli—eye opening, motor response, and verbal response—and assigns a number to each of the possible responses within these categories. The lowest possible score is 3; the highest, 15. A total score of 7 or less indicates coma.

The Glasgow Coma Scale is commonly used in the emergency department, at the scene of an accident, and for evaluating the hospitalized patient.

CHARACTERISTIC	RESPONSE/SCORE
Eye opening	■ Spontaneous—4 ■ To verbal command—3 ■ To pain—2 ■ No response—1
Best motor response	■ Obeys commands—6 ■ To painful stimuli: – Localizes pain; pushes stimulus away—5 – Flexes and withdraws—4 – Abnormal flexion—3 – Abnormal extension response—2 – No response—1
Best verbal response (Arouse patient with painful stimuli, if necessary)	■ Oriented and converses—5 ■ Disoriented and converses—4 ■ Uses inappropriate words—3 ■ Makes incomprehensible sounds—2 ■ No response—1
Total: 3 to 15	

in environment, such as admission to a hospital or other health care facility or a transfer from one unit to another, his neurologic assessment may be affected negatively. Orienting the patient to the environment and planning for other needs, such as providing adequate lighting without glare, visual and auditory clues, and appropriate assistive devices, may maximize the patient's functioning within the environment.[9]

■ Assess the patient's ability to understand and follow one-step commands that require a motor response. For example, ask him to open and close his eyes or stick out his tongue (as shown below). Note whether the patient can maintain his LOC. If you must gently shake him to keep him focused on your verbal commands, he may be neurologically compromised.

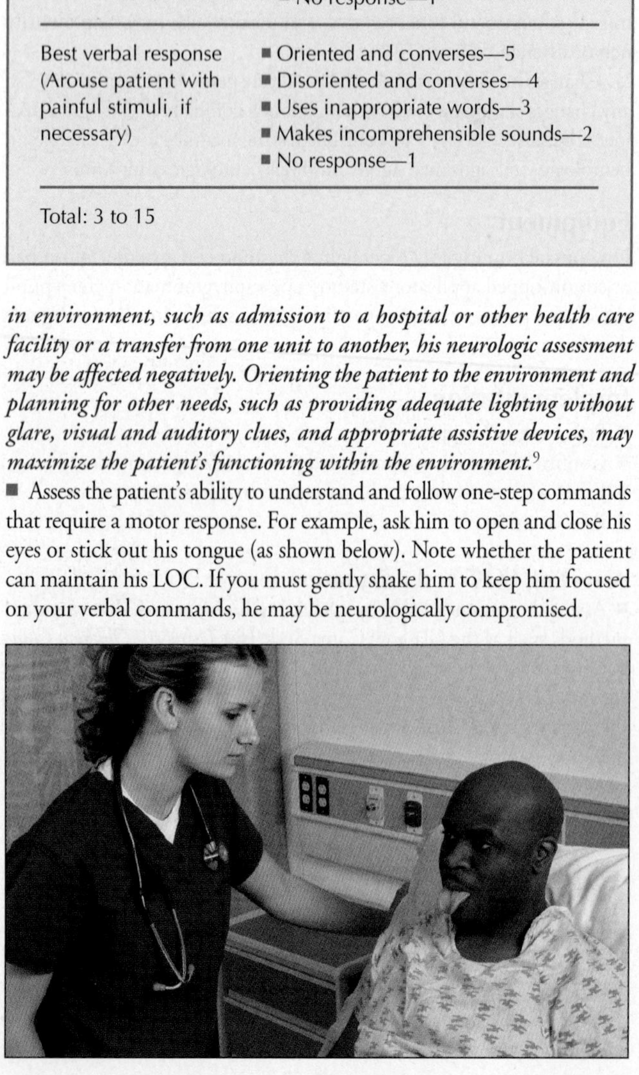

■ If the patient doesn't respond to commands or touch, apply a painful stimulus. Painful stimuli are classified as central (response via the brain) or peripheral (response via the spine). Apply a central stimulus first and note the patient's response. Acceptable central stimuli include squeezing the trapezius muscle, applying supraorbital or mandibular pressure, and rubbing the sternum. If the patient doesn't respond to central stimuli, apply a peripheral stimulus to all four extremities *to establish a baseline.* With moderate pressure, squeeze the nail beds on fingers and toes, and note his response. Check motor responses bilaterally *to rule out monoplegia (paralysis of a single area) and hemiplegia (paralysis of one side of the body).*

Examining pupils and eye movement

■ Ask the patient to open his eyes. If he doesn't respond, gently lift his upper eyelids. Inspect each pupil for size and shape, and compare the two *for equality. To evaluate pupil size more precisely,* use a chart showing the various pupil sizes (in increments of 1 mm, with the normal diameter ranging from 2 to 6 mm). Remember, pupil size varies considerably, and some patients have normally unequal pupils (anisocoria). Also see if the pupils are positioned in, or deviated from, the midline. (See *Testing the pupils.*)

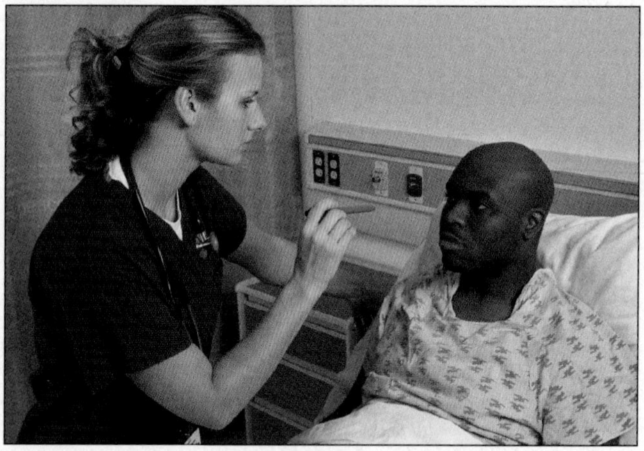

■ Test the patient's direct light response. First, darken the room. Then hold each eyelid open in turn, keeping the other eye covered. Swing the penlight from the patient's ear toward the midline of the face. Shine the light directly into the eye (as shown above). Normally, the pupil constricts immediately. When you remove the penlight, the pupil should dilate immediately. Wait about 20 seconds before testing the other pupil *to allow it to recover from reflex stimulation.*

■ Test consensual light response. Hold both eyelids open, but shine the light into one eye only. Watch for constriction in the other pupil, *which indicates proper nerve function of the optic chiasm.*

■ Brighten the room and have the conscious patient open his eyes. Observe the eyelids for ptosis or drooping. Then check extraocular movements. Hold up one finger, and ask the patient to follow it with his eyes alone. As you move the finger up, down, laterally, and obliquely, see if the patient's eyes track together to follow your finger (conjugate gaze). Watch for involuntary jerking or oscillating eye movements (nystagmus).

■ Check accommodation. Hold up one finger midline to the patient's face and several feet away. Have the patient focus on your finger. Gradually move your finger toward his nose while he focuses on your finger. *This action should cause his eyes to converge and both pupils to constrict equally.*

■ Bring a pencil or other object in from the side and have the patient state when the object enters his field of vision. *This tests his peripheral field.*

Using the Rancho Los Amigos Cognitive Scale

Widely used to classify brain-injured patients according to their behavior, the Rancho Los Amigos Cognitive Scale describes the phases of recovery—from coma to independent functioning—on a scale of I (unresponsive) to VIII (purposeful, appropriate, alert, and oriented). This chart is useful when assessing patients with posttraumatic amnesia.

LEVEL	RESPONSE	CHARACTERISTICS
I	None	The patient is unresponsive to any stimulus, including pain.
II	Generalized	The patient makes limited, inconsistent, nonpurposeful responses, often to pain only.
III	Localized	The patient can localize and withdraw from painful stimuli, can make purposeful responses and focus on presented objects, and may follow simple commands, but inconsistently and in a delayed manner.
IV	Confused and agitated	The patient is alert but agitated, confused, disoriented, and aggressive. He can't perform self-care and has no awareness of present events. Bizarre behavior is likely; agitation appears related to internal confusion.
V	Confused and inappropriate	The patient is alert and responds to commands but is easily distracted and can't concentrate on tasks or learn new information. He becomes agitated in response to external stimuli, and his behavior and speech are inappropriate. His memory is severely impaired and he can't carry over learning from one situation to another.
VI	Confused and appropriate	The patient has some awareness of himself and others but is inconsistently oriented. He can follow simple directions consistently with cueing and can relearn some old skills, such as activities of daily living, but continues to have serious memory problems (especially short-term memory).
VII	Automatic and appropriate	The patient is consistently oriented with little or no confusion but frequently appears robotic when performing daily routines. His awareness of himself and his interaction with his environment increase, but he lacks insight, judgment, problem-solving skills, and the ability to plan realistically.
VIII	Purposeful and appropriate	The patient is alert and oriented, recalls and integrates past events, learns new activities, and performs activities of daily living independently; however, deficits in stress tolerance, judgment, and abstract reasoning persist. He may function in society at a reduced level.

Testing the pupils

Slightly darken the room. Then test the pupils for direct response (reaction of the pupil you're testing) and consensual response (reaction of the opposite pupil) by holding a penlight about 20″ (51 cm) from the patient's eyes, directing the light at the eye from the side.

Next, test accommodation by placing your finger about 4″ (10 cm) from the bridge of the patient's nose. Ask him to look at a fixed object in the distance and then to look at your finger. His eyes should converge and his pupils should constrict.

Grading pupil size

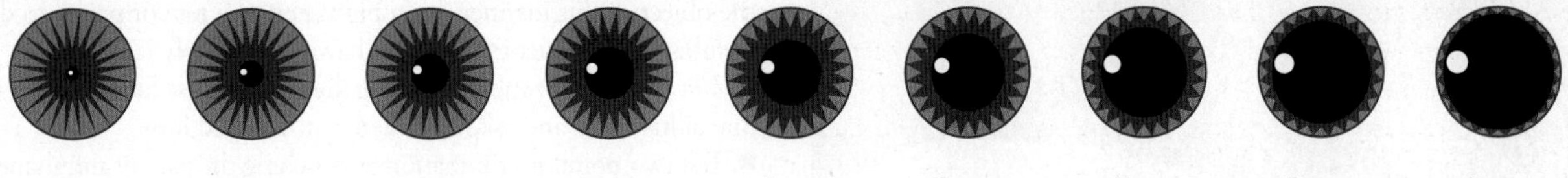

■ Test the corneal reflex by touching a wisp of cotton ball to the cornea. *This test normally causes an immediate blink reflex.* Repeat for the other eye.

NURSING ALERT *Excessive testing of the corneal reflex can cause corneal damage. Perform this assessment carefully.*

■ If the patient is unconscious, test the oculocephalic (doll's eye) reflex. Hold the patient's eyelids open. Then quickly but gently turn the patient's head to one side and then the other. If the patient's eyes move in the opposite direction from the side to which you turn the head, the reflex is intact.

NURSING ALERT *Never test the doll's eye reflex if you know or suspect that the patient has a cervical spine injury* because permanent spinal cord damage may result.

Evaluating motor function

■ If the patient is conscious, test his grip strength in both hands at the same time. Extend your hands, ask him to squeeze your fingers as hard as he can, and compare the strength of each hand. Grip strength is usually slightly stronger in the dominant hand.

- Test arm strength by having the patient close his eyes and hold his arms straight out in front of him with the palms up (as shown below). See if either arm drifts downward or pronates, *indicating muscle weakness.*

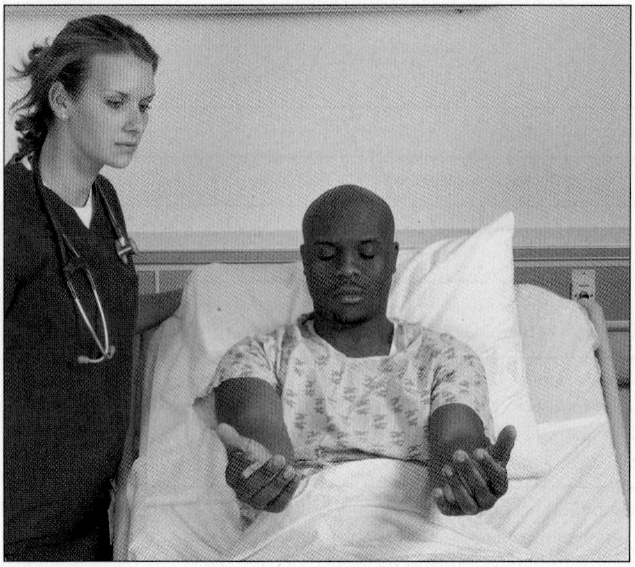

- Test leg strength by having the patient raise his legs, one at a time (as shown below), against gentle downward pressure from your hand. Gently push down on each leg at the midpoint of the thigh *to evaluate muscle strength.*

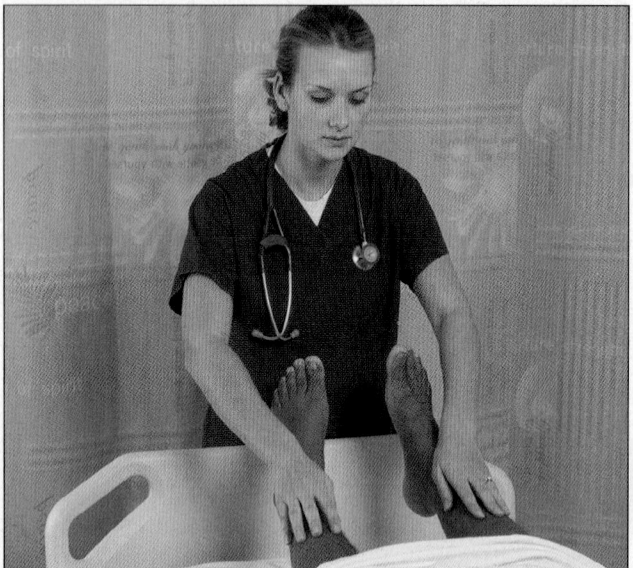

NURSING ALERT *If decorticate or decerebrate posturing develops in response to stimuli, notify the practitioner immediately.* (*See* **Identifying warning postures.**)

- Evaluate muscle tone by having the patient flex and extend the extremities on both sides.
- Test the plantar reflex. To do so, stroke the lateral aspect of the sole of the patient's foot with your thumbnail or another moderately sharp object. *Normally, this elicits flexion of all toes* (as shown on top right). Watch for a positive Babinski's sign—dorsiflexion of the great toe with fanning of the other toes—*which indicates an upper motor neuron lesion.*

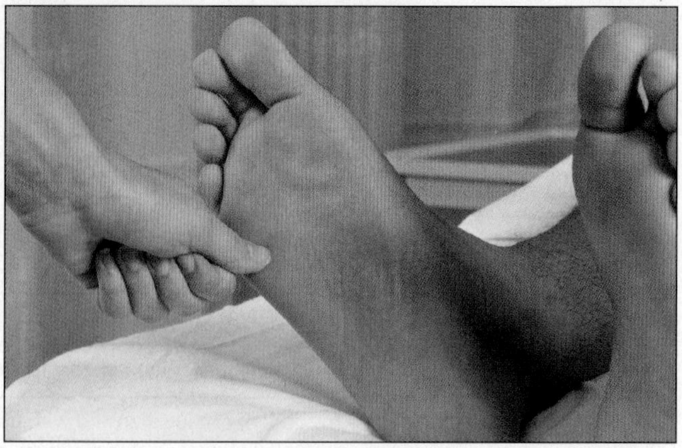

Evaluating sensory function

- To test for pain sensation, start by having the patient close his eyes. Then, using a safety pin, gently touch various areas of the patient's body, alternating between the sharp and dull end of the pin. Ask the patient "Is this sharp or dull?" as you proceed. Compare corresponding areas on the two sides of the body. Start with both shoulders and then proceed with the inner and outer aspects of the forearms, the thumbs and little fingers, the fronts of the thighs, the medial and lateral aspects of both calves, the little toes, and the medial aspect of the buttock *to test most of the dermatomes and major peripheral nerves.*[10]
- Test the patient's sense of light touch by touching his skin lightly with a wisp of cotton while his eyes remain closed. Ask him to respond whenever he feels a touch. Compare corresponding areas on the two sides of the body.[10]
- To test vibratory sense, apply a tuning fork over different bony prominences while the patient keeps his eyes closed. Tap the tuning fork on the heel of your hand and place it firmly over a distal interphalangeal joint of the patient's finger, and then over the interphalangeal joint of the big toe. Ask the patient to tell you when the sensation stops; then touch the fork to stop it.[11]
- Assess position sense (proprioception) by grasping the patient's big toe, holding it by its sides between your thumb and index finger, and then pulling it away from the other toes. Show the patient "up" and "down" as you move the toe clearly upward and downward. Then, have the patient close his eyes and ask him to tell you whether you're moving his toe up or down as you move the large toe in an arc. Repeat several times on each side.[10]
- To test stereognosis, have the patient close his eyes. Place a familiar object, such as a paperclip or key, in the patient's hand and have him identify it. If motor impairment prevents the patient from identifying the object in this manner, use a blunt end of a pen or pencil to draw a number in the patient's palm and have him identify it.[10]
- Test point localization by having the patient close his eyes; then touch one of his limbs and ask him where you touched him.
- Test two-point discrimination by touching the patient simultaneously in two contralateral areas with an opened paperclip. Find the minimal distance at which the patient can discriminate one from two points.[10]

Completing the neurologic examination

- Assess the patient's temperature, pulse, respiratory rate, and blood pressure. His pulse pressure—the difference between systolic pressure and diastolic pressure—is especially important *because widening pulse pressure can indicate increasing ICP.*
- Perform hand hygiene.[1,2,3,4,5]
- Disinfect your stethoscope and other equipment as necessary using a disinfectant pad.[12,13]
- Perform hand hygiene.[1,2,3,4,5]
- Document the procedure.[14,15,16]

Identifying warning postures

Decorticate and decerebrate postures are ominous signs of central nervous system deterioration.

Decorticate (abnormal flexion)

In the decorticate posture, the patient's arms are adducted and flexed, with the wrists and fingers flexed on the chest. The legs may be stiffly extended and internally rotated, with plantar flexion of the feet.

The decorticate posture may indicate a lesion of the frontal lobe, internal capsule, or cerebral peduncles.

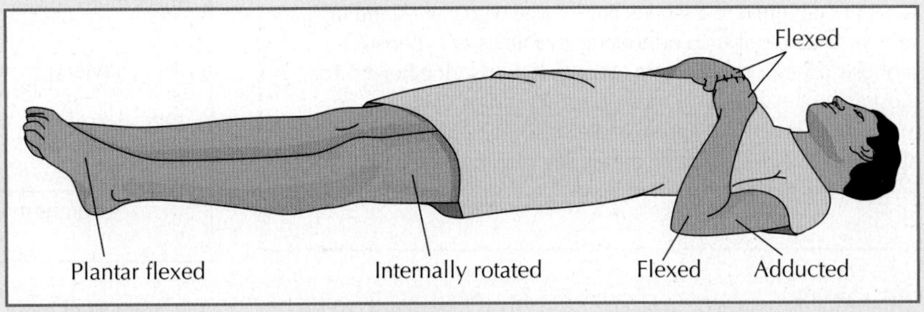

Decerebrate (extension)

In the decerebrate posture, the patient's arms are adducted and extended with the wrists pronated and the fingers flexed. One or both legs may be stiffly extended, with plantar flexion of the feet.

The decerebrate posture may indicate lesions of the upper brain stem.

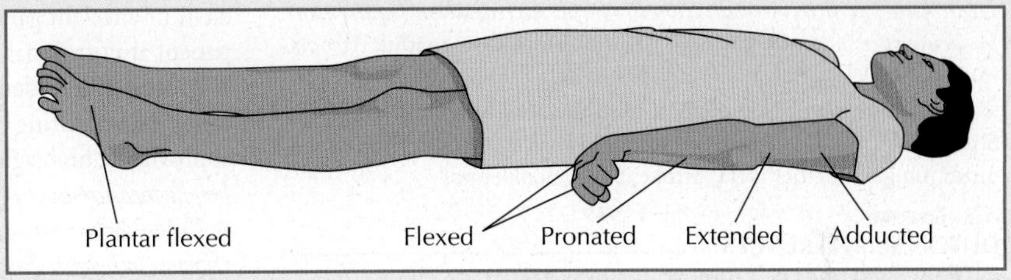

Special considerations

NURSING ALERT *If a previously stable patient suddenly develops a change in neurologic or routine vital signs, further assess his condition, and notify the practitioner immediately.* One of the earliest changes that may occur with increased ICP is a change in LOC. Changes in pulse and blood pressure do occur, but generally late in the course of increasing ICP.

- Be aware that clinical issues that commonly affect older adults may negatively influence the neurologic assessment, including fluid and electrolyte imbalances, opioid analgesia administration, fatigue, environmental changes, pain, infection, and depression.[9]
- In acute care settings, older adults are at risk for delirium, so the neurologic assessment should include an ongoing assessment using a standardized delirium assessment tool *to ensure early detection.*[9]
- If you suspect the patient is having a stroke, use the National Institutes of Health Stroke Scale *to evaluate him.*[17]

Documentation

Baseline data require detailed documentation; subsequent notes can be brief unless the patient's condition changes. Record the patient's LOC and orientation, pupillary activity, motor function, and routine vital signs. To save time while keeping complete records, you may be allowed to use abbreviations. To avoid misinterpretation, use only commonly understood abbreviations and terms, such as PERRLA (pupils equal, round, reactive to light and accommodation) and EOM (extraocular movements).

Also describe the patient's behavior—for example, "difficult to arouse by gentle shaking," "sleepy," or "unresponsive to painful stimuli."

REFERENCES

1 World Health Organization. (2009). "WHO guidelines on hand hygiene in health care: First global patient safety challenge, clean care is safer care" [Online]. Accessed May 2015 via the Web at http://whqlibdoc.who.int/publications/2009/9789241597906_eng.pdf (Level IV)

2 The Joint Commission. (2015). Standard NPSG.07.01.01. *Comprehensive accreditation manual for hospitals: The official handbook.* Oakbrook Terrace, IL: The Joint Commission. (Level VII)

3 Centers for Disease Control and Prevention. (2002). Guideline for hand hygiene in health-care settings: Recommendations of the Healthcare Infection Control Practices Advisory Committee and the HICPAC/SHEA/APIC/IDSA Hand Hygiene Task Force. *MMWR Recommendations and Reports, 51*(RR-16), 1–45. Accessed May 2015 via the Web at http://www.cdc.gov/mmwr/pdf/rr/rr5116.pdf (Level II)

4 Centers for Medicare & Medicaid Services, Department of Health and Human Services. (2014). Condition of participation: infection control. 42 C.F.R. § 482.42.

5 American Osteopathic Association. (2014). Standard 07.01.21. *Healthcare Facilities Accreditation Program: Accreditation requirements for acute care hospitals.* Chicago, IL: American Osteopathic Association. (Level VII)

6 The Joint Commission. (2015). Standard NPSG.01.01.01. *Comprehensive accreditation manual for hospitals: The official handbook.* Oakbrook Terrace, IL: The Joint Commission. (Level VII)

7 Centers for Medicare & Medicaid Services, Department of Health and Human Services. (2014). Condition of participation: Patient's rights. 42 C.F.R. § 482.13(c)(1).

8 American Osteopathic Association. (2014). Standard 15.01.16. *Healthcare Facilities Accreditation Program: Accreditation requirements for acute care hospitals.* Chicago, IL: American Osteopathic Association. (Level VII)

9 Thompson, H. J. (2009). "Neurologic assessment of the older adult: A guide for nurses" [Online]. Accessed May 2015 via the Web at http://www.aann.org/pdf/cpg/aannneuroassessmentolderadult.pdf (Level VII)

10 Bickley, L. (2013). *Bates' guide to physical examination and history taking* (11th ed.). Philadelphia, PA: Lippincott Williams & Wilkins.

11 Hickey, J. V. (2014). *The clinical practice of neurological and neurosurgical nursing* (7th ed.). Philadelphia, PA: Wolters Kluwer.

12 Rutala, W. A., et al. (2008). "Guideline for disinfection and sterilization in healthcare facilities, 2008" [Online]. Accessed May 2015 via the Web at http://www.cdc.gov/hicpac/pdf/guidelines/Disinfection_Nov_2008.pdf (Level I)

13 American Osteopathic Association. (2014). Standard 07.02.03. *Healthcare Facilities Accreditation Program: Accreditation requirements for acute care hospitals.* Chicago, IL: American Osteopathic Association. (Level VII)

14 The Joint Commission. (2015). Standard RC.01.03.01. *Comprehensive accreditation manual for hospitals: The official handbook.* Oakbrook Terrace, IL: The Joint Commission. (Level VII)

15 Centers for Medicare & Medicaid Services, Department of Health and Human Services. (2014). Condition of participation: Medical record services. 42 C.F.R. § 482.24(b).

Overcoming height measurement problems

A patient confined to a wheelchair or one who can't stand up straight because of such orthopedic problems as kyphosis or scoliosis poses a challenge to accurately measuring height. The most accurate alternative method uses a sliding caliper—the method of choice—to approximate standing height.[8] Other alternative methods include measuring recumbent length, knee height, forearm length, or demispan.[9]

16 American Osteopathic Association. (2014). Standard 10.00.03. *Healthcare Facilities Accreditation Program: Accreditation requirements for acute care hospitals.* Chicago, IL: American Osteopathic Association. (Level VII)

17 National Institute of Neurological Disorders and Stroke. (n.d.). "NIH Stroke scale" [Online]. Accessed May 2015 via the Web at http://www.ninds.nih.gov/doctors/NIH_Stroke_Scale_Booklet.pdf

ADDITIONAL REFERENCES

Iacono, L. A., et al. (2014). Standardizing neurological assessment. *Journal of Neuroscience Nursing, 46,* 125–132.

Lower, J. (2010). Using pain to assess neurologic response. *Nursing Critical Care, 5*(4), 11–12.

Rank, W. (2013). Performing a focused neurologic assessment. *Nursing, 43*(2), 37–40.

Taylor, C., et al. (2015). *Fundamentals of nursing: The art and science of nursing care* (8th ed.). Philadelphia, PA: Wolters Kluwer

NUTRITIONAL SCREENING

A patient's nutritional status is evaluated by examining information from several sources, such as the patient's medical history, physical assessment findings, and laboratory results. If nutritional screening determines the patient is at risk for a nutritional disorder, a comprehensive nutritional assessment may then be conducted to set goals and determine interventions to correct actual or potential imbalances.[1]

Nutritional screening also examines certain variables to determine the risk of problems in specific populations—such as pregnant women, elderly people, or those with certain disorders (such as cardiac disorders)—to detect deficiencies or potential imbalances.

Equipment

Scale with stadiometer ▪ nutritional screening tool ▪ Optional: chair or bed scale, tape measure.

Preparation of equipment

Select the appropriate scale—usually, a standing scale for an ambulatory patient or a chair or bed scale for an acutely ill or debilitated patient. Make sure the scale is balanced; *standing scales and, to a lesser extent, bed scales may become unbalanced when transported.*

Implementation

- Perform hand hygiene.[2,3,4,5,6]
- Confirm the patient's identity using at least two patient identifiers.[7]
- Explain the purpose of and procedure for nutritional screening to the patient.
- Ask the patient to remove his shoes and obtain his weight using a scale. *Weight provides a rough estimate of body composition.*
- Ask about unplanned or unintentional weight loss or gain. Determine how much weight the patient lost or gained and over what period of time.

Calculating BMI

Use one of the formulas below to calculate your patient's body mass index (BMI).

$$\text{BMI} = \left(\frac{\text{weight in pounds}}{\text{height in inches} \times \text{height in inches}}\right) \times 703$$

OR

$$\text{BMI} = \left(\frac{\text{weight in kilograms}}{\text{height in centimeters} \times \text{height in centimeters}}\right) \times 10{,}000$$

A weight loss of more than 5% of body weight in 30 days or 10% in 180 days, or a weight gain of 10 lb (4.5 kg) or more in 180 days places the patient at nutritional risk.

- Measure the patient's height while he's standing erect without shoes, using the measuring bar on the scale. If the patient can't stand, you can approximate his height by using an alternative method. (See *Overcoming height measurement problems.*)
- Calculate or estimate body mass index (BMI) *to evaluate weight in relation to height.* (See *Calculating BMI.*)[10]
- A BMI of 18.5 to 24.9 defines healthy weight; a BMI of 25 to 29.9 defines overweight; a BMI of 30 or more defines obesity.[11] (See *Determining BMI.*)
- Evaluate the patient's weight distribution by measuring his waist circumference around his abdomen at the level of the iliac crest. Before reading the tape measure, ensure that the tape is snug but doesn't compress the skin and is parallel to the floor. If the measurement is greater than 35″ (89 cm) for a woman or 40″ (102 cm) for a man (with a normal BMI), the patient is at greater risk for health problems.[1] People with a high distribution of fat around their waists as opposed to their hips and thighs are at greater risk for such diseases as type 2 diabetes, dyslipidemia, hypertension, and cardiovascular disease.[10,12,13]
- Question the patient about his eating habits, living environment, and functional *status to determine whether he's at risk for nutritional problems. A problem in any of these areas places the patient at risk and requires further nutritional assessment.* (See *Risk factors for malnutrition,* page 554.)
- Review the medical record and interview the patient *to determine whether his present illness or medical history places him at nutritional risk.*
- Review physical assessment findings for signs of poor nutrition. (See *Evaluating nutritional disorders,* page 555.)
- Make a referral to a registered dietitian if a nutritional screening suggests the patient is at risk for nutritional problems.[1] A registered dietitian will then perform a comprehensive nutritional assessment.
- Perform hand hygiene.[2,3,4,5,6]
- Document the procedure.[17,18,19]

Special considerations

- The nutritional screening is typically performed during the initial nursing history and physical assessment, but should be completed within 24 hours of admission.[1,20,21]
- When measuring height, note the growth of children as well as diminishing height of older adults. Growth of children may be noted on standardized charts *to assess growth patterns for possible abnormalities.* Diminishing height of older adults may be related to osteoporotic changes and should be investigated.

Documentation

Record the date and time of the nutritional screening. Place the patient's height and weight on the screening form as well as the graphic sheet or patient care flow sheet. Note the type of scale used. Complete

Determining BMI

Body mass index (BMI) measures weight in relation to height. The BMI ranges shown here are for adults. Although these ranges don't provide an exact guide for healthy or unhealthy weight, they show that health risks increase with increasing weight and obesity. To use the graph below, find the patient's weight along the bottom and then go straight up until you come to the line that matches his height. The shaded area indicates whether the patient is healthy, overweight, or obese.

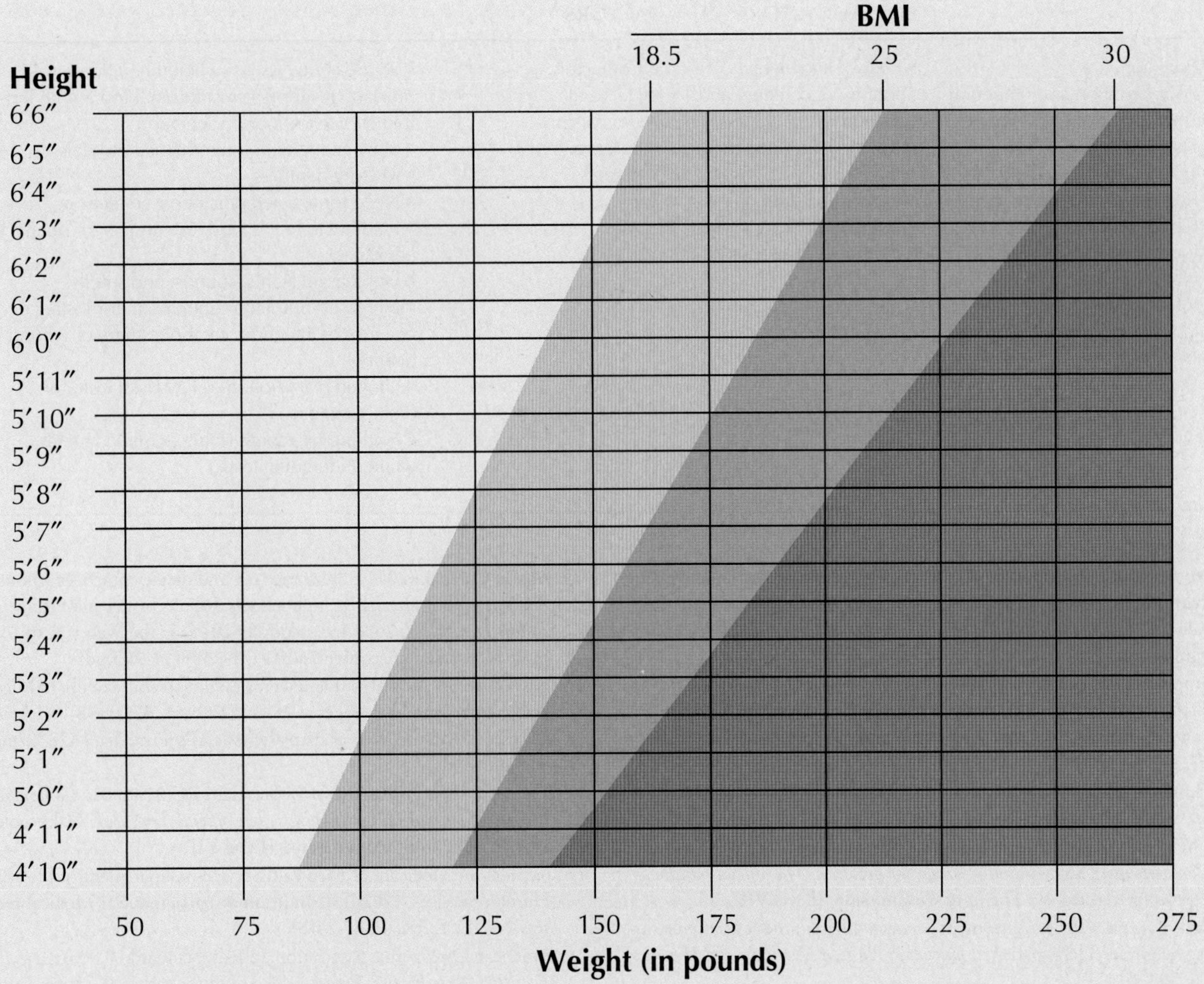

Adapted from U.S. Department of Agriculture, U.S. Department of Health and Human Services. (2010). *Dietary guidelines for Americans* (7th ed.). Washington, DC: U.S. Government Printing Office.

the screening tool as recommended. Calculate and record the patient's BMI. Use a progress note to record information that doesn't have a space on the screening tool. Record whether the patient has experienced any weight loss or significant weight gain, the time over which the loss or gain occurred, and how much weight was lost or gained.

Make sure laboratory results are documented, including the name of anyone you notified of abnormal results, and whether orders were given. Note any nutritional problems detected during the physical examination and review of the patient's medical record. Include any patient teaching provided. For patients at nutritional risk, record the date and time, names of the people notified and whether those who were notified came to see the patient, any orders received, and your nursing interventions and the patient's response.

REFERENCES

1 Mueller, C., et al. (2011). A.S.P.E.N. clinical guidelines: Nutrition screening, assessment, and intervention in adults. *Journal of Parenteral and Enteral Nutrition, 35,* 16–24. Accessed May 2015 via the Web at http://pen.sagepub.com/content/35/1/16.full.pdf (Level VII)

2 The Joint Commission. (2015). Standard NPSG.07.01.01. *Comprehensive accreditation manual for hospitals: The official handbook.* Oakbrook Terrace, IL: The Joint Commission. (Level VII)

3 Centers for Disease Control and Prevention. (2002). Guideline for hand hygiene in health-care settings: Recommendations of the Healthcare Infection Control Practices Advisory Committee and the HICPAC/SHEA/APIC/IDSA Hand Hygiene Task Force. *MMWR Recommendations and Reports, 51*(RR-16), 1–45. Accessed May 2015 via the Web at http://www.cdc.gov/mmwr/pdf/rr/rr5116.pdf (Level II)

Risk factors for malnutrition[14,15]

Several types of risk factors can place a patient at risk for malnutrition. Processes associated with aging can also lead to malnutrition, although aging itself isn't an independent risk factor. Risk factors for malnutrition include medical, lifestyle and social, psychological, and hospitalization-related.

Medical factors	Lifestyle and social factors	Psychological factors	Hospitalization-related factors
■ Poor appetite ■ Poor dentition and other oral problems ■ Dysphagia ■ Loss of taste and smell ■ Respiratory disorders ■ GI disorders ■ Endocrine disorders ■ Neurologic disorders ■ Infections ■ Physical disability and poor mobility ■ Drug interactions ■ Other disease states, such as cancer	■ Lack of knowledge about food, cooking, and nutrition ■ Isolation and loneliness ■ Poverty ■ Inability to shop or prepare food ■ Substance abuse	■ Confusion ■ Dementia ■ Depression ■ Bereavement ■ Anxiety	■ Food-service issues (when the patient's sole nutritional supply is institutional food, with limited choice or poor presentation) ■ Slow eating with limited time for meals ■ Missing dentures ■ Need for assisted or supervised feeding ■ Inability to reach food, use cutlery, or open packages ■ Unpleasant sights, sounds, and smells ■ Increased nutrient requirement (for instance, because of infection, catabolic state, or wound healing) ■ Limited provision for religious or cultural dietary needs ■ Nothing-by-mouth status or missed meals while undergoing tests

4 World Health Organization. (2009). "WHO guidelines on hand hygiene in health care: First global patient safety challenge, clean care is safer care" [Online]. Accessed May 2015 via the Web at http://whqlibdoc.who.int/publications/2009/9789241597906_eng.pdf (Level IV)

5 American Osteopathic Association. (2014). Standard 07.01.21. *Healthcare Facilities Accreditation Program: Accreditation requirements for acute care hospitals.* Chicago, IL: American Osteopathic Association. (Level VII)

6 Centers for Medicare & Medicaid Services, Department of Health and Human Services. (2014). Condition of participation: Infection control. 42 C.F.R. § 482.42.

7 The Joint Commission. (2015). Standard NPSG.01.01.01. *Comprehensive accreditation manual for hospitals: The official handbook.* Oakbrook Terrace, IL: The Joint Commission. (Level VII)

8 Frid, H., et al. (2013). Agreement between different methods of measuring height in elderly patients. *Journal of Human Nutrition and Dietetics, 26,* 504–511.

9 Froehlich-Grobe, K., et al. (2011). Measuring height without a stadiometer. *American Journal of Physical Medicine and Rehabilitation, 90,* 658–666. Accessed May 2015 via the Web at http://www.ncbi.nlm.nih.gov/pmc/articles/PMC3148840/

10 U.S. Department of Health and Human Services. (1998). "Clinical guidelines on the identification, evaluation, and treatment of overweight and obesity in adults. NIH Publication No. 98-4083" [Online]. Accessed May 2015 via the Web at http://www.nhlbi.nih.gov/guidelines/obesity/ob_gdlns.pdf

11 U.S. Department of Agriculture & the U.S. Department of Health and Human Services. (2010). "Report of the dietary guidelines advisory committee on the dietary guidelines for Americans" [Online]. Accessed May 2015 via the Web at http://www.health.gov/dietaryguidelines/dga2010/DietaryGuidelines2010.pdf

12 Huat, M., et al. (2011). Insulin resistance, low cardiorespiratory fitness, and increased exercise blood pressure: Contribution of abdominal obesity. *Hypertension, 58,* 1036–1042.

13 McEvoy, J. W., et al. (2010). Coronary artery calcium progression: An important clinical measurement? A review of published reports. *Journal of the American College of Cardiology, 56,* 1613–1622.

14 De Morais, C. et al. (2013). Nutritional risk of European elderly. *European Journal of Clinical Nutrition, 67,* 1215–1219.

15 Arcan, C., et al. (2011). Substance use and dietary practices among students attending alternative high schools: Results from a pilot study. *BMC Public Health, 11,* 263. Accessed May 2015 via the Web at http://www.biomedcentral.com/content/pdf/1471-2458-11-263.pdf

16 Bassiouny, M. A. (2013). Dental erosion due to abuse of illicit drugs and acidic carbonated beverages. *General Dentistry, 61*(2), 38–44. Accessed May 2015 via the Web at http://www.agd.org/media/142832/ma13_bassiouny.pdf

17 The Joint Commission. (2015). Standard RC.01.03.01. *Comprehensive accreditation manual for hospitals: The official handbook.* Oakbrook Terrace, IL: The Joint Commission. (Level VII)

18 Centers for Medicare & Medicaid Services, Department of Health and Human Services. (2014). Condition of participation: Medical records services. 42 C.F.R. § 482.24(b).

19 American Osteopathic Association. (2014). Standard 10.00.03. *Healthcare Facilities Accreditation Program: Accreditation requirements for acute care hospitals.* Chicago, IL: American Osteopathic Association. (Level VII)

20 The Joint Commission. (2015). Standard PC.01.02.01. *Comprehensive accreditation manual for hospitals: The official handbook.* Oakbrook Terrace, IL: The Joint Commission. (Level VII)

21 American Osteopathic Association. (2014). Standard 10.01.24. *Healthcare Facilities Accreditation Program: Accreditation requirements for acute care hospitals.* Chicago, IL: American Osteopathic Association. (Level VII)

Additional references

Boaz, M., et al. (2013). Nurses and nutrition: A survey of knowledge and attitudes regarding nutrition assessment and care of hospitalized elderly patients. *Journal of Continuing Education in Nursing, 44,* 357–364.

Caccialanza, R., et al. (2013). Serum prealbumin: An independent marker of short-term energy intake in the presence of multiple-organ disease involvement. *Nutrition, 29,* 580–582.

Craven, R.F., & Hirnle, C.J. (2012). *Fundamentals of nursing: Human health and function* (7th ed.). Philadelphia, PA: Lippincott Williams & Wilkins.

Omidvari, A. H., et al. (2013). Nutritional screening for improving professional practice for patient outcomes in hospital and primary care settings. *Cochrane Database of Systematic Reviews, 2013*(6), CD005539.

Nettina, S.M. (2014). *Lippincott manual of nursing practice* (10th ed.). Philadelphia, PA: Wolters Kluwer.

Evaluating nutritional disorders

This chart can help you interpret your nutritional assessment findings. Body systems are listed below, with signs or symptoms and the implications for each.

BODY SYSTEM OR REGION	SIGN OR SYMPTOM	IMPLICATIONS
General	■ Weakness and fatigue	■ Anemia or electrolyte imbalance
	■ Weight loss	■ Decreased calorie intake, increased calorie use, or inadequate nutrient intake or absorption
Skin, hair, and nails	■ Dry, flaky skin	■ Vitamin A, vitamin B–complex, or linoleic acid deficiency
	■ Dry skin with poor turgor	■ Dehydration
	■ Rough, scaly skin with bumps	■ Vitamin A deficiency
	■ Petechiae or ecchymoses	■ Vitamin C or K deficiency
	■ Sore that won't heal	■ Protein, vitamin C, or zinc deficiency
	■ Thinning, dry hair	■ Protein deficiency
	■ Spoon-shaped, brittle, or ridged nails	■ Iron deficiency
Eyes	■ Night blindness; corneal swelling, softening, or dryness; Bitot spots (gray triangular patches on the conjunctiva)	■ Vitamin A deficiency
	■ Red conjunctiva	■ Riboflavin deficiency
Throat and mouth	■ Cracks at the corner of the mouth	■ Riboflavin or niacin deficiency
	■ Magenta tongue	■ Riboflavin deficiency
	■ Beefy, red tongue	■ Vitamin B_{12} deficiency
	■ Soft, spongy, bleeding gums	■ Vitamin C deficiency
	■ Poor dentition	■ Overconsumption of refined sugars or acidic carbonated beverages; illicit drug use[16]
	■ Swollen neck (goiter)	■ Iodine deficiency
Cardiovascular	■ Edema ■ Third and fourth heart sounds ■ Shortness of breath ■ Cough	■ Protein deficiency
	■ Tachycardia, murmur, hypotension	■ Fluid volume deficit; anemia
GI	■ Ascites	■ Protein deficiency
Musculoskeletal	■ Bone pain and bow legs	■ Vitamin D or calcium deficiency
	■ Muscle wasting	■ Protein, carbohydrate, and fat deficiency
Neurologic	■ Altered mental status ■ Ataxia	■ Dehydration and thiamine or vitamin B_{12} deficiency
	■ Paresthesia, neuropathies	■ Vitamin B_{12}, pyridoxine, or thiamine deficiency

EQUIPMENT

How the Ommaya reservoir works

To insert an Ommaya reservoir, the practitioner drills a burr hole and inserts the device's catheter through the patient's nondominant frontal lobe into the lateral ventricle. The reservoir, which has a self-sealing silicone injection dome, rests over the burr hole under a scalp flap. This creates a slight, soft bulge on the scalp about the size of a quarter. Usually, drugs are injected into the dome with a syringe.

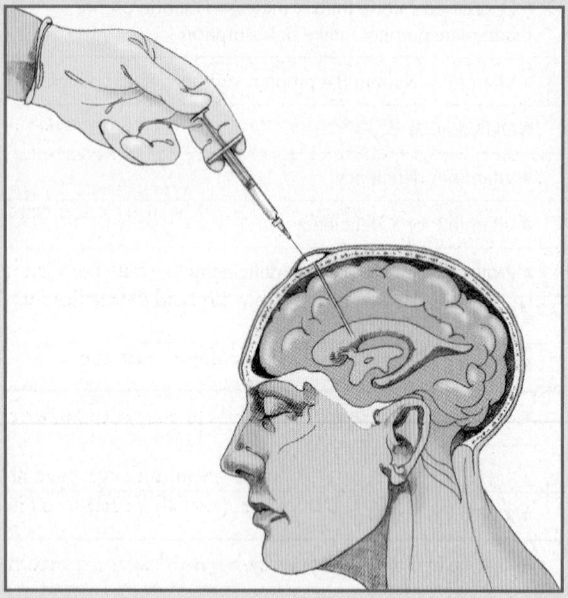

O

OMMAYA RESERVOIR DRUG INFUSION

Also known as a *subcutaneous cerebrospinal fluid (CSF) reservoir,* the Ommaya reservoir allows delivery of long-term drug therapy to the CSF by way of the brain's ventricles. It's most commonly used for chemotherapy and pain management, specifically for treating central nervous system (CNS) lymphoma, malignant CNS disease, and meningeal carcinomatosis. The reservoir spares the patient repeated lumbar punctures to administer chemotherapeutic drugs, analgesics, antibiotics, and antifungals.

The reservoir is a mushroom-shaped silicone apparatus with an attached catheter. It's surgically implanted beneath the patient's scalp, and the catheter is threaded into the ventricle through a burr hole in the skull. (See *How the Ommaya reservoir works.*) Besides providing convenient, comparatively painless access to CSF, the Ommaya reservoir permits consistent and predictable drug distribution throughout the subarachnoid space and CNS. It also allows for measurement of intracranial pressure (ICP).

Before reservoir insertion, the patient may receive a local or general anesthetic, depending on his condition and the practitioner's preference. After an X-ray confirms placement of the reservoir, a pressure dressing is applied for 24 hours. The sutures may be removed in about 10 days. However, the reservoir can be used within 48 hours to deliver drugs, obtain CSF pressure measurements, drain CSF, and withdraw CSF specimens.

The practitioner usually injects drugs into the Ommaya reservoir, but a specially trained nurse may perform this procedure if permitted by the facility and the state's nurse practice act. This sterile procedure usually takes 15 to 30 minutes.

Equipment

Equipment varies but may include the following: Preservative-free prescribed drug ■ personal protective equipment (sterile gloves, gown, mask and goggles or mask with face shield) ■ antiseptic solution (avoid antiseptics containing alcohol or acetone) ■ 10-mL syringe ■ two 3-mL syringes ■ 25G 5/8″ (1.6-cm) butterfly needle ■ 1-mL prefilled syringe containing preservative-free normal saline solution ■ sterile drape ■ sterile gauze pads ■ thermometer ■ sphygmomanometer ■ stethoscope ■ disinfectant pad ■ Optional: CSF collection tubes, label, laboratory biohazard transport bag, additional medications as prescribed.

For chemotherapy

Material safety data sheet for prescribed chemotherapy drug ■ prescribed chemotherapy medication ■ scale ■ several pairs of powder-free chemotherapy gloves ■ nonlinting, nonabsorbent disposable gown ■ face shield ■ National Institute for Occupational Safety and Health–approved respirator mask (if aerosolization is likely)[1] ■ syringes with luer-lock connector ■ chemotherapy sharps container ■ hazardous-waste container approved for cytotoxic waste ■ chemotherapy spill kit ■ booties ■ supplies for emergency treatment (soap, eyewash, sterile saline solution for irrigation) ■ emergency equipment (crash cart with cardiac medications, defibrillator, handheld resuscitation bag with mask, intubation equipment).

Preparation of equipment

Make sure that a chemotherapy spill kit and emergency equipment are readily available if chemotherapy is being administered. Also ensure that the emergency equipment is functioning properly.

Ensure that the medication to be administered is brought to room temperature as needed.

Implementation

■ Avoid distractions and interruptions when preparing and administering *medications to prevent medication administration errors.*[2,3]

Preparing for medication administration

■ Review the patient's medical record for an allergy or other contraindication to the prescribed medication. If an allergy or a contraindication is present, don't administer the medication; notify the practitioner.[4,5]

■ Verify the order on the patient's medication administration record by checking it against the practitioner's order.[4,5,6]

■ Compare the medication label with the order in the patient's medical record.[4,5,6]

■ Check the expiration date on the medication. If the medication is expired, return it to the pharmacy and obtain new medication.[4,5,6]

■ Visually inspect the solution for particles, discoloration, or other loss of integrity; don't administer the medication if its integrity is compromised.[4,5,6]

■ Discuss any unresolved concerns about the medication with the patient's practitioner.[4,5,6]

■ Perform hand hygiene.[7,8,9,10,11]

■ Confirm the patient's identity using two patient identifiers.[12]

■ If the patient is receiving the medication for the first time, teach him about the potential adverse reactions and discuss any other concerns related to the medication.[4,5,6]

■ Assess the patient's baseline vital signs, pain level, and neurologic status; if any are altered, stop the procedure and notify the practitioner.

Preparing for chemotherapy administration

■ Review the patient's medical record for initial cancer diagnosis and staging or current cancer status; recent treatments, including surgery, radiation therapy, hormone therapy, cytotoxic therapy, and complementary therapy; medical, psychiatric, and surgical history; presence of allergic or hypersensitivity reactions; pregnancy and reproductive status, including the last menstrual period if applicable; and physical examination that includes assessment of organ function appropriate for the planned treatment regimen.[13,14]

■ Check that the order is written and contains the patient's complete name and a second identifier, the date, the patient's diagnosis, any allergies, and the regimen's name and number (if applicable), including the individual drug's generic name, treatment criteria and dosage calculation method, the patient's height and weight, and any other variables used to calculate the dose. The order must also contain the dosage, the route and rate of administration, the schedule, duration of therapy, cumulative lifetime dose (if applicable), sequence of drug administration (if applicable), and any supportive care treatments appropriate for the regimen, such as premedications for hypersensitivity, nausea, and hydration if necessary. Have another practitioner qualified to prepare or administer chemotherapy do the same.[13,14]

■ Make sure that the practitioner has obtained written informed consent and that the consent form is in the patient's medical record.[13,15]

■ Become familiar with the information contained in the material safety data sheet specific to the prescribed drug.[16]

■ In collaboration with the patient's multidisciplinary team, review the patient's test results, specifically complete blood count, blood urea nitrogen level, platelet count, and liver function studies.[17]

■ Check the expiration date on the medication. If the medication is expired, return it to the pharmacy and obtain new medication.[4,5,6]

■ Visually inspect the solution for particles, discoloration, or other loss of integrity; don't administer the medication if its integrity is compromised.[4,5,6]

■ Perform hand hygiene.[7,8,9,10,11]

■ Confirm the patient's identity using at least two patient identifiers.[12]

■ Review with the patient his current medications, including over-the-counter medications and complementary and alternative therapies; notify the practitioner of any changes.[14]

■ Assess the patient's clinical and performance status.[14]

■ Verify with the patient any allergies, previous reactions, and treatment-related toxicities.[14]

■ Monitor any cumulative chemotherapy dose *to ensure that the patient hasn't reached his maximum lifetime dose.*[17]

■ Ask the patient about any psychosocial concerns or cultural or spiritual issues that may affect treatment, and take action as indicated.[14]

■ Confirm the treatment plan, drug route, and symptom management plan with the patient.[13]

■ Confirm that the patient has received written information regarding his cancer diagnosis and associated chemotherapy regimen, it's associated short- and long-term adverse effects (including fertility risks, as appropriate), goals of therapy, and the continuing care plan.[14]

■ Obtain the patient's vital signs, including pain level, *to use as a baseline for comparison.*

■ Double-check his height, weight, and body surface area.[14]

■ Recalculate the dose, as ordered, using the patient's body surface area and weight, if applicable;[17] check your calculations against the written order.

■ Verify that the drug is properly labeled when you receive it from the pharmacy and that this information includes the patient's full name and second identifier, full generic drug name, drug administration route, total dose to be given, total volume required to administer the dosage, date of administration, and date and time of preparation and expiration. Make sure that it also contains any special handling instructions and a label that clearly identifies the drug as hazardous and for intrathecal use only.[13,14]

Administering the medication or chemotherapeutic agent

■ Ensure that placement of the Ommaya reservoir has been confirmed before initial use.

■ Confirm that informed consent has been obtained and is in the patient's medical record.[15,18]

■ If required, conduct a preprocedure verification *to make sure that all relevant documentation, related information, and equipment are available and correctly identified to the patient's identifiers.*[19,20]

■ Perform hand hygiene.[7,8,9,10,11]

■ Provide privacy and explain the procedure.[6,21]

■ Determine whether the practitioner has ordered any premedications *to combat adverse effects of the prescribed medication or chemotherapeutic agent* and administer them as prescribed following safe medication administration practices.[4,5]

■ Gather the prescribed medication or chemotherapeutic agent and the appropriate equipment.

■ If your facility uses a bar code scanning system, scan your identification badge, the patient's identification bracelet, and the medication's bar code.

■ Position the patient so that he's either sitting or reclining.

■ Perform hand hygiene.[7,8,9,10,11]

■ Open a sterile tray and prepare a sterile field on a work surface close to the patient.

■ Place the prescribed medication or chemotherapeutic agent and necessary supplies on the sterile field. Make sure that all medications on and off the sterile field are clearly labeled.[22,23]

■ Wash your hands using soap and water if the drug is a chemotherapeutic agent; perform hand hygiene if it isn't.[7,8,9,10,11,13]

■ Put on personal protective equipment.[24] If you're administering a chemotherapeutic agent, wear two pairs of sterile, powder-free chemotherapy gloves, a gown, a mask, a face shield if splashing is likely, and a respirator if necessary.[1,13,25] Make sure that your inner glove cuff is worn under the gown cuff and that the outer glove cuff extends over the gown cuff *to fully protect your skin.* Inspect your *gloves to make sure that they're physically intact.*

■ Conduct a time-out immediately before starting the procedure *to perform a final assessment ensuring that the correct patient, site, positioning, and procedure are identified and, as applicable, that all relevant information and necessary equipment are available.*[26]

■ Examine the area over the reservoir for signs of infection or trauma.

■ *To confirm placement and to fill the reservoir,* gently palpate the reservoir and pump it three or four times; expect free flow of CSF from the ventricle into the reservoir.

■ Drape the reservoir site with a sterile drape and prepare the patient's scalp with an antiseptic solution, as determined by your facility, working in a circular motion from the center outward. Allow the solution to dry completely *to achieve its maximum effect.*[27]

NURSING ALERT *Chemotherapeutic drugs are considered high-alert medications* because they can cause significant patient harm if used in error. *Never administer a chemotherapeutic drug without performing an independent double-check with another practitioner who is qualified to prepare or administer chemotherapy.*[13,14,28]

NURSING ALERT *Vinca alkaloids such as vincristine are never given in an Ommaya reservoir* because of potentially lethal neurotoxicity, including coma and death.[13]

■ Verify that the prescribed medication is being administered at the proper time, in the prescribed dose, and by the correct route *to reduce the risk of medication errors.*[4,5,6] If administering a chemotherapeutic agent, have another practitioner who is qualified to prepare or administer chemotherapy perform an independent double-check *to verify the patient's identity and to make sure that the correct drug is prepared in the prescribed concentration and volume, the drug hasn't expired, the drug's indication corresponds with the patient's diagnosis, the dosage calculations are correct and the dosing formula used to derive the final dose is correct, the route of administration is safe and proper for the patient, and the drug's integrity is intact.* Both of you should sign the patient's medical record indicating that the verification took place.[13,14]

- Compare the results of the independent double-check with the other practitioner and, if no discrepancies exist, begin administering the drug. If discrepancies exist, rectify them before administering the drug.[20,29]
- Using sterile technique, attach a 10-mL syringe to the butterfly needle.
- Place the butterfly needle at a 45-degree angle, and insert it into the reservoir.
- Slowly and gently aspirate 3 mL of CSF into the attached syringe *to make sure that it's clear and doesn't contain blood.*[30] If the aspirate isn't clear, notify the practitioner before continuing.
- If laboratory studies are needed, clamp the tubing, discard the CSF and, using a new syringe, withdraw the appropriate amount of CSF needed for any studies ordered.

NURSING ALERT *Don't use a Vacutainer to aspirate CSF* because rapidly withdrawing CSF with this device could damage the ventricle's choroid plexus.

- Continue to aspirate as many milliliters of CSF as the volume of drug to be instilled. (Some facilities use the CSF instead of a preservative-free diluent to deliver the medication.)
- Detach the syringe from the needle hub.
- Attach the drug syringe.
- Instill the prescribed medication or chemotherapeutic agent slowly, monitoring the patient for headache, nausea, dizziness, or other change in neurologic status.
- Pinch the tubing, detach the syringe, attach the syringe containing preservative-free normal saline solution, and slowly flush the reservoir.
- Withdraw the needle.
- Cover the site with a sterile gauze pad, and apply gentle pressure for a moment or two until superficial bleeding stops.
- Gently pump the reservoir to distribute the medication.
- Discard the needle and syringe in an appropriate sharps disposal container; use a chemotherapy sharps container if the medication was a chemotherapeutic agent.
- If laboratory testing is ordered, place the CSF reserved for laboratory testing in the collection tubes and label the tubes in the presence of the patient *to prevent mislabeling.*[12] Then discard the syringe in an appropriate sharps container.
- Instruct the patient to lie quietly for about 15 to 30 minutes after the procedure *to prevent meningeal irritation, which can lead to nausea and vomiting.*
- Monitor the patient for adverse drug reactions and signs and symptoms of increased ICP—such as vital sign changes, nausea, vomiting, pain, and dizziness—every 30 minutes for 2 hours, every hour for 2 hours, every 4 hours for 24 hours, and then every 8 hours for the duration of care.[31]

Completing the procedure

- Remove and discard used supplies in appropriate waste receptacles.[25,32]
- Remove your personal protective equipment and discard it in an appropriate receptacle. If you administered chemotherapy, discard your equipment in the hazardous-waste container for cytotoxic waste.[25]
- Wash your hands with soap and water if you administered a chemotherapeutic agent,[9,13,14,25] or perform hand hygiene if you didn't.[7,8,9,10,11]
- Perform a comprehensive pain assessment using techniques appropriate for the patient's age, condition, and ability to understand.[33]
- Administer pain medication as needed and prescribed following safe medication administration practices.[4,5,6]
- Place labeled specimens in a laboratory transport bag, and send them to the laboratory.
- With a disinfectant pad, disinfect equipment that isn't for single-patient use.[34,35]
- Perform hand hygiene.[7,8,9,10,11]
- Document the procedure.[36,37,38]

Special considerations

- Be aware the practitioner may prescribe an antiemetic to be administered 30 minutes before the procedure *to control nausea and vomiting.*
- If the patient is scheduled to receive an Ommaya reservoir, explain the procedure before reservoir insertion. Make sure that the patient and his family understand the potential complications, and answer any questions they may have. Reassure the patient that any hair clipped for the implant will grow back and that only a coin-sized patch must remain clipped for injections. (Hair regrowth will be slower if the patient is receiving chemotherapy.)
- After the reservoir is implanted, the site is commonly left open to air after the first 24 hours.[30] Inform the patient that he may resume normal activities, but instruct him to protect the site from bumps and traumatic injury while the incision heals. Tell him that unless complications develop, the reservoir should function for years.
- Each chemotherapy agent has unique adverse effects. Assess and monitor the patient for anticipated adverse effects for the agent administered. Treatment-related toxicities should be evaluated, graded, and documented using standard definitions or criteria.[14]
- If some of the chemotherapy drug comes in contact with your skin, wash the involved area thoroughly with soap (not a germicidal agent) and water. If eye contact occurs, flood the eye with water or saline solution for at least 15 minutes while holding the eyelid open. Obtain a medical evaluation as soon as possible after accidental exposure.[13]
- If a spill occurs, use a chemotherapy spill kit to clean the area. Wear all personal protective equipment (double gloves, a gown, a face shield or goggles, booties, and a respirator if aerosolization is possible) when cleaning the spill. Post a sign to warn others. Report and document the spill appropriately.[13]

Patient teaching

Teach the patient and his family about measures to prevent health care facility–associated infections, including the importance of hand hygiene. Encourage them to remind health care workers who fail to perform hand hygiene before providing care.

Instruct the patient and his family to notify the practitioner if any signs of infection (for example, redness, swelling, tenderness, or drainage) develop at the insertion site or if the patient develops headache, neck stiffness, or fever, *which may indicate a systemic infection.*

Verify that the patient received written educational materials appropriate for his reading level and understanding that include information about his diagnosis, chemotherapy plan (if applicable), possible long- and short-term adverse effects, risks associated with the regimen, reportable signs and symptoms, monitoring, sexual relations, contraception, special precautions, and follow-up care if the patient is receiving chemotherapy.

Complications

Infection may develop but can usually be treated successfully with antibiotics injected directly into the reservoir. Persistent infection may require removal of the reservoir.

Catheter migration or blockage may cause symptoms of increased ICP, such as headache and nausea. If the practitioner suspects this problem, he may gently push and release the reservoir several times (a technique called *pumping*). With his finger on the patient's scalp, the practitioner can feel the reservoir refill. Slow filling suggests catheter migration or blockage, which must be confirmed by a computed tomography scan. Surgical correction is required.

Documentation

Document your assessment findings; the type and size of needle used; patient tolerance; CSF characteristics; medication, dose, and volume administered; amount of CSF withdrawn; specimens collected and results; and any complications. Also record the appearance of the reservoir insertion site before and after access. Note any adverse effects of the drug, the practitioner who was notified, prescribed interventions, and the patient's response to the interventions. Document any patient and family teaching and their understanding of the teaching.

References

1 Centers for Disease Control and Preventions. (2008). "Personal protective equipment for health care workers who work with hazardous drugs" [Online]. Accessed May 2015 via the Web at http://www.cdc.gov/niosh/docs/wp-solutions/2009-106/pdfs/2009-106.pdf

2 Westbrook, J., et al. (2010). Association of interruptions with an increased risk and severity of medication administration errors. *Archives of Internal Medicine, 170,* 683–690. (Level IV)

3 Institute for Safe Medication Practices. (2013). Side tracks on the safety express: Interruptions lead to errors and unfinished . . . Wait, what was I doing? *Nurse Advise-ERR, 11*(2), 1–4. Accessed May 2015 via the Web at https://www.ismp.org/Newsletters/acutecare/showarticle.aspx?id=37 (Level VII)

4 The Joint Commission. (2015). Standard MM.06.01.01. *Comprehensive accreditation manual for hospitals: The official handbook.* Oakbrook Terrace, IL: The Joint Commission. (Level VII)

5 American Osteopathic Association. (2014). Standard 16.01.03. *Healthcare Facilities Accreditation Program: Accreditation requirements for acute care hospitals.* Chicago, IL: American Osteopathic Association. (Level VII)

6 Centers for Medicare & Medicaid Services, Department of Health and Human Services. (2014). Condition of participation: Nursing services. 42 C.F.R. § 482.23(c).

7 Centers for Disease Control and Prevention. (2002). Guideline for hand hygiene in health-care settings: Recommendations of the Healthcare Infection Control Practices Advisory Committee and the HICPAC/SHEA/APIC/IDSA Hand Hygiene Task Force. *MMWR Recommendations and Reports, 51*(RR-16), 1–45. Accessed May 2015 via the Web at http://www.cdc.gov/mmwr/pdf/rr/rr5116.pdf (Level II)

8 World Health Organization. (2009). "WHO guidelines on hand hygiene in health care: First global patient safety challenge, clean care is safer care" [Online]. Accessed May 2015 via the Web at http://whqlibdoc.who.int/publications/2009/9789241597906_eng.pdf (Level IV)

9 The Joint Commission. (2015). Standard NPSG.07.01.01. *Comprehensive accreditation manual for hospitals: The official handbook.* Oakbrook Terrace, IL: The Joint Commission. (Level VII)

10 American Osteopathic Association. (2014). Standard 07.01.10. *Healthcare Facilities Accreditation Program: Accreditation requirements for acute care hospitals.* Chicago, IL: American Osteopathic Association. (Level VII)

11 Centers for Medicare & Medicaid Services, Department of Health and Human Services. (2014). Condition of participation: Infection control. 42 C.F.R. § 482.42.

12 The Joint Commission. (2015). Standard NPSG.01.01.01. *Comprehensive accreditation manual for hospitals: The official handbook.* Oakbrook Terrace, IL: The Joint Commission. (Level VII)

13 Polovich, M., et al. (Eds.). (2014). *Chemotherapy and biotherapy guidelines and recommendations for practice* (4th ed.). Pittsburgh, PA: Oncology Nursing Society.

14 Neuss, M. N., et al. (2013). 2013 updated American Society of Clinical Oncology/Oncology Nursing Society chemotherapy administration safety standards including standards for the safe administration and management of oral chemotherapy. *Oncology Nursing Forum, 40,* 225–233. Accessed May 2015 via the Web at https://www.ons.org/sites/default/files/2013chemostandards.pdf (Level VII)

15 Centers for Medicare & Medicaid Services, Department of Health and Human Services. (2014). Condition of participation: Patient's rights, 42 C.F.R. § 482.13.

16 Occupational Safety & Health Administration. (1999). "OSHA technical manual: Controlling occupational exposure to harmful drugs" [Online]. Accessed May 2015 via the Web at http://www.osha.gov/dts/osta/otm/otm_vi/otm_vi_2.html

17 Standard 62: Antineoplastic therapy. Infusion nursing standards of practice. (2011). *Journal of Infusion Nursing, 34,* S87–S88. (Level VII)

18 American Osteopathic Association. (2014). Standard 15.01.11. *Healthcare Facilities Accreditation Program: Accreditation requirements for acute care hospitals.* Chicago, IL: American Osteopathic Association. (Level VII)

19 The Joint Commission. (2015). Standard UP.01.01.01. *Comprehensive accreditation manual for hospitals: The official handbook.* Oakbrook Terrace, IL: The Joint Commission. (Level VII)

20 American Osteopathic Association. (2014). Standard 30.00.14. *Healthcare Facilities Accreditation Program: Accreditation requirements for acute care hospitals.* Chicago, IL: American Osteopathic Association. (Level VII)

21 American Osteopathic Association. (2014). Standard 15.01.16. *Healthcare Facilities Accreditation Program: Accreditation requirements for acute care hospitals.* Chicago, IL: American Osteopathic Association. (Level VII)

22 The Joint Commission. (2015). Standard NPSG.03.04.01. *Comprehensive accreditation manual for hospitals: The official handbook.* Oakbrook Terrace, IL: The Joint Commission. (Level VII)

23 American Osteopathic Association. (2014). Standard 25.01.27. *Healthcare Facilities Accreditation Program: Accreditation requirements for acute care hospitals.* Chicago, IL: American Osteopathic Association. (Level VII)

24 Siegel, J. D., et al. (2007). "2007 guideline for isolation precautions: Preventing transmission of infectious agents in healthcare settings" [Online]. Accessed May 2015 via the Web at http://www.cdc.gov/hicpac/pdf/isolation/Isolation2007.pdf (Level II)

25 National Institute for Occupational Safety and Health (NIOSH). (2004). "Preventing occupational exposure to antineoplastic and other hazardous drugs in health care settings" [Online]. Accessed May 2015 via the Web at http://www.cdc.gov/niosh/docs/2004-165/pdfs/2004-165.pdf

26 The Joint Commission. (2015). Standard UP.01.03.01. *Comprehensive accreditation manual for hospitals: The official handbook.* Oakbrook Terrace, IL: The Joint Commission. (Level VII)

27 Dailey, P. A. (2009). "Chlorhexidine or povidone-iodine: Do we follow the guidelines or the package insert?" [Online]. Accessed May 2015 via the Web at http://apicwv.org/docs/19.pdf

28 Institute for Safe Medication Practices. (2012). "ISMP's list of high-alert medications" [Online]. Accessed May 2015 via the Web at http://www.ismp.org/tools/highalertmedications.pdf

29 Institute for Safe Medication Practices. (2008). Conducting an independent double-check. *ISMP Medication Safety Alert! Nurse Advise-ERR, 6*(12), 1. Accessed May 2015 via the Web at http://www.ismp.org/newsletters/nursing/Issues/NurseAdviseERR200812.pdf (Level VII)

30 Standard 58. Intraspinal access devices. Infusion nursing standards of practice. (2011). *Journal of Infusion Nursing, 34,* S81–S82. (Level VII)

31 Aiello-Laws, L., & Rutledge, D. N. (2008). Management of adult patients receiving intraventricular chemotherapy for the treatment of leptomeningeal metastasis. *Clinical Journal of Oncology Nursing, 12,* 429–435.

32 Occupational Safety and Health Administration. (n.d.). "Bloodborne pathogens, standard number 1910.1030" [Online]. Accessed May 2015 via the Web at http://www.osha.gov/pls/oshaweb/owadisp.show_document?p_table=standards&p_id=10051 (Level VII)

33 The Joint Commission. (2015). Standard PC.01.02.07. *Comprehensive accreditation manual for hospitals: The official handbook.* Oakbrook Terrace, IL: The Joint Commission. (Level VII)

34 Rutala, W. A., et al. (2008). "Guideline for disinfection and sterilization in healthcare facilities, 2008" [Online]. Accessed May 2015 via the Web at http://www.cdc.gov/hicpac/pdf/guidelines/Disinfection_Nov_2008.pdf (Level I)

35 American Osteopathic Association. (2014). Standard 07.02.03. *Healthcare Facilities Accreditation Program: Accreditation requirements for acute care hospitals.* Chicago, IL: American Osteopathic Association. (Level VII)
36 The Joint Commission. (2015). Standard RC.01.03.01. *Comprehensive accreditation manual for hospitals: The official handbook.* Oakbrook Terrace, IL: The Joint Commission. (Level VII)
37 American Osteopathic Association. (2014). Standard 10.00.03. *Healthcare Facilities Accreditation Program: Accreditation requirements for acute care hospitals.* Chicago, IL: American Osteopathic Association. (Level VII)
38 Centers for Medicare & Medicaid Services, Department of Health and Human Services. (2014). Condition of participation: Medical record services. 42 C.F.R. § 482.24(b).

ORAL CARE

Oral care, which typically involves the nurse or patient brushing and flossing the patient's teeth and inspecting the mouth, is commonly performed in the morning, at bedtime, and after meals. Oral care removes soft plaque deposits and calculus from the teeth, cleans and massages the gums, reduces mouth odor, provides comfort, and reduces the risk of infection.

Patients who are intubated and receiving mechanical ventilation require oral care more frequently because mechanical ventilation dries the oral mucosa and affects salivary flow, increasing the risk of infection.[1] Colonization of microorganisms in the oropharynx is a factor in the development of ventilator-associated pneumonia (VAP). The microorganisms that develop on the tooth surface because of dental plaque can translocate from the mouth to the lung, which can result in VAP.[1] In addition to routine oral care, the Institute for Healthcare Improvement has added daily oral care with chlorhexidine to its VAP-prevention bundle because evidence shows that it helps prevent VAP when combined with the other bundle elements, including elevating the patient's head 30 to 45 degrees, interrupting sedation daily and assessing readiness to wean, and providing peptic ulcer disease and deep vein thrombosis prophylaxis, unless contraindicated.[2]

Other factors that can increase the risk of oral problems include cognitive impairment, swallowing difficulty, disruptive behavior or resistance to care, functional impairment, use of certain medications, previous or current radiation or chemotherapy, tobacco and alcohol use, previous history of dental problems, and lack of access to dental care.[3]

Equipment

Towel ■ facial tissues ■ gloves ■ emesis basin ■ mouthwash (preferably alcohol-free)[3] ■ toothbrush ■ toothpaste ■ plastic cup ■ drinking straw ■ dental floss or interdental cleaner ■ Optional: other personal protective equipment, oral irrigating device, tongue blade, 4″ × 4″ (10-cm × 10-cm) gauze pads, adhesive tape, penlight, dental floss holder, small mirror.

For a comatose or debilitated patient as needed

Fluid-impermeable pad ■ plastic cup ■ drinking straw ■ mouthwash ■ bite block or mouth prop[3] ■ petroleum jelly or other appropriate lubricant[3] ■ dental floss and dental floss holder ■ toothbrush ■ toothpaste ■ oral suction equipment or gauze pads ■ sponge-tipped swab ■ water, sterile water, or normal saline solution ■ gloves ■ Optional: other personal protective equipment, penlight, oral irrigating device.

For an intubated patient

Facility-approved oral assessment tool ■ fluid-impermeable pad ■ suction equipment ■ petroleum jelly ■ sponge-tipped swabs ■ sterile water[4] ■ soft-bristle toothbrush ■ toothpaste ■ gloves ■ gauze pads ■ penlight ■ Optional: chlorhexidine mouth rinse, other personal protective equipment, bite block, oropharyngeal airway.

Preparation of equipment

Bring a cup of water and other equipment to the patient's bedside. If you'll be using oral suction equipment, connect the tubing to the suction canister and suction catheter, turn on the suction apparatus, and check for correct operation.

Implementation

- Perform hand hygiene.[5,6,7,8,9]
- Put on gloves and other personal protective equipment, as needed.[10,11]
- Confirm the patient's identity using at least two patient identifiers.[12]
- Explain the procedure to the patient *to decrease anxiety and promote cooperation.*
- Provide privacy[13]
- Assess the patient's current oral hygiene regimen and self-care ability *to help determine the level of oral care necessary.*[3]
- Assess the oropharyngeal cavity, as needed.[14] Inspect the patient's lips *to see if they're dry, cracked, or caked*; if so, expect the same condition inside the oral cavity. Palpate the oropharyngeal cavity with your gloved index finger, moving along the gingival surfaces. If oral secretions are present, assess their amount, viscosity, and color. Suction the oropharyngeal cavity, as needed.

Supervising oral care

- For a bedridden patient capable of self-care, encourage the patient to perform her own mouth care.
- If permitted by the patient's condition, place the patient in the Fowler position *to promote comfort.*
- Place the overbed table in front of the patient, and arrange the equipment on it. Open the table and set up the built-in mirror, if available (as shown below), or position a small mirror on the table.

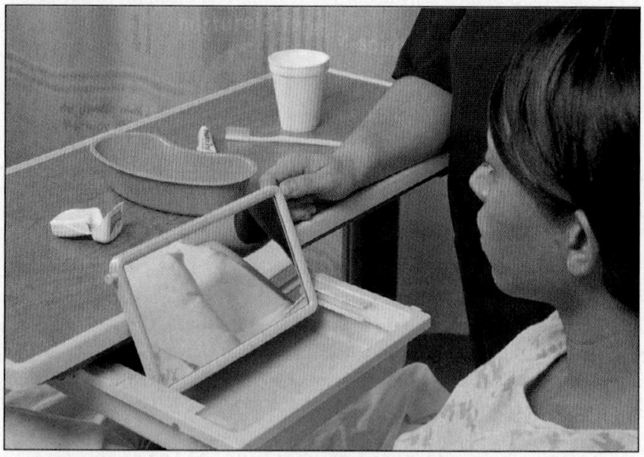

- Drape a towel over the patient's chest *to protect her gown.*
- Instruct her to floss her teeth while looking into the mirror.
- Observe the patient *to make sure she's flossing correctly,* and correct her if necessary. If the patient is using dental floss, tell her to wrap the floss around the second or third fingers of both hands. Starting with her front teeth and without injuring the gums, she should insert the floss as far as possible into the space between each pair of teeth (as shown on next page, top left). Then she should clean the surfaces of adjacent teeth by pulling the floss up and down against the side of each tooth. After the patient flosses a pair of teeth, remind her to use a clean 1″ (2.5-cm) section of floss for the next pair.

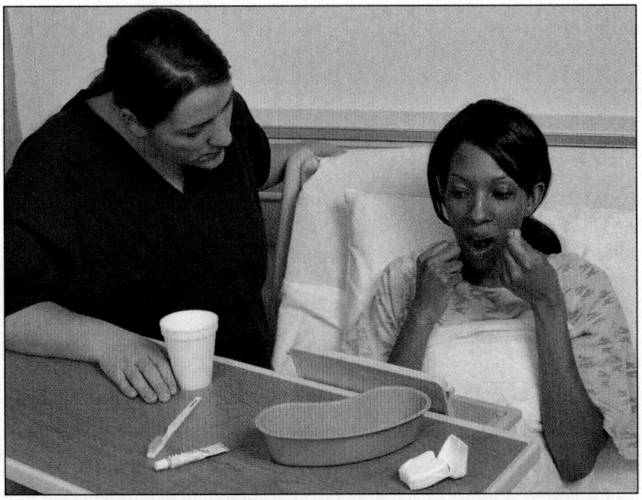

■ While the patient flosses, mix mouthwash and water in a plastic cup, place a straw in the cup, and position the emesis basin nearby.
■ Instruct the patient to brush her teeth and gums while looking into the mirror. Encourage her to rinse frequently during brushing, and provide facial tissues *for her to wipe her mouth.*

Performing oral care for a comatose or debilitated patient

■ For a comatose patient or a conscious patient incapable of self-care, you'll perform oral care.
■ If the patient is resisting oral care, obtain the assistance of an additional coworker or caregiver, as necessary, *because some patients may resist oral care because of disruptive behaviors or cognitive impairment.* Use skillful, strategic communication with the patient and, if necessary, try oral care at another time of day when the patient is more cooperative or in a more suitable environment.[3]
■ If the patient wears dentures, clean them thoroughly. (See *Denture care,* page 562.)
■ Some patients may benefit from an oral irrigating device. (See *Using an oral irrigating device,* page 563.)
■ Arrange the equipment on the overbed table or bedside stand, including the oral suction equipment, if necessary. Turn on the apparatus. If a suction apparatus isn't available, wipe the inside of the patient's mouth frequently with a moist, sponge-tipped swab.
■ Mix mouthwash and water in a plastic cup and place a straw in it.
■ Raise the bed to a comfortable working height *to prevent back strain.* Then lower the head of the bed, and position the patient on her side, with her face extended over the edge of the pillow (as shown below) *to facilitate drainage and prevent fluid aspiration.*

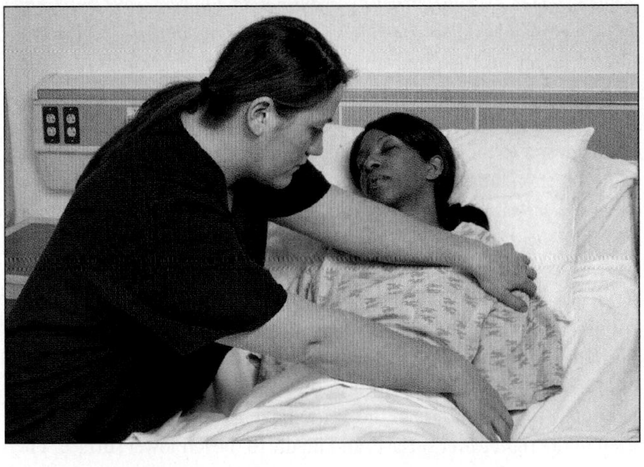

■ Place a fluid-impermeable pad under the patient's chin and an emesis basin near her cheek *to absorb or catch drainage.*
■ Lubricate the patient's oral tissues and lips with petroleum jelly (as shown below) *to prevent dryness and cracking.*[3] Reapply lubricant, as needed, during oral care.

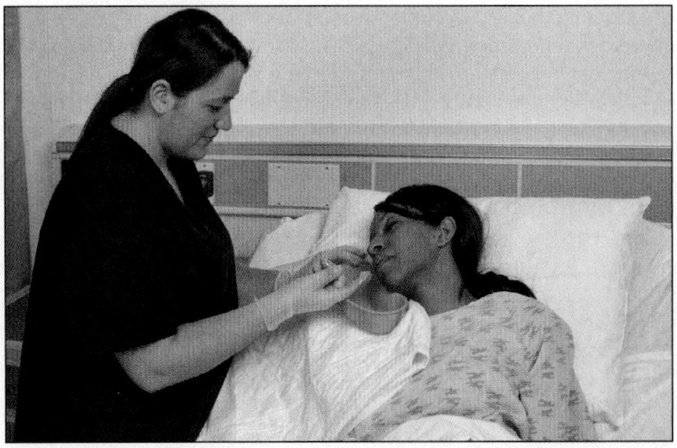

■ If necessary, insert the mouth prop *to hold the patient's mouth open during oral care.*[3]
■ Using a dental floss holder, hold the floss against each tooth and direct it as close to the gum as possible without injuring the sensitive tissues around the tooth.
■ Wet the toothbrush with water, sterile water, or normal saline solution. If necessary, use hot water *to soften the bristles.*
■ Apply toothpaste.
■ Brush the patient's lower teeth from the gum line up; the upper teeth, from the gum line down (as shown below). Place the brush at a 45-degree angle to the gum line, and press the bristles gently into the gingival sulcus. Using short, gentle strokes *to prevent gum damage,* brush the facial surfaces (toward the cheek) and the lingual surfaces (toward the tongue) of the bottom teeth. Use just the tip of the brush for the lingual surfaces of the front teeth. Then, using the same technique, brush the facial and lingual surfaces of the top teeth. Next, brush the biting surfaces of the bottom and top teeth, using a back and forth motion. If possible, ask the patient to rinse frequently during brushing by taking the mouthwash solution through the straw. Hold the emesis basin steady under the patient's cheek, and wipe her mouth and cheeks with facial tissues, as needed.

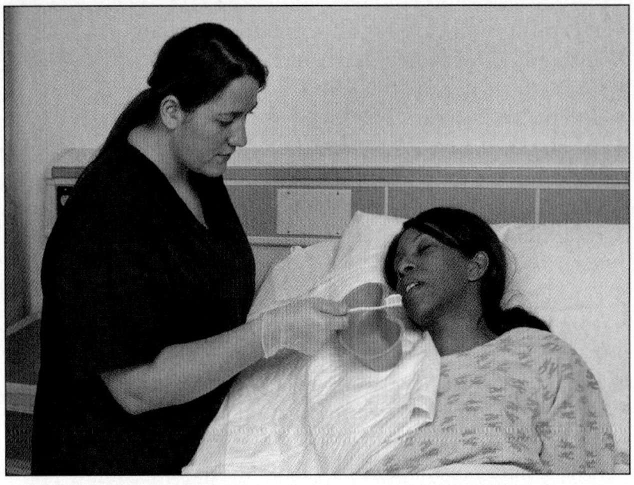

■ After brushing the patient's teeth, dip a sponge-tipped mouth swab into the mouthwash solution. Press the swab against the side of the plastic cup *to remove excess moisture.* Gently stroke the gums, buccal surfaces, palate, and tongue *to clean the mucosa and stimulate circulation.*

Denture care

Prostheses made of acrylic resins, vinyl composites, or both, dentures replace some or all of the patient's natural teeth. Dentures require proper care *to remove soft plaque deposits and calculus and to reduce mouth odor.* Such care involves removing and rinsing dentures after meals, daily brushing and removal of tenacious deposits, and soaking in a commercial denture cleaner. Dentures must be removed from the comatose or presurgical patient *to prevent possible airway obstruction.*

Equipment and preparation

Start by assembling the following equipment at the patient's bedside:

- Emesis basin
- Labeled denture cup
- Soft-bristled toothbrush or denture brush[2,14]
- Gloves
- Mild soap, denture cream, paste, or gel[2,14]
- Commercial denture cleaner if available[2,14]
- Paper towel or washcloth
- Sponge-tipped swab
- Mouthwash (preferably alcohol-free)
- Gauze
- Adhesive denture liner (optional)

Perform hand hygiene and put on gloves.[5,6,7,8,9,10,11]

Removing dentures

- To remove a full upper denture, grasp the front and palatal surfaces of the denture with your thumb and forefinger. Position the index finger of your opposite hand over the upper border of the denture and press *to break the seal between denture and palate.* Grasp the denture with gauze *because saliva can make it slippery.*
- To remove a full lower denture, grasp the front and lingual surfaces of the denture with your thumb and index finger and gently lift up.
- To remove partial dentures, first ask the patient or a caregiver how the prosthesis is retained and how to remove it. If the partial denture is held in place with clips or snaps, then exert equal pressure on the border of each side of the denture. Avoid lifting the clasps, *which easily bend or break.*

Performing oral and denture care

- After removing dentures, place them in a properly labeled denture cup. Add warm water and a commercial denture cleaner, if available, *to remove stains and hardened deposits.* Follow package directions. Avoid soaking dentures in mouthwash containing alcohol *because it may damage a soft liner.*
- If dentures are particularly dirty, you may soak them in a 50:50 solution of diluted white vinegar and cold water. They may also need chemical cleaning by a dental professional.[2]
- Instruct the patient to rinse with mouthwash *to remove food particles and reduce mouth odor.* Then stroke the palate, buccal surfaces, gums, and tongue with a soft toothbrush or sponge-tipped mouth swab *to clean the mucosa and stimulate circulation.* Inspect for irritated areas or sores *because they may indicate a poorly fitting denture.*
- Physically clean the dentures with soap or appropriate denture cream, paste, or gel and a soft-bristled toothbrush or denture brush in a basin or sink filled with water and lined with a paper towel or washcloth *to prevent denture breakage if dropped.* Don't use toothpastes intended for natural teeth *because they're too abrasive and will scratch the acrylic surface.*[2,14] Clean the dentures using only moderate pressure *to prevent scratches* and warm water *to prevent distortion.*
- Clean the denture cup, and then place the dentures in it.
- Rinse the brush.
- Clean and dry the emesis basin.
- Return all equipment to the patient's bedside stand.

Inserting dentures

- If the patient desires, apply adhesive liner to the dentures. Moisten dentures with water, if necessary, *to reduce friction and ease insertion.*
- Encourage the patient to wear the dentures *to enhance appearance, facilitate eating and speaking, and prevent changes in the gum line that may affect denture fit.*

Replace the swab as necessary for thorough cleaning. Avoid inserting the swab too deeply *to prevent gagging and vomiting.*

Performing oral care for an intubated patient

- Elicit the help of a coworker if needed.
- Gather the appropriate equipment.
- Perform hand hygiene.[5,6,7,8,9]
- Put on gloves and other personal protective equipment as needed *to comply with standard precautions.*[10,11]
- Confirm the patient's identity using at least two patient identifiers.[12]
- Explain the procedure to the patient *to decrease anxiety and promote cooperation with the procedure.*
- Provide privacy.[13]
- Turn on the suction equipment and make sure it's functioning properly.
- Raise the bed to a comfortable working position to prevent back strain.
- Place the patient in the high Fowler position *to reduce the risk of aspiration.*
- Place a fluid-impermeable pad under the patient's chin *to absorb drainage.*
- Assess the patient's level of consciousness; if the patient is unconscious or disoriented, he may reflexively bite down when something is introduced into the mouth. You may need a bite block or oropharyngeal airway *to keep the mouth open.*[4]
- Perform deep suctioning and suction the patient's oropharynx *to prevent aspiration of secretions in the oropharynx* and above the endotracheal (ET) tube cuff *because oral care stimulates additional secretions.*[4]
- Assess the patient's oropharyngeal cavity using a facility-approved oral assessment tool if necessary. If the patient's lips are dried and cracked, lubricate them with petroleum jelly before beginning your assessment.[4]
- To assess the oropharyngeal cavity, first place a gloved finger in the side of the patient's mouth between the teeth and cheek *to generate trust and demonstrate to the patient that the examination and care won't be painful.*[4] Have a penlight available *to visualize oral structures if needed.*[4] Move your gloved finger on the gingival surfaces around the mouth.[4] Moisten a single layer of a soft gauze pad and wrap it around your index finger, and move the finger from the right upper to left upper gingiva, and then from the left lower to the right lower gingiva.[4,15] Repeat your assessment in the same direction for the inside of the mouth (lingual); use the same direction *because a standardized approach avoids missing areas during your assessment.*[4] Examine the gauze for bloody drainage; if bleeding is present and copious, use a gauze-wrapped finger to brush the patient's teeth, not a toothbrush.[4]
- Gently brush the patient's teeth, gums, and tongue at least twice daily using a soft-bristle toothbrush, toothpaste,[1] and a small amount of sterile water[4] *to reduce oropharyngeal colonization and dental plaque, which increase the risk of VAP.*[16] Brush in one continuous line, starting at the left upper gingival surface of the teeth, moving to the right upper surface, then to the right lower surface, and finally to the left lower surface. Then

EQUIPMENT

Using an oral irrigating device

An oral irrigating device, such as the Water Pik, directs a pulsating jet of water around the teeth *to massage gums and remove debris and food particles*. It's especially useful for cleaning areas missed by brushing, such as around bridgework, crowns, and dental wires. *Because this device enhances oral hygiene,* it benefits patients undergoing head and neck irradiation, which can damage teeth and cause severe caries. The device also maintains oral hygiene in a patient with a fractured jaw or with mouth injuries that limit standard mouth care.

Equipment and preparation

To use the device, first assemble the following equipment:

- Oral irrigating device
- Towel
- Gloves and other personal protective equipment, as needed
- Emesis basin
- Pharyngeal suction apparatus
- Salt solution or mouthwash (alcohol-free) if ordered
- Soap

Perform hand hygiene and put on gloves.[5,6,7,8,9,10,11]

Implementation

- Insert the oral irrigating device's plug into a nearby electrical outlet.
- Remove the device's cover, turn it upside down, and fill it with lukewarm water or with a mouthwash or salt solution, as ordered. When using a salt solution, dissolve the salt beforehand in a separate container and then pour the solution into the cover. Salt solutions shouldn't be used in patients who have problems with dryness and dehydration *because salt solutions exacerbate these conditions.*
- Secure the cover to the base of the device. Remove the water hose handle from the base, and snap the jet tip into place. If necessary, wet the grooved end of the tip *to ease insertion.* Adjust the pressure dial to the setting most comfortable for the patient. If her gums are tender and prone to bleed, choose a low setting.
- Turn the patient to her side *to prevent aspiration of water.* Then place a towel under her chin and an emesis basin next to her cheek *to absorb or catch drainage.*
- Adjust the knurled knob on the handle *to direct the water jet,* place the jet tip in the patient's mouth, and turn on the device. Instruct the alert patient to keep her lips partially closed *to avoid spraying water.*
- Direct the water at a right angle to the gum line of each tooth and between teeth (as shown below). Avoid directing water under the patient's tongue *because this action may injure sensitive tissue.*

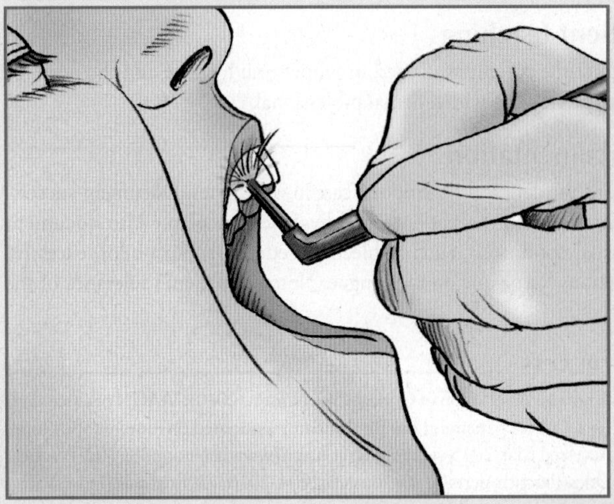

- After irrigating each tooth, pause briefly and instruct the patient to expectorate the water or solution into the emesis basin. If she's unable to do so, suction it from the sides of the mouth with the pharyngeal suction apparatus. After irrigating all teeth, turn off the device, and remove the jet tip from the patient's mouth.
- Empty the remaining water or solution from the cover, remove the jet tip from the handle, and return the handle to the base.
- Clean the jet tip with soap and water, rinse the cover, and dry them both and return them to storage.

switch to the lingual surface of the teeth, starting at the lower left, and moving through all surfaces in a set pattern.[4]

- If the patient is orally intubated, carefully clean the portion of the ET tube in the patient's oral cavity as part of oral care *because plaque and bacterial biofilm can form on the surface of the tube.*[4]
- Suction the patient's oropharynx *to remove excess fluid and debris, which helps prevent aspiration.*[4,16]
- Moisturize the oral mucosa and lips every 2 to 4 hours *to reduce oral inflammation and improve oral health.*[1]
- Use a chlorhexidine mouth rinse daily, as prescribed, *to prevent VAP.*[2] Use a chlorhexidine mouth rinse twice daily during the perioperative period for adult patients who have undergone cardiac surgery, as prescribed, *to prevent VAP.*[1]
- Reassess the patient's oropharynx *to note the effectiveness of oral care.*
- If needed to prevent biting in the orally intubated patient, insert a bite block or oropharyngeal airway by inserting it along the ET tube.[16]
- Reposition the patient for comfort, maintaining the head of the bed at 30 to 45 degrees, *to prevent aspiration and reduce the risk of VAP.*[2,17,18]
- Return the patient's bed to the low position *to maintain patient safety.*

After oral care

- Reassess the patient's mouth for cleanliness and tooth and tissue condition.
- Rinse the toothbrush and clean the emesis basin.
- Remove your gloves and any other personal protective equipment worn.
- Perform hand hygiene.[5,6,7,8,9]
- Place a clean suction catheter on the tubing.
- Return reusable equipment to the appropriate storage location.
- Discard disposable equipment in the appropriate receptacle.
- Perform hand hygiene.[5,6,7,8,9]
- Document the procedure.[19,20,21]

Special considerations

- Use sponge-tipped mouth swabs to clean the teeth of a patient with sensitive gums. *These swabs produce less friction than a toothbrush but don't clean as well.*
- Implement different strategies *to facilitate the patient's oral hygiene care plan,* as needed. For example, break down dental care tasks for the patient; consult with a practitioner for review of medications that could affect oral health; modify the patient's diet; increase the patient's fluid intake; encourage the patient to eliminate sugar-containing gum or lozenges, smoking, caffeine, and alcohol; and use different dental products, such as modified toothbrushes, mouth rinses, saliva substitutes, and spray bottles.[2]

- Don't use chlorhexidine and fluoride together *because fluoride can interfere with the action of chlorhexidine*; allow 1 to 2 hours between their use.[2]
- Prescription-strength fluoride is contraindicated for patients who can't follow directions or expectorate adequately as well as for those who tend to swallow inadvertently.[2]
- Clean the mouth of a toothless comatose patient by wrapping a gauze pad around your index finger, moistening it with mouthwash, and gently swabbing the oral tissues.
- Remember that mucous membranes dry quickly in the patient breathing through the mouth or receiving oxygen therapy. Moisten the patient's mouth and lips regularly with moistened sponge-tipped swabs or water.[1]

Patient teaching

Instruct the patient as needed in proper oral hygiene and the need for regular follow-up with a dental professional.[2]

Documentation

Record the date and time of oral care in your notes. Document successful strategies in the patient's oral hygiene care plan.[2] Also document unusual conditions, such as bleeding, edema, mouth odor, excessive secretions, or plaque on the tongue. Note the patient's tolerance of the procedure.

REFERENCES

1 American Association of Critical-Care Nurses. (2010). "AACN practice alert: Oral care for patients at risk for ventilator-associated pneumonia" [Online]. Accessed May 2015 via the Web at http://www.aacn.org:88/WD/Practice/Docs/PracticeAlerts/oral%20care%2004-2010%20final.pdf (Level VII)

2 Institute for Healthcare Improvement. (2012). *How-to-guide: Prevent ventilator-associated pneumonia.* Cambridge, MA: Institute for Healthcare Improvement. (Level VII)

3 Johnson, V. B., & Chalmers, J. (2011). "Oral hygiene care for functionally dependent and cognitively impaired older adults" [Online]. Accessed May 2015 via the Web at http://www.guideline.gov/content.aspx?id=34447 (Level VII)

4 Ames, N. J., et al. (2011). Effects of systematic oral care in critically ill patients: A multicenter study. *American Journal of Critical Care, 20,* e103–e113. Accessed May 2015 via the Web at http://www.aacn.org/wd/Cetests/media/a1120053.pdf

5 The Joint Commission. (2015). Standard NPSG.07.01.01. *Comprehensive accreditation manual for hospitals: The official handbook.* Oakbrook Terrace, IL: The Joint Commission. (Level VII)

6 World Health Organization. (2009). "WHO guidelines on hand hygiene in health care: First global patient safety challenge, clean care is safer care" [Online]. Accessed May 2015 via the Web at http://whqlibdoc.who.int/publications/2009/9789241597906_eng.pdf (Level IV)

7 Centers for Disease Control and Prevention. (2002). Guideline for hand hygiene in health-care settings: Recommendations of the Healthcare Infection Control Practices Advisory Committee and the HICPAC/SHEA/APIC/IDSA Hand Hygiene Task Force. *MMWR Recommendations and Reports, 51*(RR-16), 1–45. Accessed May 2015 via the Web at http://www.cdc.gov/mmwr/pdf/rr/rr5116.pdf (Level II)

8 Centers for Medicare & Medicaid Services, Department of Health and Human Services. (2014). Condition of participation: Infection control. 42 C.F.R. § 482.42.

9 American Osteopathic Association. (2014). Standard 07.01.21. *Healthcare Facilities Accreditation Program: Accreditation requirements for acute care hospitals.* Chicago, IL: American Osteopathic Association. (Level VII)

10 Siegel, J. D., et al. (2007). "2007 guideline for isolation precautions: Preventing transmission of infectious agents in healthcare settings" [Online]. Accessed May 2015 via the Web at http://www.cdc.gov/hicpac/pdf/isolation/Isolation2007.pdf (Level II)

11 American Osteopathic Association. (2014). Standard 07.01.10. *Healthcare Facilities Accreditation Program: Accreditation requirements for acute care hospitals.* Chicago, IL: American Osteopathic Association. (Level VII)

12 The Joint Commission. (2015). Standard.NPSG.01.01.01. *Comprehensive accreditation manual for hospitals: The official handbook.* Oakbrook Terrace, IL: The Joint Commission. (Level VII)

13 American Osteopathic Association. (2014). Standard 15.01.16. *Healthcare Facilities Accreditation Program: Accreditation requirements for acute care hospitals.* Chicago, IL: American Osteopathic Association. (Level VII)

14 American Dental Association. (2013). "Removable partial dentures: Caring for your dentures" [Online]. Accessed May 2015 via the Web at http://www.mouthhealthy.org/en/az-topics/d/dentures-partial

15 Darby, M. L., & Walsh, M. (Eds.). (2010). *Dental hygiene: Theory and practice* (3rd ed.). St Louis, MO: Saunders.

16 Lynn-McHale Wiegand, D. (Ed.). (2011). *AACN procedure manual for critical care* (6th ed.). St. Louis, MO: Saunders.

17 Klompas, M., et al. (2014). Strategies to prevent ventilator-associated pneumonia in acute care hospitals: 2014 update. *Infection Control and Hospital Epidemiology, 35,* 915–936. Accessed May 2015 via the Web at http://www.jstor.org/stable/10.1086/677144 (Level I)

18 Association of Professionals in Infection Control and Epidemiology (APIC). (2009). "An APIC guide 2009: Guide to the elimination of ventilator-associated pneumonia" [Online]. Accessed May 2015 via the Web at http://www.apic.org/Resource_/EliminationGuideForm/18e326ad-b484-471c-9c35-6822a53ee4a2/File/VAP_09.pdf (Level IV)

19 The Joint Commission. (2015). Standard RC.01.03.01. *Comprehensive accreditation manual for hospitals: The official handbook.* Oakbrook Terrace, IL: The Joint *Commission.* (Level VII)

20 Centers for Medicare & Medicaid Services, Department of Health and Human Services. (2014). Condition of participation: Medical record services. 42 C.F.R. § 482.24(b).

21 American Osteopathic Association. (2014). Standard 10.00.03. *Healthcare Facilities Accreditation Program: Accreditation requirements for acute care hospitals.* Chicago, IL: American Osteopathic Association. (Level VII)

ORAL DRUG ADMINISTRATION

Because oral administration is usually the safest, most convenient, and least expensive method, most drugs are administered by this route. Drugs for oral administration are available in many forms: tablets, enteric-coated tablets, capsules, syrups, elixirs, oils, liquids, suspensions, powders, and granules. Some require special preparation before administration, such as mixing with juice to make them more palatable; oils, powders, and granules most often require such preparation.

Sometimes oral drugs are prescribed in higher dosages than their parenteral equivalents because after absorption through the GI system, they are immediately broken down by the liver before they reach the systemic circulation.

ELDER ALERT ***Oral dosages normally prescribed for adults may be dangerous for elderly patients*** **because of decreased hepatic and renal clearance.**

Oral administration is contraindicated for unconscious patients; it may also be contraindicated in patients with nausea and vomiting and in those who can't swallow.

Make sure you understand the pharmacology behind the medications administered *to prevent potential error and patient harm.*[1]

Equipment

Patient's medication record ■ prescribed medication ■ medication cup ■ Optional: appropriate vehicle (such as pudding or applesauce) for crushed pills (commonly used with elderly patients), and juice, water, or milk for liquid medications; drinking straw; pill-crushing device; pill-cutting device (for scored tablets).

Implementation

- Avoid distractions and interruptions when preparing and administering medication to *prevent medication administration errors.*[2,3]

■ Verify the order on the patient's medication record by checking it against the practitioner's order.[4,5,6]
■ Gather the prescribed medication and the appropriate equipment.
■ Compare the medication label against the order in the patient's medical record.[4,5,6]
■ Check the patient's medical record for an allergy or a contraindication to the prescribed medication. If an allergy or a contraindication exists, don't administer the medication; notify the practitioner.[4,5,6]

NURSING ALERT *Cardiovascular agents, antibiotics, diuretics, anticoagulants, antidiabetics, steroids, opioids, anticholinergics, benzodiazepines, and nonsteroidal anti-inflammatory drugs most commonly cause drug interactions.* To avoid drug interactions, *review with the patient all current prescribed and over-the-counter medications, dietary supplements, and herbal preparations. Notify the patient's practitioner and your facility's pharmacy of any potential interactions.*[1,7,8,9,10]

■ Check the expiration date on the medication (as shown below). If the medication is expired, return it to the pharmacy and obtain new medication.[4,5,6]

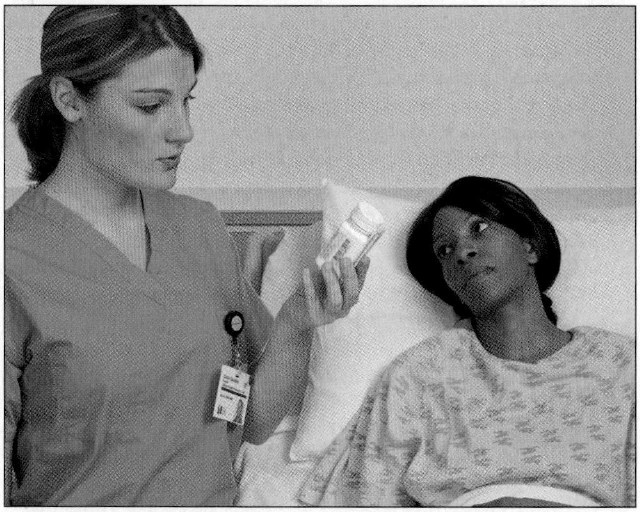

■ Visually inspect the medication for any loss of integrity; don't administer the medication if its integrity is compromised.[4,5,6]
■ Discuss any unresolved concerns about the medication with the patient's practitioner.[4,5,6]
■ Perform hand hygiene.[11,12,13,14,15]
■ Confirm the patient's identity using at least two patient identifiers.[5,16]
■ If the patient is receiving the medication for the first time, teach her about significant adverse reactions and discuss any other concerns related to the medication.[4,5,6]
■ Assess the patient's condition *to determine the need for the medication and the effectiveness of previous therapy.*
■ Carefully observe the patient for a rash, pruritus, cough, or other signs of an adverse reaction to a previously administered drug.
■ Explain the procedure to the patient.
■ Provide privacy.[17,18]
■ Verify that the medication is being administered at the proper time, in the prescribed dose, and by the correct route *to reduce the risk of medication errors.*[4,5,6]
■ If your facility uses a bar code scanning system, scan your identification badge, the patient's identification bracelet, and the medication's bar code.
■ Give the patient her medication (as shown on top right) and an appropriate vehicle or liquid, as needed, *to aid swallowing, minimize adverse effects, or promote absorption.* For example, give cyclophosphamide with adequate amounts of fluids *to force diuresis and subsequently reduce the risk of urinary tract toxicity;*[19] give antitussive cough syrup without a fluid *to avoid diluting its soothing effect on the throat.* If appropriate, crush the medication *to facilitate swallowing.*

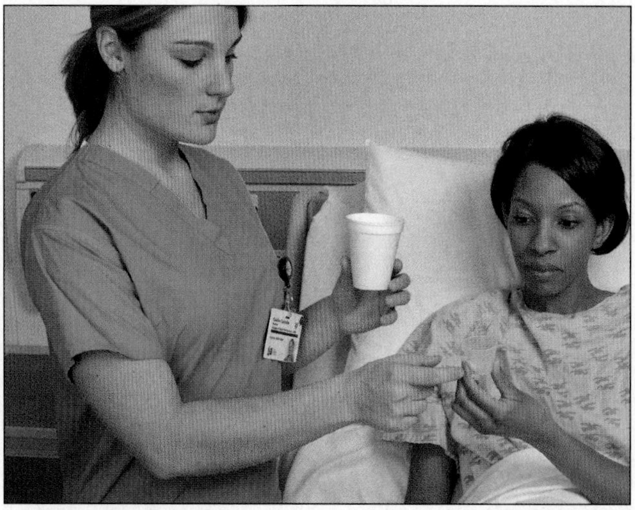

■ Stay with the patient until she has swallowed the drug. If she seems confused or disoriented, check her mouth *to make sure she has swallowed it.* Return and reassess the patient's response within 1 hour after giving the medication.[20]
■ Perform hand hygiene.[11,12,13,14,15]
■ Document the procedure.[21,22,23]

Special considerations

■ Notify the practitioner about any medication withheld.
■ Use care when measuring the prescribed dose of liquid oral medication. (See *Measuring liquid medications,* page 566.)
■ Don't give medication from a poorly labeled or unlabeled container. Don't attempt to label or reinforce drug labels yourself. *This must be done by a pharmacist.*[24,25]
■ Never give a medication prepared by someone else. Never return unwrapped or prepared medications to stock containers; instead, dispose of them or return them to the pharmacy. Keep in mind that the disposal of any controlled substance must be cosigned by another nurse, as mandated by law.
■ If the patient questions you about her medication or dosage, check the medication record again. If the medication is correct, reassure her. Make sure you tell her about any changes in the medication or dosage. Instruct her, as appropriate, about possible adverse effects. Ask her to report anything that she feels may be an adverse effect.
■ *To avoid damaging or staining the patient's teeth,* administer iron preparations through a straw.
■ An unpleasant-tasting liquid can usually be made more palatable if taken through a straw *because the liquid contacts fewer taste buds.*
■ If the patient can't swallow a whole tablet or capsule, ask the pharmacist if the drug is available in liquid form or if it can be administered by another route. If not, ask him if you can crush the tablet or open the capsule and mix it with food. Keep in mind that many enteric-coated or time-release medications and gelatin capsules shouldn't be crushed. Remember to contact the practitioner for an order to change the route of administration when necessary.

Patient teaching

Teach the patient about her oral medications, including the indication; dosage; potential interactions with other drugs, foods, and herbal and dietary supplements; adverse effects; and special administration guidelines.[7,8] Provide the patient with a completely reconciled list of her medications and with written information about those medications at

Measuring liquid medications

To pour liquids, hold the medication cup at eye level. Use your thumb to mark off the correct level on the cup (as shown below).

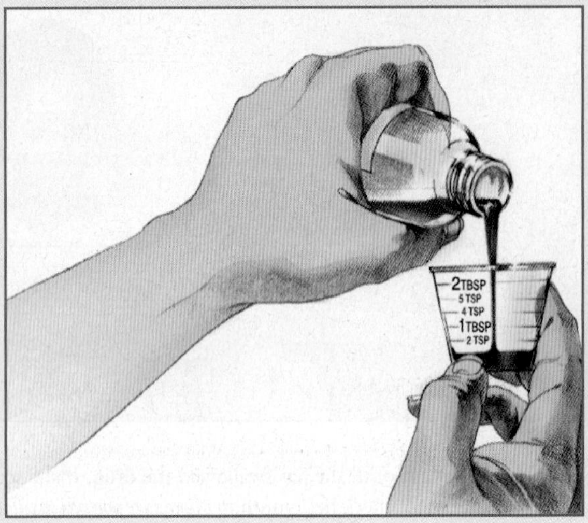

Then put the cup down and read the bottom of the meniscus, which is the curved surface of the liquid, at eye level *to ensure accuracy*. If you've poured too much medication into the cup, discard the excess. Don't return it to the bottle. Here are a few additional tips:

- Hold the container so that the medication flows from the side opposite the label *so it won't run down the container and stain or obscure the label.* Remove drips from the lip of the bottle first and then from the sides, using a clean, damp paper towel.
- For a liquid measured in drops, use only the dropper supplied with the medication.

discharge.[26,27] Make sure you meet the health literacy needs of the patient and caregiver when providing discharge instructions.[28] To assist those with functional, cognitive, or memory deficits, provide detailed medication templates or pictorial aids; assist the patient and caregiver with memory aids and dispensing devices, as needed.[29]

Take special care when teaching older patients, who are at risk for polypharmacy. (See *Reducing medication risks in older patients.*)

Documentation

Note the drug administered, the dose, the date and time, and any adverse reactions. If adverse reactions occurred, document your interventions and the patient's response to those interventions. If the patient refused a drug, document the refusal and notify the charge nurse and the patient's practitioner, as needed. Also note if a drug was omitted or withheld for other reasons, such as radiology or laboratory tests, or if, in your judgment, the drug was contraindicated at the ordered time. Verify and sign out all controlled-substances according to your controlled substances documentation system. Document patient teaching and the patient's comprehension of your teaching.

REFERENCES

1 Ndosi, M. E., & Newell, R. (2009). Nurses' knowledge of pharmacology behind drugs they commonly administer. *Journal of Clinical Nursing, 18,* 570–580.

2 Westbrook, J., et al. (2010). Association of interruptions with an increased risk and severity of medication administration errors. *Archives of Internal Medicine, 170,* 683–690. (Level IV)

3 Institute for Safe Medication Practices. (2013). Side tracks on the safety express: Interruptions lead to errors and unfinished . . . Wait, what was I doing? *Nurse Advise-ERR, 11*(2), 1–4. Accessed May 2015 via the Web at https://www.ismp.org/Newsletters/acutecare/showarticle.aspx?id=37

4 The Joint Commission. (2015). Standard MM.06.01.01. *Comprehensive accreditation manual for hospitals: The official handbook.* Oakbrook Terrace, IL: The Joint Commission. (Level VII)

5 American Osteopathic Association. (2014). Standard 16.01.03. *Healthcare Facilities Accreditation Program: Accreditation requirements for acute care hospitals.* Chicago, IL: American Osteopathic Association. (Level VII)

6 Centers for Medicare & Medicaid Services, Department of Health and Human Services. (2014). Condition of participation: Nursing services. 42 C.F.R. § 482.23(c).

7 Glaser, J., & Rolita, L. (2009). Educating the older adult in over-the-counter medication use. *Geriatrics and Aging, 12,* 103–109.

8 Boparai, M. K., & Korc-Grodzicki, B. (2011). Prescribing for older adults. *Mount Sinai Journal of Medicine, 78,* 613–626.

9 Gabe, M. E., et al. (2011). Adverse drug reactions: Treatment burdens and nurse-led medication monitoring. *Journal of Nursing Management, 19,* 377–392.

10 Woodruff, K. (2010). Preventing polypharmacy in older adults. *American Nurse Today, 5,* 10. Accessed May 2015 via the Web at http://www.americannursetoday.com/article.aspx?id=7132&fid=6852#

11 The Joint Commission. (2015). Standard NPSG.07.01.01. *Comprehensive accreditation manual for hospitals: The official handbook.* Oakbrook Terrace, IL: The Joint Commission. (Level VII)

12 Centers for Disease Control and Prevention. (2002). Guideline for hand hygiene in health-care settings: Recommendations of the Healthcare Infection Control Practices Advisory Committee and the HICPAC/SHEA/APIC/IDSA Task Force. *MMWR Recommendations and Reports, 51*(RR-16), 1–45. Accessed May 2015 via the Web at http://www.cdc.gov/mmwr/pdf/rr/rr5116.pdf (Level II)

13 World Health Organization. (2009). "WHO guidelines on hand hygiene in health care: First global patient safety challenge, clean care is safer care" [Online]. Accessed May 2015 via the Web at http://whqlibdoc.who.int/publications/2009/9789241597906_eng.pdf (Level IV)

14 American Osteopathic Association. (2014). Standard 07.01.10. *Healthcare Facilities Accreditation Program: Accreditation requirements for acute care hospitals.* Chicago, IL: American Osteopathic Association. (Level VII)

15 Centers for Medicare & Medicaid Services, Department of Health and Human Services. (2014). Condition of participation: Infection control. 42 C.F.R. § 482.42.

16 The Joint Commission. (2015). Standard NPSG.01.01.01. *Comprehensive accreditation manual for hospitals: The official handbook.* Oakbrook Terrace, IL: The Joint Commission. (Level VII)

17 Centers for Medicare & Medicaid Services, Department of Health and Human Services. (2014). Condition of participation: Patient's rights. 42 C.F.R. § 482.13(c)(1).

18 American Osteopathic Association. (2014). Standard 15.01.16. *Healthcare Facilities Accreditation Program: Accreditation requirements for acute care hospitals.* Chicago, IL: American Osteopathic Association. (Level VII)

19 Roxane Laboratories. (2013). "Cyclophosphamide capsules prescribing information" [Online]. Accessed May 2015 via the Web at http://www.accessdata.fda.gov/drugsatfda_docs/label/2013/203856s000lbl.pdf

20 The Joint Commission. (2015). Standard MM.07.01.03. *Comprehensive accreditation manual for hospitals: The official handbook.* Oakbrook Terrace, IL: The Joint Commission. (Level VII)

21 The Joint Commission. (2015). Standard RC.01.03.01. *Comprehensive accreditation manual for hospitals: The official handbook.* Oakbrook Terrace, IL: The Joint Commission. (Level VII)

22 American Osteopathic Association. (2014). Standard 10.00.03. *Healthcare Facilities Accreditation Program: Accreditation requirements for acute care hospitals.* Chicago, IL: American Osteopathic Association. (Level VII)

23 Centers for Medicare & Medicaid Services, Department of Health and Human Services. (2014). Condition of participation: Medical record services. 42 C.F.R. § 482.24(b).

Reducing medication risks in older patients[10]

To help prevent polypharmacy and other medication risks, you can help older patients manage and adhere to their medication regimens by instructing them (and caregivers, as appropriate) to take the following actions:

- Maintain an accurate list of all medications, including over-the-counter and prescribed drugs, generic and brand-name medications, dietary supplements, and herbal remedies; note dosages, dosing frequency, and the reason for taking each drug.
- Maintain a complete list of practitioners and their associated contact information.
- Bring all current medications to each practitioner's appointment.
- Post the name and telephone number of the local pharmacy where it can be easily seen.
- Adhere to dietary restrictions.
- Understand potential medication-related problems that require emergency care.
- Take medications exactly as directed.
- Link dosing schedules to routine activities of daily living.
- Use only one pharmacy to obtain medications.
- Don't share medications with others.
- Store medications in a secure, dry location away from sunlight; refrigerate medications, if necessary.
- Properly dispose of old medications.

24 The Joint Commission. (2015). Standard MM.05.01.01. *Comprehensive accreditation manual for hospitals: The official handbook.* Oakbrook Terrace, IL: The Joint Commission. (Level VII)

25 American Osteopathic Association. (2014). Standard 25.01.18. *Healthcare Facilities Accreditation Program: Accreditation requirements for acute care hospitals.* Chicago, IL: American Osteopathic Association. (Level VII)

26 American Osteopathic Association. (2014). Standard 25.02.13. *Healthcare Facilities Accreditation Program: Accreditation requirements for acute care hospitals.* Chicago, IL: American Osteopathic Association. (Level VII)

27 The Joint Commission. (2015). Standard NPSG.03.06.01. *Comprehensive accreditation manual for hospitals: The official handbook.* Oakbrook Terrace, IL: The Joint Commission. (Level VII)

28 The Joint Commission. (2010). *Advancing effective communication, cultural competence and patient- and family-centered care: A roadmap for hospitals.* Oakbrook Terrace, IL: The Joint Commission. (Level VII)

29 Hesselink, G., et al. (2012). Are patients discharged with care? A qualitative study of perceptions and experiences of patients, family members and care providers. *BMJ Quality and Safety, 21,* i39–i49.

ADDITIONAL REFERENCES

Bailey, D. G., et al. (2013). Grapefruit-medication interactions: Forbidden fruit or avoidable consequences? *Canadian Medical Association Journal, 185,* 309–316. Accessed June 2014 via the Web at http://www.cmaj.ca/content/early/2012/11/26/cmaj.120951.full.pdf

Craven, R. F., & Hirnle, C. J. (2012). *Fundamentals of nursing: Human health and function* (7th ed.). Philadelphia, PA: Lippincott Williams & Wilkins.

Nettina, S. M. (2014). *Lippincott manual of nursing practice* (10th ed.). Philadelphia, PA: Wolters Kluwer.

ORGAN DONOR, IDENTIFICATION

In 1984, the U.S. Congress passed the National Organ Transplant Act, which established the Organ Procurement and Transplant Network, a national registry for organ matching.[1] This act was created to address the critical shortage of organ donations and to improve the organ matching and placement process. With passage of this act, it's now a federal requirement for U.S. health care facilities to identify potential organ donors.

In addition to requirements of the National Organ Transplant Act, the U.S. Department of Health and Human Services requires U.S. health care facilities to report every death or imminent death to the Organ Procurement Organization (OPO) as part of the health care facility's condition of participation and eligibility to receive Medicare funds. The Joint Commission has also addressed organ donation in its accreditation requirements.[2]

As part of the process of identifying a potential organ donor, to help elicit a more positive response from the family, the practitioner should keep the family members informed about the patient's condition and provide them with information about realistic expectations for the patient's outcome.[3] The death pronouncement and the request to consider organ donation should never occur at the same time.[3] The health care facility and OPO should agree when a referral to the OPO should be made. Guidelines vary on what criteria to use, but they generally stipulate that referral to the OPO should occur when a patient scores 4 or less on the Glasgow Coma Scale[4,5] and there is an absence of brain stem reflexes.[3,5]

As the need for organ donation continues to surge, timely identification and maintenance of potential organ donors becomes even more critical to saving lives. Innovative programs are needed to provide an effective model for identifying donors, creating decision protocols, and integrating organ donation into the end-of-life continuum of care.

Equipment

Organ donation information materials ■ brain death information (commonly dictated by state laws) ■ blood sampling tubes and labels ■ Optional: personal protective equipment, equipment for monitoring vital signs and fluid status.

Preparation of equipment

Have information about organ donation and appropriate consent forms readily available. Make sure that the information is provided in a language and at a literacy level that the family members can understand.[6,7,8]

Implementation

- Determine whether the patient has an advance directive that addresses organ donation or if he is listed in a donor registry (such as on a driver's license) *because these legal documents, which are supported in most states, may influence the family's ultimate decision.*[2,6,9,10]
- Keep family members informed of the patient's medical condition *to prepare them for realistic patient outcomes.*[3]
- Arrange for an interdisciplinary meeting with the family in a quiet, nonthreatening environment, if needed, *to further help the family realize the diagnosis and prognosis.*[5]
- Consult the OPO coordinator in your area when the patient's death is imminent and before brain death testing begins *to inform the coordinator that your facility is evaluating a potential candidate for organ donation so that the coordinator can be present to guide staff members through the preparation process when appropriate.*[5]
- Collaborate with the OPO staff member *to make sure that the family's needs are met. Advance planning with the OPO helps improve donation rates.*[5,11]
- Perform hand hygiene.[12,13,14,15,16]
- Confirm the patient's identity using at least two patient identifiers.[17]
- Put on personal protective equipment, including gloves, a gown, and eye protection, if indicated.[18,19]
- Collect laboratory samples as indicated *to provide data for the assessment of organ function.* Tests may include complete blood count, liver and renal function tests, electrolyte levels, and human immunodeficiency virus tests.[3]
- Monitor vital signs and fluid status *because a patient with decreased organ perfusion may not be eligible to donate an organ.*[3]

■ Assist with examining the patient for the determination of brain death.[20]
■ As applicable, ensure that the patient's brain death has been declared and documented. Many states have certain criteria that must be followed, as well as guidelines on what type of practitioner can make the declaration, before the OPO coordinator can officially approach family members and determine their willingness to discuss organ donation.[21]
■ Contact the OPO coordinator if brain death is declared *so that a coordinator can discuss possible organ donation with the family. The OPO coordinator has the special knowledge, training, and experience to be able to deliver the appropriate message to families.*[5]
■ If the family agrees to proceed with organ donation, the OPO coordinator obtains dated and timed witnessed consent and then coordinates the process with the health care team.[6,8]
■ Encourage the family to be at the bedside as much as possible and keep them informed as procedures and preparations are taking place *to help promote family time and facilitate closure.* Assure the family that the primary focus is on the care and dignity of the patient, whether or not the donation occurs.[5]
■ Make sure that the family knows what to expect regarding end-of-life care, including when drugs are discontinued and ventilator or other therapies are withdrawn *to help prevent additional grief or anxiety.*[5]
■ Discard used supplies in the appropriate manner.[18]
■ Remove and discard your gloves and personal prote4ctive equipment[18] and perform hand hygiene.[12,13,14,15,16]
■ Document the procedure.[22,23,24]

Special considerations

■ Be aware of cultural, religious, and spiritual preferences that must also be considered when approaching the family about organ donation.[7]
■ If an ethical dilemma arises, consult your facility's ethics committee *to help clarify the decision-making process or offer viable alternatives for the family or staff members.*
■ Guidelines and practices for the determination of brain death and legislation regarding consents and procedures for organ procurement can vary based on national and state regulations as well as the patient's age.[4,20,21,25,26,27]

Complications

If communication with the OPO coordinator isn't established early enough, trust may be lost between the professional caregivers and the family, and successful organ donation may be denied. Other negative outcomes that may result include the patient's wishes not being honored, obtaining consent for organs that aren't viable, and identifying a donor who isn't medically suitable for organ donation.[3,11]

Documentation

Document any interactions you have with the family, such as multidisciplinary conferences and contact with the OPO coordinator. Document any family teaching provided and the family members' understanding of the teaching. After brain death has been determined, document the date and time of the determination as well as the name of the practitioner who made the declaration. Include all methods used to determine brain death. Document any family contact, visitation, requests, or further teaching that occurs after the organ donation process is in place.

REFERENCES

1 U.S. Department of Health & Human Services Organ Procurement and Transplantation Network. (n.d.). "Policy management: National Organ Transplant Act" [Online]. Accessed May 2015 via the Web at http://optn.transplant.hrsa.gov/policiesAndBylaws/nota.asp
2 The Joint Commission. (2015). Standard RI.01.05.01. *Comprehensive accreditation manual for hospitals: The official handbook.* Oakbrook Terrace, IL: The Joint Commission. (Level VII)
3 Lynn-McHale Wiegand, D. (Ed.). (2011). *AACN procedure manual for critical care* (6th ed.). St. Louis, MO: Saunders.
4 Rudge, C., et al. (2012). International practices of organ donation. *British Journal of Anaesthesia, 108*(Suppl. 1), i48–i55. Accessed May 2015 via the Web at http://bja.oxfordjournals.org/content/108/suppl_1/i48.full
5 National Institute for Health and Clinical Excellence (NICE). (n.d.). *Clinical guideline no. 135: Organ donation for transplantation: improving donor identification and consent rates for deceased organ donation.* London: National Institute for Health and Clinical Excellence. Accessed May 2015 via the Web at http://www.guideline.gov/content.aspx?id=36816 (Level I)
6 Centers for Medicare & Medicaid Services, Department of Health and Human Services. (2014). Condition of participation: Patient's rights. 42 C.F.R. § 482.13(b)(2).
7 The Joint Commission. (2010). "Advancing effective communication, cultural competence, and patient- and family-centered care: A roadmap for hospitals" [Online]. Oakbrook Terrace, IL: The Joint Commission. Accessed May 2015 via the Web at http://www.jointcommission.org/assets/1/6/aroadmapforhospitalsfinalversion727.pdf (Level VII)
8 American Osteopathic Association. (2014). Standard 30.01.11. *Healthcare Facilities Accreditation Program: Accreditation requirements for acute care hospitals.* Chicago, IL: American Osteopathic Association. (Level VII)
9 U.S. Department of Health and Human Services. (n.d.). "Organ donation: The process" [Online]. Accessed May 2015 via the Web at http://organdonor.gov/about/organdonationprocess.html
10 American Osteopathic Association. (2014). Standard 15.01.12. *Healthcare Facilities Accreditation Program: Accreditation requirements for acute care hospitals.* Chicago, IL: American Osteopathic Association. (Level VII)
11 Ehrle, R. (2006). Timely referral of potential organ donors. *Critical Care Nurse, 26*(2), 88–93. Accessed May 2015 via the Web at http://ccn.aacnjournals.org/content/26/2/88.full (Level V)
12 Centers for Disease Control and Prevention. (2002). Guideline for hand hygiene in health-care settings: Recommendations of the Healthcare Infection Control Practices Advisory Committee and the HICPAC/SHEA/APIC/IDSA Hand Hygiene Task Force. *MMWR Recommendations and Reports, 51*(RR-16), 1–45. Accessed May 2015 via the Web at http://www.cdc.gov/mmwr/pdf/rr/rr5116.pdf (Level II)
13 The Joint Commission. (2015). Standard NPSG.07.01.01. *Comprehensive accreditation manual for hospitals: The official handbook.* Oakbrook Terrace, IL: The Joint Commission. (Level VII)
14 World Health Organization. (2009). "WHO guidelines on hand hygiene in health care: First global patient safety challenge, clean care is safer care" [Online]. Accessed May 2015 the Web at http://whqlibdoc.who.int/publications/2009/9789241597906_eng.pdf (Level IV)
15 American Osteopathic Association. (2014). Standard 07.01.10. *Healthcare Facilities Accreditation Program: Accreditation requirements for acute care hospitals.* Chicago, IL: American Osteopathic Association. (Level VII)
16 Centers for Medicare & Medicaid Services, Department of Health and Human Services. (2014). Condition of participation: Infection control. 42 C.F.R. § 482.42.
17 The Joint Commission. (2015). Standard NPSG.01.01.01. *Comprehensive accreditation manual for hospitals: The official handbook.* Oakbrook Terrace, IL: The Joint Commission. (Level VII)
18 Siegel, J. D., et al. (2007). "2007 guideline for isolation precautions: Preventing transmission of infectious agents in healthcare settings" [Online]. Accessed May 2015 via the Web at http://www.cdc.gov/hicpac/pdf/isolation/Isolation2007.pdf (Level II)
19 American Osteopathic Association. (2014). Standard 07.01.10. *Healthcare Facilities Accreditation Program: Accreditation requirements for acute care hospitals.* Chicago, IL: American Osteopathic Association. (Level VII)
20 Wijdicks, E. F. M., et al. (2010). Evidence-based guideline update: Determining brain death in adults: Report of the Quality Standards Subcommittee of the American Academy of Neurology. *Neurology, 74,* 1911–1918. Accessed May 2015 via the Web at http://www.neurology.org/cgi/reprint/74/23/1911 (Level I)

21 U.S. Department of Health and Human Services. (2011). "State organ donation legislation" [Online]. Accessed May 2015 via the Web at http://www.organdonor.gov/legislation_micro/
22 The Joint Commission. (2015). Standard RC.01.03.01. *Comprehensive accreditation manual for hospitals: The official handbook.* Oakbrook Terrace, IL: The Joint Commission. (Level VII)
23 American Osteopathic Association. (2014). Standard 10.00.03. *Healthcare Facilities Accreditation Program: Accreditation requirements for acute care hospitals.* Chicago, IL: American Osteopathic Association. (Level VII)
24 Centers for Medicare & Medicaid Services, Department of Health and Human Services. (2014). Condition of participation: Medical record services. 42 C.F.R. § 482.24(b).
25 Wijdicks, E. F. M. (2011). The transatlantic divide over brain death determination and the debate. *Brain, 2011,* 1–11. Accessed May 2015 via the Web at http://brain.oxfordjournals.org/content/early/2011/12/24/brain.awr282.full.pdf+html
26 Nakagawa, T. A., et al. (2011). American Academy of Pediatrics: Guidelines for the determination of brain death in infants and children: An update of the 1987 task force recommendations. *Pediatrics, 128,* e720–e740. Accessed May 2015 via the Web at http://pediatrics.aappublications.org/content/128/3/e720.full (Level VII)
27 Smith, M. (2012). Brain death: Time for an international consensus. *British Journal of Anaesthesia, 108*(Suppl. 1), i6–i9. Accessed May 2015 via the Web at http://bja.oxfordjournals.org/content/108/suppl_1/i6.full.pdf+html

Oronasopharyngeal suction

Oronasopharyngeal suction removes secretions from the pharynx by a suction catheter inserted through the mouth or nostril. Used to maintain a patent airway, this procedure helps the patient who can't clear his airway effectively with coughing and expectoration, such as the unconscious or severely debilitated patient. The procedure should be performed as often as necessary, depending on the patient's condition. Including oral suctioning as part of standard oral hygiene practice in intubated patients may reduce the risk of ventilator-associated pneumonia.[1,2]

Because the catheter may inadvertently slip into the lower airway or esophagus, oronasopharyngeal suction is a sterile procedure that requires sterile equipment. However, clean technique is sufficient for a tonsil tip suction device. In fact, an alert patient can use a tonsil tip suction device himself to remove secretions.

Equipment

Wall suction or portable suction unit with connecting tubing ■ water-soluble lubricant ■ sterile normal saline solution ■ disposable sterile container ■ sterile suction catheter (a #10 to #16 French) ■ sterile gloves ■ overbed table ■ towel ■ stethoscope ■ hospital-grade disinfectant ■ Optional: tongue blade, tonsil tip suction device, nasopharyngeal or oropharyngeal airway (optional for frequent suctioning), personal protective equipment (such as a gown and mask and goggles or mask with face shield).

A commercially prepared kit contains a sterile catheter, a disposable container, and sterile gloves.

Preparation of equipment

Gather and place the suction equipment on the patient's overbed table or bedside stand. Position the table or stand on your preferred side of the bed *to facilitate suctioning.* Connect the tubing to the suctioning unit. Date and then open the bottle of normal saline solution.

Implementation

■ Verify the practitioner's order for oropharyngeal suctioning if your facility requires one.

■ Review the patient's blood gas or oxygen saturation values and vital signs. Check his history for contraindications, such as a deviated septum, nasal polyps, nasal obstruction, traumatic injury, facial trauma, epistaxis, or mucosal swelling.

■ Gather and prepare the appropriate equipment.

■ Perform hand hygiene.[3,4,5,6,7]

■ Confirm the patient's identity using at least two patient identifiers.[8]

■ Explain the procedure to the patient even if he's unresponsive. Inform him that suctioning may stimulate transient coughing or gagging, but tell him that coughing helps to mobilize secretions. If he has been suctioned before, just summarize the reasons for the procedure. Reassure him throughout the procedure *to minimize anxiety and fear, which can increase oxygen consumption.*

■ Put on personal protective equipment, as appropriate, *to comply with standard precautions.*[9,10]

■ Evaluate the patient's respiratory status and ability to cough and deep breathe *to determine his ability to move secretions up the tracheobronchial tree.*

■ If you are suctioning through the nose, determine which nostril is more patent.

■ Place the patient in the semi-Fowler or high Fowler position, if tolerated, *to promote lung expansion and effective coughing.* If the patient is unconscious, position him on his side facing you *to help promote drainage of secretions.*

■ Place a towel across the patient's chest.

■ Turn on the suction from the wall or portable unit and

■ set the pressure, typically to between 100 and 120 mm Hg; *higher pressures cause excessive trauma without enhancing secretion removal.*[11]

■ Occlude the end of the connecting tubing *to check suction pressure.*

■ Using sterile technique, open the suction catheter kit or the packages containing the sterile catheter, container, and gloves. Put on the gloves;[9] consider your dominant hand sterile and your nondominant hand nonsterile.

■ Using your nondominant hand, pour the saline solution into the sterile container.

■ With your nondominant hand, place a small amount of water-soluble lubricant on the sterile area of the catheter. *The lubricant facilitates passage of the catheter during nasopharyngeal suctioning.*

■ Pick up the catheter with your dominant (sterile) hand and attach it to the connecting tubing (as shown below). Use your nondominant hand to control the suction valve while your dominant hand manipulates the catheter.

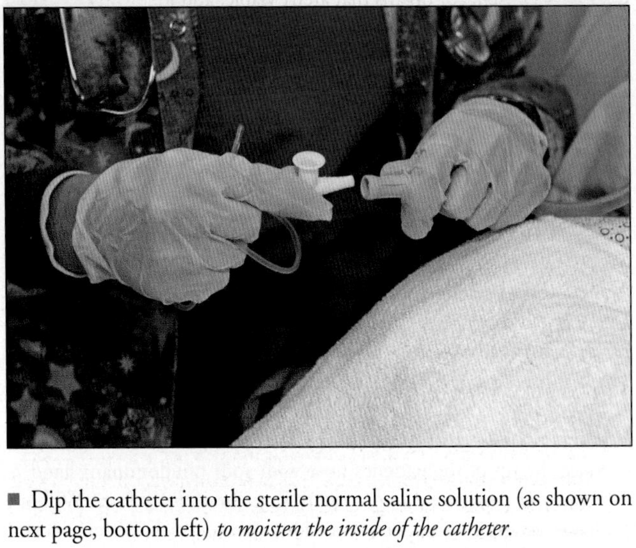

■ Dip the catheter into the sterile normal saline solution (as shown on next page, bottom left) *to moisten the inside of the catheter.*

PATIENT TEACHING

Tips on airway clearance

Deep breathing and coughing are vital for removing secretions from the lungs. Other techniques used to help clear the airways include diaphragmatic breathing and forced expiration. Here's how to teach these techniques to your patients.

Diaphragmatic breathing

First, tell the patient to lie in the supine position, with his head elevated 15 to 20 degrees on a pillow. Tell him to place one hand on his abdomen and then inhale so that he can feel his abdomen rise. Explain that this is known as "breathing with the diaphragm."

Next, instruct the patient to exhale slowly through his nose—or, even better, through pursed lips—while letting his abdomen collapse. Explain that this action decreases his respiratory rate and increases his tidal volume.

Suggest that the patient perform this exercise for 30 minutes several times a day. After he becomes accustomed to the position and has learned to breathe using his diaphragm, he may apply abdominal weights of 8.8 to 11 lb (4 to 5 kg). *The weights enhance the movement of the diaphragm toward the head during expiration.*

To enhance the effectiveness of exercise, the patient may also manually compress the lower costal margins, perform straight-leg lifts, and coordinate the breathing technique with a physical activity such as walking.

Forced expiration

Explain to the patient that forced expiration (also known as *huff coughing)* helps clear secretions while causing less traumatic injury than does a cough. To perform the technique, tell the patient to forcefully expire without closing his glottis, starting with a middle to low lung volume. Tell him to follow this expiration with a period of diaphragmatic breathing and relaxation.

Inform the patient that if his secretions are in the central airways, he may have to use a more forceful expiration or a cough to clear them.

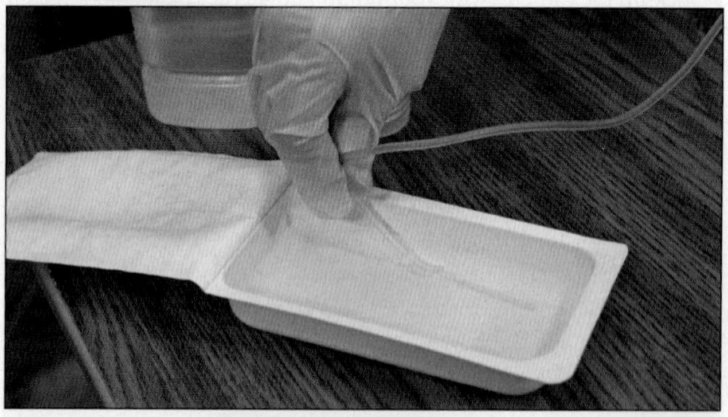

■ Instruct the patient to cough and breathe slowly and deeply several times before beginning suction. *Coughing helps loosen secretions and may decrease the amount of suction necessary, while deep breathing helps minimize or prevent hypoxia.* (See *Tips on airway clearance.*)

For nasal insertion

■ Raise the tip of the patient's nose with your nondominant hand *to straighten the passageway and facilitate insertion of the catheter.* Without applying suction, gently insert the suction catheter into the patient's nostril (as shown on top right). Roll the catheter between your fingers *to help it advance through the turbinates.* Continue to advance the catheter approximately 5″ to 6″ (13 to 15 cm) until you reach the pool of secretions or the patient begins to cough.

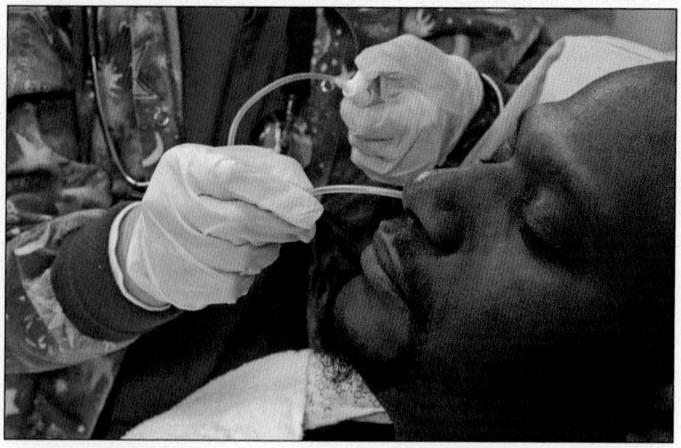

For oral insertion

■ Without applying suction, gently insert the catheter into the patient's mouth. Advance it 3″ to 4″ (7.5 to 10 cm) along the side of the patient's mouth until you reach the pool of secretions or the patient begins to cough. Suction both sides of the patient's mouth and pharyngeal area.

Completing the procedure

■ Using intermittent suction, withdraw the catheter from either the mouth or the nose with a continuous rotating motion *to minimize invagination of the mucosa into the catheter's tip and side ports.* Apply suction for no longer than 10 seconds at a time *to minimize tissue trauma.*

■ Between passes, wrap the catheter around your dominant hand *to prevent contamination.*

■ If secretions are thick, clear the lumen of the catheter by dipping it in normal saline solution and applying suction.

■ Repeat the procedure, up to three times, until gurgling or bubbling sounds stop and respirations are quiet. Allow 30 seconds to 1 minute *to allow reoxygenation and reventilation.*

■ After completing suctioning, pull your sterile glove off over the coiled catheter and discard them.[9]

■ Flush the connecting tubing with normal saline solution. Then discard the container of normal saline solution and remove your other glove.[9]

■ Remove and discard other personal protective equipment, if worn.[9]

■ Perform hand hygiene.[3,4,5,6,7]

■ Reassess the patient's respiratory status *to evaluate the patient's tolerance of the procedure.*

■ Clean and disinfect your stethoscope using a disinfectant pad.[12,13]

■ Perform hand hygiene.[3,4,5,6,7]

■ Document the procedure.[14,15,16]

Special considerations

■ If the patient has no history of nasal problems, alternate suctioning between nostrils *to minimize traumatic injury.*

■ If the patient requires repeated oronasopharyngeal suctioning, the use of a nasopharyngeal or oropharyngeal airway will help with catheter insertion, reduce traumatic injury, and promote a patent airway. (See the "Nasopharyngeal airway insertion and care" and "Oropharyngeal airway insertion and care" procedures, pages 536, 571.)

■ If the patient has excessive oral secretions, consider using a tonsil tip suction device, *which allows the patient to remove oral secretions independently.*

■ Let the patient rest after suctioning while you continue to observe him. The frequency and duration of suctioning depend on the patient's tolerance of the procedure and on complications.

Patient teaching

Oronasopharyngeal suctioning may be performed in the home using a portable suction machine. Under these circumstances, suctioning is a clean rather than a sterile procedure. Properly cleaned catheters can be reused, putting less financial strain on the patient. Whether the patient requires disposable or reusable suction equipment, make sure that the patient and his caregivers have received proper teaching and support.

Complications

Increased dyspnea caused by hypoxia and anxiety may result from this procedure. Hypoxia can result *because oxygen from the oronasopharynx is removed with the secretions.* The amount of oxygen removed varies, depending upon the duration of the suctioning, suction flow and pressure, the size of the catheter in relation to the size of the patient's airway, and the patient's physical condition.

In addition, bloody aspirate can result from prolonged or traumatic suctioning. Using water-soluble lubricant can help to minimize traumatic injury.

Documentation

Record the date, time, reason for suctioning, and technique used; the amount, color, consistency, and odor (if any) of the secretions; the patient's respiratory status before and after the procedure; any complications and the nursing actions taken; and the patient's tolerance of the procedure. Document any patient teaching and the patient's understanding of the teaching.

REFERENCES

1 Association of Professionals in Infection Control and Epidemiology. (2009). "An APIC guide 2009: Guide to the elimination of ventilator-associated pneumonia" [Online]. Accessed May 2015 via the Web at http://www.apic.org/Resource_/EliminationGuideForm/18e326ad-b484-471c-9c35-6822a53ee4a2/File/VAP_09.pdf (Level IV)

2 Sole, M. L., et al. (2011). Oronasopharyngeal secretion volume in intubated patients: The importance of oral suctioning. *American Journal of Critical Care, 20,* e141–e145. (Level IV)

3 The Joint Commission. (2015). Standard NPSG.07.01.01. *Comprehensive accreditation manual for hospitals: The official handbook.* Oakbrook Terrace, IL: The Joint Commission. (Level VII)

4 Centers for Disease Control and Prevention. (2002). Guideline for hand hygiene in health-care settings: Recommendations of the Healthcare Infection Control Practices Advisory Committee and the HICPAC/SHEA/APIC/IDSA Hand Hygiene Task Force. *MMWR Recommendations and Reports, 51*(RR-16), 1–45. Accessed May 2015 via the Web at http://www.cdc.gov/mmwr/pdf/rr/rr5116.pdf (Level II)

5 World Health Organization. (2009). "WHO guidelines on hand hygiene in health care: First global patient safety challenge, clean care is safer care" [Online]. Accessed May 2015 via the Web at http://whqlibdoc.who.int/publications/2009/9789241597906_eng.pdf (Level IV)

6 Centers for Medicare & Medicaid Services, Department of Health and Human Services. (2014). Condition of participation: Infection control. 42 C.F.R. 482.42.

7 American Osteopathic Association. (2014). Standard 07.01.21. *Healthcare Facilities Accreditation Program: Accreditation requirements for acute care hospitals.* Chicago, IL: American Osteopathic Association. (Level VII)

8 The Joint Commission. (2015). Standard NPSG.01.01.01. *Comprehensive accreditation manual for hospitals: The official handbook.* Oakbrook Terrace, IL: The Joint Commission. (Level VII)

9 Siegel, J. D., et al. (2007). "2007 guideline for isolation precautions: Preventing transmission of infectious agents in healthcare settings" [Online]. Accessed May 2015 via the Web at http://www.cdc.gov/hicpac/pdf/isolation/Isolation2007.pdf (Level II)

10 American Osteopathic Association. (2014). Standard 07.01.10. *Healthcare Facilities Accreditation Program: Accreditation requirements for acute care hospitals.* Chicago, IL: American Osteopathic Association. (Level VII)

11 Lynn-McHale Wiegand, D. (Ed.). (2011). *AACN procedure manual for critical care* (6th ed.). St. Louis, MO: Saunders.

12 Rutala, W. A., et al. (2008). "Guideline for disinfection and sterilization in healthcare facilities, 2008" [Online]. Accessed May 2015 via the Web at http://www.cdc.gov/hicpac/pdf/guidelines/Disinfection_Nov_2008.pdf (Level I)

13 American Osteopathic Association. (2014). Standard 07.02.03. *Healthcare Facilities Accreditation Program: Accreditation requirements for acute care hospitals.* Chicago, IL: American Osteopathic Association. (Level VII)

14 The Joint Commission. (2015). Standard RC.01.03.01. *Comprehensive accreditation manual for hospitals: The official handbook.* Oakbrook Terrace, IL: The Joint Commission. (Level VII)

15 Centers for Medicare & Medicaid Services, Department of Health and Human Services. (2014). Condition of participation: Medical record services. 42 C.F.R. § 482.24(b).

16 American Osteopathic Association. (2014). Standard 10.00.03. *Healthcare Facilities Accreditation Program: Accreditation requirements for acute care hospitals.* Chicago, IL: American Osteopathic Association. (Level VII)

OROPHARYNGEAL AIRWAY INSERTION AND CARE

An oropharyngeal airway, a curved plastic device, is inserted into the mouth to the posterior pharynx to establish or maintain a patent airway. In an unconscious patient, the tongue usually obstructs the posterior pharynx. The oropharyngeal airway conforms to the curvature of the palate, removing the obstruction and allowing air to pass around and through the tube. It also facilitates oropharyngeal suctioning. The oropharyngeal airway is intended for short-term use and should be used only in an unresponsive patient who can't maintain his airway. It may be left in place longer as an airway adjunct to prevent the orally intubated patient from biting the endotracheal tube.

The oropharyngeal airway isn't the airway of choice for the patient with loose or avulsed teeth or who has undergone recent oral surgery.

NURSING ALERT *Inserting this airway in an conscious or semiconscious patient may stimulate vomiting and laryngospasm; use only in unresponsive patients who don't have a cough or gag reflex.*[1]

Equipment

For inserting

Oral airway of appropriate size ▪ tongue blade ▪ padded tongue blade ▪ gloves ▪ tape ▪ stethoscope ▪ hospital-grade disinfectant ▪ oral care supplies ▪ Optional: suction equipment, resuscitation mask, handheld resuscitation bag or oxygen-powered breathing device, mask and goggles or mask with face shield.

For reflex testing

Cotton-tipped applicator.

Preparation of equipment

Select an appropriate size airway for your patient; *an oversized airway can obstruct breathing by depressing the epiglottis into the laryngeal opening.* Usually, you'll select a medium size (size 4 or 5) for the average adult and a large size (size 6) for the large adult. Be sure to confirm the correct size of the airway by placing the airway flange beside the patient's cheek, parallel to his front teeth. If the airway is the right size, the airway curve should reach to the angle of the jaw.

Implementation

- Verify the practitioner's order.
- Gather the appropriate equipment.
- Perform hand hygiene.[2,3,4,5,6]
- Confirm the patient's identity using at least two patient identifiers.[7]

EQUIPMENT

Inserting an oral airway

Unless this position is contraindicated, hyperextend the patient's head (as shown below) before using either the cross-finger or tongue blade insertion method.

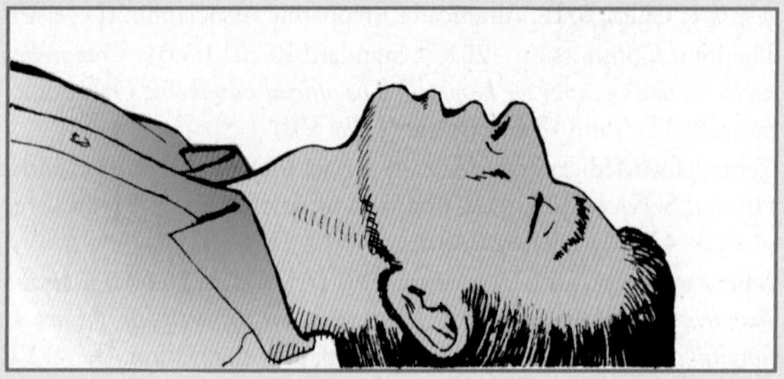

To insert an oral airway using the cross-finger method, place your thumb on the patient's lower teeth and your index finger on his upper teeth. Gently open his mouth by pushing his teeth apart (as shown below).

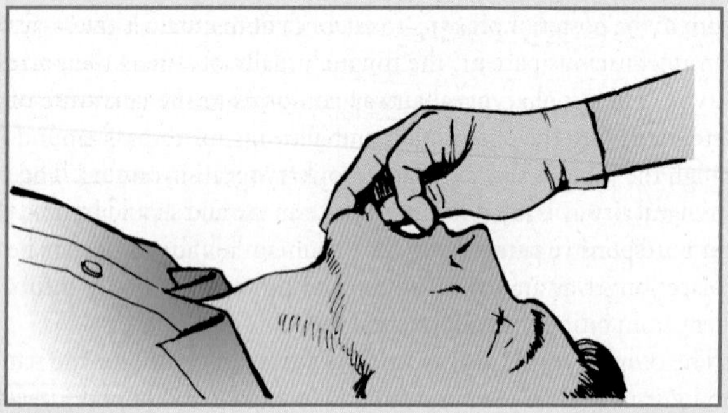

Insert the airway upside down *to avoid pushing the tongue toward the pharynx,* and slide it over the tongue toward the back of the mouth. Rotate the airway as it approaches the posterior wall of the pharynx so that it points downward (as shown below).

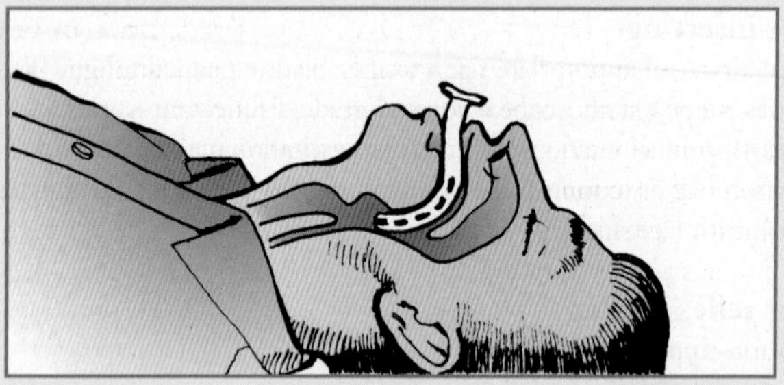

To use the tongue blade technique, open the patient's mouth and depress his tongue with the blade. Guide the airway over the back of the tongue as you did for the cross-finger technique.

- Explain the procedure to the patient even though he may not appear to be alert.
- Provide privacy.[8,9]
- Put on gloves as necessary *to comply with standard precautions.* Use a mask and goggles or a mask with face shield if secretions are copious
- If the patient is wearing dentures, remove them *so they don't cause further airway obstruction.*
- Suction the patient if necessary. (See "Oronasopharyngeal suction," page 569.)
- Place the patient in the supine position with his neck hyperextended, if this isn't contraindicated. Otherwise, use the jaw-thrust maneuver if a cervical spine injury is suspected.[1]
- Insert the airway using the cross-finger or the tongue blade technique. (See *Inserting an oral airway.*)
- Immediately after insertion, auscultate the lungs and assess the patient's respirations. If respirations are absent or inadequate, initiate artificial positive-pressure ventilation with a mouth-to-mask technique, a handheld resuscitation bag, or an oxygen-powered breathing device *to ensure adequate ventilation.* Stridor, gasping respirations, or snoring may indicate inadequate airway placement.[10]
- After you insert and secure the airway, position the patient on his side *to decrease the risk of aspiration of vomitus.*
- Frequently check the position of the airway to ensure correct placement. Make sure that the patient's lips and tongue aren't between his teeth and airway *to prevent traumatic injury.*
- Suction the patient as necessary.
- Reassess the patient's respiratory status following suctioning and at an interval determined by the patient's condition and your facility.[10]
- Perform oral care every 2 to 4 hours.[10] Remove the airway. Brush teeth, gums, and tongue at least twice per day using a soft toothbrush. Moisturize the oral mucosa and lips every 2 to 4 hours.[13,14] Reinsert the airway after oral care. (See the "Oral care" procedure, page 560.)
- While you've removed the airway for oral care, observe the mouth's mucous membranes[13,14] *because tissue irritation or ulceration can result from prolonged airway use.*
- Remove and discard your gloves.[11]
- Perform hand hygiene.[2,3,4,5,6]
- Clean and disinfect your stethoscope with a disinfectant pad.[15,16]
- Perform hand hygiene.[2,3,4,5,6]
- Document the procedure.[17,18,19]

Special considerations

- Evaluate the patient's behavior *to provide the cue for airway removal.* The patient is likely to gag or cough as he becomes more alert, indicating that he no longer needs the airway.
- When the patient regains consciousness and can swallow, remove the airway by pulling it outward and downward, following the mouth's natural curvature.
- Remove the oropharyngeal airway every 8 hours or as needed. Clean the airway according to the manufacturer's instructions and reinsert the clean airway.[10]
- After removing the airway, test the patient's cough and gag reflexes *to ensure that removal of the airway wasn't premature and that the patient can maintain his own airway.* To test for the gag reflex, use a cotton-tipped applicator to touch both sides of the posterior pharynx. To test for the cough reflex, gently touch the posterior oropharynx with the cotton-tipped applicator.

Complications

Tooth damage or loss, tissue damage, and bleeding may result from insertion. If the airway is too long, it may press the epiglottis against the entrance of the larynx, producing complete airway obstruction. If the airway isn't inserted properly, it may push the tongue posteriorly, aggravating the problem of upper airway obstruction.

If respirations are absent or inadequate immediately after inserting the airway, initiate artificial positive-pressure ventilation by using a mouth-to-mask technique, a handheld resuscitation bag, or an oxygen-powered breathing device. (See "Manual ventilation," page 489.)

Documentation

Record the date and time of the airway's insertion, size of the airway, removal and cleaning of the airway, condition of mucous membranes, any suctioning, adverse reactions and nursing actions taken, and the patient's tolerance of the procedure.

REFERENCES

1 American Heart Association. (2010). 2010 American Heart Association guidelines for cardiopulmonary resuscitation and emergency cardiovascular care. *Circulation, 122,* S729–S767. (Level II)

2 The Joint Commission. (2015). Standard NPSG.07.01.01. *Comprehensive accreditation manual for hospitals: The official handbook.* Oakbrook Terrace, IL: The Joint Commission. (Level VII)

3 Centers for Disease Control and Prevention. (2002). Guideline for hand hygiene in health-care settings: Recommendations of the Healthcare Infection Control Practices Advisory Committee and the HICPAC/SHEA/APIC/IDSA Hand Hygiene Task Force. *MMWR Recommendations and Reports, 51*(RR-16), 1–45. Accessed May 2015 via the Web at http://www.cdc.gov/mmwr/pdf/rr/rr5116.pdf (Level II)

4 World Health Organization. (2009). "WHO guidelines on hand hygiene in health care: First global patient safety challenge, clean care is safer care" [Online]. Accessed May 2015 via the Web at http://whqlibdoc.who.int/publications/2009/9789241597906_eng.pdf (Level IV)

5 Centers for Medicare & Medicaid Services, Department of Health and Human Services. (2014). Condition of participation: Infection control. 42 C.F.R. § 482.42.

6 American Osteopathic Association. (2014). Standard 07.01.21. *Healthcare Facilities Accreditation Program: Accreditation requirements for acute care hospitals.* Chicago, IL: American Osteopathic Association. (Level VII)

7 The Joint Commission. (2015). Standard NPSG.01.01.01. *Comprehensive accreditation manual for hospitals: The official handbook.* Oakbrook Terrace, IL: The Joint Commission. (Level VII)

8 Centers for Medicare & Medicaid Services, Department of Health and Human Services. (2014). Condition of participation: Patient's rights. 42 C.F.R. § 482.13(c)(1).

9 American Osteopathic Association. (2014). Standard 15.01.16. *Healthcare Facilities Accreditation Program: Accreditation requirements for acute care hospitals.* Chicago, IL: American Osteopathic Association. (Level VII)

10 Lynn-McHale Wiegand, D. (Ed.). (2011). AACN procedure manual for critical care (6th ed.). St. Louis, MO: Saunders.

11 Siegel, J. D., et al. (2007). "2007 guideline for isolation precautions: Preventing transmission of infectious agents in healthcare settings" [Online]. Accessed May 2015 via the Web at http://www.cdc.gov/hicpac/pdf/isolation/Isolation2007.pdf (Level II)

12 American Osteopathic Association. (2014). Standard 07.01.10. *Healthcare Facilities Accreditation Program: Accreditation requirements for acute care hospitals.* Chicago, IL: American Osteopathic Association. (Level VII)

13 American Association of Critical-Care Nurses. (2010). "AACN practice alert: Oral care for patients at risk for ventilator-associated pneumonia" [Online]. Accessed May 2015 via the Web at http://www.aacn.org/WD/Practice/Docs/PracticeAlerts/oral%20care%2004-2010%20final.pdf (Level VII)

14 Ames, N. J., et al. (2011). Effects of systematic oral care in critically ill patients: A multicenter study. *American Journal of Critical Care, 20,* 103–113. Accessed May 2015 via the Web at http://www.aacn.org/wd/Cetests/media/a1120053.pdf (Level VI)

15 Rutala, W. A., et al. (2008). "Guideline for disinfection and sterilization in healthcare facilities, 2008" [Online]. Accessed May 2015 via the Web at http://www.cdc.gov/hicpac/pdf/guidelines/Disinfection_Nov_2008.pdf (Level I)

16 American Osteopathic Association. (2014). Standard 07.02.03. *Healthcare Facilities Accreditation Program: Accreditation requirements for acute care hospitals.* Chicago, IL: American Osteopathic Association. (Level VII)

17 The Joint Commission. (2015). Standard RC.01.03.01. *Comprehensive accreditation manual for hospitals: The official handbook.* Oakbrook Terrace, IL: The Joint Commission. (Level VII)

18 Centers for Medicare & Medicaid Services, Department of Health and Human Services. (2014). Condition of participation: Medical record services. 42 C.F.R. § 482.24(b).

19 American Osteopathic Association. (2014). Standard 10.00.03. *Healthcare Facilities Accreditation Program: Accreditation requirements for acute care hospitals.* Chicago, IL: American Osteopathic Association. (Level VII)

ADDITIONAL REFERENCE

Taylor, C., et al. (2015). *Fundamentals of nursing: The art and science of nursing care* (7th ed.). Philadelphia, PA: Wolters Kluwer.

OXYGEN ADMINISTRATION

A patient will need oxygen therapy when hypoxemia results from a respiratory or cardiac emergency or an increase in metabolic function.

In a *respiratory emergency,* oxygen administration enables the patient to reduce his ventilatory effort. When conditions such as atelectasis or acute respiratory distress syndrome impair diffusion, or when lung volumes are decreased from alveolar hypoventilation, this procedure boosts alveolar oxygen levels.

In a *cardiac emergency,* oxygen therapy helps meet the increased myocardial workload as the heart tries to compensate for hypoxemia. Oxygen administration is particularly important for a patient whose myocardium is already compromised—for instance, from a myocardial infarction or cardiac arrhythmia.

When *metabolic demand* is high (in cases of massive trauma, burns, or high fever, for instance) oxygen administration supplies the body with enough oxygen to meet its cellular needs. This procedure also increases oxygenation in the patient with a reduced blood oxygen-carrying capacity, perhaps from carbon monoxide poisoning or sickle cell crisis.

The adequacy of oxygen therapy is determined by arterial blood gas (ABG) analysis, oximetry monitoring, and clinical examinations. The patient's disease, physical condition, and age help determine the most appropriate method of administration.

Equipment

The equipment needed depends on the type of delivery system ordered. (See *Guide to oxygen delivery systems,* page 574.) Equipment includes selections from the following list: Oxygen source (wall unit, cylinder, liquid tank, or concentrator) ■ flowmeter ■ adapter, if using a wall unit, or a pressure-reduction gauge, if using a cylinder ■ sterile humidity bottle and adapters ■ sterile distilled water ■ OXYGEN PRECAUTIONS sign ■ appropriate oxygen delivery system (nasal cannula, simple mask, or nonrebreather mask for low-flow and variable oxygen concentrations; Venturi mask, aerosol mask, T tube, tracheostomy collar, tent, or oxygen hood for high-flow and specific oxygen concentrations) ■ small-diameter or large-diameter connection tubing ■ jet adapter for Venturi mask (if adding humidity) ■ stethoscope ■ sphygmomanometer ■ pulse oximeter and probe ■ Optional: gloves, mask and goggles or mask with face shield,[1] gauze pads, tape, oxygen analyzer, ABG kit.

Preparation of equipment

Although a respiratory therapist typically is responsible for setting up, maintaining, and managing the equipment, you'll need a working knowledge of the oxygen system being used.

Check the oxygen outlet port *to verify flow.* If using a nasal cannula, pinch the tubing near the prongs *to listen for a higher-pitched sound caused by the release of increased pressure.* All oxygen delivery systems should be checked at least once each day; some systems require more frequent checks by a calibrated analyzer.[2]

Implementation

- Verify the practitioner's order for the oxygen therapy *because oxygen is considered a medication or therapy and should be prescribed.*[3]
- Gather the equipment.
- Perform hand hygiene.[4,5,6,7,8]
- Confirm the patient's identity using at least two patient identifiers.[9]

EQUIPMENT

Guide to oxygen delivery systems

Patients may receive oxygen through one of several administration systems. Each has its own benefits, drawbacks, and indications for use. The advantages and disadvantages of each system are compared below.

Nasal cannula

Oxygen is delivered through plastic cannulas in the patient's nostrils.

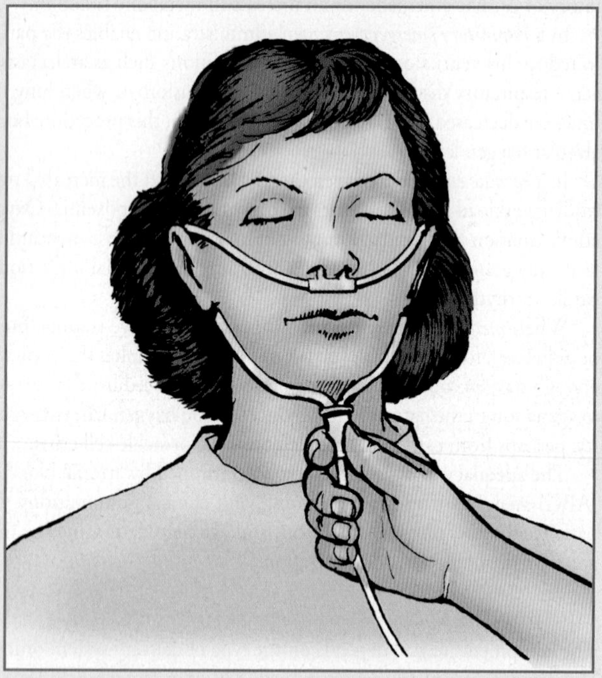

Advantages: Safe and simple; comfortable and easily tolerated; nasal prongs can be shaped to fit any face; effective for low oxygen concentrations; allows movement, eating, and talking; inexpensive and disposable.

Disadvantages: Can't deliver concentrations higher than 40%; can't be used in complete nasal obstruction; may cause headaches or dry mucous membranes if flow rate exceeds 6 L/minute;[2] can dislodge easily.

Administration guidelines: Hook the cannula tubing behind the patient's ears and under the chin. Slide the adjuster upward under the chin *to secure the tubing.* If using an elastic strap to secure the cannula, position it over the ears and around the back of the head. Don't apply it too tightly *because doing so can result in excess pressure on facial structures and cannula occlusion as well.* With a nasal cannula, oral breathers achieve the same oxygen delivery as nasal breathers. Provide humidification at a flow rate greater than 4 L/minute.[2] Use care when assigning an estimated fraction of inspired oxygen (F_{IO_2}) to patients *because this low-flow system can have great fluctuations.*[2]

Simple mask

Oxygen flows through an entry port at the bottom of the mask and exits through large holes on the sides of the mask.

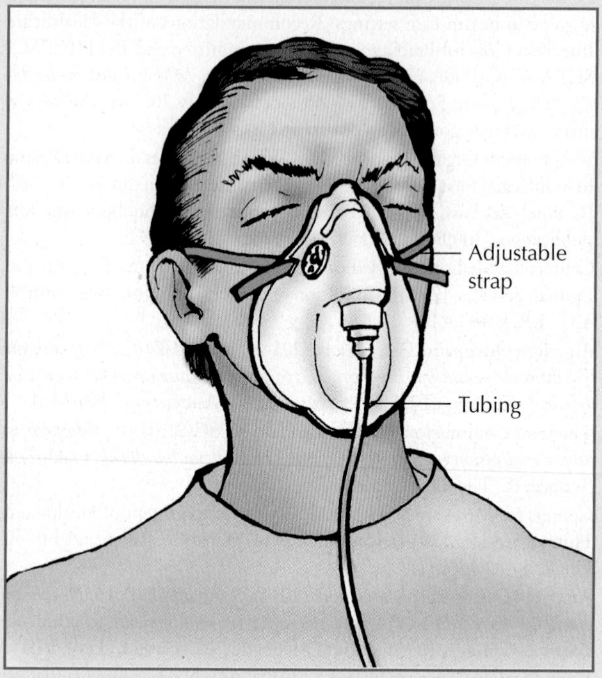

Advantages: Can deliver concentrations of 35% to 50%.[2]

Disadvantages: Hot and confining; may irritate patient's skin; tight seal, which may cause discomfort, is required for higher oxygen concentrations; interferes with talking and eating; impractical for long-term therapy because of its imprecision.

Administration guidelines: Select the mask size that offers the best fit. Place the mask over the patient's nose, mouth, and chin, and mold the flexible metal edge to the bridge of the nose. Adjust the elastic band around the head *to hold the mask firmly but comfortably over the cheeks, chin, and bridge of the nose.* For elderly or cachectic patients with sunken cheeks, tape gauze pads to the mask over the cheek area *to try to create an airtight seal. Without this seal, room air dilutes the oxygen, preventing delivery of the prescribed concentration.* A minimum of 5 L/minute is required in all masks *to flush expired carbon dioxide from the mask so that the patient doesn't rebreathe it.*[2]

- Obtain a baseline physical assessment, including vital signs, breath sounds, oxygen saturation, and physical assessment. In an emergency, verify that the patient has a patent airway before administering oxygen.
- Explain the procedure to the patient, and let him know why he needs oxygen. He will need to be able to cooperate with the oxygen administration.
- Select the most appropriate oxygen delivery device based on the order and the patient's status.
- Check the patient's room *to make sure it's safe for oxygen administration.* Whenever possible, replace electrical devices with nonelectrical ones.
- Place an OXYGEN PRECAUTIONS sign over the patient's bed and on the door to his room.
- Put on gloves and other personal protective equipment as needed *to comply with standard precautions.*[10]
- Help place the oxygen delivery device on the patient. Make sure it fits properly and is stable.

EQUIPMENT

Guide to oxygen delivery systems *(continued)*

Nonrebreather mask

On inhalation, the one-way valve opens, directing oxygen from a reservoir bag into the mask. On exhalation, gas exits the mask through the one-way expiratory valve and enters the atmosphere. The patient breathes gas only from the bag.

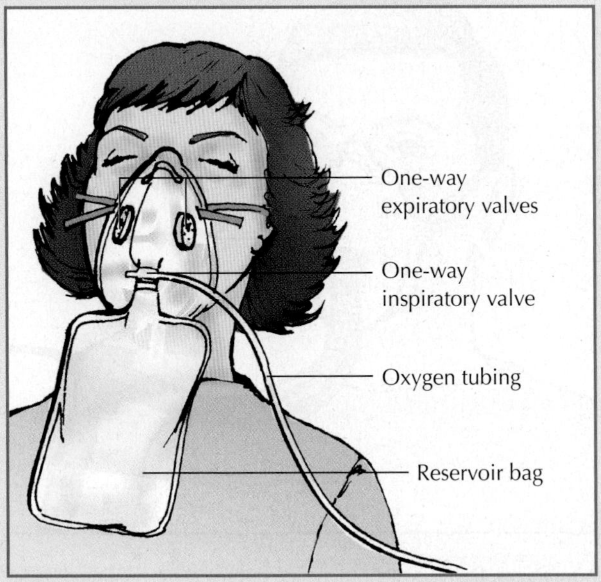

Advantages: Delivers the highest possible oxygen concentration (60% to 90%) short of intubation and mechanical ventilation; effective for short-term therapy; can be converted to a partial rebreather mask, if necessary, by removing the one-way valve.

Disadvantages: Requires a tight seal, which may be difficult to maintain and may cause discomfort; may irritate the patient's skin; interferes with talking and eating; impractical for long-term therapy.

Administration guidelines: Follow procedures listed for the simple mask. Make sure that the mask fits very snugly and that the one-way valves are secure and functioning. Provide a minimum flow rate of 10 L/minute.[2] *Because the mask excludes room air,* valve malfunction can cause carbon dioxide buildup and suffocate an unconscious patient. If the reservoir bag collapses more than slightly during inspiration, raise the flow rate until you see only a slight deflation. *Marked or complete deflation indicates an insufficient flow rate.* Keep the reservoir bag from twisting or kinking. *Ensure free expansion* by making sure the bag lies outside the patient's gown and bedcovers.

CPAP mask

This system allows the spontaneously breathing patient to receive continuous positive airway pressure (CPAP), with or without an artificial airway. A positive end-expiratory pressure valve may be fitted to the mask on the lower expiratory *port to allow expired gases to be exhaled under a fixed valve pressure.*

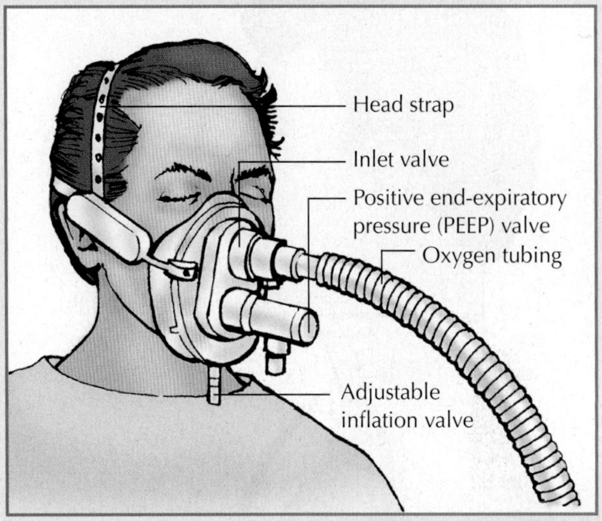

Advantages: Noninvasively improves arterial oxygenation by increasing functional residual capacity; allows the patient to avoid intubation; allows the patient to talk and cough without interrupting positive pressure.

Disadvantages: Requires a tight fit, which may cause discomfort; interferes with eating and talking; increases the risk of aspiration if the patient vomits; increases the risk of pneumothorax, diminished cardiac output, and gastric distention; must be used cautiously in patients with chronic obstructive pulmonary disease, bullous lung disease, low cardiac output, or tension pneumothorax.

Administration guidelines: Place one strap behind the patient's head and the other strap over his head *to ensure a snug fit.* Attach one latex strap to the connector prong on one side of the mask. Then, use one hand to position the mask on the patient's face while using the other hand to connect the strap to the other side of the mask. After the mask is applied, assess the patient's respiratory, circulatory, and GI function every hour. Watch for signs of pneumothorax, decreased cardiac output, a drop in blood pressure, and gastric distention.

(continued)

- Monitor the patient's response to oxygen therapy using pulse oximetry. Make sure that the alarm limits are set appropriately for the patient's current condition and that alarms are turned on, functioning properly, and audible to staff.[11,12,13,14]
- If the practitioner has ordered an ABG analysis to evaluate ventilation, acid-base balance, oxygenation status, or oxygen-carrying capacity, check values after allowing sufficient time for the patient's oxygenation to return to a steady state. (See the "Arterial puncture for blood gas analysis" procedure, page 37.) *A patient with healthy lungs may achieve a steady state within 5 minutes after a change in therapy; a patient with chronic obstructive pulmonary disease (COPD) may require 20 to 30 minutes.*[15]
- Assess the patient frequently for signs and symptoms of hypoxia, such as restlessness, decreased level of consciousness, increased heart rate, arrhythmias, perspiration, dyspnea, use of accessory muscles, yawning or flared nostrils, cyanosis, and cool, clammy skin. Obtain vital signs, as needed.
- Observe the patient's skin integrity *to prevent skin breakdown on pressure points from the oxygen delivery device.* Wipe moisture or perspiration from the patient's face and from the mask, as needed.
- Remove and discard your personal protective equipment, if worn.[10]
- Perform hand hygiene.[4,5,6,7,8]
- Clean and disinfect your stethoscope using a disinfectant pad *to prevent transmission of microorganisms.*[16,17]
- Perform hand hygiene.[4,5,6,7,8]
- Document the procedure.[18,19,20]

EQUIPMENT

Guide to oxygen delivery systems *(continued)*

Transtracheal oxygen

The patient receives oxygen through a catheter inserted into the tracheal cartilage through a small permanent opening in the base of his neck in a simple outpatient procedure.

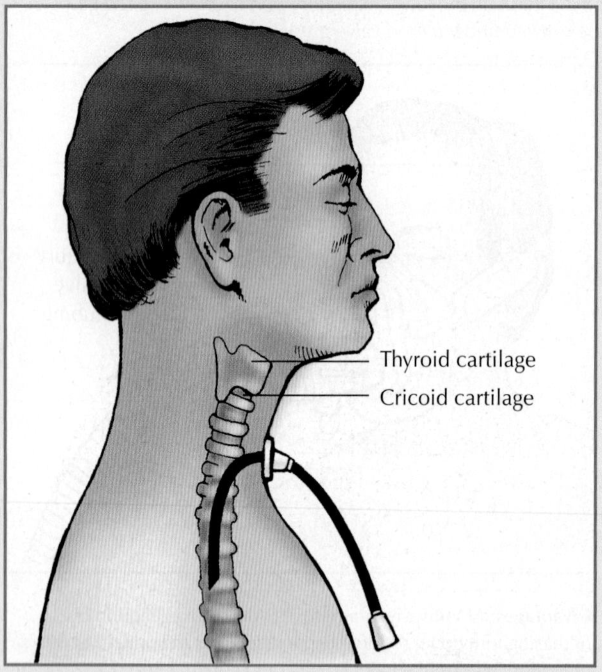

Advantages: Supplies oxygen to the lungs throughout the respiratory cycle; provides continuous oxygen without hindering mobility; doesn't interfere with eating or talking; doesn't dry mucous membranes; catheter can easily be concealed by a shirt or scarf.
Disadvantages: Not suitable for use in patients at risk for bleeding or those with severe bronchospasm, uncompensated respiratory acidosis, pleural herniation into the base of the neck, or high corticosteroid dosages.
Administration guidelines: After insertion, obtain a chest X-ray *to confirm placement.* Monitor the patient for bleeding, respiratory distress, pneumothorax, pain, coughing, or hoarseness. Don't use the catheter for about 1 week after insertion *to decrease the risk of subcutaneous emphysema.*

Venturi mask

The mask is connected to a Venturi device, which mixes a specific volume of air and oxygen.

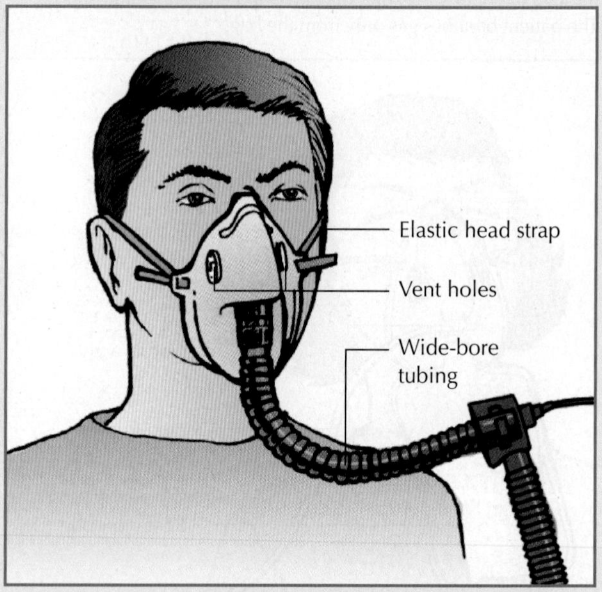

Advantages: Delivers highly accurate oxygen concentration despite patient's respiratory pattern *because the same amount of air is always entrained*; dilute jets can be changed or dial turned to change oxygen concentration; doesn't dry mucous membranes; humidity or aerosol can be added.
Disadvantages: Confining and may irritate skin; oxygen concentration may be altered if mask fits loosely, tubing kinks, oxygen intake ports become blocked, flow is insufficient, or patient is hyperpneic; interferes with eating and talking; condensate may collect and drip on the patient if humidification is used.
Administration guidelines: Make sure that the oxygen flow rate is set at the amount specified on each mask and that the Venturi valve is set for the desired FIO_2.

Special considerations

- If the patient will be receiving oxygen at a concentration above 60% for more than 24 hours, watch carefully for signs of oxygen toxicity. *Prolonged high concentrations of oxygen can cause lung injury. Surfactant activity may be impaired, and increased capillary congestion, edema, interstitial space thickening, and fibrotic changes may occur.* The patient may exhibit signs and symptoms of tracheobronchial irritation, such as coughing and substernal discomfort. Remind the patient to cough and deep-breathe frequently *to prevent atelectasis.* Also, *to prevent the development of serious lung damage,* measure ABG values repeatedly *to determine whether high oxygen concentrations are still necessary.*
- Maintain the patient's target oxygen saturation level within the recommended range, unless otherwise specified, which is 94% to 98%. If the patient has COPD or other risk factors for hypercapnic respiratory failure, a saturation of 88% to 92% may be recommended.[3]
- Be aware that flowmeters, which connect to an oxygen or compressed air source, are color-coded so that oxygen (green) isn't confused with compressed air (yellow).[3]
- Avoid interruptions in oxygen therapy for walking or transport.[2] Regularly check the content of cylinders and calculate how long they will last. This is especially important for cylinders on resuscitation carts and when transferring a patient.[3]
- The Joint Commission issued a sentinel event alert concerning medical device alarm safety *because alarm-related events have been associated with permanent loss of function or death.* Among the major contributing factors were improper alarm settings, alarms inappropriately turned off, and alarm signals not audible to staff. Make sure alarm limits are set appropriately and that alarms are turned on, functioning properly, and audible to staff. Follow facility guidelines for preventing alarm fatigue.[11]

EQUIPMENT

Guide to oxygen delivery systems *(continued)*

Aerosols

A face mask, hood, tent, or tracheostomy tube or collar is connected to wide-bore tubing that receives aerosolized oxygen from a jet nebulizer. The jet nebulizer, which is attached near the oxygen source, adjusts air entrainment in a manner similar to the Venturi device.

Advantages: Administers high humidity; gas can be heated (when delivered through an artificial airway) or cooled (when delivered through a tent).

Disadvantages: Condensate collected in the tracheostomy collar or T tube may drain into the tracheostomy; the weight of the T tube can put stress on the tracheostomy tube.

Administration guidelines: Guidelines vary with the type of nebulizer used—the ultrasonic, large-volume, small-volume, or in-line. When using a high-output nebulizer, watch for signs of overhydration, pulmonary edema, crackles, and electrolyte imbalance.

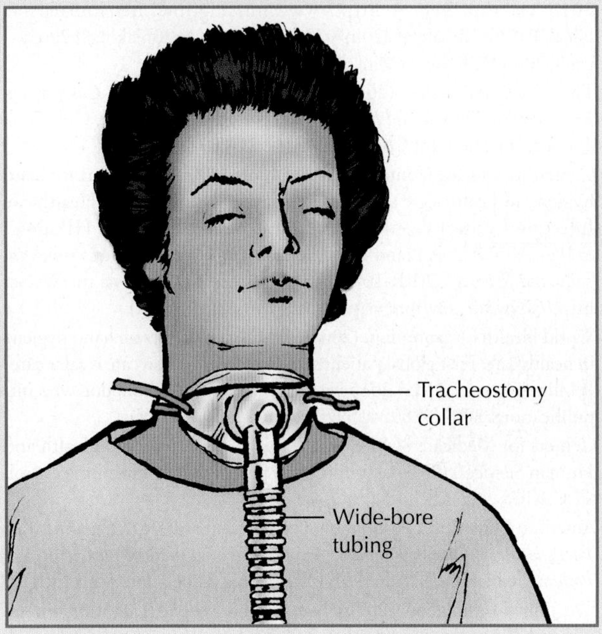

Patient teaching

Before discharging a patient who will receive oxygen therapy at home, make sure you know the types of oxygen therapy, the kinds of services that are available, and the service schedules offered by local home suppliers. Together with the practitioner and the patient, choose the device best suited to the patient. (See *Types of home oxygen therapy.*)

If the patient will be receiving transtracheal oxygen therapy, teach him how to properly clean and care for the catheter. Advise him to keep the skin surrounding the insertion site clean and dry *to prevent infection.*

No matter which device the patient uses, you'll need to evaluate the ability and motivation of the patient and family members to administer oxygen therapy at home. Make sure they understand the reason the patient is receiving oxygen and the safety issues involved in oxygen administration. Teach them how to properly use and clean the equipment and supplies.

If the patient will be discharged with oxygen for the first time, make sure his health insurance covers home oxygen. If it doesn't, find out what criteria he must meet to obtain coverage. Without a third-party payer, the patient may not be able to afford home oxygen therapy.

Types of home oxygen therapy

Oxygen therapy can be administered at home using an oxygen tank, an oxygen concentrator, or liquid oxygen.

Oxygen tank

Commonly used for patients who need oxygen on a standby basis or who need a ventilator at home, the oxygen tank has several disadvantages, including its cumbersome design and the need for frequent replacement. *Because oxygen is stored under high pressure,* the oxygen tank also poses a potential hazard.

Oxygen concentrator

The oxygen concentrator extracts oxygen molecules from room air. It can be used for low oxygen flow (less than 4 L/minute) and doesn't need to be refilled with oxygen. However, *because the oxygen concentrator runs on electricity,* it won't function during a power failure.

Liquid oxygen

This option is commonly used by patients who are oxygen-dependent but still mobile. The system includes a large liquid reservoir for home use. When the patient wants to leave the house, he fills a portable unit worn over the shoulder; this supplies oxygen for up to several hours, depending on the liter flow.

Complications

Oxygen use increases the risk of fires. Humidification systems may become contaminated, increasing the risk of infection.[2] With a fraction of inspired oxygen of greater than 50%, absorption atelectasis, oxygen toxicity, and depression of ciliary or leukocytic function may occur; ventilatory depression may occur in spontaneously breathing patients with elevated arterial carbon dioxide levels.[2]

Hypothermia and increased oxygen consumption may result from administering cool oxygen. Pressure ulcers may develop on the patient's head and face and around his nose during prolonged oxygen administration.

Documentation

Record the date and time of oxygen administration; the type of delivery device; the oxygen flow rate; the patient's vital signs,[3] skin color, respiratory effort, and lung sounds; his response before and after initiation of therapy; complications and the nursing actions taken; and any patient or family teaching.

REFERENCES

1 World Health Organization. (2009). "Glove use information leaflet" [Online]. Accessed May 2015 via the Web at http://www.who.int/gpsc/5may/Glove_Use_Information_Leaflet.pdf (Level VII)

2 American Association for Respiratory Care (AARC). (2002). AARC clinical practice guideline: Oxygen therapy for adults in the acute care

facility. *Respiratory Care, 47,* 717–720. Accessed May 2015 via the Web at http://www.rcjournal.com/cpgs/otachcpg-update.html (Level VII)
3 National Patient Safety Agency. (2010). Safety in practice: Making oxygen use safer in hospitals. *Nursing Times, 106*(19), 10–11. Accessed May 2015 via the Web at http://www.nursingtimes.net/Journals/1/Files/2010/5/18/Safety%20in%20practice%20-%20making%20oxygen%20use%20safer%20in%20hospitals.pdf
4 The Joint Commission. (2015). Standard NPSG.07.01.01. *Comprehensive accreditation manual for hospitals: The official handbook.* Oakbrook Terrace, IL: The Joint Commission. (Level VII)
5 Centers for Disease Control and Prevention. (2002). Guideline for hand hygiene in health-care settings: Recommendations of the Healthcare Infection Control Practices Advisory Committee and the HICPAC/SHEA/APIC/IDSA Hand Hygiene Task Force. *MMWR Recommendations and Reports, 51*(RR-16), 1–45. Accessed May 2015 via the Web at http://www.cdc.gov/mmwr/pdf/rr/rr5116.pdf (Level II)
6 World Health Organization. (2009). "WHO guidelines on hand hygiene in health care: First global patient safety challenge, clean care is safer care" [Online]. Accessed May 2015 via the Web at http://whqlibdoc.who.int/publications/2009/9789241597906_eng.pdf (Level IV)
7 Centers for Medicare & Medicaid Services, Department of Health and Human Services. (2014). Condition of participation: Infection control. 42 C.F.R. § 482.42.
8 American Osteopathic Association. (2014). Standard 07.01.21. *Healthcare Facilities Accreditation Program: Accreditation requirements for acute care hospitals.* Chicago, IL: American Osteopathic Association. (Level VII)
9 The Joint Commission. (2015). Standard NPSG.01.01.01. *Comprehensive accreditation manual for hospitals: The official handbook.* Oakbrook Terrace, IL: The Joint Commission. (Level VII)
10 Siegel, J. D., et al. (2007). "2007 guideline for isolation precautions: Preventing transmission of infectious agents in healthcare settings" [Online]. Accessed May 2015 via the Web at http://www.cdc.gov/hicpac/pdf/isolation/Isolation2007.pdf (Level II)
11 The Joint Commission. (2013). "Sentinel event alert: Medical device alarm safety in hospitals" [Online]. Accessed May 2015 via the Web at http://www.jointcommission.org/assets/1/18/SEA_50_alarms_4_5_13_FINAL1.PDF (Level VII)
12 The Joint Commission. (2015). Standard NPSG.06.01.01. *Comprehensive accreditation manual for hospitals: The official handbook.* Oakbrook Terrace, IL: The Joint Commission. (Level VII)
13 Graham, K. C., & Cvach, M. (2010). Monitor alarm fatigue: Standardizing use of physiological monitors and decreasing nuisance alarms. *American Journal of Critical Care, 19,* 28–37.
14 American Association of Critical-Care Nurses. (2013). "AACN practice alert: Alarm management" [Online]. Accessed May 2015 via the Web at http://www.aacn.org/wd/practice/docs/practicealerts/alarm-management-practice-alert.pdf (Level VII)
15 Kacmarek, R. M., et al. (2013). *Egan's fundamentals of respiratory care* (10th ed.). St. Louis, MO: Mosby.
16 Rutala, W. A., et al. (2008). "Guideline for disinfection and sterilization in healthcare facilities, 2008" [Online]. Accessed May 2015 via the Web at http://www.cdc.gov/hicpac/pdf/guidelines/Disinfection_Nov_2008.pdf (Level I)
17 American Osteopathic Association. (2014). Standard 07.02.03. *Healthcare Facilities Accreditation Program: Accreditation requirements for acute care hospitals.* Chicago, IL: American Osteopathic Association. (Level VII)
18 The Joint Commission. (2015). Standard RC.01.03.01. *Comprehensive accreditation manual for hospitals: The official handbook.* Oakbrook Terrace, IL: The Joint Commission. (Level VII)
19 Centers for Medicare & Medicaid Services, Department of Health and Human Services. (2014). Condition of participation: Medical record services. 42 C.F.R. § 482.24(b).
20 American Osteopathic Association. (2014). Standard 10.00.03. *Healthcare Facilities Accreditation Program: Accreditation requirements for acute care hospitals.* Chicago, IL: American Osteopathic Association. (Level VII)

ADDITIONAL REFERENCES

Nettina, S. M. (2014). *Lippincott manual of nursing practice* (10th ed.). Philadelphia, PA: Wolters Kluwer.
Taylor, C., et al. (2015). *Fundamentals of nursing: The art and science of nursing care* (8th ed.). Philadelphia, PA: Wolters Kluwer.
Ward, J. J. (2013). High-flow oxygen administration by nasal cannula for adult and perinatal patients. *Respiratory Care, 58,* 98–122. Accessed May 2015 via the Web at http://rc.rcjournal.com/content/58/1/98.full (Level V)

P

PAIN MANAGEMENT

Defined as the sensory and emotional experience associated with actual or potential tissue damage, pain includes not only the perception of an uncomfortable stimulus, but also the response to that perception.

The patient's report of pain is the most reliable indicator of the existence of pain. When a patient feels severe pain, he seeks medical help because he believes the pain signals a serious problem. This perception produces anxiety, which, in turn, increases the pain. To assess and manage pain properly, the nurse must depend on both the patient's subjective description and objective tools.

According to The Joint Commission, health care facilities are required to develop policies and procedures that support the appropriate use of analgesics and other pain-control therapies.[1] Pain should be assessed at admission and reassessed at regular intervals.[1] Pain assessment should include personal, cultural, spiritual, and ethnic beliefs. Patients and families should be educated about their role in pain management. They should also be informed about potential limitations and adverse effects of pain treatment.

Several interventions can be used to manage pain, including analgesics, emotional support, comfort measures, and complementary and alternative therapies such as cognitive techniques to distract the patient and Reiki or aromatherapy to promote relaxation. Severe pain usually requires an opioid analgesic. Invasive measures, such as epidural analgesia or patient-controlled analgesia (PCA), may also be required.

Equipment

Facility-approved pain assessment tool or scale ▪ oral hygiene supplies ▪ water ▪ soap ▪ washcloth and towel ▪ nonopioid analgesic (such as aspirin or acetaminophen) ▪ Optional: PCA device; mild opioid (such as oxycodone or codeine); strong opioid (such as morphine or hydromorphone), pillow, cold compresses, lotion, radio or other device that allows the patient to listen to music.

Implementation

- Perform hand hygiene.[2,3,4,5,6]
- Confirm the patient's identity using at least two patient identifiers.[7]
- Obtain the assistance of a medical interpreter as needed.[8,9]
- Explain to the patient how pain medications work together with other pain management therapies to provide relief. Also explain that management aims to keep pain at a low level *to permit optimal bodily function.*[10]
- Using a facility-approved pain assessment tool or scale, perform a comprehensive pain assessment using techniques appropriate for the patient's age, condition, and ability to understand. Ask key questions and note the patient's response.[1] For example, ask him to describe the pain's duration, severity, and location. Look for physiologic or behavioral clues to the pain's severity.[11] (See *How to assess pain.*)

Giving medications

- If the patient is allowed oral medications, begin with a nonopioid analgesic, such as acetaminophen or aspirin, every 4 to 6 hours as ordered.[12]

■ If the patient needs more relief than a nonopioid analgesic provides, administer a mild opioid (such as oxycodone or codeine) as ordered.[12]
■ If the patient needs still more pain relief, you may administer a strong opioid (such as morphine or hydromorphone), as ordered, following safe medication administration practices.[13,14] If possible, administer an oral form of the medication following safe medication administration practices.[12,13,14] Check the appropriate drug information for each medication given.
■ If ordered, teach the patient how to use a PCA device, *which can help the patient manage his pain and decrease his anxiety.* (See the "Patient-controlled analgesia" procedure, page 592.)
■ Reassess pain in a timely manner according to the onset of the prescribed medication. Ensure that your assessment is comprehensive and appropriate to the circumstances (type of pain, level of intervention, and care setting) *to ensure the safety and efficacy of care.*[1] Reassessment should include not only pain relief but also adverse reactions or events produced by treatment and the impact of pain and treatment on patient function and quality of life.[15]
■ If the patient is still in pain, notify the practitioner.

Providing emotional support
■ Show your concern by spending time talking with the patient. Because of his pain and his inability to manage it, the patient may be anxious and frustrated. *Such feelings can worsen his pain.*
■ Assess the patient's spiritual and cultural needs and incorporate spiritual and cultural practices as desired by the patient.
■ Use nonpharmacologic interventions when appropriate.

Performing comfort measures
■ Reposition the patient periodically *to reduce muscle spasms and tension and to relieve pressure on bony prominences.* Increasing the angle of the bed can reduce pull on an abdominal incision, diminishing pain. If appropriate, elevate a limb *to reduce swelling, inflammation, and pain.*
■ Splinting or supporting abdominal and chest incisions with a pillow when coughing or changing position helps decrease pain.
■ Apply cold compresses, as appropriate, *to decrease discomfort.*[11]
■ Give the patient a back massage *to help relax tense muscles.*[11]
■ Perform passive range-of-motion exercises *to prevent stiffness and further loss of mobility, relax tense muscles, and provide comfort.*
■ Provide oral hygiene. Keep a glass or cup of fresh water at the bedside *because many pain medications tend to dry the mouth.*
■ Wash the patient's face and hands *to soothe him, which may reduce his perception of pain.*

Using cognitive techniques
■ Help the patient enhance the effect of analgesics by using such techniques as distraction, guided imagery, deep breathing, and relaxation.[11] You can easily use these "mind-over-pain" techniques at the bedside. Choose the method the patient prefers. If possible, start these techniques when the patient feels little or no pain. If he feels persistent pain, begin with short, simple exercises. Before beginning, dim the lights, loosen or remove the patient's restrictive clothing, and eliminate noise from the environment.
■ For *distraction,* have the patient focus his attention on an enjoyable activity. For instance, have him use music as a distraction by turning on the radio or another device that lets the patient listen to music when the pain begins. Have him close his eyes and concentrate on listening to the music and raising or lowering the volume as his pain increases or subsides. Note, however, that distraction is mainly helpful in relieving pain lasting for brief episodes or for painful procedures of short duration.
■ For *imagery,* help the patient concentrate on a peaceful, pleasant image, such as walking on the beach. Encourage him to concentrate on the details of that image by asking about the associated sights, sounds, smells, tastes, and touch. *The positive emotions evoked by this exercise minimize pain.*
■ For *deep breathing,* have the patient stare at an object, then slowly inhale and exhale as he counts aloud to maintain a comfortable rate and rhythm. Have him concentrate on the rise and fall of his abdomen. Encourage him to feel more and more weightless with each breath while he concentrates on the rhythm of his breathing or on any restful image.
■ For *muscle relaxation,* have the patient focus on a particular muscle group. Then ask him to tense the muscles and note the sensation. After 5 to 7 seconds, tell him to relax the muscles and concentrate on the relaxed state. Have him note the difference between the tense and relaxed

How to assess pain

To assess pain properly, you need to consider the patient's description and your observations of the patient's physical and behavioral responses. A comprehensive, culturally sensitive pain assessment tool can help capture the effects of cultural norms on the patient's pain experiences, examine the meaning that the pain has to the patient, and determine the patient's treatment preferences (such as herbs, home remedies, complementary therapies, and the services of alternative or cultural healers).[8]

Start by asking the following questions (bearing in mind that the patient's responses will be shaped by his previous experiences, self-image, and beliefs about his condition):
■ Where's the pain located? How long does it last? How often does it occur?
■ How would you describe the pain?
■ What brings the pain on?
■ What relieves the pain or makes it worse?
■ What do you think is causing your pain?
■ What do you fear most about the pain?
■ What problems does the pain cause you?
■ Who else have you consulted about the pain? Family members? A traditional healer?
■ What treatments do you think might help you with the pain?

Ask the patient to rank his pain on a scale from 0 to 10, with 0 denoting lack of pain and 10 denoting the worst pain possible. Establish with the patient what would be considered a low pain level, usually 4 or lower on a 0-to-10 scale. Observe the patient's behavioral and physiologic responses to pain. Physiologic responses may be sympathetic or parasympathetic.

Behavioral responses
Behavioral responses include altered body position, moaning, sighing, grimacing, withdrawal, crying, restlessness, muscle twitching, and immobility.

Sympathetic responses
Sympathetic responses are commonly associated with mild to moderate pain and include pallor, elevated blood pressure, dilated pupils, skeletal muscle tension, dyspnea, tachycardia, and diaphoresis.

Parasympathetic responses
Parasympathetic responses are commonly associated with severe, deep pain and include pallor, decreased blood pressure, bradycardia, nausea, vomiting, weakness, dizziness, and loss of consciousness.

Assess pain at regular intervals, usually at least every 2 hours; during rest and activity; and throughout the night (when pain is usually heightened). Keep in mind that the ability to sleep doesn't indicate absence of pain.

Visual pain rating scale[21]

Patients with language difficulties can indicate pain using many instruments. One such instrument is the Wong-Baker FACES© Pain Rating Scale (shown below), which uses six faces to help the patient describe his level of pain.

Wong-Baker FACES Scale

Another nonverbal instrument involves the use of a smiling face and a frowning face, such as the ones shown below. Ask the patient to choose the face that describes how he's feeling—either happy because he has no pain or sad because he has pain. Alternatively, to pinpoint varying levels of pain, you can ask the patient to draw a face.

Wong-Baker FACES® Pain Rating Scale, The Wong-Baker FACES Foundation. Reprinted with permission.

states. After he tenses and relaxes one muscle group, have him proceed to another and then another until he's covered his entire body.

Completing the procedure

■ Reassess the patient's pain level and quality approximately 15 to 30 minutes after parenteral pain medication or approximately 60 minutes after oral pain medication.[1,11] If the patient is still in pain, notify the practitioner and alter the treatment plan as appropriate.

■ Work with the patient to develop a care plan using interventions appropriate to the patient's lifestyle.[16] These interventions may include prescribed medications, emotional support, comfort measures, complementary and alternative therapies such as cognitive techniques, and education about pain and its management. Emphasize the importance of maintaining good bowel habits, respiratory function, and mobility *because pain can exacerbate problems in these areas.*

■ Perform hand hygiene.[2,3,4,5,6]

■ Document your findings and interventions.[17,18,19]

Special considerations

■ During periods of intense pain, the patient's ability to concentrate diminishes. If the patient is in severe pain, help him to select a cognitive technique that's easy to use. After he selects a technique, encourage him to use it consistently. Remind the patient that results of cognitive therapy techniques improve with practice. Help him through the initial sessions.

■ Pain shouldn't be considered a normal part of the aging process. Provide pain relief for elderly patients using pharmacologic and nonpharmacologic approaches. Remember, safety is a special concern, especially the risk of falls resulting from impaired mobility due to pain and from adverse effects of pain medications.[20]

■ Identify age-related factors that affect assessment and pain management in elderly patients.[20]

NURSING ALERT Because of adverse effects, *avoid certain medications (such as meperidine) in elderly patients.*

■ Cultural remedies for pain, such as the involvement of extended family and the use of complementary therapies such as acupuncture, should be permitted and even encouraged. Research indicates that family support improves patient outcomes and that acupuncture can be effective in managing pain.[8]

■ Be aware that patients receiving opioid analgesics may be at risk for addiction, physical dependence, or tolerance.

■ *Addiction* is defined as psychological dependence characterized by a persistent pattern of dysfunctional drug use; during acute pain treatment, it occurs in less than 1% of cases.[11] Addiction is characterized by a craving for the drug to experience effects other than pain relief. A patient demonstrating such behavior usually has a preexisting problem that's exacerbated by opioid use.[11] Discuss with the practitioner an addicted patient's problem, and make appropriate referrals to experts.

■ *Physical dependence* is a physiologic state in which withdrawal signs and symptoms occur with abrupt cessation or reversal of the drug. Physical dependence doesn't mean that addiction coexists. Signs and symptoms include anxiety, irritability, chills and hot flashes, excessive salivation and tearing, rhinorrhea, sweating, nausea, vomiting, and seizures. These signs and symptoms are likely to begin within 12 hours and peak within 72 hours of discontinuing the drug. *To reduce the risk of dependence,* discontinue an opioid by decreasing the dose gradually each day.

■ *Tolerance* is a neuroadaptive response in which one or more of the drug's effects, such as analgesia or sedation, decreases over time. Tolerance and addiction may be exclusive of one another.

■ If the patient has dementia or another cognitive impairment, don't assume that he can't understand the pain scale or communicate his pain. Experiment with several pain scales to find one that works. A scale featuring faces, such as the Wong-Baker FACES© Pain Rating Scale, is a good choice for many cognitively impaired patients and those with limited language skills. (See *Visual pain rating scale.*)

Complications

The most common adverse effects of analgesics include respiratory depression (the most serious), sedation, constipation, pruritus, nausea, vomiting, and addiction.

Documentation

Document each step of the nursing process. Describe the subjective information you elicited from the patient, using his own words. Note the location, quality, and duration of the pain as well as precipitating factors.

Record the pain-relief method selected and the patient's rating of the pain before and after pain management interventions. Use a flow sheet to document pain assessment findings. Summarize your actions, including the name and dosage of any medication given and the patient's response. If the patient's pain wasn't relieved, note alternative treatments to consider the next time pain occurs. Also record any complications of drug therapy.

REFERENCES

1 The Joint Commission. (2015). Standard PC.01.02.07. *Comprehensive accreditation manual for hospitals: The official handbook.* Oakbrook Terrace, IL: The Joint Commission. (Level VII)

2 The Joint Commission. (2015). Standard NPSG.07.01.01. *Comprehensive accreditation manual for hospitals: The official handbook.* Oakbrook Terrace, IL: The Joint Commission. (Level VII)

3 Centers for Disease Control and Prevention. (2002). Guideline for hand hygiene in health-care settings: Recommendations of the Healthcare Infection Control Practices Advisory Committee and the HICPAC/SHEA/APIC/IDSA Hand Hygiene Task Force. *MMWR Recommendations and Reports, 51*(RR-16), 1–45. Accessed May 2015 via the Web at http://www.cdc.gov/mmwr/pdf/rr/rr5116.pdf (Level II)

4 World Health Organization. (2009). "WHO guidelines on hand hygiene in health care: First global patient safety challenge, clean care is safer care" [Online]. Accessed May 2015 via the Web at http://whqlibdoc.who.int/publications/2009/9789241597906_eng.pdf (Level IV)

5 Centers for Medicare & Medicaid Services, Department of Health and Human Services. (2014). Condition of participation: Infection control. 42 C.F.R. § 482.42.

6 American Osteopathic Association. (2014). Standard 07.01.21. *Healthcare Facilities Accreditation Program: Accreditation requirements for acute care hospitals.* Chicago, IL: American Osteopathic Association. (Level VII)

7 The Joint Commission. (2015). Standard NPSG.01.01.01. *Comprehensive accreditation manual for hospitals: The official handbook.* Oakbrook Terrace, IL: The Joint Commission. (Level VII)

8 Narayan, M. C. (2010). Culture's effects on pain assessment and management. *American Journal of Nursing, 110*(4), 38–47. Accessed May 2015 via the Web at http://www.nursingcenter.com/pdf.asp?AID=996206

9 The Joint Commission. (2015). Standard PC.02.01.21. *Comprehensive accreditation manual for hospitals: The official handbook.* Oakbrook Terrace, IL: The Joint Commission. (Level VII)

10 The Joint Commission. (2015). Standard PC.02.03.01. *Comprehensive accreditation manual for hospitals: The official handbook.* Oakbrook Terrace, IL: The Joint Commission. (Level VII)

11 American Society of PeriAnesthesia Nurses. (2003). ASPAN pain and comfort clinical guideline. *Journal of PeriAnesthesia Nursing, 18,* 232–236. Accessed May 2015 via the Web at http://www.aspan.org/Portals/6/docs/ClinicalPractice/Guidelines/ASPAN_ClinicalGuideline_PainComfort.pdf (Level VII)

12 World Health Organization. (n.d.). "WHO's cancer pain relief ladder for adults" [Online]. Accessed May 2015 via the Web at http://www.who.int/cancer/palliative/painladder/en/

13 Centers for Medicare & Medicaid Services, Department of Health and Human Services. (2014). Condition of participation: Nursing services. 42 C.F.R. § 482.23(c).

14 American Osteopathic Association. (2014). Standard 16.01.03. *Healthcare Facilities Accreditation Program: Accreditation requirements for acute care hospitals.* Chicago, IL: American Osteopathic Association. (Level VII)

15 Gordon, D. B., et al. (2008). Improving reassessment and documentation of pain management. *Joint Commission Journal on Quality and Patient Safety, 34,* 509–517. (Level VI)

16 Hooten, W. M., et al. Institute for Clinical Systems Improvement (ICSI). (2013). "ICSI health care guideline: Assessment and management of chronic pain" [Online]. Accessed May 2015 via the Web at https://www.icsi.org/_asset/bw798b/ChronicPain.pdf (Level VII)

17 The Joint Commission. (2015). Standard RC.01.03.01. *Comprehensive accreditation manual for hospitals: The official handbook.* Oakbrook Terrace, IL: The Joint Commission. (Level VII)

18 Centers for Medicare & Medicaid Services, Department of Health and Human Services. (2014). Condition of participation: Medical record services. 42 C.F.R. § 482.24(b).

19 American Osteopathic Association. (2014). Standard 10.00.03. *Healthcare Facilities Accreditation Program: Accreditation requirements for acute care hospitals.* Chicago, IL: American Osteopathic Association. (Level VII)

20 Harmon, J. R., et al. (2012). Efficacy of the use of evidence-based algorithmic guidelines in the acute care setting for pain assessment and management in older people: A critical review of the literature. *International Journal of Older People Nursing, 7,* 127–140. (Level V)

21 Hockenberry, M. J., & Wilson, D. (2013). Wong's essentials of pediatric nursing (9th ed.). St. Louis, MO: Mosby.

ADDITIONAL REFERENCES

American Society of Anesthesiologists. (2012). Practice guidelines for acute pain management in the perioperative setting: An updated report by the American Society of Anesthesiologists Task Force on Acute Pain Management. *Anesthesiology, 116,* 248–273. Accessed May 2015 via the Web at http://journals.lww.com/anesthesiology/Fulltext/2012/02000/Practice_Guidelines_for_Acute_Pain_Management_in.11.asp (Level VII)

Thorson, D., et al. Institute for Clinical Systems Improvement. (2014). "Health care protocol: Acute pain assessment and opioid prescribing protocol" [Online]. Accessed May 2015 via the Web at https://www.icsi.org/_asset/dyp5wm/Opioids.pdf (Level I)

PARENTERAL NUTRITION ADMINISTRATION

When a patient can't meet his nutritional needs by oral or enteral feedings, he may require IV nutritional support, or parenteral nutrition (PN). The patient's diagnosis, history, and prognosis determine the need for PN. Generally, this treatment is prescribed for any patient who can't absorb nutrients though the GI tract for more than 10 days.

More specific indications include debilitating illness lasting longer than 2 weeks; loss of 10% or more of pre-illness weight; serum albumin level below 3.5 g/dL; excessive nitrogen loss from wound infection, fistulas, or abscesses; renal or hepatic failure; or a nonfunctioning GI tract for 5 to 7 days in a severely catabolic patient.

Common illnesses that can trigger the need for PN include inflammatory bowel disease, radiation enteritis, severe diarrhea, intractable vomiting, and moderate to severe pancreatitis. A massive small-bowel resection, bone marrow transplantation, high-dose chemotherapy or radiation therapy, and major surgery can also hinder a patient's ability to absorb nutrients, requiring PN.

PN shouldn't be given to patients with a normally functioning GI tract, and it has limited value for well-nourished patients whose GI tract will resume normal function within 10 days. It also may be inappropriate for patients with a poor prognosis or if the risks of PN outweigh the benefits.

PN may be given through a peripheral or central venous (CV) access device. Depending on the solution, it may be used to boost the patient's caloric intake, supply full caloric needs, or surpass the patient's caloric requirements.

The type of PN prescribed depends on the patient's condition and metabolic needs and on the administration route. The solution usually contains protein, carbohydrates, electrolytes, vitamins, and trace minerals. A lipid emulsion provides the necessary fat. Standard IV solutions, such as dextrose 5% in water, dextrose 10% in water, and normal saline solution, are nutritionally incomplete and don't provide sufficient calories to maintain a patient's nutritional status. (See *Types of parenteral nutrition,* page 582.)

Types of parenteral nutrition

TYPE	SOLUTION COMPONENTS/LITER	USES	SPECIAL CONSIDERATIONS
Total parenteral nutrition (TPN) by way of central venous (CV) access	■ Dextrose 15% in water ($D_{15}W$) to $D_{25}W$ (1 L of dextrose 25% = 850 nonprotein calories) ■ Crystalline amino acids 2.5% to 8.5% ■ Electrolytes, vitamins, trace elements, and insulin, as ordered ■ Lipid emulsion 10% to 20% (usually infused as a separate solution)	■ For TPN lasting 2 weeks or more ■ For patients with large caloric and nutrient needs ■ Provides calories, restores nitrogen balance, and replaces essential vitamins, electrolytes, minerals, and trace elements ■ Promotes tissue synthesis, wound healing, and normal metabolic function ■ Allows bowel rest and healing; reduces activity in the gallbladder, pancreas, and small intestine ■ Improves tolerance of surgery	***Basic solution*** ■ Nutritionally complete ■ Requires minor surgical procedure for CV access insertion and radiologic placement verification ■ Highly hypertonic solution ■ May cause metabolic complications (glucose intolerance, electrolyte imbalance, essential fatty acid deficiency) ***IV lipid emulsion*** ■ May not be used effectively in severely stressed patients (especially burn patients) ■ May interfere with immune mechanisms ■ Given by way of CV access device; irritates peripheral vein in long-term use
Total nutrient admixture	■ One day's nutrients contained in a single bag (also called *3:1 solution*) ■ Combines lipid emulsion with other parenteral solution components	■ For parenteral nutrition (PN) for 2 weeks or more ■ For relatively stable patients ■ For patients with large caloric and nutrient needs ■ Provides calories, restores nitrogen balance, and replaces essential vitamins, electrolytes, minerals, and trace elements ■ Promotes tissue synthesis, wound healing, and normal metabolic function ■ Allows bowel rest and healing; reduces activity in the gallbladder, pancreas, and small intestine ■ Improves tolerance of surgery	■ Nutritionally complete ■ Requires minor surgical procedure for CV access insertion and radiologic placement verification ■ Highly hypertonic solution ■ May cause metabolic complications (glucose intolerance, electrolyte imbalance) ■ Reduces need to handle bag, reducing contamination risk ■ Decreases nursing time and reduces need for infusion sets and electronic devices, lowering facility costs, increasing patient mobility, and allowing easier adjustment to home care ■ Has limited use because not all types and amounts of components are compatible ■ Requires a 1.2-micron filter[1]
Peripheral parenteral nutrition	■ D_5W to $D_{10}W$ ■ Crystalline amino acids 2.5% to 5% ■ Electrolytes, minerals, vitamins, and trace elements, as ordered ■ Lipid emulsion 10% or 20% (1 L of dextrose 10% and amino acids 3.5% infused at the same time as 1 L of lipid emulsion = 1,440 nonprotein calories)	■ For PN lasting 2 weeks or less ■ Provides up to 2,000 calories/day ■ Maintains adequate nutritional status in patients who can tolerate relatively high fluid volume, in those who usually resume bowel function and oral feedings after a few days, and in those susceptible to infections associated with CV access device	***Basic solution*** ■ Nutritionally complete for a short time ■ Can't be used long term in nutritionally depleted patients ■ Used for weight maintenance, not weight gain ■ Avoids insertion and care of CV access device but requires adequate venous access ■ Delivers less hypertonic solutions than TPN ■ May cause phlebitis ■ Less chance of metabolic complications than with TPN ***IV lipid emulsion*** ■ As effective as dextrose for caloric source ■ Diminishes phlebitis if infused at the same time as basic nutrient solution

Total parenteral nutrition (TPN) refers to any nutrient solution, including lipids, given through a CV access device. Peripheral parenteral nutrition (PPN), which is given through a peripheral catheter, supplies full caloric needs while avoiding the risks that accompany CV access. To keep from sclerosing the vein through which it's administered, the dextrose in PPN solution must be limited to 10%.[1] Because of this, the success of PPN depends on the patient's tolerance of the large volume of fluid necessary to supply his nutritional needs.

In many cases, the patient may need an increase in the glucose content beyond the level a peripheral vein can handle. For example, most TPN solutions are six times more concentrated than blood. As a result, they must be delivered into a vein with a high blood flow rate to dilute the solution.

The most common delivery route for TPN is through a CV access device into the superior vena cava.

Equipment

Prescribed PN solution ■ sterile IV administration set for the infusion pump ■ 0.2-micron filter (or 1.2-micron filter if the solution contains lipids or albumin)[1] ■ syringe prefilled with preservative-free normal saline solution ■ disinfectant pad (alcohol, tincture of iodine, or chlorhexidine-based) ■ electronic infusion pump[1] ■ intake-and-output record ■ gloves ■ Optional: mask, glucometer, supplies for blood specimen collection, scale.

Preparation of equipment

Remove the PN solution from the refrigerator 30 minutes to 1 hour before use.[1]

Implementation

■ Verify the practitioner's order and make sure that the prescribed therapy is appropriate for the patient's age, condition, and access device. Confirm that the access device catheter tip is located as appropriate and that the dose, rate, and route are appropriate for the patient.[1,2]

■ Make sure that the solution container is labeled with the patient's identifiers, his weight and age, the administration date and time, the expiration date, the route of administration (central or peripheral), the glucose concentration, and component names and dosages. (All components should be labeled as amounts per day and listed in the same sequence and same unit of measure as the practitioner's order.) Make sure the total volume of solution and the infusion rate are included as well as the duration of the infusion (continuous or cycled) and the appropriate size filter to use.[1,2] Inspect the integrity of the container and solution and return the solution to the pharmacy if the integrity of the container is compromised, the solution is cloudy or contains particles, or the solution is expired.[1,2]

■ Perform hand hygiene.[3,4,5,6,7,8,9]

■ Confirm the patient's identity using at least two patient identifiers.[10]

■ Explain the procedure to the patient *to allay his anxiety.*

■ Compare the patient's name and second patient identifier on the solution container against the name on the patient's identification bracelet.

■ If your facility uses a bar code scanning system, scan your identification badge, the patient's identification bracelet, and the solution's bar code.

■ Put on gloves and, if required by your facility, a mask.[11,12]

■ Connect the IV infusion pump administration set and micron filter (if the tubing doesn't contain an in-line filter); insert the filter as close to the catheter insertion site as possible.[13]

■ Squeeze the IV drip chamber and, holding the drip chamber upright, insert the tubing spike into the IV bag or bottle. Then release the drip chamber.

■ Prime the administration set tubing by inverting the filter at the distal end of the tubing and then opening the roller clamp. Let the solution fill the filter and the tubing; gently tap the tubing, filter, and Y-ports *to dislodge trapped air and prevent air embolism.*[14]

■ Attach the IV administration set tubing to the infusion pump following the manufacturer's instructions, and set the infusion rate, concentration, and volume to be infused. Make sure that the infusion pump alarms are turned on and functioning. Label the container and IV tubing with the date, the time, and your initials.

■ Thoroughly disinfect the access port with a disinfectant pad using friction and allow it to dry.[15] Then verify patency of the access device by aspirating for a blood return *to reduce the risk of infiltration and extravasation.*[16,17]

■ Flush the catheter with preservative-free normal saline solution according to the catheter type.[17,18]

■ Clamp the access device before disconnecting it *to prevent air from entering the catheter.* If the catheter is a CV access device and a clamp isn't available, ask the patient to perform the Valsalva maneuver just as you change the tubing, if possible. Or, if the patient is being mechanically ventilated, change the IV tubing immediately after the machine delivers a breath at peak inspiration. *Both of these measures increase intrathoracic pressure and prevent air embolism.*[14]

■ Using sterile technique, attach the tubing to the designated luer-lock port.

■ Trace the tubing from the patient to its point of origin *to make sure that you've connected it to the proper port.*[2,16,19] After connecting the tubing, remove the clamp, if applicable. Secure all connections *to prevent harmful disconnections.*

NURSING ALERT *TPN solutions are considered high-alert medications* because they can cause significant harm when used in error.[20]

■ Before beginning the PN infusion, have another nurse perform an independent double-check, if required by your facility, to *verify the patient's identity and to make sure that the correct solution is hanging in the prescribed concentration, the solution's indication corresponds with the patient's diagnosis, the dosage calculations are correct and the dosing formula used to derive the final dose is correct, the route of administration is safe and proper for the patient, the pump settings are correct, and the infusion line is attached to the correct port.*[2,21]

■ After comparing the results of the independent double-check with the other nurse (if required), begin infusing the PN, as ordered, if there are no discrepancies. If discrepancies exist, rectify them before beginning the infusion.[21]

NURSING ALERT *Maintain PN infusions at the prescribed rate. Avoid interrupting the infusion for routine care or patient transport. Don't adjust the rate for "off-schedule" infusion starts or alter the infusion rate in response to changes in fluid needs.*[2,22]

■ Discard used supplies in the appropriate receptacles.[11,12,23]

■ Remove and discard your gloves and mask, if worn.[11,12,23]

■ Perform hand hygiene.[3,4,5,6,7,8,9]

■ Monitor the patient's glucose level according to the ordered parameters.[2] *Insulin may be added to the PN solution; however, the patient may still need additional subcutaneous doses.* (See the "Parenteral nutrition monitoring" procedure, page 587.)

■ Obtain blood specimens for laboratory analysis according to the ordered parameters.[2] Report abnormalities to the practitioner. (See the "Parenteral nutrition monitoring" procedure, page 587.)

■ Monitor intake and output and weigh the patient daily at the same time each morning, after he voids if possible.[2] Suspect fluid imbalance if the patient gains more than 1 lb (0.5 kg) daily.

■ Document the procedure.[24,25,26,27]

Special considerations

■ For patients at risk for refeeding syndrome, administer IV potassium, phosphate, and magnesium supplements, as ordered. Monitor blood levels daily or more frequently, as ordered.[22]

■ Don't perform routine site care and dressing changes if the patient has a short peripheral catheter; instead, change the dressing if it becomes damp or soiled or if it's no longer intact.[7,28]

■ If the patient has a short-term CV access device, routine dressing changes depend on the type of dressing. Change transparent semipermeable dressings at least every 7 days; change gauze dressings every 2 days. Change either type if it becomes damp or soiled or if it's no longer intact.[7,28] Dressing changes should also include cleaning the catheter-skin junction with an antiseptic solution and changing the stabilization device, if used.[28]

■ If lipids aren't being infused, change the administration tubing and filters that are used continuously no more frequently than every 96 hours; replace tubing every 24 hours if lipids are being administered continuously, or according to your facility's policy. If lipids are being administered intermittently, change the administration tubing with each new container. Change the administration tubing immediately if you suspect contamination or when the integrity of the product or system has been compromised *to reduce the risk of vascular catheter–associated infection.* Hang time for a container of PN shouldn't exceed 24 hours; for lipids, it shouldn't exceed 12 hours.[29]

TROUBLESHOOTING

Correcting common parenteral nutrition problems

Complications	Signs and symptoms	Interventions
Metabolic problems		
Hepatic dysfunction	Elevated serum aspartate aminotransferase, alkaline phosphatase, and bilirubin levels	Reduce total caloric intake and dextrose intake, making up lost calories by administering a lipid emulsion. Change to cyclical infusion. Use specific hepatic formulations only if the patient has encephalopathy.
Hypercapnia	Heightened oxygen consumption, increased carbon dioxide production, and measured respiratory quotient of 1 or greater	Reduce total caloric and dextrose intake, and balance dextrose and fat calories.
Hyperglycemia	Fatigue, restlessness, confusion, anxiety, weakness, polyuria, dehydration, elevated serum glucose levels and, in severe hyperglycemia, delirium or coma	Restrict dextrose intake by decreasing either the rate of infusion or the dextrose concentration. Compensate for calorie loss by administering lipid emulsion. Begin insulin therapy.
Hyperosmolarity	Confusion, lethargy, seizures, hyperosmolar hyperglycemic nonketotic syndrome, hyperglycemia, dehydration, and glycosuria	Discontinue dextrose infusion. Administer insulin and half-normal saline solution with 10 to 20 mEq/L of potassium *to rehydrate the patient.*
Hypocalcemia	Polyuria, dehydration, and elevated blood and urine glucose levels	Increase calcium supplements.
Hypoglycemia	Sweating, shaking, and irritability after the infusion has stopped	Increase dextrose intake or decrease exogenous insulin intake.
Hypokalemia	Muscle weakness, paralysis, paresthesia, and arrhythmias	Increase potassium supplements.
Hypomagnesemia	Tingling around the mouth, paresthesia in the fingers, mental changes, and hyperreflexia	Increase magnesium supplements.
Hypophosphatemia (refeeding syndrome)	Irritability, weakness, fluid retention, arrhythmias, cardiac failure, seizures, paresthesia, coma, and respiratory arrest accompanied by drops in potassium and magnesium levels	Increase phosphate supplements.
Metabolic acidosis	Elevated serum chloride level and reduced serum bicarbonate level	Increase acetate and decrease chloride in the parenteral nutrition (PN) solution.
Metabolic alkalosis	Reduced serum chloride level and elevated serum bicarbonate level	Decrease acetate and increase chloride in the PN solution.
Zinc deficiency	Dermatitis, alopecia, apathy, depression, taste changes, confusion, poor wound healing, and diarrhea	Increase zinc supplements.

(continued)

HOSPITAL-ACQUIRED CONDITION ALERT *Keep in mind that vascular catheter–associated infection is considered a hospital-acquired condition* because it can be reasonably prevented using best practices. *Follow infection prevention techniques (such as performing hand hygiene and following sterile technique) when administering PN* to reduce the risk of vascular catheter–associated infection.[30,31]

■ Closely monitor the catheter site for signs of catheter site infection and local tissue swelling, which may indicate infiltration.[2,32,33] *Extravasation of PN solution can lead to tissue necrosis.* (See *Correcting common parenteral nutrition problems.*)

■ Take caution when using the PN line for other functions.[1] Don't use a single-lumen CV access device to infuse blood or blood products, give a bolus injection, administer simultaneous IV solutions, measure CV pressure, or draw blood for laboratory tests without a practitioner's order. Seek compatibility information or consult the facility pharmacist before coadministration of medications with PN.[2]

TROUBLESHOOTING

Correcting common parenteral nutrition problems *(continued)*

COMPLICATIONS	SIGNS AND SYMPTOMS	INTERVENTIONS
MECHANICAL PROBLEMS		
Clotted central venous (CV) access device	Interrupted flow rate and resistance to flushing and blood withdrawal	Attempt to aspirate the clot. If unsuccessful, instill a thrombolytic agent *to clear the catheter lumen*, as ordered.
Cracked or broken tubing	Fluid leaking from the tubing	Apply a padded hemostat above the break *to prevent air from entering the line*. Change the tubing immediately.
Dislodged catheter	Catheter out of the vein	Apply pressure to the site with a sterile gauze pad.
Too-rapid infusion	Nausea, headache, and lethargy	Adjust the infusion rate and, if applicable, check the infusion pump.
OTHER PROBLEMS		
Air embolism	Apprehension, chest pain, tachycardia, hypotension, cyanosis, seizures, loss of consciousness, and cardiac arrest	Clamp the catheter. Place the patient in the left lateral decubitus position.[14] Administer oxygen, as ordered. If cardiac arrest occurs, begin cardiopulmonary resuscitation. When the catheter is removed, cover the insertion site with a dressing for 24 to 48 hours.
Extravasation	Swelling and pain around the insertion site	Stop the infusion. Aspirate fluid from the catheter with a small syringe.[32] Assess the patient for cardiopulmonary abnormalities; a chest X-ray may be required.
Phlebitis	Pain, tenderness, redness, and warmth	Apply gentle heat to the area, and elevate the insertion site if possible.
Pneumothorax and hydrothorax	Dyspnea, chest pain, cyanosis, and decreased breath sounds	Assist with chest tube insertion and apply suction, as ordered.
Septicemia	Red and swollen catheter site, chills, fever, and leukocytosis	Remove the catheter and culture the tip. Obtain a blood culture if the patient has a fever.
Thrombosis	Erythema and edema at the insertion site; ipsilateral swelling of the arm, neck, face, and upper chest; pain at the insertion site and along the vein; malaise; fever; and tachycardia	Remove the catheter promptly. If not contraindicated, systemic anticoagulation therapy may be used. Apply warm compresses to the insertion site, and elevate the affected extremity. Venous flow studies may be performed.

- Provide oral care regularly. Also provide emotional support. Keep in mind that patients commonly associate eating with positive feelings and can become disturbed when they can't eat.

Patient teaching

Patients who require prolonged or indefinite PN may be able to receive the therapy at home. Home PN reduces the need for long hospitalizations and allows the patient to resume many of his normal activities. Make a home care referral and begin patient teaching before discharge to make sure the patient knows how to perform the administration procedure and how to handle complications.

Teach the patient the potential adverse effects and complications of PN.[2] Encourage him to inspect his mouth regularly for signs of parotitis, glossitis, and oral lesions. Tell him that he may have fewer bowel movements while receiving PN therapy. Encourage him to remain physically active *to help his body use the nutrients more fully.*

Complications

Catheter-related sepsis is the most serious complication of PN. Although rare, a malpositioned subclavian or jugular vein catheter may lead to thrombosis or sepsis. An air embolism, a potentially fatal complication, can occur during IV tubing changes if the tubing is inadvertently disconnected. It may also result from undetected hairline cracks in the tubing or hub. Extravasation of PN solution can cause necrosis and then sloughing of the epidermis and dermis.

Documentation

Document the type of the access device used, the PN formulation and additives, the volume of solution administered, the condition of the catheter insertion site, your assessment findings, the patient's response to therapy, and any complications and interventions and the patient's response to those interventions. (See *Documenting parenteral nutrition,* page 586.)

Documenting parenteral nutrition[1,2,25]

When documenting parenteral nutrition (PN), make sure to include:

- the type and location of the access device, including catheter tip confirmation, as appropriate
- the condition of the insertion site
- the presence of blood return
- the verification process
- the volume and rate of the solution infused
- any additives added to the solution
- your observations of any adverse reactions and your interventions
- when you discontinue a central or peripheral IV catheter for PN
- the date and time and the type of dressing applied after PN was discontinued
- the appearance of the administration site
- any patient education.

Document any patient teaching provided and the patient's understanding of your teaching.

References

1 Standard 65. Parenteral nutrition. Infusion nursing standards of practice. (2011). *Journal of Infusion Nursing, 34,* S91–S92. (Level VII)

2 Ayers, P., et al. (2014). A.S.P.E.N. parenteral nutrition safety consensus recommendations. *Journal of Parenteral and Enteral Nutrition, 38,* 296–333. Accessed May 2015 via the Web at http://pen.sagepub.com/content/38/3/296.full.pdf (Level VII)

3 Centers for Disease Control and Prevention. (2002). Guideline for hand hygiene in health-care settings: Recommendations of the Healthcare Infection Control Practices Advisory Committee and the HICPAC/SHEA/APIC/IDSA Hand Hygiene Task Force. *MMWR Recommendations and Reports, 51*(RR-16), 1–45. Accessed May 2015 via the Web at http://www.cdc.gov/mmwr/pdf/rr/rr5116.pdf (Level II)

4 World Health Organization. (2009). "WHO guidelines on hand hygiene in health care: First global patient safety challenge, clean care is safer care" [Online]. Accessed May 2015 via the Web at http://whqlibdoc.who.int/publications/2009/9789241597906_eng.pdf (Level IV)

5 The Joint Commission. (2015). Standard NPSG.07.01.01. *Comprehensive accreditation manual for hospitals: The official handbook.* Oakbrook Terrace, IL: The Joint Commission. (Level VII)

6 Standard 19. Hand hygiene. Infusion nursing standards of practice. (2011). *Journal of Infusion Nursing, 34,* S26–S27. (Level VII)

7 Centers for Disease Control and Prevention. (2011). "Guidelines for the prevention of intravascular catheter-related infections" [Online]. Accessed May 2015 via the Web at http://www.cdc.gov/hicpac/pdf/guidelines/bsi-guidelines-2011.pdf (Level I)

8 American Osteopathic Association. (2014). Standard 07.01.10. *Healthcare Facilities Accreditation Program: Accreditation requirements for acute care hospitals.* Chicago, IL: American Osteopathic Association. (Level VII)

9 Centers for Medicare & Medicaid Services, Department of Health and Human Services. (2014). Condition of participation: Infection control. 42 C.F.R. § 482.42.

10 The Joint Commission. (2015). Standard NPSG.01.01.01. *Comprehensive accreditation manual for hospitals: The official handbook.* Oakbrook Terrace, IL: The Joint Commission. (Level VII)

11 Siegel, J. D., et al. (2007). "2007 guideline for isolation precautions: Preventing transmission of infectious agents in healthcare settings" [Online]. Accessed May 2015 via the Web at http://www.cdc.gov/hicpac/pdf/isolation/Isolation2007.pdf (Level II)

12 Occupational Safety and Health Administration. (n.d.). "Bloodborne pathogens, standard number 1910.1030" [Online]. Accessed May 2015 via the Web at http://www.osha.gov/pls/oshaweb/owadisp.show_document?p_table=STANDARDS&p_id=10051 (Level VII)

13 Standard 28. Filters. Infusion nursing standards of practice. (2011). *Journal of Infusion Nursing, 34,* S33–S34. (Level VII)

14 Standard 50. Air embolism. Infusion nursing standards of practice. (2011). *Journal of Infusion Nursing, 34,* S69–S70. (Level VII)

15 Standard 27. Needleless connectors. Infusion nursing standards of practice. (2011). *Journal of Infusion Nursing, 34,* S32–S33. (Level VII)

16 Standard 61. Parenteral medication and solution administration. Infusion nursing standards of practice. (2011). *Journal of Infusion Nursing, 34,* S86–S87. (Level VII)

17 Standard 45. Flushing and locking. Infusion nursing standards of practice. (2011). *Journal of Infusion Nursing, 34,* S59–S63. (Level VII)

18 Infusion Nurses Society. (2011). *Policies and procedures for infusion nursing* (4th ed.). Boston, MA: Infusion Nurses Society.

19 U.S. Food and Drug Administration. (n.d.). "Look. Check. Connect. Safe medical device connections save lives" [Online]. Accessed May 2015 via the Web at http://www.fda.gov/downloads/MedicalDevices/Safety/AlertsandNotices/UCM134873.pdf

20 Institute for Safe Medication Practices. (2012). "ISMP's list of high-alert medications" [Online]. Accessed May 2015 via the Web at http://www.ismp.org/tools/highalertmedications.pdf (Level VII)

21 Institute for Safe Medication Practices. (2008). Conducting an independent double-check. *ISMP Medication Safety Alert! Nurse Advise-ERR, 6*(12), 1. Accessed May 2015 via the Web at http://www.ismp.org/newsletters/nursing/Issues/NurseAdviseERR200812.pdf (Level VII)

22 Agency for Clinical Innovation. (2011). "Parenteral nutrition pocketbook: For adults." [Online]. Accessed May 2015 via the Web at http://www.aci.health.nsw.gov.au/__data/assets/pdf_file/0010/159805/aci_parenteral_nutrition_pb.pdf

23 Standard 22. Safe handling and disposal of sharps, hazardous materials, and hazardous waste. Infusion nursing standards of practice. (2011). *Journal of Infusion Nursing, 34,* S28–S29. (Level VII)

24 The Joint Commission. (2015). Standard RC.01.03.01. *Comprehensive accreditation manual for hospitals: The official handbook.* Oakbrook Terrace, IL: The Joint Commission. (Level VII)

25 Standard 14. Documentation. Infusion nursing standards of practice. (2011). *Journal of Infusion Nursing, 34,* S20–S21. (Level VII)

26 American Osteopathic Association. (2014). Standard 10.00.03. *Healthcare Facilities Accreditation Program: Accreditation requirements for acute care hospitals.* Chicago, IL: American Osteopathic Association. (Level VII)

27 Centers for Medicare & Medicaid Services, Department of Health and Human Services. (2014). Condition of participation: Medical record services. 42 C.F.R. § 482.24(b).

28 Standard 46. Vascular access device site care and dressing changes. Infusion nursing standards of practice. (2011). *Journal of Infusion Nursing, 34,* S63–S64. (Level VII)

29 Standard 43. Administration set change. Infusion nursing standards of practice. (2011). *Journal of Infusion Nursing, 34,* S55–S57. (Level VII)

30 Jarrett, N., et al. (2013). "Evidence-based guidelines for selected and previously considered hospital-acquired conditions: Final report" [Online]. Accessed May 2015 via the Web at http://www.cms.gov/Medicare/Medicare-Fee-for-Service-Payment/HospitalAcqCond/Downloads/Evidence-Based-Guidelines.pdf

31 Standard 18. Infection prevention. Infusion nursing standards of practice. (2011). *Journal of Infusion Nursing, 34,* S25–S26.

32 Standard 48. Infiltration and extravasation. Infusion nursing standards of practice. (2011). *Journal of Infusion Nursing, 34,* S66–S68. (Level VII)

33 Centers for Medicare & Medicaid Services, & The Joint Commission. (2014). "The specifications manual for national hospital inpatient quality measures (version 4.3a)" [Online]. Accessed May 2015 via the Web at http://www.qualitynet.org/dcs/ContentServer?c=Page&pagename=QnetPublic%2FPage%2FQnetTier4&cid=1228773564870

Additional references

Gilbert, K. A., & Worthington, P. H. (2012). Parenteral nutrition risks, complications, and management. *Journal of Infusion Nursing, 35,* 52–64.

Nettina, S. M. (2014). *Lippincott manual of nursing practice* (10th ed.). Philadelphia, PA: Wolters Kluwer.

Pontes-Arruda, A., et al. (2012). Is there a difference in bloodstream infections in critically ill patients associated with ready-to-use versus compounded parenteral nutrition? *Clinical Nutrition, 31,* 728–734. (Level V)

PARENTERAL NUTRITION MONITORING

Parenteral nutrition (PN) requires careful monitoring.[1,2] Because the typical patient is in a protein-wasting state, PN therapy causes marked changes in fluid and electrolyte status and in glucose, amino acid, mineral, and vitamin levels. If the patient displays an adverse reaction or signs of complications, the PN regimen can be changed, as needed.

Assessing a patient's nutritional status includes a physical examination and a review of body weight, body composition, somatic and visceral protein stores, and laboratory values. Monitoring a patient's condition during PN requires recognizing the signs and symptoms of possible complications, understanding laboratory test results, and keeping careful records.

Because the PN solution is high in glucose content, the infusion must start slowly to allow the patient's pancreatic beta cells to adapt to it by increasing insulin output. Within the first 3 to 5 days of PN, the typical adult patient can tolerate 3 L of solution daily without adverse reactions. Lipid emulsions also need close monitoring because the high fat content can cause the patient's lipid levels to rise. Because of the risk of vascular catheter–associated infection and other access device complications, the venous access device through which PN is administered also requires monitoring.[1,3]

HOSPITAL-ACQUIRED CONDITION ALERT ***Keep in mind that vascular catheter–associated infection is considered a hospital-acquired condition* because it can be reasonably prevented using best practices. *Follow infection prevention techniques (such as performing hand hygiene and following sterile technique) when administering PN* to reduce the risk of vascular catheter–associated infection.**[4,5]

Equipment

PN solution ■ infusion pump ■ administration set tubing and filter ■ blood glucose meter ■ thermometer ■ stethoscope ■ sphygmomanometer ■ watch with second hand ■ scale ■ input and output record ■ additional equipment for nutritional assessment, as ordered ■ supplies for blood specimen collection ■ Optional: face mask, gloves, sterile gloves, dressing change kit, antiseptic solution, stabilizing device.

Preparation of equipment

For information on preparing the infusion pump and PN solution, see the appropriate procedures. Make sure that each bag or bottle is labeled with the patient's identifiers, his weight, the administration date and time, the solution's expiration date, the route of administration (central or peripheral), the glucose concentration, component names, and dosages. All components should be ordered and labeled as amounts per day for adults, and amounts per kilogram per day for children. The total volume of solution and the infusion rate should be included as well as the duration of the infusion (continuous or cycled) and the appropriate size filter to use.[2] (If the bag or bottle is damaged and you don't have an immediate replacement, hang a bag of dextrose 10% in water, as prescribed, until the new container is ready.)

Implementation

- Perform hand hygiene and put on gloves or sterile gloves and mask, if required.[6,7,8,9,10,11,12]
- Confirm the patient's identity using at least two patient identifiers.[13]
- Explain the procedure to the patient *to diminish his anxiety and encourage cooperation.* Instruct him to inform you if he experiences any unusual sensations during the infusion.
- Record vital signs at least every 8 hours, or as ordered, *because temperature elevation may be a sign of intravascular catheter–related bloodstream infection.*
- Change the administration tubing and filters no more frequently than every 96 hours if lipids aren't being infused; replace tubing every 24 hours if lipids are being infused continuously Change the administration tubing immediately if contamination is suspected or if the integrity of the product or system has been compromised.[10,14]
- If the patient has a short peripheral catheter, don't perform routine site care; instead, change the dressing if it becomes damp or soiled or is no longer intact.[10,15]
- If the patient has a short-term central venous (CV) access device, routine dressing changes depend on the type of dressing. Change transparent semipermeable dressings at least every 7 days; change gauze dressings every 2 days. Change either dressing if it becomes damp or soiled or is no longer intact.[10,15] A dressing change should also include cleaning the catheter-skin junction with an antiseptic solution and replacing the stabilizing device, if used.[15]
- Assess the patient daily;[16] monitor for signs of peripheral and pulmonary edema. Inspect the vascular catheter insertion site daily, and palpate for tenderness through the intact dressing. Remove the dressing and thoroughly examine the site if fever, tenderness, or other findings that suggest a local or bloodstream infection exist.[3,10,15] If ordered, measure the patient's arm circumference and skin-fold thickness over the triceps.
- Weigh the patient in kilograms at the same time each morning (after voiding), with the patient in similar-weight clothing, and on the same scale. Compare these data with his fluid intake and output record.[16] *Weight gain, particularly early in treatment, may indicate fluid overload rather than increasing fat and protein stores.* A patient shouldn't gain more than 1.5 kg per week; a weight gain of 0.5 kg per week is a reasonable goal for most patients; suspect fluid imbalance if the patient gains more than 0.5 kg daily.
- *Monitor the patient's bowel function* by auscultating bowel sounds and assessing the number, volume, and consistency of bowel movements.[17]
- Monitor the patient for signs and symptoms of glucose metabolism disturbance, fluid and electrolyte imbalances, and nutritional aberrations.[1,2,16] Some patients may require supplemental insulin for the duration of PN; the pharmacy should add insulin directly to the PN solution.[2] Monitor electrolyte levels frequently—daily at first.[1] Monitor serum albumin levels weekly. (See *Laboratory monitoring of parenteral nutrition,* page 588.) Later, as the patient's condition stabilizes, you won't need to monitor these values quite as closely. (Be aware that in a severely dehydrated patient, albumin levels may actually drop initially as treatment restores hydration.)
- Monitor potassium, magnesium, phosphate, and calcium levels. If these electrolytes have been added to the PN solution, the dosage may need adjusting *to maintain normal serum levels.*[1]
- Monitor serum glucose levels every 6 hours initially, and then once per day or according to the ordered parameters.[2] Watch for signs and symptoms of hyperglycemia, such as thirst, hunger, and polyuria. Periodically confirm blood glucose meter readings with laboratory tests.
- Assess renal function by monitoring blood urea nitrogen and creatinine levels *because increases can indicate excess amino acid intake.* Also assess nitrogen balance with 24-hour urine collection, as ordered.[1]
- Assess liver function by periodically monitoring liver enzyme, bilirubin, triglyceride, and cholesterol levels. *Abnormal values may indicate an intolerance or excess of lipid emulsions or problems with metabolizing the protein or glucose in the PN formula.*[1]
- Provide emotional support. *Patients tend to associate eating with positive feelings and can become disturbed when eating is prohibited.*[15]
- Provide frequent oral care. (See the "Oral care," procedure, page 560.)
- Keep the patient active *to enable him to use nutrients more fully.*
- When discontinuing PN, decrease the infusion rate slowly, depending on the patient's current glucose intake, *to minimize the risk of hyperinsulinemia and resulting hypoglycemia.* Weaning usually takes place over 24 to 48 hours but can be completed in 4 to 6 hours if the patient receives sufficient oral or IV carbohydrates.
- While weaning the patient from PN, document his dietary intake and work with the nutritionist *to determine the total calorie and protein intake.* Also teach other health care staff members caring for the patient the importance of recording food intake. Use percentages of food consumed

Laboratory monitoring of parenteral nutrition

These laboratory tests are usually ordered as part of monitoring for a patient receiving parenteral nutrition (PN).

Baseline tests

Complete blood count (CBC); comprehensive metabolic panel (CMP);* cholesterol and triglycerides; liver function tests, including prothrombin time (PT), International Normalized Ratio (INR), lactate dehydrogenase, and bilirubin; and magnesium, phosphate, and transferrin levels (additional tests that may be performed upon initiation of PN include trace elements and vitamin levels)[1,18]

Daily tests

Weight, intake and output, glucose by fingerstick every 6 hours until stable, then as directed; basic metabolic panel (BMP),** magnesium and phosphate levels, and liver function tests until stable, then two to three times a week, as directed[1]

Weekly tests

CBC; CMP; cholesterol, triglycerides, and c-reactive protein (CRP) levels;[1] PT; INR; and transferrin level

Additional tests

As indicated for patients receiving long-term PN: zinc, copper, selenium, manganese, folate, vitamin B_{12}, and vitamins A, D, and E levels; bone mineral density assessment[1,19]

*CMP includes blood urea nitrogen (BUN), creatinine, sodium, chloride, carbon dioxide (CO_2), glucose, potassium, calcium, albumin, total protein, alkaline phosphatase, alanine transaminase, aspartate transaminase, and bilirubin.
**BMP includes BUN, creatinine, sodium, chloride, CO_2, glucose, and potassium levels.

(such as "ate 50% of a baked potato") instead of subjective descriptions (such as "had a good appetite") *to provide a more accurate account of patient intake.*

- Remove and discard your gloves and mask, if worn.
- Perform hand hygiene.[6,7,8,9,10,11,12]
- Document the procedure.[20,21,22,23]

Special considerations

- Always maintain strict sterile technique when handling the equipment used to administer therapy.[16] *Because the PN solution serves as a medium for bacterial growth and the CV access device provides systemic access,* the patient is at risk for infection and sepsis.
- During daily multidisciplinary rounds, discuss the patient's readiness for enteral feeding; switch to enteral feeding as soon as the patient's condition warrants. Make sure the CV access device is removed as soon as it's no longer needed *to reduce the risk of vascular catheter–related bloodstream infection.*[10,16]
- When using a filter, position it as close to the access site as possible.[24] Check the filter's porosity and psi capacity *to make sure it exceeds the psi exerted by the infusion pump.*
- Don't allow PN solutions to hang for more than 24 hours; hang time for lipids shouldn't exceed 12 hours.[16]
- Be careful when using the PN access device for other functions.[16] If using a single-lumen CV access device, don't use the device to infuse blood or blood products, give a bolus injection, administer simultaneous IV solutions, measure CV pressure, or obtain blood samples for laboratory testing without a practitioner's order. Never add medication to a PN solution container.[2] Also, don't use a three-way stopcock, if possible, *because add-on devices increase the risk of infection.*
- When a patient is severely malnourished, starting PN may spark refeeding syndrome, which includes a rapid drop in potassium, magnesium, and phosphorus levels. *To avoid compromising cardiac function,* initiate feeding slowly and monitor the patient's blood values especially closely until they stabilize.[1]

Patient teaching

Teach the patient about measures to prevent intravascular catheter–related infections, including the importance of hand hygiene.[25] Encourage the patient and his family to remind staff members if they fail to perform hand hygiene before delivering care. Teach the patient about signs and symptoms of complications and to report them immediately.

Patients who require prolonged or indefinite PN may be able to receive the therapy at home. Home PN reduces the need for long hospitalizations and allows the patient to resume many of his normal activities. Make a home care referral and begin patient teaching before discharge to make sure that the patient knows how to perform the administration procedure and how to handle complications.

Complications

Catheter-related, metabolic, and mechanical complications can occur during PN administration. (See the "Parenteral nutrition administration" procedure, page 581.)

Documentation

Document the type of access device used, the PN formulation, additives, the volume of solution, the rate of infusion, your assessment findings, and the patient's response to therapy. Record adverse effects, the date and time, the name of the practitioner notified, any prescribed interventions, and the patient's response to those interventions. Document patient teaching provided and the patient's understanding of your teaching.

References

1 Agency for Clinical Innovation. (2011). "Parenteral nutrition pocketbook: For adults" [Online]. Accessed May 2015 via the Web at http://www.aci.health.nsw.gov.au/__data/assets/pdf_file/0010/159805/aci_parenteral_nutrition_pb.pdf (Level VII)

2 Ayers, P., et al. (2014). A.S.P.E.N. parenteral nutrition safety consensus recommendations. *Journal of Parenteral and Enteral Nutrition, 38,* 296–333. Accessed May 2015 via the Web at http://pen.sagepub.com/content/38/3/296.full.pdf (Level VII)

3 Centers for Medicare & Medicaid Services, & The Joint Commission. (2014). "The specifications manual for national hospital inpatient quality measures (version 4.3a)" [Online]. Accessed May 2015 via the Web at http://www.qualitynet.org/dcs/ContentServer?c=Page&pagename=QnetPublic%2FPage%2FQnetTier4&cid=1228773564870

4 Jarrett, N., et al. (2013). "Evidence-based guidelines for selected and previously considered hospital-acquired conditions: Final report" [Online]. Accessed May 2015 via the Web at http://www.cms.gov/Medicare/Medicare-Fee-for-Service-Payment/HospitalAcqCond/Downloads/Evidence-Based-Guidelines.pdf

5 Standard 49. Infection. Infusion nursing standards of practice. (2011). *Journal of Infusion Nursing, 34,* S68–S69. (Level VII)

6 Centers for Disease Control and Prevention. (2002). Guideline for hand hygiene in health-care settings: Recommendations of the Healthcare Infection Control Practices Advisory Committee and the HICPAC/SHEA/APIC/IDSA Hand Hygiene Task Force. *MMWR Recommendations and Reports, 51*(RR–16), 1–45. Accessed May 2015 via the Web at http://www.cdc.gov/mmwr/pdf/rr/rr5116.pdf (Level II)

7 World Health Organization. (2009). "WHO guidelines on hand hygiene in health care: First global patient safety challenge, clean care is safer care" [Online]. Accessed May 2015 via the Web at http://whqlibdoc.who.int/publications/2009/9789241597906_eng.pdf (Level IV)

8 The Joint Commission. (2015). Standard NPSG.07.01.01. *Comprehensive accreditation manual for hospitals: The official handbook.* Oakbrook Terrace, IL: The Joint Commission. (Level VII)
9 Standard 19. Hand hygiene. Infusion nursing standards of practice. (2011). *Journal of Infusion Nursing, 34,* S26–S27. (Level VII)
10 Centers for Disease Control and Prevention. (2011). "Guidelines for the prevention of intravascular catheter-related infections" [Online]. Accessed May 2015 via the Web at http://www.cdc.gov/hicpac/pdf/guidelines/bsi-guidelines-2011.pdf (Level I)
11 Centers for Medicare & Medicaid Services, Department of Health and Human Services. (2014). Condition of participation: Infection control. 42 C.F.R. § 482.42.
12 American Osteopathic Association. (2014). Standard 07.01.10. *Healthcare Facilities Accreditation Program: Accreditation requirements for acute care hospitals.* Chicago, IL: American Osteopathic Association. (Level VII)
13 The Joint Commission. (2015). Standard NPSG.01.01.01. *Comprehensive accreditation manual for hospitals: The official handbook.* Oakbrook Terrace, IL: The Joint Commission. (Level VII)
14 Standard 43. Administration set change. Infusion nursing standards of practice. (2011). *Journal of Infusion Nursing, 34,* S55–S57. (Level VII)
15 Standard 46. Vascular access device site care and dressing changes. Infusion nursing standards of practice. (2011). *Journal of Infusion Nursing, 34,* S63–S64. (Level VII)
16 Standard 65. Parenteral nutrition. Infusion nursing standards of practice. (2011). *Journal of Infusion Nursing, 34,* S91–S92. (Level VII)
17 Iyer, K. R. (2013). "Short bowel syndrome: Tailoring nutritional and medical interventions to improve outcomes" [Online]. Accessed May 2015 via the Web at http://www.medscape.org/viewarticle/810558
18 Fessler, T. A. (2013). Trace elements in parenteral nutrition: A practical guide for dosage and monitoring for adult patients. *Nutrition in Clinical Practice, 28,* 722–729.
19 Staun, M., et al. (2009). ESPEN guidelines on parenteral nutrition: Home parenteral nutrition (HPN) in adult patients. *Clinical Nutrition, 28,* 467–479. Accessed May 2015 via the Web at http://espen.info/documents/0909/Home%20Parenteral%20Nutrition%20in%20adults.pdf (Level VII)
20 The Joint Commission. (2015). Standard RC.01.03.01. *Comprehensive accreditation manual for hospitals: The official handbook.* Oakbrook Terrace, IL: The Joint Commission. (Level VII)
21 Standard 14. Documentation. Infusion nursing standards of practice. (2011). *Journal of Infusion Nursing, 34,* S20–S21. (Level VII)
22 Centers for Medicare & Medicaid Services, Department of Health and Human Services. (2014). Condition of participation: Medical record services. 42 C.F.R. § 482.24(b).
23 American Osteopathic Association. (2014). Standard 10.00.03. *Healthcare Facilities Accreditation Program: Accreditation requirements for acute care hospitals.* Chicago, IL: American Osteopathic Association. (Level VII)
24 Standard 28. Filters. Infusion nursing standards of practice. (2011). *Journal of Infusion Nursing, 34,* S33–S34. (Level VII)
25 The Joint Commission. (2015). Standard NPSG.07.04.01. *Comprehensive accreditation manual for hospitals: The official handbook.* Oakbrook Terrace, IL: The Joint Commission. (Level VII)

ADDITIONAL REFERENCES

Infusion Nurses Society. (2010). *Infusion nursing: An evidence-based approach* (3rd ed.). St. Louis, MO: Saunders.
Infusion Nurses Society. (2013). *Policies and procedures for infusion nursing of the older adult* (2nd ed.). Boston, MA: Infusion Nurses Society.

PASSIVE RANGE-OF-MOTION EXERCISES

Used to move the patient's joints through as full a range of motion (ROM) as possible, passive ROM exercises improve or maintain joint mobility and help prevent contractures. Performed by a nurse, physical therapist, or caregiver of the patient's choosing, these exercises are indicated for the patient with temporary or permanent loss of mobility, sensation, or consciousness. Performed properly, passive ROM exercises require recognition of the patient's limits of motion and support of all joints during movement.

Exercises performed in the bed help with joint mobility, strength, and endurance and they prepare the patient for ambulation. When included as a component of care, ROM exercises can enhance patient outcomes, improve gas exchange, reduce rates of ventilator-associated pneumonia, shorten the duration of mechanical ventilation, and enhance long-term functional ability.[1]

During passive ROM exercises, another person moves the patient's extremities so that the joints move through a complete ROM, maximally stretching all muscle groups within each plane over each joint. The exercises described here treat all joints, but they don't have to be performed in the order presented or all at once. They can be schedules over the course of a day, whenever the patient is in the most convenient position. All exercises should be performed slowly, gently, and to the end of the normal ROM or to the point of pain, but no further. (See *Glossary of joint movements,* page 590.) Each position should be held for 1 to 2 seconds. Typically, these exercises are performed three times for each joint, at least twice a day.[2]

Passive ROM exercises are contraindicated in patients with septic joints, acute thrombophlebitis, severe arthritic joint inflammation, bone tumors or metastases, acute myocardial infarction, or recent trauma with possible hidden fractures or internal injuries.

Equipment

Optional: gloves, other personal protective equipment.

Implementation

- Determine the joints that need ROM exercises.
- Consult the practitioner or physical therapist about limitations or precautions for specific exercises.
- Perform hand hygiene.[3,4,5,6,7]
- Confirm the patient's identity using at least two patient identifiers.[8]
- Explain the procedure to the patient.
- Raise the bed to a comfortable working height and use proper upper body mechanics during ROM exercises.
- Put on gloves and other personal protective equipment, as needed, *to comply with standard precautions.*[9,10]

Exercising the neck

- While supporting the patient's head with your hands, extend her neck, flex her chin to her chest, and tilt her head laterally toward each shoulder.
- Rotate the patient's head from right to left (as shown below).

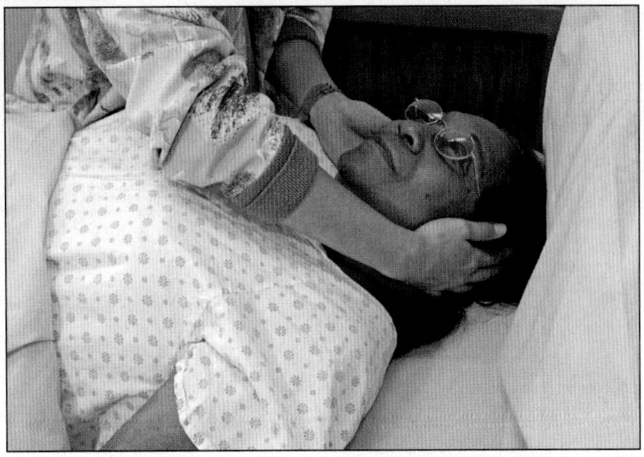

Exercising the shoulders

- Support the patient's arm in an extended, neutral position; then extend her forearm and flex it back.

Glossary of joint movements

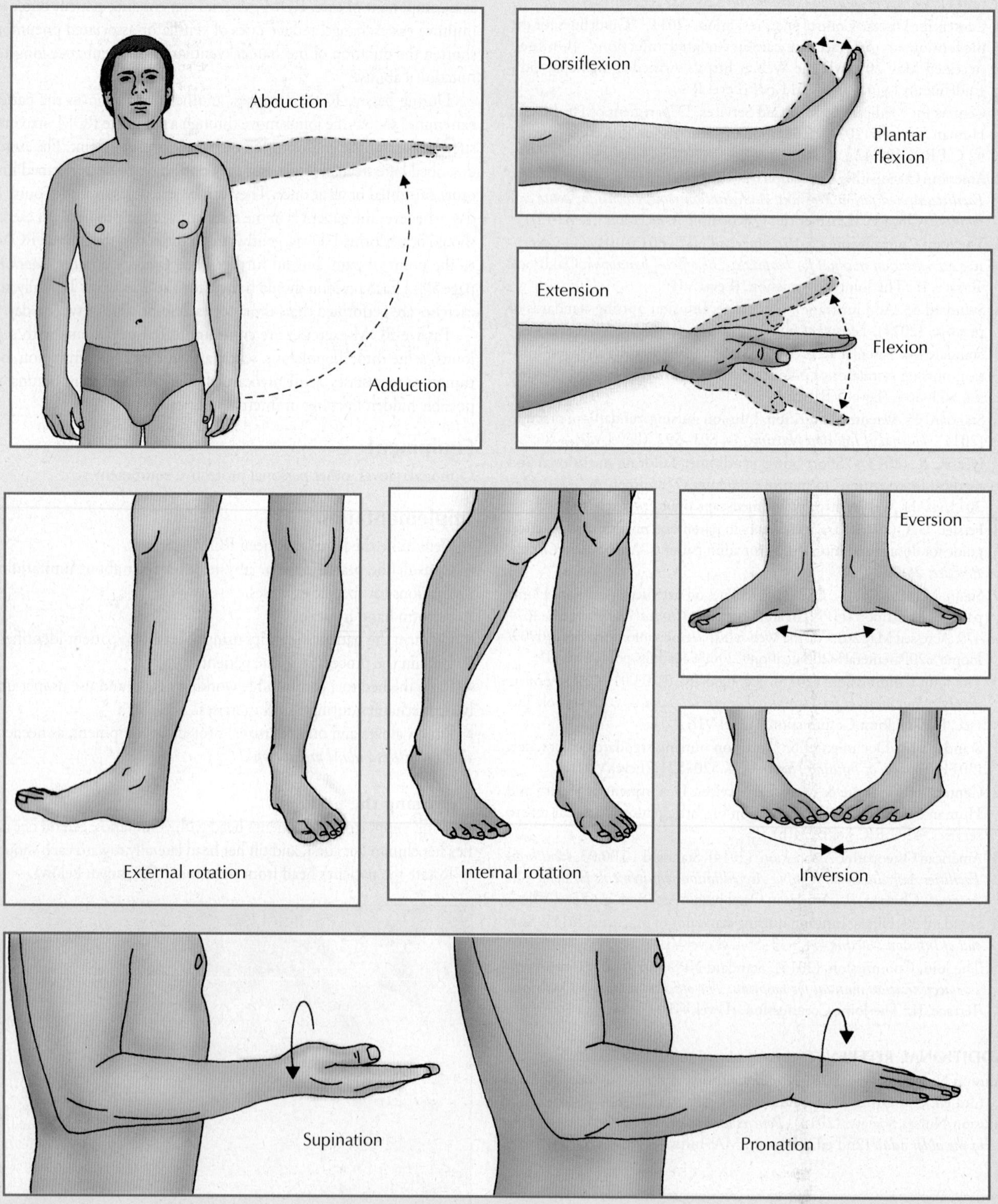

- Abduct he patient's arm outward from the side of her body, and then adduct it back to the side.
- Rotate the shoulder so that the patient's arm crosses the midline, and then bend the elbow so that the hand touches the opposite shoulder and then touches the mattress for complete internal rotation.
- Return the patient's shoulder to a neutral position and, with elbow bent, push the patient's arm backward so that the back of her hand touches the mattress for complete external rotation (as shown on next page, top left).

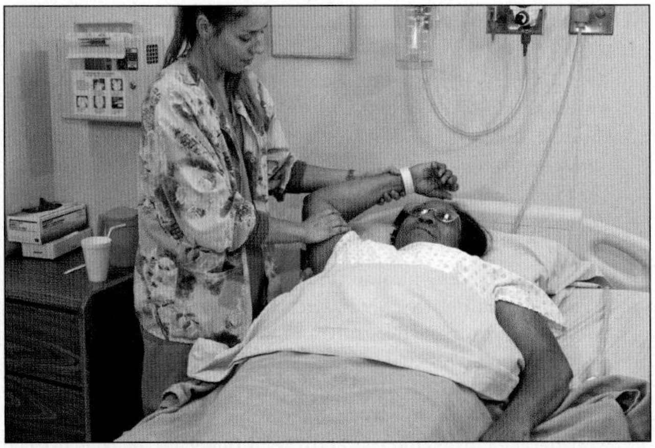

Exercising the elbow

- Place the patient's arm at her side with her palm facing up.
- Flex and extend the patient's arm at the elbow (as shown below).

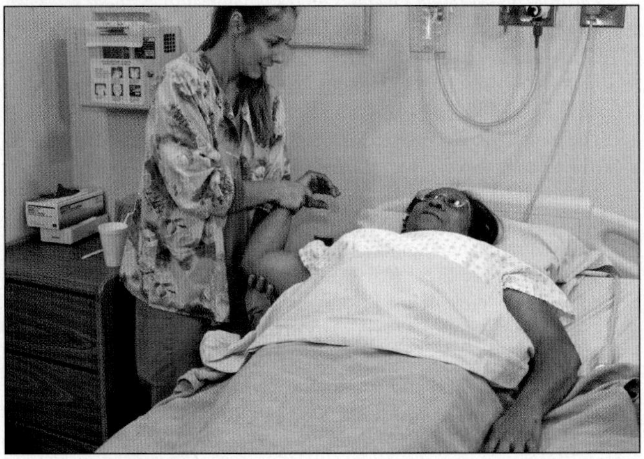

Exercising the forearm

- Stabilize the patient's elbow, and then twist her hand to bring her palm up (supination, as shown below).
- Twist it back again to bring her palm down (pronation).

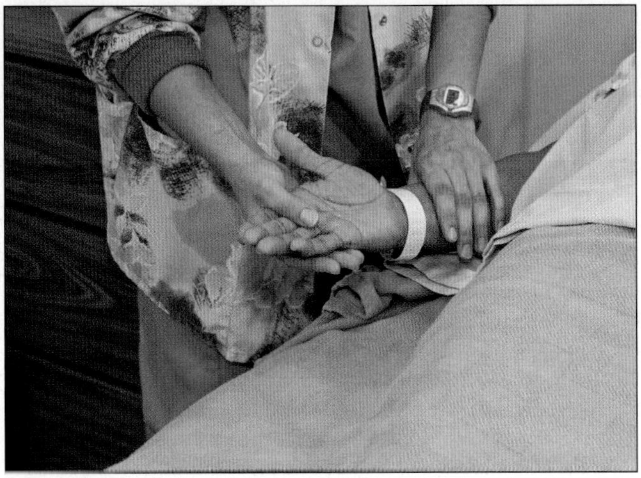

Exercising the wrist

- Stabilize the patient's forearm, and then flex and extend her wrist.
- Rock the patient's hand sideways for lateral flexion.
- Rotate the patient's hand in a circular motion (as shown on top right).

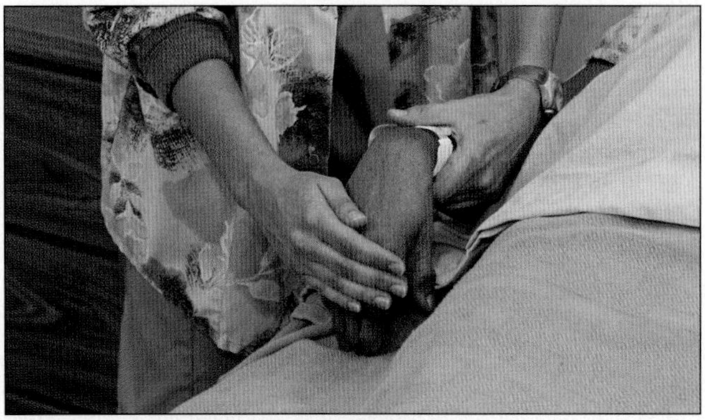

Exercising the fingers and thumb

- Extend the patient's fingers, and then flex her hand into a fist; repeat extension and flexion of each joint of each finger and thumb separately.
- Spread two adjoining fingers apart (abduction, as shown below), and then bring them together (adduction).
- Oppose each fingertip to the patient's thumb.
- Rotate the thumb and each finger in a circle.

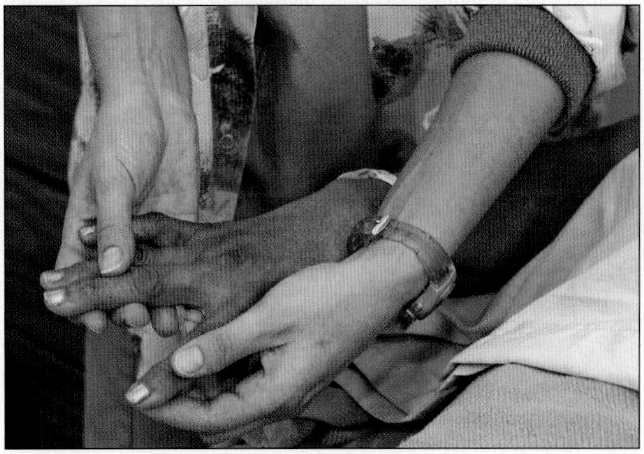

Exercising the hip and knee

- Fully extend the patient's leg, and then bend her hip and knee toward her chest, allowing full joint flexion.
- Move the patient's straight leg sideways, out and away from her other leg (abduction), and then back, over, and across it (adduction).
- Rotate the patient's straight leg internally toward the midline (as shown below), and then externally away from the midline.

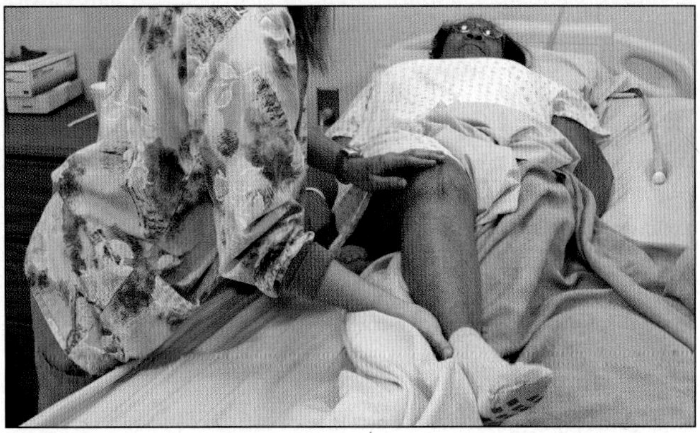

Exercising the ankle

- Bend the patient's foot so that her toes push upward (dorsiflexion), and then bend her foot so that her toes push downward (plantar flexion).

- Rotate her ankle in a circular motion.
- Invert the patient's ankle so that the sole of her foot faces the midline (as shown below), and evert her ankle so that the sole faces away from the midline.

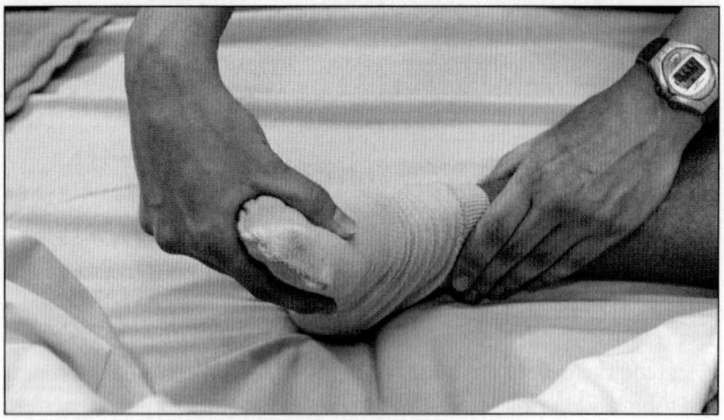

Exercising the toes

- Flex the patient's toes toward the sole, and then extend them back toward the top of her foot.
- Spread two adjoining toes apart (abduction, as shown below), and bring them together (adduction).

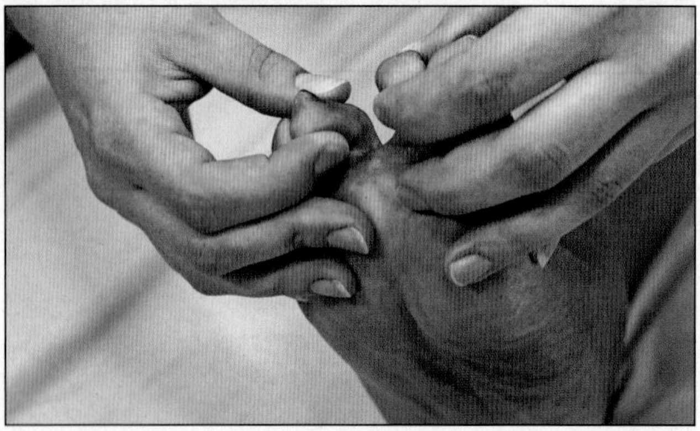

Completing the procedure

- Remove and discard your gloves and other personal protective equipment, if worn.[9]
- Perform hand hygiene.[3,4,5,6]
- Document the procedure.[11,12,13]

Special considerations

- *Because joints begin to stiffen within 24 hours of disuse,* start passive ROM exercises as soon as possible, and perform them at least once each shift, or three times a day,[1] usually while bathing or turning the patient. Use proper body mechanics, and repeat each exercise at least three times.
- Patients who experience prolonged bed rest or limited activity without profound weakness can also be taught to perform ROM exercises on their own (called *active ROM exercises*), or they may benefit from isometric exercises. (See *Learning about isometric exercises.*)
- If a disabled patient requires long-term rehabilitation after discharge, consult with a physical therapist and teach a family member or caregiver to perform passive ROM exercises.

Documentation

Record the joints exercised, the presence of edema or pressure areas, any pain resulting from the exercises, any limitation of ROM, and the patient's tolerance of the exercises.

REFERENCES

1 Vollman, K. M. (2010). Progressive mobility in the critically ill. *Critical Care Nurse, 30*(2), S3–S16. Accessed May 2015 via the Web at http://www.aacn.org/WD/CETests/Media/C102S.pdf

2 Hinkle, J. L. & Cheever, K. H. (2014). *Brunner & Suddarth's textbook of medical-surgical nursing* (13th ed.). Philadelphia, PA: Wolters Kluwer.

3 The Joint Commission. (2015). Standard NPSG.07.01.01. *Comprehensive accreditation manual for hospitals: The official handbook.* Oakbrook Terrace, IL: The Joint Commission. (Level VII)

4 Centers for Disease Control and Prevention. (2002). Guideline for hand hygiene in health-care settings: Recommendations of the Healthcare Infection Control Practices Advisory Committee and the HICPAC/SHEA/APIC/IDSA Hand Hygiene Task Force. *MMWR Recommendations and Reports, 51*(RR-16), 1–45. Accessed May 2015 via the Web at http://www.cdc.gov/mmwr/pdf/rr/rr5116.pdf (Level III)

5 World Health Organization. (2009). "WHO guidelines on hand hygiene in health care: First global patient safety challenge, clean care is safer care" [Online]. Accessed May 2015 via the Web at http://whqlibdoc.who.int/publications/2009/9789241597906_eng.pdf (Level IV)

6 American Osteopathic Association. (2012). Standard 07.01.21. *Healthcare Facilities Accreditation Program: Accreditation requirements for acute care hospitals.* Chicago, IL: American Osteopathic Association. (Level VII)

7 Centers for Medicare & Medicaid Services, Department of Health and Human Services. (2014). Condition of participation: Infection control. 42 C.F.R. § 482.42.

8 The Joint Commission. (2015). Standard NPSG.01.01.01. *Comprehensive accreditation manual for hospitals: The official handbook.* Oakbrook Terrace, IL: The Joint Commission. (Level VII)

9 Occupational Safety and Health Administration. (n.d.). "Bloodborne pathogens, standard number 1910.1030" [Online]. Accessed May 2015 via the Web at http://www.osha.gov/pls/oshaweb/owadisp.show_document?p_table=standards&p_id=10051 (Level VII)

10 American Osteopathic Association. (2014). Standard 07.01.10. *Healthcare Facilities Accreditation Program: Accreditation requirements for acute care hospitals.* Chicago, IL: American Osteopathic Association. (Level VII)

11 The Joint Commission. (2015). Standard RC.01.03.01. *Comprehensive accreditation manual for hospitals: The official handbook.* Oakbrook Terrace, IL: The Joint Commission. (Level VII)

12 Centers for Medicare & Medicaid Services, Department of Health and Human Services. (2014). Condition of participation: Medical record services. 42 C.F.R. § 482.24(b).

13 American Osteopathic Association. (2014). Standard 10.00.03. *Healthcare Facilities Accreditation Program: Accreditation requirements for acute care hospitals.* Chicago, IL: American Osteopathic Association. (Level VII)

ADDITIONAL REFERENCE

Craven, R. F., & Hirnle, C. J. (2012). *Fundamentals of nursing: Human health and function* (7th ed.). Philadelphia, PA: Lippincott Williams & Wilkins.

PATIENT-CONTROLLED ANALGESIA

Patient-controlled analgesia (PCA) is a drug delivery system providing IV analgesia, usually morphine, when the patient presses a button at the end of a cord. Analgesia is provided at the level and time needed by the patient. The device prevents the patient from accidentally overdosing by imposing a lockout time between doses, usually 6 to 10 minutes. During this interval, the patient won't receive any analgesic, even if he pushes the button.

PCA offers several advantages. It eliminates the need for IM analgesics, provides pain relief tailored to each patient's size and pain tolerance, gives the patient a sense of control over pain, and allows the patient to sleep at night with minimal daytime drowsiness. It also improves postoperative deep breathing, coughing, and ambulation and reduces opioid use compared with those who don't receive PCA.

PCA is typically given to patients postoperatively and to those with terminal cancer or other chronic diseases. To receive PCA therapy, a

Learning about isometric exercises

Patients can strengthen and increase muscle tone by contracting muscles against resistance (from other muscles or from a stationary object, such as a bed or a wall) without joint movement. These exercises require only a comfortable position—standing, sitting, or lying down—and proper body alignment. For each exercise, instruct the patient to hold each contraction for 2 to 5 seconds and to repeat it three to four times daily, below peak contraction level for the first week and at peak level thereafter.

Neck rotators

The patient places the heel of his hand above one ear. Then he pushes his head toward the hand as forcefully as possible, without moving the head, neck, or arm. He repeats the exercise on the other side.

Neck flexors

The patient places both palms on his forehead. Without moving his neck, he pushes his head forward while resisting with his palms.

Neck extensors

The patient clasps his fingers behind his head, and then pushes his head against his clasped hands without moving his neck.

Shoulder elevators

Holding his right arm straight down at his side, the patient grasps his right wrist with his left hand. He then tries to shrug his right shoulder, but prevents it from moving by holding his arm in place. He repeats this exercise, alternating arms.

Shoulder, chest, and scapular musculature

The patient places his right fist in his left palm and raises both arms to shoulder height. He pushes his fist into his palm as forcefully as possible without moving either arm. Then, with his arms in the same position, he clasps his fingers and tries to pull his hands apart. He repeats the pattern, beginning with the left fist in the right palm.

Elbow flexors and extensors

With his right elbow bent 90 degrees and his right palm facing upward, the patient places his left fist against his right palm. He tries to bend his right elbow further while resisting with the left fist. He repeats the pattern, bending his left elbow.

Abdomen

The patient assumes a sitting position and bends slightly forward, with his hands in front of the middle of his thighs. He tries to bend forward further, resisting by pressing his palms against his thighs.

Alternatively, in the supine position, he clasps his hands behind his head. Then he raises his shoulders about 1″ (2.5 cm), holding this position for a few seconds.

Back extensors

In a sitting position, the patient bends forward and places his hands under his buttocks. He tries to stand up, resisting with both hands.

Hip abductors

While standing, the patient squeezes his inner thighs together as tightly as possible. Placing a pillow between his knees supplies resistance and increases the effectiveness of this exercise.

Hip extensors

The patient squeezes his buttocks together as tightly as possible.

Knee extensors

The patient straightens his knee fully. Then he vigorously tightens the muscle above the knee so that it moves his kneecap upward. He repeats this exercise, alternating legs.

Ankle flexors and extensors

The patient pulls his toes upward, holding briefly. Then he pushes them down as far as possible, again holding briefly.

patient must be mentally alert and able to understand and comply with instructions and procedures and have no history of allergy to the analgesic.

To ensure patient safety, standardized medication concentrations and standardized or preprinted order sets for PCA or authorized agent–controlled analgesia are recommended.[1,2,3] PCA is intended to be controlled by the patient, but for patients who can't use PCA independently, authorized agent–controlled analgesia—analgesia controlled by an authorized, educated agent such as a nurse or caregiver—offers a safe alternative. To increase the safety of authorized agent–controlled analgesia, authorized agents must receive proper education, keep accurate clinical documentation, and carefully adhere to institutional guidelines, and eligible patients and agents must be carefully selected.[4] To prevent unauthorized analgesia administration, hazard warning signs should be placed on the PCA equipment, and family members and health care practitioners should be taught about the potential dangers of administering PCA without authorization.[1,2,3]

Equipment

Patient's medical and medication records ▪ PCA system and system-specific tubing ▪ syringe with prescribed medication ▪ antiseptic pads (alcohol, tincture of iodine, or chlorhexidine-based) ▪ compatible IV solution ▪ gloves ▪ tape ▪ labels ▪ naloxone ▪ oxygen administration setup and equipment ▪ Optional: pulse oximeter with probe, capnography monitoring equipment, vital signs monitoring equipment, antiemetic.

Preparation of equipment

Several types of PCA devices are available, so follow the manufacturer's instructions for setting up the device. Obtain the medication and verify the medication order. Gather equipment and bring it to the patient's bedside. Plug the PCA device into an electrical outlet. If the device is battery-operated, make sure that the battery is fully charged and working. Have oxygen and naloxone readily available *in case the patient develops respiratory depression.*[2]

Implementation

- Avoid distractions and interruptions when preparing and administering medication *to prevent medication administration errors.*[5,6]
- Verify the practitioner's order.[7,8,9]
- Compare the medication label with the order in the patient's medical record.[7,8,9]
- Check the patient's medical record for an allergy or a contraindication to the prescribed medication. If an allergy or a contraindication exists, don't administer the medication; instead, notify the practitioner.[7,8,9]
- Review the patient's medical record for risk factors, such as advanced age, morbid obesity, obstructive sleep apnea, chronic obstructive pulmonary disease, or renal insufficiency, that place the patient at risk for respiratory depression or other adverse events.[1]
- Check the expiration date on the medication. If the medication is expired, return it to the pharmacy and obtain new medication.[7,8,9]
- Visually inspect the solution for particles, discoloration, or other loss of integrity; don't administer the medication if its integrity is compromised.[7,8,9]

■ Discuss any unresolved concerns about the medication with the patient's practitioner.[7,8,9]
■ Verify that the medication is being administered at the proper time, in the prescribed dose, and by the correct route *to reduce the risk of medication errors.*[7,8,9]
■ Perform hand hygiene.[10,11,12,13,14,15,16]
■ Confirm the patient's identity using at least two patient identifiers.[17]
■ Provide privacy. Teach the patient about potential adverse reactions and discuss any other concerns related to the medication.[7,8,9,18,19] Provide education at the patient's level of understanding, avoiding medical jargon. Obtain the assistance of a medical interpreter, as needed. Teach the patient how to use the PCA device and assess the patient's comprehension by using the teach-back method. Notify the practitioner if the patient can't participate safely in PCA therapy.[1,20]
■ Obtain vital signs *to serve as a baseline for comparison.*
■ If the patient is at risk for respiratory depression, consider monitoring pulse oximetry, capnography, or both *to promptly detect respiratory depression.*[1]
■ Perform hand hygiene.[10,11,12,13,14,15,16] and put on gloves.[21]
■ Assess the patient's IV access site for pain, redness, or swelling, and aspirate for blood *to ensure patency.* If the patient doesn't have IV access, insert an appropriate device. (See the "IV catheter insertion and removal" procedure, page 446.)
■ If your facility uses a bar code scanning system, scan your identification badge, the patient's identification bracelet, and the medication's bar code.
■ Have another nurse perform an independent double-check, if required by your facility, *to verify the patient's identity and the correct medication and concentration.*[1,2,3]

NURSING ALERT *Opioids are considered a high-alert medication* because they can cause significant patient harm when used in error. *Before beginning an opioid infusion, have another nurse perform an independent double-check, if required by your facility,* to verify the patient's identity and to make sure that the correct medication is in the syringe in the prescribed concentration, the medication's indication corresponds with the patient's diagnosis, the dosage calculations are correct, the route of administration is safe and proper for the patient, the pump settings are correct, and the infusion line is attached to the correct port.[22,23]

■ Compare the results of the independent double-check with another nurse if required. If discrepancies exist, rectify them before beginning PCA.
■ Connect the device tubing to the medication syringe, and insert the syringe into the PCA device. Make sure that the markings and labels on the syringe are readily visible. Prime the tubing *to remove air from the system and reduce the risk of an air embolism.*
■ Thoroughly disinfect the needleless connection port on the patient's IV line with an antiseptic pad using friction, and allow it to dry.[14] Then connect the PCA tubing to the patient's IV line or IV access device at the lowest possible port.[2]
■ Trace the tubing from the patient to the point of origin *to make sure that it's connected to the correct port before starting the infusion.*[24]
■ Program the device to deliver the prescribed parameters, such as loading dose, basal rate, bolus amount, and bolus lockout time. Have a second nurse confirm these settings *to prevent possible errors.*[1,2]
■ Adjust the prescribed IV solution flow rate, if appropriate.
■ Label the PCA pump, PCA tubing, and IV infusion tubing.
■ Instruct the patient to push the button each time he has pain and needs relief.[3]
■ Monitor the patient's vital signs, sedation level, oxygen saturation level, and capnography (if used) frequently during the initial loading dose and at least every 4 hours throughout therapy. Monitor the patient more frequently during the first 24 hours and at night, *when hypoventilation and nocturnal hypoxia may occur.*[1,2] Be aware of the amount the patient will receive when he activates the device and the maximum amount that he can receive within a specified time (if using an adjustable device).[2]
■ Perform a comprehensive pain assessment at the start of therapy and a reassessment every 4 hours using techniques appropriate for the patient's age, condition, and ability to understand.[1,2,25,26] Notify the practitioner if the patient's pain isn't being relieved.
■ Inspect the infusion site for changes, including redness, tenderness, and swelling, at least every 4 hours;[27] check the device function, including the rate, periodically.
■ Replace the medication syringe when empty using safe medication administration practices.[7,8,9]
■ Discard used equipment appropriately.[21]
■ Remove and discard your gloves,[21] and perform hand hygiene.[10,11,12,13,14,15,16]
■ Document the procedure.[28,29,30]

Special considerations

■ Encourage the patient to cough and deep breathe *to promote ventilation.*
■ Monitor the IV insertion site for infiltration into subcutaneous tissues and for catheter occlusion, *which may cause the drug to back up into the primary IV tubing.*
■ If the analgesic nauseates the patient, administer an antiemetic, as ordered.
■ Verify PCA pump settings at the beginning of each shift and during or immediately after receiving handoff communications.[2]

Patient teaching

Before initiating PCA therapy, teach the patient how the device works.[2] Allow the patient to practice with a sample device. Reinforce that he should take enough analgesic to relieve acute pain but not enough to make him feel drowsy.

Complications

Potential complications include respiratory depression (secondary to the drug) and IV infiltration.

Documentation

Record the date and time of PCA therapy initiation; the IV access device used and its location; baseline vital signs and pain assessment; medication doses (loading dose, individual doses, and time interval); and ongoing assessments of vital signs, pain, and the IV site. Also document the patient's understanding and tolerance of the procedure and any patient teaching provided.

References

1 Standard 64. Patient-controlled analgesia. Infusion nursing standards of practice. (2011). *Journal of Infusion Nursing, 34,* S89–S91. (Level VII)
2 Institute for Safe Medication Practices. (2014). "Part II—How to prevent errors: Safety issues with patient-controlled analgesia" [Online]. Accessed May 2015 via the Web at http://www.ismp.org/newsletters/acutecare/articles/20030724.asp (Level VII)
3 Institute for Safe Medication Practices. (n.d.). "Patient controlled analgesia: Making it safer for patients" [Online]. Accessed May 2015 via the Web at http://www.ismp.org/profdevelopment/PCAMonograph.pdf (Level VII)
4 Cooney, M. F., et al. (2013). American Society for Pain Management Nursing position statement with clinical practice guidelines: Authorized agent controlled analgesia. *Pain Management Nursing, 14,* 176–181. Accessed May 2015 via the Web at http://www.aspmn.org/documents/AuthorizedAgentControlledAnalgesia_PMN_August2013.pdf (Level VII)
5 Westbrook, J., et al. (2010). Association of interruptions with an increased risk and severity of medication administration errors. *Archives of Internal Medicine, 170,* 683–690. (Level IV)

6 Institute for Safe Medication Practices. (2013). Side tracks on the safety express: Interruptions lead to errors and unfinished...Wait, what was I doing? *Nurse Advise-ERR, 11*(2), 1–4. Accessed May 2015 via the Web at https://www.ismp.org/Newsletters/acutecare/showarticle.aspx?id=37 (Level VII)

7 The Joint Commission. (2015). Standard MM.06.01.01. *Comprehensive accreditation manual for hospitals: The official handbook.* Oakbrook Terrace, IL: The Joint Commission. (Level VII)

8 American Osteopathic Association. (2014). Standard 16.01.03. *Healthcare Facilities Accreditation Program: Accreditation requirements for acute care hospitals.* Chicago, IL: American Osteopathic Association. (Level VII)

9 Centers for Medicare & Medicaid Services, Department of Health and Human Services. (2014). Condition of participation: Nursing services. 42 C.F.R. § 482.23(c).

10 The Joint Commission. (2015). Standard NPSG.07.01.01. *Comprehensive accreditation manual for hospitals: The official handbook.* Oakbrook Terrace, IL: The Joint Commission. (Level VII)

11 World Health Organization. (2009). "WHO guidelines on hand hygiene in health care: First global patient safety challenge, clean care is safer care" [Online]. Accessed May 2015 via the Web at http://whqlibdoc.who.int/publications/2009/9789241597906_eng.pdf (Level IV)

12 Centers for Disease Control and Prevention. (2002). Guideline for hand hygiene in health-care settings: Recommendations of the Healthcare Infection Control Practices Advisory Committee and the HICPAC/SHEA/APIC/IDSA Hand Hygiene Task Force. *MMWR Recommendations and Reports, 51*(RR-16), 1–45. Accessed May 2015 via the Web at http://www.cdc.gov/mmwr/pdf/rr/rr5116.pdf (Level II)

13 Standard 19. Hand hygiene. Infusion nursing standards of practice. (2011). *Journal of Infusion Nursing, 34,* S26–S27. (Level I)

14 Centers for Disease Control and Prevention. (2011). "Guidelines for the prevention of intravascular catheter-related infections" [Online]. Accessed May 2015 via the Web at http://www.cdc.gov/hicpac/pdf/guidelines/bsi-guidelines-2011.pdf (Level I)

15 American Osteopathic Association. (2014). Standard 07.01.10. *Healthcare Facilities Accreditation Program: Accreditation requirements for acute care hospitals.* Chicago, IL: American Osteopathic Association. (Level VII)

16 Centers for Medicare & Medicaid Services, Department of Health and Human Services. (2014). Conditions of participation: Infection control. 42 C.F.R. § 482.42.

17 The Joint Commission. (2014). Standard NPSG.01.01.01. *Comprehensive accreditation manual for hospitals: The official handbook.* Oakbrook Terrace, IL: The Joint Commission. (Level VII)

18 American Osteopathic Association (2014). Standard 15.01.16. *Healthcare Facilities Accreditation Program: Accreditation requirements for acute care hospitals.* Chicago, IL: American Osteopathic Association. (Level VII)

19 Centers for Medicare & Medicaid Services, Department of Health and Human Services. (2014). Condition of participation: Patient's rights. 42 C.F.R. § 482.13(c)(1).

20 The Joint Commission. (2010). *Advancing effective communication, cultural competence, and patient- and family-centered care: A roadmap for hospitals.* Oakbrook Terrace, IL: The Joint Commission. (Level VII)

21 Siegel, J. D., et al. (2007). "2007 guideline for isolation precautions: Preventing transmission of infectious agents in healthcare settings" [Online]. Accessed May 2015 via the Web at http://www.cdc.gov/hicpac/pdf/isolation/Isolation2007.pdf (Level I)

22 Institute for Safe Medication Practices. (2012). "ISMP's list of high-alert medications" [Online]. Accessed May 2015 via the Web at http://www.ismp.org/tools/highalertmedications.pdf (Level VII)

23 Institute for Safe Medication Practices. (2008). "Conducting an independent double-check" [Online]. Accessed May 2015 via the Web at http://www.ismp.org/newsletters/nursing/Issues/NurseAdviseERR200812.pdf (Level VII)

24 U.S. Food and Drug Administration. (n.d.). "Look. Check. Connect. Safe medical device connections save lives" [Online]. Accessed May 2015 via the Web at http://www.fda.gov/downloads/MedicalDevices/Safety/AlertsandNotices/UCM134873.pdf

25 The Joint Commission. (2015). Standard PC.01.02.07. *Comprehensive accreditation manual for hospitals: The official handbook.* Oakbrook Terrace, IL: The Joint Commission. (Level VII)

26 American Osteopathic Association (2014). Standard 16.02.05. *Healthcare Facilities Accreditation Program: Accreditation requirements for acute care hospitals.* Chicago, IL: American Osteopathic Association. (Level VII)

27 Infusion Nurses Society. (2012). "INS Paper: Recommendations for frequency of assessment of the short peripheral catheter site" [Online]. Accessed May 2015 via the Web at http://www.ins1.org/files/public/07_05_12_Assessment_Position_Paper_BOD_FINAL.pdf (Level VII)

28 The Joint Commission. (2015). Standard RC.01.03.01. *Comprehensive accreditation manual for hospitals: The official handbook.* Oakbrook Terrace, IL: The Joint Commission. (Level VII)

29 American Osteopathic Association. (2014). Standard 10.00.03. *Healthcare Facilities Accreditation Program: Accreditation requirements for acute care hospitals.* Chicago, IL: American Osteopathic Association. (Level VII)

30 Centers for Medicare & Medicaid Services, Department of Health and Human Services. (2014). Condition of participation: Medical record services. 42 C.F.R. § 482.24(b). (Level VII)

PERICARDIOCENTESIS, ASSISTING

Pericardiocentesis is a needle aspiration of pericardial fluid. This procedure is both therapeutic and diagnostic. It can be performed as an emergency measure to relieve cardiac tamponade; it can also provide a fluid sample to confirm and identify the cause of pericardial effusion (excess pericardial fluid) to help determine appropriate therapy.

Normally, small amounts of plasma-derived fluid within the pericardium lubricate the heart, reducing friction for the beating heart. Excess pericardial fluid may accumulate after inflammation, cardiac surgery, rupture, or penetrating trauma (such as a gunshot or stab wound) of the pericardium. Rapidly forming effusions, such as those that develop after cardiac surgery or penetrating trauma, may induce cardiac tamponade, a potentially lethal syndrome marked by increased intrapericardial pressure that prevents complete ventricular filling and thus reduces cardiac output. Slowly forming effusions such as those that occur in pericarditis typically pose less immediate danger because they allow the pericardium more time to adapt to the accumulating fluid and may be better managed medically or surgically.[1,2]

The pericardium normally contains 15 to 30 mL of sterile fluid.[2] Pericardial fluid is clear and straw-colored, without evidence of pathogens, blood, or malignant cells. The white blood cell count in the fluid is usually less than 1,000/mm^3. Its glucose concentration should approximate the glucose levels in blood. Pericardial effusions are typically classified as transudates or exudates. (See *Pericardial effusions: Transudates and exudates,* page 596.)

Equipment

Prepackaged pericardiocentesis tray ■ vital signs monitoring equipment ■ oxygen source ■ supplemental oxygen delivery equipment ■ pulse oximeter ■ Kelly clamp ■ two-dimensional echocardiography equipment and echocontrast medium ■ defibrillator and emergency drugs ■ laboratory request form ■ sterile gloves ■ sterile marker ■ sterile labels ■ gloves ■ protective eyewear ■ surgical caps ■ sterile gowns ■ electrocardiograph (ECG) or bedside monitor ■ prescribed sedative ■ Optional: clippers, hemodynamic monitoring equipment, nasogastric tube, suction apparatus, alcohol pad.

If a prepackaged equipment tray isn't available, you'll need the following: Antiseptic solution (2% chlorhexidine-based solution) ■ 1% lidocaine for local anesthetic ■ sterile needles (25G for anesthetic and 14G, 16G, and 18G 4″ or 5″ [10- or 13-cm] cardiac or spinal needles)[2,3] ■ 50- or 60-mL syringe with luer-lock tip ■ sterile specimen containers for culture ■ laboratory biohazard transport bags ■ sterile drapes and towels ■ 4″ × 4″ (10-cm × 10-cm) sterile gauze pads ■ sterile occlusive dressing ■ three-way stopcock.

Pericardial effusions: Transudates and exudates

Transudates are protein-poor effusions that usually arise from mechanical factors altering fluid formation or resorption, such as increased hydrostatic pressure, decreased plasma oncotic pressure, or obstruction of the pericardial lymphatic drainage system by a tumor.

Most exudates result from inflammation and contain large amounts of protein. Inflammation damages the capillary membrane, allowing protein molecules to leak into the pericardial fluid. Both effusion types occur in pericarditis, neoplasms, acute myocardial infarction, tuberculosis, rheumatoid disease, and systemic lupus erythematosus.

Preparation of equipment

Echocardiography generally guides needle insertion.[2,3,4,5] Connect the patient to the bedside monitor, which is set to read lead V_1. Connect the patient to a pulse oximeter. Make sure that the defibrillator and other emergency equipment are functioning and readily available. Check the expiration date on each sterile package and inspect each for tears. Assist the practitioner with arterial catheter insertion for hemodynamic monitoring, as required.[2]

Implementation

- Verify the practitioner's order.
- Gather the appropriate equipment.
- Conduct a preprocedure verification *to make sure that all relevant documentation, related information, and equipment are available and correctly identified to the patient's identifiers.*[6,7]
- Verify that the laboratory and imaging studies are complete, as ordered, and that the results are in the patient's medical record. Notify the practitioner of any unexpected results.[8]
- Confirm that informed consent has been obtained and that the consent is in the patient's medical record.[9,10,11]
- Perform hand hygiene.[12,13,14,15,16]
- Confirm the patient's identity using at least two patient identifiers.[17]
- Explain the procedure to the patient *to ease his anxiety and ensure his cooperation.* Inform the patient that he may feel some pressure when the needle is inserted into the pericardial sac. Answer any questions he may have.
- Check the patient's health history for hypersensitivity to latex or to the local anesthetic.
- If the patient's condition allows, confirm his nothing-by-mouth status before the procedure for sufficient time to allow for gastric emptying *to prevent pulmonary aspiration*; minimum fasting recommendations are 2 hours for clear liquids, 4 hours for breast milk, 6 hours for infant formula, 6 or more hours for a light meal or nonhuman milk, and 8 hours or more for fried or fatty foods or meat.[18]
- Verify patent IV access *in case fluids and medications are needed during the procedure.*
- Obtain the patient's vital signs, cardiac rhythm, heart sounds, oxygen saturation, respiratory status, and neurologic status *to serve as a baseline for comparison during and after the procedure.*[4]
- Confirm that the correct procedure has been identified for the correct patient at the correct site.[6,7]
- Administer supplemental oxygen, as ordered.[3]
- Administer sedation as ordered, following safe medication administration practices.[19,20,21]
- Immediately before the procedure, provide privacy.[22,23]
- Perform hand hygiene.[12,13,14,15,16]
- Insert a nasogastric tube, as ordered and as time allows, *to decompress the stomach and decrease the risk of gastric perforation.* (See the "Nasogastric tube insertion and removal" procedure, page 531.)[3]
- Prepare a sterile field by carefully opening up the equipment tray on the overbed table. Be careful not to contaminate the sterile field as you open the wrapper.[24] Label all medications, medication containers, and other solutions on and off the sterile field, maintaining the sterility of the sterile field.[25,26]
- Provide adequate lighting at the puncture site, and adjust the height of the patient's bed *to allow the practitioner to perform the procedure comfortably.*
- Place the patient in the supine position with the head of the bed elevated 30 to 60 degrees if not contraindicated *to facilitate breathing and reduce the risk of aspiration of fluids.*[2,4,27] Attach the cardiac monitoring leads, if not already attached.
- Perform hand hygiene[12,13,14,15,16] and assist the practitioner, as necessary, with putting on protective eyewear, a mask, a cap, a sterile gown, and sterile gloves. Then put on the same equipment.[28,29]
- The practitioner cleans the skin with sterile gauze pads soaked in antiseptic solution from the left costal margin to the xiphoid process. You may need to clip the hair from the area before applying the antiseptic solution.[24]
- Conduct a time-out immediately before starting the procedure *to ensure that the correct patient, site, positioning, and procedure are identified and that, as applicable, all relevant information and necessary equipment are available.*[30]
- If the anesthetic is only available in a multidose vial, clean the injection port of the vial with an alcohol pad. Then invert the vial 45 degrees so that the practitioner can insert a 25G needle and syringe and withdraw the anesthetic for injection.
- Before the practitioner injects the anesthetic, tell the patient that he'll experience a transient burning sensation and local pain.
- The practitioner attaches a 50- or 60-mL syringe to one end of a three-way stopcock and the cardiac or spinal needle to the other end.[4]
- Assist the practitioner and the echocardiogram technician, as needed. The practitioner may inject echocontrast medium *to verify needle placement.*
- The practitioner inserts the needle through the chest wall into the pericardial sac, maintaining gentle aspiration until fluid appears in the syringe. He angles the needle 35 to 45 degrees toward the tip of the right scapula between the left costal margin and the xiphoid process. *This subxiphoid approach minimizes the risk of lacerating the coronary vessels or the pleura.*
- Carefully observe the ECG tracing when the practitioner inserts the needle; *ST-segment elevation indicates that the needle has reached the epicardial surface, and the practitioner should retract it slightly; an abnormally shaped QRS complex may indicate perforation of the myocardium. Premature ventricular contractions usually indicate that the needle has touched the ventricular wall.*
- When the practitioner has positioned the needle properly, he attaches a Kelly clamp to the skin surface *so that it won't advance any further.*
- Assist the practitioner during aspiration of the pericardial fluid and labeling and numbering of the specimen containers. (See *Aspirating pericardial fluid.*)
- If bacterial culture and sensitivity tests are scheduled, record on the laboratory request any antimicrobial drugs the patient is receiving. If you suspect anaerobic organisms, consult the laboratory about proper collection technique *to avoid exposing the aspirate to air.* Label all specimens in the presence of the patient with the patient's name, identification number, and the date and time of the collection *to prevent mislabeling.*[17] Make sure that the containers are clearly labeled with the source of the specimen. Send them to the laboratory immediately in a laboratory biohazard transport bag.[28]
- When the practitioner withdraws the needle, immediately apply pressure to the site with sterile gauze pads for 3 to 5 minutes. Clean the area around the site with an antiseptic solution and then apply a sterile occlusive dressing.[4]

Aspirating pericardial fluid

In pericardiocentesis, a needle and syringe assembly is inserted through the chest wall into the pericardial sac (as illustrated below). Electrocardiographic (ECG) monitoring, with a leadwire attached to the needle and electrodes placed on the limbs (right arm [RA], right leg [RL], left arm [LA], and left leg [LL]), helps ensure proper needle placement and avoids damage to the heart.

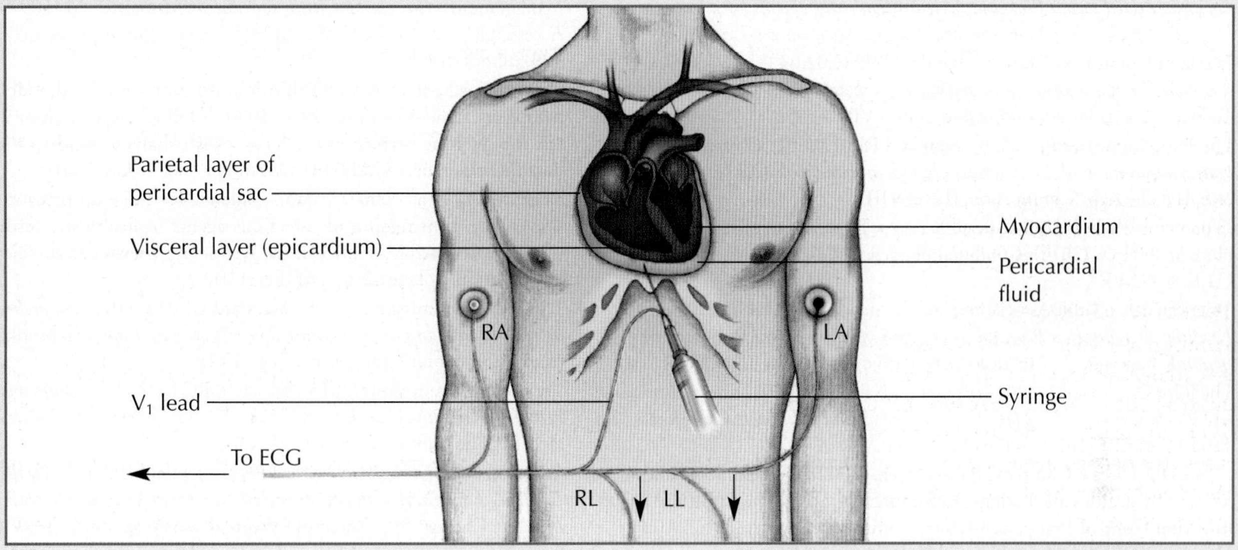

■ Remove and discard personal protective equipment[28,29] and perform hand hygiene.[12,13,14,15,16]

■ Obtain a portable chest X-ray immediately after the procedure *to assess for pneumothorax and hemothorax,* as ordered.[4]

■ Monitor blood pressure, pulse, respirations, oxygen saturation level, and heart sounds every 15 minutes until stable *to assess for complications.*[4] Your facility may require more frequent monitoring. Reassure the patient that such monitoring is routine.

■ Monitor the puncture site for bleeding every 15 minutes until the patient's condition stabilizes and then every 4 hours for 24 hours.[4]

■ Monitor continually for cardiac arrhythmias and document rhythm strips.

■ Monitor hemoglobin, hematocrit, and coagulation levels, as ordered and indicated, *to assess for effusion recurrence or bleeding at the pericardiocentesis site.*[4]

■ Notify the practitioner of critical test results within the time frame determined by your facility *to prevent treatment delays.* Notify the practitioner of any changes in vital signs, cardiac rhythm, or patient condition.[8]

■ Return all equipment to the proper location and dispose of used supplies in appropriate receptacles.[28]

■ Perform hand hygiene.[12,13,14,15,16]

■ Document the procedure.[31,32,33]

Special considerations

■ Watch for grossly bloody fluid aspirate, *which may indicate inadvertent puncture of a cardiac chamber.*

■ After the procedure, be alert for respiratory and cardiac distress. Watch especially for signs of cardiac tamponade, which include muffled and distant heart sounds, distended jugular veins, paradoxical pulse, and shock. Cardiac tamponade may result from rapid accumulation of pericardial fluid or puncture of a coronary vessel, causing bleeding into the pericardial sac.[27]

■ Depending on the patient's condition, the practitioner may place a catheter in the pericardium *to enable continuous drainage.* Monitor and record the amount and appearance of any drainage collected.[2,27]

Complications

Pericardiocentesis should be performed cautiously because of the risk of potentially fatal complications, such as laceration of a coronary artery or the myocardium. Other possible complications include ventricular fibrillation or vasovagal arrest; pleural infection; accidental puncture of the lung (pneumothorax or hemothorax), liver, or stomach; recurrence of pericardial effusion; and cardiac tamponade.

To minimize the risk of complications, echocardiography should precede pericardiocentesis to determine the effusion site. Generally, surgical drainage and biopsy are safer than pericardiocentesis.

Documentation

Record the initiation and completion time of the procedure, the patient's response, vital signs, cardiac rhythm, and any medications administered. Also record and document ECG recording strips from before, during, and after the procedure. Document the amount, color, and consistency of the fluid; the number of specimen containers collected; and the time of transport to the laboratory. Document any complications and interventions performed. Document patient and family teaching provided and their understanding of your teaching.

References

1 Lee, T. H., et al. (2013). Pericardiocentesis in trauma: A systematic review. *Journal of Trauma and Acute Care Surgery, 75,* 543–549. (Level I)

2 Fitch, M. T., et al. (2012). Emergency pericardiocentesis. *New England Journal of Medicine, 36,* e17–e21. Accessed May 2015 via the Web at http://www.nejm.org/doi/pdf/10.1056/NEJMvcm0907841

3 Shlamovitz, G. Z. (2013). "Pericardiocentesis" [Online]. Accessed May 2015 via the Web at http://emedicine.medscape.com/article/80602-overview#a09

4 Lynn-McHale Wiegand, D. (Ed.). (2011). *AACN procedure manual for critical care* (6th ed.). St. Louis, MO: Saunders.

5 Salazar, M., et al. (2012). Use of contrast echocardiography to detect displacement of the needle during pericardiocentesis. *Echocardiography, 29,* E60–E61. (Level VI)
6 The Joint Commission. (2015). Standard UP.01.01.01. *Comprehensive accreditation manual for hospitals: The official handbook.* Oakbrook Terrace, IL: The Joint Commission. (Level VII)
7 American Osteopathic Association. (2014). Standard 30.00.14. *Healthcare Facilities Accreditation Program: Accreditation requirements for acute care hospitals.* Chicago, IL: American Osteopathic Association. (Level VII)
8 The Joint Commission. (2015). Standard NPSG.02.03.01. *Comprehensive accreditation manual for hospitals: The official handbook.* Oakbrook Terrace, IL: The Joint Commission. (Level VII)
9 The Joint Commission. (2015). Standard RI.01.03.01. *Comprehensive accreditation manual for hospitals: The official handbook.* Oakbrook Terrace, IL: The Joint Commission. (Level VII)
10 Centers for Medicare & Medicaid Services, Department of Health and Human Services. (2014). Condition of participation: Patient's rights. 42 C.F.R. § 482.13.
11 American Osteopathic Association. (2014). Standard 15.01.11. *Healthcare Facilities Accreditation Program: Accreditation requirements for acute care hospitals.* Chicago, IL: American Osteopathic Association. (Level VII)
12 The Joint Commission. (2015). Standard NPSG.07.01.01. *Comprehensive accreditation manual for hospitals: The official handbook.* Oakbrook Terrace, IL: The Joint Commission. (Level VII)
13 Centers for Disease Control and Prevention. (2002). Guideline for hand hygiene in health-care settings: Recommendations of the Healthcare Infection Control Practices Advisory Committee and the HICPAC/SHEA/APIC/IDSA Hand Hygiene Task Force. *MMWR Recommendations and Reports, 51*(RR-16), 1–45. Accessed May 2015 via the Web at http://www.cdc.gov/mmwr/pdf/rr/rr5116.pdf (Level II)
14 World Health Organization. (2009). "WHO guidelines on hand hygiene in health care: First global patient safety challenge, clean care is safer care" [Online]. Accessed May 2015 via the Web at http://whqlibdoc.who.int/publications/2009/9789241597906_eng.pdf (Level IV)
15 American Osteopathic Association. (2014). Standard 07.01.10. *Healthcare Facilities Accreditation Program: Accreditation requirements for acute care hospitals.* Chicago, IL: American Osteopathic Association. (Level VII)
16 Centers for Medicare & Medicaid Services, Department of Health and Human Services. (2014). Condition of participation: Infection control. 42 C.F.R. § 482.42.
17 The Joint Commission. (2015). Standard NPSG.01.01.01. *Comprehensive accreditation manual for hospitals: The official handbook.* Oakbrook Terrace, IL: The Joint Commission. (Level VII)
18 American Society for Anesthesiologists. (2011). "Practice guidelines for preoperative fasting and the use of pharmacologic agents to reduce the risk of pulmonary aspiration: Application to healthy patients undergoing elective procedures" [Online]. Accessed May 2015 via the Web at http://journals.lww.com/anesthesiology/Fulltext/2011/03000/Practice_Guidelines_for_Preoperative_Fasting_and.13.aspx (Level V)
19 American Osteopathic Association. (2014). Standard 16.01.03. *Healthcare Facilities Accreditation Program: Accreditation requirements for acute care hospitals.* Chicago, IL: American Osteopathic Association. (Level VII)
20 The Joint Commission. (2015). Standard MM.06.01.01. *Comprehensive accreditation manual for hospitals: The official handbook.* Oakbrook Terrace, IL: The Joint Commission. (Level VII)
21 Centers for Medicare & Medicaid Services, Department of Health and Human Services. (2014). Condition of participation: Nursing services. 42 C.F.R. § 482.23(c).
22 American Osteopathic Association. (2014). Standard 15.01.16. *Healthcare Facilities Accreditation Program: Accreditation requirements for acute care hospitals.* Chicago, IL: American Osteopathic Association. (Level VII)
23 Centers for Medicare & Medicaid Services, Department of Health and Human Services. (2014). Condition of participation: Patient's rights. 42 C.F.R. § 482.13(c)(1).
24 The Joint Commission. (2015). Standard NPSG.07.05.01. *Comprehensive accreditation manual for hospitals: The official handbook.* Oakbrook Terrace, IL: The Joint Commission. (Level VII)
25 The Joint Commission. (2015). Standard NPSG.03.04.01. *Comprehensive accreditation manual for hospitals: The official handbook.* Oakbrook Terrace, IL: The Joint Commission. (Level VII)
26 American Osteopathic Association. (2014). Standard 25.01.27. *Healthcare Facilities Accreditation Program: Accreditation requirements for acute care hospitals.* Chicago, IL: American Osteopathic Association. (Level VII)
27 Shiavone, W. A. (2013). Cardiac tamponade: 12 pearls in diagnosis and management. *Cleveland Clinic Journal of Medicine, 80,* 109–116. Accessed May 2015 via the Web at http://www.ccjm.org/content/80/2/109.full.pdf+html
28 Occupational Safety and Health Administration. (n.d.). "Bloodborne pathogens, standard number 1910. 1030" [Online]. Accessed May 2015 via the Web at http://www.osha.gov/pls/oshaweb/owadisp.show_document?p_table=STANDARDS&p_id=10051 (Level VII)
29 Siegel, J. D., et al. (2007). "2007 guideline for isolation precautions: Preventing transmission of infectious agents in healthcare settings" [Online]. Accessed May 2015 via the Web at http://www.cdc.gov/hicpac/pdf/isolation/Isolation2007.pdf (Level II)
30 The Joint Commission. (2015). Standard UP.01.03.01. *Comprehensive accreditation manual for hospitals: The official handbook.* Oakbrook Terrace, IL: The Joint Commission. (Level VII)
31 The Joint Commission. (2015). Standard RC.01.03.01. *Comprehensive accreditation manual for hospitals: The official handbook.* Oakbrook Terrace, IL: The Joint Commission. (Level VII)
32 American Osteopathic Association. (2014). Standard 10.00.03. *Healthcare Facilities Accreditation Program: Accreditation requirements for acute care hospitals.* Chicago, IL: American Osteopathic Association. (Level VII)
33 Centers for Medicare & Medicaid Services, Department of Health and Human Services. (2014). Condition of participation: Medical record services. 42 C.F.R. § 482.24(b).

ADDITIONAL REFERENCE

Visweswaran, G. K., et al. (2013). Novel use of a disposable digital pressure transducer to increase the safety of pericardiocentesis. *Catheter and Cardiovascular Interventions, 81,* E68–E71. (Level VI)

PERINEAL CARE

Perineal care, which includes care of the external genitalia and the anal area, should be performed during the daily bath and, if the patient is incontinent, at bedtime and after urination and bowel movements. The procedure promotes cleanliness and prevents infection. It also removes irritating and odorous secretions, such as smegma, a cheeselike substance that collects under the foreskin of the penis. For a patient with perineal skin breakdown, frequent bathing followed by application of a moisture-barrier skin protectant aids healing.

Standard precautions must be followed when providing perineal care, with great consideration for the patient's privacy.[1]

Equipment

Gloves ▪ bath blanket ▪ bathing supplies (disposable cleaning cloths, prepackaged bath product, or washcloths; a towel; mild soap or pH-balanced skin cleaner) ▪ fluid-impermeable pad ▪ Optional: facility-approved disinfectant, bath basin, perineal bottle, moisture-barrier skin protectant, absorbent underpad or brief.

After genital or rectal surgery, you may need to use sterile supplies, including sterile gloves, gauze, and cotton balls.

Preparation of equipment

If you're using a basin, fill it two-thirds full with warm water.

NURSING ALERT Studies have shown that patients' bath basins are a reservoir for bacteria and may be a source of transmission of health care facility–acquired infections.[2] *Clean and disinfect the basin with a facility-approved disinfectant after use.*[3]

Implementation

- Gather the equipment at the patient's bedside.
- Perform hand hygiene and put on gloves.[4,5,6,7,8]
- Confirm the patient's identity using at least two patient identifiers.[9]
- Provide privacy.[10,11]
- Explain the procedure to the patient *to enhance cooperation.*
- Adjust the bed to a comfortable working height *to prevent back strain,* and lower the head of the bed, if allowed.
- Put on gloves *to comply with standard precautions.*[1,12]
- Help the patient into the supine position. Place a fluid-impermeable pad under the patient's buttocks *to protect the bed from stains and moisture.*
- Drape the patient's legs, using a bath blanket, *to minimize exposure and embarrassment* and expose the genital area.
- Wet the washcloth with warm water from a running spigot or the bath basin and apply mild soap. If you're using disposable cleaning cloths or a prepackaged bath product, open the packages and obtain the wet cloths.

NURSING ALERT *A pH-balanced skin cleaner is more effective than soap in preventing and treating incontinence-associated dermatitis* because soap is alkaline and can strip the skin of natural oils, leading to secondary infection from fungi and bacteria.[13,14]

For a female patient

- Ask the patient to bend her knees slightly and to spread her legs.
- Assess the patient's perineal area for color changes, skin breakdown, drainage, discharge, or tenderness. Notify the practitioner and the wound ostomy continence nurse, as needed.
- Separate the patient's labia with one hand and wash with the other, using gentle downward strokes from the front to the back of the perineum *to prevent intestinal organisms from contaminating the urethra or vagina.* Avoid the area around the anus, and use a clean section of washcloth for each stroke by folding each used section inward. *This method prevents the spread of contaminated secretions or discharge.*
- If you're using soap and water, wet a clean washcloth and rinse thoroughly from front to back *because soap residue can cause skin irritation.* Pat the area dry with a bath towel *because moisture can also cause skin irritation and discomfort.*
- Turn the patient on her side to the Sims position, if possible, *to expose the anal area.*
- Clean, rinse, and dry the anal area, starting at the posterior vaginal opening and wiping from front to back.
- After cleaning the perineum, apply a moisture-barrier skin protectant, as needed (cream, ointment, or film-forming skin protectant) *to protect and maintain intact skin or to treat nonintact skin.*[15]

For a male patient

- Hold the shaft of the penis with one hand and wash with the other, beginning at the tip and working in a circular motion from the center to the periphery (as shown on top right) *to avoid introducing microorganisms into the urethra.* Use a clean section of washcloth for each stroke *to prevent the spread of contaminated secretions or discharge.*
- If you're using soap and water, wet a clean washcloth and rinse thoroughly, using the same circular motion.
- For an uncircumcised patient, gently retract the foreskin and clean beneath it. If appropriate, rinse well but don't dry *because moisture provides lubrication and prevents friction when replacing the foreskin.* Replace the foreskin *to avoid constriction of the penis, which causes edema and tissue damage.*
- Wash the rest of the penis, using downward strokes toward the scrotum. If appropriate, rinse well and pat dry with a towel.
- Clean the top and sides of the scrotum; if appropriate, rinse thoroughly and pat dry. Handle the scrotum gently *to avoid causing discomfort.*

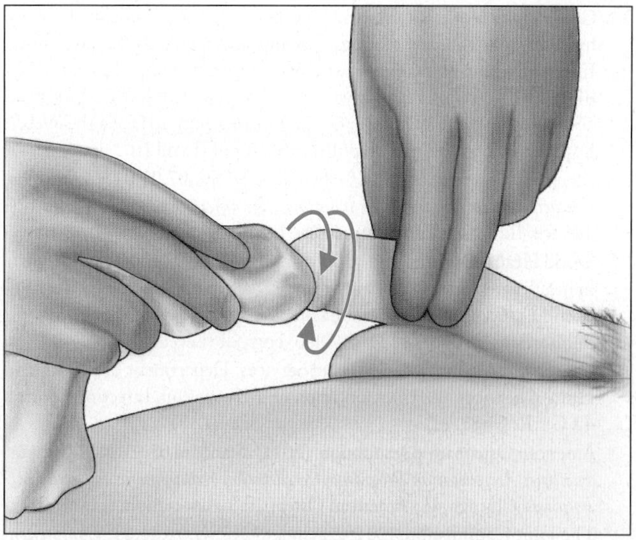

- Turn the patient on his side. Clean the bottom of the scrotum and the anal area. If appropriate, rinse well and pat dry.
- After cleaning the perineum, apply a moisture-barrier skin protectant (cream, ointment, or film-forming skin protectant), as needed, *to protect and maintain intact skin or to treat nonintact skin.*[15]

Completing the procedure

- Reposition the patient comfortably.
- Remove the bath blanket and fluid-impermeable pad, and then replace the bed linens.
- If you're using a bath basin, clean and disinfect it using a facility-approved disinfectant.[3,16]
- Dispose of soiled articles in the appropriate receptacle.[17]
- Remove and discard your gloves.[1]
- Perform hand hygiene.[4,5,6,7,8]
- Document the procedure.[18,19,20]

Special considerations

- Provide perineal care to a patient of the opposite gender in a matter-of-fact way *to minimize embarrassment.*
- If the patient is incontinent, gently clean the skin with water or pH-balanced skin cleaner. Avoid excessive friction and scrubbing, *which can further traumatize the patient's skin.*[15]
- If the patient is incontinent, select an absorbent underpad or brief *to wick incontinence moisture away from the skin rather than trapping moisture against the skin, which can cause maceration.*

Documentation

Record perineal care and any special treatment in your notes. Document the need for continued treatment, if necessary. Describe perineal skin condition and odor or discharge.

REFERENCES

1 Siegel, J. D., et al. (2007). "2007 guideline for isolation precautions: Preventing transmission of infectious agents in healthcare settings" [Online]. Accessed May 2015 via the Web at http://www.cdc.gov/hicpac/pdf/isolation/Isolation2007.pdf (Level II)

2 Johnson, D., et al. (2009). Patient's bath basins as potential sources of infection: A multicenter sampling study. *American Journal of Critical Care, 18,* 31–40. Accessed May 2015 via the Web at http://ajcc.aacnjournals.org/content/18/1/31.full (Level IV)

3 Rutala, W. A., et al. (2008). "Guideline for disinfection and sterilization in healthcare facilities, 2008" [Online]. Accessed May 2015 via the Web at http://www.cdc.gov/hicpac/guidelines/Disinfection_Nov_2008.pdf (Level I)

4 Centers for Disease Control and Prevention. (2002). Guideline for hand hygiene in health-care settings: Recommendations of the Healthcare Infection Control Practices Advisory Committee and the HICPAC/SHEA/APIC/IDSA Hand Hygiene Task Force. *MMWR Recommendations and Reports, 51*(RR–16), 1–45. Accessed May 2015 via the Web at http://www.cdc.gov/mmwr/pdf/rr/rr5116.pdf (Level II)

5 The Joint Commission. (2015). Standard NPSG.07.01.01. *Comprehensive accreditation manual for hospitals: The official handbook.* Oakbrook Terrace, IL: The Joint Commission. (Level VII)

6 World Health Organization. (2009). "WHO guidelines on hand hygiene in health care: First global patient safety challenge, clean care is safer care" [Online]. Accessed May 2015 via the Web at http://whqlibdoc.who.int/publications/2009/9789241597906_eng.pdf (Level IV)

7 Centers for Medicare & Medicaid Services, Department of Health and Human Services. (2014). Condition of participation: Infection control. 42 C.F.R. § 482.42.

8 American Osteopathic Association. (2014). Standard 07.01.21. *Healthcare Facilities Accreditation Program: Accreditation requirements for acute care hospitals.* Chicago, IL: American Osteopathic Association. (Level VII)

9 The Joint Commission. (2015). Standard NPSG.01.01.01. *Comprehensive accreditation manual for hospitals: The official handbook.* Oakbrook Terrace, IL: The Joint Commission. (Level VII)

10 Centers for Medicare & Medicaid Services, Department of Health and Human Services. (2014). Condition of participation: Patient's rights. 42 C.F.R. § 482.13(c)(1).

11 American Osteopathic Association. (2014). Standard 15.01.16. *Healthcare Facilities Accreditation Program: Accreditation requirements for acute care hospitals.* Chicago, IL: American Osteopathic Association. (Level VII)

12 American Osteopathic Association. (2014). Standard 07.01.10. *Healthcare Facilities Accreditation Program: Accreditation requirements for acute care hospitals.* Chicago, IL: American Osteopathic Association. (Level VII)

13 Langemo, D., et al. (2011). Incontinence and incontinence-associated dermatitis. *Advances in Skin and Wound Care, 24,* 126–139. Accessed May 2015 via the Web at http://www.nursingcenter.com/pdf.asp?AID=1126332

14 Beeckman, D., et al. (2010). What is the most effective method of preventing and treating incontinence associated dermatitis? *Nursing Times, 106*(38), 22–25.

15 Institute for Clinical Systems Improvement. (2012; reviewed 2014). "Health care protocol: Pressure ulcer prevention and treatment protocol (3rd ed.)" [Online]. Accessed May 2015 via the Web at https://www.icsi.org/_asset/6t7kxy/PresUlcerTrmt-Interactive0112.pdf (Level VII)

16 American Osteopathic Association. (2014). Standard 07.02.03. *Healthcare Facilities Accreditation Program: Accreditation requirements for acute care hospitals.* Chicago, IL: American Osteopathic Association. (Level VII)

17 Occupational Safety and Health Administration. (n.d.). "Bloodborne pathogens, standard number 1910.1030" [Online]. Accessed May 2015 via the Web at http://www.osha.gov/pls/oshaweb/owadisp.show_document?p_table=STANDARDS&p_id=10051 (Level VII)

18 The Joint Commission. (2015). Standard RC.01.03.01. *Comprehensive accreditation manual for hospitals: The official handbook.* Oakbrook Terrace, IL: The Joint Commission. (Level VII)

19 Centers for Medicare & Medicaid Services, Department of Health and Human Services. (2014). Condition of participation: Medical record services. 42 C.F.R. § 482.24(b).

20 American Osteopathic Association. (2014). Standard 10.00.03. *Healthcare Facilities Accreditation Program: Accreditation requirements for acute care hospitals.* Chicago, IL: American Osteopathic Association. (Level VII)

PERIPHERALLY INSERTED CENTRAL CATHETER USE

For patients who need long-term central venous (CV) infusion therapy or require repeated venous access, a peripherally inserted central catheter (PICC) may be the best option. The PICC provides safe, reliable access for drug administration and blood sampling and helps avoid complications that can occur with a CV access device.

A practitioner may order a PICC if the patient has suffered trauma or burns resulting in chest injury or if the patient has respiratory compromise due to chronic obstructive pulmonary disease, a mediastinal mass, cystic fibrosis, or pneumothorax. PICCs are also used for patients receiving home care. Infusions commonly given by PICC include total parenteral nutrition, chemotherapy, antibiotics, intermittent inotropics, fluids, and analgesics.

PICCs are made of silicone or polyurethane and vary in diameter and length. They're available in single, double, and triple-lumen versions; a PICC with the minimum number of lumens necessary to manage the patient's care should be used.[1] The type and size of PICC used depends on the patient's size and anatomic measurements as well as the therapy required. Power injection–capable PICCs are also available for patients who require injection of contrast media for computed tomography and other studies.

Most PICCs are manufactured with smooth, rounded tips to reduce trauma to the vein wall during insertion. To avoid the need to trim a PICC, the best option is to select a catheter length that's as close to the desired length measurement as possible. Groshong PICCs can't be trimmed; the catheter length needs to be subtracted from the total length of the PICC, with any extra length left outside the insertion site, safely secured.

Most PICCs have a preloaded stylet wire inside the catheter to add stiffness to the soft catheter, easing its advancement through the vein. The stylet terminates 1 to 2 cm away from the catheter tip. If the catheter length does require trimming, the stylet must be withdrawn and repositioned 1 to 2 cm from the cut end. The stylet should never be cut; it's removed after insertion.

PICC devices are easier to insert than other CV devices. A single catheter may be used for the entire course of therapy, resulting in greater convenience and reduced cost. If the state nurse practice act permits, a nurse trained in PICC insertion may perform the procedure, although competency may need to demonstrated yearly.

Veins to consider for PICC insertion include the basilic, median cubital, cephalic, and brachial. When selecting a site, avoid areas that are painful on palpation; veins compromised by bruising, infiltration, phlebitis, sclerosing, or cording; and forearm and upper arm veins that could be used for vascular access in patients with stage 4 or 5 chronic kidney disease. In patients who have had breast surgery with axillary node dissection, avoid using arm veins on the affected side; also avoid veins on the affected side in stroke patients, those with lymphedema, and those undergoing radiation therapy.[2] Use an ultrasound device to guide insertion *to increase your rate of success and reduce the risk of insertion-related complications.*[3] When inserted, the catheter is advanced until it reaches the superior vena cava near the junction of the right atrium.[3]

HOSPITAL-ACQUIRED CONDITION ALERT ***Keep in mind that a vascular catheter–associated infection is considered a hospital-acquired condition because it can be reasonably prevented using best practices. Make sure that infection-prevention techniques (such as performing hand hygiene, using maximal barrier precautions, following sterile technique, and properly preparing the insertion site) are followed during insertion to*** **reduce the risk of vascular catheter–associated infection.**[4,5,6,7,8]

PICCs may be inserted with a modified Seldinger technique (discussed here), or with a through-the-introducer technique.

PICC infusion and associated site care, including flushing of the catheter, may be performed by a nurse or appropriately trained parent or guardian. A PICC dressing should be changed at least every 7 days. Although a transparent semipermeable dressing is preferred,[9,10] a gauze dressing should be used if the patient is diaphoretic or the site is bleeding or oozing. A gauze dressing should be changed every 2 days; either dressing should be replaced immediately if it becomes damp, loosened, or visibly soiled to reduce the risk of infection, or if further assessment is needed because of drainage, infection, or inflammation.[9,10] Because the immune system's defense against infection declines with age, older patients are more susceptible to infection; comorbid disease may also increase their risk of vascular catheter–associated bloodstream infections.[11] Changes in sensorium and cognition may cause older patients to accidently manipulate the PICC device and dressings, increasing the risk of infection. For these reasons, older patients may require more frequent dressing changes.

PICCs are commonly used to administer drugs, such as opioids, analgesics, antibiotics, parenteral nutrition, and chemotherapy. Because older patients commonly have compromised cardiac, hepatic, or renal systems, they're at risk for complications associated with parenteral drug administration. Such patients may not be able to articulate their symptoms because of such underlying conditions as stroke, intubation, tracheotomy, dementia, and delirium. Older patients who receive large volumes of fluid or fluid at a rapid rate may quickly develop cardiac failure, shock, and cardiac arrest, so frequent monitoring during infusions is essential.

Speed shock—a condition that results from rapid administration of a bolus medication or infusion—also poses a risk to older patients; they may be unable to articulate such symptoms as dizziness or headache because of their rapid onset. These early symptoms can rapidly progress to chest tightness, hypotension, irregular pulse, and anaphylactic shock. To reduce the risk of speed shock, older patients require a carefully controlled rate of administration and need close monitoring.[6]

To prevent catheter-related bloodstream infections, the injection surface should be wiped with an antiseptic pad using friction and allowed it air-dry each time it's accessed.[1] PICCs are removed as soon as therapy is complete, when the catheter becomes damaged or broken and can't be repaired, when the patient has discomfort or pain, when a central line–associated bloodstream infection is suspected and, possibly, when the catheter becomes occluded. The catheter should be measured after removal to ensure that it was removed intact.[12]

Equipment

For insertion

PICC insertion kit ▪ PICC catheter ▪ PICC insertion checklist ▪ antiseptic swabs (chlorhexidine-based [preferred], tincture of iodine, povidone-iodine, or alcohol) ▪ sterile and clean measuring tape ▪ preservative-free normal saline solution ▪ syringes and needles of appropriate size ▪ fluid-impermeable pad ▪ sterile drapes ▪ disposable skin marker ▪ single-patient-use tourniquet ▪ sterile marker ▪ sterile labels ▪ clean gloves ▪ sterile gloves ▪ sterile gown ▪ masks ▪ protective eyewear ▪ head covers ▪ 1% lidocaine without epinephrine ▪ catheter securement device, sterile tape, or sterile surgical strips ▪ sterile transparent semipermeable dressing ▪ sterile 2″ × 2″ (5-cm × 5-cm) gauze pads ▪ hospital-grade disinfectant ▪ Optional: bedside ultrasound equipment, sterile and clean disposable ultrasound probe cover, ultrasound gel, locator system, echogenic needle, heparin (10 units/mL), single-patient-use scissors or surgical clippers with disposable head, soap and basin of water, needleless connector.

Use an all-inclusive insertion kit or cart that contains all of the necessary components for maintaining sterile technique during catheter insertion *to reduce the risk of catheter-related bloodstream infection.*[9,13]

For flushing

Gloves ▪ 10 mL-syringe prefilled with preservative-free normal saline solution[15] ▪ antiseptic pads (alcohol, tincture of iodine, or chlorhexidine-based) ▪ Optional: syringe of facility-approved locking solution, prescribed IV fluid.

For a dressing change

Gloves ▪ sterile gloves ▪ masks ▪ sterile drape ▪ antiseptic swabs (chlorhexidine-based [preferred], tincture of iodine, povidone-iodine, or alcohol)[1,9,10] ▪ sterile disposable tape measure ▪ sterile tape, sterile surgical strips, or securement device ▪ label ▪ transparent semipermeable dressing or sterile 4″ × 4″ (10-cm × 10-cm) gauze pads ▪ Optional: adhesive remover, chlorhexidine-impregnated sponge dressing, skin preparation adhesive.

Many facilities stock commercially prepared or facility-prepared sterile dressing change kits that contains the necessary supplies.

For drug administration

Patient's medication administration record ▪ gloves ▪ prescribed medication in an IV container with administration set (for infusion) or in a syringe (for IV bolus) ▪ two 10-mL syringes prefilled with preservative-free normal saline solution ▪ antiseptic pads (alcohol, tincture of iodine, or chlorhexidine-based).

For removal

Gloves ▪ fluid-impermeable pad ▪ sterile occlusive dressing ▪ petroleum-based ointment ▪ tape ▪ sterile gauze pads ▪ tape measure ▪ Optional: other personal protective equipment, single-patient-use tourniquet, suture removal kit.

Implementation

Inserting a PICC

- Verify the practitioner's order for PICC insertion.
- Gather the appropriate equipment.
- Ensure that informed consent has been obtained and that the consent form is in the patient's medical record.[14,16,17,18]
- Conduct a preprocedure verification *to make sure that all relevant documentation, related information, and equipment are available and correctly identified to the patient's identifiers.*[19]
- Check the patient's allergy status *to prevent anaphylaxis.*
- Obtain the assistance of a second nurse or appropriate assistant who's been properly trained *to make sure that sterile technique is maintained during the procedure.*[20]
- Perform hand hygiene.[1,13,21,22,23,24,25,26]
- Confirm the patient's identity using at least two patient identifiers.[27]
- Provide the patient with information related to the PICC insertion procedure, including the benefits, management, and potential risks. Teach the patient and his family about measures to prevent central line–associated bloodstream infections, including the importance of hand hygiene. Encourage them to remind staff members to perform hand hygiene and to follow infection prevention practices when providing care.[13]
- Use an insertion checklist *to help adhere to infection prevention and safety practices during insertion.*[9,13,20,21] Have your assistant stop the procedure immediately if any breaks in sterile technique are observed.
- Assess the patient's upper extremities and chest for a contraindication to PICC placement.[5,6]
- If you're using ultrasound, place a clean disposable cover on the bedside ultrasound probe. Then place a single-patient-use tourniquet on the patient's selected upper arm, and examine the arm and use the ultrasound probe *to locate appropriate veins.* Mark the expected insertion site with a disposable skin marker and then remove the tourniquet.
- Using a clean measuring tape, measure the distance from the intended insertion site to the desired terminal tip location *to determine insertion depth.*[6,7]
- Measure the midarm circumference of the selected extremity *to provide a baseline measurement.*[6,7]
- Close the door to the room and put a sign on the door that reads STERILE PROCEDURE IN PROGRESS. DO NOT ENTER.[5]

■ Put on a surgical head cover, protective eyewear, and a mask. Have the second person do the same.[1,3,20,28]
■ Perform hand hygiene.[1,13,21,22,23,24,25,26]
■ Disinfect your work area using a hospital-grade disinfectant, and then allow it to dry.[5,6]
■ For upper extremity insertion, position the patient in the semi-Fowler position with the arm abducted. Place a fluid-impermeable pad under the arm.
■ Clean the intended insertion site with soap and water if it's visibly soiled.[3,6,7,20]
■ If necessary, remove excess hair from the insertion site using clippers or scissors.[3,5,6,20]
■ Prepare a sterile field using a sterile drape, and set up the PICC supplies on the sterile field.
■ Prepare the lidocaine and preservative-free normal saline flush syringes.
■ Label all medications, medication containers, and other solutions on and off the sterile field using a sterile marker and labels.[29]
■ Perform hand hygiene; a 3-minute scrub from fingertips to elbows is recommended for PICC insertion.[5,6]
■ Put on a sterile gown and sterile gloves.[5,6]
■ Follow the manufacturer's recommendations and guidelines for altering the device length if the device requires trimming. Don't use scissors to adjust PICC length *because trimming with scissors causes rough, irregular surfaces.*[30]
■ Prepare the catheter according to the manufacturer's recommendations and flush the device with preservative-free normal saline solution.[6,7]
■ Place the catheter on the sterile field.
■ Place a sterile drape under the patient's arm.
■ Prepare the insertion site by scrubbing with chlorhexidine swabs using a back-and-forth motion for about 30 seconds. Allow the area to dry. Don't touch the intended insertion site.[1,3,6,7] If a contraindication to chlorhexidine exists, prepare the site with another recommended antiseptic following the manufacturer's instructions. For povidone-iodine, apply with swabs beginning at the intended insertion site and moving outward in concentric circles; allow the povidone-iodine to remain on the skin for at least 2 minutes if needed *to dry completely.*[5,6]
■ If using ultrasound, place a sterile probe cover on the ultrasound probe *to prevent cross-contamination between patients.* If using a locator system, follow the manufacturer's directions for use.
■ Remove and discard your gloves.[6,7]
■ Perform hand hygiene.[1,13,21,22,23,24,25,26]
■ Reapply the tourniquet about 4″ (10 cm) above the antecubital fossa. Make sure that an arterial pulse is easily palpable distal to the tourniquet.[31]
■ Put on a new pair of sterile gloves.[5,6]
■ Place a full body drape over the patient from head to toe. Cover everything except the insertion site *to comply with maximal barrier precautions, which reduces the risk of central line–related bloodstream infection.*[3,5,6]
■ Conduct a time-out immediately before starting the procedure *to determine that the correct patient, site, positioning, and procedure are identified and to confirm, as applicable, that relevant information and necessary equipment are available.*[32]
■ Anesthetize the area with lidocaine *to provide for patient comfort during insertion.*[6,7]
■ If using ultrasound, apply sterile ultrasound gel to the probe and use it *to locate the appropriate vein as well as the adjacent artery and nerve.*[5,6]
■ Perform a venipuncture using the appropriate device provided in the insertion kit. (An echogenic needle is used with ultrasound guidance.) Observe for blood return.[5,6]
■ Firmly grasp the device using your thumb and forefinger. If using an over-the-needle device, remove the stylet.[5,6]
■ Insert the guide wire into the device and carefully advance it; stop advancing the guide wire if you meet resistance, and don't advance it past the axilla.[5,6]
■ Gently remove the catheter or needle, taking care not to dislodge or damage the guide wire.[5,6] If necessary, make a small skin nick at the insertion site *to facilitate the advancement of the introducer or dilator.*
■ Remove the tourniquet.[5,6]
■ Thread the introducer or dilator over the guide wire until you're sure the tip is well within the vein. After successful vein entry, you should see blood return.
■ Carefully remove the guide wire and place it on the sterile field.[5,6] Advance the introducer the rest of the way into the vein.
■ Confirm the preinsertion measurement for the desired catheter insertion depth.[5,6]
■ Carefully separate and remove the dilator from the introducer while holding the introducer still.[5,6] *To minimize blood loss,* try applying finger pressure on the vein just beyond the distal end of the introducer sheath or place a finger over the opening of the introducer.
■ If using a locator system, activate it now and follow the manufacturer's directions. Advance the catheter at a slow, steady pace until it's in position at the premeasured length.[5,6]
■ Grasp the tabs of the introducer sheath and flex them toward its distal end *to split the sheath.* Peel the introducer away from the catheter while pulling away from the insertion site.[5,6]
■ Check for blood return, and if present, flush the catheter with preservative-free normal saline solution; assess for complications.[5,6]
■ Attach a needleless connector to the end of the catheter.[5]
■ Clean the site and secure the catheter with a catheter securement device, sterile tape, or sterile surgical strips.[33]
■ Lock the catheter with heparin as prescribed or according to facility protocol.[5,6]
■ If necessary, apply a sterile 2″ × 2″ (5-cm × 5-cm) gauze pad directly over the site and a sterile transparent semipermeable dressing over the gauze pad.[10] Leave this dressing in place for 24 hours.
■ Dispose of used items properly.[28,34,35]
■ Remove and discard your personal protective equipment.[5,6]
■ Perform hand hygiene.[1,13,21,22,23,24,25,26]
■ Label the dressing with the date, the time, the gauge and length of the PICC, and your initials.[5,10]
■ Obtain a chest X-ray *to verify proper placement before initiating an infusion,* if ordered.[3,5]
■ Perform hand hygiene.[1,13,21,22,23,24,25,26]
■ Document the procedure.[36,37,38,39]

Flushing a PICC

■ Review the patient's medical records *to confirm the type and size of the catheter and the location of the catheter tip because the flush protocol depends on the type and size of the catheter.*
■ Gather the appropriate equipment
■ Perform hand hygiene.[1,13,21,22,23,24,25,26]
■ Confirm the patient's identity using at least two patient identifiers.[27]
■ Put on gloves.[6,8,9]
■ Thoroughly disinfect the needleless connector with an antiseptic pad using friction, and then allow the connector to dry.[1,5,6,40]
■ Maintaining sterility of the syringe tip, attach the 10-mL syringe of preservative-free normal saline solution.[6,7]
■ Open the clamp and slowly aspirate until you obtain a brisk blood return.[6,7,41]
■ Slowly inject preservative-free normal saline solution into the catheter.
■ Remove and discard the syringe.[5,6]
■ Thoroughly disinfect the needleless connector with an antiseptic pad using friction and then allow it to dry.[5,6,40]

■ Administer IV fluid through the catheter as prescribed, or proceed with locking the device if indicated.

Locking a PICC

■ Maintaining sterility of the syringe tip, attach the syringe of facility-approved locking solution (heparin flush or preservative-free normal saline solution), as required, to the needleless connector.
■ Slowly inject the solution into the catheter.[5,6,40]
■ Clamp the device according to the type of needleless connector used.
■ For a positive-pressure needleless connector, disconnect the syringe and then clamp the catheter. For a negative-pressure needleless connector, clamp the catheter while maintaining pressure on the syringe plunger and then disconnect the syringe. For a neutral needleless connector, clamp the catheter before or after removing the syringe.[5,6,40]
■ Double-check all connections *to prevent tubing misconnections and air embolism.*[42]

Completing the procedure

■ Discard the syringe and other used supplies in appropriate receptacles.[28]
■ Remove and discard your gloves.[5,6]
■ Perform hand hygiene.[1,13,21,22,23,24,25,26]
■ Document the procedure.[36,37,38,39]

Performing a PICC dressing change

■ Gather the necessary equipment.
■ Perform hand hygiene.[1,13,21,22,23,24,25,26]
■ Confirm the patient's identity using at least two patient identifiers.[27]
■ Explain the procedure to the patient.
■ Put on a mask.[1,2]
■ Assemble your supplies on a sterile field.[5,6]
■ Position the patient with his arm extended away from his body *to gain access to the insertion site* and so that the insertion site is below heart level *to reduce the risk of air embolism.*[5,6]
■ Assess the insertion site before dressing removal for drainage, inflammation, tenderness, and redness.[5,6]
■ Remove the existing dressing beginning at the device hub and gently pulling the dressing perpendicular to the skin toward the insertion site *to prevent catheter dislodgment and tearing or stripping of fragile skin.*[5,6]
■ If the patient had a chlorhexidine-impregnated sponge dressing *to provide sustained antimicrobial action at the insertion site,* remove and discard it in the appropriate receptacle.
■ Remove the securement device and discard it.[5,6]
■ Inspect the integrity of the catheter and hub *to detect any defects, such as cracks or splits.*[2]
■ Remove and discard your gloves.[5,6]
■ Perform hand hygiene.[1,13,21,22,23,24,25,26]
■ Put on sterile gloves.[3,5,6,28]
■ Use a sterile tape measure to measure the external length of the catheter from hub to skin entry *to make sure that the catheter hasn't migrated.*[5,6]
■ Clean the catheter insertion site with an antiseptic following the manufacturer's instructions. Apply chlorhexidine (preferred) with an applicator using a back-and-forth motion for at least 30 seconds. Allow the solution to dry completely.[5,6] For povidone-iodine, apply it with swabs in concentric circles, beginning at the insertion site and moving outward. Allow the solution to remain on the skin for at least 2 minutes or longer if needed *to dry completely.*[5,6]
■ If applicable, apply a chlorhexidine-impregnated sponge dressing at the catheter base.[2,5,6] Position the chlorhexidine dressing with the catheter resting on or near the radial slit of the disk. The edges of the slit must touch *to maximize antimicrobial action.* Always follow the manufacturer's directions.
■ Apply a securement device, surgical strips, or sterile tape.[7,43]
■ Apply a transparent semipermeable (or gauze and tape) dressing to the insertion site.[1,2]
■ Discard used supplies in appropriate receptacles.[28,34,35]
■ Remove and discard your gloves and mask.
■ Perform hand hygiene.[1,13,21,22,23,24,25,26]
■ Label the dressing with the date and time and your initials.[2]
■ Perform hand hygiene.[1,13,21,22,23,24,25,26]
■ Document the procedure.[36,37,38,39]

Administering drugs using a PICC

■ Avoid distractions and interruptions when preparing and administering medications *to prevent medication errors.*[44,45]
■ Review the patient's medical record for confirmation of catheter type, size, and tip location. Review laboratory test results and assess the appropriateness of therapy.[5,6]
■ Gather the appropriate equipment, including a prefilled syringe of the prescribed medication or a prepared infusion container with the prescribed medication.
■ Verify the practitioner's order; make sure it contains the type of fluid and volume, medication and dosage, route of administration, and frequency and duration.[5,6,46,47]
■ Compare the medication label with the practitioner's order *to verify the correct medication, indication, dose, route, and time of administration.*[46,47,48]
■ Check the expiration date on the medication. If the medication has expired, return it to the pharmacy and obtain new medication.[5,6,46,47,48]
■ Visually inspect the solution for particles, discoloration, and other signs of loss of integrity; don't administer the medication if its integrity is compromised.[5,6,46,47,48]
■ Check the patient's medical record for an allergy or a contraindication to the prescribed medication. If one exists, don't administer the medication; notify the practitioner.[47,48]
■ Discuss any unresolved concerns about the medication with the patient's practitioner.[48]
■ Verify that the medication is being administered at the proper time, in the prescribed dose, and by the correct route *to reduce the risk of medication errors.*[47,48]
■ Perform hand hygiene.[1,13,21,22,23,24,25,26]
■ Confirm the patient's identity using at least two patient identifiers.[27]
■ Explain the procedure to the patient. If the patient is receiving the medication for the first time, teach him or his family about potential adverse reactions and discuss any other concerns related to the medication.[48]
■ Obtain the patient's vital signs and assess his condition if applicable.[5,6]
■ Put on gloves.[5,6,28]
■ Thoroughly disinfect the needleless connector with an antiseptic pad using friction and allow it to dry. [5,6]
■ While maintaining sterility of the syringe tip, attach a prefilled syringe containing preservative-free normal saline solution to the needleless connector (a 10-mL syringe should be used to assess PICC patency *to prevent catheter damage* unless a smaller flush syringe that's designed to generate lower amounts of pressure is used), unclamp the catheter, and slowly aspirate until you obtain a brisk, positive blood return *to confirm the patency of the access device.* If you don't obtain a blood return, troubleshoot the device and then notify the patient's practitioner *because the catheter tip may have migrated*; arrange for a chest X-ray to verify placement, as ordered.[5,6]
■ Slowly inject preservative-free normal saline solution into the PICC, noting any resistance during injection; if you note resistance, stop the injection; don't inject against resistance. Further evaluate the device if you're unable to flush it freely.[5,6]

- Remove and discard the syringe in the appropriate container.[5,6,35]
- Thoroughly disinfect the needleless connector with an antiseptic pad using friction and then allow it to dry.[5,6]
- If your facility uses a bar code scanning system, scan your identification badge, the patient's identification bracelet, and the medication's bar code.

Administering an IV bolus injection

- Attach the syringe containing the prescribed medication for IV bolus injection to the needleless connector.[5,6]
- Inject the medication into the PICC at the rate indicated on the medication label. Consult with the pharmacist if a rate isn't specified.[5,6]
- Remove and discard the syringe in the appropriate container.[5,6]

Administering an infusion

- Spike the IV infusion container and prime the IV tubing and insert the tubing into the IV infusion pump.
- Clamp the PICC.
- Connect the IV administration set tubing to the PICC.
- Trace the tubing from the patient to its point of origin *to make sure that you're connecting the tubing to the correct port.*[49]
- Set the electronic infusion pump according to the practitioner's order. Make sure that the alarm limits are set appropriately and that the alarms are turned on, functioning properly, and audible to staff.[50,51,52]
- Unclamp the PICC and administration set tubing; begin the infusion, as ordered. When the infusion is complete, clamp the catheter and disconnect the administration set tubing.

Completing the procedure

- Remove and discard your gloves.[5,6]
- Perform hand hygiene.[1,13,21,22,23,24,25,26]
- Document the procedure.[36,37,38,39]

Removing a PICC

- Verify the practitioner's order to discontinue the catheter.[1]
- Gather and prepare the necessary supplies.
- Perform hand hygiene.[1,13,21,22,23,24,25,26]
- Confirm the patient's identity using at least two patient identifiers.[27]
- Explain the procedure to the patient *to reduce anxiety and promote cooperation.*[5,6]
- Instruct the patient in how to perform the Valsalva maneuver during removal *to prevent air embolism;*[1,5,6] if contraindicated, have him exhale instead.[5,6,43]
- Put on gloves and other personal protective equipment, as indicated.[3,5,6,28]
- Position the patient in the Trendelenburg position when possible.[42] If not possible, assist the patient to a recumbent position so that the insertion site is at or below heart level *to reduce the risk of air embolism.*[5,6]
- Discontinue all infusions and document the volume infused in the patient's intake and output record.[5,6]
- Place a fluid-impermeable pad under the patient's arm.
- Stabilize the catheter at the hub with one hand.
- Carefully remove the dressing, beginning at the device hub and gently pulling the dressing perpendicular to the skin toward the insertion site *to prevent skin tearing or stripping.*[5,6]
- If the catheter is secured with a securement device, remove the device. If the catheter is secured with sutures, carefully cut and remove them.[5]
- Assess the site for signs of infection, including swelling, drainage, redness, and inflammation.[1]
- Apply gauze to the insertion site; with your dominant hand, slowly withdraw the catheter using gentle, even pressure (as shown on top right).[5,6]

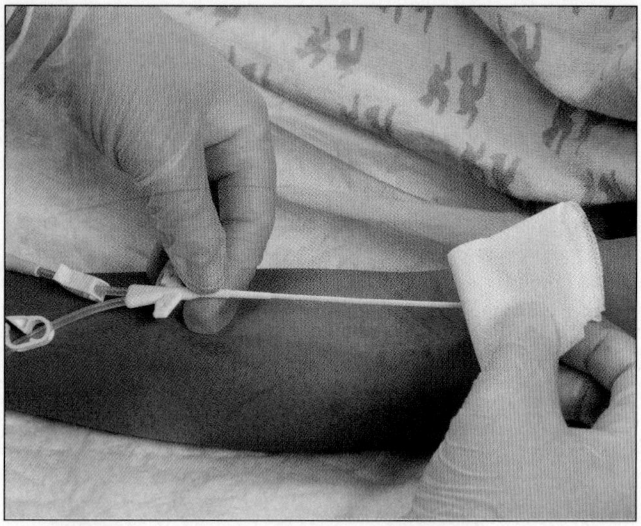

- Note that the catheter should come out easily. If you feel resistance, stop and notify the practitioner.[1,5,6]
- After successful removal of the catheter, apply manual pressure to the site with a sterile gauze pad until hemostasis is achieved. (1 to 5 minutes is recommended.)[42]
- Cover the site with petroleum-based ointment, a sterile gauze pad, and a sterile occlusive dressing *to seal the skin-to-vein tract and reduce the risk of air embolus.*[1,5,6,42,43]
- Assess the integrity of the removed catheter. Compare the length of the catheter with the original insertion length (as shown below) *to ensure that the entire catheter has been removed.*[5,6] If you note any damage, notify the practitioner and assess the patient for signs and symptoms of catheter embolism (palpitations, arrhythmia, dyspnea, cough, and thoracic pain). Note that a chest X-ray may be needed *for further evaluation.*[5,6]

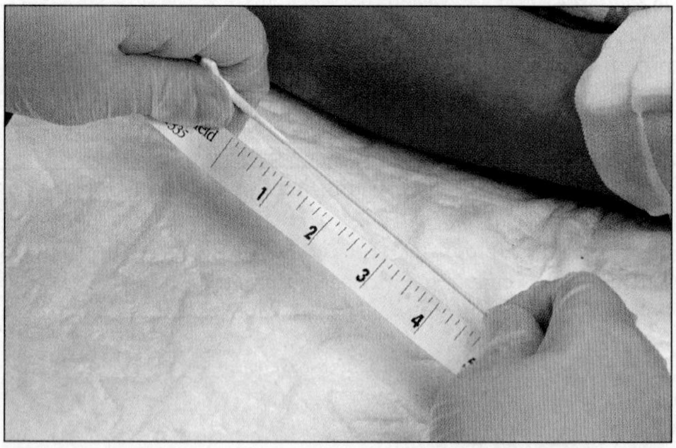

NURSING ALERT *If a PICC isn't intact after removal, apply a tourniquet to the upper arm, above the insertion site, close to the axilla, to prevent the advancement of the broken piece into the right atrium. Maintain the patient on strict bed rest, notify the practitioner, and monitor the patient closely for signs of distress. Have emergency resuscitative equipment available. If radiographic extraction of the catheter embolus is necessary, explain the procedure to the patient.*[5,6]

- Instruct the patient to remain lying recumbent for 30 minutes after removal.[6,43]
- Dispose of used supplies in the appropriate receptacles.[28]
- Remove and discard your gloves and any other personal protective equipment worn.
- Perform hand hygiene.[1,13,21,22,23,24,25,26]
- Document the procedure.[36,37,38,39]

Special considerations

- The Joint Commission issued a sentinel event alert concerning medical device alarm safety *because alarm-related events have been associated with permanent loss of function or death.* Among the major contributing factors were improper alarm settings, alarms turned off, and alarm signals not audible to staff. Make sure alarm limits are set appropriately, and that alarms are turned on, functioning properly, and audible to staff. Follow facility guidelines for preventing alarm fatigue.[50,51,52]
- Always use a 10-mL or larger syringe *to prevent catheter rupture.*
- PICC therapy works best when introduced early in treatment; it shouldn't be considered a last resort for patients with sclerotic or repeatedly punctured veins.
- Confirm a venous blood return and catheter patency before initiating any infusion.
- For catheters that aren't being used routinely, flush nonvalved catheters at least every 24 hours and valved catheters at least weekly.[41] Flush the catheter with preservative-free normal saline solution; lock with heparin (10 units/mL) if the catheter is to be heparin locked.[41]
- If necessary, use a declotting agent to clear a clotted PICC, but make sure you read the manufacturer's recommendations first. (See *Troubleshooting a PICC,* page 606.)
- Inspect and palpate the catheter insertion site daily *to discern tenderness through the transparent semipermeable dressing.*[1,10] Look at the catheter and cannula pathway, and check for bleeding, redness, drainage, and swelling. *Although oozing is common for the first 24 hours after insertion, excessive bleeding after that period should be evaluated.*
- Ask the patient whether he is having pain associated with therapy.
- Assess catheter necessity daily during multidisciplinary rounds and discontinue it as soon as it's no longer needed *to reduce the risk of central line–associated bloodstream infection.*[1,12,20,53]
- Change the PICC site dressing, and assess the site every 24 hours until healing has occurred.[5,6]

Report catheter defects to risk management, the manufacturer, and regulatory agencies, as directed by your facility.

- If the you inadvertently withdraw the catheter a significant amount during a dressing change, measure from the exit site to the hub and reapply a sterile dressing. Notify the practitioner, and prepare for a chest X-ray to determine the position of the PICC tip.
- When a medication is incompatible with preservative-free normal saline solution, flush the device with dextrose 5% in water and then follow by flushing with preservative-free normal saline solution, heparin flush solution, or both. Dextrose 5% in water should be flushed from the catheter *because it provides nutrients for biofilm growth, which increases the risk of vascular catheter–associated infection.*[41]
- Follow the PICC manufacturer's flushing instructions after the administration of contrast media.[54]

Patient teaching

If the patient will be discharged with a PICC line, teach the patient or family members the proper technique for flushing the line and changing the dressing if it becomes soiled. Have the patient or family member perform return demonstrations of these procedures.

Complications

PICC therapy causes fewer and less severe complications than conventional CV access devices. Catheter breakage on removal is a potential complication. Other possible adverse effects of PICC insertion are infection and thrombosis.[55,56] Air embolism—always a potential risk of venipuncture—poses less danger with PICC therapy than with traditional CV access devices *because the line is inserted below heart level.* Regardless, be alert for sudden onset of dyspnea, continued coughing, breathlessness, chest pain, hypotension, jugular vein distention, tachyarrhythmias, wheezing, tachypnea, altered mental status, altered speech, changes in facial appearance, numbness, and paralysis.[43,42] If any of these signs or symptoms occurs, place the patient in a left lateral decubitus position with his head down and administer 100% oxygen.[42] Apply pressure to the site after removal until bleeding has stopped.

Catheter tip migration may occur with vigorous flushing. Patients receiving chemotherapy are most vulnerable to this complication *because of frequent nausea and vomiting and subsequent changes in intrathoracic pressure.*

Because infection is always a risk with a PICC, watch for such signs as swelling, redness, and drainage at the site or increased temperature. Thrombosis, local skin irritation, catheter migration, and accidental catheter removal are other complications associated with a PICC dressing change.[55,56]

Complications during removal include venospasm, thrombosis, and catheter breakage. With venospasm and thrombosis, you will feel resistance during removal.

Documentation

Document the entire procedure, including site preparation, infection prevention, and safety precautions taken; the date and time of insertion; the number and location of insertion attempts; functionality of the device; local anesthetic used; method of insertion; and any problems with catheter placement. Also document the gauge length and type of catheter as well as the insertion location. Record the external length of the catheter at the time of placement. Note the lot number and manufacturer. Document unexpected outcomes and your interventions. Document that the anatomic location of the catheter tip was confirmed by X-ray before initial use. Complete the insertion checklist.[14]

Document the time, type, and amount of flush solution used as well as any resistance to flushing. Document whether the patient experienced any pain or discomfort during flushing.

For dressing change documentation, include the condition and length of the external catheter, the appearance of the site, stabilization device type, and any reports of pain or tenderness. Record the date and the time of the dressing change, any unexpected outcomes, and your interventions.

Document the medication, route, dose, rate, and time of administration; the condition of the insertion site before and after administration; and the patient's response to the medication.

Document PICC removal interventions and the condition, length, and site of the catheter.

Document any teaching provided to the patient and his family and their understanding of the teaching.

REFERENCES

1 Centers for Disease Control and Prevention. (2011). "Guidelines for the prevention of intravascular catheter-related infections" [Online]. Accessed May 2015 via the Web at http://www.cdc.gov/hicpac/pdf/guidelines/bsi-guidelines-2011.pdf (Level I)

2 Standard 33. Site selection. Infusion nursing standards of practice. (2011). *Journal of Infusion Nursing, 34,* S40–S43. (Level VII)

3 Standard 35. Vascular access site preparation and device management. Infusion nursing standards of practice. (2011). *Journal of Infusion Nursing, 34,* S44–S46. (Level VII)

4 Jarrett, N., et al. (2013). "Evidence-based guidelines for selected and previously considered hospital-acquired conditions: Final report" [Online]. Accessed May 2015 via the Web at http://www.cms.gov/Medicare/Medicare-Fee-for-Service-Payment/HospitalAcqCond/Downloads/Evidence-Based-Guidelines.pdf

5 Infusion Nurses Society. (2011). *Policies and procedures for infusion nursing* (4th ed.). Boston, MA: Infusion Nurses Society.

6 Infusion Nurses Society. (2013). *Policies and procedures for infusion nursing of the older adult* (2nd ed.). Boston, MA: Infusion Nurses Society.

7 American Osteopathic Association. (2014). Standard 07.01.02. *Healthcare Facilities Accreditation Program: Accreditation requirements for acute care hospitals.* Chicago, IL: American Osteopathic Association. (Level VII)

TROUBLESHOOTING

Troubleshooting a PICC

PROBLEM	INTERVENTION
Inability to flush or draw blood	■ Examine the peripherally inserted central catheter (PICC) *to ensure that clamps (if used or as part of extension tubing) are open, and to confirm the catheter isn't kinked.* ■ If sutures are present, make sure they aren't causing obstruction. ■ Assess for catheter occlusion, which may result from the patient's position; external or internal mechanical obstruction (kinked catheter under the dressing, catheter migration, precipitation, thrombosis); nonthrombotic factors such as drug precipitates; thrombotic factors, such as fibrin deposits or blood clots; catheter pinch-off resulting from an area of compression between the first rib and clavicle; or the medication itself and its compatibilities. ■ Note when the catheter was last functioning and when the last blood return was documented. ■ Extend or raise the patient's arm over his head. *This may help move the catheter away from the vessel wall.* If the catheter remains positional, notify the practitioner. An X-ray may be needed to determine tip placement. ■ If you suspect occlusion from precipitation, attempt to aspirate *to clear the catheter.* If successful, flush the catheter with preservative-free normal saline solution between all medications. If unsuccessful, obtain a practitioner's order for an agent to treat the precipitates. Consult with the pharmacy and determine who is permitted to perform this procedure in your facility. The instilled volume of the solution to clear precipitates shouldn't exceed the internal volume of the catheter *to avoid pushing precipitate into the bloodstream.* Instillation, aspiration, and flushing should be done using a method that doesn't exceed the catheter manufacturer's maximum pressure limits *to avoid line rupture.* ■ If occlusion is due to thrombosis, obtain a practitioner's order for a thrombolytic declotting agent; follow the manufacturer's recommendations, and determine who is permitted to administer the declotting agent in your facility.
Infiltration or extravasation (suspected or actual)	■ Always assess along the path of the catheter when performing IV site assessments. ■ Assess the extent of infiltration or extravasation using a standardized scale.[29] ■ Discontinue the infusion and remove the administration set, but don't remove the PICC. Aspirate fluid from the catheter using a small syringe. ■ Notify the practitioner of the extravasation or infiltration; report the solution or medications infusing at the time of the complication, the estimated volume of fluid that escaped into the tissue, and the site's appearance. ■ Obtain a practitioner's order, in collaboration with the pharmacy, for an agent to treat the infiltration or extravasation if needed. Treatment depends on the properties of the infiltrated medication or solution, the manufacturer's guidelines for that agent, and the severity of the problem.
Phlebitis	■ Encourage limitation of movement at the PICC site. ■ Apply warm, moist soaks to the extremity *to ease discomfort.* ■ If signs or symptoms increase or if streak formation or a palpable cord is present, notify the practitioner. ■ If pain at the access site and erythema or edema accompany the phlebitis, the PICC may need to be removed.
Catheter PICC migration (suspected or actual)	■ Be aware that catheter migration may be caused by excessive sneezing, coughing, or vomiting. Suspect migration of the PICC distally if the patient complains of chest pain or hears a noise during flushing of the PICC. ■ If migration is internal, or if external PICC migration is greater than 2 cm, notify the practitioner. ■ Obtain an order for an X-ray *to confirm tip placement.* ■ Be aware that external migration may necessitate replacement of a PICC or a change in therapy; internal migration requires manipulation or removal.
Leaking or damaged catheter	■ Clamp and secure the catheter *to prevent migration and possible embolization of a catheter fragment.* Catheter embolization is an emergency and may require surgical intervention. ■ Determine the extent and location of damage. ■ A registered nurse competent in this procedure using the manufacturer's repair kit and guidelines may repair the PICC line. Note that not all PICC manufacturers provide repair kits; repair with other materials may lead to catheter separation and migration or embolization. ■ Be aware that inability to repair the PICC necessitates its removal. ■ Report a defective catheter using the proper channels established by your facility.
Bleeding at insertion site	■ Apply a gauze dressing after initial placement of the PICC, and change the first dressing in 24 hours. Be aware that mild bleeding at the site may occur for the first 24 hours after PICC placement. ■ Limit movement of the extremity using an arm board as necessary. ■ If bleeding increases or persists past the first 24 hours, notify the practitioner.

8 American Osteopathic Association. (2014). Standard 07.01.19. *Healthcare Facilities Accreditation Program: Accreditation requirements for acute care hospitals.* Chicago, IL: American Osteopathic Association. (Level VII)

9 Standard 35. Vascular access site preparation and device management. Infusion nursing standards of practice. (2011). *Journal of Infusion Nursing, 34,* S44–S46. (Level VII)

10 Standard 46. Vascular access device site care and dressing changes. Infusion nursing standards of practice. (2011). *Journal of Infusion Nursing, 34,* S63–S64. (Level VII)

11 Azar, A., & Ballas, Z. K. Immune function in older adults. (2012). In: *UpToDate,* Stiehm, R. E., & Feldweg, A. M. (Eds.). Accessed May 2015 via http://www.uptodate.com/contents/search

12 Standard 44. Vascular access device removal. Infusion nursing standards of practice. (2011). *Journal of Infusion Nursing, 34,* S57–S59. (Level VII)

13 The Joint Commission. (2015). Standard NPSG.07.04.01. *Comprehensive accreditation manual for hospitals: The official handbook.* Oakbrook Terrace, IL: The Joint Commission. (Level VII)

14 The Joint Commission. (2015). Standard RI.01.03.01. *Comprehensive accreditation manual for hospitals: The official handbook.* Oakbrook Terrace, IL: The Joint Commission. (Level VII)

15 Medcomp. (2011). "1.9F & 2.9F Peripherally inserted central vein access catheter instructions for use" [Online]. Accessed May 2015 via the Web at http://www.medcompnet.com/products/pediatrics/pediatric_vascu-picc.html#ifu

16 Standard 12. Informed consent. Infusion nursing standards of practice. (2011). *Journal of Infusion Nursing, 34,* S17–S18. (Level VII)

17 Centers for Medicare & Medicaid Services, Department of Health and Human Services. (2014). Condition of participation: Patient's rights. 42 C.F.R. § 482.13.

18 American Osteopathic Association. (2014). Standard 15.01.11. *Healthcare Facilities Accreditation Program: Accreditation requirements for acute care hospitals.* Chicago, IL: American Osteopathic Association. (Level VII)

19 The Joint Commission. (2015). Standard UP.01.01.01. *Comprehensive accreditation manual for hospitals: The official handbook.* Oakbrook Terrace, IL: The Joint Commission. (Level VII)

20 Marschall, J., et al. (2014). SHEA/IDSA practice recommendation: Strategies to prevent central line-associated bloodstream infections in acute care hospitals. *Infection Control and Hospital Epidemiology, 35,* 753–771. Accessed May 2015 via the Web at http://www.jstor.org/stable/10.1086/676533 (Level I)

21 The Joint Commission. (2015). Standard NPSG.07.01.01. *Comprehensive accreditation manual for hospitals: The official handbook.* Oakbrook Terrace, IL: The Joint Commission. (Level VII)

22 Centers for Disease Control and Prevention. (2002). Guideline for hand hygiene in health-care settings: Recommendations of the Healthcare Infection Control Practices Advisory Committee and the HICPAC/SHEA/APIC/IDSA Hand Hygiene Task Force. *MMWR Recommendations and Reports, 51*(RR-16), 1–45. Accessed May 2015 via the Web at http://www.cdc.gov/mmwr/pdf/rr/rr5116.pdf (Level II)

23 World Health Organization. (2009). "WHO guidelines on hand hygiene in health care: First global patient safety challenge, clean care is safer care" [Online]. Accessed May 2015 via the Web at http://whqlibdoc.who.int/publications/2009/9789241597906_eng.pdf (Level IV)

24 Standard 19. Hand hygiene. Infusion nursing standards of practice. (2011). *Journal of Infusion Nursing, 34,* S26–S27. (Level VII)

25 American Osteopathic Association. (2014). Standard 07.01.21. *Healthcare Facilities Accreditation Program: Accreditation requirements for acute care hospitals.* Chicago, IL: American Osteopathic Association. (Level VII)

26 Centers for Medicare & Medicaid Services, Department of Health and Human Services. (2014). Condition of participation: Infection control. 42 C.F.R. § 482.42.

27 The Joint Commission. (2015). Standard NPSG.01.01.01. *Comprehensive accreditation manual for hospitals: The official handbook.* Oakbrook Terrace, IL: The Joint Commission. (Level VII)

28 Occupational Safety and Health Administration. (n.d.). "Bloodborne pathogens, standard number 1910.1030" [Online]. Accessed May 2015 via the Web at http://www.osha.gov/pls/oshaweb/owadisp.show_document?p_table=STANDARDS&p_id=10051 (Level VII)

29 The Joint Commission. (2015). Standard NPSG.03.04.01. *Comprehensive accreditation manual for hospitals: The official handbook.* Oakbrook Terrace, IL: The Joint Commission. (Level VII)

30 Standard 32. Vascular access device selection. Infusion nursing standards of practice. (2011). *Journal of Infusion Nursing, 34,* S37–S40. (Level VII)

31 Standard 31. Tourniquets. Infusion nursing standards of practice. (2011). *Journal of Infusion Nursing, 34,* S36. (Level VII)

32 The Joint Commission. (2015). Standard UP.01.03.01. *Comprehensive accreditation manual for hospitals: The official handbook.* Oakbrook Terrace, IL: The Joint Commission. (Level VII)

33 Standard 36. Vascular access device stabilization. Infusion nursing standards of practice. (2011). *Journal of Infusion Nursing, 34,* S46–S47. (Level VII)

34 Standard 18. Infection prevention. Infusion nursing standards of practice. (2011). *Journal of Infusion Nursing, 34,* S25–S26. (Level VII)

35 Standard 22. Safe handling and disposal of sharps, hazardous materials, and hazardous waste. Infusion nursing standards of practice. (2011). *Journal of Infusion Nursing, 34,* S28–S29. (Level VII)

36 The Joint Commission. (2015). Standard RC.01.03.01. *Comprehensive accreditation manual for hospitals: The official handbook.* Oakbrook Terrace, IL: The Joint Commission. (Level VII)

37 Standard 14. Documentation. Infusion nursing standards of practice. (2011). *Journal of Infusion Nursing, 34,* S20–S21. (Level VII)

38 American Osteopathic Association. (2014). Standard 10.00.03. *Healthcare Facilities Accreditation Program: Accreditation requirements for acute care hospitals.* Chicago, IL: American Osteopathic Association. (Level VII)

39 Centers for Medicare & Medicaid Services, Department of Health and Human Services. (2014). Condition of participation: Medical record services. 42 C.F.R. § 482.24(b).

40 Standard 27. Needleless connectors. Infusion nursing standards of practice. (2011). *Journal of Infusion Nursing, 34,* S32–S33. (Level VII) Infusion Nurses Society. (2008). Flushing protocols. Boston, MA: Infusion Nurses Society. (Level VII)

41 Standard 45. Flushing and locking. Infusion nursing standards of practice. (2011). *Journal of Infusion Nursing, 34,* S59–S63. (Level VII)

42 Feil, M. (2012). Reducing risk of air embolism associated with central venous access devices. *Pennsylvania Patient Safety Advisory, 9,* 58–65. Accessed May 2015 via the Web at http://patientsafetyauthority.org/ADVISORIES/AdvisoryLibrary/2012/Jun;9(2)/documents/58.pdf

43 Standard 50. Air embolism. Infusion nursing standards of practice. (2011). *Journal of Infusion Nursing, 34,* S69–S70. (Level VII)

44 Westbrook, J., et al. (2010). Association of interruptions with an increased risk and severity of medication administration errors. *Archives of Internal Medicine, 170,* 683–690.

45 Institute for Safe Medication Practices. (2013). Side tracks on the safety express: Interruptions lead to errors and unfinished...Wait, what was I doing? *Nurse Advise-ERR, 11*(2), 1–4. Accessed May 2015 via the Web at https://www.ismp.org/Newsletters/acutecare/showarticle.aspx?id=37

46 Standard 61. Parenteral medication and solution administration. Infusion nursing standards of practice. (2011). *Journal of Infusion Nursing, 34,* S86–S87. (Level VII)

47 American Osteopathic Association. (2014). Standard 16.01.03. *Healthcare Facilities Accreditation Program: Accreditation requirements for acute care hospitals.* Chicago, IL: American Osteopathic Association. (Level VII)

48 The Joint Commission. (2015). Standard MM.06.01.01. *Comprehensive accreditation manual for hospitals: The official handbook.* Oakbrook Terrace, IL: The Joint Commission. (Level VII)

49 U.S. Food and Drug Administration. (n.d.). "Look. Check. Connect. Safe medical device connections save lives" [Online]. Accessed May 2015 via the Web at http://www.fda.gov/downloads/MedicalDevices/Safety/AlertsandNotices/UCM134873.pdf

50 The Joint Commission. (2013). "Sentinel event alert: Medical device alarm safety in hospitals" [Online]. Accessed May 2015 via the Web at http://www.jointcommission.org/assets/1/18/SEA_50_alarms_4_5_13_FINAL1.PDF (Level VII)

51 The Joint Commission. (2015). Standard NPSG.06.01.01. *Comprehensive accreditation manual for hospitals: The official handbook.* Oakbrook Terrace, IL: The Joint Commission. (Level VII)

52 Graham, K. C., & Cvach, M. (2010). Monitor alarm fatigue: Standardizing use of physiological monitors and decreasing nuisance alarms. *American Journal of Critical Care, 19,* 28–37.
53 Association of Professionals in Infection Control and Epidemiology (APIC). (2009). "An APIC guide 2009: Guide to the elimination of catheter-related bloodstream infections" [Online]. Accessed May 2015 via the Web at http://www.apic.org/Resource_/EliminationGuideForm/259c0594-17b0-459d-b395-fb143321414a/File/APIC-CRBSI-Elimination-Guide.pdf (Level IV)
54 American College of Radiology (ACR) Committee on Drugs and Contrast Media. (2013). "ACR manual on contrast media: Version 9" [Online]. Accessed May 2015 via the Web at http://www.acr.org/~/media/ACR/Documents/PDF/QualitySafety/Resources/Contrast%20Manual/2013_Contrast_Media.pdf
55 Chopra, V., et al. (2012). Bloodstream infection, venous thrombosis, and peripherally inserted central catheters: Reappraising the evidence. *American Journal of Medicine, 125,* 733–741.
56 Liem, T. K., et al. (2012). Peripherally inserted central catheter usage patterns and associated symptomatic upper extremity venous thrombosis. *Journal of Vascular Surgery, 55,* 761–767.

PERIPHERAL NERVE STIMULATION

Peripheral nerve stimulation assesses and monitors the depth of neuromuscular blockade in patients receiving neuromuscular-blocking drugs, which are administered to produce paralysis.[1] Neuromuscular-blocking drugs may be given to help synchronize breathing and mechanical ventilation in patients with severe lung injury; assist with the treatment of severe muscle spasms in patients with seizures, tetanus, or drug overdose; and help in the management of increased intracranial pressure in patients with head injury.

A peripheral nerve stimulator (PNS) is used to evaluate the level of neuromuscular blockade and determine the lowest therapeutic dose of the neuromuscular-blocking drug needed to produce paralysis. The PNS works by stimulating a peripheral nerve with a series of brief electrical pulses to produce a muscle response or twitch.

The train of four (TOF) is the most commonly used method for monitoring neuromuscular blockade. In this method, a series of four electrical impulses are delivered to a particular peripheral nerve. If four twitches occur, then 75% or less of the receptors are blocked. Three twitches occur when 80% of the receptors are blocked. One or two twitches indicate 85% to 90% neuromuscular blockade.[1] After the neuromuscular-blocking drug is administered, it's titrated so that each set of four electrical impulses produces one or two muscle twitches. The absence of twitches may indicate that 100% of the receptors are blocked, exceeding the desired level of neuromuscular blockade.[1]

Equipment

PNS ■ two electrode gel patches ■ two leadwires ■ alcohol pads ■ Optional: clippers.

Implementation

■ Verify the practitioner's order.
■ Perform hand hygiene *to reduce the transmission of microorganisms.*[2,3,4,5,6]
■ Confirm the patient's identity using at least two patient identifiers.[7]
■ Explain the reasons for neuromuscular blockade and peripheral nerve stimulation to the patient and family *to increase their understanding and reduce anxiety.*
■ Select a site for electrode placement that's accessible and free from edema, wounds, catheters, and dressings *to ensure optimum placement for conduction of stimulating current.* The preferred monitoring site is the ulnar nerve, but if it isn't accessible, other sites may be used.
■ If the patient has excessive hair where an electrode is to be placed, remove the hair with clippers *to improve contact of the pad with the skin.*

Ulnar nerve stimulation

■ Use an alcohol pad to clean the site on the patient's arm where the electrodes are to be placed and allow it to dry *to reduce skin resistance.*
■ Place the patient's arm in a relaxed position with the palm up *so that the ulnar nerve is easily accessible.*
■ Place one electrode over the ulnar nerve at the crease of the wrist and the other electrode 1 to 2 cm away, parallel to the carpi ulnaris tendon (as shown below) *to ensure stimulation of the ulnar nerve.*

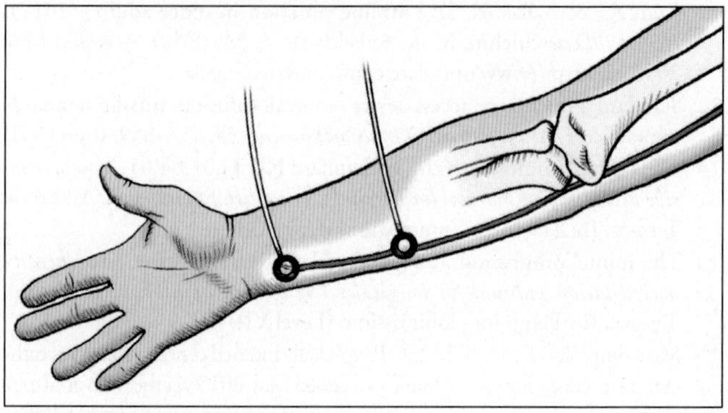

■ Attach the leadwires to the PNS.
■ Connect the black lead (negative) to the electrode nearest the wrist and the red lead (positive) to the electrode on the forearm.
■ Turn on the PNS on and choose a low amplitude—commonly 10 to 20 milliampere (mA)—*because higher current can cause overstimulation of the nerve and rhythmic nerve firing.*[1]
■ Press the TOF button to initiate the four impulses. Count the number of thumb adductions or twitches that the stimulator produces while lightly feeling for twitches. Don't count finger movement that's caused by muscle stimulation.
■ Turn off the PNS.
■ Perform hand hygiene.[2,3,4,5,6]

Facial nerve stimulation

■ Use an alcohol pad to clean the site on the patient's face where the electrodes are to be placed and allow it to dry *to improve contact of the electrode with the skin.*
■ Place one electrode near the outer canthus of the eye and a second electrode 2 cm below and at the level of the tragus of the ear (as shown below) *to ensure stimulation of the facial nerve.*

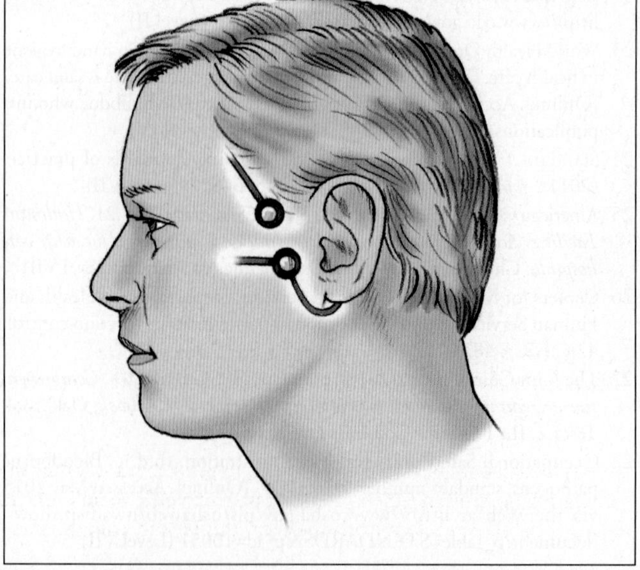

■ Attach the leadwires to the PNS
■ Connect the black lead (negative) to the electrode nearest the tragus and the red lead (positive) to the electrode near the outer canthus of the eye.
■ Turn on the PNS on and choose a low amplitude—commonly 10 to 20 mA—*because higher current can cause overstimulation of the nerve and rhythmic nerve firing.*
■ Press the TOF button to initiate the four impulses. Count the number of twitches you observe while lightly feeling for twitches.
■ Turn off the PNS.
■ Perform hand hygiene.[2,3,4,5,6]

Posterior tibial nerve stimulation

■ Use an alcohol pad to clean the site on the patient's foot where the electrodes are to be placed and allow it to dry *to improve contact of the electrode with the skin.*
■ Place one electrode 2 cm behind the medial malleolus and a second electrode 2 cm above the first electrode (as shown below) *to ensure stimulation of the posterior tibial nerve.*

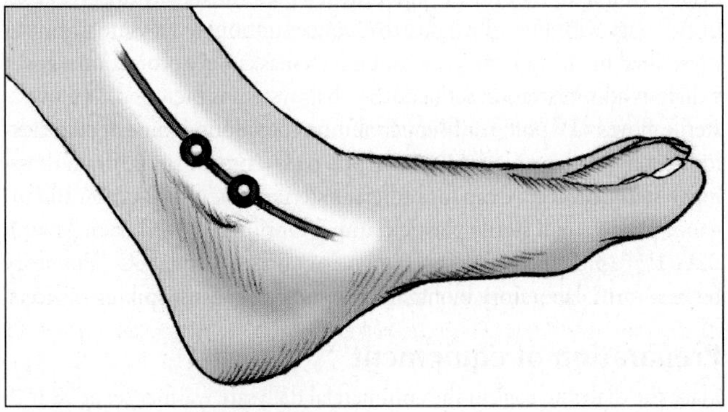

■ Attach the leadwires to the PNS.
■ Connect the black lead (negative) to the electrode behind the medial malleolus and the red lead (positive) to the electrode above the first.
■ Turn on the PNS on and choose a low mA—commonly 10 to 20 mA—*because higher current can cause overstimulation of the nerve and rhythmic nerve firing.*
■ Press the TOF button to initiate the four impulses. Note plantar flexion of the great toe and count the number of twitches that the stimulation produces.
■ Turn off the PNS.
■ Perform hand hygiene.[2,3,4,5,6]

Establishing supramaximal stimulation

■ *To determine the baseline amplitude setting for a patient who hasn't received neuromuscular blockade,* set the amplitude to 5 mA and press the TOF button to initiate the stimulus.[1]
■ Note the number of twitches produced.
■ Increase the amplitude 5 mA at a time until four muscle twitches are produced by the TOF stimulation. *This step establishes the amount of current that should be used for peripheral nerve stimulation and enhances the reliability of testing.*[1]

Establishing TOF after neuromuscular blockade

■ Determine the TOF 10 to 15 minutes following a bolus dose or any change in neuromuscular drug administration *to assess the level of neuromuscular blockade.*
■ If no twitches occur, troubleshoot the equipment. Next, increase the stimulating current and then retest another nerve. If there's still no response, check the neuromuscular blocker infusion rate, concentration, and dose, and then hold the bolus dose or reduce the infusion rate, as ordered. Retest the TOF in 10 to 15 minutes.[10]
■ If one or two twitches occur, continue the current rate of the infusion.
■ If three or four twitches occur, increase the rate of the neuromuscular blockade and then retest the TOF in 10 to 15 minutes.

Ongoing care

■ Perform respiratory, cardiovascular, and neurologic assessments before any increase in the level of neuromuscular blockade.
■ Perform neurovascular assessments hourly.
■ Change electrodes daily, or more frequently if they become loose or the gel has dried out *to ensure optimum conduction.*[1]
■ Assess the skin under the electrodes for signs of irritation or breakdown, *which could impede conduction.*
■ Reevaluate the level of neuromuscular blockade every 4 to 8 hours during therapy with neuromuscular-blocking drugs, as ordered, after the patient is stable and an adequate level of neuromuscular blockade is reached.[1]
■ Perform hand hygiene.[2,3,4,5,6]
■ Document the procedure.[11,12,13]

Special considerations

■ *Because neuromuscular-blocking drugs don't produce amnesia, sedation, or analgesia,* sedative and analgesic drugs should always be administered before giving a neuromuscular-blocking drug.[7]
■ Assess the patient's baseline electrolyte, blood urea nitrogen, and creatinine levels *because imbalances may potentiate the effects of neuromuscular-blocking drugs.*[10]
■ *To avoid complications of neuromuscular blockade,* the patient will require routine frequent oral care and suctioning, deep vein thrombosis prophylaxis (as ordered), GI prophylaxis (as ordered), eye lubrication, and footdrop prevention measures.[10]
■ Peripheral nerve stimulators are unreliable for discerning the degree of neuromuscular recovery necessary for spontaneous ventilation and tracheal extubation. *To assess readiness for tracheal extubation,* more precise medical devices are needed such as neuromuscular monitors that provide objective responses to nerve stimulation. Such monitors use different methods to measure the evoked muscle responses to electrical nerve stimulation.[14]
■ If the patient has hemiplegia, hemiparesis, or peripheral neuropathy (from diabetes or other conditions), keep in mind that the motor response to PNS may not be as pronounced, which may lead to the incorrect belief that a higher dose of neuromuscular-blocking drugs is needed. With hemiplegia and hemiparesis, place the electrodes on the unaffected limb, if possible.
■ Check the site of electrode placement carefully *because incorrect placement can lead to muscle, rather than nerve, stimulation.*[1]
■ If no twitches are elicited at a level that previously elicited a response, troubleshoot the PNS before decreasing the level of neuromuscular blockade. Check the polarity of the leads, battery charge, electrode contact with the skin, condition of electrode gel pads, and leadwire connections.

Complications

Excessive neuromuscular blockade can cause protracted paralysis and muscle weakness. During TOF testing, the patient may experience mild discomfort. Skin irritation and breakdown can occur under the electrode pads. Cardiac arrhythmias can result if the PNS leadwires come in contact with an external pacing catheter or leadwire.

Documentation

Record the date and time of the assessment. Record the initial TOF assessment, amplitude used, and dose of neuromuscular-blocking drug being administered. Document each subsequent TOF assessment on the appropriate flow sheet as a ratio of twitches per four stimulations—for example, 0/4, 1/4, 2/4, 3/4, 4/4.

Note the current used as well as any bolus doses or changes in the rate of infusion of the neuromuscular-blocking drug. Record respiratory, cardiovascular, and neurologic assessments on a frequent assessment form. Note any adverse effects of neuromuscular blockade, the time and name of the practitioner notified, orders given, nursing interventions performed, and the patient's response. Include any patient and family teaching and their understanding of the teaching.

REFERENCES

1 Lynn-McHale Wiegand, D. (Ed.). (2011). *AACN procedure manual for critical care* (6th ed.). St. Louis, MO: Saunders.

2 The Joint Commission. (2015). Standard NPSG.07.01.01. *Comprehensive accreditation manual for hospitals: The official handbook.* Oakbrook Terrace, IL: The Joint Commission. (Level VII)

3 Centers for Disease Control and Prevention. (2002). Guideline for hand hygiene in health-care settings: Recommendations of the Healthcare Infection Control Practices Advisory Committee and the HICPAC/SHEA/APIC/IDSA Hand Hygiene Task Force. *MMWR Recommendations and Reports, 51*(RR-16), 1–45. Accessed May 2015 via the Web at http://www.cdc.gov/mmwr/pdf/rr/rr5116.pdf (Level II)

4 World Health Organization. (2009). "WHO guidelines on hand hygiene in health care: First global patient safety challenge, clean care is safer care" [Online]. Accessed May 2015 via the Web at http://whqlibdoc.who.int/publications/2009/9789241597906_eng.pdf (Level IV)

5 Centers for Medicare & Medicaid Services, Department of Health and Human Services. (2014). Condition of participation: Infection control. 42 C.F.R. § 482.42.

6 American Osteopathic Association. (2014). Standard 07.01.21. *Healthcare Facilities Accreditation Program: Accreditation requirements for acute care hospitals.* Chicago, IL: American Osteopathic Association. (Level VII)

7 The Joint Commission. (2015). Standard NPSG.01.01.01. *Comprehensive accreditation manual for hospitals: The official handbook.* Oakbrook Terrace, IL: The Joint Commission. (Level VII)

8 Centers for Medicare & Medicaid Services, Department of Health and Human Services. (2014). Condition of participation: Patient's rights. 42 C.F.R. § 482.13(c)(1).

9 American Osteopathic Association. (2014). Standard 15.01.16. *Healthcare Facilities Accreditation Program: Accreditation requirements for acute care hospitals.* Chicago, IL: American Osteopathic Association. (Level VII)

10 Saenz, A. D. (2013). "Peripheral nerve stimulator: Train of four monitoring" [Online]. Accessed May 2015 via the Web at http://emedicine.medscape.com/article/2009530-overview

11 The Joint Commission. (2015). Standard RC.01.03.01. *Comprehensive accreditation manual for hospitals: The official handbook.* Oakbrook Terrace, IL: The Joint Commission. (Level VII)

12 Centers for Medicare & Medicaid Services, Department of Health and Human Services. (2014). Condition of participation: Medical record services. 42 C.F.R. § 482.24(b).

13 American Osteopathic Association. (2014). Standard 10.00.03. *Healthcare Facilities Accreditation Program: Accreditation requirements for acute care hospitals.* Chicago, IL: American Osteopathic Association. (Level VII)

14 Brull, S. J., & Murphy, G. S. (2010). Residual neuromuscular block: Lessons unlearned. Part II: Methods to reduce the risk of residual weakness. *Anesthesia & Analgesia, 111,* 129–140. Accessed May 2015 via the Web at http://journals.lww.com/anesthesia-analgesia/Fulltext/2010/07000/Residual_Neuromuscular_Block_Lessons_Unlearned_.25.aspx

PERITONEAL DIALYSIS

Peritoneal dialysis is indicated for patients with stage 5 chronic kidney disease[1] who are looking for an alternative to renal replacement therapy. Peritoneal dialysis can also be used in patients with vascular access issues, chronic heart failure, and ischemic heart disease.[2] In this procedure, dialysate—the solution instilled into the peritoneal cavity by a catheter—draws waste products, excess fluid, and electrolytes from the blood across the semipermeable peritoneal membrane. (See *How peritoneal dialysis works.*)

After a prescribed period, the dialysate is drained from the peritoneal cavity, removing impurities with it. The dialysis procedure is then repeated, using a new dialysate each time, until waste removal is complete and fluid, electrolyte, and acid-base balance has been restored. The procedure is also known as the *dialysis cycle,* consisting of the dialysate instillation time, the dialysate dwell time, and the dialysate drain time.

Peritoneal dialysis is usually contraindicated in patients who have had extensive abdominal or bowel surgery or extensive abdominal trauma, who are obese, or who have severe vascular disease or respiratory distress.

The catheter may be inserted in the operating room or under sterile conditions on the nursing unit. Dialysis can be performed either manually or using an automatic or semiautomatic cycle machine. (See *Comparing peritoneal dialysis catheters,* page 612.)

Equipment

Scale ■ vital signs monitoring equipment ■ prescribed dialysate (1-L, 2-L, or 3-L bags with prescribed dextrose concentration) ■ dialysate warmer ■ prescribed medication ■ sterile container ■ masks ■ eye protection ■ gown ■ dialysis administration set (a double-bag system is preferred)[1] ■ gloves ■ sterile gloves ■ IV pole ■ antiseptic solution (povidone-iodine or chlorhexidine) ■ hypoallergenic tape ■ antiseptic pads ■ precut sterile drain dressings ■ sterile protective cap for catheter ■ sterile 4″ × 4″ (10-cm × 10-cm) gauze pads ■ small sterile plastic clamp ■ Optional: 10-mL syringe with 22G 1½″ (3.8 cm) needle, specimen containers with labels, laboratory request form, laboratory biohazard transport bag, assist spiking device.

Preparation of equipment

Place the dialysate bags in the commercial dialysate warmer set at 98.6° F (37° C) for about 1 hour *to ensure the dialysate is at body temperature. Warming the dialysate decreases the patient's discomfort during the procedure and reduces vasoconstriction of the peritoneal capillaries. Dilated capillaries enhance blood flow to the peritoneal membrane surface, increasing waste clearance into the peritoneal cavity.* Add prescribed medications to the dialysate bag immediately before the dialysate will be hung and used.

Implementation

- Verify the practitioner's order.
- Review recent laboratory results (blood urea nitrogen, serum creatinine, albumin, bicarbonate, glucose, potassium, and hemoglobin levels; hematocrit; and white blood cell and platelet counts).[1]
- Gather the equipment at the patient's bedside.
- Perform hand hygiene.[3,4,5,6,7]
- Confirm the patient's identity using at least two patient identifiers.[8]
- Provide privacy.[9,10]
- Explain the procedure to the patient to *allay his fear and enhance cooperation.* If the patient previously received peritoneal dialysis, ask about his response to previous reatment.[1]
- Obtain the patient's baseline vital signs (supine and upright blood pressure, apical pulse rate and rhythm, and rate and depth of respirations).[1] Assess the patient's respiratory and abdominal status.[11]
- Place the patient in the supine position if the patient's catheter is newly implanted.[1]
- Put on a gown, a mask, eye protection, and gloves *to comply with standard precautions.*[12,13]
- Inspect the warmed dialysate, which should appear clear and colorless.
- Add any prescribed medication to the dialysate using strict sterile technique *to avoid contaminating the solution.*[11]
- Prepare the dialysis administration set. (See *Setup for peritoneal dialysis.*)

How peritoneal dialysis works

Peritoneal dialysis works through a combination of diffusion and osmosis.

Diffusion
In diffusion, particles move through a semipermeable membrane from an area of high-solute concentration to an area of low-solute concentration. In peritoneal dialysis, the water-based dialysate being infused contains glucose, sodium chloride, calcium, magnesium, acetate or lactate, and no waste products. Therefore, the waste products and excess electrolytes in the blood cross through the semipermeable peritoneal membrane into the dialysate. Removing the waste-filled dialysate and replacing it with fresh solution keeps the waste concentration low and encourages further diffusion.

Osmosis
In osmosis, fluids move through a semipermeable membrane from an area of low-solute concentration to an area of high-solute concentration. In peritoneal dialysis, dextrose is added to the dialysate to give it a higher solute concentration than the blood, creating a high osmotic gradient. Water migrates from the blood through the membrane at the beginning of each infusion, when the osmotic gradient is highest.

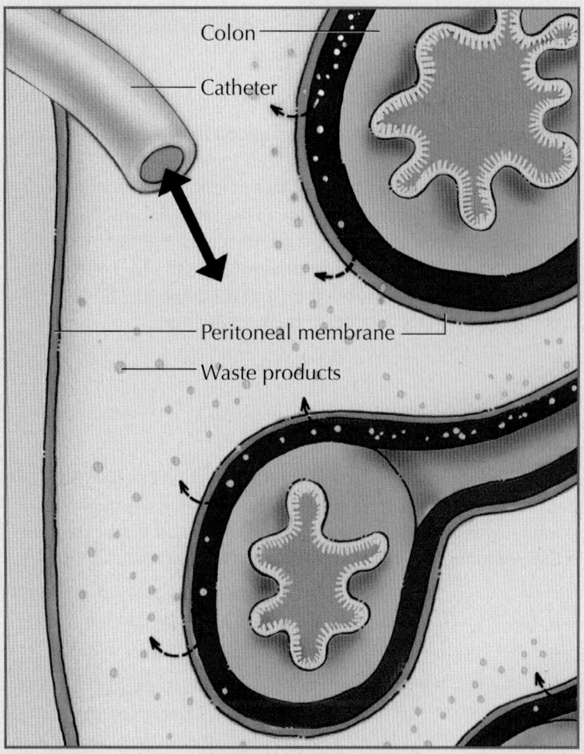

■ Close the clamps on all the lines.
■ Place the drainage bag below the patient *to facilitate gravity drainage* and connect the drainage line to it. Connect the dialysate infusion lines to the first bag of dialysate using sterile technique. Avoid manual spiking as much as possible *to reduce the risk of peritonitis*; if spiking can't be avoided, use an assist device, if available.[14] Hang the bag on the IV pole at the patient's bedside.
■ Prime the tubing by opening the infusion lines and allowing the solution to flow until all the lines are primed. Close the clamp.
■ Prepare the sterile field.[11]
■ Open the sterile container and pour the antiseptic solution into it.[11]
■ Open the sterile 4″ × 4″ (10-cm × 10-cm) gauze pads.[11]
■ Remove and discard your gloves,[12] perform hand hygiene,[3,4,5,6,7] and put on sterile gloves.[11,12]
Saturate a sterile gauze pad with antiseptic solution. Scrub the catheter connection end for 1 minute and then allow it to dry *to reduce transmission of microorganisms.*[11]
■ Connect the dialysis administration set to the catheter using sterile technique *to prevent contamination of the catheter and the solution, which could cause peritonitis.*
■ Trace the tubing from the patient to its point of origin t*o make sure that you're connecting the tubing to the correct port before beginning the dialysate instillation.*[15]
■ Unclamp the line to the patient. Rapidly instill 500 mL of dialysate into the peritoneal cavity *to test the catheter's patency.*
■ Reclamp the line to the patient.
■ Immediately unclamp the line to the drainage bag *to allow fluid to drain into the bag.* Outflow should be brisk.
■ Having established the catheter's patency, clamp the lines to the drainage bag and unclamp the lines to the patient to infuse the prescribed volume of solution over a period of 5 to 10 minutes, or as ordered.

Setup for peritoneal dialysis

This illustration shows the proper setup for peritoneal dialysis.

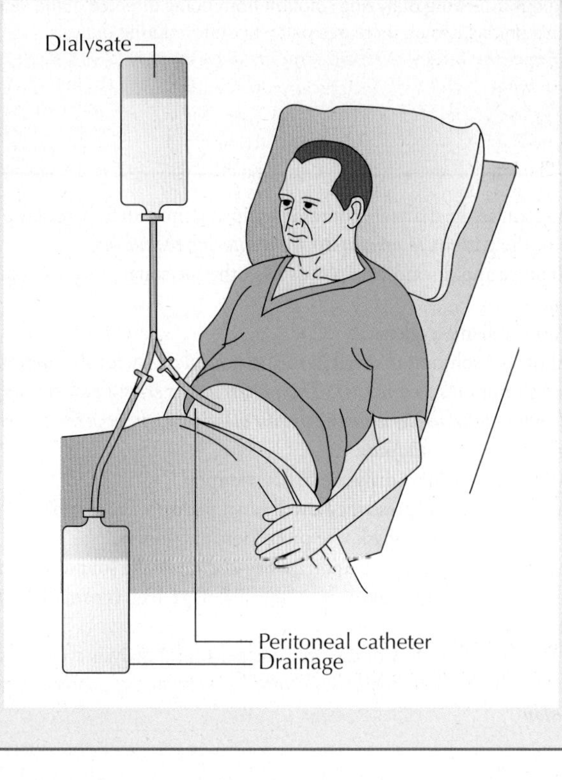

EQUIPMENT

Comparing peritoneal dialysis catheters

The first step in any type of peritoneal dialysis is insertion of a catheter *to allow instillation of dialyzing solution*. The surgeon may insert one of the three catheters described here.

Tenckhoff catheter

To implant a Tenckhoff catheter, the surgeon inserts the first 17 cm (6¾″) of the catheter into the patient's abdomen. The next 7-cm (2¾″) segment, which may have a Dacron cuff at one or both ends, is imbedded subcutaneously. Within a few days after insertion, the patient's tissues grow around the cuffs, forming a tight barrier against bacterial infiltration. The remaining 10 cm (3⅞″) of the catheter extends outside of the abdomen and is equipped with a metal adapter at the tip that connects to dialyzer tubing.

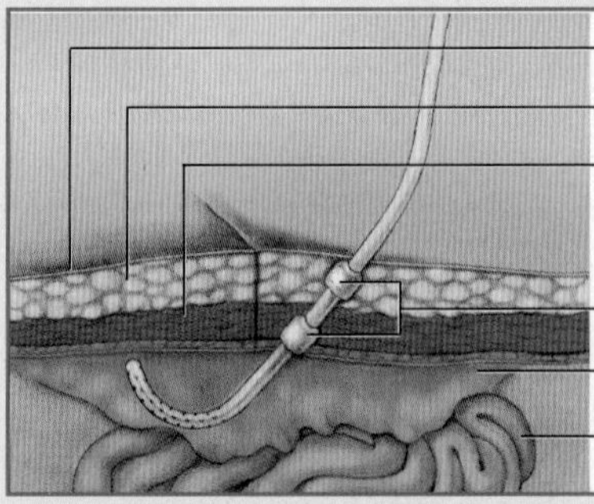

Flanged-collar catheter

To insert this kind of catheter, the surgeon positions its flanged collar just below the skin so that the device extends through the abdominal wall. He keeps the distal end of the cuff from extending into the peritoneum, where it could cause adhesions.

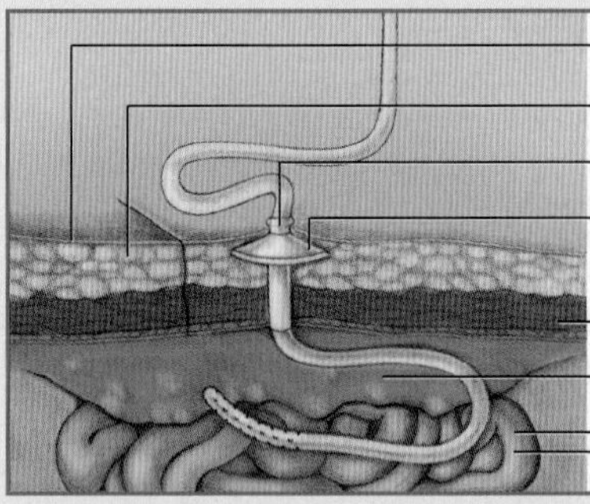

Column-disk peritoneal catheter

To insert a column-disk peritoneal catheter (CDPC), the surgeon rolls up the flexible disk section of the implant, inserts it into the peritoneal cavity, and retracts it against the abdominal wall. The implant's first cuff rests just outside the peritoneal membrane, and its second cuff rests just underneath the skin.

Because the CDPC doesn't float freely in the peritoneal cavity, it keeps inflowing dialyzing solution from being directed at the sensitive organs, which increases patient comfort during dialysis.

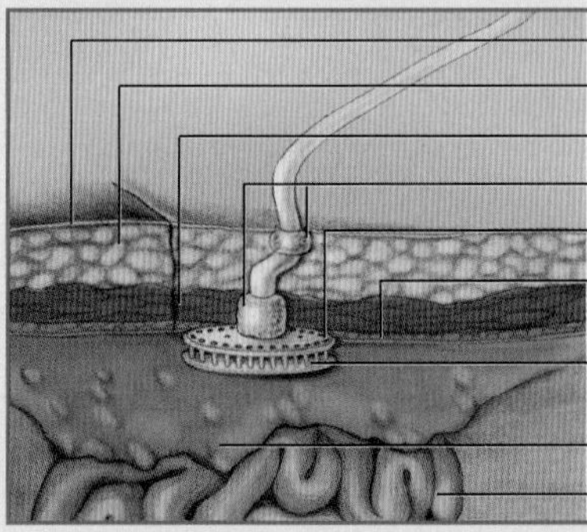

- As soon as the dialysate container empties, immediately reclamp the line to the patient *to prevent air from entering the tubing.*
- Remove and discard your gloves and other personal protective equipment.[12]
- Perform hand hygiene.[3,4,5,6,7]
- Allow the solution to dwell in the peritoneal cavity for the prescribed time (10 minutes to 4 hours). *This process allows excess fluid, electrolytes, and accumulated wastes to move from the blood through the peritoneal membrane and into the dialysate.*
- Make sure the next dialysate bag is warming.
- At the end of the prescribed dwell time, perform hand hygiene[3,4,5,6,7] and put on a gown, a mask, eye protection, and gloves.[12]
- Unclamp the line to the drainage bag and allow the solution to drain from the peritoneal cavity into the drainage bag (normally 20 to 30 minutes).
- Observe the outflow of the previous peritoneal dialysis cycle *to make sure that the fluid has completely drained before beginning another dialysate infusion.*
- Repeat the infusion-dwell-drain cycle immediately after the dialysate drains until the prescribed number of fluid exchanges has been completed.
- If the practitioner requires a dialysate specimen, collect one after every 10 infusion-dwell-drain cycles (always during the drain phase) and after every 24-hour period, or as ordered. To do this, thoroughly disinfect the injection port with antiseptic solution and then allow it to dry. Attach the 10-mL syringe to the 22G 1½″ (3.8-cm) needle, insert it into the injection port on the drainage line using strict sterile technique, and aspirate the drainage sample. Transfer the sample to the specimen container, label it in the presence of the patient *to prevent* mislabeling,[8] and send it to the laboratory in a laboratory biohazard transport bag[16] with a laboratory request form.
- Remove and discard your gloves.[12]
- Perform hand hygiene.[3,4,5,6,7]
- After completing the prescribed number of exchanges, clamp the catheter.
- Perform hand hygiene.[3,4,5,6,7]
- Put on sterile gloves.[12]

■ Disconnect the dialysis administration set from the peritoneal catheter, and place a sterile protective cap over the catheter's connection end.[11]
■ Securely tape the catheter to the patient's abdomen *to prevent accidental dislodgment.*[11]
■ Dispose of all used supplies in appropriate receptacles.[11,12]
■ Remove and discard your gloves and other personal protective equipment.[12]
■ Perform hand hygiene.[3,4,5,6,7]
■ Document the procedure.[17,18,19]

Special considerations

■ Change the catheter dressing at an interval determined by your facility or whenever it becomes wet or soiled.
■ *To prevent protein depletion,* the practitioner may order a high-protein diet or a protein supplement. He will also monitor serum albumin levels.
■ *To prevent respiratory distress,* place the patient in a position that maximizes his lung expansion. Promote lung expansion through turning and deep-breathing exercises. In some patients, decreasing the dialysate volume may be necessary.

NURSING ALERT *If the patient suffers severe respiratory distress during the dwell phase of dialysis, immediately drain the peritoneal cavity and notify the practitioner. Carefully monitor any patient on peritoneal dialysis who's being weaned from a ventilator.*

■ Dialysate is available in three concentrations—4.25% dextrose, 2.5% dextrose, and 1.5% dextrose. The 4.25% solution usually removes the largest amount of fluid from the blood *because its glucose concentration is highest.* If your patient receives this concentrated solution, monitor him carefully *to prevent excess fluid loss.* Also, some of the glucose in the 4.25% solution may enter the patient's bloodstream, causing hyperglycemia severe enough to require an insulin injection or an insulin addition to the dialysate.
■ Patients with low serum potassium levels may require the addition of potassium to the dialysate solution *to prevent further losses.*
■ Heparin is sometimes added to the dialysate *to prevent occlusion of fibrin in the dialysis catheter.*[11]
■ *To reduce the risk of peritonitis,* use strict sterile technique during the catheter insertion, dialysate exchanges, and dressing changes. Ensure all personnel and the patient wear masks in the room whenever the dialysis system is opened or entered.[11]
■ Monitor the patient's hemodynamic status. Note his fluid balance at the end of each infusion-dwell-drain cycle (the patient's fluid balance is positive if he retains fluid at the end of an exchange and negative if you recover more fluid than was instilled with the exchange). Notify the practitioner if the patient retains 500 mL or more of fluid for three consecutive cycles or if he loses 1 L of fluid for three consecutive cycles.
■ Weigh the patient daily using the same scale *to help determine how much fluid is being removed during dialysis treatment.*[11] Note the time and any variations in the weighing technique next to his weight on his chart.
■ If dialysate instillation or drainage is slow or absent, check all of the tubing for kinks. You can also try raising the IV pole or repositioning the patient *to increase the inflow rate.* Repositioning the patient or applying manual pressure to the lateral aspects of the patient's abdomen may also help increase drainage. If these maneuvers fail, notify the practitioner. The catheter may be improperly positioned or an accumulation of fibrin may obstruct the catheter.
■ Always examine the drained fluid from each exchange (effluent) for color and clarity. Normally, the fluid is clear or pale yellow, but pink-tinged effluent may appear during the first three or four cycles. If the effluent remains pink-tinged or if it's grossly bloody, suspect bleeding into the peritoneal cavity and notify the practitioner. Also notify the practitioner if the effluent contains feces, which suggests bowel perforation, or if it's cloudy, which suggests peritonitis. Obtain a specimen for culture and Gram stain. Send the specimen in a labeled specimen container to the laboratory with a laboratory request form.
■ Expect patient discomfort at the start of the procedure. If the patient experiences pain during the procedure, determine when it occurs, its quality and duration, and whether it radiates to other body parts, and notify the practitioner. Pain during infusion usually results from a dialysate that's too cool or acidic. Pain may also result from rapid instillation. Slowing the inflow rate may reduce the pain. Severe, diffuse pain with rebound tenderness and cloudy effluent may indicate peritoneal infection. Pain that radiates to the shoulder often results from air accumulation under the diaphragm. Severe, persistent perineal or rectal pain can result from improper catheter placement.
■ Remember that a patient undergoing peritoneal dialysis commonly requires a great deal of assistance in his daily care. *To minimize his discomfort,* perform daily care during a drain phase in the cycle, when the abdomen is less distended.
■ During and after dialysis, monitor the patient and assess his abdominal and respiratory status and response to treatment.
■ Monitor the patient's vital signs according to his condition and at an interval determined by your facility; *there's no evidence-based research to indicate best practice for frequency of vital signs assessment.*[20] Notify the practitioner of any abrupt changes in the patient's condition.
■ Monitor the patient's fluid and electrolyte status. Report unexpected results to the practitioner and administer fluids and electrolytes, as prescribed.
■ Check whether your facility has a clearly developed curriculum for peritoneal dialysis training.[14]
■ Support the patient with his potential alteration in body image and ability to live a satisfying lifestyle as a peritoneal dialysis patient. Encourage the patient and caregiver to build and use available support systems.[21,22]

Patient teaching

If the patient or a caregiver is to perform peritoneal dialysis in the home, begin teaching the purpose and indication for it; appropriate techniques for preparation, installation, and drainage of dialysate; and methods to troubleshoot complications. Ensure that the patient is aware of the importance of infection control, proper diet and hydration, routine care and maintenance of the catheter and insertion site, and compliance with the prescribed regimen. Review potential complications and instruct the patient or caregiver to immediately report cloudy effluent, abdominal pain, and fever and to save any drained, cloudy dialysate to bring to the dialysis clinic.[23] Give the patient contact information to report complications and additional educational information and resources as indicated.

Complications

Peritonitis, the most common complication, usually follows contamination of the dialysate, but it may develop if solution leaks from the catheter exit site and flows back into the catheter tract. Respiratory distress may result when dialysate in the peritoneal cavity increases pressure on the diaphragm, which decreases lung expansion.

Protein depletion may result from the diffusion of protein in the blood into the dialysate solution through the peritoneal membrane. As much as 14 g of protein may be lost daily—more in patients with peritonitis.

Constipation is a major cause of inflow-outflow problems and the patient may require laxatives or stool softeners.

Excessive fluid loss from the use of 4.25% solution can cause hypovolemia, hypotension, and shock. Excessive fluid retention may lead to blood volume expansion, hypertension, peripheral edema, and even pulmonary edema and heart failure.

Other possible complications include electrolyte imbalance and hyperglycemia, which can be identified by frequent blood tests.

Documentation

Record the amount of dialysate infused and drained, any medications added to the dialysate solution, and the color and character of the effluent. Record the patient's daily weight and fluid balance. Use a peritoneal dialysis flowchart to compute total fluid balance after each exchange. Note the patient's vital signs and tolerance of the treatment as well as other pertinent observations. Note any complications and nursing actions taken as well as home instruction provided.

REFERENCES

1 American Nephrology Nurses' Association. (2011). *Nephrology nursing: Scope and standards of practice* (7th ed.). Pitman, NJ: American Nephrology Nurses' Association.

2 National Kidney Foundation. (2006). "2006 Updates: Clinical practice guidelines and clinical practice recommendations: Hemodialysis adequacy, peritoneal dialysis adequacy, vascular access" [Online]. Accessed May 2015 via the Web at http://www2.kidney.org/professionals/kdoqi/pdf/12-50-0210_JAG_DCP_Guidelines-VA_Oct06_SectionC_ofC.pdf (Level VII)

3 Centers for Disease Control and Prevention. (2002). Guideline for hand hygiene in health-care settings: Recommendations of the Healthcare Infection Control Practices Advisory Committee and the HICPAC/SHEA/APIC/IDSA Hand Hygiene Task Force. *MMWR Recommendations and Reports, 51*(RR-16), 1–45. Accessed May 2015 via the Web at http://www.cdc.gov/mmwr/pdf/rr/rr5116.pdf (Level II)

4 World Health Organization. (2009). "WHO guidelines on hand hygiene in health care: First global patient safety challenge, clean care is safer care" [Online]. Accessed May 2015 via the Web at http://whqlibdoc.who.int/publications/2009/9789241597906_eng.pdf (Level IV)

5 The Joint Commission. (2015). Standard NPSG.07.01.01. *Comprehensive accreditation manual for hospitals: The official handbook.* Oakbrook Terrace, IL: The Joint Commission. (Level VII)

6 Centers for Medicare & Medicaid Services, Department of Health and Human Services. (2014). Condition of participation: Infection control. 42 C.F.R. § 482.42.

7 American Osteopathic Association. (2014). Standard 07.01.21. *Healthcare Facilities Accreditation Program: Accreditation requirements for acute care hospitals.* Chicago, IL: American Osteopathic Association. (Level VII)

8 The Joint Commission. (2015). Standard NPSG.01.01.01. *Comprehensive accreditation manual for hospitals: The official handbook.* Oakbrook Terrace, IL: The Joint Commission. (Level VII)

9 Centers for Medicare & Medicaid Services, Department of Health and Human Services. (2014). Condition of participation: Patient's rights. 42 C.F.R. § 482.13(c)(1).

10 American Osteopathic Association. (2014). Standard 15.01.16. *Healthcare Facilities Accreditation Program: Accreditation requirements for acute care hospitals.* Chicago, IL: American Osteopathic Association. (Level VII)

11 Lynn-McHale Wiegand, D. (Ed.). (2011). *AACN procedure manual for critical care* (6th ed.). St. Louis, MO: Saunders.

12 Siegel, J. D., et al. (2007). "2007 guideline for isolation precautions: Preventing transmission of infectious agents in healthcare settings" [Online]. Accessed May 2015 via the Web at http://www.cdc.gov/hicpac/pdf/isolation/Isolation2007.pdf (Level II)

13 American Osteopathic Association. (2014). Standard 07.01.10. *Healthcare Facilities Accreditation Program: Accreditation requirements for acute care hospitals.* Chicago, IL: American Osteopathic Association. (Level VII)

14 Piraino, B., et al. (2011). ISPD position statement on reducing the risks of peritoneal dialysis–related infections. *Peritoneal Dialysis International, 31,* 614–630. Accessed May 2015 via the Web at http://ispd.org/media/pdf/Perit_Dial_Int-2011-Piraino-614-30.pdf (Level VII)

15 U.S. Food and Drug Administration. (n.d.). "Look. Check. Connect. Safe medical device connections save lives" [Online]. Accessed May 2015 via the Web at http://www.fda.gov/downloads/MedicalDevices/Safety/AlertsandNotices/UCM134873.pdf

16 Occupational Safety and Health Administration. (n.d.). "Bloodborne pathogens, standard number 1910.1030" [Online]. Accessed May 2015 via the Web at http://www.osha.gov/pls/oshaweb/owadisp.show_document?p_table=STANDARDS&p_id=10051 (Level VII)

17 The Joint Commission. (2015). Standard RC.01.03.01. *Comprehensive accreditation manual for hospitals: The official handbook.* Oakbrook Terrace, IL: The Joint Commission. (Level VII)

18 Centers for Medicare & Medicaid Services, Department of Health and Human Services. (2014). Condition of participation: Medical record services. 42 C.F.R. § 482.24(b).

19 American Osteopathic Association. (2014). Standard 10.00.03. *Healthcare Facilities Accreditation Program: Accreditation requirements for acute care hospitals.* Chicago, IL: American Osteopathic Association. (Level VII)

20 American Society of PeriAnesthesia Nurses. (2012). *2012–2014 Perianesthesia nursing standards, practice recommendations and interpretive statements.* Cherry Hill, NJ: American Society of PeriAnesthesia Nurses. (Level VII)

21 Moore, R., & Teitelbaum, I. (2009). Preventing burnout in peritoneal dialysis patients. *Advances in Peritoneal Dialysis, 25,* 92–95. Accessed May 2015 via the Web at http://www.advancesinpd.com/adv09/308a-Moore-Final.pdf (Level V)

22 Burkart, J. M. Patient information: Peritoneal dialysis (beyond the basics). (2014). In: *UpToDate,* Golper, T. A., & Sheridan, A. M. (Eds.). Accessed May 2015 via the Web at http://www.uptodate.com/contents/search

23 Li, P. K., et al. (2010). ISPD guidelines/recommendations: Peritoneal dialysis-related infections. Recommendations: 2010 update. *Peritoneal Dialysis International, 30,* 393–423. Accessed May 2015 via the Web at http://www.pdiconnect.com/content/30/4/393.full.pdf+html (Level VII)

ADDITIONAL REFERENCES

Hagen, S. M., et al. (2014). A systematic review and meta-analysis of the influence of peritoneal catheter type on complication rate and catheter survival. *Kidney International, 85,* 920–932. (Level I)

Hinkle, J. L., & Cheever, K. H. (2014). *Brunner & Suddarth's textbook of medical-surgical nursing* (13th ed.). Philadelphia, PA: Wolters Kluwer.

Nettina, S. M. (2014). *Lippincott manual of nursing practice* (10th ed.). Philadelphia, PA: Wolters Kluwer.

PERITONEAL LAVAGE, ASSISTING

Peritoneal lavage may be used for both diagnostic and therapeutic purposes.[1] It's used mainly as a diagnostic tool in patients with blunt abdominal trauma to help detect bleeding in the peritoneal cavity. It's used therapeutically in patients with hypothermia to warm the abdominal cavity, in those with peritonitis or intra-abdominal abscess to provide irrigation, and in cancer patients to obtain cytology specimens.

The procedure may involve several steps. Initially, the practitioner inserts a catheter through the abdominal wall into the peritoneal cavity and aspirates the peritoneal fluid with a syringe. If he can't see blood in the aspirated fluid, he infuses a balanced saline solution and siphons the fluid from the cavity. He inspects the siphoned fluid for blood and also sends fluid samples to the laboratory for microscopic examination. When possible, the practitioner may have abdominal ultrasound performed before peritoneal lavage to assess fluid in the abdominal cavity, or during the procedure to assist with catheter placement.

The medical team maintains strict sterile technique throughout this procedure to avoid introducing microorganisms into the peritoneum and causing peritonitis. (See *Tapping the peritoneal cavity.*)

Peritoneal lavage is contraindicated in a patient who has had multiple abdominal surgeries, has an abdominal wall hematoma, is unstable and needs immediate surgery, has coagulopathies, or can't be catheterized before the procedure. The procedure requires great caution and a different technique if the patient is pregnant.

Equipment

Equipment for vital signs measurement ▪ indwelling urinary catheter insertion equipment ▪ nasogastric (NG) tube insertion equipment ▪

Tapping the peritoneal cavity

After preparing the patient's skin with an antiseptic solution and administering a local anesthetic *to numb the area near the patient's navel*, the surgeon will make a small incision (about 3/4″ [2 cm]) through the skin and subcutaneous tissues of the abdominal wall. He'll retract the tissue, ligate several blood vessels, and use sterile 4″ × 4″ (10-cm × 10-cm) gauze pads to absorb and keep incisional blood from entering the wound and producing a false-positive test result. Next, he'll direct the trocar through the incision into the pelvic midline until the instrument enters the peritoneum. Then he'll advance the peritoneal catheter (via the trocar) 6″ to 8″ (15 to 20 cm) into the pelvis.

Using a syringe attached to the catheter, the practitioner will aspirate fluid from the peritoneal cavity and look for blood or other abnormal findings.

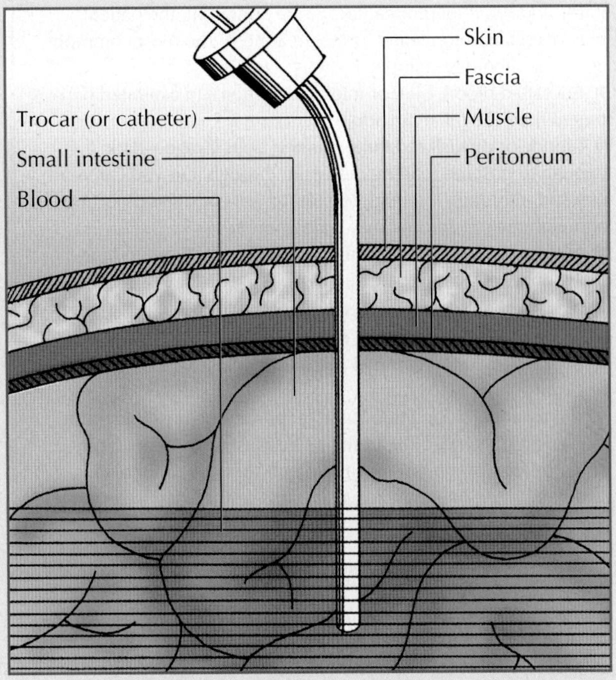

gastric suction machine ▪ hair clippers ▪ IV pole ▪ macrodrip IV tubing ▪ IV solutions (1 L of warmed, lactated Ringer's solution or normal saline solution) ▪ peritoneal dialysis tray ▪ gloves ▪ sterile gloves ▪ gowns ▪ masks and goggles or masks with face shields ▪ antiseptic solution (povidone-iodine or chlorhexidine) ▪ 3-mL syringe with 25G 1″ (2.5-cm) needle ▪ 1% lidocaine with epinephrine ▪ 8″ (20.3-cm) #14 intracatheter extension tubing and a small sterile hemostat (to clamp tubing) ▪ 30-mL syringe ▪ 20G 1½″ (3.8-cm) needle ▪ sterile towels ▪ three containers for specimen collection, including one sterile tube for a culture and sensitivity specimen ▪ labels ▪ sterile 4″ × 4″ (10-cm × 10-cm) gauze pads ▪ alcohol pads ▪ 1″ (2.5-cm) hypoallergenic tape ▪ 2-0 and 3-0 sutures ▪ laboratory biohazard transport bag ▪ Optional: prescribed analgesia or sedation, dressings and tape specially formulated for fragile skin.

If using a commercially prepared peritoneal dialysis kit (containing a #15 peritoneal dialysis catheter, trocar, and extension tubing with roller clamp), make sure the macrodrip IV tubing doesn't have a reverse-flow (or backcheck) valve that prevents infused fluid from draining out of the peritoneal cavity.

Preparation of equipment

Check the expiration date on each sterile package and inspect each for tears. Replace any items as needed.

Implementation

- Confirm that written informed consent is obtained and that the consent is in the patient's medical record.[2,3,4]
- Check the patient's medical history for allergies to medications or latex.
- Conduct a preprocedure verification *to make sure that all relevant documentation, related information, and equipment are available and correctly identified to the patient's identifiers.*[5,6]
- Verify that the laboratory and imaging studies have been completed as ordered and that the results are in the patient's medical record. Notify the practitioner of any abnormal results.
- Perform hand hygiene.[7,8,9,10,11]
- Confirm the patient's identity using at least two patient identifiers.[12]
- Provide privacy.[13,14]
- Reinforce the practitioner's explanation of the procedure, and answer the patient's questions.
- Confirm that the correct procedure has been identified for the correct patient at the correct site.[5]
- Obtain the patient's vital signs *to serve as a baseline for comparison during and after the procedure.*
- If family members remain present for the procedure, ask them to perform hand hygiene and to put on gowns, gloves, masks, and goggles.[15]
- Advise the patient to expect a sensation of abdominal fullness. Also inform him that he may experience a chill if the lavage solution isn't warmed or doesn't reach his body temperature.
- Insert an indwelling urinary catheter and attach it to a drainage bag, as ordered, *to decrease the risk of the practitioner accidentally perforating the bladder during the procedure.*
- Insert an NG tube, as ordered. (See the "Nasogastric tube insertion and removal" procedure, page 531.) Attach this tube to the gastric suction machine (set for low intermittent suction) *to drain the patient's stomach contents. Decompressing the stomach prevents vomiting and subsequent aspiration and minimizes the possibility of bowel perforation during trocar or catheter insertion.* Make sure an X-ray is obtained *to verify placement of the NG tube.*
- Clip the hair, as ordered, from the area between the patient's umbilicus and pubis.
- Set up the IV pole. Attach the macrodrip tubing to the lavage solution container, and clear air from the tubing *to avoid introducing air into the peritoneal cavity during lavage.*
- Place the patient in the supine position.[1]
- Administer analgesia or sedatives, if ordered and indicated, following safe medication administration practices.[16,17] *Analgesia or sedation may be indicated if the patient is in pain or agitated to facilitate patient comfort, safety, and cooperation.*

Interpreting peritoneal lavage results

If test findings in peritoneal lavage are abnormal, the patient may need laparotomy and further treatment. The most common abnormal findings include:

- unclotted blood, bile, or intestinal contents in aspirated peritoneal fluid (20 mL in an adult)
- bloody or pinkish red fluid returned from lavage—dark enough to obscure reading newsprint through it (if you can read newsprint through the fluid, test results are considered negative, although the practitioner may order more tests)
- green, cloudy, turbid, or milky peritoneal fluid return (normally appears clear to pale yellow)
- red blood cell count exceeding 100,000/mm^3
- white blood cell count exceeding 500/mm^3
- bacteria in fluid (identified by culture and sensitivity testing or Gram stain).

If the patient's condition is stable, borderline positive results may suggest the need for additional tests, such as echography and arteriography. If test results are questionable or inconclusive, the practitioner may leave the catheter in place to repeat the procedure.

- Put on a gown, a mask and goggles or a mask with face shield, and gloves *to comply with standard precautions.*[18,19,20]
- Using sterile technique, open the peritoneal dialysis tray. Label all medications, medication containers, and other solutions on and off the sterile field.[21,22]
- Help the practitioner put on personal protective equipment. The practitioner will prepare the patient's abdomen from the costal margin to the pubic area and from flank to flank with the antiseptic solution and allow it to dry. He'll drape the area with sterile towels from the dialysis tray *to create a sterile field.*
- Conduct a time-out immediately before starting the procedure *to perform a final assessment that the correct patient, site, positioning, and procedure are identified and, as applicable, that relevant information and necessary equipment are available.*[23]
- Using sterile technique, hand the practitioner the 3-mL syringe and the 25G 1″ (2.5-cm) needle. If the peritoneal dialysis tray doesn't contain a sterile ampule of anesthetic, disinfect the top of a multidose vial of 1% lidocaine with epinephrine with an alcohol pad and allow it to dry, and invert the vial at a 45-degree angle *to allow the practitioner to insert the needle and withdraw the anesthetic without touching the nonsterile vial.*
- The practitioner injects the anesthetic directly below the umbilicus (or at an adjacent site if the patient has a surgical scar). After the area is anesthetized, he makes an incision, inserts the catheter or trocar, withdraws fluid, and checks the findings. The fluid sample is then sent for laboratory analysis. If findings are positive, the procedure will end and you'll prepare the patient for laparotomy and further measures. Even if retrieved fluid looks normal, lavage will continue. (See *Interpreting peritoneal lavage results.*)
- Trace the catheter extension tubing to its point of origin;[24] connect it to the IV tubing, if ordered; and instill 700 to 1,000 mL (10 mL/kg body weight) of the warmed IV solution into the peritoneal cavity over 10 to 15 minutes. Then clamp the tubing with the hemostat.[1]
- Unless contraindicated by the patient's injuries (such as a spinal cord injury, fractured ribs, or unstable pelvic fracture), gently tilt the patient from side to side *to distribute the fluid throughout the peritoneal cavity.* If the patient's condition contraindicates tilting, the practitioner may gently palpate the sides of the abdomen *to distribute the fluid.*[1]
- After 5 to 10 minutes, place the IV container below the level of the patient's body, and open the clamp on the IV tubing. *Lowering the container helps excess fluid to drain.* Gently drain as much of the fluid as possible from the peritoneal cavity to the container. Be careful not to disconnect the tubing from the catheter. The peritoneal cavity may take 20 to 30 minutes to drain completely.
- *To obtain a fluid specimen,* while maintaining sterile technique, thoroughly disinfect the port on the IV tubing using an alcohol pad, and allow it to dry. Withdraw between 25 and 30 mL of fluid from a port in the IV tubing, using a 30-mL syringe. Disinfect the top of each specimen container with an alcohol pad and allow it to dry. Deposit fluid specimens in the containers for culture and sensitivity analysis, Gram stain, red and white blood cell counts, amylase and bile level determinations, and spun-down sediment evaluation. *Note:* If you didn't obtain the culture and sensitivity specimen first, change the needle before drawing this fluid sample *to avoid contaminating the specimen.*
- Label all the specimens in the presence of the patient *to prevent mislabeling*[12] and send them to the laboratory immediately in a laboratory biohazard transport bag.[20] With positive test results, the practitioner will usually perform a laparotomy. If test results are normal, the practitioner will close the incision with sutures.
- Remove and discard your gloves.[18,20]
- Perform hand hygiene.[7,8,9,10,11]
- Put on sterile gloves[18,20] and dress the incision with a sterile 4″ × 4″ (10-cm × 10-cm) gauze pad secured with 1″ (2.5-cm) hypoallergenic tape.

NURSING ALERT ***If the patient has fragile skin, use dressings and tape specially formulated for fragile skin* to prevent skin stripping and tearing during removal.**[25]

- Remove and discard your gloves and other personal protective equipment.[18,20]
- Perform hand hygiene.[7,8,9,10,11]
- Monitor vital signs according to the patient's condition and at an interval determined by your facility; *there's no evidence-based research to indicate best practice for frequency of vital signs assessment.*[26] Report signs and symptoms of shock (tachycardia, decreased blood pressure, diaphoresis, dyspnea or shortness of breath, and vertigo) immediately. Assess the incisional site frequently for bleeding.
- Perform a comprehensive pain assessment using techniques appropriate for the patient's age, condition, and ability to understand.[27] Administer pain medication, as needed and ordered, following safe medication administration practices.[16,17]
- Discard used supplies in the appropriate receptacle.[20]
- Return reusable equipment to the appropriate department for cleaning and sterilization.[28,29]
- Perform hand hygiene.[7,8,9,10,11]
- Document the procedure.[30,31,32]

Special considerations

- If the practitioner orders abdominal X-rays, they will probably precede peritoneal lavage. *X-ray films taken after lavage may be unreliable because of air introduced into the peritoneal cavity.*

Complications

Bleeding from lacerated blood vessels may occur at the incisional site or intra-abdominally. A visceral perforation causes peritonitis and requires laparotomy for repair. If the patient has respiratory distress, infusion of a balanced saline solution may cause additional stress and trigger respiratory arrest.

The bladder may be lacerated or punctured if it isn't emptied completely before peritoneal lavage. Infection may develop at the incision site without strict sterile technique.

Documentation

Record the type and size of the peritoneal dialysis catheter used, the type and amount of solution instilled and withdrawn from the peritoneal cavity, and the amount and color of fluid returned. Document whether the fluid flowed freely into and out of the abdomen. Note which specimens were obtained and sent to the laboratory. Document X-rays obtained and results. Also note any complications encountered and any nursing actions taken to handle them.

REFERENCES

1 Lynn-McHale Wiegand, D. (Ed.). (2011). *AACN procedure manual for critical care* (6th ed.). St. Louis, MO: Saunders.

2 The Joint Commission. (2015). Standard RI.01.03.01. *Comprehensive accreditation manual for hospitals: The official handbook.* Oakbrook Terrace, IL: The Joint Commission. (Level VII)

3 Centers for Medicare & Medicaid Services, Department of Health and Human Services. (2014). Condition of participation: Patient's rights. 42 C.F.R. § 482.13(b)(2).

4 American Osteopathic Association. (2014). Standard 15.01.11. *Healthcare Facilities Accreditation Program: Accreditation requirements for acute care hospitals.* Chicago, IL: American Osteopathic Association. (Level VII)

5 The Joint Commission. (2015). Standard UP.01.01.01. *Comprehensive accreditation manual for hospitals: The official handbook.* Oakbrook Terrace, IL: The Joint Commission. (Level VII)

6 American Osteopathic Association. (2014). Standard 30.00.14. *Healthcare Facilities Accreditation Program: Accreditation requirements for acute care hospitals.* Chicago, IL: American Osteopathic Association. (Level VII)

7 Centers for Disease Control and Prevention. (2002). Guideline for hand hygiene in health-care settings: Recommendations of the Healthcare Infection Control Practices Advisory Committee and the HICPAC/SHEA/APIC/IDSA Hand Hygiene Task Force. *MMWR Recommendations and Reports, 51*(RR-16), 1–45. Accessed May 2015 via the Web at http://www.cdc.gov/mmwr/pdf/rr/rr5116.pdf (Level II)

8 World Health Organization. (2009). "WHO guidelines on hand hygiene in health care: First global patient safety challenge, clean care is safer care" [Online]. Accessed May 2015 via the Web at http://whqlibdoc.who.int/publications/2009/9789241597906_eng.pdf (Level IV)

9 The Joint Commission. (2015). Standard NPSG.07.01.01. *Comprehensive accreditation manual for hospitals: The official handbook.* Oakbrook Terrace, IL: The Joint Commission. (Level VII)

10 Centers for Medicare & Medicaid Services, Department of Health and Human Services. (2014). Condition of participation: Infection control. 42 C.F.R. § 482.42.

11 American Osteopathic Association. (2014). Standard 07.01.21. *Healthcare Facilities Accreditation Program: Accreditation requirements for acute care hospitals.* Chicago, IL: American Osteopathic Association. (Level VII)

12 The Joint Commission. (2015). Standard NPSG.01.01.01. *Comprehensive accreditation manual for hospitals: The official handbook.* Oakbrook Terrace, IL: The Joint Commission. (Level VII)

13 Centers for Medicare & Medicaid Services, Department of Health and Human Services. (2014). Condition of participation: Patient's rights. 42 C.F.R. § 482.13(c)(1).

14 American Osteopathic Association. (2014). Standard 15.01.16. *Healthcare Facilities Accreditation Program: Accreditation requirements for acute care hospitals.* Chicago, IL: American Osteopathic Association. (Level VII)

15 American Association of Critical-Care Nurses. (2010). "AACN practice alert: Family presence during resuscitation and invasive procedures" [Online]. Accessed May 2015 via the Web at http://www.aacn.org/wd/practice/docs/practicealerts/family-presence-during-resuscitation-invasive-procedures.pdf (Level VII)

16 Centers for Medicare & Medicaid Services, Department of Health and Human Services. (2014). Condition of participation: Nursing services. 42 C.F.R. § 482.23(c).

17 American Osteopathic Association. (2014). Standard 16.01.03. *Healthcare Facilities Accreditation Program: Accreditation requirements for acute care hospitals.* Chicago, IL: American Osteopathic Association. (Level VII)

18 Siegel, J. D., et al. (2007). "2007 guideline for isolation precautions: Preventing transmission of infectious agents in healthcare settings" [Online]. Accessed May 2015 via the Web at http://www.cdc.gov/hicpac/pdf/isolation/Isolation2007.pdf (Level II)

19 American Osteopathic Association. (2014). Standard 07.01.10. *Healthcare Facilities Accreditation Program: Accreditation requirements for acute care hospitals.* Chicago, IL: American Osteopathic Association. (Level VII)

20 Occupational Safety and Health Administration. (n.d.). "Bloodborne pathogens, standard number 1910.1030" [Online]. Accessed May 2015 via the Web at http://www.osha.gov/pls/oshaweb/owadisp.show_document?p_table=STANDARDS&p_id=10051 (Level VII)

21 The Joint Commission. (2015). Standard NPSG.03.04.01. *Comprehensive accreditation manual for hospitals: The official handbook.* Oakbrook Terrace, IL: The Joint Commission. (Level VII)

22 American Osteopathic Association. (2014). Standard 25.01.27. *Healthcare Facilities Accreditation Program: Accreditation requirements for acute care hospitals.* Chicago, IL: American Osteopathic Association. (Level VII)

23 The Joint Commission. (2015). Standard UP.01.03.01. *Comprehensive accreditation manual for hospitals: The official handbook.* Oakbrook Terrace, IL: The Joint Commission. (Level VII)

24 U.S. Food and Drug Administration. (n.d.). "Look. Check. Connect. Safe medical device connections save lives" [Online]. Accessed May 2015 via the Web at http://www.fda.gov/downloads/MedicalDevices/Safety/AlertsandNotices/UCM134873.pdf

25 LeBlanc, K., et al. (2013). International skin tear advisory panel: A tool kit to aid in the prevention, assessment, and treatment of skin tears using a simplified classification system. Advances in Skin & Wound Care, 26, 459–476. (Level IV)

26 American Society of PeriAnesthesia Nurses. (2012). *2012-2014 Perianesthesia nursing standards, practices and interpretative statements.* Cherry Hill, NJ: American Society of PeriAnesthesia Nurses. (Level VII)

27 The Joint Commission. (2015). Standard PC.01.02.07. *Comprehensive accreditation manual for hospitals: The official handbook.* Oakbrook Terrace, IL: The Joint Commission. (Level VII)

28 Rutala, W. A., et al. (2008). "Guideline for disinfection and sterilization in healthcare facilities, 2008" [Online]. Accessed May 2015 via the Web at http://www.cdc.gov/hicpac/pdf/guidelines/Disinfection_Nov_2008.pdf (Level I)

29 American Osteopathic Association. (2014). Standard 07.02.03. *Healthcare Facilities Accreditation Program: Accreditation requirements for acute care hospitals.* Chicago, IL: American Osteopathic Association. (Level VII)

30 The Joint Commission. (2015). Standard RC.01.03.01. *Comprehensive accreditation manual for hospitals: The official handbook.* Oakbrook Terrace, IL: The Joint Commission. (Level VII)

31 Centers for Medicare & Medicaid Services, Department of Health and Human Services. (2014). Condition of participation: Medical record services. 42 C.F.R. § 482.24(b).

32 American Osteopathic Association. (2014). Standard 10.00.03. *Healthcare Facilities Accreditation Program: Accreditation requirements for acute care hospitals.* Chicago, IL: American Osteopathic Association. (Level VII)

ADDITIONAL REFERENCES

Jagminas, L. (2014). "Diagnostic peritoneal lavage" [Online]. Accessed May 2015 via the Web at http://emedicine.medscape.com/article82888-overview

Mezhir, J. J., et al. (2013). Prospective clinical trial of diagnostic peritoneal cytology in patients with a gastric cancer. *Journal of Surgical Oncology, 107,* 794–798. (Level IV)

PERMANENT PACEMAKER CARE

Designed to operate for 3 to 20 years, a permanent pacemaker is a self-contained device that provides electrical stimulation to the myocardium. The surgeon implants the pacemaker in a pocket beneath the patient's skin. This procedure is usually done in the operating room or cardiac catheterization laboratory. Nursing responsibilities involve monitoring the electrocardiogram (ECG) and maintaining sterile technique.

Understanding pacemaker codes

A permanent pacemaker's three-letter (or sometimes five-letter) code simply refers to how it's programmed. The first letter represents the chamber that is paced; the second letter, the chamber that is sensed; and the third letter, how the pulse generator responds. The fourth letter describes rate modulation, and the fifth letter specifies the location or absence of multisite pacing. Typically, only the first three letters are shown.

First letter	Second letter	Third letter
A = atrium V = ventricle D = dual (both chambers) O = not applicable S = single	A = atrium V = ventricle D = dual (both chambers) O = not applicable S = single	I = inhibited T = triggered D = dual (inhibited and triggered) O = not applicable

Fourth letter	Fifth letter
R = rate modulation—a sensor adjusts the programmed heart rate in response to patient activity. O = none	O = none A = atrium or atria V = ventricle or ventricles D = dual site

Examples of two common programming codes:

DDD
Pace: atrium and ventricle
Sense: atrium and ventricle
Response: inhibited and triggered
This is a fully automatic, or universal, pacemaker.

VVI
Pace: ventricle
Sense: ventricle
Response: inhibited
This is a demand pacemaker, inhibited.

Permanent pacemakers function in the demand mode, allowing the patient's heart to beat on its own but preventing it from falling below a preset rate. Pacing electrodes can be placed in the atria, the ventricles, or both chambers (atrioventricular [AV] sequential, dual chamber). (See *Understanding pacemaker codes.*) The most common pacing codes are VVI for single-chamber pacing and DDD for dual-chamber pacing.

Candidates for permanent pacemakers include patients with symptomatic sinus node dysfunction, acquired AV block, chronic bifascicular block, persistent AV block after the acute phase of myocardial infarction, hypersensitive carotid sinus syndrome, neurocardiogenic syncope, bradycardia or syncope after cardiac transplantation, detection and determination of symptomatic recurrent supraventricular tachycardia, hypertrophic cardiomyopathy with sinus node dysfunction or AV block, and congenital heart disease.[1]

A biventricular pacemaker is effective in patients with heart failure who have intraventricular conductor defects. This device differs from a standard pacemaker in that it has three leads instead of one or two. One lead is placed in the right atrium and the others are placed in each of the ventricles, where they simultaneously stimulate the right and left ventricle. This allows the ventricles to coordinate their pumping action, making the heart more efficient.

Equipment

Patient's medical record ■ sphygmomanometer or electronic blood pressure machine ■ stethoscope ■ pulse oximeter and probe ■ ECG monitor and recorder ■ gloves ■ clippers ■ sterile gauze dressing ■ hypoallergenic tape ■ IV catheter insertion equipment ■ IV fluid ■ hospital-grade disinfectant pads ■ prescribed antibiotics ■ prescribed sedation ■ programmer specific to the selected pacemaker device ■ backup pacing, defibrillation, and resuscitation equipment[2] ■ Optional: prescribed analgesic, prescribed antiseptic ointment, pacemaker literature for patient teaching.

Preparation of equipment

Ensure that backup pacing, defibrillation, and resuscitation equipment are readily available *in the event of pacemaker failure.*[2]

Implementation

Preoperative care

- Verify the practitioner's order.
- Perform hand hygiene.[3,4,5,6,7]
- Confirm the patient's identity using at least two patient identifiers.[8]
- Explain the procedure to the patient. Provide and review literature from the manufacturer or from the American Heart Association *so that the patient can learn about the pacemaker and how it works.* Emphasize that the pacemaker merely augments his natural heart rate.
- Confirm that written informed consent has been obtained and that the consent is in the patient's medical record.[9,10,11]
- Ask the patient whether he's allergic to anesthetics or iodine.
- Conduct a preprocedure verification process *to make sure that all relevant documentation, related information, and equipment are available and correctly identified to the patient's identifiers.*[12,13]
- Verify that laboratory and imaging studies are complete, as ordered, and that the results are in the patient's medical record. Notify the practitioner of any unexpected results.[12]
- Perform hand hygiene[3,4,5,6,7] and put on gloves.[14,15]
- For pacemaker insertion, use clippers to remove chest hair from the axilla to the midline and from the clavicle to the nipple line on the side selected by the surgeon, if necessary.
- Insert an IV catheter and begin infusing IV fluid at the ordered rate. (See the "IV catheter insertion and removal" procedure, page 446.)
- Obtain vital signs, oxygen saturation level,[16] and an ECG *to serve as a baseline for comparison during and after the procedure.*
- Confirm the patient's nothing-by-mouth status before the procedure; minimum fasting recommendations include 2 hours for clear liquids, 4 hours for breast milk, 6 hours for infant formula, 6 or more hours for

a light meal or nonhuman milk, and 8 hours or more for fried or fatty foods or meat.[17]

- Administer antibiotics, as ordered, following safe medication administration practices.[18,19,20,21]
- Administer sedation, as ordered, following safe medication administration practices.[19,20,21]
- Discard all used supplies appropriately.[14,15]
- Remove and discard your gloves[14,15] and perform hand hygiene.[3,4,5,6,7]
- Disinfect your stethoscope using a disinfectant pad.[22]
- Perform hand hygiene.[3,4,5,6,7]
- Provide handoff communication to the health care team member who will be assuming care of the patient during the procedure; allow the opportunity to ask questions.[23,24]
- Document the procedure.[25,26,27]

Postoperative care

- Perform hand hygiene[3,4,5,6,7] and put on gloves.[14,15]
- Confirm the patient's identity using at least two patient identifiers.[8]
- Verify and document the pacemaker settings and parameters.[28]
- Monitor the patient's ECG *to check for arrhythmias and to ensure correct pacemaker functioning.*[29]
- Monitor for pacemaker malfunction, such as pulse generator failure, failure to sense, failure to capture, or decreased cardiac output.
- Obtain a chest X-ray *to verify lead placement and to check for lead fragmentation, dislodgment of the generator leads, or heart enlargement.*[30]
- Obtain a 12-lead ECG, if ordered.
- Monitor the IV flow rate; the IV catheter is usually kept in place for 24 to 48 hours postoperatively *to allow for possible treatment of arrhythmias.*
- Inspect the dressing for signs of bleeding, and regularly assess the incision site for signs of infection (swelling, redness, or exudate).[31,32,33]
- Change the dressing and apply antiseptic ointment to the incision line, as ordered.[28] If the dressing becomes soiled or the site is exposed to air, change the dressing immediately.
- Monitor the patient's vital signs as required by the patient's condition and your facility; *there's no evidence-based research to indicate best practice for frequency of vital signs assessment.*[34]
- Monitor the patient's level of consciousness, cardiac status, and respiratory status, as required by your facility and the patient's condition.

ELDER ALERT ***Confused elderly patients with second-degree heart block won't show immediate improvement in level of consciousness.***

- Perform a comprehensive pain assessment using techniques appropriate for the patient's age, condition, and ability to understand.[35] Administer an analgesic, as ordered and indicated.[19,20,21]
- Discard all used supplies appropriately.[14,15]
- Remove and discard your gloves[14,15] and perform hand hygiene.[3,4,5]
- Disinfect your stethoscope using a disinfectant pad.[22,36]
- Perform hand hygiene.[3,4,5,6,7]
- Document the procedure.[25,26,27]

Special considerations

- Electronic interference may occur with implanted devices; take the necessary precautions *to prevent interference.*

Patient teaching

Teach the patient and family about pacemaker precautions and care. Tell them to report syncope or near syncope, muscle twitching over the pacemaker site, frequent hiccups, a pulse rate lower than the pacemaker's lowest preset limit, and any redness, pain, swelling, or discharge from incision sites or over the pacemaker pocket. Tell them that if they aren't able to palpate the pacemaker at the insertion site, then the pacemaker may have migrated and follow-up medical care is necessary.

Instruct the patient to avoid close contact with machinery and to avoid placing cellular devices directly over the pacemaker because of electromagnetic interference. Explain that pacemakers require regular follow-up care to assess battery and pacemaker function.[29] The practitioner can perform assessments during follow-up visits or through transtelephonic monitoring. (See *Teaching the patient who has a permanent pacemaker,* page 620.)

Provide the patient with an identification card that lists the pacemaker type and manufacturer, serial number, pacemaker rate setting, date implanted, and the practitioner's name; tell him he should carry the card with him at all times.

Complications

NURSING ALERT *Watch for signs and symptoms of a perforated ventricle, with resultant cardiac tamponade: persistent hiccups, distant heart sounds, pulsus paradoxus, hypotension with narrow pulse pressure, increased venous pressure, cyanosis, distended jugular veins, decreased urine output, restlessness, or complaints of fullness in the chest. If the patient develops any of these, notify the practitioner immediately.*

Insertion of a permanent pacemaker also places the patient at risk for infection, lead displacement, or a lead fracture and disconnection.[37]

Documentation

Document the type of pacemaker used, the serial number and the manufacturer's name, the pacing rate, the date of implantation, and the surgeon's name. Note whether the pacemaker successfully treated the patient's arrhythmias and the condition of the incision site. Document the patient's vital signs, cardiac status, respiratory status, and ECG results.

REFERENCES

1 Tracy, C. M., et al. (2012). 2012 ACCF/AHA/HRS focused update of the 2008 guidelines for device-based therapy of cardiac rhythm abnormalities: A report of the American College of Cardiology Foundation/American Heart Association Task Force on Practice Guidelines and the Heart Rhythm Society. *Circulation, 126,* 1784–1800. Accessed May 2015 via the Web at http://circ.ahajournals.org/content/126/14/1784.full.pdf+html (Level VII)

2 American Society of Anesthesiologists Task Force on Perioperative Management of Patients with Cardiac Implanted Electronic Devices. (2011). Practice advisory for the perioperative management of patients with cardiac implanted electronic devices. *Anesthesiology, 114,* 247–261. Accessed May 2015 via the Web at http://www.guideline.gov/content.aspx?id=34403 (Level VII)

3 Centers for Disease Control and Prevention. (2002). Guideline for hand hygiene in health-care settings: Recommendations of the Healthcare Infection Control Practices Advisory Committee and the HICPAC/SHEA/APIC/IDSA Hand Hygiene Task Force. *MMWR Recommendations and Reports, 51*(RR-16), 1–45. Accessed May 2015 via the Web at http://www.cdc.gov/mmwr/pdf/rr/rr5116.pdf (Level II)

4 The Joint Commission. (2015). Standard NPSG.07.01.01. *Comprehensive accreditation manual for hospitals: The official handbook.* Oakbrook Terrace, IL: The Joint Commission. (Level VII)

5 World Health Organization. (2009). "WHO guidelines on hand hygiene in health care: First global patient safety challenge, clean care is safer care" [Online]. Accessed May 2015 via the Web at http://whqlibdoc.who.int/publications/2009/9789241597906_eng.pdf (Level IV)

6 American Osteopathic Association. (2014). Standard 07.01.10. *Healthcare Facilities Accreditation Program: Accreditation requirements for acute care hospitals.* Chicago, IL: American Osteopathic Association. (Level VII)

7 Centers for Medicare & Medicaid Services, Department of Health and Human Services. (2014). Condition of participation: Infection Control. 42 C.F.R. § 482.42

8 The Joint Commission. (2015). Standard NPSG.01.01.01. *Comprehensive accreditation manual for hospitals: The official handbook.* Oakbrook Terrace, IL: The Joint Commission. (Level VII)

PATIENT TEACHING

Teaching the patient who has a permanent pacemaker

If your patient is going home with a permanent pacemaker, teach him about daily care, safety and activity guidelines, and other precautions.

Daily care

- Clean your pacemaker site gently with soap and water when you take a shower or a bath. Leave the incision exposed to the air.
- Inspect your skin around the incision. A slight bulge is normal, but call your practitioner if you feel discomfort or notice swelling, redness, a discharge, or other problems.[18]
- Check your pulse for 1 minute as your nurse or practitioner showed you—on the side of your neck, inside your elbow, or on the thumb side of your wrist. Your pulse rate should be the same as your pacemaker rate or faster. Contact your practitioner if you think your heart is beating too fast or too slow.
- Take your medications, including those for pain, as prescribed. Even with a pacemaker, you still need the medication that your practitioner ordered.

Safety and activity

- Keep your pacemaker instruction booklet handy, and carry your pacemaker identification card at all times. This card has your pacemaker model number and other information needed by health care personnel who treat you.
- You can resume most of your usual activities when you feel comfortable doing so, but don't drive until the practitioner gives you permission. Also avoid heavy lifting and stretching exercises for at least 6 weeks or as directed by your practitioner.
- Use both arms equally to prevent stiffness. Check with your practitioner before you golf, swim, play tennis, or perform other strenuous activities.

Electromagnetic interference

- Today's pacemakers are designed and insulated to eliminate most electrical interference. You can safely operate common household electrical devices, including microwave ovens, razors, and sewing machines. And you can ride in or operate a motor vehicle without it affecting your pacemaker.
- Take care to avoid direct contact with large running motors, high-powered CB radios and other similar equipment, welding machinery, and radar devices.
- If your pacemaker activates the metal detector in an airport, show your pacemaker identification card to the security official.
- Because the metal in your pacemaker makes you ineligible for certain diagnostic studies, such as magnetic resonance imaging, be sure to inform your practitioners, dentist, and other health care personnel that you have a pacemaker.

Special precautions

- If you feel light-headed or dizzy when you're near any electrical equipment, moving away from the device should restore normal pacemaker function. Ask your practitioner about particular electrical devices.
- Notify your practitioner if you experience any signs or symptoms of pacemaker failure, such as palpitations, a fast heart rate, a slow heart rate (5 to 10 beats less than the pacemaker's setting), dizziness, fainting, shortness of breath, swollen ankles or feet, anxiety, forgetfulness, or confusion.
- If you feel like you're going to faint, immediately call 911 and lie down to prevent falling.

Checkups

- Be sure to schedule a follow-up visit, and keep regular checkup appointments with your practitioner.
- If your practitioner monitors your pacemaker status remotely by wireless telemetry, keep your transmission schedule and instructions handy.[1]

9 The Joint Commission. (2014). Standard RI.01.03.01. *Comprehensive accreditation manual for hospitals: The official handbook.* Oakbrook Terrace, IL: The Joint Commission. (Level VII)

10 Centers for Medicare & Medicaid Services, Department of Health and Human Services. (2014). Condition of participation: Patients' rights. 42 C. F. R. § 482.13.

11 American Osteopathic Association. (2014). Standard 30.01.11. *Healthcare Facilities Accreditation Program: Accreditation requirements for acute care hospitals.* Chicago, IL: American Osteopathic Association. (Level VII)

12 The Joint Commission. (2015). Standard UP.01.01.01. *Comprehensive accreditation manual for hospitals: The official handbook.* Oakbrook Terrace, IL: The Joint Commission. (Level VII)

13 American Osteopathic Association. (2014). Standard 30.00.14. *Healthcare Facilities Accreditation Program: Accreditation requirements for acute care hospitals.* Chicago, IL: American Osteopathic Association. (Level VII)

14 Siegel, J. D., et al. (2007). "2007 guideline for isolation precautions: Preventing transmission of infectious agents in healthcare settings" [Online]. Accessed May 2015 via the Web at http://www.cdc.gov/hicpac/pdf/isolation/Isolation2007.pdf (Level II)

15 Occupational Safety and Health Administration. (n.d.). "Bloodborne pathogens, standard number 1910.1030." [Online]. Accessed May 2015 via the Web at http://www.osha.gov/pls/oshaweb/owadisp.show_document?p_table=STANDARDS&p_id=10051 (Level VII)

16 American Society of Anesthesiologists Task Force on Sedation and Analgesia by Non-Anesthesiologists. (2002). Practice guidelines for sedation and analgesia by non-anesthesiologists. *Anesthesiology, 96,* 1004–1017. (Level VII)

17 American Society of Anesthesiologists. (2011). Practice guidelines for preoperative fasting and the use of pharmacologic agents to reduce the risk of pulmonary aspiration: Application to healthy patients undergoing elective procedures. *Anesthesiology, 114*(3), 495-511. (Level VII)

18 Baddour, L. M., et al. (2010). Update on cardiovascular implantable electronic device infections and their management: A scientific statement from the American Heart Association. *Circulation, 121,* 458–477. (Level VII)

19 American Osteopathic Association. (2014). Standard 16.01.03. *Healthcare Facilities Accreditation Program: Accreditation requirements for acute care hospitals.* Chicago, IL: American Osteopathic Association. (Level VII)

20 The Joint Commission. (2015). Standard MM.06.01.01. *Comprehensive accreditation manual for hospitals: The official handbook.* Oakbrook Terrace, IL: The Joint Commission. (Level VII)

21 Centers for Medicare & Medicaid Services, Department of Health and Human Services. (2014). Condition of participation: Nursing services. 42 C.F.R. § 482.23(c).

22 Rutala, W. A., et al. (2008). "Guideline for disinfection and sterilization in healthcare facilities, 2008" [Online]. Accessed May 2015 via the Web at http://www.cdc.gov/hicpac/pdf/guidelines/Disinfection_Nov_2008.pdf (Level I)

23 The Joint Commission. (2015). Standard PC.02.02.01. *Comprehensive accreditation manual for hospitals: The official handbook.* Oakbrook Terrace, IL: The Joint Commission. (Level VII)

24 Joint Commission Center for Transforming Healthcare. (2010). "Improving transitions of care: Hand-off communications" [Online]. Accessed May 2015 via the Web at http://www.centerfortransforminghealthcare.org/assets/4/6/CTH_Hand-off_commun_set_final_2010.pdf (Level V)

25 The Joint Commission. (2015). Standard RC.01.03.01. *Comprehensive accreditation manual for hospitals: The official handbook.* Oakbrook Terrace, IL: The Joint Commission. (Level VII)

26 American Osteopathic Association. (2014). Standard 10.00.03. *Healthcare Facilities Accreditation Program: Accreditation requirements for acute care hospitals.* Chicago, IL: American Osteopathic Association. (Level VII)

27 Centers for Medicare & Medicaid Services, Department of Health and Human Services. (2014). Condition of participation: Medical record services. 42 C.F.R. § 482.24(b).

28 Ellenbogen, K. A., et al. (2011). *Clinical cardiac pacing, defibrillation, and resynchronization therapy* (4th ed.). St. Louis, MO: Saunders.

29 Lynn-McHale Wiegand, D. (Ed.). (2011). *AACN procedure manual for critical care* (6th ed.). St. Louis, MO: Saunders.

30 Dissman, R., et al. (2013). Double left ventricular pacing following accidental malpositioning of the right ventricular electrode during implantation of a cardiac resynchronization therapy device. *Journal of Cardiothoracic Surgery, 8,* 162. Accessed May 2015 via the Web at http://www.cardiothoracicsurgery.org/content/pdf/1749-8090-8-162.pdf

31 The Joint Commission. (2015). Standard NPSG.07.05.01. *Comprehensive accreditation manual for hospitals: The official handbook.* Oakbrook Terrace, IL: The Joint Commission. (Level VII)

32 Centers for Medicare & Medicaid Services, & The Joint Commission. (2014). "The specifications manual for national hospital inpatient quality measures (version 4.3a)" [Online]. Accessed May 2015 via the Web at http://www.qualitynet.org/dcs/ContentServer?c=Page&pagename=QnetPublic%2FPage%2FQnetTier4&cid=1228773564870

33 Centers for Medicare & Medicaid Services, Department of Health and Human Services. (2012). "Hospital-acquired conditions" [Online]. Accessed May 2015 via the Web at http://www.cms.gov/Medicare/Medicare-Fee-for-Service-Payment/HospitalAcqCond/Hospital-Acquired_Conditions.html

34 American Society of PeriAnesthesia Nurses. (2012). *2012–2014 Perianesthesia nursing standards, practice recommendations and interpretive statements.* Cherry Hill, NJ: American Society of PeriAnesthesia Nurses.

35 The Joint Commission. (2015). Standard PC.01.02.07. *Comprehensive accreditation manual for hospitals: The official handbook.* Oakbrook Terrace, IL: The Joint Commission. (Level VII)

36 American Osteopathic Association. (2014). Standard 07.02.03. *Healthcare Facilities Accreditation Program: Accreditation requirements for acute care hospitals.* Chicago, IL: American Osteopathic Association. (Level VII)

37 Gillis, A. M., et al. (2012). HRS/ACCF expert consensus statement on pacemaker device and mode selection. *Heart Rhythm, 9,* 1344–1365. Accessed May 2015 via the Web at http://www.guideline.gov/content.aspx?id=39248 (Level VII)

PERSONAL PROTECTIVE EQUIPMENT

Isolation precautions may be implemented to prevent the spread of infection from patient to patient, from patients to health care workers, or from health care workers to patients.[1,2,3] Central to the success of these procedures is the selection of the proper personal protective equipment and adequate training of those who use it.

Equipment

Materials required for isolation typically include personal protective equipment, an isolation cart or anteroom for storing equipment, and a door card or sign alerting staff members and others entering the room that isolation precautions are in effect.

Personal protective equipment

Fluid-resistant gowns ▪ gloves ▪ goggles or face shield ▪ masks or respirator (each staff member must be trained in their proper use).

Preparation of equipment

Remove the cover from the isolation cart if necessary, and set up the work area. Check the cart or anteroom *to make sure an adequate amount of the proper isolation supplies are available for the designated isolation category.*

Implementation

- Remove your watch (or push it well up on your arm) and your rings if required by your facility. *These actions help to prevent the spread of microorganisms hidden under your watch or rings.*
- Perform hand hygiene.[4,5,6,7,8]
- Pick up the gown and allow it to unfold in front of you without touching areas of your body that may be contaminated *to minimize the transmission of microorganisms.* Put on the gown and wrap it around the back of your uniform, making sure it overlaps and completely covers your uniform *to prevent contact with the patient or his environment.*[9] Tie the strings or fasten the snaps or pressure-sensitive tabs at the neck. Then tie the waist strings.
- Place the mask snugly over your nose and mouth. Secure the ear loops around your ears or tie the strings at the middle of the back of your head and neck *so the mask won't slip off.* If the mask has a metal strip, squeeze it to fit your nose firmly but comfortably.[9] (See *Putting on a face mask,* page 622.) If you wear eyeglasses, tuck the upper edge of the mask under the lower edge of the glasses.
- Choose eye protection according to your risk of exposure. Although goggles provide eye protection, they don't protect the rest of the face from splashing of potentially infectious substances. Wear a face shield for any procedures that may involve spraying or splashing of respiratory secretions or other body fluids.[9]
- Select gloves according to your hand size *to make sure they fit securely.* Put on the gloves and pull them over the cuffs of your gown *to cover the edges of the gown's sleeves.*[9]

Special considerations

- If airborne precautions are required, an N95 or higher level particulate respirator approved by the Occupational Safety and Health Administration should be worn rather than a surgical mask.[9,10] (See the "Airborne precautions" procedure, page 10.) Employees who wear respirators must be properly fit-tested initially, and then periodically thereafter according to federal, state, and local regulations.[11]
- Always perform hand hygiene before putting on gloves *to avoid contaminating the gloves with microorganisms from your hands.*[4,5,6,7,8]
- Use gloves only once.[9] Be aware that isolation garb loses its effectiveness when wet *because moisture permits organisms to seep through the material.* Change masks and gowns as soon as moisture is noticeable or according to the manufacturer's recommendations or your facility's guidelines.[12]
- Keep isolation supplies stocked *so they're readily available for those who must enter the patient's room.*

Documentation

None needed.

REFERENCES

1 The Joint Commission. (2015). Standard IC.02.01.01. *Comprehensive accreditation manual for hospitals: The official handbook.* Oakbrook Terrace, IL: The Joint Commission. (Level VII)

2 Centers for Medicare & Medicaid Services, Department of Health and Human Services. (2014). Condition of participation: Patient's rights. 42 C.F.R. § 482.13(b)(2).

3 American Osteopathic Association. (2014). Standard 07.01.10. *Healthcare Facilities Accreditation Program: Accreditation requirements for acute care hospitals.* Chicago, IL: American Osteopathic Association. (Level VII)

4 The Joint Commission. (2015). Standard NPSG.07.01.01. *Comprehensive accreditation manual for hospitals: The official handbook.* Oakbrook Terrace, IL: The Joint Commission. (Level VII)

5 Centers for Disease Control and Prevention. (2002). Guideline for hand hygiene in health-care settings: Recommendations of the Healthcare Infection Control Practices Advisory Committee and the HICPAC/SHEA/APIC/IDSA Hand Hygiene Task Force. *MMWR Recommenda-*

Putting on a face mask

To avoid spreading airborne particles, wear a face mask. Position the mask to cover your nose and mouth, and secure it high enough *to ensure stability*. Tie the top strings at the back of your head above the ears. Then tie the bottom strings at the base of your neck. Alternatively, if the mask has ear loops, secure them around your ears.[9]

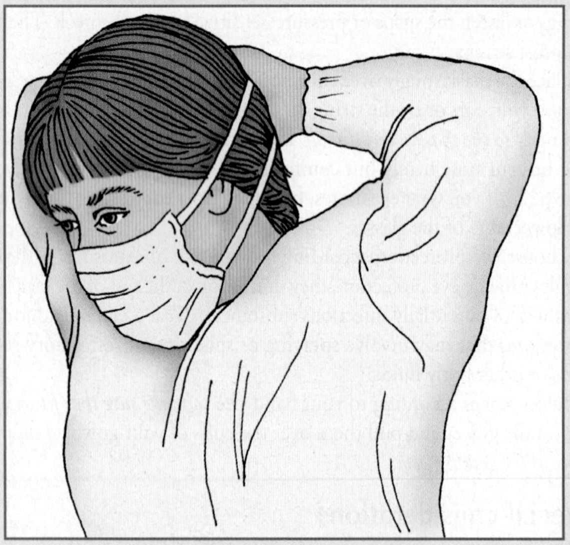

Adjust the metal nose strip if the mask has one.[9]

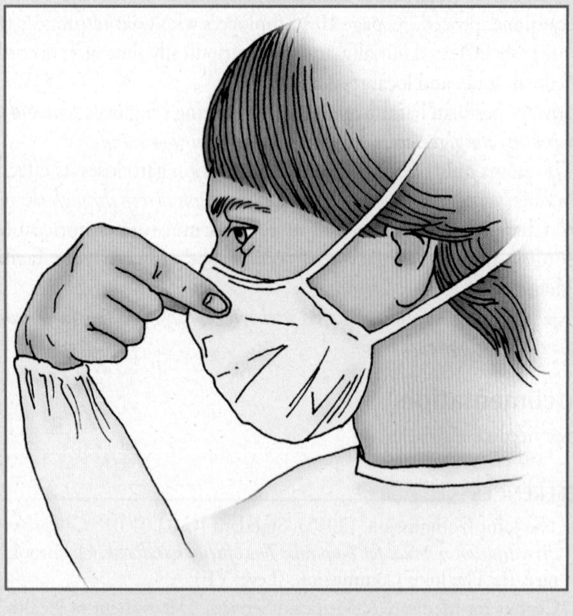

tions and Reports, 51(RR-16), 1–45. Accessed May 2015 via the Web at http://www.cdc.gov/mmwr/pdf/rr/rr5116.pdf (Level II)

6 World Health Organization. (2009). "WHO guidelines on hand hygiene in health care: First global patient safety challenge, clean care is safer care" [Online]. Accessed May 2015 via the Web at http://whqlibdoc.who.int/publications/2009/9789241597906_eng.pdf (Level IV)

7 American Osteopathic Association (2014). Standard 07.01.21. *Healthcare Facilities Accreditation Program: Accreditation requirements for acute care hospitals.* Chicago, IL: American Osteopathic Association. (Level VII)

8 Centers for Medicare & Medicaid Services, Department of Health and Human Services. (2014). Condition of participation: Infection control. 42 C.F.R. § 482.42.

9 Siegel, J. D., et al. (2007). "2007 guideline for isolation precautions: Preventing transmission of infectious agents in healthcare settings" [Online]. Accessed May 2015 via the Web at http://www.cdc.gov/hicpac/pdf/isolation/Isolation2007.pdf (Level II)

10 Occupational Safety and Health Administration. (n.d.). "Respiratory protection, standard number 1910.134" [Online]. Accessed May 2015 via the Web at http://www.osha.gov/pls/oshaweb/owadisp.show_document?p_table=STANDARDS&p_id=12716 (Level VII)

11 Jensen, P., et al. (2005). Guidelines for preventing the transmission of *Mycobacterium tuberculosis* in health-care settings, 2005. *MMWR Recommendations and Reports, 54*(RR-17), 1–141. Accessed May 2015 via the Web at http://www.cdc.gov/mmwr/pdf/rr/rr5417.pdf (Level II)

12 Occupational Health and Safety Administration. (n.d.). "Bloodborne pathogens, standard number 1910.1030" [Online]. Accessed May 2015 via the Web at http://www.osha.gov/pls/oshaweb/owadisp.show_document?p_table=STANDARDS&p_id=10051 (Level VII)

POSTMORTEM CARE

After a patient dies, care includes preparing the body for family viewing, arranging transportation to the morgue or funeral home, and determining the disposition of the patient's belongings. In addition, postmortem care entails comforting and supporting the patient's family and friends and providing for their privacy. Postmortem care usually begins after a practitioner certifies the patient's death. If the patient died violently or under suspicious circumstances, postmortem care may be postponed until the medical examiner completes an autopsy.

Equipment

Gauze or soft string ties ■ gloves ■ chin straps ■ abdominal pads ■ cotton balls ■ plastic shroud or body wrap ■ three identification tags ■ adhesive bandages ■ plastic bag ■ water-filled basin ■ soap ■ towels ■ washcloths ■ stretcher ■ Optional: tape, personal protective equipment, written patient information on the processes that are followed after death.

A commercial morgue pack usually contains gauze or string ties, chin straps, a shroud, and identification tags.

Implementation

- Notify the appropriate facility personnel, such as the nursing supervisor, that the patient has been pronounced dead.
- Notify the clergyperson or social worker, as needed, *to assist the family.*
- Notify the local organ procurement agency of the patient's death, as indicated.[2,3]
- Provide privacy and maintain patient dignity.[1,4]
- Offer age-appropriate support to family members who are present.[1]
- Put on gloves and other personal protective equipment as needed *to comply with standard precautions,* or maintain isolation precautions if they were being used. Offer personal protective equipment to other staff and family members as required *to ensure the health and safety of all people coming in contact with the body.*[1,5,6]
- Place the body in the supine position, with the arms at the sides and the head on a pillow. Then elevate the head of the bed 30 degrees *to prevent discoloration from blood settling in the face.*
- If the patient wore dentures, gently insert them; then close the mouth.
- Close the eyes by gently pressing on the lids with your fingertips. If they don't stay closed, place moist cotton balls on the eyelids for a few minutes, and then try again to close them.
- Place a folded towel under the chin *to keep the jaw closed.*
- Remove any tape, catheters, and any other tubes that the patient has in place if an autopsy isn't being performed; if an autopsy is required, keep them in place, as indicated.

■ Apply adhesive bandages to all puncture sites and replace soiled dressings.
■ Ask the family if they would prefer to leave the patient's jewelry on the body and collect all the patient's valuables *to prevent loss.* If you're unable to remove a ring, cover it with gauze, tape it in place, and tie the gauze to the wrist *to prevent slippage and subsequent loss.*
■ If family members wish to remain with and assist with caring for the body or perform after-death rituals because of ethnic, religious, or cultural requirements, allow them to do so.[1,7]
■ Clean the body thoroughly, using soap, a water-filled basin, and washcloths.
■ Place one or more abdominal pads between the buttocks *to absorb rectal discharge or drainage.*
■ Cover the body up to the chin with a clean sheet.
■ Offer comfort and emotional support to the family and intimate friends. Ask if they wish to see the patient. If they do, allow them to do so in privacy.
■ After the family leaves, remove the towel from under the chin of the deceased patient. Pad the chin, and wrap chin straps under the chin and tie them loosely on top of the head. Then, pad the wrists and ankles *to prevent bruises,* and tie them together with gauze or soft string ties.
■ Fill out the three identification tags. Each tag should include the deceased patient's name, room and bed numbers, date and time of death, and the practitioner's name. Tie one tag to the deceased patient's hand or foot, but don't remove his identification bracelet *to ensure correct identification.*
■ Notify the morgue or security that the patient is being transferred to the morgue.
■ Prepare the body on the stretcher. Place a shroud or body wrap on the morgue stretcher and, with assistance, transfer the body to the stretcher. Wrap the body, and tie the shroud or wrap with the string provided. Attach another identification tag to the front of the shroud or wrap; then cover the shroud or wrap with a clean sheet. If a shroud or wrap isn't available, dress the deceased patient in a clean gown and cover the body with a sheet.
■ Place the deceased patient's personal belongings, including valuables, in a bag and attach the third identification tag to it.
■ If the patient required isolation precautions, use your facility's method for identifying them.[5,6]
■ Remove and discard your gloves and any other personal protective equipment worn.
■ Perform hand hygiene.[8,9,10,11]
■ Close the doors of adjacent rooms if possible. Then take the body to the morgue, using corridors that aren't crowded and, if possible, a service elevator.
■ Document the procedure.[12,13,14]

Special considerations

■ Honor the spiritual or cultural wishes of the deceased patient and his family and caregivers while ensuring that legal obligations are met.[1]
■ Give the deceased patient's personal belongings to his family or bring them to the morgue. If you give the family jewelry or money, make sure a coworker is present as a witness. Obtain the signature of an adult family member *to verify receipt of valuables or to state their preference that jewelry remain on the patient.*
■ When a patient's family members can't view the body within the designated time frame on the health care facility unit, make arrangements for viewing the body at another appropriate location, if desired.[1]

Patient teaching

Provide the family with written information on the processes to be followed after death and the role of such people and resources as funeral homes, social workers, and bereavement support agencies. Allow an opportunity for the family to ask questions.[1]

Documentation

Document that postmortem care was provided. Although the extent of documentation varies among facilities, always record the disposition of the patient's possessions, especially jewelry and money. Also note the date and time the deceased patient was transported to the morgue and the name of the person who received the body.

REFERENCES

1 National End of Life Care Programme and National Nurse Consultant Group (Palliative Care). (2011). "Guidance for staff responsible for care after death (last offices)" [Online]. Accessed May 2015 via the Web at http://www.nhsiq.nhs.uk/media/2426968/care_after_death___guidance.pdf

2 Centers for Medicare & Medicaid Services, Department of Health and Human Services. (2014). Condition of participation: Organ, tissue, and eye procurement. 42 C.F.R. § 482.45.

3 American Osteopathic Association. (2014). Standard 14.00.01. *Healthcare Facilities Accreditation Program: Accreditation requirements for acute care hospitals.* Chicago, IL: American Osteopathic Association. (Level VII)

4 American Osteopathic Association. (2014). Standard 15.01.16. *Healthcare Facilities Accreditation Program: Accreditation requirements for acute care hospitals.* Chicago, IL: American Osteopathic Association. (Level VII)

5 Centers for Medicare & Medicaid Services, Department of Health and Human Services. (2014). Condition of participation: Infection control. 42 C.F.R. § 482.42.

6 American Osteopathic Association. (2014). Standard 07.01.10. *Healthcare Facilities Accreditation Program: Accreditation requirements for acute care hospitals.* Chicago, IL: American Osteopathic Association. (Level VII)

7 National Institute on Aging. (2012). "Things to do after someone dies" [Online]. Accessed May 2015 via the Web at http://www.nia.nih.gov/health/publication/end-life-helping-comfort-and-care/things-do-after-someone-dies

8 The Joint Commission. (2015). Standard NPSG.07.01.01. *Comprehensive accreditation manual for hospitals: The official handbook.* Oakbrook Terrace, IL: The Joint Commission. (Level VII)

9 Centers for Disease Control and Prevention. (2002). Guideline for hand hygiene in health-care settings: Recommendations of the Healthcare Infection Control Practices Advisory Committee and the HICPAC/SHEA/APIC/IDSA Hand Hygiene Task Force. *MMWR Recommendations and Reports, 51*(RR-16), 1–45. Accessed May 2015 via the Web at http://www.cdc.gov/mmwr/pdf/rr/rr5116.pdf (Level II)

10 World Health Organization. (2009). "WHO guidelines on hand hygiene in health care: First global patient safety challenge, clean care is safer care" [Online]. Accessed May 2015 via the Web at http://whqlibdoc.who.int/publications/2009/9789241597906_eng.pdf (Level IV)

11 American Osteopathic Association. (2014). Standard 07.01.21. *Healthcare Facilities Accreditation Program: Accreditation requirements for acute care hospitals.* Chicago, IL: American Osteopathic Association. (Level VII)

12 The Joint Commission. (2015). Standard RC.01.03.01. *Comprehensive accreditation manual for hospitals: The official handbook.* Oakbrook Terrace, IL: The Joint Commission. (Level VII)

13 Centers for Medicare & Medicaid Services, Department of Health and Human Services. (2014). Condition of participation: Medical record services. 42 C.F.R. § 482.24(b).

14 American Osteopathic Association. (2014). Standard 10.00.03. *Healthcare Facilities Accreditation Program: Accreditation requirements for acute care hospitals.* Chicago, IL: American Osteopathic Association.

ADDITIONAL REFERENCES

Craven, R.F., & Hirnle, C.J. (2012). *Fundamentals of nursing: Human health and function* (7th ed.). Philadelphia, PA: Lippincott Williams & Wilkins.

Taylor, C., et al. (2015). *Fundamentals of nursing: The art and science of nursing care* (7th ed.). Philadelphia, PA: Wolters Kluwer.

POSTOPERATIVE CARE

Postoperative care begins when the patient arrives on the postanesthesia care unit (PACU) and continues as he moves to the short procedure unit, medical-surgical unit, or critical care area. The purpose of postoperative care is to minimize postoperative complications, such as pain, inadequate oxygenation, or adverse physiologic effects of sudden movement, through early detection and prompt treatment.[1]

Recovery from general anesthesia takes longer than its induction because the anesthetic is retained in fat and muscle. Because fat has a meager blood supply, it releases the anesthetic slowly, providing enough anesthesia to maintain adequate blood and brain levels during surgery. The patient's recovery time varies with his amount of body fat, his overall condition, his premedication regimen, and the type, dosage, and duration of anesthesia.

Equipment

Gloves ▪ thermometer ▪ watch or clock ▪ stethoscope ▪ sphygmomanometer ▪ blood pressure equipment ▪ pulse oximeter ▪ facility-approved assessment tools ▪ blood glucose monitor ▪ prescribed medications and fluids ▪ disinfectant pad ▪ Optional: transfer board, oxygen delivery equipment, suction equipment, other personal protective equipment, cardiac monitor, end-tidal carbon dioxide monitor.

Implementation

- Gather the necessary equipment at the patient's bedside.
- Perform hand hygiene.[2,3,4,5,6]
- Put on gloves and other personal protective equipment, as needed.[7,8]
- Confirm the patient's identity using at least two patient identifiers.[9]
- Receive hand-off communication from the perianesthesia nurse *to obtain information about the patient's intraoperative status, immediate postoperative condition before admission to the PACU, and condition during his stay in PACU.* This report should include relevant preoperative status, operative procedure, estimated fluid and blood loss and replacement, medications administered, anesthesia or sedation technique and agents administered, length of time anesthesia or sedation was administered, complications that occurred during the course of anesthesia and treatment for those complications (including the time at which reversal agents were given), pain and comfort management interventions and plan, and emotional status.[10] You should also be given the opportunity to ask questions and seek clarification about any aspect of the patient's care that might be unclear.[10,11]
- Transfer the patient from the PACU stretcher to the bed, and position him properly. Get a coworker to help, if necessary. When moving the patient, keep transfer movements smooth *to minimize pain and postoperative complications and avoid back strain among team members.* Use a transfer board as needed.[12]
- Raise the bed's side rails *to ensure the patient's safety.*

NURSING ALERT *If the patient has had orthopedic surgery, always get a coworker to help transfer him. Ask the coworker to move only the affected extremity. If the patient is in skeletal traction, you may receive special orders for moving him. If you must move him, have one coworker move the weights as you and another coworker move the patient.*

- Monitor the patient's respiratory status by assessing his airway for movement, depth of respirations, breath sounds, and oxygen saturation level. Provide oxygen, as ordered, *for patients at risk for hypoxemia.*[13] Simple face masks are generally used until the patient is more awake. Monitor the patient's vital signs at a frequency determined by your facility and the patient's condition; *there's no evidence-based research to indicate best practice for frequency of vital signs assessment.*[14]
- Monitor the patient's pulse rate. It should be strong and easily palpable. The heart rate should be within 20% of the preoperative heart rate. Monitor the patient's cardiac rhythm, if indicated.[13]
- Compare postoperative blood pressure with preoperative blood pressure. It should be within 20% of the preoperative level unless the patient suffered a hypotensive episode during surgery.
- Elevate the head of the bed, if not contraindicated, *to improve ventilation and to prevent aspiration of secretions.*[12]
- At frequent intervals, assess the patient's level of consciousness, skin color, and mucous membranes. *A patient who's somnolent or disoriented is unable to protect his airway or interact properly with the environment and is at risk of aspiration, hypoventilation, poor pain management, and falls.*
- Obtain the patient's core body temperature *because anesthesia lowers body temperature.* If the patient has a temperature lower than 96.8°F (36°C) or is shivering or demonstrating other signs of hypothermia, use active rewarming measures and assess the patient's temperature and thermal comfort level at a minimum of every 15 minutes until he reaches normothermia.[15] *Hypothermia adversely affects many systems and inhibits the metabolism of inhaled, IV, and regional anesthetics.*[14,15,16,17]
- Perform a neurologic assessment, particularly in a patient who has undergone a surgical procedure involving components of the neurologic system.
- Monitor blood glucose levels, if ordered. *Postoperative control of blood glucose levels is linked to surgical site infection prevention, especially after cardiac surgery.*[17]

HOSPITAL-ACQUIRED CONDITION ALERT *Keep in mind that a surgical site infection after certain cardiac surgeries, bariatric surgeries, or orthopedic procedures is considered a hospital-acquired condition* because it can be reasonably prevented using best practices. *Make sure that infection prevention techniques (such as performing hand hygiene, monitoring blood glucose levels postoperatively, and maintaining normothermia) are followed* to reduce the risk of surgical site infection.[18,19,20,21]

- Complete a GI assessment and verify the patency of any nasogastric or orogastric drainage tubes present. Also verify whether they should be connected to suction; after connecting to suction, if ordered, trace the tubing from the patient to its point of origin *to make sure that you've connected it to the proper port.*[22] Assess the patient's bowel sounds, especially if the patient underwent surgery involving the abdomen.
- Assess for nausea as soon as the patient awakens and regularly thereafter. If the patient is nauseous, quantify the severity using a facility-approved assessment tool. *Nausea and vomiting should be treated early and aggressively.*[13,23,24]
- Perform a genitourinary assessment. If the patient has an indwelling urinary catheter, assess the color, quantity, and quality of urine. Remove the catheter as ordered or according to facility protocol as soon as it's no longer needed *to reduce the risk of catheter-associated urinary tract infection.*[25,26,27,28]
- If the patient has had urinary tract surgery, he may have continuous bladder irrigation *to control bleeding and reduce the chance of blockage or clots forming in the bladder.* If so, maintain continuous bladder irrigation as ordered by the practitioner.[29]
- Perform a comprehensive pain assessment using techniques appropriate for the patient's age, condition, and ability to understand.[30] Evaluate the pain using a facility-approved pain assessment tool. Assess pain type, location, frequency, and duration. Also assess other sources of discomfort, such as nausea, vomiting, positioning, and anxiety. As appropriate, follow a multimodal pain management approach that may include opioid and nonopioid therapy, positioning, cold or heat application, and treatment for anxiety.[31] (See the "Pain management" procedure, page 578.)
- Administer pain medication as ordered and indicated following safe medication administration practices.[32,33] Assess the patient's pain level before and after administration.
- For patient's receiving IV opioid medication, frequently monitor the patient's respiratory rate, oxygen saturation level by pulse oximetry, end-tidal carbon dioxide level by capnography, and sedation levels using a

standardized sedation scale, to decrease the risk of adverse events associated with IV opioid use.[32,34]

■ For patient's receiving IV opioid medication, explain to the patient and family members about the assessment and monitoring process and tell them to alert staff if breathing problems or sedation occur.[32,34]

■ Assess the patient's infusion sites for redness, pain, swelling, or drainage. *These findings indicate infiltration and require discontinuing the IV line and restarting it at another site.*[35] Trace the line from the patient to its point of origin *to make sure it's attached to the proper port to prevent dangerous misconnections.*[22]

■ Assess surgical wound dressings; they should be clean and dry. If they're soiled, assess the characteristics of the drainage and outline the soiled area. Note the date and time of assessment on the dressing. Assess the soiled area frequently; if it enlarges, reinforce the dressing and alert the practitioner.[36]

■ Note the presence and condition of any drains and tubes. Note the color, type, odor, and amount of drainage. Make sure all drains are properly connected and free from kinks and obstructions.

■ If the patient has had vascular or orthopedic surgery, assess the appropriate extremity—or all extremities—depending on the surgical procedure. Perform a neurovascular assessment, including color, temperature, sensation, movement, and presence and quality of pulses, and notify the practitioner of any abnormalities.

■ Continue venous thromboembolism (VTE) prophylaxis, such as using sequential compression sleeves or boots, according to the practitioner's order or facility protocol.[25]

HOSPITAL-ACQUIRED CONDITION ALERT *Keep in mind that VTE after total knee or hip replacement is considered a hospital-acquired condition* because it can be reasonably prevented using best practices. *Make sure that VTE prevention techniques (such as using sequential compression sleeves or boots) are followed* to reduce the risk of VTE.[20,37]

■ Encourage coughing and deep-breathing exercises (unless the patient has just had nasal, ophthalmic, or neurologic surgery) and incentive spirometry use, if indicated and prescribed.[38]

■ Administer IV fluids[4] and medications, such as antibiotics, analgesics, antiemetics, or reversal agents, as ordered and appropriate following safe medication administration practices.[25]

■ If the patient was receiving a beta-adrenergic blocker before surgery, collaborate with the patient's practitioner to make sure that he receives it during the perioperative period, as appropriate.[25]

■ If administering IV fluids or medications through an infusion pump, make sure that alarm limits are set according to the patient's current condition and that the alarms are turned on, functioning properly, and audible to staff. [39,40,41]

■ Assess and address the patient's safety needs.[14]

■ Remove all fluids from the patient's bedside until he is alert enough to eat and drink. Before giving him liquids, assess his gag reflex *to prevent aspiration.* To do this, lightly touch the back of his throat with a cotton swab; the patient will gag if the reflex has returned. Do this test quickly *to prevent a vagal reaction.*

■ Monitor the patient's intake and output.

■ Remove and discard your gloves and other personal protective equipment, if worn.[7]

■ Perform hand hygiene.[2,3,4,5,6]

■ Clean and disinfect your stethoscope using a disinfectant pad.[42,43]

■ Perform hand hygiene.[2,3,4,5,6]

■ Document the procedure.[44,45,46]

Special considerations

■ The Joint Commission has issued a sentinel event alert concerning medical device alarm safety *because alarm-related events have been associated with permanent loss of function or death.* Among the major contributing factors were improper alarm settings, alarms inappropriately turned off, and alarm signals not audible to staff. Make sure that alarm limits are set appropriately and that alarms are turned on and audible to staff. Follow facility guidelines for preventing alarm fatigue.[47]

■ Fear, pain, anxiety, hypothermia, confusion, and immobility can upset the patient and jeopardize his safety and postoperative status. Offer emotional support to the patient and his family. Keep in mind that the patient who has lost a body part or who has been diagnosed with an incurable disease will need ongoing emotional support. Refer him and his family for counseling as needed.

■ As the patient recovers from general anesthesia, reflexes appear in reverse order to that in which they disappeared. Hearing recovers first, so avoid holding inappropriate conversations.

■ A patient under general anesthesia can't protect his own airway *because of muscle relaxation.* As he recovers, his cough and gag reflexes reappear. If he can lift his head without assistance, he's usually able to breathe on his own.

■ If the patient received spinal anesthesia, he may need to remain in the supine position with the bed adjusted to between 0 and 20 degrees for at least 6 hours *to reduce the risk of spinal headache from leakage of cerebrospinal fluid.* The patient won't be able to move his legs, so reassure him that sensation and mobility will return. (See *Assessing level of blockade from spinal anesthesia,* page 626.)

■ If the patient has had an epidural analgesia infusion for postoperative pain control, monitor his respiratory status closely. *Respiratory arrest may result from the respiratory depressant effects of the opioid.* Also monitor the patient's blood pressure, heart rate, and arterial oxygen saturation at an interval determined by your facility or the patient's condition. He may also suffer from nausea, vomiting, or itching. Epidural analgesia may also include administering a local anesthetic with the opioid. (See the "Epidural analgesic administration" procedure, page 295.) Assess the patient's lower-extremity motor strength every 2 to 4 hours. If sensorimotor loss occurs (numbness or weakness of the legs), notify the practitioner *because the dosage may need to be decreased.*

ELDER ALERT *If the patient is older, be aware of age-related changes that will alter your assessment. Monitor cardiovascular status carefully* because blood loss, pain, bed rest, and fluid and electrolyte imbalances can alter it. *Also carefully monitor respiratory status* because ventilation and oxygenation can be altered by age-related changes or years of smoking or chronic diseases. *Closely monitor level of consciousness and pain* because mental status changes can affect these and make pain control more difficult. Drug metabolism slows with age, *so monitor the older adult's risk of drug reactions, toxicity, and interactions. Monitor intake and output carefully and watch for urinary tract infections* because of decreased renal functioning and bladder capacity. *Position the older patient carefully, and prevent postoperative falls* because the patient may have osteoporosis and may be prone to fractures. *Also monitor for signs and symptoms of infection* because the risk of infection increases with age.

Complications

Postoperative complications may include cardiac arrhythmias, hypotension, hypovolemia, septicemia, septic shock, atelectasis, pneumonia, thrombophlebitis, pulmonary embolism, urine retention, wound infection, wound dehiscence, evisceration, abdominal distention, paralytic ileus, constipation, altered body image, and postoperative psychosis.

Recovery from anesthesia isn't a linear progression. Patients can, and often do, regress to a less awake status, have occluded airways, become unstable because of slow bleeding or sepsis, have spikes or dips in blood pressure and heart rate due to peaking or wearing off of medication, or become suddenly nauseated with severe emesis that puts them at risk for aspiration. Hypothermia, hypoxemia, hypoventilation, and airway obstruction are the primary complications monitored for on the PACU.[48]

Assessing level of blockade from spinal anesthesia

Spinal anesthesia produces a sympathetic, sensory, and motor block. If the patient received spinal anesthesia, be ready to assess the downward progression of the level of blockade. Using a dermatome chart aids this assessment. Each dermatome represents a specific body area supplied with nerve fibers from an individual spinal root (cervical, thoracic, lumbar, or sacral). To document the patient's sensory and motor function, mentally divide his body into dermatomes. Anatomic reference points include the nipple line at T4, xiphoid at T6, umbilicus at T10, and groin at L1.

Anterior view **Posterior view**

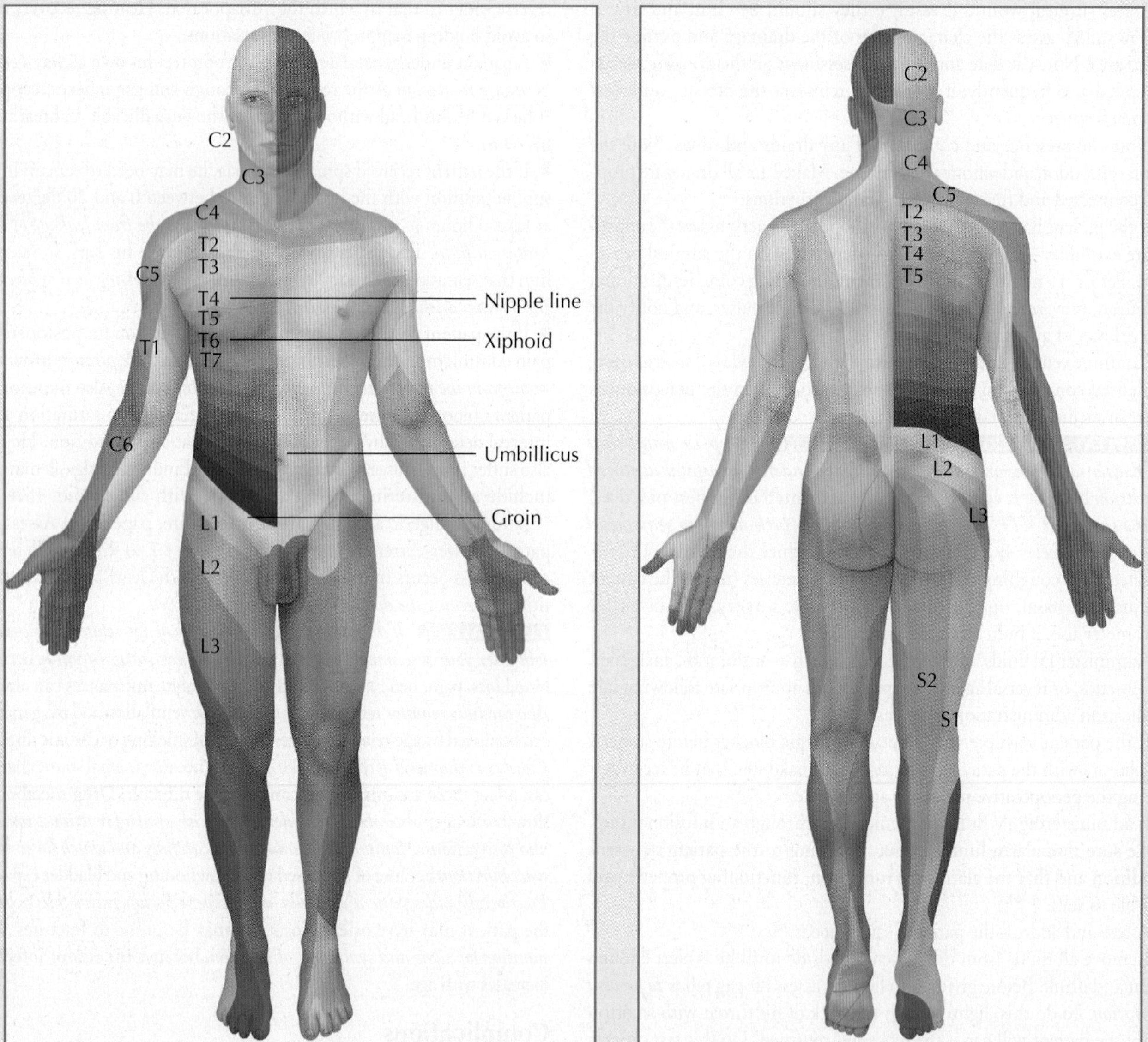

Documentation

Document vital signs according to your facility's documentation format. Record the condition of dressings and drains and characteristics of drainage. Document all interventions taken to alleviate pain and anxiety and the patient's responses to them. Document any complications and interventions taken.

REFERENCES

1 The Joint Commission. (2015). Standard PC.03.01.07. *Comprehensive accreditation manual for hospitals: The official handbook.* Oakbrook Terrace, IL: The Joint Commission. (Level VII)

2 The Joint Commission. (2015). NPSG.07.01.01. *Comprehensive accreditation manual for hospitals: The official handbook.* Oakbrook Terrace, IL: The Joint Commission. (Level VII)

3 Centers for Disease Control and Prevention. (2002). Guideline for hand hygiene in health-care settings: Recommendations of the Healthcare Infection Control Practices Advisory Committee and the HICPAC/SHEA/APIC/IDSA Hand Hygiene Task Force. *MMWR Recommendations and Reports, 51*(RR-16), 1–45. Accessed May 2015 via the Web at http://www.cdc.gov/mmwr/pdf/rr/rr5116.pdf (Level II)

4 World Health Organization. (2009). "WHO guidelines on hand hygiene in health care: First global patient safety challenge, clean care is safer care"

[Online]. Accessed May 2015 via the Web at http://whqlibdoc.who.int/publications/2009/9789241597906_eng.pdf (Level IV)

5 Centers for Medicare & Medicaid Services, Department of Health and Human Services. (2014). Condition of participation: Infection control. 42 C.F.R. § 482.42.

6 American Osteopathic Association. (2014). Standard 07.01.21. *Healthcare Facilities Accreditation Program: Accreditation requirements for acute care hospitals.* Chicago, IL: American Osteopathic Association. (Level VII)

7 Siegel, J. D., et al. (2007). "2007 guideline for isolation precautions: Preventing transmission of infectious agents in healthcare settings" [Online]. Accessed May 2015 via the Web at http://www.cdc.gov/hicpac/pdf/isolation/Isolation2007.pdf (Level II)

8 American Osteopathic Association. (2014). Standard 07.01.10. *Healthcare Facilities Accreditation Program: Accreditation requirements for acute care hospitals.* Chicago, IL: American Osteopathic Association. (Level VII)

9 The Joint Commission. (2015). Standard NPSG.01.01.01. *Comprehensive accreditation manual for hospitals: The official handbook.* Oakbrook Terrace, IL: The Joint Commission. (Level VII)

10 Recommended practices for transfer of patient care information. (2014). In R. Conner, et al. (Eds.), *Perioperative standards and recommended practices 2014.* Denver, CO: AORN, Inc. (Level VII)

11 The Joint Commission. (2015). Standard PC.02.02.01. *Comprehensive accreditation manual for hospitals: The official handbook.* Oakbrook Terrace, IL: The Joint Commission. (Level VII)

12 AORN guidance statement: Safe patient handling and movement in the perioperative setting. (2014). In R. Conner, et al. (Eds.), *Perioperative standards and recommended practices 2014.* Denver, CO: AORN, Inc. (Level VII)

13 American Society of Anesthesiologists Task Force on Postanesthetic Care. (2013). Practice guidelines for postanesthetic care: An updated report by the American Society of Anesthesiologists Task Force on Postanesthetic Care. *Anesthesiology, 18,* 291–307. Accessed May 2015 via the Web at http://anesthesiology.pubs.asahq.org/article.aspx?articleid=1918686 (Level VII)

14 American Society of PeriAnesthesia Nurses. (2012). *2012-2014 Perianesthesia nursing standards, practice recommendations and interpretive statements.* Cherry Hill, NJ: American Society of PeriAnesthesia Nurses. (Level VII)

15 American Society of PeriAnesthesia Nurses. (2010). ASPAN's evidence-based clinical practice guideline for the promotion of perioperative normothermia: Second edition. *Journal of PeriAnesthesia Nursing, 25,* 346–365. Accessed May 2015 via the Web at http://www.aspan.org/Portals/6/docs/ClinicalPractice/Guidelines/Normothermia_Guideline_12-10_JoPAN.pdf (Level VII)

16 Recommended practices for the prevention of unplanned perioperative hypothermia. (2014). In R. Conner, et al. (Eds.), *Perioperative standards and recommended practices 2014.* Denver, CO: AORN, Inc. (Level VII)

17 Institute for Healthcare Improvement. (2012). *How to guide: Prevent surgical site infections.* Cambridge, MA: Institute for Healthcare Improvement. (Level V)

18 The Joint Commission. (2015). Standard NPSG.07.05.01. *Comprehensive accreditation manual for hospitals: The official handbook.* Oakbrook Terrace, IL: The Joint Commission. (Level VII)

19 American Osteopathic Association. (2012). Standard 07.01.20. *Healthcare Facilities Accreditation Program: Accreditation requirements for acute care hospitals.* Chicago, IL: American Osteopathic Association. (Level VII)

20 Jarrett, N., et al. (2013). "Evidence-based guidelines for selected and previously considered hospital-acquired conditions: Final report" [Online]. Accessed May 2015 via the Web at http://www.cms.gov/Medicare/Medicare-Fee-for-Service-Payment/HospitalAcqCond/Downloads/Evidence-Based-Guidelines.pdf (Level VII)

21 Anderson, D. J., et al. (2014). SHEA/IDSA practice recommendation: Strategies to prevent surgical site infections in acute care hospitals: 2014 update. *Infection Control and Hospital Epidemiology, 35,* 605–627. Accessed May 2015 via the Web at http://www.jstor.org/stable/10.1086/676022 (Level II)

22 U.S. Food and Drug Administration. (n.d.). "Look. Check. Connect. Safe medical device connections save lives." [Online]. Accessed May 2015 via the Web at http://www.fda.gov/downloads/MedicalDevices/Safety/AlertsandNotices/UCM134873.pdf

23 Habib, A. S., et al. (2006). Postoperative nausea and vomiting following inpatient surgeries in a teaching hospital: A retrospective database analysis. *Current Medical Research and Opinion, 22,* 1093–1099. (Level IV)

24 American Society of PeriAnesthesia Nurses. (2006). ASPAN'S evidence-based clinical practice guideline for the prevention and/or management of PONV/PDNV. *Journal of PeriAnesthesia Nursing, 21,* 230–250. Accessed May 2015 via the Web at www.aspan.org/Portals/6/docs/ClinicalPractice/Guidelines/PONV-PDNV_Clinical_Guideline_Aug_2006_JoPAN.pdf (Level VII)

25 Centers for Medicare & Medicaid Services, & The Joint Commission. (2014). "The specifications manual for national hospital inpatient quality measures (version 4.3b)" [Online]. Accessed May 2015 via the Web at http://www.qualitynet.org/dcs/ContentServer?c=Page&pagename=QnetPublic%2FPage%2FQnetTier4&cid=1228773564870 (Level VII)

26 Association of Professionals in Infection Control and Epidemiology (APIC). (2014). "APIC Implementation Guide: Guide to preventing catheter-associated urinary tract infections" [Online]. Accessed May 2015 via the Web at http://apic.org/Resource_/EliminationGuideForm/6473ab9b-e75c-457a-8d0f-d57d32bc242b/File/APIC_CAUTI_web_0603.pdf (Level IV)

27 Healthcare Infection Control Practices Advisory Committee. (2010). "Guideline for prevention of catheter-associated urinary tract infections, 2009" [Online]. Accessed May 2015 via the Web at http://www.cdc.gov/hicpac/pdf/CAUTI/CAUTIguideline2009final.pdf

28 The Joint Commission. (2014). Standard NPSG.07.06.01. *Comprehensive accreditation manual for hospitals: The official handbook.* Oakbrook Terrace, IL: The Joint Commission. (Level VII)

29 Feliciano, T., et al. (2008). A retrospective, descriptive, exploratory study evaluating incidence of postoperative urinary retention after spinal anesthesia and its effect on PACU discharge. *Journal of Perianesthesia Nursing, 23,* 394–400. (Level IV)

30 The Joint Commission. (2015). Standard PC.01.02.07. *Comprehensive accreditation manual for hospitals: The official handbook.* Oakbrook Terrace, IL: The Joint Commission. (Level VII)

31 American Society of Anesthesiologists. (2012). Practice guidelines for acute pain management in the perioperative setting: An updated report by the American Society of Anesthesiologists Task Force on Acute Pain Management. *Anesthesiology, 116,* 248–273. (Level VII)

32 Centers for Medicare & Medicaid Services, Department of Health and Human Services. (2014). Condition of participation: Nursing services. 42 C.F.R. § 482.23(c).

33 American Osteopathic Association. (2014). Standard 16.01.03. *Healthcare Facilities Accreditation Program: Accreditation requirements for acute care hospitals.* Chicago, IL: American Osteopathic Association. (Level VII)

34 Centers for Medicare & Medicaid Services. (2014). "Requirements for hospital medication administration, particularly intravenous (IV) medications and post-operative care of patients receiving IV opioids" [Online]. Accessed May 2015 via the Web at http://www.cms.gov/Medicare/Provider-Enrollment-and-Certification/SurveyCertificationGenInfo/Downloads/Survey-and-Cert-Letter-14-15.pdf

35 Standard 48. Infiltration and extravasation. Infusion nursing standards of practice. (2011). *Journal of Infusion Nursing, 34,* S66–S68. (Level VII)

36 The Joint Commission. (2015). Standard NPSG.07.05.01. *Comprehensive accreditation manual for hospitals: The official handbook.* Oakbrook Terrace, IL: The Joint Commission. (Level VII)

37 American Osteopathic Association. (2014). Standard 16.02.02. *Healthcare Facilities Accreditation Program: Accreditation requirements for acute care hospitals.* Chicago, IL: American Osteopathic Association. (Level VII)

38 Restrepo, R. D., et al. (2011). AARC clinical practice guideline: Incentive spirometry, 2011. *Respiratory Care, 56,* 1600–1604. Accessed May 2015 via the Web at http://rc.rcjournal.com/content/56/10/1600.full.pdf (Level VII)

39 American Association of Critical-Care Nurses. (2013). "AACN Practice Alert: Alarm management" [Online]. Accessed May 2015 via the Web at http://www.aacn.org/wd/practice/docs/practicealerts/alarm-management-practice-alert.pdf (Level VII)

40 The Joint Commission. (2015). Standard NPSG.06.01.01. *Comprehensive accreditation manual for hospitals: The official handbook.* Oakbrook Terrace, IL: The Joint Commission. (Level VII)
41 Graham, K. C., & Cvach, M. (2010). Monitor alarm fatigue: Standardizing use of physiological monitors and decreasing nuisance alarms. *American Journal of Critical Care, 19,* 28–35.
42 Rutala, W. A., et al. (2008). "Guideline for disinfection and sterilization in healthcare facilities, 2008" [Online]. Accessed May 2015 via the Web at http://www.cdc.gov/hicpac/pdf/guidelines/Disinfection_Nov_2008.pdf (Level I)
43 American Osteopathic Association. (2014). Standard 07.02.03. *Healthcare Facilities Accreditation Program: Accreditation requirements for acute care hospitals.* Chicago, IL: American Osteopathic Association. (Level VII)
44 The Joint Commission. (2015). Standard RC.01.03.01. *Comprehensive accreditation manual for hospitals: The official handbook.* Oakbrook Terrace, IL: The Joint Commission. (Level VII)
45 Centers for Medicare & Medicaid Services, Department of Health and Human Services. (2014). Condition of participation: Medical record services. 42 C.F.R. § 482.24(b).
46 American Osteopathic Association. (2014). Standard 10.00.03. *Healthcare Facilities Accreditation Program: Accreditation requirements for acute care hospitals.* Chicago, IL: American Osteopathic Association. (Level VII)
47 The Joint Commission. (2013). "Sentinel event alert: Medical device alarm safety in hospitals" [Online]. Accessed May 2015 via the Web at http://www.jointcommission.org/assets/1/18/SEA_50_alarms_4_5_13_FINAL1.PDF (Level VII)
48 Flockton, E., et al. (2008). Reversal of rocuronium-induced neuromuscular block with sugammadex is faster than reversal of cisatracurium-induced block with neostigmine. *British Journal of Anaesthesia, 100,* 622–630. (Level II)

PREOPERATIVE CARE

Preoperative care begins when surgery is planned and ends with the administration of anesthesia. This phase of care includes a preoperative interview and assessment to collect baseline subjective and objective data from the patient and his family; diagnostic tests such as urinalysis, electrocardiography (ECG), and chest radiography; preoperative teaching; informed consent from the patient; and physical preparation.

If the patient is having same-day surgery, he'll need instructions before the day of surgery that cover the time he's to arrive at the facility, the need to leave all jewelry and valuables at home, the need to have someone accompany him to and stay with him after surgery, fasting guidelines, medication use, and any prescribed surgical preparation, such as showering with an antimicrobial cleaner.

Equipment

Thermometer ■ sphygmomanometer ■ stethoscope ■ pulse oximetry monitor ■ watch with second hand ■ scale ■ tape measure ■ patient gown ■ facility-approved pain assessment scale ■ preoperative checklist ■ prescribed medications ■ prescribed IV fluids ■ patient education materials ■ blood glucose monitoring supplies ■ disinfectant pad ■ Optional: gloves, IV insertion kit, cardiac monitor, specimen collection supplies, clippers.

Implementation

Before the day of surgery

- Verify the practitioner's orders.
- Gather the appropriate equipment.
- Review the patient's preadmission assessment findings, including X-ray examinations, laboratory test results, and other preoperative tests, as indicated.[1,2,3]
- Perform hand hygiene.[4,5,6,7,8]
- Put on personal protective equipment as needed *to comply with standard precautions.*[9,10]
- Confirm the patient's identity using at least two patient identifiers.[11]
- If the patient is having same-day surgery, make sure the patient has arranged for someone to accompany him home after surgery.
- Obtain a health history, including previous surgery, skin condition, history of multiple drug-resistant organisms, external or implanted medical devices, sensory limitations, and home use of noninvasive positive-pressure ventilation or apnea monitors.[12,13] Use your facility's preoperative surgical assessment database, if available, to gather this information.
- Assess the patient's knowledge, perceptions, and expectations about the planned surgery.[1,2]
- Ask the patient whether he has allergies to latex, medications, food, or other *substances to determine the risk of an allergic reaction.*[12,13]
- Ask the patient whether he or any family member has ever had a serious reaction to anesthesia.[12]
- Obtain a complete list of medications the patient uses, including prescription drugs, over-the-counter medications, herbal preparations and supplements, alcohol, tobacco, and illicit drugs.[12,13,14,15] *It may be necessary to adjust or continue medications whose sudden cessation may provoke a withdrawal syndrome.*[16]
- If the patient was receiving a beta-adrenergic blocker, collaborate with the patient's practitioner to make sure he receives it during the perioperative period, as appropriate.[17]
- Ask whether the patient has an advance directive.[18,19] Provide information about advance directives as appropriate. (See the "Advance directives" procedure, page 7.)
- Obtain the patient's height, weight, vital signs, and oxygen saturation level.[12,13]
- Perform a comprehensive pain assessment using techniques appropriate for the patient's age, condition, and ability to understand.[13,20]
- Obtain a pain and analgesic history; ask about measures that have been effective in relieving or controlling pain in the past. Also ask about expectations for controlling pain after surgery. *By obtaining a thorough pain history preoperatively, the health care team may be able to better control pain postoperatively.*[1,12,13]
- Perform educational, socioeconomic, cultural, and spiritual assessments *to determine the patient's level of understanding about the surgical procedure and whether he has special needs while in the facility.*[12,13]
- Assess for mobility limitations and disabilities, including mental and physical impairments, *which may require the use of additional equipment or supplies.* Assess and address the patient's safety needs, including the risk of falling, and implement fall prevention interventions as needed.[12,13,15,21]
- Assess the patient's risk of postoperative nausea and vomiting (PONV) so that PONV prophylaxis can be considered *to decrease postoperative discomfort.* Consider the patient's history of PONV, the duration of surgery, and the type of surgery being performed in your assessment.[12,13]
- Assess the patient's cognitive, mental, and cardiopulmonary status;[15,22] skin condition; functional and sensory limitations; and use of any hearing or visual aids and assistive or prosthetic devices.
- Obtain other assessment data as pertinent to the surgical procedure.[2,12,13]
- Identify risk factors that may interfere with a positive expected outcome. Consider age, general health, medications, mobility, nutritional status, fluid and electrolyte disturbances, and lifestyle. Also consider the location, nature, and extent of the surgical procedure.[13]

ELDER ALERT ***Be aware that the development of postoperative delirium is a common complication of surgery in older patients.***[15]

- Provide patient education using methods appropriate to the patient's and caregiver's preference and level of understanding. Include typical events that the patient can expect. Explain the typical incision, dressings, and staples or sutures that will be used. *Preoperative teaching can help reduce postoperative anxiety and pain, increase patient compliance, hasten recovery, and decrease length of stay.*[13,23]

■ Teach the patient how to use a pain assessment scale that's appropriate for the patient's age, condition, and ability to understand; to rate and report pain; and discuss analgesic tools and methods such as patient-controlled analgesia.[13,16,24,25]
■ Teach the patient and family about behavioral pain control techniques, such as biofeedback and progressive relaxation, *to help the patient manage perioperative pain and anxiety.*[13,16]
■ Discuss equipment that may be used postoperatively, such as nasogastric tubes and IV equipment. Determine whether the patient will require home health care services and, if so, help him make the necessary arrangements.[12,13]
■ Tell the patient about exercises that he may be expected to perform after surgery, such as deep breathing, coughing (while splinting the incision if necessary), extremity exercises and movement, and early ambulation *to minimize respiratory and circulatory complications.*[13,26]

NURSING ALERT ***Be aware that, if the patient is undergoing ophthalmic or neurologic surgery, he won't be asked to cough*** **because coughing increases intracranial pressure.**

■ Talk the patient through the sequence of events from the operating room, to the postanesthesia care unit, and back to the patient's room or to an intensive care unit or surgical care unit, as appropriate, *to allay the patient's anxiety.*[13]
■ When discussing transfer procedures and techniques, describe sensations the patient will experience. Tell him that he'll be taken to the operating room on a stretcher and transferred from the stretcher to an operating room table. Explain that, for his own safety, he'll be held securely to the table with soft straps.
■ Tell the patient that the operating room may feel cool.
■ Explain that the operating room nurses will check his vital signs frequently, and electrodes may be put on his chest *to monitor his heart rate during surgery.*
■ Describe the drowsy, floating sensation he'll feel as the anesthetic takes effect. Tell him it's important that he relax at this time.
■ Tell the patient that he'll be required to fast before the procedure according to the practitioner's order *to reduce vomiting and the risk of aspiration.* Minimum fasting recommendations include 2 hours for clear liquids, 6 or more hours for a light meal or nonhuman milk, and 8 hours or more for fried or fatty foods or meat.[27]
■ If ordered by the practitioner, administer a combination of parenteral and oral antimicrobial agents *to reduce the risk of surgical site infection after colorectal surgery.* If ordered, administer mechanical bowel preparation in combination with oral antimicrobial agents *because data supporting the use of oral antimicrobials to reduce the risk of surgical site infection has been studied in combination with mechanical bowel preparation.*[28]
■ Advise the patient not to shave or remove hair at or near the surgical site before surgery *to prevent the risk of surgical site infection.*[29] Also tell the patient to clean his skin the night before or the morning of surgery; *some studies support the use of 2% chlorhexidine cloths wiped on the surgical site the night before and the morning of surgery for specific procedures, such as cardiothoracic and total joint procedures.*[2,30]
■ Remove and discard your personal protective equipment if worn.[9,10]
■ Perform hand hygiene.[4,5,6,7,8]
■ Clean and disinfect your stethoscope with a disinfectant pad.[31,32]
■ Perform hand hygiene.[4,5,6,7,8]
■ Document the procedure.[33,34]

On the day of surgery

■ Verify the practitioner's orders.
■ Perform hand hygiene.[4,5,6,7,8]
■ Confirm that written informed consent is obtained and that the consent is in the patient's medical record.[35,36,37]
■ Conduct a preprocedure verification *to make sure that all documentation, related information, and equipment are available and correctly identified to the patient's identifiers.*[3,38]
■ Verify that the laboratory and imaging studies have been completed, as ordered, and that the results are in the patient's medical record. Notify the practitioner of any unexpected results.
■ Collect additional laboratory specimens and perform other tests as indicated, such as an ECG.[12]
■ Assess vital signs *to serve as a baseline for comparison during and after the procedure.*
■ Ensure patent IV access.
■ Take these measures *to prevent surgical site infection:* Don't remove hair at the operative site unless the presence of hair will interfere with the operative procedure. If hair removal is necessary, remove the hair using clippers; don't use a razor.[28] Administer the prescribed prophylactic antibiotic within 1 hour before incision *to maximize tissue concentration;* administer fluoroquinolones and vancomycin within 2 hours before incision.[28] Obtain the patient's blood glucose level, as ordered, *to identify hyperglycemia;* initiate treatment as needed and ordered.[29]

HOSPITAL-ACQUIRED CONDITION ALERT ***Keep in mind that a surgical site infection following certain cardiac surgeries, bariatric surgeries, or orthopedic procedures is considered a hospital-acquired condition*** **because it can be reasonably prevented using best practices.** ***Make sure that infection prevention techniques (such as using clippers for hair removal, administering antibiotics 1 hour before incision, and monitoring for hyperglycemia) are followed*** **to reduce the risk of surgical site infection.**[30,39,40]

■ Administer ordered preoperative medications, including analgesics as part of a multimodal analgesic pain-management program.[16]
■ Complete the preoperative checklist.
■ Provide support to the patient and his family.
■ Notify the surgeon and anesthesia care provider as needed regarding abnormal assessment findings, and document responding orders.[12]
■ Assess the patient's retention of preoperative teaching and reinforce education as indicated.[12,13]
■ Make sure that the patient has a responsible adult who will transport him home and assume his care after discharge.[12]
■ Allow loved ones time to be with the patient before surgery *so that the patient feels comforted and supported from the physical and emotional presence of the family preoperatively.*[41]

Just before moving the patient to the surgical area

■ Make sure the patient is wearing a hospital gown, has his identification bracelet in place, and has his vital signs recorded. Check to see that all hairpins, nail polish, and jewelry have been removed. Note whether dentures, contact lenses, or prosthetic devices have been removed or left in place.
■ Verify with the patient that the correct surgical site has been marked.[38,42]
■ Provide face-to-face hand-off communication about the patient's status and care to the person who will assume responsibility for the patient in the operating room. Allow time for questions and to clarify any information.[27,44,45]
■ Perform hand hygiene.[4,5,6,7,8]
■ Clean and disinfect your stethoscope with a disinfectant pad.[31,32]
■ Perform hand hygiene.[4,5,6,7,8]
■ Document the procedure.[33,34,46]

Special considerations

■ The patient may benefit from a tour of the areas he will see during perioperative events.
■ Preoperative medications must be given on time *to enhance the effect of ordered anesthesia.* Don't give oral medications unless prescribed. Be sure to raise the bed's side rails immediately after giving preoperative medications.[1]
■ If family members or others are present, direct them to the appropriate waiting area and offer support as needed.[14]

Documentation

Complete the preoperative checklist used by your facility. Record all nursing care measures performed, preoperative medications administered, results of diagnostic tests, and the time the patient is transferred to the surgical area. Make sure the patient's medical record and the surgical checklist accompany the patient to surgery.

REFERENCES

1 Preoperative patient care in the ambulatory surgery setting. (2014). In Conner, R., et al. (Eds.), *Perioperative standards and recommended practices 2014.* Denver, CO: AORN, Inc. (Level VII)

2 Institute for Clinical Systems Improvement. (2012). "Preoperative evaluation" [Online]. Accessed May 2015 via the Web at http://www.guideline.gov/content.aspx?id=38289 (Level VII)

3 The Joint Commission. (2015). Standard UP.01.01.01. *Comprehensive accreditation manual for hospitals: The official handbook.* Oakbrook Terrace, IL: The Joint Commission. (Level VII)

4 Centers for Disease Control and Prevention. (2002). Guideline for hand hygiene in health-care settings: Recommendations of the Healthcare Infection Control Practices Advisory Committee and the HICPAC/SHEA/APIC/IDSA Hand Hygiene Task Force. *MMWR Recommendations and Reports, 51*(RR-16), 1–45. Accessed May 2015 via the Web at http://www.cdc.gov/mmwr/pdf/rr/rr5116.pdf (Level II)

5 World Health Organization. (2009). "WHO guidelines on hand hygiene in health care: First global patient safety challenge, clean care is safer care" [Online]. Accessed May 2015 via the Web at http://whqlibdoc.who.int/publications/2009/9789241597906_eng.pdf (Level IV)

6 The Joint Commission. (2015). Standard NPSG.07.01.01. *Comprehensive accreditation manual for hospitals: The official handbook.* Oakbrook Terrace, IL: The Joint Commission. (Level VII)

7 Centers for Medicare & Medicaid Services, Department of Health and Human Services. (2014). Condition of participation: Infection control. 42 C.F.R. § 482.42.

8 American Osteopathic Association. (2014). Standard 07.01.21. *Healthcare Facilities Accreditation Program: Accreditation requirements for acute care hospitals.* Chicago, IL: American Osteopathic Association. (Level VII)

9 Siegel, J. D., et al. (2007). "2007 guideline for isolation precautions: Preventing transmission of infectious agents in healthcare settings" [Online]. Accessed May 2015 via the Web at http://www.cdc.gov/hicpac/pdf/isolation/Isolation2007.pdf (Level II)

10 American Osteopathic Association. (2014). Standard 07.01.10. *Healthcare Facilities Accreditation Program: Accreditation requirements for acute care hospitals.* Chicago, IL: American Osteopathic Association. (Level VII)

11 The Joint Commission. (2015). Standard NPSG.01.01.01. *Comprehensive accreditation manual for hospitals: The official handbook.* Oakbrook Terrace, IL: The Joint Commission. (Level VII)

12 American Society of PeriAnesthesia Nurses. (2012). *2012-2014 Perianesthesia nursing standards, practice recommendations and interpretative statements.* Cherry Hill, NJ: American Society of PeriAnesthesia Nurses. (Level VII)

13 The Joint Commission. (2015). Standard PC.03.01.03. *Comprehensive accreditation manual for hospitals: The official handbook.* Oakbrook Terrace, IL: The Joint Commission. (Level VII)

14 The Joint Commission. (2015). Standard NPSG.03.06.01. *Comprehensive accreditation manual for hospitals: The official handbook.* Oakbrook Terrace, IL: The Joint Commission. (Level VII)

15 American College of Surgeons National Surgical Quality Improvement Program. (2012). "ACS NSQIP/AGS best practice guidelines: Optimal preoperative assessment of the geriatric surgical patient" [Online]. Accessed May 2015 via the Web at http://site.acsnsqip.org/wp-content/uploads/2011/12/ACS-NSQIP-AGS-Geriatric-2012-Guidelines.pdf (Level VII)

16 American Society of Anesthesiologists. (2012). Practice guidelines for acute pain management in the perioperative setting: An updated report by the American Society of Anesthesiologists Task Force on Acute Pain Management. *Anesthesiology, 116,* 248–273. (Level VII)

17 Centers for Medicare & Medicaid Services, & The Joint Commission. (2014). "The specifications manual for national hospital inpatient quality measures (version 4.3a)" [Online]. Accessed May 2015 via the Web at http://www.qualitynet.org/dcs/ContentServer?c=Page&pagename=QnetPublic%2FPage%2FQnetTier4&cid=1228773564870

18 The Joint Commission. (2015). Standard RI.01.05.01. *Comprehensive accreditation manual for hospitals: The official handbook.* Oakbrook Terrace, IL: The Joint Commission. (Level VII)

19 American Osteopathic Association. (2014). Standard 15.01.12. *Healthcare Facilities Accreditation Program: Accreditation requirements for acute care hospitals.* Chicago, IL: American Osteopathic Association. (Level VII)

20 The Joint Commission. (2015). Standard PC.01.02.07. *Comprehensive accreditation manual for hospitals: The official handbook.* Oakbrook Terrace, IL: The Joint Commission. (Level VII)

21 The Joint Commission. (2015). Standard PC.01.02.08. *Comprehensive accreditation manual for hospitals: The official handbook.* Oakbrook Terrace, IL: The Joint Commission. (Level VII)

22 American College of Cardiology and American Heart Association Task Force on Practice Guidelines. (2007). ACC/AHA 2007 guidelines on perioperative cardiovascular evaluation and care for noncardiac surgery. *Circulation, 116,* e418–e500. (Level VII)

23 Devine, E. C., & Cook, T. D. (1983). A meta-analytic analysis of effects of psychoeducational interventions on length of postsurgical hospital stay. *Nursing Research, 32,* 267–274. (Level I)

24 American Society of PeriAnesthesia Nurses. (2003). ASPAN pain and comfort clinical guideline. *Journal of PeriAnesthesia Nursing, 18,* 232–236. Accessed May 2015 via the Web at http://www.aspan.org/Portals/6/docs/ClinicalPractice/Guidelines/ASPAN_ClinicalGuideline_PainComfort.pdf (Level VII)

25 The Joint Commission. (2015). Standard PC.01.02.07. *Comprehensive accreditation manual for hospitals: The official handbook.* Oakbrook Terrace, IL: The J (Level VII)

26 Clarke, H. D., et al. (2012). Preoperative patient education reduces in-hospital falls after total knee arthroplasty. *Clinical Orthopaedics and Related Research, 470,* 244–249. (Level III)

27 American Society of Anesthesiologists. (2011). "Practice guidelines for preoperative fasting and the use of pharmacologic agents to reduce the risk of pulmonary aspiration: Application to healthy patients undergoing elective procedures" [Online]. Accessed May 2015 via the Web at http://journals.lww.com/anesthesiology/Fulltext/2011/03000/Practice_Guidelines_for_Preoperative_Fasting_and.13.aspx (Level VII)

28 Anderson, D. J., et al. (2014). SHEA/IDSA practice recommendation: Strategies to prevent surgical site infections in acute care hospitals: 2014 update. *Infection Control and Hospital Epidemiology, 35,* 605–627. Accessed May 2015 via the Web at http://www.jstor.org/stable/10.1086/676022

29 Institute for Healthcare Improvement. (2012). *How-to-guide: Prevent surgical site infections.* Cambridge, MA: Institute for Healthcare Improvement. (Level VII)

30 The Joint Commission. (2015). Standard NPSG.07.05.01. *Comprehensive accreditation manual for hospitals: The official handbook.* Oakbrook Terrace, IL: The Joint Commission. (Level VII)

31 Rutala, W. A., et al. (2008). "Guideline for disinfection and sterilization in healthcare facilities, 2008" [Online]. Accessed May 2015 via the Web at http://www.cdc.gov/hicpac/pdf/guidelines/Disinfection_Nov_2008.pdf (Level I)

32 American Osteopathic Association. (2014). Standard 07.02.03. *Healthcare Facilities Accreditation Program: Accreditation requirements for acute care hospitals.* Chicago, IL: American Osteopathic Association. (Level VII)

33 Centers for Medicare & Medicaid Services, Department of Health and Human Services. (2014). Condition of participation: Medical record services. 42 C.F.R. § 482.24(b).

34 American Osteopathic Association. (2014). Standard 10.00.03. *Healthcare Facilities Accreditation Program: Accreditation requirements for acute care hospitals.* Chicago, IL: American Osteopathic Association. (Level VII)

35 American Osteopathic Association. (2014). Standard 30.01.11. *Healthcare Facilities Accreditation Program: Accreditation requirements for acute care hospitals.* Chicago, IL: American Osteopathic Association. (Level VII)

36 The Joint Commission. (2015). Standard RI.01.03.01. *Comprehensive accreditation manual for hospitals: The official handbook.* Oakbrook Terrace, IL: The Joint Commission. (Level VII)

37 Centers for Medicare & Medicaid Services, Department of Health and Human Services. (2014). Condition of participation: Patient's rights. 42 C.F R. § 482.13.

38 American Osteopathic Association. (2014). Standard 30.00.14. *Healthcare Facilities Accreditation Program: Accreditation requirements for acute care hospitals.* Chicago, IL: American Osteopathic Association. (Level VII)

39 Jarrett, N., et al. (2013). "Evidence-based guidelines for selected and previously considered hospital-acquired conditions: Final report" [Online]. Accessed May 2015 via the Web at http://www.cms.gov/Medicare/Medicare-Fee-for-Service-Payment/HospitalAcqCond/Downloads/Evidence-Based-Guidelines.pdf (Level VII)

40 American Osteopathic Association. (2014). Standard 07.01.20. *Healthcare Facilities Accreditation Program: Accreditation requirements for acute care hospitals.* Chicago, IL: American Osteopathic Association. (Level VII)

41 Trimm, D. R., & Sanford, J. T. (2010). The process of family waiting during surgery. *Journal of Family Nursing, 16,* 435–461. Accessed May 2015 via the Web at http://jfn.sagepub.com/content/16/4/435.full.pdf+html (Level VI)

42 The Joint Commission. (2015). Standard UP.01.02.01. *Comprehensive accreditation manual for hospitals: The official handbook.* Oakbrook Terrace, IL: The Joint Commission. (Level VII)

43 Recommended practices for transfer of patient care information. (2014). In R. Conner, et al. (Eds.), *Perioperative standards and recommended practices 2014.* Denver, CO: AORN, Inc. (Level VII)

44 The Joint Commission. (2015). Standard PC.02.02.01. *Comprehensive accreditation manual for hospitals: The official handbook.* Oakbrook Terrace, IL: The Joint Commission. (Level VII)

45 Joint Commission Center for Transforming Healthcare. (2010). Improving transitions of care: Hand-off communications. Oakbrook Terrace, IL: The Joint Commission. (Level VII)

46 The Joint Commission. (2015). Standard RC.01.03.01. *Comprehensive accreditation manual for hospitals: The official handbook.* Oakbrook Terrace, IL: The Joint Commission. (Level VII)

PREOPERATIVE SKIN PREPARATION

Proper preparation of the patient's skin for surgery renders it as free as possible from microorganisms, which reduces the risk of infection at the incision site.[1]

Unless contraindicated, before an open class 1 surgical procedure below the chin, the patient should have two preoperative baths or showers with 4% chlorhexidine gluconate to reduce the number of microorganisms on the skin and to decrease the risk of contaminating the surgical incision.[2] After each preoperative shower, the patient's skin should be thoroughly rinsed to remove residual chlorhexidine gluconate, which may cause skin irritation. The patient's skin should be dried with a fresh, clean, dry towel and the patient should put on clean clothing to reduce the risk of reintroducing microorganisms to clean skin.[1]

Patients undergoing surgery of the head should be instructed in or assisted with performing two preoperative shampoos with chlorhexidine shampoo. Contact with the eyes, ears, and other mucous membranes should be avoided.[2] Conditioners and other hair care products shouldn't be used because a chemical reaction between the chlorhexidine and the hair care product may impede the antiseptic effectiveness of chlorhexidine.[1]

Only hair interfering with the surgical procedure should be removed because hair removal may increase the risk of infection. If hair removal is necessary, electric clippers should be used.[3] The hair should be clipped on the day of surgery in a location outside of the operating or procedure room to decrease the risk of surgical site infection.[1,4,5]

The area of preparation always exceeds that of the expected incision to minimize the number of microorganisms in the areas adjacent to the proposed incision and to allow surgical draping of the patient without contamination.[1] The procedure described here doesn't duplicate or replace the full sterile preparation that immediately precedes surgery. Instead, it covers preparation of the skin when preoperative showers haven't been performed. Because the efficacy of antiseptic agents depends on the cleanliness of the skin, superficial soil, debris, and transient microbes should be removed first to reduce the risk of wound contamination.[1]

Equipment

Antiseptic skin cleaner (4% chlorhexidine gluconate) ▪ gloves ▪ tap water ▪ bath blanket ▪ towels ▪ fluid-impermeable pad ▪ adjustable light ▪ Optional: 4″ × 4″ (10-cm × 10-cm) gauze pads; basin; cotton-tipped applicators; nail polish remover; trash bag; electric or battery-operated clippers for single use or with a reusable head that can be disinfected; depilatory cream; antiseptic soap solution; personal protective equipment; pulse lavage (with protective shield), high-pressure parallel water jet, or brush-suction irrigation.

Preparation of equipment

Use warm tap water *because heat reduces the skin's surface tension and facilitates removal of soil and hair.* Pour plain warm water into the basin *for rinsing.*

Implementation

- Verify the practitioner's order.
- Review the patient's medical record for an allergy or a sensitivity to skin preparation agents. Use an alternative antiseptic agent if indicated.[1]
- Gather the appropriate equipment.
- Perform hand hygiene.[6,7,8]
- Confirm the patient's identity using at least two patient identifiers.[9]
- Explain the procedure to the patient, including the reason for the extensive preparations, *to decrease his anxiety.*
- Provide privacy and put on gloves and, if needed, other personal protective equipment.
- Place the patient in a comfortable position, drape him with the bath blanket, and expose the preparation area; *to ensure privacy and avoid chilling the patient,* expose only one small area at a time while performing skin preparation.
- Place a fluid-impermeable pad beneath the patient *to catch spills and avoid linen changes.* Adjust the light *to illuminate the preparation area.*
- Assess skin condition in the preparation area, and report a rash, an abrasion, or a laceration to the practitioner before beginning the procedure. *Any break in the skin increases the risk of infection and could cause cancellation of planned surgery.*[1]
- Have the patient remove all jewelry.[1]
- Remove cosmetics using a nonirritating agent *to facilitate securing an endotracheal tube, if needed, and for other reasons identified by the surgical team.*[1]
- Clean under the patient's fingernails and remove nail polish, if necessary. If the patient is having hand or wrist surgery, make sure that the nails are short and natural, with no artificial nail surfaces, such as extensions, overlays, acrylic, silk wraps, or enhancements.[1]
- If hair would interfere with the surgical procedure, remove it using electric or battery-operated clippers for single use or with a reusable head that can be disinfected between patients. *Clipping hair, if necessary, the day of surgery reduces the risk of surgical site infection.* As possible, limit the amount of clipping *to reduce the risk of microscopic nicks, which increase the risk of surgical site infection.*[1,5]
- Wash the skin around the surgical site *to remove gross contaminants and oils that might block the penetration of the antiseptic agent.*[1] Carefully clean skin folds and crevices *because they harbor greater numbers of microorganisms.* Clean anatomic areas that contain more debris separately *to prevent the distribution of microorganisms from these areas to the surgical site.*[1]

■ If the patient is having abdominal surgery, clean the umbilicus. If necessary, instill antiseptic solution into the umbilicus *to soften debris.* Then remove the debris using a cotton-tipped applicator *because debris within the umbilicus is a contaminant and can't be adequately disinfected.*[1]
■ If an intestinal or urinary stoma is within the surgical field, clean the area gently and separately from the rest of the prepped area *to remove organic material that might interfere with the effectiveness of the antiseptic agent.*[1]
■ For a surgical field that includes the penis, retract the foreskin, if present, and then gently clean the penis *because organic material and microorganisms accumulate under the foreskin.* After cleaning the foreskin, pull it back over the glans *to prevent circulatory compromise.*[1]
■ Dry the area with a clean towel, and remove the fluid-impermeable pad.
■ Give the patient any special instructions for care of the prepared area, and remind him to keep the area clean for surgery. Make sure that the patient is comfortable.
■ Dispose of used supplies appropriately.
■ Remove and discard your gloves and any other personal protective equipment worn.
■ Perform hand hygiene.[6,7,8]
■ Document the procedure.[10]

Special considerations

■ In cases of head surgery, verify the surgical site before hair removal. *Identifying the surgical site before the time-out ensures that the correct site is prepped, reducing the risk of wrong-site surgery.*
■ Scalp hair removal is usually performed in the operating room, but if you're required to prepare the patient's scalp, put all hair in a plastic or paper bag and store it with the patient's possessions.
■ Depilatory cream can also be used to remove hair. Although this method produces clean, intact skin without risking lacerations or abrasions, it can cause skin irritation or rash, especially in the groin area.[1] Before doing so, perform a skin test *to determine whether the cream irritates the skin.*[1] If possible, cut long hairs with scissors before applying the cream *because the remaining hair will require less cream;* then use a glove to apply the cream in a ½" (1.3-cm) thick layer. After about 10 minutes, remove the cream with moist gauze pads. Then wash the area with antiseptic soap solution, rinse, and pat dry.
■ Traumatic orthopedic wounds with exposed bone may be cleaned using pulse lavage, high-pressure parallel water jet, or brush-suction irrigation. Use sterile normal saline solution and cautiously irrigate the wound *to prevent aerosolization of contaminants;* a pulse lavage protective shield may be beneficial.[1]

Complications

Rashes, nicks, lacerations, and abrasions are the most common complications of skin preparation. They also increase the risk of postoperative infection.

Documentation

Documentation should include the product used, date, time, and area prepared as well as the condition of the skin before and after preparation. Include documentation about hair removal, if performed, including the time, method, and area of removal.[1]

REFERENCES

1 Recommended practices for preoperative patient skin antisepsis. (2014). In R. Conner, et al. (Eds.), *Perioperative standards and recommended practices 2014.* Denver, CO: AORN, Inc. (Level VII)
2 Barzoloski-O'Connor, B. (2011). Surgical site infection: New solutions for an old problem. *OR Nurse, 5*(1), 8–9.
3 Tanner, J., et al. (2011). Preoperative hair removal to reduce surgical site infection. *Cochrane Database of Systematic Reviews, 2011*(11), CD004122.
4 Anderson, D. J., et al. (2014). SHEA/IDSA practice recommendation: Strategies to prevent surgical site infections in acute care hospitals: 2014 update. *Infection Control and Hospital Epidemiology, 35,* 605–627. Accessed May 2015 via the Web at http://www.jstor.org/stable/10.1086/676022 (Level I)
5 Institute for Healthcare Improvement. (2012). *5 Million Lives Campaign. Getting started kit: Prevent surgical site infections.* Cambridge, MA: Institute for Healthcare Improvement. (Level V)
6 Centers for Disease Control and Prevention. (2002). Guideline for hand hygiene in health-care settings: Recommendations of the Healthcare Infection Control Practices Advisory Committee and the HICPAC/SHEA/APIC/IDSA Hand Hygiene Task Force. *MMWR Recommendations and Reports, 51* (RR-16), 1–45. Accessed May 2015 via the Web at http://www.cdc.gov/mmwr/pdf/rr/rr5116.pdf (Level II)
7 The Joint Commission. (2015). Standard NPSG.07.01.01. *Comprehensive accreditation manual for hospitals: The official handbook.* Oakbrook Terrace, IL: The Joint Commission. (Level VII)
8 World Health Organization (2009). "WHO guidelines on hand hygiene in health care: First global patient safety challenge, clean care is safer care" [Online]. Accessed May 2015 via the Web at http://whqlibdoc.who.int/publications/2009/9789241597906_eng.pdf (Level IV)
9 The Joint Commission. (2015). Standard NPSG.01.01.01. *Comprehensive accreditation manual for hospitals: The official handbook.* Oakbrook Terrace, IL: The Joint Commission. (Level VII)
10 The Joint Commission. (2015). Standard RC.01.03.01. *Comprehensive accreditation manual for hospitals: The official handbook.* Oakbrook Terrace, IL: The Joint Commission. (Level VII)

PRESSURE DRESSING APPLICATION

For effective control of capillary or small-vein bleeding, temporary application of pressure directly over a wound may be achieved with a bulk dressing held by a glove-protected hand, bound into place with a pressure bandage, or held under pressure by an inflated air splint. A pressure dressing requires frequent checks for wound drainage to determine its effectiveness in controlling bleeding. The wound shouldn't be cleaned until the bleeding stops.

Equipment

Two or more sterile gauze pads ■ roller gauze ■ adhesive tape ■ gloves ■ metric ruler ■ Optional: clean cloth.

Preparation of equipment

Obtain the pressure dressing quickly *to avoid excessive blood loss.* Use clean cloth for the dressing if sterile gauze pads are unavailable.

Implementation

■ Perform hand hygiene.[1,2,3,4]
■ Put on gloves and other personal protective equipment as needed *to comply with standard precautions.*[3]
■ Quickly explain the procedure to the patient *to help decrease his anxiety.*
■ Elevate and immobilize the injured body part *to help reduce bleeding.*
■ Place enough gauze pads over the wound to cover it.
■ For an extremity or a trunk wound, hold the dressing firmly over the wound and wrap the roller gauze tightly across it and around the body part *to provide pressure on the wound.* Secure the bandage with adhesive tape.
■ To apply a dressing to the neck, the shoulder, or another location that can't be tightly wrapped, don't use roller gauze. Instead, apply tape directly over the dressings *to provide the necessary pressure at the wound site.*
■ Assess pulse, temperature, and skin condition distal to the wound site *because excessive pressure can obstruct normal circulation.*

■ Inspect the dressing frequently *to monitor wound drainage.* Use the metric standard of measurement to determine the amount of drainage, and document these serial measurements for later reference. Don't circle a potentially wet dressing with ink *because such markings don't provide permanent documentation in the medical record and also risk contaminating the dressing.*
■ If the dressing becomes saturated, don't remove it; *removal would interfere with the pressure.* Instead, apply an additional dressing over the saturated one and continue to monitor and record drainage.
■ Obtain additional medical care as soon as possible.
■ Remove and discard your gloves[3] and any other personal protective equipment worn.
■ Perform hand hygiene.[1,2,4,5]
■ Document the procedure.[6,7]

Special considerations

■ Apply pressure directly to the wound with your gloved hand if sterile gauze pads and clean cloth are unavailable.
■ Avoid using an elastic bandage to bind the dressing *because it can't be wrapped tightly enough to create pressure on the wound site.*

Complications

A pressure dressing that's applied too tightly can impair circulation.

Documentation

When the bleeding is controlled, record the date and time of dressing application, site of the wound, presence or absence of distal pulses, integrity of distal skin, amount of wound drainage, and complications.

REFERENCES

1 The Joint Commission. (2015). Standard NPSG.07.01.01. *Comprehensive accreditation manual for hospitals: The official handbook.* Oakbrook Terrace, IL: The Joint Commission. (Level VII)
2 Centers for Disease Control and Prevention. (2002). Guideline for hand hygiene in health-care settings: Recommendations of the Healthcare Infection Control Practices Advisory Committee and the HICPAC/SHEA/APIC/IDSA Hand Hygiene Task Force. *MMWR Recommendations and Reports, 51*(RR-16), 1–45. Accessed May 2015 via the Web at http://www.cdc.gov/mmwr/pdf/rr/rr5116.pdf (Level II)
3 Siegel, J. D., et al. (2007). "2007 guideline for isolation precautions: Preventing transmission of infectious agents in healthcare settings" [Online]. Accessed June 2014 via the Web at http://www.cdc.gov/hicpac/pdf/isolation/Isolation2007.pdf (Level II)
4 American Osteopathic Association. (2014). Standard 07.01.10. *Healthcare Facilities Accreditation Program: Accreditation requirements for acute care hospitals.* Chicago, IL: American Osteopathic Association. (Level VII)
5 World Health Organization. (2009). "WHO guidelines on hand hygiene in health care: First global patient safety challenge, clean care is safer care" [Online]. Accessed May 2015 via the Web at http://whqlibdoc.who.int/publications/2009/9789241597906_eng.pdf (Level IV)
6 The Joint Commission. (2015). Standard RC.01.03.01. *Comprehensive accreditation manual for hospitals: The official handbook.* Oakbrook Terrace, IL: The Joint Commission. (Level VII)
7 American Osteopathic Association. (2014). Standard 10.00.03. *Healthcare Facilities Accreditation Program: Accreditation requirements for acute care hospitals.* Chicago, IL: American Osteopathic Association. (Level VII)

PRESSURE ULCER CARE

As the name implies, pressure ulcers result when pressure—applied with great force for a short period or with less force over a long period—impairs circulation, depriving tissues of oxygen and other life-sustaining nutrients. This process damages skin and underlying structures. Untreated, resulting ischemic lesions can lead to serious infection.

Most pressure ulcers develop over bony prominences, where friction and shearing force combine with pressure to break down skin and underlying tissues. Persistent pressure on bony prominences obstructs capillary blood flow, leading to tissue necrosis. Common sites include the sacrum, coccyx, ischial tuberosities, and greater trochanters. Other common sites include the skin over the vertebrae, scapulae, elbows, knees, and heels in bedridden and relatively immobile patients.

Successful pressure ulcer treatment involves relieving pressure, restoring circulation, promoting adequate nutrition and, if possible, resolving or managing related disorders. Typically, the effectiveness and duration of treatment depend on the pressure ulcer's characteristics.[1] (See *Staging pressure ulcers,* page 634.)

Ideally, prevention is the key to avoiding extensive therapy. Preventive measures include off-loading pressure, maintaining adequate nourishment, and ensuring mobility to relieve pressure and promote circulation.[2] A risk assessment is part of an overall prevention plan.[2] (See *Braden scale: Predicting pressure ulcer risk,* page 636.)[3,4,5]

When a pressure ulcer develops despite preventive efforts, treatment includes methods to decrease pressure, such as frequent repositioning to shorten pressure duration and the use of special equipment to reduce pressure intensity. Treatment also may involve pressure-reducing devices, such as special beds, mattresses, mattress overlays, and chair cushions.

Equipment

Facility-approved skin assessment tool ■ pressure-redistribution devices ■ pillows ■ appropriate skin cleaner and bath supplies ■ lotion ■ protective moisture barrier ■ Optional: gloves, trapeze bar, heel protection devices, absorbent underpads or undergarments.

Implementation

■ Perform hand hygiene.[6,7,8,9,10]
■ Confirm the patient's identity using at least two patient identifiers.[11]
■ Explain the procedure to the patient.
■ Provide privacy.[12,13,14]
■ Put on gloves, as indicated.[15,16]
■ Perform a comprehensive skin assessment using a facility-approved skin assessment tool; *a comprehensive skin assessment may be the first step in pressure ulcer prevention.*[17,18]
■ Turn and reposition the patient every 1 to 2 hours or more frequently, as required, unless contraindicated. For patients with limited mobility, use a pressure-redistribution device, such as air, gel, or a 4″ (10-cm) foam mattress overlay.[19,20] The patient's condition may indicate the need for low- or high-air-loss bed therapy *to redistribute excessive pressure and promote evaporation of excess moisture.*
■ When turning the patient, lift him rather than slide him *because sliding increases friction and shear.*[2,21] Use a turning sheet and get help from coworkers, if necessary.

NURSING ALERT *Avoid placing the patient directly on his trochanter.*[2] *Instead, place him on his side, at about a 30-degree angle.*[21,22]

■ Use pillows and other pressure-redistribution devices *to position the patient and increase his comfort.* (See the "Alignment and pressure-reducing devices" procedure, page 15.)
■ Eliminate sheet wrinkles *that could increase pressure and cause discomfort.* Make sure the patient's heels don't rest on the bed.[21]
■ Work with the patient and multidisciplinary team to implement a regular repositioning routine, *because patients at risk for pressure ulcers require teaching and encouragement to perform regular repositioning movements that redistribute pressure, preventing the buildup of pressure around areas at risk.*[23] Post a repositioning schedule at the patient's bedside. Adapt position changes to his situation. Emphasize the importance of regular position changes to the patient and his family, and encourage their participation in the treatment and prevention of pressure ulcers by having them perform a position change correctly, after you have demonstrated how.[23]

Staging pressure ulcers[1]

Pressure ulcer staging reflects the depth and extent of tissue involvement. The classification system developed by the National Pressure Ulcer Advisory Panel is the most widely used system and categorizes pressure ulcers into four stages and two additional categories—suspected deep tissue injury and unstageable pressure ulcers.

Suspected deep tissue injury

Deep tissue injury is characterized by a purple or maroon localized area of intact skin or blood-filled blister caused by damage to underlying soft tissue from pressure or shear. It may be preceded by tissue that's painful, firm, mushy, boggy, or warm or cool compared with adjacent tissue. The depth of the suspected deep tissue injury is unknown. It may be difficult to detect in patients with darkly pigmented skin. It may initially appear as a thin blister over a dark wound bed.

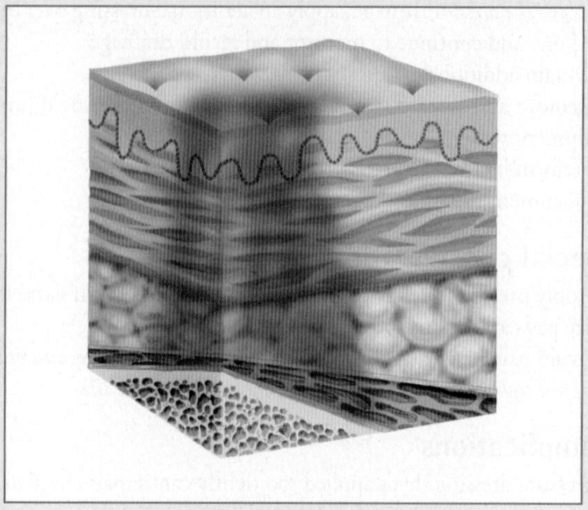

Stage I

A stage I pressure ulcer involves intact skin with nonblanchable redness of a localized area, usually over a bony prominence. The area may be warmer or cooler than adjacent tissue or painful and firm or soft. Darkly pigmented skin may not have visible blanching, but its color and temperature may differ from the surrounding area.

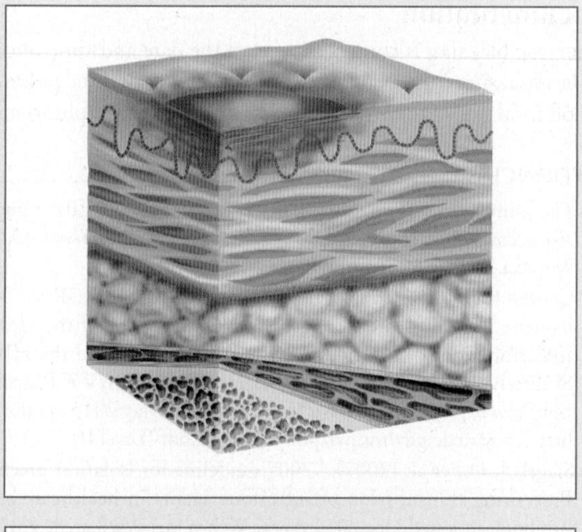

Stage II

A stage II pressure ulcer exhibits a partial-thickness loss of the dermis, appearing as a shallow, open ulcer with a red-pink wound bed without slough. It may also present as an intact or open serum-filled blister. This stage shouldn't be used to describe skin tears, tape burns, excoriation, perineal dermatitis, or maceration.

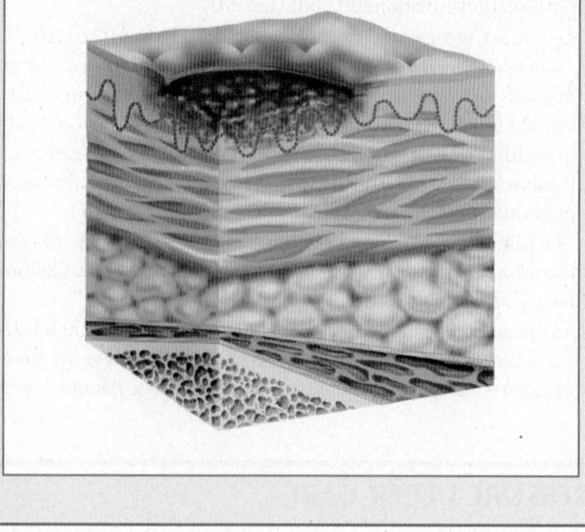

Staging pressure ulcers *(continued)*

Stage III

A stage III pressure ulcer exhibits full-thickness tissue loss. Subcutaneous fat may be visible, but bone, tendon, and muscle aren't exposed. Slough may be present, but it doesn't obscure the depth of tissue loss. Undermining and tunneling may be present. The depth of a stage III ulcer varies by anatomic location.

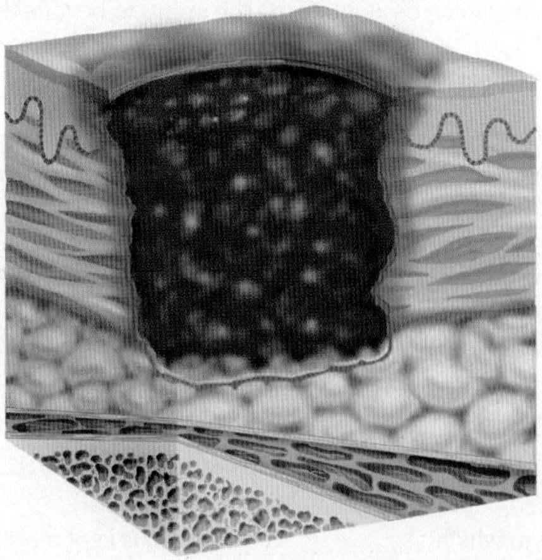

Stage IV

A stage IV pressure ulcer involves full-thickness tissue loss with exposed bone, tendon, or muscle. Slough or eschar may be present on some parts of the wound bed. Undermining and tunneling are also common. The depth of a stage IV ulcer varies by anatomic location.

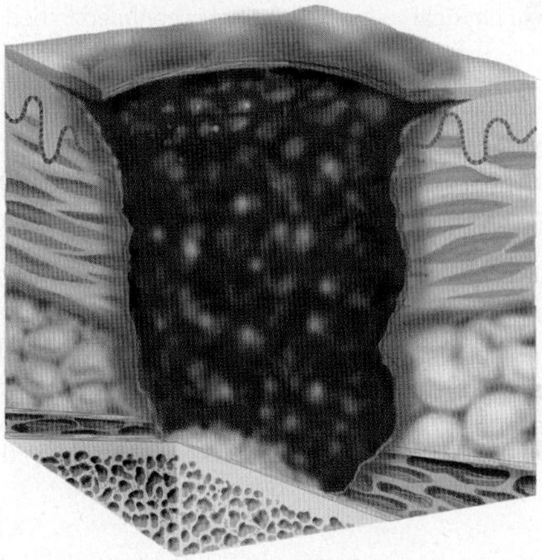

Unstageable

An unstageable ulcer is characterized by full-thickness tissue loss, in which the base of the ulcer in the wound bed is covered by slough, eschar, or both. Until enough slough or eschar is removed to expose the base of the wound, the true depth, and therefore stage, can't be determined.

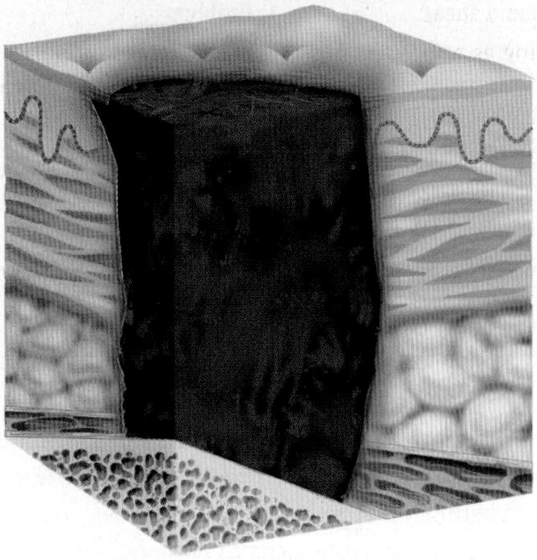

Braden scale: Predicting pressure ulcer risk

The Braden scale, shown here, is the most reliable of several instruments used to assess the risk of developing pressure ulcers. The numbers to the left of each description are the points to be tallied; the lower the score, the greater the risk.

Patient's name: ______________________

Evaluator's name: ______________________

Sensory perception Ability to respond meaningfully to pressure-related discomfort	**1. Completely limited** Patient is unresponsive (doesn't moan, flinch, or grasp in response) to painful stimuli because of diminished level of consciousness or sedation. OR Patient has a limited ability to feel pain over most of body's surface.	**2. Very limited** Patient responds only to painful stimuli; can't communicate discomfort except through moaning or restlessness. OR Patient has a sensory impairment that limits ability to feel pain or discomfort over half of body.
Moisture Degree to which skin is exposed to moisture	**1. Constantly moist** Patient's skin is kept moist almost constantly by perspiration or urine; dampness is detected every time he's moved or turned.	**2. Very moist** Patient's skin is usually but not always moist; linen must be changed at least once per shift.
Activity Degree of physical activity	**1. Bedfast** Patient is confined to bed.	**2. Chairfast** Patient's ability to walk is severely limited or nonexistent; can't bear own weight and must be assisted into a chair or wheelchair.
Mobility Ability to change and control body position	**1. Completely immobile** Patient doesn't make even slight changes in body or extremity position without assistance.	**2. Very limited** Patient makes occasional slight changes in body or extremity position but can't make frequent or significant changes independently.
Nutrition Usual food intake pattern	**1. Very poor** Patient never eats a complete meal; rarely eats more than one-third of any food offered; eats two servings or less of protein (meat or dairy products) per day; takes fluids poorly; doesn't take a liquid dietary supplement. OR Patient is NPO or maintained on clear liquids or IV fluids for more than 5 days.	**2. Probably inadequate** Patient rarely eats a complete meal and generally eats only about one-half of any food offered; protein intake includes only three servings of meat or dairy products per day; occasionally will take a dietary supplement. OR Patient receives less than optimum amount of liquid diet or tube feeding.
Friction and shear	**1. Problem** Patient requires moderate to maximum assistance in moving; complete lifting without sliding against sheets is impossible; frequently slides down in bed or chair, requiring frequent repositioning with maximum assistance; spasticity, contractures, or agitation leads to almost constant friction.	**2. Potential problem** Patient moves feebly or requires minimum assistance during a move; skin probably slides to some extent against sheets, chair restraints, or other devices; maintains relatively good position in chair or bed most of the time but occasionally slides down.

- As appropriate, implement active or passive range-of-motion exercises *to redistribute pressure and promote circulation. To save time,* combine these exercises with bathing, if applicable.
- Direct a patient confined to a chair or wheelchair to shift his weight every 15 minutes *to promote blood flow to compressed tissues.*[2,5,21]
- Show a paraplegic patient how to shift his weight by doing push-ups in the wheelchair. If the patient needs your help, sit next to him and help him shift his weight to one buttock for 60 seconds; then repeat the procedure on the other side. Provide him with pressure-redistribution cushions, as appropriate. However, avoid seating the patient on a rubber or plastic doughnut, *which can increase localized pressure at vulnerable points.*

NURSING ALERT *The Wound, Ostomy and Continence Nurses Society (WOCN) recommends avoiding the use of doughnuts, foam rings, foam cut-outs, and synthetic sheepskin.*[5]

- If a patient confined to a chair or wheelchair can stand, assist the patient into a standing position every hour, if possible.[23]
- Adjust or pad appliances, casts, or splints, as needed, *to ensure proper fit and avoid increased pressure and impaired circulation.*

Date of Assessment: ____________________

3. Slightly limited Patient responds to verbal commands but can't always communicate discomfort or the need to be turned. OR Patient has some sensory impairment that limits ability to feel pain or discomfort in one or two extremities.	**4. No impairment** Patient responds to verbal commands; has no sensory deficit that would limit ability to feel or voice pain or discomfort.	**Score**
3. Occasionally moist Patient's skin is occasionally moist; linen requires an extra change approximately once per day.	**4. Rarely moist** Patient's skin is usually dry; linen requires changing only at routine intervals.	**Score**
3. Walks occasionally Patient walks occasionally during the day, but for very short distances, with or without assistance; spends majority of each shift in a bed or chair.	**4. Walks frequently** Patient walks outside room at least twice per day and inside room at least once every 2 hours during waking hours.	**Score**
3. Slightly limited Patient makes frequent (although slight) changes in body or extremity position independently.	**4. No limitations** Patient makes major and frequent changes in body or extremity position without assistance.	**Score**
3. Adequate Patient eats more than one-half of most meals; eats four servings of protein (meat and dairy products) per day; occasionally refuses a meal but will usually take a supplement if offered. OR Patient is on a tube feeding or total parenteral nutrition regimen that probably meets most nutritional needs.	**4. Excellent** Patient eats most of every meal and never refuses a meal; usually eats four or more servings of meat and dairy products per day; occasionally eats between meals; doesn't require supplementation.	**Score**
3. No apparent problem Patient moves in bed and in chair independently and has sufficient muscle strength to lift up completely during move; maintains good position in bed or chair at all times.		**Score**
	Total Score	

■ Apply heel protection devices, as required, *to prevent heel pressure ulcers.* The devices should completely offload pressure from the heels. If placing pillows under calves to decrease pressure, place the pillow longitudinally underneath the calf with the heel suspended in air.[5]

■ Tell the patient to avoid hot water, drying bar soaps, and irritating cleaning agents, such as those with fragrance or alcohol, *because they dry the skin.*[5] Applying lotion after bathing will help keep his skin hydrated.[2] Also tell him to avoid vigorous massage *because it can damage capillaries.*

■ If diarrhea develops or if the patient is incontinent, clean and dry soiled skin following each episode. Then apply a protective moisture barrier *to prevent incontinence-associated dermatitis.*[2] (See the "Incontinence management, fecal" and "Incontinence management, urinary" procedures, pages 387, 388.)[2,5]

■ If the patient's condition permits, recommend a diet that includes adequate calories, protein, and vitamins.[2] Dietary therapy may involve nutritional consultation, food supplements, enteral feeding, or total parenteral nutrition.[24,25]

■ Consult with your facility's wound, continence, and ostomy nurse; nutritionist or registered dietician; and physical or occupational therapist, as indicated, *because pressure ulcer prevention requires a multidisciplinary approach.*[17,23,26]
■ Remove and discard your gloves.[15,16]
■ Perform hand hygiene.[6,7,8,9,10]
■ Document the procedure.[27,28,29]

Special considerations

■ Comprehensive skin assessment shouldn't be a one-time event limited to admission. Repeat it regularly *to determine whether changes in skin condition have occurred.* Perform a comprehensive skin assessment when the patient is admitted to the unit, daily while he's on the unit, and when he's transferred or discharged. In some settings, the patient may need assessments as frequently as every shift. The admission assessment is particularly important when the patient arrives at the emergency department, operating room, and recovery room. You may need to conduct more frequent assessments on units where pressure ulcers may develop rapidly, such as the critical care unit. Staff members on each unit should know how frequently they should perform comprehensive skin assessments.[17,30]
■ Except for brief periods, avoid raising the head of the bed more than 30 degrees *to prevent shearing forces.*[2]
■ Avoid using elbow and heel protectors that fasten with a single narrow strap. *The strap may impair neurovascular function in the involved hand or foot.*
■ In incontinent patients, use absorbent underpads or undergarments that wick moisture away from the skin. The WOCN also recommends establishing a bowel and bladder management retraining program and possibly using a pouching system or a bowel or fecal containment device *to contain excessive stool output and protect the skin.* They also suggest considering use of an indwelling urinary catheter for patients with severe urinary incontinence that has contributed to or may contaminate a pressure ulcer.[5]
■ Depending on the patient's needs, repair of stage III and stage IV pressure ulcers may require surgical intervention, such as direct closure, skin grafting, and flaps.

Patient teaching

Make sure the patient, family members, and caregivers learn pressure ulcer prevention and treatment strategies so that they understand the importance of care, the available choices, the rationales for treatments, and their own role in selecting goals and shaping the care plan.[2,23]

Complications

If left untreated, pressure ulcers may produce ischemia and local infection. Advancing infection or cellulitis can lead to septicemia. Severe erythema may signal worsening cellulitis, which indicates that the offending organisms have invaded the tissue and are no longer localized.

Documentation

Update the care plan, as required. On the clinical record, document a complete skin assessment and interventions used to prevent pressure ulcers and the patient's response. If a pressure ulcer develops, note changes in the condition or size of the pressure ulcer and elevations of skin temperature. Document when the practitioner was notified of pertinent abnormal observations.

References

1 National Pressure Ulcer Advisory Panel. (2007). "Pressure ulcer stages revised by NPUAP" [Online]. Accessed May 2015 via the Web at http://www.npuap.org/pr2.htm (Level V)

2 Institute for Clinical Systems Improvement. (2012, reaffirmed 2014). "Health care protocol: Pressure ulcer prevention and treatment protocol (3rd ed.)" [Online]. Accessed May 2015 via the Web at https://www.icsi.org/_asset/6t7kxy/ (Level V)

3 Moore, Z. E., & Cowman, S. (2014). Risk assessment tools for the prevention of pressure ulcers. *Cochrane Database of Systematic Reviews, 2014*(2), CD006471. (Level I)

4 Agency for Healthcare Research and Quality. (2013). "Pressure ulcer risk assessment and prevention: Comparative effectiveness" [Online]. Accessed May 2015 via the Web at http://effectivehealthcare.ahrq.gov/ehc/products/309/1490/pressure-ulcer-prevention-executive-130508.pdf (Level I)

5 Wound, Ostomy and Continence Nurses Society. (2010). "Guideline for prevention and management of pressure ulcers" [Online]. Accessed May 2015 via the Web at http://guideline.gov/content.aspx?id=23868 (Level VII)

6 Centers for Disease Control and Prevention. (2002). Guideline for hand hygiene in health-care settings: Recommendations of the Healthcare Infection Control Practices Advisory Committee and the HICPAC/SHEA/APIC/IDSA Hand Hygiene Task Force. *MMWR Recommendations and Reports, 51*(RR-16), 1–45. Accessed May 2015 via the Web at http://www.cdc.gov/mmwr/pdf/rr/rr5116.pdf (Level II)

7 World Health Organization. (2009). "WHO guidelines on hand hygiene in health care: First global patient safety challenge, clean care is safer care" [Online]. Accessed May 2015 via the Web at http://whqlibdoc.who.int/publications/2009/9789241597906_eng.pdf (Level IV)

8 The Joint Commission. (2015). Standard NPSG.07.01.01. *Comprehensive accreditation manual for hospitals: The official handbook.* Oakbrook Terrace, IL: The Joint Commission. (Level VII)

9 American Osteopathic Association. (2014). Standard 07.01.21. *Healthcare Facilities Accreditation Program: Accreditation requirements for acute care hospitals.* Chicago, IL: American Osteopathic Association. (Level VII)

10 Centers for Medicare & Medicaid Services, Department of Health and Human Services. (2014). Condition of participation: Infection control. 42 C.F.R. § 482.42.

11 The Joint Commission. (2015). Standard NPSG.01.01.01. *Comprehensive accreditation manual for hospitals: The official handbook.* Oakbrook Terrace, IL: The Joint Commission. (Level VII)

12 American Osteopathic Association. (2014). Standard 15.01.16. *Healthcare Facilities Accreditation Program: Accreditation requirements for acute care hospitals.* Chicago, IL: American Osteopathic Association. (Level VII)

13 The Joint Commission. (2015). Standard RI.01.01.01. *Comprehensive accreditation manual for hospitals: The official handbook.* Oakbrook Terrace, IL: The Joint Commission. (Level VII)

14 Centers for Medicare & Medicaid Services, Department of Health and Human Services. (2014). Condition of participation: Patient's rights. 42 C.F.R. § 482.13(c)(1).

15 Siegel, J. D., et al. (2007). "2007 guideline for isolation precautions: Preventing transmission of infectious agents in healthcare settings" [Online]. Accessed May 2015 via the Web at http://www.cdc.gov/hicpac/pdf/isolation/Isolation2007.pdf (Level II)

16 American Osteopathic Association. (2014). Standard 16.02.02. *Healthcare Facilities Accreditation Program: Accreditation requirements for acute care hospitals.* Chicago, IL: American Osteopathic Association. (Level VII)

17 Agency for Healthcare Quality and Research. (2011). "Preventing pressure ulcers in hospitals: A toolkit for improving quality of care" [Online]. Accessed May 2015 via the Web at http://www.ahrq.gov/research/ltc/pressureulcertoolkit/putoolkit.pdf

18 American Osteopathic Association. (2014). Standard 07.01.21. *Healthcare Facilities Accreditation Program: Accreditation requirements for acute care hospitals.* Chicago, IL: American Osteopathic Association. (Level VII)

19 McInnes, E., et al. (2011). Support surfaces for pressure ulcer prevention. *Cochrane Database of Systematic Reviews, 2011*(4), CD001735.

20 Wong, V. (2011). Skin blood flow response to 2-hour repositioning in long-term care residents: A pilot study. *Journal of Wound, Ostomy and Continence Nursing, 38,* 529–537.

21 National Pressure Ulcer Advisory Panel and European Pressure Ulcer Advisory Panel. (2009). "Prevention and treatment of pressure ulcers: Clinical

practice guidelines" [Online]. Accessed May 2015 via the Web at http://www.npuap.org/Final_Quick_Prevention_for_web_2010.pdf (Level VII)
22 Knox, D. M., et al. (1994). Effects of different turn intervals on skin of healthy older adults. *Advances in Wound Care, 7,* 48–56.
23 Schofield, R., et al. (2013). "Reviewing the literature on the effectiveness of pressure relieving movements" [Online]. Accessed May 2015 via the Web at http://www.hindawi.com/journals/nrp/2013/124095/
24 Sernekos, L. (2013). Nutritional treatment of pressure ulcers: What is the evidence? *Journal of the American Association of Nurse Practitioners, 25,* 281–288. Accessed May 2015 via the Web at http://onlinelibrary.wiley.com/doi/10.1002/2327-6924.12025/pdf
25 Doley, J. (2010). Nutrition management of pressure ulcers. *Nutrition in Clinical Practice, 25,* 50–60.
26 Dorner, B., et al. (2009). "The role of nutrition in pressure ulcer prevention and treatment: National Pressure Ulcer Advisory Panel white paper" [Online]. Accessed May 2015 via the Web at http://www.npuap.org/wp-content/uploads/2012/03/Nutrition-White-Paper-Website-Version.pdf
27 The Joint Commission. (2015). Standard RC.01.03.01. *Comprehensive accreditation manual for hospitals: The official handbook.* Oakbrook Terrace, IL: The Joint Commission. (Level VII)
28 Centers for Medicare & Medicaid Services, Department of Health and Human Services. (2014). Condition of participation: Medical record services. 42 C.F.R. § 482.24(b).
29 American Osteopathic Association. (2014). Standard 10.00.03. *Healthcare Facilities Accreditation Program: Accreditation requirements for acute care hospitals.* Chicago, IL: American Osteopathic Association. (Level VII)
30 American Osteopathic Association. (2014). Standard 10.01.24. *Healthcare Facilities Accreditation Program: Accreditation requirements for acute care hospitals.* Chicago, IL: American Osteopathic Association. (Level VII)

ADDITIONAL REFERENCE

Doughty, D. (2012). Differential assessment of trunk wounds: Pressure ulceration versus incontinence associated dermatitis versus intertriginous dermatitis. *Ostomy Wound Management, 58*(4), 20–22.

PROGRESSIVE AMBULATION

After surgery or a period of bed rest, patients must begin the gradual return to full ambulation. When it's begun promptly and properly, progressive ambulation thwarts many of the complications of prolonged inactivity.

The American Academy of Orthopaedic Surgeons recommends early progressive ambulation after hip and knee arthroplasty to prevent venous thromboembolism.[1] Other complications prevented by early progressive ambulation include respiratory stasis and hypostatic pneumonia; urine retention, urinary tract infection, urinary stasis, and calculus formation; abdominal distention, constipation, and decreased appetite; and sensory deprivation. Progressive ambulation also helps restore the patient's sense of equilibrium and enhances his self-confidence and self-image.[2] In hip replacement patients, early dangling and ambulation result in excellent postoperative pain management and a shortened length of stay.[3]

Progressive ambulation begins with dangling the patient's feet over the edge of the bed and progresses to seating him in an armchair or wheelchair, walking around the room with him, and then walking with him in the halls until he can walk by himself. (See *Helping a patient regain mobility.*) The patient's progress depends on his physical condition and his tolerance. Successful return to full ambulation requires correct body mechanics, careful patient observation, and open communication among patient, practitioner, and nurse.

Helping a patient regain mobility

Use the tips below to help a patient regain mobility as he sits in a chair and then progresses to walking.

Sitting
Seat the patient in a chair with armrests and a straight back, with his lower back against the rear of the chair, feet flat on the floor, hips and knees at right angles, and upper body straight. Rest his forearms on the armrests.

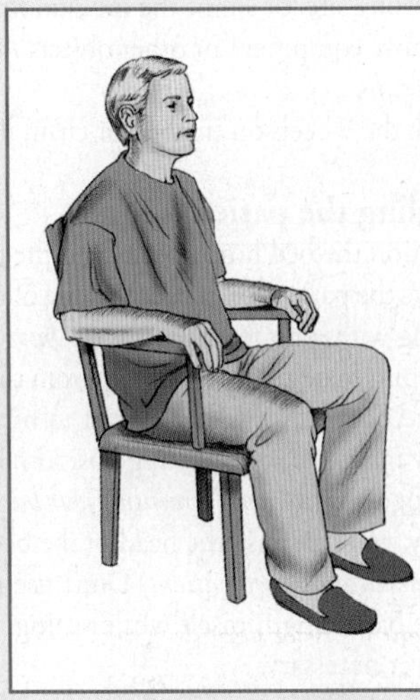

Walking
Provide a path unimpeded by equipment and other objects, and avoid overexertion. If necessary, hold the patient *so you can control his upper and lower body and any lateral movements.* Alternatively, use a gait belt if the patient is at risk for falling *because it provides a secure grasping surface to aid with patient transfer and ambulation.*[4]

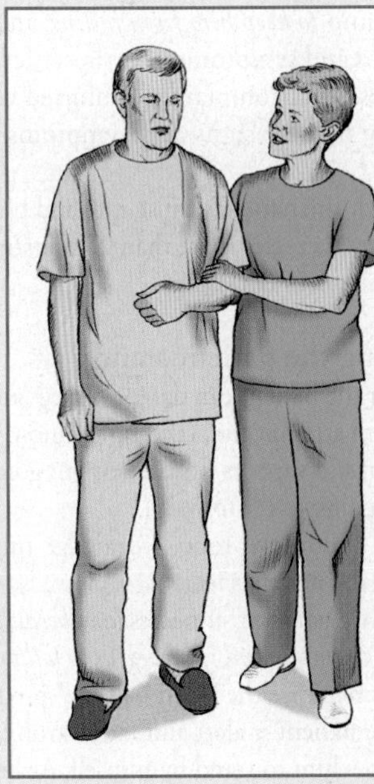

Equipment

Robe ■ chair or wheelchair ■ slippers for sitting; hard-soled shoes for walking ■ Optional: assistive device (cane, crutches, walker), prescribed analgesic, blood pressure cuff and stethoscope or automated blood pressure device, gait belt.

If the patient requires an assistive device, the physical therapist usually selects the appropriate one and teaches its use.

Implementation

- Check the patient's history, diagnosis, and therapeutic regimen.
- Gather the appropriate equipment.
- Perform hand hygiene.[5,6,7,8,9]
- Confirm the patient's identity using at least two patient identifiers.[10]
- Perform a comprehensive pain assessment using techniques appropriate for the patient's age, condition, and ability to understand.[11]
- Administer an analgesic, as needed and ordered, following safe medication practices, and wait 30 to 60 minutes for it to take effect before attempting ambulation.

NURSING ALERT *A medicated patient may develop hypotension, dizziness, or drowsiness.*

- Explain the goal of ambulation. Provide encouragement *because the patient may be hesitant or fearful;* reassure him that he need not attempt more than he can reasonably do. If he fears pain in an incision, show him how to support the incision by placing a hand alongside or gently over the dressing site, or splint the incision for him.
- Remove equipment or other objects *to provide a clear path and to help prevent falls.*
- Lock the wheels on the bed or chair, if appropriate.

Dangling the patient's legs

- Position the bed horizontally and the patient laterally, facing you.
- Move the patient's legs over the side of the bed and grasp his shoulders, standing with your feet apart *so you have a wide base of support.*
- Ask him to help by pushing up from the bed with his arms. Then shift your weight from the foot closest to his head to the other foot as you steadily raise him to the sitting position. Pull with your whole body, not just your arms, *to avoid straining your back and jostling the patient.* Alternatively, you can raise the head of the bed to a 45-degree angle *to allow easier elevation of the patient.* Don't use this method if the patient has trouble balancing himself while sitting. Ask a coworker for assistance whenever necessary.
- While the patient adjusts to an upright position, continue to stand facing him *to keep him from falling,* and observe him closely. Be alert for signs and symptoms of orthostatic hypotension, such as fainting, dizziness, and complaints of blurred vision. Be prepared to respond quickly if these signs and symptoms develop *to prevent him from falling.*
- Check the patient's pulse rate and blood pressure, as needed. If the pulse rate increases more than 20 beats/minute, allow the patient to rest before slowly progressing.

Helping the patient stand

- After the patient can dangle his legs and support his weight on them, have him attempt the standing position. Help the patient put on a robe and nonskid slippers first (if he's not going to walk) or hard-soled shoes (if he's going to try to walk).
- Don't allow the robe, a drainage tube, or anything else to dangle around the patient's feet.
- Apply a gait belt, if necessary,[4] *because it can help you safely lower the patient to the ground if he begins to fall or loses balance during transfer or ambulation.* (See the "Gait belt use" procedure, page 333.)
- If the patient is alert and fairly strong, place his feet flat on the floor and allow him to stand by himself. As he stands, place one hand under his axilla and the other hand around his waist *to prevent falls.* Help him stand fully erect. Encourage him to look forward and not at the floor *to help maintain his balance.*
- If the patient needs help standing up, face him and position your knees at either side of his knees. Bend your knees, put your arms around his waist, and instruct him to push up from the bed with his arms. Then straighten your knees and pull the patient with you while rising to an erect position. *This technique helps you avoid back strain.*

Helping the patient sit or walk

- After the patient stands, you can pivot and lower him into an armchair or wheelchair, or you can begin to walk with him.
- If you've decided to seat him, make sure you've applied the wheelchair's brakes or that the chair is secure and won't slip as you lower the patient into it. Place his lower back against the rear of the chair and his feet flat on the floor. Position his hips and knees at right angles, and keep his upper body straight. Then flex his elbows and place his forearms on the arms of the chair.
- If the patient can walk safely only with your assistance, stand to the side and slightly behind him, placing one hand under his axilla and the other hand around his waist. If the patient has weakness or paralysis on one side, stand on the affected side and stabilize him by putting one arm around his waist.
- If necessary, ask a coworker to help you. Stand on opposite sides of the patient and place one hand under his arm or on his elbow.
- Give the patient verbal and tactile cues *to encourage him.* Stay close to a railed wall or another supportive structure.

Completing the procedure

- Perform hand hygiene.[5,6,7,8,9]
- Document the procedure.[12,13,14]

Special considerations

- Patients receiving medications such as beta-adrenergic blockers and vasodilators may be subject to episodes of bradycardia and hypotension.
- If early ambulation is impossible, encourage bed exercises.
- Don't let the use of catheters and IV tubing discourage ambulation; secure these devices *so they are easily portable,* and check dressings and tubes carefully afterward *for proper position and changes in drainage.*
- If the patient begins to fall, try to break his fall by easing him to the bed, chair, or floor, making sure he doesn't strike his head. Then summon help. Don't leave the patient alone—he needs your comfort and reassurance.
- If the patient experiences dyspnea, diaphoresis, or orthostatic hypotension, stabilize his position and take vital signs. Place him in the semi-Fowler position *to facilitate breathing.* If his condition doesn't improve rapidly, notify the practitioner.

Documentation

Record the type of transfer and assistance needed; the duration of sitting, standing, or walking; the distance walked, if appropriate; the patient's response to ambulation; and any significant changes in blood pressure, pulse, and respiration.

REFERENCES

1 American Academy of Orthopaedic Surgeons. (2011). *Preventing venous thromboembolic disease in patients undergoing elective hip and knee arthroplasty: Evidence-based guideline and evidence report* (2nd ed.). Rosemont, IL: American Academy of Orthopaedic Surgeons. Accessed May 2015 via the Web at http://www.aaos.org/research/guidelines/VTE/VTE_full_guideline.pdf (Level I)

2 Killey, B., & Watt, E. (2006). The effect of extra walking on the mobility, independence and exercise self-efficacy of elderly hospital in-patients: A pilot study. *Contemporary Nurse, 22,* 120–133.

3 Morris, B. A., et al. (2010). Clinical practice guidelines for early mobilization hours after surgery. *Orthopaedic Nursing, 29,* 290–316. Accessed May 2015 via the Web at http://www.nursingcenter.com/lnc/CEArticle?an=00006416-201009000-00003&Journal_ID=403341&Issue_ID=1092086 (Level IV)

4 Degelau, J., et al. (2012). "Institute for Clinical Systems Improvement: Health care protocol: Prevention of falls (acute care) (3rd ed.)" [Online]. Accessed May 2015 via the Web at https://www.icsi.org/_asset/dcn15z/Falls-Interactive0412.pdf

5 The Joint Commission. (2015). Standard NPSG.07.01.01. *Comprehensive accreditation manual for hospitals: The official handbook.* Oakbrook Terrace, IL: The Joint Commission. (Level VII)

6 Centers for Disease Control and Prevention. (2002). Guideline for hand hygiene in health-care settings: Recommendations of the Healthcare Infection Control Practices Advisory Committee and the HICPAC/SHEA/APIC/IDSA Hand Hygiene Task Force. *MMWR Recommendations and Reports, 51*(RR-16), 1–45. Accessed May 2015 via the Web at http://www.cdc.gov/mmwr/pdf/rr/rr5116.pdf (Level II)

7 World Health Organization. (2009). "WHO guidelines on hand hygiene in health care: First global patient safety challenge, clean care is safer care" [Online]. Accessed May 2015 via the Web at http://whqlibdoc.who.int/publications/2009/9789241597906_eng.pdf (Level IV)
8 Centers for Medicare & Medicaid Services, Department of Health and Human Services. (2014). Condition of participation: Infection control. 42 C.F.R. § 482.42.
9 American Osteopathic Association. (2014). Standard 07.01.21. *Healthcare Facilities Accreditation Program: Accreditation requirements for acute care hospitals.* Chicago, IL: American Osteopathic Association.
10 The Joint Commission. (2015). Standard NPSG.01.01.01. *Comprehensive accreditation manual for hospitals: The official handbook.* Oakbrook Terrace, IL: The Joint Commission. (Level VII)
11 The Joint Commission. (2015). Standard PC.01.02.07. *Comprehensive accreditation manual for hospitals: The official handbook.* Oakbrook Terrace, IL: The Joint Commission. (Level VII)
12 The Joint Commission. (2015). Standard RC.01.03.01. *Comprehensive accreditation manual for hospitals: The official handbook.* Oakbrook Terrace, IL: The Joint Commission. (Level VII)
13 Centers for Medicare & Medicaid Services, Department of Health and Human Services. (2014). Condition of participation: Medical record services. 42 C.F.R. § 482.24.
14 American Osteopathic Association. (2014). Standard 10.00.03. *Healthcare Facilities Accreditation Program: Accreditation requirements for acute care hospitals.* Chicago, IL: American Osteopathic Association.

PRONE POSITIONING

Prone positioning is a therapeutic maneuver to improve oxygenation and pulmonary mechanics in patients with acute lung injury or mechanically ventilated patients with acute respiratory distress syndrome (ARDS) who require high concentrations of inspired oxygen. Also known as *proning*, the procedure involves physically turning a patient from a supine position (on the back) to a face-down position (prone position).

The recommended criteria for using prone positioning include patients with ARDS who require high plateau pressure or a high fraction of inspired oxygen, which make mechanical ventilation potentially damaging to the lungs.[1]

The physical challenges of prone positioning have been a traditional barrier to its use. However, equipment innovations (such as a lightweight, cushioned frame that straps to the front of the patient before turning) have helped to minimize the risks associated with moving patients and maintaining them in the prone position for several hours at a time. Several bed manufacturers have also developed automated systems designed to provide multiple intervals of prone therapy automatically over an extended time. With the appropriate equipment, prone positioning may promote better movement of the diaphragm by allowing the abdomen to expand more fully.

Prone positioning is usually performed for 6 or more hours a day, for as long as 10 days, until the requirement for a high concentration of inspired oxygen resolves. Aside from early intervention, factors that predict how patients will respond aren't consistent among studies, and a patient's initial response doesn't always predict his subsequent responses. Patients with extrapulmonary ARDS (such as ARDS due to multiple trauma) appear to respond consistently to prone positioning.[2] Although research has demonstrated improved oxygenation with proning, it's unclear whether the survival rate is increased.[3]

Prone positioning can be accomplished by manually turning the patient or by using an automated proning device, such as the RotoProne™ Therapy System. Prone positioning is contraindicated in patients whose heads can't be supported in a face-down position as well as in those who can't tolerate a head-down position. Relative contraindications include increased intracranial pressure; unstable spine, chest, or pelvis; unstable bone fractures; left-sided heart failure (nonpulmonary respiratory failure); shock; abdominal compartment syndrome; abdominal surgery; extreme obesity (greater than 300 lb [136 kg]); and pregnancy. Thorough evaluation of hemodynamically unstable patients (systolic blood pressure less than 90 mm Hg), despite aggressive fluid resuscitation and vasopressors, is essential before initiating prone positioning.

Contraindications specific to RotoProne™ Therapy include unstable cervical, thoracic, lumbar, pelvic, skull, or facial fractures; cervical or skeletal traction; uncontrolled intracranial pressure; body weight below 88 lb (40 kg) or above 350 lb (159 kg); or height less than 54 inches (137 cm) or greater than 78 inches (198 cm).[4]

Equipment

Hospital bed, specialty bed, or automated prone-positioning device ▪ small towels ▪ small pillows or rolled towels ▪ drawsheet ▪ suction equipment ▪ oral care supplies (see the "Oral care" procedure, page 560) ▪ monitoring equipment, as indicated (such as cardiac monitor, hemodynamic monitoring setup, stethoscope, pulse oximeter, and capnography monitor) ▪ emergency equipment (crash cart with cardiac medications, defibrillator, handheld resuscitation bag with mask, intubation equipment) ▪ hospital-grade disinfectant ▪ arterial blood sampling equipment ▪ Optional: gloves, other personal protective equipment, wound and ostomy care supplies, tape, bite block, eye lubricant.

Preparation of equipment

Turn off the patient's enteral tube feeding 1 hour before prone positioning *to reduce the risk of aspiration during the turning process.*[1] Make sure that emergency equipment is readily available and functioning properly.[1] Using a hospital-grade disinfectant, clean and disinfect the positioner between positioning turns and when discontinuing prone positioning.[5,6]

Implementation

- Verify the practitioner's order.
- Perform hand hygiene.[7,8,9,10,11]
- Confirm the patient's identity using at least two patient identifiers.[12]

Assessing the patient

- Assess the patient's hemodynamic status *to determine whether the patient can tolerate the prone position.*
- Assess the patient's neurologic status before prone positioning. Typically, the patient will be sedated heavily. Although agitation isn't a contraindication for the procedure, you must manage it effectively.
- Determine whether the patient's size and weight will allow turning a 180 degrees on a narrow critical care bed. If needed, consider obtaining a wider specialty bed or the RotoProne™ Therapy System.
- Explain the procedure to the patient and family members and answer all questions *to allay their anxiety and promote cooperation.*

Before turning the patient

- Gather the equipment.
- Perform hand hygiene[7,8,9,10,11] and put on gloves or other protective equipment as needed.[13,14]
- Provide eye care, including lubrication and horizontal taping of eyelids, if indicated.[1]
- Ensure that the patient's tongue is inside the mouth; if it's edematous or protruding, insert a bite block.[1]
- Secure the patient's endotracheal (ET) tube or tracheotomy tube *to prevent accidental dislodgment.*[1]
- Perform anterior body wound care and dressing changes.[1]
- Empty ileostomy or colostomy drainage bags.[1]
- Remove anterior chest wall electrocardiogram (ECG) monitoring leads while ensuring the ability to monitor the patient's cardiac rate and rhythm. You'll position these leads on the patient's back after the patient is in the prone position.[1]
- Ensure that the bed's brake is engaged.

Turning the patient manually

■ Position up to six staff members appropriately on either side of the bed and at the head of the bed, depending on the size and complexity of the patient.[1,4]

NURSING ALERT *The staff member at the head of the bed is responsible for monitoring the ET tube and mechanical ventilator tubing.*

■ Adjust all patient tubing and invasive monitoring lines *to prevent dislodgment, kinking, disconnection, or contact with the patient's body during the turning procedure and while the patient remains in the prone position.*

NURSING ALERT *Place all lines inserted in the upper torso over the right or left shoulder, with the exception of chest tubes, which are placed at the foot of the bed. Position all lines inserted in the lower torso at the foot of the bed.*[1]

■ Turn the patient's face away from the ventilator, placing the ET tubing on the side of the patient's face that's turned away from the ventilator.[1] Loop the remaining tubing above the patient's head to *prevent disconnection of the ventilator tubing or kinking of the ET tube.*

■ Lower the side rails of the bed and move the patient to the edge of the bed farthest away from the ventilator using a drawsheet. The person closest to the patient maintains body contact with the bed at all times, serving as a side rail.[1]

■ Tuck the patient's arm and hand that are resting in the center of the bed under the buttocks. Cross the leg closest to the edge of the bed over the opposite leg at the ankle, *which will help with forward motion when the turning process begins.*[1]

NURSING ALERT *If you can't straighten and tuck the patient's arm under the buttocks, tuck the arm into the open space between the chest and pelvic pads.*

■ Turn the patient toward the ventilator, first turning the patient onto the side, and then roll the patient into the prone position.[1]

NURSING ALERT *Always turn the patient in the direction of the mechanical ventilator.*

■ Gently move the patient's tucked arm and hand *so they're parallel to the body,* and then flex them to a comfortable position.[1] Alternatively, place one of the patient's arms up and one down, as in a swimmer's position.[1,4]

■ Support the patient's ankles and feet with a pillow or towel roll *to provide correct flexion while prone.*[1]

■ Pad the patient's elbows with small towels *to prevent ulnar nerve compression.*

■ Replace ECG monitoring leads on the patient's back.

Turning the patient using the RotoProne™ Therapy system[1]

■ Ask a coworker to help you position the patient on the RotoProne™ Therapy System.

■ Secure ventilator tubes and other upper body lines into the tube management system at the head of the bed.

■ Secure all lower body tubes and lines through the circular opening at the foot of the bed.

■ Make sure all tubes have enough slack and that they can slide freely without being pinched or compressed by the tube management system during turning.

NURSING ALERT *Don't hang or attach any equipment to the side of the RotoProne™ Therapy System support frame.*[4]

■ Secure the patient into the system following the manufacturer's instructions:

■ Secure the patient within the side packs *to prevent shear or friction injuries during turning.*

■ Secure the abdominal support mesh over the patient's abdomen.

■ Position the lower leg packs, pelvic pack, and chest pack appropriately.

■ Make sure the patient's head is secure within the headpiece.

■ Place the face pack on the patient's face, making sure the top pad is above the eyebrows and the side pieces are around the mouth.

■ Remove all equipment from around the RotoProne™ Therapy System before turning *to prevent patient or caregiver injury.*[4]

■ Use the RotoProne™ touch screen *to turn the patient prone following the manufacturer's instructions.*

■ Using the touch screen, place the patient in the reverse Trendelenburg position *to elevate the head of the bed, decrease edema, and prevent aspiration.*[1]

■ Open back hatches and replace ECG monitoring leads.

Monitoring the patient

■ Monitor the patient's response to the prone position by assessing vital signs, oxygen saturation level (by pulse oximeter), and capnography. The patient's vital signs should return to normal within 10 minutes of initiating the prone position. Obtain an arterial sample for blood gas analysis, as ordered, within 30 minutes of a position change.[1]

■ Reposition the patient's head hourly while in the prone position *to prevent facial breakdown.* As one person lifts the patient's head, the second person moves the headpieces *to provide head support in a different position.*[1]

■ Perform range-of-motion exercises to the shoulders, arms, and legs every 2 hours.

■ If the patient was manually turned prone, adjust his position frequently *to prevent skin breakdown.*[4]

■ Give frequent oral care and suction the patient's airway, as needed. *The prone position promotes postural drainage.*

■ After the patient is prone, restart the patient's tube feeding, as ordered and tolerated; *prone position involves minimal risk of aspiration because the patient is in a head-down position.*[1]

■ Assess the security of the ET tube or tracheostomy tube and all lines and tubes.[4]

■ Monitor the length of time the patient is prone. *The maximum recommended time to remain prone is 3 hours and 15 minutes, alternating with 45 minutes of supine positioning.*[1,4]

■ Remove and discard your gloves and any other personal protective equipment worn,[13] and perform hand hygiene.[7,8,9,10,11]

Returning the patient to the supine position

■ Perform hand hygiene[7,8,9,10,11]

■ Put on gloves and other personal protective equipment as needed *to comply with standard precautions.*[13,14]

■ Remove the posterior chest ECG leads while ensuring the ability to monitor the patient's cardiac rate and rhythm; you'll reposition the leads on the patient's chest once the patient is supine.

Manually returning the patient to the supine position

■ Position the patient on the edge of the bed closest to the ventilator.[1]

■ Adjust all patient tubing and monitoring lines *to prevent dislodging.*[1]

■ Position up to six staff members appropriately on either side of the patient and at the head of the bed, depending on the size and complexity of the patient.[1,4]

■ Straighten the patient's arms and rest them on either side. Cross the leg closest to the edge of the bed over the opposite leg.[1]

■ Turn the patient onto his side and then onto his back.

■ Position his arms parallel to his body.

Returning the patient in the RotoProne™ Therapy System to the supine position

■ Use the touch screen and follow the manufacturer's instructions to return the patient to the supine position.

■ Insert the locking pin.[1]

■ Remove the face pack.

■ Using the touch screen, place the patient in the reverse Trendelenburg position *to elevate the head of the bed, decrease edema, and prevent aspiration.*[1]

Completing the procedure

- Replace ECG leads onto the patient's chest.
- Assess the patient's response.
- Remove and discard your gloves and other personal protective equipment worn.[13,14]
- Perform hand hygiene.[7,8,9,10,11]
- Document the procedure.[15,16,17]

Special considerations

- You'll usually need a practitioner's order before prone positioning of a critically ill patient.
- The procedure requires special training and established guidelines *to ensure patient safety.*
- Not all patients with ARDS respond favorably to prone positioning, and the benefit sometimes decreases over time.
- The patient may not have an immediate positive response to the prone position. Maximum response to the position may take up to 6 hours in some patients.[1]
- Some patients may require increased sedation during the procedure.
- *To reduce the risk of aspirating gastric contents during the turning procedure,* it's recommended that tube feedings be turned off 1 hour before initiating the position. You can safely restart tube feedings after positioning the patient.[1,18]
- The prone-positioning schedule is generally determined by the patient's ability to maintain improvements in partial pressure of arterial oxygen while in the prone position.[1]
- Use capnography, if possible, *to detect dislodgement of the ET tube.*
- Discontinue the procedure when the patient no longer demonstrates improved oxygenation with the position change.

NURSING ALERT *Lateral rotation therapy is strongly recommended with prone positioning.*

Complications

Potential complications of prone positioning include inadvertent ET extubation; airway obstruction; decreased oxygen saturation; apical atelectasis; obstructed chest tube; pressure injuries on the weight-bearing parts of the body, including the knees and chest; hemodynamic instability; dislodgment of central venous access; transient arrhythmias; reversible dependent edema of the face (forehead, eyelids, conjunctiva, lips, and tongue) and anterior chest wall; contractures; enteral feeding intolerance; aspiration of enteral feeding when repositioned; and corneal ulceration.

NURSING ALERT *Critically ill patients with active intra-abdominal processes, regardless of position, are at risk for sepsis and septic shock.*

Documentation

Document the patient's response to therapy, ability to tolerate the turning procedure, length of time in the position, and positioning schedule. Also document monitoring, any complications during or after the procedure, and any nursing interventions. Record patient and family teaching and their understanding of your teaching.

REFERENCES

1 Lynn-McHale Wiegand, D. (Ed.) (2011). *AACN procedure manual for critical care* (6th ed.). Philadelphia, PA: Saunders.

2 Alsaghir, A. H., & Martin, C. M. (2008). Effect of prone positioning in patients with acute respiratory distress syndrome: A meta-analysis. *Critical Care Medicine, 36,* 603–609. (Level I)

3 Sud, S., et al. (2008). Effect of mechanical ventilation in the prone position on clinical outcomes in patients with acute hypoxemic respiratory failure: A systematic review and meta-analysis. *Canadian Medical Association Journal, 178,* 1153–1161. (Level I)

4 Arjohuntleigh, Inc. (2013) "RotoProne™ Therapy System therapy guidelines" [Online]. Accessed May 2015 via the Web at http://www.arjolibrary.com/ExternalLink/ShowFile.aspx?Id=4ae0ee34-7fb3-4178-99b4-c2bed0a659a7

5 Rutala, W. A., et al. (2008). "Guideline for disinfection and sterilization in healthcare facilities, 2008" [Online]. Accessed May 2015 via the Web at http://www.cdc.gov/hicpac/pdf/guidelines/Disinfection_Nov_2008.pdf (Level I)

6 American Osteopathic Association. (2014). Standard 07.02.03. *Healthcare Facilities Accreditation Program: Accreditation requirements for acute care hospitals.* Chicago, IL: American Osteopathic Association. (Level VII)

7 Centers for Disease Control and Prevention. (2002). Guideline for hand hygiene in health-care settings: Recommendations of the Healthcare Infection Control Practices Advisory Committee and the HICPAC/SHEA/APIC/IDSA Hand Hygiene Task Force. *MMWR Recommendations and Reports, 51*(RR-16), 1–45. Accessed May 2015 via the Web at http://www.cdc.gov/mmwr/pdf/rr/rr5116.pdf (Level II)

8 World Health Organization. (2009). "WHO guidelines on hand hygiene in health care: First global patient safety challenge, clean care is safer care" [Online]. Accessed May 2015 via the Web at http://whqlibdoc.who.int/publications/2009/9789241597906_eng.pdf (Level IV)

9 The Joint Commission. (2015). Standard NPSG.07.01.01. *Comprehensive accreditation manual for hospitals: The official handbook.* Oakbrook Terrace, IL: The Joint Commission. (Level VII)

10 American Osteopathic Association. (2014). Standard 07.01.21. *Healthcare Facilities Accreditation Program: Accreditation requirements for acute care hospitals.* Chicago, IL: American Osteopathic Association. (Level VII)

11 Centers for Medicare & Medicaid Services, Department of Health and Human Services. (2014). Condition of participation: Infection control. 42 C.F.R. § 482.42.

12 The Joint Commission. (2015). Standard NPSG.01.01.01. *Comprehensive accreditation manual for hospitals: The official handbook.* Oakbrook Terrace, IL: The Joint Commission. (Level VII)

13 Siegel J. D., et al. (2007). "2007 guideline for isolation precautions: Preventing transmission of infectious agents in healthcare settings" [Online]. Accessed May 2015 via the Web at http://www.cdc.gov/hicpac/pdf/isolation/Isolation2007.pdf (Level II)

14 American Osteopathic Association. (2014). Standard 07.01.10. *Healthcare Facilities Accreditation Program: Accreditation requirements for acute care hospitals.* Chicago, IL: American Osteopathic Association. (Level VII)

15 The Joint Commission. (2015). Standard RC.01.03.01. *Comprehensive accreditation manual for hospitals: The official handbook.* Oakbrook Terrace, IL: The Joint Commission. (Level VII)

16 American Osteopathic Association. (2014). Standard 10.00.03. *Healthcare Facilities Accreditation Program: Accreditation requirements for acute care hospitals.* Chicago, IL: American Osteopathic Association. (Level VII)

17 Centers for Medicare & Medicaid Services, Department of Health and Human Services. (2014). Condition of participation: Medical record services. 42 C.F.R. § 482.24(b).

18 Reignier, J., et al. (2010). Before-after study of a standardized ICU protocol for early enteral feeding in patients turned in the prone position. *Clinical Nutrition, 29,* 210–216. (Level VI)

ADDITIONAL REFERENCES

Dirkes, S., et al. (2012), Prone positioning: Is it safe and effective? *Critical Care Nursing Quarterly, 35*(1), 64–75.

Guérin, C., et al. (2013). Prone positioning in severe acute respiratory distress syndrome. *New England Journal of Medicine, 368,* 2159–2168. (Level IV)

PROTECTIVE ENVIRONMENT GUIDELINES

The Centers for Disease Control and Prevention recommends that patients undergoing allogenic hematopoietic stem cell transplant (in which bone marrow is taken from a person other than the recipient) be placed in a protective environment room for the prevention of fungal infections.[1,2] An effective protective environment requires a positive-pressure room with the door kept closed to maintain the proper air pressure balance between the isolation room and the adjoining hallway (12 air exchanges per hour). Positive air pressure must be monitored and documented daily with smoke tubes or flutter strips.[3] The incoming air is filtered through high-efficiency particulate air (HEPA) filtration before circulation.[4,5]

Equipment

Gloves ▪ gowns ▪ masks ▪ N95 respirator masks ▪ positive-pressure room with HEPA filter ▪ Optional: new thermometer, blood pressure cuff, stethoscope.

Equipment should be restricted to the patient's room.

Preparation of equipment

Ensure that all equipment taken into the room is properly cleaned with facility- and Environmental Protection Agency–approved disinfectant before entering the room. Follow the manufacturer's guidelines for disinfectant use. *Products have different contact times and are effective only if the product remains on the item to be cleaned for the appropriate amount of time.*[5,6]

Implementation

- Gather the necessary equipment.
- Review the patient's medical record and verify the need for a protective environment.
- Perform hand hygiene before putting on gloves, after removing gloves, and as indicated during patient care.[1,5,7,8,9,10,11]
- Wear gloves, a gown, and a mask according to standard precautions and other precautions (droplet, contact, and airborne) as indicated.[2,12]
- Confirm the patient's identity using at least two patient identifiers.[13]
- Place the patient in the protective environment room and explain the protective environment requirements to the patient and his family *to reduce patient anxiety and promote cooperation.*
- Keep the patient's door (and the anteroom door, if applicable) closed at all times *to maintain the proper air pressure balance between the protective environment room and the adjoining hallway.*[2] Put a protective environment precautions sign on the door *to notify anyone entering the room of the protective environment and associated requirements.*
- Screen visitors *to prevent anyone with a known or suspected infection from entering the room.*
- Ensure daily room cleaning with techniques that minimize dust, such as wet-dusting horizontal surfaces.[5]
- Avoid transporting the patient out of the room; if the patient must be moved, make sure he wears an N95 mask *to protect the patient from breathing in small particles that may cause infection.*[3] Also, notify the receiving department that the patient is on protective environment requirements and that the patient must be returned to his room promptly.
- Prohibit fresh or dried flowers or potted plants in protective environment rooms or areas *because standing water supports growth of microorganisms and soil harbors fungus.*[15]
- Document the procedure.[16,17,18]

Special considerations

- If the patient requires airborne precautions, implement them in the protective environment room if an anteroom is present. *Air in the anteroom is filtered by a portable HEPA filtration unit.* If there isn't an anteroom, place the patient in an airborne infection isolation room with portable ventilation units and HEPA filters *to increase the filtration of fungal spores.*[2]

Documentation

Record the need for a protective environment in the nursing care plan and as otherwise indicated by your facility. Document initiation and maintenance, the patient's tolerance of the procedure, and any patient or family teaching provided. Also document the date the protective environment was discontinued.

REFERENCES

1 Duffy, L. (2009). Care of immunocompromised patients in hospital. *Nursing Standard, 23*(36), 35–41.

2 Siegel, J. D., et al. (2007). "2007 Guideline for isolation precautions: Preventing transmission of infectious agents in healthcare settings" [Online]. Accessed May 2015 via the Web at http://www.cdc.gov/hicpac/pdf/isolation/Isolation2007.pdf (Level II)

3 Sehulster, L., & Chinn, R. Y. W. (2003). Guidelines for environmental infection control in health-care facilities: Recommendations of CDC and the Healthcare Infection Control Practices Advisory Committee (HICPAC). *MMWR Recommendations and Reports, 52*(RR-10), 1–42. Accessed May 2015 via the Web at http://www.cdc.gov/mmwr/preview/mmwrhtml/rr5210a1.htm (Level I)

4 Carrico, R., et al. (Eds.). (2009). *APIC text of infection control and epidemiology: Volume 1.* Washington, DC: Association for Professionals in Infection Control and Epidemiology.

5 Riley, M., & Flood, A. (2009). Are your isolation precautions up-to-date? *Nursing Critical Care, 4*(3), 8–10.

6 Centers for Disease Control and Prevention. (2008). "Guideline for disinfection and sterilization in healthcare facilities: Surface disinfection" [Online]. Accessed May 2015 via the Web at http://www.cdc.gov/hicpac/disinfection_sterilization/3_4surfacedisinfection.html (Level I)

7 Centers for Disease Control and Prevention. (2002). Guideline for hand hygiene in health-care settings: Recommendations of the Healthcare Infection Control Practices Advisory Committee and the HICPAC/SHEA/APIC/IDSA Hand Hygiene Task Force. *MMWR Recommendations and Reports, 51*(RR-16), 1–45. Accessed May 2015 via the Web at http://www.cdc.gov/mmwr/pdf/rr/rr5116.pdf (Level II)

8 World Health Organization. (2009). "WHO guidelines on hand hygiene in health care: First global patient safety challenge, clean care is safer care" [Online]. Accessed May 2015 via the Web at http://whqlibdoc.who.int/publications/2009/9789241597906_eng.pdf (Level IV)

9 The Joint Commission. (2015). Standard NPSG.07.01.01. *Comprehensive accreditation manual for hospitals: The official handbook.* Oakbrook Terrace, IL: The Joint Commission. (Level VII)

10 American Osteopathic Association. (2014). Standard 07.01.21. *Healthcare Facilities Accreditation Program: Accreditation requirements for acute care hospitals.* Chicago, IL: American Osteopathic Association. (Level VII)

11 Centers for Medicare & Medicaid Services, Department of Health and Human Services. (2014). Condition of participation: Infection control. 42 C.F.R. § 482.42.

12 American Osteopathic Association. (2014). Standard 07.01.10. *Healthcare Facilities Accreditation Program: Accreditation requirements for acute care hospitals.* Chicago, IL: American Osteopathic Association. (Level VII)

13 The Joint Commission. (2015). Standard NPSG.01.01.01. *Comprehensive accreditation manual for hospitals: The official handbook.* Oakbrook Terrace, IL: The Joint Commission. (Level VII)

14 Zitella, L. J., et al. (2006). Putting evidence into practice: Prevention of infection. *Clinical Journal of Oncology Nursing, 10,* 739–750.

15 Craven, R. F., & Hirnle, C. J. (2012). *Fundamentals of nursing: Human health and function* (7th ed.). Philadelphia, PA: Lippincott Williams & Wilkins.

16 The Joint Commission. (2015). Standard RC 01.03.01. *Comprehensive accreditation manual for hospitals: The official handbook.* Oakbrook Terrace, IL: The Joint Commission. (Level VII)

17 Centers for Medicare & Medicaid Services, Department of Health and Human Services. (2014). Condition of participation: Medical record services. 42 C.F.R. § 482.24(b).

18 American Osteopathic Association. (2014). Standard 10.00.03. *Healthcare Facilities Accreditation Program: Accreditation requirements for acute care hospitals.* Chicago, IL: American Osteopathic Association. (Level VII)

PULMONARY ARTERY PRESSURE AND PULMONARY ARTERY WEDGE PRESSURE MONITORING

Continuous pulmonary artery pressure (PAP) and intermittent pulmonary artery wedge pressure (PAWP) measurements provide important information about left ventricular function and preload. PAWP may also be referred to as *pulmonary artery occlusion pressure.*[1] This information is useful not only for monitoring but also for aiding diagnosis, refining assessments, guiding interventions, and projecting patient outcomes.

All acutely ill patients are candidates for PAP monitoring, especially those who are hemodynamically unstable, who need fluid management or continuous cardiopulmonary assessment, or who are receiving multiple or frequently administered cardioactive drugs. A pulmonary artery (PA) catheter is recommended for many clinical conditions and can be used to assess intravascular volume, particularly in patients with severe pulmonary edema, heart failure, or oliguric renal failure; guide therapy in severe refractory shock or multiple-organ-dysfunction syndrome; and guide therapy to maximize oxygen delivery to tissues in some selected patients.

PA catheters can have up to six lumens, allowing more hemodynamic information to be gathered. In addition to distal and proximal lumens used to measure pressures, a PA catheter has a balloon inflation lumen that inflates the balloon for PAWP measurement and a thermistor connector lumen that allows cardiac output measurement. Some catheters also have a pacemaker wire lumen that provides a port for pacemaker electrodes and measures continuous mixed venous oxygen saturation. (See *PA catheters: From basic to complex,* page 646.)

The PA catheter is inserted into the heart's right side with the distal tip lying in the pulmonary artery. Left-sided pressures can be assessed indirectly.

No specific contraindications for PAP monitoring exist. However, some patients require special precautions, including elderly patients with pulmonary hypertension, those with left bundle-branch heart block, and those for whom a systemic infection would be life-threatening.

Equipment

1.5-mL syringe attached to balloon port or catheter.

Implementation

- Verify the practitioner's order for PAP monitoring.
- Perform hand hygiene.[2,3,4,5,6]
- Confirm the patient's identity using at least two patient identifiers.[7,8]
- Explain the procedure to the patient.
- Place the patient in the supine position, with the head of the bed elevated no more than 45 degrees.[1] Then wait 5 to 15 minutes before taking measurements *so that the patient can stabilize after the position change.*[9]

Obtaining a PAP measurement

- After the catheter has been inserted, record initial pressure and subsequent PAP values and monitor waveforms. These values will be used to calculate other important hemodynamic indices. *To ensure accurate values,* make sure the transducer is properly leveled and zeroed at the phlebostatic axis, located at the fourth intercostal space at one-half of the anterior-posterior diameter of the chest.[9]
- Perform a dynamic response measurement or square wave test and document it at the start of each shift, with a change in the waveform configuration, or when the system is opened to air.[9,10] (See *Square wave test,* page 647.)
- Always obtain PAP values at end expiration (when the patient completely exhales).[9] *At this time, intrathoracic pressure approaches atmospheric pressure and has the least effect on PAP.*[1] If you obtain a reading during other phases of the respiratory cycle, respiratory interference may occur. For instance, during inspiration, when intrathoracic pressure drops, PAP may be falsely low because the negative pressure is transmitted to the catheter. During expiration, when intrathoracic pressure rises, PAP may be falsely high.
- Use a simultaneous electrocardiogram (ECG) *to facilitate correct PAP measurements* (dual-channel strip of the ECG and PA waveform). Digital readouts may reflect pressures obtained throughout respiration and may not be accurate. Alternatively, you can use the monitor cursor line if simultaneous graphic recording of the ECG and PA waveform isn't possible, you can use the monitor cursor line.[11]
- Make sure that the scale of the PAP tracing is set appropriately on the monitor. Most PA scales are commonly set at 40 mm Hg.
- Align the QT interval with the PA waveform. The peak of the PA waveform is the PA systolic pressure.
- Align the end of the QRS complex with the PA waveform. Measure the PA diastolic pressure at the point of the intersection of the QRS complex and the PA waveform.
- Perform hand hygiene.[2,3,4,5,6]
- Document the procedure.[12,13,14]

Obtaining a PAWP measurement

- PAWP is recorded by inflating the balloon and letting it float in a distal artery. Some facilities allow only practitioners or specially trained nurses to take a PAWP reading *because of the risk of pulmonary artery rupture,* a rare but life-threatening complication. If your facility permits you to perform this procedure, do so with extreme caution and make sure you're thoroughly familiar with intracardiac waveform interpretation.
- To begin, verify that the transducer is properly leveled and zeroed. Detach the syringe from the balloon inflation hub. Draw 1.5 mL of air into the syringe, and then reattach the syringe to the hub. Being running a dual-chamber recording of the ECG and PA waveform. Watching the monitor, inject the air through the hub slowly and smoothly. When you see a wedge tracing on the monitor, immediately stop inflating the balloon. (See *Observing the PAWP waveform,* page 647.)

NURSING ALERT ***Never inflate the balloon beyond the volume needed to obtain a wedge tracing. Never inflate the balloon for more than 15 seconds (two to four respiratory cycles) or leave the balloon inflated*** **because this may cause a pulmonary infarction and rupture.**[1]

- Take the pressure reading at end expiration. Note the amount of air needed to change the PA tracing to a wedge tracing (normally, 1.25 to 1.5 mL). If the wedge tracing appeared with the injection of less than 1.25 mL, suspect that the catheter has migrated into a more distal branch and requires repositioning. If the balloon is in a more distal branch, the tracings may move up the oscilloscope, indicating that the catheter tip is recording balloon pressure rather than PAWP, which may lead to PA rupture.
- Detach the syringe from the balloon inflation port and allow the balloon to deflate on its own. Observe the waveform tracing and make sure the tracing returns from the wedge tracing to the normal PA tracing.
- In looking at the dual-channel recorded strip, identify the *a* wave of the PAWP waveform. The *a* wave represents atrial contraction and correlates with the end of the QRS complex. Measure the mean of the *a* wave *to obtain an accurate PAWP measurement.*[1]

Completing the procedure

- Perform hand hygiene.[2,3,4,5,6]
- Document the procedure.[12,13,14]

Special considerations

- Advise the patient to use caution when moving about in bed *to avoid dislodging the catheter.*

EQUIPMENT

PA catheters: From basic to complex

Depending on the intended use, a pulmonary artery (PA) catheter may be basic or complex. The basic PA catheter has a distal and proximal lumen, a thermistor, and a balloon inflation gate valve. The distal lumen, which exits in the pulmonary artery, monitors PA pressure. Its hub usually is marked PA DISTAL or is color-coded yellow. The proximal lumen exits in the right atrium or vena cava, depending on the size of the patient's heart. It monitors right atrial pressure and can be used as the injected solution lumen for cardiac output determination and for infusing solutions. The proximal lumen hub usually is marked PROXIMAL or is color-coded blue.

The thermistor, located about 1½" (4 cm) from the distal tip, measures temperature (aiding core temperature evaluation) and allows cardiac output measurement. The thermistor connector attaches to a cardiac output connector cable and then to a cardiac output monitor. Typically, the thermistor connector is red. The balloon inflation gate valve is used for inflating the balloon tip with air. A stopcock connection, typically color-coded red, may be used.

Additional lumens

Some PA catheters have additional lumens used to obtain other hemodynamic data or permit certain interventions. For instance, a proximal infusion port, which exits in the right atrium or vena cava, allows additional fluid administration. A right ventricular lumen, exiting in the right ventricle, allows fluid administration, right ventricular pressure measurement, or use of a temporary ventricular pacing lead.

Some catheters have additional right atrial and right ventricular lumens for atrioventricular pacing. A right ventricular ejection fraction test-response thermistor, with PA and right ventricular sensing electrodes, allows volumetric and ejection fraction measurements.

Fiber-optic filaments, such as those used in pulse oximetry, exit into the pulmonary artery and permit measurement of continuous mixed venous oxygen saturation.

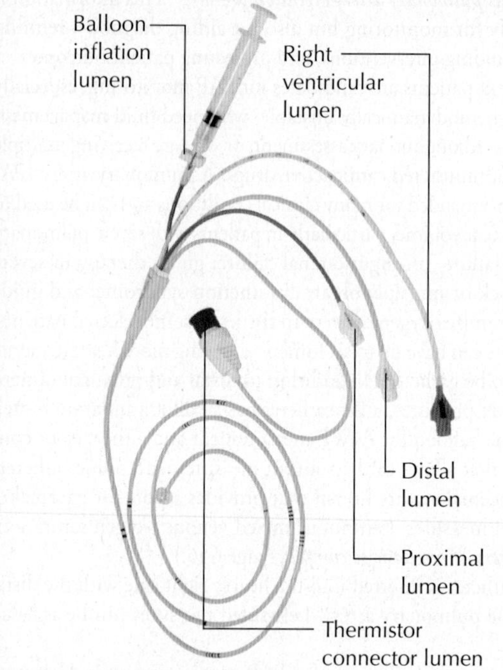

■ Use ECG tracings simultaneously *to help identify waveforms.*[8]

■ Never inflate the balloon with more than the recommended air volume (specified on the catheter shaft) *because this action may cause loss of elasticity or balloon rupture.* With appropriate inflation volume, the balloon floats easily through the heart chambers and rests in the main branch of the pulmonary artery, producing accurate waveforms. Never inflate the balloon with fluids *because they may not be able to be retrieved from inside the balloon, preventing deflation.*

■ Be aware that the catheter may slip back into the right ventricle. *Because the tip may irritate the ventricle and cause arrhythmias,* check the monitor for a right ventricular waveform to detect this problem promptly.

■ *To minimize valvular trauma,* make sure the balloon is deflated whenever the catheter is withdrawn from the pulmonary artery to the right ventricle or from the right ventricle to the right atrium.

■ Never flush the PA catheter for longer than 2 seconds *because PA rupture may occur with prolonged flushing of high-pressure fluids.*[1]

■ If you find a close correlation between the PA diastolic pressure and the PA occlusive pressure, follow the diastolic pressure *to minimize the number of times the PA catheter balloon is inflated.*

■ Change the dressing whenever it's moist or every 48 hours for a gauze dressing and at least every 7 days for a transparent dressing.[15,16] Change the pressure tubing and flush solution every 96 hours, or as needed.[16,17]

Complications

Complications of PA catheter insertion include pulmonary artery perforation, pulmonary infarction, catheter knotting, local or systemic infection, cardiac arrhythmias, and heparin-induced thrombocytopenia (if heparin is used in the flush solution).

Documentation

Document the date and time the measurements were taken, the results of the dynamic response or square wave test, the measurement results, the amount of air needed to obtain a wedge pressure tracing, and the patient's response.

REFERENCES

1 Lynn-McHale Wiegand, D. (Ed.). (2011). *AACN procedure manual for critical care* (6th ed.). St. Louis, MO: Saunders.

2 The Joint Commission. (2015). Standard NPSG.07.01.01. *Comprehensive accreditation manual for hospitals: The official handbook.* Oakbrook Terrace, IL: The Joint Commission. (Level VII)

3 Centers for Disease Control and Prevention. (2002). Guideline for hand hygiene in health-care settings: Recommendations of the Healthcare Infection Control Practices Advisory Committee and the HICPAC/SHEA/APIC/IDSA Hand Hygiene Task Force. *MMWR Recommendations and Reports, 51*(RR-16), 1–45. Accessed May 2015 via the Web at http://www.cdc.gov/mmwr/pdf/rr/rr5116.pdf (Level II)

4 World Health Organization. (2009). "WHO guidelines on hand hygiene in health care: First global patient safety challenge, clean care is safer care" [Online]. Accessed May 2015 via the Web at http://whqlibdoc.who.int/publications/2009/9789241597906_eng.pdf (Level IV)

5 American Osteopathic Association. (2014). Standard 07.01.10. *Healthcare Facilities Accreditation Program: Accreditation requirements for acute care hospitals.* Chicago, IL: American Osteopathic Association. (Level VII)

Square wave test[10]

When using a pressure monitoring system, you must ensure and document the system's accuracy. Along with leveling and zeroing the system to atmospheric pressure at the phlebostatic axis and interpreting waveforms, you can ensure accuracy by performing the square wave test (or dynamic response test). To perform the test, take the following steps:

- Activate the fast-flush device for 1 second, and then release. Obtain a graphic printout.
- Observe for the desired response: The pressure wave rises rapidly, squares off, and is followed by a series of oscillations. (See illustration below.)
- Know that these oscillations should have an initial downstroke, which extends below the baseline and just 1 to 2 oscillations after the initial downstroke. Usually, but not always, the first upstroke is about one-third the height of the initial downstroke.
- Be aware that the intervals between oscillations should be no more than 0.08 second (2 small boxes).

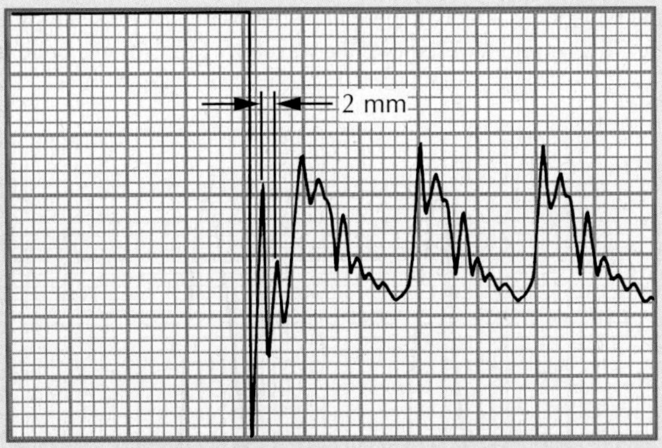

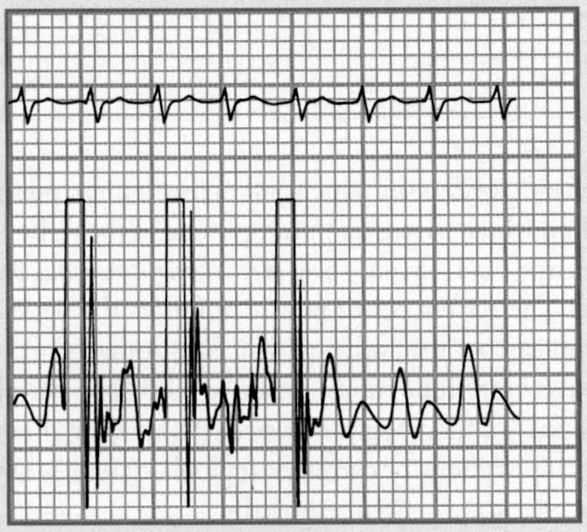

Underdamped square wave

If you observe extra oscillations after the initial downstroke or more than 0.08 second between oscillations, the waveform is underdamped. (See illustration below.) This can cause falsely high pressure readings and artifact in the waveforms. It can be corrected by:

- removing excess tubing or extra stopcocks from the system
- inserting a damping device (available from pressure tubing companies).

Repeat the square wave test and read the pressure waveform.

Overdamped square wave

If you observe a slurred upstroke at the beginning of the square wave and a loss of oscillations after the initial downstroke, the waveform is overdamped. (See illustration below.) This can cause falsely low pressure readings, and you can lose the sharpness of waveform peaks and the dicrotic notch. It can be corrected by:

- clearing the line of any blood or air
- checking to make sure there are no kinks or obstructions in the line
- ensuring that you're using short, low-compliance tubing.

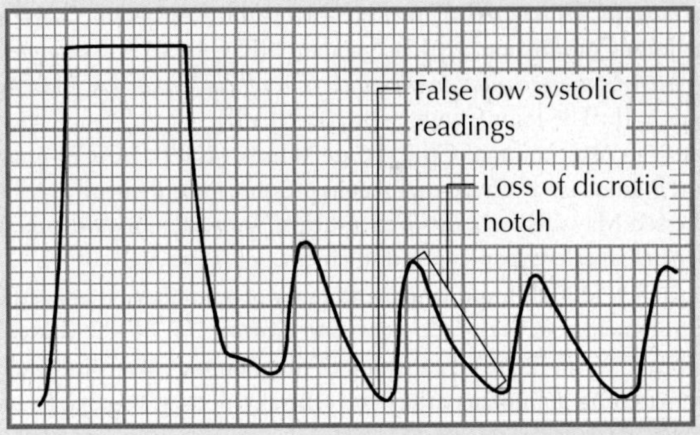

Observing the PAWP waveform

Upon balloon inflation, you should see the normal pulmonary artery pressure (PAP) waveform flatten to the characteristic pulmonary artery wedge pressure (PAWP) waveform. Balloon inflation should be halted upon observation of this waveform. Upon balloon deflation, the PAP waveform should immediately reappear.

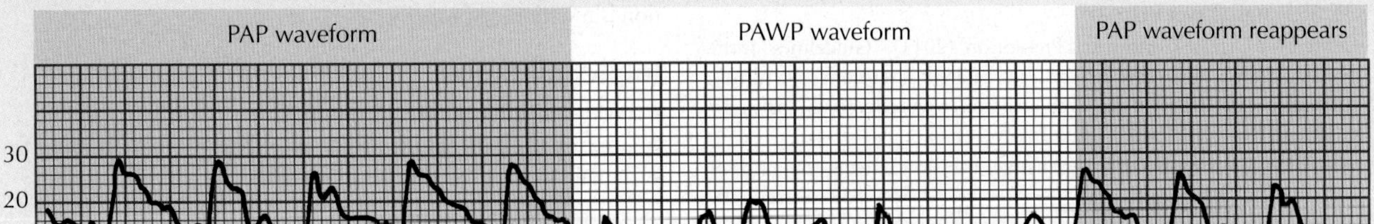

Identifying a normal pulse amplitude waveform

If the patient has adequate peripheral perfusion, the pulse amplitude monitor will usually display a normal waveform, like the one shown here. This waveform resembles the waveform seen when a patient has an arterial line.

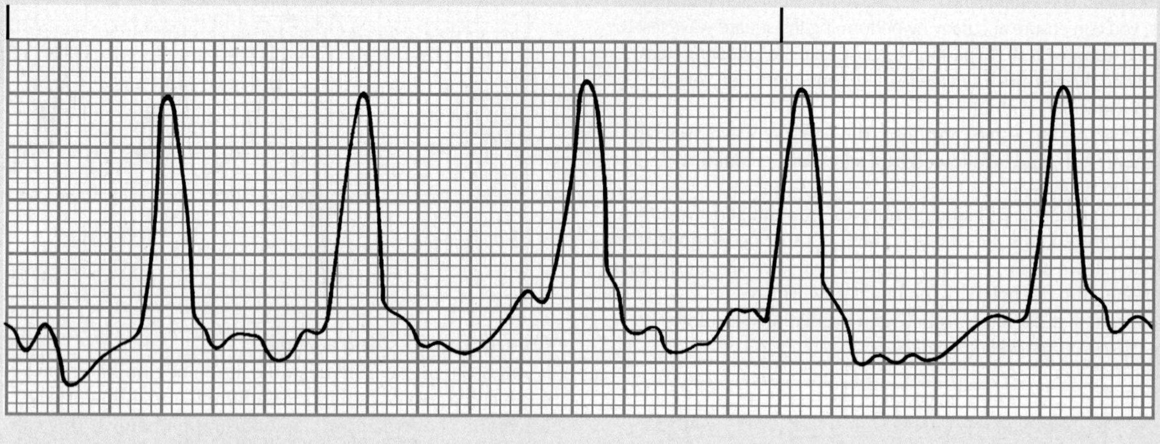

6 Centers for Medicare & Medicaid Services, Department of Health and Human Services. (2014). Condition of participation: Infection control. 42 C.F.R. § 482.42.

7 American Osteopathic Association. (2014). Standard 30.00.14. *Health-care Facilities Accreditation Program: Accreditation requirements for acute care hospitals.* Chicago, IL: American Osteopathic Association. (Level VII)

8 The Joint Commission. (2015). Standard NPSG.01.01.01. *Comprehensive accreditation manual for hospitals: The official handbook.* Oakbrook Terrace, IL: The Joint Commission. (Level VII)

9 American Association of Critical Care Nurses. (2009). "AACN practice alert: Pulmonary artery/central venous pressure measurement" [Online]. Accessed May 2015 via the Web at http://www.aacn.org/wd/practice/docs/practicealerts/pap-cvp-measurement.pdf (Level VII)

10 Quaal, S. J. (2001). Improving the accuracy of pulmonary artery catheter measurements. *Journal of Cardiovascular Nursing, 15,* 71–82. (Level VI)

11 Pasion, E., et al. (2010). Evaluation of the monitor cursor-line method for measuring pulmonary artery and central venous pressures. *American Journal of Critical Care, 19,* 511–521.

12 The Joint Commission. (2015). Standard RC.01.03.01. *Comprehensive accreditation manual for hospitals: The official handbook.* Oakbrook Terrace, IL: The Joint Commission. (Level VII)

13 American Osteopathic Association. (2014). Standard 10.00.03. *Health-care Facilities Accreditation Program: Accreditation requirements for acute care hospitals.* Chicago, IL: American Osteopathic Association. (Level VII)

14 Centers for Medicare & Medicaid Services, Department of Health and Human Services. (2014). Condition of participation: Medical record services. 42 C.F.R. § 482.24(b).

15 Standard 46. Vascular access device site care and dressing changes. Infusion nursing standards of practice. (2011). *Journal of Infusion Nursing, 34,* S63–S64. (Level VII)

16 Centers for Disease Control and Prevention. (2011). "Guidelines for the prevention of intravascular catheter-related infections" [Online]. Accessed May 2015 via the Web at http://www.cdc.gov/hicpac/pdf/guidelines/bsi-guidelines-2011.pdf (Level I)

17 Standard 43. Administration set change. Infusion nursing standards of practice. (2011). *Journal of Infusion Nursing, 34,* S55–S57. (Level VII)

PULSE AMPLITUDE MONITORING

Determining the presence and strength of peripheral pulses, an essential part of cardiovascular assessment, helps you to evaluate the adequacy of peripheral perfusion. A pulse amplitude monitor simplifies this procedure. A sensor taped to the patient's skin over a pulse point sends signals to a monitor, which measures the amplitude of the pulse and displays it as a waveform on a screen. (See *Identifying a normal pulse amplitude waveform.*) The system continuously monitors the patient's peripheral pulse so you can perform other patient care duties.

The pulse amplitude monitor can be used after peripheral vascular reconstruction on the upper or lower extremities or after percutaneous transluminal peripheral or coronary angioplasty (either with the sheaths in place or after they've been removed).

Because the sensor monitors only relatively flat pulse points, it can't be used for the posterior tibial pulse point. Also, movement distorts the waveform, so the patient must stay as still as possible during monitoring. The patient shouldn't have lesions on the skin where the pulse will be monitored because the sensor must be placed directly on this site; the sensor and tape could irritate the lesion, or the lesion could impair transmission of the pulse amplitude. If the patient has a strong peripheral pulse, you'll see an adequate waveform.

Equipment

Pulse amplitude display monitor with sensor ■ hospital-grade disinfectant.

Preparation of equipment

Plug the monitor into a grounded outlet. Turn on the monitor and allow it to warm up, which may take up to 10 seconds. Plug the sensor cable into the monitor; then tap the sensor gently. If tapping causes interference on the display screen, you can assume the sensor-monitor connection is functioning properly.

Implementation

- Perform hand hygiene.[1,2,3,4,5]
- Confirm the patient's identity using at least two patient identifiers.[6,7]
- Explain to the procedure to the patient.

Initiating monitor use

- Locate the pulse you want to monitor. Tell the patient that you'll tape the sensor to a selected site, usually the foot.
- Place the sensor over the strongest point of the pulse you're going to monitor. While observing the display screen, move the sensor until you see a strong upright waveform.

■ Without moving the sensor from this site, peel off the adhesive strips and affix the sensor securely to the patient's foot. *The sensor must maintain proper skin contact,* so be sure to tape it firmly.
■ Adjust the height of the pulse wave signal to half the height of the display screen. *This will give the waveform room to fluctuate as the pulse amplitude increases and decreases.*
■ Set the low and high waveform amplitude alarms *so you'll be alerted to any waveform changes.*
■ Print out a strip of the patient's waveform.

Discontinuing monitor use

■ Print out a strip of the patient's waveform.
■ Peel the sensor tapes from the patient's skin and discard them.
■ Turn the machine off but keep it plugged in.
■ Perform hand hygiene.[1,2,3,4,5]
■ Disinfect the monitor using a hospital-grade disinfectant.[8,9]

Completing the procedure

■ Perform hand hygiene.[1,2,3,4,5]
■ Place the strip printout in the patient's medical record.
■ Document the procedure.[10,11,12]

Special considerations

■ Be aware that, although the waveform displayed by a pulse amplitude monitor may resemble an electrocardiogram or blood pressure waveform, it's not the same.
■ Don't apply much pressure on the pulse sensor film or press on it with a sharp object *because such stress may warp or destroy the sensor.*
■ Never place the sensor over an open wound or on ulcerated skin.
■ If waveform amplitude decreases, assess the patient's leg for capillary refill time, temperature, color, and sensation. The amplitude change may stem from a malfunction in the monitor itself (such as a low battery) or from a thrombus, hematoma, or significant change in the patient's hemodynamic status.
■ If the display screen is blank when you turn on the machine, make sure that the monitor is plugged in. If it's plugged in but the screen remains blank, the screen may need repair.
■ If the screen is functioning but no waveform appears on it, first check the sensor-monitor connection. Then check the sensor by gently tapping it *to see if interference appears on the screen.* If the sensor is working properly, relocate the peripheral pulse on the patient's foot, and reapply the sensor. If your interventions don't work, the screen may need servicing.

Complications

Local irritation from the sensor adhesive tape may occur.

Documentation

Print out a strip of the patient's waveform, and place the strip in the patient's medical record during every shift and whenever you note a change in the waveform or the patient's condition. Along the left side of the strip, you'll see a reference scale used to measure pulse amplitude height. Include this scale in your documentation. Indicate the site where the sensor was placed.

REFERENCES

1 The Joint Commission. (2015). Standard NPSG.07.01.01. *Comprehensive accreditation manual for hospitals: The official handbook.* Oakbrook Terrace, IL: The Joint Commission. (Level VII)

2 Centers for Disease Control and Prevention. (2002). Guideline for hand hygiene in health-care settings: Recommendations of the Healthcare Infection Control Practices Advisory Committee and the HICPAC/SHEA/APIC/IDSA Hand Hygiene Task Force. *MMWR Recommendations and Reports, 51*(RR-16), 1–45. Accessed May 2015 via the Web at http://www.cdc.gov/mmwr/pdf/rr/rr5116.pdf (Level II)

3 World Health Organization. (2009). "WHO guidelines on hand hygiene in health care: First global patient safety challenge, clean care is safer care" [Online]. Accessed May 2015 via the Web at http://whqlibdoc.who.int/publications/2009/9789241597906_eng.pdf (Level IV)

4 American Osteopathic Association. (2014). Standard 07.01.21. *Healthcare Facilities Accreditation Program: Accreditation requirements for acute care hospitals.* Chicago, IL: American Osteopathic Association. (Level VII)

5 Centers for Medicare & Medicaid Services, Department of Health and Human Services. (2014). Condition of participation: Infection control. 42 C.F.R. § 482.42.

6 The Joint Commission. (2015). Standard NPSG.01.01.01. *Comprehensive accreditation manual for hospitals: The official handbook.* Oakbrook Terrace, IL: The Joint Commission. (Level VII)

7 American Osteopathic Association. (2014). Standard 30.00.14. *Healthcare Facilities Accreditation Program: Accreditation requirements for acute care hospitals.* Chicago, IL: American Osteopathic Association. (Level VII)

8 Rutala, W. A., et al. (2008). "Guideline for disinfection and sterilization in healthcare facilities, 2008" [Online]. Accessed May 2015 via the Web at http://www.cdc.gov/hicpac/pdf/guidelines/Disinfection_Nov_2008.pdf (Level I)

9 American Osteopathic Association. (2014). Standard 07.02.03. *Healthcare Facilities Accreditation Program: Accreditation requirements for acute care hospitals.* Chicago, IL: American Osteopathic Association. (Level VII)

10 The Joint Commission. (2015). Standard RC.01.03.01. *Comprehensive accreditation manual for hospitals: The official handbook.* Oakbrook Terrace, IL: The Joint Commission. (Level VII)

11 American Osteopathic Association. (2014). Standard 10.00.03. *Healthcare Facilities Accreditation Program: Accreditation requirements for acute care hospitals.* Chicago, IL: American Osteopathic Association. (Level VII)

12 Centers for Medicare & Medicaid Services, Department of Health and Human Services. (2014). Condition of participation: Medical record services. 42 C.F.R. § 482.24(b).

PULSE ASSESSMENT

Blood pumped into an already-full aorta during ventricular contraction creates a fluid wave that travels from the heart to the peripheral arteries. This recurring wave—called a *pulse*—is palpable at locations on the body where an artery crosses over bone or firm tissue. The radial artery in the wrist is the most common palpation site in adults and children older than 3. (See *Pulse points,* page 650.) In infants and children younger than age 3, a stethoscope is used to listen to the heart itself rather than palpating a pulse. Because auscultation is done at the heart's apex, this is called the apical pulse.

An apical-radial pulse is taken by simultaneously counting apical and radial beats—the first by auscultation at the apex of the heart, the second by palpation at the radial artery. Some heartbeats detected at the apex can't be detected at peripheral sites. When this occurs, the apical pulse rate is higher than the radial; the difference is the pulse deficit.

Pulse taking involves determining the rate (number of beats per minute), rhythm (pattern or regularity of the beats), and volume (amount of blood pumped with each beat). If the pulse is faint or weak, use a Doppler ultrasound blood flow detector if available.

Equipment

Watch with second hand ■ Optional: blanket or sheet, stethoscope, disinfectant pad.

Preparation of equipment

If you aren't using your own stethoscope, disinfect the earpieces with a disinfectant pad before and after use *to prevent cross-contamination.*[1,2]

Pulse points

Shown below are anatomic locations where an artery crosses bone or firm tissue and can be palpated for a pulse.

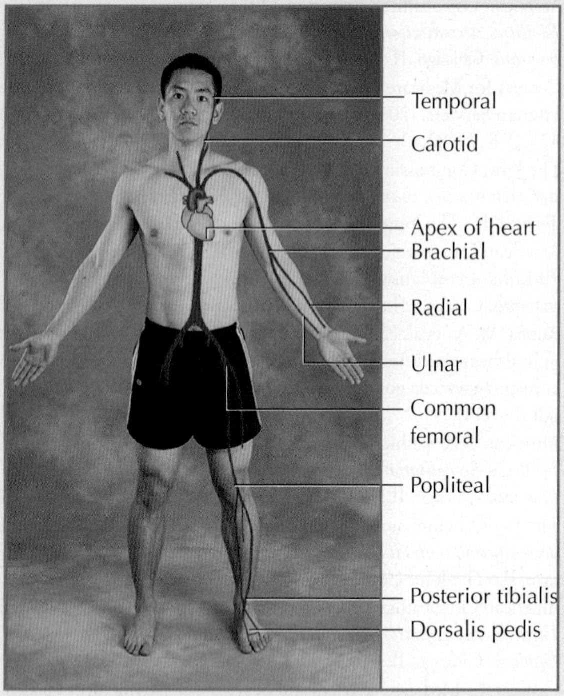

Implementation

- Gather and prepare the appropriate equipment.
- Perform hand hygiene.[3,4,5,6,7]
- Confirm the patient's identity using at least two patient identifiers.[8]
- Tell the patient that you intend to take his pulse.
- Make sure the patient is comfortable and relaxed *because an awkward, uncomfortable position may affect the heart rate.*

Taking a radial pulse

- Place the patient in a sitting or supine position, with his arm at his side or across his chest.
- Gently press your index, middle, and ring fingers on the radial artery, inside the patient's wrist, using moderate pressure (as shown below); *excessive pressure may obstruct blood flow distal to the pulse site.* Don't use your thumb to take the patient's pulse *because your thumb's own strong pulse may be confused with the patient's pulse.*

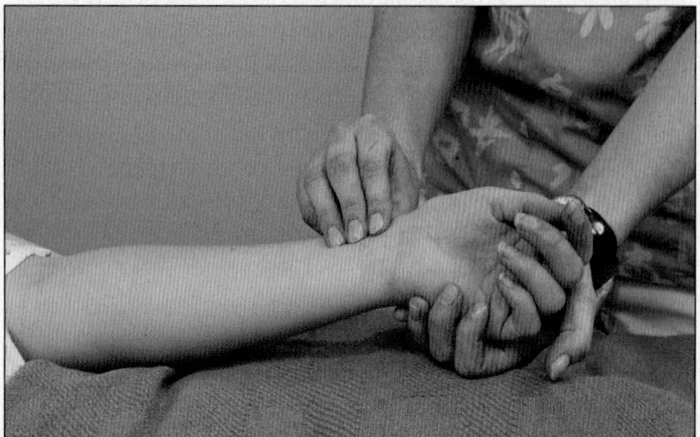

- After locating the pulse, if the rhythm is regular and the rate seems normal, count for 30 and then multiply by 2. If the rate is unusually fast or slow, count for 60 seconds.
- While counting the rate, assess pulse rhythm and amplitude. If the pulse is irregular, note whether the irregularity occurs in a pattern or randomly. If you aren't sure, use your stethoscope to obtain an apical pulse.[9] (See *Identifying pulse patterns.*)

Taking an apical pulse

- Help the patient to the supine position.
- Drape the patient with a blanket or sheet, if necessary.
- Warm the diaphragm or bell of the stethoscope in your hand. *Placing a cold stethoscope against the skin may startle the patient and momentarily increase the heart rate.* Keep in mind that the bell transmits low-pitched sounds more effectively than the diaphragm does.
- Place the diaphragm or bell of the stethoscope over the apex of the heart (normally located at the fifth intercostal space left of the midclavicular line). Then insert the earpieces into your ears. Count the beats for 60 seconds (as shown below), and note their rhythm, volume, and intensity (loudness).

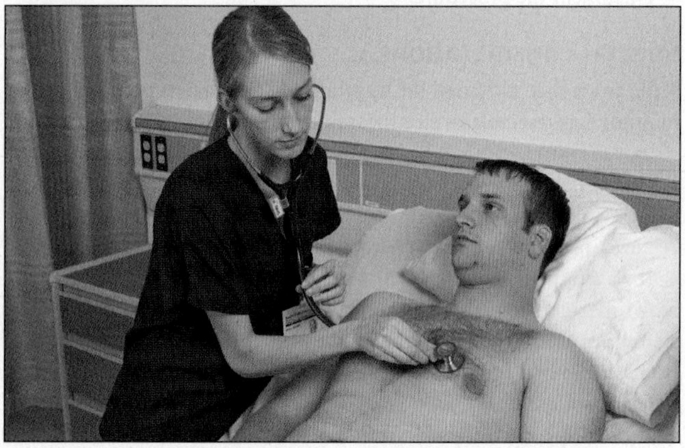

- Remove the stethoscope and make the patient comfortable.
- Perform hand hygiene.[3,4,5,6,7]
- Clean the stethoscope with an alcohol pad *to prevent cross-contamination.*[1,2]

Taking an apical-radial pulse

- Work with another nurse to obtain the apical-radial pulse; one person palpates the radial pulse while the other auscultates the apical pulse with a stethoscope. Both must use the same watch when counting beats.
- Help the patient to the supine position.
- Drape the patient, if necessary.
- Locate the apical or radial pulse, while the other nurse locates the other pulse.
- Determine a time to begin counting.
- Count beats for 60 seconds, starting at the appropriate time.
- Perform hand hygiene.[3,4,5,6,7]
- Clean and disinfect the stethoscope with a disinfectant pad *to prevent cross-contamination.*[1,2]

Completing the procedure

- Perform hand hygiene.[3,4,5,6,7]
- Document the procedure.[10,11,12]

Special considerations

- When the pulse is faint or weak, use a Doppler ultrasound blood flow detector if available. (See the "Doppler use" procedure, page 248.) Note that a rapid, weak, or faint pulse may indicate dehydration.

Identifying pulse patterns

TYPE	RATE	RHYTHM (PER 3 SECONDS)	CAUSES AND INCIDENCE
Normal	60 to 100 beats/minute; in neonates, 120 to 140 beats/ minute	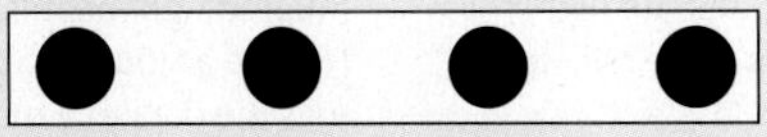	■ Varies with such factors as age, physical activity, and gender (men usually have lower pulse rates than women)
Tachycardia	More than 100 beats/ minute	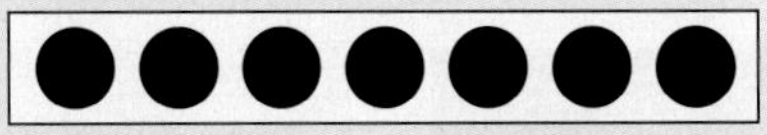	■ Accompanies stimulation of the sympathetic nervous system by emotional stress, such as anger, fear, or anxiety, or by the use of certain drugs such as caffeine ■ May result from exercise and from certain health conditions, such as heart failure, anemia, and fever (which increases oxygen requirements and therefore pulse rate)
Bradycardia	Less than 60 beats/minute	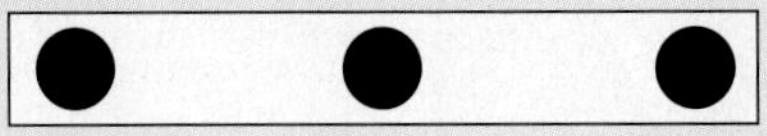	■ Accompanies stimulation of the parasympathetic nervous system by drug use, especially digoxin, and such conditions as cerebral hemorrhage and heart block ■ May also be present in fit athletes
Irregular	Uneven time intervals between beats (for example, periods of regular rhythm interrupted by pauses or premature beats)	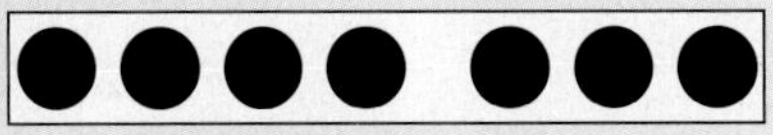	■ May indicate cardiac irritability, hypoxia, digoxin toxicity, potassium imbalance, or sometimes more serious arrhythmias if premature beats occur frequently ■ Occasional premature beats are normal

■ If another nurse isn't available for an apical-radial pulse, hold the stethoscope in place with the hand that holds the watch while palpating the radial pulse with the other hand. You can then feel any discrepancies between the apical and radial pulses.

Documentation

Record the pulse rate, rhythm, and volume as well as the time of measurement. Describe the amplitude as diminished, brisk, or bounding. When recording the apical pulse, also include intensity of heart sounds. When recording the apical-radial pulse, document the rate according to the pulse site—for example, A/R 80/76.

REFERENCES

1 Rutala, W. A., et al. (2008). "Guideline for disinfection and sterilization in healthcare facilities, 2008" [Online]. Accessed May 2015 via the Web at http://www.cdc.gov/hicpac/pdf/guidelines/Disinfection_Nov_2008.pdf (Level I)

2 American Osteopathic Association. (2014). Standard 07.02.03. *Healthcare Facilities Accreditation Program: Accreditation requirements for acute care hospitals.* Chicago, IL: American Osteopathic Association. (Level VII)

3 The Joint Commission. (2015). Standard NPSG.07.01.01. *Comprehensive accreditation manual for hospitals: The official handbook.* Oakbrook Terrace, IL: The Joint Commission. (Level VII)

4 World Health Organization. (2009). "WHO guidelines on hand hygiene in health care: First global patient safety challenge, clean care is safer care" [Online]. Accessed May 2015 via the Web at http://whqlibdoc.who.int/publications/2009/9789241597906_eng.pdf (Level IV)

5 Centers for Disease Control and Prevention. (2002). Guideline for hand hygiene in health-care settings: Recommendations of the Healthcare Infection Control Practices Advisory Committee and the HICPAC/SHEA/APIC/IDSA Hand Hygiene Task Force. *MMWR Recommendations and Reports, 51*(RR-16), 1–45. Accessed May 2015 via the Web at http://www.cdc.gov/mmwr/pdf/rr/rr5116.pdf (Level II)

6 American Osteopathic Association. (2014). Standard 07.01.21. *Healthcare Facilities Accreditation Program: Accreditation requirements for acute care hospitals.* Chicago, IL: American Osteopathic Association. (Level VII)

7 Centers for Medicare & Medicaid Services, Department of Health and Human Services. (2014). Condition of participation: Infection control. 42 C.F.R. § 482.42.

8 The Joint Commission. (2015). Standard NPSG.01.01.01. *Comprehensive accreditation manual for hospitals: The official handbook.* Oakbrook Terrace, IL: The Joint Commission. (Level VII)

9 Bickley, L. (2013). *Bates' guide to physical examination and health history taking* (11th ed.). Philadelphia, PA: Lippincott Williams & Wilkins.

10 The Joint Commission. (2015). Standard RC.01.03.01. *Comprehensive accreditation manual for hospitals: The official handbook.* Oakbrook Terrace, IL: The Joint Commission. (Level VII)

11 Centers for Medicare & Medicaid Services, Department of Health and Human Services. (2014). Condition of participation: Medical record services. 42 C.F.R. § 482.24(b).

12 American Osteopathic Association. (2014). Standard 10.00.03. *Healthcare Facilities Accreditation Program: Accreditation requirements for acute care hospitals.* Chicago, IL: American Osteopathic Association. (Level VII)

ADDITIONAL REFERENCE

Kobayashi, H. (2013). Effect of measurement duration on accuracy of pulse-counting. *Ergonomics, 56,* 1940–1944. Accessed May 2015 via the Web at http://www.ncbi.nlm.nih.gov/pmc/articles/PMC3877911/ (Level VI).

PULSE OXIMETRY

Performed intermittently or continuously, pulse oximetry is a relatively simple procedure used to monitor arterial oxygen saturation noninvasively. Pulse oximeters usually denote arterial oxygen saturation values with the symbol Spo_2, whereas invasively measured arterial oxygen saturation values are denoted by the symbol Sao_2. Pulse oximetry can aid

EQUIPMENT

How oximetry works

The pulse oximeter allows noninvasive monitoring of arterial oxygen saturation (SpO_2) levels, by measuring the absorption (amplitude) of light waves as they pass through areas of the body that are highly perfused by arterial blood. Oximetry also monitors pulse rate and amplitude.

Light-emitting diodes in a transducer (photodetector) attached to the patient's body (shown below on the index finger) send red and infrared light beams through tissue. The photodetector records the relative amount of each color absorbed by arterial blood and transmits the data to a monitor, which displays the information with each heartbeat. If the SpO_2 level or pulse rate varies from preset limits, the monitor triggers visual and audible alarms.

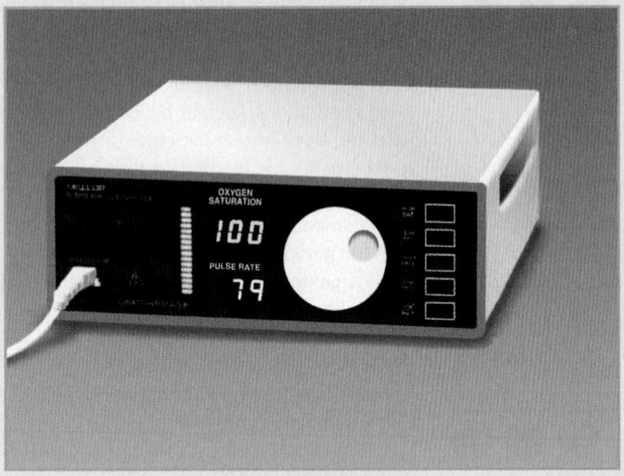

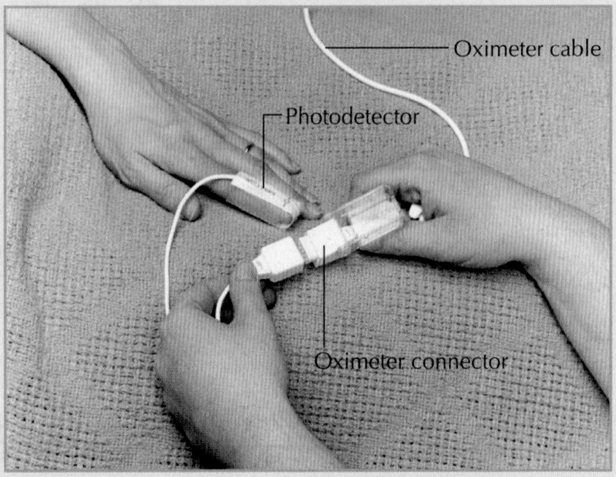

clinical decision-making; however, it isn't a substitute for a clinical assessment. Arterial blood gas (ABG) measurements, obtained by arterial puncture, are the gold standard for measuring oxygen saturation level.[1]

In this procedure, two diodes send red and infrared light through a pulsating arterial vascular bed, like the one in the fingertip. A photodetector slipped over the finger measures the transmitted light as it passes through the vascular bed, detects the relative amount of color absorbed by arterial blood, and calculates the SpO_2 without interference from surrounding venous blood, skin, connective tissue, or bone. Using the ear probe, oximetry works by monitoring the transmission of light waves through the vascular bed of a patient's earlobe. Results will be inaccurate if the patient's earlobe is poorly perfused, as from a low cardiac output. If a patient is hemodynamically unstable, a forehead sensor may be a better alternative for obtaining an accurate reading because the forehead is reasonably resistant to the vasoconstrictive effects of the sympathetic nervous system.[2] (See *How oximetry works.*)

Equipment

Oximeter ▪ finger, ear probe, forehead sensor (preferably a disposable, adhesive sensor)[3] ▪ hospital-grade disinfectant wipe or pad ▪ Optional: warming blankets, nail polish remover, nail clippers, supplemental oxygen delivery equipment.

Preparation of equipment

Follow the manufacturer's guidelines for proper operation of pulse oximeters, probes, and sensors.[4] Set alarm limits according to the manufacturer's instructions and the patient's clinical condition and medical history. Ensure that the alarms are turned on, functioning properly, and audible to staff *to reach a balance between actionable and false-positive alarms*[3,5,6]

Implementation

- Perform hand hygiene.[7,8,9,10,11]
- Confirm the patient's identity using at least two patient identifiers.[12]
- Explain the procedure to the patient.
- Warm the patient with blankets, as needed; *the patient should be kept warm to exclude motion artifact caused by shivering.*[4]

Using a finger probe

- Select a finger for the test. Although the index finger is commonly used, a smaller finger may be selected if the patient's fingers are too large for the equipment. Make sure the patient isn't wearing false fingernails, and remove any nail polish from the test finger. Place the transducer (photodetector) probe over the patient's finger so that light beams and sensors oppose each other. If the patient has long fingernails, position the probe perpendicular to the finger, if possible, or clip the fingernail. Always position the patient's hand at heart level *to eliminate venous pulsations and to promote accurate readings.*
- Turn on the power switch (as shown below). If the device is working properly, a beep will sound, a display will light momentarily, and the pulse searchlight will flash. The SpO_2 and pulse rate displays will show stationary zeros. After four to six heartbeats, the SpO_2 and pulse rate displays will supply information with each beat, and the pulse amplitude indicator will begin tracking the pulse.

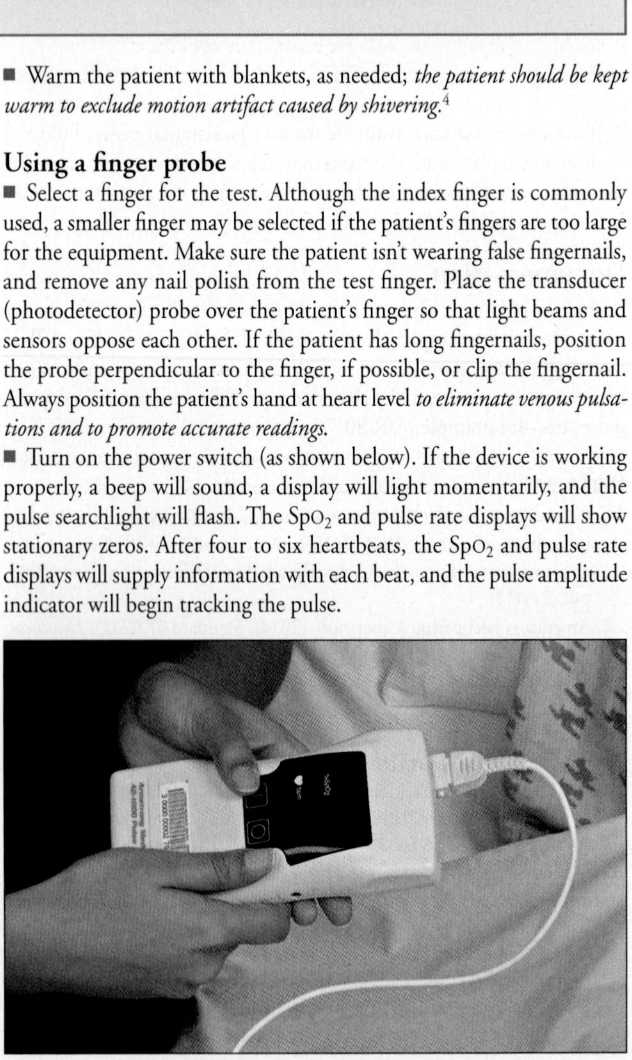

Using an ear probe

■ Using an alcohol pad, massage the patient's earlobe for 10 to 20 seconds (as shown below) and allow it to dry. Mild erythema indicates adequate vascularization.

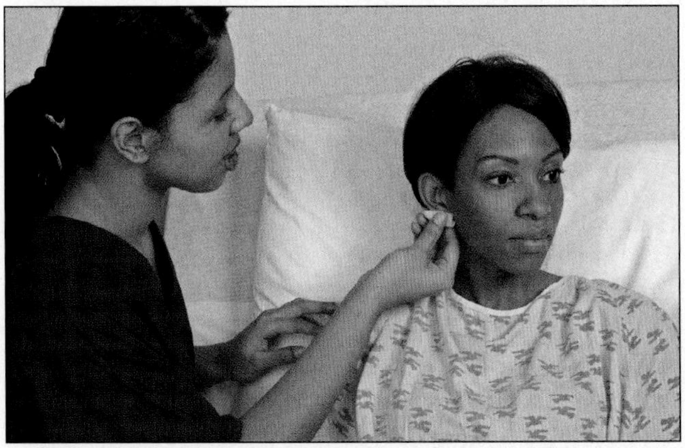

■ Following the manufacturer's instructions, attach the ear probe to the patient's earlobe or pinna. Use the ear probe stabilizer for prolonged or exercise testing. Be sure to establish good contact on the ear; *an unstable probe may set off the low-perfusion alarm.*
■ After the probe has been attached for a few seconds, a saturation reading and pulse waveform will appear on the oximeter's screen.
■ Leave the ear probe in place for 3 or more minutes until readings stabilize at the highest point, or take three separate readings and average them. Make sure you revascularize the patient's earlobe each time.

Using a forehead sensor

■ Make sure the patient's forehead is clean and dry.
■ Following the manufacturer's instructions, attach the forehead sensor to the patient's forehead.
■ Turn on the device.
■ After the probe has been attached for a few seconds, a saturation reading and pulse waveform will appear on the oximeter's screen.

Completing the procedure

■ If monitoring continuous pulse oximetry, confirm that alarm limits are set appropriately for the patient's current condition and that the alarms are turned on, functioning properly, and audible to staff.[3,6,13]
■ If the pulse oximeter alarms, assess the patient's respiratory status and make sure the sensor remains attached properly.
■ If you detect and confirm low saturation levels, administer supplemental oxygen, as needed and prescribed.
■ Check and document the pulse oximeter reading and the skin under the probe regularly. Change the sensor site as needed or at an interval established by your facility.
■ When the practitioner orders monitoring to be discontinued, remove the probe, turn off and unplug the unit and, if using a reusable probe, clean it by gently rubbing it with a disinfectant wipe or pad.[14,15]
■ Perform hand hygiene.[7,8,9,10,11]
■ Document the procedure.[16,17,18]

Special considerations

■ The pulse rate on the pulse oximeter should correspond with the patient's actual pulse. If the rates don't correspond, the saturation reading can't be considered accurate. Assess the patient, check the oximeter, and reposition the probe, if necessary.[19]
■ Collaborate with an interprofessional team, including biomedical engineering, to determine the best delay and threshold settings.[3]
■ Use disposable, adhesive sensors (if available), and replace the sensors when they no longer adhere properly to the patient's skin.[3]
■ If you've performed oximetry properly, readings are typically accurate to within plus-or-minus 2% of SpO_2 at higher levels, but may reflect SpO_2 less accurately when SpO_2 falls below 80%.[20,21]
■ Certain factors may interfere with accuracy, including elevated carboxyhemoglobin or methemoglobin levels (such as occur in heavy smokers and city dwellers), which can cause a falsely elevated SpO_2 reading; certain intravascular substances, such as lipid emulsions and dyes; excessive light (for example, from phototherapy, surgical lamps, direct sunlight, and excessive ambient lighting); excessive patient movement; excessive ear pigment; hypothermia; hypotension; vasoconstriction; poor perfusion; and severe sepsis or septic shock.[1,4,21]
■ Forehead sensors are a good alternative for patients with poor peripheral circulation and in patients under general anesthesia whose extremities aren't readily accessible.[4]
■ If you're using SpO_2 to guide weaning the patient from forced inspiratory oxygen, obtain samples for ABG analysis occasionally to correlate SpO_2 readings with SaO_2 levels.
■ If you're using an automatic blood pressure cuff on the same extremity used for measuring SpO_2, the cuff will interfere with SpO_2 readings during inflation.
■ If light is a problem, cover the probes; if patient movement is a problem, move the probe or select a different probe; and if ear pigment is a problem, reposition the probe, revascularize the site, or use a finger probe. (See *Diagnosing pulse oximeter problems*, page 654.)
■ Normal SpO_2 levels for pulse oximetry are 95% to 100% for adults. An SpO_2 of 92% or less suggests hypoxemia.[1] For such patients, follow your facility's protocol or the practitioner's orders, which may include increasing oxygen therapy. If SpO_2 levels decrease suddenly, you may need to resuscitate the patient immediately. Notify the practitioner of any significant change in the patient's condition.
■ The Joint Commission issued a sentinel event alert concerning medical device alarm safety *because alarm-related events have been associated with permanent loss of function or death.* Among the major contributing factors were improper alarm settings, alarms inappropriately turned off, and alarm signals not audible to staff. Make sure alarm limits are set appropriately and that alarms are turned on, functioning properly, and audible to staff. Follow facility guidelines for preventing alarm fatigue.[22]

Patient teaching

Explain to the patient and family why you're using pulse oximetry, how it works, and what the readings indicate in language that they can comprehend. Also explain the factors that can lead to false alarms and the importance of frequent site assessment and rotation.[4]

Documentation

Document the date, time, procedure type, patient's activity level and position, probe site, amount of supplemental oxygen and oxygen saturation as well as any action taken. Record readings on appropriate flowcharts if indicated.

REFERENCES

1 Mohammad, Y., et al. (2010). "Clinical use of pulse oximetry: A pocket reference" [Online]. Accessed May 2015 via the Web at http://www.copd-alert.com/OximetryPG.pdf
2 Lynn-McHale Wiegand, D. (Ed.). (2011). *AACN procedure manual for critical care* (6th ed.). St. Louis, MO: Saunders.
3 American Association of Critical-Care Nurses. (2013). "AACN practice alert: Alarm management" [Online]. Accessed May 2015 via the Web at http://www.aacn.org/wd/practice/docs/practicealerts/alarm-management-practice-alert.pdf (Level VII)

TROUBLESHOOTING

Diagnosing pulse oximeter problems

To maintain a continuous display of arterial oxygen saturation (SpO_2) levels, keep the monitoring site clean and dry. Make sure the skin doesn't become irritated from adhesives used to keep disposable probes in place. You may need to change the site if this happens. Disposable probes that irritate the skin also can be replaced by nondisposable models.

Another common problem with pulse oximeters is the failure of the devices to obtain a signal. If the device you're using fails to obtain a signal, first assess the patient's vital signs. If they're sufficient to produce a signal, check for a poor connection, inadequate or intermittent blood flow to the site, or equipment malfunctions.

Poor connection

To check for a poor connection, make sure that the sensors are properly aligned properly. Make sure that wires are intact and securely fastened and that the pulse oximeter is plugged into a power source.

Inadequate or intermittent blood flow to the site

To determine inadequate or intermittent blood flow to the site, assess the patient's pulse rate and capillary refill time. If blood flow to the site is decreased, take corrective action by loosening restraints, removing tight-fitting clothes, taking off a blood pressure cuff, or assessing arterial and IV catheters. If none of these interventions works, you may need to find an alternate site. Finding a site with proper circulation may also prove challenging when a patient is receiving vasoconstrictive drugs. Refer to the manufacturer's recommendations regarding the effects of low perfusion states on pulse oximeter performance.[1]

Equipment malfunctions

If you suspect an equipment malfunction, remove the pulse oximeter from the patient, set the alarm limits, and try the instrument on yourself or another healthy person. This test will tell you if the equipment is working correctly.

4 Valdez-Lowe, C., et al. (2009). Pulse oximetry in adults. *American Journal of Nursing, 109*(6), 52–59. Accessed May 2015 via the Web at http://www.nursingcenter.com/prodev/ce_article.asp?tid=864063

5 Taenzer, A. H., et al. (2010). Impact of pulse oximetry surveillance on rescue events and intensive care unit transfers: A before-and-after concurrence study. *Anesthesiology, 112,* 282–287. Accessed May 2015 via the Web at http://journals.lww.com/anesthesiology/Fulltext/2010/02000/Impact_of_Pulse_Oximetry_Surveillance_on_Rescue.10.aspx/

6 The Joint Commission. (2015). Standard NPSG.06.01.01. *Comprehensive accreditation manual for hospitals: The official handbook.* Oakbrook Terrace, IL: The Joint Commission. (Level VII)

7 Centers for Disease Control and Prevention. (2002). Guideline for hand hygiene in health-care settings: Recommendations of the Healthcare Infection Control Practices Advisory Committee and the HICPAC/SHEAP/APIC/IDSA Hand Hygiene Task Force. *MMWR Recommendations and Reports, 51*(RR-16), 1–45. Accessed May 2015 via the Web at http://www.cdc.gov/mmwr/pdf/rr/rr5116.pdf (Level II)

8 World Health Organization. (2009). "WHO guidelines on hand hygiene in health care: First global patient safety challenge, clean care is safer care" [Online]. Accessed May 2015 via the Web at http://whqlibdoc.who.int/publications/2009/9789241597906_eng.pdf (Level IV)

9 The Joint Commission. (2015). Standard NPSG.07.01.01. *Comprehensive accreditation manual for hospitals: The official handbook.* Oakbrook Terrace, IL: The Joint Commission. (Level VII)

10 Centers for Medicare & Medicaid Services, Department of Health and Human Services. (2014). Condition of participation: Infection control. 42 C.F.R. § 482.42.

11 American Osteopathic Association. (2014). Standard 07.01.21. *Healthcare Facilities Accreditation Program: Accreditation requirements for acute care hospitals.* Chicago, IL: American Osteopathic Association. (Level VII)

12 The Joint Commission. (2015). Standard NPSG.01.01.01. *Comprehensive accreditation manual for hospitals: The official handbook.* Oakbrook Terrace, IL: The Joint Commission. (Level VII)

13 Graham, K. C., & Cvach, M. (2010). Monitor alarm fatigue: Standardizing use of physiological monitors and decreasing nuisance alarms. *American Journal of Critical Care, 19,* 28–37.

14 Rutala, W. A., et al. (2008). "Guideline for disinfection and sterilization in healthcare facilities, 2008" [Online]. Accessed May 2015 via the Web at http://www.cdc.gov/hicpac/pdf/guidelines/Disinfection_Nov_2008.pdf

15 American Osteopathic Association. (2014). Standard 07.02.03. *Healthcare Facilities Accreditation Program: Accreditation requirements for acute care hospitals.* Chicago, IL: American Osteopathic Association. (Level VII)

16 The Joint Commission. (2015). Standard RC.01.03.01. *Comprehensive accreditation manual for hospitals: The official handbook.* Oakbrook Terrace, IL: The Joint Commission. (Level VII)

17 Centers for Medicare & Medicaid Services, Department of Health and Human Services. (2014). Condition of participation: Medical record services. 42 C.F.R. § 482.24(b).

18 American Osteopathic Association. (2014). Standard 10.00.03. *Healthcare Facilities Accreditation Program: Accreditation requirements for acute care hospitals.* Chicago, IL: American Osteopathic Association. (Level VII)

19 World Health Organization. (2011). "Pulse oximetry training manual" [Online]. Accessed May 2015 via the Web at http://www.who.int/patientsafety/safesurgery/pulse_oximetry/who_ps_pulse_oxymetry_training_manual_en.pdf

20 Casey, G. (2011). Pulse oximetry: What are we really measuring? *Nursing New Zealand, 17*(3), 24–29.

21 Wilson, B. J., et al. (2010). The accuracy of pulse oximetry in emergency department patients with severe sepsis and septic shock: A retrospective cohort study. *BMC Emergency Medicine, 10,* 9. Accessed May 2015 via the Web at http://www.ncbi.nlm.nih.gov/pmc/articles/PMC2876142/pdf/1471-227X-10-9.pdf (Level III)

22 The Joint Commission. (2013). "Sentinel event alert: Medical device alarm safety in hospitals" [Online]. Accessed May 2015 via the Web at http://www.jointcommission.org/assets/1/18/SEA_50_alarms_4_5_13_FINAL1.PDF (Level VII)

R

Radiation implant therapy

For this treatment, also called *brachytherapy,* the practitioner uses implants of radioactive isotopes (encapsulated in seeds, needles, or sutures)[1] to deliver ionizing radiation within a body cavity or interstitially to a tumor site. Implants can deliver a continuous radiation dose over several hours or days to a specific site while minimizing exposure to adjacent tissues. The implants may be permanent or temporary. Isotopes such as cesium-137 and -131, gold-198, iodine-125, iridium-192, palladium-103, and phosphorus-32 are used to treat cancers. (See *Radioisotopes and their uses.*)

Common implant sites include the brain, breast, cervix, endometrium, lung, neck, oral cavity, prostate, and vagina. Radiation implant therapy is commonly combined with external radiation therapy (teletherapy) for increased effectiveness.

Radioisotopes and their uses

Unstable elements, radioisotopes emit three kinds of energy particles as they decay to a stable state. These particles are ranked by their penetrating power. *Alpha particles* possess the lowest energy level and are easily stopped by a sheet of paper. More powerful *beta particles* can be stopped by the skin's surface. *Gamma rays,* the most powerful, can be stopped only by dense shielding, such as lead. Some isotopes commonly used in cancer treatments are listed below.

RADIOISOTOPE	KEY FACTS	NURSING INTERVENTIONS
Cesium-137 (^{137}Cs) Gynecologic cancers, head and neck cancers, rectal cancers, and esophageal cancers	■ 30-year half-life ■ Emits gamma particles ■ Encased in steel capsules placed temporarily in the patient in the operating room	■ Elevate the head of the bed no more than 45 degrees. ■ Encourage fluids and implement a low-residue diet. ■ Encourage quiet activities; enforce strict bed rest, as ordered.
Iodine-125 (^{125}I) Localized or unresectable tumors, slow-growing tumors, and recurrent disease	■ 60-day half-life ■ Emits gamma particles ■ Permanently implanted as tiny seeds or sutures directly into the tumor or tumor bed	■ *Because seeds may become dislodged,* no linens, body fluids, instruments, or utensils may leave the patient's room until they're monitored. ■ If a seed is dislodged and found, call the radiation oncology department; use long-handled forceps to put it in a lead-lined container in the room. ■ Monitor body fluids *to detect displaced seeds.* Give the patient a 24-hour urine container that can be closed.
Iridium-192 (^{192}Ir) Gynecologic cancers and tumors of the prostate, brain, head, neck, rectum, and breast	■ 74-day half-life ■ Emits gamma particles ■ Temporarily implanted as seeds strung inside special catheters implanted around the tumor	■ If a catheter is dislodged, call the radiation oncology department; use long-handled forceps to put the implant in a lead-lined container in the room.
Palladium-103 (^{103}Pd) Prostate cancer	■ 17-day half-life ■ Emits gamma particles ■ Permanently implanted as seeds in the tumor or tumor bed	■ *Because seeds may become dislodged,* no linens, body fluids, instruments, or utensils may leave the patient's room until they're monitored. ■ If a seed is dislodged and found, call the radiation oncology department; use long-handled forceps to put it in a lead-lined container in the room. ■ Monitor body fluids *to detect displaced seeds.* Give the patient a 24-hour urine container that can be closed.
Phosphorus-32 (^{32}P) Polycythemia, leukemia, bone metastasis, and malignant ascites	■ 14-day half-life ■ Emits beta particles ■ Used as an IV solution rather than an implant *because of its low energy level*	■ No shielding is required other than a lucite syringe shield. ■ Patients receiving ^{32}P are placed in a private room with a separate bathroom.
Gold-198 (^{198}Au) Localized male genitourinary tumors	■ 3-day half-life ■ Emits gamma particles ■ Permanently implanted as tiny seeds directly into the tumor or tumor bed	■ If you find a dislodged seed, call the radiation oncology department for disposal.
Cesium-131(^{131}Cs) Prostate, liver, head, and neck tumors	■ 10-day half-life ■ Permanently implanted as tiny seeds directly into the tumor bed ■ Emits gamma particles	■ If you find a dislodged seed, call the radiation oncology department for disposal.

For treatment, the patient is usually placed in a private room (with its own bathroom) located as far away from high-traffic areas as practical. If monitoring shows an increased radiation hazard, adjacent rooms and hallways may also need to be restricted. Consult your facility's radiation safety guidelines.

Equipment

Patient medical record ■ film badge or pocket dosimeter ■ RADIATION PRECAUTION sign for door ■ RADIATION PRECAUTION warning labels ■ masking tape ■ lead-lined container ■ long-handled forceps ■ Optional: lead shield and lead strip.

For implants inserted in the oral cavity or neck

Emergency tracheotomy tray.

For implants inserted in the anal cavity or vagina

Male T-binder ■ sanitary napkins.

Preparation of equipment

Place the lead-lined container and long-handled forceps in a corner of the patient's room. Mark a "safe line" on the floor with masking tape 6′ (1.8 M) from the patient's bed *to warn visitors to keep clear of the patient to minimize their radiation exposure.* If desired, place a portable lead shield in the back of the room *to use when providing care.*

Place an emergency tracheotomy tray in the room if an implant will be inserted in the oral cavity or neck.

Implementation

- Confirm that written informed consent has been obtained and is documented in the patient's medical record.[2,3,4,5]
- Perform hand hygiene.[6,7,8,9,10]
- Confirm the patient's identity using at least two patient identifiers.[11]
- Explain the treatment and its goals to the patient. Before treatment begins, review your facility's radiation safety and visitation procedures, potential adverse effects, and interventions for those effects. Also review long-term concerns and home care issues.
- Make sure that all laboratory tests are performed before beginning treatment.

After radiation implantation

- Place the RADIATION PRECAUTION sign on the patient's door.
- If laboratory studies are required during treatment, a technician (equipped with a film badge) should obtain the specimen and label the specimen with the patient's name, identification number, and date and time of collection in the presence of the patient *to prevent mislabeling*[11] and affix it with a RADIATION PRECAUTION label, and then alert laboratory personnel before taking the samples to the laboratory. If urine tests are needed for phosphorus-32 therapy, ask the radiation oncology department or a laboratory technician about how to safely transport these specimens.
- Affix a RADIATION PRECAUTION warning label to the patient's identification wristband.
- Alert staff members that the patient is receiving radiation implant therapy by placing a RADIATION PRECAUTION warning in the patient's medical record *to prevent accidental exposure to radiation.*
- Wear a film badge or dosimeter at or above waist level during the entire shift. Turn in the radiation badge monthly or according to your facility's protocol. *Pocket dosimeters measure immediate exposures. In many facilities, these measurements aren't part of the permanent exposure record but are used to ensure that nurses receive the lowest possible exposure.*
- Each nurse must have a personal, nontransferable film badge or ring badge that's worn only within the work environment.[13] *Badges document each person's cumulative lifetime radiation exposure.* Only primary caregivers are badged and allowed into the patient's room.
- *To minimize exposure to radiation,* use the three principles of time, distance, and shielding: Time—Limit the amount of time spent near the radiation source,[13] and plan to give care in the shortest time possible *because less time equals less exposure.* Distance—Work as far away from the radiation source as possible; give care from the side opposite the implant or from a position allowing the greatest working distance possible *because the intensity of radiation exposure varies inversely as the square of the distance from the source.* Shielding—Add a protective barrier between yourself and the radioactive source if needed and desired; the type of shielding used depends on the type of radiation.[13]
- Provide essential nursing care only, limiting time in the patient's room. Make sure that perineal wipes, sanitary pads, and similar items are bagged correctly and monitored. (Refer to your facility's radiation guideline.)
- Keep soiled linens in the patient's room until scanned and cleared by the radiation officer.[13]
- Dressing changes over an implanted area must be supervised by the radiation technician or another designated caregiver.
- Before discharge, a patient's temporary implant must be removed and properly stored by the radiation oncology department. A patient with a permanent implant may not be released until his radioactivity level is less than 5 millirems/hour at a distance of 1 M.
- Perform hand hygiene.[6,7,8,9,10]
- Document the procedure.[14,15,16]

Special considerations

- Nurses and visitors who are pregnant or trying to conceive or father a child must not care for patients receiving radiation implant therapy *because the gonads and developing embryo and fetus are highly susceptible to the damaging effects of ionizing radiation.*
- If the patient must be moved out of his room, notify the appropriate department of the patient's status *to give receiving personnel time to make appropriate preparations to receive the patient.* When moving the patient, make sure that the route is clear of equipment and other people and that the elevator (if there is one) is keyed and ready to receive the patient. Move the patient in a bed or wheelchair, accompanied by two caregivers equipped with badges. If the patient is delayed along the way, stand as far away from the bed as possible until you can continue.
- The patient's room must be monitored daily by the radiation oncology department, and disposables must be monitored and removed according to facility guidelines.
- If a code is called on a patient with an implant, follow your facility's code procedures as well as these steps: Notify the code team of the patient's radioactive status *to exclude any team member who is pregnant or trying to conceive or father a child.* Also notify the radiation oncology department. Cover the implant site with a strip of lead shielding if possible. Don't allow anything to leave the patient's room until it's monitored for radiation. Limit those entering the room to personnel essential to performing code procedures. The primary care nurse must remain in the room (as far away from the patient as possible) *to act as a resource person for the patient and to provide film badges or dosimeters to code team members.*
- If an implant becomes dislodged, notify the radiation oncology department staff members and follow their instructions. Typically, the dislodged implant is collected with long-handled forceps and placed in a lead-shielded container.
- Tell the patient who has had a cervical implant to expect slight to moderate vaginal bleeding after being discharged. This flow normally changes color from pink to brown to white. Instruct her to notify the practitioner if bleeding increases, persists for more than 48 hours, or has a foul odor. Explain to the patient that she may resume most normal activities but should avoid sexual intercourse and the use of tampons until after her follow-up visit to the practitioner (about 6 weeks after discharge). Instruct her to take showers rather than baths for 2 weeks, to avoid douching unless allowed by the practitioner, and to avoid activities that cause abdominal strain for 6 weeks.
- Refer the patient for sexual or psychological counseling if needed.
- If a patient with an implant dies on the unit, notify the radiation oncology department *so they can remove a temporary implant and store it properly.* If the implant was permanent, radiation oncology staff members will determine which precautions to follow before postmortem care can be provided and before the body can be moved to the morgue.

Patient teaching

Teach the patient about radiation therapy, the need for temporary isolation, adverse effects, and complications. Help the patient and family consider visitation through media formats, such as phone calls, social media, video chat, and e-mail. Tell the patient that full benefits of treatment may not occur for several months. Assure the patient and family that radiation exposure isn't measurable once the patient is discharged.

Complications

Depending on the implant site and total radiation dose, complications of implant therapy may include dislodgment of the radiation source or applicator, tissue fibrosis, xerostomia, radiation pneumonitis, muscle atrophy, sterility, vaginal dryness or stenosis, fistulas, hypothyroidism, altered bowel habits, infection, airway obstruction, diarrhea, cystitis, myelosuppression, neurotoxicity, and secondary cancers. Encourage the patient and family members to keep in contact with the radiation oncology department and to call them if concerns or physical changes occur.

Documentation

Record radiation precautions taken during treatment, adverse effects of therapy, teaching provided to the patient and his family and their responses to it, the patient's tolerance of isolation procedures and the family's compliance with procedures, and referrals to local cancer services.

REFERENCES

1 Bruner, D., et al. (Eds.). (2011). *Manual for radiation oncology nursing practice and education* (4th ed.). Pittsburgh, PA: Oncology Nursing Society.

2 The Joint Commission. (2015). Standard RI.01.03.01. *Comprehensive accreditation manual for hospitals: The official handbook.* Oakbrook Terrace, IL: The Joint Commission. (Level VII)

3 Centers for Medicare & Medicaid Services, Department of Health and Human Services. (2014). Condition of participation: Patient's rights. 42 C. F. R. § 482.13.

4 American College of Radiology. (2010). "ACR-ASTRO practice guideline for the performance of high-dose-rate brachytherapy" [Online]. Accessed May 2015 via the Web at http://www.acr.org/~/media/ACR/Documents/PGTS/guidelines/High_Dose_Rate_Brachy.pdf (Level II)

5 American Osteopathic Association. (2014). Standard 15.01.11. *Healthcare Facilities Accreditation Program: Accreditation requirements for acute care hospitals.* Chicago, IL: American Osteopathic Association. (Level VII)

6 Centers for Disease Control and Prevention. (2002). Guideline for hand hygiene in health-care settings: Recommendations of the Healthcare Infection Control Practices Advisory Committee and the HICPAC/SHEA/APIC/IDSA Hand Hygiene Task Force. *MMWR Recommendations and Reports, 51*(RR–16), 1–45. Accessed May 2015 via the Web at http://www.cdc.gov/mmwr/pdf/rr/rr5116.pdf (Level II)

7 World Health Organization. (2009). "WHO guidelines on hand hygiene in health care: First global patient safety challenge, clean care is safer care" [Online]. Accessed May 2015 via the Web at http://whqlibdoc.who.int/publications/2009/9789241597906_eng.pdf (Level IV)

8 The Joint Commission. (2015). Standard NPSG.07.01.01. *Comprehensive accreditation manual for hospitals: The official handbook.* Oakbrook Terrace, IL: The Joint Commission. (Level VII)

9 American Osteopathic Association. (2014). Standard 07.01.21. *Healthcare Facilities Accreditation Program: Accreditation requirements for acute care hospitals.* Chicago, IL: American Osteopathic Association. (Level VII)

10 Centers for Medicare & Medicaid Services, Department of Health and Human Services. (2014). Condition of participation: Infection control. 42 C.F.R. § 482.42.

11 The Joint Commission. (2015). Standard NPSG.01.01.01. *Comprehensive accreditation manual for hospitals: The official handbook.* Oakbrook Terrace, IL: The Joint Commission. (Level VII)

12 American Osteopathic Association. (2014). Standard 30.00.14. *Healthcare Facilities Accreditation Program: Accreditation requirements for acute care hospitals.* Chicago, IL: American Osteopathic Association. (Level VII)

13 Polovich, M., et al., (Eds.). (2014). *Chemotherapy and biotherapy guidelines and recommendations for practice* (4th ed.). Pittsburgh, PA: Oncology Nursing Society.

14 The Joint Commission. (2015). Standard RC.01.03.01. *Comprehensive accreditation manual for hospitals: The official handbook.* Oakbrook Terrace, IL: The Joint Commission. (Level VII)

15 American Osteopathic Association. (2014). Standard 10.00.03. *Healthcare Facilities Accreditation Program: Accreditation requirements for acute care hospitals.* Chicago, IL: American Osteopathic Association. (Level VII)

16 Centers for Medicare & Medicaid Services, Department of Health and Human Services. (2014). Condition of participation: Medical record services. 42 C.F.R. § 482.24(b).

RADIATION THERAPY, EXTERNAL

About 60% of all cancer patients are treated with some form of external radiation therapy. Also called radiotherapy, this treatment delivers radiation—X-rays or gamma rays—directly to the cancer site.

Radiation doses are based on the type, stage, and location of the tumor as well as on the patient's size, condition, and overall treatment goals. Doses are given in increments, usually 3 to 5 times a week, until the total dose is reached.

The goals of radiation therapy include *cure,* in which the cancer is completely destroyed and not expected to recur; *control,* in which the cancer doesn't progress or regress but is expected to progress at some later time; or *palliation,* in which radiation is given to relieve signs and symptoms (such as bone pain, seizures, bleeding, and headache) caused by the cancer.

External beam radiation therapy is delivered by machines that aim a concentrated beam of high-energy particles (photons and gamma rays) at the target site. Two types of machines are commonly used: units containing cobalt or cesium as radioactive sources for gamma rays, and linear accelerators that use electricity to produce X-rays. Linear accelerators produce high energy with great penetrating ability.

Radiation therapy may be augmented by chemotherapy, radiation implant therapy (brachytherapy), or surgery, as needed.

Equipment

Radiation therapy machine.

Implementation

- Verify the practitioner's order.
- Confirm that written informed consent has been obtained and is in the patient's medical record.[1,2,3]
- Perform hand hygiene.[4,5,6,7,8]
- Confirm the patient's identity using at least two patient identifiers.[9,10]
- Explain the treatment to the patient and his family. Review the treatment goals, and discuss the range of potential adverse effects as well as interventions to minimize them. Also discuss possible long-term complications and treatment issues. Educate the patient and his family about local cancer services.
- Review the patient's clinical record for recent laboratory and imaging results, and alert the radiation oncology staff to any abnormalities or pertinent results (such as myelosuppression, paraneoplastic syndromes, oncologic emergencies, and tumor progression).
- Reassure the patient as he begins therapy; he'll first undergo simulation (treatment planning), in which the target area is mapped out on his body using a machine similar to the radiation therapy machine. Then the target area is tattooed or marked in ink on his body *to ensure accurate treatments.*
- The practitioner and radiation oncologist determine the duration and frequency of treatments, depending on the patient's body size, size of portal, extent and location of cancer, and treatment goals.
- The patient is positioned on the treatment table beneath the machine.[11] Treatments last from a few seconds to a few minutes. Reassure the patient that he won't feel anything and that he won't be radioactive.
- After treatment is complete, the patient may return home or to his room.
- Perform hand hygiene.[4,5,6,7,8]
- Document the procedure.[12,13,14]

Special considerations

■ Emphasize the importance of keeping all scheduled radiation treatment appointments *because missed appointments may affect treatment outcomes.* Make sure that the patient is aware of how to prepare for his specified treatment, such as having a full bladder for prostate radiation or learning to hold his breath for respiratory gating.[15]

■ Emphasize the importance of keeping follow-up appointments *so that the practitioner can address treatment outcomes and resolution of signs and symptoms.*

■ Tell the patient to avoid the use of lotions, topical medications, deodorants, perfumes, and powders before treatment.

■ Encourage the patient to avoid sun exposure for 1 year after treatment and to use a sunblock with a sun protection factor of 15 or higher.

■ Refer the patient to a support group, such as a local chapter of the American Cancer Society.

Patient teaching

Teach the patient and his family proper skin care and management of the possible adverse effects of treatment. Explain to the patient that the full benefit of radiation treatments may not occur until several weeks or months after treatments begin. Instruct him to report any long-term adverse effects.

Instruct the patient about the importance of leaving the target area markings intact *to ensure treatment accuracy.*

Complications

Adverse effects arise gradually and diminish gradually after treatments. They may be acute, subacute (accumulating as treatment progresses), chronic (following treatment), or long-term (arising months to years after treatment). Adverse effects are localized to the area of treatment, and their severity depends on the total radiation dosage, underlying organ sensitivity, and the patient's overall condition.

Common acute and subacute adverse effects can include altered skin integrity, altered GI and genitourinary function, altered fertility and sexual function, altered bone marrow production, anxiety, fatigue, sleep disturbances, and alopecia.

Long-term complications or adverse effects may include radiation pneumonitis, neuropathy, skin and muscle atrophy, telangiectasia, fistulas, altered endocrine function, and secondary cancers. Other long-term treatment complications include headache, alopecia, xerostomia, dysphagia, stomatitis, altered skin integrity (wet or dry desquamation), nausea, vomiting, heartburn, diarrhea, cystitis, and fatigue.

Documentation

Record radiation precautions taken during treatment, interventions used and evaluation of the interventions, grading of adverse effects, and teaching given to the patient and family and their understanding of your teaching. Also document the patient's tolerance of isolation procedures and the family's compliance with procedures, discharge plans and teaching, and referrals to local cancer services, if applicable.

References

1 Centers for Medicare & Medicaid Services, Department of Health and Human Services. (2014). Condition of participation: Patient's rights. 42 C.F.R. § 482.13.

2 The Joint Commission. (2014). Standard RI.01.03.01. *Comprehensive accreditation manual for hospitals: The official handbook.* Oakbrook Terrace, IL: The Joint Commission. (Level VII)

3 American Osteopathic Association. (2014). Standard 15.01.11. *Healthcare Facilities Accreditation Program: Accreditation requirements for acute care hospitals.* Chicago, IL: American Osteopathic Association. (Level VII)

4 Centers for Disease Control and Prevention. (2002). Guideline for hand hygiene in health-care settings: Recommendations of the Healthcare Infection Control Practices Advisory Committee and the HICPAC/SHEA/APIC/IDSA Hand Hygiene Task Force. *MMWR Recommendations and Reports, 51*(RR-16), 1–45. Accessed May 2015 via the Web at http://www.cdc.gov/mmwr/pdf/rr/rr5116.pdf (Level II)

5 World Health Organization. (2009). "WHO guidelines on hand hygiene in health care: First global patient safety challenge, clean care is safer care" [Online]. Accessed May 2015 via the Web at http://whqlibdoc.who.int/publications/2009/9789241597906_eng.pdf (Level IV)

6 The Joint Commission. (2015). Standard NPSG.07.01.01. *Comprehensive accreditation manual for hospitals: The official handbook.* Oakbrook Terrace, IL: The Joint Commission. (Level VII)

7 American Osteopathic Association. (2014). Standard 07.01.21. *Healthcare Facilities Accreditation Program: Accreditation requirements for acute care hospitals.* Chicago, IL: American Osteopathic Association. (Level VII)

8 Centers for Medicare & Medicaid Services, Department of Health and Human Services. (2014). Condition of participation: Infection control. 42 C.F.R. § 482.42.

9 The Joint Commission. (2015). Standard NPSG.01.01.01. *Comprehensive accreditation manual for hospitals: The official handbook.* Oakbrook Terrace, IL: The Joint Commission. (Level VII)

10 American Osteopathic Association. (2014). Standard 30.00.14. *Healthcare Facilities Accreditation Program: Accreditation requirements for acute care hospitals.* Chicago, IL: American Osteopathic Association. (Level VII)

11 American College of Radiology. (2011). "ACR-ASTRO practice guideline for 3D external beam radiation planning and conformal therapy" [Online]. Accessed May 2015 via the Web at http://www.acr.org/Quality-Safety/Standards-Guidelines/Practice-Guidelines-by-Modality/~/media/ACR/Documents/PGTS/guidelines/3D_External_Beam.pdf (Level I)

12 The Joint Commission. (2015). Standard RC.01.03.01. *Comprehensive accreditation manual for hospitals: The official handbook.* Oakbrook Terrace, IL: The Joint Commission. (Level VII)

13 American Osteopathic Association. (2014). Standard 10.00.03. *Healthcare Facilities Accreditation Program: Accreditation requirements for acute care hospitals.* Chicago, IL: American Osteopathic Association. (Level VII)

14 Centers for Medicare & Medicaid Services, Department of Health and Human Services. (2014). Condition of participation: Medical record services. 42 C.F.R. § 482.24(b).

15 Bruner, D., et al. (Eds.). (2011). *Manual for radiation oncology nursing practice and education* (4th ed.). Pittsburgh, PA: Oncology Nursing Society.

Additional reference

Zaorsky, N. G., et al. (2013). Stereotactic body radiation therapy for prostate cancer: Is the technology ready to be the standard of care? *Cancer Treatment Reviews, 39,* 212–218. (Level II)

Radioactive iodine therapy

Because the thyroid gland concentrates iodine, radioactive iodine-131 (^{131}I) can be used to treat thyroid cancer. Usually administered orally, this isotope is used to treat postoperative residual cancer, recurrent disease, inoperable primary thyroid tumors, invasion of the thyroid capsule, and thyroid ablation as well as cancers that have metastasized to cervical or mediastinal lymph nodes or other distant sites.

Because ^{131}I is absorbed systemically, all body secretions, especially urine, must be considered radioactive. For ^{131}I treatments, the patient usually is placed in a private room (with its own bathroom) located as far away from high-traffic areas as practical. Adjacent rooms and hallways may also need to be restricted. Consult your facility's radiation safety guidelines.

In lower doses, ^{131}I also may be used to treat hyperthyroidism. Most patients receive this treatment on an outpatient basis and are sent home with appropriate home care instructions.

Equipment

Patient's medical record ■ film badges, pocket dosimeters, or ring badges ■ RADIATION PRECAUTION sign for door ■ RADIATION PRECAUTION warning labels ■ waterproof gowns ■ gloves ■ hazardous-waste containers ■ sealable leak-proof bags ■ plastic wrap ■ absorbent plastic-lined pads ■ masking tape ■ radioresistant gloves ■ emergency tracheotomy tray ■ Optional: portable lead shield, nondisposable radioresistant gloves.

Preparation of equipment

Assemble all necessary equipment in the patient's room. Keep an emergency tracheotomy tray just outside the room or in a handy place at the nurses' station *because of the potential for neck swelling following treatment.* Place the RADIATION PRECAUTION sign on the door. Place an alert in the patient's medical record *to ensure staff awareness of the patient's radioactive status.*

Keep a hazardous-waste container lined with a clear and then a red leak-proof bag in the patient's room. Keep sealable leak-proof bags in the patient's room for containing linens. Keep objects in the patient's room until they've been scanned and cleared by the radiation safety officer.[1,2]

Notify the dietitian to supply foods and beverages only in disposable containers and to provide disposable utensils.

Implementation

■ Review the patient's health history for vomiting, diarrhea, productive cough, and sinus drainage, *which could increase the risk of radioactive secretions.*

■ Confirm that written informed consent has been obtained and is in the patient's medical record.[2,3,4,5]

■ Perform hand hygiene.[6,7,8,9,10]

■ Confirm the patient's identity using at least two patient identifiers.[11,12]

■ Explain the procedure and review treatment goals with the patient and his family. Before treatment begins, review with the patient your facility's radiation safety and visitation procedures, potential adverse effects, interventions, and home care procedures.

■ Check for allergies to iodine-containing substances, such as contrast media or shellfish. Review the patient's medication history for thyroid-containing or thyroid-altering drugs and for lithium carbonate, *which may increase* ^{131}I *uptake.*

■ Ensure that all ordered laboratory tests are performed before beginning treatment.[2]

■ If necessary, remove the patient's dentures *to avoid contaminating them and to reduce radioactive secretions.* Tell him they'll be returned 48 hours after treatment.

After the treatment

■ Affix a RADIATION PRECAUTION label to the patient's identification band.

■ Encourage the patient to use the toilet rather than a bedpan or urinal and to flush it three times after each use *to reduce radiation levels.*[2] *To help avoid splash and aerosol contamination,* close the lid or cover the toilet before flushing.

■ Tell the patient to remain in his room except for tests or procedures.[2] Allow him to ambulate.

■ Unless contraindicated, instruct the patient to increase his fluid intake to 3 qt (3 L) daily.

■ Encourage the patient to chew or suck on hard candy *to keep salivary glands stimulated and prevent them from becoming inflamed (which may develop in the first 24 hours).*

■ If laboratory testing is required, a laboratory technician equipped with a radiation badge obtains the specimen; labels it with the patient's name, identification number, and the date and time of the collection in the presence of the patient *to prevent mislabeling;*[11] affixes the specimen with a RADIATION PRECAUTION warning label; and alerts laboratory department personnel before transporting it. If urine tests are needed, ask the radiation oncology department or laboratory technician how to transport the specimens safely.

■ Wear a film badge or dosimeter at or above waist level during the entire shift. Turn in the radiation badge monthly or as directed by your facility and be sure to record your exposures accurately. *Pocket dosimeters measure immediate exposures. These measurements may not be part of the permanent exposure record, but they help ensure that nurses receive the lowest possible exposure.*

■ Each nurse must have a personal, nontransferable film badge or ring badge. *Badges document each person's cumulative lifetime radiation exposure.* Only primary caregivers are badged and allowed into the patient's room.[1]

■ Wear gloves to touch the patient or objects in his room.

■ Wear a waterproof gown and gloves when handling the patient's body secretions (for example, when moving his emesis basin).

■ Allow visitors to stay no more than 30 minutes every 24 hours with the patient.[2] Stress that no visitors who are pregnant or trying to conceive or father a child will be allowed to visit the patient.

PEDIATRIC ALERT *Visitors younger than age 18 shouldn't be permitted.*

■ Restrict direct contact to no more than 30 minutes or 20 millirems per day. If the patient is receiving 200 millicuries of ^{131}I, remain with him only 2 to 4 minutes and stand no closer than 1′ (30 cm) away. If standing 3′ (1 M) away, the time limit is 20 minutes; if standing 5′ (1.5 M) away, the limit is 30 minutes.

■ Perform only essential nursing care, limiting time in the room. Make sure that perineal wipes, sanitary pads, and similar items are bagged correctly.

■ If the patient vomits or urinates on the floor, notify the nuclear medicine department and use nondisposable radioresistant gloves when cleaning the floor. After cleanup, wash your gloved hands, remove the gloves and leave them in the room, and then rewash your hands.

■ If the patient must be moved from his room, notify the appropriate department of his status *so that receiving personnel can make appropriate arrangements to receive him.* When moving the patient, ensure that the route is clear of equipment and other people and that the elevator (if there is one) is keyed and ready to receive the patient. Move the patient in a bed or wheelchair, accompanied by two badged caregivers. If delayed, stand as far away from him as possible until you can continue.

■ The patient's room must be cleaned by the radiation oncology department, not by housekeeping. The room must be monitored daily, and disposables must be monitored and removed according to your facility's guidelines.

■ At discharge, schedule the patient for a follow-up examination. Also arrange for a whole-body scan approximately 7 to 10 days after ^{131}I treatment.

■ Inform the patient and family of community support services for cancer patients.

■ Perform hand hygiene.[6,7,8,9,10]

■ Document the procedure.[13,14,15]

Special considerations

■ Nurses and visitors who are pregnant or trying to conceive or father a child must not attend or visit patients receiving ^{131}I therapy *because the gonads and developing embryo and fetus are highly susceptible to the damaging effects of ionizing radiation.*

■ If a code is called on a patient undergoing ^{131}I therapy, follow your facility's code procedures as well as these steps. Notify the code team of the patient's radioactive status *to exclude any team member who is pregnant or trying to conceive or father a child.* Also notify the radiation oncology department. Don't allow anything out of the patient's room until it's monitored. Limit those entering the room to personnel essential to

PATIENT TEACHING

What to do after ^{131}I treatment

- Instruct the patient to report any long-term adverse reactions. In particular, review signs and symptoms of hypothyroidism and hyperthyroidism. Also ask him to report any signs and symptoms of thyroid cancer, such as enlarged lymph nodes, dyspnea, bone pain, nausea, vomiting, and abdominal discomfort.
- Although the patient's radiation level at discharge will be safe, suggest that he take extra precautions during the first week, such as using separate eating utensils, sleeping in a separate bedroom, and avoiding body contact.
- Sexual intercourse may be resumed 1 week after ^{131}I treatment. However, urge a female patient to avoid pregnancy for 6 months after treatment, and tell a male patient to avoid impregnating his partner for 3 months after treatment.

performing code procedures. The primary care nurse must remain in the room (as far as possible from the patient) *to act as a resource person and to provide film badges or dosimeters to code team members.*

- If the patient dies on the unit, notify the radiology safety officer, who will determine which precautions to follow before postmortem care is provided and before the body can be removed to the morgue.

Patient teaching

Teach the patient about precautions that will need to be followed when he returns home. (See *What to do after ^{131}I treatment.*)

Complications

Myelosuppression is common in patients who undergo repeated ^{131}I treatments. Radiation pulmonary fibrosis may develop if extensive lung metastasis was present when ^{131}I was administered.

Other complications may include nausea, vomiting, headache, radiation thyroiditis, fever, sialadenitis, and pain and swelling.

Documentation

Record radiation precautions taken during treatment, teaching provided to the patient and his family, the patient's tolerance of (and the family's compliance with) isolation procedures, and referrals to local cancer counseling services.

References

1 Polovich, M., et al., (Eds.). (2014). *Chemotherapy and biotherapy guidelines and recommendations for practice* (4th ed.). Pittsburgh, PA: Oncology Nursing Society.

2 American College of Radiology (ACR). (2010). "ACR-ASTRO practice guideline for the performance of therapy with unsealed radiopharmaceutical sources" [Online]. Accessed May 2015 via the Web at http://www.acr.org/~/media/ACR/Documents/PGTS/guidelines/Unsealed_Radiopharms.pdf (Level I)

3 Centers for Medicare & Medicaid Services, Department of Health and Human Services. (2014). Condition of participation: Patient's rights. 42 C.F.R. § 482.13.

4 The Joint Commission. (2015). Standard RI.01.03.01. *Comprehensive accreditation manual for hospitals: The official handbook.* Oakbrook Terrace, IL: The Joint Commission. (Level VII)

5 American Osteopathic Association. (2014). Standard 15.01.11. *Healthcare Facilities Accreditation Program: Accreditation requirements for acute care hospitals.* Chicago, IL: American Osteopathic Association. (Level VII)

6 Centers for Disease Control and Prevention. (2002). Guideline for hand hygiene in health-care settings: Recommendations of the Healthcare Infection Control Practices Advisory Committee and the HICPAC/SHEA/APIC/IDSA Hand Hygiene Task Force. *MMWR Recommendations and Reports, 51*(RR-16), 1–45. Accessed May 2015 via the Web at http://www.cdc.gov/mmwr/pdf/rr/rr5116.pdf (Level II)

7 World Health Organization. (2009). "WHO guidelines on hand hygiene in health care: First global patient safety challenge, clean care is safer care" [Online]. Accessed May 2015 via the Web at http://whqlibdoc.who.int/publications/2009/9789241597906_eng.pdf (Level IV)

8 The Joint Commission. (2015). Standard NPSG.07.01.01. *Comprehensive accreditation manual for hospitals: The official handbook.* Oakbrook Terrace, IL: The Joint Commission. (Level VII)

9 American Osteopathic Association. (2014). Standard 07.01.21. *Healthcare Facilities Accreditation Program: Accreditation requirements for acute care hospitals.* Chicago, IL: American Osteopathic Association. (Level VII)

10 Centers for Medicare & Medicaid Services, Department of Health and Human Services. (2014). Condition of participation: Infection control. 42 C.F.R. § 482.42.

11 The Joint Commission. (2015). Standard NPSG.01.01.01. *Comprehensive accreditation manual for hospitals: The official handbook.* Oakbrook Terrace, IL: The Joint Commission. (Level VII)

12 American Osteopathic Association. (2014). Standard 30.00.14. *Healthcare Facilities Accreditation Program: Accreditation requirements for acute care hospitals.* Chicago, IL: American Osteopathic Association. (Level VII)

13 The Joint Commission. (2015). Standard RC.01.03.01. *Comprehensive accreditation manual for hospitals: The official handbook.* Oakbrook Terrace, IL: The Joint Commission. (Level VII)

14 American Osteopathic Association. (2014). Standard 10.00.03. *Healthcare Facilities Accreditation Program: Accreditation requirements for acute care hospitals.* Chicago, IL: American Osteopathic Association. (Level VII)

15 Centers for Medicare & Medicaid Services, Department of Health and Human Services. (2014). Condition of participation: Medical record services. 42 C.F.R. § 482.24(b).

Additional references

Ejeh, J. E., et al. (2013). Effectiveness of fixed dose radioactive iodine (RAI) for the treatment of hyperthyroidism: Experience of a teaching hospital in South West Nigeria. *Molecular Imaging and Radionuclide Therapy, 22*(2), 36–41.

Nettina, S. M. (2014). *Lippincott manual of nursing practice* (10th ed.). Philadelphia, PA: Wolters Kluwer.

Occupational Safety and Health Administration. (n.d.). "Ionizing radiation, standard number 1910.1096" [Online]. Accessed May 2015 via the Web at http://www.osha.gov/pls/oshaweb/owadisp.show_document?p_table=STANDARDS&p_id=10098 (Level I)

Rectal suppositories and ointments

A rectal suppository is a small, solid, medicated mass, usually cone-shaped, with a cocoa butter or glycerin base. It may be inserted to stimulate peristalsis and defecation or to relieve pain, vomiting, and local irritation. Rectal suppositories commonly contain drugs that reduce fever and induce relaxation but can't be given orally because they interact poorly with digestive enzymes, or have an offensive taste. They're also useful when a patient can't take medications orally because of nausea, vomiting, or another GI condition. Rectal suppositories melt at body temperature and are absorbed slowly.

Because insertion of a rectal suppository may stimulate the vagus nerve, this procedure is contraindicated in patients with potential cardiac arrhythmias. It may also be contraindicated in patients with active rectal bleeding or recent rectal or prostate surgery because of the risk of local trauma or discomfort during insertion.

An ointment is a semisolid medication used to produce local effects. It may be applied externally to the anus or internally to the rectum with an applicator. Rectal medications may also be used when a patient is vomiting, unable to swallow, or unconscious.

Equipment

Rectal suppository or ointment ■ applicator ■ patient's medical and medication records ■ gloves ■ water-soluble lubricant ■ 4″ × 4″ (10-cm × 10-cm) gauze pads ■ Optional: bedpan, soap and water.

Preparation of equipment

Store rectal suppositories in the refrigerator until needed *to prevent softening and, possibly, decreased effectiveness of the medication. A softened suppository is also difficult to handle and insert.* To harden a softened suppository, hold it (in its wrapper) under cold running water.

Implementation

■ Avoid distractions and interruptions when preparing and administering medications *to prevent medication administration errors.*[1,2]
■ Verify the practitioner's order.[3]
■ Compare the medication label with the order in the patient's medical record.[3,4]
■ Check the expiration date on the medication. If the medication is expired, return it to the pharmacy and obtain a new medication.[3,4]
■ Visually inspect the medication for discoloration or any other loss of integrity; don't administer the medication if its integrity is compromised.[3,4]
■ Discuss any unresolved concerns about the medication with the patient's practitioner.[3,4]
■ Perform hand hygiene.[5,6,7,8,9]
■ Confirm the patient's identity using at least two patient identifiers.[10,11]
■ Explain the procedure to the patient.
■ If the patient is receiving the medication for the first time, teach him about potential adverse reactions and discuss any other concerns related to administering the medication.[3]
■ Verify that the medication is being administered at the proper time, in the prescribed dose, and by the correct route *to reduce the risk of medication errors.*[3,4]
■ If your facility uses a bar code scanning system, scan your identification badge, the patient's identification bracelet, and the medication's bar code.
■ Provide privacy.
■ Put on gloves.[12,13]
■ Position the patient on his left side in the Sims position. Drape him with the bedcovers *to expose only the buttocks.*

Rectal suppository administration

■ Remove the suppository from its wrapper and lubricate it with water-soluble lubricant.
■ Lift the patient's upper buttock with your nondominant hand *to expose the anus.*
■ Instruct the patient to take several deep breaths through his mouth *to help relax the anal sphincters and reduce anxiety or discomfort during insertion.*
■ Using the index finger of your dominant hand, insert the suppository—tapered end first—about 1″ (2.5 cm), until you feel it pass the internal anal sphincter.[14] Try to direct the tapered end toward the side of the rectum *so that it contacts the membranes.* (See *How to administer a rectal suppository.*)
■ Ensure the patient's comfort. Encourage him to lie quietly and, if applicable, to squeeze or hold his buttocks together *to retain the suppository for the appropriate length of time.* The patient should retain a suppository administered to relieve constipation as long as possible (at least 20 minutes) to be effective.

Rectal ointment administration

■ *To apply externally,* use gloves or a gauze pad to spread medication over the anal area.

How to administer a rectal suppository

When inserting a suppository, direct its tapered end toward the side of the rectum *so that it contacts the membranes, encouraging absorption of the medication.*

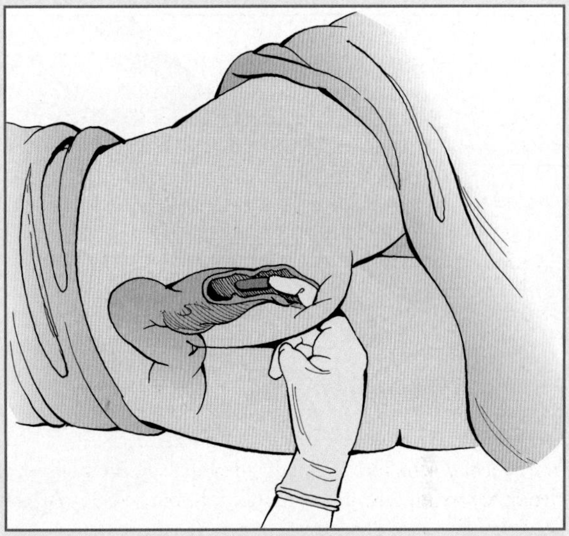

■ *To apply internally,* expect to use about 1″ (2.5 cm) of ointment. *To gauge how much pressure to use during application,* squeeze a small amount from the tube before you attach the applicator. Then attach the applicator to the tube of ointment and coat the applicator with water-soluble lubricant.
■ Lift the patient's upper buttock with your nondominant hand *to expose the anus.*
■ Instruct the patient to take several deep breaths through his mouth *to relax the anal sphincters and reduce anxiety or discomfort during insertion.*
■ Gently insert the applicator, directing it toward the umbilicus. (See *How to administer rectal ointment,* page 662.)
■ Slowly squeeze the tube *to eject the medication.*
■ Remove the applicator and place a folded 4″ × 4″ (10-cm × 10-cm) gauze pad between the patient's buttocks *to absorb excess ointment.*
■ Detach the applicator from the tube and recap the tube. Then clean the applicator thoroughly with soap and warm water.

Completing the procedure

■ Remove and discard your gloves and perform hand hygiene.[5,6,7,8,9]
■ Document the procedure.[15,16,17]

Special considerations

■ *Because the intake of food and fluid stimulates peristalsis,* a suppository for relieving constipation should be inserted about 30 minutes before mealtime *to help soften the feces in the rectum and facilitate defecation.* A medicated retention suppository should be inserted between meals.
■ Instruct the patient to avoid expelling the suppository. If he has difficulty retaining it, have a bedpan close by *to place underneath the patient.*
■ Make sure the patient's call light is handy, and watch for his signal *because he may be unable to suppress the urge to defecate.* For example, a patient with proctitis has a highly sensitive rectum and may not be able to retain a suppository for long.
■ Inform the patient that the suppository may discolor his next bowel movement. For example, hydrocortisone suppositories can give feces a silver-gray, pasty appearance.

How to administer rectal ointment

When applying a rectal ointment internally, be sure to lubricate the applicator *to minimize pain on insertion.* Direct the applicator tip toward the patient's umbilicus.

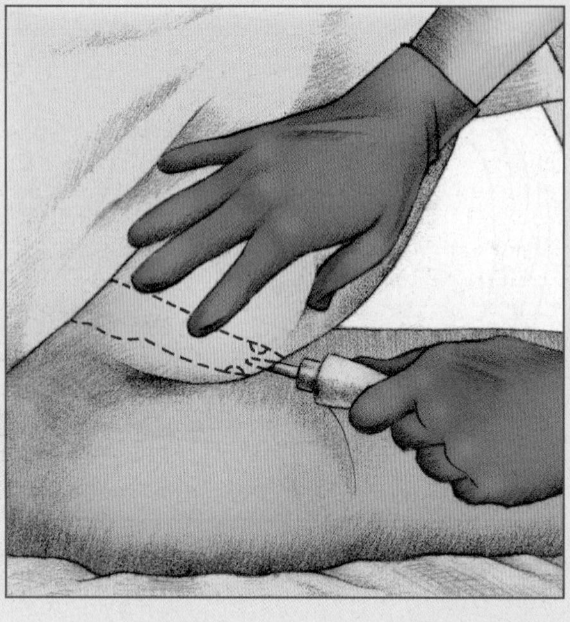

- Advise the patient to report any increase in itching or burning in the rectal area. *This may indicate increased irritation.*

Patient teaching

Some rectal suppositories and ointments are available over the counter. Teach the patient how to self-administer the suppositories or ointment if appropriate.

Complications

Complications may be related to the action of the medication. Occasionally, vagal nerve stimulation may occur, causing a vagal reaction. Irritation of the rectal area may occur.

Documentation

Record the administration time, dosage, medication name, and patient response to the medication. Document patient teaching and the patient's understanding of your teaching. Note any adverse reactions and record interventions required and the patient's response to those interventions.

REFERENCES

1 Westbrook, J., et al. (2010). Association of interruptions with an increased risk and severity of medication administration errors. *Archives of Internal Medicine, 170,* 683–690. (Level IV)

2 Institute for Safe Medication Practices. (2013). Side tracks on the safety express: Interruptions lead to errors and unfinished...Wait, what was I doing? *Nurse Advise-ERR, 11*(2), 1–4. Accessed May 2015 via the Web at https://www.ismp.org/Newsletters/acutecare/showarticle.aspx?id=37

3 The Joint Commission. (2015). Standard MM.06.01.01. *Comprehensive accreditation manual for hospitals: The official handbook.* Oakbrook Terrace, IL: The Joint Commission. (Level VII)

4 American Osteopathic Association. (2014). Standard 16.01.03. *Healthcare Facilities Accreditation Program: Accreditation requirements for acute care hospitals.* Chicago, IL: American Osteopathic Association. (Level VII)

5 The Joint Commission. (2015). Standard NPSG.07.01.01. *Comprehensive accreditation manual for hospitals: The official handbook.* Oakbrook Terrace, IL: The Joint Commission. (Level VII)

6 Centers for Disease Control and Prevention. (2002). Guideline for hand hygiene in health-care settings: Recommendations of the Healthcare Infection Control Practices Advisory Committee and the HICPAC/SHEA/APIC/IDSA Hand Hygiene Task Force. *MMWR Recommendations and Reports, 51*(RR-16), 1–45. Accessed May 2015 via the Web at http://www.cdc.gov/mmwr/pdf/rr/rr5116.pdf (Level II)

7 World Health Organization. (2009). "WHO guidelines on hand hygiene in health care: First global patient safety challenge, clean care is safer care" [Online]. Accessed May 2015 via the Web at http://whqlibdoc.who.int/publications/2009/9789241597906_eng.pdf (Level IV)

8 American Osteopathic Association. (2014). Standard 07.01.21. *Healthcare Facilities Accreditation Program: Accreditation requirements for acute care hospitals.* Chicago, IL: American Osteopathic Association. (Level VII)

9 Centers for Medicare & Medicaid Services, Department of Health and Human Services. (2014). Condition of participation: Infection control. 42 C.F.R. § 482.42.

10 The Joint Commission. (2015). Standard NPSG.01.01.01. *Comprehensive accreditation manual for hospitals: The official handbook.* Oakbrook Terrace, IL: The Joint Commission. (Level VII)

11 American Osteopathic Association. (2014). Standard 30.00.14. *Healthcare Facilities Accreditation Program: Accreditation requirements for acute care hospitals.* Chicago, IL: American Osteopathic Association. (Level VII)

12 Siegel, J. D., et al. (2007). "2007 guideline for isolation precautions: Preventing transmission of infectious agents in healthcare settings" [Online]. Accessed May 2015 via the Web at http://www.cdc.gov/hicpac/pdf/isolation/Isolation2007.pdf (Level II)

13 American Osteopathic Association. (2014). Standard 07.01.10. *Healthcare Facilities Accreditation Program: Accreditation requirements for acute care hospitals.* Chicago, IL: American Osteopathic Association. (Level VII)

14 Craven, R. F., & Hirnle, C. J. (2012). *Fundamentals of nursing: Human health and function* (7th ed.). Philadelphia, PA: Lippincott Williams & Wilkins.

15 The Joint Commission. (2015). Standard RC.01.03.01. *Comprehensive accreditation manual for hospitals: The official handbook.* Oakbrook Terrace, IL: The Joint Commission. (Level VII)

16 American Osteopathic Association. (2014). Standard 10.00.03. *Healthcare Facilities Accreditation Program: Accreditation requirements for acute care hospitals.* Chicago, IL: American Osteopathic Association. (Level VII)

17 Centers for Medicare & Medicaid Services, Department of Health and Human Services. (2014). Condition of participation: Medical record services. 42 C.F.R. § 482.24(b).

ADDITIONAL REFERENCE

Nettina, S. M. (2014). *Lippincott manual of nursing practice* (10th ed.). Philadelphia, PA: Wolters Kluwer.

RECTAL TUBE INSERTION AND REMOVAL

Whether GI hypomotility simply slows the normal release of gas and feces or results in paralytic ileus, inserting a rectal tube may relieve the discomfort of distention and flatus. Decreased motility may result from various medical or surgical conditions, certain medications (such as atropine and opioids), or even swallowed air. Conditions that contraindicate using a rectal tube include recent rectal or prostatic surgery, recent myocardial infarction, and diseases of the rectal mucosa.

Equipment

Stethoscope ▪ fluid-impermeable pads ▪ drape ▪ water-soluble lubricant ▪ commercial kit or #22 to #34 French rectal tube of soft rubber or plastic ▪ container ▪ tape ▪ gloves ▪ equipment for performing perineal care ▪ disinfectant pad ▪ Optional: other personal protective equipment.

Implementation

- Verify the practitioner's order.
- Bring all the equipment at the patient's bedside.
- Provide privavy.[1,2]
- Perform hand hygiene.[3,4,5,6,7]
- Confirm the patient's identity using at least two patient identifiers.[8]
- Explain the procedure to the patient *to enhance cooperation and relieve anxiety.*
- Check for abdominal distention. Using the stethoscope, auscultate for bowel sounds.
- Put on gloves and other personal protective equipment as needed *to comply with standard precautions.*[9,10]
- Place the fluid-impermeable pads under the patient's buttocks *to absorb any drainage that may leak from the tube.*
- Position the patient in the left-lateral Sims position *to facilitate rectal tube insertion.*
- Drape the patient's exposed buttocks.
- Lubricate the rectal tube tip with water-soluble lubricant *to ease insertion and prevent rectal irritation.*
- Lift the patient's right buttock *to expose the anus.*
- Insert the rectal tube tip into the anus, advancing the tube 2″ to 4″ (5 to 10 cm) into the rectum (as shown below). Direct the tube toward the umbilicus along the anatomic course of the large intestine.

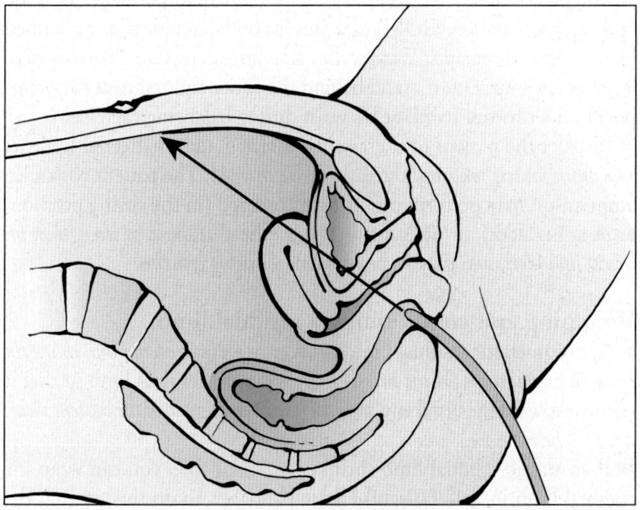

- As you insert the tube, tell the patient to breathe slowly and deeply, or suggest that he bear down as he would for a bowel movement *to relax the anal sphincter and ease insertion.* Never force the tube if you feel an obstruction.
- Using tape, secure the rectal tube to the buttocks. Then attach the tube to the container *to collect possible leakage.*
- Remove the tube after 20 minutes. If the patient reports continued discomfort or if gas wasn't expelled, you can repeat the procedure in 2 or 3 hours if ordered.
- Clean the patient, and replace soiled linens and the fluid-impermeable pad. Make sure the patient feels as comfortable as possible.
- Check for abdominal distention and listen for bowel sounds.
- Discard used equipment appropriately. Alternatively, clean and store useable equipment appropriately.
- Remove and discard your gloves and any other personal protective equipment worn.[9,10]
- Perform hand hygiene.[3,4,5,6,7]
- Clean and disinfect your stethoscope using a disinfectant pad.[11,12]
- Perform hand hygiene.[3,4,5,6,7]
- Document the procedure.[13,14,15]

Special considerations

- Fastening a plastic bag to the external end of the tube lets you observe gas expulsion (like a balloon).
- Repeat insertion periodically *to stimulate GI activity.* If the tube fails to relieve distention, notify the practitioner.

Complications

- Leaving a rectal tube in place indefinitely does little to promote peristalsis, can reduce sphincter responsiveness, and may lead to permanent sphincter damage or pressure necrosis of the mucosa.

Documentation

Record the date and time that you inserted the tube. Write down the amount, color, and consistency of any evacuated matter. Describe the patient's abdomen—hard, distended, soft, or drumlike on percussion. Note bowel sounds before and after insertion and the patient's tolerance of the procedure.

REFERENCES

1 Centers for Medicare & Medicaid Services, Department of Health and Human Services. (2014). Condition of participation: Patient's rights. 42 C.F.R. § 482.13(c)(1).

2 American Osteopathic Association. (2014). Standard 15.01.16. *Healthcare Facilities Accreditation Program: Accreditation requirements for acute care hospitals.* Chicago, IL: American Osteopathic Association. (Level VII)

3 World Health Organization. (2009). "WHO guidelines on hand hygiene in health care: First global patient safety challenge, clean care is safer care" [Online]. Accessed May 2015 via the Web at http://whqlibdoc.who.int/publications/2009/9789241597906_eng.pdf (Level IV)

4 Centers for Disease Control and Prevention. (2002). Guideline for hand hygiene in health-care settings: Recommendations of the Healthcare Infection Control Practices Advisory Committee and the HICPAC/SHEA/APIC/IDSA Hand Hygiene Task Force. *MMWR Recommendations and Reports, 51*(RR-16), 1–45. Accessed May 2015 via the Web at http://www.cdc.gov/mmwr/pdf/rr/rr5116.pdf (Level II)

5 The Joint Commission. (2015). Standard NPSG.07.01.01. *Comprehensive accreditation manual for hospitals: The official handbook.* Oakbrook Terrace, IL: The Joint Commission. (Level VII)

6 Centers for Medicare & Medicaid Services, Department of Health and Human Services. (2014). Condition of participation: Infection control. 42 C.F.R. § 482.42.

7 American Osteopathic Association. (2014). Standard 07.01.21. *Healthcare Facilities Accreditation Program: Accreditation requirements for acute care hospitals.* Chicago, IL: American Osteopathic Association. (Level VII)

8 The Joint Commission. (2015). Standard NPSG.01.01.01. *Comprehensive accreditation manual for hospitals: The official handbook.* Oakbrook Terrace, IL: The Joint Commission. (Level VII)

9 Siegel, J. D., et al. (2007). "2007 guideline for isolation precautions: Preventing transmission of infectious agents in healthcare settings" [Online]. Accessed May 2015 via the Web at http://www.cdc.gov/hicpac/pdf/isolation/Isolation2007.pdf (Level II)

10 American Osteopathic Association. (2014). Standard 07.01.10. *Healthcare Facilities Accreditation Program: Accreditation requirements for acute care hospitals.* Chicago, IL: American Osteopathic Association. (Level VII)

11 Rutala, W. A., et al. (2008). "Guideline for disinfection and sterilization in healthcare facilities, 2008" [Online]. Accessed May 2015 via the Web at http://www.cdc.gov/hicpac/pdf/guidelines/Disinfection_Nov_2008.pdf (Level I)

12 American Osteopathic Association. (2014). Standard 07.02.03. *Healthcare Facilities Accreditation Program: Accreditation requirements for acute care hospitals.* Chicago, IL: American Osteopathic Association. (Level VII)

13 The Joint Commission. (2015). Standard RC.01.03.01. *Comprehensive accreditation manual for hospitals: The official handbook.* Oakbrook Terrace, IL: The Joint Commission. (Level VII)

14 American Osteopathic Association. (2014). Standard 10.00.03. *Healthcare Facilities Accreditation Program: Accreditation requirements*

for acute care hospitals. Chicago, IL: American Osteopathic Association. (Level VII)

15 Centers for Medicare & Medicaid Services, Department of Health and Human Services. (2014). Condition of participation: Medical record services. 42 C.F.R. § 482.24(b).

ADDITIONAL REFERENCES

Nettina, S.M. (2014). *Lippincott manual of nursing practice* (10th ed.). Philadelphia, PA: Wolters Kluwer.

Popek, S., & Senegore, A. (2013). Indwelling rectal tubes: An unusual cause of significant rectal bleeding in two critically ill patients. *American Surgeon, 79,* 219–220.

Taylor, C., et al. (2015). *Fundamentals of nursing: The art and science of nursing care* (7th ed.). Philadelphia, PA: Wolters Kluwer.

RESIDUAL LIMB CARE

Patient care immediately after limb amputation includes monitoring drainage from the residual limb, controlling pain, reducing edema, positioning the affected limb, assisting with exercises prescribed by a physical therapist, and wrapping and conditioning the residual limb. Postoperative care of the residual limb will vary slightly, depending on the amputation site (arm or leg) and the type of dressing applied to the residual limb (elastic bandage or plaster cast).

After the residual limb heals, it requires daily care, including proper hygiene and continued muscle-strengthening exercises. As the patient recovers from the physical and psychological trauma of amputation, he will need to learn correct procedures for routine daily care of the residual limb.

Equipment

For postoperative residual limb care

Gloves ■ pressure dressing ■ abdominal pad ■ overhead trapeze ■ 1″ (2.5-cm) adhesive tape or bandage clips ■ trochanter roll (for a leg) ■ elastic residual limb shrinker or 4″ (10-cm) elastic bandage ■ Optional: tourniquet, prescribed skin and wound care products.

For ongoing residual limb care

Mild soap ■ residual limb socks or athletic tube socks ■ two washcloths ■ two towels.

Implementation

- Perform hand hygiene.[1,2,3,4,5]
- Confirm the patient's identity using at least two patient identifiers.[6]
- Provide privacy.[7,8,9]
- Explain the procedure to the patient *to enhance cooperation and reduce anxiety.*
- Put on gloves *to reduce to transmission of microorganisms.*[10,11]
- Perform routine postoperative care. Frequently assess the patient's respiratory status and level of consciousness, monitor IV infusions, assess tube patency, and provide for the patient's comfort, pain management, and safety. Monitor vital signs at an interval determined by your facility and the patient's condition; *there's no evidence-based research to indicate best practice for frequency of monitoring vital signs.* (See the "Postoperative care" procedure, page 624.)[12]

Monitoring residual limb drainage

- *Because gravity causes fluid to accumulate at the residual limb,* frequently inspect the dressing to assess the amount of blood and drainage on the dressing. Notify the practitioner if accumulations of drainage or blood increase rapidly. If excessive bleeding occurs, notify the practitioner immediately and apply a pressure dressing or compress the appropriate pressure points. If this doesn't control bleeding, use a tourniquet only as a last resort.
- Tape the abdominal pad over the moist part of the dressing as necessary. *Doing so provides a dry area to help prevent bacterial infection.*

Positioning the extremity

- Elevate the extremity for the first 24 hours, as ordered, *to reduce swelling and promote venous return.*[13,14]
- For an arm amputation, position the patient's arm with his elbow extended and his shoulder abducted *to prevent contractures.*
- For a leg amputation, elevate the foot of the bed slightly and place a trochanter roll against the patient's hip *to prevent external rotation.*

NURSING ALERT ***Don't place a pillow under the thigh to flex the hip*** **because this positioning can cause hip flexion contracture.** ***For the same reason, tell the patient to avoid prolonged sitting.***[13]

- After a below-the-knee amputation, maintain knee extension *to prevent hamstring muscle contractures.*
- After any level of leg amputation, place the patient on a firm surface in the prone position for at least 2 hours a day, with his legs close together and without pillows under his stomach, hips, knees, or residual limb, unless this position is contraindicated.[14] *This position helps prevent hip flexion, contractures, and abduction; it also stretches the flexor muscles.*

Assisting with prescribed exercises

- After arm amputation, encourage the patient to exercise the remaining arm *to prevent muscle contractures.* Help the patient perform isometric and range-of-motion (ROM) exercises for both shoulders, as prescribed by the physical therapist, *because use of a prosthesis requires both shoulders.*
- After leg amputation, stand behind the patient and, if necessary, support him with your hands at his waist during balancing exercises.
- Instruct the patient to exercise the affected and unaffected limbs *to maintain muscle tone and increase muscle strength.* The patient with a leg amputation may perform push-ups, as ordered (in the sitting position, arms at his sides), or pull-ups on the overhead trapeze *to strengthen his arms, shoulders, and back in preparation for using crutches.*

Wrapping and conditioning a residual limb

- Apply an elastic residual limb shrinker *to prevent edema and shape the limb in preparation for the prosthesis.*[14] Wrap the residual limb so that it narrows toward the distal end *to help ensure comfort when the patient wears the prosthesis.*
- If an elastic residual limb shrinker isn't available, you can wrap the residual limb in a 4″ (10-cm) elastic bandage. To do this, stretch the bandage to about two-thirds its maximum length as you wrap it diagonally around the residual limb, with the greatest pressure distally. (Depending on the size of the leg, you may need to use two 4″ [10-cm] bandages.) Secure the bandage with clips or adhesive tape. Make sure the bandage covers the residual limb smoothly *because wrinkles or exposed areas encourage skin breakdown.* (See *Wrapping a residual limb.*)
- To wrap an amputated arm, follow the same technique as described for the leg using a 4″ (10-cm) elastic bandage and wrapping the patient's remaining arm using figure-eight turns until the entire residual limb is covered. Pass the bandage wrap across the patient's back and shoulders *to anchor it,* and then secure the bandage with clips or adhesive tape.
- If the patient experiences throbbing after the residual limb is wrapped, the bandage may be too tight; remove the bandage immediately and reapply it less tightly. *Throbbing indicates impaired circulation.*
- Unwrap the residual limb every 4 to 6 hours for the first 2 days postoperatively, as prescribed, and then at least once daily.[13] Assess for signs and symptoms of infection and skin irritation or breakdown. Assess the color, temperature, and most-proximal pulse on the residual limb before rewrapping it, comparing findings with the contralateral extremity.[13] Report your findings to the practitioner.
- After removing the bandage to rewrap it, massage the residual limb gently, always pushing toward the suture line rather than away from it.

Wrapping a residual limb

Proper residual limb care helps protect the limb, reduces swelling, and prepares the limb for a prosthesis. As you perform the procedure, teach it to the patient.

Start by elevating the residual limb *to reduce edema and vascular stasis.*[13] Obtain two 4″ (10-cm) elastic bandages and center the end of the first 4″ (10-cm) bandage at the top of the patient's thigh. Unroll the bandage downward over the residual limb and to the back of the leg.

Make three figure-eight turns to adequately cover the ends of the residual limb. As you wrap, be sure to include the roll of flesh in the groin area. Use enough pressure to ensure that the residual limb narrows toward the end *so that it fits comfortably into the prosthesis*.

Use the second 4″ (10-cm) bandage *to anchor the first bandage around the waist.* For a below-the-knee amputation, use the knee *to anchor the bandage in place.* Secure the bandage with clips or adhesive tape. Check the residual limb bandage regularly, and rewrap it if it bunches at the end.

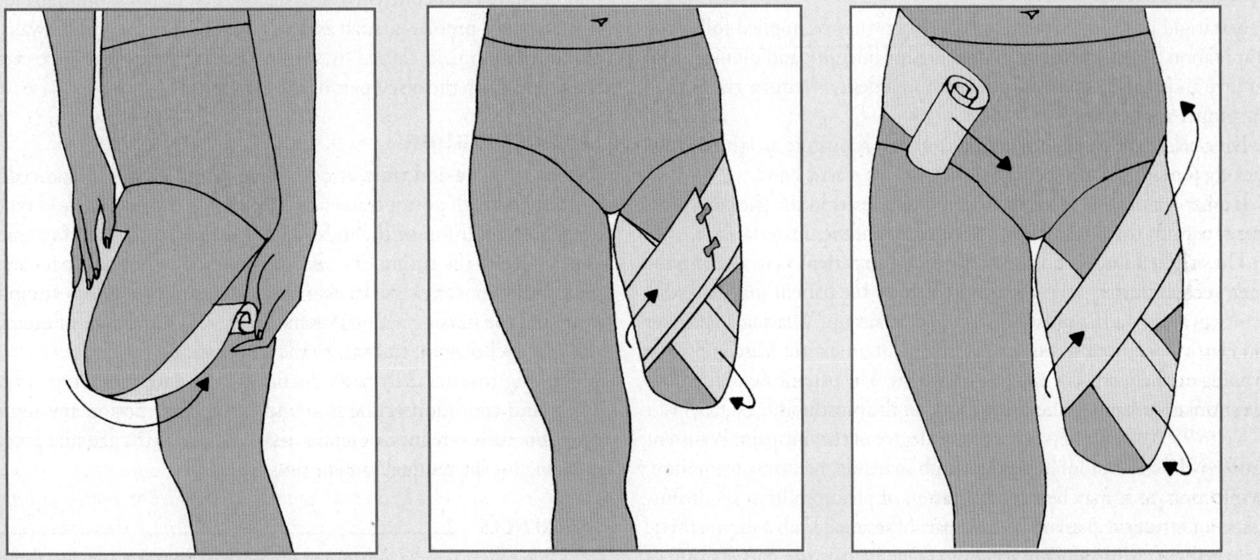

Massage stimulates circulation and prevents scar tissue from adhering to the bone.

- Perform residual limb skin care and wound care as needed and prescribed.[13]
- When healing begins, instruct the patient to push the residual limb against a pillow. Then have him progress gradually to pushing against harder surfaces, such as a padded chair, and then a hard chair. *These conditioning exercises will help the patient adjust to experiencing pressure and sensation in the residual limb.*

Caring for the healed residual limb

- *To shape the residual limb,* have the patient wear an elastic bandage 24 hours a day except while bathing.
- *To prevent infection,* bathe the residual limb but never shave it. If possible, bathe the residual limb at the end of the day *because the warm water may cause swelling, making reapplication of the prosthesis difficult.* Don't soak the residual limb for long periods.[14]
- Avoid applying lotions, oils, or creams to the residual limb, unless prescribed; *these may clog follicles, which increases the risk of infection.*[13,14]
- Inspect the residual limb for redness, swelling, irritation, and calluses. Report any of these to the practitioner. Tell the patient to avoid putting weight on the residual limb. (The skin should be firm but not taut over the bony end of the limb.)
- Continue muscle-strengthening exercises *so that the patient can build the strength he'll need to control the prosthesis.*
- Change and wash the patient's elastic bandages or sock every day *to avoid exposing the skin to excessive perspiration, which can be irritating.* Wash the elastic bandages in warm water and gentle, nondetergent soap; lay them flat on a towel to dry. *Machine washing or drying may shrink the elastic bandages.*
- Remove and discard your gloves.
- Perform hand hygiene.[1,2,3,4,5]
- Document the procedure.[18,19,20]

Caring for the plastic prosthesis

- Wipe the plastic socket of the prosthesis with a damp cloth and mild soap *to prevent bacterial accumulation.*

NURSING ALERT *Soap left in the socket or liner can cause rashes, so patients should make sure that the socket and liners are completely free from soap after washing.*[15]

- Wipe the insert (if the prosthesis has one) with a dry cloth.
- Dry the prosthesis thoroughly; if possible, allow it to dry overnight.
- Maintain and lubricate the prosthesis, as instructed by the manufacturer.
- Check for malfunctions and adjust or repair the prosthesis as necessary *to prevent further damage.*
- Check the condition of the shoe on a foot prosthesis frequently, and change it as necessary.

Applying the prosthesis

- Inspect the residual limb before and after prosthetic use. Assess for signs and symptoms of infection, skin irritation, or skin breakdown. Assess the color, temperature, and most-proximal pulse on the residual limb before reapplying the prosthesis, comparing findings with the contralateral extremity.[14,15,16]

■ Apply a clean prosthetic sock or liner. *Any part of the interface that touches the skin—socket, prosthetic sock, or liner—should undergo a thorough washing every day with hot water and antibacterial soap.*[15] Keep the seams away from bony prominences.
■ If the prosthesis has an insert, remove it from the socket, place it over the residual limb, and insert the residual limb into the prosthesis.
■ If it has no insert, slide the prosthesis over the residual limb. Secure the prosthesis onto the residual limb according to the manufacturer's directions. Ensure a good fit. *Improper socket fit can increase pressure and accelerate skin breakdown.*[17]
■ Perform hand hygiene.[1,2,3,4,5]
■ Document the procedure.[18,19,20]

Special considerations

■ Semirigid or rigid residual limb dressings may be applied following amputation. Assess the surgical dressing for integrity and drainage and remove and replace them as ordered. Some designs require training in the proper application.[13,14]
■ For a below-the-knee amputation, you may substitute an athletic tube sock for a residual limb sock by cutting off the elastic band.
■ If a known irritant or allergic component exists in the patient's prosthesis, consult the prosthetist to switch it to another material.[17]
■ The residual limb tends to swell when the patient isn't wearing the liner, such as during sleep. As a consequence, the patient may have difficulty putting on the prosthesis after he wakes up. Wearing a shrinker (an elastic sock used to control swelling) or an elastic bandage while sleeping can help prevent swelling overnight. The patient should remove the shrinker or bandage before putting on the prosthesis.[15]
■ Up to 95% of amputees report some degree of chronic pain. Persistent pain may be a symptom of residual limb ischemia, neuroma formation, or infection, or it may be a manifestation of phantom limb syndrome. Assess and treat the patient's pain as part of residual limb and prosthetic management. Multimodality pain management is the cornerstone of successful amputation rehabilitation and consists of a combination of epidural, IV, and oral analgesics.[21]

Patient teaching

Emphasize to the patient that proper care of his residual limb can speed healing. Tell him to inspect his residual limb carefully every day, using a mirror, and to continue proper daily residual limb care. Instruct him to call the practitioner if the incision appears to be opening, looks red or swollen, feels warm, is painful to touch, or is seeping drainage.

Make sure the patient knows the signs and symptoms that indicate problems in the residual limb. Explain that a 10-lb (4.5-kg) change in body weight will alter his residual limb size and require a new prosthesis socket to ensure a correct fit. He should wash the residual limb with unscented, uncolored antibacterial soap at least once a day.

Tell the patient to massage the residual limb toward the suture line to mobilize the scar and prevent its adherence to bone. Advise him to avoid exposing the skin around the residual limb to excessive perspiration, which can be irritating. Tell him to change his elastic bandages or residual limb sock daily to avoid this irritation.

Tell the patient that he may experience twitching, spasms, or phantom limb sensations (such as pain, warmth, cold, or itching) as his residual limb muscles adjust to amputation. Tell the patient that phantom pain usually peaks about 1 month after amputation, but a second peak may occur about 1 year after amputation.[22] Measures such as imagery, biofeedback, and distraction may help relieve phantom limb pain or other sensations. Advise him that he can decrease these symptoms with heat, massage, or gentle pressure. If his residual limb is sensitive to touch, tell him to rub it with a dry washcloth for 4 minutes three times a day.

Inform the patient that exercise of the remaining muscles in an amputated limb must begin the day after surgery. A physical therapist will direct these exercises. For example, arm exercises progress from isometrics to assisted ROM to active ROM. Leg exercises include rising from a chair, balancing on one leg, and ROM exercises of the knees and hips.

Stress the importance of performing prescribed exercises to help minimize complications, maintain muscle strength and tone, prevent contractures, and promote independence. Also stress the importance of positioning to prevent contractures and edema.

Complications

The most common postoperative complications include hemorrhage, infection, contractures, and a swollen or flabby residual limb. Complications that may develop at any time after an amputation include hematoma formation; skin breakdown or irritation from lack of ventilation; bone erosion or osteomyelitis; a sebaceous cyst or boil from tight socks; psychological problems, such as denial, depression, or withdrawal; and phantom limb pain caused by stimulation of nerves that once carried sensations from the distal part of the extremity.

Documentation

Record the date and time of observations and of specific procedures performed for all postoperative care, including the amount and type of drainage, condition of the dressing, need for dressing reinforcement, appearance of the suture line and surrounding tissue, and pain assessment. Also note any signs of skin irritation or infection, any complications and the nursing actions taken, the patient's tolerance of exercises, and his psychological reaction to the amputation.

During routine daily care, document the date, time, type of care given, and condition of the skin and suture line, noting any signs of irritation, such as redness or tenderness. Also record the patient's progress in caring for the residual limb or prosthesis.

REFERENCES

1 Centers for Disease Control and Prevention. (2002). Guideline for hand hygiene in health-care settings: Recommendations of the Healthcare Infection Control Practices Advisory Committee and the HICPAC/SHEA/APIC/IDSA Hand Hygiene Task Force. *MMWR Recommendations and Reports, 51*(RR-16), 1–45. Accessed May 2015 via the Web at http://www.cdc.gov/mmwr/pdf/rr/rr5116.pdf (Level II)
2 World Health Organization. (2009). "WHO guidelines on hand hygiene in health care: First global patient safety challenge, clean care is safer care" [Online]. Accessed May 2015 via the Web at http://whqlibdoc.who.int/publications/2009/9789241597906_eng.pdf (Level IV)
3 The Joint Commission. (2015). Standard NPSG.07.01.01. *Comprehensive accreditation manual for hospitals: The official handbook.* Oakbrook Terrace, IL: The Joint Commission. (Level VII)
4 Centers for Medicare & Medicaid Services, Department of Health and Human Services. (2014). Condition of participation: Infection control. 42 C.F.R. § 482.42.
5 American Osteopathic Association. (2014). Standard 07.01.21. *Healthcare Facilities Accreditation Program: Accreditation requirements for acute care hospitals.* Chicago, IL: American Osteopathic Association. (Level VII)
6 The Joint Commission. (2015). Standard NPSG.01.01.01. *Comprehensive accreditation manual for hospitals: The official handbook.* Oakbrook Terrace, IL: The Joint Commission. (Level VII)
7 The Joint Commission. (2015). Standard RI.01.01.01. *Comprehensive accreditation manual for hospitals: The official handbook.* Oakbrook Terrace, IL: The Joint Commission. (Level VII)
8 Centers for Medicare & Medicaid Services, Department of Health and Human Services. (2014). Condition of participation: Patient's rights. 42 C.F.R. § 482.13(c)(1).
9 American Osteopathic Association. (2014). Standard 15.01.16. *Healthcare Facilities Accreditation Program: Accreditation requirements for acute care hospitals.* Chicago, IL: American Osteopathic Association. (Level VII)
10 Siegel, J. D., et al. (2007). "2007 guideline for isolation precautions: Preventing transmission of infectious agents in healthcare settings"

[Online]. Accessed May 2015 via the Web at http://www.cdc.gov/hicpac/pdf/isolation/Isolation2007.pdf (Level II)

11 American Osteopathic Association. (2014). Standard 07.01.10. *Healthcare Facilities Accreditation Program: Accreditation requirements for acute care hospitals.* Chicago, IL: American Osteopathic Association. (Level VII)

12 American Society of PeriAnesthesia Nurses. (2015). *2015-2017 Perianesthesia nursing standards, practice recommendations and interpretive statements.* Cherry Hill, NJ: American Society of PeriAnesthesia Nurses. (Level VII)

13 Pullen, R. L. (2010). Clinical queries: Caring for a patient after amputation. *Nursing, 40*(1), 15.

14 Society for Vascular Nursing. (2014). "Circulating the facts about peripheral artery disease: Lower extremity amputations" [Online]. Accessed May 2015 via the Web at http://svnnet.org/uploads/File/PatientEd/AmputationBk.pdf

15 Porter, R. S., & Kaplan, J. L. (Eds.). (2010). *The Merck manual online.* Whitehouse Station, NJ: Merck & Co. Accessed May 2015 via the Web at http://www.merckmanuals.com/professional/

16 British Association of Chartered Physiotherapists in Amputee Rehabilitation. (2012). "Evidence based clinical guidelines for the physiotherapy management of adults with lower limb prostheses" [Online]. Accessed May 2015 via the Web at http://www.csp.org.uk/publications/clinical-guidelines-physiotherapy-management-adults-lower-limb-prostheses (Level VII)

17 Highsmith, M. J., et al. (2011). Identifying and managing skin issues with lower-limb prosthetic use. *InMotion, 21*(1), 41–43. Accessed May 2015 via the Web at http://www.amputee-coalition.org/inmotion/jan_feb_11/skin_issues_lower.pdf

18 The Joint Commission. (2015). Standard RC.01.03.01. *Comprehensive accreditation manual for hospitals: The official handbook.* Oakbrook Terrace, IL: The Joint Commission. (Level VII)

19 Centers for Medicare & Medicaid Services, Department of Health and Human Services. (2014). Condition of participation: Medical record services. 42 C.F.R. § 482.24(b).

20 American Osteopathic Association. (2014). Standard 10.00.03. *Healthcare Facilities Accreditation Program: Accreditation requirements for acute care hospitals.* Chicago, IL: American Osteopathic Association. (Level VII)

21 Kalapatapu, V. Lower extremity amputation. (2013). In: *UpToDate,* Collins, K. A. (Ed.). Accessed May 2015 via the Web at http://www.uptodate.com/contents/lower-extremity-amputation

22 Schley, M. T., et al. (2008). Painful and nonpainful phantom and stump sensations in acute traumatic amputees. *Journal of Trauma and Acute Care Surgery, 65,* 858–864. (Level VI)

RESPIRATION ASSESSMENT

Controlled by the respiratory center in the lateral medulla oblongata, respiration is the exchange of oxygen and carbon dioxide between the atmosphere and body cells. External respiration, or breathing, is accomplished by the diaphragm and chest muscles and delivers oxygen to the lower respiratory tract and alveoli.

Four measures of respiration—rate, rhythm, depth, and sound—reflect the body's metabolic state, diaphragm and chest-muscle condition, and airway patency. Respiratory rate is recorded as the number of cycles (with one cycle consisting of inspiration and expiration) per minute; rhythm, as the regularity of these cycles; depth, as the volume of air inhaled and exhaled with each respiration; and sound, as the audible digression from normal, effortless breathing. Normal respiratory rates for an adult range from 12 to 20 breaths/minute;[1] however, it's important to know the patient's normal baseline respiratory rate so that you can detect changes in the patient's condition.

The best time to assess the patient's respirations is immediately after taking the pulse rate.

Equipment

Watch with second hand ▪ stethoscope ▪ disinfectant pad.

Implementation

- Perform hand hygiene.[2,3,4,5,6] (If you performed hand hygiene before taking the patient's pulse, you don't need to repeat this step.)
- Confirm the patient's identity using at least two patient identifiers.[7]
- Place your fingertips over the patient's radial artery, and don't tell the patient you're counting respirations. *If you tell him, he'll become conscious of his respirations and the rate may change.*
- Count respirations by observing the rise and fall of the patient's chest during breathing. Alternatively, position the patient's opposite arm across his chest and count respirations by feeling its rise and fall. Consider one rise and one fall as one respiration.
- If the patient's respirations are regular, count his respirations for 30 seconds and multiply by two *to determine the respiratory rate.* Alternatively, count the patient's respirations for 60 seconds if respirations are irregular *to account for variations in respiratory rate and pattern.*[8]
- As you count respirations, be alert for and record such breath sounds as stertor, stridor, wheezing, and expiratory grunting. *Stertor* is a snoring sound resulting from secretions in the trachea and large bronchi. Listen for it in patients with neurologic disorders and in those who are comatose. *Stridor* is an inspiratory crowing sound that occurs with upper airway obstruction in laryngitis, croup, or the presence of a foreign body. *Wheezing* is caused by partial obstruction in the smaller bronchi and bronchioles. This high-pitched, musical sound is common in patients with emphysema or asthma. *Expiratory grunting* is a deep, low-pitched sound heard at the end of each breath that coincides with the closure of the glottis and may indicate respiratory distress.

ELDER ALERT ***In older patients, an expiratory grunt may result from partial airway obstruction or neuromuscular reflex.***

- Observe chest movements for depth of respirations. If the patient inhales a small volume of air, record this as shallow; record the inhalation of a large volume as deep.
- Listen to breathing *to determine the rhythm and sound of respirations.* (See *Identifying respiratory patterns,* page 668.)
- To detect breath sounds—such as crackles and rhonchi—or the lack of sound in the lungs, use a stethoscope. *Crackles* are discontinuous sounds heard on inspiration and indicate fluid in the alveoli or airway or the opening of collapsed alveoli. *Rhonchi* are low-pitched rumbling sounds that indicate secretions in the airway.
- Observe the patient for use of accessory muscles, such as the scalene, sternocleidomastoid, trapezius, and latissimus dorsi. *Use of these muscles reflects a weakness of the diaphragm and the external intercostal muscles, the primary muscles of respiration.*
- Clean and disinfect your stethoscope using a disinfectant pad.[9,10]
- Perform hand hygiene.[2,3,4,5,6]
- Document your findings.[11,12,13]

Special considerations

- When assessing the patient's respiratory status, consider his personal and family history. Ask if the patient smokes; if he says yes, find out how many years he's smoked and how many packs a day.
- If the patient's respiratory rate suddenly increases, assess him for other signs of respiratory distress, such as anxiety, nasal flaring, accessory muscle use, abnormal breath sounds, grunting, and cyanosis. *To detect cyanosis,* look for characteristic bluish discoloration under the tongue and in the nail beds or lips, buccal mucosa, or conjunctiva. Report your findings to the patient's practitioner.
- If the patient's respiratory rate suddenly decreases, assess for an underlying cause and notify the patient's practitioner, as needed.[1]
- If the patient becomes apneic or he's only gasping, activate the emergency response system and assess his circulation, airway, and breathing. Begin cardiopulmonary resuscitation.[14]

Identifying respiratory patterns

TYPE	CHARACTERISTICS	PATTERN	POSSIBLE CAUSES
Apnea	Periodic absence of breathing		▪ Mechanical airway obstruction ▪ Conditions affecting the brain's respiratory center
Apneustic	Prolonged, gasping inspiration followed by extremely short, inefficient expiration	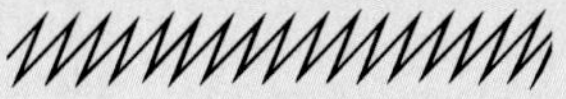	▪ Lesions of the respiratory center
Bradypnea	Slow, regular respirations of equal depth	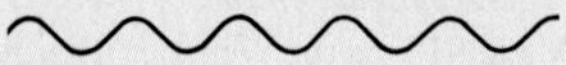	▪ Normal pattern during sleep ▪ Conditions affecting the respiratory center, such as tumors, metabolic disorders, and respiratory decompensation ▪ Use of opiates and alcohol
Cheyne-Stokes	Rapid, deep respirations punctuated by periods of apnea lasting 20 to 60 seconds	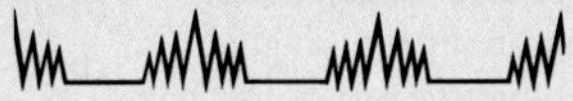	▪ Increased intracranial pressure ▪ Severe heart failure ▪ Kidney failure ▪ Meningitis ▪ Drug overdose ▪ Cerebral anoxia
Eupnea	Normal rate and rhythm	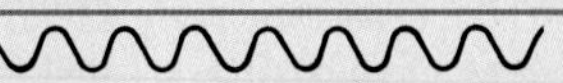	▪ Normal respiration
Kussmaul	Rapid (over 20 breaths/minute), deep (resembling sighs), labored respirations without pause	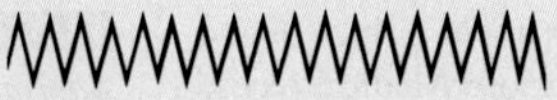	▪ Kidney failure or metabolic acidosis, particularly diabetic ketoacidosis
Tachypnea	Rapid respirations; rate increase corresponds with body temperature–about four breaths/minute for every 1°F (0.6°C) above normal	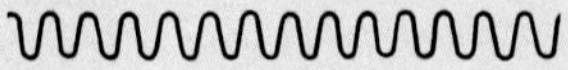	▪ Pneumonia ▪ Compensatory respiratory alkalosis ▪ Respiratory insufficiency ▪ Lesions in the respiratory center ▪ Salicylate poisoning

Documentation

Record the rate, depth, rhythm, and sound of the patient's respirations.

REFERENCES

1 Hunter, J. & Rawlings-Anderson, K. (2008). Respiratory assessment. *Nursing Standard, 22*(41), 41–43.

2 The Joint Commission. (2015). Standard NPSG.07.01.01. *Comprehensive accreditation manual for hospitals: The official handbook.* Oakbrook Terrace, IL: The Joint Commission. (Level VII)

3 World Health Organization. (2009). "WHO guidelines on hand hygiene in health care: First global patient safety challenge, clean care is safer care" [Online]. Accessed May 2015 via the Web at http://whqlibdoc.who.int/publications/2009/9789241597906_eng.pdf (Level IV)

4 Centers for Disease Control and Prevention. (2002). Guideline for hand hygiene in health-care settings: Recommendations of the Healthcare Infection Control Practices Advisory Committee and the HICPAC/SHEA/APIC/IDSA Hand Hygiene Task Force. *MMWR Recommendations and Reports, 51*(RR-16), 1–45. Accessed May 2015 via the Web at http://www.cdc.gov/mmwr/pdf/rr/rr5116.pdf (Level II)

5 American Osteopathic Association. (2014). Standard 07.01.21. *Healthcare Facilities Accreditation Program: Accreditation requirements for acute care hospitals.* Chicago, IL: American Osteopathic Association. (Level VII)

6 Centers for Medicare & Medicaid Services, Department of Health and Human Services. (2014). Condition of participation: Infection control. 42 C.F.R. § 482.42.

7 The Joint Commission. (2015). Standard NPSG.01.01.01. *Comprehensive accreditation manual for hospitals: The official handbook.* Oakbrook Terrace, IL: The Joint Commission. (Level VII)

8 Lockwood, C., et al. (2004). Vital signs. *JBI Reports, 2,* 207–230.

9 Rutala, W. A., et al. (2008). "Guideline for disinfection and sterilization in healthcare facilities, 2008" [Online]. Accessed May 2015 via the Web at http://www.cdc.gov/hicpac/pdf/guidelines/Disinfection_Nov_2008.pdf (Level I)

10 American Osteopathic Association. (2014). Standard 07.02.03. *Healthcare Facilities Accreditation Program: Accreditation requirements for acute care hospitals.* Chicago, IL: American Osteopathic Association. (Level VII)

11 The Joint Commission. (2015). Standard RC.01.03.01. *Comprehensive accreditation manual for hospitals: The official handbook.* Oakbrook Terrace, IL: The Joint Commission. (Level VII)

12 American Osteopathic Association. (2014). Standard 10.00.03. *Healthcare Facilities Accreditation Program: Accreditation requirements for acute care hospitals.* Chicago, IL: American Osteopathic Association. (Level VII)

13 Centers for Medicare & Medicaid Services, Department of Health and Human Services. (2014). Condition of participation: Medical record services. 42 C.F.R. § 482.24(b).

14 American Heart Association. (2010). 2010 American Heart Association guidelines for cardiopulmonary resuscitation and emergency cardiovascular care. *Circulation, 122,* S685–S705. (Level II)

RESTRAINT APPLICATION

The Centers for Medicare & Medicaid Services (CMS) and The Joint Commission define restraints as devices that immobilize or reduce the ability of a patient to move the arms, legs, body, or head freely, except in situations involving orthopedic devices, surgical bandages, and similar devices required for the patient's care.[1,2] The Healthcare Facilities Accreditation Program (HFAP) defines physical restraint as any manual method, physical or mechanical device, material, or equipment attached or adjacent to the patient that restricts freedom of movement or normal access to one's body.[3]

A vest restraint can be used to prevent self-injury due to falls or to immobilize a patient to assist medical treatment. It's applied to a patient's torso over his hospital gown or clothing. The straps are then secured to the patient's bed frame or chair.

A limb restraint is a device consisting of a cuff, typically made of padded fabric or foam, applied to a patient's wrists or ankles with straps that are secured to the patient's bed frame or chair. Limb restraints are used to prevent self-injury or the removal of therapeutic equipment, such as IV lines, indwelling catheters, and nasogastric tubes.

A mitt restraint is a pocket enclosure that's applied over a patient's hand to prevent self-injury or the removal of therapeutic equipment, such as IV lines, indwelling catheters, and nasogastric tubes. Mitt restraints may be padded or rigid and may include finger separators or leave the fingers exposed. Optional straps that can be secured to the patient's bed frame or chair may be included with the device or may need to be ordered separately if indicated. Most mitt restraints can be applied to either hand.

A belt restraint consists of a strip of material—usually cotton fabric or mesh—that's applied over a patient's gown or clothing, around the waist or lap. The straps are then secured to the patient's bed frame or chair. Belt restraints can be used to prevent self-injury from falling or to immobilize a patient, if needed, during medical treatment.

A leather or leather-like restraint is made of leather or a synthetic substitute for leather, such as polyurethane or vinyl. The restraint is applied to a patient's wrists or ankles and then secured to a bed frame or chair. Leather restraints are used to prevent self-injury or injury to others and to immobilize a patient for medical treatment. Although some facilities prefer to use traditional leather restraints because of the perceived strength of the material, synthetic materials offer the advantage of being easier to clean and disinfect.

The CMS, The Joint Commission, and HFAP recognize the rights of patients to be free from restraint or seclusion, of any form, imposed as a means of coercion, discipline, convenience, or retaliation by staff members. Restraint or seclusion may only be used to ensure the immediate physical safety of the patient, a staff member, or others and should be used only when all other methods have failed to keep the patient from harming himself or others. This standard has been established with the intent of reducing the overall use of restraint. If restraint must be used, the health care provider must choose a restraint that's the least restrictive to the patient and discontinue restraint use at the earliest possible time.[1,2,3]

Only staff members trained in the use of restraints as well as less restrictive techniques aimed at avoiding restraint are permitted to evaluate the need for restraint, apply restraints, and monitor patients who are restrained.[4,5,6]

Interventions that can reduce the need for restraint include pain management techniques, conversation with the patient, exercise, activity involvement, meditation, prayer, contact with familiar people or places, and such therapies as massage, therapeutic touch, aromatherapy, music therapy, pet therapy, and reminiscence therapy.[7]

Equipment

Restraint device (vest, limb, mitt, belt, or leather) ■ Optional: gloves, gown, mask, eye protection, straps, key, cuff liners (if recommended by the manufacturer).

Preparation of equipment

Because there are various types of body restraints, refer to the manufacturer's preparation and application instructions. Some vest restraints wrap around the patient with the straps crossing in the front, whereas other types close with a zipper at the patient's back. Check to see that you have obtained the correct size for the patient's build and weight. Some devices require that the straps be fed through the cuff before application. *Because there are various types of belt restraints,* make sure you've chosen a restraint that's appropriate for your patient. For example, a restraint may hold a patient in a stationary position or allow the patient to roll from side to side, may wrap around the pelvis in addition to the waist for additional security when sitting up, or be padded or unpadded. Some belt restraints wrap around the patient with the straps crossing in the back; others have straps that cross in the front.

If using leather restraints, make sure the straps are unlocked and the key fits the lock. If indicated by the manufacturer, apply cuff liners to the restraint cuffs *to reduce friction between the patient's skin and the restraint, which helps prevent skin irritation and breakdown.*

Check the device for damage before use; obtain a new device if necessary.

Implementation

■ Obtain a practitioner's order for the restraint. In an emergency situation, obtain an order as soon as possible after applying the restraint.[1,8,9]

NURSING ALERT *If the patient is being restrained because of violent or self-destructive behavior that jeopardizes his physical safety or that of staff members or others, the doctor, clinical psychologist, or other licensed independent practitioner responsible for the patient's care must conduct an in-person evaluation within 1 hour of initiation of the restraint. A specially trained nurse or physician's assistant may perform the face-to-face evaluation; however, the nurse or physician's assistant must consult the attending doctor, clinical psychologist, or other licensed independent practitioner who's responsible for the care of the patient as soon as possible after completing the 1-hour face-to-face evaluation.*[1,9,10]

■ Gather the appropriate equipment.

■ Perform hand hygiene.[11,12,13,14,15]

■ Put on gloves and personal protective equipment as needed *to comply with standard precautions.*[14,15]

■ If the patient's condition allows, confirm the patient's identity using at least two patient identifiers.[16]

■ Tell the patient that you're applying a restraint. Assure him that the restraint is being used to protect him from injury rather than to punish him. Emphasize that the restraint will be removed as soon as it is safe to do so, and tell him the criteria you'll use for discontinuing restraint.

■ If necessary, obtain the assistance of additional staff members to apply the restraint.

Applying a criss-cross vest restraint

■ If the patient's condition permits, assist the patient to a sitting position. If the patient is unable to sit, apply the vest restraint by rolling the patient side-to-side.

■ Smooth out the patient's gown or clothing, removing as many wrinkles as possible *to prevent skin breakdown.*

■ Slip the vest over the patient's gown or clothing.

■ Assist the patient in putting his arms through the armholes with the V-shape neck in front. Criss-cross the straps in the front of the vest. *Never criss-cross the flaps in the back because doing so may cause the patient to choke if he tries to squirm out of the vest.*

■ Feed the straps through the holes in the front of the vest, as indicated by manufacturer's instructions.

Applying a zipper vest restraint

■ Place the vest over the patient with the zipper in back.
■ Assist the patient in placing her arms through the armholes.
■ Zip up the back of the restraint.

Applying a limb restraint

■ Position the patient's wrist or ankle in the soft padded cuff portion of the restraint by slipping the cuff over the patient's hand or foot. If using a wrap-type device, wrap the wrist or ankle so that the fasteners are on the outside of the device.
■ If indicated, fasten the buckle or Velcro fastener.
■ Adjust the straps for a snug fit that doesn't compromise the patient's circulation. You should be able to slip one or two fingers between the restraint and the patient's skin. *Applying the restraint too tightly may impair circulation distal to the restraint.*

Applying a mitt restraint

■ Assess for baseline hand and finger circulation *to determine the appropriateness of the device and to determine whether circulatory changes may occur after application.*
■ Insert the patient's hand into the mitt with his palm facing down according to the manufacturer's instructions. If finger separators are available in the device, separate each finger into its own slot.
■ Wrap the strap over the mitt and around the patient's wrist *to secure the mitt to the patient.*
■ Secure the strap with the device's fastener, which may be Velcro or some other type of fastener.
■ Adjust the straps for a snug fit that doesn't compromise the patient's circulation. You should be able to slip one or two fingers between the restraint and the patient's skin. *Applying the restraint too tightly may impair circulation distal to the restraint.*

Applying a belt restraint

Restraining a patient in a chair or wheelchair

■ Position the patient as far back in the seat as possible. If the patient is in a wheelchair, make sure that the wheels are locked.
■ Wrap the device around the patient's hips and over his smoothed-out gown or clothing so that the straps end up at the back of the chair.
■ If the belt is padded, place the padded side toward the patient.
■ If the device includes a pelvic holder, place the narrow side to the back of the chair and bring the wide part of the holder up between the patient's legs and connect the straps.
■ Criss-cross the straps at the back of the chair *for added security.*

Restraining a patient in a bed

■ Position the belt under the patient at waist level.
■ Thread the straps through the slots at either the front or back of the patient according to the manufacturer's directions and the desired movement limitation.

Applying a leather restraint

■ *Ensure the safety of the patient and staff members* by having enough trained staff members available to assist in properly applying restraints. *Never attempt to apply leather restraints to a patient alone.* Give each staff member a specific task to immobilize the patient before applying the restraints.[17,18]
■ Place the patient on the bed in the supine position, with each arm and leg securely held down *to minimize combative behavior and to prevent injury to the patient and others.* Immobilize the patient's arms and legs above and below the joints—knee, ankle, shoulder, and wrist—*to minimize his movement without exerting excessive force.*
■ For each restraint, wrap the restraint around the extremity and adjust it to fit. Apply the restraint securely but not too tightly. You should be able to slip one finger between the restraint and the patient's skin. *A tight restraint can compromise circulation; a loose one can slip off or move up the patient's arm or leg, causing skin irritation and breakdown.*
■ Secure the locking mechanism and make sure that it clicks. Tug it gently *to be sure it's secure.*
■ Attach the connecting strap to the restraint, and then secure the strap to the bed frame, out of the patient's reach. Flex the patient's arm or leg slightly before locking the strap *to allow room for movement and to prevent frozen joints and dislocations.*
■ Once the restraint is secure, allow the coworker to release the arm or leg. Then recheck the restraint *for proper fit.*
■ Repeat the procedure for each restraint.
■ Place the key in an accessible location at the nurse's station.

Completing the procedure

■ Tie all the straps of the restraints securely to the frame of the bed, chair, or wheelchair and out of the patient's reach. Never secure the restraint to a bed rail. Use a bow or knot that you can release quickly and easily in an emergency. (See *Tying a quick-release knot.*) Never tie a regular knot to secure the straps. Leave 1″ to 2″ (2.5 to 5 cm) of slack in the straps *to allow room for movement.*
■ Monitor the patient's physical and psychological well-being, including (but not limited to) vital signs, respiratory and circulatory status, skin integrity, and any special requirements identified during the practitioner's assessment, at a frequency determined by your facility, the patient's condition, and the type of device used.[1,17] Be alert for complications, such as impaired breathing and circulation, skin breakdown, and psychological distress. Make sure that the restraint doesn't tighten with the patient's movements. Adjust the fit if necessary. Notify the practitioner if signs and symptoms persist.
■ If the patient consented to have family members (or another significant person) informed about care, notify them of the use of restraint, the patient monitoring that will be used during restraint, and the criteria for discontinuing restraint.[1,17]
■ Assist the restrained patient with nutrition, hydration, hygiene, elimination, pain control, and comfort measures.[18]
■ *To prevent pressure ulcers,* reposition the patient regularly, pad bony prominences and other vulnerable areas, and keep the skin clean and dry.[19,20]
■ If you can do so safely and while continually monitoring the patient, release the restraint regularly as required by your facility *to allow the patient to participate in care, perform range-of-motion (ROM) exercises, turn, stretch, and breathe deeply.* Have a coworker assist as needed when releasing the restraint.
■ Continue to reassess the need for restraint, and release the restraints as soon as the patient's condition permits, according to the practitioner's order.[18,10,21]
■ Debrief the patient after removal of the restraint *to identify what led to use of the restraint and what could have been done differently,* and counsel the patient for physical or psychological trauma that may have resulted from the use of the restraint.[20]
■ Remove and discard your gloves and personal protection equipment, if worn.[14]
■ Perform hand hygiene.[11,12,13,14,15]
■ Document the procedure.[21,22,23,24]

Special considerations

■ Follow the U.S. Food and Drug Administration's recommendations regarding bed safety, and be alert for a restrained patient's potential for entrapment and serious injury.[25]
■ Use a vest restraint should with caution in a patient with heart failure or respiratory disorder.

Tying a quick-release knot

A quick-release knot allows you to quickly release the knot, using one hand, if the patient is in distress or has an emergency. Follow the steps below to tie a quick-release knot.

1. Wrap the attachment strap once around the bed frame, leaving at least an 8" (20-cm) tail. Fold the loose end in half *to create a loop*.

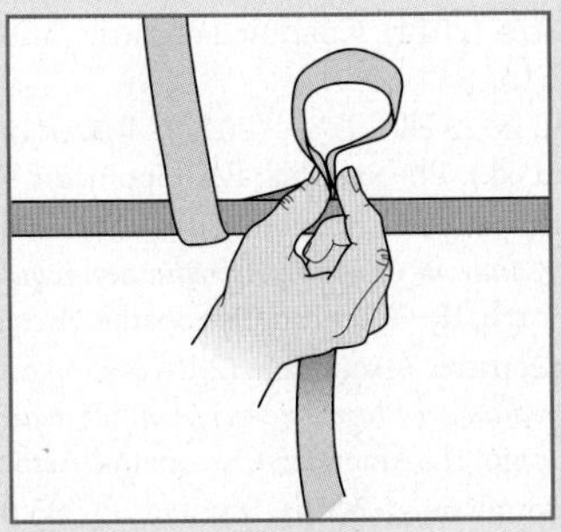

2. Cross the loop over the other end of the tie.

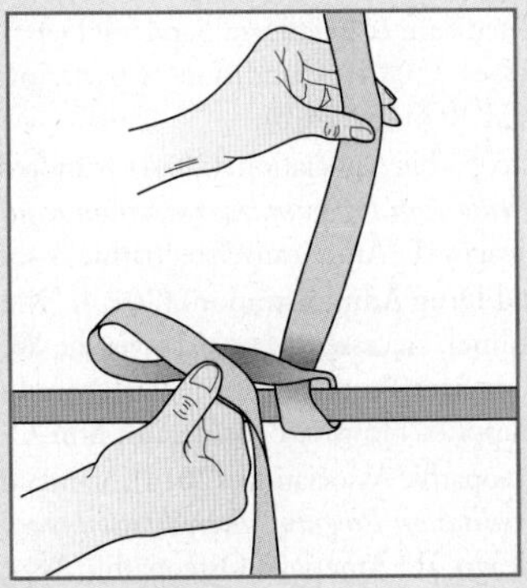

3. Insert the folded strap where the straps cross over each other. This step will feel like when you are tying your shoes.

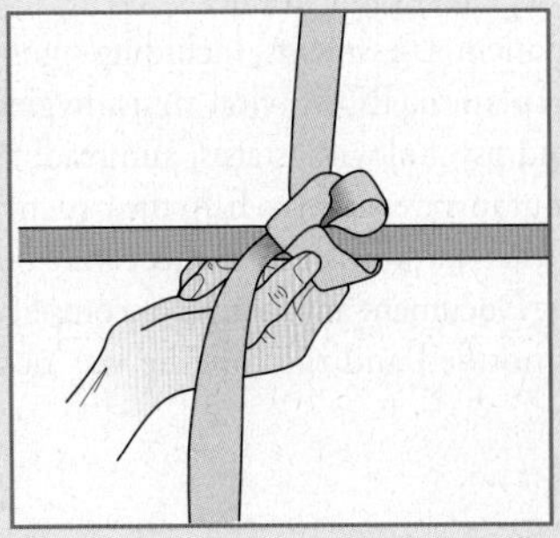

4. Pull on the loop to tighten.

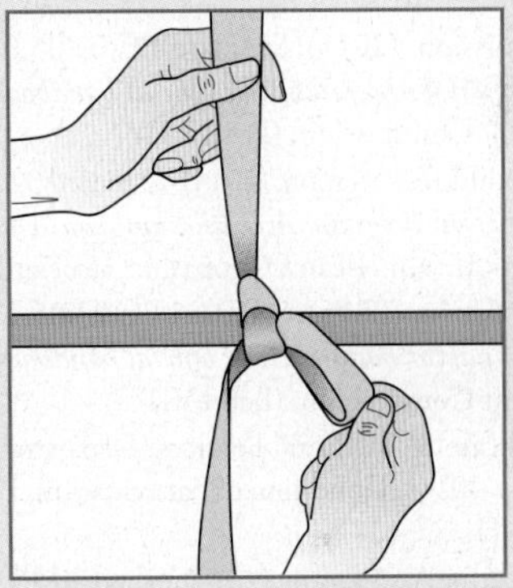

■ When the patient is at high risk for aspiration, restrain him on his side. Never secure all four restraints to one side of the bed *because the patient may fall out of bed.*

■ Don't apply a limb or mitt restraint above an IV site *because the constriction may occlude the infusion or cause infiltration into surrounding tissue.*

■ Never secure restraints to the side rails *because someone might inadvertently lower the rail before noticing the attached restraint. This movement may jerk the patient's limb or body, causing him discomfort and trauma.* Never secure restraints to the fixed frame of the bed if you must change the patient's position.[25]

■ Don't restrain a patient in the prone position. *This position limits his field of vision, intensifies feelings of helplessness and vulnerability, and impairs respiration, especially if the patient has been sedated.*

■ If the patient continues to require restraint, obtain a new order from the practitioner in accordance with your facility's policy and at least within 24 hours of the previous order. The practitioner will need to evaluate the patient before writing a new restraint order.

■ If the patient is being restrained because of violent or self-destructive behavior, follow The Joint Commission or HFAP and CMS guidelines for order limits[1,8,26] (unless your facility has more restrictive guidelines): 4 hours for adults, 2 hours for children and adolescents ages 9 to 17, and 1 hour for children younger than age 9.

■ Note that the doctor, clinical psychologist, or other licensed practitioner responsible for the patient's care may renew orders for patient restraint because of violent or self-destructive behavior to the above time limits for a maximum of 24 consecutive hours. After 24 hours, the practitioner must write a new order for restraint use.[1,8,26]

■ Follow your facility's channels for reporting to CMS any death that occurs while a patient is in restraint or within 24 hours of restraint removal.[27,28,29]

■ After removing restraints, disinfect them according to the manufacturer's instructions. You may wash synthetic restraints by machine or wipe them down with a disinfectant. You may clean soiled leather restraints with a disinfectant; however, you must discard leather restraints if they were exposed to blood or other body fluids.[30,31]

Complications

Some patients resist restraint and, in the course of resisting, may injure themselves or others.

Excessively tight limb restraints can reduce peripheral circulation. Apply restraints carefully and check them regularly. Skin breakdown can occur under limb restraints. To prevent this complication, make sure that the restraint is padded around the patient's wrists and ankles, loosen or remove the restraints frequently, and provide regular skin care.

Long periods of immobility can predispose the patient to pneumonia, urine retention, constipation, and sensory deprivation. Reposition the patient and attend to his elimination requirements as needed.

Serious injury, entrapment, and even death may result from inappropriate use of restraint.

Documentation

Document each episode of the use of restraint, including the date and time of initiation of restraint use as well as the total number of minutes of physical restraint use.[32] Document the patient's signs and symptoms, the less restrictive interventions you tried first, your assessment of the need for restraint, and the name of the doctor or other licensed independent practitioner who evaluated the patient and ordered the restraint, as required by your facility. Document the patient's response to the restraints. Include the conditions or behaviors necessary for discontinuing the restraint and whether these conditions were communicated to the patient.[33,34,35]

Document each in-person evaluation by the doctor, clinical psychologist, or licensed independent practitioner.

Record regular patient assessments, including signs of injury, nutrition, hydration, circulation, ROM, vital signs, hygiene, elimination, comfort, physical and psychological status, and readiness for removing restraints. Record your interventions to help the patient meet the conditions for removing the restraint. A flow sheet may be used to record frequent assessments. Document any injuries or complications, the name of the practitioner notified and the time he was notified, and your actions.

REFERENCES

1 Centers for Medicare & Medicaid Services, Department of Health and Human Services. (2014). Condition of participation: Patient's rights. 42 C.F.R. § 482.13(e).

2 The Joint Commission. (2015). Standard PC.03.05.01. *Comprehensive accreditation manual for hospitals: The official handbook.* Oakbrook Terrace, IL: The Joint Commission. (Level VII)

3 American Osteopathic Association. (2014). Standard 32.02.01. *Healthcare Facilities Accreditation Program: Accreditation requirements for acute care hospitals.* Chicago, IL: American Osteopathic Association. (Level VII)

4 The Joint Commission. (2015). Standard PC.03.05.17. *Comprehensive accreditation manual for hospitals: The official handbook.* Oakbrook Terrace, IL: The Joint Commission. (Level VII)

5 Centers for Medicare & Medicaid Services, Department of Health and Human Services. (2014). Condition of participation: Patient's rights. 42 C.F.R. § 482.13(f).

6 American Osteopathic Association. (2014). Standard 15.02.34. *Healthcare Facilities Accreditation Program: Accreditation requirements for acute care hospitals.* Chicago, IL: American Osteopathic Association. (Level VII)

7 American Nurses Association. (2012). "Position statements: Reduction of patient restraint and seclusion in health care settings" [Online]. Accessed May 2015 via the Web at http://www.nursingworld.org/restraintposition

8 The Joint Commission. (2015). Standard PC.03.05.05. *Comprehensive accreditation manual for hospitals: The official handbook.* Oakbrook Terrace, IL: The Joint Commission. (Level VII)

9 American Osteopathic Association. (2014). Standard 15.02.10. *Healthcare Facilities Accreditation Program: Accreditation requirements for acute care hospitals.* Chicago, IL: American Osteopathic Association. (Level VII)

10 The Joint Commission. (2015). Standard PC.03.05.11. *Comprehensive accreditation manual for hospitals: The official handbook.* Oakbrook Terrace, IL: The Joint Commission. (Level VII)

11 The Joint Commission. (2015). Standard NPSG.07.01.01. *Comprehensive accreditation manual for hospitals: The official handbook.* Oakbrook Terrace, IL: The Joint Commission. (Level VII)

12 Centers for Disease Control and Prevention. (2002). Guideline for hand hygiene in health-care settings: Recommendations of the Healthcare Infection Control Practices Advisory Committee and the HICPAC/SHEA/APIC/IDSA Hand Hygiene Task Force. *MMWR Recommendations and Reports, 51*(RR-16), 1–45. Accessed May 2015 via the Web at http://www.cdc.gov/mmwr/pdf/rr/rr5116.pdf (Level II)

13 World Health Organization. (2009). "WHO guidelines on hand hygiene in health care: First global patient safety challenge, clean care is safer care" [Online]. Accessed May 2015 via the Web at http://whqlibdoc.who.int/publications/2009/9789241597906_eng.pdf (Level IV)

14 Centers for Medicare & Medicaid Services, Department of Health and Human Services. (2014). Condition of participation: Infection control. 42 C.F.R. § 482.42.

15 American Osteopathic Association. (2014). Standard 07.01.10. *Healthcare Facilities Accreditation Program: Accreditation requirements for acute care hospitals.* Chicago, IL: American Osteopathic Association. (Level VII)

16 The Joint Commission. (2015). Standard NPSG.01.01.01. *Comprehensive accreditation manual for hospitals: The official handbook.* Oakbrook Terrace, IL: The Joint Commission. (Level VII)

17 The Joint Commission. (2015). Standard PC.03.05.07. *Comprehensive accreditation manual for hospitals: The official handbook.* Oakbrook Terrace, IL: The Joint Commission. (Level VII)

18 Centers for Medicare & Medicaid Services, Department of Health and Human Services. (2014). Condition of participation: Patient's rights. 42 C.F.R. § 482.13.

19 Baranoski, S., & Ayello, E. A. (2012). *Wound care essentials: Practice principles* (3rd ed.). Philadelphia, PA: Lippincott Williams & Williams.

20 American Osteopathic Association. (2014). Standard 16.02.02. *Healthcare Facilities Accreditation Program: Accreditation requirements for acute care hospitals.* Chicago, IL: American Osteopathic Association. (Level VII)

21 American Osteopathic Association. (2014). Standard 15.02.16. *Healthcare Facilities Accreditation Program: Accreditation requirements for acute care hospitals.* Chicago, IL: American Osteopathic Association. (Level VII)

22 The Joint Commission. (2015). Standard PC.03.05.15. *Comprehensive accreditation manual for hospitals: The official handbook.* Oakbrook Terrace, IL: The Joint Commission. (Level VII)

23 Centers for Medicare & Medicaid Services, Department of Health and Human Services. (2014). Condition of participation: Medical record services. 42 C.F.R. § 482.24(b).

24 American Osteopathic Association. (2014). Standard 10.00.03. *Healthcare Facilities Accreditation Program: Accreditation requirements for acute care hospitals.* Chicago, IL: American Osteopathic Association. (Level VII)

25 U.S. Food and Drug Administration. (2013). "Medical devices: Hospital beds" [Online]. Accessed May 2015 via the Web at http://www.fda.gov/MedicalDevices/ProductsandMedicalProcedures/GeneralHospitalDevicesandSupplies/HospitalBeds/default.htm

26 American Osteopathic Association. (2014). Standard 15.02.13. *Healthcare Facilities Accreditation Program: Accreditation requirements for acute care hospitals.* Chicago, IL: American Osteopathic Association. (Level VII)

27 The Joint Commission. (2015). Standard PC.03.05.19. *Comprehensive accreditation manual for hospitals: The official handbook.* Oakbrook Terrace, IL: The Joint Commission. (Level VII)

28 Centers for Medicare & Medicaid Services, Department of Health and Human Services. (2014). Condition of participation: Patient's rights. 42 C.F.R. 482.13(g).

29 American Osteopathic Association. (2014). Standard 15.02.41. *Healthcare Facilities Accreditation Program: Accreditation requirements for acute care hospitals.* Chicago, IL: American Osteopathic Association. (Level VII)

30 American Osteopathic Association. (2014). Standard 15.02.26. *Healthcare Facilities Accreditation Program: Accreditation requirements for acute care hospitals.* Chicago, IL: American Osteopathic Association. (Level VII)

31 American Osteopathic Association. (2014). Standard 15.02.27. *Healthcare Facilities Accreditation Program: Accreditation requirements for acute care hospitals.* Chicago, IL: American Osteopathic Association. (Level VII)

32 The Joint Commission. (2013). "Specifications manual for Joint Commission national quality measures (version 2014a)" [Online]. Accessed May 2015 via the Web at http://manual.jointcommission.org/releases/TJC2014A/MIF0117.html

33 American Osteopathic Association. (2014). Standard 15.02.25. *Healthcare Facilities Accreditation Program: Accreditation requirements for acute care hospitals.* Chicago, IL: American Osteopathic Association. (Level VII)

34 American Osteopathic Association. (2014). Standard 15.02.28. *Healthcare Facilities Accreditation Program: Accreditation requirements for acute care hospitals.* Chicago, IL: American Osteopathic Association. (Level VII)

35 American Osteopathic Association. (2014). Standard 15.02.24. *Healthcare Facilities Accreditation Program: Accreditation requirements for acute care hospitals.* Chicago, IL: American Osteopathic Association. (Level VII)

RING REMOVAL

A ring can become excessively tight on a patient's finger after an injury such as a sprain, or from some other cause of swelling such as the swelling that can occur in a localized allergic reaction. Very tight-fitting rings can obstruct lymphatic drainage, causing swelling and further constriction. Removal may be necessary to relieve chronic or acute edema and to prevent vascular compromise in a finger or toe constricted by a ring or metal or plastic band.

Equipment

Ice ■ soap and water ■ towel ■ lubricant (petroleum jelly, lotion) ■ rubber tourniquet or Penrose drain ■ Optional: local anesthetic without epinephrine, syringe, needles, alcohol pads, gloves, prescribed pain medication, cold packs, sterile dressing, tetanus immunization.

Coiled-string method

String, umbilical tape, ribbon gauze, or thick suture material ■ Optional: hemostat.

Ring-cutter method

Lubricant (some cutters require a water-soluble lubricant) ■ ring cutter (manual, battery, or electric-powered) ■ pliers, hemostat, or ring spreader ■ protective eyewear ■ 20-mL syringe filled with water.

Implementation

■ Perform hand hygiene.[1,2,3,4,5]
■ Confirm the patient's identity using at least two patient identifiers.[6]
■ Explain the procedure to the patient.
■ Put on gloves as needed *to comply with standard precautions*.[7,8]
■ Inspect the digit for wounds, lacerations, fractures, or dislocations. Assess the digit's capillary refill, sensation, and movement.

NURSING ALERT *If vascular compromise is present, the ring should be removed with a ring cutter as quickly as possible.*

■ Perform a comprehensive pain assessment using techniques appropriate for the patient's age, condition, and ability to understand.[9] Intervene as necessary.
■ Arrange for an X-ray of the digit, if ordered, and report abnormal findings to the practitioner.
■ *To limit further swelling,* apply ice and elevate the affected extremity above heart level. You can also wrap a rubber tourniquet or Penrose drain circumferentially in a distal-to-proximal direction *to reduce swelling.* Leave the wrap in place for 5 minutes, and then remove it.
■ Lubricate the skin beneath the ring with soap and water or a lubricant *to allow the ring to be slipped off of the finger or toe.* Hold the ring with a towel, and pull with a rocking motion in an attempt to remove the ring.

NURSING ALERT *Even if the patient tells you he has tried to remove the object from the finger at home, it's generally worthwhile to attempt removal with soap and water or a lubricant before trying other techniques. The pain from constriction often prevents the patient from applying adequate circular traction to remove the ring.*

■ If the ring can't be removed, use one of the methods below.

Using the coiled-string method

NURSING ALERT *Don't use the coiled-string method if the patient has any lacerations, fractures, or dislocations involving the affected digit; instead, use a ring cutter.*

■ While the affected digit is elevated, slip the end of a long strip of string under the ring. Use a hemostat, if necessary, to thread the string under the ring.
■ Anchor the string with your nondominant hand, or ask the patient to anchor it.
■ Wrap the string around the digit, beginning adjacent to the ring margin. Wrap the string in a snug, smooth, single layer in a clockwise fashion, slightly overlapping the previous layer, progressing from proximal to distal until it covers the area of greatest swelling. *Because the area of the proximal interphalangeal joint is the most difficult area to slip the ring over,* make sure that you wrap this area firmly (as shown below).

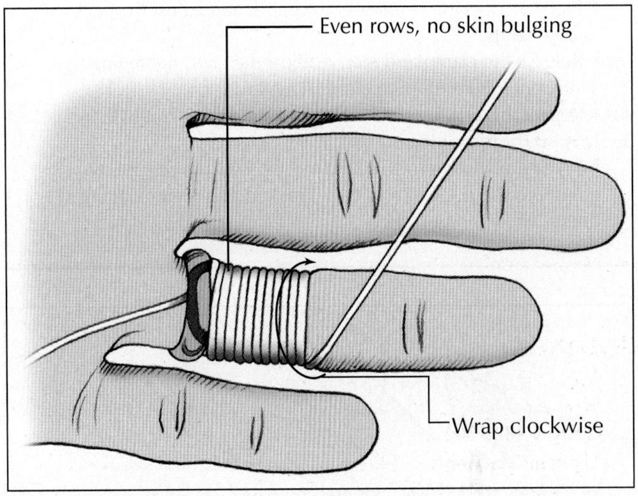

■ When the wrapping is complete, pull the proximal end of the string against the ring and then start to unwrap the string in a clockwise direction, moving the ring toward the tip of the finger (as shown below). If needed, place a small amount of lubricant over the string *to facilitate sliding the ring.*

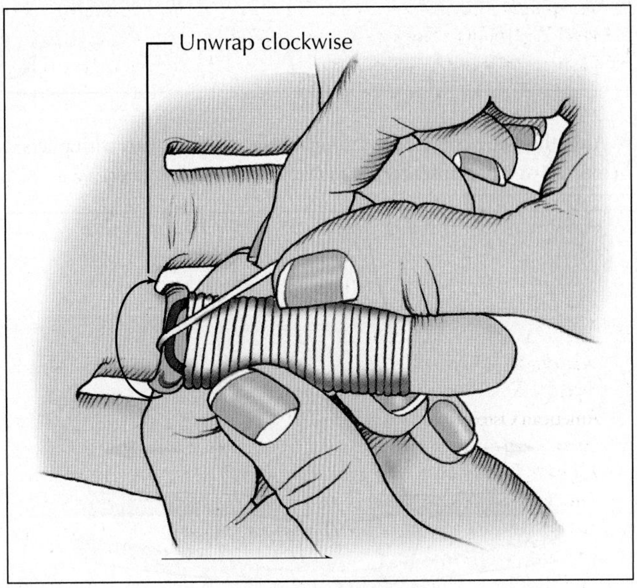

NURSING ALERT *Moving the ring over the proximal interphalangeal joint will be the most difficult and may cause the most pain to the patient. It's not uncommon to cause abrasions to the skin during this procedure.*

Using the manual ring-cutter method

■ Obtain written consent for cutting and removing the ring.
■ Put on protective eyewear *to avoid possible injury caused by metal fragments.*
■ Slip the curved finger guard of the ring cutter under the ring. Use lubricant if necessary. Rotate the ring, if possible, so that the thinnest part of the band is located under the saw blade (as shown on next page, top left).
■ Clamp the cutting disk down firmly on the ring, and use the turnkey to manually turn the cutting disk until the ring is severed.

Using locking pliers

Tungsten carbide, ceramic, and natural stone rings made of onyx or jade are removed by cracking them into pieces with standard locking pliers. Follow these steps:

- Place the locking pliers over the band, and adjust the jaws to clamp lightly.
- Release the clamp and then readjust the jaws, tightening the screw one-quarter turn to clamp it again.
- Repeat this process until you hear a crack. The ring will break into two or more pieces.
- Take care when removing the pieces. *Because the cracked edges are sharp,* don't rotate the cracked ring on the patient's finger.

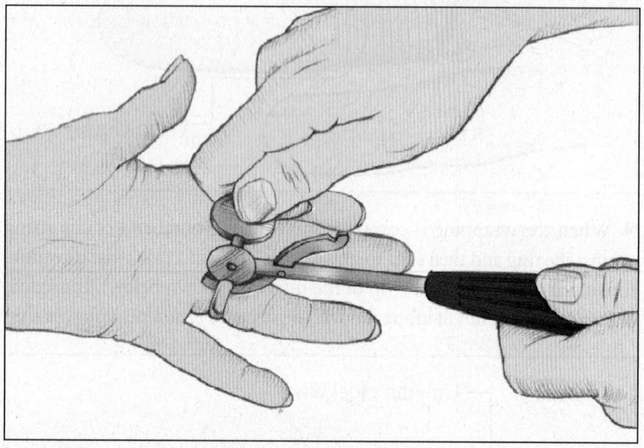

- After the ring has been cut through, bend the ring apart with pliers, a hemostat, or a ring spreader (as shown below) *to allow removal.*

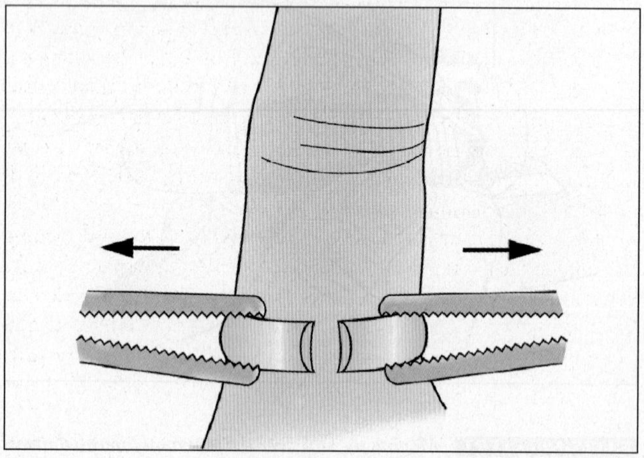

- If the ring is a wide band, it may be necessary to make a second cut *to remove a wedge from the ring.*
- Remove the ring.
- Irrigate the skin with water *to remove any metal particles.*
- Remove protective eyewear.

Using the battery- or electric-powered ring-cutter method

- Obtain written consent for cutting and removing the ring.
- Put on protective eyewear *to avoid possible injury caused by metal fragments.*
- Ensure that the correct cutting blade is in place. *Some manufacturers supply different blades for different types of metals.* Always follow the manufacturer's instructions.
- Place the finger guard of the ring cutter under the ring. Use lubricant if necessary. Rotate the ring, if possible, so that the thinnest part of the band is located under the saw blade.
- Turn on the power to the cutting blade so that it's rotating before it makes contact with the ring.
- Apply gentle pressure to make contact between the rotating blade and the ring.

NURSING ALERT *The friction caused by cutting may produce an uncomfortable amount of heat in the ring and the patient's hand. Ask the patient if he's comfortable, and regularly check the temperature of the ring and cutter blade with your fingers. Stop briefly to allow the ring and cutter to cool down if necessary.*

- After you've cut through the ring, bend the ring apart with pliers, a hemostat, or a ring spreader *to allow removal* or make a second cut on the opposite side of the ring and remove the wedge.
- Remove the ring.
- Irrigate the skin with water *to remove any metal particles.*
- Remove your protective eyewear.

Completing the procedure

- Reassess the neurovascular status of the digit.
- Elevate the digit and apply cold packs, as ordered.
- Discard the supplies in the appropriate receptacle.
- Remove and discard your gloves, if worn.
- Perform hand hygiene.[1,2,3,4,5]
- Document the procedure.[10,11,12]

Special considerations

- Some rings are made of tungsten carbide, ceramic, or natural stone; these rings can be removed with locking pliers (vise-grip pliers). (See *Using locking pliers.*)
- Return all pieces of the removed ring to the patient.
- If required, assist the practitioner with administering digital anesthesia using a local anesthetic without epinephrine.

NURSING ALERT *Never use products containing epinephrine on a finger or toe because epinephrine exerts a vasoconstrictive effect.*

- Reassess the neurovascular status frequently after ring removal. Notify the practitioner immediately of any abnormalities.
- Assess the patient's pain level, and administer analgesics as ordered, following safe medication administration practices.
- Clean any open wounds, and cover them with a sterile dressing *to prevent infection.*
- Administer tetanus immunization, as indicated and ordered, following safe medication administration practices.
- When removing rings or other objects from children, use age-appropriate terms. Allow the child's parents or guardian to stay and hold the child during the procedure. Allow the child to examine the equipment, if appropriate.

Patient teaching

Inform the patient that pain should dissipate in 1 to 2 hours and that edema should resolve within 24 hours (or as indicated by initial trauma to the digit). Usually, all signs and symptoms should resolve within 48 hours. Tell the patient that no follow-up is needed unless complications arise. Instruct him to apply an ice pack to the digit for 20 minutes four times daily for 36 to 48 hours *to relieve edema and pain.* Caution the patient to avoid wearing constricting objects on fingers and toes and to remove rings from digits whenever edema is possible. Instruct the patient to contact the practitioner promptly if he experiences signs and symptoms of infection (warmth, increased edema, and pain).

Complications

If a ring remains in place on an injured finger, the constricting effects of the circumferential object can lead to obstruction of lymphatic drainage, which in turn leads to more swelling and further constriction. Venous and, eventually, arterial circulation can be compromised by this constriction. Skin on the affected digit can be cut by the coiled-string technique or by a ring cutter.

Documentation

Document your assessment findings, including the skin condition and neurovascular status of the digit before and after ring removal. Document the methods used to facilitate removal of the ring, the success achieved, and the disposition of the ring. Record the patient's pain status and interventions provided. Record any patient teaching and discharge instructions provided, questions asked by the patient and your responses, and the patient's understanding of digit care.[10]

REFERENCES

1 Centers for Disease Control and Prevention. (2002). Guideline for hand hygiene in health-care settings: Recommendations of the Healthcare Infection Control Practices Advisory Committee and the HICPAC/SHEA/APIC/IDSA Hand Hygiene Task Force. *MMWR Recommendations and Reports, 51*(RR-16), 1–45. Accessed May 2015 via the Web at http://www.cdc.gov/mmwr/pdf/rr/rr5116.pdf (Level II)

2 The Joint Commission. (2015). Standard NPSG.07.01.01. *Comprehensive accreditation manual for hospitals: The official handbook.* Oakbrook Terrace, IL: The Joint Commission. (Level VII)

3 World Health Organization. (2009). "WHO guidelines on hand hygiene in health care: First global patient safety challenge, clean care is safer care" [Online]. Accessed May 2015 via the Web at http://whqlibdoc.who.int/publications/2009/9789241597906_eng.pdf (Level IV)

4 American Osteopathic Association. (2014). Standard 07.01.21. *Healthcare Facilities Accreditation Program: Accreditation requirements for acute care hospitals.* Chicago, IL: American Osteopathic Association. (Level VII)

5 Centers for Medicare & Medicaid Services, Department of Health and Human Services. (2014). Condition of participation: Infection control. 42 C.F.R. § 482.42.

6 The Joint Commission. (2015). Standard NPSG.01.01.01. *Comprehensive accreditation manual for hospitals: The official handbook.* Oakbrook Terrace, IL: The Joint Commission. (Level VII)

7 American Osteopathic Association. (2014). Standard 07.01.10. *Healthcare Facilities Accreditation Program: Accreditation requirements for acute care hospitals.* Chicago, IL: American Osteopathic Association. (Level VII)

8 Siegel J. D., et al. (2007). "2007 guideline for isolation precautions: Preventing transmission of infectious agents in healthcare settings" [Online]. Accessed May 2015 via the Web at http://www.cdc.gov/hicpac/pdf/isolation/Isolation2007.pdf (Level II)

9 The Joint Commission. (2015). Standard PC 01.02.07. *Comprehensive accreditation manual for hospitals: The official handbook.* Oakbrook Terrace, IL: The Joint Commission. (Level VII)

10 The Joint Commission. (2015). Standard RC 03.01.01. *Comprehensive accreditation manual for hospitals: The official handbook.* Oakbrook Terrace, IL: The Joint Commission. (Level VII)

11 American Osteopathic Association. (2014). Standard 10.00.03. *Healthcare Facilities Accreditation Program: Accreditation requirements for acute care hospitals.* Chicago, IL: American Osteopathic Association. (Level VII)

12 Centers for Medicare & Medicaid Services, Department of Health and Human Services. (2014). Condition of participation: Medical record services. 42 C.F.R. § 482.24(b).

ADDITIONAL REFERENCE

Nelson, A. J., & Manzo, R. L. (2012). "How to safely remove a ring" [Online]. Accessed May 2015 via the Web at http://www.assh.org/Public/Safety/Pages/How-to-Get-Ring-Off.aspx

ROTATION BEDS

Rotation beds—such as the RotoRest™ Delta—promote postural drainage and peristalsis and help prevent ventilator-associated pneumonia and complications of immobility.[1,2,3,4] According to the Food and Drug Administration, the RotoRest™ bed is intended to treat or prevent pressure ulcers; treat severe, extensive burns; and aid circulation.[5] Because the bed holds the patient motionless, it's especially helpful for a patient with spinal cord injury, multiple trauma, stroke, multiple sclerosis, coma, severe burns, hypostatic pneumonia, atelectasis, or other unilateral lung involvement causing poor ventilation and perfusion.

Rotation beds turn in an arc up to 90 degrees and can be set to pause on either side for up to 30 minutes. They can accommodate cervical traction devices and tongs. Arm and leg hatches on the bed fold down to allow for range-of-motion (ROM) exercises. Other bed features include a fan, access for X-rays, and supports and clips for chest tubes, catheters, and drains. Racks beneath the bed hold X-ray plates in place for chest and spinal films. (See *Understanding the RotoRest™ Delta therapy system,* page 676.)

Rotation beds are contraindicated for pregnant patients and patients who have severe claustrophobia, an open chest, multiple rib fractures, persistent intracranial hypertension, bronchospasm,[6] an unstable pelvis, or an unstable cervical fracture without neurologic deficit and the complications of immobility. Patient transfer and positioning on the bed should be performed by at least two people to ensure the patient's safety.

Equipment

Rotation bed with appropriate accessories ▪ pillowcases or fluid-impermeable pads ▪ flat sheet or padding ▪ Optional: gloves.

Preparation of equipment

When using the RotoRest™ Delta therapy system, carefully inspect the bed and run it through a complete cycle in both automatic and manual modes *to ensure that it's working properly.* Check the tightness of the set screws at the head of the bed, if applicable for that model.

To prepare the bed for the patient, remove the counterbalance weights from the keel and place them in the base frame's storage area. Release the connecting arm by pulling down on the cam handle and depressing the lower side of the footboard. Next, lock the table in the horizontal position, and place all side supports in the extreme lateral position by loosening the cam handles on the underside of the table. Slide the supports off the bed. Note that all supports and packs are labeled RIGHT or LEFT on the bottom *to facilitate reassembly.*

Remove the knee packs by depressing the snap button and rotating and pulling the packs from the tube. Then remove the abductor packs by depressing and sliding them toward the head of the bed. Next, loosen the foot and knee assemblies by lifting the cam handle at its base, and slide them to the foot of the bed. Last, loosen the shoulder clamp assembly and knobs; swing the shoulder clamps to the vertical position and retighten them.

If applicable for the bed model, remove the cervical, thoracic, and perineal packs. Cover them with pillowcases or fluid-impermeable pads, smooth all wrinkles, and replace the packs. Cover the upper half of the bed, which is a solid unit, with padding or a sheet. Install new disposable foam cushions for the patient's head, shoulders, and feet.

Implementation

- Perform hand hygiene.[7,8,9,10,11]
- Put on gloves if needed *to comply with standard precautions.*[12,13]
- Confirm the patient's identity using at least two patient identifiers.[14]
- If possible, show the patient the bed before use. Explain and demonstrate its operation and reassure the patient that the bed will hold him securely.

EQUIPMENT

Understanding the RotoRest™ Delta therapy system

Various companies make several types and models of rotation beds and each may vary slightly. Be sure to follow the instructions specific to the type of bed you're using. The instructions below apply to the RotoRest™ Delta therapy system.

Driven by a silent motor, the RotoRest™ Delta turns the immobilized patient slowly and continuously. The motion provides constant passive exercise and peristaltic stimulation without depriving the patient of sleep or risking further injury. The bed is radiolucent, permitting X-rays to be taken through it without moving the patient. It also has a built-in cooling fan, and allows access for surgery on patients with multiple trauma without disrupting spinal alignment or traction.

The bed's hatches give access to various parts of the patient's body. Arm hatches permit full range of motion and have holes for chest tubes. Leg hatches allow full hip extension. The perineal hatch provides access for bowel and bladder care, the thoracic hatch for chest auscultation and lumbar puncture, and the cervical hatch for wound care, bathing, and shampooing.

Top view

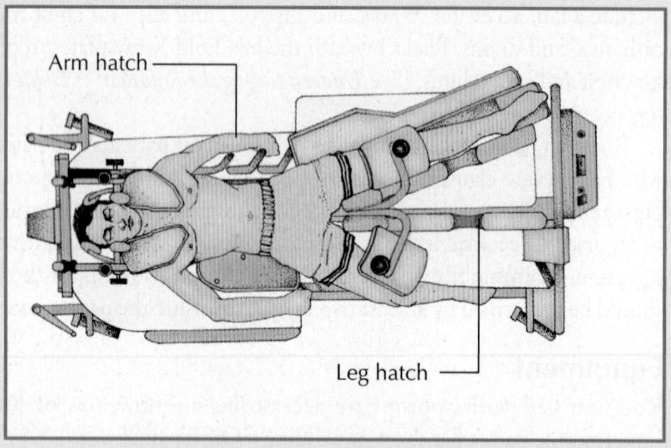

Back view

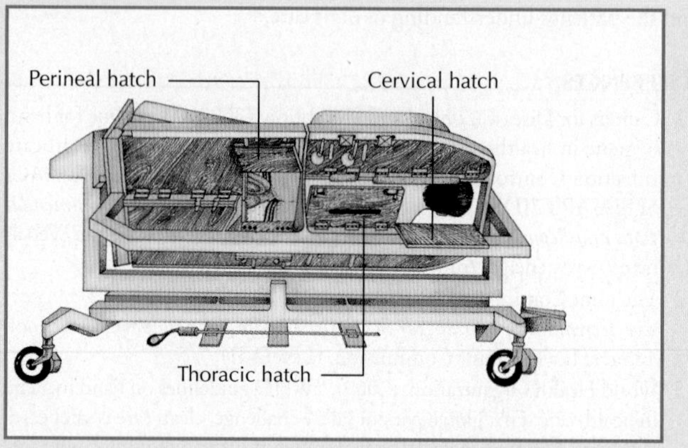

■ Before positioning the patient on the bed, make sure it's turned off. Then, place and lock the bed in the horizontal position, out of gear. Latch all hatches and lock the wheels *to ensure patient safety.*

■ Obtain assistance and transfer the patient. Move him gently to the center of the bed *to prevent contact with the pillar posts and to ensure proper balance during bed operation.* Smooth the pillowcase or fluid-impermeable pad beneath his hips and other bony prominences. Then place any tubes through the appropriate notches in the hatches and ensure that any traction weights hang freely.

■ Insert the thoracic side supports in their posts. Adjust the patient's longitudinal position to allow a 1″ (2.5-cm) space between the axillae and the supports *to avoid pressure on the axillary blood vessels and the brachial plexus.* Push the supports against his chest and lock the cam arms securely *to provide support and ensure patient safety.*

■ Place the disposable supports under the patient's legs *to remove pressure from his heels and prevent pressure ulcers.*

■ Install and adjust the foot supports so that the patient's feet lie in the normal anatomic position, *which helps prevent footdrop.* The foot supports should be in position for only 2 hours every shift *to prevent excessive pressure on the soles and toes.*

■ Place the abductor packs in the appropriate supports, allowing a 6″ (15-cm) space between the packs and the patient's groin. Tighten the knobs on the bed's underside at the base of the support tubes.

■ Install the leg side supports snugly against the patient's hips, and tighten the cam arms. Position the knee assemblies slightly above his knees and tighten the cam arms. Then place your hand on the patient's knee and move the knee pack until it rests lightly on the top of your hand. Repeat for the other knee.

■ Loosen the retaining rings on the crossbar, and slide the head and shoulder assembly laterally. *The retaining rings maintain correct lateral position of the shoulder clamp assembly and head support pack.*

■ Carefully lower the head and shoulder assembly into place and slide it to touch the patient's head.

■ Place your hand on the patient's shoulder, and move the shoulder pack until it touches your hand. Tighten it in place. Repeat for the other shoulder. *The 1″ (2.5-cm) clearance between the shoulders and the packs prevents excess pressure, which can lead to pressure ulcers.*

■ Place the head pack close to, but not touching, the patient's ears (or tongs) *to prevent pressure ulcers.*

■ Tighten the head and shoulder assembly securely *so it won't lift off the bed.* Position the restraining rings next to the shoulder assembly bracket and tighten them.

■ Place the patient's arms on the disposable supports. Install the side arm supports and secure the safety straps, placing one across the shoulder assembly and the other over the thoracic supports *to prevent falls and injury.* If necessary, cover the patient with a flat sheet.

Balancing the bed

■ Place one hand on the footboard *to prevent the bed from turning rapidly if it's unbalanced.* Then remove the locking pin. If the bed rotates to one side, reposition the patient in its center; if it tilts to the right, gently turn it slightly to the left and slide the packs on the right side toward the patient; if it tilts to the left, reverse the process. If a large imbalance exists, you may have to adjust the packs on both sides.

■ After the patient is centered, gently turn the bed into position.

■ Measure the space between the patient's chest, hip, and thighs and the inside of the packs. If the space appears too tight, slide both packs outward. *Excessively loose packs cause the patient to slide from side to side during turning, possibly resulting in unnecessary movement at fracture sites, skin irritation from shearing force, and bed imbalance. Overly tight packs can place pressure on the patient during turning.*

■ After adjusting the packs, check the bed; balance it and make any necessary adjustments.

Initiating automatic bed rotation

■ Ensure that all packs are securely in place. Then hold the footboard firmly and remove the locking pin *to start the bed's motor.* The bed will continue to rotate until the pin is reinserted.

■ Raise the connecting arm cam handle until the connecting assembly snaps into place, locking the bed into automatic rotation.

■ Remain with the patient for at least three complete turns from side to side *to evaluate his comfort and safety.* Observe his response and offer him emotional support.

■ Perform hand hygiene.[7,8,9,10,11]

■ Document the procedure.[15,16,17]

Special considerations

■ If the patient goes into cardiac arrest while on the bed, perform cardiopulmonary resuscitation after taking the bed out of gear, locking it in horizontal position, removing the side arm support and the thoracic pack, lifting the shoulder assembly, and dropping the arm pack. Doing all these steps takes only 5 to 10 seconds. *You won't need a cardiac board because of the bed's firm surface.*

■ If the electricity fails, lock the bed in horizontal or lateral position and rotate it manually every 30 minutes *to prevent pressure ulcers.* If cervical traction causes the patient to slide upward, place the bed in the reverse Trendelenburg position; if extremity traction causes the patient to migrate toward the foot of the bed, use the Trendelenburg position.

■ Lock the bed in the extreme lateral position for access to the back of the head, thorax, and buttocks through the appropriate hatches.

■ Clean the mattress and nondisposable packs during patient care, and rinse them thoroughly *to remove all soap residue.*

■ When replacing the packs and hatches, take care not to pinch the patient's skin between the packs, *which can cause pain and tissue necrosis.*

■ Expect increased drainage from any pressure ulcers for the first few days the patient is on the bed *because the motion helps debride necrotic tissue and improves local circulation.*

■ Perform or schedule daily ROM exercises, as ordered, *because the bed allows full access to all extremities without disturbing spinal alignment.* Drop the arm hatch for shoulder rotation, remove the thoracic packs for shoulder abduction, and drop the leg hatch and remove leg and knee packs for hip rotation and full leg motion.

■ For a female patient, tape an indwelling urinary catheter to the thigh before bringing it through the perineal hatch. For a male patient with spinal cord lesions, tape the catheter to the abdomen and then to the thigh *to facilitate gravity drainage.* Hang the drainage bag on the clips provided, and make sure it doesn't become caught between the bed frames during rotation.

■ If the patient has a tracheal or endotracheal tube and is on mechanical ventilation, attach the tube support bracket between the cervical pack and the arm packs. Tape the connecting T tubing to the support and run it beside the patient's head and off the center of the table *to help prevent reflux of condensation.*

■ For a patient with pulmonary congestion or pneumonia, suction secretions more often during the first 12 to 24 hours on the bed *because the motion will increase drainage.*

Documentation

Document the preparation of the bed and the transfer of the patient into the bed. Record changes in the patient's condition and his response to therapy in your progress notes. Note turning times and ongoing care on the flowchart.

REFERENCES

1 Coppadora, A., et al. (2012). Novel preventive strategies for ventilator-associated pneumonia. *Critical Care, 16,* 210.

2 Staudinger, T., et al. (2010). Continuous lateral rotation therapy to prevent ventilator-associated pneumonia. *Critical Care Medicine, 38,* 486–490. (Level II)

3 Swadener-Culpepper, L., et al. (2008). The impact of continuous lateral rotation therapy in overall clinical and financial outcomes of critically ill patients. *Critical Care Nursing Quarterly, 31,* 270–279. (Level II)

4 Goldhill, D. R., et al. (2007). Rotational bed therapy to prevent and treat respiratory complications: A review and meta-analysis. *American Journal of Critical Care, 16,* 50–61. (Level II)

5 U.S. Food and Drug Administration. (2013). "CFR code of federal regulations title 21: Physical medicine devices: Manual patient rotation bed" [Online]. Accessed May 2015 via the Web at http://www.accessdata.fda.gov/scripts/cdrh/cfdocs/cfcfr/CFRSearch.cfm?fr=890.5180&SearchTerm=890%2E5180

6 ArjoHuntleigh. (2013)." RotoRest™ Delta therapy system" [Online]. Accessed May 2015 via the Web at http://www.arjolibrary.com/ExternalLink/ShowFile.aspx?Id=09956523-b188-41a1-84e0-96a6e9520852

7 The Joint Commission. (2015). Standard NPSG.07.01.01. *Comprehensive accreditation manual for hospitals: The official handbook.* Oakbrook Terrace, IL: The Joint Commission. (Level VII)

8 Centers for Disease Control and Prevention. (2002). Guideline for hand hygiene in health-care settings: Recommendations of the Healthcare Infection Control Practices Advisory Committee and the HICPAC/SHEA/APIC/IDSA Hand Hygiene Task Force. *MMWR Recommendations and Reports, 51*(RR-16), 1–45. Accessed May 2015 via the Web at http://www.cdc.gov/mmwr/pdf/rr/rr5116.pdf (Level II)

9 World Health Organization. (2009). "WHO guidelines on hand hygiene in health care: First global patient safety challenge, clean care is safer care" [Online]. Accessed May 2015 via the Web at http://whqlibdoc.who.int/publications/2009/9789241597906_eng.pdf (Level IV)

10 Centers for Medicare & Medicaid Services, Department of Health and Human Services. (2014). Condition of participation: Infection control. 42 C.F.R. § 482.42.

11 American Osteopathic Association. (2014). Standard 07.01.21. *Healthcare Facilities Accreditation Program: Accreditation requirements for acute care hospitals.* Chicago, IL: American Osteopathic Association. (Level VII)

12 Siegel, J. D., et al. (2007). "2007 guideline for isolation precautions: Preventing transmission of infectious agents in healthcare settings" [Online]. Accessed May 2015 via the Web at http://www.cdc.gov/hicpac/pdf/isolation/Isolation2007.pdf (Level II)

13 American Osteopathic Association. (2014). Standard 07.01.10. *Healthcare Facilities Accreditation Program: Accreditation requirements for acute care hospitals.* Chicago, IL: American Osteopathic Association. (Level VII)

14 The Joint Commission. (2015). Standard NPSG 01.01.01. *Comprehensive accreditation manual for hospitals: The official handbook.* Oakbrook Terrace, IL: The Joint Commission. (Level VII)

15 The Joint Commission. (2015). Standard RC.01.03.01. *Comprehensive accreditation manual for hospitals: The official handbook.* Oakbrook Terrace, IL: The Joint Commission. (Level VII)

16 Centers for Medicare & Medicaid Services, Department of Health and Human Services. (2014). Condition of participation: Medical record services. 42 C.F.R. § 482.24(b).

17 American Osteopathic Association. (2014). Standard 10.00.03. *Healthcare Facilities Accreditation Program: Accreditation requirements for acute care hospitals.* Chicago, IL: American Osteopathic Association. (Level VII)

ADDITIONAL REFERENCE

Simonis, G., et al. (2012). A prospective, randomized trial of continuous lateral rotation ("kinetic therapy") in patients with cardiogenic shock. *Clinical Research in Cardiology, 101,* 955–962. (Level VI)

SAFE MEDICATION ADMINISTRATION PRACTICES, GENERAL

An *adverse drug event* (ADE) is defined as harm to the patient, including mental harm, physical harm, or loss of function, that results from a medication error. A *medication error* is a mistake that occurs during the medication administration process. If a mistake occurs, it doesn't matter whether the patient was harmed or whether there was only a potential for injury; it's still considered a medication error.[1] An ADE is a more direct measure of harm to the patient than a medication error.

ADEs can be further defined as preventable or nonpreventable. A *preventable ADE* occurs as a result of a clinician error or a systematic error and thus could have been prevented. A *nonpreventable ADE* results from a drug's pharmacologic properties.[1] A potential ADE is also known as a *near miss or close call* because, although the patient wasn't harmed, the potential for risk or harm was averted because of actions taken by the patient or clinician.[1]

To promote a culture of safety and to prevent medication errors, nurses must avoid distractions and interruptions when preparing and administering medications[2,3] and adhere to the "five rights" of medication administration: identify the right patient by using at least two patient-specific identifiers; select the right medication; administer the right dose; administer the medication at the right time; and administer the medication by the right route. Recent literature identifies nine rights of medication administration, which in addition to the five rights includes the right documentation, the right action (or appropriate reason for prescribing the medication), the right form, and the right response.[4]

Equipment

Patient's medical record ▪ patient's medication reconciliation form or list ▪ medication order sheets, preprinted or plain ▪ regular or electronic medication administration record ▪ Optional: conversion weight chart.

Implementation

- Avoid distractions and interruptions when preparing and administering medication *to prevent medication errors.*[2,3]

Verifying the medication order

- Follow a written or typed order or an order entered into a computer order-entry system *because these types of orders are less likely to result in error or misunderstanding.*[5]
- Make sure that the prescriber's order contains a diagnosis, a condition, or an indication for the medication.[4,6,7]
- Verify that other essential elements of the medication order are present, including the patient's name, age, and weight (preferably in kilograms); the date and time the order was written; the name of the drug to be administered; the drug dosage; the route of administration; the frequency of administration; dose calculation requirements (when applicable); the exact strength or concentration of the drug (when applicable); the quantity of the drug or duration of administration (when applicable); specific instructions for use (when applicable); and the signature of the person writing the information.[4,7]

Identifying the patient

- Check the patient's medical record *to make sure that all the required documents, medication information, sensitivities, history, physical examination, diagnoses, and laboratory results are present and up to date.*[8]
- Perform hand hygiene.[9,10,11,12,13]
- Confirm the patient's identity using at least two patient identifiers *to minimize the potential for a medication error related to patient misidentification.* Compare the information with the regular or electronic medication administration record.[14]
- Explain to the patient the name and purpose of each medication and when and how it will be administered. Discuss important and common adverse effects of each medication and what to do if the patient experiences signs or symptoms of an adverse reaction. Discuss any possible drug-drug, drug-food, or drug-disease interactions.[7,15,16,17]

Obtaining an accurate medication listing

- Ensure that you have complete list of the patient's current medications—including all prescription and over-the-counter medications and dietary supplements—as well as a history of known drug or food allergies.[8,15] If possible, involve the patient in creating this medication list. If the patient can't participate in creating the list, obtain help from an immediate family member or another authorized person. If the list was obtained before the patient's date of admission, update it *to provide the most accurate listing of the medications that the patient is taking.*[8]
- Ensure that the medication list is available in the patient's medical record and that it's reviewed by his health care providers. *This practice helps reduce the risk of drug interactions, allergic reactions, and dose-related errors and helps identify contraindications.*
- Send a copy of the patient's medication list and new medication orders to the pharmacy *so that the pharmacy can check the appropriateness of the new medication against the patient's current medications; this helps prevent drug interactions, allergic reactions, improper routes of administration, duplication of medications or types or classes of medications, and administration of a contraindicated medication.*[18,19]

Checking for medication contraindications

- Obtain and update the patient's allergy information and current medications during each admission or transfer *to ensure that all health care providers have access to the most up-to-date information.*[20]
- Communicate the patient's current allergy information to all members of the health care team.
- Send medication orders to the pharmacy before the medication is administered *so that the pharmacy can check the medication against the patient's current active medications.*[18,19]
- Have all health care providers review the listing of current medications and allergies at each patient encounter *to determine the appropriateness of each medication for the intended condition.*[1,15]
- If any health care team member has questions about a medication, whether it's a new drug or part of the patient's existing regimen, that team member should contact the pharmacist on duty before administering it.[1]

Ensuring accurate dosage calculations

- Make sure that the patient's most recent weight (in kilograms) is documented in the medical record *to allow for accurate weight-related dosage calculations.*[21]
- Have a conversion chart readily available in case weight is documented in only one unit of measure.
- Calculate the correct dosage of medications that are ordered using weight-based dose schedules. Have two licensed practitioners verify these calculations.
- Use automated dosage calculations whenever possible, especially with IV infusion pumps, *to eliminate dosage calculation errors for drugs with narrow therapeutic dose ranges.*

Administering high-alert medications

- Identify high-alert medications based on your facility's approved list.[4,22] High-alert medications include anticoagulants, antidiabetic agents, sedatives, and chemotherapeutic drugs.[1,23]

■ Monitor medication dosing carefully, especially if dosing adjustments are necessary because of narrow therapeutic windows.[1]

■ Obtain and review any laboratory values required for dosing adjustments; collaborate with the practitioner if values are out of the therapeutic range; watch for adverse effects.[1]

NURSING ALERT *If a patient is receiving an IV opioid, frequently monitor his respiratory rate, sedation level, and oxygen saturation level by continuous pulse oximetry or continuous capnography to monitor exhaled carbon dioxide* to decrease the risk of adverse events associated with IV opioid use. *If adverse reactions occur, respond promptly to prevent treatment delays.*[24]

NURSING ALERT *Before administering a high-alert medication, if required by your facility, ask another nurse to perform an independent double-check* to verify the patient's identity and to make sure that the right medication is on hand, that the medication's indication corresponds with the patient's diagnosis, that dosage calculations are correct, that the route of administration is safe and proper for the patient, and that, if giving an infusion, the pump settings are correct and the infusion line is attached to the correct port.[25]

Handling verbal orders

■ Minimize the use of verbal orders *because verbal orders are especially susceptible to error.*[46]

■ Have the prescriber repeat and verify the verbal order.[26]

■ Record the verbal order in the patient's medical record, and make sure you include the date and name of the prescriber who gave the verbal order, your name as the person who received and recorded the order, and the name of the person who implemented the order.

■ Read back the order to the prescriber as you have written it down *to confirm correct documentation.*[4,27]

Administering scheduled medications in a timely manner[28]

■ Keep in mind that maintenance doses administered according to a standard repeated cycle of frequency, such as every 4 hours or 3 times per day, are considered scheduled medications.

■ Identify a time-critical list of common scheduled medications specific to the patient population of the facility unit, such as the oncology unit.

■ Identify a time-critical list of scheduled medications that might be used on all units. Examples of time-critical scheduled medications include antibiotics, anticoagulants, insulin, anticonvulsants, immunosuppressive agents, non-IV pain medications, medications prescribed for administration within a specific time of the medication order, medications that must be administered apart from other medications for optimal therapeutic effect, and medications prescribed more frequently than every 4 hours.[4]

■ Establish guidelines to facilitate the administration of time-critical medications that must be administered 30 minutes before or after the regular scheduled times for medications.

■ Establish guidelines to facilitate the administration of non–time-critical daily, weekly, and monthly medications that are to be administered 2 hours before or after the scheduled time.

■ Give medications that are administered more frequently than daily but less frequently than every 4 hours (for instance, twice daily or three times per day) no more than 1 hour before or after the scheduled time.

Completing the procedure

■ Monitor and document the effectiveness of all medications administered.[29,30,31]

■ Document any medication errors or adverse effects according to your facility's event-reporting system.[4,32]

■ Dispose of all containers *to avoid cross-contamination.* Keep in mind that after a medication is removed from its original container, it should be used for one patient only.

■ Perform hand hygiene.[9,10,11,12,13]

Evaluating the medication management process

■ Make sure that there's a defined method for reviewing and updating any preprinted order sheets or standing orders. Routinely review this process *to look for points of failure that could contribute to a medication error.*[33]

■ Make sure that the pharmacy annually reviews the high-risk medications and look-alike and sound-alike medications it stores and uses. *The pharmacy should remove medications if they aren't being used.*[34,35]

■ Make sure that a list of "Do Not Use" abbreviations, symbols, and acronyms is updated regularly and is posted prominently where medications are prepared. (See *Abbreviations to avoid* and *Additional abbreviations to avoid,* page 680.)[33]

Special considerations

■ Maintain a nonpunitive culture for reporting medication errors *to encourage reporting compliance.*

■ Adjust dosages as needed based on the patient's age or if renal insufficiency is identified. *Pediatric patients, patients with identified renal dysfunction, and patients older than age 80 are at higher risk for ADEs.*[15]

■ Perform a medication reconciliation at transition points, such as during admission, discharge, and transfer between units.[6,37]

■ Your facility should establish standards for a medication delivery process and develop ways to ensure ongoing review and evaluation.

■ Use smart pump technology and standardized medication concentrations when available *to reduce the risk of IV medication infusion errors.*

■ Make sure that the infusion pump alarm limits are set according to the patient's current condition and that the alarms are turned on, functioning properly, and audible to staff.[38,39,40,41]

■ In addition to the computerized physician order entry and electronic medication administration record, use a bar code scanning system (if available) to scan the bar codes on medications and the patient's identification bracelet (as shown below) *to reduce medication administration errors and as a final step to intercept a medication error before drug administration.*[15] (See *Using a bar code scanning system below.*)

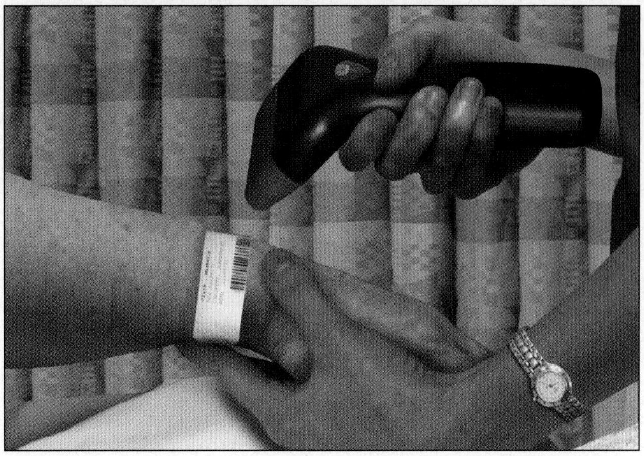

■ If indicated, include the patient's age and weight in the patient's medical and medication records.

■ When possible, medications should be prescribed electronically.[1,15]

■ Handle medications brought by the patient from home as directed by your facility.[4,42]

■ If any questions arise about a prescribed medication, collaborate with the prescriber or pharmacist.[6,7,17]

Abbreviations to avoid[36]

To reduce the risk of medical errors, The Joint Commission has created a "Do Not Use" list of abbreviations. The list applies to all orders and medication-related documentation that's handwritten, part of a free-text computer entry, or on preprinted forms.

Abbreviation	Potential problem	Preferred term
U (for "unit")	Mistaken as zero, four, or cc.	Write "unit."
IU (for "international unit")	Mistaken as IV (intravenous) or 10 (ten).	Write "international unit."
Q.D., Q.O.D, QD, QOD, q.d., q.o.d., qd, qod (Latin abbreviations for "once daily" and "every other day")	Mistaken for each other. The period after the "Q" can be mistaken for an "I" and the "O" can be mistaken for "I."	Write "daily" and "every other day."
Trailing zero (X.0 mg) (Note: Prohibited only for medication-related notations); lack of leading zero (.X mg)	Decimal point is missed.	Never write a zero by itself after a decimal point (X mg), and always use a zero before a decimal point (0.X mg).
MS MSO4 MgSO4	Confused for one another. Can mean "morphine sulfate" or "magnesium sulfate."	Write "morphine sulfate" or "magnesium sulfate."

Additional abbreviations to avoid

Below are additional abbreviations that may be included in the "Do not use list" in the future.

Do not use	Use instead
>	Write "greater than."
<	Write "less than."
Abbreviations for drug names	Write out the full drug name.
Apothecary units	Use metric units.
@	Write "at."
cc	Write "mL" or "ml," or spell out "milliliters" (mL is preferred).
μ	Write "mcg" or "micrograms."

Adapted with permission from The Joint Commission.

- Be especially alert during high-risk situations, such as when you're stressed, tired, or angry, or when supervising inexperienced personnel. Monitor and modify work schedules *to minimize work- or fatigue-related medication errors.*
- If an automated dispensing cabinet is used to dispense medications, follow the manufacturer's instructions for use.
- Report all medication errors and adverse effects; this includes preventable ADEs, close calls, and hazardous conditions.[4,6,43]

Patient teaching

Teach the patient to keep a current list of his medications. This list should include all prescription medications, over-the-counter or nonprescription medications, herbal supplements, vitamins, and minerals. The patient should familiarize himself with the list and directions for the proper use of the medications. He should also understand any possible adverse effects and what to do if he experiences such effects.[15]

Encourage the patient and family or caregiver to ask questions about any medications that the patient is taking, especially if it's a newly prescribed drug. The patient shouldn't take any medication without knowing its purpose. Tell the patient that it's acceptable to ask for written instructions about medications *to use as a reference.*[15]

Complications

With any medication use, there's the potential for an ADE or medication error. Familiarize yourself with all medications that you administer and be aware of potential ADEs. Know the required antidotes if indicated. Resources should be readily available to confirm any potential ADE if you aren't familiar with the medications being used. Report any medication errors, adverse drug reactions, and medication incompatibilities immediately to the attending practitioner or clinical psychologist.[32]

Documentation

Document all medications administered in the patient's regular or electronic medication administration record. If a medication wasn't administered, document the reason why, any interventions taken, when the practitioner was notified, and the patient's response to interventions.

If the patient experiences an ADE or medication error, document the event as required by your facility. Your facility may require that you submit a medication error report to the National Medication Errors Reporting Program operated by the Institute for Safe Medication Practices, a patient safety organization certified by the Agency for Healthcare Research and Quality. The Medication Errors Reporting Program is a confidential, voluntary medication error reporting program that performs expert analysis of system-based causes of medication errors.[43]

References

1 Zhu, J., & Weingart, S. N. Prevention of adverse drug events in hospitals. (2014). In: *UpToDate*, Gandhi, T. K., & Lin, F. H. (Eds.). Accessed May 2015 via the Web at http://www.uptodate.com/contents/search

2 Westbrook, J., et al. (2010). Association of interruptions with an increased risk and severity of medication administration errors. *Archives of Internal Medicine, 170,* 683–690.

3 Institute for Safe Medication Practices. (2012). Side tracks on the safety express: Interruptions lead to errors and unfinished...Wait, what was I doing? *Nurse Advise-ERR, 11*(2), 1–4. Accessed May 2015 via the Web at https://www.ismp.org/Newsletters/acutecare/showarticle.aspx?id=37

4 Centers for Medicare & Medicaid Services, Department of Health and Human Services. (2014). Condition of participation: Nursing services. 42 C.F.R. § 482.23(c).

5 Taylor, C. R., et al. (2015). *Fundamentals of nursing: The art and science of nursing care* (8th ed.). Philadelphia, PA: Wolters Kluwer.

6 The Joint Commission. (2015). Standard MM.04.01.01. *Comprehensive accreditation manual for hospitals: The official handbook.* Oakbrook Terrace, IL: The Joint Commission. (Level VII)

7 American Osteopathic Association. (2014). Standard 16.01.03. *Healthcare Facilities Accreditation Program: Accreditation requirements for acute care hospitals.* Chicago, IL: American Osteopathic Association. (Level VII)

8 The Joint Commission. (2015). Standard NPSG.03.06.01. *Comprehensive accreditation manual for hospitals: The official handbook.* Oakbrook Terrace, IL: The Joint Commission. (Level VII)

9 The Joint Commission. (2015). Standard NPSG.07.01.01. *Comprehensive accreditation manual for hospitals: The official handbook.* Oakbrook Terrace, IL: The Joint Commission. (Level VII)

10 World Health Organization. (2009). "WHO guidelines on hand hygiene in health care: First global patient safety challenge, clean care is safer care" [Online]. Accessed May 2015 via the Web at http://whqlibdoc.who.int/publications/2009/9789241597906_eng.pdf (Level IV)

11 Centers for Disease Control and Prevention. (2002). Guideline for hand hygiene in health-care settings: Recommendations of the Healthcare Infection Control Practices Advisory Committee and the HICPAC/SHEA/APIC/IDSA Hand Hygiene Task Force. *MMWR Recommendations and Reports, 51*(RR-16), 1–45. Accessed May 2015 via the Web at http://www.cdc.gov/mmwr/pdf/rr/rr5116.pdf (Level II)

12 Centers for Medicare & Medicaid Services, Department of Health and Human Services. (2014). Condition of participation: Infection control. 42 C.F.R. § 482.42.

13 American Osteopathic Association. (2014). Standard 07.01.21. *Healthcare Facilities Accreditation Program: Accreditation requirements for acute care hospitals.* Chicago, IL: American Osteopathic Association. (Level VII)

14 The Joint Commission. (2015). Standard NPSG.01.01.01. *Comprehensive accreditation manual for hospitals: The official handbook.* Oakbrook Terrace, IL: The Joint Commission. (Level VII)

15 Institute of Medicine of the National Academies Committee on Identifying and Preventing Medication Errors, Board on Health Care Services. (2007). *Preventing medication errors: Quality chasm series.* Washington, DC: National Academies Press.

16 The Joint Commission. (2015). Standard PC.02.03.01. *Comprehensive accreditation manual for hospitals: The official handbook.* Oakbrook Terrace, IL: The Joint Commission. (Level VII)

17 The Joint Commission. (2015). Standard MM.06.01.01. *Comprehensive accreditation manual for hospitals: The official handbook.* Oakbrook Terrace, IL: The Joint Commission. (Level VII)

18 The Joint Commission. (2015). Standard MM.05.01.01. *Comprehensive accreditation manual for hospitals: The official handbook.* Oakbrook Terrace, IL: The Joint Commission. (Level VII)

19 Centers for Medicare & Medicaid Services, Department of Health and Human Services. (2014). Condition of participation: Pharmaceutical services. 42 C.F.R. § 482.25 (b).

20 The Joint Commission. (2015). Standard MM.01.01.01. *Comprehensive accreditation manual for hospitals: The official handbook.* Oakbrook Terrace, IL: The Joint Commission. (Level VII)

21 Institute for Safe Medication Practices. (2014). "2014-15 targeted medication safety best practices for hospitals" [Online]. Accessed May 2015 via the Web at http://www.ismp.org/tools/bestpractices/TMSBP-for-Hospitals.pdf

22 The Joint Commission. (2015). Standard MM.01.01.03. *Comprehensive accreditation manual for hospitals: The official handbook.* Oakbrook Terrace, IL: The Joint Commission. (Level VII)

23 Institute for Safe Medication Practices. (2014). "ISMP list of high-alert medications in acute care settings" [Online]. Accessed May 2015 via the Web at http://www.ismp.org/Tools/highalertmedications.pdf (Level VII)

24 Centers for Medicare & Medicaid Services. (2014). "Requirements for hospital medication administration, particularly intravenous (IV) medications and post-operative care of patients receiving IV opioids" [Online]. Accessed May 2015 via the Web at http://www.cms.gov/Medicare/Provider-Enrollment-and-Certification/SurveyCertificationGenInfo/Downloads/Survey-and-Cert-Letter-14-15.pdf

25 Institute for Safe Medication Practices. (2008). Conducting an independent double-check. *ISMP Medication Safety Alert! Nurse Advise-ERR, 6*(12), 1. Accessed May 2015 via the Web at http://www.ismp.org/newsletters/nursing/Issues/NurseAdviseERR200812.pdf (Level VII)

26 Centers for Medicare & Medicaid Services, Department of Health and Human Services. (2014). Condition of participation: Nursing services. 42 C.F.R. § 482.23.

27 The Joint Commission. (2015). Standard PC.02.01.03. *Comprehensive accreditation manual for hospitals: The official handbook.* Oakbrook Terrace, IL: The Joint Commission. (Level VII)

28 Institute for Safe Medication Practices. (2011). "ISMP acute care guidelines for timely administration of scheduled medications" [Online]. Accessed May 2015 via the Web at http://www.ismp.org/tools/guidelines/acutecare/tasm.pdf (Level VII)

29 The Joint Commission. (2015). Standard RC.01.03.01. *Comprehensive accreditation manual for hospitals: The official handbook.* Oakbrook Terrace, IL: The Joint Commission. (Level VII)

30 American Osteopathic Association. (2014). Standard 10.00.03. *Healthcare Facilities Accreditation Program: Accreditation requirements for acute care hospitals.* Chicago, IL: American Osteopathic Association. (Level VII)

31 Centers for Medicare & Medicaid Services, Department of Health and Human Services. (2014). Condition of participation: Medical record services. 42 C.F.R. § 482.24(b).

32 The Joint Commission. (2015). Standard MM.07.01.03. *Comprehensive accreditation manual for hospitals: The official handbook.* Oakbrook Terrace, IL: The Joint Commission. (Level VII)

33 Institute for Safe Medication Practices. (2010). "ISMP's guidelines for standard order sets" [Online]. Accessed May 2015 via the Web at http://www.ismp.org/tools/guidelines/StandardOrderSets.pdf (Level VII)

34 Institute for Safe Medication Practices. (2014). "ISMP's list of error-prone abbreviations, symbols and dose-designations" [Online]. Accessed May 2015 via the Web at http://www.ismp.org/tools/errorproneabbreviations.pdf (Level VII)

35 The Joint Commission. (2015). Standard MM.01.02.01. *Comprehensive accreditation manual for hospitals: The official handbook.* Oakbrook Terrace, IL: The Joint Commission. (Level VII)

36 The Joint Commission. (2013). "Facts about the official 'Do Not Use' list" [Online]. Accessed May 2015 via the Web at http://www.jointcommission.org/assets/1/18/Do_Not_Use_List.pdf (Level VII)

37 American Osteopathic Association. (2014). Standard 25.02.13. *Healthcare Facilities Accreditation Program: Accreditation requirements for acute care hospitals.* Chicago, IL: American Osteopathic Association. (Level VII)

38 American Association of Critical-Care Nurses. (2013). "AACN Practice Alert: Alarm management" [Online]. Accessed May 2015 via the Web at http://www.aacn.org/wd/practice/docs/practicealerts/alarm-management-practice-alert.pdf (Level VII)

39 Graham, K. C., & Cvach, M. (2010). Monitor alarm fatigue: Standardizing use of physiological monitors and decreasing nuisance alarms. *American Journal of Critical Care, 19,* 28–37.

40 The Joint Commission. (2015). Standard NPSG.06.01.01. *Comprehensive accreditation manual for hospitals: The official handbook.* Oakbrook Terrace, IL: The Joint Commission. (Level VII)

41 The Joint Commission. (2013). "Sentinel event alert: Medical device alarm safety in hospitals" [Online]. Accessed May 2015 via the Web at http://www.jointcommission.org/assets/1/18/SEA_50_alarms_4_5_13_FINAL1.PDF (Level VII)

Classifying seizure types

Developed by the International League Against Epilepsy (ILAE), this seizure classification system can help health care workers caring for patients with epilepsy use terms more consistently and communicate more effectively.

Partial (or focal) seizures

Arising from a localized area in the brain, partial seizures cause specific signs and symptoms associated with the specific area of the brain affected. Partial seizures are characterized as *simple partial, complex partial,* and *secondarily generalized.*[1] The ILAE has proposed reclassifying partial (or focal) seizures according to their features, such as aura, motor, autonomic, or responsiveness.[2]

Simple partial seizures

A simple partial seizure can present in several ways, depending on the focal point of the seizure in the brain. Simple partial seizures don't cause altered consciousness; the patient is alert and oriented but can't control his signs and symptoms. An aura, or warning of an impending seizure, is actually a simple partial seizure.[1] Some of the ways that a simple partial seizure can manifest include:

- motor signs (jerking of the thumb or the cheek)
- somatosensory symptoms (visual, vestibular, gustatory, olfactory, or auditory hallucinations or sensations)
- autonomic signs (such as tachycardia, sweating, and pupillary dilation)
- psychic symptoms (such as feelings of déjà-vu or dreamy states).[1]

Complex partial seizures

Consciousness becomes altered with a complex partial seizure.[1] During this type of seizure, the patient isn't aware of his environment. A simple partial seizure may precede a complex partial seizure. Characteristics vary and depend on the location of the abnormal discharge. During a complex partial seizure, the patient may experience automatic purposeless movements, such as lip-smacking, eye-blinking, picking at clothing, and walking aimlessly.[1]

Secondarily generalized seizures

Beginning in a focal or localized part of the brain, a secondarily generalized seizure may progress to a generalized seizure as both hemispheres of the brain become involved. Loss of consciousness may occur immediately or in 1 to 2 minutes as seizure activity progresses.[1]

Primary generalized seizures

As the term suggests, primary generalized seizures cause a general electrical abnormality involving both sides of the brain; there isn't a localized or focal onset of the abnormal activity. Primary generalized seizures include *absence, myoclonic, tonic-clonic, atonic, tonic,* and *clonic* seizures.

Absence seizures

An absence seizure occurs commonly in children, but may also affect adults. It usually begins with a brief change in the level of consciousness, indicated by blinking or swallowing or a blank stare, and slight mouth movements.[1] Typically, the seizure comes on suddenly and is brief; the impairment may be so brief that the patient may be unaware of it.[1] If not properly treated, these seizures can recur as often as 100 times per day and may result in learning difficulties.

Myoclonic seizures

A myoclonic seizure is marked by abrupt muscle contractions of the body extremities. Seizure activity may occur in the face or be generalized.[1]

Tonic-clonic (grand mal) seizures

Typically, a tonic-clonic seizure begins with a loss of consciousness that's followed by tonic and clonic activity. The body stiffens (tonic phase) and then alternates between episodes of muscle spasm and relaxation (clonic phase).[1] Tongue biting, incontinence, labored breathing, apnea, and subsequent cyanosis may also occur. The seizure stops in 2 to 5 minutes, when abnormal electrical conduction of the neurons is completed. The patient then regains consciousness but may be somewhat confused and may have difficulty talking. If he can talk, he may complain of drowsiness, fatigue, headache, muscle soreness, and arm or leg weakness. He may fall into a deep sleep after the seizure.

Atonic seizures

Atonic seizures, characterized by a general loss of muscle tone and a temporary loss of consciousness, occur in young children. They're sometimes called a *drop attacks* because they causes the patient to fall forward.[1]

Tonic seizures

Tonic seizures involve stiffening of the extremities; they may be associated with falling.[1]

Clonic seizures

During a clonic seizure. The patient experiences symmetrical limb jerking.[1]

42 The Joint Commission. (2014). Standard MM.03.01.05. *Comprehensive accreditation manual for hospitals: The official handbook.* Oakbrook Terrace, IL: The Joint Commission. (Level VII)

43 Institute for Safe Medication Practices. (n.d.). "The National Medication Errors Reporting Program (ISMP MERP)" [Online]. Accessed May 2015 via the Web at https://www.ismp.org/orderforms/reporterrortoismp.asp

SEIZURE MANAGEMENT

Seizures are paroxysmal events associated with abnormal electrical discharges of neurons in the brain. Partial seizures are usually unilateral, involving a localized or focal area of the brain. Generalized seizures involve the entire brain. (See *Classifying seizure types.*) When a patient has a generalized seizure, nursing care aims to protect him from injury and prevent serious complications. Appropriate care also includes observation of seizure characteristics to help determine the area of the brain involved.

Patients considered at risk for seizures are those with a history of seizures and those with conditions that predispose them to seizures. These conditions include metabolic abnormalities, such as hypocalcemia and pyridoxine deficiency; brain tumors or other space-occupying lesions; infections, such as meningitis, encephalitis, and brain abscess; traumatic injury, especially if the dura mater was penetrated; ingestion of toxins, such as mercury, lead, or carbon monoxide; genetic abnormalities, such as tuberous sclerosis and phenylketonuria; perinatal injuries; and stroke. Patients at risk for seizures need precautionary measures to help prevent injury if a seizure occurs. (See *Precautions for generalized seizures.*)

Equipment

Stethoscope ▪ sphygmomanometer ▪ pulse oximeter ▪ gloves ▪ side rail pads or bath blankets ▪ adhesive tape ▪ disinfectant pad ▪ Optional: pillow, blanket, oral or nasal airway, suction equipment, emergency equipment (crash cart with emergency medications and endotracheal intubation equipment), seizure activity record, IV catheter insertion equipment, normal saline solution, oxygen administration equipment, IV intermittent infusion device.

Preparation of equipment

If the patient is at risk for seizures, place an oral airway and suction equipment at the patient's bedside and pad his side rails with side rail pads, if available (use bath blankets if pads aren't available). Make sure emergency equipment is readily available and in working condition.

Implementation

- Gather and prepare the necessary equipment.
- Perform hand hygiene.[3,4,5,6,7]
- Confirm the patient's identify using at least two patient identifiers.[8]

During a seizure

- If you are with a patient when he experiences an aura, help him into bed, raise the side rails, and adjust the bed *so that the patient lies flat.* If he's away from his room, lower him to the floor and place a pillow, blanket, or other soft material under his head *to protect his head from hitting the floor.*
- Put on gloves *to comply with standard precautions.*[9,10]
- Provide privacy, if possible.[11,12]
- Stay with the patient during the seizure, and be ready to intervene if complications such as airway obstruction develop.[1] If necessary, have another staff member obtain the appropriate equipment and notify the practitioner of the obstruction.
- Assess the patient's airway for patency. If necessary, turn the patient on his side *to allow secretions to drain and his tongue to fall forward.*

NURSING ALERT ***Don't try to hold the patient's mouth open or place your hands inside his mouth because he may bite you. After the patient's jaw becomes rigid, don't force an airway into place*** **because you may break his teeth or cause another injury.**

- Move hard or sharp objects out of the patient's way and loosen his clothing.
- Don't forcibly restrain the patient or restrict his movements during the seizure *because the force of the patient's movements against restraints could cause muscle strain or even joint dislocation.*
- Assess the patient during the seizure, including level of consciousness (LOC). Observe the earliest sign, such as head or eye deviation, as well as how the seizure progresses, what form it takes, and how long it lasts. *Your description may help determine the seizure's type and cause.*[1]
- If this is the patient's first seizure, notify the practitioner immediately. If the patient has had seizures before, notify the practitioner only if the seizure activity is prolonged or if the patient fails to regain consciousness. (See *Understanding status epilepticus.*)
- If ordered, insert an IV catheter and infuse normal saline solution at a keep-vein-open rate.

NURSING ALERT ***Don't attempt to insert an IV catheter during an active seizure unless absolutely necessary*** **because doing so can cause injuries.**

- If the seizure is prolonged and the patient becomes hypoxemic, administer oxygen as ordered. Some patients may require endotracheal intubation. Attach the patient to a pulse oximeter *to monitor oxygen saturation levels.*
- For a patient known to be diabetic, administer 50 mL of dextrose 50% by IV push as ordered, following safe medication administration

Precautions for generalized seizures

By taking appropriate precautions, you can help protect a patient from injury, aspiration, and airway obstruction should he have a seizure. Plan your precautions using information obtained from the patient's history. What kind of seizure has the patient had before? Is he aware of exacerbating factors? Sleep deprivation, missed doses of anticonvulsants, even upper respiratory tract infections can increase seizure frequency in some people who have had seizures. Was his previous seizure an acute episode, or did it result from a chronic condition?

Gather the equipment

Based on answers provided in the patient's history, you can tailor your precautions to his needs. Start by gathering the appropriate equipment, including a hospital bed with full-length side rails, side rail pads (or bath blankets if side rail pads aren't available), adhesive tape, an oral airway, and oral or nasal suction equipment.

Bedside preparations

Carry out the precautions you think appropriate for the patient. Remember that a patient with preexisting seizures who's being admitted for a change in medication, treatment of an infection, or detoxification may have an increased risk of seizures.

- Explain the reasons for the precautions to the patient.
- *To protect the patient's limbs, head, and feet from injury if he has a seizure while in bed,* cover the side rails, headboard, and footboard with side rail pads or bath blankets. If you use blankets, keep them in place with adhesive tape. Keep the side rails raised while the patient is in bed *to prevent falls.* Keep the bed in a low position *to minimize any injuries that may occur if the patient climbs over the rails.*
- Place an airway at the patient's bedside, or tape it to the wall above the bed. Keep suction and oxygen equipment nearby *in case you need to establish a patent airway.* Explain to the patient how you'll use the airway.
- If the patient has frequent or prolonged seizures, prepare an IV intermittent infusion device *to facilitate administration of emergency medications.*

Understanding status epilepticus

Status epilepticus is defined as recurrent seizures without complete recovery of consciousness between attacks. If the patient has virtually continuous seizure activity for more than 30 minutes, with or without impaired consciousness, it may also be classified as status epilepticus.[1] The most serious and life-threatening type is *generalized tonic-clonic status epilepticus.*[1]

Always an emergency, status epilepticus is accompanied by respiratory distress. It can result from abrupt withdrawal of anticonvulsant medications, hypoxic or metabolic encephalopathy, acute head trauma, or septicemia secondary to encephalitis or meningitis.

Emergency treatment of status epilepticus usually consists of diazepam, phenytoin, or phenobarbital; dextrose 50% IV (when seizures are secondary to hypoglycemia); and thiamine IV (in the presence of alcohol use disorder or alcohol withdrawal).

practices.[13,14,15] For a patient known to have alcohol use disorder, the practitioner may order IV thiamine.

After a seizure

- Turn the patient on his side and apply suction if necessary *to facilitate drainage of secretions and maintain a patent airway.* Insert an oral or nasal airway if needed.
- Assess the patient for injuries.
- Reorient and reassure the patient, as necessary.
- Place the bed in its lowest position with the brakes engaged and pad the side rails with side rail pads or bath blankets *in case the patient experiences another seizure.*
- Monitor the patient's vital signs and oxygen saturation and conduct a neurologic assessment, including LOC, motor strength, pupillary activity, ability to speak and remember, and orientation, at a frequency determined by the patient's condition or as ordered.
- Ask the patient about his aura and activities preceding the seizure. *The type of aura (auditory, visual, olfactory, gustatory, or somatic) helps pinpoint the site in the brain where the seizure originated.*
- Remove and discard your gloves.[9]
- Perform hand hygiene.[3,4,5,6,7]
- Clean and disinfect your stethoscope using a disinfectant pad.[16,17]
- Perform hand hygiene.[3,4,5,6,7]
- Document the procedure.[18,19,20]

Special considerations

- Because a seizure can indicate an underlying disorder, such as meningitis or a metabolic (especially hypoglycemic) or electrolyte (especially hyponatremia) imbalance, the practitioner will order a complete diagnostic workup if the cause of the seizure isn't evident.[21]
- When a patient with a known seizure history is hospitalized, insert an IV catheter *so IV access is available to administer seizure medication, if needed.*

Patient teaching

Caution the patient who has epileptic seizures and other sudden-onset seizures about ascending heights, working with fire or cooking, using power tools, taking unsupervised baths, swimming, and driving. State laws may restrict operation of motorized vehicles, so consult your state law. Encourage the use of helmets to prevent head trauma while biking, skiing, riding a motorcycle, or participating in other activities, as indicated, based on the patient's lifestyle and type and degree of seizure control.[22] Review with the patient and his family first-aid for seizures in the home and strategies to prevent injury.[23,24] Review the patient's medication regimen, and reinforce the importance of complying with laboratory testing to determine therapeutic drug levels, as indicated.[25]

Make sure the patient understands that abrupt withdrawal of an antiseizure medication can trigger status epilepticus. When there's a need for reduction, discontinuation, or substitution of the medication, explain that he should do so gradually and under the practitioner's care.

Tell the patient that various stimuli can trigger seizures and to be aware that he may have a seizure when exposed to them. If he does have a seizure, he should avoid exposure to the stimulus as much as possible and maintain a seizure diary.

Instruct the patient to tell all of his practitioners about his seizure disorder and the medications that he's taking before any medical or dental treatment or surgery. Recommend that he wear a medical identification bracelet or necklace stating that he has a seizure disorder or is taking antiseizure medication.

Complications

The patient who experiences a seizure may experience an injury, respiratory difficulty, and decreased mental capability. Common injuries include scrapes and bruises suffered when the patient hits objects during the seizure and traumatic injury to the tongue caused by biting. If you suspect a serious injury, such as a fracture or deep laceration, notify the practitioner and arrange for appropriate evaluation and treatment.

Changes in respiratory function may include aspiration, airway obstruction, and hypoxemia. After the seizure, complete a respiratory assessment and notify the practitioner if you suspect a problem. Expect most patients to experience a postictal period of decreased mental status lasting 30 minutes to 24 hours. Reassure the patient that this doesn't indicate incipient brain damage.

Documentation

Document that the patient requires seizure precautions, and record all precautions taken.

If a seizure occurs, document the event on a seizure activity record (if used in your facility) or other appropriate location in the patient's medical record. Document the date and time the seizure began as well as its duration and any precipitating factors. Identify any sensation that may be considered an aura. If the seizure was preceded by an aura, have the patient describe what he experienced.

Record involuntary behavior that occurred at the onset, such as lip smacking, chewing movements, or hand and eye movements. Describe where the behavior began and the parts of the body involved. Note the progression or pattern to the activity. Document whether the patient's eyes deviated to one side and if the pupils changed in size, shape, equality, or reaction to light. Note if the patient's teeth were clenched or open. Record any incontinence, vomiting, or salivation that occurred during the seizure.

Note the patient's response to the seizure. Was the patient aware of what happened? Did he fall into a deep sleep following the seizure? Was he upset or ashamed? Also note any medications the patient received, complications he experienced during the seizure, and interventions you performed. Finally, note the patient's postseizure vital signs, oxygen saturation level, and neurologic status.

Document instructions provided regarding seizure management and injury prevention.

References

1 Fisher, R. E., & Long, L. (2007, revised 2009). "AANN clinical practice guideline series: Care of the patient with seizures (2nd ed.)" [Online]. Accessed May 2015 via the Web at http://www.aann.org/pdf/cpg/aann-seizures.pdf (Level VII)

2 Berg, A. T., et al. (2010). "Revised terminology and concepts for organizations of seizures and epilepsies: Report of the ILAE Commission on Classification and Terminology, 2005–2009" [Online]. Accessed May 2015 via the Web at http://www.ilae.org/Visitors/Centre/ctf/documents/ClassificationReport_2010_000.pdf (Level VII)

3 The Joint Commission. (2015). Standard NPSG.07.01.01. *Comprehensive accreditation manual for hospitals: The official handbook.* Oakbrook Terrace, IL: The Joint Commission. (Level VII)

4 Centers for Disease Control and Prevention. (2002). Guideline for hand hygiene in health-care settings: Recommendations of the Healthcare Infection Control Practices Advisory Committee and the HICPAC/SHEA/APIC/IDSA Hand Hygiene Task Force. *MMWR Recommendations and Reports, 51*(RR-16), 1–45. Accessed May 2015 via the Web at http://www.cdc.gov/mmwr/pdf/rr/rr5116.pdf (Level II)

5 World Health Organization. (2009). "WHO guidelines on hand hygiene in health care: First global patient safety challenge, clean care is safer care" [Online]. Accessed May 2015 via the Web at http://whqlibdoc.who.int/publications/2009/9789241597906_eng.pdf (Level IV)

6 Centers for Medicare & Medicaid Services, Department of Health and Human Services. (2014). Condition of participation: Infection control. 42 C.F.R. § 482.42.

7 American Osteopathic Association. (2014). Standard 07.01.21. *Healthcare Facilities Accreditation Program: Accreditation requirements for acute care hospitals.* Chicago, IL: American Osteopathic Association. (Level VII)
8 The Joint Commission. (2015). Standard NPSG.01.01.01. *Comprehensive accreditation manual for hospitals: The official handbook.* Oakbrook Terrace, IL: The Joint Commission. (Level VII)
9 Siegel, J. D., et al. (2007). "2007 guideline for isolation precautions: Preventing transmission of infectious agents in healthcare settings" [Online]. Accessed May 2015 via the Web at http://www.cdc.gov/hicpac/pdf/isolation/Isolation2007.pdf (Level II)
10 American Osteopathic Association. (2014). Standard 07.01.10. *Healthcare Facilities Accreditation Program: Accreditation requirements for acute care hospitals.* Chicago, IL: American Osteopathic Association. (Level VII)
11 Centers for Medicare & Medicaid Services, Department of Health and Human Services. (2014). Condition of participation: Patient's rights. 42 C.F.R. § 482.13(c)(1).
12 American Osteopathic Association. (2014). Standard 15.01.16. *Healthcare Facilities Accreditation Program: Accreditation requirements for acute care hospitals.* Chicago, IL: American Osteopathic Association. (Level VII)
13 The Joint Commission. (2015). Standard MM.06.01.01. *Comprehensive accreditation manual for hospitals: The official handbook.* Oakbrook Terrace, IL: The Joint Commission. (Level VII)
14 American Osteopathic Association. (2014). Standard 16.01.03. *Healthcare Facilities Accreditation Program: Accreditation requirements for acute care hospitals.* Chicago, IL: American Osteopathic Association. (Level VII)
15 Centers for Medicare & Medicaid Services, Department of Health and Human Services. (2014). Condition of participation: Nursing services. 42 C.F.R. § 482.23(c).
16 Rutala, W. A., et al. (2008). "Guideline for disinfection and sterilization in healthcare facilities, 2008" [Online]. Accessed May 2015 via the Web at http://www.cdc.gov/hicpac/pdf/guidelines/Disinfection_Nov_2008.pdf (Level I)
17 American Osteopathic Association. (2014). Standard 07.02.03. *Healthcare Facilities Accreditation Program: Accreditation requirements for acute care hospitals.* Chicago, IL: American Osteopathic Association. (Level VII)
18 The Joint Commission. (2015). Standard RC.01.03.01. *Comprehensive accreditation manual for hospitals: The official handbook.* Oakbrook Terrace, IL: The Joint Commission. (Level VII)
19 Centers for Medicare & Medicaid Services, Department of Health and Human Services. (2014). Condition of participation: Medical record services. 42 C.F.R. § 482.24(b).
20 American Osteopathic Association. (2014). Standard 10.00.03. *Healthcare Facilities Accreditation Program: Accreditation requirements for acute care hospitals.* Chicago, IL: American Osteopathic Association. (Level VII)
21 Krumholz, A., et al. (2007). Practice parameter: Evaluating an apparent unprovoked first seizure in adults. *Neurology, 69,* 1996–2007. Accessed May 2015 via the Web at http://www.neurology.org/content/69/21/1996.full.pdf (Level VII)
22 Ko, D. Y. (2014). "Epilepsy and seizures" [Online]. Accessed May 2015 via the Web at http://emedicine.medscape.com/article/1184846-overview
23 Epilepsy Foundation. (2014). "Seizure first aid" [Online]. Accessed May 2015 via the Web at http://www.epilepsy.com/get-help/seizure-first-aid
24 Epilepsy Foundation. (2013). "Staying safe" [Online]. Accessed May 2015 via the Web at http://www.epilepsy.com/get-help/staying-safe
25 St. Louis, E. K. (2009). Monitoring antiepileptic drugs: A level-headed approach. *Current Neuropharmacology, 7,* 115–119. Accessed May 2015 via the Web at http://www.ncbi.nlm.nih.gov/pmc/articles/PMC2730002/

SELF-CATHETERIZATION

Self-catheterization is performed by many patients who have some form of impaired or absent bladder function. This form of intermittent catheterization is preferable to an indwelling urinary catheter because intermittent self-catheterization has a lower risk of infection and other complications.[1,2] The two major advantages of self-catheterization are that the patient maintains independence and regains bladder control. Self-catheterization also allows normal sexual intimacy without the fear of incontinence, decreases the chance of urinary reflux, reduces the use of aids and appliances and, in many cases, allows the patient to return to work.

The patient should be taught how to self-catheterize and will need to receive periodic follow-up care to maintain compliance.[1] At home, the patient will use clean technique for self-catheterization.[3] In the health care facility, nurses and the patient can use either clean or sterile technique.

Equipment

Sterile catheter (of appropriate material, diameter, and length)[1] ■ washcloths ■ soap and water ■ small packet of water-soluble lubricant ■ gloves ■ Optional: calibrated drainage container, paper towels, fluid-impermeable pads, gooseneck lamp, catheterization record, mirror.

Implementation

- Review the patient's medical record for contraindications to the procedure and any allergy or sensitivity to latex.
- Verify the practitioner's order.
- Gather the necessary equipment.
- Perform hand hygiene.[3,4,5,6,7,8]
- Confirm the patient's identity using at least two patient identifiers.[9]
- Explain the procedure in the language, reading level, and format appropriate for the patient's level of understanding. Obtain the assistance of a medical interpreter, as needed.[10,11]
- Provide privacy.[12,13,14]
- Tell the patient to begin by trying to urinate into the toilet or, if a toilet isn't available or the patient needs to measure urine quantity, into a calibrated drainage container. Then have the patient perform thorough hand hygiene using soap and water.[15]
- Put on gloves.[16,17]
- Demonstrate how the patient should perform the catheterization, explaining each step clearly and carefully. Position a gooseneck lamp nearby if room lighting is inadequate *to make the urinary meatus clearly visible.* Arrange the patient's clothing so that it's out of the way.

Teaching the male patient

- Tell the patient to wash and rinse the end of his penis thoroughly with soap and water, pulling back the foreskin, if appropriate. As applicable, he should keep the foreskin pulled back during the procedure.
- Show him how to squeeze lubricant onto a paper towel and have him roll the first 6″ to 8″ (15 to 20 cm) of the catheter in the lubricant. *Tell him that copious lubrication will make the procedure more comfortable for him.* Then show him how to insert the catheter. (See *Teaching the male patient self-catheterization,* page 686.)
- When the urine stops draining, tell him to remove the catheter slowly and, if necessary, pull the foreskin forward again.
- Have him get dressed.

Teaching the female patient

- Demonstrate and explain to the patient that she should separate the vaginal folds as widely as possible with the fingers of her nondominant hand *to obtain a full view of the urinary meatus.* She may need to use a mirror *to visualize the meatus.* Ask if she's right- or left-handed and, if necessary, tell her which is her nondominant hand.
- Instruct the patient to hold her labia open with the nondominant hand and then to use the dominant hand to wash the perineal area thoroughly with a soapy washcloth, using downward strokes. Tell her to rinse the soap from the area with another clean wet or damp washcloth using downward strokes as well.
- Show her how to squeeze some lubricant onto the first 2″ to 4″ (5 to 10 cm) of the catheter and then how to insert the catheter. (See *Teaching the female patient self-catheterization,* page 686.)

PATIENT TEACHING

Teaching the male patient self-catheterization

Teach the patient to find a comfortable position (some men prefer to stand for the procedure but it can be done just as easily in the sitting position)[18] and hold his penis in his nondominant hand, at a right angle to his body. He should hold the catheter in his dominant hand as if it were a pencil or a dart and slowly insert it 6″ to 8″ (15.2 to 20.3 cm) into the urethra until urine begins flowing. If resistance is felt at the passage of the catheter at the prostatic urethra, instruct the patient to apply firm, gently, steady pressure to the pelvic floor muscles and the muscles should relax, allowing the catheter to pass.[18] Then he should gently advance the catheter about 1″ (2.5 cm) further, allowing all urine to drain into the toilet or drainage container.

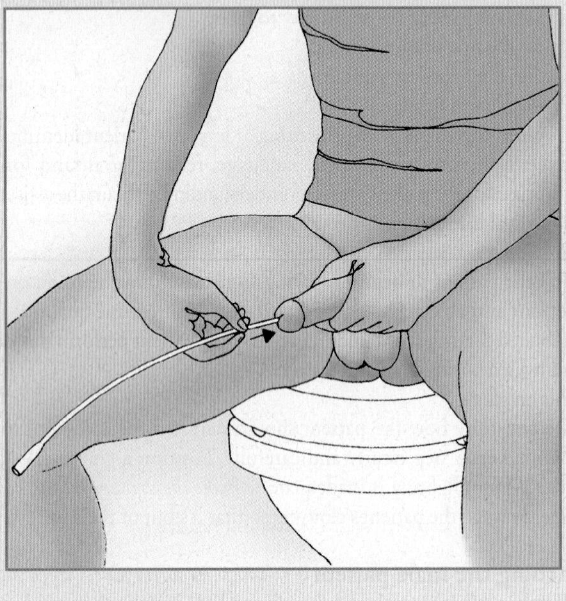

PATIENT TEACHING

Teaching the female patient self-catheterization

Instruct the female patient to hold the catheter in her dominant hand as if it were a pencil or a dart, about ½″ (1.3 cm) from its tip. Keeping the vaginal folds separated, tell her to slowly insert the lubricated catheter about 2″ to 4″ (5 to 10 cm) into the urethra. Inform her if she feels resistance, she should apply, firm, gentle, steady pressure to the pelvic floor muscles; the muscles should then relax, allowing the catheter to pass.[18] Tell her to press down with her abdominal muscles *to empty the bladder,* allowing all urine to drain through the catheter and into the toilet or drainage container.

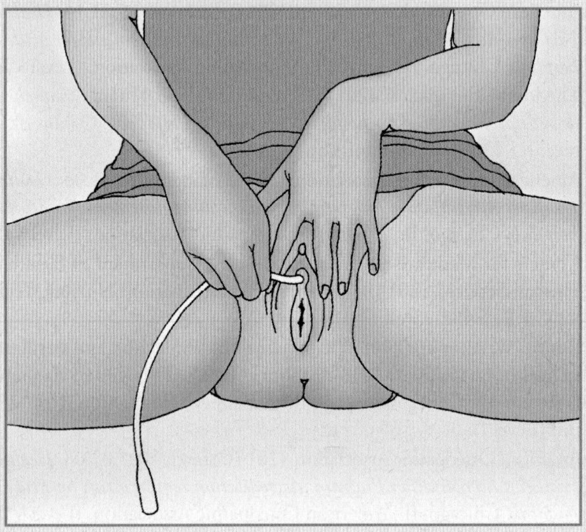

■ When the urine stops draining, tell her to remove the catheter slowly and get dressed.

Completing the procedure

■ Tell the patient to dispose of equipment appropriately and to perform hand hygiene.
■ Remove and discard your gloves.[16,17]
■ Perform hand hygiene.[4,5,6,7,8]
■ Document the procedure.[19,20,21]

Special considerations

■ Avoid latex exposure in patients who require frequent catheterization.[22]
■ Hydrophilic catheters might be preferable to standard catheters for patients requiring intermittent catheterization.[4] Catheter choice more often depends on the patient's general clinical situation, such as injury, manual dexterity, visual impairment, urethral sensibility, and age, than on the cause of the bladder dysfunction.[1]
■ A female patient may prefer a shorter catheter of 6″ to 12″ (15 cm to 30 cm), which is easier to grasp and manipulate, *because women have shorter urethras than men and a shorter catheter won't loop or kink, allowing urine to more easily drain through the catheter.*[1]
■ Catheters with lengths of approximately 16″ (about 40 cm) allow for adequate passage through a male urethra.[1]
■ Curved and olive-tipped catheters are available as needed for certain clinical conditions, such as urethral strictures or enlarged prostates. Closed intermittent catheterization systems are also available and have been designed to reduce contamination of the bladder *because the catheter never comes in direct contact with the inserter's hands.*[1]
■ Follow the manufacturer's instructions for catheter use. Single-use devices shouldn't be reused in any setting.[1] Instruct the patient to keep a supply of catheters at home and to use a new catheter each time.
■ Explain to the patient that the timing of catheterization is critical *to prevent overdistention of the bladder, which can lead to infection.* Self-catheterization is usually performed every 4 to 6 hours around the clock (or more often at first).
■ Stress the importance of regulating fluid intake, as ordered, *to prevent incontinence while maintaining adequate hydration.* However, explain that incontinent episodes may occur occasionally. For managing incontinence, the practitioner or a home health care nurse can help develop a plan such as more frequent catheterizations. After an incontinent episode, tell the patient to wash with soap and water, pat the area dry with a towel, and expose the skin to the air for as long as possible. Bedding and furniture can be protected by covering them with rubber or plastic sheets and then covering the rubber or plastic with fabric.
■ Stress the importance of taking medications as ordered *to increase urine retention and help prevent incontinence.*
■ Explain that if the patient can't pass the catheter and can feel that the bladder is full, the patient should contact the practitioner immediately.[18]

Patient teaching

At discharge, give the patient individualized written instructions regarding home care.[15,23] *To prevent urinary tract infections (UTIs) associated with catheterization,* emphasize the importance of hand and perineal hygiene. Also instruct the patient to perform catheterization after voiding (if the patient maintains the capacity to void spontaneously),[1] before a bowel movement *to minimize bacterial contamination of the urethra,* and right before bed *to minimize nocturia.*[15] Encourage the female patient to clean the perineal area immediately after vaginal intercourse and to avoid the use of spermicidal lubricants *because these products may alter vaginal and urethral flora.*[1] Advise the patient to keep a voiding diary to help evaluate bladder emptying over time.[15] If the patient has difficulty practicing self-catheterization because of limited mobility, vision, or dexterity, family members and caregivers can be taught the procedure.[2] Provide the patient and family with contact information for appropriate follow-up and peer support *to enhance compliance.*[15]

Complications

Overdistention of the bladder can lead to a UTI and urine leakage. Long-term complications may include such urethral- and bladder-related conditions as bleeding, kidney stone formation, urethritis, stricture, and creation of a false passage.[1] Improper hand washing or equipment cleaning can also lead to a UTI.

Documentation

Record the date and time of catheterization, the characteristics of the urine (color, odor, clarity, and presence of particles or blood), the amount of urine (increased, decreased, or no change), and any problems encountered during the procedure. Note whether the patient has difficulty performing a return demonstration.

REFERENCES

1 Newman, D. K., & Wilson, M. M. (2011). Review of intermittent catheterization and current best practices. *Urology Nursing, 31,* 12–28. Accessed May 2015 via the Web at http://www.suna.org/sites/default/files/download/education/2013/article3101229.pdf

2 Herter, R., & Wallace-Kazer, M. (2010). Best practices in urinary catheter care. *Home Healthcare Nurse, 28,* 342–349. Accessed May 2015 via the Web at http://journals.lww.com/homehealthcarenurseonline/Fulltext/2010/06000/Best_Practices_in_Urinary_Catheter_Care.5.aspx

3 Healthcare Infection Control Practices Advisory Committee. (2010). "Guideline for prevention of catheter-associated urinary tract infections, 2009" [Online]. Accessed May 2015 via the Web at http://www.cdc.gov/hicpac/pdf/CAUTI/CAUTIguideline2009final.pdf (Level I)

4 Centers for Disease Control and Prevention. (2002). Guideline for hand hygiene in health-care settings: Recommendations of the Healthcare Infection Control Practices Advisory Committee and the HICPAC/SHEA/APIC/IDSA Hand Hygiene Task Force. *MMWR Recommendations and Reports, 51*(RR-16), 1–45. Accessed May 2015 via the Web at http://www.cdc.gov/mmwr/pdf/rr/rr5116.pdf (Level II)

5 World Health Organization. (2009). "WHO guidelines on hand hygiene in health care: First global patient safety challenge, clean care is safer care" [Online]. Accessed May 2015 via the Web at http://whqlibdoc.who.int/publications/2009/9789241597906_eng.pdf (Level IV)

6 The Joint Commission. (2015). Standard NPSG.07.01.01. *Comprehensive accreditation manual for hospitals: The official handbook.* Oakbrook Terrace, IL: The Joint Commission. (Level VII)

7 American Osteopathic Association. (2014). Standard 07.01.21. *Healthcare Facilities Accreditation Program: Accreditation requirements for acute care hospitals.* Chicago, IL: American Osteopathic Association. (Level VII)

8 Centers for Medicare & Medicaid Services, Department of Health and Human Services. (2014). Condition of participation: Infection control. 42 C.F.R. § 482.42.

9 The Joint Commission. (2015). Standard NPSG.01.01.01. *Comprehensive accreditation manual for hospitals: The official handbook.* Oakbrook Terrace, IL: The Joint Commission. (Level VII)

10 The Joint Commission. (2015). Standard PC.04.01.05. *Comprehensive accreditation manual for hospitals: The official handbook.* Oakbrook Terrace, IL: The Joint Commission. (Level VII)

11 The Joint Commission. (2010). *Advancing effective communication, cultural competence, and patient-, and family-centered care: A roadmap for hospitals.* Oakbrook Terrace, IL: The Joint Commission. Accessed May 2015 via the Web at http://www.jointcommission.org/assets/1/6/ARoadmapforHospitalsfinalversion727.pdf (Level VII)

12 The Joint Commission. (2015). Standard RI.01.01.01. *Comprehensive accreditation manual for hospitals: The official handbook.* Oakbrook Terrace, IL: The Joint Commission. (Level VII)

13 Centers for Medicare & Medicaid Services, Department of Health and Human Services. (2014). Condition of participation: Patient's rights. 42 C.F.R. § 482.13(c)(1).

14 American Osteopathic Association. (2014). Standard 15.01.16. *Healthcare Facilities Accreditation Program: Accreditation requirements for acute care hospitals.* Chicago, IL: American Osteopathic Association. (Level VII)

15 Vahr, S., et al. (2013). *Catheterisation. Urethral intermittent in adults: Dilatation, urethral intermittent in adults.* Arnhem: European Association of Urology Nurses. (Level VII)

16 American Osteopathic Association. (2014). Standard 07.01.10. *Healthcare Facilities Accreditation Program: Accreditation requirements for acute care hospitals.* Chicago, IL: American Osteopathic Association. (Level VII)

17 Siegel, J. D., et al. (2007). "2007 guideline for isolation precautions: Preventing transmission of infectious agents in healthcare settings" [Online]. Accessed May 2015 via the Web at http://www.cdc.gov/hicpac/pdf/isolation/Isolation2007.pdf (Level II)

18 Society for Urologic Nurses and Associates. (2006). "Clinical practice guidelines: Adult clean intermittent catheterization" [Online]. Accessed May 2015 via the Web at http://www.suna.org/resources/adultCICGuide.pdf (Level VII)

19 The Joint Commission. (2015). Standard RC.01.03.01. *Comprehensive accreditation manual for hospitals: The official handbook.* Oakbrook Terrace, IL: The Joint Commission. (Level VII)

20 Centers for Medicare & Medicaid Services, Department of Health and Human Services. (2014). Condition of participation: Medical record services. 42 C.F.R. § 482.24(b).

21 American Osteopathic Association. (2014). Standard 10.00.03. *Healthcare Facilities Accreditation Program: Accreditation requirements for acute care hospitals.* Chicago, IL: American Osteopathic Association. (Level VII)

22 Sussman, G., & Gold, M. (1996). *Guidelines for the management of latex allergies and safe latex use in health care facilities.* Ottawa: CHA Press. Accessed May 2015 via the Web at http://www.sussmanresearch.com/wp-content/uploads/2014/01/Guidlines-For-The-Management-Of-Latex-Allergies-And-Safe-Latex-Use-In-Healthcare-Facilities.pdf (Level VII)

23 Centers for Medicare & Medicaid Services, Department of Health and Human Services. (2014). Condition of participation: Discharge planning. 42 C.F.R. § 482.43.

SEQUENTIAL COMPRESSION THERAPY

Sequential compression therapy helps prevent venous thromboembolism, a disorder that includes deep vein thrombosis (DVT) and pulmonary embolism in patients at risk. This safe, effective, noninvasive therapy massages the legs in a wavelike, milking motion that promotes blood flow in the lower extremities to decrease the risk of thrombosis. A study of 2,270 postsurgical patients found a 60% reduction in DVT compared with a control group without prophylaxis.[1]

HOSPITAL-ACQUIRED CONDITION ALERT *Venous thromboembolism in patients who underwent total knee or hip replacement is considered a hospital-acquired condition because using best practices can reasonably prevent the condition.*[2,3] *Prevention practices, such as the use of mechanical compression devices, including antiembolism stockings and intermittent pneumatic compression devices (also known as sequential compression therapy); early ambulation; and pharmacologic prophylaxis, reduce the risk of venous thromboembolism.*[4]

Sequential compression therapy is used in combination with anticoagulant medications to prevent DVT in low- to moderate-risk patients. However, sequential compression is used without anticoagulants for patients at high risk for bleeding.[5,6,7] Preventive measures continue for as long as the patient remains at risk.

Both antiembolism stockings and sequential compression sleeves are commonly used preoperatively and postoperatively because blood clots tend to form during surgery. About 20% of blood clots form in the femoral vein; sequential compression therapy counteracts blood stasis and coagulation changes, two of the three major factors that promote DVT. It reduces stasis by increasing peak blood flow velocity, which helps empty the femoral vein's valve cusps of pooled or static blood., The compressions also cause an anticlotting effect by increasing fibrinolytic activity, which stimulates the release of a plasminogen activator.

Studies show that as many as 81% of patients at risk for developing DVT don't comply with sequential compression therapy.[6] Explaining the procedure to patients, including the importance of complying with therapy, can promote compliance.

Sequential compression therapy shouldn't be used in patients with acute DVT (or DVT diagnosed within the last 6 months), serious arterial insufficiency, ischemic vascular disease, massive edema of the legs resulting from pulmonary edema or heart failure, or any local condition that the compression sleeves would aggravate, such as dermatitis, wound infection, cellulitis, gangrene, or vein ligation (immediate postoperative).[8,9] It's also unlikely to benefit patients with pronounced leg deformities.

Equipment

Measuring tape and sizing chart for the brand of sleeves you're using ▪ pair of compression sleeves in correct size ▪ connecting tubing ▪ compression controller ▪ hospital-grade disinfectant.

Implementation

Initiating compression therapy

- Verify the practitioner's order.
- Perform hand hygiene.[10,11,12,13,14]
- Confirm the patient's identity using at least two patient identifiers.[15,16]
- Explain the procedure to the patient *to increase cooperation and compliance.*

Determining the proper sleeve size

- Measure the circumference of the upper thigh while the patient rests in bed by placing the measuring tape under the thigh at the gluteal furrow (as shown below).

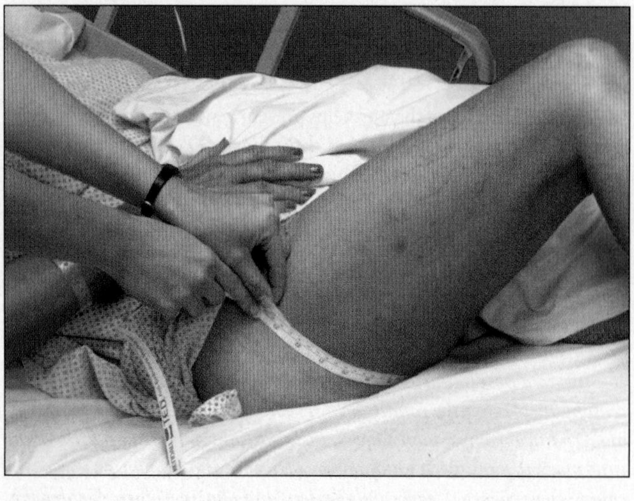

- Hold the tape snugly, but not tightly, around the patient's leg. Note the exact circumference.
- Find the patient's thigh measurement on the sizing chart, and locate the corresponding size of compression sleeves.
- Remove the compression sleeves from the package and unfold them.
- Lay the unfolded sleeves on a flat surface with the cotton lining facing up (as shown below).

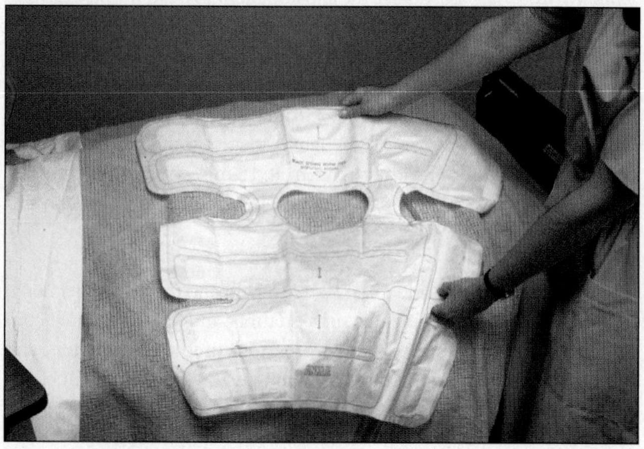

- Note the markings on the lining denoting the ankle and the area behind the knee at the popliteal pulse point. Use these markings to position the sleeve at the appropriate landmarks.

Applying the sleeves

- Place the patient's leg on the sleeve lining. Position the back of the knee over the popliteal opening.
- Make sure that the back of the ankle is over the ankle marking.
- Starting at the side opposite the clear plastic tubing, wrap the sleeve snugly around the patient's leg.
- Fasten the sleeve securely with the Velcro fasteners. *For the best fit,* first secure the ankle and calf sections, and then the thigh.
- The sleeve should fit snugly, but not tightly. Check the fit by inserting two fingers between the sleeve and the patient's leg at the knee opening. Loosen or tighten the sleeve by readjusting the Velcro fastener.
- Using the same procedure, apply the second sleeve (as shown below).

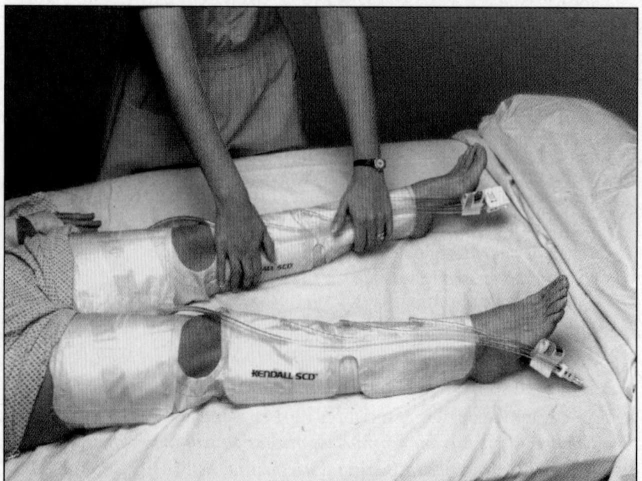

Operating the system

- Connect each sleeve to the tubing leading to the controller. (Some devices require that both sleeves be attached to the controller for the controller to function.) Line up the blue arrows on the sleeve connector with the arrows on the tubing connectors, and push the ends together firmly. Listen for a click, signaling a firm connection. Make sure that the tubing is not kinked.

- Plug the compression controller into the proper wall outlet. Turn on the power. If your controller can function with one or both sleeves attached, be sure to turn on the sleeves that are needed. The controller automatically sets the compression sleeve pressure at 45 mm Hg, which is the midpoint of the normal range (35 to 55 mm Hg).
- Observe to see how well the patient tolerates the therapy and to make sure the controller is working properly as the system completes its first cycle.
- Check the AUDIBLE ALARM key. The green light should be lit, indicating that the alarm is working.[17]
- Perform hand hygiene.[10,11,12,13,14]
- Document the procedure.[18,19,20]

Discontinuing compression therapy

- Verify the practitioner's order.
- Perform hand hygiene.[10,11,12,13,14]
- Confirm the patient's identity using at least two patient identifiers.[15,16]
- Explain the procedure to the patient *to increase compliance.*
- Turn off the power.
- Open the Velcro fasteners on the sleeves and remove them from the extremity.
- Depress the latches on each side of the connector and pull them apart *to disconnect the tubing from the compressor.*
- Clean and disinfect the tubing and compressor using a hospital-grade disinfectant.[21,22]
- Store the tubing and compressor as determined by your facility *because this equipment isn't disposable.*
- Perform hand hygiene.[10,11,12,14]
- Document the procedure.[18,19,20]

Special considerations

- The compression sleeves should function continuously (24 hours daily) until the patient is fully ambulatory. Check the sleeves at least once each shift *to ensure proper fit and inflation.*[17]
- Remove the sleeves when the patient is walking, bathing, or leaving the room for tests or other procedures by undoing the Velcro fasteners. Reapply them immediately after any of these activities.[17]
- Remove the sleeves and assess and document skin integrity every 8 hours *to avoid skin breakdown,* especially in patients with decreased sensation or who are unresponsive.
- Assess the extremities for peripheral pulses, edema, changes in sensation, and movement at least once each shift.
- Knee-length sleeves are also available. Measure the patient's calf circumference to determine the proper size. Application is similar to thigh-length sleeves.
- The compression controller also has a mechanism to help cool the patient.
- If you're applying only one sleeve—for example, if the patient has a cast—leave the unused sleeve folded in the plastic bag. Cut a small hole in the bag's sealed bottom edge, and pull the sleeve connector (the part that holds the connecting tubing) through the hole. Then you can join both sleeves to the compression controller.
- If a malfunction triggers the instrument's alarm, you'll hear beeping. The system shuts off whenever the alarm is activated. To respond to the alarm, follow the instructions provided by the manufacturer.

Patient teaching

Teach the patient about the compression device and the importance of compliance with the therapy.

Complications

The most common complication of compression therapy is skin irritation, which usually results from sweating.

Documentation

Document the procedure, the patient's response to and understanding of the procedure, and the status of the alarm and cooling settings.

REFERENCES

1 Urbankova, J., et al. (2005). "Intermittent pneumatic compression and deep vein thrombosis prevention: A meta-analysis in postoperative patients" [Online]. Accessed May 2015 via the Web at http://venoushealth.com/wp-content/uploads/2011/06/DVT_Web_IPC-and-DVT-prevention.pdf (Level I)

2 Centers for Medicare & Medicaid Services, Department of Health and Human Services. (2012). "Hospital-acquired conditions" [Online]. Accessed May 2015 via the Web at http://www.cms.gov/Medicare/Medicare-Fee-for-Service-Payment/HospitalAcqCond/Hospital-Acquired_Conditions.html

3 National Hospital Inpatient Quality Reporting Measures Specifications Manual. (2013). "Release Notes Version: 4.3b" [Online]. Accessed May 2015 via the Web at http://www.qualitynet.org/dcs/ContentServer?c=Page&pagename=QnetPublic%2FPage%2FQnetTier4&cid=1228773564870

4 Jarrett, N., et al. (2013). "Evidence-based guidelines for selected and previously considered hospital-acquired conditions: Final report" [Online]. Accessed May 2015 via the Web at http://www.cms.gov/Medicare/Medicare-Fee-for-Service-Payment/HospitalAcqCond/Downloads/Evidence-Based-Guidelines.pdf

5 Ennis, R. S. (2011). "Deep venous thrombosis prophylaxis in orthopedic surgery" [Online]. Accessed May 2015 via the Web at http://emedicine.medscape.com/article/1268573-overview#a1

6 American Association of Critical-Care Nurses. (2010). "AACN practice alert: Venous thromboembolism prevention" [Online]. Accessed May 2015 via the Web at http://www.aacn.org/WD/Practice/Docs/PracticeAlerts/VTE%20Prevention%2004-2010%20final.pdf (Level II)

7 Meyer, S. (2010). Leg compression and pharmacologic prophylaxis for venous thromboembolism prevention in high-risk patients. *American Family Physician, 81,* 284–285. (Level I)

8 Centers for Medicare & Medicaid Services. (2001). "Decision memo for pneumatic compression pumps for venous insufficiency" [Online]. Accessed May 2015 via the Web at http://cms.hhs.gov/medicare-coverage-database/details/nca-decision-memo.aspx?NCAId=63&NcaName=Pneumatic+Compression+Pumps+for+Venous+Insufficiency&NCDId=225&ncdver=1&IsPopup=y&bc=AAAAAAAACAAAAA%3D%3D&

9 Kendall. (n.d.). "Model 7325 operation and service manual: SCD response compression system" [Online]. Accessed May 2015 via the Web at http://www.meql.com/Manuals/Kendall-Response-7325-Manual.pdf

10 The Joint Commission. (2015). Standard NPSG.07.01.01. *Comprehensive accreditation manual for hospitals: The official handbook.* Oakbrook Terrace, IL: The Joint Commission. (Level VII)

11 Centers for Disease Control and Prevention. (2002). Guideline for hand hygiene in health-care settings: Recommendations of the Healthcare Infection Control Practices Advisory Committee and the HICPAC/SHEA/APIC/IDSA Hand Hygiene Task Force. *MMWR Recommendations and Reports, 51*(RR-16), 1–45. Accessed May 2015 via the Web at http://www.cdc.gov/mmwr/pdf/rr/rr5116.pdf (Level II)

12 World Health Organization. (2009). "WHO guidelines on hand hygiene in health care: First global patient safety challenge, clean care is safer care" [Online]. Accessed May 2015 via the Web at http://whqlibdoc.who.int/publications/2009/9789241597906_eng.pdf (Level IV)

13 American Osteopathic Association. (2014). Standard 07.01.21 *Healthcare Facilities Accreditation Program: Accreditation requirements for acute care hospitals.* Chicago, IL: American Osteopathic Association. (Level VII)

14 Centers for Medicare & Medicaid Services, Department of Health and Human Services. (2014). Condition of participation: Infection control. 42 C.F.R. § 482.42.

15 The Joint Commission. (2015). Standard NPSG.01.01.01. *Comprehensive accreditation manual for hospitals: The official handbook.* Oakbrook Terrace, IL: The Joint Commission. (Level VII)
16 American Osteopathic Association. (2014). Standard 30.00.14. *Healthcare Facilities Accreditation Program: Accreditation requirements for acute care hospitals.* Chicago, IL: American Osteopathic Association. (Level VII)
17 Association of Perioperative Registered Nurses (AORN). (2013). *Perioperative standards and recommended practices.* Denver, CO: AORN, Inc. (Level I)
18 The Joint Commission. (2015). Standard RC.01.03.01. *Comprehensive accreditation manual for hospitals: The official handbook.* Oakbrook Terrace, IL: The Joint Commission. (Level VII)
19 American Osteopathic Association. (2014). Standard 10.00.03. *Healthcare Facilities Accreditation Program: Accreditation requirements for acute care hospitals.* Chicago, IL: American Osteopathic Association. (Level VII)
20 Centers for Medicare & Medicaid Services, Department of Health and Human Services. (2013). Condition of participation: Medical record services. 42 C.F.R. § 482.24(b).
21 Rutala, W. A., et al. (2008). "Guideline for disinfection and sterilization in healthcare facilities, 2008" [Online]. Accessed May 2015 via the Web at http://www.cdc.gov/hicpac/pdf/guidelines/Disinfection_Nov_2008.pdf (Level I)
22 American Osteopathic Association. (2014). Standard 07.02.03. *Healthcare Facilities Accreditation Program: Accreditation requirements for acute care hospitals.* Chicago, IL: American Osteopathic Association. (Level VII)

ADDITIONAL REFERENCES

American Congress of Obstetricians and Gynecologists (ACOG) Committee on Practice Bulletins. (2011). ACOG practice bulletin number 123: Thromboembolism in pregnancy. *Obstetrics and Gynecology, 118,* 718–729.
Boelig, M. M., et al. (2011). Are sequential compression devices commonly associated with in-hospital falls? A myth-busters review using the patient safety net database. *Journal of Patient Safety, 7,* 77–79. (Level IV)
Craven, R. F., & Hirnle, C. J. (2012). *Fundamentals of nursing: Human health and function* (7th ed.). Philadelphia, PA: Lippincott Williams & Wilkins.
Guyatt, G. H., et al. (2012). Executive summary: Antithrombotic and thrombolytic therapy, 9th ed.: American College of Chest Physicians evidence-based clinical practice guidelines. *Chest, 141,* 7S–47S. (Level I)
Qaseem, A., et al. (2011). "Venous thromboembolism prophylaxis in hospitalized patients: A clinical practice guideline from the American College of Physicians" [Online]. Accessed May 2015 via the Web at http://www.annals.org/content/155/9/625.full.pdf+html (Level I)

SEXUAL ASSAULT EXAMINATION

Each facility or agency has a specific protocol for specimen collection in cases involving sexual assault. Collected from various sources, specimens can include blood, hair, nails, tissues, and such body fluids as urine, semen, saliva, and vaginal secretions. In addition, evidence can be obtained from the results of diagnostic tests, such as computed tomography and radiography. Regardless of the protocol or specimen source, accurate and precise specimen collection is essential in conjunction with thorough, objective documentation because in many cases this information will be used as evidence in legal proceedings.

Many facilities have a Sexual Assault Nurse Examiner (SANE) available to care for patients who are victims of sexual assault. The SANE is a skilled professional who can provide comprehensive care to the sexual assault patient and collect evidence. The SANE may also be called upon at a later date to testify in legal proceedings.

If you're responsible for collecting specimens in a sexual assault, follow these important guidelines:

- Know your facility's method for specimen collection in sexual assault cases.
- When obtaining specimens, collect them from the victim and, if possible, from the suspect.
- Inform local law enforcement about the suspected assault after consent for release of information has been obtained from the patient.[1,2]
- Check with local law enforcement agencies about additional specimens they may need; for example, such trace evidence as soot, grass, gravel, glass, or other debris.
- Wear gloves and change them frequently; use disposable equipment and instruments if possible.[3]
- Avoid coughing, sneezing, or talking over specimens or touching your face, nose, or mouth when collecting specimens.
- Include the victim's clothing as part of the collection procedure.
- Place all items collected in a paper bag.[3]

NURSING ALERT *Never allow a specimen or item considered as evidence to be left unattended.*

- Document each item or specimen collected.
- Label each specimen in the presence of the patient *to prevent mislabeling.*[4]
- Obtain photographs of all injuries *for documentation.*[3]
- Include written documentation of the victim's physical and psychological condition on the first encounter, throughout specimen collection, and afterward.

Equipment

Powder-free, nonlubricated gloves ■ Wood lamp ■ sexual assault evidence collection kit that typically includes examination paper, tweezers, tape, nail clippers and scrapers, saline solution or distilled water, clean paper bags (one for each article of clothing), envelopes, scissors, sterile containers, pencil or pen, swabs for specimen collection, comb, ethylenediaminetetra acetic acid (EDTA) blood collection tube or blood collection filter paper, slides, envelope, deoxyribonucleic acid (DNA) stain card (contents can vary; some jurisdictions have a customized kit)[3] ■ supplies for venipuncture (see the "Venipuncture," procedure page 821) ■ supplies for urine specimen collection ■ camera ■ Optional: colposcope, anoscope,[3] tetanus toxoid, hepatitis B vaccination, antibiotics, sexually transmitted infection (STI) prophylaxis, human immunodeficiency virus (HIV) prophylaxis, emergency contraception.[5]

Preparation of equipment

Make sure that the sexual assault collection kit contains the necessary items for specimen collection, based on the evidence required by the local crime laboratory. The kit contains a form that must be completed, signed, and dated by the examiner.

Implementation

- Perform hand hygiene.[6,7,8,9,10]
- Ensure patient privacy throughout the collection procedure.[3]
- Confirm the patient's identity using at least two patient identifiers.[4]
- Assess the patient's ability to undergo the specimen collection procedure.
- Explain the procedures that the patient will undergo, explain what specimens will be collected and from where, and obtain consent as required.[3]
- Provide emotional support throughout the procedure. Obtain the assistance of a social worker or patient advocate as indicated.[3]
- Inform the patient that the presence of family members, friends, and others offering personal support during the examination may influence or be perceived as influencing the patient's statements. If the patient chooses to have anyone else present despite this knowledge, those present should not actively participate in the process.[3]
- Obtain a detailed forensic history from the patient, which is intended to guide the forensic examination, evidence collection, and the patient's medical treatment.[3]
- Put on powder-free, nonlubricated gloves.[11,12]

■ If the patient can stand, ask the patient to stand on a clean piece of examination paper; if the patient can't stand, then have the patient remain on the examination table or bed.
■ Have the patient remove each article of clothing, one at a time. Place each article in a separate, clean paper bag.[3]
■ If the clothing is wet, allow it to dry first before placing the item into the paper bag.
NURSING ALERT *Don't use plastic bags to collect clothing.* Plastic promotes bacterial growth and can destroy DNA evidence.[3]
■ Fold the examination paper onto itself and place it into a clean paper bag.
■ Fold over, seal, label, and initial each bag.
■ Before obtaining specimens, inspect the genital area using a Wood lamp. *This device uses long-wave ultraviolet light to scan the area for secretions and helps identify areas of trauma.*
NURSING ALERT *In some jurisdictions, toluidine blue dye may be used to highlight areas of trauma, but its use is controversial* because it may be perceived by the court as changing the appearance of the tissue. *Therefore, it isn't universally used. When employed, toluidine blue dye should be applied using a cotton swab before an internal or digital speculum examination is performed.*[3]

Collecting vaginal or cervical secretions
■ Keep in mind when collecting specimens that the quality of the swabs collected is specific to the type of specimen. For moist secretions, typically a one-swab technique is used; if secretions are dry, then a two-swab technique is used.
■ Swab the vaginal area thoroughly with four swabs, or according to local jurisdiction; swab the cervical area with two swabs, making sure to keep the vaginal swabs separate from the cervical swabs.
■ Gently roll each vaginal swab over a slide and allow the slides and swabs to air-dry; do the same for the cervical swabs.
■ Place the vaginal swabs in the swab container and close it; place the slides in the cardboard sleeve, close it, and tape it shut; repeat this procedure for the cervical swabs.
■ Place the swab container and cardboard sleeve into the envelope, and seal it securely.
■ Complete the information requested on the front of the envelope; if vaginal and cervical swabs are obtained, use a separate envelope for each.

Collecting anal secretions
■ Moisten the provided swabs with sterile water.
■ Insert each swab gently, approximately 1¼″ (3.2 cm) into the patient's rectum.
■ Rotate the swab gently, and then remove it.
■ Allow the swabs to air-dry and then place them in an envelope.
■ Seal and label the envelope appropriately.

Collecting penile secretions
■ Moisten the provided swabs with sterile water.
■ Swab the entire external surface of the penis.
■ Repeat this at least one more time (so that you obtain at least two swabs).
■ Allow the swabs to air-dry and then place them in an envelope.
■ Seal and label the envelope appropriately.

Collecting pubic hair
■ Place the provided collection paper under the patient's buttocks and, using the comb provided in the kit, comb through the pubic hair.[3] *The purpose is to collect any debris, trace evidence, or hair from the suspect that may be present.*
■ Fold the collection paper containing the comb, hair, and other debris, and place it in an envelope. Seal and label the envelope appropriately.
■ Alternatively, if requested in your local jurisdiction, obtain 20 to 30 plucked hairs from the patient as reference samples; allow the patient the option of plucking his or her own pubic hair.
■ Place the plucked hair in the envelope; seal and label it appropriately.

Collecting blood samples
■ After performing a venipuncture, obtain at least 5 mL of blood in an EDTA tube.
■ Write the patient's name and date on the label of the tube.
■ Remove the DNA stain card from the kit and label it with the patient's name.
■ Withdraw 1 mL of blood from the EDTA blood collection tube, and apply blood to each of the four circles on the card, completely filling each circle if possible.
■ Let the card air-dry and then place the card in the envelope.
■ Seal and label the envelope appropriately.
■ Place the blood tube into the tube holder supplied in the kit, and seal the holder with the tape supplied in the kit (may be referred to as evidence tape).
■ Place the tube and holder in the zippered bag provided.
■ Collect additional blood samples to test for pregnancy; STIs, such as HIV and syphilis; or toxicology, as appropriate, and send them to the laboratory immediately.

Collecting urine specimens
■ Obtain a random urine specimen from the patient. Remind the patient not to use cleaning wipes *to avoid destroying possible evidence.*
■ Obtain a urine specimen for drug screening immediately if it's suspected that the patient was given drugs to facilitate the sexual assault and if the examination takes place within 96 hours of the assault.[3]

Storing and transporting specimens
■ Place blood samples inside the evidence collection envelope, which must be refrigerated while maintaining the chain of custody.[3]
■ You can store evidence collection envelopes without blood samples at room temperature while maintaining the chain of custody.[3]
■ Remove and discard your gloves and perform hand hygiene.[6,7,8,9,10]
■ Give all the specimens to the police when they arrive.
■ Carefully document the handoff *to ensure proper chain of custody.*[3]
■ Document the procedure.[13,14,15]

Special considerations
■ Follow the directions in the sexual assault evidence collection kit precisely *to ensure that the proper chain of custody is followed.*
■ If a female or transgender male patient is menstruating, collect tampons and sanitary napkins. Air dry them as much as possible, and then place them in a separate paper collection bag.[3]
■ Provide culturally sensitive follow-up counseling and support to the patient. Provide referrals as necessary.[3]
■ If necessary, administer ordered medications, such as tetanus toxoid, antibiotics for STI prophylaxis, emergency contraceptives, and HIV prophylaxis.[5]
■ Assess the patient's hepatitis B immunization status; vaccinate the patient, as needed and prescribed.[5]
■ Make sure a support person is available to accompany the patient home.
■ Arrange for a referral to a local support group or a trained counselor for follow-up.
■ Report cases of suspected child abuse in accordance with state guidelines.[5]

Patient teaching

At the initial examination and, if indicated, at follow-up examinations, counsel the patient about the signs and symptoms of STIs, the need for immediate examination if signs and symptoms occur, and the importance of abstaining from sexual intercourse until STI prophylaxis is completed.[5] Provide discharge instructions that include planning for safety. Discuss examination payment and reimbursement information, steps and options in the criminal justice process, community resources that are available to sexual assault victims, and procedures for patients to access their medical records and applicable law enforcement reports.[3]

Documentation

For each specimen collected, document the type of specimen, the area from which you collected the specimen, the time, the patient's name and identification number, and other relevant information. Include photographs as appropriate, making sure to also include relevant information about each photo. Regardless of the protocol or specimen source, collect all specimens accurately and precisely, and document thoroughly and objectively because, in many cases, this information will be used as evidence in legal proceedings.

References

1 The Joint Commission. (2015). Standard RI.01.06.03. *Comprehensive accreditation manual for hospitals: The official handbook.* Oakbrook Terrace, IL: The Joint Commission. (Level VII)

2 The Joint Commission. (2015). Standard PC.01.02.09. *Comprehensive accreditation manual for hospitals: The official handbook.* Oakbrook Terrace, IL: The Joint Commission. (Level VII)

3 U.S. Department of Justice, Office on Violence Against Women. (2013). "A national protocol for sexual assault medical forensic examinations" [Online]. Accessed May 2015 via the Web at https://www.ncjrs.gov/pdffiles1/ovw/241903.pdf (Level VII)

4 The Joint Commission. (2015). Standard NPSG.01.01.01. *Comprehensive accreditation manual for hospitals: The official handbook.* Oakbrook Terrace, IL: The Joint Commission. (Level VII)

5 Centers for Disease Control and Prevention. (2010). "Sexual assault and STDs. Sexually transmitted diseases: Treatment guidelines, 2010" [Online]. Accessed May 2015 via the Web at http://www.cdc.gov/std/treatment/2010/sexual-assault.htm (Level II)

6 The Joint Commission. (2015). Standard NPSG.07.01.01. *Comprehensive accreditation manual for hospitals: The official handbook.* Oakbrook Terrace, IL: The Joint Commission. (Level VII)

7 Centers for Disease Control and Prevention. (2002). Guideline for hand hygiene in health-care settings: Recommendations of the Healthcare Infection Control Practices Advisory Committee and the HICPAC/SHEA/APIC/IDSA Hand Hygiene Task Force. *MMWR Recommendations and Reports, 51*(RR-16), 1–45. Accessed May 2015 via the Web at http://www.cdc.gov/mmwr/pdf/rr/rr5116.pdf (Level II)

8 World Health Organization. (2009). "WHO guidelines on hand hygiene in health care: First global patient safety challenge, clean care is safer care" [Online]. Accessed May 2015 via the Web at http://whqlibdoc.who.int/publications/2009/9789241597906_eng.pdf (Level IV)

9 American Osteopathic Association. (2014). Standard 07.01.21. *Healthcare Facilities Accreditation Program: Accreditation requirements for acute care hospitals.* Chicago, IL: American Osteopathic Association. (Level VII)

10 Centers for Medicare & Medicaid Services, Department of Health and Human Services. (2014). Condition of participation: Infection control. 42 C.F.R. § 482.42.

11 Siegel J. D., et al. (2007). "2007 guideline for isolation precautions: Preventing transmission of infectious agents in healthcare settings" [Online]. Accessed May 2015 via the Web at http://www.cdc.gov/hicpac/pdf/isolation/Isolation2007.pdf (Level II)

12 American Osteopathic Association. (2014). Standard 07.01.10. *Healthcare Facilities Accreditation Program: Accreditation requirements for acute care hospitals.* Chicago, IL: American Osteopathic Association. (Level VII)

13 The Joint Commission. (2015). Standard RC.01.03.01. *Comprehensive accreditation manual for hospitals: The official handbook.* Oakbrook Terrace, IL: The Joint Commission. (Level VII)

14 American Osteopathic Association. (2014). Standard 10.00.03. *Healthcare Facilities Accreditation Program: Accreditation requirements for acute care hospitals.* Chicago, IL: American Osteopathic Association. (Level VII)

15 Centers for Medicare & Medicaid Services, Department of Health and Human Services. (2014). Condition of participation: Medical record services. 42 C.F.R. § 482.24(b).

Sharp debridement

Debridement involves removing necrotic tissue or contaminated foreign debris from a wound. As necrotic tissue develops, it becomes a barrier to wound healing and a medium for bacterial growth. Removing this tissue decreases the risk of infection, accelerates wound healing, and prevents further complications associated with tissue destruction. Surgical debridement is recommended for large or deep wounds. However, when surgical debridement isn't appropriate for the patient's condition, sharp, chemical (or enzymatic), mechanical, autolytic, or biosurgical debridement may be used.[1]

Sharp debridement involves using a scalpel, scissors, or other sharp instrument to excise a wound's necrotic material up to the viable tissue.[1] It's the most rapid form of debridement and can be combined with other forms of debridement, as needed. A practitioner, physical therapist, or specially trained nurse may perform sharp debridement.[2,3]

Sharp debridement should be used cautiously in patients with a compromised immune system, compromised vascular supply to the limb, or sepsis.[2] Relative contraindications for sharp debridement include anticoagulant therapy and bleeding disorders.[2]

Equipment

Prescribed analgesic ■ two pairs of sterile gloves[4,5] ■ two sterile gowns ■ mask ■ goggles[6] ■ cap ■ wound measuring device ■ sterile scissors or scalpel ■ sterile forceps ■ prescribed cleaning solutions and medications ■ sterile 4″ × 4″ (10-cm × 10-cm) gauze pads ■ dressings ■ Optional: camera, hemostatic agent, calcium alginate dressing.

Implementation

■ Review the patient's medical record and check his history for hypersensitivity to latex or analgesics.

■ Confirm that the practitioner has obtained written informed consent and that the consent is in the patient's medical record.[7,8,9]

■ Conduct a preprocedure verification *to make sure that all relevant documentation, related information, and equipment are available and correctly identified to the patient identifiers.*[10,11]

■ Verify that laboratory studies are complete, as ordered, and that the results are in the patient's medical record. Notify the practitioner of any unexpected results.[10,11]

■ Perform hand hygiene.[12,13,14,15,16]

■ Confirm the patient's identity using at least two patient identifiers according to your facility's policy.[17]

■ Provide privacy and explain the procedure to the patient and answer his questions *to allay his fears and enhance cooperation.*

■ Teach him distraction and relaxation techniques, if possible, *to minimize his discomfort.*

■ Perform a comprehensive pain assessment using techniques appropriate for the patient's age, condition, and ability to understand.[18,19,20]

■ Administer an analgesic, following safe medication administration practices, at an appropriate time before debridement begins based on the onset and peak of the medication prescribed, or give an IV analgesic immediately before the procedure, as ordered.[1,2,6,20,21,22]

- Keep the patient warm. Expose only the area to be debrided *to prevent chilling and fluid and electrolyte loss.*
- If the wound to be debrided is on a lower extremity, perform a neurovascular assessment before beginning the procedure *to obtain baseline information.*[1,2] *Inadequate perfusion may result in wound extension.*[6]
- Prepare a sterile field. Using sterile technique, set up the supplies on the sterile field.[4,5]
- Label all medications, medication containers, and solutions on and off the sterile field.[23,24]
- Perform hand hygiene[12,13,14,15,16] and put on a cap, a mask, goggles, a sterile gown, and sterile gloves.[4,5,25,26]
- Conduct a time-out immediately before starting the procedure *to ensure that the correct patient, site, positioning, and procedure are identified and, as applicable, that all relevant information and necessary equipment are available.*[27]
- Gently remove the dressings and clean the wound.[20] (For detailed directions for burn dressings see the "Burn care" procedure, page 105.)
- Measure the wound *to determine how wound healing is progressing.* If applicable, photograph the wound *for additional documentation.*[2]
- Remove and discard your gown and gloves,[25,26] perform hand hygiene,[12,13,14,15,16] and put on another sterile gown and sterile gloves.[25,26]
- Lift the necrotic tissue with forceps. Use the scalpel or scissors to cut the tissue. Keep the scalpel or scissors parallel to or angled away from the wound bed.
- Replace the dressing over the wound.
- Dispose of all equipment in the appropriate receptacle.[25,26]
- Remove and discard your gloves and remove your personal protective equipment.[25,26]
- Perform hand hygiene.[12,13,14,15,16]
- Perform a comprehensive pain assessment using techniques appropriate for the patient's age, condition, and ability to understand; respond to the patient's pain appropriately.[18,28]
- Perform hand hygiene.[12,13,14,15,16]
- Document the procedure.[29,30,31]

Special considerations

- *Because debridement removes dead tissue,* bleeding should be minimal. If bleeding occurs, apply gentle pressure on the wound with sterile 4″ × 4″ (10-cm × 10-cm) gauze pads. Then apply a hemostatic agent or calcium alginate dressing, as ordered.[20] If bleeding persists, notify the practitioner, and maintain pressure on the wound until the practitioner arrives. Excessive bleeding or spurting vessels may require ligation.

Complications

Infection may develop despite the use of sterile technique and equipment. Bleeding, the most common complication, may occur if debridement exposes an eroded blood vessel or if you inadvertently cut a vessel. Fluid and electrolyte imbalances may result from exudate lost during the procedure.

Documentation

Record the date and time of wound debridement, the area debrided, and solutions and medications used. Describe the wound's condition, noting signs of infection or skin breakdown. Record the patient's tolerance of and reaction to the procedure. Note indications for additional therapy. Record the administration of preprocedure pain medication and pain assessment before and after the procedure.

REFERENCES

1 Institute for Clinical Systems Improvement. (2012). "Health care protocol: Pressure ulcer prevention and treatment protocol (3rd ed.)" [Online]. Accessed May 2015 via the Web at http://www.icsi.org/_asset/6t7kxy/PressureUlcer.pdf (Level VII)

2 National Pressure Ulcer Advisory Panel and European Pressure Ulcer Advisory Panel. (2009). *Pressure ulcer prevention and treatment: Clinical practice guidelines.* Washington, DC: National Pressure Ulcer Advisory Panel. (Level VII)

3 Harris, R. J. (2009). The nursing practice of conservative sharp wound debridement: Promotion, education, and proficiency. *Wound Care Canada, 7*(1), 22–30. Accessed May 2015 via the Web at http://cawc.net/images/uploads/wcc/harris.pdf

4 Wound, Ostomy and Continence Nurses Society. (2005). "Position statement: Clean versus sterile: Management of chronic wounds" [Online]. Accessed May 2015 via the Web at http://c.ymcdn.com/sites/www.wocn.org/resource/resmgr/archives/clvst.pdf (Level VII)

5 Wound, Ostomy and Continence Nurses Society Wound Committee & the Association for Professionals in Infection Control and Epidemiology, Inc. (2012). Clean vs. sterile dressing techniques for management of chronic wounds: A fact sheet. *Journal of Wound, Ostomy and Continence Nursing, 39*(Suppl. 2), S30–S34. Accessed May 2015 via the Web at http://www.nursingcenter.com/lnc/journalarticle?Article_ID=1320693 (Level VII)

6 Lynn-McHale Wiegand, D. (Ed.). (2011). *AACN procedure manual for critical care* (6th ed.). St. Louis, MO: Saunders.

7 Centers for Medicare & Medicaid Services, Department of Health and Human Services. (2014). Condition of participation: Patient's rights. 42 C.F.R. § 482.13.

8 The Joint Commission. (2015). Standard RI.01.03.01. *Comprehensive accreditation manual for hospitals: The official handbook.* Oakbrook Terrace, IL: The Joint Commission. (Level VII)

9 American Osteopathic Association. (2014). Standard 15.01.11. *Healthcare Facilities Accreditation Program: Accreditation requirements for acute care hospitals.* Chicago, IL: American Osteopathic Association. (Level VII)

10 The Joint Commission. (2015). Standard UP.01.01.01. *Comprehensive accreditation manual for hospitals: The official handbook.* Oakbrook Terrace, IL: The Joint Commission. (Level VII)

11 American Osteopathic Association. (2014). Standard 30.00.14. *Healthcare Facilities Accreditation Program: Accreditation requirements for acute care hospitals.* Chicago, IL: American Osteopathic Association. (Level VII)

12 Centers for Disease Control and Prevention. (2002). Guideline for hand hygiene in health-care settings: Recommendations of the Healthcare Infection Control Practices Advisory Committee and the HICPAC/SHEA/APIC/IDSA Hand Hygiene Task Force. *MMWR Recommendations and Reports, 51*(RR-16), 1–45. Accessed May 2015 via the Web at http://www.cdc.gov/mmwr/pdf/rr/rr5116.pdf (Level II)

13 World Health Organization. (2009). "WHO guidelines on hand hygiene in health care: First global patient safety challenge, clean care is safer care" [Online]. Accessed May 2015 via the Web at http://whqlibdoc.who.int/publications/2009/9789241597906_eng.pdf (Level IV)

14 The Joint Commission. (2015). Standard NPSG.07.01.01. *Comprehensive accreditation manual for hospitals: The official handbook.* Oakbrook Terrace, IL: The Joint Commission. (Level VII)

15 Centers for Medicare & Medicaid Services, Department of Health and Human Services. (2014). Condition of participation: Infection control. 42 C.F.R. § 482.42.

16 American Osteopathic Association. (2014). Standard 07.01.21. *Healthcare Facilities Accreditation Program: Accreditation requirements for acute care hospitals.* Chicago, IL: American Osteopathic Association. (Level VII)

17 The Joint Commission. (2015). Standard NPSG.01.01.01. *Comprehensive accreditation manual for hospitals: The official handbook.* Oakbrook Terrace, IL: The Joint Commission. (Level VII)

18 The Joint Commission. (2015). Standard PC.01.02.07. *Comprehensive accreditation manual for hospitals: The official handbook.* Oakbrook Terrace, IL: The Joint Commission. (Level VII)

19 American Osteopathic Association. (2014). Standard 16.02.01. *Healthcare Facilities Accreditation Program: Accreditation requirements for acute care hospitals.* Chicago, IL: American Osteopathic Association. (Level VII)

20 Woo, K. Y., & Ibbald, R. G. (2010). Local wound care for malignant and palliative wounds. *Advances in Skin and Wound care, 23,* 417–428.

21 Centers for Medicare & Medicaid Services, Department of Health and Human Services. (2014). Condition of participation: Nursing services. 42 C.F.R. § 482.23(c).

22 American Osteopathic Association. (2014). Standard 16.01.03. *Healthcare Facilities Accreditation Program: Accreditation requirements for acute care hospitals.* Chicago, IL: American Osteopathic Association. (Level VII)

23 The Joint Commission. (2015). Standard NPSG.03.04.01. *Comprehensive accreditation manual for hospitals: The official handbook.* Oakbrook Terrace, IL: The Joint Commission. (Level VII)

24 American Osteopathic Association. (2014). Standard 25.01.27. *Healthcare Facilities Accreditation Program: Accreditation requirements for acute care hospitals.* Chicago, IL: American Osteopathic Association. (Level VII)

25 Siegel, J. D., et al. (2007). "2007 guideline for isolation precautions: Preventing transmission of infectious agents in healthcare settings" [Online]. Accessed May 2015 via the Web at http://www.cdc.gov/hicpac/pdf/isolation/Isolation2007.pdf (Level II)

26 American Osteopathic Association. (2014). Standard 07.01.10. *Healthcare Facilities Accreditation Program: Accreditation requirements for acute care hospitals.* Chicago, IL: American Osteopathic Association. (Level VII)

27 The Joint Commission. (2015). Standard UP.01.03.01. *Comprehensive accreditation manual for hospital: The official handbook.* Oakbrook Terrace, IL: The Joint Commission. (Level VII)

28 American Osteopathic Association. (2014). Standard 16.02.05. *Healthcare Facilities Accreditation Program: Accreditation requirements for acute care hospitals.* Chicago, IL: American Osteopathic Association. (Level VII)

29 The Joint Commission. (2015). Standard RC.01.03.01. *Comprehensive accreditation manual for hospitals: The official handbook.* Oakbrook Terrace, IL: The Joint Commission. (Level VII)

30 Centers for Medicare & Medicaid Services, Department of Health and Human Services. (2014). Condition of participation: Medical record services. 42 C.F.R. § 482.24(b).

31 American Osteopathic Association. (2014). Standard 10.00.03. *Healthcare Facilities Accreditation Program: Accreditation requirements for acute care hospitals.* Chicago, IL: American Osteopathic Association. (Level VII)

Additional references

Baranoski, S., & Ayello, E.A. (2012). *Wound care essentials: Practice principles* (3nd ed.). Philadelphia, PA: Lippincott Williams & Williams.

Fleck, C., & Chakravarthy, D. (2010). Newer debridement methods for wound bed preparation. *Advances in Skin and Wound Care, 23*(7), 313–315.

Wound, Ostomy and Continence Nurses Society. (2011). *Guideline for management of wounds in patients with lower-extremity venous disease.* Glenview, IL: WOCN. (Level VII)

Shaving

Performed with a safety or electric razor, shaving is part of the male patient's usual daily care. Besides reducing bacterial growth on the face, shaving promotes patient comfort by removing facial hair that can itch and irritate the skin and produce an unkempt appearance. Because nicks and cuts occur more frequently with a safety razor, shaving with an electric razor is indicated for a patient with a clotting disorder or a patient undergoing anticoagulant therapy. Shaving may be contraindicated in the patient with a facial skin disorder or wound.

Equipment

For a safety razor

Shaving kit containing a razor and soap container ▪ gloves ▪ soap or shaving cream ▪ towel ▪ washcloth ▪ basin ▪ Optional: aftershave lotion, antiseptic lotion.

For an electric razor

Electric razor ▪ bath towel ▪ gloves ▪ light source ▪ Optional: preshave and aftershave lotions, mirror, grounded three-pronged plug.

Preparation of equipment

For a safety razor, make sure the blade is sharp, clean, even, and rust-free. If necessary, insert a new blade securely into the razor. A razor may be used more than once, but only for the same patient. If the patient is bedridden, gather the equipment on the bedside stand or overbed table; if he's ambulatory, gather it at the sink.

For an electric razor, check its cord for fraying or other damage that could create an electrical hazard. If the razor isn't double-insulated or battery operated, use a grounded three-pronged plug. Examine the razor head for sharp edges and dirt. Read the manufacturer's instructions, if available. Gather the equipment at the bedside.

Implementation

- Perform hand hygiene.[1,2,3,4,5]
- Tell the patient that you're going to shave him, and provide privacy.[6] Ask him to assist you as much as possible *to promote his independence.*
- Unless contraindicated, place the conscious patient in the high Fowler or semi-Fowler position. If the patient is unconscious, elevate his head *to prevent soap and water or facial hair from running behind it.*
- Direct bright light onto the patient's face, but not into his eyes.
- Put on gloves.[7,8,9]

Using a safety razor

- Drape a bath towel around the patient's shoulders, and tuck it under his chin *to protect the bed from moisture and to catch falling facial hair.*
- Fill the basin with warm water. Using the washcloth, wet the patient's entire beard with warm water. Let the warm cloth soak the beard for at least 1 minute *to soften facial hair.*
- Apply shaving cream to the beard. Or, if you're using soap, rub it *to form a lather.*
- Gently stretch the patient's skin taut with one hand and shave with the other, holding the razor firmly. Ask the patient to puff his cheeks or turn his head, as necessary, *to shave hard-to-reach areas.*
- Begin at the patient's sideburns and work toward his chin using short, firm, downward strokes in the direction of hair growth (as shown below). *This method reduces skin irritation and helps prevent nicks and cuts.*

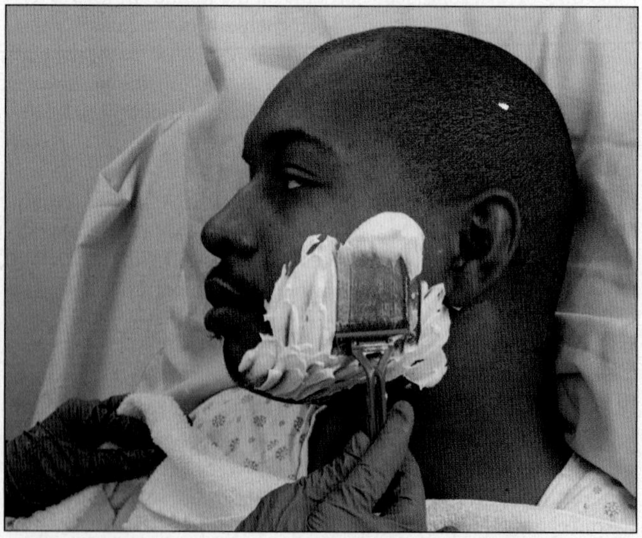

- Rinse the razor often *to remove facial hair.* Apply more warm water or shaving cream to the patient's face, as needed, *to maintain adequate lather.*
- Shave across the patient's chin and up the neck and throat. Use short, gentle strokes for the neck and the area around the nose and mouth *to avoid skin irritation.*

■ Change the water, and rinse any remaining lather and facial hair from the patient's face. Then dry his face with a bath towel and, if the patient desires, apply aftershave lotion.
■ Rinse the razor, rinse and disinfect the basin as indicated,[10,11] and then return the razor to its storage area or dispose of it in a sharps container.[7]

Using an electric razor

■ Drape a bath towel around the patient's shoulders and tuck it under his chin *to catch falling facial hair.*
■ Plug in the razor and apply preshave lotion, if available, *to remove skin oils.* If the razor head is adjustable, select the appropriate setting.
■ Using a circular motion and pressing the razor firmly against the skin, shave each area of the patient's face until smooth.
■ If the patient desires, apply aftershave lotion.
■ Clean the razor head, and return the razor to its storage area.[10,11]

Completing the procedure

■ Remove and discard your gloves[7,8,9] and perform hand hygiene.[1,2,3,4,5]
■ Document the procedure.[12,13,14]

Special considerations

■ If the patient is conscious, find out his usual shaving routine. Although shaving in the direction of hair growth is most common, the patient may prefer the opposite direction.
■ Don't interchange patients' shaving equipment *to prevent cross-contamination.*
■ Shaving may be contraindicated if the patient is on anticoagulant therapy (for example, tissue plasminogen activator or heparin).
■ A safety inspection by medical maintenance may need to be performed before using an electric razor brought from home.

Complications

Cuts and abrasions are the most common complications of shaving and can require application of antiseptic lotion.

Documentation

If applicable, record nicks or cuts resulting from shaving.

REFERENCES

1 The Joint Commission. (2015). Standard NPSG.07.01.01. *Comprehensive accreditation manual for hospitals: The official handbook.* Oakbrook Terrace, IL: The Joint Commission. (Level VII)
2 Centers for Disease Control and Prevention. (2002). Guideline for hand hygiene in health-care settings: Recommendations of the Healthcare Infection Control Practices Advisory Committee and the HICPAC/SHEA/APIC/IDSA Hand Hygiene Task Force. *MMWR Recommendations and Reports, 51*(RR-16), 1–45. Accessed May 2015 via the Web at http://www.cdc.gov/mmwr/pdf/rr/rr5116.pdf (Level II)
3 World Health Organization. (2009). "WHO guidelines on hand hygiene in health care: First global patient safety challenge, clean care is safer care" [Online]. Accessed May 2015 via the Web at http://whqlibdoc.who.int/publications/2009/9789241597906_eng.pdf (Level IV)
4 American Osteopathic Association. (2012). Standard 07.01.21. *Healthcare Facilities Accreditation Program: Accreditation requirements for acute care hospitals.* Chicago, IL: American Osteopathic Association. (Level VII)
5 Centers for Medicare & Medicaid Services, Department of Health and Human Services. (2014). Condition of participation: Infection control. 42 C.F.R. § 482.42.
6 American Osteopathic Association. (2014). Standard 15.01.16. *Healthcare Facilities Accreditation Program: Accreditation requirements for acute care hospitals.* Chicago, IL: American Osteopathic Association. (Level VII)
7 Occupational Safety and Health Administration. (n.d.). "Bloodborne pathogens, standard number 1910.1030" [Online]. Accessed May 2015 via the Web at http://www.osha.gov/pls/oshaweb/owadisp.show_document?p_table=standards&p_id=10051 (Level VII)
8 American Osteopathic Association. (2012). Standard 07.01.10. *Healthcare Facilities Accreditation Program: Accreditation requirements for acute care hospitals.* Chicago, IL: American Osteopathic Association. (Level VII)
9 Siegel, J. D., et al. (2007). "2007 guideline for isolation precautions: Preventing transmission of infectious agents in healthcare settings" [Online]. Accessed May 2015 via the Web at http://www.cdc.gov/hicpac/pdf/isolation/Isolation2007.pdf (Level II)
10 Rutala, W. A. (2008). "Guideline for disinfection and sterilization in healthcare facilities, 2008" [Online]. Accessed May 2015 via the Web at http://www.cdc.gov/hicpac/pdf/guidelines/Disinfection_Nov_2008.pdf (Level I)
11 American Osteopathic Association. (2014). Standard 07.02.03. *Healthcare Facilities Accreditation Program: Accreditation requirements for acute care hospitals.* Chicago, IL: American Osteopathic Association.
12 Centers for Medicare & Medicaid Services, Department of Health and Human Services. (2014). Condition of participation: Medical record services. 42 C.F.R. § 482.24(b).
13 American Osteopathic Association. (2012). Standard 10.00.03. *Healthcare Facilities Accreditation Program: Accreditation requirements for acute care hospitals.* Chicago, IL: American Osteopathic Association.
14 The Joint Commission. (2015). Standard RC.01.03.01. *Comprehensive accreditation manual for hospitals: The official handbook.* Oakbrook Terrace, IL: The Joint Commission. (Level VII)

ADDITIONAL REFERENCE

Craven, R. F., & Hirnle, C. J. (2012). *Fundamentals of nursing: Human health and function* (7th ed.). Philadelphia, PA: Lippincott Williams & Wilkins.

SITZ BATH

A sitz bath involves immersion of the pelvic area in warm or hot water. It is used to relieve discomfort, especially after perineal or rectal surgery or childbirth. The bath promotes wound healing by cleaning the perineum and anus, increasing circulation, and reducing inflammation. It also helps relax local muscles.

To be performed correctly, the sitz bath requires frequent checks of water temperature to ensure safety, comfort, and therapeutic effects. Correct draping of the patient during and prompt dressing after the bath help prevent vasoconstriction.

Equipment

Sitz tub, portable sitz bath, or regular bathtub ■ bath mat ■ rubber mat ■ bath (utility) thermometer ■ two bath blankets ■ towels ■ patient gown ■ hospital-grade disinfectant ■ gloves ■ Optional: rubber ring, footstool, overbed table, IV pole (to hold irrigation bag), wheelchair or stretcher, dressings, personal protective equipment, blood pressure monitoring device, stethoscope, watch or clock with a second hand.

A portable sitz bath kit is available in a commercial disposable kit for single-patient use. The kit includes a plastic basin that fits over a commode and an irrigation bag with tubing and clamp.

Preparation of equipment

Make sure the sitz tub, portable sitz bath, or regular bathtub is clean and disinfected. As an alternative, obtain a disposable sitz bath kit from the central supply department.

Sitz bath and regular bathtub

Position the bath mat next to the bathtub, sitz tub, or commode. If you're using a tub, place the rubber mat on its surface *to prevent falls.* Place the rubber ring on the bottom of the tub *to serve as a seat for the patient,* and cover the ring with a towel *for comfort.* Keep the patient elevated *to improve water flow over the wound site and to avoid unnecessary pressure on tender tissues.*

Fill the sitz tub or bathtub one-third to one-half full *so that the water will reach the seated patient's umbilicus.* Use warm water (94° to 98°F [34.4° to 36.7°C]) for relaxation or wound cleaning and healing and hot water (110° to 115°F [43.3° to 46.1°C]) for heat application. Run the water slightly warmer than desired *because it will cool while the patient prepares for the bath.* Measure the water temperature using the bath thermometer.

Commercial sitz bath kit

Open the package and familiarize yourself with the equipment.

Fill the basin to the specified line with water at the prescribed temperature. Place the basin under the commode seat, clamp the irrigation tubing to block water flow, and fill the irrigation bag with water of the same temperature as that in the basin. To create flow pressure, hang the bag above the patient's head on a hook, towel rack, or IV pole.

Implementation

- Verify the practitioner's order.
- Perform hand hygiene.[1,2,3,4,5]
- Confirm the patient's identity using at least two patient identifiers.[6,7]
- Explain the procedure to the patient.
- Put on gloves and other personal protective equipment as necessary.[4,8,9]
- Assess the patient's condition.
- Instruct the patient to void.
- Assist the patient to the bath area, provide privacy, and make sure the area is warm and free of drafts. Help the patient undress, as needed.
- Remove and dispose of any soiled dressings.[9] If a dressing adheres to a wound, allow it to soak off in the water.
- Assist the patient into the tub or onto the commode, as needed. Instruct him to use the safety rail *for balance.* Explain that the sensation may be unpleasant initially *because the wound area is already tender.* Assure him that this discomfort will soon be relieved by the warm water.
- For any apparatus except a regular bathtub, if the patient's feet don't reach the floor and the weight of his legs presses against the edge of the equipment, place a small stool under the patient's feet *to decrease pressure on local blood vessels.* Also place a folded towel against the patient's lower back *to prevent discomfort and promote correct body alignment.*
- Drape the patient's shoulders and knees with bath blankets *to avoid chills that may cause vasoconstriction.*
- If you're using a sitz tub or bathtub, check the water temperature frequently with the bath thermometer. If the temperature drops significantly, add warm water. For maximum safety, first help the patient stand up slowly *to prevent dizziness and loss of balance.* Then, with the patient holding the safety rail *for support,* run warm water into the tub. Check water temperature. When the water reaches the correct temperature, help the patient sit down again to resume the bath.
- If you're using a commercial sitz bath kit, open the clamp on the irrigation tubing *to allow a stream of water to flow continuously over the wound site.* Refill the bag with water of the correct temperature as needed, and encourage the patient to regulate the flow himself. Place the patient's overbed table in front of him *to provide support and comfort.*
- If necessary, stay with the patient during the bath. If you must leave, place the call light within his reach, show him how to use it, and ensure his privacy.
- Assess the patient's color and general condition frequently. If he complains of feeling weak, faint, or nauseated or shows signs of cardiovascular distress, discontinue the bath, check the patient's pulse and blood pressure, and assist him back to bed. Use a wheelchair or stretcher to transport the patient to his room if necessary, and notify the practitioner.
- When the prescribed sitz bath time has elapsed—usually 15 to 20 minutes—tell the patient to use the safety rail *for balance,* and help him to a standing position slowly *to prevent dizziness and to allow him to regain his equilibrium.*
- If necessary, help the patient dry himself.
- Remove and discard your gloves,[8,9] perform hand hygiene,[1,2,3,4] and put on a new pair of gloves.[8,9]
- Re-dress the wound as needed.
- Provide the patient with a clean gown, and help him dress and return to bed or back to his room.
- Dispose of soiled materials properly.[9]
- Empty, clean, and disinfect the sitz tub, bathtub, or portable sitz bath using a hospital-grade disinfectant s required by your facility.[10,11] Return the commercial sitz bath kit to the patient's bedside for later use.
- Remove and discard your gloves and other personal protective equipment, if worn[8,9] and perform hand hygiene.[1,2,3,4,5]
- Document the procedure.[12,13,14]

Special considerations

- Use a regular bathtub only if a sitz tub, portable sitz bath, or commercial sitz bath kit is unavailable. A regular bathtub is less effective for local treatment than a sitz device and should be avoided *because the application of heat to the extremities causes vasodilation and draws blood away from the perineal area,*
- If the patient will be sitting in a bathtub with his extremities immersed in the hot water, check his pulse before, during, and after the bath *to help detect vasodilation that could make him feel faint when he stands up.*
- Tell the patient never to touch an open wound *because of the risk of infection.*

Patient teaching

Teach the patient how to perform a sitz bath and how to care for the equipment if he will continue sitz baths at home.

Complications

Weakness or faintness can result from heat or the exertion of changing position during a sitz bath. An irregular or accelerated pulse may indicate cardiovascular distress.

Documentation

Record the date, time, duration, and temperature of the bath; wound condition before and after treatment, including color, odor, and amount of drainage; any complications; and the patient's response to treatment.

REFERENCES

1 The Joint Commission. (2015). Standard NPSG.07.01.01. *Comprehensive accreditation manual for hospitals: The official handbook.* Oakbrook Terrace, IL: The Joint Commission. (Level VII)

2 Centers for Disease Control and Prevention. (2002). Guideline for hand hygiene in health-care settings: Recommendations of the Healthcare Infection Control Practices Advisory Committee and the HICPAC/SHEA/APIC/IDSA Hand Hygiene Task Force. *MMWR Recommendations and Reports, 51*(RR-16), 1–45. Accessed May 2015 via the Web at http://www.cdc.gov/mmwr/pdf/rr/rr5116.pdf (Level II)

3 World Health Organization. (2009). "WHO guidelines on hand hygiene in health care: First global patient safety challenge, clean care is safer care" [Online]. Accessed May 2015 via the Web at http://whqlibdoc.who.int/publications/2009/9789241597906_eng.pdf (Level IV)

4 American Osteopathic Association. (2012). Standard 07.01.21. *Healthcare Facilities Accreditation Program: Accreditation requirements for acute care hospitals.* Chicago, IL: American Osteopathic Association. (Level VII)

5 Centers for Medicare & Medicaid Services, Department of Health and Human Services. (2014). Condition of participation: Infection control. 42 C.F.R. § 482.42.

6 The Joint Commission. (2015). Standard NPSG.01.01.01. *Comprehensive accreditation manual for hospitals: The official handbook.* Oakbrook Terrace, IL: The Joint Commission. (Level VII)

7 American Osteopathic Association. (2012). Standard 30.00.14. *Healthcare Facilities Accreditation Program: Accreditation requirements for acute care hospitals.* Chicago, IL: American Osteopathic Association. (Level VII)

8 Siegel, J. D., et al. (2007). "2007 Guideline for isolation precautions: Preventing transmission of infectious agents in healthcare settings" [Online]. Accessed May 2015 via the Web at http://www.cdc.gov/hicpac/pdf/isolation/Isolation2007.pdf (Level II)

9 Occupational Safety and Health Administration. (n.d.). "Bloodborne pathogens, standard number 1910.1030" [Online]. Accessed May 2015 via the Web at http://www.osha.gov/pls/oshaweb/owadisp.show_document?p_table=STANDARDS&p_id=10051 (Level VII)

10 Rutala, W. A., et al. (2008). "Guideline for disinfection and sterilization in healthcare facilities, 2008" [Online]. Accessed May 2015 via the Web at http://www.cdc.gov/hicpac/pdf/guidelines/Disinfection_Nov_2008.pdf (Level I)

11 American Osteopathic Association. (2014). Standard 07.02.03. *Healthcare Facilities Accreditation Program: Accreditation requirements for acute care hospitals.* Chicago, IL: American Osteopathic Association. (Level VII)

12 The Joint Commission. (2015). Standard RC.01.03.01. *Comprehensive accreditation manual for hospitals: The official handbook.* Oakbrook Terrace, IL: The Joint Commission. (Level VII)

13 American Osteopathic Association. (2014). Standard 10.00.03. *Healthcare Facilities Accreditation Program: Accreditation requirements for acute care hospitals.* Chicago, IL: American Osteopathic Association. (Level VII)

14 Centers for Medicare & Medicaid Services, Department of Health and Human Services. (2014). Condition of participation: Medical record services. 42 C.F.R. § 482.24(b).

ADDITIONAL REFERENCES

Craven, R. F., & Hirnle, C. J. (2012). *Fundamentals of nursing: Human health and function* (7th ed.). Philadelphia, PA: Lippincott Williams & Wilkins.

Taylor, C., et al. (2015). *Fundamentals of nursing: The art and science of nursing care* (8th ed.). Philadelphia, PA: Wolters Kluwer.

SKIN BIOPSY

Skin biopsy is a diagnostic test in which a small piece of tissue is removed, under local anesthesia, from a lesion that's suspected of being malignant or from another dermatosis.

One of three techniques may be used: shave biopsy, punch biopsy, or excisional biopsy. *Shave biopsy* cuts the lesion above the skin line, which allows further biopsy of the site. *Punch biopsy* removes an oval or round core plug from the center of the lesion. *Excisional biopsy* removes the entire lesion and is indicated for rapidly expanding lesions; malignant or dysplastic tissue; cases in which the margins of the skin surrounding the lesion need to be clear; sclerotic, bullous, or atrophic lesions; and examining the border of a lesion surrounding normal skin.

Lesions suspected of being malignant usually have changed in color, size, or appearance or have failed to heal properly. (See *The ABCDEs of malignant melanoma.*)[1] Fully developed lesions should be selected for biopsy whenever possible because they provide more diagnostic information than lesions that are resolving or in early stages of development. For example, if the skin shows blisters, the biopsy should include the most mature blisters.

Normal skin consists of squamous epithelium (epidermis) and fibrous connective tissue (dermis). Benign growths include cysts, seborrheic keratoses, warts, pigmented nevi (moles), keloids, dermatofibromas, and neurofibromas. Malignant tumors include dysplastic nevi, basal cell carcinoma, squamous cell carcinoma, and malignant melanoma.

Equipment

Gloves ▪ sterile gloves ▪ #15 scalpel for shave or excisional biopsy ▪ antiseptic agent (isopropyl alcohol, povidone-iodine solution, or chlorhexidine) ▪ punch for punch biopsy ▪ local anesthetic ▪ sterile specimen

The ABCDEs of malignant melanoma[1]

Keep in mind the ABCDE rule to help you remember the warning signs of malignant melanoma.

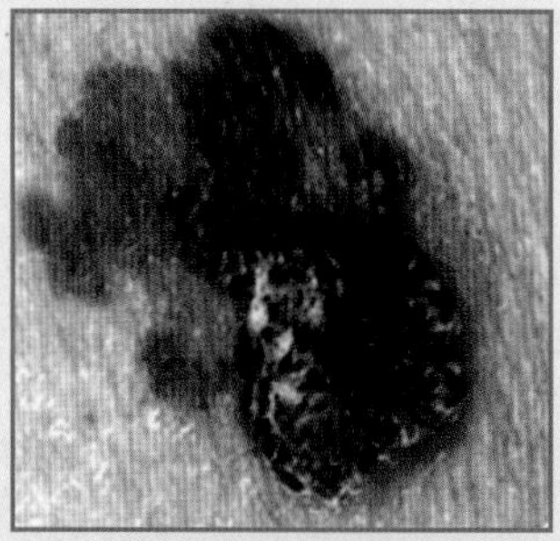

Asymmetry: One half of a mole or birthmark doesn't match the other.

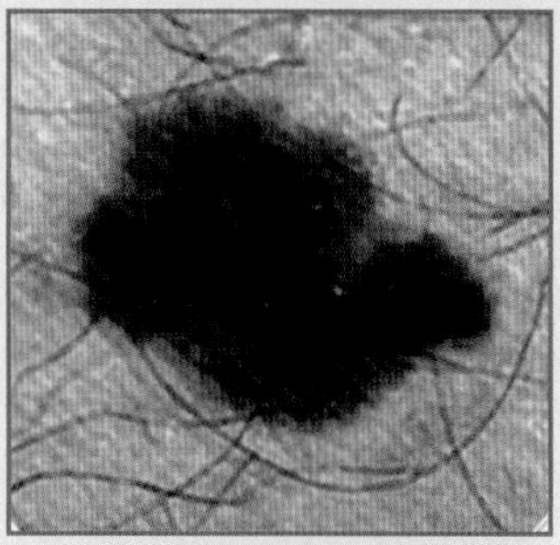

Border: The edges are irregular, ragged, notched, or blurred.

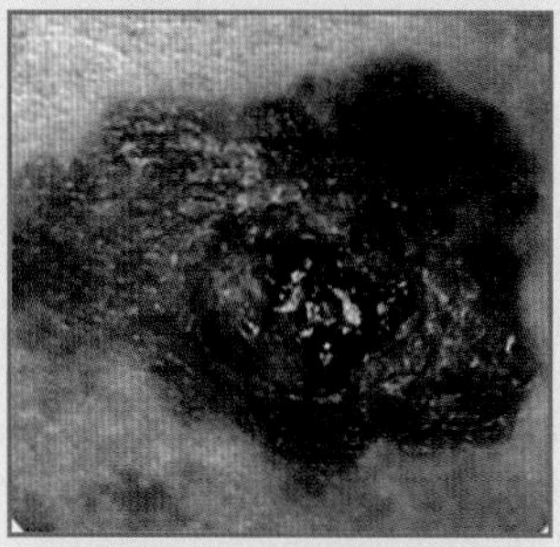

Color: The pigmentation isn't uniform; it may have varying degrees of brown, black, or occasionally red.

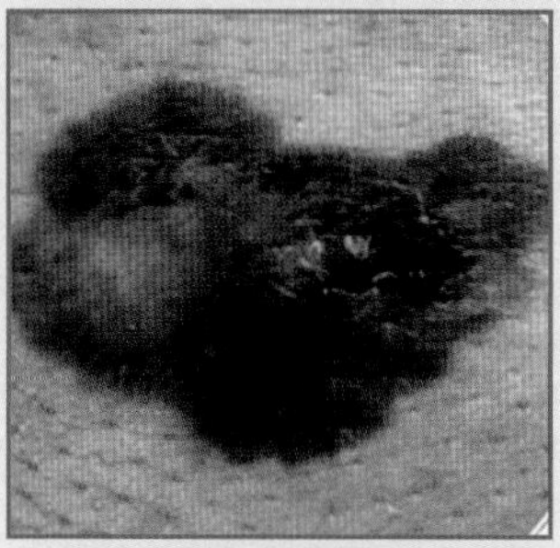

Diameter: The diameter is greater than 1/4" (6 mm), about the size of a pencil eraser. There's a sudden or progressive increase in size.

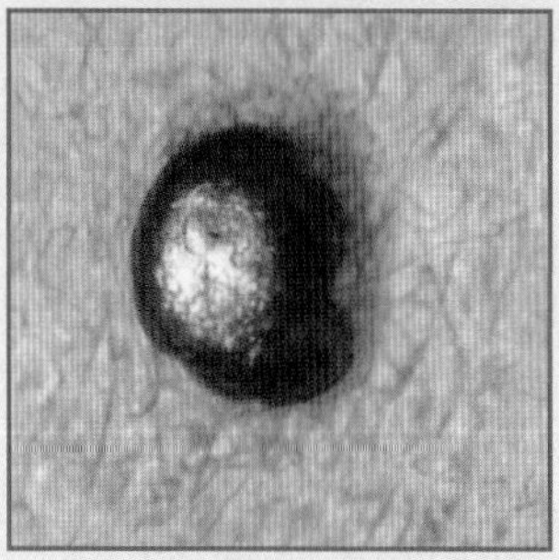

Evolving: The size, shape, color, elevation, or another trait has changed, or a new sign or symptom, such as bleeding, itching, or crusting, has developed.

bottle containing 10% formaldehyde solution or other preservative[2] ▪ 3-0, 4-0, or 5-0 sutures for punch or excisional biopsy ▪ adhesive bandage ▪ forceps ▪ scissors ▪ adhesive strips ▪ Optional: topical hemostatic agent, antibiotic ointment, analgesics as ordered, transparent wound dressings.[2]

Preparation of equipment

Some biopsy specimens require special fixation techniques and may need to be delivered to the laboratory in different preservative fluids. Consult your facility's pathologist if you are unsure of any required techniques.[2]

Implementation

- Verify the practitioner's order.
- Confirm that the patient's informed consent has been obtained and that the consent form is in the patient's medical record.[3,4,5]
- Check the patient's history for hypersensitivity to latex or to the local anesthetic.
- Gather the appropriate equipment.
- Perform hand hygiene.[6,7,8,9,10]
- Confirm the patient's identity using at least two patient identifiers.[11]
- Reinforce the practitioner's explanation of the procedure. Explain to the patient that the biopsy provides a skin specimen for microscopic study. Describe the procedure, and tell the patient who will perform it. Answer any questions that the patient may have *to ease anxiety and ensure cooperation.*
- Inform the patient that he doesn't need to restrict food or fluids.
- Tell him that he'll receive a local anesthetic for pain.
- Inform him that the biopsy will take about 15 minutes and that the test results are usually available within 7 days, depending on the facility.
- Put on gloves.
- Label all medications, medication containers, and other solutions on and off the sterile field.[12]
- Position the patient comfortably, and clean the skin with an antiseptic agent, such as isopropyl alcohol, povidone-iodine solution, or chlorhexidine,[13] before the practitioner administers the local anesthetic.
- Assist with the biopsy procedure, as needed.
- For a shave biopsy, the practitioner cuts the growth off at the skin line with a #15 scalpel and immediately places the tissue in a properly labeled specimen bottle containing 10% formaldehyde solution. Apply pressure to the biopsy area *to stop bleeding.* Apply an adhesive bandage.
- For a punch biopsy, the practitioner pulls the skin surrounding the lesion taut, introduces the punch into the lesion firmly, and rotates the punch *to obtain a tissue specimen.* He lifts the plug with forceps or a needle and severs as deeply into the fat layer as possible. He then places the specimen in a properly labeled specimen bottle containing 10% formaldehyde solution or a sterile container if indicated. After the procedure the practitioner closes the wound according to the size of the punch; the wound may require an adhesive bandage alone or sutures.
- For an excisional biopsy, the practitioner uses a #15 scalpel *to excise the lesion;* he makes the incision as wide and as deep as necessary. The practitioner removes the tissue specimen and places it immediately in a properly labeled specimen bottle containing 10% formaldehyde solution. He applies pressure to the site *to stop bleeding* and then he closes the wound according to the location of the biopsy. If the incision is large, it may need skin grafting; if it's small, adhesive strips may be sufficient.

NURSING ALERT ***Handle biopsy specimens carefully* to minimize injury and excess tissue drying that may interfere with histopathologic evaluation.[2]**

- Check the biopsy site for bleeding. Apply a topical hemostatic agent as needed.[2]
- Remove and discard your gloves and perform hand hygiene.[6,7,8]
- Label the specimen container in the presence of the patient *to prevent mislabeling* and send it to the laboratory immediately.[11]
- If the patient experiences pain, administer analgesics as prescribed following safe medication administration practices.
- Perform hand hygiene.[6,7,8,9,10]
- Document the procedure.[14,15,16]

Special considerations

- Shave biopsies aren't recommended for suspected melanomas.

Patient teaching

Advise the patient going home with sutures to keep the area clean and as dry as possible for 24 hours. Tell him that facial sutures will be removed in 3 to 5 days and trunk sutures in 7 to 14 days. Instruct the patient with adhesive strips to leave them in place for 14 to 21 days or until they fall off. After a shave biopsy, instruct the patient to apply an antibiotic ointment daily until the wound heals or to use transparent wound dressings.[2] Instruct the patient to report signs and symptoms of infection—including redness, swelling, pain, discharge from the wound, and skin that's warm or hot—to his practitioner as soon as possible.

Complications

Possible complications may include bleeding and infection of the surrounding tissue as well as subsequent scar formation.

Documentation

Document the time of the biopsy, the site from which the specimen was obtained, the appearance of the specimen and site, and whether bleeding occurred at the biopsy site. Document patient teaching provided.

References

1 The Skin Cancer Foundation. (2014). "Warning signs: The ABCDEs of melanoma" [Online]. Accessed May 2015 via the Web at http://www.skincancer.org/skin-cancer-information/melanoma

2 Zuber, T. J. (2012). Skin biopsy techniques: When and how to perform shave and excisional biopsy. *Consultant360, 52,* 522–526. Accessed May 2015 via the Web at http://www.consultant360.com/article/skin-biopsy-techniques-when-and-how-perform-shave-and-excisional-biopsy

3 American Osteopathic Association. (2014). Standard 30.01.11. *Healthcare Facilities Accreditation Program: Accreditation requirements for acute care hospitals.* Chicago, IL: American Osteopathic Association. (Level VII)

4 Centers for Medicare & Medicaid Services, Department of Health and Human Services. (2014). Condition of participation: Patient's rights. 42 C.F.R. § 482.13(b)(2).

5 The Joint Commission. (2015). Standard RI.01.03.01. *Comprehensive accreditation manual for hospitals: The official handbook.* Oakbrook Terrace, IL: The Joint Commission. (Level VII)

6 The Joint Commission. (2015). Standard NPSG.07.01.01. *Comprehensive accreditation manual for hospitals: The official handbook.* Oakbrook Terrace, IL: The Joint Commission. (Level VII)

7 Centers for Disease Control and Prevention. (2002). Guideline for hand hygiene in health-care settings: Recommendations of the Healthcare Infection Control Practices Advisory Committee and the HICPAC/SHEA/APIC/IDSA Hand Hygiene Task Force. *MMWR Recommendations and Reports, 51*(RR-16), 1–45. Accessed May 2015 via the Web at http://www.cdc.gov/mmwr/pdf/rr/rr5116.pdf (Level II)

8 World Health Organization. (2009). "WHO guidelines on hand hygiene in health care: First global patient safety challenge, clean care is safer care" [Online]. Accessed May 2015 via the Web at http://whqlibdoc.who.int/publications/2009/9789241597906_eng.pdf (Level IV)

9 American Osteopathic Association. (2014). Standard 07.01.21. *Healthcare Facilities Accreditation Program: Accreditation requirements for acute care hospitals.* Chicago, IL: American Osteopathic Association. (Level VII)

10 Centers for Medicare & Medicaid Services, Department of Health and Human Services. (2014). Condition of participation: Infection control. 42 C.F.R. § 482.42.

11 The Joint Commission. (2015). Standard NPSG.01.01.01. *Comprehensive accreditation manual for hospitals: The official handbook.* Oakbrook Terrace, IL: The Joint Commission. (Level VII)

How to care for a donor graft site

Autografts are usually taken from another area of the patient's body with a dermatome, an instrument that cuts uniform, split-thickness skin portions—typically, about 0.013 to 0.05 cm thick. Autografting makes the donor site a partial-thickness wound, which may bleed, drain, and cause pain.

The donor site needs scrupulous care *to prevent infection, which could convert the site to a full-thickness wound.* Depending on the graft's thickness, tissue may be obtained from the donor site again in as few as 10 days.

A donor site dressing is applied intraoperatively. An outer gauze dressing may also be used and can be taken off on the first postoperative day; the inner dressing will protect the new epithelial proliferation. In addition to the inner dressing, the donor site may be dressed in antibiotic-impregnated gauze or a synthetic skin substitute.

Care for the donor site as you would the autograft, using dressing changes at the initial stages *to prevent infection and promote healing*. To dressing the wound, follow these steps:

- Perform hand hygiene[7,8,9,10,11] and put on sterile gloves.[12,13]
- Remove the outer gauze dressings within 24 hours. Inspect the inner dressing for signs of infection, and then leave it open to the air *to speed drying and healing.*
- Leave small amounts of fluid accumulation alone. Using sterile technique, aspirate larger amounts through the dressing with a small-gauge needle and syringe.
- Don't apply any creams to the donor site until it's dry.
- When dry, you may apply a thin layer of cream, according to the practitioner's preference, daily *to keep the skin tissue pliable.*
- As the donor site heals, different types of dressings may be required based on the amount of exudate and level of re-epithelialization.[2]

12 The Joint Commission. (2015). Standard NPSG.03.04.01. *Comprehensive accreditation manual for hospitals: The official handbook.* Oakbrook Terrace, IL: The Joint Commission. (Level VII)

13 Zuber, T. J. (2012). Skin biopsy techniques: When and how to perform punch biopsy. *Consultant360, 52*(6). Accessed May 2015 via the Web at http://www.consultant360.com/article/skin-biopsy-techniques-when-and-how-perform-punch-biopsy

14 The Joint Commission. (2015). Standard RC.01.03.01. *Comprehensive accreditation manual for hospitals: The official handbook.* Oakbrook Terrace, IL: The Joint Commission. (Level VII)

15 Centers for Medicare & Medicaid Services, Department of Health and Human Services. (2014). Condition of participation: Medical records services. 42 C.F.R. § 482.24(b).

16 American Osteopathic Association. (2014). Standard 10.00.03. *Healthcare Facilities Accreditation Program: Accreditation requirements for acute care hospitals.* Chicago, IL: American Osteopathic Association. (Level VII)

SKIN GRAFT CARE

A skin graft consists of healthy skin taken either from the patient (autograft) or a donor (allograft) and applied to the patient's body to resurface an area damaged by burns, traumatic injury, or surgery. The procedures for caring for both types of grafts are essentially the same. However, an autograft requires care for two sites: the graft site and the donor site.

The graft itself may be one of several types: split-thickness, full-thickness, or pedicle-flap. (See *Understanding types of grafts.*) Successful grafting depends on various factors, including clean wound granulation with adequate vascularization, complete contact of the graft with the wound bed, sterile technique to prevent infection, adequate graft immobilization, and skilled care.

The size and depth of the patient's burns determine whether the burns will require grafting. Grafting usually occurs at the completion of wound debridement. The goal is to cover all wounds with an autograft or allograft within 2 weeks. With enzymatic debridement, grafting may be performed 5 to 7 days after debridement is complete; with surgical debridement, grafting can occur the same day as the surgery.

A practitioner or a specially trained nurse may change graft dressings. The dressings usually stay in place for 3 to 5 days after surgery *to avoid disturbing the graft site.* Traditionally, petroleum jelly gauze dressings have been used to cover skin graft or donor sites, but this practice isn't currently recommended because these dressings form a poor bacterial barrier, increasing the risk of infection.[1] Various dressings materials have been evaluated based on their clinical efficacy, number of dressing changes required for optimal healing, patient reports of pain with application and removal, and health care provider preference. Examples include paraffin gauze–based, hydrocolloid, alginate, semipermeable film, silicone, and hydrofiber.[1,2,3,4,5] Initial skin graft dressings are applied in the operating room and covered with elastic gauze or a compression bandage to promote hemostasis and minimize exudate. Splints may also be applied, if needed, to immobilize and protect the grafted area.[6]

The skin graft donor site also requires diligent care. (See *How to care for a donor graft site.*)

Understanding types of grafts

A burn patient may receive one or more of the graft types described below.

Split-thickness

A split-thickness graft is used most commonly for covering open burns. This graft includes the epidermis and part of the dermis. It may be applied as a sheet (usually on the face or neck *to preserve the cosmetic result*) or as a mesh. A mesh graft has tiny slits cut in it, which allow the graft to expand up to nine times its original size. Mesh grafts prevent fluids from collecting under the graft and typically are used over extensive full-thickness burns.

Full-thickness

A full-thickness graft includes the epidermis and the entire dermis. Consequently, the graft contains hair follicles, sweat glands, and sebaceous glands, which typically aren't included in split-thickness grafts. Full-thickness grafts usually are used for small burns that cause deep wounds.

Pedicle-flap

A pedicle-flap graft includes not only skin and subcutaneous tissue, but also subcutaneous blood vessels *to ensure a continued blood supply to the graft.* Pedicle-flap grafts may be used during reconstructive surgery *to cover previous defects.*

Equipment

Prescribed analgesic ▪ gloves ▪ sterile gloves ▪ sterile gown ▪ cap ▪ mask ▪ sterile forceps ▪ sterile scissors ▪ sterile 4″ × 4″ (10-cm × 10-cm) gauze pads ▪ prescribed skin graft dressing ▪ elastic gauze or compression bandage ▪ warm normal saline solution ▪ moisturizing cream ▪ topical

Evacuating fluid from a sheet graft

When a small pocket of fluid (called a *bleb*) accumulates beneath a sheet graft, the practitioner or specially trained nurse will need to evacuate the fluid using a sterile scalpel and sterile cotton-tipped applicators. First, using the scalpel, carefully make a small nick in the sheet graft directly over the area of the bleb (as shown below). Express the fluid by rolling sterile cotton-tipped applicators gently over the graft toward the nick *to express the fluid.* Then gently dab away the expressed fluid using a sterile gauze pad moistened with normal saline solution.[26]

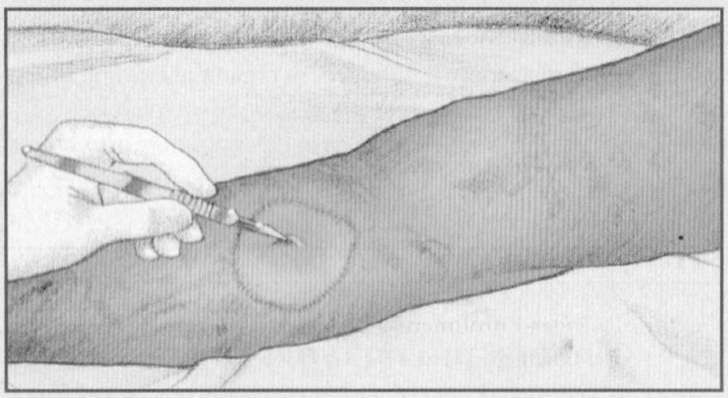

medication (such as micronized silver sulfadiazine cream) ■ Optional: sterile cotton-tipped applicators, sterile scalpel, sterile skin compresses, supplies for wound specimen collection, small-gauge needle and syringe, negative-pressure wound therapy equipment.

Implementation

- Verify the practitioner's order.
- Gather the equipment.
- Perform hand hygiene.[7,8,9,10,11,12]
- Prepare a sterile field. Using sterile technique, set up the supplies on the sterile field.[12,13]
- Label all medications, medication containers, and solutions on and off the sterile field.[14,15]
- Confirm the patient's identity using at least two patient identifiers.[16]
- Provide privacy and explain the procedure to the patient *to allay fears and enhance cooperation.*[17,18,19]
- Perform a comprehensive pain assessment using techniques appropriate for the patient's age, condition, and ability to understand.[20,21]
- Following safe medication administration practices, administer an analgesic, as ordered, at an appropriate time (depending on the medication's peak and onset of action) before beginning the procedure. Alternatively, give an IV analgesic immediately before the procedure.[22,23,24]
- If the patient is receiving IV opioid medication, frequently monitor his vital signs, respiratory status, and sedation level *to promptly recognize and treat oversedation and respiratory depression related to IV opioid use.* Explain the monitoring process to the patient and his family (including that it may be necessary to awaken the patient to assess the effects of medication). Advise the patient and his family to alert a staff member immediately if breathing problems or other changes occur that might be a reaction to the medication.[24,25]
- Remove the patient's splint if worn.[6]
- Perform hand hygiene.[7,8,9,10,11]
- Put on a cap, a sterile gown, a mask, and gloves.[12,13]
- Gently lift off all outer dressings. Soak the middle dressings with warm saline solution. Remove these carefully and slowly *to avoid disturbing the graft site.*
- Remove and discard your gloves.[12,13]
- Perform hand hygiene.[7,8,9,10,11]
- Put on the sterile gloves.[12,13]
- Assess the condition of the graft. Estimate the percentage of skin graft that has adhered successfully to the wound bed.[2] Also assess for signs of infection. Notify the practitioner if you note purulent drainage. Obtain a wound culture if ordered. (See the "Swab specimen collection" procedure, page 734.)
- If ordered, remove the inner graft dressing with sterile forceps, and clean the area gently. If necessary, soak the dressing with warm normal saline solution *to ease removal.*[26]
- Inspect an allograft for signs of rejection, such as infection and delayed healing. Inspect a sheet graft frequently for blebs. If ordered, evacuate them carefully with a sterile scalpel. If the sheet graft has been in place for less than 48 hours and the fluid is near the edge of the graft, gently roll the fluid to the edge and out from under the graft using sterile cotton-tipped applicators.[26] (See *Evacuating fluid from a sheet graft.*)
- Apply topical medication if ordered following safe medication administration practices.[22,23,24]
- If you removed the dressing, replace with a new prescribed dressing over the site *to promote wound healing and prevent infection.*[26] Use sterile scissors to cut the appropriate size.
- Cover the inner dressing with sterile 4″ × 4″ (10-cm × 10-cm) gauze and elastic gauze dressing or a compression bandage.
- Assess the donor site.
- Clean any completely healed areas, and apply prescribed moisturizing cream to them *to keep the skin pliable and to retard scarring.*[26]
- Discard used equipment and supplies in appropriate receptacles.[12,13]
- Remove and discard your gloves, gown, mask, and cap.[12,13]
- Perform hand hygiene.[7,8,9,10,11]
- Reassess the patient's pain and respond appropriately.[20,27]
- Document the procedure.[28,29,30]

Special considerations

- Discontinue hydrotherapy 3 to 4 days after grafting as ordered by the practitioner *to avoid dislodging the graft.* Avoid using a blood pressure cuff over the graft. Don't tug or pull dressings during dressing changes. Keep the patient from lying on the graft.
- If the graft dislodges, apply sterile skin compresses *to keep the area moist until the surgeon reapplies the graft.* If the graft affects an arm or a leg, elevate the affected extremity *to reduce postoperative edema.* Check for bleeding and signs and symptoms of neurovascular impairment, such as increasing pain, numbness or tingling, coolness, and pallor.
- Apply negative pressure to the graft site, if ordered, *because recent research demonstrates that applying topical negative pressure increases the quantity and quality of split skin graft success compared with traditional dressings.*[31,32] (See Negative pressure wound therapy, page 541.)
- The patient is generally allowed to shower after the fifth postoperative day at the practitioner's discretion.

Patient teaching

Teach the patient about graft and donor site care, including how to apply moisturizing cream to healed areas. Stress the importance of using a sunscreen containing titanium dioxide or oxybenzone and with a sun protection factor of 20 or higher on all grafted areas *to avoid sunburn and discoloration.*[1]

Complications

Graft failure may result from traumatic injury, hematoma or seroma formation, infection, an inadequate graft bed, rejection, or compromised nutritional status.

Documentation

Record the time and date of all dressing changes. Document all medications used, and note the patient's response to the medications and pain assessment. Describe the condition of the graft, and note any signs and symptoms of infection or rejection. Record any additional treatment, and note the patient's reaction to the graft. Document any patient teaching provided.

REFERENCES

1 Edwards, J. (2007). Focus: Management of skin grafts and donor sites. *Nursing Times, 103*(43), 52–53.

2 Beldon, P. (2007). What you need to know about skin grafts and donor site wounds. *Wound Essentials, 2007,* 149–155. Accessed May 2015 via the Web at http://www.woundsinternational.com/pdf/content_196.pdf

3 Canadian Agency for Drugs and Technologies in Health (CADTH). (2013). *Dressings and care of skin graft sites: A review of clinical evidence and guidelines.* Ottawa, ON: CADTH.

4 Jeong, H. S., et al. (2011). Hydrocolloid dressings in skin grafting for immobilization and compression. *Dermatologic Surgery, 37,* 320–324.

5 Kaiser, D., et al. (2013). Alginate dressing and polyurethane film versus paraffin gauze in the treatment of split-thickness skin graft donor sites: A randomized controlled pilot study. *Advances in Skin & Wound Care, 26,* 67–73. (Level II)

6 Foster, K., & Richey, K. (2008). Wound wise: The story on partial-thickness skin grafts. *Nursing Made Incredibly Easy, 6*(2), 19–21. Accessed May 2015 via the Web at http://www.nursingcenter.com/lnc/pdfjournal?AID=774634&an=00152258-200803000-00005&Journal_ID=&Issue_ID=

7 Centers for Disease Control and Prevention. (2002). Guideline for hand hygiene in health-care settings: Recommendations of the Healthcare Infection Control Practices Advisory Committee and the HICPAC/SHEA/APIC/IDSA Hand Hygiene Task Force. *MMWR Recommendations and Reports 51*(RR-16), 1–45. Accessed May 2015 via the Web at http://www.cdc.gov/mmwr/pdf/rr/rr5116.pdf (Level II)

8 World Health Organization. (2009). "WHO guidelines on hand hygiene in health care: First global patient safety challenge, clean care is safer care" [Online]. Accessed May 2015 via the Web at http://whqlibdoc.who.int/publications/2009/9789241597906_eng.pdf (Level IV)

9 The Joint Commission. (2015). Standard NPSG.07.01.01. *Comprehensive accreditation manual for hospitals: The official handbook.* Oakbrook Terrace, IL: The Joint Commission. (Level VII)

10 American Osteopathic Association. (2014). Standard 07.01.21. *Healthcare Facilities Accreditation Program: Accreditation requirements for acute care hospitals.* Chicago, IL: American Osteopathic Association. (Level VII)

11 Centers for Medicare & Medicaid Services, Department of Health and Human Services. (2014). Condition of participation: Infection control. 42 C.F.R. § 482.42.

12 Siegel, J. D., et al. (2007). "2007 guideline for isolation precautions: Preventing transmission of infectious agents in healthcare settings" [Online]. Accessed May 2015 via the Web at http://www.cdc.gov/hicpac/pdf/isolation/Isolation2007.pdf (Level II)

13 American Osteopathic Association. (2014). Standard 07.01.10. *Healthcare Facilities Accreditation Program: Accreditation requirements for acute care hospitals.* Chicago, IL: American Osteopathic Association. (Level VII)

14 The Joint Commission. (2015). Standard NPSG.03.04.01. *Comprehensive accreditation manual for hospitals: The official handbook.* Oakbrook Terrace, IL: The Joint Commission. (Level VII)

15 American Osteopathic Association. (2014). Standard 25.01.27. *Healthcare Facilities Accreditation Program: Accreditation requirements for acute care hospitals.* Chicago, IL: American Osteopathic Association. (Level VII)

16 The Joint Commission. (2015). Standard NPSG.01.01.01. *Comprehensive accreditation manual for hospitals: The official handbook.* Oakbrook Terrace, IL: The Joint Commission. (Level VII)

17 The Joint Commission. (2015). Standard RI.01.01.01. *Comprehensive accreditation manual for hospitals: The official handbook.* Oakbrook Terrace, IL: The Joint Commission. (Level VII)

18 American Osteopathic Association. (2014). Standard 15.01.16. *Healthcare Facilities Accreditation Program: Accreditation requirements for acute care hospitals.* Chicago, IL: American Osteopathic Association. (Level VII)

19 Centers for Medicare & Medicaid Services, Department of Health and Human Services. (2014). Condition of participation: Patient's rights. 42 C.F.R. § 482.13(c)(1).

20 The Joint Commission. (2015). Standard PC.01.02.07. *Comprehensive accreditation manual for hospitals: The official handbook.* Oakbrook Terrace, IL: The Joint Commission. (Level VII)

21 American Osteopathic Association. (2014). Standard 16.02.01. *Healthcare Facilities Accreditation Program: Accreditation requirements for acute care hospitals.* Chicago, IL: American Osteopathic Association. (Level VII)

22 The Joint Commission. (2015). Standard MM.06.01.01. *Comprehensive accreditation manual for hospitals: The official handbook.* Oakbrook Terrace, IL: The Joint Commission. (Level VII)

23 American Osteopathic Association. (2014). Standard 16.01.03. *Healthcare Facilities Accreditation Program: Accreditation requirements for acute care hospitals.* Chicago, IL: American Osteopathic Association. (Level VII)

24 Centers for Medicare & Medicaid Services, Department of Health and Human Services. (2014). Condition of participation: Nursing services. 42 C.F.R. § 482.23(c).

25 Centers for Medicare & Medicaid Services. (2014). "Requirements for hospital medication administration, particularly intravenous (IV) medications and post-operative care of patients receiving IV opioids" [Online]. Accessed May 2015 via the Web at http://www.cms.gov/Medicare/Provider-Enrollment-and-Certification/SurveyCertificationGenInfo/Downloads/Survey-and-Cert-Letter-14-15.pdf

26 Lynn-McHale Wiegand, D. (Ed.). (2011). *AACN procedure manual for critical care* (6th ed.). St. Louis, MO: Saunders.

27 American Osteopathic Association. (2014). Standard 16.02.05. *Healthcare Facilities Accreditation Program: Accreditation requirements for acute care hospitals.* Chicago, IL: American Osteopathic Association. (Level VII)

28 The Joint Commission. (2015). Standard RC.01.03.01. *Comprehensive accreditation manual for hospitals: The official handbook.* Oakbrook Terrace, IL: The Joint Commission. (Level VII)

29 Centers for Medicare & Medicaid Services, Department of Health and Human Services. (2014). Condition of participation: Medical record services. 42 C.F.R. § 482.24(b).

30 American Osteopathic Association. (2014). Standard 10.00.03. *Healthcare Facilities Accreditation Program: Accreditation requirements for acute care hospitals.* Chicago, IL: American Osteopathic Association. (Level VII)

31 Azzopardi, E. A., et al. (2013). Application of topical negative pressure (vacuum-assisted closure) to split-thickness skin grafts: A structured evidence-based review. *Annals of Plastic Surgery, 70,* 23–29.

32 Petkar, K. S., et al. (2011). A prospective randomized controlled trial comparing negative pressure dressing and conventional dressing methods on split-thickness skin grafts in burned patients. *Burns, 37,* 925–929. (Level II)

ADDITIONAL REFERENCES

Hernandez, J. L., et al. (2013). Use of continuous local anesthetic infusion in the management of postoperative split-thickness skin graft donor site pain. *Journal of Burn Care & Research, 34,* e257–e262. (Level VI)

Kagan, R. J., et al. (2013). Surgical management of the burn wound and use of skin substitutes: An expert panel white paper. *Journal of Burn Care & Research, 34,* e60–e79. (Level VII)

SKIN STAPLE AND CLIP REMOVAL

A practitioner may use skin staples or clips instead of standard sutures to close lacerations or surgical wounds. Because they can secure a wound more quickly than sutures, they may substitute for surface sutures where cosmetic results aren't a prime consideration, such as in abdominal closure. When properly placed, staples and clips distribute tension evenly along the suture line with minimal tissue trauma and compression, promoting healing and minimizing scarring. Because staples and clips are made from surgical stainless steel, tissue reaction to them is minimal. Practitioners typically remove skin staples and

Removing a staple

To remove a staple, position the extractor's lower jaws beneath the span of the first staple. Squeeze the handles until they're completely closed, and then lift the staple away from the skin. The extractor changes the shape of the staple and pulls the prongs out of the intradermal tissue (as shown below).

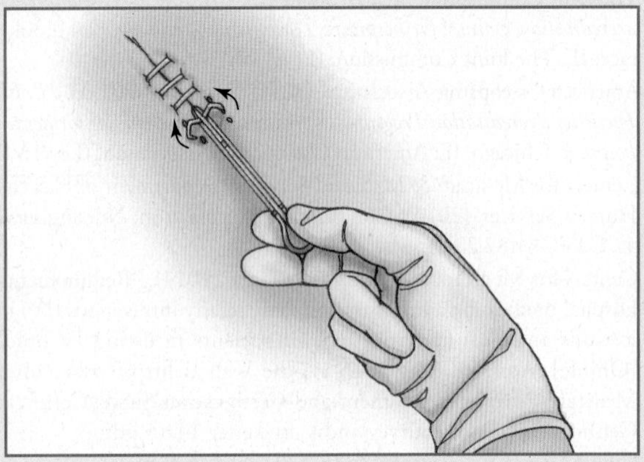

clips, but some facilities permit qualified nurses to perform this procedure.

Skin staples and clips are contraindicated when the wound's location requires cosmetically superior results or when the incision site makes it impossible to maintain at least a 5-mm distance between the staple and the underlying bone, vessels, or internal organs.

Equipment

Gloves ■ sterile 4″ × 4″ (10-cm × 10-cm) gauze pads ■ tape ■ waterproof trash container ■ sterile gloves ■ sterile barrier or drape to make a sterile field ■ sterile staple or clip extractor ■ antiseptic cleaning agents (pads or swabs) ■ Optional: butterfly or regular adhesive strips.

Prepackaged, sterile, disposable staple or clip extractors are available.

Implementation

- If your facility allows you to remove skin staples and clips, verify the practitioner's order *to confirm the exact timing and details for this procedure.*[1] The practitioner may want you to remove only alternate staples or clips initially and to leave others in place for an additional day or two *to support the incision.*
- Check the patient's medical record for a history of allergies, especially to adhesive tape and topical solutions or medications.
- Gather the equipment in the patient's room.
- Check the expiration date on each sterile package and inspect them for tears. If the integrity is compromised, obtain new supplies.
- Perform hand hygiene.[2,3,4,5,6]
- Confirm the patient's identity using at least two patient identifiers.[7]
- Provide privacy.[8,9,10]
- Explain the procedure to the patient. Tell him that he may feel a slight pulling or tickling sensation, but little discomfort, during staple removal. Reassure him that, because his incision is healing properly, removing the supporting staples or clips won't weaken the incision line.
- Place the patient in a comfortable position that doesn't place undue tension on the incision.
- Perform hand hygiene.[2,3,4]
- Place the trash container near the patient's bed, and position it properly *to avoid reaching across the sterile field or the wound when disposing of soiled articles.*
- If the patient's wound has a dressing, put on gloves and carefully remove it. Discard the dressing and the gloves in the waterproof trash bag.[11,12]
- Perform hand hygiene.[2,3,4,5,6]
- Assess the patient's incision. Notify the practitioner of gaping, drainage, inflammation, and other signs of infection.
- Establish a sterile work area with all the equipment and supplies you'll need for removing staples or clips and for cleaning and dressing the incision. Open the package containing the sterile staple or clip extractor, maintaining asepsis. Put on sterile gloves.[11,12]
- Wipe the incision gently with antiseptic pads or swabs, working from the inner aspect to the outer aspect of the wound *to remove surface encrustations and reduce the risk of infection.*[1]
- Pick up the sterile staple or clip extractor. Then, starting at one end of the incision, remove the staple or clip. (See *Removing a staple.*) Holding the extractor over the waterproof trash container, release the handle *to discard the staple or clip.*
- Repeat the procedure for each staple or clip until you've removed them all.
- Apply a sterile gauze dressing, if needed, *to prevent infection and irritation from clothing.*
- Remove and discard your gloves[11,12] and perform hand hygiene.[2,3,4,5,6]
- Properly clean or dispose of soiled equipment and supplies.[11,12,13,14]
- Perform hand hygiene.[2,3,4,5,6]
- Document the procedure.[15,16,17]

Special considerations

- When removing a staple or clip, place the extractor's jaws carefully between the patient's skin and the staple or clip *to avoid patient discomfort.* If extraction is difficult, notify the practitioner; *staples or clips placed too deeply within the skin or left in place too long may resist removal.*
- If the wound dehisces after you remove staples or clips, apply butterfly or regular adhesive strips *to approximate and support the edges,* and call the practitioner immediately to repair the wound.[1] (See *Types of adhesive skin closures.*)
- You may also apply butterfly or regular adhesive strips after removing staples or clips even if the wound is healing normally *to give added support to the incision and prevent lateral tension from forming a wide scar.* Leave the strips in place for 3 to 5 days.[1]

Patient teaching

If the patient is being discharged, teach him how to remove the dressing and care for the wound. Instruct him to call the practitioner immediately if he observes wound discharge, gaping, or inflammation. Tell him the redness surrounding the incision should gradually disappear, and that after a few weeks only a thin line should show. Encourage the patient to use sunblock products on the wound for 3 to 6 months *to aid healing and reduce scar formation.*[18]

Complications

Complications of staple removal include infection, missing a staple, and incomplete healing on removal, which may require application of adhesive strips.

Documentation

Record the date and time of staple or clip removal, the number of staples or clips removed, the appearance of the incision, dressings or butterfly strips applied, signs of wound complications, the patient's tolerance of the procedure, and any patient teaching provided.

REFERENCES

1 Lynn-McHale Wiegand, D. (Ed.). (2011). *AACN procedure manual for critical care* (6th ed.). St. Louis, MO: Saunders.

2 Centers for Disease Control and Prevention. (2002). Guideline for hand hygiene in health-care settings: Recommendations of the Healthcare Infection Control Practices Advisory Committee and the HICPAC/SHEA/APIC/IDSA Hand Hygiene Task Force. *MMWR Recommendations and Reports, 51*(RR-16), 1–45. Accessed May 2015 via the Web at http://www.cdc.gov/mmwr/pdf/rr/rr5116.pdf (Level II)

3 World Health Organization. (2009). "WHO guidelines on hand hygiene in health care: First global patient safety challenge, clean care is safer care" [Online]. Accessed May 2015 via the Web at http://whqlibdoc.who.int/publications/2009/9789241597906_eng.pdf (Level IV)

4 The Joint Commission. (2015). Standard NPSG.07.01.01. *Comprehensive accreditation manual for hospitals: The official handbook.* Oakbrook Terrace, IL: The Joint Commission. (Level VII)

5 Centers for Medicare & Medicaid Services, Department of Health and Human Services. (2014). Condition of participation: Infection control. 42 C.F.R. § 482.42.

6 American Osteopathic Association. (2014). Standard 07.01.21. *Healthcare Facilities Accreditation Program: Accreditation requirements for acute care hospitals.* Chicago, IL: American Osteopathic Association. (Level VII)

7 The Joint Commission. (2015). Standard NPSG.01.01.01. *Comprehensive accreditation manual for hospitals: The official handbook.* Oakbrook Terrace, IL: The Joint Commission. (Level VII)

8 Centers for Medicare & Medicaid Services, Department of Health and Human Services. (2014). Condition of participation: Patient's rights. 42 C.F.R. § 482.13(c)(1).

9 The Joint Commission. (2015). Standard RI.01.01.01. *Comprehensive accreditation manual for hospitals: The official handbook.* Oakbrook Terrace, IL: The Joint Commission. (Level VII)

10 American Osteopathic Association. (2014). Standard 15.01.16. *Healthcare Facilities Accreditation Program: Accreditation requirements for acute care hospitals.* Chicago, IL: American Osteopathic Association. (Level VII)

11 Siegel, J. D., et al. (2007). "2007 guideline for isolation precautions: Preventing transmission of infectious agents in healthcare settings" [Online]. Accessed May 2015 via the Web at http://www.cdc.gov/hicpac/pdf/isolation/Isolation2007.pdf (Level II)

12 American Osteopathic Association. (2014). Standard 07.01.10. *Healthcare Facilities Accreditation Program: Accreditation requirements for acute care hospitals.* Chicago, IL: American Osteopathic Association. (Level VII)

13 Rutala, W. A., et al. (2008). "Guideline for disinfection and sterilization in healthcare facilities, 2008" [Online]. Accessed May 2015 via the Web at http://www.cdc.gov/hicpac/pdf/guidelines/Disinfection_Nov_2008.pdf (Level I)

14 American Osteopathic Association. (2014). Standard 07.02.03. *Healthcare Facilities Accreditation Program: Accreditation requirements for acute care hospitals.* Chicago, IL: American Osteopathic Association. (Level VII)

15 The Joint Commission. (2015). Standard RC.01.03.01. *Comprehensive accreditation manual for hospitals: The official handbook.* Oakbrook Terrace, IL: The Joint Commission. (Level VII)

16 Centers for Medicare & Medicaid Services, Department of Health and Human Services. (2014). Condition of participation: Medical record services. 42 C.F.R. § 482.24(b).

17 American Osteopathic Association. (2014). Standard 10.00.03. *Healthcare Facilities Accreditation Program: Accreditation requirements for acute care hospitals.* Chicago, IL: American Osteopathic Association. (Level VII)

18 Nicks, B. A., et al. (2010). Acute wound management: Revisiting the approach to assessment, irrigation, and closure considerations. *International Journal of Emergency Medicine, 3,* 399–407. Accessed May 2015 via the Web at http://www.ncbi.nlm.nih.gov/pmc/articles/PMC3047833/

ADDITIONAL REFERENCES

Baudoin, L. M., & Mayeaux, E. J. (2014). A guide to better wound closures. *Journal of Family Practice, 63,* 181–186. Accessed May 2015 via the Web at http://www.jfponline.com/fileadmin/qhi/jfp/pdfs/6304/JFP_06304_Article1.pdf

Craven, R. F., & Hirnle, C. J. (2012). *Fundamentals of nursing: Human health and function* (7th ed.). Philadelphia, PA: Lippincott Williams & Wilkins.

Nettina, S. M. (2014). *Lippincott manual of nursing practice* (10th ed.). Philadelphia, PA: Wolters Kluwer.

Nuthalapaty, F. S., et al. (2013). A randomized controlled trial of early versus delayed skin staple removal following caesarean section in the obese patient. *Journal of Obstetrics and Gynaecology Canada, 35,* 426–433. (Level II)

Taylor, C., et al. (2015). *Fundamentals of nursing: The art and science of nursing care* (8th ed.). Philadelphia, PA: Wolters Kluwer.

EQUIPMENT

Types of adhesive skin closures

Adhesive strips made of thin strips of sterile, nonwoven, porous fabric tape are a primary means of keeping a wound closed after staple or clip removal.

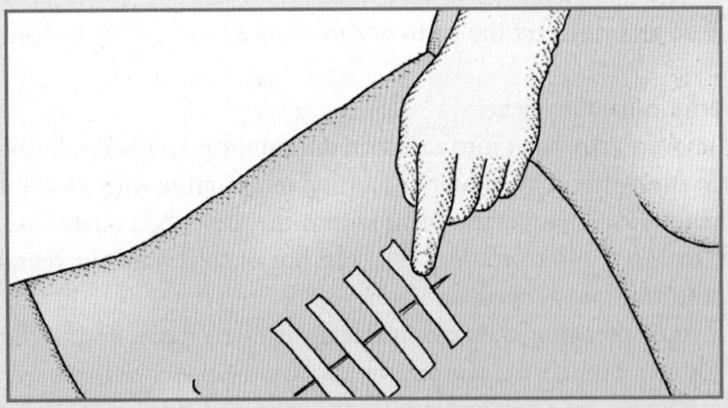

Butterfly adhesive strips consist of wider sterile, waterproof adhesive strips that are connected by a narrow, nonadhesive bridge. These strips help close small wounds and assist healing after staple or clip removal.

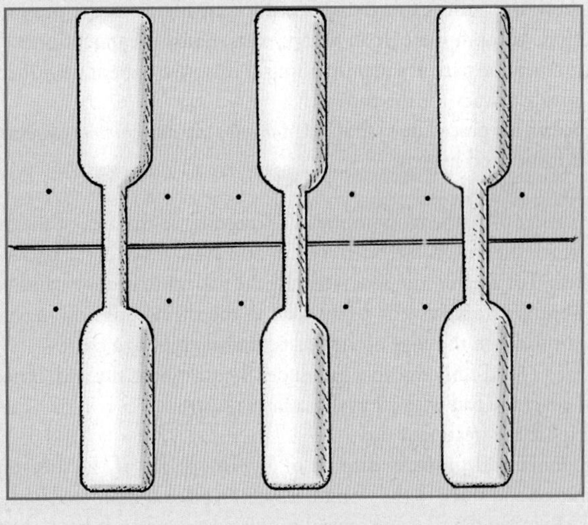

SOAKS

A soak involves immersion of a body part in warm water or a medicated solution. This treatment helps to soften exudates, facilitate debridement, enhance suppuration, clean wounds or burns, rehydrate wounds, apply medication to infected areas, and increase local blood supply and circulation.

Most soaks are applied with clean tap water and clean technique. Sterile solution and sterile equipment are required for treating wounds, burns, and other breaks in the skin.

Equipment

Basin, or arm or foot tub ▪ bath (utility) thermometer ▪ warm tap water or prescribed solution ▪ cup ▪ pitcher ▪ fluid-impermeable pad ▪ overbed table ▪ footstool ▪ pillows ▪ towels ▪ gauze pads and other dressing materials ▪ gloves ▪ hospital-grade disinfectant ▪ Optional: sterile gloves.

Preparation of equipment

- Perform hand hygiene.[1,2,3,4,5]
- Clean and disinfect the basin or tub using a hospital-grade disinfectant.[6,7]
- Perform hand hygiene.[1,2,3,4,5]
- Run warm tap water into a pitcher, or heat the prescribed solution, as applicable. Measure the water or solution temperature with a bath thermometer. If the temperature isn't within the prescribed range (usually 105° to 110°F [40.6° to 43.3°C]), add hot or cold water, or reheat or cool the solution, as needed.

If you're preparing the soak outside the patient's room, heat the liquid slightly above the correct temperature *to allow for cooling during transport.* If the solution for a medicated soak isn't premixed, prepare the solution and heat it to the prescribed temperature.

Implementation

- Verify the practitioner's order.
- Check the patient's medical record for an allergy to the prescribed solution, as appropriate. If an allergy exists, notify the practitioner.
- Confirm the patient's identity using at least two patient identifiers.[8]
- Provide privacy for the patient.[9,10]
- Explain the procedure to the patient *to allay fear and enhance cooperation.*
- Perform hand hygiene.[1,2,3,4,5]
- Put on gloves.[11,12]
- Position the patient appropriately, according to the area of the body for which the soak is intended: For an arm soak, instruct the patient to sit erect. For a leg or foot soak, instruct the patient to lie down and bend the appropriate knee. For a foot soak in the sitting position, have the patient to sit on the edge of the bed or transfer him to a chair.
- Place a fluid-impermeable pad under the treatment site and, if necessary, cover the pad with a towel *to absorb spillage.*
- Expose the treatment site.
- Remove and properly dispose of any dressing.[11] If the dressing is encrusted and stuck to the wound, leave it in place and proceed with the soak. Remove the dressing several minutes later, when it has begun to soak free.
- Position the soak basin under the treatment site on the bed, overbed table, footstool, or floor, as appropriate. If the soak basin or tub will be placed in the bed, make sure that the bed is flat beneath it *to prevent spills.*
- Pour the heated liquid into the soak basin or tub.
- Lower the patient's affected area into the basin or tub gradually *to allow adjustment to the temperature change.* Make sure the soak solution covers the treatment site.
- Make the patient comfortable, and ensure proper body alignment. Support other body parts with pillows or towels as needed *to prevent discomfort and muscle strain.*
- Remove and discard your gloves.[11,12]
- Check the temperature of the soak solution with the bath thermometer every 5 minutes. If the temperature drops below the prescribed range, remove some of the cooled solution with a cup, lift the patient's arm or leg from the basin *to avoid burns,* and add hot water or solution to the basin. Mix the liquid thoroughly and then recheck the temperature. If the temperature is within the prescribed range, lower the affected area back into the basin.
- Observe the patient for signs of tissue intolerance, including extreme redness at the treatment site, excessive drainage, bleeding, and maceration. If such signs develop or the patient complains of pain, discontinue the treatment and notify the practitioner.
- After 15 to 20 minutes, or as ordered, perform hand hygiene[1,2,3,4,5] and put on a new pair of gloves,[11,12] lift the patient's treatment area from the basin or tub, and remove the basin or tub.
- Dry the area thoroughly with a towel. If the patient has a wound, dry the skin around it without touching the wound.
- While the skin is hydrated from the soak, use gauze pads to remove loose scales or crusts.
- Observe the treatment area for general appearance, degree of swelling, debridement, suppuration, and healing.
- Remove the towel and fluid-impermeable pad, and make the patient comfortable in bed.
- If the patient's wound requires redressing, remove and discard your gloves,[11,12] perform hand hygiene,[1,2,3,4,5] put on new gloves, and then redress the wound.[11,12]
- Discard the soak solution and dispose of soiled materials in appropriate receptacles.[11]
- Remove and discard your gloves.[11,12]
- Perform hand hygiene.[1,2,3,4,5]
- Put on new gloves.[11,12]
- Clean and disinfect the basin or tub using a hospital-grade disinfectant.[6,7]
- Remove and discard your gloves.[11,12]
- Perform hand hygiene.[1,2,3,4,5]
- If the soak treatment is to be repeated, store the equipment in the patient's room, out of his reach; otherwise, return it to the central supply department.
- Document the procedure.[13,14,15]

Special considerations

- To treat large areas, particularly burns, a soak may be administered in a whirlpool or Hubbard tank.

Complications

Tissue intolerance is a complication of soaks; its signs and symptoms include extreme redness, excessive drainage, bleeding, maceration, and pain at the treatment site.

Documentation

Record the date, time, and duration of the soak; the treatment site; the solution used and its temperature; skin and wound appearance before, during, and after treatment; and the patient's tolerance of treatment.

References

1 The Joint Commission. (2015). Standard NPSG.07.01.01. *Comprehensive accreditation manual for hospitals: The official handbook.* Oakbrook Terrace, IL: The Joint Commission. (Level VII)

2 Centers for Disease Control and Prevention. (2002). Guideline for hand hygiene in health-care settings: Recommendations of the Healthcare Infection Control Practices Advisory Committee and the HICPAC/SHEA/APIC/IDSA Hand Hygiene Task Force. *MMWR Recommendations and Reports, 51*(RR-16), 1–45. Accessed May 2015 via the Web at http://www.cdc.gov/mmwr/pdf/rr/rr5116.pdf (Level II)

3 World Health Organization. (2009). "WHO guidelines on hand hygiene in health care: First global patient safety challenge, clean care is safer care" [Online]. Accessed May 2015 via the Web at http://whqlibdoc.who.int/publications/2009/9789241597906_eng.pdf (Level IV)

4 American Osteopathic Association. (2014). Standard 07.01.21. *Healthcare Facilities Accreditation Program: Accreditation requirements for acute care hospitals.* Chicago, IL: American Osteopathic Association. (Level VII)

5 Centers for Medicare & Medicaid Services, Department of Health and Human Services. (2014). Condition of participation: Infection control. 42 C.F.R. § 482.42.

6 Rutala, W. A., et al. (2008). "Guideline for disinfection and sterilization in healthcare facilities, 2008" [Online]. Accessed May 2015 via the Web at http://www.cdc.gov/hicpac/pdf/guidelines/Disinfection_Nov_2008.pdf (Level I)
7 American Osteopathic Association. (2014). Standard 07.02.03. *Healthcare Facilities Accreditation Program: Accreditation requirements for acute care hospitals.* Chicago, IL: American Osteopathic Association. (Level VII)
8 The Joint Commission. (2015). Standard NPSG.01.01.01. *Comprehensive accreditation manual for hospitals: The official handbook.* Oakbrook Terrace, IL: The Joint Commission. (Level VII)
9 American Osteopathic Association. (2014). Standard 15.01.16. *Healthcare Facilities Accreditation Program: Accreditation requirements for acute care hospitals.* Chicago, IL: American Osteopathic Association. (Level VII)
10 Centers for Medicare & Medicaid Services, Department of Health and Human Services. (2014). Condition of participation: Patient's rights. 42 C.F.R. § 482.13(c)(1).
11 Siegel, J. D., et al. (2007). "2007 guideline for isolation precautions: Preventing transmission of infectious agents in healthcare settings" [Online]. Accessed May 2015 via the Web at http://www.cdc.gov/hicpac/pdf/isolation/Isolation2007.pdf (Level II)
12 American Osteopathic Association. (2014). Standard 07.01.10. *Healthcare Facilities Accreditation Program: Accreditation requirements for acute care hospitals.* Chicago, IL: American Osteopathic Association. (Level VII)
13 The Joint Commission. (2015). Standard RC.01.03.01. *Comprehensive accreditation manual for hospitals: The official handbook.* Oakbrook Terrace, IL: The Joint Commission. (Level VII)
14 American Osteopathic Association. (2014). Standard 10.00.03. *Healthcare Facilities Accreditation Program: Accreditation requirements for acute care hospitals.* Chicago, IL: American Osteopathic Association. (Level VII)
15 Centers for Medicare & Medicaid Services, Department of Health and Human Services. (2014). Condition of participation: Medical record services. 42 C.F.R. § 482.24(b).

ADDITIONAL REFERENCE

Craven, R. F., & Hirnle, C. J. (2012). *Fundamentals of nursing: Human health and function* (7th ed.). Philadelphia, PA: Lippincott Williams & Wilkins.

SPIRITUAL CARE

Religious beliefs can profoundly influence a patient's recovery rate, attitude toward treatment, and overall response to hospitalization. In certain religious groups, beliefs can preclude diagnostic tests and therapeutic treatments, require dietary restrictions, or prohibit organ donation and artificial prolongation of life. (See *Beliefs and practices of selected religions,* page 706.)

Consequently, effective patient care requires recognition of and respect for the patient's religious beliefs.[1] Recognizing his beliefs and need for spiritual care may require close attention to his nonverbal cues or to seemingly casual remarks that express his spiritual concerns. Respecting his beliefs may require setting aside your own beliefs to help the patient follow his. Providing spiritual care may require contacting an appropriate member of the clergy in the facility or community, gathering equipment needed to help the patient perform rites and administer sacraments, and preparing him for a pastoral visit.

Equipment

Optional: Clean towels (one or two), teaspoon or medicine cup, container of water (for emergency baptism), other supplies specific to the patient's religious affiliation.

Some facilities, particularly those with a religious affiliation, provide baptismal trays. The clergy member may bring holy water, holy oil, or other religious articles to minister to the patient.

Preparation of equipment

For baptism, cover a small table with a clean towel. Fold a second towel and place it on the table, along with the teaspoon or medicine cup. For communion and anointing, cover the bedside stand with a clean towel.

Implementation

- Check the patient's admission record *to determine his religious affiliation.* Remember that some patients may claim no religious beliefs. However, even an agnostic may wish to speak with a clergy member, so watch and listen carefully for subtle expressions of this desire.
- Perform hand hygiene.[2,3,4,5,6]
- Confirm the patient's identity using at least two patient identifiers.[7]
- Assess the patient's spiritual needs, resources, and preferences.[8] Evaluate the patient's behavior for signs of loneliness, anxiety, or fear, *emotions that may signal his need for spiritual counsel.* Also consider whether the patient is facing a health crisis, which may occur with chronic illness and before childbirth, surgery, or impending death. Remember that a patient may feel acutely distressed because of his inability to participate in religious observances. Help such a patient verbalize his beliefs *to relieve stress.* Listen to him and let him express his concerns, but carefully refrain from imposing your beliefs on him *to avoid conflict and further stress.*[8]
- If the patient requests, arrange a visit by an appropriate member of the clergy. Consult this clergy member if you need more information about the patient's beliefs.
- If your patient faces the possibility of abortion, amputation, transfusion, or other medical procedures with important religious implications, try to discover his spiritual attitude. Also, try to determine your patient's attitude toward the importance of laying on of hands, confession, communion, observance of holy days (such as the Sabbath), and restrictions in diet or physical appearance. *Helping the patient continue his normal religious practices during hospitalization can help reduce stress.*
- If the patient is pregnant, find out her beliefs concerning infant baptism and circumcision, and comply with them after birth.

PEDIATRIC ALERT *If a neonate is in critical condition and the family requests it, call an appropriate clergy member immediately. In an extreme emergency, you can perform a Roman Catholic baptism using a container of any available water. If you do so, be sure to notify the priest when he arrives* because this sacrament must be administered only once.

- If a Jewish woman delivers a male infant prematurely or by cesarean birth, ask her whether she plans to observe the rite of circumcision, or a bris, a significant ceremony performed on the 8th day after birth. (*Because a patient who delivers a healthy, full-term baby vaginally is usually discharged quickly,* this ceremony is normally performed outside the facility.) For a bris, ensure privacy and, if requested, sterilize the instruments.
- If the patient requests communion, prepare him for it before the clergy member arrives. First, place him in the Fowler or semi-Fowler position if his condition permits. Otherwise, allow him to remain supine. Tuck a clean towel under his chin and straighten the bed linens.
- If a terminally ill patient requests the Sacrament of the Sick (Last Rites) or special treatment of his body after death, call an appropriate clergy member. For the Roman Catholic patient, call a Roman Catholic priest to administer the sacrament, even if the patient is unresponsive or comatose. *To prepare the patient for this sacrament,* uncover his arms and fold back the top linens *to expose his feet.* After the clergy member anoints the patient's forehead, eyes, nose, mouth, hands, and feet, straighten and retuck the bed linens.
- Perform hand hygiene.[2,3,4,5,6]
- Document the procedure.[9,10,11]

Special considerations

- Handle the patient's religious articles carefully *to avoid damage or loss.*
- Become familiar with religious resources in your facility. Some facilities employ one or more clergy members who counsel patients and staff members and link patients to other pastoral resources.

Beliefs and practices of selected religions

A patient's religious beliefs can affect his attitudes toward illness and traditional medicine. By trying to accommodate the patient's religious beliefs and practices in your plan of care, you can increase his willingness to learn and comply with treatment regimens. *Because religious beliefs may vary within particular sects,* individual practices may differ from those described here.

Adventist
- *Birth and death rituals:* None (baptism of adults only)
- *Dietary restrictions:* Alcohol, coffee, tea, opioids, stimulants, and meat or animal products (in some groups)
- *Practices in health crisis:* Communion, baptism, divine healing and anointing with oil (in some groups), prayer, and Saturday Sabbath (in some groups)

Baptist
- *Birth and death rituals:* At birth, none (baptism of believers only); before death, counseling by clergy member and prayer
- *Dietary restrictions:* Alcohol, coffee, and tea (in some groups)
- *Practices in health crisis*: Healing by laying on of hands (in some groups) as well as resistance to medical therapy (occasionally approved)

Christian Scientist
- *Birth and death rituals:* At birth, none; before death, counseling by a Christian Science practitioner
- *Dietary restrictions:* Alcohol, coffee, and tobacco
- *Practices in health crisis:* Refusal of all treatments (most groups), including drugs, biopsies, physical examination, and blood transfusions; vaccination permitted only when required by law; alteration of thoughts believed to cure illness; hypnotism and psychotherapy prohibited (Christian Scientist nurses and nursing homes honor these beliefs)

Church of Christ
- *Birth and death rituals:* None (baptism at age 8 or older)
- *Dietary restrictions:* Alcohol discouraged
- *Practices in health crisis:* Communion, anointing with oil, laying on of hands, and counseling (all performed by a minister)

Eastern Orthodox
- *Birth and death rituals:* At birth, baptism and confirmation; before death, last rites; for members of the Russian Orthodox Church, arms are crossed after death, fingers set in cross, and unembalmed body clothed in natural fiber
- *Dietary restrictions:* For members of the Russian Orthodox Church and usually the Greek Orthodox Church, no meat or dairy products on Wednesday or Friday or during Lent
- *Practices in health crisis:* Anointing of the sick; for members of the Russian Orthodox Church, cross necklace is replaced immediately after surgery and shaving of male patients is prohibited except in preparation for surgery; for members of the Greek Orthodox Church, communion and Sacrament of Holy Unction

Episcopalian
- *Birth and death rituals:* At birth, baptism; before death, occasional last rites
- *Dietary restrictions:* For some members, abstention from meat on Friday, fasting before communion (which may be daily)
- *Practices in health crisis:* Communion, prayer, and counseling (all performed by a minister)

Jehovah's Witnesses
- *Birth and death rituals:* None
- *Dietary restrictions:* Abstention from foods to which blood has been added
- *Practices in health crisis:* Typically, no blood transfusions permitted; a court order may be required for emergency transfusion

Judaism
- *Birth and death rituals:* Ritual circumcision on 8th day after birth; burial of dead fetus; ritual washing of dead; burial (including organs and other body tissues) occurs as soon as possible; no autopsy or embalming
- *Dietary restrictions:* For Orthodox and Conservative Jews, kosher dietary laws (for example, pork and shellfish prohibited); for Reform Jews, usually no restrictions
- *Practices in health crisis:* Rabbinical consultation required for donation or transplantation of organs; for Orthodox and Conservative Jews, medical procedures possibly prohibited on the Sabbath (from sundown Friday to sundown Saturday) and on special holidays

Lutheran
- *Birth and death rituals:* Baptism usually performed 6 to 8 weeks after birth
- *Dietary restrictions:* None
- *Practices in health crisis:* Communion, prayer, and counseling (all performed by a minister)

Mormon
- *Birth and death rituals:* At birth, none (baptism at age 8 or older); before death, baptism and gospel preaching
- *Dietary restrictions:* Alcohol, tobacco, tea, and coffee prohibited; meat intake limited
- *Practices in health crisis:* Belief in divine healing through the laying on of hands; communion on Sunday; refusal of medical treatment by some members; special undergarment worn by many

Muslim
- *Birth and death rituals:* If spontaneous abortion occurs before 130 days, fetus treated as discarded tissue; after 130 days, fetus treated as a human being; before death, confession of sins with family present; after death, only relatives or friends may touch the body
- *Dietary restrictions:* Pork prohibited; daylight fasting during 9th month of Islamic calendar
- *Practices in health crisis*: Faith healing (for the patient's morale only); conservative members reject medical therapy

Orthodox Presbyterian
- *Birth and death rituals:* Infant baptism; scripture reading and prayer before death
- *Dietary restrictions:* None
- *Practices in health crisis:* Communion, prayer, and counseling (all performed by a minister)

Beliefs and practices of selected religions *(continued)*

Pentecostal Assembly of God, Foursquare Church

■ *Birth and death rituals:* None (baptism only after age of accountability)

■ *Dietary restrictions:* Abstention from alcohol, tobacco, meat slaughtered by strangling, any food to which blood has been added, and sometimes pork

■ *Practices in health crisis:* Divine healing through prayer, anointing with oil, laying on of hands

Roman Catholic

■ *Birth and death rituals:* Infant baptism, including baptism of aborted fetus without sign of clinical death (tissue necrosis); before death, anointing of the sick

■ *Dietary restrictions:* Fasting or abstention from meat on Ash Wednesday and on Fridays during Lent (practice usually waived for the hospitalized)

■ *Practices in health crisis:* Burial of major amputated limb (sometimes) in consecrated ground; donation or transplantation of organs allowed if the benefit to recipient outweighs the donor's potential harm; Sacrament of the Sick also performed when patients are ill, not just before death, and sometimes performed shortly after admission

United Methodist

■ *Birth and death rituals:* None (baptism of children and adults only)

■ *Dietary restrictions:* None

■ *Practices in health crisis:* Communion before surgery or similar crisis; donation of body parts encouraged

■ If the patient tries to convert you to his personal beliefs, tell him that you respect his beliefs but are content with your own. Likewise, avoid attempts to convert the patient to your personal beliefs.[8]

Documentation

If baptism was performed, complete a baptismal form and attach it to the patient's record; send a copy of the form to the appropriate clergy member. Record the rites of circumcision and Last Rites in the patient's medical record.

REFERENCES

1 The Joint Commission. (2015). Standard RI.01.01.01. *Comprehensive accreditation manual for hospitals: The official handbook.* Oakbrook Terrace, IL: The Joint Commission. (Level VII)

2 Centers for Disease Control and Prevention. (2002). Guideline for hand hygiene in health care settings: Recommendations of the Healthcare Infection Control Practices Advisory Committee and the HICPAC/SHEA/APIC/IDSA Hand Hygiene Task Force. *MMWR Recommendations and Reports, 51*(RR-16), 1–45. Accessed May 2015 via the Web at http://www.cdc.gov/mmwr/pdf/rr/rr5116.pdf (Level II)

3 World Health Organization. (2009). "WHO guidelines on hand hygiene in health care: First global patient safety challenge, clean care is safer care" [Online]. Accessed May 2015 via the Web at http://whqlibdoc.who.int/publications/2009/9789241597906_eng.pdf (Level IV)

4 The Joint Commission. (2015). Standard NPSG.07.01.01. *Comprehensive accreditation manual for hospitals: The official handbook.* Oakbrook Terrace, IL: The Joint Commission. (Level VII)

5 American Osteopathic Association. (2012). Standard 07.01.21. *Healthcare Facilities Accreditation Program: Accreditation requirements for acute care hospitals.* Chicago, IL: American Osteopathic Association. (Level VII)

6 Centers for Medicare & Medicaid Services, Department of Health and Human Services. (2014). Condition of participation: Infection control. 42 C.F.R. § 482.42.

7 The Joint Commission. (2015). Standard NPSG.01.01.01. *Comprehensive accreditation manual for hospitals: The official handbook.* Oakbrook Terrace, IL: The Joint Commission. (Level VII)

8 Taylor, E. J. (2011). Spiritual care: Evangelism at the bedside? *Journal of Christian Nursing, 28,* 194–202. Accessed May 2015 via the Web at http://www.nursingcenter.com/pdf.asp?AID=1233832

9 The Joint Commission. (2015). Standard RC.01.03.01. *Comprehensive accreditation manual for hospitals: The official handbook.* Oakbrook Terrace, IL: The Joint Commission. (Level VII)

10 Centers for Medicare & Medicaid Services, Department of Health and Human Services. (2014). Condition of participation: Medical record services. 42 C.F.R. § 482.24(b).

11 American Osteopathic Association. (2014). Standard 10.00.03. *Healthcare Facilities Accreditation Program: Accreditation requirements for acute care hospitals.* Chicago, IL: American Osteopathic Association. (Level VII)

SPLINT APPLICATION

By immobilizing the site of an injury, a splint alleviates pain and allows the injury to heal in proper alignment. It also minimizes possible complications, such as excessive bleeding into tissues and restricted blood flow caused by bone pressing against vessels. In cases of multiple serious injuries, a splint allows caretakers to move the patient without risking further damage to bones, muscles, nerves, blood vessels, and skin.

Splints have traditionally been made of plaster of Paris; however, in recent years, many different types of splinting materials have become available. Types of splints include air splints, vacuum splints, and those made from preformed plaster, fiberglass, padded fiberglass, and aluminum. Preformed, rigid commercial splints are available for use on various body parts, come in multiple sizes, and are usually made of hard plastic and Velcro.[1] Commercial splints may be removed to enable skin assessment; however, repeated removal by the patient may delay healing or cause additional injury.[1]

A practitioner may order a splint to immobilize a simple or compound fracture, dislocation, or subluxation.[2] (See *Rigid splint,* page 708.)

Equipment

Rigid splint ■ tape measure ■ padding ■ Velcro straps, 2″ (5-cm) roller gauze, or 2″ (5-cm) cloth strips ■ tape ■ pillows ■ vital signs monitoring equipment ■ Optional: gloves and other personal protective equipment, ice, prescribed pain medication.

A practitioner may prefer to use an air splint (an inflatable, semirigid splint) to secure an injured extremity. (See *Using an air splint,* page 708.) You can use Velcro straps, roller gauze, or cloth strips as bindings for a rigid or air splint. However, avoid using twine or rope, if possible, *because they can restrict circulation.*

Implementation

■ Perform hand hygiene.[3,4,5,6,7]

■ Put on gloves and other personal protective equipment, as needed.[8,9]

■ Confirm the patient's identity using at least two patient identifiers.[10]

EQUIPMENT

Rigid splint

A rigid splint, as shown below, can help immobilize a fracture or dislocation in an extremity. Ideally, two people should apply a rigid splint to an extremity.

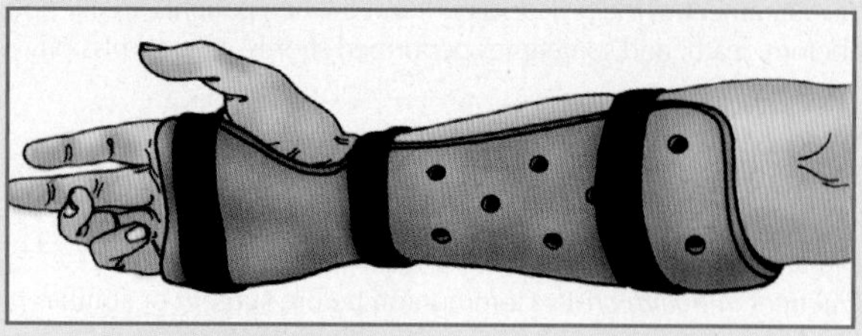

EQUIPMENT

Using an air splint

In an emergency, you can apply an air splint, shown below, *to immobilize a fracture or control bleeding,* especially from a forearm or lower leg. This compact, comfortable splint is made of double-walled plastic and provides gentle, diffuse pressure over an injured area. After choosing the appropriate splint wrap it around the affected extremity, secure it with Velcro or other strips, and then inflate it. Inflate the splint only to the point where you can slip a finger between the splint and the skin *so that it fits snugly enough to immobilize the extremity without impairing circulation.*[2]

An air splint may actually control bleeding better than a local pressure bandage. Its clear plastic construction simplifies inspection of the affected site for bleeding, pallor, or cyanosis. An air splint also allows the patient to be moved without further damage to the injured limb.

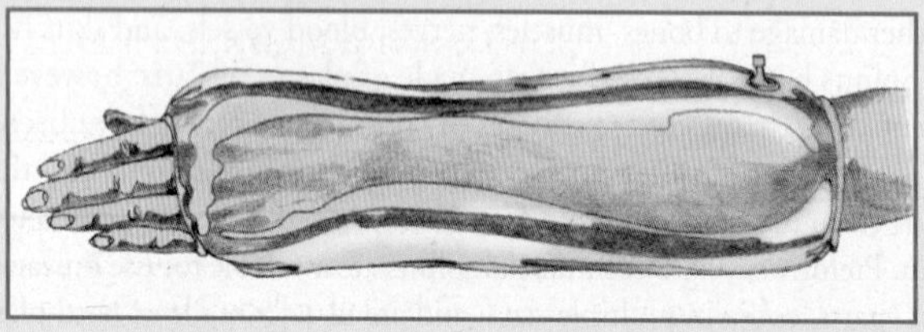

- Obtain a history of the circumstances surrounding the injury (including the time and mechanism of injury) and significant medical history, including alcohol use, medications, allergies, and tetanus immunization status if known. Ask the time of the patient's last oral intake, and keep the patient on nothing-by-mouth status if procedural sedation or surgical intervention is possible. (See the "Moderate sedation" procedure, page 505.)[2]
- Explain the procedure to the patient and provide emotional support *to allay his fears.*
- Provide privacy.[11,12,13]
- If necessary, remove or cut away the patient's clothing and remove jewelry if the injury involves the hand or foot and the patient is wearing jewelry on the extremity.[2]
- Begin a thorough head-to-toe assessment, inspecting for obvious deformities, swelling, or bleeding.
- Perform a comprehensive pain assessment using techniques appropriate for the patient's age, condition, and ability to understand.[14,15]
- Administer pain medications, as ordered and indicated, following safe medication administration practices.[16,17,18] Make sure the patient has adequate analgesia during and after splinting *because splint application may involve painful movement of the injured limb.*[19]
- Assess the affected extremity's range of motion (ROM).
- Inspect and gently palpate the injured area for evidence of fracture or dislocation.
- Assess neurovascular integrity distal to the injury site.[2]
- If possible, align the injured extremity in its normal anatomic position.
- Don't attempt to straighten a dislocation *to avoid damaging misplaced vessels and nerves.*
- Measure the uninjured side *to determine the proper splint size.* Choose a splint that will immobilize the joints above and below the fracture.[20]
- Pad the splint, as needed, *to protect bony prominences.*
- Support the injured extremity above and below the fracture site while applying firm, gentle traction.[20]
- Have an assistant place the splint under, beside, or on top of the extremity.
- Have the assistant apply the bindings to secure the splint, being careful not to compromise the circulation; the splint should fit snugly but not be constrictive.[20]
- Assess the neurovascular status of the extremity. If it's impaired by the bindings, release and reapply them.
- Elevate the injured extremity, keeping in mind that excessive elevation may compromise arterial circulation.[2,20]
- Monitor the patient's vital signs frequently *to detect signs of shock.* Fractured bones may cause significant bleeding into surrounding tissues.
- Monitor the patient's neurovascular status by assessing skin color, temperature of the extremities, the presence of paresthesia, and pulses as well as the patient's ability to move his extremities. *Numbness or paralysis distal to an injury indicates nerve injury.* (See *Assessing neurovascular status.*)
- Reassess for pain, and respond appropriately.[14,21]
- Apply ice to the injury, as needed, *to minimize swelling.*[2]
- Assess the patient for signs of skin breakdown on an ongoing basis; *skin breakdown may result from contact with the splint or immobility.*
- Remove and discard your gloves and other personal protective equipment if worn.[8,9]
- Perform hand hygiene.[3,4,5,6,7]
- Document the procedure.[22,23,24]

Special considerations

- If a commercially prepared splint isn't available, the practitioner, physical therapist, or occupational therapist may develop a customized splint for the patient.
- Another body part may serve as a temporary splint. To splint a leg in this manner, pad the inner aspect and secure it to the other leg with roller gauze or cloth strips.
- Collaborate with the practitioner, physical therapist, or occupational therapist about the splint application and removal schedule, the activities permitted, and recommended ROM and strengthening exercises.
- Under a practitioner's direct supervision, apply gentle traction, and carefully remove a splint if there's evidence of improper application or vascular impairment.

Patient teaching

Teach the patient how to remove and apply the splint properly and the schedule he should follow. Also review permissible activities while wearing the splint. Tell the patient to check his skin beneath the splint several times a day and to report numbness, tingling, pain, a change in skin temperature, and skin breakdown in the affected extremity. Instruct the patient never to place foreign objects between the splinting material and the skin.

Complications

Multiple transfers and repeated manipulation of a fracture may cause fat embolism. This complication usually occurs within 36 hours of an injury or manipulation.[25] Signs and symptoms of fat embolism include dyspnea, agitation, hypoxia, changes in mental status, and a petechial rash. Other possible complications include pressure ulcers or contact dermatitis beneath the splint, neurovascular compromise, and decreased ROM.[19]

Documentation

Record the circumstances surrounding the injury, including the time and mechanism of injury. Document the patient's complaints, noting whether his symptoms are localized. Record the neurovascular assessment before and after applying the splint. Note the type of wound and the type and amount of any drainage. Note the time of splint application. Be sure to note if the bone end slips into surrounding tissue or if transportation causes a change in the degree of dislocation.

REFERENCES

1 Kronfol, R. Splinting of musculoskeletal injuries. (2014). In: *UpToDate*, Fields, K. B., et al. (Eds.). Accessed May 2015 via the Web at www.uptodate.com/contents/search

2 Emergency Nurses Association. (2012). *Sheehy's emergency nursing principles and practice* (7th ed.). St. Louis, MO: Mosby.

3 Centers for Disease Control and Prevention. (2002). Guideline for hand hygiene in health-care settings: Recommendations of the Healthcare Infection Control Practices Advisory Committee and the HICPAC/SHEA/APIC/IDSA Hand Hygiene Task Force. *MMWR Recommendations and Reports, 51*(RR-16), 1–45. Accessed May 2015 via the Web at http://www.cdc.gov/mmwr/pdf/rr/rr5116.pdf (Level II)

4 World Health Organization. (2009). "WHO guidelines on hand hygiene in health care: First global patient safety challenge, clean care is safer care" [Online]. Accessed May 2015 via the Web at http://whqlibdoc.who.int/publications/2009/9789241597906_eng.pdf (Level IV)

5 The Joint Commission. (2015). Standard NPSG.07.01.01. *Comprehensive accreditation manual for hospitals: The official handbook.* Oakbrook Terrace, IL: The Joint Commission. (Level VII)

6 Centers for Medicare & Medicaid Services, Department of Health and Human Services. (2014). Condition of participation: Infection control. 42 C.F.R. § 482.42.

7 American Osteopathic Association. (2014). Standard 07.01.21. *Healthcare Facilities Accreditation Program: Accreditation requirements for acute care hospitals.* Chicago, IL: American Osteopathic Association. (Level VII)

8 Siegel, J. D., et al. (2007). "2007 guideline for isolation precautions: Preventing transmission of infectious agents in healthcare settings" [Online]. Accessed May 2015 via the Web at http://www.cdc.gov/hicpac/pdf/isolation/Isolation2007.pdf (Level II)

9 American Osteopathic Association. (2014). Standard 07.01.10. *Healthcare Facilities Accreditation Program: Accreditation requirements for acute care hospitals.* Chicago, IL: American Osteopathic Association. (Level VII)

10 The Joint Commission. (2015). Standard NPSG.01.01.01. *Comprehensive accreditation manual for hospitals: The official handbook.* Oakbrook Terrace, IL: The Joint Commission. (Level VII)

11 Centers for Medicare & Medicaid Services, Department of Health and Human Services. (2014). Condition of participation: Patient's rights. 42 C.F.R. § 482.13(c)(1).

12 American Osteopathic Association. (2014). Standard 15.01.16. *Healthcare Facilities Accreditation Program: Accreditation requirements for acute care hospitals.* Chicago, IL: American Osteopathic Association. (Level VII)

13 The Joint Commission. (2015). Standard RI.01.01.01. *Comprehensive accreditation manual for hospitals: The official handbook.* Oakbrook Terrace, IL: The Joint Commission. (Level VII)

14 The Joint Commission. (2015). Standard PC.01.02.07. *Comprehensive accreditation manual for hospitals: The official handbook.* Oakbrook Terrace, IL: The Joint Commission. (Level VII)

15 American Osteopathic Association. (2014). Standard 16.02.01. *Healthcare Facilities Accreditation Program: Accreditation requirements for acute care hospitals.* Chicago, IL: American Osteopathic Association. (Level VII)

Assessing neurovascular status

When assessing an injured extremity, include these steps and compare your findings bilaterally.

- Inspect the color of the patients fingers or toes.
- *To detect edema,* note the size of the patient's digits.
- Simultaneously touch the digits of the affected and unaffected extremities and compare temperature.
- Check capillary refill by pressing on the distal tip of one digit until it's white. Then release the pressure and note how soon the normal color returns. It should return quickly in both the affected and unaffected extremities.
- Check sensation by touching the fingers or toes and asking the patient how they feel. Note reports of any numbness or tingling.
- *To check proprioception,* tell the patient to close his eyes; then move one of his digits and ask him which position it's in.
- *To test movement,* tell the patient to wiggle his toes or move his fingers.
- Palpate the distal pulses *to assess vascular patency.*

Record your findings for the affected and the unaffected extremities, using standard terminology *to avoid ambiguity.* Warmth, free movement, rapid capillary refill, and normal color, sensation, and proprioception indicate sound neurovascular status.

16 Centers for Medicare & Medicaid Services, Department of Health and Human Services. (2014). Condition of participation: Nursing services. 42 C.F.R. § 482.23(c).

17 The Joint Commission. (2015). Standard MM.06.01.01. *Comprehensive accreditation manual for hospitals: The official handbook.* Oakbrook Terrace, IL: The Joint Commission. (Level VII)

18 American Osteopathic Association. (2014). Standard 16.01.03. *Healthcare Facilities Accreditation Program: Accreditation requirements for acute care hospitals.* Chicago, IL: American Osteopathic Association. (Level VII)

19 Bentley, S. (2013). "Posterior long leg splinting" [Online]. Accessed May 2015 via the Web at http://emedicine.medscape.com/article/1355131-overview

20 Proehl, J. A. (2009). *Emergency nursing procedures* (4th ed.). Philadelphia, PA: Saunders.

21 American Osteopathic Association. (2014). Standard 16.02.05. *Healthcare Facilities Accreditation Program: Accreditation requirements for acute care hospitals.* Chicago, IL: American Osteopathic Association. (Level VII)

22 The Joint Commission. (2015). Standard RC.01.03.01. *Comprehensive accreditation manual for hospitals: The official handbook.* Oakbrook Terrace, IL: The Joint Commission. (Level VII)

23 Centers for Medicare & Medicaid Services, Department of Health and Human Services. (2014). Condition of participation: Medical record services. 42 C.F.R. § 482.24(b).

24 American Osteopathic Association. (2014). Standard 10.00.03. *Healthcare Facilities Accreditation Program: Accreditation requirements for acute care hospitals.* Chicago, IL: American Osteopathic Association. (Level VII)

25 Porpodis, K., et al. (2012). Fat embolism due to bilateral femoral fracture: A case report. *International Journal of General Medicine, 2012*(5), 59–63.

SPONGE BATH

A sponge bath with tepid water reduces fever by dilating superficial blood vessels, which releases heat and lowers body temperature. It may lower systemic temperature when routine fever treatments fail. Tepid-water sponge baths are no longer recommended for children; they can lead to extreme chilling and shock (because children's nervous systems are still immature) and they offer little advantage antipyretics.[1]

Equipment

Basin of tepid water, about 80° to 93°F (27° to 34°C) ■ bath (utility) thermometer ■ bath blanket ■ fluid-impermeable pad ■ washcloths ■ patient thermometer ■ towel ■ clean hospital gown (for patient) ■ hospital-grade disinfectant ■ Optional: gloves, antipyretics, ice bag and cover.

Preparation of equipment

Prepare an ice bag and cover; *the cover prevents skin irritation and tissue damage.*[2] Then place the bath thermometer in a basin, and run water over it until the temperature reaches the high end of the tepid range (93°F [34°C]) *because the water will cool during the bath.* Immerse the washcloths in the tepid solution until saturated.

Implementation

- Verify the practitioner's order.
- Gather and prepare the necessary equipment.
- Perform hand hygiene.[3,4,5,6,7]
- Confirm the patient's identity using at least two patient identifiers.[8,9]
- Check the patient's medication record for recent administration of an antipyretic *because this type of drug can affect the patient's response to the bath.*
- Explain the procedure to the patient.
- Provide privacy, and make sure the room is warm and free from drafts.[10,11]
- Put on gloves as needed *to comply with standard precautions.*[5]
- Place a fluid-impermeable pad under the patient *to catch any spills* and a bath blanket on top of him *for privacy.* Then remove the patient's gown. Also remove the top bed linen *to avoid wetting it.*
- Obtain the patient's temperature, pulse, and respirations *to serve as baselines.*
- Place a covered ice bag on his head *to prevent headache and nasal congestion that occur as the rest of the body cools.*
- Wring out each washcloth before sponging the patient *so that the water doesn't drip and cause discomfort.*
- Place moist washcloths over the major superficial blood vessels in the axillae, groin, and popliteal areas *to accelerate cooling.* Change the washcloths as they warm.
- Bathe each extremity separately for about 5 minutes; then sponge the chest and abdomen for 5 minutes. Turn the patient, and bathe his back and buttocks for 5 to 10 minutes. Keep the patient covered except for the body part you're sponging.
- Pat each area dry after sponging but avoid rubbing with the towel *because rubbing increases cell metabolism and produces heat.*
- Add tepid water to the basin as necessary *to maintain the desired water temperature.*
- Monitor the patient's temperature, pulse, and respirations every 10 minutes or as needed. Notify the practitioner if the patient's temperature doesn't fall within 30 minutes.
- Observe the patient for chills, shivering, pallor, mottling, cyanosis of the lips or nail beds, and changes in vital signs—especially a rapid, weak, or irregular pulse—*because such signs may indicate an emergency.* If any of these signs occur, discontinue the bath, cover the patient lightly, and notify the practitioner.
- If no adverse effects occur, bathe the patient for at least 30 minutes or until the patient's temperature reaches 1° to 2°F (0.6° to 1°C) above the desired level *because his temperature will continue to fall naturally.* Continue to monitor his temperature until it stabilizes.
- After the bath, make sure the patient is dry and comfortable. Dress him in a fresh gown and cover him lightly.
- Dispose of used supplies in the appropriate receptacles.[12]
- Remove and discard your gloves, if worn.[6,12]
- If the treatment will be repeated, clean and disinfect the equipment using a hospital-grade disinfectant,[13,14] and store the equipment in the patient's room.
- Perform hand hygiene.[3,4,5,6,7]
- Obtain the patient's temperature, pulse, and respirations 30 minutes after the bath *to determine the treatment's effectiveness.*
- Perform hand hygiene.[3,4,5,6,7]
- Document the procedure.[15,16,17]

Special considerations

- If ordered, administer an antipyretic 15 to 20 minutes before the sponge bath *to achieve more rapid fever reduction.*
- Consider covering the patient's trunk with a wet towel for 15 minutes *to speed cooling.* Resaturate the towel as necessary.
- Refrain from bathing the breasts of a postpartum patient *because they could become overly dry or develop fissures.*
- Take a rectal temperature, unless contraindicated, *for accuracy.*

Complications

Accelerated temperature reduction can provoke seizure activity.

Documentation

Record the date, time, and duration of the bath; the temperature of the water; the patient's temperature, pulse, and respirations before, during, and after the procedure; any complications and interventions; and the patient's tolerance to the treatment.

References

1 Pillitteri, A. (2014). *Maternal and child health nursing: Care of the childbearing and childrearing family* (7th ed.). Philadelphia, PA: Wolters Kluwer.

2 Craven, R. F., & Hirnle, C. J. (2012). *Fundamentals of nursing: Human health and function* (7th ed.). Philadelphia, PA: Lippincott Williams & Wilkins.

3 The Joint Commission. (2015). Standard NPSG.07.01.01. *Comprehensive accreditation manual for hospitals: The official handbook.* Oakbrook Terrace, IL: The Joint Commission. (Level VII)

4 Centers for Disease Control and Prevention. (2002). Guideline for hand hygiene in health-care settings: Recommendations of the Healthcare Infection Control Practices Advisory Committee and the HICPAC/SHEA/APIC/IDSA Hand Hygiene Task Force. *MMWR Recommendations and Reports, 51*(RR-16), 1–45. Accessed May 2015 via the Web at http://www.cdc.gov/mmwr/pdf/rr/rr5116.pdf (Level II)

5 World Health Organization. (2009). "WHO guidelines on hand hygiene in health care: First global patient safety challenge, clean care is safer care" [Online]. Accessed May 2015 via the Web at http://whqlibdoc.who.int/publications/2009/9789241597906_eng.pdf (Level IV)

6 American Osteopathic Association. (2014). Standard 07.01.21. *Healthcare Facilities Accreditation Program: Accreditation requirements for acute care hospitals.* Chicago, IL: American Osteopathic Association. (Level VII)

7 Centers for Medicare & Medicaid Services, Department of Health and Human Services. (2014). Condition of participation: Infection control. 42 C.F.R. § 482.42.

8 The Joint Commission. (2015). Standard NPSG.01.01.01. *Comprehensive accreditation manual for hospitals: The official handbook.* Oakbrook Terrace, IL: The Joint Commission. (Level VII)

9 American Osteopathic Association. (2014). Standard 30.00.14. *Healthcare Facilities Accreditation Program: Accreditation requirements for acute care hospitals.* Chicago, IL: American Osteopathic Association. (Level VII)

10 American Osteopathic Association. (2014). Standard 15.01.16. *Healthcare Facilities Accreditation Program: Accreditation requirements for acute care hospitals.* Chicago, IL: American Osteopathic Association. (Level VII)

11 Centers for Medicare & Medicaid Services, Department of Health and Human Services. (2014). Condition of participation: Patient's rights. 42 C.F.R. § 482.13(c)(1).

12 Siegel, J. D., et al. (2007). "2007 guideline for isolation precautions: Preventing transmission of infectious agents in healthcare settings" [Online]. Accessed May 2015 via the Web at http://www.cdc.gov/hicpac/pdf/isolation/Isolation2007.pdf (Level II)

13 Rutala, W. A., et al. (2008). "Guideline for disinfection and sterilization in healthcare facilities, 2008" [Online]. Accessed May 2015 via the Web at http://www.cdc.gov/hicpac/pdf/guidelines/Disinfection_Nov_2008.pdf (Level I)
14 American Osteopathic Association. (2014). Standard 07.02.03. *Healthcare Facilities Accreditation Program: Accreditation requirements for acute care hospitals.* Chicago, IL: American Osteopathic Association. (Level VII)
15 The Joint Commission. (2015). Standard RC.01.03.01. *Comprehensive accreditation manual for hospitals: The official handbook.* Oakbrook Terrace, IL: The Joint Commission. (Level VII)
16 American Osteopathic Association. (2014). Standard 10.00.03. *Healthcare Facilities Accreditation Program: Accreditation requirements for acute care hospitals.* Chicago, IL: American Osteopathic Association. (Level VII)
17 Centers for Medicare & Medicaid Services, Department of Health and Human Services. (2014). Condition of participation: Medical record services. 42 C.F.R. § 482.24(b).

ADDITIONAL REFERENCES

Nettina, S. M. (2014). *Lippincott manual of nursing practice* (10th ed.). Philadelphia, PA: Wolters Kluwer.
Taylor, C., et al. (2015). *Fundamentals of nursing: The art and science of nursing care* (8th ed.). Philadelphia, PA: Wolters Kluwer.

SPUTUM COLLECTION

Secreted by mucous membranes lining the bronchioles, bronchi, and trachea, sputum helps protect the respiratory tract from infection. When expelled from the respiratory tract, sputum carries saliva, nasal and sinus secretions, dead cells, and normal oral bacteria from the respiratory tract. Sputum specimens may be cultured for identification of respiratory pathogens. Laboratory examination of sputum helps in the diagnosis and treatment of such conditions as pneumonia and tuberculosis (TB). It's easiest to collect sputum specimens early in the morning because secretions usually accumulate overnight.

Sputum specimens collected by expectoration are commonly used for cytology, culture and sensitivity, and acid-fast bacilli testing. Cytologic examination helps identify abnormal cells. Culture and sensitivity testing identifies specific microorganisms and antibiotic sensitivity. Smear specimens that test positive for acid-fast bacilli must also undergo culture and sensitivity testing to confirm TB.

When a patient is unable to produce an adequate specimen, additional treatments may be needed to help mobilize secretions. These treatments include nebulizer use, hydration, deep breathing exercises, chest percussion, and postural drainage. Tracheal suctioning involves removing secretions from the trachea or bronchi using a catheter inserted through the nose. Sputum collection by tracheal suctioning is contraindicated within 1 hour of eating and in patients with esophageal varices, nausea, facial or basilar skull fractures, increased intracranial pressure, laryngospasm, or bronchospasm. It should be performed cautiously in patients with heart disease because it can precipitate cardiac arrhythmias.

Equipment

For expectoration

Sterile specimen container with tight-fitting cap ▪ gloves ▪ specimen label ▪ laboratory request form and laboratory biohazard transport bag ▪ mask ▪ goggles or face shield ▪ supplies for oral hygiene ▪ stethoscope ▪ Optional: gown, respirator (such as an N95) if TB or other airborne pathogens are suspected, small-volume nebulizer, pillow (for splinting), prescribed solution for aerosolization (hypertonic saline, N-acetylcysteine,[1] propylene glycol, or sterile or distilled water).

For tracheal suctioning

#12 to #14 French sterile suction catheter ▪ water-soluble lubricant ▪ laboratory request form and laboratory biohazard transport bag ▪ specimen label ▪ sterile gloves ▪ mask ▪ goggles or face shield ▪ sterile in-line specimen trap (Lukens trap) ▪ sterile container with sterile normal saline solution ▪ suction source with regulator ▪ suction canister ▪ oxygen therapy equipment ▪ supplies for oral care ▪ stethoscope ▪ Optional: gown, nasopharyngeal airway (if frequent suctioning is needed),[2] respirator (such as an N95) if TB or other airborne pathogens are suspected, pulse oximeter.

Commercial suction kits are available but the equipment in them varies. Check the package label when gathering equipment.

Preparation of equipment

If using tracheal suction to obtain the sputum specimen, set up the suction equipment and make sure that it's functioning properly. Adjust the suction pressure to the lowest level necessary to remove secretions, usually 110 to 150 mm Hg for adults. Suctioning with excessive negative pressure can cause atelectasis, hypoxia, and mucosal damage.[3] Verify the suction pressure before performing the procedure.

Implementation

- Verify the practitioner's order.
- Gather the appropriate equipment.
- Perform hand hygiene.[4,5,6,7,8]
- Confirm the patient's identity using at least two patient identifiers.[9]
- Explain the procedure and the need to collect a specimen of sputum (not saliva) *to promote cooperation.*
- Have all supplies within reach.
- Instruct the patient to sit in a chair or at the edge of the bed. If he can't sit up, place him in the high Fowler position. *These positions help the patient exert a greater force when coughing, increasing the likelihood of gathering an adequate sample.*
- Perform hand hygiene.[4,5,6,7,8]
- Put on a mask, eye protection, gloves, and a gown if necessary.[10,11]

NURSING ALERT *If the patient is on airborne precautions, wear a fit-tested N95 or higher level disposable respirator when caring for the patient; put on the respirator before entering the room and remove it after exiting the room. If you anticipate substantial spraying of respiratory fluids, wear gloves and a gown as well as goggles or a face shield.*[11]

- Perform treatment as ordered (such as nebulizer use, chest percussion, and postural drainage) *to assist specimen production,* as needed. (See the "Nebulizer therapy" and "Chest physiotherapy" procedures, pages 537, 171.)

Sputum collection by expectoration

- Ask the patient to rinse his mouth with water *to reduce specimen contamination.* (Avoid mouthwash or toothpaste *because they may affect the mobility of organisms in the sputum sample.*)
- If the patient has a surgical incision or localized area of discomfort, have him place his hands firmly over the affected area or place a pillow over the area *to provide splinting, which reduces tension during coughing.*
- Instruct the patient to take three slow, deep breaths and to then cough deeply from a maximal inspiration. Repeat the procedure as necessary until he produces sputum. Allow rest periods between each maneuver.
- When sputum is mobilized, instruct the patient to expectorate directly into the specimen container without touching the inside or rim of the container. Have the patient continue producing sputum until the amount totals at least 5 mL if possible.
- Cap the container and, if necessary, clean its exterior.

NURSING ALERT *If the patient has asthma or chronic bronchitis, watch for aggravated bronchospasms with the use of sodium chloride or acetylcysteine aerosols in concentrations higher than 10%.*

Sputum collection by tracheal suctioning

- Inform the patient of the need to collect a sputum specimen, and explain the procedure, including physiologic responses that might occur

EQUIPMENT

Attaching a specimen trap to a suction catheter

Wearing gloves, push the suction tubing onto the male adapter of the in-line specimen trap.

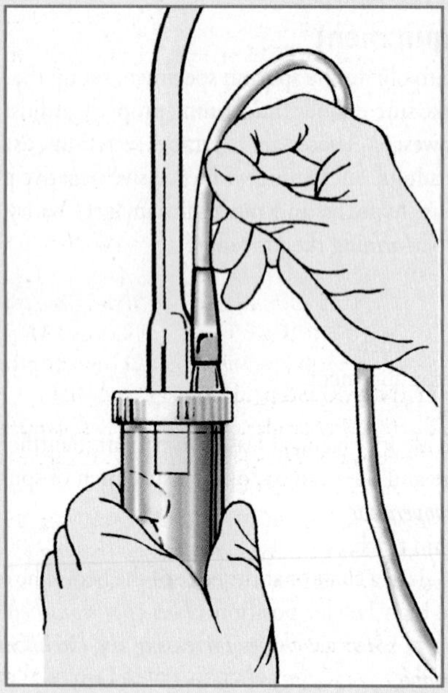

Insert the suction catheter into the rubber tubing of the trap.

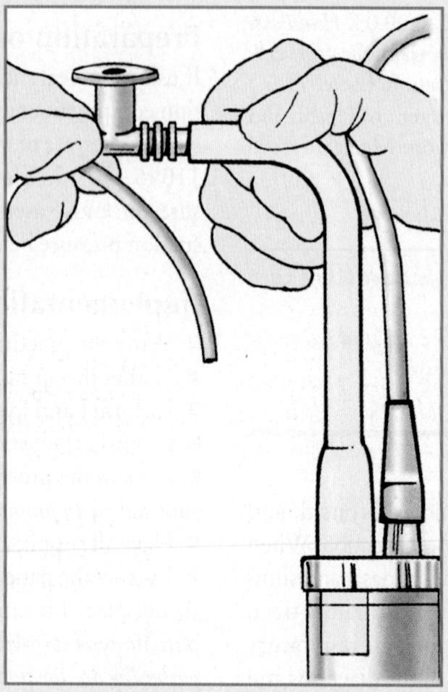

After suctioning, disconnect the in-line trap from the suction tubing and catheter. *To seal the container,* connect the rubber tubing to the male adapter of the trap

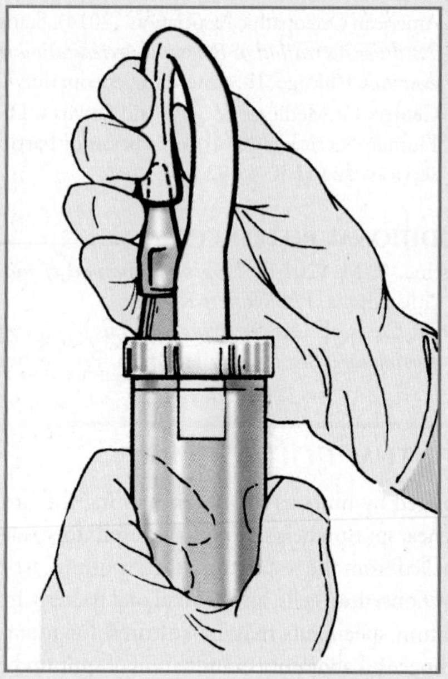

during the procedure, such as the need to cough or gag and shortness of breath, *to promote cooperation.*

- Administer oxygen to the patient before beginning the procedure, as ordered.
- Position the patient in the high or semi-Fowler position *to promote lung expansion and to facilitate the patient's ability to cough.*
- Assess the patient's respiratory status, including respiratory rate, depth, and pattern, and the color of the nail beds and mucous membranes.
- Perform hand hygiene.[4,5,6,7,8]
- Put on personal protective equipment, as appropriate.[10,11]
- Put on sterile gloves. Consider the suction catheter hand sterile and your other hand clean *to prevent cross-contamination.*[12]
- Connect the suction tubing to the male adapter of the in-line specimen trap. Attach the sterile suction catheter to the rubber tubing of the trap. (See *Attaching a specimen trap to a suction catheter.*)
- Lubricate the catheter with normal saline solution or water-soluble lubricant.
- Gently pass the catheter through the patient's nostril, directing it toward the septum and floor of the nasal cavity, without applying suction.[2,3,12] Gently twist the catheter if you feel resistance in the nostril. If twisting doesn't help, withdraw the catheter and insert it in the other nostril.[2]
- When the catheter reaches the larynx, have the patient assume a "sniffing" position (flexion of the neck on the body and extension of the head on the neck) *to help align the opening of the larynx with the lower pharynx, easing passage of the catheter through the larynx.* Advance the catheter into the trachea until the patient coughs or you feel resistance.[2] Tell him to take several deep breaths through his mouth *to ease insertion.*
- To obtain the specimen, suction for 5 to 10 seconds, but never for longer than 15 seconds *because prolonged suctioning can cause atelectasis and hypoxia.* If the procedure must be repeated, administer oxygen and wait at least 1 minute *to allow the patient time to return to his preprocedure condition.*[2]
- When collection is completed, discontinue the suction, gently remove the catheter, and administer oxygen.
- Administer oxygen, as ordered.
- Verify that the patient is in stable condition.
- Turn off the suction source.
- Detach the catheter from the in-line specimen trap, gather it up in your dominant hand, and pull your glove cuff inside out and down around the used catheter *to enclose it for disposal.*
- Detach the trap from the tubing connected to the suction device. Seal the trap tightly by connecting the rubber tubing to the male adapter of the trap.
- Clear the suction tubing with normal saline solution.
- Examine the specimen *to make sure you obtained an adequate sample.*

Completing the procedure

- Remove and discard your gloves and any other personal protective equipment worn.
- Perform hand hygiene.[4,5,6,7,8]
- Label the specimen container in the presence of the patient *to prevent mislabeling.*[9] Include on the laboratory request form whether the patient was febrile or taking antibiotics and whether sputum was induced *because such specimens commonly appear watery and may resemble saliva.*
- Send the specimen to the laboratory immediately in a laboratory biohazard transport bag.[13] *A delay in transport of the sample to the laboratory could damage the specimen and alter the accuracy of the results.*
- Offer the patient oral care.
- Perform hand hygiene.[4,5,6,7,8]
- Document the procedure.[14,15,16]

Special considerations

- If possible, collect the specimen early in the morning, before breakfast, *because secretions accumulate overnight, making collection easier.*
- If normal maximal cough efforts fail to produce a specimen, consider having the patient attempt the forced expiratory technique, also known as huff coughing, which consists of one or two huffs (forced expirations) from mid- to low-lung volumes with the glottis open. Have the patient repeat the process until he obtains maximal bronchial clearance; he can reinforce the process by compressing his chest wall using a brisk adduction movement of the upper arms.[15]
- Before sending the specimen to the laboratory, examine it *to make sure it's actually sputum, not saliva; saliva will produce inaccurate test results.*
- *Because expectorated sputum is contaminated by normal mouth flora,* tracheal suctioning provides a more reliable specimen for diagnosis.
- If the patient is suspected of having TB, don't use more than 20% propylene glycol with water when inducing a sputum specimen *because a higher concentration inhibits growth of the pathogen and causes erroneous test results.* If propylene glycol isn't available, use 10% to 20% acetylcysteine with water or sodium chloride.
- Sputum induction increases TB case detection; it's useful for patients who have negative results on spontaneous smear microscopy or who can't expectorate spontaneously. It's well-tolerated by children and adults.[17]
- As many as three consecutive morning specimens may be required if the suspected organism is *Mycobacterium tuberculosis.*
- If TB is suspected, place the patient on airborne precautions in an airborne infection isolation room *to reduce the risk of transmission.*[11,18]

Complications

Patients with cardiac disease may develop arrhythmias during the procedure as a result of vagus nerve stimulation caused by coughing. Because of the increased intrathoracic pressure associated with forced coughing, neurologic symptoms such as light-headedness and headache may occur.[19]

Documentation

Document the collection method used; the time and date of collection; the patient's tolerance of the procedure; the color, volume, and consistency of the specimen; and the specimen's proper disposition.[14]

REFERENCES

1 Balsamo, R., et al. (2010). Mucoactive drugs. *European Respiratory Review, 19,* 127–133. Accessed May 2015 via the Web at http://err.ersjournals.com/content/19/116/127.full.pdf

2 Kacmarek, R. M., et al. (2013). *Egan's fundamentals of respiratory care* (10th ed.). St Louis, MO: Mosby.

3 American Association for Respiratory Care (AARC). (2004). AARC clinical practice guideline: Nasotracheal suctioning—2004 revision & update. *Respiratory Care, 49,* 1080–1084. (Level VII)

4 Centers for Disease Control and Prevention. (2002). Guideline for hand hygiene in health-care settings: Recommendations of the Healthcare Infection Control Practices Advisory Committee and the HICPAC/SHEA/APIC/IDSA Hand Hygiene Task Force. *MMWR Recommendations and Reports, 51*(RR-16), 1–45. Accessed May 2015 via the Web at http://www.cdc.gov/mmwr/pdf/rr/rr5116.pdf (Level II)

5 The Joint Commission. (2015). Standard NPSG.07.01.01. *Comprehensive accreditation manual for hospitals: The official handbook.* Oakbrook Terrace, IL: The Joint Commission. (Level VII)

6 World Health Organization. (2009). "WHO guidelines on hand hygiene in health care: First global patient safety challenge, clean care is safer care" [Online]. Accessed May 2015 via the Web at http://whqlibdoc.who.int/publications/2009/9789241597906_eng.pdf (Level IV)

7 American Osteopathic Association. (2014). Standard 07.01.21. *Healthcare Facilities Accreditation Program: Accreditation requirements for acute care hospitals.* Chicago, IL: American Osteopathic Association. (Level VII)

8 Centers for Medicare & Medicaid Services, Department of Health and Human Services. (2014). Condition of participation: Infection control. 42 C.F.R. § 482.42.

9 The Joint Commission. (2015). Standard NPSG.01.01.01. *Comprehensive accreditation manual for hospitals: The official handbook.* Oakbrook Terrace, IL: The Joint Commission. (Level VII)

10 American Osteopathic Association. (2014). Standard 07.01.10. *Healthcare Facilities Accreditation Program: Accreditation requirements for acute care hospitals.* Chicago, IL: American Osteopathic Association. (Level VII)

11 Siegel, J. D., et al. (2007). "2007 guideline for isolation precautions: Preventing transmission of infectious agents in healthcare settings" [Online]. Accessed May 2015 via the Web at http://www.cdc.gov/hicpac/pdf/isolation/Isolation2007.pdf (Level II)

12 Centers for Disease Control and Prevention. (2004). Guidelines for preventing health-care-associated pneumonia, 2003: Recommendations of CDC and the Healthcare Infection Control Practices Advisory Committee. MMWR Recommendations and Reports, 53(RR-3), 1–32. Accessed May 2015 via the Web at http://www.cdc.gov/mmwr/pdf/rr/rr5303.pdf (Level II)

13 Occupational Safety and Health Administration. (n.d.). "Bloodborne pathogens, standard number 1910.1030" [Online]. Accessed May 2015 via the Web at http://www.osha.gov/pls/oshaweb/owadisp.show_document?p_table=STANDARDS&p_id=10051(Level VII)

14 The Joint Commission. (2015). Standard RC.01.03.01. *Comprehensive accreditation manual for hospitals: The official handbook.* Oakbrook Terrace, IL: The Joint Commission. (Level VII)

15 American Osteopathic Association. (2014). Standard 10.00.03. *Healthcare Facilities Accreditation Program: Accreditation requirements for acute care hospitals.* Chicago, IL: American Osteopathic Association. (Level VII)

16 Centers for Medicare & Medicaid Services, Department of Health and Human Services. (2014). Condition of participation: Medical record services. 42 C.F.R. § 482.24(b).

17 Hepple, P., et al. (2012). Microscopy compared to culture for the diagnosis of tuberculosis in induced sputum samples: A systematic review. *International Journal of Tuberculosis and Lung Disease, 16,* 579–588. Accessed May 2015 via the Web at http://tbevidence.org/documents/sysrev/specimen/Hepple%20Ford%20Mcnerney%20-%202012.pdf (Level V)

18 Centers for Disease Control and Prevention. (2005). Guidelines for preventing the transmission of *Mycobacterium tuberculosis* in health-care settings, 2005. *MMWR Recommendations and Reports, 54*(RR-17), 1–141. Accessed May 2015 via the Web at http://www.cdc.gov/mmwr/PDF/rr/rr5417.pdf (Level I)

19 American Association for Respiratory Care (AARC). (1993). AARC clinical practice guideline: Directed cough. *Respiratory Care, 38,* 495–499. (Level VII)

ADDITIONAL REFERENCES

Craven, R. F., & Hirnle, C. J. (2012). *Fundamentals of nursing: Human health and function* (7th ed.). Philadelphia, PA: Lippincott Williams & Wilkins.

Nettina, S. M. (2014). *Lippincott manual of nursing practice* (10th ed.). Philadelphia, PA: Wolters Kluwer.

STANDARD PRECAUTIONS

Standard precautions were developed by the Centers for Disease Control and Prevention (CDC) to protect against the transmission of infection. CDC officials recommend that health care workers assume that all patients are potentially infected or colonized (carriers of an organism without signs or symptoms of infection) with an organism that could be transmitted in the health care setting, regardless of their diagnosis.[1]

Part of routine control practices, standard precautions includes wearing gloves for situations involving known or anticipated contact with blood, body fluids, tissue, mucous membranes, or nonintact skin.[1] If the task or procedure being performed may result in splashing or splattering of blood or body fluids to the face, a mask and goggles or face shield

Transmission-based precautions[1]

These precautions may be necessary in addition to standard precautions, depending on the patient's condition.

PRECAUTION TYPE	INDICATIONS	NURSING ACTIONS
Airborne	To prevent the spread of infection when a patient is suspected of or known to have an infection that's spread by the airborne route	■ Place the patient in an airborne infection isolation room with monitored negative pressure, if available. ■ Make sure that all people who enter the room wear a respirator mask (N95).[1]
Contact	To prevent the spread of epidemiologically important infectious organisms through direct or indirect contact with the patient or his environment	■ Place the patient in a single-patient room, if possible. ■ Wear a gown and gloves for all interactions with the patient or the patient's environment. ■ Follow your facility's infection-control plan *to determine when to initiate contact precautions.*[3] ■ Designate patient care equipment if possible.[1]
Droplet	To prevent the spread of infectious organisms through close respiratory or mucous membrane contact with respiratory secretions from an infected patient	■ Place the patient in a single-patient room, if possible. ■ Put on a mask before entering the patient's room when coming within 3′ (1 M) of the patient. ■ Designate patient care equipment if possible.[1]

should be worn. If the task or procedure being performed may result in splashing or splattering of blood or body fluids to the body, a fluid-resistant gown or apron should be worn.[1,2] Additional protective clothing such as shoe covers may be appropriate to protect the feet in situations that may expose the health care worker to large amounts of blood or body fluids (or both), such as when caring for a trauma patient in the operating room or emergency department.

Standard precautions should be combined with transmission-based precautions for patients with confirmed or suspected infection with highly transmissible pathogens.[1,3,4] (See *Transmission-based precautions* as well as the "Airborne precautions," "Contact precautions," and "Droplet precautions" procedures, pages 10, 209, 249.)

NURSING ALERT ***Because of the evolving situation surrounding Ebola virus disease, please refer to the latest recommendations from the CDC, found at http://www.cdc.gov/vhf/ebola/hcp/index.html, when caring for a patient with known or suspected Ebola.***

Equipment

Gloves ■ masks ■ N95 fit-tested disposable respirator ■ mask and goggles or mask with face shield ■ gown ■ resuscitation bag ■ hospital-grade disinfectant ■ bags for specimens ■ Optional: shoe covers, apron.

Implementation

■ Gather the appropriate equipment.

■ Wash your hands immediately if they become contaminated with blood or body fluids, excretions, secretions, or drainage.[2,5,6,7,8]

■ Perform hand hygiene before and after patient care and before and after putting on and removing gloves. *Hand hygiene removes microorganisms from your skin.*[5,6,7,8] If your hands aren't visibly soiled, use an alcohol-based hand sanitizer for routine decontamination.[1,5,6,7,8]

■ Wear gloves if you will or could come in contact with blood, specimens, tissue, body fluids, secretions or excretions, mucous membrane, broken skin, or contaminated surfaces or objects.[1,2]

■ Change your gloves and perform hand hygiene when moving from a contaminated to a clean site during patient care and in between patient contacts *to avoid cross-contamination.*[1,5,6,7,8]

■ Wear a fluid-resistant gown as well as a mask and goggles or a mask with face shield during procedures likely to generate splash or splatter of blood or body fluids, such as surgery, endoscopic procedures, dialysis, catheter insertion, and intubation or manipulation of arterial lines.[1,2]

■ Wear a mask during lumbar puncture procedures, such as a myelogram and spinal or epidural anesthesia. The health care worker performing the procedure should wear a mask with a face shield.[1]

■ Follow safe injection practices; whenever possible, use single-dose vials instead of multidose vials. Use a sterile, single-use disposable needle and syringe for each injection.[1] Use safety needles if they're available.[2]

■ Handle used needles and other sharp instruments carefully. Don't bend or break them, reinsert them into their original sheaths, remove needles from syringes, or unnecessarily handle them. Activate any safety mechanisms immediately after use. Discard the instruments intact immediately after use into a puncture-resistant sharps disposal container. Use tools to pick up broken glass or other sharp objects. *These measures reduce the risk of accidental injury or infection.* Use a needleless IV system whenever possible.[1,2]

■ Immediately notify your employee health provider (or the provider's designee) of all needle-stick or other sharp-object injuries, mucosal splashes, or contamination of open wounds or nonintact skin with blood or body fluids *to allow investigation of the incident and appropriate care and documentation.* Complete all follow-up screening and care as recommended by your employee health provider.[2]

■ Properly label all specimens collected from patients in the presence of the patient *to prevent mislabeling* and place them in plastic bags at the collection site.[9] Attach requisition slips to the outside of the bags.[2]

■ Place all items that have come in direct contact with the patient's secretions, excretions, blood, drainage, or body fluids—such as nondisposable utensils or instruments—in a single impervious bag or container labelled biohazardous before removal from the room. Place linens and trash in single bags of sufficient thickness to contain the contents.[1,2]

■ While wearing the appropriate personal protective equipment, promptly clean all blood and body fluid spills. Blot the spill with an absorbent material (such as a paper towel) first, and then clean the area with detergent and water. Notify the environmental services department of the spill *so they can properly clean the area.*[2]

■ If you have an exudative lesion, avoid all direct patient contact until the condition has resolved and you've been cleared by the employee health provider.[10]

■ If you have dermatitis or another condition resulting in broken skin on your hands, avoid situations where you may have contact with blood and body fluids (even though gloves could be worn) until the condition has resolved and you've been cleared by the employee health care provider.

■ Following the manufacturer's instructions, properly clean and disinfect or sterilize reusable equipment with hospital-grade disinfectant before using it for another patient.[1,11,12]

■ Teach patients, family members, and visitors about respiratory hygiene and cough etiquette. Provide a mask for anyone who presents with signs or symptoms of respiratory infection. Tell people to cover their mouths and noses with a tissue when coughing or sneezing, dispose of the tissue promptly, and then perform hand hygiene.[1,5,6,7,8]

■ Document the type of isolation in the patient's medical record.[13,14]

Special considerations

■ Keep mouthpieces, resuscitation bags, and other ventilation devices nearby *to eliminate the need for emergency mouth-to-mouth resuscitation, which in turn reduces the risk of exposure to body fluids.*

■ Be aware that disposable food trays and dishes aren't necessary for standard precautions.[1]

NURSING ALERT Because you may not always know which organisms may be present in every clinical situation, *you must use standard precautions for every contact with blood, body fluids, secretions, excretions, drainage, mucous membranes, and nonintact skin.[1] Use your judgment in individual cases about whether to implement additional isolation precautions, such as airborne, droplet, or contact precautions or a combination of them. In addition, if your work requires you to be exposed to blood, you should receive the hepatitis B virus vaccine series.*

Complications

Failure to follow standard precautions may lead to exposure to bloodborne pathogens or other infectious agents and to all the complications they may cause.

Documentation

Record any isolation precautions that may be needed in addition to standard precautions.

REFERENCES

1 Siegel, J. D., et al. (2007). "2007 guideline for isolation precautions: Preventing transmission of infectious agents in healthcare settings" [Online]. Accessed May 2015 via the Web at http://www.cdc.gov/hicpac/pdf/isolation/Isolation2007.pdf (Level I)

2 Occupational Safety and Health Administration. (n.d.). "Bloodborne pathogens, standard number 1910.1030" [Online]. Accessed May 2015 via the Web at http://www.osha.gov/pls/oshaweb/owadisp.show_document?p_table=standards&p_id=10051 (Level I)

3 The Joint Commission. (2015). Standard IC.02.01.01. *Comprehensive accreditation manual for hospitals: The official handbook.* Oakbrook Terrace, IL: The Joint Commission. (Level VII)

4 American Osteopathic Association. (2014). Standard 07.01.10. *Healthcare Facilities Accreditation Program: Accreditation requirements for acute care hospitals.* Chicago, IL: American Osteopathic Association. (Level VII)

5 Centers for Disease Control and Prevention. (2002). Guideline for hand hygiene in health care settings: Recommendations of the Healthcare Infection Control Practices Advisory Committee and the HICPAC/SHEA/APIC/IDSA Hand Hygiene Task Force. *MMWR Recommendations and Reports, 51*(RR-16), 1–45. Accessed May 2015 via the Web at http://www.cdc.gov/mmwr/pdf/rr/rr5116.pdf (Level II)

6 The Joint Commission. (2015). Standard NPSG.07.01.01. *Comprehensive accreditation manual for hospitals: The official handbook.* Oakbrook Terrace, IL: The Joint Commission. (Level VII)

7 World Health Organization. (2009). "WHO guidelines on hand hygiene in health care: First global patient safety challenge, clean care is safer care" [Online]. Accessed May 2015 via the Web at http://whqlibdoc.who.int/publications/2009/9789241597906_eng.pdf (Level IV)

8 American Osteopathic Association. (2014). Standard 07.01.21. *Healthcare Facilities Accreditation Program: Accreditation requirements for acute care hospitals.* Chicago, IL: American Osteopathic Association. (Level VII)

9 The Joint Commission. (2015). Standard NPSG.01.01.01. *Comprehensive accreditation manual for hospitals: The official handbook.* Oakbrook Terrace, IL: The Joint Commission. (Level VII)

10 The Joint Commission. (2015). Standard IC.02.03.01. *Comprehensive accreditation manual for hospitals: The official handbook.* Oakbrook Terrace, IL: The Joint Commission. (Level VII)

11 Rutala, W. A., et al. (2008). "Guideline for disinfection and sterilization in healthcare facilities, 2008" [Online]. Accessed May 2015 via the Web at http://www.cdc.gov/hicpac/pdf/guidelines/Disinfection_Nov_2008.pdf (Level I)

12 The Joint Commission. (2015). Standard IC.02.02.01. *Comprehensive accreditation manual for hospitals: The official handbook.* Oakbrook Terrace, IL: The Joint Commission. (Level VII)

13 American Osteopathic Association. (2014). Standard 10.00.03. *Healthcare Facilities Accreditation Program: Accreditation requirements for acute care hospitals.* Chicago, IL: American Osteopathic Association. (Level VII)

14 Centers for Medicare & Medicaid Services, Department of Health and Human Services. (2014). Condition of participation: Medical record services. 42 C.F.R. § 482.24(b).

STERILE TECHNIQUE, BASIC

Sterile technique is used to prevent contamination with microbes, preventing infection. It's used in conjunction with other procedures and isn't a procedure in itself. Sterile technique should be followed whenever a patient's skin is intentionally perforated, during procedures that involve entry into a sterile body cavity, or when contact with nonintact skin resulting from trauma or surgery is possible.

Procedures requiring sterile technique include any surgical procedure; vaginal birth; invasive radiologic procedures; vascular access insertion, care, and maintenance; and preparation of total parenteral nutrition and chemotherapeutic agents.[1] Other procedures, such as urinary catheter insertion, tracheostomy care, and surgical or wound irrigation and dressing changes, may also require sterile technique depending on the patient's condition and facility protocols.

Certain patients with compromised immune systems (such as those with burns or recent organ transplants and those receiving chemotherapy or radiation therapy) may require sterile technique more often, even for some procedures that would normally require only clean technique.

Equipment

Sterile gloves ■ personal protective equipment ■ sterile supplies, as required by the procedure to be performed ■ Optional: sterile bowl, sterile normal saline solution, sterile drape.

Many procedures have commercially prepared kits that provide all of the necessary components.

Preparation of equipment

Gather all the necessary equipment in the patient's room. Check each package carefully and discard any that has a hole or tear or is wet.[2] Note the expiration date and discard any packages that are expired.[2] Ensure that the sterilization tape has turned the appropriate color (see your facility's guidelines; color depends on the product used and sterilization method). Prepare a clean surface to set up the equipment for the sterile procedure.

Implementation

■ Verify the practitioner's order *to ensure that the right procedure is being performed on the right patient at the right time.*[3]

■ If required, confirm that written informed consent has been obtained and that the consent form is in the patient's medical record.[4,5,6]
■ Perform hand hygiene.[7,8,9,10,11]
■ Confirm the patient's identity using at least two patient identifiers.[12]
■ Explain the procedure to the patient and family *to relieve anxiety and ensure understanding and cooperation.*
■ Assess the patient's level of pain using techniques appropriate for the patient's age, condition, and ability to understand.[13] Administer an analgesic 20 to 30 minutes before the procedure, as needed, *to promote patient comfort,* following safe medication administration practices.
■ Remove you rings, watch, and bracelets.
■ Perform hand hygiene.[7,8,9,10,11]
■ Follow standard precautions by putting on the necessary personal protective equipment for the procedure.[14,15] (See the "Standard precautions" procedure, page 713.)

Opening sterile kits

■ Remove the plastic outer wrapper from the procedure kit, if one is present.
■ Place the inner wrapped kit on a clean, dry, flat surface *because any moisture on the table could be absorbed through the wrapper and contaminate the sterile supplies.*
■ Position the kit so that the tip of the triangle-pointed wrapper is toward you *so you don't have to reach over the sterile contents after the other flaps are opened.*
■ Grasp the outer portion of this outermost flap *to avoid contaminating the sterile field.*[2]
■ Open the flap away from your body, keeping your arm outstretched to the side (as shown below) *so it doesn't cross over the sterile field.*[2]

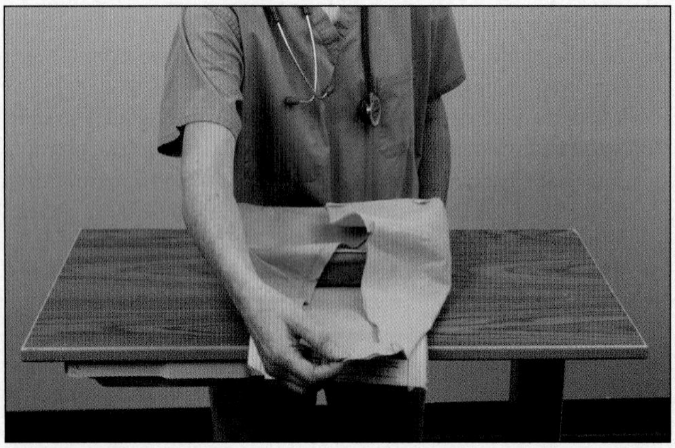

■ Grasp the outer surface of the first side flap with your hand on the same side as the flap (as shown below) *to avoid crossing over the sterile field.* Open the flap fully *to prevent the wrapper from falling back into place.*

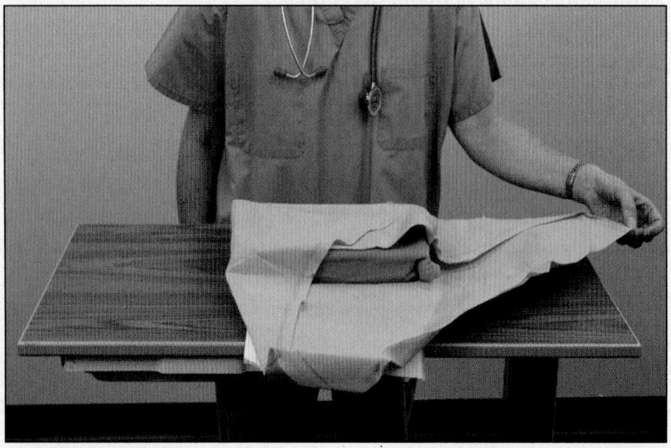

■ Grasp the outer surface of the second side flap and open it with your hand on the same side as the flap (as shown below).

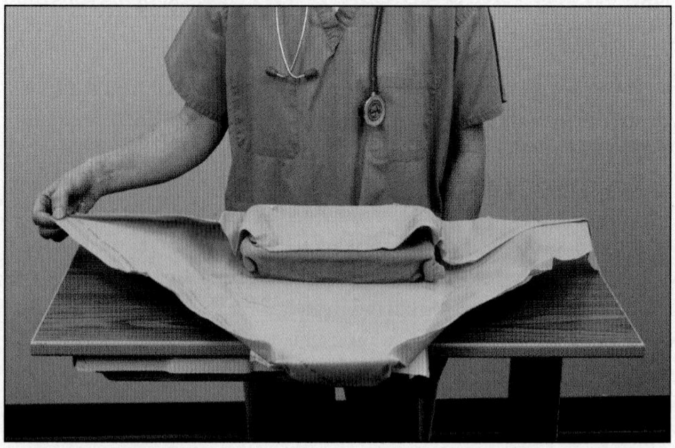

■ Grasp the outer surface of the innermost flap and open it toward your body (as shown below).[2]

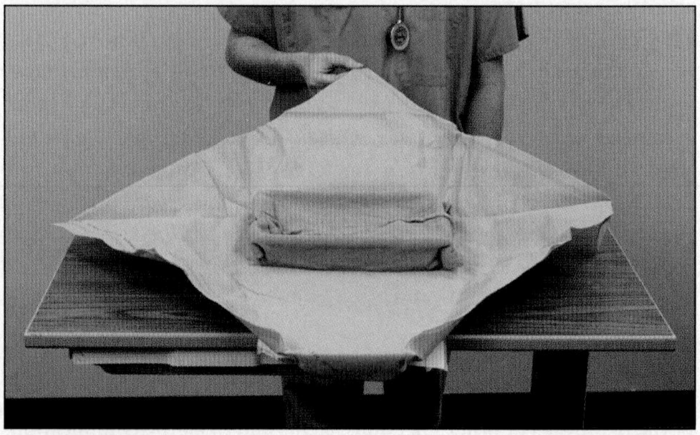

Opening wrapped sterile items

■ Grasp the sterile item wrapped in paper or linen in your nondominant hand.
■ Break the sterilization tape.
■ Use your dominant hand to grasp the outer surface of the top outermost flap *to avoid touching a sterile surface.*
■ Open the flap away from your body.
■ Grasp the outer surface of the first side flap and open it fully to the side.
■ Repeat with the other side flap.
■ Secure all flaps in your nondominant hand *to avoid dangling and contaminating the sterile field.*
■ Grasp the outer surface of the inner flap and open it toward you.
■ Place the item on the sterile field, ensuring that only sterile surfaces touch other sterile surfaces *to avoid contamination.*[2]
■ Make sure the item is at least 1″ (2.5 cm) from the edge of the sterile field *because any closer to the edge is considered unsterile.*

Opening peel-pack containers or pouches

■ Grasp the unsealed corner of the wrapper and pull it toward you.
■ Open a peel-pack pouch (such as gloves and syringes) by grasping each side of the unsealed edge with the thumb side of each hand parallel to the seal and pulling apart gently.
■ Hold the sides back so the wrap covers your hands and exposes the sterile item.
■ If the item is light, drop it onto the sterile field. Don't allow the item to slide across the package side when dropping the item onto the sterile field. Give heavy items to a scrubbed person or open on a separate surface.[2]

Pouring sterile solutions

■ Open the wrapped package containing the sterile bowl as described above *to avoid contaminating the sterile field.* Label the bowl with the name of the solution to be poured into it.[16]

■ Place the bowl on the edge of the sterile field but inside of the 1″ (2.5-cm) safety margin *so that solution can be poured without reaching across the sterile field.*

■ Unwrap the seal on the sterile solution bottle.

■ Unscrew the cap without touching the edges of the bottle.

■ Pour the solution into the bowl without reaching over the sterile field *to reduce the risk of touching sterile surfaces.*[2]

■ Pour slowly *to avoid splashing onto the drape and contaminating the sterile field.*[2]

■ Discard any unused solution.[2] *The edge of the container is considered contaminated after the contents have been poured.*

Opening and putting on sterile gloves

■ Open the package containing the sterile gloves, touching only the outer side of the glove wrapper. Keep in mind that some commercially prepared kits (such as the kit for inserting an indwelling urinary catheter) include a pair of sterile gloves; if gloves are included they will be the uppermost item in the pack.

■ Grasp the paper glove wrapper and place it on a clean, dry, flat surface.

■ Open the inner package, touching only the outer edges of the wrapper (as shown below).

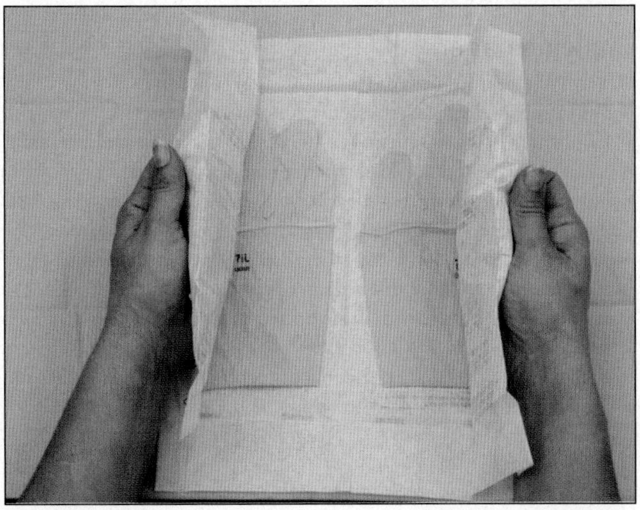

■ Use the thumb and fingers of your nondominant hand to grasp the folded inner surface portion of the glove for the dominant hand, touching only the inner portion of the glove (as shown below) *to avoid contaminating the outer portion of the glove.*

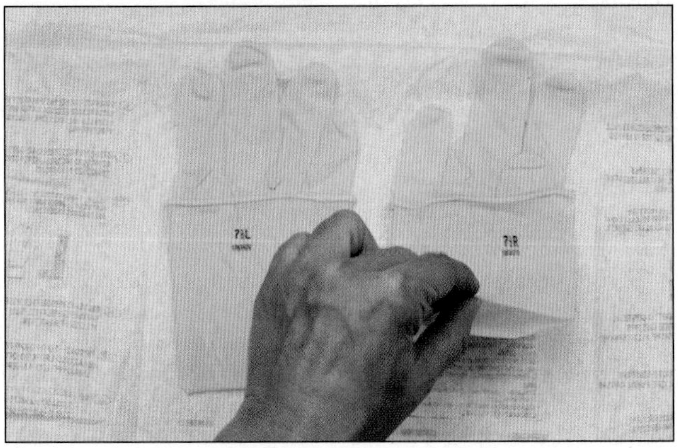

■ Lift up the glove and insert your dominant hand into the glove, palm side up (as shown below).

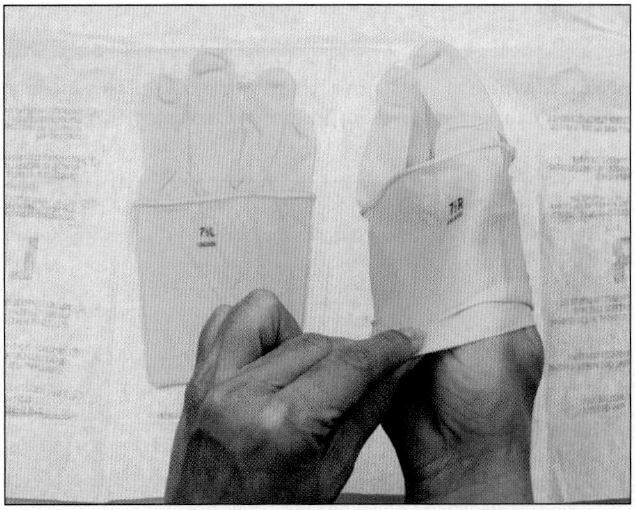

■ Pull down the cuff by touching only the inner surface of the glove. Gently stretch the glove over your hand. Make sure the outside of the glove doesn't touch the nonsterile surface.[17]

■ Insert the four fingers of your dominant gloved hand into the sterile outer cuff of the other glove, keeping your thumb pulled back out of the way (as shown below).

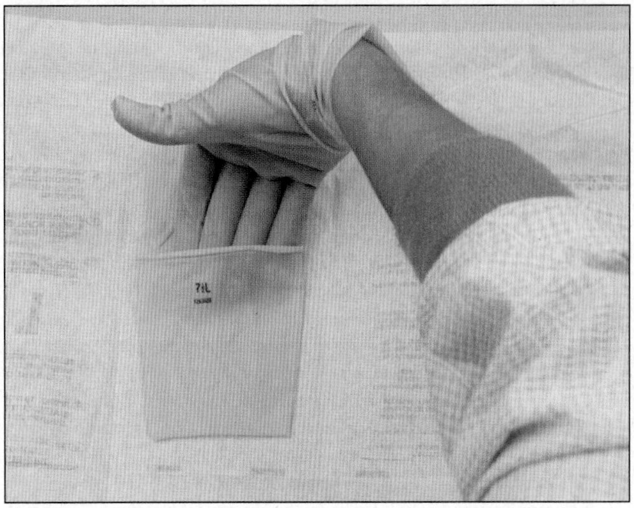

■ Lift up the glove and insert the nondominant hand into the glove. Allow the cuff to come uncuffed as you finish putting it on, but don't touch the skin of the arm with your gloved hand.

■ Adjust the fingers of the gloves after both your hands are gloved.

■ Keep your hands above waist level *to decrease the potential for contamination.*[17]

Special considerations

■ Be sure to open supplies away from the already setup sterile field *to avoid contaminating the field.*[18] Hold the opened additional supplies above the sterile field and drop them onto the field.[2]

■ Be aware that medical asepsis, also called *clean technique,* isn't the same as sterile technique. Medical asepsis is focused on the absence of pathogenic organisms and doesn't require items to be sterile. Sterile technique and surgical asepsis are focused on the elimination of all microorganisms.

Complications

Infection may result from failure to properly follow sterile technique.

Documentation

Document the procedure that was performed, using guidelines for that procedure. Within this documentation, note the sterile supplies used and that sterile technique was followed. Note the date and time of the procedure.

REFERENCES

1 World Health Organization. (n.d.). "Glove use information leaflet" [Online]. Accessed May 2015 via the Web at http://www.who.int/gpsc/5may/Glove_Use_Information_Leaflet.pdf

2 Recommended practices for maintaining a sterile field. (2014). In R. Conner, et al. (Eds.), *Perioperative standards and recommended practices 2014*. Denver, CO: AORN, Inc. (Level VII)

3 The Joint Commission. (2015). Standard UP.01.01.01. *Comprehensive accreditation manual for hospitals: The official handbook.* Oakbrook Terrace, IL: The Joint Commission. (Level VII)

4 American Osteopathic Association. (2014). Standard 15.01.11. *Healthcare Facilities Accreditation Program: Accreditation requirements for acute care hospitals.* Chicago, IL: American Osteopathic Association. (Level VII)

5 The Joint Commission. (2015). Standard RI.01.03.01. *Comprehensive accreditation manual for hospitals: The official handbook.* Oakbrook Terrace, IL: The Joint Commission. (Level VII)

6 Centers for Medicare & Medicaid Services, Department of Health and Human Services. (2014). Condition of participation: Patient's rights. 42 C.F.R. § 482.13(b)(2).

7 The Joint Commission. (2015). Standard NPSG.07.01.01. *Comprehensive accreditation manual for hospitals: The official handbook.* Oakbrook Terrace, IL: The Joint Commission. (Level VII)

8 Centers for Disease Control and Prevention. (2002). Guideline for hand hygiene in health-care settings: Recommendations of the Healthcare Infection Control Practices Advisory Committee and the HICPAC/SHEA/APIC/IDSA Hand Hygiene Task Force. *MMWR Recommendations and Reports, 51*(RR-16), 1–45. Accessed May 2015 via the Web at http://www.cdc.gov/mmwr/pdf/rr/rr5116.pdf (Level II)

9 World Health Organization. (2009). "WHO guidelines on hand hygiene in health care: First global patient safety challenge, clean care is safer care" [Online]. Accessed May 2015 via the Web at http://whqlibdoc.who.int/publications/2009/9789241597906_eng.pdf (Level IV)

10 American Osteopathic Association. (2014). Standard 07.01.21. *Healthcare Facilities Accreditation Program: Accreditation requirements for acute care hospitals.* Chicago, IL: American Osteopathic Association. (Level VII)

11 Centers for Medicare & Medicaid Services, Department of Health and Human Services. (2014). Condition of participation: Infection control. 42 C.F.R. § 482.42.

12 The Joint Commission. (2015). Standard NPSG.01.01.01. *Comprehensive accreditation manual for hospitals: The official handbook.* Oakbrook Terrace, IL: The Joint Commission. (Level VII)

13 The Joint Commission. (2015). Standard PC.01.02.07. *Comprehensive accreditation manual for hospitals: The official handbook.* Oakbrook Terrace, IL: The Joint Commission. (Level VII)

14 American Osteopathic Association. (2014). Standard 07.01.10. *Healthcare Facilities Accreditation Program: Accreditation requirements for acute care hospitals.* Chicago, IL: American Osteopathic Association. (Level VII)

15 Siegel, J. D., et al. (2007). "2007 guideline for isolation precautions: Preventing transmission of infectious agents in healthcare settings" [Online]. Accessed May 2015 via the Web at http://www.cdc.gov/hicpac/pdf/isolation/Isolation2007.pdf (Level II)

16 The Joint Commission. (2015). Standard NPSG.03.04.01. *Comprehensive accreditation manual for hospitals: The official handbook.* Oakbrook Terrace, IL: The Joint Commission. (Level VII)

17 Timby, B. K. (2012). *Fundamental nursing skills and concepts* (10th ed.). Philadelphia, PA: Lippincott Williams & Wilkins.

18 Taylor, C. R., et al. (2015). *Fundamentals of nursing: The art and science of nursing care* (8th ed.). Philadelphia, PA: Lippincott Williams & Wilkins.

ADDITIONAL REFERENCE

Craven, R. F., & Hirnle, C. J. (2012). *Fundamentals of nursing: Human health and function* (7th ed.). Philadelphia, PA: Lippincott Williams & Wilkins.

STOOL SPECIMEN COLLECTION

Stool is collected to determine the presence of blood, ova and parasites, pathogens, or such substances as ingested drugs. Gross examination of stool characteristics, including color, consistency, and odor, can reveal such conditions as GI bleeding and steatorrhea.

Stool specimens may be collected over a specific time period, such as 48, 72, or 96 hours. Typically, timed specimens are used to test for fat, porphyrins, urobilinogen, nitrogen, and electrolytes. Because stool specimens can't be obtained on demand, proper collection requires careful instructions to the patient to ensure an uncontaminated specimen.

Equipment

Sample container with lid ▪ gloves ▪ tongue blade ▪ paper towel ▪ bedpan or portable commode ▪ laboratory biohazard transport bag ▪ laboratory request form ▪ specimen label ▪ Optional: fluid-impermeable pad, absorbent adult brief, enema equipment (see the "Enema administration" procedure, page 289), patient care reminder that says SAVE ALL STOOLS.

Commercial kits are available for stool specimen collection, preservation, and transport, depending on the specific testing requirements. Follow the manufacturer's instructions for use.

Implementation

- Verify the practitioner's order for the stool collection.
- Perform hand hygiene *to prevent cross-contamination.*[1,2,3,4,5]
- Confirm the patient's identity using at least two patient identifiers.[6]
- Explain the procedure to the patient and his family, if possible, *to ensure their cooperation and prevent inadvertent disposal of timed stool samples.*
- Tell the patient to notify you when he has the urge to defecate. Have him defecate into a clean, dry bedpan or commode. Instruct him not to contaminate the sample with urine or toilet tissue *because urine inhibits fecal bacterial growth and toilet tissue contains bismuth, which interferes with test results.* If the patient is female, as appropriate, instruct her not to contaminate the sample with menstrual blood, *which may interfere with test results.*
- Put on gloves.[7,8]

Random stool collection

- If the patient is incontinent, collect a stool sample from a fluid-impermeable pad or an absorbent adult brief.
- Using a tongue blade, transfer the most representative stool sample from the bedpan or commode to the container, and place the lid on the container.
- If the patient passes blood, mucus, or pus with the stool, include it with the specimen.
- Wrap the tongue blade in a paper towel and discard it in the appropriate receptacle.[7,8]

Timed stool collection

- Place a patient care reminder that says SAVE ALL STOOLS over the patient's bed and in his bathroom.
- Tell the patient to notify you when he has the urge to defecate. At that time, have him defecate into a clean, dry bedpan or commode. Instruct him not to contaminate the specimen with urine or toilet tissue *because urine inhibits fecal bacterial growth and toilet tissue contains bismuth, which interferes with test results.* As appropriate, instruct a female patient to avoid contaminating the specimen with menstrual blood.

■ Begin timing with the passage of this first stool.
■ Collect the first specimen by using a tongue blade to transfer the stool from the bedpan or commode to the container and include it in the total specimen.
■ Continue to collect stools passed, remembering to transfer all stool to the specimen container.
■ If stool must be obtained with an enema, use only tap water or normal saline solution.
■ If ordered, immediately send each stool specimen to the laboratory with a laboratory request form. Alternatively, if permitted, refrigerate the specimens collected during the test period and send them to the laboratory when the collection is completed.[9]

Completing the procedure

■ Remove and discard your gloves[7,8] and perform hand hygiene *to prevent cross-contamination.*[1,2,3,4,5]
■ Make sure that the patient is comfortable after the procedure and that he has the opportunity to thoroughly clean his hands and perianal area.
■ Label the specimen in the presence of the patient *to prevent mislabeling.*[6]
■ Send the specimen to the laboratory in a laboratory biohazard transport bag[9] with the laboratory request form.
■ Perform hand hygiene.[1,2,3,4,5]
■ Document the procedure.[10,11,12]

Special considerations

■ Never place a stool specimen in a refrigerator that contains food or medication *to prevent contamination.*
■ If testing for *Clostridium difficile,* collect only diarrheal (unformed) stool unless ileus due to infection is suspected.[13]
■ Notify the practitioner if the stool specimen looks unusual.
■ Certain drugs and substances render stool specimens unsatisfactory for laboratory testing. If possible, collect specimens before these substances are administered; otherwise, wait to collect specimens until after the effects have passed. Such drugs and substances include antacids, kaolin, mineral oil and other oily materials, nonabsorbable antidiarrheal preparations, barium or bismuth (which need 7 to 10 days for effects to clear), antimicrobial agents (which need 2 to 3 weeks), and gallbladder dyes (which need 3 weeks).[14]

Patient teaching

If the patient is to collect a specimen at home, instruct him to collect it in a clean container with a tight-fitting lid, wrap the container in a paper bag, and keep it in the refrigerator (separate from food items) until it can be transported.

Documentation

Record the date and time you collected the specimen and sent it to the laboratory. Record the stool's color, odor, and consistency as well as any unusual characteristics; also note whether the patient had difficulty passing the stool.

References

1 The Joint Commission. (2015). Standard NPSG.07.01.01. *Comprehensive accreditation manual for hospitals: The official handbook.* Oakbrook Terrace, IL: The Joint Commission. (Level VII)
2 Centers for Disease Control and Prevention. (2002). Guideline for hand hygiene in health-care settings: Recommendations of the Healthcare Infection Control Practices Advisory Committee and the HICPAC/SHEA/APIC/IDSA Hand Hygiene Task Force. *MMWR Recommendations and Reports, 51*(RR-16), 1–45. Accessed May 2015 via the Web at http://www.cdc.gov/mmwr/pdf/rr/rr5116.pdf (Level II)
3 World Health Organization. (2009). "WHO guidelines on hand hygiene in health care: First global patient safety challenge, clean care is safer care" [Online]. Accessed May 2015 via the Web at http://whqlibdoc.who.int/publications/2009/9789241597906_eng.pdf (Level IV)
4 American Osteopathic Association. (2014). Standard 07.01.21. *Healthcare Facilities Accreditation Program: Accreditation requirements for acute care hospitals.* Chicago, IL: American Osteopathic Association. (Level VII)
5 Centers for Medicare & Medicaid Services, Department of Health and Human Services. (2014). Condition of participation: Infection control. 42 C.F.R. § 482.42.
6 The Joint Commission. (2015). Standard NPSG.01.01.01. *Comprehensive accreditation manual for hospitals: The official handbook.* Oakbrook Terrace, IL: The Joint Commission. (Level VII)
7 Siegel, J. D., et al. (2007). "2007 guideline for isolation precautions: Preventing transmission of infectious agents in healthcare settings" [Online]. Accessed May 2015 via the Web at http://www.cdc.gov/hicpac/pdf/isolation/Isolation2007.pdf (Level II)
8 American Osteopathic Association. (2014). Standard 07.01.10. *Healthcare Facilities Accreditation Program: Accreditation requirements for acute care hospitals.* Chicago, IL: American Osteopathic Association. (Level VII)
9 Occupational Safety and Health Administration. (n.d.). "Bloodborne pathogens, standard number 1910.1030" [Online]. Accessed May 2015 via the Web at http://www.osha.gov/pls/oshaweb/owadisp.show_document?p_table=STANDARDS&p_id=10051 (Level VII)
10 The Joint Commission. (2015). Standard RC.01.03.01. *Comprehensive accreditation manual for hospitals: The official handbook.* Oakbrook Terrace, IL: The Joint Commission. (Level VII)
11 Centers for Medicare & Medicaid Services, Department of Health and Human Services. (2014). Condition of participation: Medical record services. 42 C.F.R. § 482.24(b).
12 American Osteopathic Association. (2014). Standard 10.00.03. *Healthcare Facilities Accreditation Program: Accreditation requirements for acute care hospitals.* Chicago, IL: American Osteopathic Association. (Level VII)
13 Dubberke, E. R., et al. (2014). Strategies to prevent *Clostridium difficile* infections in acute care hospitals: 2014 update. *Infection Control and Hospital Epidemiology, 35,* S48–S65. Accessed May 2015 via the Web at http://www.jstor.org/stable/10.1086/676023 (Level II)
14 Centers for Disease Control and Prevention. (2013). "Diagnostic procedures: Stool specimens" [Online]. Accessed May 2015 via the Web at http://www.cdc.gov/dpdx/diagnosticProcedures/stool/specimencoll.html

Additional references

Centers for Disease Control and Prevention. (2013). "Foodborne outbreaks: Guidelines for specimen collection" [Online]. Accessed May 2015 via the Web at http://www.cdc.gov/foodsafety/outbreaks/investigating-outbreaks/specimen-collection.html (Level VII)
Craven, R. F., & Hirnle, C. J. (2012). *Fundamentals of nursing: Human health and function* (7th ed.). Philadelphia, PA: Lippincott Williams & Wilkins.
Nettina, S. M. (2014). *Lippincott manual of nursing practice* (10th ed.). Philadelphia, PA: Wolters Kluwer.

ST-SEGMENT MONITORING

A sensitive indicator of myocardial damage, the ST segment is normally flat or isoelectric. A depressed ST segment may result from cardiac glycosides, myocardial ischemia, or a subendocardial infarction. An elevated ST segment suggests myocardial infarction.

Continuous ST-segment monitoring is helpful for patients with acute coronary syndromes and for those who have received thrombolytic therapy or have undergone coronary angioplasty or cardiac surgery.[1] ST-segment monitoring allows early detection of reocclusion. It's also useful for patients who have had previous episodes of cardiac ischemia without chest pain, for those who have difficulty distinguishing cardiac pain from pain associated with other sources, and for those who have difficulty communicating.[2] It gives the practitioner the ability to identify and reverse ischemia by starting early interventions.[3]

Changes in the ST segment

Closely monitoring the ST segment on a patient's ECG can help you detect ischemia or injury before the infarction develops.

ST-segment depression

An ST segment is considered depressed when it's 0.5 mm or more below the baseline. A depressed ST segment may indicate myocardial ischemia or digoxin toxicity.

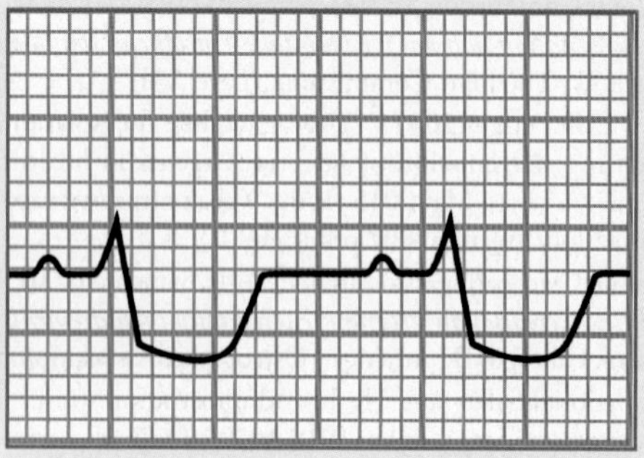

ST-segment elevation

An ST segment is considered elevated when it's 1 mm or more above the baseline. An elevated ST segment may indicate myocardial injury.

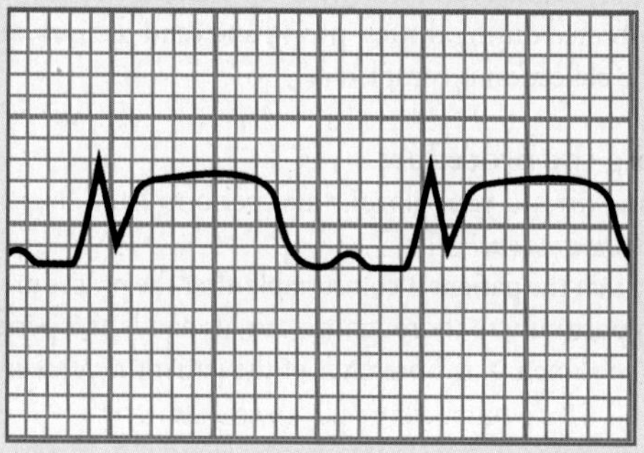

Because ischemia typically occurs in only one portion of the heart muscle, not all electrocardiogram (ECG) leads detect it. Select the most appropriate lead by examining ECG tracings obtained during an ischemic episode. The leads showing ischemia are the same leads to use for ST-segment monitoring.

ST-segment monitoring isn't useful for patients with left or right bundle-branch block or a ventricular paced rhythm or for those who are very restless.[3]

Equipment

ECG electrodes ▪ ECG monitor cable ▪ leadwires ▪ cardiac monitor programmed for ST-segment monitoring ▪ soap and water or cleaning pads ▪ towel ▪ alcohol pads ▪ gauze pad or wash cloth ▪ Optional: gloves, clippers, black indelible ink marker.

Preparation of equipment

Bring the equipment to the patient's bedside, plug the cardiac monitor into an electrical outlet, and turn the monitor on *to warm up the machine.*

Implementation

- Verify the practitioner's order.
- Gather and prepare the necessary equipment.
- Perform hand hygiene[4,5,6,7,8] and put on gloves, as needed, *to comply with standard precautions.*[9,10]
- Confirm the patient's identity using at least two patient identifiers.[11]
- Explain the procedure to the patient.
- Provide privacy.[12,13]
- Place the patient in the supine position.[14,15]
- If the patient isn't already on a monitor, turn on the device and attach the cables. (See the "Electrocardiogram, 12-lead" procedure, page 265.)
- Select the sites for electrode placement. Properly prepare the patient's skin for attachment as you would for continuous cardiac monitoring or a 12-lead ECG by cleaning the intended sites with soap and water or cleaning pads and drying them thoroughly *to enhance electrode contact.* Rub the skin at the intended sites with a gauze pad, washcloth, or sandpaper on the electrode *to roughen a small area of the skin and promote electrode adherence.* Don't use alcohol *because it can dry out the skin.*[16] If necessary, remove excess hair from intended sites with clippers *to ensure good skin contact with the electrodes.*[17]
- If possible, mark the intended sites with black indelible ink when electrode placement has been determined *to prevent inaccurate electrode placement if an electrode needs to be replaced.*[15,17]
- Attach the leadwires to the electrodes and position the electrodes appropriately on the patient's skin.
- Activate ST-segment monitoring by pressing the MONITORING PROCEDURES key and then the ST key. Activate individual ST parameters by pressing the ON/OFF parameter key.
- Select the appropriate ECG for each ST channel to be monitored by pressing the PARAMETERS key and then the key labeled ECG. If monitoring only one lead, choose the lead most likely to show arrhythmias and ST-segment changes.[3,15] Lead III is sensitive to inferior ischemia, and V_3 is sensitive to anterior or posterior ischemia.
- Identify the ECG complex landmarks, as prompted by the monitor.[17]
- Adjust the ST point to 60 milliseconds after the J point (as shown below).[3,15]

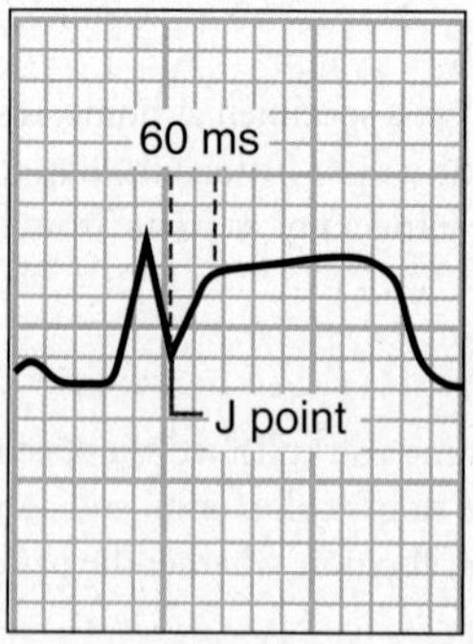

- Set the alarm limits for each ST-segment parameter by manipulating the high- and low-limit keys. Set the alarm parameter 1 to 2 mm above and below the patient's baseline ST segment.[15,17] Make sure the alarms are turned on, functioning properly, and audible to staff.[16,18,19,20]
- Press the key labeled STANDARD DISPLAY *to return to the display screen.*
- Assess the waveform shown on the monitor.
- Evaluate the ST-segment waveform depression or elevation. (See *Changes in the ST segment.*)
- Remove and discard your gloves, if worn.[9,10]

- Perform hand hygiene.[4,5,6,7,8]
- Document the procedure.[21,22,23]

Special considerations

- The Joint Commission issued a sentinel event alert concerning medical device alarm safety *because alarm-related events have been associated with permanent loss of function or death.* Among the major contributing factors were improper alarm settings, alarms inappropriately turned off, and alarm signals not audible to staff. Make sure that alarm limits are set appropriately, and that alarms are turned on, functioning properly, and audible to staff. Follow facility guidelines for preventing alarm fatigue.[19]
- Verify the patient's ST-segment limit parameters with the practitioner. Commonly, when a limit is surpassed for more than 1 minute, visual and audible alarms are activated.
- If you note ischemia, obtain a 12-lead ECG and assess the patient for signs and symptoms of acute ischemia, such as arrhythmias, angina, and hemodynamic changes.

Complications

Complications include skin irritation at the electrode sites.

Documentation

Document in the patient's medical record the leads being monitored and the ST-segment measurement points. Document the initial ECG strip and baseline ST-segment monitoring and any strips that suggest ST-segment changes.

REFERENCES

1 Yan, A. T., et al. (2007). Long-term prognostic value and therapeutic implications of continuous ST-segment monitoring in acute coronary syndrome. *American Heart Journal, 153,* 500–506. (Level IV)

2 Drew, B. J., et al. (2002). Frequency, characteristics, and clinical significance of transient ST segment elevation in patients with acute coronary syndromes. *European Heart Journal, 23,* 941–947. (Level V)

3 Drew, B. J., et al. (2004). AHA scientific statement: Practice standards for electrocardiographic monitoring in hospital settings. *Journal of Cardiovascular Nursing, 20,* 76–106. (Level II)

4 World Health Organization. (2009). "WHO guidelines on hand hygiene in health care: First global patient safety challenge, clean care is safer care" [Online]. Accessed May 2015 via the Web at http://whqlibdoc.who.int/publications/2009/9789241597906_eng.pdf (Level IV)

5 Centers for Disease Control and Prevention. (2002). Guideline for hand hygiene in health care settings: Recommendations of the Healthcare Infection Control Practices Advisory Committee and the HICPAC/SHEA/APIC/IDSA Hand Hygiene Task Force. *MMWR Recommendations and Reports, 51*(RR-16), 1–45. Accessed May 2015 via the Web at http://www.cdc.gov/mmwr/pdf/rr/rr5116.pdf (Level II)

6 Centers for Medicare & Medicaid Services, Department of Health and Human Services. (2014). Condition of participation: Infection control. 42 C.F.R. § 482.42.

7 The Joint Commission. (2015). Standard NPSG.07.01.01. *Comprehensive accreditation manual for hospitals: The official handbook.* Oakbrook Terrace, IL: The Joint Commission. (Level VII)

8 American Osteopathic Association. (2014). Standard 07.01.21. *Healthcare Facilities Accreditation Program: Accreditation requirements for acute care hospitals.* Chicago, IL: American Osteopathic Association. (Level VII)

9 Siegel, J. D., et al. (2007). "2007 guideline for isolation precautions: Preventing transmission of infectious agents in healthcare settings" [Online]. Accessed May 2015 via the Web at http://www.cdc.gov/hicpac/pdf/isolation/Isolation2007.pdf (Level II)

10 American Osteopathic Association. (2014). Standard 07.01.10. *Healthcare Facilities Accreditation Program: Accreditation requirements for acute care hospitals.* Chicago, IL: American Osteopathic Association. (Level VII)

11 The Joint Commission. (2015). Standard NPSG.01.01.01. *Comprehensive accreditation manual for hospitals: The official handbook.* Oakbrook Terrace, IL: The Joint Commission. (Level VII)

12 American Osteopathic Association. (2014). Standard 15.01.16. *Healthcare Facilities Accreditation Program: Accreditation requirements for acute care hospitals.* Chicago, IL: American Osteopathic Association. (Level VII)

13 Centers for Medicare & Medicaid Services, Department of Health and Human Services. (2014). Condition of participation: Patient's rights. 42 C.F.R. § 482.13(c)(1).

14 Fox, L., et al. (2010). Continuous ST-segment monitoring in the intensive care unit. *Critical Care Nurse, 30*(5), 33–44.

15 American Association of Critical-Care Nurses. (2009). "AACN practice alert: ST segment monitoring" [Online]. Accessed May 2015 via the Web at http://www.aacn.org/WD/Practice/Docs/PracticeAlerts/ST_Segment_Monitoring_05-2009.pdf (Level I)

16 American Association of Critical-Care Nurses. (2013). "AACN practice alert: Alarm management" [Online]. Accessed May 2015 via the Web at http://www.aacn.org/wd/practice/docs/practicealerts/alarm-management-practice-alert.pdf (Level VII)

17 Lynn-McHale Wiegand, D. (Ed.). (2011). *AACN procedure manual for critical care* (6th ed.). St. Louis, MO: Saunders.

18 The Joint Commission. (2015). Standard NPSG.06.01.01. *Comprehensive accreditation manual for hospitals: The official handbook.* Oakbrook Terrace, IL: The Joint Commission. (Level VII)

19 The Joint Commission. (2013). "Sentinel event alert: Medical device alarm safety in hospitals" [Online]. Accessed May 2015 via the Web at http://www.jointcommission.org/assets/1/18/SEA_50_alarms_4_5_13_FINAL1.PDF (Level VII)

20 Graham, K. C., & Cvach, M. (2010). Monitor alarm fatigue: Standardizing use of physiological monitors and decreasing nuisance alarms. *American Journal of Critical Care, 19,* 28–37.

21 The Joint Commission. (2015). Standard RC.01.03.01. *Comprehensive accreditation manual for hospitals: The official handbook.* Oakbrook Terrace, IL: The Joint Commission. (Level VII)

22 American Osteopathic Association. (2014). Standard 10.00.03. *Healthcare Facilities Accreditation Program: Accreditation requirements for acute care hospitals.* Chicago, IL: American Osteopathic Association. (Level VII)

23 Centers for Medicare & Medicaid Services, Department of Health and Human Services. (2014). Condition of participation: Medical record services. 42 C.F.R. § 482.24(b).

SUBCUTANEOUS INJECTION

Subcutaneous injection delivers a drug into the adipose (fatty) tissue beneath the skin. This method allows the drug to move into the bloodstream more rapidly than when given by mouth because it's absorbed mainly through capillaries. When compared with IM injection, subcutaneous injection provides slower, more sustained drug delivery; minimizes tissue trauma; and carries little risk of striking large blood vessels and nerves.

Drugs recommended for subcutaneous injection include nonirritating aqueous solutions and suspensions contained in 0.5 to 2 mL of fluid. Heparin and insulin, for example, are usually administered subcutaneously. Some diabetic patients may benefit from an insulin infusion pump. (See *Types of insulin infusion pumps,* page 722.)

Subcutaneous injections are performed using a relatively short needle. The most common subcutaneous injection sites are the outer aspect of the upper arm, the anterior thigh, loose tissue of the lower abdomen, the upper hips, the buttocks, and the upper back. (See *Locating subcutaneous injection sites,* page 723.) Subcutaneous injection is contraindicated in sites that are inflamed, edematous, scarred, or covered by a mole, birthmark, or other lesion. It may also be contraindicated in patients with impaired coagulation mechanisms.

Equipment

Prescribed medication in a single-dose ampule or a single-dose or multidose vial ■ patient's medical and medication records ■ 25G to 27G ½"

EQUIPMENT

Types of insulin infusion pumps

Open-loop system

The open-loop pump (shown below) is used most commonly. It infuses insulin but can't respond to changes in the patient's serum glucose levels. These portable, self-contained, programmable insulin pumps are small and unobtrusive.

The pump delivers insulin in small (basal) doses every few minutes and large (bolus) doses that the patient sets manually. The system consists of a reservoir containing the insulin syringe, a small pump, an infusion-rate selector that allows insulin release adjustments, a battery, and a plastic catheter with an attached needle leading from the syringe to the subcutaneous injection site. The needle is typically held in place with waterproof tape. The patient can wear the pump on his belt or in his pocket—practically anywhere as long as the infusion line has a clear path to the injection site.

The infusion-rate selector automatically releases about one-half the total daily insulin requirement. The patient releases the remainder in bolus doses before meals and snacks. He must change the syringe daily and the needle, catheter, and injection site every other day.

Closed-loop system

The self-contained closed-loop system detects and responds to changing serum glucose levels. A typical closed-loop system includes a glucose sensor, a programmable computer, a power supply, a pump, and an insulin reservoir. The computer triggers continuous insulin delivery in appropriate amounts from the reservoir.

Nonneedle catheter system

In a nonneedle delivery system, a tiny plastic catheter is inserted into the skin over a needle using a special insertion device (shown below). The needle is then withdrawn, leaving the catheter in place. This catheter can be placed in the abdomen, thigh, or flank and should be changed every 2 to 3 days.

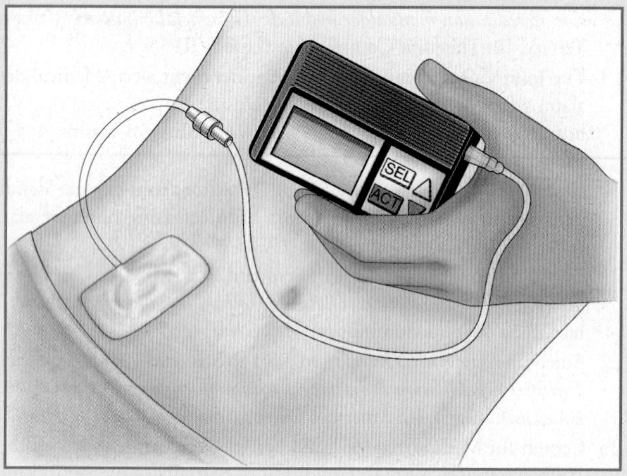

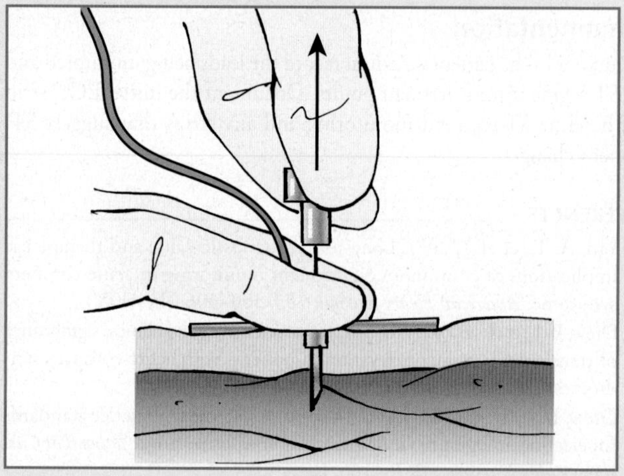

(1.3-cm) to 5/8″ (1.6-cm) needle ■ 1- to 3-mL syringe ■ antiseptic pads ■ gauze pads ■ Optional: gloves, ice pack, filter needle, antiseptic cleaning agent, insulin syringe.

Implementation

■ Avoid distractions and interruptions when preparing and administering medication *to prevent medication errors.*[1,2,3]

■ Verify the practitioner's order.[3,4,5]

■ Compare the medication label with the order in the patient's medication administration record.[3,4,5]

■ Review the patient's medical record for allergies or contraindications to the prescribed medication. If an allergy or a contraindication exists, don't administer the medication; instead, notify the practitioner.[3,4,5]

■ Check the expiration date on the medication. If the medication is expired, return it to the pharmacy and obtain new medication.[3,4,5]

■ Visually inspect the medication for particles, discoloration, and other signs of loss of integrity; don't administer the medication if its integrity is compromised.[3,4,5]

■ Discuss any unresolved concerns about the medication with the patient's practitioner.[3,4,5]

■ Choose equipment appropriate to the prescribed medication and injection site, and make sure it works properly.

■ Calculate the dosage and have another nurse verify it, if necessary.

NURSING ALERT ***Insulin and heparin are considered high-alert medications*** **because they can cause significant patient harm when used in error.** ***Before administering either medication, have another nurse perform an independent double-check if required by your facility*** **to verify the patient's identity and to make sure that the correct medication is being administered in the prescribed concentration, the medication's indication corresponds with the patient's diagnosis, the dosage calculations are correct and the dosing formula used to derive the final dose is correct, and the route of administration is safe and appropriate for the patient.** ***Compare your results with the results of the independent double-check and, if no discrepancies exist, administer the medication. If discrepancies exist, rectify them before administering the drug.***[6,7]

■ Perform hand hygiene.[8,9,10,11,12]

Drawing up medication from a single-dose ampule

■ Wrap a gauze pad around the ampule's neck and snap off the top, directing the force away from your body. Attach a filter needle to the syringe and withdraw the medication, keeping the needle's bevel tip below the level of the solution. Tap the syringe *to clear air from it.* Cover the needle with the needle sheath. Read the label again as you draw up the medication for injection.[4]

■ Before discarding the ampule, check the medication label against the patient's medication administration record.[4]

■ Detach the filter needle and discard the filter needle and ampule in a puncture-resistant sharps container. Attach the appropriate needle to the syringe.

Drawing up medication from a single-dose or multidose vial

■ Reconstitute powdered drugs according to instructions. Make sure all crystals have dissolved in the solution. Warm the vial by rolling it between your palms *to help the drug dissolve faster.*
■ Clean the vial's rubber stopper with an alcohol pad. Pull the syringe plunger back until the volume of air in the syringe equals the volume of drug to be withdrawn from the vial.
■ Without inverting the vial, insert the needle into the vial. Inject the air, invert the vial, and keep the needle's bevel tip below the level of the solution as you withdraw the prescribed amount of medication. Read the label again as you draw up the medication for injection.[4] Cover the needle with the needle sheath. Tap the syringe *to clear any air from it.*
■ Check the medication label against the patient's medication record before discarding the single-dose vial or returning the multidose vial to the shelf.[4]

Administering the subcutaneous injection

■ Confirm the patient's identity using at least two patient identifiers.[13]
■ Explain the procedure to the patient.
■ If the patient is receiving the medication for the first time, teach him about potential adverse reactions and discuss any other concerns related to the medication.[3,4]
■ Verify that the medication is being administered at the proper time, in the prescribed dose, and by the correct route *to reduce the risk of medication errors.*[3,4,5]
■ If your facility uses a bar code scanning system, scan your identification badge, the patient's identification bracelet, and the medication's bar code, or follow the procedure for your facility's bar code system.
■ Assess the patient's condition *to determine the need for the medication and the effectiveness of previous therapy.*
■ Carefully observe the patient for a rash, pruritus, cough, or other signs of an adverse reaction to a previously administered drug.
■ Select an appropriate injection site. Rotate sites according to a schedule for repeated injections, using different areas of the body unless contraindicated (heparin, for example, should be injected only in the abdomen if possible).
■ Provide privacy.[14,15]
■ Position the patient and expose the injection site.
■ Put on gloves if contact with blood or body fluids is likely or if your skin or the patient's skin isn't intact; *gloves aren't required for routine subcutaneous injections because they don't protect against needlestick injury.*[16,17,18,19,20]
■ Clean the injection site with an antiseptic pad, beginning at the center of the site and moving outward in a circular motion. Allow the skin to dry before injecting the drug *to avoid a stinging sensation from introducing alcohol into subcutaneous tissues.*
■ Loosen the protective needle sheath.
■ Holding the syringe in your dominant hand, grasp the skin around the injection site firmly with your nondominant hand *to elevate the subcutaneous tissue,* forming a 1" (2.5-cm) fat fold.[21]
■ Insert the loosened needle sheath between the fourth and fifth fingers of your nondominant hand while still pinching the skin around the injection site. Pull back the syringe with your dominant hand *to uncover the needle by grasping the syringe like a pencil.* Don't touch the needle.
■ Position the needle with its bevel up.
■ Tell the patient he'll feel a needle prick.
■ Insert the needle quickly in one motion at a 45- or 90-degree angle. (See *Technique for subcutaneous injections,* page 724.) Release the patient's skin *to avoid injecting the drug into compressed tissue and irritating nerve fibers.*
■ Inject the medication.
■ Remove the needle gently but quickly at the same angle used for insertion and, if present, activate the safety mechanism *to prevent accidental needle-stick injury.*[16]

Locating subcutaneous injection sites

Subcutaneous injection sites (highlighted below) include the fat pads on the abdomen, upper hips, upper back, and lateral upper arms and thighs. For subcutaneous injections administered repeatedly, such as insulin, rotate sites. Choose one injection site in one area, move to a corresponding injection site in the next area, and so on. When returning to an area, choose a new site in that area.

Preferred injection sites for insulin are the arms, abdomen, thighs, and buttocks. The preferred injection site for heparin is the lower abdominal fat pad, just below the umbilicus.

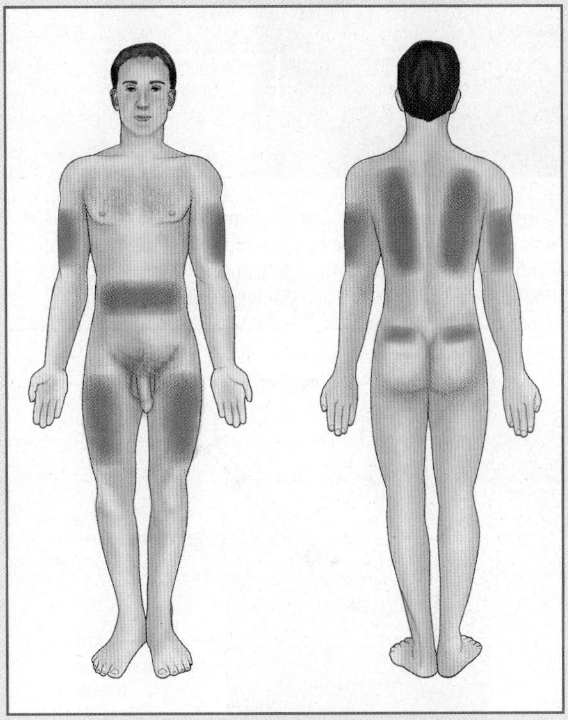

■ Cover the site with a gauze pad, and apply gentle pressure. Don't massage the site.[22]
■ Remove and discard the gauze pad.[16]
■ Check the injection site for bleeding and bruising.
■ Properly dispose of the injection equipment. *To avoid needle-stick injuries,* don't resheath the needle.[16,19]
■ Remove and discard your gloves, if worn.[16,19,20]
■ Perform hand hygiene.[8,9,10,11,12]
■ Document the procedure.[23,24,25]

Special considerations

■ Aspiration for blood is no longer recommended *because administration into the bloodstream with subcutaneous injections is rare.*[22] Aspiration for blood also isn't recommended for the administration of immunizations and vaccines.[26]
■ If the medication isn't going to be administered immediately, clearly label the medication syringe *to prevent a medication error.* An immediately administered medication is one that's prepared, taken directly to the patient, and administered without any break in the process.[27,28,29] Vaccine doses shouldn't be drawn up into a syringe until immediately before administration.[30]
■ When using prefilled syringes, adjust the angle and depth of insertion according to needle length.

Technique for subcutaneous injections

Before giving the injection, elevate the subcutaneous tissue at the site by grasping it firmly.

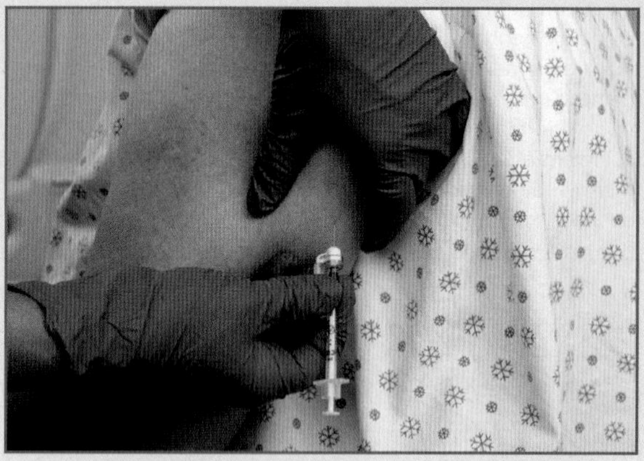

Insert the needle at a 45- or 90-degree angle to the skin surface, depending on needle length and the amount of subcutaneous tissue at the site. Some medications, such as heparin, should always be injected at a 90-degree angle.

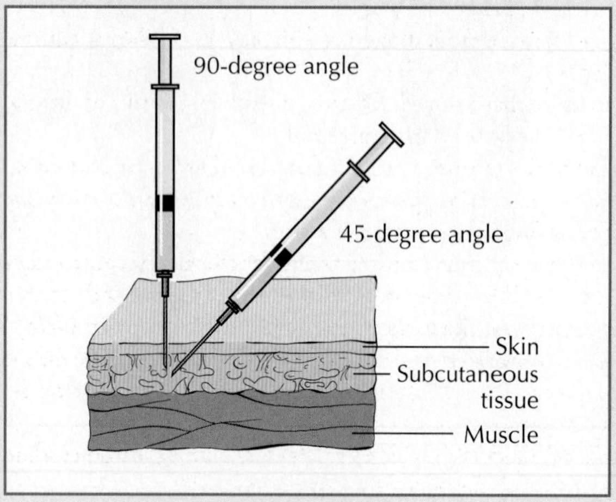

For insulin injections

- *To establish more consistent blood insulin levels,* rotate insulin injection sites within anatomic regions. Preferred insulin injection sites are the arms, abdomen, thighs, and buttocks.
- Make sure the type of insulin, unit dosage, and syringe are correct.
- When combining insulins in a syringe, make sure they're compatible. Follow your facility's guidelines regarding which type of insulin to draw up first.
- Before drawing up insulin suspension, gently roll and invert the bottle. Don't shake the bottle *because shaking can cause foam or bubbles to develop in the syringe.*
- Insulin may be administered through an inserted insulin pump. However, before administering the drug, make sure the patient doesn't already have a pump in place.

For heparin injections

- The preferred site for a heparin injection is the lower abdominal fat pad, 2″ (5 cm) beneath the umbilicus, between the right and left iliac crests. *Injecting heparin into this area, which isn't involved in muscle activity, reduces the risk of local capillary bleeding.* Always rotate the sites from one side to the other.
- Inject the drug slowly into the fat pad. Leave the needle in place for 10 seconds after injection, and then withdraw it.[31]
- Don't administer any injections within 2″ (5 cm) of a scar, a bruise, or the umbilicus.
- Don't rub or massage the site after the injection *because doing so can cause localized minute hemorrhages and bruises.*
- If the patient bruises easily, apply ice to the site for the first 5 minutes after the injection *to minimize local hemorrhage,* and then apply pressure.

Patient teaching

Teach the patient about the medication and how to perform the injection if he'll be self-administering at home. Have the patient perform a return demonstration *to determine medication administration competency.*

Complications

Concentrated or irritating solutions may cause sterile abscesses to form. Repeated injections in the same site can cause lipodystrophy, a localized reaction affecting adipose tissue.

Documentation

Record the time and date of the injection, the medication and dose administered, the injection site and route, and the patient's response.

REFERENCES

1 Westbrook, J., et al. (2010). Association of interruptions with an increased risk and severity of medication administration errors. *Archives of Internal Medicine, 170,* 683–690. (Level IV)

2 Institute for Safe Medication Practices. (2013). Side tracks on the safety express: Interruptions lead to errors and unfinished...Wait, what was I doing? *Nurse Advise-ERR, 11*(2), 1–4. Accessed May 2015 via the Web at https://www.ismp.org/Newsletters/acutecare/showarticle.aspx?id=37

3 American Osteopathic Association. (2014). Standard 16.01.03. *Healthcare Facilities Accreditation Program: Accreditation requirements for acute care hospitals.* Chicago, IL: American Osteopathic Association. (Level VII)

4 The Joint Commission. (2015). Standard MM.06.01.01. *Comprehensive accreditation manual for hospitals: The official handbook.* Oakbrook Terrace, IL: The Joint Commission. (Level VII)

5 Centers for Medicare & Medicaid Services, Department of Health and Human Services. (2014). Condition of participation: Nursing services. 42 C.F.R. § 482.23(c).

6 Institute for Safe Medication Practices. (2012). "ISMP's list of high-alert medications" [Online]. Accessed May 2015 via the Web at http://www.ismp.org/tools/highalertmedications.pdf

7 Institute for Safe Medication Practices. (2008). Conducting an independent double-check. *ISMP Medication Safety Alert! Nurse Advise-ERR, 6*(12), 1. Accessed May 2015 via the Web at http://www.ismp.org/newsletters/nursing/Issues/NurseAdviseERR200812.pdf

8 The Joint Commission. (2015). Standard NPSG.07.01.01. *Comprehensive accreditation manual for hospitals: The official handbook.* Oakbrook Terrace, IL: The Joint Commission. (Level VII)

9 Centers for Disease Control and Prevention. (2002). Guideline for hand hygiene in health-care settings: Recommendations of the Healthcare Infection Control Practices Advisory Committee and the HICPAC/SHEA/APIC/IDSA Hand Hygiene Task Force. *MMWR Recommendations and Reports, 51*(RR-16), 1–45. Accessed May 2015 via the Web at http://www.cdc.gov/mmwr/pdf/rr/rr5116.pdf (Level II)

10 World Health Organization. (2009). "WHO guidelines on hand hygiene in health care: First global patient safety challenge, clean care is safer care" [Online]. Accessed May 2015 via the Web at http://whqlibdoc.who.int/publications/2009/9789241597906_eng.pdf (Level IV)

11 American Osteopathic Association. (2014). Standard 07.01.21. *Healthcare Facilities Accreditation Program: Accreditation requirements for acute care hospitals.* Chicago, IL: American Osteopathic Association. (Level VII)

12 Centers for Medicare & Medicaid Services, Department of Health and Human Services. (2014). Condition of participation: Infection control. 42 C.F.R. § 482.42.

13 The Joint Commission. (2014). Standard NPSG.01.01.01. *Comprehensive accreditation manual for hospitals: The official handbook.* Oakbrook Terrace, IL: The Joint Commission. (Level VII)

14 American Osteopathic Association. (2014). Standard 15.01.16. *Healthcare Facilities Accreditation Program: Accreditation requirements for acute care hospitals.* Chicago, IL: American Osteopathic Association. (Level VII)

15 Centers for Medicare & Medicaid Services, Department of Health and Human Services. (2014). Condition of participation: Patient's rights. 42 C.F.R. § 482.13(c)(1).

16 Occupational Safety and Health Administration. (n.d.). "Bloodborne pathogens, standard number 1910.1030" [Online]. Accessed May 2015 via the Web at http://www.osha.gov/pls/oshaweb/owadisp.show_document?p_table=STANDARDS&p_id=10051 (Level VII)

17 Centers for Disease Control and Prevention. (n.d.). "Vaccine administration" [Online]. Accessed May 2015 via the Web at http://www.cdc.gov/vaccines/pubs/pinkbook/downloads/appendices/D/vacc_admin.pdf

18 World Health Organization. (2010). "WHO best practices for injections and related procedures toolkit" [Online]. Accessed May 2015 via the Web at http://whqlibdoc.who.int/publications/2010/9789241599252_eng.pdf (Level IV)

19 Siegel, J. D., et al. (2007). "2007 guideline for isolation precautions: Preventing transmission of infectious agents in healthcare settings" [Online]. Accessed May 2015 via the Web at http://www.cdc.gov/hicpac/pdf/isolation/Isolation2007.pdf (Level II)

20 American Osteopathic Association. (2014). Standard 07.01.10. *Healthcare Facilities Accreditation Program: Accreditation requirements for acute care hospitals.* Chicago, IL: American Osteopathic Association. (Level VII)

21 Peragallo-Dittko, V. (1995). Aspiration of the subcutaneous insulin injection: Clinical evaluation of needle size and amount of subcutaneous fat. *Diabetes Educator, 21,* 291–296. (Level VI)

22 Craven, R. F., & Hirnle, C. J. (2012). *Fundamentals of nursing: Human health and function* (7th ed.). Philadelphia, PA: Lippincott Williams & Wilkins.

23 The Joint Commission. (2015). Standard RC.01.03.01. *Comprehensive accreditation manual for hospitals: The official handbook.* Oakbrook Terrace, IL: The Joint Commission. (Level VII)

24 American Osteopathic Association. (2014). Standard 10.00.03. *Healthcare Facilities Accreditation Program: Accreditation requirements for acute care hospitals.* Chicago, IL: American Osteopathic Association. (Level VII)

25 Centers for Medicare & Medicaid Services, Department of Health and Human Services. (2014). Condition of participation: Medical record services. 42 C.F.R. § 482.24(b).

26 Petousis-Harris, H. (2008). Vaccine injection technique and reactogenicity—Evidence for practice. *Vaccine, 26,* 6299–6304. (Level V)

27 The Joint Commission. (2015). Standard MM.05.01.09. *Comprehensive accreditation manual for hospitals: The official handbook.* Oakbrook Terrace, IL: The Joint Commission. (Level VII)

28 The Joint Commission. (2015). Standard NPSG.03.04.01. *Comprehensive accreditation manual for hospitals: The official handbook.* Oakbrook Terrace, IL: The Joint Commission. (Level VII)

29 American Osteopathic Association. (2014). Standard 25.01.18. *Healthcare Facilities Accreditation Program: Accreditation requirements for acute care hospitals.* Chicago, IL: American Osteopathic Association. (Level VII)

30 Centers for Disease Control and Prevention. (2011). General recommendations on immunization: Recommendations of the Advisory Committee on Immunization Practices (ACIP). *MMWR Recommendations and Reports, 60*(RR-02), 1–60. Accessed May 2015 via the Web at http://www.cdc.gov/mmwr/pdf/rr/rr6002.pdf (Level II)

31 Zaybak, A., & Khorshid, L. (2008). A study on the effect of the duration of subcutaneous heparin injection on bruising and pain. *Journal of Clinical Nursing, 17,* 378–385. (Level VI)

ADDITIONAL REFERENCES

Black, L. (2013). Ditch the pinch: Bilateral exposure injuries during subcutaneous injection. *American Journal of Infection Control, 41,* 815–819. (Level IV)

Nettina, S. M. (2014). *Lippincott manual of nursing practice* (10th ed.). Philadelphia, PA: Wolters Kluwer.

Saltiel-Berzin, R., et al. (2012). Translating the research in insulin injection technique: Implications for practice. *Diabetes Educator, 38,* 635–643. (Level IV)

SUBDERMAL DRUG IMPLANTS

A method of drug delivery, subdermal implants come in the form of flexible capsules or rods, which are placed under the skin. This method is most commonly used to inject various hormones (such as contraceptive hormones) that diffuse slowly and are absorbed into the bloodstream.

Equipment

Patient's medical record and medication administration record ■ sterile surgical drapes ■ sterile gloves ■ antiseptic solution ■ local anesthetic ■ prescribed implants (some medications include an implantation kit with insertion tool)[1,2] ■ needles ■ 5-ml syringe ■ #11 scalpel ■ #10 trocar ■ forceps ■ sterile absorbable sutures or sterile adhesive surgical strips ■ sterile gauze ■ tape ■ gloves.

Implementation

- Avoid distractions and interruptions when preparing and administering the medication to prevent medication errors.[3,4]
- Verify the practitioner's order.[4,5,6]
- Compare the medication label with the order in the patient's medical record.[4,5,6]
- Confirm that written informed consent is obtained and that the consent is in the patient's medical record.[1,7,8,9]
- Conduct a preprocedure verification *to make sure that all relevant documentation, related information, and equipment are available and correctly identified to the patient's identifiers.*[9,10]
- Check the patient's medical record for allergies or contraindications to the prescribed medication. If an allergy or a contraindication exists, don't administer the medication; instead, notify the practitioner.[4,5,6]
- Check the expiration date on the medication. Don't give the medication if it has expired; instead, return it to the pharmacy and obtain new medication.[4,5,6]
- Visually inspect the medication for loss of integrity; don't administer the medication if its integrity is compromised.[4,5,6]
- Discuss any unresolved concerns about the medication with the patient's practitioner.[4,5,6]
- Perform hand hygiene.[11,12,13,14,15]
- Confirm the patient's identity using at least two patient identifiers.[9,16]
- Reinforce the practitioner's explanation of the procedure, and answer the patient's questions.
- Check the patient's history for hypersensitivity to latex or to the local anesthetic.
- If the patient is receiving the medication for the first time, teach about potential adverse reactions and discuss any other concerns related to the medication.[4,5,6]
- Verify that the medication is being administered at the proper time, in the prescribed dose, and by the correct route *to reduce the risk for medication errors.*[4,5,6]
- Put on gloves.[17,18,19]
- Assist the patient into the supine position on the examination table.
- If appropriate, make sure that the insertion site is marked as required by your facility.[9,20]
- During the procedure, stay and provide support, as necessary, while the practitioner inserts the implants.
- The practitioner performs hand hygiene and then puts on sterile gloves.[11,12,13,17]

■ The practitioner cleans the site with antiseptic solution and then drapes the site with sterile drapes.
■ Conduct a time-out immediately before starting the procedure to perform a final assessment *to ensure that the correct patient, site, positioning, and procedure are identified and, as applicable, that all relevant information and necessary equipment are available.*[9,21]
■ After anesthetizing the upper portion of the nondominant arm, the practitioner uses a #10 trocar or insertion tool to insert each capsule through a 2-mm incision.
■ After insertion, the practitioner removes the trocar or insertion tool and palpates the area *to verify the presence of the implant.* If the practitioner can't palpate the implant, the insertion tool (if used) should be checked *to see whether it still contains the implant.* Implant placement can also be verified using X-ray, computed tomography, ultrasonography, or magnetic resonance imaging.[12]
■ The practitioner closes the incision with sterile absorbable sutures or sterile adhesive surgical strips and covers it with sterile gauze and tape.
■ Discard used supplies and sharps in appropriate receptacles.[17,18,19]
■ Remove and discard your gloves.[17,18,19]
■ Perform hand hygiene.[11,12,13,14,15]
■ Document the procedure.[22,23,24]

Special considerations

■ If the implant is a contraceptive and it becomes dislodged, the patient will need an alternative form of birth control until the implant is replaced.
■ If the implant is a contraceptive, confirm that the patient isn't pregnant before implant insertion.[1]

Patient teaching

Tell the patient to resume normal activities but to protect the site during the first few days after implantation. Advise the patient not to bump the insertion site and to keep the area dry and covered with a gauze bandage for 3 days. Tell the patient to report signs of bleeding or infection at the insertion site. Instruct the patient to notify the practitioner immediately if one of the implants falls out before the skin heals.

Documentation

Document the name of the drug, insertion or administration site, date and time of insertion, and patient's response to the procedure. Note the date when the implant should be removed and a new implant should be inserted. Document patient teaching and the patient's comprehension of your teaching

REFERENCES

1 Merck and Company, Inc. (2012). "Nexplanon: Highlights of prescribing information" [Online]. Accessed May 2015 via the Web at http://www.merck.com/products/usa/pi_circulars/n/nexplanon/nexplanon_pi.pdf
2 Endo Pharmaceuticals Solutions Inc. (2011). "VANTAS: Highlights of prescribing information" [Online]. Accessed May 2015 via the Web at http://www.vantasimplant.com/pdf/VANTAS-Prescribing-Information.pdf
3 Westbrook, J., et al. (2010). Association of interruptions with an increased risk and severity of medication administration errors. *Archives of Internal Medicine, 170,* 683–690.
4 American Osteopathic Association. (2014). Standard 16.01.03. *Healthcare Facilities Accreditation Program: Accreditation requirements for acute care hospitals.* Chicago, IL: American Osteopathic Association. (Level VII)
5 The Joint Commission. (2014). Standard MM.06.01.01. *Comprehensive accreditation manual for hospitals: The official handbook.* Oakbrook Terrace, IL: The Joint Commission. (Level VII)
6 Centers for Medicare & Medicaid Services, Department of Health and Human Services. (2014). Condition of participation: Nursing services. 42 C.F.R. § 482.23(c).
7 The Joint Commission. (2015). Standard RI.01.03.01. *Comprehensive accreditation manual for hospitals: The official handbook.* Oakbrook Terrace, IL: The Joint Commission. (Level VII)
8 Centers for Medicare & Medicaid Services, Department of Health and Human Services. (2014). Condition of participation: Patient's rights. 42 C.F.R. § 482.13.
9 American Osteopathic Association. (2014). Standard 30.00.14. *Healthcare Facilities Accreditation Program: Accreditation requirements for acute care hospitals.* Chicago, IL: American Osteopathic Association. (Level VII)
10 The Joint Commission. (2015). Standard UP.01.01.01. *Comprehensive accreditation manual for hospitals: The official handbook.* Oakbrook Terrace, IL: The Joint Commission. (Level VII)
11 The Joint Commission. (2015). Standard NPSG.07.01.01. *Comprehensive accreditation manual for hospitals: The official handbook.* Oakbrook Terrace, IL: The Joint Commission. (Level VII)
12 Centers for Disease Control and Prevention. (2002). Guideline for hand hygiene in health-care settings: Recommendations of the Healthcare Infection Control Practices Advisory Committee and the HICPAC/SHEA/APIC/IDSA Hand Hygiene Task Force. *MMWR Recommendations and Reports, 51*(RR-16), 1–45. Accessed May 2015 via the Web at http://www.cdc.gov/mmwr/pdf/rr/rr5116.pdf (Level II)
13 World Health Organization. (2009). "WHO guidelines on hand hygiene in health care: First global patient safety challenge, clean care is safer care" [Online]. Accessed May 2015 via the Web at http://whqlibdoc.who.int/publications/2009/9789241597906_eng.pdf (Level IV)
14 American Osteopathic Association. (2014). Standard 07.01.21. *Healthcare Facilities Accreditation Program: Accreditation requirements for acute care hospitals.* Chicago, IL: American Osteopathic Association. (Level VII)
15 Centers for Medicare & Medicaid Services, Department of Health and Human Services. (2014). Condition of participation: Infection control. 42 C.F.R. § 482.42.
16 The Joint Commission. (2015). Standard NPSG.01.01.01. *Comprehensive accreditation manual for hospitals: The official handbook.* Oakbrook Terrace, IL: The Joint Commission. (Level VII)
17 Siegel, J. D., et al. (2007). "2007 guideline for isolation precautions: Preventing transmission of infectious agents in healthcare settings" [Online]. Accessed May 2015 via the Web at http://www.cdc.gov/hicpac/pdf/isolation/Isolation2007.pdf (Level II)
18 Occupational Safety and Health Administration. (n.d.). "Bloodborne pathogens, standard number 1910.1030" [Online]. Accessed May 2015 via the Web at http://www.osha.gov/pls/oshaweb/owadisp.show_document?p_table=STANDARDS&p_id=10051 (Level VII)
19 American Osteopathic Association. (2014). Standard 07.01.10. *Healthcare Facilities Accreditation Program: Accreditation requirements for acute care hospitals.* Chicago, IL: American Osteopathic Association. (Level VII)
20 The Joint Commission. (2015). Standard UP.01.02.01. *Comprehensive accreditation manual for hospitals: The official handbook.* Oakbrook Terrace, IL: The Joint Commission. (Level VII)
21 The Joint Commission. (2015). Standard UP.01.03.01. *Comprehensive accreditation manual for hospitals: The official handbook.* Oakbrook Terrace, IL: The Joint Commission. (Level VII)
22 The Joint Commission. (2015). Standard RC.01.03.01. *Comprehensive accreditation manual for hospitals: The official handbook.* Oakbrook Terrace, IL: The Joint Commission. (Level VII)
23 American Osteopathic Association. (2014). Standard 10.00.03. *Healthcare Facilities Accreditation Program: Accreditation requirements for acute care hospitals.* Chicago, IL: American Osteopathic Association. (Level VII)
24 Centers for Medicare & Medicaid Services, Department of Health and Human Services. (2014). Condition of participation: Medical record services. 42 C.F.R. § 482.24(b).

SURGICAL DRAIN REMOVAL

Surgical drains are important adjuncts to postoperative care because they promote wound healing by providing an exit site for fluid that accumulates in or near the wound bed. Drains should be removed when they malfunction or when drainage becomes minimal. Drains commonly inserted during surgery include a closed drainage system, a bulb suction drain, and Penrose drain.

Equipment

Sterile 4″ × 4″ (10-cm × 10-cm) gauze pads ■ tape (paper or silicone for frail skin)[1] ■ gown ■ gloves ■ sterile gloves ■ Optional: suture-removal kit, prescribed pain medication, sterile specimen swabs, sterile specimen containers, laboratory transport bags, mask, face shield, nonadherent contact layers, nonadherent or silicone foam dressing, other topical dressing specifically formulated for fragile skin.

Implementation

■ Verify the practitioner's order.
■ Review the patient's medical record to determine the type of drain to be removed, its location, and the method used to secure it *to ensure proper removal.*
■ Verify whether a surgical drain, drain tip, or drainage culture is needed to be sent for culturing upon drain removal.
■ Perform hand hygiene.[2,3,4,5,6]
■ Confirm the patient's identity using at least two patient identifiers.[7]
■ Explain the procedure to the patient *to allay his fear and anxiety.*
■ Perform a comprehensive pain assessment using techniques appropriate for the patient's age, condition, and ability to understand.[8]
■ Administer pain medications, as ordered, following safe medication administration practices.[9]
■ Put on gloves and a gown; also put on a mask and a face shield, if necessary, *to protect yourself from splashing.*[10,11]
■ Position the patient comfortable and in a manner that provides you with adequate access to the surgical site.
■ If the drain contains suction from its initial closure, release the suction from the drain.
■ Note the volume, color, consistency, and odor of drainage within the drain.
■ Remove the drain dressing *to gain access to the exit site.* Remove the dressing and tape carefully *to prevent skin tears.* Dispose of it in an appropriate receptacle.
■ Remove and discard your gloves.[10]
■ Perform hand hygiene[2,3,4,5,6] and put on sterile gloves.[2,3,10]
■ Open the sterile gauze pads and suture-removal kit if necessary.
■ Place a sterile gauze pad close to the exit site *to absorb any remaining drainage while you remove the drain.*[12]
■ Have the patient breathe deeply and smoothly. Grasp the drain close to the skin.[13]
■ Gently withdraw the drain using smooth, steady traction. If you feel resistance, stop the procedure and notify the practitioner.[9,12]
■ Check that you've removed the entire drain. Examine the drain tip for irregularities or other signs of breakage. The drain should have a clean-cut edge and not appear jagged or torn.[13] Dispose of it in an appropriate receptacle.[10]
■ If the tip is required for culture, cut it with sterile scissors and place it in a sterile specimen container. Label the specimen container in the presence of the patient *to prevent mislabeling.*[7] Place the specimen in a laboratory transport bag and send it to the laboratory.
■ Assess the patient's skin integrity at the exit site for signs of infection, such as redness, swelling, a foul odor, or purulent drainage, and for signs of fluid accumulation.[12]
■ If purulent drainage and inflammation are present at the exit site, obtain a swab specimen. Place the swab in its container and then label the container in the presence of the patient *to prevent mislabeling.*[7] Place the specimen container in a laboratory transport bag and send it to the laboratory.
■ Maintain pressure over the drain site with a gauze pad until drainage or bleeding is minimal.
■ Remove and discard your gloves,[10] perform hand hygiene,[2,3,4,5,6] and put on new sterile gloves.[10]
■ Place a sterile gauze pad over the drain exit site and secure it with tape. Alternately, if the patient has frail skin, cover the site with nonadherent contact layers, a nonadherent or silicone foam dressing, or other topical dressing specifically formulated for fragile skin. Secure the dressing with paper or silicone tape *to prevent skin stripping or tearing.*[1] Label the dressing with the date, the time, and your initials.[12]
■ Discard used materials in an appropriate receptacle.[10]
■ Reassess the patient's pain assessment and respond appropriately.[8]
■ Remove and discard your gloves and any other personal protective equipment worn.[10]
■ Perform hand hygiene.[2,3,4,5,6]
■ Document the procedure.[14,15,16]

Special considerations

■ Drainage from the exit site should be minimal and should cease within 24 hours of drain removal. If drainage continues, notify the practitioner *because fluid may be accumulating beneath the skin and require evacuation.*[12]

Patient teaching

Teach the patient about the signs and symptoms of infection, such as fever, chills, nausea, vomiting, or evidence of redness, swelling, purulent drainage, or odor from the drain site. Tell him to notify the practitioner if these signs and symptoms develop or if a sudden increase in pain at the drain site occurs.

Complications

Pain may accompany drain removal and persist after removal. Impaired wound healing may be a complication if fluid accumulates beneath the skin. Infection and injury to adjacent tissues may also occur.

Documentation

Document the date and time of drain removal, the type of drain removed, the condition of the exit site, and the presence and characteristics of drainage. Document your pain assessments and any medications given as well as any specimens collected and sent for microbiologic examination. Document the patient's tolerance of the procedure, patient teaching performed, and the patient's understanding of the teaching.

REFERENCES

1 LeBlanc, K., et al. (2013). International skin tear advisory panel: A tool kit to aid in the prevention, assessment, and treatment of skin tears using a simplified classification system. *Advances in Skin & Wound Care, 26,* 459–476.

2 Centers for Disease Control and Prevention. (2002). Guideline for hand hygiene in health-care settings: Recommendations of the Healthcare Infection Control Practices Advisory Committee and the HICPAC/SHEA/APIC/IDSA Hand Hygiene Task Force. *MMWR Recommendations and Reports, 51*(RR-16), 1–45. Accessed May 2015 via the Web at http://www.cdc.gov/mmwr/pdf/rr/rr5116.pdf (Level II)

3 The Joint Commission. (2015). Standard NPSG.07.01.01. *Comprehensive accreditation manual for hospitals: The official handbook.* Oakbrook Terrace, IL: The Joint Commission. (Level VII)

4 World Health Organization. (2009). "WHO guidelines on hand hygiene in health care: First global patient safety challenge, clean care is safer care" [Online]. Accessed May 2015 via the Web at http://whqlibdoc.who.int/publications/2009/9789241597906_eng.pdf (Level IV)

5 Centers for Medicare & Medicaid Services, Department of Health and Human Services. (2014). Condition of participation: Infection control. 42 C.F.R. § 482.42.

Tailoring wound care to wound color

To promote healing in any wound, keep it moist, clean, and free of debris. For an open wound, use wound color to guide the specific management approach and to assess how well the wound is healing.

Red wounds

Red, the color of healthy granulation tissue, indicates normal healing. When a wound begins to heal, a layer of pale pink granulation tissue covers the wound bed. As this layer thickens, it becomes beefy red. Cover a red wound, keep it moist and clean, and protect it from trauma. Use a transparent dressing, hydrocolloid dressing, or gauze dressing moistened with sterile normal saline solution or impregnated with petroleum jelly or an antibiotic.

Yellow wounds

Yellow is the color of exudate produced by microorganisms in an open wound. When a wound heals without complications, the immune system removes microorganisms. However, if there are too many microorganisms to remove, exudate accumulates and becomes visible. Exudate usually appears whitish yellow, creamy yellow, yellowish green, or beige. Dry exudate appears darker.

If the patient has a yellow wound, clean it and remove exudate using irrigation; then cover it with a moist dressing. Use absorptive products or a moist gauze dressing with or without an antibiotic. You may also use hydrotherapy with whirlpool or high-pressure irrigation.

Black wounds

Black, the least healthy color, signals necrosis. Dead, avascular tissue slows healing and provides a site for microorganisms to proliferate.

A black wound should be debrided. After removing dead tissue, apply a dressing to keep the wound moist and guard against external contamination. As ordered, use enzyme products, surgical debridement, hydrotherapy with whirlpool or irrigation, or a moist gauze dressing.

Multicolored wounds

You may note two or even all three colors in a wound. In this case, classify the wound according to the least healthy color present. For example, if your patient's wound is both red and yellow, classify it as a yellow wound.

6 American Osteopathic Association. (2014). Standard 07.01.21. *Healthcare Facilities Accreditation Program: Accreditation requirements for acute care hospitals.* Chicago, IL: American Osteopathic Association. (Level VII)

7 The Joint Commission. (2014). Standard NPSG.01.01.01. *Comprehensive accreditation manual for hospitals: The official handbook.* Oakbrook Terrace, IL: The Joint Commission. (Level VII)

8 The Joint Commission. (2015). Standard PC.01.02.07. *Comprehensive accreditation manual for hospitals: The official handbook.* Oakbrook Terrace, IL: The Joint Commission. (Level VII)

9 Durai, R., & Ng, P. C. H. (2010). Surgical vacuum drains: Types, uses, and complications. *AORN, 91,* 266–271.

10 Siegel, J. D., et al. (2007). "2007 guideline for isolation precautions: Preventing transmission of infectious agents in healthcare settings" [Online]. Accessed May 2015 via the Web at http://www.cdc.gov/hicpac/pdf/isolation/Isolation2007.pdf (Level II)

11 American Osteopathic Association. (2014). Standard 07.01.10. *Healthcare Facilities Accreditation Program: Accreditation requirements for acute care hospitals.* Chicago, IL: American Osteopathic Association. (Level VII)

12 Lynn-McHale Wiegand, D. (Ed.). (2011). *AACN procedure manual for critical care* (6th ed.). Philadelphia, PA: Saunders.

13 Walker, J. (2007). Patient preparation for safe removal of surgical drains. *Nursing Standard, 21*(49), 39–41

14 The Joint Commission. (2015). Standard RC.01.03.01. *Comprehensive accreditation manual for hospitals: The official handbook.* Oakbrook Terrace, IL: The Joint Commission. (Level VII)

15 Centers for Medicare & Medicaid Services, Department of Health and Human Services. (2014). Condition of participation: Medical record services. 42 C.F.R. § 482.24(b).

16 American Osteopathic Association. (2014). Standard 10.00.03. *Healthcare Facilities Accreditation Program: Accreditation requirements for acute care hospitals.* Chicago, IL: American Osteopathic Association. (Level VII)

Surgical wound management

When caring for a patient with a surgical wound, the nurse carries out procedures that help prevent infection by stopping pathogens from entering the wound. Besides promoting patient comfort, such procedures protect the skin surface from maceration and excoriation caused by contact with irritating drainage. They also allow for measurement of wound drainage to monitor fluid balance.

The two primary methods used to manage a draining surgical wound are dressing and drainage collection pouching. Dressing is preferred, unless caustic or excessive drainage is compromising the patient's skin integrity. Usually, lightly seeping wounds with drains and wounds with minimal purulent drainage can be managed with packing and gauze dressings. If the patient has a surgical wound, you must monitor him and choose the appropriate dressing.

Dressing a wound calls for sterile technique and sterile supplies to prevent contamination. The color of the wound can help determine which type of dressing to apply. (See *Tailoring wound care to wound color.*) Change the dressing often enough to keep the skin dry, and always follow standard precautions set by the Centers for Disease Control and Prevention.

Equipment

Patient's medical record ■ gloves ■ sterile gloves ■ sterile 4″ × 4″ (10-cm × 10-cm) gauze pads ■ sterile dressing set ■ prescribed antiseptic cleaning agent ■ adhesive or other tape ■ soap and water ■ sterile scissors ■ sterile 4″ × 4″ (10-cm × 10-cm) precut drain dressings or tracheostomy pads ■ Optional: gown and face shield or goggles, surgical mask, wound irrigant and irrigation supplies, sterile forceps, sterile cotton-tipped applicators, skin protectant, large absorbent dressings, collodion spray or acetone-free adhesive remover, prescribed topical medication, sterile normal saline solution, graduated container, and Montgomery straps or a T-binder, fishnet tube elasticized dressing support.

Implementation

- Verify the practitioner's order for specific wound care and medication instructions.
- Ask the patient about allergies, especially to tape, topical solutions, or medications.
- Gather all equipment in the patient's room.
- Check the expiration date on each sterile package, and inspect for tears.
- Perform hand hygiene.[1,2,3,4,5]
- Confirm the patient's identity using at least two patient identifiers.[6]
- Explain the procedure to the patient *to allay his fears and ensure his cooperation.*
- Perform a comprehensive pain assessment using techniques appropriate for the patient's age, condition, and ability to understand. Administer pain medications, as needed and as ordered, before dressing application.[7]

Removing the old dressing

- Note the location of surgical drains *to avoid dislodging them during the procedure.*

■ Provide privacy[8,9] and position the patient, as necessary. *To avoid chilling him,* expose only the wound site.
■ Put on a gown and a face shield or goggles, if necessary. Then put on clean gloves.[10,11]
■ Assess the patient's condition.
■ Loosen the soiled dressing by holding the patient's skin and pulling the tape or dressing toward the wound. *This protects the newly formed tissue and prevents stress on the incision.* Moisten the tape with acetone-free adhesive remover, if necessary, *to make the tape removal less painful (particularly if the skin is hairy).* Don't apply solvents to the incision *because they could contaminate the wound.*

ELDER ALERT *Remove adhesive tape carefully* to prevent skin tears in elderly patients.

■ Slowly remove the soiled dressing. If the gauze adheres to the wound, loosen the gauze by moistening it with sterile normal saline solution.
■ Observe the dressing for the amount, type, color, and odor of drainage.
■ Discard the dressing and your gloves in the appropriate receptacle.[10,11,12]

Caring for the wound

■ Perform hand hygiene.[1,2,3,4,5]
■ Establish a sterile field with all the equipment and supplies you'll need for suture-line care and the dressing change, including a sterile dressing set and antiseptic cleaning agent. If the practitioner has ordered ointment, squeeze the needed amount onto the sterile field. If you're using an antiseptic from an unsterile bottle, pour the antiseptic cleaning agent into a sterile container *so you won't contaminate your gloves after putting them on.*
■ Put on sterile gloves.[10,11]
■ Saturate the sterile gauze pads with the prescribed antiseptic cleaning agent. Avoid using cotton balls *because they may shed fibers in the wound, causing irritation, infection, or adhesion.*
■ If ordered, irrigate the wound, using the specified solution. (See the "Wound irrigation" procedure, page 840.)
■ Pick up the moistened gauze pad, and squeeze out the excess solution.
■ For an open wound, clean the wound in a full or half circle, beginning in the center and working outward. Use a new swab or pad for each circle (as shown below). Clean to at least 1″ (2.5 cm) beyond the end of the new dressing.

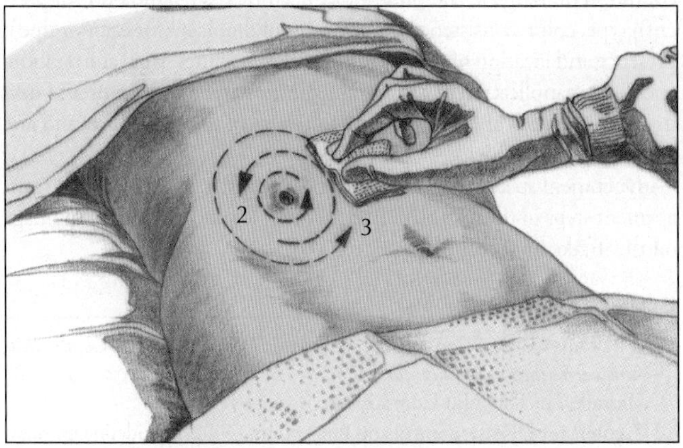

■ For a linear incision, work from the top of the incision, wipe once to the bottom, and then discard the gauze pad. With a second moistened pad, wipe from top to bottom in a vertical path next to the incision. Continue to work outward from the incision in lines running parallel to it (as shown on top right). Always wipe from the clean area toward the less clean area (usually from top to bottom). Use each gauze pad for only one stroke *to avoid tracking wound exudate and normal body flora from surrounding skin to the clean areas.* Remember that the suture line is cleaner than the adjacent skin and the top of the suture line is usually cleaner than the bottom *because more drainage collects at the bottom of the wound.*

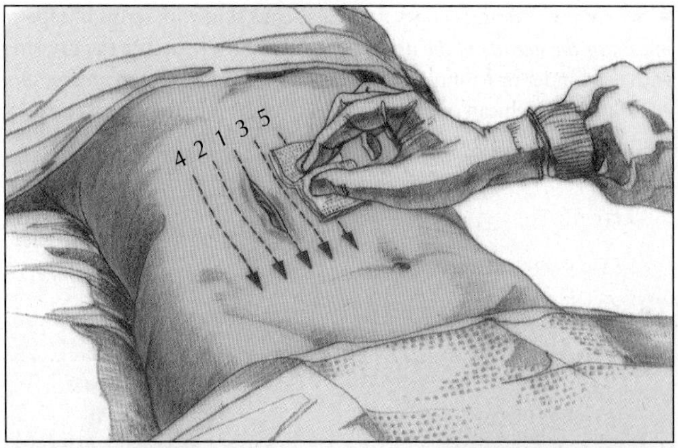

■ Use sterile cotton-tipped applicators for efficient cleaning of tight-fitting wire sutures, deep and narrow wounds, and wounds with pockets. Remember to wipe only once with each applicator.
■ Clean the patient's surgical drain surface last. *Because moisture promotes bacterial growth,* the drain is the most contaminated area. Clean the skin around the drain by wiping in half or full circles from the drain site outward.
■ Clean all areas of the wound *to wash away debris, pus, blood, and necrotic material.* Try not to disturb sutures or irritate the incision. Clean to at least 1″ (2.5 cm) beyond the end of the new dressing. Check to make sure the edges of the incision are lined up properly, and check for signs of infection (heat, redness, swelling, induration, and odor), dehiscence, and evisceration. If you observe such signs or if the patient reports pain at the wound site, notify the practitioner.
■ Wash the skin surrounding the wound with soap and water, and pat it dry using a sterile 4″ × 4″ (10-cm × 10-cm) gauze pad. Avoid oil-based soap *because it may interfere with tape adherence.* If ordered, obtain a wound culture. (See the "Swab specimen collection" procedure, page 734.)
■ Apply a skin protectant, if needed.
■ If ordered, pack the wound with gauze pads or strips folded to fit, using a sterile forceps. Avoid using cotton-lined gauze pads *because cotton fibers can adhere to the wound surface and cause complications.* Pack the wound, using the wet-to-damp method. *Soaking the packing material in solution and wringing it out so that it's slightly moist provides a moist wound environment that absorbs debris and drainage without disrupting new tissue when the packing is removed.*

Applying a fresh gauze dressing

■ Gently place sterile 4″ × 4″ (10-cm × 10-cm) gauze pads at the center of the wound, and move progressively outward to the edges of the wound site. Extend the gauze at least 1″ (2.5 cm) beyond the incision in each direction, and cover the wound evenly with enough sterile dressings (usually two or three layers) to absorb all drainage until the next dressing change. Use large absorbent dressings to form outer layers, if needed, *to provide greater absorbency.*

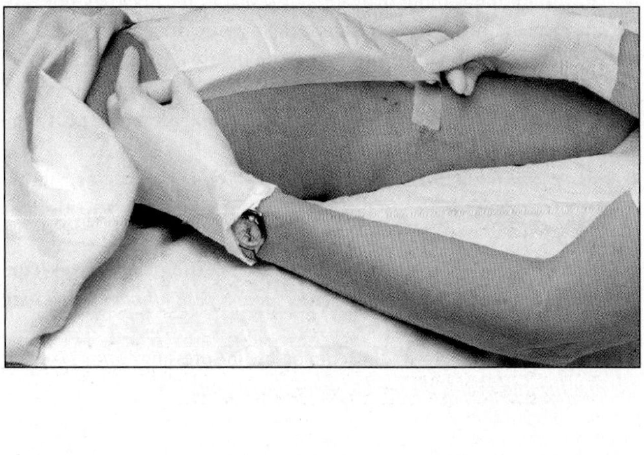

■ Secure the dressing's edges to the patient's skin with strips of tape *to maintain the sterility of the wound site.* Alternatively, secure the dressing with a T-binder or Montgomery straps (as shown below) *to prevent skin excoriation,* which can occur with repeated tape removal necessitated by frequent dressing changes.

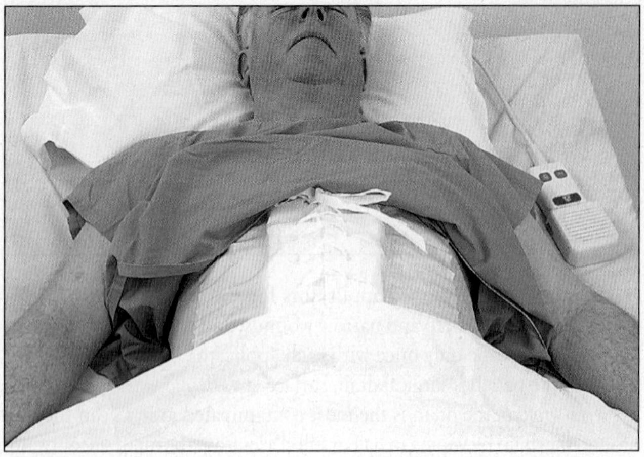

■ If the wound is on a limb, secure the dressing with a fishnet tube elasticized dressing support.

Dressing a wound with a drain

■ Use commercially precut sterile gauze dressings; gently press one drain dressing close to the skin around the drain *so that the tubing fits into the slit.* Press the second drain dressing around the drain from the opposite direction *so that the two dressings encircle the drain.*

■ Layer as many uncut, sterile 4″ × 4″ (10-cm × 10-cm) gauze pads or large absorbent dressings around the tubing as needed *to absorb expected drainage.*

■ Tape the dressing in place, or use a T-binder or Montgomery straps.

Completing the procedure

■ Make sure the patient is comfortable.

■ Discard all used supplies in appropriate receptacles.[10,11,12]

■ Remove and discard your gloves.[10,11,12]

■ Perform hand hygiene.[1,2,3,4,5]

■ Document the procedure.[13,14,15]

Special considerations

■ If the patient has two wounds in the same area, cover each wound separately with layers of sterile 4″ × 4″ (10-cm × 10-cm) gauze pads. Then cover each site with a large absorbent dressing secured to the patient's skin with tape. Don't use a single large absorbent dressing to cover both sites *because drainage quickly saturates a pad, promoting cross-contamination.*

■ If a wound drains more than about 1½ oz (50 mL) per day not captured by the drain, apply a pouch to collect excess drainage.

■ When packing a wound, don't pack it too tightly *because this compresses adjacent capillaries and may prevent the wound edges from contracting.* Avoid overlapping damp packing onto surrounding skin *because it macerates the intact tissue.*

■ *To save time when dressing a wound with a drain,* use precut tracheostomy pads or drain dressings instead of custom-cutting gauze pads to fit around the drain.

■ If your patient is sensitive to adhesive tape, use paper or silk tape *because it's less likely to cause a skin reaction and peels off more easily than adhesive tape does.*

■ Use a surgical mask to cradle a chin or jawline dressing; *doing so secures the dressing and avoids the need to shave the patient's hair.*

■ If ordered, use a collodion spray or similar topical protectant instead of a gauze dressing. Moisture- and contaminant-proof, this covering dries in a clear, impermeable film that leaves the wound visible for observation and avoids the friction caused by a dressing.

■ *Because many practitioners prefer to change the first postoperative dressing themselves to check the incision,* don't change the first dressing unless you have specific instructions to do so. If you have no such order and drainage comes through the dressings, reinforce the dressing with fresh sterile gauze. Request an order to change the dressing, or ask the practitioner to change it as soon as possible. A reinforced dressing shouldn't remain in place longer than 24 hours *because it's an excellent medium for bacterial growth.*

■ For a recent postoperative patient or a patient with complications, check the dressing every 15 to 30 minutes, or as ordered. For the patient with a properly healing wound, check the dressing at least once every 8 hours.

■ If the dressing becomes wet from the outside (for example, from spilled drinking water), replace it as soon as possible *to prevent wound contamination.*

Patient teaching

If your patient will need wound care after discharge, provide appropriate teaching. If he'll be caring for the wound himself, stress the importance of using sterile technique, and teach him how to examine the wound for signs of infection and other complications. Also show him how to change dressings, and give him written instructions for all procedures to be performed at home.

Complications

A major complication of a dressing change is an allergic reaction to an antiseptic cleaning agent, a prescribed topical medication, or adhesive tape. This reaction may lead to skin redness, rash, excoriation, or infection. Skin tears are also a potential complication.

Documentation

Document the date, time, and type of wound management procedure; amount of soiled dressing and packing removed; wound appearance (size, condition of margins, and presence of necrotic tissue) and odor (if present); type, color, consistency, and amount of drainage (for each wound); presence and location of drains; additional procedures, such as irrigation, packing, or application of a topical medication; type and amount of new dressing or pouch applied; patient's tolerance of the procedure; and any patient teaching provided.

Document special or detailed wound care instructions and pain management steps in the care plan. Record the color and amount of drainage on the intake-and-output sheet.

REFERENCES

1 The Joint Commission. (2015). Standard NPSG.07.01.01. *Comprehensive accreditation manual for hospitals: The official handbook.* Oakbrook Terrace, IL: The Joint Commission. (Level VII)

2 Centers for Disease Control and Prevention. (2002). Guideline for hand hygiene in health-care settings: Recommendations of the Healthcare Infection Control Practices Advisory Committee and the HICPAC/SHEA/APIC/IDSA Hand Hygiene Task Force. *MMWR Recommendations and Reports, 51*(RR–16), 1–45. Accessed May 2015 via the Web at http://www.cdc.gov/mmwr/pdf/rr/rr5116.pdf (Level II)

3 World Health Organization. (2009). "WHO guidelines on hand hygiene in health care: First global patient safety challenge, clean care is safer care" [Online]. Accessed May 2015 via the Web at http://whqlibdoc.who.int/publications/2009/9789241597906_eng.pdf (Level IV)

4 American Osteopathic Association. (2014). Standard 07.01.21. *Healthcare Facilities Accreditation Program: Accreditation requirements for acute care hospitals.* Chicago, IL: American Osteopathic Association. (Level VII)

5 Centers for Medicare & Medicaid Services, Department of Health and Human Services. (2014). Condition of participation: Infection control. 42 C.F.R. § 482.42.
6 The Joint Commission. (2015). Standard NPSG.01.01.01. *Comprehensive accreditation manual for hospitals: The official handbook.* Oakbrook Terrace, IL: The Joint Commission. (Level VII)
7 The Joint Commission. (2015). Standard PC.01.02.07. *Comprehensive accreditation manual for hospitals: The official handbook.* Oakbrook Terrace, IL: The Joint Commission. (Level VII)
8 American Osteopathic Association. (2014). Standard 15.01.16. *Healthcare Facilities Accreditation Program: Accreditation requirements for acute care hospitals.* Chicago, IL: American Osteopathic Association. (Level VII)
9 Centers for Medicare & Medicaid Services, Department of Health and Human Services. (2014). Condition of participation: Patient's rights. 42 C.F.R. § 482.13(c)(1).
10 Siegel, J. D., et al. (2007). "2007 guideline for isolation precautions: Preventing transmission of infectious agents in healthcare settings" [Online]. Accessed May 2015 via the Web at http://www.cdc.gov/hicpac/pdf/isolation/Isolation2007.pdf (Level II)
11 American Osteopathic Association. (2014). Standard 07.01.10. *Healthcare Facilities Accreditation Program: Accreditation requirements for acute care hospitals.* Chicago, IL: American Osteopathic Association. (Level VII)
12 Occupational Safety and Health Administration. (n.d.). "Bloodborne pathogens, standard number 1910.1030" [Online]. Accessed May 2015 via the Web at http://www.osha.gov/pls/oshaweb/owadisp.show_document?p_table=STANDARDS&p_id=10051 (Level VII)
13 The Joint Commission. (2015). Standard RC.01.03.01. *Comprehensive accreditation manual for hospitals: The official handbook.* Oakbrook Terrace, IL: The Joint Commission. (Level VII)
14 American Osteopathic Association. (2014). Standard 10.00.03. *Healthcare Facilities Accreditation Program: Accreditation requirements for acute care hospitals.* Chicago, IL: American Osteopathic Association. (Level VII)
15 Centers for Medicare & Medicaid Services, Department of Health and Human Services. (2014). Condition of participation: Medical record services. 42 C.F.R. § 482.24(b).

ADDITIONAL REFERENCES

Baranoski, S., & Ayello, E. A. (2012). *Wound care essentials: Practice principles* (3rd ed.). Philadelphia, PA: Lippincott Williams & Williams.
Craven, R. F., & Hirnle, C. J. (2012). *Fundamentals of nursing: Human health and function* (7th ed.). Philadelphia, PA: Lippincott Williams & Wilkins.
Hess, C. T. (2012). *Clinical guide to skin & wound care* (7th ed.). Philadelphia, PA: Lippincott Williams & Wilkins.

SUTURE REMOVAL

The goal of this procedure is to remove skin sutures from a healed wound without damaging newly formed tissue. The timing of suture removal depends on the shape, size, and location of the sutured incision; the absence of inflammation, drainage, and infection; and the patient's general condition. Usually, for a sufficiently healed wound, sutures are removed 7 to 10 days after insertion.

The specific technique used for removal depends on the method of suturing; however, all require sterile technique to prevent contamination. Although sutures usually are removed by a practitioner, in many facilities, a nurse may remove them on the practitioner's order.

Equipment

Gloves ■ sterile 4″ × 4″ (10-cm × 10-cm) dressing ■ tape ■ waterproof trash container ■ sterile drape ■ sterile gloves ■ sterile scissors ■ sterile forceps or sterile hemostat ■ sterile gauze pads ■ antiseptic cleaning agent ■ Optional: normal saline solution, butterfly or regular adhesive strips.

Prepackaged, sterile suture-removal trays are available.

Implementation

■ If your facility allows you to remove sutures, check the practitioner's order *to confirm the details of this procedure.* If the patient has interrupted sutures or an incompletely healed suture line, remove only those sutures specified by the practitioner. He may want to leave some sutures in place for an additional day or two *to support the suture line.*

■ Check the patient's medical record for a history of allergies, especially to adhesive tape and povidone-iodine or other topical solutions or medications.[1,2,3]

■ Gather the equipment in the patient's room.

■ Check the expiration date on each sterile package and inspect for tears. If the integrity is compromised, obtain new supplies.

■ Perform hand hygiene.[4,5,6,7,8]

■ Confirm the patient's identity using at least two patient identifiers.[9]

■ Explain the procedure to the patient *to allay his fears and enhance cooperation.* Assure him that this procedure typically is painless but that he may feel a tickling sensation as the sutures come out. Reassure him that, because his wound is healing properly, removing the sutures won't weaken the incision.

■ Provide privacy.[10,11,12]

■ Position the patient so he's comfortable without placing undue tension on the suture line. *Because some patients experience nausea or dizziness during the procedure,* have the patient recline if possible. Adjust the light to have it shine directly on the suture line.

■ Place the trash container near the patient's bed. Position the container properly *to avoid reaching across the sterile field or the suture line when disposing of soiled articles.*

■ If the patient's wound has a dressing, perform hand hygiene and put on clean gloves, remove the dressing carefully, and discard it in the waterproof trash container.[13,14]

■ Inspect the patient's wound for possible gaping, drainage, inflammation, signs of infection, and embedded sutures. Notify the practitioner if the wound has failed to heal properly. *The absence of a healing ridge under the suture line 5 to 7 days after the incision indicates that the line needs continued support and protection during the healing process.*

■ Remove and discard your gloves[13,14] and perform hand hygiene.[4,5,6,7,8]

■ Establish a sterile work area with all the equipment and supplies you'll need for suture removal and wound care. Open the suture-removal tray and put on sterile gloves.

■ Using sterile technique, clean the suture line *to decrease the number of microorganisms present and reduce the risk of infection.* The cleaning process should also moisten the sutures sufficiently *to ease removal.* Soften them further, if needed, with normal saline solution.

■ Proceed according to the type of suture you're removing. (See *Methods for removing sutures,* page 732.) *Because the visible part of a suture is exposed to skin bacteria and considered contaminated,* be sure to cut sutures at the skin surface on one side of the visible part of the suture. Remove the suture by lifting and pulling the visible end off the skin *to avoid drawing this contaminated portion back through subcutaneous tissue.*

■ If ordered, remove every other suture *to maintain some support for the incision.* Then go back and remove the remaining sutures.

■ After removing sutures, wipe the incision gently with gauze pads soaked in an antiseptic cleaning agent. Apply a light sterile gauze dressing, if needed, *to prevent infection and irritation from clothing.*

■ Remove and discard your gloves.[13,14]

■ Perform hand hygiene.[4,5,6,7,8]

■ Properly dispose of the solutions and clean or dispose of soiled equipment and supplies.[13,14,15,16]

■ Perform hand hygiene.[4,5,6,7,8]

■ Document the procedure.[17,18,19]

Methods for removing sutures

Removal techniques usually depend on the type of sutures to be removed. The first two illustrations below show how to cut and grasp sutures; the remaining illustrations show how to remove four common suture types. Keep in mind that for all suture types, it's important to grasp and cut sutures in the correct place *to avoid pulling the exposed (and thus contaminated) suture material through subcutaneous tissue*.

Cutting the suture

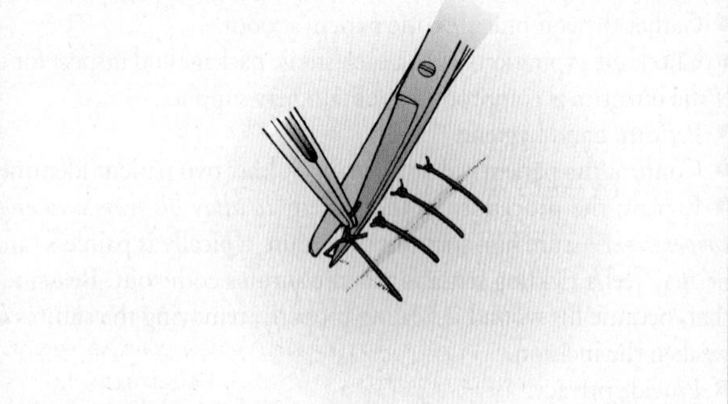

Plain interrupted sutures

Using sterile forceps, grasp the knot of the first suture and raise it off the skin. *Doing so exposes a small portion of the suture that was below skin level.* Place the rounded tips of sterile curved-tip suture scissors against the skin, and cut through the exposed portion of the suture.

Grasping the suture

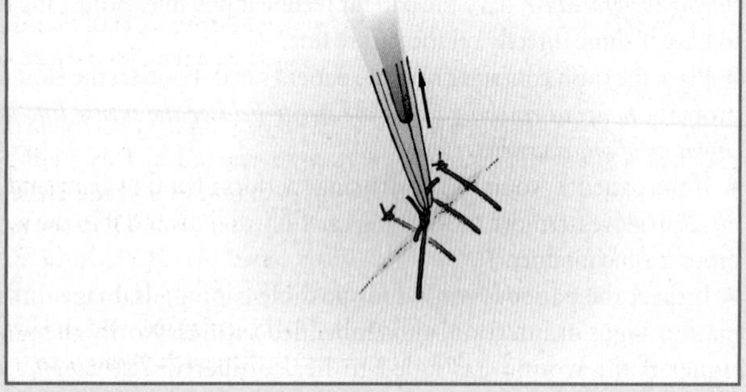

Then, still holding the knot with the forceps, pull the cut suture up and out of the skin in a smooth, continuous motion to *avoid causing the patient pain.*

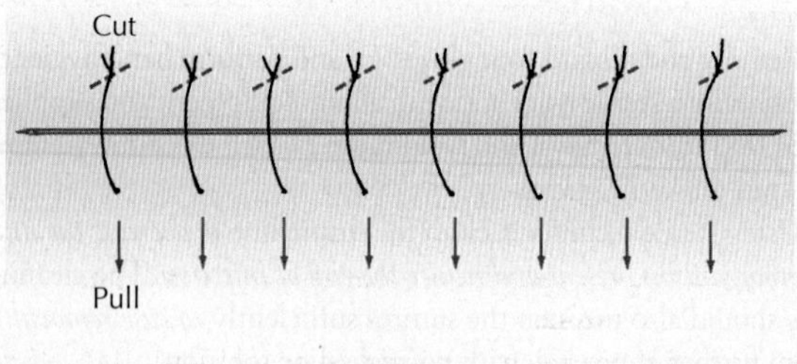

Discard the suture. Repeat the process for every other suture (alternating sutures) initially; if the wound doesn't gape, you can then remove the remaining sutures as ordered.

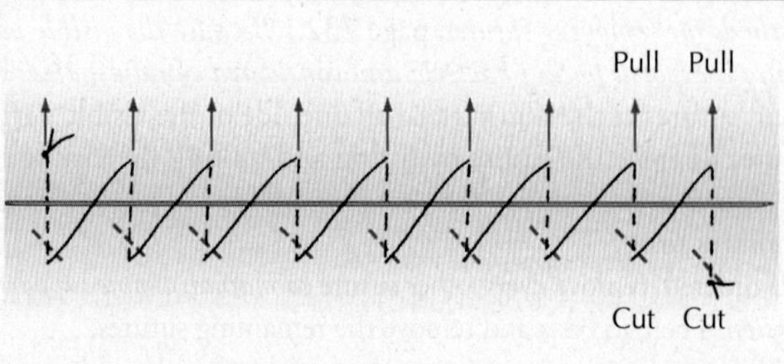

Plain continuous sutures

Cut the first suture on the side opposite the knot. Next, cut the same side of the next suture in line. Then lift the first suture out in the direction of the knot. Proceed along the suture line, grasping each suture where you grasped the knot on the first one.

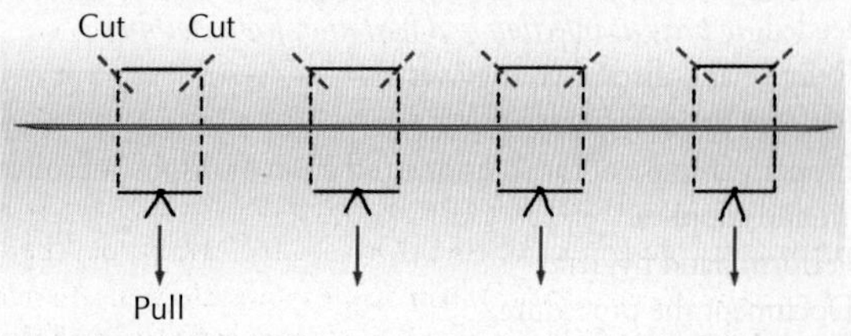

Mattress interrupted sutures

If possible, remove the small, visible portion of the suture opposite the knot by cutting it at each visible end and lifting the small piece away from the skin *to prevent pulling it through and contaminating subcutaneous tissue.* Then remove the rest of the suture by pulling it out in the direction of the knot. If the visible portion is too small to cut twice, cut it once and pull the entire suture out in the opposite direction. Repeat these steps for the remaining sutures, and monitor the incision carefully for infection.

(continued)

Methods for removing sutures *(continued)*

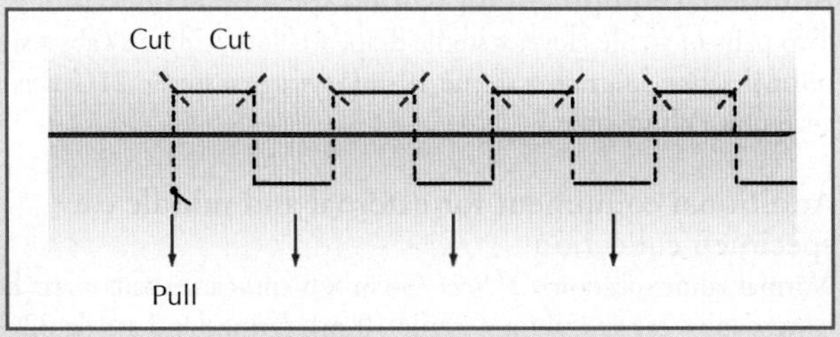

Mattress continuous sutures

Follow the procedure for removing mattress interrupted sutures, first removing the small visible portion of the suture, if possible, *to prevent pulling it through and contaminating subcutaneous tissue.* Then extract the rest of the suture in the direction of the knot.

Special considerations

- Check the practitioner's order for the time of suture removal. Usually, you'll remove sutures on the head and neck 3 to 5 days after insertion; on the chest and abdomen, 5 to 7 days after insertion; and on the lower extremities, 7 to 10 days after insertion.
- If the patient has retention and regular sutures in place, check the practitioner's order for the sequence in which they are to be removed. *Because retention sutures link underlying fat and muscle tissue and give added support to the obese or slow-healing patient,* they usually remain in place for 14 to 21 days.
- Be particularly careful to clean the suture line before attempting to remove mattress sutures *to decrease the risk of infection when the visible, contaminated part of the stitch is too small to cut twice for sterile removal and must be pulled through the tissue.* After you have removed mattress sutures this way, monitor the suture line carefully *for subsequent infection.*
- According to the practitioner's preference, inform the patient that he may shower in 1 or 2 days if the incision is dry and heals well after suture removal.
- If the wound dehisces during suture removal, apply butterfly or regular adhesive strips *to support and approximate the edges,* and call the practitioner immediately to repair the wound.
- Apply butterfly or regular adhesive strips after any suture removal, if desired, *to give added support to the incision line and prevent lateral tension on the wound from forming a wide scar.* Leave the strips in place for 3 to 5 days, as ordered.

Patient teaching

If the patient is being discharged, teach him how to remove the dressing and care for the wound. Instruct him to call the practitioner immediately if he observes wound discharge, gaping, or inflammation. Tell him that the redness surrounding the incision should gradually disappear, and only a thin line should show after a few weeks. Encourage the patient to use sunblock products on the wound for 3 to 6 months *to aid healing and reduce scar formation.*[20]

Complications

Complications of suture removal include infection, missed removal of a suture, and incomplete healing resulting from removing the sutures too soon.

Documentation

Record the date and time of suture removal, type and number of sutures, appearance of the suture line, signs of wound complications, dressings or butterfly or regular adhesive strips applied, the patient's tolerance of the procedure, and any patient teaching provided.

REFERENCES

1 American Osteopathic Association. (2014). Standard 16.01.03. *Healthcare Facilities Accreditation Program: Accreditation requirements for acute care hospitals.* Chicago, IL: American Osteopathic Association. (Level VII)

2 The Joint Commission. (2015). Standard MM.06.01.01. *Comprehensive accreditation manual for hospitals: The official handbook.* Oakbrook Terrace, IL: The Joint Commission. (Level VII)

3 Centers for Medicare & Medicaid Services, Department of Health and Human Services. (2014). Condition of participation: Nursing services. 42 C.F.R. § 482.23(c).

4 Centers for Disease Control and Prevention. (2002). Guideline for hand hygiene in health-care settings: Recommendations of the Healthcare Infection Control Practices Advisory Committee and the HICPAC/SHEA/APIC/IDSA Hand Hygiene Task Force. *MMWR Recommendations and Reports, 51*(RR-16), 1–45. Accessed May 2015 via the Web at http://www.cdc.gov/mmwr/pdf/rr/rr5116.pdf (Level II)

5 World Health Organization. (2009). "WHO guidelines on hand hygiene in health care: First global patient safety challenge, clean care is safer care" [Online]. Accessed May 2015 via the Web at http://whqlibdoc.who.int/publications/2009/9789241597906_eng.pdf (Level IV)

6 The Joint Commission. (2015). Standard NPSG.07.01.01. *Comprehensive accreditation manual for hospitals: The official handbook.* Oakbrook Terrace, IL: The Joint Commission. (Level VII)

7 American Osteopathic Association. (2014). Standard 07.01.21. *Healthcare Facilities Accreditation Program: Accreditation requirements for acute care hospitals.* Chicago, IL: American Osteopathic Association. (Level VII)

8 Centers for Medicare & Medicaid Services, Department of Health and Human Services. (2014). Condition of participation: Infection control. 42 C.F.R. § 482.42.

9 The Joint Commission. (2015). Standard NPSG.01.01.01. *Comprehensive accreditation manual for hospitals: The official handbook.* Oakbrook Terrace, IL: The Joint Commission. (Level VII)

10 American Osteopathic Association. (2014). Standard 15.01.16. *Healthcare Facilities Accreditation Program: Accreditation requirements for acute care hospitals.* Chicago, IL: American Osteopathic Association. (Level VII)

11 The Joint Commission. (2015). Standard RI.01.01.01. *Comprehensive accreditation manual for hospitals: The official handbook.* Oakbrook Terrace, IL: The Joint Commission. (Level VII)

12 Centers for Medicare & Medicaid Services, Department of Health and Human Services. (2014). Condition of participation: Patient's rights. 42 C.F.R. § 482.13(c)(1).

13 Siegel, J. D., et al. (2007). "2007 guideline for isolation precautions: Preventing transmission of infectious agents in healthcare settings" [Online]. Accessed May 2015 via the Web at http://www.cdc.gov/hicpac/pdf/isolation/Isolation2007.pdf (Level II)

14 American Osteopathic Association. (2014). Standard 07.01.10. *Healthcare Facilities Accreditation Program: Accreditation requirements for acute care hospitals.* Chicago, IL: American Osteopathic Association. (Level VII)

15 Rutala, W. A., et al. (2008). "Guideline for disinfection and sterilization in healthcare facilities, 2008" [Online]. Accessed May 2015 via the Web

at http://www.cdc.gov/hicpac/pdf/guidelines/Disinfection_Nov_2008.pdf (Level I)

16 American Osteopathic Association. (2014). Standard 07.02.03. *Healthcare Facilities Accreditation Program: Accreditation requirements for acute care hospitals.* Chicago, IL: American Osteopathic Association. (Level VII)

17 The Joint Commission. (2015). Standard RC.01.03.01. *Comprehensive accreditation manual for hospitals: The official handbook.* Oakbrook Terrace, IL: The Joint Commission. (Level VII)

18 Centers for Medicare & Medicaid Services, Department of Health and Human Services. (2014). Condition of participation: Medical record services. 42 C.F.R. § 482.24(b).

19 American Osteopathic Association. (2014). Standard 10.00.03. *Healthcare Facilities Accreditation Program: Accreditation requirements for acute care hospitals.* Chicago, IL: American Osteopathic Association. (Level VII)

20 Nicks, B. A., et al. (2010). Acute wound management: Revisiting the approach to assessment, irrigation, and closure considerations. *International Journal of Emergency Medicine, 3,* 399–407. Accessed May 2015 via the Web at http://www.ncbi.nlm.nih.gov/pmc/articles/PMC3047833/

ADDITIONAL REFERENCES

Baudoin, L. M., & Mayeaux, E. J. (2014). A guide to better wound closures. *Journal of Family Practice, 63,* 181–186. Accessed May 2015 via the Web at http://www.jfponline.com/fileadmin/qhi/jfp/pdfs/6304/JFP_06304_Article1.pdf

Craven, R. F., & Hirnle, C. J. (2012). *Fundamentals of nursing: Human health and function* (7th ed.). Philadelphia, PA: Lippincott Williams & Wilkins.

MacDonald, P., et al. (2012). Are patients willing to remove, and capable of removing, their own nonabsorbable sutures? *Canadian Journal of Emergency Medicine, 14,* 218–223. (Level III)

Taylor, C., et al. (2015). *Fundamentals of nursing: The art and science of nursing care* (8th ed.). Philadelphia, PA: Wolters Kluwer.

SWAB SPECIMEN COLLECTION

Correct collection and handling of swab specimens helps laboratory staff members identify pathogens accurately with a minimum of contamination from normal bacterial flora.

Collection methods vary depending on the type of specimen being collected. For instance, collection of throat, nasopharyngeal, external ear, and eye specimens usually involves sampling inflamed tissues and exudates, typically using sterile swabs of cotton or other absorbent material; wound exudate may also be aspirated into a syringe. Wound specimen collection normally involves sampling wound tissues and exudates expressed from the wound with sterile swabs of cotton or another absorbent material.

Collection of fluid from the middle ear is performed by a practitioner using a needle and syringe to withdraw fluid from the middle ear through the tympanic membrane; this method is referred to as *tympanocentesis.*

Inflammatory eye conditions can result from a number of diseases, and various organisms can cause eye infections. Aerobes, anaerobes, fungi, mycobacteria, viruses, parasites, and *Chlamydia trachomatis* can all be recovered using appropriate collection techniques.

Normal bacterial flora in stool includes several potentially pathogenic organisms. Bacteriologic examinations help identify pathogens that cause overt GI disease—such as typhoid and dysentery—and carrier states. A sensitivity test may follow isolation of the pathogen. Correctly identifying the causative organism is vital for treating the patient, helping to prevent possible fatal complications (especially in a debilitated patient), and preventing the spread of a severe infectious disease.

Equipment

Gloves[1] ▪ penlight[1] ▪ sterile swab (cotton wool or synthetic fiber)[1] ▪ sterile culture tube with transport medium or commercial collection kit ▪ specimen label ▪ laboratory request form ▪ laboratory biohazard transport bag ▪ Optional: mask and other personal protective equipment.[2]

Additional equipment for throat and nasopharyngeal specimen collection

Tongue blade.[1]

Additional equipment for wound specimen collection

Two pairs of sterile gloves ▪ sterile drape ▪ chlorhexidine swabs ▪ sterile normal saline solution ▪ sterile 10-mL syringe ▪ sterile 21G needle ▪ anaerobic culture tube.

Additional equipment for external and middle ear specimen collection

Normal saline solution ▪ 2″ × 2″ (5-cm × 5-cm) gauze pads ▪ wax hook ▪ otoscope ▪ ear speculum ▪ sterile 10-mL syringe and sterile 22G 1″ (2.5 cm) needle ▪ Optional: culture swabs.

Additional equipment for eye specimen collection

Sterile normal saline solution ▪ two sterile 2″ × 2″ (5-cm × 5-cm) gauze pads ▪ sterile wire culture loop (for corneal scraping).

Additional equipment for rectal specimen collection

Soap and water ▪ washcloth ▪ normal saline solution or sterile broth medium.

Implementation

- Verify the practitioner's order.
- Perform hand hygiene.[3,4,5,6,7]
- Confirm the patient's identity using at least two patient identifiers.[8]
- Explain the procedure to the patient *to ease his anxiety and ensure cooperation.*

Throat specimen collection

- Tell the patient that he may gag during the swabbing but that the procedure will probably take less than 1 minute.
- Instruct the patient to sit erect at the edge of the bed or in a chair, facing you.
- Put on gloves and other personal protective equipment, as needed.[1,2,9,10]
- Ask the patient to tilt back his head.
- Depress his tongue with the tongue blade, and illuminate his throat with the penlight *to check for inflamed areas.*[1]
- If the patient starts to gag, withdraw the tongue blade and tell him to breathe deeply. After he's relaxed, reinsert the tongue blade but not as deeply as before. Encourage the patient to close his eyes or stare at the ceiling *to promote cooperation.*
- Open and remove the swab, taking care not to touch the tip with your hands *because the swab is sterile.*[1] If you touch the swab, discard it and obtain a new swab.
- Using the swab, wipe the tonsillar areas from side to side, including inflamed or purulent sites. Make sure you don't touch the tongue, cheeks, saliva, or teeth with the swab *to avoid contaminating it with oral bacteria.*[1]
- Move the swab into the posterior pharynx and wipe the area using a gentle side-to-side sweeping motion.
- Withdraw the swab and immediately place it in the culture tube.[1] If you're using a commercial kit, crush the ampule of culture medium at the bottom of the tube, and then push the swab into the medium *to keep the swab moist.*

Nasopharyngeal specimen collection

- Tell the patient that he may gag or feel the urge to sneeze during the swabbing but that the procedure takes less than 1 minute.
- Have the patient sit erect at the edge of the bed or in a chair, facing you.

■ Put on gloves, a mask, and other personal protective equipment as necessary.[1,9,10]
■ Ask the patient to blow his nose *to clear his nasal passages.* Then check his nostrils *for patency* with a penlight.
■ Determine the more patent nostril by having the patient exhale and occlude one nostril first and then the other.
■ While it's still in the package, bend the sterile swab in a curve; then open the package without contaminating the swab.
■ Ask the patient to cough *to bring organisms to the nasopharynx for a better specimen.*
■ Ask the patient to tilt his head back.
■ Gently pass the swab through the more patent nostril about 3″ to 4″ (7.5 to 10 cm) into the nasopharynx, keeping the swab near the septum and floor of the nose. Rotate the swab quickly and remove it. (See *Obtaining a nasopharyngeal specimen.*)
■ Alternatively, depress the patient's tongue with a tongue blade, and pass the bent swab up behind the uvula. Rotate the swab and withdraw it.
■ Remove the cap from the culture tube, insert the swab, and break off the contaminated end.
■ Close the tube tightly.

Obtaining a nasopharyngeal specimen

When the swab passes into the nasopharynx, gently but quickly rotate it *to collect a specimen.* Then remove the swab, taking care not to injure the nasal mucous membrane.

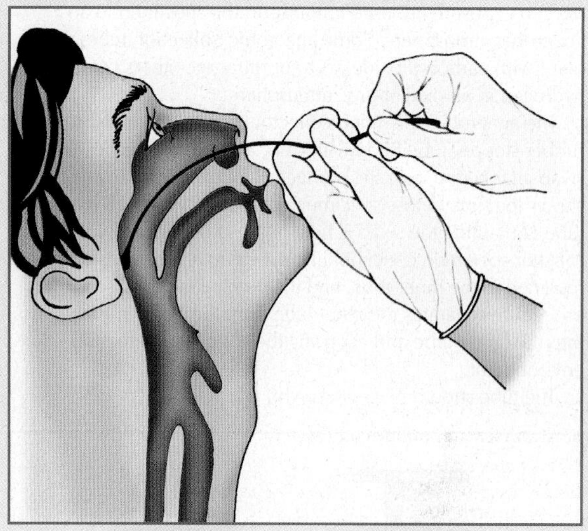

Wound specimen collection
■ Carefully remove the dressing to expose the wound. Dispose of the soiled dressings properly.[9]
■ Remove and discard your gloves and perform hand hygiene.[3,4,5,6,7]
■ Prepare a sterile field and put on sterile gloves.
■ Clean the wound with sterile normal saline solution to remove old drainage *to prevent specimen contamination.*[11]
■ Clean the area around the wound with a chlorhexidine swab *to reduce the risk of contaminating the specimen with skin bacteria.* Then allow the area to dry.[12]
■ For an aerobic culture of a deep wound, identify a 1-cm^2 area of clean wound tissue.[13] Moisten the swab with sterile normal saline solution.[13] Using the swab, apply light pressure to the identified area; then rotate the swab *to try to produce exudate.*[13] Remove the swab from the wound and immediately place it in an aerobic culture tube.[13]
■ For an anaerobic culture of a deep wound, identify a 1-cm^2 area of clean wound tissue. Moisten the swab with sterile normal saline solution.[13] Using the swab, apply light pressure to the identified area; then rotate the swab *to try to produce exudate.*[13] Remove the swab from the wound.[13] Immediately place the swab in an anaerobic culture tube and press the plunger with continuous gentle force *to create an anaerobic environment inside the culture tube.*[13] (See *Understanding anaerobic specimen collection,* page 736.)
NURSING ALERT *Make sure the quality of the specimen you obtain is adequate for a culture and Gram stain. Note that the culture must come from the cleanest tissue possible—not pus, slough, eschar, or necrotic material. Never collect exudate from the skin.*[14]

External ear specimen collection
■ Gently clean excess debris from the patient's ear with normal saline solution and gauze pads.
■ Insert the sterile swab into the ear canal, and rotate it gently along the walls of the canal *to avoid damaging the eardrum.*
■ Withdraw the swab, being careful not to touch other surfaces *to avoid contaminating the specimen.*
■ Place the swab in the sterile culture tube with transport medium.

Middle ear specimen collection
■ Clean the patient's outer ear with normal saline solution and gauze pads.
■ Assist with wax removal as indicated.
■ The practitioner visualizes and punctures the eardrum with a needle and aspirates fluid into the syringe. He may also collect a specimen using a sterile culture swab.[15]
■ The practitioner places the fluid in the sterile specimen container.

Eye specimen collection
■ Gently clean excess debris from the outside of the patient's eye with sterile normal saline solution and sterile gauze pads, wiping from the inner to the outer canthus.
■ Retract the lower eyelid *to expose the conjunctival sac.* Gently rub the sterile swab over the conjunctiva, being careful not to touch other surfaces. Move from the inner canthus to the outer canthus. Hold the swab parallel to the eye, rather than pointed directly at it *to prevent corneal irritation or trauma due to sudden movement.* (If a corneal scraping is required, this procedure is performed by a practitioner, using a wire culture loop.)
■ Immediately place the swab or wire loop in the culture tube with transport medium.

Rectal swab specimen collection
■ Clean the area around the patient's anus using a washcloth and soap and water *to minimize contamination of the specimen.*
■ Insert the swab, moistened with normal saline solution or sterile broth medium, through the anus and advance it about 1½″ (4 cm). While withdrawing the swab, gently rotate it against the walls of the lower rectum *to sample a large area of the rectal mucosa.*
■ Place the swab in a culture tube with transport medium.

Completing the procedure
■ Remove and discard your gloves, and perform hand hygiene.[3,4,5,6,7]
■ Label the specimen in the presence of the patient *to prevent mislabeling.*[1,8]
■ On the laboratory request form, indicate whether any organism is strongly suspected, especially *Corynebacterium diphtheriae* (requires two swabs and special growth medium) and *Neisseria meningitidis* (requires enriched selective media).

Understanding anaerobic specimen collection tubes

Some anaerobes die when exposed to toxic amounts of oxygen. *To facilitate anaerobic collection and culturing,* tubes that limit oxygen exposure are used to transport the specimen in an anaerobic atmosphere. Some anaerobic collection tubes are filled with carbon dioxide (CO_2) or nitrogen; others contain hydrogen in an oxygen-free atmosphere.

The anaerobic specimen collector shown here consists of a rubber-stopper tube filled with CO_2, a small inner tube, and a swab attached to a plastic plunger. The drawing below (left) shows the tube before specimen collection. The small inner tube containing the swab is held in place by the rubber stopper.

After specimen collection (below right), the swab is quickly replaced in the inner tube, and the plunger is depressed. This procedure separates the inner tube from the stopper, forcing it into the larger tube and exposing the specimen to the CO_2-rich environment.

The tube should be kept upright.

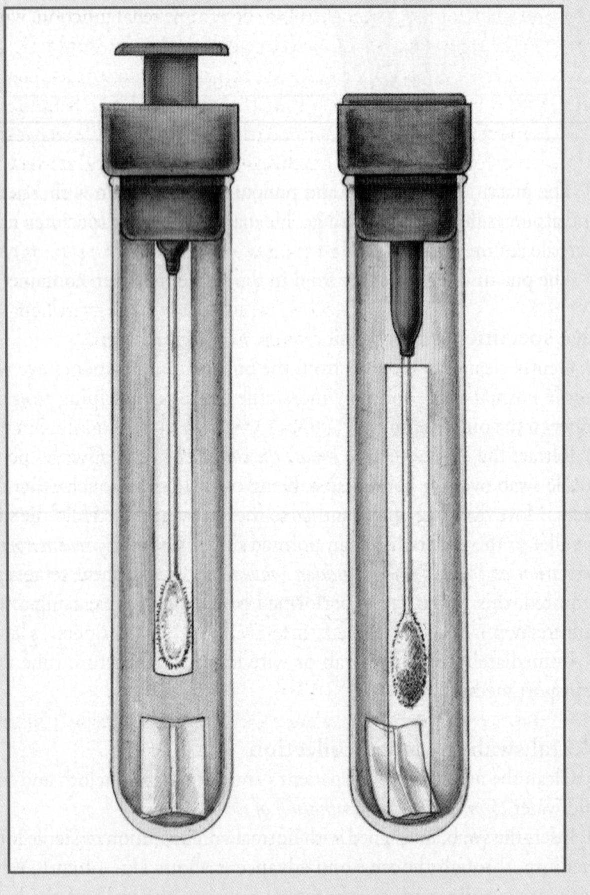

- Place the specimen in a laboratory biohazard transport bag and send it to the laboratory immediately *to prevent growth or deterioration of microbes.*[9]
- Remove and discard your gloves and perform hand hygiene.[3,4,5,6,7]
- Document the procedure.[16,17,18]

Special considerations

- Note recent antibiotic therapy on the laboratory request form.
- If possible, obtain a specimen before starting antimicrobial therapy.
- Check with the laboratory for special instructions for viral studies.
- *To maximize sensitivity for a large number of viruses,* collection of combined nasopharyngeal and oropharyngeal specimens is the most effective approach.[19]
- *Because throat swabs and anterior nasal swabs have unacceptably low rates of deoxyribonucleic acid recovery,* don't use them for pertussis diagnosis.[20]
- Instruct the patient to avoid antiseptic mouthwash before the procedure.
- *To avoid stimulating the gag reflex during the procedure and possibly causing the patient to vomit,* it's advisable to wait 1 hour after a meal before conducting the procedure.
- Notify the practitioner if the patient shows signs or symptoms of a systemic infection or has difficulty breathing because of swelling of the tongue or throat.
- For infants and young children, use specially designed midturbinate nasal flocked swabs that have a collar that prevents them from being inserted too deeply.[21]
- Although you would normally clean the area around a wound to prevent contamination by normal skin flora, don't clean a perineal wound with alcohol or chlorhexidine *because it could irritate sensitive tissues.* Also, make sure that antiseptic doesn't enter the wound. The Levine technique for wound specimen collection has greater accuracy and specificity in diagnosing an infection than tissue biopsy and culture.[13]
- When collecting an eye specimen, don't use an antiseptic before culturing *to avoid irritating the eye and inhibiting growth of organisms in the culture.* If the patient is a child or an uncooperative adult, ask a coworker to restrain the patient's head *to prevent eye trauma resulting from sudden movement.*
- Collect each eye specimen separately *to avoid cross-contamination.*
- Don't refrigerate eye specimens.
- If a specimen is needed for anal-rectal cancer screening, you may need to advance the swab 2″ to 2½″ (5 cm to 6 cm).[22]

Patient teaching

- Instruct the patient about the importance of respiratory hygiene, cough etiquette, hand hygiene, and other infection-control measures used to control the spread of respiratory infections.[16]

Complications

Laryngospasm may occur after the culture is obtained if the patient has epiglottiditis or diphtheria. Keep resuscitation equipment nearby.

Documentation

Record the time, date, and site of specimen collection and recent or current antibiotic therapy. Also note whether the specimen has an unusual appearance or odor. Document the patient's tolerance of the procedure. Document any patient teaching and the patient's understanding of that teaching.

REFERENCES

1 Kotloff, K., & Van Beneden, C. (2008). "Standardization of epidemiologic protocols for surveillance of acute diseases caused by *Streptococcus pyogenes*: Pharyngitis, impetigo, and invasive diseases" [Online]. Accessed May 2015 via the Web at http://www.niaid.nih.gov/topics/strepThroat/Documents/acutegroupastrep.pdf

2 World Health Organization. (2006). "Collecting, preserving and shipping specimens for the diagnosis of avian influenza A (H5N1) virus infection: Guide for field operations" [Online]. Accessed May 2015 via the Web at http://www.who.int/csr/resources/publications/surveillance/WHO_CDS_EPR_ARO_2006_1.pdf (Level VII)

3 Centers for Disease Control and Prevention. (2002). Guideline for hand hygiene in health care settings: Recommendations of the Healthcare Infection Control Practices Advisory Committee and the HICPAC/SHEA/APIC/IDSA Hand Hygiene Task Force. *MMWR Recommendations*

and Reports, 51(RR-16), 1–45. Accessed May 2015 via the Web at http://www.cdc.gov/mmwr/pdf/rr/rr5116.pdf (Level II)

4 The Joint Commission. (2015). Standard NPSG.07.01.01. *Comprehensive accreditation manual for hospitals: The official handbook.* Oakbrook Terrace, IL: The Joint Commission. (Level VII)

5 World Health Organization. (2009). "WHO guidelines on hand hygiene in health care: First global patient safety challenge, clean care is safer care" [Online]. Accessed May 2015 via the Web at http://whqlibdoc.who.int/publications/2009/9789241597906_eng.pdf (Level IV)

6 American Osteopathic Association. (2014). Standard 07.01.21. *Healthcare Facilities Accreditation Program: Accreditation requirements for acute care hospitals.* Chicago, IL: American Osteopathic Association. (Level VII)

7 Centers for Medicare & Medicaid Services, Department of Health and Human Services. (2014). Condition of participation: Infection control. 42 C.F.R. § 482.42.

8 The Joint Commission. (2015). Standard NPSG.01.01.01. *Comprehensive accreditation manual for hospitals: The official handbook.* Oakbrook Terrace, IL: The Joint Commission. (Level VII)

9 Occupational Safety and Health Administration. (n.d.). "Bloodborne pathogens, standard number 1910.1030" [Online]. Accessed May 2015 via the Web at http://www.osha.gov/pls/oshaweb/owadisp.show_document?p_table=STANDARDS&p_id=10051 (Level VII)

10 American Osteopathic Association. (2014). Standard 07.01.10. *Healthcare Facilities Accreditation Program: Accreditation requirements for acute care hospitals.* Chicago, IL: American Osteopathic Association. (Level VII)

11 Craven, R. F., & Hirnle, C. J. (2012). *Fundamentals of nursing: Human health and function* (7th ed.). Philadelphia, PA: Lippincott Williams & Wilkins.

12 Carrico, R., et al. (Eds.). (2009). *APIC text of infection control and epidemiology* (3rd ed.). Washington, DC: Association for Professionals in Infection Control and Epidemiology.

13 Bryant, R. A., & Nix, D. P. (2012). *Acute & chronic wounds: Current management concepts* (4th ed.). St Louis, MO: Mosby.

14 Centers for Disease Control and Prevention. (2010, updated 2012). "Get smart for healthcare: Clinician guide" [Online]. Accessed May 2015 via the Web at http://www.cdc.gov/getsmart/healthcare/learn-from-others/resources/clinician-guide.html

15 Adoga, A. S., et al. (2010). Swab and aspiration specimen collection methods and antibiogram in chronic suppurative otitis media at Jos University Teaching Hospital: Which is superior? *Annals of African Medicine, 9,* 230–234. Accessed May 2015 via the Web at http://www.ajol.info/index.php/aam/article/viewFile/67171/55274

16 The Joint Commission. (2015). Standard RC.01.03.01. *Comprehensive accreditation manual for hospitals: The official handbook.* Oakbrook Terrace, IL: The Joint Commission. (Level VII)

17 American Osteopathic Association. (2012). Standard 10.00.03. *Healthcare Facilities Accreditation Program: Accreditation requirements for acute care hospitals.* Chicago, IL: American Osteopathic Association. (Level VII)

18 Centers for Medicare & Medicaid Services, Department of Health and Human Services. (2014). Condition of participation: Medical record services. 42 C.F.R. § 482.24(b).

19 Kim, C., et al. (2011). Comparison of nasopharyngeal and oropharyngeal swabs for the diagnosis of eight respiratory viruses by real-time reverse transcription-PCR assays. *PLoS ONE, 6*(6), e21610. Accessed May 2015 via the Web at http://www.plosone.org/article/info%3Adoi%2F10.1371%2Fjournal.pone.0021610

20 Centers for Disease Control and Prevention. (2012). "Best practices for health care professionals on the use of polymerase chain reaction (PCR) for diagnosing pertussis" [Online]. Accessed May 2015 via the Web at http://www.cdc.gov/pertussis/clinical/downloads/diagnosis-pcr-best-practices.pdf

21 Siegel, J. D., et al. (2007). "2007 guideline for isolation precautions: Preventing transmission of infectious agents in healthcare settings" [Online]. Accessed May 2015 via the Web at http://www.cdc.gov/hicpac/pdf/isolation/Isolation2007.pdf (Level II)

22 Bean, S. M., & Chhieng, D. C. (2010). Anal-rectal cytology: The other Pap test. *LabMedicine, 41,* 168–171. Accessed May 2015 via the Web at http://labmed.ascpjournals.org/content/41/3/168.full.pdf+html

SYNCHRONIZED CARDIOVERSION

Synchronized cardioversion delivers an electrical charge to the myocardium that's timed with the QRS complex. This charge causes immediate depolarization, interrupting reentry circuits and allowing the sinoatrial node to resume control. Synchronizing the electrical charge with the QRS complex prevents delivery during the relative refractory period of the cardiac cycle, when a shock would lead to ventricular fibrillation.[1]

Synchronized cardioversion is the treatment of choice for arrhythmias, such as unstable supraventricular tachycardia resulting from reentry, unstable atrial flutter, unstable atrial fibrillation, and unstable monomorphic ventricular tachycardia with a pulse that doesn't respond to vagal maneuvers (the Valsalva maneuver or carotid sinus massage) or drug therapy.[1] The procedure can be elective or urgent depending on the patient tolerance of the arrhythmia.[1] For example, if the patient is hemodynamically unstable (altered mental status, shock or hypotension, and chest pain), immediate cardioversion is necessary.[2]

Synchronized cardioversion should be performed according to the 2010 American Heart Association guidelines and should follow an assessment of the patient's cardiac and metabolic status.[1] Assessment should include electrolyte levels, particularly potassium levels, which should be in the normal range; creatinine levels to determine renal function, which helps guide the dosage of adjunctive medications; and serum digoxin levels, which should be in the nontoxic range. If the patient has chronic lung disease, arterial blood gas (ABG) analysis may also be helpful.

Contraindications to synchronized cardioversion include tachycardia related to digoxin toxicity, sinus tachycardia, and multifocal atrial tachycardia. Atrial fibrillation increases the patient's risk for stroke, thus cardioversion is contraindicated in patients with atrial fibrillation who aren't receiving anticoagulation unless transesophageal imaging is performed to rule out thrombus formation.[3,4] Anticoagulation therapy is recommended for 3 weeks before elective cardioversion to convert hemodynamically stable atrial fibrillation to normal sinus rhythm.[5]

Equipment

Cardioverter-defibrillator ▪ self-adhesive cardioversion-defibrillation pads or anterior, posterior, or transverse paddles and conductive gel pads ▪ cardiac monitor with recording system ▪ 12-lead electrocardiogram (ECG) machine ▪ oxygen administration equipment ▪ artificial airway ▪ handheld resuscitation bag ▪ emergency pacing equipment ▪ emergency cardiac medications ▪ stethoscope ▪ automatic blood pressure device ▪ pulse oximeter ▪ disinfectant pad ▪ hospital-grade disinfectant ▪ Optional: sedative or analgesia, IV catheter insertion equipment, clippers, gloves.

Preparation of equipment

Have emergency equipment available at the patient's bedside, and make sure that it's functioning properly.

Implementation

- Verify the practitioner's orders. Check to see whether cardiac medications have been prescribed for administration before the procedure.
- Check the patient's medical record for recent serum potassium and magnesium levels and ABG results. Also check the most recent digoxin level if ordered. *Electrolyte imbalances, acid-base disturbances, and digoxin toxicity increase the risk of arrhythmias.*[5] Notify the practitioner of critical test results within your facility's established time frame *so that the patient can be treated promptly.*[6]
- Confirm that written informed consent is obtained and that the consent is in the patient's medical record.[5,7,8,9]
- Gather the appropriate equipment.
- Conduct a preprocedure verification *to make sure that all relevant documentation, related information, and equipment are available and correctly identified to the patient's identifiers.*[10]

■ Perform hand hygiene.[11,12,13,14,15]
■ Put on gloves if needed *to comply with standard precautions.*[16,17]
■ Confirm the patient's identity using at least two patient identifiers.[18]
■ Provide privacy and explain the procedure to the patient and his family *to allay their fears and anxiety.*[19,20]
■ If the patient's condition allows, have him maintain nothing-by-mouth status before the procedure; minimum fasting recommendations are 2 hours for clear liquids, 6 hours or more for a light meal, and 8 hours or more for fried or fatty foods or meat.[21]
■ Make sure that the patient is attached to a cardiac monitor, pulse oximeter, and automatic blood pressure device. Make sure that the alarm limits are set appropriately for the patient's current condition and that the alarms are turned on, functioning properly, and audible to staff.[22,23,24,25]
■ Obtain the patient's vital signs and oxygen saturation level, and assess his neurologic, cardiovascular, and respiratory status to *determine whether immediate cardioversion is necessary.*[2,5]
■ If the patient's oxygenation is inadequate or he shows signs of labored breathing, notify the practitioner and administer supplemental oxygen, as prescribed.[2]
■ Make sure that the patient has patent IV access; if he doesn't, insert an IV catheter. (See the "IV catheter insertion and removal" procedure, page 446.)
■ Obtain a 12-lead ECG *to better define the patient's heart rhythm and to serve as a baseline for comparison.* If the patient is unstable, don't delay immediate cardioversion to obtain the ECG.[2,5]
■ Administer cardiac medications, if prescribed, following safe medication administration practices.[26,27]
■ Remove all metal objects from the patient *because metal conducts electricity and could cause burns during cardioversion.*[5]
■ If the patient has dentures, a partial plate, or another oral prosthesis, determine whether the device supports airway patency or has the potential to obstruct it. Remove the device if it increases the risk of airway obstruction.[5]
■ Make sure that the patient is in a dry environment and that his chest is dry *because if the rescuer or patient comes in contact with water, a conductor of electricity, the rescuer can receive a shock or the patient can receive a skin burn.*[5]
■ Place the patient in the supine position *to provide access to the patient's chest during the procedure.*[5]
■ If necessary, clip hair from the patient's chest *to make sure that the electrodes adhere properly.*[5]
■ Remove transdermal medication patches from the patient's chest, if present, or make sure that the cardioversion-defibrillation pads or paddles don't touch the patches during the procedure *to prevent a chest burn during cardioversion.*[5]
■ If the patient isn't already receiving supplemental oxygen, consider preoxygenating him before cardioversion *to promote myocardial oxygenation and to reduce the risk of cerebral and cardiac complications.*[5]
■ A specially trained health care provider will administer moderate sedation or anesthesia if time allows and the patient's condition permits.
■ Monitor the patient's heart rate, blood pressure, and respiratory rate *to promptly detect changes in the patient's condition and prevent treatment delays.*
■ Conduct a time-out before starting the procedure, if time allows, *to perform a final assessment that the correct patient and procedure are identified and that all relevant information and necessary equipment are available.*[28]
■ Turn on the cardioverter-defibrillator.[5]
■ Attach the patient to the monitoring leadwires on the cardioverter-defibrillator *because the device must be able to sense the R wave to provide synchronized cardioversion.*[5]
■ Apply the self-adhesive cardioversion-defibrillation pads according to the manufacturer's directions; for anterolateral placement, place one pad at the heart's apex just left of the nipple at the midaxillary line and the other pad just below the right clavicle to the right of the sternum. Alternatively, remove the paddles from the machine and place the paddles and the conductive gel pads using anterolateral placement.[1,5] Depending on the patient, you can use alternative pad positions, such as the anteroposterior, anterior-left infrascapular, and anterior-right infrascapular.[1] Don't place the self-adhesive cardioversion-defibrillation pads or paddles over a female patient's breast *because doing so decreases transthoracic resistance.*[5]
■ Turn on the ECG recording device to obtain a continuous printout *to document the patient's response to cardioversion.*[5]
■ Push the SYNC button *to synchronize the machine with the patient's QRS complex.* Assess the cardioverter-defibrillator waveform and make sure that the SYNC button flashes with each of the patient's QRS complexes; listen for audible beeps. *Synchronization with the patient's QRS complex prevents the random discharge of electrical charges, which may cause ventricular fibrillation.*[5]
■ Set the energy level to the prescribed dose. Advanced cardiac life support protocols call for an initial shock of 50 to 100 joules for a patient with unstable supraventricular tachycardia, 120 to 200 joules for a patient with atrial fibrillation, 50 to 100 joules for a patient with atrial flutter, and 100 joules for a patient with monomorphic ventricular tachycardia with a pulse.[1]
■ Charge the cardioverter-defibrillator.
■ Disconnect the oxygen source before cardioversion *to decrease the risk of combustion in the presence of electrical current.*[5]
■ Confirm that all personnel are clear of the patient and his bed. If you're using cardioversion-defibrillation pads, push the discharge button. If you're using paddles, apply firm pressure (approximately 25 to 30 lb [11.3 to 13.6 kg])[29] to each paddle against the patient's chest wall, push the discharge button, and wait for the energy to be discharged. Keep in mind that the machine has to synchronize the discharge with the QRS complex.

NURSING ALERT ***Don't touch the bed, the patient, or any equipment attached to the patient while cardioversion is being administered* to prevent transfer of the electrical current to health care workers.**

■ Assess the patient's cardiac rhythm on the monitor.
■ If the arrhythmia fails to convert after the initial shock, repeat the procedure, increasing the energy dose in a stepwise fashion[1] or as instructed by the practitioner. Check that the synchronization mode is active after each cardioversion attempt *because many defibrillators automatically default to the unsynchronized mode.*
■ When the patient's rhythm converts, monitor his vital signs, oxygen saturation level, and cardiovascular, neurologic, and respiratory status *to evaluate his response to the procedure.*[5] Reconnect the patient to the oxygen source as appropriate.
■ Turn off the continuous ECG recording device.
■ Obtain a follow-up 12-lead ECG, as ordered.
■ Inspect the patient's chest for electrical burns; treat burns as needed and prescribed.[5]
■ Perform a comprehensive pain assessment using techniques appropriate for the patient's age, condition, and ability to understand.[30] Administer analgesia as ordered and indicated using safe medication administration practices.[26,27]
■ Discard used supplies in appropriate receptacles.[16]
■ Remove and discard your gloves if worn.[16]
■ Perform hand hygiene.[11,12,13,14,15]
■ Document the procedure.[33,34,35]

Special considerations

■ Be aware that synchronized cardioversion must sense the R wave to deliver the current outside of the heart's vulnerable period. Make sure that the synchronization markers are clearly visible on the monitor and that their location is consistent from beat to beat. If necessary, adjust the lead or size settings *to yield the best display.*[36]

■ If the patient has a permanent pacemaker or an implantable cardioverter-defibrillator, don't place the pads or paddles over the device *because doing so can impair current flow to the patient's heart and damage the device.*[5]

■ The Joint Commission has issued a sentinel event alert concerning medical device alarm safety *because alarm-related events have been associated with permanent loss of function or death.* Among the contributing factors are improper alarm settings, alarms inappropriately turned off, and alarm signals not audible to staff. Make sure that alarm limits are set appropriately and that alarms are turned on, functioning properly, and audible to staff. Follow facility guidelines for preventing alarm fatigue.[22]

Complications

Common complications following synchronized cardioversion are skin burns, pulmonary edema, hypotension, embolism, and transient, harmless arrhythmias, such as atrial, ventricular, and junctional premature beats. Serious ventricular arrhythmias such as ventricular fibrillation can also occur; however, this type of arrhythmia is more likely to result from high amounts of electrical energy, digoxin toxicity, severe heart disease, electrolyte imbalance, or improper synchronization with the R wave.

Documentation

Document the procedure, including the voltage delivered with each attempt, rhythm strips before and after the procedure, medications administered, and the patient's tolerance of the procedure. Note any emergency interventions required and the patient's response to these interventions. Record the patient's vital signs and your assessment findings. Document any patient teaching and the patient's understanding of your teaching.

REFERENCES

1 American Heart Association. (2010). 2010 American Heart Association guidelines for cardiopulmonary resuscitation and emergency cardiovascular care. *Circulation, 122,* S706–S719. (Level II)

2 American Heart Association. (2010). 2010 American Heart Association guidelines for cardiopulmonary resuscitation and emergency cardiovascular care. *Circulation, 122,* S729–S776. (Level II)

3 Beinart, S. C. (2013). "Synchronized electrical cardioversion" [Online]. Accessed May 2015 via the Web at http://emedicine.medscape.com/article/1834044-overview#a05

4 Marchiondo, K. (2007). Transesophageal imaging and interventions: Nursing implications. *Critical Care Nurse, 27*(2), 25–36. (Level V)

5 Lynn-McHale Wiegand, D. (Ed.). (2011). *AACN procedure manual for critical care* (6th ed.). St. Louis, MO: Saunders.

6 The Joint Commission. (2015). Standard NPSG.02.03.01. *Comprehensive accreditation manual for hospitals: The official handbook.* Oakbrook Terrace, IL: The Joint Commission. (Level VII)

7 The Joint Commission. (2015). Standard RI.01.03.01. *Comprehensive accreditation manual for hospitals: The official handbook.* Oakbrook Terrace, IL: The Joint Commission. (Level VII)

8 Centers for Medicare & Medicaid Services, Department of Health and Human Services. (2014). Condition of participation: Patient's rights. 42 C.F.R. § 482.13(b)(2).

9 American Osteopathic Association. (2014). Standard 30.01.11. *Healthcare Facilities Accreditation Program: Accreditation requirements for acute care hospitals.* Chicago, IL: American Osteopathic Association. (Level VII)

10 The Joint Commission. (2015). Standard UP.01.01.01. *Comprehensive accreditation manual for hospitals: The official handbook.* Oakbrook Terrace, IL: The Joint Commission. (Level VII)

11 The Joint Commission. (2015). Standard NPSG.07.01.01. *Comprehensive accreditation manual for hospitals: The official handbook.* Oakbrook Terrace, IL: The Joint Commission. (Level VII)

12 Centers for Disease Control and Prevention. (2002). Guideline for hand hygiene in health-care settings: Recommendations of the Healthcare Infection Control Practices Advisory Committee and the HICPAC/SHEA/APIC/IDSA Hand Hygiene Task Force. *MMWR Recommendations and Reports, 51*(RR-16), 1–45. Accessed May 2015 via the Web at http://www.cdc.gov/mmwr/pdf/rr/rr5116.pdf (Level II)

13 World Health Organization. (2009). "WHO guidelines on hand hygiene in health care: First global patient safety challenge, clean care is safer care" [Online]. Accessed May 2015 via the Web at http://whqlibdoc.who.int/publications/2009/9789241597906_eng.pdf (Level IV)

14 Centers for Medicare & Medicaid Services, Department of Health and Human Services. (2014). Condition of participation: Infection control. 42 C.F.R. § 482.42.

15 American Osteopathic Association. (2014). Standard 07.01.21. *Healthcare Facilities Accreditation Program: Accreditation requirements for acute care hospitals.* Chicago, IL: American Osteopathic Association. (Level VII)

16 Siegel, J. D., et al. (2007). "2007 guideline for isolation precautions: Preventing transmission of infectious agents in healthcare settings" [Online]. Accessed May 2015 via the Web at http://www.cdc.gov/hicpac/pdf/isolation/Isolation2007.pdf (Level II)

17 American Osteopathic Association. (2014). Standard 07.01.10. *Healthcare Facilities Accreditation Program: Accreditation requirements for acute care hospitals.* Chicago, IL: American Osteopathic Association. (Level VII)

18 The Joint Commission. (2015). Standard NPSG.01.01.01. *Comprehensive accreditation manual for hospitals: The official handbook.* Oakbrook Terrace, IL: The Joint Commission. (Level VII)

19 Centers for Medicare & Medicaid Services, Department of Health and Human Services. (2013). Condition of participation: Patient's rights. 42 C.F.R. § 482.13(c)(1).

20 American Osteopathic Association. (2014). Standard 15.01.16. *Healthcare Facilities Accreditation Program: Accreditation requirements for acute care hospitals.* Chicago, IL: American Osteopathic Association. (Level VII)

21 American Society of Anesthesiologists. (2011). Practice guidelines for preoperative fasting and the use of pharmacologic agents to reduce the risk of pulmonary aspiration: Application to healthy patients undergoing elective procedures. *Anesthesiology, 114,* 495–511. (Level VII)

22 The Joint Commission. (2013). "Sentinel event alert: Medical device alarm safety in hospitals" [Online]. Accessed May 2015 via the Web at http://www.jointcommission.org/assets/1/18/SEA_50_alarms_4_5_13_FINAL1.PDF (Level VII)

23 The Joint Commission. (2015). Standard NPSG.06.01.01. *Comprehensive accreditation manual for hospitals: The official handbook.* Oakbrook Terrace, IL: The Joint Commission. (Level VII)

24 Graham, K. C. & Cvach, M. (2010). Monitor alarm fatigue: Standardizing use of physiological monitors and decreasing nuisance alarms. *American Journal of Critical Care, 19,* 28–37.

25 American Association of Critical-Care Nurses. (2013). "AACN practice alert: Alarm management" [Online]. Accessed May 2015 via the Web at http://www.aacn.org/wd/practice/docs/practicealerts/alarm-management-practice-alert.pdf (Level VII)

26 Centers for Medicare & Medicaid Services, Department of Health and Human Services. (2014). Condition of participation: Preparation and administration of drugs. 42 C.F.R. § 482.23(c).

27 American Osteopathic Association. (2014). Standard 16.01.03. *Healthcare Facilities Accreditation Program: Accreditation requirements for acute care hospitals.* Chicago, IL: American Osteopathic Association. (Level VII)

28 The Joint Commission. (2015). Standard UP.01.03.01. *Comprehensive accreditation manual for hospitals: The official handbook.* Oakbrook Terrace, IL: The Joint Commission. (Level VII)

29 McKean, S. C., et al. (Eds.). (2012). *Principles and practice of hospital medicine.* New York, NY: McGraw Hill.

30 The Joint Commission. (2015). Standard PC.01.02.07. *Comprehensive accreditation manual for hospitals: The official handbook.* Oakbrook Terrace, IL: The Joint Commission. (Level VII)

31 Rutala, W. A., et al. (2008). "Guideline for disinfection and sterilization in healthcare facilities, 2008" [Online]. Accessed May 2015 via the Web at http://www.cdc.gov/hicpac/pdf/guidelines/Disinfection_Nov_2008.pdf (Level I)

32 American Osteopathic Association. (2014). Standard 07.02.3. *Healthcare Facilities Accreditation Program: Accreditation requirements for acute care hospitals.* Chicago, IL: American Osteopathic Association. (Level VII)

33 The Joint Commission. (2015). Standard RC.01.03.01. *Comprehensive accreditation manual for hospitals: The official handbook.* Oakbrook Terrace, IL: The Joint Commission. (Level VII)
34 Centers for Medicare & Medicaid Services, Department of Health and Human Services. (2014). Condition of participation: Medical record services. 42 C.F.R. § 482.24(b).
35 American Osteopathic Association. (2014). Standard 10.00.03. *Healthcare Facilities Accreditation Program: Accreditation requirements for acute care hospitals.* Chicago, IL: American Osteopathic Association. (Level VII)
36 ZOLL Medical Corporation. (2010). "Zoll M series operator's guide" [Online]. Accessed May 2015 via the Web at http://www.zoll.us/download/zoll_m_series_operators_guide.pdf

ADDITIONAL REFERENCES

Chen, W. S., et al. (2013). Comparison of pharmacological and electrical cardioversion in permanent atrial fibrillation after prosthetic cardiac valve replacement: A prospective randomized trial. *Journal of International Medical Research, 41,* 1067–1073. (Level II)

Nettina, S. M. (2014). *Lippincott manual of nursing practice* (10th ed.). Philadelphia, PA: Wolters Kluwer.

T

TEMPERATURE ASSESSMENT

Normal body temperature ranges vary by site, with higher temperatures at the core of the body and lower temperatures at the periphery.[1] Core body temperature can only be measured invasively, commonly with a pulmonary artery catheter; however, even though it's considered the gold standard, pulmonary artery temperature can only be monitored in specialized clinical settings. An esophageal probe or an indwelling urinary catheter with a temperature probe can also be used to measure temperature invasively.[2]

The American College of Critical Care and the Infectious Diseases Society of America recommend using the most accurate and reliable method to measure temperature, taking into consideration the clinical circumstances of the patient. They state that temperature is most accurately measured using invasive measures, followed by rectal, oral, and temporal membrane measurement. Axillary temperature measurement, temporal artery estimates, and chemical dot thermometers shouldn't be used on the intensive care unit, and rectal temperature measurements should be avoided in neutropenic patients.[2,3]

Normal body temperature is commonly thought of as 98.6°F (37°C). In healthy patients, this temperature may vary by about 0.3° to 0.6°F (0.5° to 1°C), according to the patient's circadian rhythm and menstrual cycle. Mean temperature is lower in older adults. With strenuous exercise, temperature can rise about 1° to 1.5°F (2°C to 3°C).

Not only biological process, but also environmental factors can alter body temperature, including hot lights, specialized mattresses, air conditioning, dialysis, cardiopulmonary bypass, peritoneal lavage, and continuous hemofiltration. Medications or damage to the central or autonomic nervous system can also alter a patient's ability to regulate temperature. With so many factors potentially influencing temperature, it may be difficult to determine whether a change results from a physiologic process, a medication, or an environmental influence.[1,2]

This procedure covers noninvasive methods for measuring temperature, such as rectal, oral, and temporal membrane measurement. When selecting the best temperature measuring system for the patient, choose one that provides reliable, reproducible values safely and conveniently. For example, oral temperature measurement is safe, convenient, and familiar for alert and cooperative patients.[2]

Because temperature can vary greatly among methods and sites, use the same method and site consistently throughout an episode of care, if possible, and document it in the patient's medical record.[4,5] If a patient develops a new fever, note trends in the patient's temperature data and evaluate other vital signs; don't make clinical decisions based on a single temperature reading.[2,5]

Equipment

Electronic thermometer (standard or tympanic) ■ disposable thermometer sheath or probe cover ■ disinfectant pad ■ Optional: gloves, water-soluble lubricant, wipe, facial tissue, washcloth, toilet paper.

Preparation of equipment

Make sure that any device used to measure temperature is maintained and calibrated appropriately. Follow the manufacturer's instructions for use and cover the thermometer probe with a cover or sheath, as needed.

Implementation

- Perform hand hygiene.[6,7,8,9,10]
- Confirm the patient's identity using at least two patient identifiers.[11]
- Explain the procedure to the patient.

Assessing rectal temperature

- Provide privacy.[12,13]
- Put on gloves.[14,15]
- Assist the patient to a side-lying position with the top leg flexed.
- Lubricate about 1½″ (4 cm) of the tip of the covered probe *to ease insertion,* unless a prelubricated sheath is available.[16]
- Lift the patient's upper buttock, and gently insert the lubricated thermometer probe into the anus about 1½″ (4 cm).[16]
- Hold the thermometer in place for the duration of time indicated by the manufacturer *to ensure that the maximum temperature is displayed.* Read the temperature display.
- Carefully remove the thermometer probe.
- Remove and dispose of the rectal probe cover or sheath.
- Clean the lubricant from the patient's anal area if necessary.
- Remove and discard your gloves.
- Perform hand hygiene.[6,7,8,9,10]
- Assist the patient to a comfortable position.

Assessing oral temperature

- If the patient has recently had hot or cold liquids, chewed gum, or smoked, wait 15 minutes before taking an oral temperature.[17]
- Position the tip of the thermometer under the patient's tongue in the posterior sublingual pocket *because the external carotid artery perfuses the area, reflecting changes in core temperature.*[1,4,18]
- Instruct the patient to close the lips but to avoid biting down.
- Leave the thermometer in place for the duration of time indicated by the manufacturer *to ensure that the maximum temperature is displayed.* Read the temperature display.
- Remove and discard the oral probe cover or sheath.

Assessing tympanic membrane temperature

- Make sure the tympanic lens is clean before using the thermometer; *a dirty lens may produce inaccurate temperature measurements.*[2]
- If the patient has been lying with the ear on a pillow, allow 20 minutes to elapse *to allow the temperature to normalize.*[3]
- Examine the patient's ear *because cerumen may reduce the accuracy of readings.*[4] Choose the other ear or an alternative method for measuring the patient's temperature if cerumen is present.

■ Stabilize the patient's head and gently pull the ear up and back (for adults), as shown below.

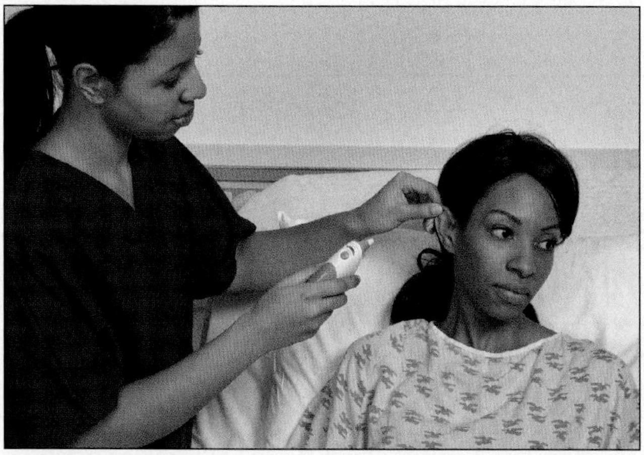

■ Insert the thermometer into the patient's ear following the manufacturer's instructions. *Depending on the thermometer's design, some thermometers require a light seal, where others require a full seal and a twist of the thermometer.*[1]
■ Press the activation button and hold the thermometer in place for the duration of time indicated by the manufacturer *to ensure that the maximum temperature is displayed.* Read the temperature display.
■ Remove and discard the probe cover.

Completing the procedure
■ Perform hand hygiene.[6,7,8,910]
■ Clean and disinfect the thermometer after use[19,20] *to prevent cross-contamination* and then return it to the charging base *so that it is ready for the next use.*
■ Perform hand hygiene.[6,7,8,9,10]
■ Document the procedure.[21,22,23]

Special considerations
■ Keep in mind that the accuracy of a temperature measurement is influenced by the equipment and your technique; closely follow the manufacturer's instructions for use.[1]
■ Mouth breathing, heated supplemental gases, and hot or cold fluids can distort oral temperature measurements.[2]
■ Rectal temperature measurement has been implicated in the spread of enteric pathogens such as *Clostridium difficile* or vancomycin-resistant enterococci through the device or health care worker. Make sure the thermometer and probe are properly cleaned and disinfected between use and that other infection-prevention guidelines are followed *to prevent the spread of infection.*[2]

Complications
Inaccurate technique may lead to a delay in treatment or inappropriate treatment. Rectal trauma or perforation may occur with rectal temperature assessment. Oral temperature assessment may cause damage to the oral mucosa, especially in patients with abnormal mucosa due to trauma, thermal injury, infection, surgery, cancer, or cytotoxic medications. Tympanic membrane temperature assessment may cause trauma to the tympanic membrane.[2]

Documentation
Record the time, site, device, and temperature in the patient's medical record. Document prescribed interventions and the patient's response to those interventions. Record any patient teaching and the patient's comprehension of your teaching.

REFERENCES

1 Davie, A., & Amoore, J. (2010). Best practice in the measurement of body temperature. *Nursing Standard, 24*(42), 42–49. Accessed May 2015 via the Web at http://nursingstandard.rcnpublishing.co.uk/archive/article-best-practice-in-the-measurement-of-body-temperature
2 O'Grady, N. P., et al. (2008). Guidelines for evaluation of new fever in critically ill adult patients: 2008 update from the American College of Critical Care Medicine and the Infectious Disease Society of America. *Critical Care Medicine, 36,* 1330–1349. (Level II)
3 Bridges, E., & Thomas, K. (2009). Noninvasive measurement of body temperature in critically ill patients. *Critical Care Nurse, 29*(3), 94–97.
4 McCallum, L., & Higgins, D. (2012). Measuring body temperature. *Nursing Times, 108*(45), 20–22.
5 Makic, M. B., et al. (2011). Evidence-based practice habits: Putting more sacred cows out to pasture. *Critical Care Nurse, 31*(2), 38–62.
6 The Joint Commission. (2015). Standard NPSG.07.01.01. *Comprehensive accreditation manual for hospitals: The official handbook.* Oakbrook Terrace, IL: The Joint Commission. (Level VII)
7 Centers for Disease Control and Prevention. (2002). Guideline for hand hygiene in health-care settings: Recommendations of the Healthcare Infection Control Practices Advisory Committee and the HICPAC/SHEA/APIC/IDSA Hand Hygiene Task Force. *MMWR Recommendations and Reports, 51*(RR-16), 1–45. Accessed May 2015 via the Web at http://www.cdc.gov/mmwr/pdf/rr/rr5116.pdf (Level II)
8 World Health Organization. (2009). "WHO guidelines on hand hygiene in health care: First global patient safety challenge, clean care is safer care" [Online]. Accessed May 2015 via the Web at http://whqlibdoc.who.int/publications/2009/9789241597906_eng.pdf (Level IV)
9 Centers for Medicare & Medicaid Services, Department of Health and Human Services. (2014). Condition of participation: Infection control. 42 C.F.R. § 482.42.
10 American Osteopathic Association. (2014). Standard 07.01.21. *Healthcare Facilities Accreditation Program: Accreditation requirements for acute care hospitals.* Chicago, IL: American Osteopathic Association. (Level VII)
11 The Joint Commission. (2015). Standard NPSG.01.01.01. *Comprehensive accreditation manual for hospitals: The official handbook.* Oakbrook Terrace, IL: The Joint Commission. (Level VII)
12 Centers for Medicare & Medicaid Services, Department of Health and Human Services. (2014). Condition of participation: Patient's rights. 42 C.F.R. § 482.13(c)(1).
13 American Osteopathic Association. (2014). Standard 15.01.16. *Healthcare Facilities Accreditation Program: Accreditation requirements for acute care hospitals.* Chicago, IL: American Osteopathic Association. (Level VII)
14 Siegel, J. D., et al. (2007). "2007 guideline for isolation precautions: Preventing transmission of infectious agents in healthcare settings" [Online]. Accessed May 2015 via the Web at http://www.cdc.gov/hicpac/pdf/isolation/Isolation2007.pdf (Level II)
15 American Osteopathic Association. (2014). Standard 07.01.10. *Healthcare Facilities Accreditation Program: Accreditation requirements for acute care hospitals.* Chicago, IL: American Osteopathic Association. (Level VII)
16 Taylor, C. R., et al. (2015). *Fundamentals of nursing: The art and science of nursing care* (8th ed.). Philadelphia, PA: Lippincott Williams & Wilkins.
17 Quatrara, B., et al. (2007). The effect of respiratory rate and ingestion of hot and cold beverages on the accuracy of oral temperatures measured by electronic thermometers. *MedSurg Nursing, 16,* 100, 105–108. (Level II)
18 Sund-Levander, M., & Grodzinsky, E. (2009). Time for a change to assess and evaluate body temperature in clinical practice. *International Journal of Nursing Practice, 15,* 241–249.
19 Rutala, W. A., et al. (2008). "Guideline for disinfection and sterilization in healthcare facilities, 2008" [Online]. Accessed May 2015 via the Web at http://www.cdc.gov/hicpac/pdf/guidelines/Disinfection_Nov_2008.pdf (Level I)
20 American Osteopathic Association. (2014). Standard 07.02.03. *Healthcare Facilities Accreditation Program: Accreditation requirements for acute care hospitals.* Chicago, IL: American Osteopathic Association. (Level VII)

Comparing therapeutic baths

TYPE	AGENTS	PURPOSE
Antibacterial	■ Acetic acid ■ Potassium permanganate ■ Povidone-iodine	Used to treat infected eczema, dirty ulcerations, furunculosis, and pemphigus
Colloidal	■ Aveeno colloidal oatmeal ■ Aveeno colloidal oatmeal, oilated ■ Soybean complex ■ Starch and baking soda	Used to relieve pruritus and to soothe and coat irritated skin; indicated for any irritated or oozing condition, such as atopic eczema
Emollient	■ Bath oils ■ Chamomile ■ Mineral oil	Used to clean and hydrate the skin; indicated for any dry skin condition
Tar	■ Bath oils with tar ■ Coal tar concentrate	Used to treat scaly dermatoses, sometimes in combination with ultraviolet light therapy; loosens scales and relieves pruritus

21 The Joint Commission. (2015). Standard RC.01.03.01. *Comprehensive accreditation manual for hospitals: The official handbook.* Oakbrook Terrace, IL: The Joint Commission. (Level VII)
22 Centers for Medicare & Medicaid Services, Department of Health and Human Services. (2014). Condition of participation: Medical record services. 42 C.F.R. § 482.24(b).
23 American Osteopathic Association. (2014). Standard 10.00.03. *Healthcare Facilities Accreditation Program: Accreditation requirements for acute care hospitals.* Chicago, IL: American Osteopathic Association. (Level VII)

THERAPEUTIC BATH

Also referred to as *balneotherapy,* the therapeutic bath combines water and additives to soothe and relax the patient; relieve fatigue, sore muscles and joints, and inflammation and pruritus; clean the skin; and soften and remove crusts, scales, debris, and old medications. Used primarily for their antipruritic and emollient actions, these baths coat irritated skin with a soothing, protective film. Because they constrict surface blood vessels, they also have an anti-inflammatory effect.

The addition of oatmeal powder, soluble cornstarch, or soybean complex to water creates a colloid bath, which has a soothing effect and is used to treat generalized itching. Oil baths are useful for lubricating dry skin and easing eczematous eruptions. Sodium bicarbonate added to water produces an alkaline bath that has a cooling effect and helps relieve pruritus. A medicated tar bath may be used to treat psoriasis. The film of tar left on the skin works in combination with ultraviolet light to inhibit the rapid cell turnover characteristic of psoriasis. (See *Comparing therapeutic baths.*)

A bedridden patient may benefit from a local soak with the therapeutic additive instead of a therapeutic tub bath. (See the "Soaks" procedure, page 703.)

Equipment

Bathtub ■ bath mat ■ rubber mat ■ bath (utility) thermometer ■ therapeutic additive ■ measuring device ■ colander or sieve for oatmeal powder ■ two washcloths ■ two towels ■ patient gown or loose-fitting cotton pajamas ■ gloves ■ hospital-grade disinfectant ■ Optional: lubricating cream or ointment, plastic apron or protective gown.

Preparation of equipment

Gather the supplies. Make sure the tub is clean and disinfected *because a patient with skin breakdown is particularly vulnerable to infection.* Place the bath mat next to the tub and the rubber mat on the bottom of the tub *to prevent falls; the therapeutic additive may make the tub exceptionally slippery.*

If you are giving a tar bath, wear a plastic apron or protective gown *because tar preparations stain clothing.*

Implementation

■ Verify the practitioner's order.
■ Draw the bath before bringing the patient to the bath area *to prevent chilling him.* Fill the tub with 6″ to 8″ (15 cm to 20 cm) of water at 95° to 100°F (35° to 38°C).
■ Measure the correct amount of therapeutic additive, according to the practitioner's order or package instructions. As the tub is filling, perform hand hygiene and thoroughly mix the additive in the water. Add most substances directly to the water, but place oatmeal powder in a sieve or colander under the tub faucet *to help it dissolve.* Begin with 2 tbs (about 30 mL) of oatmeal powder; then add more powder or water as needed to regulate the thickness of the oatmeal bath.
■ Perform hand hygiene.[2,3,4,5,6]
■ Confirm the patient's identity using at least two patient identifiers.[7]
■ Explain the procedure to the patient.
■ Have the patient void, if needed.
■ Escort the patient to the bath area.
■ Close the door *to provide privacy and eliminate drafts.*

NURSING ALERT *Make sure that the bathroom is well ventilated. Some patients may experience allergic reactions or hypersensitivity to the additive in the water or to the smell of the additive. If a reaction occurs, limit the patient's time in the bath and notify the practitioner. If a skin reaction to the additive occurs, gently wash the additive from the skin and notify the practitioner.*

■ Put on gloves.
■ Check the water temperature using a bath thermometer. Help the patient undress, and then help him into the tub, if necessary. Advise him to use the safety rails *to prevent falls.*
■ Tell him that the bath may feel unpleasant at first *because his skin is irritated,* but assure him that the medication will soon coat and soothe his skin.

■ Ask the patient to stretch out in the tub and submerge his body up to the chin. Support his head and neck, if needed. If he's capable, give him a washcloth to apply the bath solution gently to his face and other body areas not immersed if these areas require treatment.

NURSING ALERT *If the patient is taking a tar bath, tell him not to get the bath solution in his eyes* because tar is an eye irritant.

■ Warn the patient against scrubbing his skin *to prevent further irritation.*

■ Add warm water to the bath as needed *to maintain a comfortable temperature.*

■ Remove and discard your gloves[8,9] and perform hand hygiene.[2,3,4,5,6]

■ Allow the patient to soak for 15 to 30 minutes. *Periods of soaking longer than this may cause skin softening and damage to the skin.* If you stay with him, pull the bath curtain *to give him some privacy and protect him from drafts.* If you must leave the room, show the patient how to use the call light, and ensure his privacy.

■ After the bath, assist the patient from the tub. Have him use the safety rails *to prevent falls.*

■ Help the patient pat his skin dry with towels. Don't rub the skin *because rubbing removes some solutes and oils clinging to the skin and produces friction, worsening pruritus.*

■ Put on new gloves.[8,9]

■ Apply lubricating cream or ointment, if ordered, *to help hold water in the newly hydrated skin.*

■ Provide a fresh patient gown or loose-fitting cotton pajamas. *Tight clothing and scratchy or synthetic materials can aggravate skin conditions by causing friction and increasing perspiration.*

■ Escort the patient to his room and make sure he's comfortable.

■ Drain the bath water, and clean and disinfect the tub using hospital-grade disinfectant.[1,10] If you've given an oatmeal powder bath, drain and rinse the tub immediately or the powder will cake, making later removal difficult.

■ Discard used materials in the appropriate receptacles.[8,9]

■ Remove and discard your gloves,[8,9] and perform hand hygiene.[2,3,4,5,6]

■ Document the procedure.[11,12,13]

Special considerations

■ The treatment's purpose and type of additive used will determine the water temperature. Cool to lukewarm water is used for relieving pruritus and when adding tar or starch. Warm baths soothe, but warmer than 100°F (38°C) causes vasodilation, *which could aggravate pruritus.*

■ *Because pruritus seems worse at night,* a therapeutic bath is best before bedtime, unless ordered otherwise, *to promote restful sleep. Because the patient with a skin disorder may be self-conscious,* maintain eye contact during conversation and avoid staring at his skin. Also avoid nonverbal expressions and gestures that show revulsion. If the patient wishes, allow him to talk about his condition and how it affects his self-esteem.

■ Refrain from using soap during a therapeutic bath *because its drying effect counteracts the bath emollient.*

■ *A patient with skin breakdown chills easily,* so protect him from drafts. But after the bath, avoid covering or dressing him too warmly *because perspiration aggravates pruritus.* Instruct the patient not to scratch his skin *to prevent excoriation and infection.*

■ If the patient is confined to bed, you can place the therapeutic additive in a basin of water at 95° to 100°F (35° to 38°C) and apply it with a washcloth, using light, gentle strokes.

Patient teaching

Instruct the patient to bathe only as often as prescribed. Explain that excessive bathing can dry the skin. Advise the patient to purchase commercial bath oil because salad or cooking oils may give clothes an unpleasant odor, and mineral oil mixes poorly with water. Tell the patient to follow manufacturer's instructions for commercially prepared colloid preparations. Colloid for an oatmeal bath can be made at home by putting ½ cup (about 118 mL) of raw oatmeal into a blender and blending at medium-high speed until the material has the consistency of flour, and then sifting it to remove unground pieces. Advise the patient to avoid wearing pajamas, underwear, or other clothing that isn't cotton and loose-fitting.

Complications

The patient may experience an allergic reaction or hypersensitivity to the additive.

Documentation

Record the date, time, and duration of the bath. Note the water temperature, type and amount of additive, skin appearance before and after the bath, the patient's tolerance of the treatment, and the bath's effectiveness. Document patient teaching and the patient's understanding of your teaching.

REFERENCES

1 Rutala, W. A., et al. (2008). "Guideline for disinfection and sterilization in healthcare facilities, 2008" [Online]. Accessed May 2015 via the Web at http://www.cdc.gov/hicpac/pdf/guidelines/Disinfection_Nov_2008.pdf (Level I)

2 The Joint Commission. (2015). Standard NPSG.07.01.01. *Comprehensive accreditation manual for hospitals: The official handbook.* Oakbrook Terrace, IL: The Joint Commission. (Level VII)

3 Centers for Disease Control and Prevention. (2002). Guideline for hand hygiene in health-care settings: Recommendations of the Healthcare Infection Control Practices Advisory Committee and the HICPAC/SHEA/APIC/IDSA Hand Hygiene Task Force. *MMWR Recommendations and Reports, 51*(RR-16), 1–45. Accessed May 2015 via the Web at http://www.cdc.gov/mmwr/pdf/rr/rr5116.pdf (Level II)

4 World Health Organization. (2009). "WHO guidelines on hand hygiene in health care: First global patient safety challenge, clean care is safer care" [Online]. Accessed May 2015 via the Web at http://whqlibdoc.who.int/publications/2009/9789241597906_eng.pdf (Level IV)

5 American Osteopathic Association. (2014). Standard 07.01.21. *Healthcare Facilities Accreditation Program: Accreditation requirements for acute care hospitals.* Chicago, IL: American Osteopathic Association. (Level VII)

6 Centers for Medicare & Medicaid Services, Department of Health and Human Services. (2014). Condition of participation: Infection control. 42 C.F.R. § 482.42.

7 The Joint Commission. (2015). Standard NPSG.01.01.01. *Comprehensive accreditation manual for hospitals: The official handbook.* Oakbrook Terrace, IL: The Joint Commission. (Level VII)

8 Siegel J. D., et al. (2007). "2007 guideline for isolation precautions: Preventing transmission of infectious agents in healthcare settings" [Online]. Accessed May 2015 via the Web at http://www.cdc.gov/hicpac/pdf/isolation/Isolation2007.pdf (Level II)

9 American Osteopathic Association. (2014). Standard 07.01.10. *Healthcare Facilities Accreditation Program: Accreditation requirements for acute care hospitals.* Chicago, IL: American Osteopathic Association. (Level VII)

10 American Osteopathic Association. (2014). Standard 07.02.03. *Healthcare Facilities Accreditation Program: Accreditation requirements for acute care hospitals.* Chicago, IL: American Osteopathic Association. (Level VII)

11 The Joint Commission. (2015). Standard RC.01.03.01. *Comprehensive accreditation manual for hospitals: The official handbook.* Oakbrook Terrace, IL: The Joint Commission. (Level VII)

12 American Osteopathic Association. (2014). Standard 10.00.03. *Healthcare Facilities Accreditation Program: Accreditation requirements for acute care hospitals.* Chicago, IL: American Osteopathic Association. (Level VII)

13 Centers for Medicare & Medicaid Services, Department of Health and Human Services. (2014). Condition of participation: Medical record services. 42 C.F.R. § 482.24(b).

Positioning for thoracentesis

The choice of the position may vary. Usually, the patient is sitting upright and leaning forward. If the patient is sitting on the edge of the bed, support his legs and have him lean forward and rest his head and arms on a pillow on the overbed table (as shown). If the patient can't sit, turn him on the unaffected side and position him at the edge of the bed[1,17] with the arm of the affected side raised comfortably above his head. The head of the bed may be elevated 30 to 45 degrees unless contraindicated. Recumbent thoracentesis may be performed with ultrasound guidance.[22] *Proper positioning stretches the chest or back and allows easier access to the intercostal spaces.*

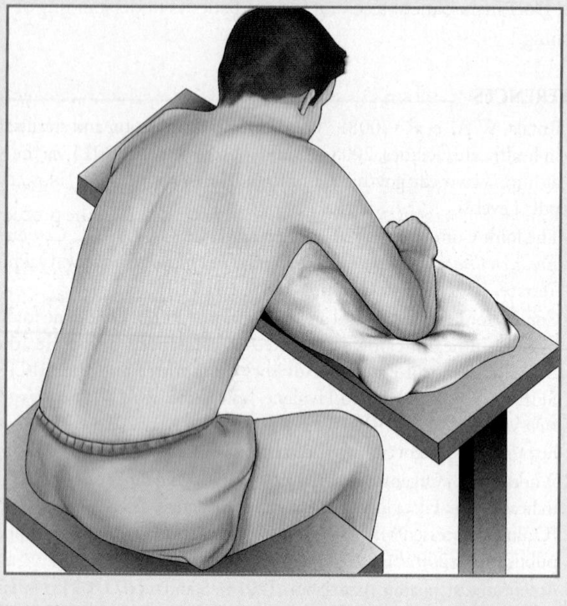

THORACENTESIS, ASSISTING

Thoracentesis involves aspiration of fluid or air from the pleural space. It relieves pulmonary compression and respiratory distress by removing accumulated air or fluid that results from injury or such conditions as tuberculosis, cancer, and heart failure. It also provides a specimen of pleural fluid or tissue for analysis and allows instillation of chemotherapeutic agents or other medications into the pleural space.

Thoracentesis is contraindicated in patients with bleeding disorders and chest wall cellulitis at the point of puncture.[1] It should be used cautiously in patients who are uncooperative, who have uncontrolled coughing, whose pleural fluid location is uncertain, who have only one functional lung, or who are on positive end-expiratory pressure mechanical ventilation.[2]

Equipment

Most facilities use a prepackaged thoracentesis tray that typically includes the following:

Sterile gloves ▪ sterile drapes ▪ 1% or 2% lidocaine ▪ 5-mL syringe with 21G and 25G needles for anesthetic injection ▪ 17G thoracentesis needle for aspiration or Teflon over-the-needle catheters ▪ 50-mL syringe ▪ three-way stopcock and tubing ▪ sterile specimen containers ▪ sterile hemostat ▪ sterile 4″ × 4″ (10-cm × 10-cm) gauze pads ▪ antiseptic cleaning swabs.

You'll also need the following:

Sterile marker ▪ sterile labels ▪ sphygmomanometer or electronic vital signs monitor ▪ pulse oximeter ▪ thermometer ▪ gowns ▪ masks and goggles or masks with face shields ▪ gloves ▪ stethoscope ▪ laboratory request forms ▪ specimen collection bottles ▪ laboratory biohazard transport bag ▪ tape ▪ biopsy needle ▪ prescribed local anesthetic with 3-mL syringe and 21G needle ▪ drainage container ▪ prescribed analgesic or sedation ▪ disinfectant pad ▪ emergency equipment (crash cart with cardiac medications, defibrillator, handheld resuscitation bag with mask, and intubation equipment) ▪ Optional: hair clippers, multidose vial of local anesthetic, alcohol pad.

Preparation of equipment

Check the expiration date on each sterile package, and inspect for tears. Prepare the necessary laboratory request form. List current antibiotic therapy on the laboratory forms *because this factor will be considered in analyzing the specimens.*

Implementation

- Verify the practitioner's orders.
- Check the patient's medical history for any allergies, especially to latex, antiseptic cleaning solution, or the local anesthetic.
- Gather and prepare the equipment at the patient's bedside or in the treatment area.
- Confirm that an informed consent has been obtained and that the consent in the patient's medical record.[3,4,5]
- Conduct a preprocedure verification *to make sure that all relevant documentation, related information, and equipment are available and correctly identified to the patient's identifiers.*[6,7]
- Verify that the laboratory and imaging studies have been completed as ordered and that the results are in the patient's medical record. Notify the practitioner of any unexpected results.
- Perform hand hygiene.[8,9,10,11,12]
- Confirm the patient's identity using at least two patient identifiers.[13]
- Reinforce the practitioner's explanation of the procedure, and answer the patient's questions. Inform him that he may feel some discomfort and pressure during the needle insertion.
- Allow the patient's family members to remain throughout the procedure if the patient permits it and they wish to do so.[14] Assist them in putting on personal protective equipment.
- Provide privacy and emotional support.[3,15]
- If required by your facility, make sure that the procedure site is marked.[7,16]
- Obtain the patient's vital signs, oxygen saturation level, and pain level and assess respiratory function *to serve as a baseline for comparison during and after the procedure.*[17,18]
- Auscultate the patient's breath sounds.
- Administer the prescribed sedative or analgesia as ordered following safe medication administration practices.[1,19,20,21]
- Position the patient appropriately *to ease the withdrawal of pleural fluid.*[17] Make sure that he's firmly supported and comfortable. (See *Positioning for thoracentesis.*)
- Remind the patient not to cough, breathe deeply, or move suddenly during the procedure *to avoid puncture of the visceral pleura or lung.* If the patient coughs, the practitioner will briefly halt the procedure and withdraw the needle slightly *to prevent puncture.*
- Expose the patient's entire chest or back as appropriate.
- Clip hair from the aspiration site if needed.
- Perform hand hygiene.[8,9,10,11,12]
- Put on a gown, a mask and goggles or mask with face shield, and gloves.[23,24]
- Using sterile technique, open the thoracentesis tray. Label all medications, medication containers, and other solutions on and off the sterile field.[25,26]
- Assist the practitioner as necessary in disinfecting the site and allowing it to dry.

■ Conduct a time-out immediately before starting the procedure *to perform a final assessment to ensure that the correct patient, site, positioning, and procedure are identified and that, as applicable, all relevant information and necessary equipment are available.*[7,27]
■ If an ampule of local anesthetic isn't included in the sterile tray and a multidose vial of local anesthetic is to be used, assist the practitioner by disinfecting the rubber stopper with an alcohol pad, allowing it to dry, and holding the inverted vial while the practitioner withdraws the anesthetic solution.
■ After draping the patient and injecting the local anesthetic, the practitioner attaches a three-way stopcock with tubing to the aspirating needle. He opens the stopcock valve between the syringe and the needle *to allow for the aspiration of pleural fluid during needle insertion and to prevent air from entering the pleural space.*[17]
■ Attach the other end of the tubing to the drainage container.
■ The practitioner inserts the needle into the pleural space and attaches a 50-mL syringe to the needle's stopcock. A hemostat may be used *to hold the needle in place and prevent a pleural tear or lung puncture.* Alternatively, the practitioner may introduce a Teflon catheter into the needle, remove the needle, and attach a stopcock and syringe or drainage tubing to the catheter *to reduce the risk of pleural puncture by the needle.*
■ Reassure the patient throughout the procedure, assessing for signs of anxiety. Keep him informed of each step.
■ Monitor vital signs regularly during the procedure. Continually observe the patient for signs and symptoms of distress such as pallor, vertigo, faintness, weak and rapid pulse, decreased blood pressure, dyspnea, tachypnea, diaphoresis, chest pain, blood-tinged mucus, and excessive coughing. Alert the practitioner if any of these develop *because they may indicate complications such as hypovolemic shock or tension pneumothorax.*
■ Assist the practitioner as necessary in specimen collection, fluid drainage, and site dressing.
■ Label the specimens with the patient's name, identification number, and the date and time of collection in the presence of the patient *to prevent mislabeling,* and send them to the laboratory in a laboratory biohazard transport bag.[28]
■ After the practitioner withdraws the needle or catheter, apply pressure to the puncture site using a sterile 4″ × 4″ (10-cm × 10-cm) gauze pad. Then apply a new sterile gauze pad and secure it with tape.
■ Place the patient in a comfortable position.
■ Assess his respiratory status, and examine the dressing for drainage.[17] Monitor his vital signs at a frequency determined by the patient's condition and your facility *because there's no evidence-based research available to indicate best practice for frequency of assessing vital signs after a procedure.*[29]
■ Perform a comprehensive pain assessment using techniques appropriate for the patient's age, condition, and ability to understand.[18] Administer pain medication, as needed and ordered, following safe medication administration practices.[19,20,21]
■ Discard used supplies in the appropriate receptacles.[28] Clean nondisposable items, and return them for sterilization.
■ Obtain a chest X-ray as ordered after the procedure.[17,30]
■ Remove and discard your gloves and personal protective equipment.[23,24]
■ Perform hand hygiene.[8,9,10,11,12]
■ Clean and disinfect your stethoscope with a disinfectant pad.[31,32]
■ Perform hand hygiene.[8,9,10,11,12]
■ Document the procedure.[33,34,35]

Special considerations

■ *To prevent pulmonary edema and hypovolemic shock after thoracentesis,* the practitioner removes the fluid slowly—no more than 1,000 mL of fluid during the first 30 minutes.[36] *Removing the fluid increases negative intrapleural pressure, which can lead to edema if the lung doesn't reexpand to fill the space.*
■ Some coughing is common as the lung reexpands.
■ Pleuritic or shoulder pain may indicate pleural irritation by the needle point.
■ The practitioner may decide to place a small-bore (pigtail) chest tube for continued drainage of a large effusion.[22]

Complications

Pneumothorax (possibly leading to mediastinal shift and requiring chest tube insertion) can occur if the needle punctures the lung and air enters the pleural cavity. Hemoptysis may also occur if the lung is punctured. Pyogenic infection can result from contamination during the procedure. Hemothorax may occur if the thoracentesis needle punctures one of the intercostal vessels. Laceration of the liver or spleen may also occur.[1] Other potential difficulties include pain, cough, anxiety, dry taps, and subcutaneous hematoma and vasovagal syncope.

Documentation

Record the date and time of thoracentesis and the name of the practitioner performing the procedure. Include the location of the puncture site; volume and description (color, viscosity, and odor) of the fluid withdrawn; whether specimens were sent to the laboratory; vital signs, pain level, and respiratory assessments before, during, and after the procedure; any postprocedure tests such as chest X-ray; any complications and nursing actions taken; and the patient's reaction to the procedure. If later signs and symptoms of pneumothorax, subcutaneous emphysema, or infection occur, notify the practitioner immediately and document your observations and interventions in the patient's medical record.

REFERENCES

1 Brauner, M. E. (2013). "Thoracentesis" [Online]. Accessed May 2015 via the Web at http://emedicine.medscape.com/article/80640-overview#a01
2 Goligher, E. C. (2011). "Utility and safety of draining pleural effusions in mechanically ventilated patients: A systematic review and meta-analysis" [Online]. Accessed May 2015 via the Web at http://www.ncbi.nlm.nih.gov/pmc/articles/PMC3221976/pdf/cc10009.pdf (Level I)
3 Centers for Medicare & Medicaid Services, Department of Health and Human Services. (2014). Condition of participation: Patient's rights. 42 C.F.R. § 482.13.
4 The Joint Commission. (2015). Standard RI.01.03.01. *Comprehensive accreditation manual for hospitals: The official handbook.* Oakbrook Terrace, IL: The Joint Commission. (Level VII)
5 American Osteopathic Association. (2014). Standard 15.01.11. *Healthcare Facilities Accreditation Program: Accreditation requirements for acute care hospitals.* Chicago, IL: American Osteopathic Association. (Level VII)
6 The Joint Commission. (2015). Standard UP.01.01.01. *Comprehensive accreditation manual for hospitals: The official handbook.* Oakbrook Terrace, IL: The Joint Commission. (Level VII)
7 American Osteopathic Association. (2014). Standard 30.00.14. *Healthcare Facilities Accreditation Program: Accreditation requirements for acute care hospitals.* Chicago, IL: American Osteopathic Association. (Level VII)
8 The Joint Commission. (2015). Standard NPSG.07.01.01. *Comprehensive accreditation manual for hospitals: The official handbook.* Oakbrook Terrace, IL: The Joint Commission. (Level VII)
9 World Health Organization. (2009). "WHO guidelines on hand hygiene in health care: First global patient safety challenge, clean care is safer care" [Online]. Accessed May 2015 via the Web at http://whqlibdoc.who.int/publications/2009/9789241597906_eng.pdf (Level IV)
10 Centers for Disease Control and Prevention. (2002). Guideline for hand hygiene in health-care settings: Recommendations of the Healthcare Infection Control Practices Advisory and the HICPAC/SHEA/APIC/IDSA Hand Hygiene Task force. *MMWR Recommendations and Reports, 51*(RR-16), 1–45. Accessed May 2015 via the Web at http://www.cdc.gov/mmwr/pdf/rr/rr5116.pdf (Level II)

11 Centers for Medicare & Medicaid Services, Department of Health and Human Services. (2014). Condition of participation: Infection control. 42 C.F.R. § 482.42.

12 American Osteopathic Association. (2014). Standard 07.01.21. *Healthcare Facilities Accreditation Program: Accreditation requirements for acute care hospitals.* Chicago, IL: American Osteopathic Association. (Level VII)

13 The Joint Commission. (2014). Standard NPSG.01.01.01. *Comprehensive accreditation manual for hospitals: The official handbook.* Oakbrook Terrace, IL: The Joint Commission. (Level VII)

14 American Association of Critical-Care Nurses. (2010). "AACN practice alert: Family presence during resuscitation and invasive procedures" [Online]. Accessed May 2015 via the Web at http://www.aacn.org/wd/practice/docs/practicealerts/family%20presence%2004-2010%20final.pdf (Level VII)

15 American Osteopathic Association. (2014). Standard 15.01.16. *Healthcare Facilities Accreditation Program: Accreditation requirements for acute care hospitals.* Chicago, IL: American Osteopathic Association. (Level VII)

16 The Joint Commission. (2015). Standard UP.01.02.01. *Comprehensive accreditation manual for hospitals: The official handbook.* Oakbrook Terrace, IL: The Joint Commission. (Level VII)

17 Lynn-McHale Wiegand, D. (Ed.). (2011). *AACN procedure manual for critical care* (6th ed.). Philadelphia, PA: Saunders.

18 The Joint Commission. (2015). Standard PC.01.02.07. *Comprehensive accreditation manual for hospitals: The official handbook.* Oakbrook Terrace, IL: The Joint Commission. (Level VII)

19 The Joint Commission. (2015). Standard MM.06.01.01. *Comprehensive accreditation manual for hospitals: The official handbook.* Oakbrook Terrace, IL: The Joint Commission. (Level VII)

20 Centers for Medicare & Medicaid Services, Department of Health and Human Services. (2014). Condition of participation: Nursing services. 42 C.F.R. § 482.23(c).

21 American Osteopathic Association. (2014). Standard 16.01.03. *Healthcare Facilities Accreditation Program: Accreditation requirements for acute care hospitals.* Chicago, IL: American Osteopathic Association. (Level VII)

22 Liu, Y., et al. (2010). Ultrasound-guided pigtail catheters for drainage of various pleural diseases. *American Journal of Emergency Medicine, 28,* 915–921. (Level IV)

23 Siegel, J. D., et al. (2007). "2007 guideline for isolation precautions: Preventing transmission of infectious agents in healthcare settings" [Online]. Accessed May 2015 via the Web at http://www.cdc.gov/hicpac/pdf/isolation/Isolation2007.pdf (Level II)

24 American Osteopathic Association. (2014). Standard 07.01.10. *Healthcare Facilities Accreditation Program: Accreditation requirements for acute care hospitals.* Chicago, IL: American Osteopathic Association. (Level VII)

25 The Joint Commission. (2015). Standard NPSG.03.04.01. *Comprehensive accreditation manual for hospitals: The official handbook.* Oakbrook Terrace, IL: The Joint Commission. (Level VII)

26 American Osteopathic Association. (2014). Standard 25.01.27. *Healthcare Facilities Accreditation Program: Accreditation requirements for acute care hospitals.* Chicago, IL: American Osteopathic Association. (Level VII)

27 The Joint Commission. (2015). Standard UP.01.03.01. *Comprehensive accreditation manual for hospitals: The official handbook.* Oakbrook Terrace, IL: The Joint Commission. (Level VII)

28 Occupational Safety and Health Administration. (n.d.). "Bloodborne pathogens, standard number 1910.1030" [Online]. Accessed May 2015 via the Web at http://www.osha.gov/pls/oshaweb/owadisp.show_document?p_table=STANDARDS&p_id=10051 (Level VII)

29 American Society of PeriAnesthesia Nurses. (2015). *2015-2017 Perianesthesia nursing standards, practice recommendations and interpretive statements.* Cherry Hill, NJ: American Society of PeriAnesthesia Nurses.

30 National Heart, Lung, and Blood Institute. (2012). "What is thoracentesis?" [Online]. Accessed May 2015 via the Web at http://www.nhlbi.nih.gov/health/health-topics/topics/thor/

31 Rutala, W. A., et al. (2008). "Guideline for disinfection and sterilization in healthcare facilities, 2008" [Online]. Accessed May 2015 via the Web at http://www.cdc.gov/hicpac/pdf/guidelines/Disinfection_Nov_2008.pdf (Level I)

32 American Osteopathic Association. (2014). Standard 07.02.03. *Healthcare Facilities Accreditation Program: Accreditation requirements for acute care hospitals.* Chicago, IL: American Osteopathic Association. (Level VII)

33 The Joint Commission. (2015). Standard RC.01.03.01. *Comprehensive accreditation manual for hospitals: The official handbook.* Oakbrook Terrace, IL: The Joint Commission. (Level VII)

34 Centers for Medicare & Medicaid Services, Department of Health and Human Services. (2014). Condition of participation: Medical record services. 42 C.F.R. § 482.24(b).

35 American Osteopathic Association. (2014). Standard 10.00.03. *Healthcare Facilities Accreditation Program: Accreditation requirements for acute care hospitals.* Chicago, IL: American Osteopathic Association. (Level VII)

36 Feller-Kopman, D., et al. (2007). Large-volume thoracentesis and the risk of reexpansion pulmonary edema. *Annals of Thoracic Surgery, 84,* 1656–1661. (Level VI)

THORACIC ELECTRICAL BIOIMPEDANCE MONITORING

A noninvasive alternative for tracking hemodynamic status, thoracic electrical bioimpedance monitoring, also known as *impedance cardiography,* provides information about a patient's cardiac index, preload, afterload, contractibility, cardiac output, and blood flow. In this procedure, electrodes are placed on the patient's thorax. The electrodes have two purposes: to send harmless low-level electricity through the patient's body and to detect return electrical signals. These signals, which are interruptions in the electrical flow, come from changes in the volume and velocity of blood as it flows through the aorta. The bioimpedance monitor interprets the signals as a waveform. Cardiac output is then computed from this waveform and the electrocardiogram (ECG).

Thoracic electrical bioimpedance monitoring eliminates the risk of infection, bleeding, pneumothorax, emboli, and arrhythmias associated with traditional invasive monitoring. The accuracy of results obtained by this method is comparable to results obtained by thermodilution; the bioimpedance monitor also automatically updates information every 2nd to 10th heartbeat.[1]

Equipment

Thoracic electrical bioimpedance unit ▪ color-coded ECG leadwires ▪ connecting cable ▪ four sets of thoracic electrical bioimpedance electrodes ▪ three ECG electrodes ▪ sterile 3″ × 3″ (7.6-cm × 7.6-cm) or 4″ × 4″ (10-cm × 10-cm) gauze pads ▪ tape measure ▪ Optional: gloves.

Implementation

- Perform hand hygiene and, as necessary, put on gloves.[2,3,4,5,6]
- Confirm the patient's identity using at least two patient identifiers.[7]
- Explain the procedure to the patient.
- Plug the thoracic electrical bioimpedance unit into a power supply.
- Press the POWER button.
- Enter information as prompted by the initial display screen appearing on the unit.
- Assist the patient onto his back with the head of the bed elevated no more than 30 degrees.
- Provide privacy,[10,11] and expose the patient's chest.
- Wet some sterile 4″ × 4″ (10-cm × 10-cm) or 3″ × 3″ (7.6-cm × 7.6-cm) gauze pads with warm water and clean the skin on each side of his neck from the base of the neck to 2″ (5 cm) above the base. Also clean the skin on both sides of the chest at the midaxillary line directly across the xiphoid process. *To ensure that you've cleaned a large enough area for electrode placement,* clean at least two fingerbreadths above and below the site.
- Place one electrode set vertically on the side of the neck in line with the ear. Make sure that the bottom of the electrode set isn't lower than the junction of the shoulder at the base of the neck.

■ Place the second set of electrodes on the opposite side of the neck in line with the ear and about 180 degrees from the first set.
■ Place the remaining two sets of electrodes on either side of the patient's chest. *To determine the correct location,* draw a line with your finger from the xiphoid process to the midaxillary line on one side of the chest. This is the site for the first chest electrode. Ensure that the top portion of the electrode is at the level of the xiphoid process.
■ Attach the ECG leadwires and try different lead selections until you obtain a consistent QRS signal. Don't remove the patient from the primary monitor *because the regular system must be maintained to ensure monitoring at the central station and to keep the alarms intact.*
■ Attach the leadwires of the bioimpedance harness to the thoracic electrical bioimpedance electrodes and the ECG electrodes.
■ Measure the distance between the bottom of an electrode set on one side of the patient's neck and the top of an electrode set on the same side of his chest. This distance, the *thorax length,* is the numeric value required by the monitor's computer to calculate accurate stroke volume. Enter this value on the patient-data screen. Then return to the waveform screen.
■ Begin monitoring the results provided by the thoracic electrical bioimpedance unit.
■ Remove and discard your gloves if worn.[8,9]
■ Perform hand hygiene.[2,3,4,5,6]
■ Document the procedure.[12,13,14]

Special considerations

■ Baseline bioimpedance values may be reduced in patients who have conditions characterized by increased fluid in the chest, such as pulmonary edema and pleural effusion.
■ Bioimpedance values may be lower than thermodilution values in patients with tachycardia and other arrhythmias.

Documentation

Note the waveforms and values on the monitor and document the values by pressing PRINT on the waveform screen to print a strip containing all the values monitored. Place the strip in the patient's chart.

REFERENCES

1 Gujjar, A. R., et al. (2008). Non-invasive cardiac output by transthoracic electrical bioimpedence in post-cardiac surgery patients: Comparison with thermodilution method. *Journal of Clinical Monitoring and Computing, 22,* 175–180. (Level VI)
2 The Joint Commission. (2015). Standard NPSG.07.01.01. *Comprehensive accreditation manual for hospitals: The official handbook.* Oakbrook Terrace, IL: The Joint Commission. (Level VII)
3 Centers for Disease Control and Prevention. (2002). Guideline for hand hygiene in health-care settings: Recommendations of the Healthcare Infection Control Practices Advisory Committee and the HICPAC/SHEA/APIC/IDSA Hand Hygiene Task Force. *MMWR Recommendations and Reports, 51*(RR-16), 1–45. Accessed May 2015 via the Web at http://www.cdc.gov/mmwr/pdf/rr/rr5116.pdf (Level II)
4 World Health Organization. (2009). "WHO guidelines on hand hygiene in health care: First global patient safety challenge, clean care is safer care" [Online]. Accessed May 2015 via the Web at http://whqlibdoc.who.int/publications/2009/9789241597906_eng.pdf (Level IV)
5 American Osteopathic Association. (2014). Standard 07.01.21. *Healthcare Facilities Accreditation Program: Accreditation requirements for acute care hospitals.* Chicago, IL: American Osteopathic Association. (Level VII)
6 Centers for Medicare & Medicaid Services, Department of Health and Human Services. (2014). Condition of participation: Infection control. 42 C.F.R. § 482.42.
7 The Joint Commission. (2015). Standard NPSG.01.01.01. *Comprehensive accreditation manual for hospitals: The official handbook.* Oakbrook Terrace, IL: The Joint Commission. (Level VII)
8 Siegel, J. D., et al. (2007). "2007 guideline for isolation precautions: Preventing transmission of infectious agents in healthcare settings" [Online]. Accessed May 2015 via the Web at http://www.cdc.gov/hicpac/pdf/isolation/Isolation2007.pdf (Level II)
9 American Osteopathic Association. (2014). Standard 07.01.10. *Healthcare Facilities Accreditation Program: Accreditation requirements for acute care hospitals.* Chicago, IL: American Osteopathic Association. (Level VII)
10 American Osteopathic Association. (2014). Standard 15.01.16. *Healthcare Facilities Accreditation Program: Accreditation requirements for acute care hospitals.* Chicago, IL: American Osteopathic Association. (Level VII)
11 Centers for Medicare & Medicaid Services, Department of Health and Human Services. (2013). Condition of participation: Patient's rights. 42 C.F.R. § 482.13(c)(1).
12 The Joint Commission. (2015). Standard RC.01.03.01. *Comprehensive accreditation manual for hospitals: The official handbook.* Oakbrook Terrace, IL: The Joint Commission. (Level VII)
13 American Osteopathic Association. (2014). Standard 10.00.03. *Healthcare Facilities Accreditation Program: Accreditation requirements for acute care hospitals.* Chicago, IL: American Osteopathic Association. (Level VII)
14 Centers for Medicare & Medicaid Services, Department of Health and Human Services. (2014). Condition of participation: Medical record services. 42 C.F.R. § 482.24(b).

TILT TABLE

A tilt table—a padded table or bed-length board that can be raised gradually from a horizontal to a vertical position—can help prevent the complications of prolonged bed rest. Used for a patient with a spinal cord injury, brain damage, orthostatic hypotension, or other condition that prevents free standing, a tilt table increases tolerance for the upright position, conditions the cardiovascular system, stretches muscles, and helps prevent contractures, bone demineralization, and urinary calculus formation.[1,2,3,4]

Tilting a patient with a tilt table is performed once or twice per day, usually in a separate room, depending on the patient's tolerance. In patients with orthostatic hypotension and postural orthostatic tachycardia, the tilt table is used as part of a diagnostic test meant to produce signs and symptoms characteristic of the disease.

Equipment

Tilt table with footboard and safety straps ■ sphygmomanometer and stethoscope or electronic vital signs monitor ■ antiembolism stockings or elastic bandages ■ Optional: electrocardiogram (ECG) monitor, gloves, abdominal binder, wooden block, stretcher.

Implementation

■ Perform hand hygiene.[5,6,7,8,9]
■ Confirm the practitioner's order.
■ Confirm the patient's identity using at least two patient identifiers.[10]
■ Explain the use and benefits of the tilt table to the patient.
■ Apply antiembolism stockings *to restrict vessel walls and help prevent blood pooling and edema.* If necessary, apply an abdominal binder *to avoid pooling of blood in the splanchnic region, which contributes to insufficient cerebral circulation and orthostatic hypotension.*
■ Make sure the tilt table is locked in the horizontal position.
■ Summon assistance and transfer the patient to the table, placing him in the supine position with feet flat against the footboard.
■ If the patient can't bear weight on one leg, place a wooden block between the footboard and the weight-bearing foot, permitting the leg that can't bear weight to dangle freely.
■ Fasten the safety straps.
■ Take the patient's blood pressure and pulse rate.
■ Tilt the table slowly in 15- to 30-degree increments, evaluating the patient constantly.[11] Obtain his blood pressure every 3 to 5 minutes

because movement from the supine to the upright position decreases systolic pressure. Be alert for signs and symptoms of insufficient cerebral circulation: dizziness, nausea, pallor, diaphoresis, tachycardia, or a change in mental status. If the patient experiences any of these signs or symptoms, or develops hypotension or seizures, return the table immediately to the horizontal position.

NURSING ALERT *Never leave the patient unattended on the tilt table* **because marked physiologic changes, such as hypotension or severe headache, can occur suddenly.**

- If the patient tolerates the position shift, continue to tilt the table until reaching the desired angle, usually 45 to 80 degrees. A 60-degree tilt gives the patient the physiologic effects and sensations of standing upright.
- The patient may remain tilted for 5 to 45 minutes, as ordered, or until he becomes symptomatic. Signs and symptoms may include nausea, light-headedness, diaphoresis, tachycardia, low blood pressure, and anxiety.
- Gradually return the patient to the horizontal position while checking his vital signs.
- Obtain assistance and transfer the patient onto a stretcher for transport back to his room.
- Perform hand hygiene.[5,6,7,8,9]
- Document the procedure.[12,13,14]

Special considerations

- If the tilt table is being used for diagnostic purposes, a cardiologist will be present and the patient should be on continuous ECG monitoring.
- Let the patient's response determine the angle of tilt and duration of elevation, but avoid prolonged upright positioning (greater than 45 minutes) *because it may lead to venous stasis.*
- In some instances, the patient may need to fast for up to 4 hours before the test.

Complications

Use of a tilt table can lead to sudden hypotension, severe headache, and other dramatic physiologic changes.

Documentation

Record the angle and duration of elevation; changes in the patient's pulse rate, blood pressure, and physical and mental status; and his response to treatment.

REFERENCES

1 Reybrouck, T., & Ector, H. (2006). Tilt training: A new challenge in the treatment of neurally mediated syncope. *Acta Cardiologica, 61,* 183–189.

2 Trees, D. (2007). Tilting in a patient's favor: Early mobilization emphasizes upright positioning and weight bearing. *Advance for Physical Therapy & Rehab Medicine, 18*(10), 29.

3 Trees, D. W., et al. (2013). Innovative mobility strategies for the patient with intensive care unit–acquired weakness: A case report. *Physical Therapy, 93,* 237–247.

4 Labandz, S. (2012). Upward and onward: Adding standing to your current practice can benefit patients of all ages. *Advance for Physical Therapy & Rehab Medicine, 23*(11), 20. Accessed May 2015 via the Web at http://physical-therapy.advanceweb.com/Archives/Article-Archives/Upward-and-Onward.aspx

5 The Joint Commission. (2015). Standard NPSG.07.01.01. *Comprehensive accreditation manual for hospitals: The official handbook.* Oakbrook Terrace, IL: The Joint Commission. (Level VII)

6 Centers for Disease Control and Prevention. (2002). Guideline for hand hygiene in health-care settings: Recommendations of the Healthcare Infection Control Practices Advisory Committee and the HICPAC/SHEA/APIC/IDSA Hand Hygiene Task Force. *MMWR Recommendations and Reports, 51*(RR-16), 1–45. Accessed May 2015 via the Web at http://www.cdc.gov/mmwr/pdf/rr/rr5116.pdf (Level II)

7 World Health Organization. (2009). "WHO guidelines on hand hygiene in health care: First global patient safety challenge, clean care is safer care" [Online]. Accessed May 2015 via the Web at http://whqlibdoc.who.int/publications/2009/9789241597906_eng.pdf (Level IV)

8 American Osteopathic Association. (2014). Standard 07.01.21. *Healthcare Facilities Accreditation Program: Accreditation requirements for acute care hospitals.* Chicago, IL: American Osteopathic Association. (Level VII)

9 Centers for Medicare & Medicaid Services, Department of Health and Human Services. (2014). Condition of participation: Infection control. 42 C.F.R. § 482.42.

10 The Joint Commission. (2015). Standard NPSG.01.01.01. *Comprehensive accreditation manual for hospitals: The official handbook.* Oakbrook Terrace, IL: The Joint Commission. (Level VII)

11 Hinkle, J. L. & Cheever, K. H. (2014). *Brunner & Suddarth's textbook of medical-surgical nursing* (13th ed.). Philadelphia, PA: Wolters Kluwer.

12 The Joint Commission. (2015). Standard RC.01.03.01. *Comprehensive accreditation manual for hospitals: The official handbook.* Oakbrook Terrace, IL: The Joint Commission. (Level VII)

13 American Osteopathic Association. (2014). Standard 10.00.03. *Healthcare Facilities Accreditation Program: Accreditation requirements for acute care hospitals.* Chicago, IL: American Osteopathic Association. (Level VII)

14 Centers for Medicare & Medicaid Services, Department of Health and Human Services. (2014). Condition of participation: Medical record services. 42 C.F.R. § 482.24(b).

TOPICAL SKIN DRUG APPLICATION

Topical drugs are applied directly to the skin surface or mucous membranes. They include lotions, pastes, ointments, creams, powders, shampoos, and aerosol sprays. Topical medications are absorbed through the epidermal layer into the dermis. The extent of absorption depends on the vascularity of the region.

Nitroglycerin, fentanyl, nicotine, and certain supplemental hormone replacements are used for systemic effects. Most other topical medications are used for local effects. Ointments have a fatty base, which is an ideal vehicle for such drugs as antimicrobials and antiseptics. Typically, topical medications should be applied two or three times a day to achieve their therapeutic effect.

Equipment

Patient's medication administration record and medical record ▪ prescribed medication ▪ gloves ▪ sterile 4″ × 4″ (10-cm × 10-cm) gauze pads ▪ transparent semipermeable dressing ▪ adhesive tape ▪ Optional: solvent (such as cottonseed oil), sterile gloves, white cotton gloves, terry cloth slippers, towels, hair brush or fine-toothed comb, clean basin.

Implementation

- Avoid distractions and interruptions when preparing and administering the medication *to prevent medication errors.*[1,2]
- Verify the practitioner's order.[3,4,5]
- Compare the medication label with the order in the patient's medical record.[3,4,5]
- Check the patient's medical record for an allergy or a contraindications to the prescribed medication. If an allergy or a contraindication exists, don't administer the medication; instead notify the practitioner.[3,4,5]
- Check the expiration date on the medication. If the medication is expired, return it to the pharmacy and obtain new medications.[3,4]
- Visually inspect the medication for loss of integrity; don't administer the medication if its integrity is compromised.[3,4,5]
- Discuss any unresolved concerns about the medication with the patient's practitioner.[3,4,5]
- Perform hand hygiene.[6,7,8,9,10]
- Confirm the patient's identity using at least two patient identifiers.[11]
- Provide privacy and explain the procedure to the patient.[12,13]

■ If the patient is receiving the medication for the first time, teach him about potential adverse reactions and discuss any other concerns related to the medication.[3,4,5]

■ Verify that the medication is being administered at the proper time, in the prescribed dose, and by the correct route *to reduce the risk of medication errors.*[3,4,5]

■ If your facility uses a bar code scanning system, scan your identification badge, the patient's identification bracelet, and the medication's bar code.

■ Put on gloves.[14,15]

■ Help the patient assume a comfortable position that provides access to the area to be treated.

■ Expose the area to be treated. Make sure the skin or mucous membrane is intact (unless the medication has been ordered to treat a skin lesion, such as an ulcer). *Applying medication to broken or abraded skin may cause unwanted systemic absorption and result in further irritation.*

■ If necessary, clean the skin of debris, including crusts, epidermal scales, and old medication. You may have to change your gloves if they become soiled.

Applying paste, cream, or ointment

■ Open the container. Place the lid or cap upside down *to prevent contamination of the inside surface.*

■ Apply the medication to the affected area with long, smooth strokes that follow the direction of hair growth using your gloved hands (as shown below). *This technique avoids forcing medication into hair follicles, which can cause irritation and lead to folliculitis.* Avoid excessive pressure when applying the medication *because it could abrade the skin.*

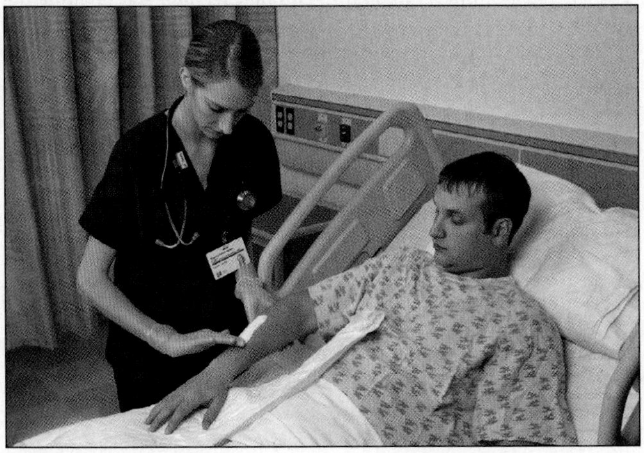

Removing ointment

■ Perform hand hygiene[6,7,8,9,10] and put on gloves.[14,15]

■ Rub solvent on your gloves and apply it liberally to the treated area in the direction of hair growth. Alternatively, saturate a sterile gauze pad with the solvent and use this pad to gently remove the ointment. Remove excess oil by gently wiping the area with a sterile gauze pad. Don't rub too hard to remove the medication *because you could irritate the skin.*

Applying other topical medications

■ To apply shampoos, follow package directions. (See *Using medicated shampoos.*)

■ To apply aerosol sprays, shake the container, if indicated, *to completely mix the medication.* Hold the container 6" to 12" (15 to 30 cm) from the skin, or follow the manufacturer's recommendation. Spray a thin film of medication evenly over the treatment area.

■ To apply powders, dry the skin surface with the gauze pads, making sure to spread skin folds where moisture collects. Then apply a thin layer of powder over the treatment area.

Using medicated shampoos

Medicated shampoos include keratolytic and cytostatic agents, coal tar preparations, and lindane (gamma benzene hexachloride) solutions. They can be used to treat such conditions as dandruff, psoriasis, and head lice. However, they're contraindicated in patients with broken or abraded skin.

Because application instructions may vary among brands, check the label on the shampoo before starting the procedure *to ensure use of the correct amount.* Keep the shampoo away from the patient's eyes. If any shampoo should accidentally get in his eyes, irrigate promptly with water. Selenium sulfide, used in cytostatic agents, is extremely toxic if ingested.

To apply a medicated shampoo, follow these steps:

■ Perform hand hygiene and put on gloves.[6,7,8,9,10,14,15]

■ Prepare the patient for shampoo treatment.

■ Shake the bottle of shampoo well *to mix the solution evenly.*

■ Wet the patient's hair thoroughly and wring out excess water.

■ Apply the proper amount of shampoo, as directed on the label.

■ Work the shampoo into a lather, adding water as necessary. Part the hair and work the shampoo into the scalp, taking care not to use your fingernails.

■ Leave the shampoo on the scalp and hair for as long as instructed (usually 5 to 10 minutes). Then rinse the hair thoroughly.

■ Towel-dry the patient's hair.

■ After the hair is dry, comb or brush it. Use a fine-tooth comb to remove nits if necessary.

■ Remove and discard your gloves, and perform hand hygiene.[6,7,8,9,10]

■ *To protect applied medications and prevent them from soiling the patient's clothes,* tape an appropriate number of sterile gauze pads or a transparent semipermeable dressing over the treated area. With certain medications (such as topical steroids), semipermeable dressings may be contraindicated. Check medication information and cautions. If you're applying a topical medication to the patient's hands or feet, cover the hands with white cotton gloves and the feet with terry cloth slippers.

Completing the procedure

■ Assess the patient's skin for signs of irritation, allergic reaction, or breakdown.

■ Dispose of uses supplies and dressings in the appropriate receptacle.[14,15]

■ Remove and discard your gloves,[14] and perform hand hygiene.[6,7,8,9,10]

■ Document the procedure.[16,17,18]

Special considerations

■ Never apply medication without first removing previous applications *to prevent skin irritation from an accumulation of medication.*

■ Be sure to wear gloves *to prevent absorption by your own skin.* If the patient has an infectious skin condition, use sterile gloves and dispose of old dressings appropriately.

■ Don't apply ointments to mucous membranes as liberally as you would to skin *because mucous membranes are usually moist and absorb ointment more quickly than skin does.* Also, don't apply too much ointment to any skin area *because it might cause irritation and discomfort, stain clothing and bedding, and make removal difficult.*

■ Never apply ointment to the eyelids or ear canal unless ordered. *The ointment may congeal and occlude the tear duct or ear canal.*

■ Inspect the treated area frequently for signs of an adverse reaction, such as an allergic reaction.

- When applying an aerosol spray or powder, make sure to prevent direct inhalation of the medication by the patient.

Patient teaching

Teach the patient how to apply the medication, if appropriate. Teach about the medication's potential adverse effects.

Complications

Skin irritation, a rash, or an allergic reaction may occur.

Documentation

Document the name of the medication, the dose, and the date and time it was administered in the patient's medication administration record. Include the route and site used. Document the appearance and integrity of the skin before administration. Record the presence or absence of adverse reactions and whether the practitioner was notified. Document the patient's response to and tolerance of therapy. Include any patient teaching.

REFERENCES

1 Westbrook, J., et al. (2010). Association of interruptions with an increased risk and severity of medication administration errors. *Archives of Internal Medicine, 170,* 683–690. (Level IV)

2 Institute for Safe Medication Practices. (2013). Side tracks on the safety express: Interruptions lead to errors and unfinished...Wait, what was I doing? *Nurse Advise-ERR, 11*(2), 1–4. Accessed May 2015 via the Web at https://www.ismp.org/Newsletters/acutecare/showarticle.aspx?id=37

3 American Osteopathic Association. (2014). Standard 16.01.03. *Healthcare Facilities Accreditation Program: Accreditation requirements for acute care hospitals.* Chicago, IL: American Osteopathic Association. (Level VII)

4 The Joint Commission. (2015). Standard MM.06.01.01. *Comprehensive accreditation manual for hospitals: The official handbook.* Oakbrook Terrace, IL: The Joint Commission. (Level VII)

5 Centers for Medicare & Medicaid Services, Department of Health and Human Services. (2014). Condition of participation: Nursing services. 42 C.F.R. § 482.23(c).

6 The Joint Commission. (2015). Standard NPSG.07.01.01. *Comprehensive accreditation manual for hospitals: The official handbook.* Oakbrook Terrace, IL: The Joint Commission. (Level VII)

7 Centers for Disease Control and Prevention. (2002). Guideline for hand hygiene in health-care settings: Recommendations of the Healthcare Infection Control Practices Advisory Committee and the HICPAC/SHEA/APIC/IDSA Hand Hygiene Task Force. *MMWR Recommendations and Reports, 51*(RR-16), 1–45. Accessed May 2015 via the Web at http://www.cdc.gov/mmwr/pdf/rr/rr5116.pdf (Level II)

8 World Health Organization. (2009). "WHO guidelines on hand hygiene in health care: First global patient safety challenge, clean care is safer care" [Online]. Accessed May 2015 via the Web at http://whqlibdoc.who.int/publications/2009/9789241597906_eng.pdf (Level IV)

9 American Osteopathic Association. (2014). Standard 07.01.21. *Healthcare Facilities Accreditation Program: Accreditation requirements for acute care hospitals.* Chicago, IL: American Osteopathic Association. (Level VII)

10 Centers for Medicare & Medicaid Services, Department of Health and Human Services. (2014). Condition of participation: Infection control. 42 C.F.R. § 482.42.

11 The Joint Commission. (2015). Standard NPSG.01.01.01. *Comprehensive accreditation manual for hospitals: The official handbook.* Oakbrook Terrace, IL: The Joint Commission. (Level VII)

12 Centers for Medicare & Medicaid Services, Department of Health and Human Services. (2014). Condition of participation: Patient's rights. 42 C.F.R. § 482.13(c)(1).

13 American Osteopathic Association. (2014). Standard 15.01.16. *Healthcare Facilities Accreditation Program: Accreditation requirements for acute care hospitals.* Chicago, IL: American Osteopathic Association. (Level VII)

14 Siegel, J. D., et al. (2007). "2007 guideline for isolation precautions: Preventing transmission of infectious agents in healthcare settings" [Online]. Accessed May 2015 via the Web at http://www.cdc.gov/hicpac/pdf/isolation/Isolation2007.pdf (Level II)

15 American Osteopathic Association. (2014). Standard 07.01.10. *Healthcare Facilities Accreditation Program: Accreditation requirements for acute care hospitals.* Chicago, IL: American Osteopathic Association. (Level VII)

16 The Joint Commission. (2015). Standard RC.01.03.01. *Comprehensive accreditation manual for hospitals: The official handbook.* Oakbrook Terrace, IL: The Joint Commission. (Level VII)

17 American Osteopathic Association. (2014). Standard 10.00.03. *Healthcare Facilities Accreditation Program: Accreditation requirements for acute care hospitals.* Chicago, IL: American Osteopathic Association. (Level VII)

18 Centers for Medicare & Medicaid Services, Department of Health and Human Services. (2014). Condition of participation: Medical record services. 42 C.F.R. § 482.24(b).

ADDITIONAL REFERENCE

Nettina, S. M. (2014). *Lippincott manual of nursing practice* (10th ed.). Philadelphia, PA: Wolters Kluwer.

TRACHEAL CUFF–PRESSURE MEASUREMENT

When inflated properly, an endotracheal (ET) or tracheostomy cuff provides a closed system for mechanical ventilation, allowing the delivery of the desired tidal volume to the patient's lungs. To function properly, the cuff must exert enough pressure on the tracheal wall to seal the airway without compromising the blood supply to the tracheal mucosa.

The ideal pressure (known as *minimal occlusive volume*) is the lowest amount needed to seal the airway. Many authorities recommend maintaining a cuff pressure lower than capillary perfusion pressure, which typically ranges from 25 to 30 mm Hg; they recommend inflating the cuff to 20 to 25 mm Hg.[1,2,3]

When cuff pressure is inadequate, oropharyngeal secretions can leak around the cuff, increasing the risk of ventilator-associated pneumonia.[3] Overinflation of the cuff can cause tracheal necrosis, tracheomalacia, tracheoinnominate artery fistula, tracheal ulceration, tracheal fibrosis, tracheal stenosis, and tracheoesophageal fistula.[4] Malpositioning the tracheostomy or ET tube or inserting a tube that's too small in diameter can also cause high cuff pressure, resulting in overfilling the cuff to achieve a seal in the trachea.[5] Actual cuff pressure varies with each patient, the type of tracheostomy tube, and the mode of ventilation.[6] To keep pressure within safe limits, minimal occlusive volume should be measured at least once each shift or at an interval determined by the facility. A nurse or respiratory therapist can measure cuff pressure.

Equipment

10-mL syringe ▪ three-way stopcock ▪ cuff pressure manometer ▪ stethoscope ▪ suction equipment ▪ handheld resuscitation bag ▪ oxygen source and tubing ▪ gloves ▪ hospital-grade disinfectant.

Preparation of equipment

Assemble all equipment at the patient's bedside. If measuring with a blood pressure manometer, attach the syringe to one stopcock port; then attach the tubing from the manometer to another port of the stopcock. Turn off the stopcock port where you'll be connecting the pilot balloon cuff *so that air can't escape from the cuff.* Use the syringe to instill air into the manometer tubing until the pressure reading reaches 10 mm Hg. *Doing so prevents sudden cuff deflation when you open the stopcock to the cuff and the manometer.*

Implementation

- Verify the practitioner's order.
- Gather and prepare the equipment.
- Perform hand hygiene.[7,8,9,10,11]
- Put on gloves.[12,13]

■ Confirm the patient's identity using at least two patient identifiers.[14]
■ Explain the procedure to the patient *to allay his fears and enhance cooperation.*
■ Hyperoxygenate the patient, if necessary. *Hyperoxygenation is recommended in critically ill patients who require full ventilator support; however, its benefit is unclear in patients who don't require full support.*[4,15]
■ Suction the ET or tracheostomy tube and the patient's oropharynx *to remove accumulated secretions above the cuff.*[6,16,17] (See the "Tracheal suctioning, intubated patient" procedure, page 752.)
■ Attach the cuff pressure manometer to the pilot balloon port.
■ Place the diaphragm of the stethoscope over the trachea and listen for an air leak (as shown below). Keep in mind that a smooth, hollow sound indicates a sealed airway; a loud, gurgling sound indicates an air leak.

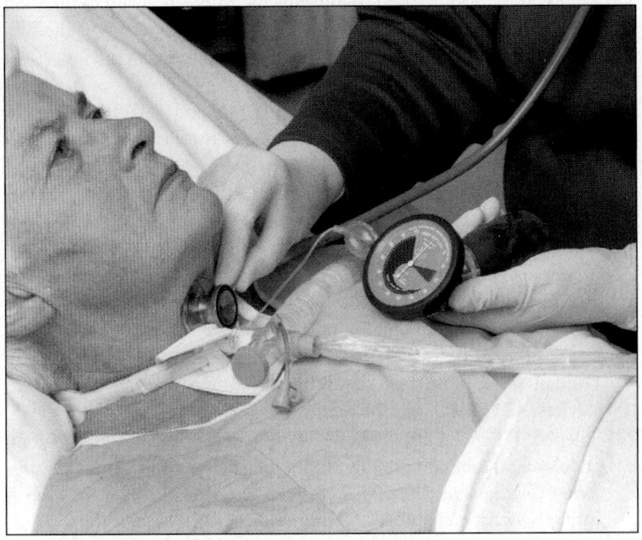

■ If you don't hear an air leak, press the red button under the dial of the cuff pressure manometer to slowly release air from the balloon on the tracheal tube (as shown below). Auscultate for an air leak.

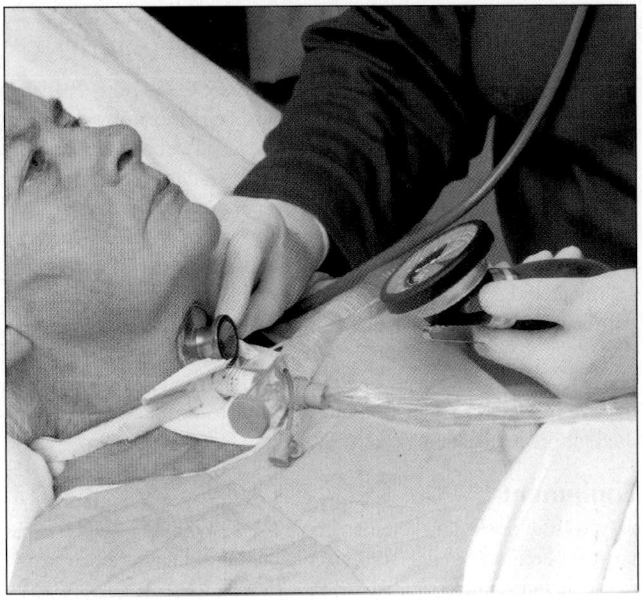

■ As soon as you hear an air leak, release the red button and gently squeeze the handle of the cuff pressure manometer to inflate the cuff (as shown on top right). Continue to add air to the cuff until you no longer hear an air leak.

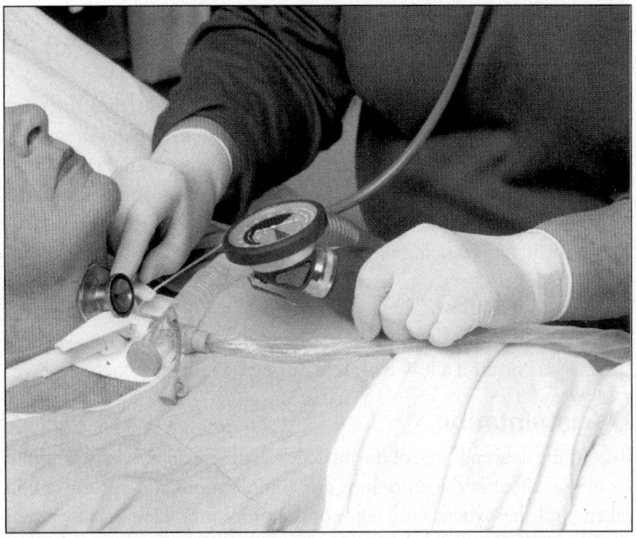

■ When the air leak ceases, read the dial on the cuff pressure manometer (as shown below). This number is the minimal pressure required to effectively occlude the trachea around the tracheal tube. In many cases, this pressure will fall within 20 to 25 mm Hg on the manometer dial.[6]

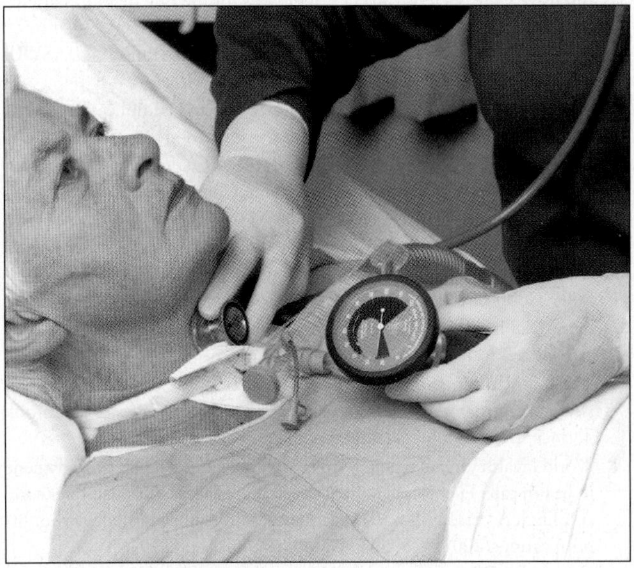

■ Disconnect the cuff pressure manometer from the pilot balloon port.
■ Remove and discard your gloves.[12]
■ Perform hand hygiene.[7,8,9,10,11]
■ Clean and disinfect your stethoscope and manometer 18 using a disinfectant pad.[19,20]
■ Perform hand hygiene.[7,8,9,10,11]
■ Document the procedure.[21,22,23]

Special considerations

■ Note that cuff pressure values vary and decrease over time. Unless continuous monitoring is performed or an automatic regulating device is attached, they can be difficult to maintain within the therapeutic range because of changes in body position, head alignment, tube migration, coughing, lung compliance, and airway and intrathoracic pressures.[24] Frequent routine assessments of cuff pressure are recommended, but optimal frequency hasn't been determined.[25]
■ Keep in mind that some patients require less pressure, whereas others require more pressure. Maintaining the cuff pressure at the lowest possible level will minimize cuff-related problems.

■ When measuring cuff pressure, keep the connection between the measuring device and the pilot balloon port tight *to avoid an air leak that could compromise cuff pressure.*
■ If you're using a stopcock, don't leave the manometer in the OFF position *because air will leak from the cuff if the syringe accidentally comes off.*
■ Note the volume of air needed to inflate the cuff. A gradual increase in this volume indicates tracheal dilation or erosion. A sudden increase in volume indicates rupture of the cuff and requires immediate reintubation if the patient is being ventilated.

Complications

Aspiration of upper airway secretions, underventilation, or coughing spasms may occur if a leak is created during cuff pressure measurement.

Documentation

Record the date and time of the procedure, cuff pressure, total amount of air in the cuff after the procedure, any complications and nursing action taken, and the patient's tolerance of the procedure. Document patient teaching performed and the patient's understanding of that teaching.

References

1 Kacmarek, R. M., et al. (2013). *Egan's fundamentals of respiratory care* (10th ed.). St. Louis, MO: Mosby.
2 Intensive Care Society. (2011). "Standards for the care of adult patients with a temporary tracheostomy: Standards and guidelines" [Online]. Accessed May 2015 via the Web at http://www.aeo.org.ec/GUIASYREVISIONES/TRAQUEOSTOMIA.pdf (Level VII)
3 Morris, L. L., et al. (2013). Tracheostomy care and complications in the intensive care unit. *Critical Care Nurse, 33*(5), 18–31.
4 Morris, L. L., & Afifi, M. S. (Eds.). (2010). *Tracheostomies: The complete guide.* New York, NY: Springer Publishing Company.
5 Regan, E. N., & Dallachiesa, L. (2009). How to care for a patient with a tracheostomy. *Nursing, 39*(8), 34–39. Accessed May 2015 via the Web at http://www.nursingcenter.com/lnc/pdf?AID=926437&an=00152193-200908000-00016&Journal_ID=54016&Issue_ID=926406
6 Lynn-McHale Wiegand, D. (Ed.). (2011). *AACN procedure manual for critical care* (6th ed.). St. Louis, MO: Saunders.
7 The Joint Commission. (2015). Standard NPSG.07.01.01. *Comprehensive accreditation manual for hospitals: The official handbook.* Oakbrook Terrace, IL: The Joint Commission. (Level VII)
8 World Health Organization. (2009). "WHO guidelines on hand hygiene in health care: First global patient safety challenge, clean care is safer care" [Online]. Accessed May 2015 via the Web at http://whqlibdoc.who.int/publications/2009/9789241597906_eng.pdf (Level IV)
9 Centers for Disease Control and Prevention. (2002). Guideline for hand hygiene in health-care settings: Recommendations of the Healthcare Infection Control Practices Advisory Committee and the HICPAC/SHEA/APIC/IDSA Hand Hygiene Task Force. *MMWR Recommendations and Reports, 51*(RR-16), 1–45. Accessed May 2015 via the Web at http://www.cdc.gov/mmwr/pdf/rr/rr5116.pdf (Level II)
10 American Osteopathic Association. (2014). Standard 07.01.21. *Healthcare Facilities Accreditation Program: Accreditation requirements for acute care hospitals.* Chicago, IL: American Osteopathic Association. (Level VII)
11 Centers for Medicare & Medicaid Services, Department of Health and Human Services. (2014). Condition of participation: Infection control. 42 C.F.R. § 482.42.
12 Siegel, J. D., et al. (2007). "2007 guideline for isolation precautions: Preventing transmission of infectious agents in healthcare settings" [Online]. Accessed May 2015 via the Web at http://www.cdc.gov/hicpac/pdf/isolation/Isolation2007.pdf (Level II)
13 American Osteopathic Association. (2014). Standard 07.01.10. *Healthcare Facilities Accreditation Program: Accreditation requirements for acute care hospitals.* Chicago, IL: American Osteopathic Association. (Level VII)
14 The Joint Commission. (2015). Standard NPSG.07.01.01. *Comprehensive accreditation manual for hospitals: The official handbook.* Oakbrook Terrace, IL: The Joint Commission. (Level VII)
15 American Association for Respiratory Care (AARC). (2010). AARC clinical practice guidelines: Endotracheal suctioning of mechanically ventilated patients with artificial airways 2010. *Respiratory Care, 55,* 758–764. Accessed May 2015 via the Web at http://www.rcjournal.com/cpgs/pdf/06.10.0758.pdf (Level VII)
16 American Association of Critical-Care Nurses. (2008). "AACN practice alert: Ventilator associated pneumonia" [Online]. Accessed May 2015 via the Web at http://www.aacn.org/WD/Practice/Docs/PracticeAlerts/Ventilator%20Associated%20Pneumonia%201-2008.pdf (Level VII)
17 American Osteopathic Association. (2014). Standard 07.01.02. *Healthcare Facilities Accreditation Program: Accreditation requirements for acute care hospitals.* Chicago, IL: American Osteopathic Association. (Level VII)
18 Spiegel, J. E. (2010). "Endotracheal tube cuffs: Design and function" [Online]. Accessed May 2015 via the Web at http://www.csen.com/cuff.pdf
19 Rutala, W. A., et al. (2008). "Guideline for disinfection and sterilization in healthcare facilities, 2008" [Online]. Accessed May 2015 via the Web at http://www.cdc.gov/hicpac/pdf/guidelines/Disinfection_Nov_2008.pdf (Level I)
20 American Osteopathic Association. (2014). Standard 07.02.03. *Healthcare Facilities Accreditation Program: Accreditation requirements for acute care hospitals.* Chicago, IL: American Osteopathic Association. (Level VII)
21 The Joint Commission. (2015). Standard RC.01.03.01. *Comprehensive accreditation manual for hospitals: The official handbook.* Oakbrook Terrace, IL: The Joint Commission. (Level VII)
22 American Osteopathic Association. (2014). Standard 10.00.03. *Healthcare Facilities Accreditation Program: Accreditation requirements for acute care hospitals.* Chicago, IL: American Osteopathic Association. (Level VII)
23 Centers for Medicare & Medicaid Services, Department of Health and Human Services. (2014). Condition of participation: Medical record services. 42 C.F.R. § 482.24(b).
24 Sole, M. L., et al. (2011). Evaluation of an intervention to maintain endotracheal tube cuff pressure within therapeutic range. *American Journal of Critical Care, 20,* 109–117. Accessed May 2015 via the Web at http://www.aacn.org/WD/CETests/Media/A1120023.pdf (Level II)
25 Rose, L., & Redl, L. (Ed.). (2008). Survey of cuff management practices in intensive care units in Australia and New Zealand. *American Journal of Critical Care, 17,* 428–435. Accessed May 2015 via the Web at http://ajcc.aacnjournals.org/content/17/5/428.full.pdf+html (Level VI)

TRACHEAL SUCTIONING, INTUBATED PATIENT

Tracheal suction is used to remove pulmonary secretions from a patient's artificial airway to prevent obstruction. Maintaining a patent airway is essential to promote the optimal exchange of oxygen and carbon dioxide and to prevent pneumonia, which can result from the pooling of secretions.[1,2]

According to the American Association for Respiratory Care (AARC) guidelines, the patient should be hyperoxygenated with 100% oxygen for 30 to 60 seconds before tracheal suctioning is performed using sterile technique.[1,3] Each suctioning event, which includes the placement and withdrawal of the suction catheter, should take no longer than 15 seconds.[3] Suction pressure should be set at the lowest possible level that clears secretions effectively.[4] After suctioning, the patient should be hyperoxygenated again for 1 minute or longer, using the same technique used for preoxygenation.[3]

Equipment

Oxygen source ■ handheld resuscitation bag with tubing ■ suction apparatus ■ collection container ■ connecting tubing ■ suction catheter kit (a sterile suction catheter, one sterile glove, one clean glove, goggles, and a disposable sterile solution container) ■ 1-L bottle of sterile water or normal saline solution ■ disinfectant pad ■ stethoscope ■ blood pressure monitoring equipment ■ pulse oximeter ■ Optional: gown, mask and goggles or mask with face shield, sterile towel, 10-mL syringe, positive end-expiratory pressure (PEEP) valve, extra suction catheter, sterile gloves.

Preparation of equipment

Choose an appropriately sized suction catheter. The catheter diameter should be no larger than half the inside diameter of the tracheostomy or endotracheal (ET) tube *to minimize hypoxia during suctioning.* (A #12 or #14 French catheter may be used for an 8-mm or larger tube.)[3,4,5,6] Place the suction equipment on the patient's overbed table or bedside stand. Position the table or stand on your preferred side of the bed *to facilitate suctioning.*

Attach the collection container to the suction apparatus and the connecting tube to the collection container. Label and date the normal saline solution or sterile water bottle. Attach the handheld resuscitation bag to the oxygen source, and make sure it's readily available. Attach the PEEP valve to the handheld resuscitation bag if indicated.

Implementation

- Verify the practitioner's order, if needed.
- Gather the appropriate equipment.
- Perform hand hygiene.[1,7,8,9,10,11]
- Confirm the patient's identity using at least two patient identifiers.[12]
- Assess the patient's vital signs, breath sounds, and general appearance, and observe for copious secretions *to establish a baseline for comparison after tracheal suctioning.* Review the patient's arterial blood gas values and oxygen saturation levels, if available. Attach the patient to a pulse oximeter *to assess oxygen saturation before and after the procedure.*[3] Evaluate the patient's ability to cough and deep-breathe *to help move secretions up the tracheobronchial tree.*[3]
- Explain the procedure to the patient, even if he's unresponsive. Tell him that suctioning usually causes transient coughing or gagging but that coughing helps to remove secretions. Continue to reassure the patient throughout the procedure *to minimize anxiety, promote relaxation, and decrease oxygen demand.*
- Put on a mask and goggles or mask with face shield and other personal protective equipment as appropriate.[3,13,14]
- Unless contraindicated, elevate the head of the bed at a 30- to 45-degree angle *to promote lung expansion and productive coughing and to prevent aspiration.*[2,15,16,17]
- Remove the top from the bottle of normal saline solution or water.
- Open the package containing the sterile solution container.
- Using strict sterile technique, open the suction catheter kit and put on the gloves. If using individual supplies, open the suction catheter and the gloves, placing first the clean (nonsterile) glove on your nondominant hand and then the sterile glove on your dominant hand.[1,3]
- Using your nondominant (nonsterile) hand, pour the normal saline solution or sterile water into the disposable sterile solution container.
- Place a sterile towel over the patient's chest, if desired, *to provide an additional sterile area.*
- Using your dominant (sterile) hand, remove the catheter from its wrapper. Keep it coiled *to prevent it from touching a nonsterile object.*
- Using your nondominant hand to manipulate the connecting tubing, attach the suction catheter to the tubing (as shown below).

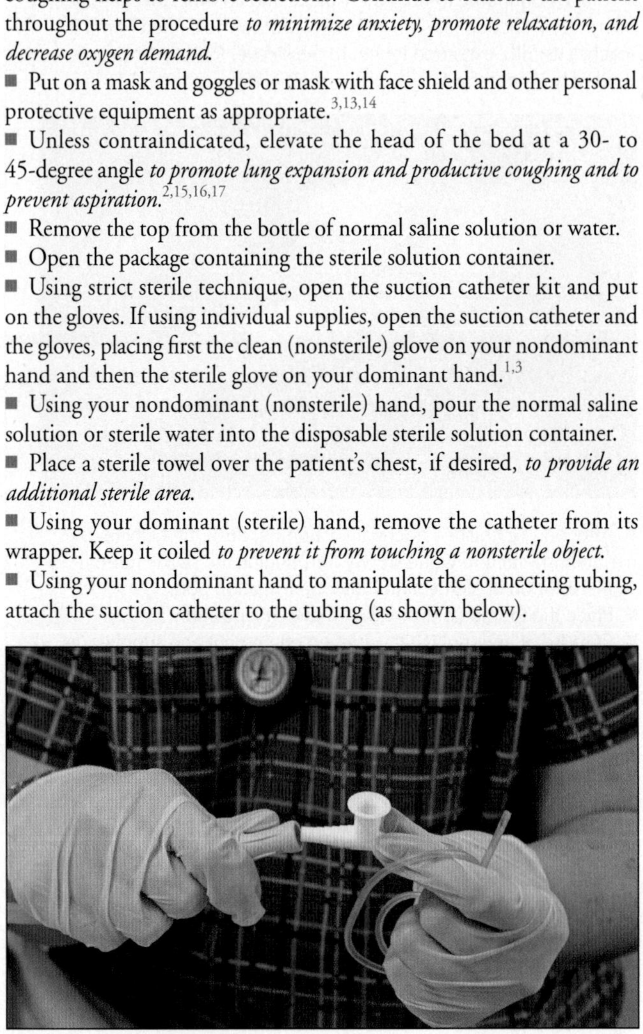

- Using your nondominant hand, set the suction pressure. Pressure should be set at the lowest possible level that clears secretions effectively.[3,4] *Higher pressures don't enhance secretion removal and may cause traumatic injury.* Occlude the suction port *to assess suction pressure.*[3]

NURSING ALERT *Experts recommend using suction pressures of up to 120 mm Hg for open tracheal suction systems and of up to 150 mm Hg for closed systems.*[3,6]

- Dip the catheter tip in the normal saline solution or sterile water (as shown below) *to lubricate the outside of the catheter and reduce tissue trauma during insertion.*

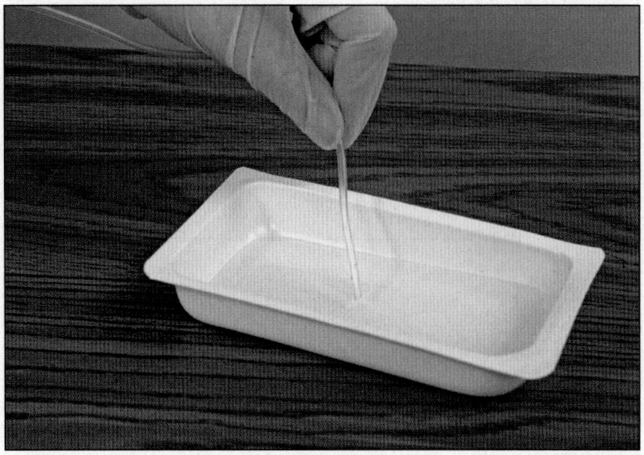

- With the catheter tip in the sterile normal saline solution or sterile water, occlude the suction control valve with the thumb of your nondominant hand (as shown below). Suction a small amount of solution or water through the catheter *to lubricate the inside of the catheter, which facilitates passage of secretions through it.*

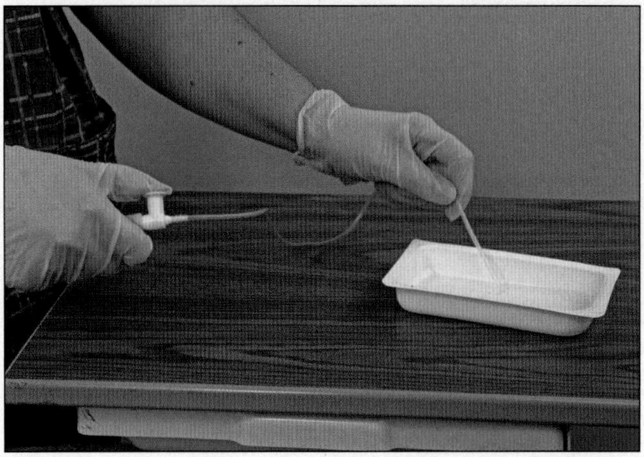

- If you're using a closed tracheal suction system, see *Closed tracheal suctioning.*
- Hyperoxygenate the patient with 100% oxygen for 30 to 60 seconds.[2,3,4,18] You can hyperoxygenate the patient using a ventilator by pressing the hyperoxygenate button or by increasing the baseline fraction of inspired oxygen (FIO_2) level. If these methods aren't available, disconnect the ventilator from the tracheostomy tube, attach the handheld resuscitation bag to the tracheostomy tube, and administer five to six breaths over 30 seconds.[18]
- Using your nondominant hand, disconnect the patient from the ventilator.
- Using your dominant hand, advance the suction catheter gently to the premeasured distance needed for insertion (generally, the length of the adapter plus the length of the tracheostomy tube) without applying

Closed tracheal suctioning

A closed tracheal suction system can ease removal of secretions and reduce patient complications. The system—which consists of a sterile suction catheter in a clear plastic sleeve—allows the patient to remain connected to the ventilator during suctioning, letting the ventilator maintain tidal volume, oxygen concentration, and positive end-expiratory pressure, which reduces the risk of suction-induced hypoxemia.

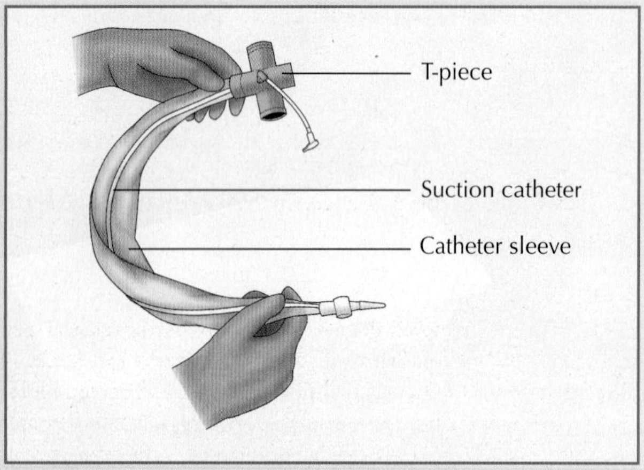

Because the catheter remains in a protective sleeve, this system also reduces risk of infection, even when the same catheter is used many times.[1,2] The caregiver doesn't need to touch the catheter, and the ventilator circuit remains closed. Closed tracheal suctioning doesn't increase or decrease the occurrence of ventilator-associated pneumonia[3] and it also reduces the risk of spraying of respiratory secretions, especially during suction-induced coughing.[18]

In patients receiving intermittent mandatory mechanical ventilation, closed tracheal suctioning may reduce arterial desaturation and eliminate the need for preoxygenation.[3]

Research doesn't suggest the best practice for closed or open suctioning technique, nor does determine that a closed system is better or worse than an open system for reducing bacterial colonization and ventilator-associated pneumonia.[19] Closed tracheal suctioning also may produce increased negative airway pressure when certain ventilatory modes are used, increasing the risk of atelectasis and hypoxemia.

Implementation

To perform the procedure, gather the equipment for the closed tracheal suction system, which consists of a suction control valve, a T-piece to connect the artificial airway to the ventilator breathing circuit, and a catheter sleeve that encloses the catheter and has connections at each end for the control valve and the T-piece. Then follow these steps:

- Perform hand hygiene.[1,7,8,9,10,11]
- Put on gloves.[13,14]
- Remove the closed suction system from its wrapping.
- Attach the control valve to the connecting tubing.
- Depress the suction control valve, and keep it depressed while setting the suction pressure to the desired level.
- Connect the T-piece to the ventilator breathing circuit; make sure that the irrigation port is closed. Then connect the T-piece to the patient's ET or tracheostomy tube.
- Hyperoxygenate the patient with 100% oxygen for 30 to 60 seconds.[2,3,4,18]
- Steadying the T-piece, use the thumb and index finger of the other hand to advance the catheter through the ET or tracheostomy tube and into the patient's tracheobronchial tree (as shown). It may be necessary to gently retract the catheter sleeve as you advance the catheter.

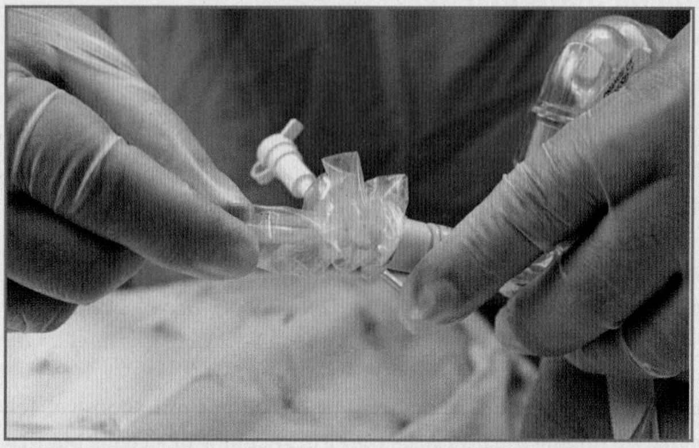

- While continuing to hold the T-piece and control valve, apply intermittent suction (as shown) and withdraw the catheter until it reaches its fully extended length in the sleeve. Repeat the procedure only if necessary.

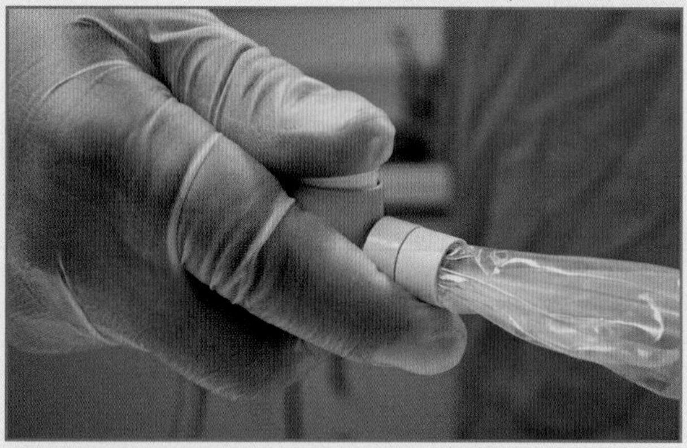

- After you've finished tracheal suctioning, flush the catheter by maintaining suction while slowly introducing the sterile normal saline solution or sterile water into the irrigation port.
- Place the thumb control valve in the OFF position.
- Dispose of and replace the suction equipment and supplies, as needed.
- Remove and discard your gloves.[13,14]
- Perform hand hygiene.[1,7,8,9,10,11]

suction. *Measuring the depth ensures that the suction catheter doesn't extend beyond the end of the tracheostomy or ET tube, which may cause trauma to the tracheal mucosa.*[3,20]

NURSING ALERT *Deep tracheal suctioning hasn't been shown to be superior to shallow tracheal suctioning and may be associated with more adverse events.*[3]

- After inserting the suction catheter, apply suction intermittently by removing and replacing the thumb of your nondominant hand over the suction control valve. Simultaneously use your dominant hand to withdraw the catheter as you roll it between your thumb and forefinger. *This rotating motion prevents the catheter from pulling tissue into the tube as it exits, avoiding tissue trauma.*

■ Use your nondominant hand to stabilize the tip of the tracheostomy tube as you withdraw the catheter *to prevent mucous membrane irritation or accidental extubation.* The suctioning event should take no longer than 15 seconds.[3]

■ Resume oxygen delivery by reconnecting the source of oxygen or ventilation and hyperoxygenating the patient's lungs with 100% oxygen for 30 to 60 seconds before continuing tracheal suctioning *to prevent or relieve hypoxia.*[2,3,18]

■ Observe the patient, and allow him to rest for a few minutes before the next tracheal suctioning. The timing of each suctioning and the length of each rest period depend on the patient's tolerance of the procedure and the absence of complications. Encourage the patient to cough between suctioning attempts *to enhance secretion removal.*

■ Observe the secretions. Normal sputum is watery and tends to be sticky. If the secretions are thick, clear the catheter periodically by dipping the tip in the sterile normal saline solution or sterile water and applying suction. Tenacious or thick sputum usually indicates dehydration. Also observe for color variations. Normal sputum is white or translucent; discolored secretions (yellow, green) may indicate infection, brown usually indicates old blood, and red indicates fresh blood. When sputum contains blood, note whether it's streaked or well mixed. Also, note how often blood appears.

■ If the patient's heart rate and rhythm are being monitored, observe for arrhythmias. If they occur, stop suctioning and ventilate the patient.

■ After tracheal suctioning, hyperoxygenate the patient with 100% oxygen for at least 1 minute using the same technique described earlier.[2,3,18]

■ Readjust the FIO_2 and, for ventilated patients, the parameters and alarms to the ordered settings. Set alarm limits according to the patient's condition, an ensure that the alarms are turned on, functioning properly, and audible to staff.[21,22,23]

■ After suctioning the lower airway, assess the patient's need for upper airway suctioning. (See the "Oronasopharyngeal suction" procedure, page 569.) Always change the suction catheter and sterile glove before resuctioning the lower airway, if necessary, *to avoid introducing microorganisms into the lower airway.*[1]

■ Clear the connecting tubing by aspirating the remaining sterile normal saline solution or sterile water.

■ Remove your gloves and other personal protective equipment and discard used supplies in the appropriate receptacles.[13] Replace supplies as needed.

■ Perform hand hygiene.[1,7,8,9,10,11]

■ Maintain the head of the patient's bed at 30 to 45 degrees, if the patient's condition allows, *to prevent ventilator-associated pneumonia.*[15,16,24]

■ Auscultate the patient's breath sounds bilaterally, obtain vital signs, and monitor oxygen saturation levels, if indicated, *to assess the procedure's effectiveness.*

■ Perform hand hygiene.[1,7,8,9,10,11]

■ Clean and disinfect your stethoscope using a disinfectant pad.[25,26]

■ Perform hand hygiene.[1,7,8,9,10,11]

■ Document the procedure.[27,28,29]

Special considerations

■ The Joint Commission has issued a sentinel event alert concerning medical device alarm safety *because alarm-related events have been associated with permanent loss of function or death.* Among the major contributing factors noted were improper alarm settings, alarms inappropriately turned off, and alarm signals not audible to staff. Ensure that alarm limits are set appropriately and that alarms are turned on, functioning properly, and audible to staff. Follow facility guidelines for preventing alarm fatigue.[30]

■ Studies show that instillation of normal saline solution into the trachea before suctioning may stimulate the patient's cough but doesn't liquefy his secretions. Keeping the patient adequately hydrated and using bronchial hygiene techniques seem to have a greater effect on mobilizing secretions. Instilling normal saline solution may also decrease arterial and mixed venous oxygenation and contribute to lower airway contamination, increasing the risk of ventilator-associated pneumonia.[3,4,6,18]

■ Don't allow the collection container on the suction machine to become more than three-quarters full *to keep from damaging the machine.*

■ Change the suction catheter and sleeve and ventilator circuit tubing only when visibly soiled *to avoid frequent disruptions in the closed circuit, which increase the risk of ventilator-associated pneumonia.*[16]

■ If the cuff of the ET or tracheostomy tube is inflated and needs to be deflated, suction the lower airway using the above procedure, then suction the upper airway before deflating the cuff using a syringe.[12]

Patient teaching

Teach the patient and his family about measures to prevent ventilator-associated pneumonia, and involve them in maintaining the head of the bed at 30 to 45 degrees.[17] If the patient will be discharged with an artificial airway, educate the patient and his family members on performing tracheal suctioning.

Complications

Because oxygen is removed along with secretions during tracheal suctioning, the patient may experience hypoxemia and dyspnea. Anxiety may alter respiratory patterns during the procedure. Cardiac arrhythmias can result from hypoxia and stimulation of the vagus nerve in the tracheobronchial tree. Tracheal or bronchial trauma can result from traumatic or prolonged suctioning.

Patients with compromised cardiovascular or pulmonary status are at risk for hypoxemia, arrhythmias, hypertension, or hypotension. Patients who are taking anticoagulants, have undergone a tracheostomy recently, have a blood dyscrasia, or who have a history of nasopharyngeal bleeding are at increased risk for bleeding as a result of tracheal suctioning. Use caution when suctioning patients who have increased intracranial pressure because suction may further increase pressure.

If the patient experiences laryngospasm or bronchospasm (rare complications) during tracheal suctioning, disconnect the suction catheter from the connecting tubing and allow the catheter to act as an airway. Discuss with the patient's practitioner the use of bronchodilators or lidocaine to reduce the risk of this complication.

Documentation

Record the date and time of the procedure; the technique used; the reason for tracheal suctioning; the amount, color, consistency, and odor (if any) of the secretions; your assessment findings; any complications and nursing actions taken; and pertinent data regarding the patient's subjective response to the procedure. Document any teaching provided to the patient and family. If the patient will be performing the procedure at home, document return demonstration and the patient's and family members' understanding of the teaching provided.

REFERENCES

1 Centers for Disease Control and Prevention. (2004). Guidelines for preventing health-care–associated pneumonia, 2003: Recommendations of CDC and the Healthcare Infection Control Practices Advisory Committee. *MMWR Recommendations and Reports, 53*(RR-3), 1–32. Accessed May 2015 via the Web at http://www.cdc.gov/mmwr/pdf/rr/rr5303.pdf (Level II)

2 American Association of Critical-Care Nurses. (2008). "AACN practice alert: Ventilator associated pneumonia" [Online]. Accessed May 2015 via the Web at http://www.aacn.org/WD/Practice/Docs/PracticeAlerts/Ventilator%20Associated%20Pneumonia%201-2008.pdf (Level VII)

3 American Association for Respiratory Care (AARC). (2010). AARC clinical practice guidelines: Endotracheal suctioning of mechanically ventilated patients with artificial airways 2010. *Respiratory Care, 55,*

758–764. Accessed May 2015 via the Web at http://www.rcjournal.com/cpgs/pdf/06.10.0758.pdf (Level VII)
4 Mackenzie, S. et al. (2011). "Intensive Care Society Standards: Standards for the care of adult patients with a temporary tracheostomy" [Online]. Accessed May 2015 via the Web at http://www.aeo.org.ec/GUIASYREVISIONES/TRAQUEOSTOMIA.pdf (Level VII)
5 Morris, L. L., & Afifi, M. S. (Eds.). (2010). *Tracheostomies: The complete guide.* New York, NY: Springer.
6 Nance-Floyd, B. (2011). Tracheostomy care: An evidence-based guide to suctioning and dressing changes. *American Nurse Today, 6*(7), 14–16. Accessed May 2015 via the Web http://www.americannursetoday.com/assets/0/434/436/440/7986/7988/7992/8022/f17622e4-1fc4-4a5c-88b7-3cd329777cb7.pdf
7 Centers for Disease Control and Prevention. (2002). Guideline for hand hygiene in health-care settings: Recommendations of the Healthcare Infection Control Practices Advisory Committee and the HICPAC/SHEA/APIC/IDSA Hand Hygiene Task Force. *MMWR Recommendations and Reports, 51*(RR-16), 1–45. Accessed May 2015 via the Web at http://www.cdc.gov/mmwr/pdf/rr/rr5116.pdf (Level II)
8 The Joint Commission. (2015). Standard NPSG.07.01.01. *Comprehensive accreditation manual for hospitals: The official handbook.* Oakbrook Terrace, IL: The Joint Commission. (Level VII)
9 World Health Organization. (2009). "WHO guidelines on hand hygiene in health care: First global patient safety challenge, clean care is safer care" [Online]. Accessed May 2015 via the Web at http://whqlibdoc.who.int/publications/2009/9789241597906_eng.pdf (Level IV)
10 Centers for Medicare & Medicaid Services, Department of Health and Human Services. (2014). Condition of participation: Infection control. 42 C.F.R. § 482.42.
11 American Osteopathic Association. (2014). Standard 07.01.21. *Healthcare Facilities Accreditation Program: Accreditation requirements for acute care hospitals.* Chicago, IL: American Osteopathic Association. (Level VII)
12 The Joint Commission. (2015). Standard NPSG.01.01.01. *Comprehensive accreditation manual for hospitals: The official handbook.* Oakbrook Terrace, IL: The Joint Commission. (Level VII)
13 Siegel, J. D., et al. (2007). "2007 guideline for isolation precautions: Preventing transmission of infectious agents in healthcare settings" [Online]. Accessed May 2015 via the Web at http://www.cdc.gov/hicpac/pdf/isolation/Isolation2007.pdf (Level II)
14 American Osteopathic Association. (2014). Standard 07.01.10. *Healthcare Facilities Accreditation Program: Accreditation requirements for acute care hospitals.* Chicago, IL: American Osteopathic Association. (Level VII)
15 Association of Professionals in Infection Control and Epidemiology. (2009). "An APIC guide 2009: Guide to the elimination of ventilator-associated pneumonia" [Online]. Accessed May 2015 via the Web at http://www.apic.org/Resource_/EliminationGuideForm/18e326ad-b484-471c-9c35-6822a53ee4a2/File/VAP_09.pdf (Level IV)
16 Klompas, M., et al. (2014). Strategies to prevent ventilator-associated pneumonia in acute care hospitals: 2014 update. *Infection Control and Hospital Epidemiology, 35,* 915–936. Accessed May 2015 via the Web at http://www.jstor.org/stable/10.1086/677144 (Level II)
17 American Osteopathic Association. (2014). Standard 07.01.02. *Healthcare Facilities Accreditation Program: Accreditation requirements for acute care hospitals.* Chicago, IL: American Osteopathic Association. (Level VII)
18 Lynn-McHale Wiegand, D. (Ed.). (2011). *AACN procedure manual for critical care* (6th ed.). St. Louis, MO: Saunders.
19 Kjonegaard, R., et al. (2010). Current practices in airway management: A descriptive evaluation. *American Journal of Critical Care, 19,* 168–173. (Level VI)
20 Pedersen, C. M., et al. (2009). Endotracheal suctioning of the adult intubated patient—What is the evidence? *Intensive and Critical Care Nursing, 25,* 21–30. (Level V)
21 American Association of Critical-Care Nurses. (2013). "AACN practice alert: Alarm management" [Online]. Accessed May 2015 via the Web at http://www.aacn.org/wd/practice/docs/practicealerts/alarm-management-practice-alert.pdf (Level VII)
22 Graham, K. C., & Cvach, M. (2010). Monitor alarm fatigue: Standardizing use of physiological monitors and decreasing nuisance alarms. *American Journal of Critical Care, 19,* 28–37.
23 The Joint Commission. (2015). Standard NPSG.06.01.01. *Comprehensive accreditation manual for hospitals: The official handbook.* Oakbrook Terrace, IL: The Joint Commission. (Level VII)
24 Institute for Healthcare Improvement. (2012). *How-to guide: Prevent ventilator-associated pneumonia.* Cambridge, MA: Institute for Healthcare Improvement. (Level VII)
25 Rutala, W. A., et al. (2008). "Guideline for disinfection and sterilization in healthcare facilities, 2008" [Online]. Accessed May 2015 via the Web at http://www.cdc.gov/hicpac/pdf/guidelines/Disinfection_Nov_2008.pdf (Level I)
26 American Osteopathic Association. (2014). Standard 07.02.03. *Healthcare Facilities Accreditation Program: Accreditation requirements for acute care hospitals.* Chicago, IL: American Osteopathic Association. (Level VII)
27 The Joint Commission. (2015). Standard RC.01.03.01. *Comprehensive accreditation manual for hospitals: The official handbook.* Oakbrook Terrace, IL: The Joint Commission. (Level VII)
28 Centers for Medicare & Medicaid Services, Department of Health and Human Services. (2014). Condition of participation: Medical record services. 42 C.F.R. § 482.24(b).
29 American Osteopathic Association. (2014). Standard 10.00.03. *Healthcare Facilities Accreditation Program: Accreditation requirements for acute care hospitals.* Chicago, IL: American Osteopathic Association. (Level VII)
30 The Joint Commission. (2013). "Sentinel event alert: Medical device alarm safety in hospitals" [Online]. Accessed May 2015 via the Web at http://www.jointcommission.org/assets/1/18/SEA_50_alarms_4_5_13_FINAL1.PDF (Level VII)

ADDITIONAL REFERENCE

Morris, L. L., et al. (2013). Tracheostomy care and complications in the intensive care unit. *Critical Care Nurse, 33*(5), 18–31.

TRACHEOSTOMY AND VENTILATOR SPEAKING VALVE

Patients with a conventional tracheostomy tube can't speak because the cuffed tracheostomy tube that directs air into the lungs on inspiration expels air through the tracheostomy tube rather than the vocal cords, mouth, and nose. Providing a means of communication for such patients is crucial for their physical and emotional well-being. Nonverbal means of communicating, such as writing, lip-reading, alphabet boards, and gestures, can be frustrating for the patient and family members as well as for health care personnel.

The Passy-Muir tracheostomy and ventilator speaking valve (PMV) allows the ventilator-dependent patient to speak. The PMV is a positive-closure, one-way speaking valve developed by David Muir (a ventilator-dependent patient). It opens upon inspiration to allow the patient to inspire through the tracheostomy tube and then closes after inspiration, redirecting the exhaled air around the tube, through the vocal cords, and out of the mouth. Other speaking valves, such as the Montgomery Ventrach, the Shiley Phonate, are also available. Some have a closed valve like the PMV; others have different types of valves.[1]

Ideally, the tracheostomy should be cuffless; however, if the tube is cuffed, it must be *completely* deflated to enable the patient to exhale and to function safely.[1,2] For maximum airflow around the tube, the tube should be no larger than two-thirds the size of the tracheal lumen.

Short- and long-term adult, pediatric, and infant tracheostomy and ventilator-dependent patients may benefit from the use of a PMV. The PMV 005 is most commonly used by nonventilated tracheostomy patients, but it can be used by ventilator patients with rubber, nondisposable ventilator tubing. The PMV 007 fits easily into the ventilator tubing used by mechanically ventilated tracheostomy patients.[1] Both valves fit the 15-mm hub of adult, pediatric, and neonatal tracheostomy tubes and can be used by patients either on or off the ventilator.

Two other PMV valves are available: the PMV 2000 and the PMV 2001. Both of these valves are low-profile and low-resistance, feature the positive-closure design, and can be used on or off the ventilator. The PMV 2000 is clear in color and is used more readily in the home care setting because it's less noticeable. The PMV 2001 is a bright purple color and is used more often in health care facilities because the color is more noticeable. These valves also include safety ties that prevent valve loss if the patient inadvertently coughs the PMV out of the tracheostomy tube.

A PMV oxygen adapter is now available for use with the PMV 2000 series speaking valves. This adapter allows improved mobility and comfort for patients who require a tracheostomy tube, speaking valve, and low-flow supplemental oxygen.

PMV use is contraindicated in patients requiring significant ventilator support, such as those with a high respiratory rate and minute ventilation requirements, high fraction of inspired oxygen, positive end-expiratory pressure greater than 5 cm H_2O, respiratory distress, frequent bronchospasm, or air-trapping problems. It's also contraindicated in patients with pneumothorax with or without air leaks if there's a potential for increased lung pressures; a larger-diameter tracheostomy tube; a tracheostomy tube with inflated cuff or foam cuff; airway obstruction above the tracheostomy, such as bilateral vocal cord paralysis, severe tracheal or laryngeal stenosis, or tumor obstruction; copious, excessive, or thick secretions; paralysis of the lips, tongue, and other muscles involved in speech; or laryngectomy.[1,3,4]

PMV use requires a multidisciplinary team approach. A practitioner's order is required for placement of the PMV and sometimes for cuff deflation. The nurse, speech language pathologist, and respiratory therapist are responsible for monitoring and assessing the patient while he's using the PMV.[2] Ventilator adjustments for the ventilator-dependent tracheostomy patient are the respiratory therapist's responsibility. A speech-language pathologist should assess the patient's cognitive, language, and oral motor function and may also evaluate swallowing status and the risk for aspiration. The patient must also be involved in the decision about whether to use the PMV.

An initial trial assesses the patient's tolerance. He must understand how the PMV functions and what to expect during the trial. If he's anxious, especially during cuff deflation, he may be unwilling to use the valve, so he'll need emotional support. The patient shouldn't be left unsupervised with the valve in place until tolerance is determined.[1]

If the patient can't tolerate the PMV initially, the team should troubleshoot to determine the cause. Problem-solving to increase patient tolerance of the one-way speaking valve may include tracheostomy tube downsizing or continued therapeutic trials with implementation of strengthening programs to address respiration, voice, and swallowing.[2] Some patients are only able to wear the PMV for a few minutes at a time, building up time gradually, as tolerated. If repeated trials fail, the speech-language pathologist should assess the patient for other communication options.

Equipment

Appropriate-sized PMV ■ gloves ■ stethoscope ■ pulse oximeter ■ equipment to measure vital signs ■ suction equipment ■ handheld resuscitation bag ■ oxygen source ■ 10-mL luer-lock syringe ■ PMV instruction booklet ■ disinfectant pad ■ cuff-deflation warning sign.

Keep in mind that the PMV 005 is for a more ambulatory tracheostomy patient and can be used with flexible rubber tubing. The PMV 007 and PMV 2001 are more convenient to use with disposable ventilator tubing. Their color, which is different from the ventilator tubing, makes it easier to identify their position in the ventilator circuitry.

Preparation of equipment

Make sure that the oxygen source and handheld resuscitation bag are readily available at the patient's bedside.

Implementation

- Verify the practitioner's order.
- Gather the appropriate equipment.
- Perform hand hygiene.[5,6,7,8,9]
- Put on gloves.[10,11]
- Confirm the patient's identity using at least two patient identifiers.[12]
- Explain the procedure to the patient, and make sure that he's comfortable with the procedure before beginning. Provide him with written instructions included in the PMV booklet. Allay any fear and anxiety he might feel before proceeding. If this is the patient's first experience, coordinate the trial with the respiratory therapist and speech-language pathologist.[2]
- Elevate the head of the patient's bed about 45 degrees.
- Assess the patient's vital signs, oxygen saturation level, breath sounds, level of consciousness, work of breathing, and tracheal and oral secretions.[3]
- Perform tracheal and oral suctioning *to clear the airway of pooled secretions that could leak past the cuff after the cuff is deflated, increasing the patient's risk of pneumonia.*[3]
- Deflate the cuff slowly *so the patient can become accustomed to using his upper airways again.* Do this by attaching a 10-mL syringe to the tracheostomy tube's pilot balloon and removing the air until air can no longer be extracted and a vacuum is created (as shown below).

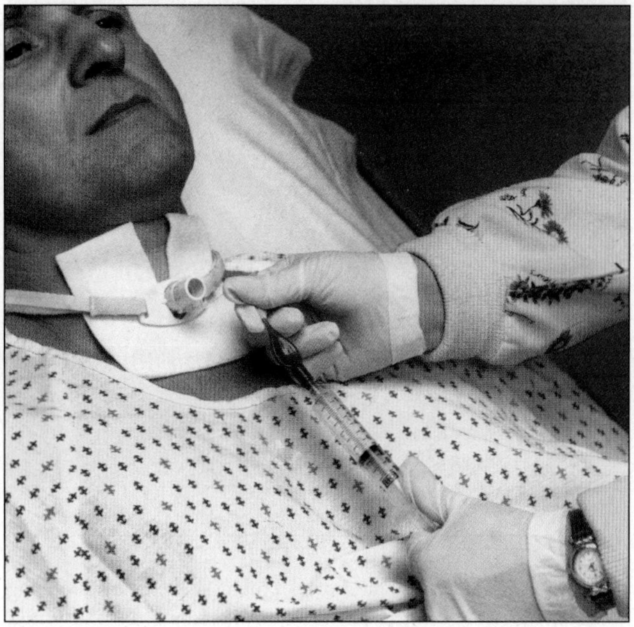

- Suction the trachea and oral cavity as needed. The tracheostomy cuff *must* be completely deflated before the PMV is placed.

NURSING ALERT ***Never place the PMV on the tracheostomy tube before deflating the cuff*** because the patient won't be able to breathe.

- Hold the PMV between your fingers. For a patient who isn't ventilator-dependent, attach the PMV to the hub of the existing tracheostomy hub with a quarter-turn twist (as shown on next page, top left).

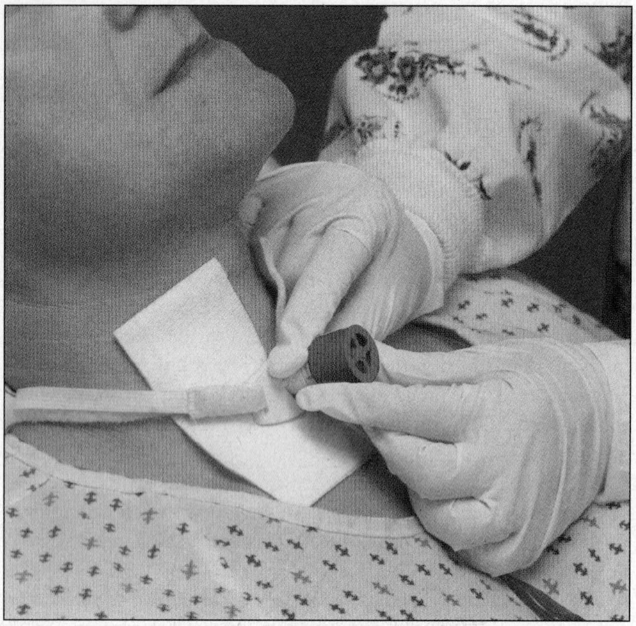

■ For the patient who is ventilator-dependent insert the PMV into the end of the wide-mouth, short-flex tubing (as shown below).

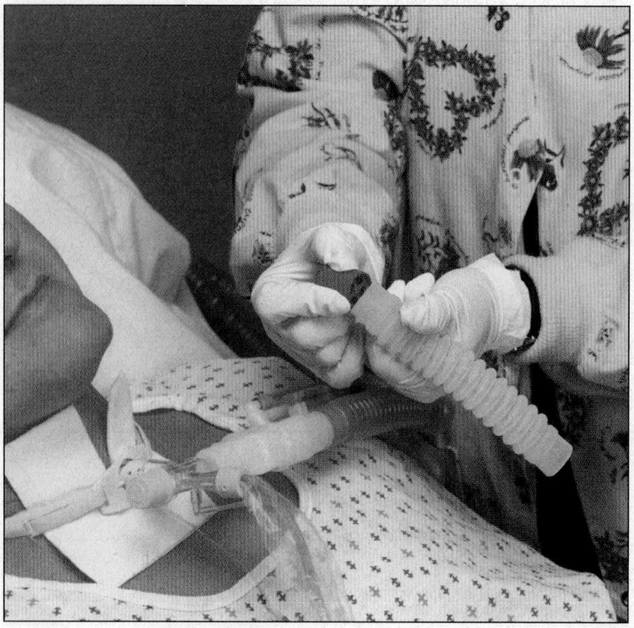

■ Connect the other end of the short-flex tubing to the ventilator tubing.
■ Attach the PMV (connected to the short-flex tubing) and the ventilator tubing to the closed-suction system (as shown on top right). Alternatively, attach the PMV between the swivel adapter and the short-flex tubing and ventilator tubing.
■ Adjust ventilator settings as needed. Make sure that the ventilator alarms are set appropriately for the patient's current condition and that the alarms are turned on, functioning properly, and audible to staff.[13,14,15]
■ After the PMV is in place, encourage the patient to relax, and tell him to notice how his lungs fill with air when the machine delivers a breath of air. Instruct him to breathe out through his nose and mouth.
■ Coach the patient to take a breath in first, then speak. Tell him to initially try vocalizing simple sounds, such as "Ahhhh," or to count "1, 2, 3, 4."[4]
■ Provide reassurance as needed; the speech-language pathologist can help facilitate voice production and speech as needed.

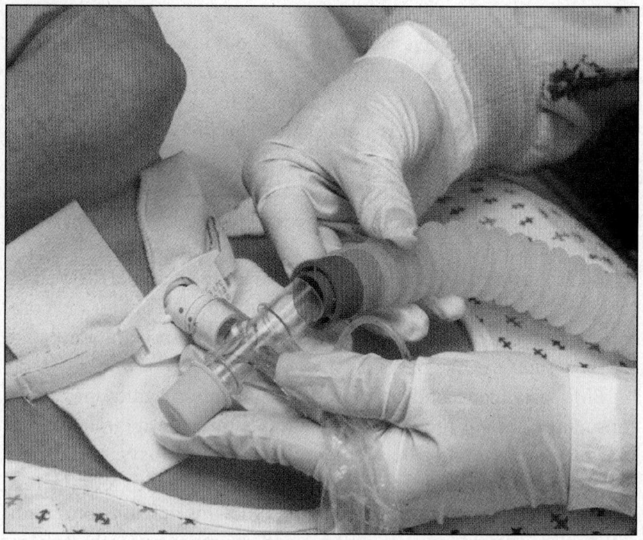

■ Evaluate the patient's response during PMV use. Monitor blood pressure, heart rate, and respiratory status.[2]
■ Monitor the patient's oxygen saturation level by pulse oximetry; maintain a level of at least 90% (or as ordered), and be alert for signs of respiratory distress.[4]

NURSING ALERT *Remove the PMV at once if the patient shows signs and symptoms of distress, such as a significant change in blood pressure or heart rate, increased respiratory rate, dyspnea, diaphoresis, anxiety, uncontrollable coughing, or arterial oxygen saturation less than 90%. Reassess the patient before trying the valve again.*[2,3]

■ Remove the valve and suction as needed *to maintain a patent airway.*[4]

NURSING ALERT *Secretions can obstruct air passage outside the tube, causing respiratory distress and valve intolerance. Although a one-way speaking valve can improve the strength of the cough, it may be difficult for the patient to cough secretions up to the mouth with the valve in place* because of the small space between the tube and the trachea, thicker secretions, inability to take deep breaths, and weak cough.[4]

■ Post cuff-deflation warning signs in the room.
■ Label the tracheostomy pilot balloon *to remind health care providers to reinflate the pilot balloon after removing the PMV.*[3]
■ Gently twist the PMV to remove it. Only when it's removed and the original setup is in place should you return the ventilator settings to their original levels and reinflate the pilot balloon cuff. Always remember to reinflate the tracheostomy cuff *after* removing the PMV.
■ Remove and discard your gloves.[10,11]
■ Perform hand hygiene.[5,6,7,8,9]
■ Clean and disinfect your stethoscope using a disinfectant pad *to prevent transmission of microorganisms.*[16,17]
■ Perform hand hygiene.[5,6,7,8,9]
■ Document the procedure.[18,19,20]

Special considerations

■ The PMV 007 and PMV 2001 are more convenient to use on patients who are ventilator-dependent *because they are tapered to fit into disposable ventilator tubing.*
■ The Joint Commission has issued a sentinel event alert concerning medical device alarm safety *because alarm-related events have been associated with permanent loss of function or death.* Among the major contributing factors were improper alarm settings, alarms inappropriately turned off, and alarm signals not audible to staff. Make sure that alarm limits are set appropriately and that alarms are turned on, functioning properly, and audible to staff. Follow facility guidelines for preventing alarm fatigue.[21]

■ Remove the PMV before administering medicated nebulizer treatments. If the PMV is inadvertently used during a nebulizer treatment, remove it immediately and rinse it thoroughly *to remove the medication residue.*[3,4]

■ Remove the valve when the patient is sleeping.[4]

■ If the patient's tracheostomy tube has a disposable inner cannula with a grasp ring, you may need to remove the inner cannula if the grasp ring extends beyond the tracheostomy tube hub.[3]

■ A PMV may be used 48 to 72 hours after a tracheotomy in a non-ventilator-dependent patient if tracheal edema and secretions from the surgical procedure have decreased.[3]

■ PMV use may need to be delayed for 48 to 72 hours after a tracheostomy tube change if tracheal swelling or bronchospasm occurs as a result of the procedure.[3]

Complications

Complications of ventilator valve use may include aspiration of secretions and respiratory distress.

Documentation

Document the type of PMV used and the time the device was placed. Document the patient's response to the procedure, including the amount of time the PMV is in place, respiratory and hemodynamic status, secretion management, and ability to vocalize. Document patient teaching and the patient's understanding of the teaching.

REFERENCES

1 Morris, L. L., & Afifi, M. S. (Eds.). (2010). *Tracheostomies: The complete guide.* New York, NY: Springer Publishing Company.

2 Windhorst, C., et al. (2009). "Patients requiring tracheostomy and mechanical ventilation. A model for interdisciplinary decision-making" [Online]. Accessed May 2015 via the Web at http://www.asha.org/Publications/leader/2009/090120/f090120a/

3 Passy-Muir, Inc. (2008). "Passy-Muir tracheostomy and ventilator swallowing and speaking valves instruction booklet" [Online]. Accessed May 2015 via the Web at http://www.passy-muir.com/sites/default/files/pdf/instructbklt.pdf

4 Grossbach, I., et al. (2011). Promoting effective communication for patients receiving mechanical ventilation. *Critical Care Nurse, 31*(3), 46–60. Accessed May 2015 via the Web at http://ccn.aacnjournals.org/content/31/3/46.full.pdf+html

5 World Health Organization. (2009). "WHO guidelines on hand hygiene in health care: First global patient safety challenge, clean care is safer care" [Online]. Accessed May 2015 via the Web at http://whqlibdoc.who.int/publications/2009/9789241597906_eng.pdf (Level IV)

6 The Joint Commission. (2015). Standard NPSG.07.01.01. *Comprehensive accreditation manual for hospitals: The official handbook.* Oakbrook Terrace, IL: The Joint Commission. (Level VII)

7 Centers for Disease Control and Prevention. (2002). Guideline for hand hygiene in health-care settings: Recommendations of the Healthcare Infection Control Practices Advisory Committee and the HICPAC/SHEA/APIC/IDSA Hand Hygiene Task Force. *MMWR Recommendations and Reports, 51*(RR-16), 1–45. Accessed May 2015 via the Web at http://www.cdc.gov/mmwr/pdf/rr/rr5116.pdf (Level II)

8 Centers for Medicare & Medicaid Services, Department of Health and Human Services. (2014). Condition of participation: Infection control. 42 C.F.R. § 482.42.

9 American Osteopathic Association. (2014). Standard 07.01.21. *Healthcare Facilities Accreditation Program: Accreditation requirements for acute care hospitals.* Chicago, IL: American Osteopathic Association. (Level VII)

10 Siegel, J. D., et al. (2007). "2007 guideline for isolation precautions: Preventing transmission of infectious agents in healthcare settings" [Online]. Accessed May 2015 via the Web at http://www.cdc.gov/hicpac/pdf/isolation/Isolation2007.pdf (Level II)

11 American Osteopathic Association. (2014). Standard 07.01.10. *Healthcare Facilities Accreditation Program: Accreditation requirements for acute care hospitals.* Chicago, IL: American Osteopathic Association. (Level VII)

12 The Joint Commission. (2014). Standard NPSG.01.01.01. *Comprehensive accreditation manual for hospitals: The official handbook.* Oakbrook Terrace, IL: The Joint Commission. (Level VII)

13 American Association of Critical-Care Nurses. (2013). "AACN practice alert: Alarm management" [Online]. Accessed May 2015 via the Web at http://www.aacn.org/wd/practice/docs/practicealerts/alarm-management-practice-alert.pdf (Level VII)

14 The Joint Commission. (2015). Standard NPSG.06.01.01. *Comprehensive accreditation manual for hospitals: The official handbook.* Oakbrook Terrace, IL: The Joint Commission (Level VII)

15 Graham, K. C., & Cvach, M. (2010). Monitor alarm fatigue: Standardizing use of physiological monitors and decreasing nuisance alarms. American Journal of Critical Care, 19, 28–37.

16 Rutala, W. A., et al. (2008). "Guideline for disinfection and sterilization in healthcare facilities, 2008" [Online]. Accessed May 2015 via the Web at http://www.cdc.gov/hicpac/pdf/guidelines/Disinfection_Nov_2008.pdf (Level I)

17 American Osteopathic Association. (2014). Standard 07.02.03. *Healthcare Facilities Accreditation Program: Accreditation requirements for acute care hospitals.* Chicago, IL: American Osteopathic Association. (Level VII)

18 The Joint Commission. (2015). Standard RC.01.03.01. *Comprehensive accreditation manual for hospitals: The official handbook.* Oakbrook Terrace, IL: The Joint Commission. (Level VII)

19 American Osteopathic Association. (2014). Standard 10.00.03. *Healthcare Facilities Accreditation Program: Accreditation requirements for acute care hospitals.* Chicago, IL: American Osteopathic Association. (Level VII)

20 Centers for Medicare & Medicaid Services, Department of Health and Human Services. (2014). Condition of participation: Medical record services. 42 C.F.R. § 482.24(b).

21 The Joint Commission. (2013). "Sentinel event alert: Medical device alarm safety in hospitals" [Online]. Accessed May 2015 via the Web at http://www.jointcommission.org/assets/1/18/SEA_50_alarms_4_5_13_FINAL1.PDF (Level VII)

ADDITIONAL REFERENCES

Fisher, D. F., et al. (2013). Tracheostomy tube change before day 7 is associated with earlier use of speaking valve and earlier oral intake. *Respiratory Care, 58,* 257–263. Accessed May 2015 via the Web at http://rc.rcjournal.com/content/58/2/257.full.pdf (Level IV)

Nettina, S. M. (2014). *Lippincott manual of nursing practice* (10th ed.). Philadelphia, PA: Wolters Kluwer.

Passy-Muir, Inc. (2003). "Passy-Muir tracheostomy and ventilator speaking valve resource guide" [Online]. Accessed May 2015 via the Web at http://www.passy-muir.com/sites/default/files/pdf/resource_guide.pdf

Passy-Muir, Inc. (2008). "Passy-Muir tracheostomy and ventilator swallowing and speaking valves patient education handbook" [Online]. Accessed May 2015 via the Web at http://www.passy-muir.com/sites/default/files/pdf/patienthdbk.pdf

Speed, L., & Harding, K. E. (2013). Tracheostomy teams reduce total tracheostomy time and increase speaking valve use: A systematic review and meta-analysis. *Journal of Critical Care, 28,* 216.e1–216.e10. (Level I)

TRACHEOSTOMY CARE

Whether a tracheotomy is performed in an emergency situation or after careful preparation, as a permanent measure or as temporary therapy, tracheostomy care has identical goals: to ensure airway patency by keeping the tube free of mucus buildup, to maintain mucous membrane and skin integrity, to prevent infection, and to provide psychological support.

The patient may have one of three types of tracheostomy tube—uncuffed, cuffed, or fenestrated. Tube selection depends on the patient's condition and the practitioner's preference.

An *uncuffed tube,* which may be plastic or metal, allows air to flow freely around the tracheostomy tube and through the larynx, reducing the risk of tracheal damage. A *cuffed tube,* made of plastic, is disposable. The cuff and the tube won't separate accidentally inside the trachea because the cuff is bonded to the tube. A cuffed tube doesn't require

EQUIPMENT

Types of tracheostomy tubes

Cuffed and uncuffed tracheostomy tubes each have both advantages and disadvantages. Cuffed tubes help seal the area between the tube and trachea, decreasing the patient's risk of aspiration. However, if the cuff pressure isn't regularly monitored, this type of tube can erode the trachea. Also, if the cuff is inflated, the patient can't talk and needs an alternate means of communication.

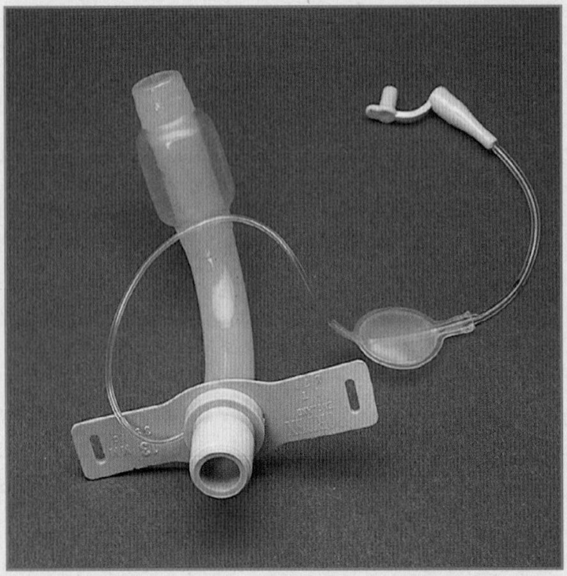

Uncuffed tubes allow the patient to eat and talk. However, this type of tube can't be used in a patient who is receiving mechanical ventilation *because oxygen may escape from around the tube.*

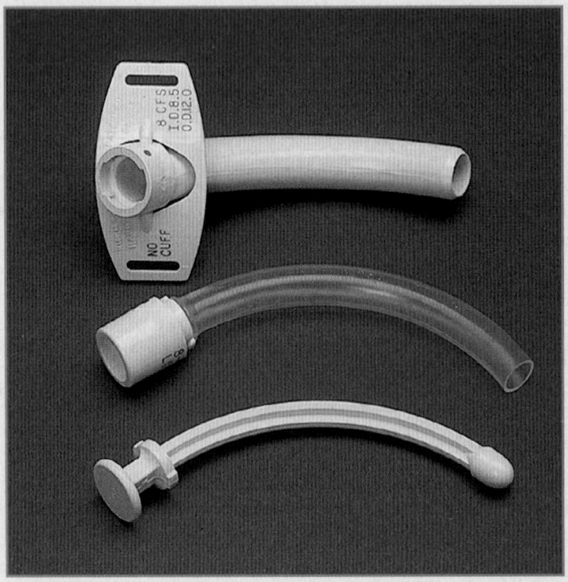

periodic deflating to lower pressure because cuff pressure is low and evenly distributed against the tracheal wall. A plastic *fenestrated tube* permits speech through the upper airway when the external opening is capped and the cuff is deflated. It also allows easy removal of the inner cannula for cleaning. However, a fenestrated tube may become occluded. (See *Types of tracheostomy tubes.*)

The maximum acceptable tracheostomy tube cuff pressure is 25 mm Hg.[1,2] When cuff pressure is inadequate, oropharyngeal secretions can leak around the cuff, increasing the risk of ventilator-associated pneumonia.[3] Overinflation of the cuff can cause tracheal necrosis, tracheomalacia, tracheoinnominate artery fistula, tracheal ulceration, fibrosis, tracheoesophageal fistula, and tracheal stenosis.[4] High cuff pressure can also be caused by malposition of the tracheostomy or insertion of a tube that's too small in diameter, resulting in overfilling of the cuff to achieve a seal in the trachea.[1] Actual cuff pressure varies with each patient, however. To keep the pressure within safe limits, cuff pressure should be measured at least once each shift or at an interval determined by the facility. (See the "Tracheal cuff–pressure measurement" procedure, page 750.) Tracheal cuff pressure can be maintained and measured by a respiratory therapist or a nurse.

To prevent infection, tracheostomy care should be performed using sterile technique until the stoma has healed. For recently performed tracheotomies, sterile gloves should be worn for all manipulations at the tracheostomy site. When the stoma has healed, clean gloves may be substituted for sterile ones.

Changing tracheostomy ties helps prevent infection and the skin underneath the ties from becoming excoriated and wet. Two types of tracheostomy ties may be used to secure tracheostomy tubes: twill tape or a commercially prepared tracheostomy tube holder. A commercially prepared tracheostomy tube holder is recommended because it protects the patient from pressure on the back of his neck and is easily adjustable.[2]

Tracheostomy cuffs need to be deflated to allow the patient to eat or drink, to remove the tube, to secure a decannulation cap, and when a speaking valve is attached to the tube.[2]

Equipment

For cuff inflation and deflation

10-mL syringe ▪ gloves ▪ stethoscope ▪ disinfectant pad ▪ handheld resuscitation bag ▪ Optional: other personal protective equipment.

For tracheostomy ties change

30″ (76-cm) length of tracheostomy twill tape or a commercially prepared tracheostomy tube holder with Velcro ties ▪ bandage scissors ▪ gloves ▪ hemostat ▪ extra tracheostomy tube and obturator ▪ Optional: sterile, precut tracheostomy dressing, other personal protective equipment.

For tracheostomy tube cannula and stoma care

Disposable inner cannula ▪ two or three sterile solution containers ▪ sterile normal saline solution or sterile water ▪ sterile cotton-tipped applicators ▪ sterile 4″ × 4″ (10-cm × 10-cm) gauze pads ▪ sterile gloves ▪ clean gloves ▪ prepackaged sterile tracheostomy dressing ▪ sterile nylon brush ▪ suctioning supplies ▪ oral care supplies ▪ handheld resuscitation bag connected to an oxygen source ▪ extra tracheostomy tubes and obturator ▪ stethoscope ▪ disinfectant pad Optional: skin barrier, sterile pipe cleaners, tracheostomy ties, other personal protective equipment (gown, mask and goggles or mask with face shield), extra inner cannula, foam tracheostomy dressing, water-soluble lubricant or topical antibiotic cream.

Note: Commercially prepared tracheostomy care kits are available.

Preparation of equipment

For tracheostomy tube cannula and stoma care

Make sure the extra tracheostomy tubes and obturator and the handheld resuscitation bag attached to an oxygen source are readily available in case of an emergency. Check the expiration date on each sterile package, and inspect for tears.

Place equipment and supplies on a clean table or stand near the patient's bed. Open the tracheostomy care kit (if available in your facility), using sterile technique. Using sterile technique, pour sterile normal saline solution or sterile water into one of the sterile solution containers, and then pour sterile normal saline solution or sterile water into the second sterile container for rinsing. For inner cannula care, you may use a third sterile solution container to hold the gauze pads and cotton-tipped applicators saturated with normal saline solution. Hydrogen peroxide is no longer recommended for cleaning inner cannulas or tracheostomy sites.[4,5]

If you'll be replacing the disposable inner cannula, open the package containing the new inner cannula while maintaining sterile technique.[5] Obtain or prepare new tracheostomy ties if indicated.

Implementation

- Gather and prepare the appropriate equipment.
- Read the cuff manufacturer's instructions *because cuff types and procedures vary widely.*
- Perform hand hygiene.[6,7,8,9,10]
- Put on gloves and other personal protective equipment as needed *to comply with standard precautions.*[11,12]
- Confirm the patient's identity using at least two patient identifiers.[13]
- Explain the procedure to the patient *to allay his fears and enhance cooperation.*
- Provide privacy.[14,15]
- Assess the patient's respiratory status *for baseline comparison.*[5]
- Help the patient into the semi-Fowler position, if possible, or place him in the supine position with the head of the bed elevated as tolerated *to prevent aspiration of secretions and to promote oxyenation.*[5,16]
- Hyperoxygenate the patient for 30 to 60 seconds, and then perform oropharyngeal suctioning *to remove accumulated secretions from above the cuff; these secretions have been implicated in the development of ventilator-associated pneumonia.*[3,17,18,19]

For cuff inflation and deflation

- Remove the ventilation device or humidified oxygen.
- Insert a 10-mL syringe into the cuff pilot balloon. Ventilate the patient with a handheld resuscitation bag and slowly withdraw air from the cuff until you hear a small leak with a stethoscope over the larynx during inspiration. *Slow deflation allows positive lung pressure to push secretions upward from the bronchi. Cuff deflation may also stimulate the patient's cough reflex, producing additional secretions.*
- Reinflate the cuff using the minimal occlusive volume technique or the minimal-leak technique *to help gauge the proper inflation point.*
- *To reinflate the cuff using the minimal occlusive volume technique:* Insert an air-filled 10-mL syringe into the cuff pilot balloon. If you hear a leak initially, slowly add air to the cuff until you've eliminated the leak. If you don't hear a leak initially, ventilate the patient with a handheld resuscitation bag and slowly withdraw air from the cuff in 0.1-mL increments until you hear a small leak. Slowly add air into the cuff until you can no longer hear the leak over the larynx on inspiration.[5]
- *To reinflate the cuff using the minimal leak technique:* Insert an air-filled 10-mL syringe into the cuff pilot balloon. If you hear a leak initially, slowly add air to the cuff until you've eliminated the leak. If you don't hear a leak initially, place your stethoscope over the patient's larynx. Slowly withdraw air from the cuff in 0.1-mL increments until you hear a small leak over the larynx on inspiration.[5]
- *To reinflate the cuff using a tracheal cuff–pressure manometer,* see the "Tracheal cuff–pressure measurement" procedure. Don't exceed 25 mm Hg when inflating the cuff using the manometer.[1,2]
- Remove the syringe *because leaving the syringe on the cuff pilot balloon may allow air to escape, causing the cuff to deflate.*[5]
- Reattach the ventilation device or humidified oxygen.
- Reassess the patient's respiratory status.[5]
- Note the exact amount of air used to inflate the cuff *to detect tracheomalacia if more air is consistently needed.*

For ties change

- Obtain assistance from another nurse or a respiratory therapist *because of the risk of accidental tube dislodgement.*[20]

NURSING ALERT *Research overwhelmingly recommends a two-person technique for changing a tracheostomy tube securing device to prevent tube dislodgment. In the two-person technique, one person holds the tracheostomy tube in place while the other person changes the securing device.*[20]

Ties change using twill tape

- If you aren't using a commercially packaged tracheostomy tube holder, prepare new ties from a 30″ (76-cm) length of twill tape by folding one end back 1″ (2.5 cm) on itself. Then, with the bandage scissors, cut a ½″ (1.3-cm) slit down the center of the tape from the folded edge.
- Prepare the other end of the tape the same way.
- Hold both ends together and, using scissors, cut the resulting circle of tape so that one piece is approximately 10″ (25 cm) long and the other is about 20″ (51 cm) long.
- Instruct the assistant to put on gloves and hold the tracheostomy tube in place; then cut the soiled tracheostomy ties with the bandage scissors or untie them and discard the ties. Be careful not to cut the tube of the pilot balloon.
- Thread the slit end of one new tie a short distance through the eye of one tracheostomy tube flange from the underside; use the hemostat, if needed, to pull the tie through. Then thread the other end of the tie completely through the slit end, and pull it taut so it loops firmly through the flange. *This technique avoids knots that can cause throat discomfort, tissue irritation, pressure, and necrosis of the patient's throat.*
- Fasten the second tie to the opposite flange in the same manner.
- Instruct the patient to flex his neck while you bring the ties around to the side, and tie them together with a square knot. *Flexion produces the same neck circumference as coughing and helps prevent an overly tight tie.* Instruct your assistant to place one finger under the tapes as you tie them *to ensure that they're tight enough to avoid slippage but loose enough to prevent choking or jugular vein constriction.*[3,4] *Placing the closure on the side allows easy access and prevents pressure necrosis at the back of the neck when the patient is recumbent.*
- Assess the patient's skin underneath the tape.[3]
- After securing the ties, cut off the excess tape with the scissors and instruct the assistant to release the tracheostomy tube.

Ties change using a commercially prepared tube holder with Velcro ties

- Instruct the assistant to put on gloves and then hold the tracheostomy tube in place *to prevent its expulsion during replacement of the ties.*[4,5]
- Remove the old tracheostomy tube holder by opening the Velcro tabs.
- Thread one Velcro tab through the flange and secure it.
- Bring the loose end of the tracheostomy tube holder around the back of the patient's neck.
- Assess the patient's skin underneath the tube holder.[4]
- Thread the remaining Velcro tab through the other flange and secure it.
- Adjust the right and left Velcro tabs as needed to ensure that only one finger can slide under the tie.[4] *Fastening too tightly can lead to skin breakdown and vascular obstruction; fastening too loosely can lead to tube expulsion.*[3]
- Check tracheostomy tie tension frequently on a patient with traumatic injury, radical neck dissection, or cardiac failure *because neck diameter can increase from swelling and cause constriction;* also check a restless patient frequently *because ties can loosen and cause tube dislodgment.*
- If necessary, apply a sterile, precut tracheostomy dressing by sliding the dressing under the flanges of the tracheostomy tube, starting at the bottom and moving to the top.

NURSING ALERT *Use a manufactured split dressing; don't cut a gauze pad* because loose fibers around the stoma or tracheostomy tube can cause irritation and increase the risk of infection.[20]

For tracheostomy tube cannula and stoma care

■ Remove and discard your gloves and perform hand hygiene.[6,7,8,9,10]
■ Put on gloves and other personal protective equipment as needed *to comply with standard precautions.*[11,12] Use a mask with face shield or mask and goggles if spraying of respiratory secretions is likely.[17]
■ Assess the need for suctioning.[5]
■ Hyperoxygenate the patient for 30 to 60 seconds before suctioning (if needed) by adjusting the fraction of inspired oxygen on the mechanical ventilator or using the temporary oxygen-enrichment program available on the ventilator to prevent hypoxemia.[17]
■ If needed, suction the tracheostomy tube by inserting the suction catheter to a premeasured distance[5,20] *to clear the airway of any secretions that may hinder oxygenation.* Determine the volume of secretions and assess them for color, consistency, and odor. (See the "Tracheal suctioning, intubated patient" procedure, page 752.)
■ With your nondominant hand, reconnect the patient to the humidifier or ventilator if necessary.
■ Hyperoxygenate the patient for at least 1 minute following suctioning.[5,17]
■ Remove the patient's tracheostomy dressing, inspect it for drainage, and then discard it.[5]
■ Assess the patient's cardiac and respiratory status *to evaluate his response to suctioning.*[1,17]
■ Remove and discard your gloves.[5,11,12]
■ Perform hand hygiene.[6,7,8,9,10]

Cleaning a nondisposable inner cannula

■ Put on sterile gloves.[5,11,12]
■ Using your nondominant hand, disconnect the ventilator or humidification device and unlock the tracheostomy tube's inner cannula by rotating it counterclockwise (as shown below).[5]

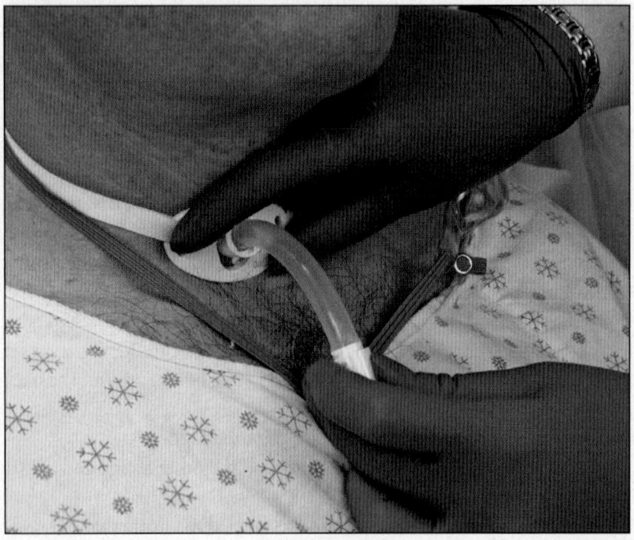

■ Remove the inner cannula and place it in the container of sterile normal saline solution or sterile water, but don't allow it to soak.
■ Place the ventilator oxygen device or humidification device over or near the outer cannula *to maintain the oxygen supply.*
■ Working quickly, use your dominant hand to scrub the cannula with the sterile nylon brush (as shown on top right).[5] You may also use a sterile pipe cleaner (provided in a commercially prepared tracheostomy care kit) if necessary to clean the inner cannula.[1]

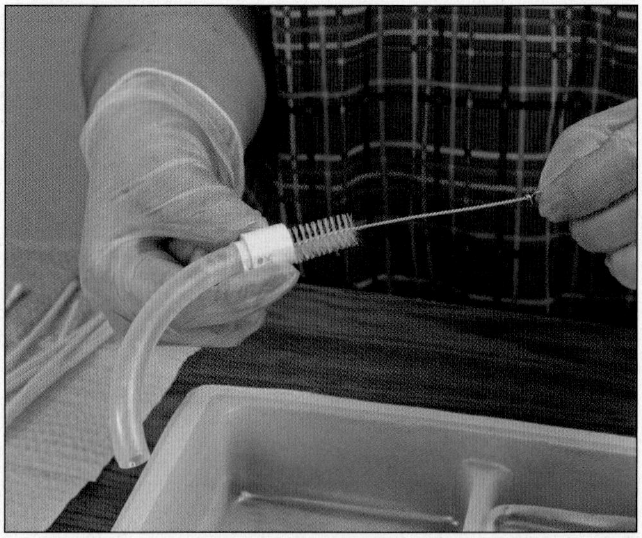

■ Immerse the cannula in the container of normal saline solution or sterile water (as shown below), and agitate it for about 10 seconds *to rinse it thoroughly.*

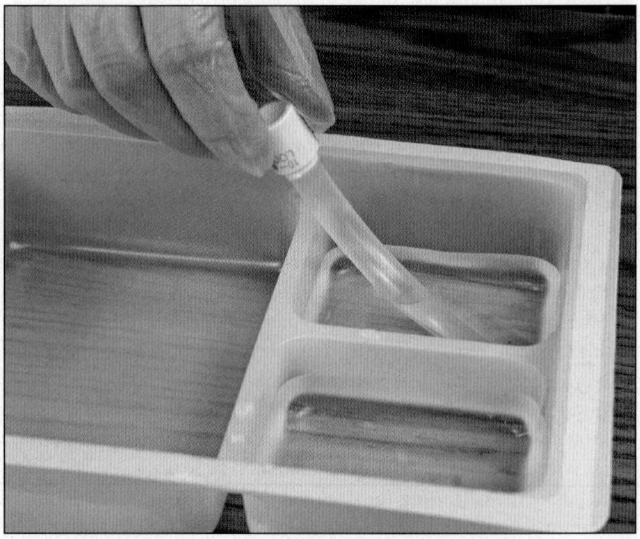

■ Inspect the cannula for cleanliness. Repeat the cleaning process if necessary. When it's clean, tap it gently against the inside edge of the sterile container *to remove excess liquid and prevent aspiration.* Alternatively, you can use a pipe cleaner to dry the inside of the inner cannula.[3] Don't dry the outer surface *because a thin film of moisture acts as a lubricant during insertion.*
■ Reinsert the inner cannula into the patient's tracheostomy tube (as shown on next page, top left). Lock it in place and then gently pull on it to make sure it's positioned securely. Reconnect the mechanical ventilator or humidification device.[5]
■ If the patient can't tolerate being disconnected from the ventilator for the time it takes to clean the inner cannula, replace the existing inner cannula with a clean one and reattach the mechanical ventilator. Then clean the cannula that you just removed from the patient and store it in a sterile container for the next time.[5]
■ Remove and discard your gloves.[11,12]

Caring for a disposable inner cannula

■ Put on clean gloves.[5,11,12]
■ Using your dominant hand, remove the patient's inner cannula.[5] After evaluating the secretions in the cannula, discard it properly.

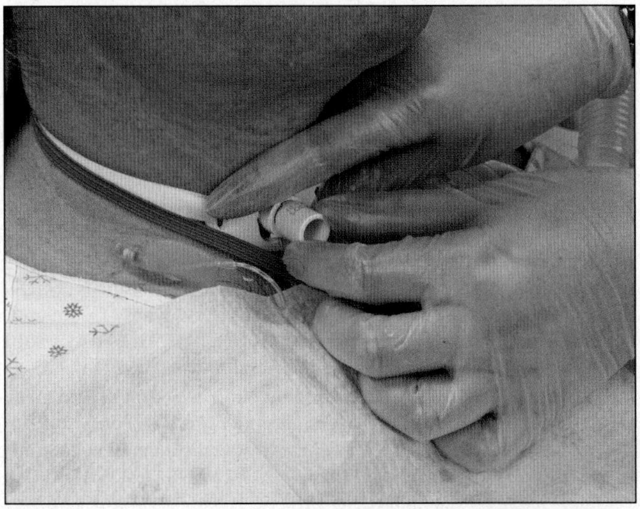

■ Pick up the new inner cannula, touching only the outer locking portion. Insert the cannula into the tracheostomy and, following the manufacturer's instructions, lock it securely.[5]
■ Replace any humidification or ventilation device.[5]
■ Remove and discard your gloves.[11,12]

Cleaning the stoma and outer cannula

■ Perform hand hygiene.[6,7,8,9,10]
■ Put on clean gloves.[5,11,12]
■ With your dominant hand, moisten a sterile gauze pad with the sterile normal saline solution or sterile water. Squeeze out the excess liquid *to prevent accidental aspiration.* Then wipe the patient's neck under the tracheostomy tube flanges and the twill tape or commercially prepared tracheostomy tube holder.
■ Assess the stoma site and surrounding skin for redness, swelling, and drainage, *which may indicate infection.*[1,4]
■ Use a sterile cotton-tipped applicator and a sterile gauze pad *to clean the stoma site and the tube's flanges.* Wipe only once with each applicator or gauze pad and then discard it *to prevent contamination of a clean area with a soiled applicator or pad.*[5]
■ Rinse debris with one or more sterile 4″ × 4″ (10-cm × 10-cm) gauze pads dampened in sterile normal saline solution or sterile water.
■ Dry the area thoroughly with additional sterile gauze pads; apply a skin barrier, as needed.[18]
■ Apply a new sterile tracheostomy dressing.[1,3] Sites with excessive moisture may require a foam tracheostomy dressing.[20]

NURSING ALERT *Always use a manufactured split dressing; don't cut a gauze pad* because loose fibers around the stoma or tracheostomy tube can cause irritation and increase the risk of infection.[18,20]

Completing the procedure

■ Make sure that the patient is comfortable, the head of the patient's bed is elevated 30 to 45 degrees *to prevent ventilator-associated pneumonia,*[21,22] and the patient can easily reach the call light and communication aids.
■ Properly clean or dispose of all equipment and supplies in the appropriate receptacles.
■ Remove and discard your gloves and any other personal protective equipment worn.[5,11,12]
■ Make sure all necessary supplies are readily available at the bedside.
■ Perform hand hygiene.[6,7,8,9,10]
■ As needed, clean and disinfect your stethoscope using a disinfectant pad.[23,24]
■ Perform hand hygiene.[6,7,8,9,10]
■ Document the procedure.[25,26,27]

Special considerations

■ Follow your facility's guidelines regarding the correct procedure if a tracheostomy tube is expelled or if the outer cannula becomes blocked. If the patient's breathing is obstructed—for example, when the tube is blocked with mucus that can't be removed by suctioning or by withdrawing the inner cannula—call the appropriate code and provide manual resuscitation with a handheld resuscitation bag or reconnect the patient to the ventilator. Don't remove the tracheostomy tube entirely *because removal may allow the airway to completely close.* Use extreme caution when attempting to reinsert an expelled tracheostomy tube *because of the risk of tracheal trauma, perforation, compression, and asphyxiation.*
■ Note that commercially prepared tracheostomy tube holders are typically more comfortable and easier to apply than ties made from twill tape; however, they may degrade over time, especially when washed with hot water.[4]
■ Refrain from changing tracheostomy ties unnecessarily during the immediate postoperative period before the stoma track is well formed (usually 4 days) *to avoid accidental dislodgement and expulsion of the tube.*[3,5]
■ Don't change a single-cannula tracheostomy tube or the outer cannula of a double-cannula tube. *Because of the risk of tracheal complications,* the practitioner typically changes the cannula; the frequency of change depends on the patient's condition.
■ If the patient's neck or stoma is excoriated or infected, consult the practitioner or a wound, ostomy, and continence nurse for an individualized care plan.[1] Apply a water-soluble lubricant or topical antibiotic cream as ordered. Don't use a powder or an oil-based substance on or around a stoma *because aspiration can cause infection and abscess.*
■ The optimal frequency for cleaning the inner cannula hasn't been determined.[3,4] Clean or change the inner cannula when needed and inspect it regularly, at least two times per day.[3,4]
■ Clean the stoma site every 4 to 8 hours.[4]
■ Change the dressing frequently whenever secretions begin to collect *because a wet dressing with exudate or secretions predisposes the patient to skin excoriation, breakdown, and infection.*[4]
■ If you accidentally remove the outer cannula of a cuffed tracheostomy tube or the patient coughs it out, never use hydrogen peroxide to clean it. *Using hydrogen peroxide may affect the integrity of the cuff.* Instead, replace it with a new tracheostomy tube.
■ Replace all equipment, including solutions, regularly according to your facility's policy *to reduce the risk of health care–acquired infections.*

Patient teaching

If the patient is being discharged with a tracheostomy, start self-care teaching as soon as he's receptive. Teach the patient how to change and clean the tube. If he's being discharged with suction equipment, make sure he and his family understand the equipment and feel comfortable using it.

Teach the patient and his family about measures to prevent ventilator-associated pneumonia, including maintaining the head of the bed at 30 to 45 degrees, and encourage them to alert staff members when the bed doesn't appear to be positioned correctly.[16,21]

Complications

Secretions that collect under dressings can encourage skin excoriation and infection. Hardened mucus or a slipped cuff can occlude the cannula opening and obstruct the airway. Tube displacement can stimulate the cough reflex if the tip rests on the carina, or it can cause blood vessel erosion and hemorrhage. Just the presence of the tube or excessive cuff pressure can produce tracheal erosion and necrosis. The cuff can rupture from overinflation or the tube can dislodge during deflation.

Complications associated with changing tracheostomy ties include dislodgement of the tube. Skin breakdown and vascular obstruction can occur if the ties are too tight. Expulsion of the tube can occur if the ties are too loose.

Documentation

Record the date and time of the procedure; the type of procedure; the amount, consistency, color, and odor of secretions; stoma and skin condition; the patient's respiratory status; changing of the tracheostomy tube by the practitioner; the duration of any cuff deflation; the amount of any cuff inflation; and cuff pressure readings and specific body position. Note complications and nursing actions taken, patient or family teaching and their comprehension of the teaching and progress, and the patient's tolerance of the treatment.

References

1 Regan, E. N., & Dallachiesa, L. (2009). How to care for a patient with a tracheostomy. *Nursing, 39*(8), 34–39. Accessed May 2015 via the Web at http://www.nursingcenter.com/pdf.asp?AID=926437

2 Intensive Care Society. (2011). "Standards for the care of adult patients with a temporary tracheostomy: Standards and guidelines" [Online]. Accessed May 2015 via the Web at http://www.aeo.org.ec/GUIASYREVISIONES/TRAQUEOSTOMIA.pdf

3 Morris, L. L., & Afifi, M. S. (Eds.). (2010). *Tracheostomies: The complete guide.* New York, NY: Springer Publishing Company.

4 Morris, L. L., et al. (2013). Tracheostomy care and complications in the intensive care unit. *Critical Care Nurse, 33*(5), 18–31.

5 Lynn-McHale Wiegand, D. (Ed.). (2011). *AACN procedure manual for critical care* (6th ed.). St. Louis, MO: Saunders.

6 World Health Organization. (2009). "WHO guidelines on hand hygiene in health care: First global patient safety challenge, clean care is safer care" [Online]. Accessed May 2015 via the Web at http://whqlibdoc.who.int/publications/2009/9789241597906_eng.pdf (Level IV)

7 The Joint Commission. (2015). Standard NPSG.07.01.01. *Comprehensive accreditation manual for hospitals: The official handbook.* Oakbrook Terrace, IL: The Joint Commission. (Level VII)

8 Centers for Disease Control and Prevention. (2002). Guideline for hand hygiene in health-care settings: Recommendations of the Healthcare Infection Control Practices Advisory Committee and the HICPAC/SHEA/APIC/IDSA Hand Hygiene Task Force. *MMWR Recommendations and Reports, 51*(RR-16), 1–45. Accessed May 2015 via the Web at http://www.cdc.gov/mmwr/pdf/rr/rr5116.pdf (Level II)

9 American Osteopathic Association. (2014). Standard 07.01.21. *Healthcare Facilities Accreditation Program: Accreditation requirements for acute care hospitals.* Chicago, IL: American Osteopathic Association. (Level VII)

10 Centers for Medicare & Medicaid Services, Department of Health and Human Services. (2014). Condition of participation: Infection control. 42 C.F.R. § 482.42.

11 Siegel, J. D., et al. (2007). "2007 guideline for isolation precautions: Preventing transmission of infectious agents in healthcare settings" [Online]. Accessed May 2015 via the Web at http://www.cdc.gov/hicpac/pdf/isolation/Isolation2007.pdf (Level II)

12 American Osteopathic Association. (2014). Standard 07.01.10. *Healthcare Facilities Accreditation Program: Accreditation requirements for acute care hospitals.* Chicago, IL: American Osteopathic Association. (Level VII)

13 The Joint Commission. (2015). Standard NPSG.01.01.01. *Comprehensive accreditation manual for hospitals: The official handbook.* Oakbrook Terrace, IL: The Joint Commission. (Level VII)

14 American Osteopathic Association. (2014). Standard 15.01.16. *Healthcare Facilities Accreditation Program: Accreditation requirements for acute care hospitals.* Chicago, IL: American Osteopathic Association. (Level VII)

15 Centers for Medicare & Medicaid Services, Department of Health and Human Services. (2014). Condition of participation: Patient's rights. 42 C.F.R. § 482.13(c)(1).

16 American Osteopathic Association. (2014). Standard 07.01.02. *Healthcare Facilities Accreditation Program: Accreditation requirements for acute care hospitals.* Chicago, IL: American Osteopathic Association. (Level VII)

17 American Association for Respiratory Care (AARC). (2010). AARC clinical practice guidelines: Endotracheal suctioning of mechanically ventilated patients with artificial airways 2010. *Respiratory Care, 55,* 758–764. Accessed May 2015 via the Web at http://www.rcjournal.com/cpgs/pdf/06.10.0758.pdf (Level VII)

18 American Association of Critical-Care Nurses . (2008). "AACN practice alert: Ventilator associated pneumonia" [Online]. Accessed May 2015 via the Web at http://www.aacn.org/WD/Practice/Docs/PracticeAlerts/Ventilator%20Associated%20Pneumonia%201-2008.pdf (Level VII)

19 Centers for Disease Control and Prevention. (2004). Guidelines for preventing health-care-associated pneumonia, 2003: Recommendations of CDC and the Healthcare Infection Control Practices Advisory Committee. *MMWR Recommendations and Reports, 53*(RR-3), 1–32. Accessed May 2015 via the Web at http://www.cdc.gov/mmwr/pdf/rr/rr5303.pdf (Level II)

20 Nance-Floyd, B. (2011). Tracheostomy care: An evidence-based guide to suctioning and dressing changes. *American Nurse Today, 6*(7), 14–16. Accessed May 2015 via the Web athttp://www.americannursetoday.com/assets/0/434/436/440/7986/7988/7992/8022/f17622e4-1fc4-4a5c-88b7-3cd329777cb7.pdf (Level VII)

21 Institute for Healthcare Improvement. (2012). *How-to guide: Prevent ventilator-associated pneumonia.* Cambridge, MA: Institute for Healthcare Improvement. (Level VII)

22 Association of Professionals in Infection Control and Epidemiology. (2009). "An APIC guide 2009: Guide to the elimination of ventilator-associated pneumonia" [Online]. Accessed May 2015 via the Web at http://www.apic.org/Resource_/EliminationGuideForm/18e326ad-b484-471c-9c35-6822a53ee4a2/File/VAP_09.pdf (Level IV)

23 Rutala, W. A., et al. (2008). "Guideline for disinfection and sterilization in healthcare facilities, 2008" [Online]. Accessed May 2015 via the Web at http://www.cdc.gov/hicpac/pdf/guidelines/Disinfection_Nov_2008.pdf (Level I)

24 American Osteopathic Association. (2014). Standard 07.02.03. *Healthcare Facilities Accreditation Program: Accreditation requirements for acute care hospitals.* Chicago, IL: American Osteopathic Association. (Level VII)

25 The Joint Commission. (2015). Standard RC.01.03.01. *Comprehensive accreditation manual for hospitals: The official handbook.* Oakbrook Terrace, IL: The Joint Commission. (Level VII)

25 Centers for Medicare & Medicaid Services, Department of Health and Human Services. (2014). Condition of participation: Medical record services. 42 C.F.R. § 482.24(b).

27 American Osteopathic Association. (2014). Standard 10.00.03. *Healthcare Facilities Accreditation Program: Accreditation requirements for acute care hospitals.* Chicago, IL: American Osteopathic Association. (Level VII)

Tracheotomy, Assisting

A tracheotomy involves surgically creating of an external opening—called a *tracheostomy*—into the trachea and inserting an indwelling tube to maintain the airway's patency. If all other attempts to establish an airway have failed, a practitioner may perform a tracheotomy at a patient's bedside. This procedure may be necessary when an airway obstruction results from laryngeal edema, foreign-body obstruction, or a tumor. An emergency tracheotomy also may be performed when endotracheal intubation is contraindicated.

Use of a cuffed tracheostomy tube provides and maintains a patent airway, prevents an unconscious or paralyzed patient from aspirating food or secretions, allows removal of tracheobronchial secretions from the patient unable to cough, replaces an endotracheal tube, and permits the use of positive-pressure ventilation.

When laryngectomy accompanies a tracheostomy, the practitioner may insert a laryngectomy tube, a shorter version of a tracheostomy tube. In addition, the patient's trachea is sutured to the skin surface. Consequently, with a laryngectomy, accidental tube expulsion doesn't precipitate immediate closure of the tracheal opening. When healing occurs, the patient has a permanent neck stoma through which respiration takes place.

Although tracheostomy tubes come in plastic and metal, plastic tubes are much more commonly used because they have a universal adapter for respiratory support equipment, such as a mechanical ventilator, and a cuff to allow positive-pressure ventilation.

Equipment

Appropriate-sized tracheostomy tube with obturator ▪ sterile tracheotomy tray (typically contains tracheal dilator, vein retractor, hemostats, and clamps) ▪ sutures and needles ▪ 4″ × 4″ (10-cm ×10-cm) gauze pads ▪ sterile drapes ▪ sterile gloves ▪ gloves ▪ gown ▪ mask with face shield or mask and goggles ▪ sterile gown ▪ sterile bowls ▪ stethoscope ▪ disinfectant pad ▪ prepackaged, sterile tracheostomy dressing ▪ blanket or towel ▪ tracheostomy ties ▪ suction apparatus and tubing ▪ alcohol pad ▪ antiseptic cleaning solution ▪ sterile water ▪ 5-mL syringe with 22G needle ▪ local anesthetic ▪ prescribed sedative ▪ oxygen therapy device ▪ oxygen source ▪ humidification source or device ▪ syringe for cuff inflation ▪ manometer (or other cuff pressure measurement device) ▪ cardiac monitor ▪ pulse oximeter ▪ end-tidal carbon dioxide detector ▪ vital signs monitoring equipment ▪ emergency equipment (crash cart with cardiac medications, defibrillator, handheld resuscitation bag, intubation equipment) ▪ Optional: IV catheter insertion kit, mechanical ventilator.

Many facilities use prepackaged, sterile tracheotomy trays.

Preparation of equipment

Perform hand hygiene and then, maintaining sterile technique, open the tray.[1,2,3,4,5] Take the tracheostomy tube from its container and place it on the sterile field. If necessary, set up the suction equipment and make sure it works. When the practitioner opens the sterile bowls, pour in the antiseptic cleaning solution.

Implementation

- Have one person stay with the patient while another obtains the necessary equipment.
- Perform hand hygiene.[1,2,3,4,5]
- Confirm the patient's identity using at least two patient identifiers.[6]
- Provide privavy.[7,8]
- Explain the procedure to the patient even if he's unresponsive.
- If possible, confirm that written informed consent has been obtained and is in the patient's medical record.[9,10,11]
- Check the patient's medical record for allergies, especially to anesthetics or latex.
- Conduct a preprocedure verification *to make sure that all relevant documentation, related information, and equipment are available and correctly identified to the patient's identifiers.*[12,13]
- Assess the patient's condition.
- Put on a gown, a mask with face shield or a mask and goggles, and gloves.[14]
- Maintain ventilation until the tracheotomy is performed.
- Make sure the patient has patent IV access; insert an IV catheter if necessary.[15]
- Sedate the patient for the procedure, as ordered, following safe medication administration practices *to decrease pain and anxiety.*[16,17,18]
- Monitor the patient's cardiac rhythm, oxygen saturation level, blood pressure, and exhaled carbon dioxide throughout the procedure.[15] Make sure that the alarm limits are appropriately set for the patient's current condition and that the alarms are turned on, functioning properly, and audible to staff.[19,20,21]
- Roll a blanket or towel to form a shoulder roll and place it under the patient's shoulders and neck *to extend his neck.* If the patient is in respiratory distress and optimal neck extension isn't tolerated, place the patient in the semi-Fowler position.[15]
- Conduct a time-out immediately before starting the procedure *to perform a final assessment that the correct patient, site, positioning, and procedure are identified and that, as applicable, all relevant information and necessary equipment are available during and after the procedure.*[13,22]
- Disinfect the top of the local anesthetic vial with an alcohol pad and then allow it to dry. Invert the vial so that the practitioner can withdraw the anesthetic using the 22G needle attached to the 5-mL syringe.
- The practitioner will put on a sterile gown, a mask with face shield or a mask and goggles, and sterile gloves.[14] Assist with the procedure as needed. (See *Assisting with a tracheotomy,* page 766.)
- When the tube is in position, attach it to the appropriate oxygen therapy device, which is connected to an oxygen source.
- Provide adequate humidification of inspired oxygen *because when a tracheostomy bypasses the upper airway, alternative methods of conditioning inspired air must be used to avoid airway damage and thickening of mucosal secretions.*[23,24]
- Inject air into the distal cuff port *to inflate the cuff.*

NURSING ALERT *Limit tracheostomy tube cuff pressure to 25 mm Hg to prevent ischemia and mucosal injury.*[25]

- Auscultate the patient's breath sounds using a stethoscope.
- Remove and discard your gloves,[14,26] perform hand hygiene,[1,2,3,4,5] and put on sterile gloves.[14]
- Apply the sterile tracheostomy dressing under the tracheostomy tube flange. Place the tracheostomy ties through the openings of the tube flanges and tie them on the side of the patient's neck. *Doing so allows easy access and prevents pressure necrosis at the back of the neck.*[25,27]
- Clean used equipment or dispose of it in appropriate receptacles. Replenish all supplies as needed.
- Assess the patient's vital signs and respiratory status at an interval determined by your facility or the patient's condition; *there's no evidence-based research to indicate best practice for frequency of vital signs monitoring, so it should be determined by each facility.*[28]
- Make sure the head of the patient's bed is elevated 30 to 45 degrees (unless contraindicated) *to prevent ventilator-associated pneumonia and to make sure that the patient is comfortable and can easily reach the call light.*[29,30]
- Obtain a chest X-ray *to confirm tube placement.*
- Remove and discard your gloves and other personal protective equipment.[14,26]
- Perform hand hygiene.[1,2,3,4,5]
- Clean and disinfect your stethoscope using a disinfectant pad.[3,13]
- Perform hand hygiene.[1,2,3,4,5]
- Document the procedure.[33,34,35]

Special considerations

- The Joint Commission issued a sentinel event alert concerning medical device alarm safety *because alarm-related events have been associated with permanent loss of function and death.* Among the major contributing factors were improper alarm settings, alarms inappropriately turned off, and alarm signals not audible to staff. Make sure that alarm limits are appropriately set and are turned on and audible to staff. Follow facility guidelines for preventing alarm fatigue.[37]
- Monitor the patient carefully for signs of infection. Ideally, the tracheotomy should be performed using sterile technique as described; however, in an emergency, this may not be possible, *increasing the risk of infection.*
- Make sure the following equipment is always at the patient's bedside: suctioning equipment *because the patient may need his airway cleared at any time;* the sterile obturator used to insert the tracheostomy tube *in case the tube is expelled;* a sterile tracheostomy tube and obturator (the same size as the one used) *in case the tube must be replaced quickly;* a spare, sterile inner cannula *that can be used if the cannula is expelled;* a sterile tracheostomy tube and obturator one size smaller than the one used, *which may be needed if the tube is expelled and the trachea begins to close;* and a sterile tracheal dilator or sterile hemostats *to maintain an open airway before inserting a new tracheostomy tube.*

Assisting with a tracheotomy

After preparing the skin with an antiseptic and allowing it to dry, the practitioner will make a horizontal or vertical incision into the skin. (A vertical incision helps avoid arteries, veins, and nerves on the lateral borders of the trachea.) Then he'll dissect subcutaneous fat and muscle and move the muscle aside with vein retractors *to locate the tracheal rings*. He'll make an incision between the second and third tracheal rings, using hemostats *to control bleeding*.

The practitioner will inject a local anesthetic into the tracheal lumen *to suppress the cough reflex* and create a stoma in the trachea. When this is done, carefully apply suction *to remove blood and secretions that may obstruct the airway or be aspirated into the lungs*. The practitioner will then insert the tracheostomy tube and obturator into the stoma (as shown below). After inserting the tube, he'll remove the obturator.

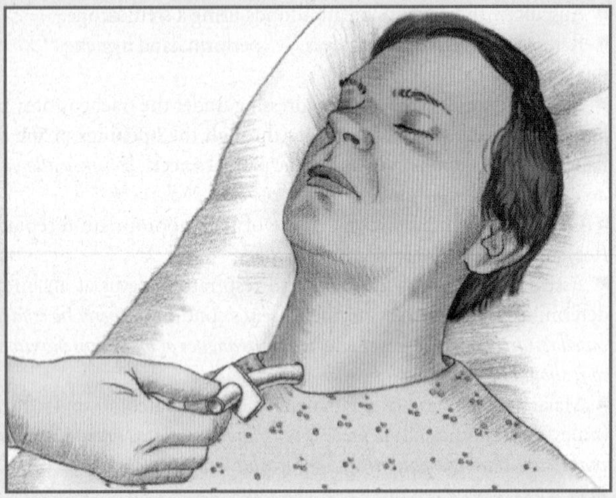

Apply a sterile tracheostomy dressing, and anchor the tube with tracheostomy ties (as shown on top right). Check for air movement through the tube and auscultate breath sounds *to ensure proper placement*.

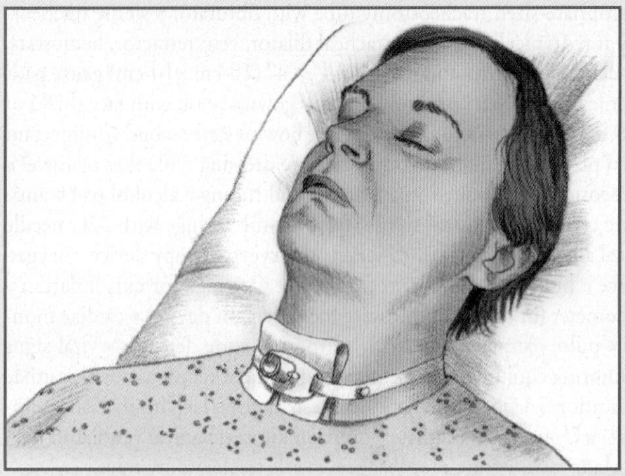

An alternative approach

A minimally invasive percutaneous tracheotomy may also be performed at the bedside. Unlike the surgical technique, this method dilates rather than cuts the tissue structures. During this procedure, the practitioner passes a needle into the trachea and then threads a dilator over a guide wire, which progressively dilates until a tracheostomy tube can be placed. This method has a similar success rate compared with the surgical approach.[27,36]

After the skin is prepared and anesthetized, the practitioner makes a 1-cm midline incision. When the stoma reaches the desired size, the practitioner inserts the tracheostomy tube. After the tube is in place, inflate the cuff, secure the tube, and check the patient's breath sounds. The practitioner will suture the corners of the incision. Then obtain a portable chest X-ray.

- Review emergency first-aid measures. When a blocked tube can't be cleared by suctioning or withdrawing the inner cannula, your facility may require you to stay with the patient while someone else calls the practitioner or the appropriate code. Continue trying to ventilate the patient with whatever method works such as a handheld resuscitation bag. Don't remove the tracheostomy tube entirely; *doing so may close the airway completely*.
- Use extreme caution if you try to reinsert an expelled tracheostomy tube *to avoid tracheal trauma, perforation, compression, and asphyxiation*.

Complications

A tracheotomy can cause an airway obstruction (from improper tube placement), hemorrhage, edema, a perforated esophagus, subcutaneous or mediastinal emphysema, aspiration of secretions, tracheal necrosis (from cuff pressure), infection, or lacerations of arteries, veins, or nerves.

Documentation

Record the reason for the procedure, the date and time it took place, the patient's respiratory status before and after the procedure, and the results of the chest X-ray. Note the type and size of tube used. Include any complications that occurred during the procedure, the amount of cuff pressure, and the respiratory therapy initiated after the procedure. Also note the patient's response to respiratory therapy.

References

1 The Joint Commission. (2015). Standard NPSG.07.01.01. *Comprehensive accreditation manual for hospitals: The official handbook.* Oakbrook Terrace, IL: The Joint Commission. (Level VII)

2 Centers for Disease Control and Prevention. (2002). Guideline for hand hygiene in health-care settings: Recommendations of the Healthcare Infection Control Practices Advisory Committee and the HICPAC/SHEA/APIC/IDSA Hand Hygiene Task Force. *MMWR Recommendations and Reports, 51*(RR-16), 1–45. Accessed May 2015 via the Web at http://www.cdc.gov/mmwr/pdf/rr/rr5116.pdf (Level II)

3 World Health Organization. (2009). "WHO guidelines on hand hygiene in health care: First global patient safety challenge, clean care is safer care" [Online]. Accessed May 2015 via the Web at http://whqlibdoc.who.int/publications/2009/9789241597906_eng.pdf (Level IV)

4 Centers for Medicare & Medicaid Services, Department of Health and Human Services. (2014). Condition of participation: Infection control. 42 C.F.R. § 482.42.

5 American Osteopathic Association. (2014). Standard 07.01.21. *Healthcare Facilities Accreditation Program: Accreditation requirements for acute care hospitals.* Chicago, IL: American Osteopathic Association. (Level VII)

6 The Joint Commission. (2015). Standard NPSG.01.01.01. *Comprehensive accreditation manual for hospitals: The official handbook.* Oakbrook Terrace, IL: The Joint Commission. (Level VII)

7 American Osteopathic Association. (2014). Standard 15.01.16. *Healthcare Facilities Accreditation Program: Accreditation requirements for acute care hospitals.* Chicago, IL: American Osteopathic Association. (Level VII)

8 Centers for Medicare & Medicaid Services, Department of Health and Human Services. (2014). Condition of participation: Patient's rights. 42 C.F.R. § 482.13(c)(1).

9 The Joint Commission. (2015). Standard RI.01.03.01. *Comprehensive accreditation manual for hospitals: The official handbook.* Oakbrook Terrace, IL: The Joint Commission. (Level VII)

10 Centers for Medicare & Medicaid Services, Department of Health and Human Services. (2014). Condition of participation: Patient's rights. 42 C.F.R. § 482.13 (b)(2).

11 American Osteopathic Association. (2014). Standard 15.01.11. *Healthcare Facilities Accreditation Program: Accreditation requirements for acute care hospitals.* Chicago, IL: American Osteopathic Association. (Level VII)

12 The Joint Commission. (2015). Standard UP.01.01.01. *Comprehensive accreditation manual for hospitals: The official handbook.* Oakbrook Terrace, IL: The Joint Commission. (Level VII)

13 American Osteopathic Association. (2014). Standard 30.00.14. *Healthcare Facilities Accreditation Program: Accreditation requirements for acute care hospitals.* Chicago, IL: American Osteopathic Association. (Level VII)

14 Siegel, J. D., et al. (2007). "2007 guideline for isolation precautions: Preventing transmission of infectious agents in healthcare settings" [Online]. Accessed May 2015 via the Web at http://www.cdc.gov/hicpac/pdf/isolation/Isolation2007.pdf (Level II)

15 Morris, L. L., & Afifi, M. S. (Eds.). (2010). *Tracheostomies: The complete guide.* New York, NY: Springer Publishing Company.

16 The Joint Commission. (2015). Standard MM.06.01.01. *Comprehensive accreditation manual for hospitals: The official handbook.* Oakbrook Terrace, IL: The Joint Commission. (Level VII)

17 American Osteopathic Association. (2014). Standard 16.01.03. *Healthcare Facilities Accreditation Program: Accreditation requirements for acute care hospitals.* Chicago, IL: American Osteopathic Association. (Level VII)

18 Centers for Medicare & Medicaid Services, Department of Health and Human Services. (2014). Condition of participation: Nursing services. 42 C.F.R. § 482.23(c).

19 Graham, K. C., & Cvach, M. (2010). Monitor alarm fatigue: Standardizing use of physiological monitors and decreasing nuisance alarms. *American Journal of Critical Care, 19,* 28–37.

20 American Association of Critical-Care Nurses. (2013). "AACN practice alert: Alarm management" [Online]. Accessed May 2015 via the Web at http://www.aacn.org/wd/practice/docs/practicealerts/alarm-management-practice-alert.pdf (Level VII)

21 The Joint Commission. (2015). Standard NPSG.06.01.01. *Comprehensive accreditation manual for hospitals: The official handbook.* Oakbrook Terrace, IL: The Joint Commission. (Level VII)

22 The Joint Commission. (2015). Standard UP.01.03.01. *Comprehensive accreditation manual for hospitals: The official handbook.* Oakbrook Terrace, IL: The Joint Commission. (Level VII)

23 Regan, K., & Hunt, K. (2008). Tracheostomy management. *Continuing Education in Anaesthesia, Critical Care & Pain, 8,* 31–35. Accessed May 2015 via the Web at http://www.medscape.com/viewarticle/574271

24 American Association for Respiratory Care (AARC). (2002). AARC clinical practice guideline: Oxygen therapy for adults in the acute care facility—2002 revision & update. *Respiratory Care, 47,* 717–720. Accessed May 2015 via the Web at http://www.rcjournal.com/cpgs/otachcpg-update.html (Level VII)

25 Regan, E. N., & Dallachiesa, L. (2009). How to care for a patient with a tracheostomy. *Nursing, 39*(8), 34–39. Accessed May 2015 via the Web at http://www.nursingcenter.com/lnc/pdf?AID=926437&an=00152193-200908000-00016&Journal_ID=54016&Issue_ID=926406

26 American Osteopathic Association. (2014). Standard 07.01.10. *Healthcare Facilities Accreditation Program: Accreditation requirements for acute care hospitals.* Chicago, IL: American Osteopathic Association. (Level VII)

27 Lynn-McHale Wiegand, D. (Ed.). (2011). *AACN procedure manual for critical care* (6th ed.). St. Louis, MO: Saunders.

28 American Society of PeriAnesthesia Nurses. (2015). *2015-2017 Perianesthesia nursing standards, practice recommendations and interpretive statements.* Cherry Hill, NJ: American Society of PeriAnesthesia Nurses. (Level VII)

29 Klompas, M., et al. (2014). Strategies to prevent ventilator-associated pneumonia in acute care hospitals: 2014 update. *Infection Control and Hospital Epidemiology, 35,* 915–936. Accessed May 2015 via the Web at http://www.jstor.org/stable/10.1086/677144 (Level II)

30 American Osteopathic Association. (2014). Standard 07.01.02. *Healthcare Facilities Accreditation Program: Accreditation requirements for acute care hospitals.* Chicago, IL: American Osteopathic Association. (Level VII)

31 Rutala, W. A., et al. (2008). "Guideline for disinfection and sterilization in healthcare facilities, 2008" [Online]. Accessed May 2015 via the Web at http://www.cdc.gov/hicpac/pdf/guidelines/Disinfection_Nov_2008.pdf (Level I)

32 American Osteopathic Association. (2014). Standard 07.02.03. *Healthcare Facilities Accreditation Program: Accreditation requirements for acute care hospitals.* Chicago, IL: American Osteopathic Association. (Level VII)

33 The Joint Commission. (2015). Standard RC.01.03.01. *Comprehensive accreditation manual for hospitals: The official handbook.* Oakbrook Terrace, IL: The Joint Commission. (Level VII)

34 American Osteopathic Association. (2014). Standard 10.00.03. *Healthcare Facilities Accreditation Program: Accreditation requirements for acute care hospitals.* Chicago, IL: American Osteopathic Association. (Level VII)

35 Centers for Medicare & Medicaid Services, Department of Health and Human Services. (2014). Condition of participation: Medical record services. 42 C.F.R. § 482.24(b).

36 Dempsey, G. A., et al. (2010). Percutaneous tracheostomy: A 6 yr prospective evaluation of the single tapered dilator technique. *British Journal of Anaesthesia, 105,* 1–7. Accessed May 2015 via the Web at http://bja.oxfordjournals.org/content/early/2010/09/02/bja.aeq238.ful (Level IV)

37 The Joint Commission. (2013). "Sentinel event alert: Medical device alarm safety in hospitals" [Online]. Accessed May 2015 via the Web at http://www.jointcommission.org/assets/1/18/SEA_50_alarms_4_5_13_FINAL1.PDF (Level VII)

ADDITIONAL REFERENCES

Morris, L. L., et al. (2013). Tracheostomy care and complications in the intensive care unit. *Critical Care Nurse, 33*(5), 18–31.

Rayess, H. M., et al. (2013). Predictive factors for patient outcomes following open bedside tracheotomy. *Laryngoscope, 123,* 923–928. (Level IV)

TRANSABDOMINAL TUBE FEEDING AND CARE

To access the stomach, duodenum, or jejunum, a practitioner may place a tube through a patient's abdominal wall. This procedure may be done surgically or percutaneously.

A gastrostomy or jejunostomy tube is usually inserted during intra-abdominal surgery. The tube may be used for feeding during the immediate postoperative period or it may provide long-term enteral access, depending on the type of surgery. Typically, the practitioner sutures the tube in place to prevent gastric contents from leaking.

In contrast, a percutaneous endoscopic gastrostomy (PEG) or percutaneous endoscopic jejunostomy (PEJ) tube can be inserted endoscopically without the need for laparotomy or general anesthesia. Typically, the insertion is done in the endoscopy suite or at the patient's bedside. Ultrasound can be used to confirm placement. A PEG or PEJ tube may be used for nutrition, drainage, and decompression. Contraindications to endoscopic placement include obstruction (such as an esophageal stricture or duodenal blockage), previous gastric surgery, morbid obesity, and ascites. These conditions necessitate surgical placement. Long-term feeding devices should be considered when the need for enteral feeding is at least 4 weeks in adults, children, and infants of term age.[1]

With either type of tube placement, feedings may begin after 24 hours (or when peristalsis resumes). Intermittent feedings are commonly administered using a feeding container or bag with or without an enteral feeding pump.[1]

Nursing care for patients receiving intermittent enteral feeding through a PEG or PEJ tube includes providing skin care at the tube site, maintaining the feeding tube, administering feedings, monitoring the patient's response to feedings, adjusting the feeding schedule, and preparing the patient for self-care after discharge.

Equipment

For intermittent or continuous feeding

Feeding formula ▪ large-bulb or catheter-tip syringe ▪ water ▪ alcohol pad ▪ enteral administration set ▪ IV pole ▪ oral care supplies ▪ gloves ▪ warning labels that say WARNING! FOR ENTERAL USE ONLY—NOT FOR IV USE ▪ Optional: enteral feeding pump, sterile water, promotility agent.

For site care

4″ × 4″ (10-cm × 10-cm) gauze pads ▪ soap and water or normal saline solution ▪ water ▪ cotton-tipped applicators ▪ hypoallergenic tape ▪ gloves ▪ Optional: external stabilization device, sterile gauze or foam dressing, skin protectant.

Preparation of equipment

Always check the expiration date on commercially prepared feeding formulas. Compare the label on the enteral feeding with the practitioner's order. If the formula has been prepared by a dietitian or pharmacist, check the label for correct patient identification, correct formula, and preparation time and date.[1] Discard any unused reconstituted formula within 24 hours of preparation.[1]

Perform hand hygiene.[1,2,3,4,5,6] Prepare the enteral administration set and administration equipment. Make sure the formula is room temperature *because cold formula can cause cramping.* Fill the feeding bag, and then purge any air from the administration tubing. If a prefilled container is available, attach it to the administration set and then purge any air from the tubing.[1]

NURSING ALERT *Make sure that the feeding bag or container is clearly labeled with a statement such as WARNING! FOR ENTERAL USE ONLY—NOT FOR IV USE* to prevent administration errors.[1]

To avoid contamination, hang only a 4-hour supply of reconstituted formula at a time. Sterile, decanted formula can hang for 8 hours. Closed-system formulas can hang for 24 to 48 hours, according to the manufacturer's guidelines.[1]

Implementation

- Verify the practitioner's order for enteral feeding, which should include the formula type, delivery site, and method and rate of administration.[1]
- Review the patient's medical record *to make sure that catheter placement was confirmed before beginning the feeding.*
- Gather and prepare the necessary equipment and the enteral feeding formula.
- Perform hand hygiene.[1,2,3,4,5,6]
- Put on gloves.[7,8]
- Confirm the patient's identity using at least two patient identifiers.[9]
- Provide privacy.[10,11]
- Explain the procedure to the patient. Tell him that feedings usually start at a slow rate of administration, with the rate increasing as tolerated. After the patient tolerates continuous feedings, he may progress to intermittent feedings as ordered.
- Assess the patient *to determine his risk for aspiration.*[1]
- Check the external length of the catheter *to determine whether the catheter has migrated.*[1] If you suspect catheter migration, don't administer the feeding; notify the practitioner.
- Have the patient sit, or elevate the head of the bed at least 30 degrees (45 degrees is preferred) unless contraindicated by the patient's condition.[1,12] *These positions help to prevent esophageal reflux and pulmonary aspiration of formula.* If the patient can't tolerate an elevation of this type, use reverse the Trendelenburg position unless contraindicated.[1]
- Remove and discard your gloves.[7,8]
- Perform hand hygiene.[1,2,3,4,5,6]
- Put on new gloves.[7,8]

For an intermittent or a continuous feeding

- Thoroughly disinfect the feeding tube hub with an alcohol pad and then allow it to dry *to prevent contamination that may occur when accessing the feeding tube hub.*[1]
- Flush the feeding tube with 30 mL of water; use sterile water if the patient is immunocompromised or critically ill.[1]
- Connect the administration set to the feeding tube. Trace the tubing from the patient to its point of origin *to make sure it's connected to the proper port before beginning the tube feeding.*[13]
- Open the flow clamp and regulate the flow to the desired rate; *commonly, an intermittent feeding period lasts 30 to 45 minutes.*[1] Follow the manufacturer's instructions for setting the flow rate if using an enteral infusion pump. *Most patients receive small volumes initially and then gradually increase as tolerated.*
- If using an enteral feeding pump, make sure that the feeding pump alarm limits are set according to the patient's current condition and that the alarms are turned on, functioning properly, and audible to staff.[14,15,16]
- Route the tubing using a standardized approach; for example, route the tube feeding administration set and enteral tube feeding pump toward the patient's feet and the IV tubing toward the patient's head *to prevent misconnections.*[1,13,17] If different access sites are used, label each tubing at both the distal (near the patient connection) and proximal (near the source container) ends *to distinguish different tubing and prevent misconnections.*[17]
- Assess for GI intolerance to tube feedings every 4 hours by assessing for abdominal distention, monitoring for complaints of abdominal pain, observing for passage of flatus and stool, and monitoring gastric residual volumes as ordered.[1,12]
- When the feeding is complete, flush the feeding tube with 30 mL of water *to maintain patency and provide hydration.*[1]
- Cap the tube *to prevent leakage.*
- Perform oral care routinely *to decrease oral bacterial colonization and subsequently reduce the risk of health care–acquired pneumonia.*
- Monitor the patient's fluid and electrolyte status *to anticipate and detect fluid and electrolyte imbalances.*

For site care

- Remove the dressing gently. Don't cut away the dressing over the catheter *because you might cut the tube or the sutures holding the tube in place.*
- Remove and discard your gloves.[7,8]
- Perform hand hygiene.[2,3,4,5,6]
- Put on a new pair of gloves.

For a gastrostomy or jejunostomy tube

- Assess the tube exit site for signs of skin breakdown, redness, edema, or the presence of purulent drainage.
- Inspect the tube for wear and tear. *A tube that wears out needs to be replaced.*
- Until healing occurs, clean the skin immediately around the gastrostomy or jejunostomy tube's exit site daily (and as needed) using a cotton-tipped applicator moistened with normal saline solution. Next, using a 4″ × 4″ (10-cm × 10-cm) gauze pad soaked in normal saline solution, clean the adjacent skin and pat it dry using another gauze pad. When the exit site has healed, wash the skin around it with soap and water daily. Rinse the area with water, and pat it dry.
- Apply skin protectant, if necessary, *to prevent skin maceration.*
- Secure the gastrostomy or jejunostomy tube to the skin with hypoallergenic tape or other external stabilization device *to prevent peristaltic migration of the tube and tension on the suture that anchors the tube in place.*

Caring for a PEG or PEJ site

The exit site of a percutaneous endoscopic gastrostomy (PEG) or percutaneous endoscopic jejunostomy (PEJ) tube requires routine observation and care. Follow these care guidelines:

■ Slide the tube's outer bumper carefully away from the skin about ½″ (1.3 cm). Depress the skin surrounding the tube gently, and inspect for leakage. *Minimal wound drainage, which appears initially after implantation, should subside in about 1 week.*

■ Assess the skin at the exit site for signs of infection, such as redness, edema, and purulent drainage.

■ Inspect the tube for wear and tear. *A tube that wears out needs to be replaced.*

■ Clean the exit site with soap and water-moistened gauze pads, and allow it to dry.

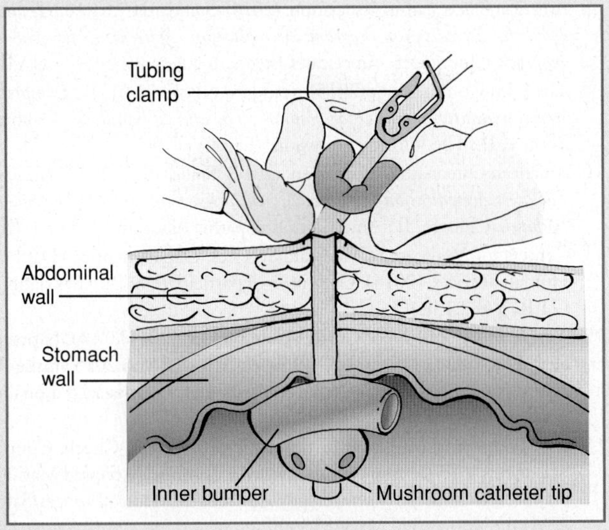

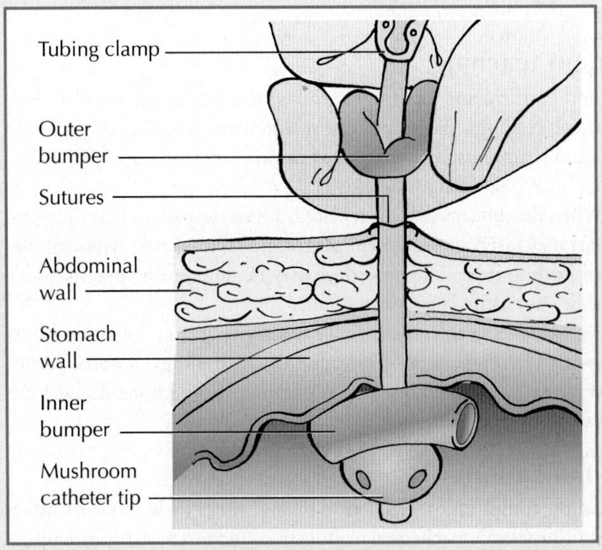

■ Rotate the outer bumper 90 degrees *to avoid applying the same tension to the same skin area and to prevent pressure ulcer formation at the exit site*, and slide the bumper back over the exit site. Ensure that the outer bumper isn't resting too tightly against the skin; one finger's breadth should fit between the skin and the outer bumper.

■ If leakage appears at the PEG tube exit site or if the patient risks dislodging the tube, apply a sterile gauze or foam dressing and an external stabilization device around the site, as needed. Apply the dressing over the outer bumper *because applying it underneath the outer bumper creates pressure on the gastrostomy tube tract, which could lead to wound abscess.*

■ Label the dressing with the date, the time, and your initials.

■ Coil the tube, if necessary, and tape it to the abdomen *to prevent pulling and contamination of the tube.* Rotate the taping site *to prevent skin damage.* (See *Caring for a PEG or PEJ site.*)

Completing the procedure

■ Remove and discard your gloves.[7,8]

■ Perform hand hygiene.[2,3,4,5,6]

■ Document the procedure.[18,19,20]

Special considerations

■ The Joint Commission issued a sentinel event alert concerning medical device alarm safety *because alarm-related events have been associated with permanent loss of function and death.* Among the major contributing factors were improper alarm settings, alarms inappropriately turned off, and alarm signals not audible to staff. Make sure that alarm limits are appropriately set and that alarms are turned on, functioning properly, and audible to staff. Follow facility guidelines for preventing alarm fatigue.[21]

■ Replace administration sets for open-system enteral feedings at least every 24 hours; for closed systems, follow the manufacturer's guidelines.[1]

■ Be aware that an enteral feeding pump is generally required for small-bowel feedings and is preferred for gastric feedings in critically ill patients.[1]

■ Check gastric residual volume every 4 hours during the first 48 hours for gastrically fed patients. After the enteral feeding goal rate is achieved, check gastric residual volume every 6 to 8 hours unless the patient is critically ill; in this case, continue to monitor every 4 hours.[1]

■ If gastric residual volume is 250 mL or greater after a second residual check, notify the practitioner; a promotility agent may be needed. Hold the feeding if gastric residual volume is greater than 500 mL; reassess the patient's tolerance by assessing GI status and glycemic control. Minimize the use of sedation, if possible, and administer a promotility agent as prescribed.[1]

■ If administering medications through the enteral feeding tube, don't mix them together *because of the risk of physical and chemical incompatibilities.*[1] Administer liquid dosage forms when available; only immediate-release solid dosage forms may be substituted. Grind tablets into a fine powder and mix them with sterile water; open capsules and mix the powder with sterile water before administration.[1]

■ If the patient vomits, complains of nausea, feels too full, or regurgitates, stop the feeding immediately and assess his condition.[1] Flush the feeding tube and attempt to restart the feeding in 1 hour. (Measure the residual gastric contents first.) You may have to decrease the volume or rate of feedings. If the patient develops signs and symptoms of dumping syndrome, which include nausea, vomiting, cramps, pallor, and diarrhea, the feedings may have been administered too quickly.

- Before administering medication, stop the feeding and flush the tube with at least 15 mL of water. Administer the medication and then flush the tube again with at least 15 mL of water, taking into consideration the patient's fluid status. Repeat with each subsequent medication. Restart the feeding within 30 minutes when withholding the feeding is necessary to prevent interference with drug bioavailability *to prevent compromising the patient's nutritional status.*[1]

Patient teaching

Teach the patient and his family members or other caregivers all aspects of enteral feedings, including tube maintenance and site care. Specify signs and symptoms to report to the practitioner, define emergency situations, and review actions to take.

When the tube needs to be replaced, advise the patient that the practitioner may insert a replacement gastrostomy button after removing the initial feeding tube. The procedure may be done in the practitioner's office or your facility's endoscopy suite.

As the patient's tolerance of tube feeding improves, he may wish to try syringe feedings rather than intermittent feedings. If appropriate, teach him how to feed himself by the syringe method. (See *Teaching the patient about syringe feeding.*)

Complications

Common complications related to enteral tubes include GI or other systemic problems, mechanical malfunction, and metabolic disturbances. Cramping, nausea, vomiting, bloating, and diarrhea may be related to a medication; rapid infusion rate (dumping syndrome); formula contamination, osmolarity, or temperature (too cold or too warm); fat malabsorption; or intestinal atrophy from malnutrition. Constipation can result from inadequate hydration or insufficient exercise.

Systemic problems may be caused by pulmonary aspiration, infection at the tube exit site, or contaminated formula.

Typical mechanical problems include tube dislodgment, obstruction, or impairment. For example, a PEG or PEJ tube may migrate if the external bumper loosens. Occlusion may result from incompletely crushed and liquefied medication particles or inadequate tube flushing. The tube may also rupture or crack from age, drying, or frequent manipulation.

Other complications include vitamin and mineral deficiencies, impaired glucose tolerance, and fluid and electrolyte imbalances, which may follow bouts of diarrhea or constipation.

Documentation

On the intake and output record, note the date, time, and amount of each feeding and the water volume instilled. Maintain total volumes for nutrients and water separately to allow calculation of nutrient intake. In your notes, document the type of formula, the infusion method and rate, the patient's tolerance of the procedure and formula, and the amount of residual gastric contents. Also record complications and abdominal assessment findings. Note patient-teaching topics covered and the patient's progress in self-care. Note the date and time site care was performed. Record the appearance of the site, including any signs of infection, such as redness, swelling, and drainage.

REFERENCES

1 Bankhead, R., et al. (2009). A.S.P.E.N. enteral nutrition practice recommendations. *Journal of Parenteral & Enteral Nutrition, 33,* 122–167. Accessed May 2015 via the Web at http://www.ismp.org/tools/articles/ASPEN.pdf (Level IV)

2 Centers for Disease Control and Prevention. (2002). Guideline for hand hygiene in health-care settings: Recommendations of the Healthcare Infection Control Practices Advisory Committee and the HICPAC/SHEA/APIC/IDSA Hand Hygiene Task Force. *MMWR Recommendations and Reports, 51*(RR-16), 1–45. Accessed May 2015 via the Web at http://www.cdc.gov/mmwr/pdf/rr/rr5116.pdf (Level II)

3 The Joint Commission. (2015). Standard NPSG.07.01.01. *Comprehensive accreditation manual for hospitals: The official handbook.* Oakbrook Terrace, IL: The Joint Commission. (Level VII)

4 World Health Organization. (2009). "WHO guidelines on hand hygiene in health care: First global patient safety challenge, clean care is safer care" [Online]. Accessed May 2015 via the Web at http://whqlibdoc.who.int/publications/2009/9789241597906_eng.pdf (Level IV)

5 Centers for Medicare & Medicaid Services, Department of Health and Human Services. (2014). Condition of participation: Infection control. 42 C.F.R. § 482.42.

6 American Osteopathic Association. (2014). Standard 07.01.21. *Healthcare Facilities Accreditation Program: Accreditation requirements for acute care hospitals.* Chicago, IL: American Osteopathic Association. (Level VII)

7 Siegel, J. D., et al. (2007). "2007 guideline for isolation precautions: Preventing transmission of infectious agents in healthcare settings" [Online]. Accessed May 2015 via the Web at http://www.cdc.gov/hicpac/pdf/isolation/Isolation2007.pdf (Level II)

8 American Osteopathic Association. (2014). Standard 07.01.10. *Healthcare Facilities Accreditation Program: Accreditation requirements for acute care hospitals.* Chicago, IL: American Osteopathic Association. (Level VII)

9 The Joint Commission. (2015). Standard NPSG.01.01.01. *Comprehensive accreditation manual for hospitals: The official handbook.* Oakbrook Terrace, IL: The Joint Commission. (Level VII)

10 American Osteopathic Association. (2014). Standard 15.01.16. *Healthcare Facilities Accreditation Program: Accreditation requirements for acute care hospitals.* Chicago, IL: American Osteopathic Association. (Level VII)

11 Centers for Medicare & Medicaid Services, Department of Health and Human Services. (2014). Condition of participation: Patient's rights. 42 C.F.R. § 482.13(c)(1).

12 American Association of Critical-Care Nurses. (2011). "AACN practice alert: Prevention of aspiration" [Online]. Accessed May 2015 via the Web at http://www.aacn.org/WD/practice/docs/practicealerts/aacn-aspiration-practice-alert.pdf (Level VII)

13 U.S. Food and Drug Administration. (n.d.). "Look. Check. Connect. Safe medical device connections save lives" [Online]. Accessed May 2015 via the Web at http://www.fda.gov/downloads/MedicalDevices/Safety/AlertsandNotices/UCM134873.pdf

14 American Association of Critical-Care Nurses. (2013). "AACN practice alert: Alarm management" [Online]. Accessed May 2015 via the Web at http://www.aacn.org/wd/practice/docs/practicealerts/alarm-management-practice-alert.pdf

15 The Joint Commission. (2015). Standard NPSG.06.01.01. *Comprehensive accreditation manual for hospitals: The official handbook.* Oakbrook Terrace, IL: The Joint Commission. (Level VII)

16 Graham, K. C., & Cvach, M. (2010). Monitor alarm fatigue: Standardizing use of physiological monitors and decreasing nuisance alarms. *American Journal of Critical Care, 19,* 28–37.

17 The Joint Commission. (2015). "Sentinel event alert: Managing risk during transition to new ISO tubing connector standards" [Online]. Accessed May 2015 via the Web at http://www.jointcommission.org/assets/1/18/SEA_53_Connectors_8_19_14_FINAL.pdf (Level VII)

18 The Joint Commission. (2015). Standard RC.01.03.01. *Comprehensive accreditation manual for hospitals: The official handbook.* Oakbrook Terrace, IL: The Joint Commission. (Level VII)

19 Centers for Medicare & Medicaid Services, Department of Health and Human Services. (2014). Condition of participation: Medical record services. 42 C.F.R. § 482.24(b).

20 American Osteopathic Association. (2014). Standard 10.00.03. *Healthcare Facilities Accreditation Program: Accreditation requirements for acute care hospitals.* Chicago, IL: American Osteopathic Association. (Level VII)

21 The Joint Commission. (2013). "Sentinel event alert: Medical device alarm safety in hospitals" [Online]. Accessed May 2015 via the Web at http://www.jointcommission.org/assets/1/18/SEA_50_alarms_4_5_13_FINAL1.PDF

ADDITIONAL REFERENCE

Nettina, S. M. (2014). *Lippincott manual of nursing practice* (10th ed.). Philadelphia, PA: Wolters Kluwer.

PATIENT TEACHING

Teaching the patient about syringe feeding

If the patient plans to feed himself by syringe when he returns home, you'll need to teach him how to do this before he's discharged. Here are some points to emphasize.

Initial instructions

First, show the patient how to clamp the feeding tube, remove the syringe's bulb or plunger, and place the tip of the syringe into the feeding tube (as shown below). Then tell him to instill between 30 and 60 mL of water into the feeding tube *to make sure it stays open and patent.*

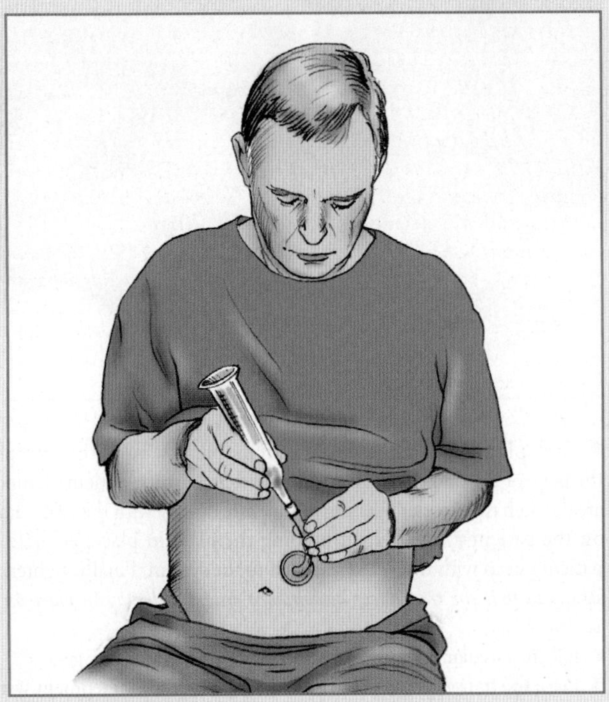

Next, tell him to pour the feeding solution into the syringe and begin the feeding (as shown on top right). As the solution flows into the stomach, show him how to tilt the syringe *to allow air bubbles to escape.* Describe the discomfort that air bubbles may cause.

Tips for free flow

When about one-fourth of the feeding solution remains, direct the patient to refill the syringe. Caution him to avoid letting the syringe empty completely *because doing so may result in abdominal cramping and gas.*

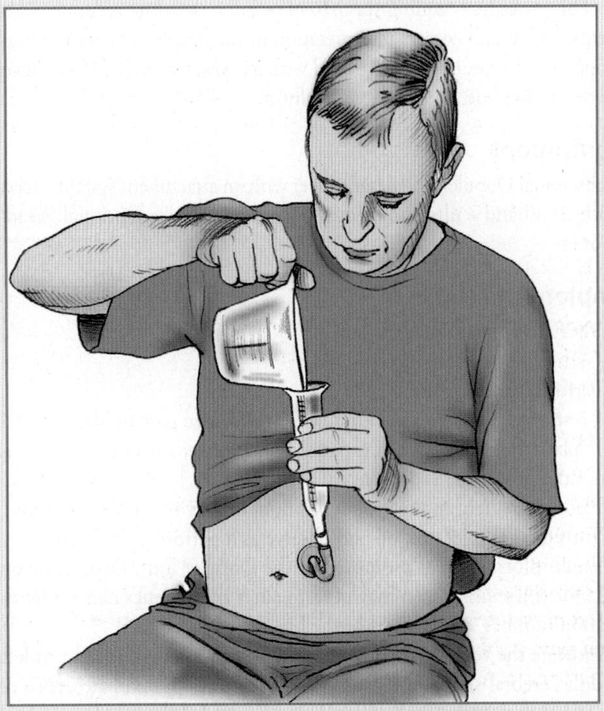

Show the patient how to increase and decrease the solution's flow rate by raising or lowering the syringe. Explain that he may need to dilute a thick solution *to promote free flow.*

Finishing up

Inform the patient that the feeding infusion process should take at least 15 minutes. If the process takes less than 15 minutes, dumping syndrome may result.

Show the patient the steps needed to finish the feeding, including how to flush the tube with water, clamp the tube, and clean the equipment for later use. If he's using disposable gear, urge him to discard it properly. Review instructions for storing unused feeding solution as appropriate.

TRANSCRANIAL DOPPLER MONITORING

Transcranial Doppler ultrasonography is a noninvasive method of monitoring blood flow in the intracranial vessels, specifically the circle of Willis.[1] This procedure is used on the intensive care unit to monitor patients who have experienced cerebrovascular disorders, such as stroke, head trauma, or subarachnoid hemorrhage. It can help detect intracranial stenosis, vasospasm, and arteriovenous malformations as well as assess collateral pathways. Because it displays a continuous waveform, it can be used in intraoperative monitoring of cerebral circulation.

Transcranial Doppler ultrasonography is also used to monitor the effect of intracranial pressure changes on the cerebral circulation, to monitor patient response to various medications, and to evaluate carbon dioxide reactivity, which may be impaired or lost from arterial obstruction or trauma. It has also been used to confirm brain death.

The transcranial Doppler unit transmits pulses of high-frequency ultrasound, which are then reflected back to the transducer by the red blood cells moving in the vessel being monitored. This information is then processed by the instrument into an audible signal and a velocity waveform, which is displayed on the monitor. The displayed waveform is actually a moving graph of blood flow velocities with *time* displayed along the horizontal axis, *velocity* displayed along the vertical axis, and *amplitude* represented by various colors or intensities within the waveform. The heart's contractions speed up the movement of blood cells during systole and slow it down during diastole, resulting in a waveform that varies in velocity over the cardiac cycle.

The major benefits of transcranial Doppler monitoring are that it provides instantaneous, real-time information about cerebral blood flow and that it's noninvasive and painless for the patient. Also, the unit itself is portable and easy to use. The major disadvantage is that it relies on the ability of the ultrasound waves to penetrate thin areas of the cranium; this is difficult if the patient has thickening of the temporal bone, which increases with age.

This procedure requires specialized training to ensure accurate vessel identification and correct interpretation of the signals. The transcranial Doppler unit should always be used with its power set at the lowest level needed to provide an adequate waveform.

Equipment

Transcranial Doppler unit ▪ transducer with an attachment system ▪ terry cloth headband ▪ ultrasonic coupling gel ▪ marker ▪ Optional: headphones.

Implementation

- Verify the practitioner's order.
- Gather the necessary equipment,
- Perform hand hygiene.[2,3,4,5,6]
- Confirm the patient's identity using at least two patient identifiers.[7]
- Explain the procedure to the patient, and answer any questions he has about the procedure as completely as possible.
- Place the patient in the proper position, usually the supine position.
- Turn the Doppler unit on and observe as it performs a self-test.
- Enter information as prompted by the Doppler unit. Depending on the unit you're using, you may need to enter the patient's name, identification number, or diagnosis or the practitioner's name.
- Indicate the vessel that you wish to monitor, usually the right or left middle cerebral artery. You'll also need to set the approximate depth of the vessel within the skull (50 mm to 56 mm for the middle cerebral artery).
- Increase the power level to 100% to initially locate the signal. You can later decrease the level as needed, depending on the thickness of the patient's skull.
- Examine the temporal region of the patient's head, and mentally identify the three windows of the transtemporal access route: posterior, middle, and anterior (as shown below).

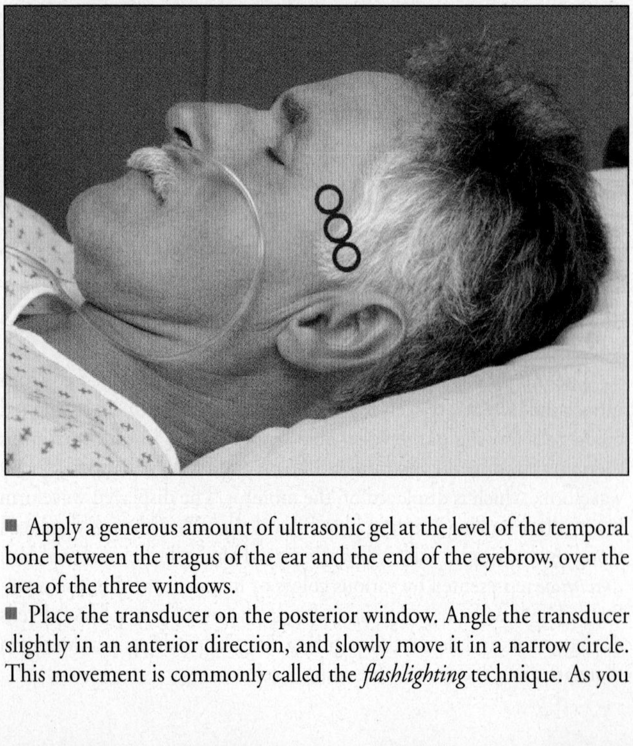

- Apply a generous amount of ultrasonic gel at the level of the temporal bone between the tragus of the ear and the end of the eyebrow, over the area of the three windows.
- Place the transducer on the posterior window. Angle the transducer slightly in an anterior direction, and slowly move it in a narrow circle. This movement is commonly called the *flashlighting* technique. As you hold the transducer at an angle and perform flashlighting, also begin to very slowly move the transducer forward across the temporal area. As you do this, listen for the audible signal with the highest pitch. This sound corresponds to the highest velocity signal, which corresponds to the signal of the vessel you are assessing. You can also use headphones *to let you better evaluate the audible signal and provide patient privacy.*
- After you've located the highest-pitched signal, use a marker to draw a circle around the transducer head on the patient's temple (as shown below). Note the angle of the transducer *so that you can duplicate it after the transducer attachment system is in place.*

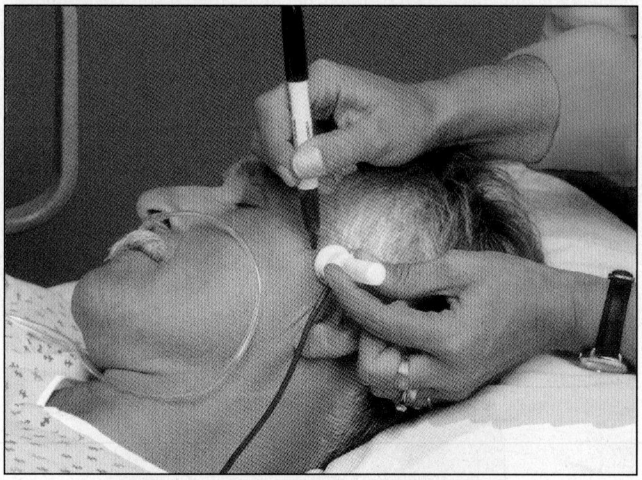

- Next, place the transducer system on the patient. To do this, first place the plate of the transducer attachment system over the patient's temporal area; match the circular opening in the plate exactly with the circle drawn on the patient's head. Then, holding the plate in place, encircle the patient's head with the straps attached to the system. Finally, tighten the straps *so that the transducer attachment system will stay in place on the patient's head.*
- Fill the circular opening in the plate with the ultrasonic gel.
- Place the transducer in the gel-filled opening in the attachment system plate. Using the plastic screws provided, loosely secure the two plates together *to hold the transducer in place but allow it to rotate for the best angle.*
- Adjust the position and angle of the transducer until you again hear the highest-pitched audible signal. When you hear this signal, look at the waveform on the monitor screen. You should see a clear waveform with a bright white line (called an *envelope*) at the upper edge of the waveform. The envelope exactly follows the contours of the waveform itself.
- If the envelope doesn't follow the waveform's contours, adjust the gain setting. If the signal is wrapping around the screen, increase the scale to drop the baseline.
- When you've determined that you have the strongest, highest-pitched signal and the best waveform, lock the transducer in place by tightening the plastic screws (as shown on next page, top left). The tightened plates will hold the transducer at the angle you've chosen. Disconnect the transducer handle.
- Place a wide terry cloth headband over the transducer attachment system, and secure it around the patient's head *to provide additional stability for the transducer.*
- Look at the monitor screen. You should be able to see a waveform and read the numeric values of the peak, mean velocities, and pulsatility index (PI+) above the displayed waveform. The shape of the waveform reveals more information. (See *Comparing velocity waveforms.*)
- Perform hand hygiene.[2,3,4,5,6]
- Document the procedure.[8,9,10]

Comparing velocity waveforms

A normal transcranial Doppler signal is usually characterized by mean velocities that fall within the normal reported values. Additional information can be gathered by evaluating the shape of the velocity waveform.

Effect of significant proximal vessel obstruction

A delayed systolic upstroke can be seen in a waveform when significant proximal vessel obstruction is present.

Normal | **Proximal vessel obstruction**

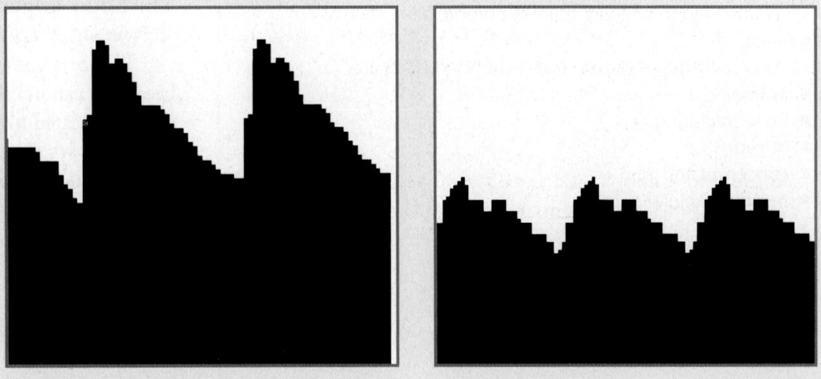

Effect of increased cerebrovascular resistance

Changes in cerebrovascular resistance, such as those that occur with increased intracranial pressure, cause a decrease in diastolic flow.

Normal | **Increased resistance**

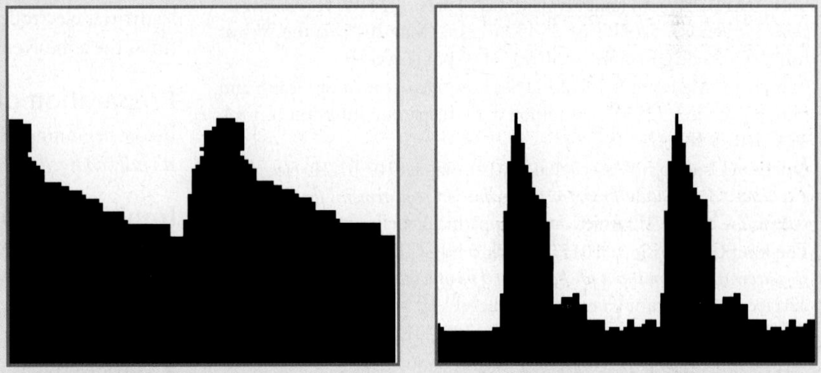

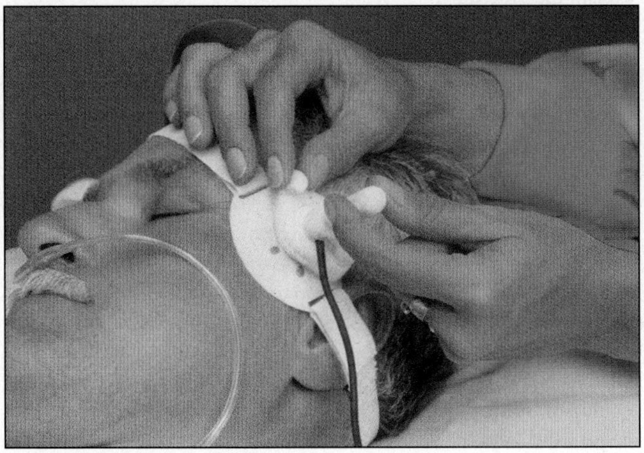

Special considerations

■ Velocity changes in the transcranial Doppler signal correlate with changes in cerebral blood flow. The parameter that most clearly reflects this change is the mean velocity. To determine this, first establish a baseline for the mean velocity. Then, as the patient's velocity increases or decreases, the value (%) will change negatively or positively from the baseline.

■ Emboli appear as high-intensity transients occurring randomly during the cardiac cycle. Emboli make a distinctive clicking, chirping, or plunking sound. You can set up an emboli counter to count either the total number of emboli aggregates or the rate of embolic events per minute.

■ Various screens can be stored on the system's hard drive and then recalled or printed.

■ Before using the transcranial Doppler system, remove turban head dressings or thick dressings over the test site.

Documentation

Record the date and the time that the monitoring began and which artery is being monitored. Document any patient teaching as well as the patient's tolerance of the procedure.

REFERENCES

1 Oliveira-Filho, J., & Koroshetz, W. J. Neuroimaging of acute ischemic stroke. (2013). In: *UpToDate*, Kasner, S. E., et al. (Eds.). Accessed May 2015 via the Web at http://www.uptodate.com/contents/search

2 World Health Organization. (2009). "WHO guidelines on hand hygiene in health care: First global patient safety challenge, clean care is safer care" [Online]. Accessed May 2015 via the Web at http://whqlibdoc.who.int/publications/2009/9789241597906_eng.pdf (Level IV)

3 The Joint Commission. (2015). Standard NPSG.07.01.01. *Comprehensive accreditation manual for hospitals: The official handbook.* Oakbrook Terrace, IL: The Joint Commission. (Level VII)

4 Centers for Disease Control and Prevention. (2002). Guideline for hand hygiene in health-care settings: Recommendations of the Healthcare Infection Control Practices Advisory Committee and the HICPAC/

Current uses of TENS

A practitioner must prescribe transcutaneous electrical nerve stimulation (TENS); it's most successful if administered and taught to the patient by a therapist skilled in its use. TENS has been helpful in temporary relief of acute pain, such as postoperative pain, and in ongoing relief of chronic pain, such as sciatica.

Among the types of pain that respond to TENS are:

- arthritis
- bone fracture pain
- bursitis
- cancer-related pain
- musculoskeletal pain
- myofascial pain
- neuralgias and neuropathies
- phantom limb pain
- postoperative incision pain
- sciatica
- whiplash.

SHEA/APIC/IDSA Hand Hygiene Task Force. *MMWR Recommendations and Reports, 51*(RR-16), 1–45. Accessed May 2015 via the Web at http://www.cdc.gov/mmwr/pdf/rr/rr5116.pdf (Level II)

5 Centers for Medicare & Medicaid Services, Department of Health and Human Services. (2014). Condition of participation: Infection control. 42 C.F.R. § 482.42.

6 American Osteopathic Association. (2014). Standard 07.01.21. *Healthcare Facilities Accreditation Program: Accreditation requirements for acute care hospitals.* Chicago, IL: American Osteopathic Association. (Level VII)

7 The Joint Commission. (2015). Standard NPSG.01.01.01. *Comprehensive accreditation manual for hospitals: The official handbook.* Oakbrook Terrace, IL: The Joint Commission. (Level VII)

8 The Joint Commission. (2015). Standard RC.01.03.01. *Comprehensive accreditation manual for hospitals: The official handbook.* Oakbrook Terrace, IL: The Joint Commission. (Level VII)

9 American Osteopathic Association. (2014). Standard 10.00.03. *Healthcare Facilities Accreditation Program: Accreditation requirements for acute care hospitals.* Chicago, IL: American Osteopathic Association. (Level VII)

10 Centers for Medicare & Medicaid Services, Department of Health and Human Services. (2014). Condition of participation: Medical record services. 42 C.F.R. § 482.24(b).

ADDITIONAL REFERENCES

Naqvi, J. et al. (2013). "Transcranial Doppler ultrasound: A review of the physical principles and major applications in critical care" [Online]. Accessed May 2015 via the Web at http://www.hindawi.com/journals/ijvm/2013/629378/

Tsivguolis, G., et al. (2013). Real-time validation of transcranial Doppler criteria in assessing recanalization during intra-arterial procedures for acute ischemic stroke: An international, multicenter study. *Stroke, 44,* 394–400. (Level VI)

TRANSCUTANEOUS ELECTRICAL NERVE STIMULATION

Transcutaneous electrical nerve stimulation (TENS) is the application of electrical stimulation to the skin for pain relief. It's based on the gate-control theory of pain, which proposes that painful impulses pass through a "gate" in the brain. TENS is performed with a portable, battery-powered device that transmits painless electrical current to peripheral nerves or directly to a painful area over relatively large nerve fibers. This treatment effectively alters the patient's perception of pain by blocking painful stimuli traveling over smaller fibers.

Used for postoperative patients and those with chronic pain, TENS reduces the need for analgesic drugs and may allow the patient to resume normal activities. Typically, a course of TENS treatments lasts 3 to 5 days. Some conditions such as phantom limb pain may require continuous stimulation; other conditions such as a painful arthritic joint require shorter periods (3 to 4 hours). TENS has also been found to decrease knee pain associated with osteoarthritis. However, recent studies have shown TENS isn't helpful in patients with chronic lower back pain.[1] (See *Current uses of TENS.*)

TENS is contraindicated for patients with cardiac pacemakers because it can interfere with pacemaker function. The procedure is also contraindicated for pregnant patients because its effect on the fetus is unknown. It's also contraindicated in patients with dementia. TENS should be used cautiously in all patients with cardiac disorders. TENS electrodes shouldn't be placed on the head or neck of patients with vascular or seizure disorders.

Equipment

TENS device ■ pregelled, self-stick electrodes ■ warm water and soap ■ washcloth ■ towel ■ leadwires ■ charged battery pack ■ battery recharger ■ Optional: alcohol pads, hypoallergenic tape.

Commercial TENS kits are available. They include the stimulator, leadwires, electrodes, spare battery pack, battery recharger, and sometimes the adhesive patch.

Preparation of equipment

Before beginning the procedure, always test the battery pack *to make sure it's fully charged.*

Implementation

- Verify the practitioner's order.
- Gather and prepare the equipment.
- Perform hand hygiene.[2,3,4,5,6]
- Confirm the patient's identity using at least two patient identifiers.[7]
- Provide privacy.[8,9]
- If the patient has never seen a TENS unit, show him the device and explain the procedure.

Before TENS treatment

- Using soap and water, thoroughly clean the skin where you'll apply the electrodes. Dry the skin before application. Use an alcohol pad, if necessary, *to remove excess oil or lotion.*
- Apply the ordered number of electrodes on the proper skin area, leaving at least 2″ (5 cm) between them. (See *Positioning TENS electrodes.*) If necessary, secure them with hypoallergenic tape. Tape all sides evenly *so that the electrodes are firmly attached to the skin.*
- Plug the pin connectors into the electrode sockets. *To protect the cords,* hold the connectors—not the cords themselves—during insertion.
- Turn the channel controls to the OFF position or as recommended in the operator's manual.
- Plug the leadwires into the jacks in the control box.
- Turn the amplitude and rate dials slowly as the manual directs. (The patient should feel a tingling sensation.) Then adjust the controls on this device to the prescribed settings or to settings that are most comfortable for the patient. Most patients select stimulation frequencies of 60 to 100 Hz.
- Attach the TENS control box to part of the patient's clothing, such as a belt, pocket, or bra.
- *To make sure the device is working effectively,* monitor the patient for signs of excessive stimulation, such as muscle twitches, and for signs of inadequate stimulation, signaled by the patient's inability to feel a mild tingling sensation.

EQUIPMENT

Positioning TENS electrodes

With transcutaneous electrical nerve stimulation (TENS), electrodes placed around peripheral nerves (or an incisional site) transmit mild electrical pulses to the brain. The current is thought to block pain impulses. The patient can influence the level and frequency of his pain relief by adjusting the controls on the device.

Typically, electrode placement varies, even though patients may have similar complaints. You can place electrodes:

- to cover the painful area or surround it, as with painful joints or muscle tenderness or spasm
- to "capture" the painful area between electrodes, as with incisional pain
- to evoke "sensory analgesia" at trigger points.[10]

In peripheral nerve injury, place electrodes proximal to the injury (between the brain and the injury site) *to avoid increasing pain*. Placing electrodes in a hypersensitive area also increases pain. In an area lacking sensation, place electrodes should on adjacent dermatomes.

The illustrations show combinations of electrode placement (red squares) and areas of nerve stimulation (shaded pink) for lower back and leg pain.

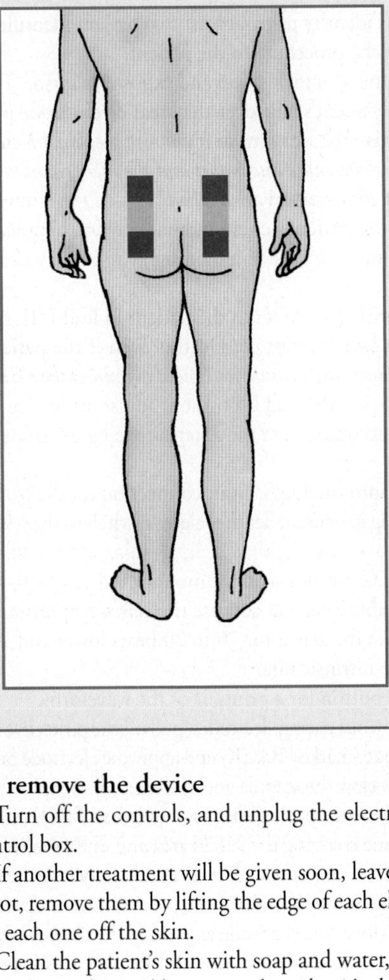

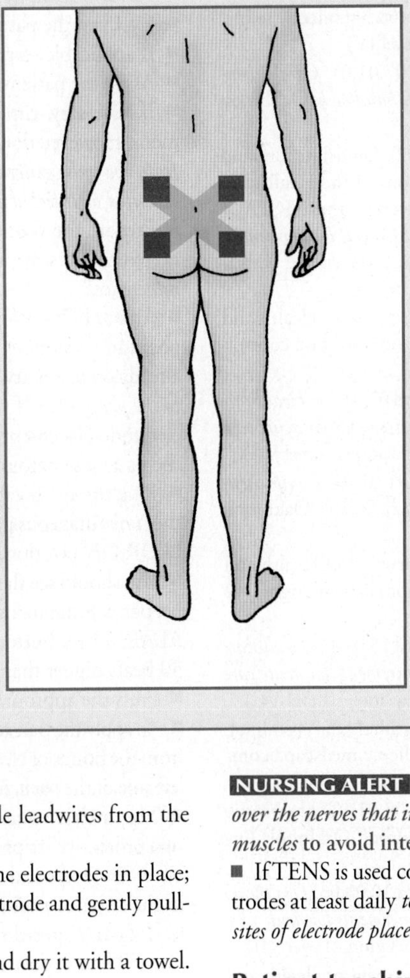

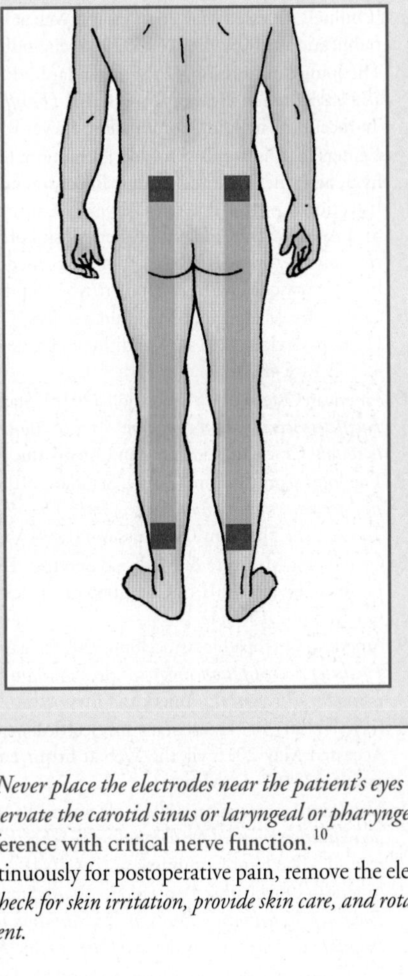

To remove the device

- Turn off the controls, and unplug the electrode leadwires from the control box.
- If another treatment will be given soon, leave the electrodes in place; if not, remove them by lifting the edge of each electrode and gently pulling each one off the skin.
- Clean the patient's skin with soap and water, and dry it with a towel.
- Recharge the used battery pack *so that it's always ready for use.*

Completing the procedure

- Perform hand hygiene.[2,3,4,5,6]
- Document the procedure.[11,12,13]

Special considerations

- If you must move the electrodes during the procedure, turn off the controls first. Follow the practitioner's orders regarding electrode placement and control settings. *Incorrect placement of the electrodes will result in inappropriate pain control.*
- Keep in mind that setting the controls too high can cause pain and setting them too low will fail to relieve pain.

NURSING ALERT *Never place the electrodes near the patient's eyes or over the nerves that innervate the carotid sinus or laryngeal or pharyngeal muscles* to avoid interference with critical nerve function.[10]

- If TENS is used continuously for postoperative pain, remove the electrodes at least daily *to check for skin irritation, provide skin care, and rotate sites of electrode placement.*

Patient teaching

If appropriate, let the patient study the operator's manual. Teach him how to place the electrodes properly and how to take care of the TENS unit.

Documentation

On the patient's medical record and the nursing care plan, record the electrode sites and the control settings. Document the patient's tolerance of treatment. Also evaluate pain control, and record the location of pain and how the patient rates his pain using a pain scale. Document patient teaching and the patient's understanding of the teaching.

REFERENCES

1 Dubinsky, R. M., & Miyasaki, J. (2010). Assessment: Efficacy of transcutaneous electric nerve stimulation in the treatment of pain in neurologic disorders (an evidence-based review). *Neurology, 74,* 173–176. (Level I)

Indications for transcutaneous pacing[1]

The American Heart Association recommends transcutaneous pacing for these class IIa indications:

- Bradycardia with hemodynamic instability unresponsive to atropine while preparing for emergent transvenous pacing
- High-degree block (Mobitz type II second-degree block or third-degree atrioventricular block)
- Symptomatic bradycardia
- Sinus arrest

2 World Health Organization. (2009). "WHO guidelines on hand hygiene in health care: First global patient safety challenge, clean care is safer care" [Online]. Accessed May 2015 via the Web at http://whqlibdoc.who.int/publications/2009/9789241597906_eng.pdf (Level IV)

3 The Joint Commission. (2015). Standard NPSG.07.01.01. *Comprehensive accreditation manual for hospitals: The official handbook.* Oakbrook Terrace, IL: The Joint Commission. (Level VII)

4 Centers for Disease Control and Prevention. (2002). Guideline for hand hygiene in health-care settings: Recommendations of the Healthcare Infection Control Practices Advisory Committee and the HICPAC/SHEA/APIC/IDSA Hand Hygiene Task Force. *MMWR Recommendations and Reports, 51*(RR-16), 1–45. Accessed May 2015 via the Web at http://www.cdc.gov/mmwr/pdf/rr/rr5116.pdf (Level II)

5 Centers for Medicare & Medicaid Services, Department of Health and Human Services. (2014). Condition of participation: Infection control. 42 C.F.R. § 482.42.

6 American Osteopathic Association. (2014). Standard 07.01.21. *Healthcare Facilities Accreditation Program: Accreditation requirements for acute care hospitals.* Chicago, IL: American Osteopathic Association. (Level VII)

7 The Joint Commission. (2015). Standard NPSG.01.01.01. *Comprehensive accreditation manual for hospitals: The official handbook.* Oakbrook Terrace, IL: The Joint Commission. (Level VII)

8 Centers for Medicare & Medicaid Services, Department of Health and Human Services. (2014). Condition of participation: Patient's rights. 42 C.F.R. § 482.13(c)(1).

9 American Osteopathic Association. (2014). Standard 15.01.16. *Healthcare Facilities Accreditation Program: Accreditation requirements for acute care hospitals.* Chicago, IL: American Osteopathic Association. (Level VII)

10 Kaye, V. (2013). "Transcutaneous electrical nerve stimulation" [Online]. Accessed May 2015 via the Web at http://emedicine.medscape.com/article/325107-overview#a1

11 The Joint Commission. (2015). Standard RC.01.03.01. *Comprehensive accreditation manual for hospitals: The official handbook.* Oakbrook Terrace, IL: The Joint Commission. (Level VII)

12 American Osteopathic Association. (2014). Standard 10.00.03. *Healthcare Facilities Accreditation Program: Accreditation requirements for acute care hospitals.* Chicago, IL: American Osteopathic Association. (Level VII)

13 Centers for Medicare & Medicaid Services, Department of Health and Human Services. (2014). Condition of participation: Medical record services. 42 C.F.R. § 482.24(b).

TRANSCUTANEOUS PACING

Transcutaneous pacing is a method of external electrical stimulation of the heart through a set of electrode pads. It isn't as efficient as transvenous pacing because the electrical stimulus (the pad) isn't in direct contact with the heart muscle. In a life-threatening situation, when time is critical, a transcutaneous pacemaker is the best choice. (See *Indications for transcutaneous pacing.*)

Transcutaneous pacing works by sending an electrical impulse from the pulse generator to the patient's heart by way of two electrodes, which are placed on the front and back of the patient's chest. Transcutaneous pacing is quick and effective, but it's used only until the practitioner can institute transvenous pacing.

Transcutaneous pacing is recommended by the 2010 American Heart Association Guidelines for Cardiopulmonary Resuscitation and Emergency Cardiovascular Care for symptomatic bradycardia when a pulse is present. It isn't recommended for cardiac arrest because research shows that it's ineffective in this situation.[1]

Equipment

Transcutaneous pacing generator ■ transcutaneous pacing electrodes ■ cardiac monitor ■ electrocardiogram (ECG) electrodes ■ 12-lead ECG machine ■ ECG cables and monitor ■ cardiac monitor output cable ■ washcloth ■ towel ■ nonemollient soap ■ blood pressure monitor ■ Optional: clippers, prescribed analgesic or sedative.

Implementation

- Perform hand hygiene[2,3,4,5,6]
- Confirm the patient's identity using at least two patient identifiers.[7]
- If applicable, explain the procedure to the patient.
- Assist the patient to the supine position and expose his torso.[8]
- If necessary, clip the patient's hair over the areas of electrode placement. However, don't shave the area *because if you nick the skin, the current from the pulse generator could cause discomfort and the nicks could become irritated or infected after the electrodes are applied.*[8]
- Prepare the skin on the patient's chest and back by washing it with nonemollient soap and water; dry the skin thoroughly *to improve electrode adherence.*[8]
- Attach ECG monitoring electrodes to the patient in lead I, II, or III position *to monitor the patient's rhythm.* Do this even if the patient is already on telemetry monitoring *because you'll need to connect the electrodes to the pacemaker.* If you select the lead II position, adjust the left leg (LL) electrode placement to accommodate the anterior pacing electrode and the patient's anatomy.
- Plug the ECG cable into the ECG input connection on the front of the transcutaneous pacing generator. Set the selector switch to the MONITOR ON position.
- You should see the ECG waveform on the monitor. Adjust the R-wave beeper volume to a suitable level and activate the alarm by pressing the ALARM ON button. Set the alarm for 10 to 20 beats lower and 20 to 30 beats higher than the intrinsic rate.
- Press the appropriate button for a printout of the waveform.
- To apply the transcutaneous pacing electrodes, pull off the protective strip from the posterior electrode (marked BACK) and apply the electrode on the left side of the back, just below the scapula and to the left of the spine.[8]
- The anterior transcutaneous pacing electrode (marked FRONT) has two protective strips—one covering the jellied area and one covering the outer rim. Expose the jellied area of the electrode and apply it to the skin in the anterior position—to the left side of the precordium in the usual lead V_2 to V_5 position. Move this electrode around to get the best waveform. Then expose the electrode's outer rim and firmly press it to the skin. (See *Transcutaneous electrode placement.*)
- You're ready to pace the heart. After making sure the energy output in milliamperes (mA) is on 0, connect the electrode cable to the monitor output cable.
- Check the waveform, looking for a tall QRS complex in lead II.
- Next, turn the selector switch to PACER ON. Tell the patient that he may feel a thumping or twitching sensation. Reassure him that you'll give him medication if he can't tolerate the discomfort.
- Set the rate dial to a rate that adequately maintains cardiac output. Look for pacer artifact or spikes, which will appear as you increase the rate. Some pacemakers have a default setting, such as 80 beats/minute, that can be adjusted as needed.[8]
- Slowly increase the amount of energy delivered to the heart by adjusting the OUTPUT mA dial. Do this until capture is achieved—you'll see a pacer spike followed by a widened QRS complex that resembles a

premature ventricular contraction. This is the pacing threshold. *To ensure consistent capture,* increase output by 10%. Don't go any higher *because you could cause the patient needless discomfort.*

- With full capture, the patient's heart rate should be approximately the same as the pacemaker rate set on the machine. The usual pacing threshold is between 40 and 80 mA. Be sure to check the patient's pulse *to ensure adequate blood flow with paced complexes;*[8] don't just rely on the monitor to determine heart rate.
- Assess the patient's vital signs, skin color, level of consciousness, and peripheral pulses *to determine the effectiveness of the paced rhythm.*
- Perform a 12-lead ECG *to serve as a baseline,* and then perform additional ECGs as required by your facility or with clinical changes.
- Perform a comprehensive pain assessment using techniques appropriate for the patient's age, condition, and ability to understand.[9] Administer an analgesic or sedative as ordered and indicated.[8]
- Perform hand hygiene.[2,3,4,5,6]
- Document the procedure.[10,11,12]

Special considerations

- If a patient is hemodynamically unstable and his back is difficult to access, the posterior electrode may be placed in the anterior-lateral position at the second or third intercostal space over the right sternal area.[8]
- Not all pacing electrodes have two protective strips as described earlier. Follow the manufacturer's instructions for electrode application
- Take care to prevent microshock, including warning the patient not to use any electrical equipment that isn't grounded, such as landline telephones, electric shavers, televisions, and lamps.
- Don't place the electrodes over a bony area *because bone conducts current poorly.* With female patients, place the anterior electrode under the patient's breast but not over her diaphragm.
- Obtain a rhythm strip before, during, and after pacemaker placement; any time that pacemaker settings are changed; and whenever the patient receives treatment for a complication due to the pacemaker.
- Monitor the ECG reading continuously, noting capture, sensing, rate, intrinsic beats, and competition of paced and intrinsic rhythms. If the pacemaker is sensing correctly, the sense indicator on the pulse generator should flash with each beat.

Complications

Complications associated with pacemaker therapy include microshock, equipment failure, and competitive or fatal arrhythmias. Transcutaneous pacemakers may also cause skin breakdown as well as muscle pain and twitching when the pacemaker fires.

Documentation

Record the reason for transcutaneous pacing, the date and time it started, the type of pacemaker used, and the locations of the electrodes. Also record the pacemaker settings. Note the patient's response to the procedure, along with any complications and interventions implemented. If possible, obtain rhythm strips before, during, and after pacemaker placement; whenever pacemaker settings are changed; and when the patient receives treatment for a complication caused by the pacemaker.

Transcutaneous electrode placement

For a noninvasive temporary pacemaker, the two pacing electrodes are placed at heart level on the patient's chest (anterior) and back (posterior), as shown below. You can apply this type of pacemaker quickly in an emergency; however, it's uncomfortable for the patient.

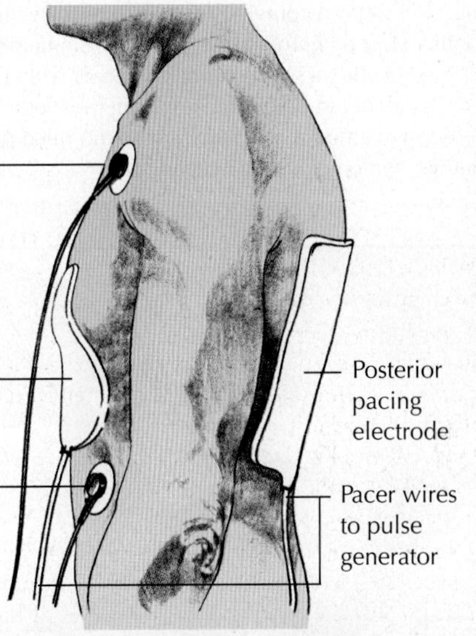

REFERENCES

1 American Heart Association. (2010). 2010 American Heart Association guidelines for cardiopulmonary resuscitation and emergency cardiovascular care. *Circulation, 122,* S706–S767. (Level II)

2 The Joint Commission. (2015). Standard NPSG.07.01.01. *Comprehensive accreditation manual for hospitals: The official handbook.* Oakbrook Terrace, IL: The Joint Commission. (Level VII)

3 Centers for Disease Control and Prevention. (2002). Guideline for hand hygiene in health-care settings: Recommendations of the Healthcare Infection Control Practices Advisory Committee and the HICPAC/SHEA/APIC/IDSA Hand Hygiene Task Force. *MMWR Recommendations and Reports, 51*(RR–16), 1–45. Accessed May 2015 via the Web at http://www.cdc.gov/mmwr/pdf/rr/rr5116.pdf (Level II)

4 World Health Organization. (2009). "WHO guidelines on hand hygiene in health care: First global patient safety challenge, clean care is safer care" [Online]. Accessed May 2015 via the Web at http://whqlibdoc.who.int/publications/2009/9789241597906_eng.pdf (Level IV)

5 American Osteopathic Association. (2014). Standard 07.01.21. *Healthcare Facilities Accreditation Program: Accreditation requirements for acute care hospitals.* Chicago, IL: American Osteopathic Association. (Level VII)

6 Centers for Medicare & Medicaid Services, Department of Health and Human Services. (2014). Condition of participation: Infection control. 42 C.F.R. § 482.42.

7 The Joint Commission. (2015). Standard NPSG.01.01.01. *Comprehensive accreditation manual for hospitals: The official handbook.* Oakbrook Terrace, IL: The Joint Commission. (Level VII)

8 Lynn-McHale Wiegand, D. (Ed.). (2011). *AACN procedure manual for critical care* (6th ed.). St. Louis, MO: Saunders.

9 The Joint Commission. (2015). Standard PC.01.02.07. *Comprehensive accreditation manual for hospitals: The official handbook.* Oakbrook Terrace, IL: The Joint Commission. (Level VII)

10 The Joint Commission. (2015). Standard RC.01.03.01. *Comprehensive accreditation manual for hospitals: The official handbook.* Oakbrook Terrace, IL: The Joint Commission. (Level VII)

11 American Osteopathic Association. (2014). Standard 10.00.03. *Healthcare Facilities Accreditation Program: Accreditation requirements for acute care hospitals.* Chicago, IL: American Osteopathic Association. (Level VII)

12 Centers for Medicare & Medicaid Services, Department of Health and Human Services. (2014). Condition of participation: Medical record services. 42 C.F.R. § 482.24(b).

ADDITIONAL REFERENCE

Woods, S., et al. (2010). *Cardiac nursing* (6th ed.). Philadelphia, PA: Lippincott Williams & Wilkins.

Applying nitroglycerin ointment

Unlike most topical medications, nitroglycerin ointment is used for its transdermal systemic effect. It's used to dilate the veins and arteries, improving cardiac perfusion in a patient with cardiac ischemia or angina pectoris.

To apply nitroglycerin ointment, start by taking the patient's baseline blood pressure *so that you can compare it with later readings.* Remove any previously applied nitroglycerin ointment. Gather your equipment. Nitroglycerin ointment, which is prescribed by the inch or centimeter, comes with a rectangular piece of ruled paper to be used in applying the medication. Squeeze the prescribed amount of ointment onto the ruled paper (as shown below). Put on gloves, if needed.

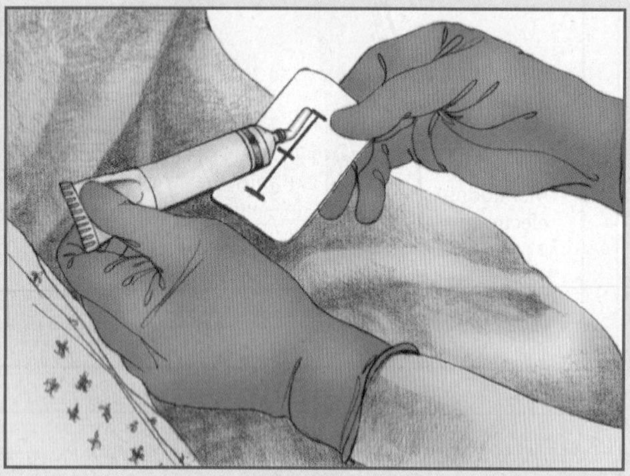

After measuring the correct amount of ointment, tape the ruled measuring paper—drug side down—directly to the skin (as shown below). (Some facilities require you to use the paper to apply the medication to the patient's skin, usually on the chest or arm. This is done by spreading a thin layer of the ointment over an area of 3" [7.6 cm].) For increased absorption, the practitioner may request that you cover the site with a transparent semipermeable dressing.

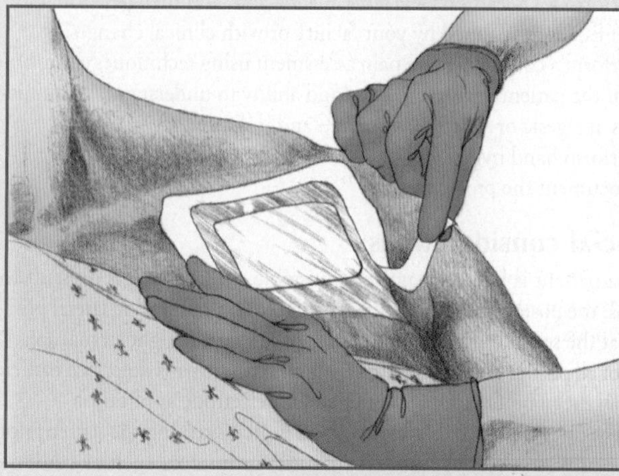

After 5 minutes, record the patient's blood pressure. If his blood pressure has dropped significantly and he has a headache (from vasodilation of blood vessels in his head), notify the practitioner immediately; the practitioner may reduce the dose. If the patient's blood pressure has dropped but he has no symptoms, instruct him to lie still until it returns to normal.

TRANSDERMAL DRUG APPLICATION

Through a measured dose of ointment or an adhesive patch applied to the skin, transdermal drugs deliver constant, controlled medication directly into the bloodstream for a prolonged systemic effect.

Nitroglycerin, one of the more common transdermal ointments, dilates coronary vessels for up to 4 hours. (See *Applying nitroglycerin ointment.*) Medications available as transdermal patches include scopolamine, used to treat motion sickness; estradiol, used for postmenopausal hormone replacement; clonidine, used to treat hypertension; nicotine, used for smoking cessation; and fentanyl, an opioid analgesic used to control chronic pain. Transdermal scopolamine can relieve motion sickness for as long as 72 hours, transdermal estradiol lasts for up to 1 week, transdermal clonidine and nicotine last for 24 hours, and transdermal fentanyl can last for up to 72 hours.

Contraindications for transdermal drug application include skin allergies or skin reactions to the drug. Transdermal drugs shouldn't be applied to broken or irritated skin, which would increase irritation, or to scarred or callused skin, which might impair absorption.

NURSING ALERT *Don't apply heat over a fentanyl transdermal system or its surrounding area* because an increase in temperature increases fentanyl release, which may result in overdose and death.[1]

Equipment

Patient's medication administration record and medical record ■ prescribed medication ■ application strip or ruled measuring paper (for nitroglycerin ointment) ■ adhesive tape ■ Optional: gloves, semipermeable dressing, clippers, equipment for assessing blood pressure.

Implementation

- Avoid distractions and interruptions when preparing and administering the medication *to prevent medication errors.*[2,3,4]
- Verify the practitioner's order order.[4,5,6]
- Compare the medication label with the order in the patient's medical record and verify that the medication is correct.[4,5,6]
- Check the patient's medical record for allergies or contraindications to the prescribed medication. If an allergy or a contraindication exists, don't administer the medication; notify the practitioner.[4,5,6]
- Check the expiration date on the medication. If the medication has expired, return it to the pharmacy and obtain new medication.[4,5,6]
- Visually inspect the medication for loss of integrity; don't administer the medication if its integrity has been compromised.[4,5,6]
- Discuss any unresolved concerns about the medication with the practitioner.[4,5,6]
- Perform hand hygiene.[7,8,9,10,11]
- Confirm the patient's identity using at least two patient identifiers.[12]
- Explain the procedure to the patient and provide privacy.[13,14]
- If the patient is receiving the medication for the first time, teach him about potential adverse reactions and discuss any other concerns related to the medication.[4,5,6]
- Verify that the medication is being administered at the correct time, in the prescribed dose, and by the correct route *to reduce the risk of medication errors.*[4,5,6]
- If your facility uses a bar code scanning system, scan your identification badge, the patient's identification bracelet, and the medication's bar code.
- Put on gloves if needed *to comply with standard precautions.*[15,16]

Applying transdermal ointment

- Remove any previously applied transdermal ointment.
- Place the prescribed amount of ointment on the application strip or measuring paper, taking care not to get any on your skin.
- Apply the application strip or ruled measuring paper to any dry, hairless area of the body as ordered. Don't rub the ointment into the skin.
- Tape the strip or ruled measuring paper and ointment to the skin. Alternatively, cover the application strip with a transparent semipermeable dressing.

Applying a transdermal patch

- Open the package and remove the patch.
- Without touching the adhesive surface, remove the clear plastic backing.
- Apply the patch to a dry, hairless area—behind the ear, for example, as with scopolamine.
- Write the date, the time, and your initials on the dressing

Completing the procedure

- Store the medication, as ordered.
- Instruct the patient to keep the area around the ointment or patch as dry as possible.
- Remove and discard your gloves, if worn,[15,16] and perform hand hygiene.[7,8,9,10,11]
- Document the procedure.[17,18,19]

Special considerations

- Reapply transdermal medications at the same time every day *to ensure a continuous effect,* but alternate the application sites *to avoid skin irritation.*
- Before reapplying nitroglycerin ointment, remove the application strip and any remaining ointment from the patient's skin at the previous site.
- Avoid shaving an area to apply the ointment. *Shaving removes the top layer of skin, which may cause the medication to absorb faster than with unshaved skin.* If necessary, use clippers to remove excess hair.
- When applying a scopolamine or fentanyl patch, instruct the patient not to drive or operate machinery until his response to the drug has been determined.
- Warn a patient using a clonidine patch to check with his practitioner before taking an over-the-counter cough preparation *because such drugs may counteract clonidine's effects.*

Patient teaching

Teach the patient how to apply the patch. (See *Applying a transdermal medication patch.*)

Complications

Topical medications may cause skin irritation, such as pruritus and a rash. The patient may also suffer adverse effects of the specific drug administered. For example, transdermal nitroglycerin may cause headaches and, in elderly patients, orthostatic hypotension. Adverse effects of scopolamine include dry mouth and drowsiness (most common); for estradiol, increased risk of endometrial cancer, thromboembolic disease, and birth defects; and for clonidine, possible severe rebound hypertension, especially if withdrawn suddenly. Anaphylactic reaction to the medication may occur. Monitor for signs and symptoms of this complication.

Documentation

Document the name of the medication, the dose, and the date and time it was administered in the patient's medication administration record. Include the route and site used. Document the appearance and integrity of the skin before administration. Record the presence or absence of adverse effects and whether the practitioner was notified of their presence. Document the patient's response to and tolerance of therapy. Document any patient teaching, the patient's understanding of the teaching, and whether you gave the patient written information about the prescribed medication.

PATIENT TEACHING

Applying a transdermal medication patch

If the patient will be receiving medication by transdermal patch, instruct him in its proper use. Explain to the patient that the patch consists of several layers. The layer closest to his skin contains a small amount of the drug and allows prompt introduction of the drug into the bloodstream. The next layer controls release of the drug from the main portion of the patch. The third layer contains the main dose of the drug. The outermost layer consists of an aluminized polyester barrier.

Teach the patient to apply the patch to appropriate skin areas, such as the upper arm or chest or behind the ear. Warn him to avoid touching the gel or surrounding tape. Tell him to use a different site for each application to *avoid skin irritation.* If necessary, he can clip the hair at the site. Caution him to avoid any area that may cause uneven absorption, such as skin folds, scars, and calluses, or any irritated or damaged skin areas. Also, tell him not to apply the patch below the elbow or knee.

Instruct the patient to wash his hands after application *to remove any medication that may have rubbed off.*

Warn the patient not to get the patch wet. Tell him to discard it if it leaks or falls off and then to clean the site and apply a new patch at a different site. If the transdermal patch contains fentanyl, warn the patient to avoid applying heat over the fentanyl transdermal system or its surrounding area *because an increase in temperature increases fentanyl release, which may result in overdose and death.*[1]

Instruct the patient to apply the patch at the same time at the prescribed interval *to ensure continuous drug delivery. Bedtime application is ideal because body movement is reduced during the night.* Lastly, tell him not to forget to remove the old patch and to dispose of it properly.

REFERENCES

1 Janssen Pharmaceuticals, Inc. (2012). Duragesic (fentanyl transdermal system) prescribing information [Online]. Accessed May 2015 via the Web at http://www.duragesic.com/sites/default/files/pdf/duragesic_0.pdf

2 Westbrook, J., et al. (2010). Association of interruptions with an increased risk and severity of medication administration errors. *Archives of Internal Medicine, 170,* 683–690. (Level IV)

3 Institute for Safe Medication Practices. (2013). Side tracks on the safety express: Interruptions lead to errors and unfinished...Wait, what was I doing? *Nurse Advise-ERR, 11*(2), 1–4. Accessed May 2015 via the Web at https://www.ismp.org/Newsletters/acutecare/showarticle.aspx?id=37

4 American Osteopathic Association. (2014). Standard 16.01.03. *Healthcare Facilities Accreditation Program: Accreditation requirements for acute care hospitals.* Chicago, IL: American Osteopathic Association. (Level VII)

5 The Joint Commission. (2015). Standard MM.06.01.01. *Comprehensive accreditation manual for hospitals: The official handbook.* Oakbrook Terrace, IL: The Joint Commission. (Level VII)

6 Centers for Medicare & Medicaid Services, Department of Health and Human Services. (2014). Condition of participation: Nursing services. 42 C.F.R. § 482.23(c).

7 The Joint Commission. (2015). Standard NPSG.07.01.01. *Comprehensive accreditation manual for hospitals: The official handbook.* Oakbrook Terrace, IL: The Joint Commission. (Level VII)

8 Centers for Disease Control and Prevention. (2002). Guideline for hand hygiene in health-care settings: Recommendations of the Healthcare Infection Control Practices Advisory Committee and the HICPAC/SHEA/APIC/IPSA Hand Hygiene Task Force. *MMWR Recommendations and Reports, 51*(RR-16), 1–45. Accessed May 2015 via the Web at http://www.cdc.gov/mmwr/pdf/rr/rr5116.pdf (Level II)
9 World Health Organization. (2009). "WHO guidelines on hand hygiene in health care: First global patient safety challenge, clean care is safer care" [Online]. Accessed May 2015 via the Web at http://whqlibdoc.who.int/publications/2009/9789241597906_eng.pdf (Level IV)
10 American Osteopathic Association. (2014). Standard 07.01.21. *Healthcare Facilities Accreditation Program: Accreditation requirements for acute care hospitals.* Chicago, IL: American Osteopathic Association. (Level VII)
11 Centers for Medicare & Medicaid Services, Department of Health and Human Services. (2014). Condition of participation: Infection control. 42 C.F.R. § 482.42.
12 The Joint Commission. (2015). Standard NPSG.01.01.01. *Comprehensive accreditation manual for hospitals: The official handbook.* Oakbrook Terrace, IL: The Joint Commission. (Level VII)
13 Centers for Medicare & Medicaid Services, Department of Health and Human Services. (2014). Condition of participation: Patient's rights. 42 C.F.R. § 482.13(c)(1).
14 American Osteopathic Association. (2014). Standard 15.01.16. *Healthcare Facilities Accreditation Program: Accreditation requirements for acute care hospitals.* Chicago, IL: American Osteopathic Association. (Level VII)
15 Siegel, J. D., et al. (2007). "2007 guideline for isolation precautions: Preventing transmission of infectious agents in healthcare settings" [Online]. Accessed May 2015 via the Web at http://www.cdc.gov/hicpac/pdf/isolation/Isolation2007.pdf (Level II)
16 American Osteopathic Association. (2014). Standard 07.01.10. *Healthcare Facilities Accreditation Program: Accreditation requirements for acute care hospitals.* Chicago, IL: American Osteopathic Association. (Level VII)
17 The Joint Commission. (2015). Standard RC.01.03.01. *Comprehensive accreditation manual for hospitals: The official handbook.* Oakbrook Terrace, IL: The Joint Commission. (Level VII)
18 American Osteopathic Association. (2014). Standard 10.00.03. *Healthcare Facilities Accreditation Program: Accreditation requirements for acute care hospitals.* Chicago, IL: American Osteopathic Association. (Level VII)
19 Centers for Medicare & Medicaid Services, Department of Health and Human Services. (2014). Condition of participation: Medical record services. 42 C.F.R. § 482.24(b).

ADDITIONAL REFERENCE

Nettina, S. M. (2014). *Lippincott manual of nursing practice* (10th ed.). Philadelphia, PA: Wolters Kluwer.

TRANSDUCER SYSTEM SETUP

Transducer systems detect intravascular and intracardiac pressures and convert them to an electrical signal that's transmitted to a monitor. The exact type of transducer system used depends on the patient's needs and the practitioner's preference. Some systems monitor pressure continuously, whereas others monitor pressure intermittently. Single-pressure transducers monitor only one type of pressure—for example, pulmonary artery pressure (PAP). Multiple-pressure transducers can monitor two or more types of pressure, such as PAP and central venous pressure.

Equipment

Bag of flush solution (usually 500 mL of normal saline solution) ▪ pressure infusion bag ▪ preassembled disposable pressure tubing with flush device and disposable transducer ▪ monitor and monitor cable ▪ pressure module ▪ IV pole with transducer mount ▪ leveling device (carpenter's level or laser) ▪ sterile, nonvented stopcock caps ▪ labels ▪ Optional: 500 to 1,000 units of heparin, gloves.

Preparation of equipment

For initial setup, turn on the monitor before gathering the equipment *to give it time to warm up.* Make sure that the monitor has the correct pressure module in place. Plug the pressure cable into the appropriate pressure module. Turn on the correct parameters (for example, pulmonary artery, right atrial, or arterial pressure) *to visualize the correct waveforms.* Set the appropriate scale for the pressure monitored *to obtain accurate pressure readings.*[1]

Implementation

Setting up the system

- Verify the practitioner's orders.
- Gather the appropriate equipment
- Perform hand hygiene.[2,3,4,5,6]
- Confirm the patient's identity using at least two patient identifiers.[7]
- Explain the procedure to the patient and his family.
- If used in your facility, add the heparin to the flush solution—usually, 1 to 2 units of heparin per milliliter of solution.

NURSING ALERT *Although heparin may prevent thrombosis, its use has been associated with thrombocytopenia and other hematologic risks. Because the risks outweigh the benefits, many facilities no longer use it in flush solutions.*[1,8]

- Label the IV flush solution bag with the date and time the solution was prepared, the dose of heparin (if added), and your initials.[1]
- Remove the preassembled pressure tubing from the package. If necessary, connect the pressure tubing to the transducer. Tighten all tubing connections *to prevent dangerous disconnections.*[9]
- Spike the outlet port of the flush solution bag with the pressure tubing spike, invert the bag, and open the roller clamp. Then compress the tubing's drip chamber, filling it halfway with the flush solution *to help prevent air bubbles from entering the tubing.*[1] Roll the roller clamp to the closed position.
- Place the flush solution bag into the pressure infuser bag. To do this, hang the pressure infuser bag on the IV pole, and then position the flush solution bag inside the pressure infuser bag. Don't inflate the pressure bag *because priming the tubing under pressure can cause air bubbles to enter the system.*[1]
- Open the tubing's roller clamp, uncoil the tube if you haven't already done so, and remove the protective cap at the end of the pressure tubing. Squeeze the continuous flush device slowly *to prime the entire system,* including the stopcock ports, with the flush solution *to eliminate air from the system.*
- As the solution nears the disposable transducer, hold the transducer at a 45-degree angle (as shown below). *This forces the solution to flow*

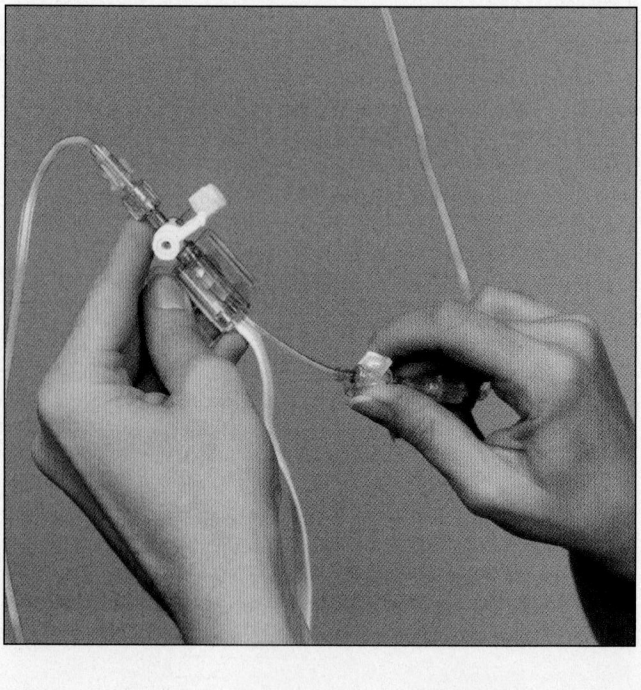

upward to the transducer. In doing so, the solution forces any air out of the system.

■ When the solution nears a stopcock, open the stopcock to air, allowing the solution to flow into the stopcock (as shown below). When the stopcock fills, close it to air and turn it open to the remainder of the tubing.

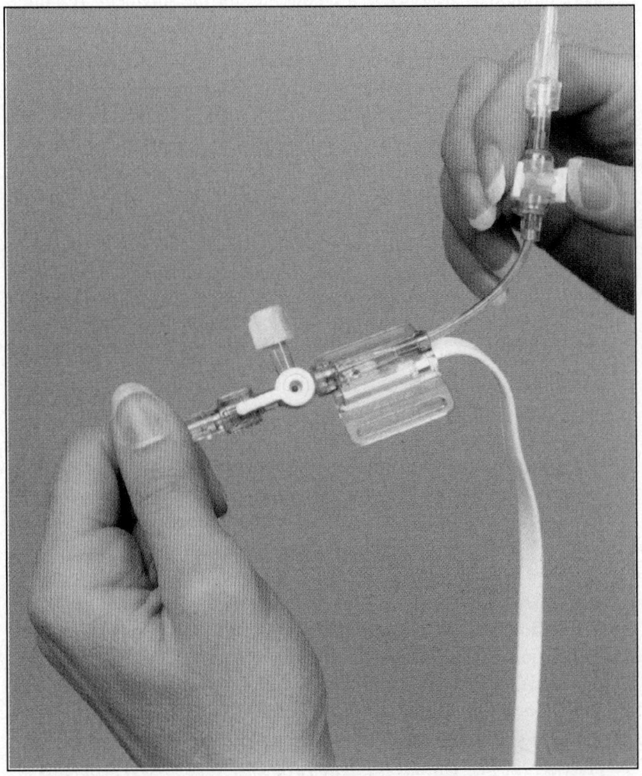

■ After removing the air from the stopcock, replace the vented cap with a sterile, nonvented cap *to prevent air from entering the system.*

■ After you've completely primed the system, replace the protective cap at the end of the tubing.

■ Inflate the pressure infuser bag to 300 mm Hg *to allow delivery of 1 to 3 mL/hour of flush solution through the catheter, minimizing cloth formation and maintaining catheter patency.*[1] Make sure that the drip chamber doesn't completely fill with fluid as you inflate the pressure bag.

■ Insert the device into the pole mount holder *to secure the transducer,* if indicated.[1]

■ Label the pressure tubing with the date, the time, and your initials *to help identify when the pressure tubing needs to be changed.*[1]

■ Before connecting the pressure monitoring system to the patient's catheter, level and zero the transducer. Zero the system during initial setup or before catheter insertion if disconnection occurs between the monitoring cable and monitor and when the values obtained don't correlate with the patient's clinical condition.[1]

Leveling and zeroing the system

■ Place the patient in the supine position with the head of the bed elevated up to 60 degrees.[10,11,12] If the patient can't tolerate such positioning, use a prone or a 20 , 30 , or 90 degree lateral position, as appropriate.[1,10]

■ Next, use the leveling device to position the air-reference stopcock or the air-fluid interface of the transducer level with the phlebostatic axis (midway between the posterior chest and the sternum at the fourth intercostal space, midaxillary line), if the patient is in the supine or prone position.[1,10] If the patient is in a lateral position, reference the stopcock or the air-fluid interface of the transducer at the lateral angle-specific reference.[10]

■ After leveling the transducer, turn the stopcock next to the transducer off to the patient and open to air. Remove the cap to the stopcock port.

■ Zero the transducer following the manufacturer's directions for zeroing.

■ When you've finished zeroing the transducer, turn the stopcock so that it's in a monitoring position with the stopcock closed to air and open to the side of the tubing that will go to the patient. Place a new, sterile, nonvented cap on the stopcock *to maintain sterility.* Now you've assembled a single-pressure transducer system (as shown below).

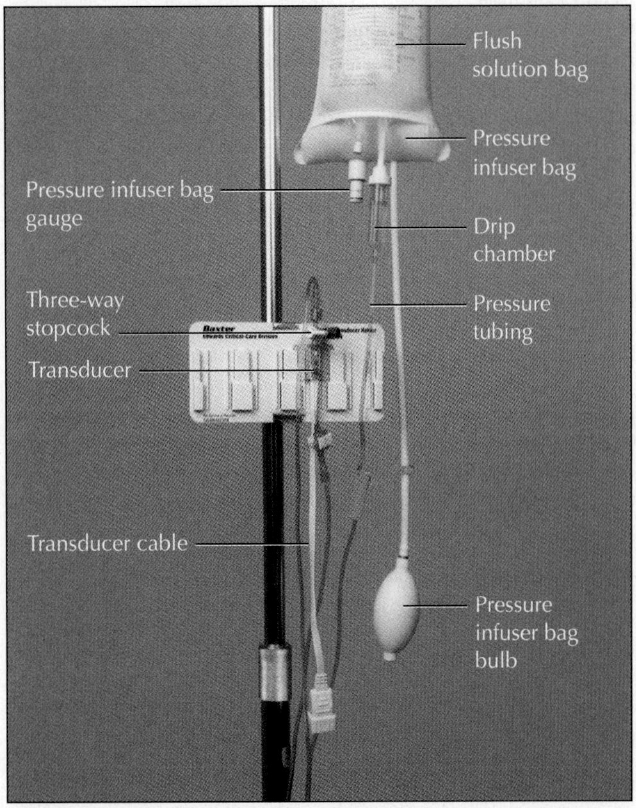

Connecting the pressure tubing to the appropriate catheter port

■ Put on gloves if necessary *to comply with standard precautions.*[13]

■ Using sterile technique, remove the cap at the end of the pressure tubing and then connect the end of the pressure tubing to the appropriate catheter port (pulmonary artery, right atrial, or arterial) *to enable pressure monitoring.*[1]

■ Trace the tubing from the patient to its point of origin *to make sure that you've connected it to the proper port.*[9]

■ Activate the fast flush device *to make sure that the flush system is functioning properly.* Assess the pressure waveforms *to make sure that the system is functioning properly.*

■ Make sure that the hemodynamic monitoring system alarms are turned on, that alarm limits are appropriate for the patient's present condition, and that alarms are audible to staff.[14]

■ Remove and discard your gloves, if worn.

Completing the procedure

■ Perform hand hygiene.[2,3,4,5,6]

■ Document the procedure.[15,16,17]

Special considerations

■ The Joint Commission has issued a sentinel event alert concerning medical device alarm safety *because alarm-related events have been associated with permanent loss of function or death.* Among the major contributing factors were improper alarm settings, alarms improperly turned off, and alarm signals not audible to staff. Make sure that alarm limits are set appropriately and that alarms are turned on and audible to staff. Follow facility guidelines for preventing alarm fatigue.[14]

■ You may use any of several methods to set up a multiple-pressure transducer system. The easiest way is to add to the single-pressure system. You'll also need another bag of heparin flush solution in a second pressure infuser bag. Then you'll prime the tubing, mount the second transducer, and connect an additional cable to the monitor. Lastly, you'll zero the second transducer.

■ Alternatively, your facility may use a Y-type tubing setup with two attached pressure transducers. This method requires only one bag of flush solution. To set up the system, proceed as you would for a single transducer, with this exception: First, prime one branch of the Y-type tubing and then the other. Next, attach two cables to the monitor in the modules for each pressure that you'll be measuring. Lastly, zero each transducer.

■ Minimize the number of manipulations and entries into the pressure monitoring system *to reduce the risk of infection.*[18]

■ If you must access the pressure monitoring system through a diaphragm instead of a stopcock, thoroughly disinfect the diaphragm with an antiseptic pad using friction before accessing the system.[18]

■ Regularly assess the transducer system *to make sure that the flush solution bag contains fluid, the system is free of air bubbles, the pressure infuser bag pressure is maintained at 300 mm Hg, and all connections are secured tightly.*[1]

■ Change the flush bag, tubing, and other components of the system every 96 hours, immediately when contamination is suspected or when the integrity of the product or system is compromised, or as required by your facility.[18,19]

Documentation

Document the patient's position for leveling and zeroing so that other health care team members can replicate the positioning. Document the type of flush solution used and the date and time of tubing changes. Record any unexpected outcomes and your interventions. Document patient and family teaching and their comprehension of the teaching.[1]

REFERENCES

1 Lynn-McHale Wiegand, D. (Ed.). (2011). *AACN procedure manual for critical care* (6th ed.). St. Louis, MO: Saunders.

2 The Joint Commission. (2015). Standard NPSG.07.01.01. *Comprehensive accreditation manual for hospitals: The official handbook.* Oakbrook Terrace, IL: The Joint Commission. (Level VII)

3 Centers for Disease Control and Prevention. (2002). Guideline for hand hygiene in health-care settings: Recommendations of the Healthcare Infection Control Practices Advisory Committee and the HICPAC/SHE/APIC/IDSA Hand Hygiene Task Force. *MMWR Recommendations and Reports, 51*(RR-16), 1–45. Accessed May 2015 via the Web at http://www.cdc.gov/mmwr/pdf/rr/rr5116.pdf (Level II)

4 World Health Organization. (2009). "WHO guidelines on hand hygiene in health care: First global patient safety challenge, clean care is safer care" [Online]. Accessed May 2015 via the Web at http://whqlibdoc.who.int/publications/2009/9789241597906_eng.pdf (Level IV)

5 American Osteopathic Association. (2014). Standard 07.01.21. *Healthcare Facilities Accreditation Program: Accreditation requirements for acute care hospitals.* Chicago, IL: American Osteopathic Association. (Level VII)

6 Centers for Medicare & Medicaid Services, Department of Health and Human Services. (2014). Condition of participation: Infection control. 42 C.F.R. § 482.42.

7 The Joint Commission. (2015). Standard NPSG.01.01.01. *Comprehensive accreditation manual for hospitals: The official handbook.* Oakbrook Terrace, IL: The Joint Commission. (Level VII)

8 Warkentin, T. E., & Greinacher, A. (2004). Heparin-induced thrombocytopenia: Recognition, treatment, and prevention. *Chest, 126,* S311–S337.

9 U.S. Food and Drug Administration. (n.d.). "Look. Check. Connect. Safe medical device connections save lives" [Online]. Accessed May 2015 via the Web at http://www.fda.gov/downloads/MedicalDevices/Safety/AlertsandNotices/UCM134873.pdf

10 American Association of Critical-Care Nurses. (2009). "AACN practice alert: Pulmonary artery/central venous pressure measurement" [Online]. Accessed May 2015 via the Web at http://www.aacn.org/wd/practice/docs/pap-measurement.pdf

11 Laulive, J. (1982). Pulmonary artery pressure and position changes in the critically ill adult. *Dimensions in Critical Care Nursing, 1,* 28–34.

12 Woods, S., & Mansfield, L. (1976). Effect of body position upon pulmonary artery pulmonary capillary wedge pressures in noncritically ill patients. *Heart and Lung, 5,* 83–90.

13 American Osteopathic Association. (2014). Standard 07.01.10. *Healthcare Facilities Accreditation Program: Accreditation requirements for acute care hospitals.* Chicago, IL: American Osteopathic Association. (Level VII)

14 The Joint Commission. (2013). "Sentinel event alert: Medical device alarm safety in hospitals" [Online]. Accessed May 2015 via the Web at http://www.jointcommission.org/assets/1/18/SEA_50_alarms_4_5_13_FINAL1.PDF (Level VII)

15 The Joint Commission. (2015). Standard RC.01.03.01. *Comprehensive accreditation manual for hospitals: The official handbook.* Oakbrook Terrace, IL: The Joint Commission. (Level VII)

16 American Osteopathic Association. (2014). Standard 10.00.03. *Healthcare Facilities Accreditation Program: Accreditation requirements for acute care hospitals.* Chicago, IL: American Osteopathic Association. (Level VII)

17 Centers for Medicare & Medicaid Services, Department of Health and Human Services. (2014). Condition of participation: Medical record services. 42 C.F.R. § 482.24(b).

18 Centers for Disease Control and Prevention. (2002). "Guidelines for the prevention of intravascular catheter-related infections" [Online]. Accessed May 2015 via the Web at http://www.cdc.gov/hicpac/pdf/guidelines/bsi-guidelines-2011.pdf (Level I)

19 Standard 43. Administration set change. Infusion nursing standards of practice. (2011). *Journal of Infusion Nursing, 34,* S55–S57. (Level I)

TRANSFER WITHIN A FACILITY

Patient transfer requires thorough preparation and documentation. Preparation includes an explanation of the transfer to the patient and his family and discussion of the patient's condition and care plan with staff members on the receiving unit.[1] Documentation of the patient's condition before and during transfer and adequate communication between the nursing staff from each unit ensures continuity of nursing care and provides legal protection for the transferring unit and its staff members.[2]

Equipment

Admission inventory of belongings ■ patient's medical and medication records ■ medications ■ patient belongings bag or suitcase ■ wheelchair, bed, or stretcher.

Implementation

■ Verify the practitioner's order for transfer.

■ If the patient is being transferred from or to an intensive care unit, your facility may require new care orders from the patient's practitioner. If so, review the new orders with the nursing staff at the receiving unit.[2,3]

■ Perform hand hygiene.[4,5,6,7,8]

■ Confirm the patient's identity using at least two patient identifiers.[9]

■ Explain the transfer to the patient and his family. If the patient is anxious about the transfer or his condition precludes patient teaching, explain the reason for the transfer to his family, especially if the transfer is the result of a serious change in the patient's condition.[1]

■ Assess the patient's physical condition *to determine the means of transfer, such as a wheelchair, bed, or stretcher.*[10]

■ If the patient requires continuous oxygen or mechanical ventilation, arrange for the respiratory therapy department to provide support during the transfer.[3]

■ Using the admissions inventory of belongings as a checklist, collect the patient's property. Check the entire room, including the closet, bedside stand, overbed table, and bathroom.

■ Gather the patient's medications stored outside of the automated dispensing machine and send them to the receiving unit upon transfer.

■ Notify the business office, the dietary department, the pharmacy, the facility telephone operator, and other appropriate departments of the transfer.[3]

■ Provide the nursing staff members on the receiving unit with a detailed handoff communication about the patient's condition and drug regimen and review the patient's nursing care plan with them *to ensure continuity of care.* Allow an opportunity for questions.[3,11,12] Use a handoff communication technique, such as the Situation-Background-Assessment-Recommendation or other facility-approved technique, *to improve communication and reduce errors.*[12,13]

■ Make sure that the reconciled list of the patient's medications has been communicated to the next practitioner who will be caring for the patient and that the communication is documented in the patient's medical record *to reduce the risk of transition-related adverse medication events.*[14,15]

■ Take or send the patient's medical record, accurate medication reconciliation list, laboratory request forms, special equipment, and other required materials to the receiving unit.[3]

■ Use a wheelchair to transport the ambulatory patient to the newly assigned room unless it's on the same unit as his present one, in which case he may be allowed to walk. Use a stretcher or bed to transport a patient whose condition doesn't permit transfer in a wheelchair.

■ Introduce the patient to the nursing staff members at the receiving unit. Then take the patient to his room and, depending on his condition, place him in the bed or seat him in a chair.

■ Introduce him to his new roommate, if appropriate, and tell him about any unfamiliar equipment such as the call light.

■ Perform hand hygiene.[4,5,6,7,8]

■ Document the procedure.[16,17,18]

Special considerations

■ Before the patient is transferred, make sure none of these patient care measures have been omitted: suctioning of airway, administering prescribed medications, completing scheduled procedures, changing soiled dressing, bathing an incontinent patient, and emptying drainage collection devices.

Documentation

Record the time and date of transfer, the patient's condition during transfer, the name of the receiving unit, and the mode of transportation. Include equipment accompanying the patient, such as IV lines and pumps, surgical drains, and oxygen therapy. Note the name and title of the person you gave your report to; also include the names of staff or family members accompanying the patient.

REFERENCES

1 The Joint Commission. (2015). Standard PC.04.01.05. *Comprehensive accreditation manual for hospitals: The official handbook.* Oakbrook Terrace, IL: The Joint Commission. (Level VII)

2 The Joint Commission. (2015). Standard PC.04.01.01. *Comprehensive accreditation manual for hospitals: The official handbook.* Oakbrook Terrace, IL: The Joint Commission. (Level VII)

3 The Joint Commission. (2015). Standard PC.04.02.01. *Comprehensive accreditation manual for hospitals: The official handbook.* Oakbrook Terrace, IL: The Joint Commission. (Level VII)

4 Centers for Disease Control and Prevention. (2002). Guideline for hand hygiene in health-care settings: Recommendations of the Healthcare Infection Control Practices Advisory Committee and the HICPAC/SHEA/APIC/IDSA Hand Hygiene Task Force. *MMWR Recommendations and Reports, 51*(RR-16), 1–45. Accessed May 2015 via the Web at http://www.cdc.gov/mmwr/pdf/rr/rr5116.pdf (Level II)

5 World Health Organization. (2009). "WHO guidelines on hand hygiene in health care: First global patient safety challenge, clean care is safer care" [Online]. Accessed May 2015 via the Web at http://whqlibdoc.who.int/publications/2009/9789241597906_eng.pdf (Level IV)

6 The Joint Commission. (2015). Standard NPSG.07.01.01. *Comprehensive accreditation manual for hospitals: The official handbook.* Oakbrook Terrace, IL: The Joint Commission. (Level VII)

7 American Osteopathic Association. (2014). Standard 07.01.21. *Healthcare Facilities Accreditation Program: Accreditation requirements for acute care hospitals.* Chicago, IL: American Osteopathic Association. (Level VII)

8 Centers for Medicare & Medicaid Services, Department of Health and Human Services. (2014). Condition of participation: Infection control. 42 C.F.R. § 482.42

9 The Joint Commission. (2015). Standard NPSG.01.01.01. *Comprehensive accreditation manual for hospitals: The official handbook.* Oakbrook Terrace, IL: The Joint Commission. (Level VII)

10 The Joint Commission. (2015). Standard PC.04.01.03. *Comprehensive accreditation manual for hospitals: The official handbook.* Oakbrook Terrace, IL: The Joint Commission. (Level VII)

11 The Joint Commission. (2015). Standard PC.02.02.01. *Comprehensive accreditation manual for hospitals: The official handbook.* Oakbrook Terrace, IL: The Joint Commission. (Level VII)

12 Joint Commission Center for Transforming Healthcare. (2012). "Targeted solutions tool: Improving hand-off communications" [Online]. Accessed May 2015 via the Web at http://www.jointcommission.org/assets/1/6/TST_HOC_Persp_08_12.pdf (Level IV)

13 Institute for Healthcare Improvement. (2011). *SBAR technique for communication: A situational briefing model.* Cambridge, MA: Institute for Healthcare Improvement. (Level V)

14 The Joint Commission. (2015). Standard NPSG.03.06.01. *Comprehensive accreditation manual for hospitals: The official handbook.* Oakbrook Terrace, IL: The Joint Commission. (Level VII)

15 American Osteopathic Association. (2014). Standard 25.02.13. *Healthcare Facilities Accreditation Program: Accreditation requirements for acute care hospitals.* Chicago, IL: American Osteopathic Association. (Level VII)

16 The Joint Commission. (2015). Standard RC.01.03.01. *Comprehensive accreditation manual for hospitals: The official handbook.* Oakbrook Terrace, IL: The Joint Commission. (Level VII)

17 Centers for Medicare & Medicaid Services, Department of Health and Human Services. (2014). Condition of participation: Medical record services. 42 C.F.R. § 482.24(b).

18 American Osteopathic Association. (2014). Standard 10.00.03. *Healthcare Facilities Accreditation Program: Accreditation requirements for acute care hospitals.* Chicago, IL: American Osteopathic Association. (Level VII)

ADDITIONAL REFERENCES

Clarke, D., et al. (2012). Achieving the 'perfect handoff' in patient transfers: Building teamwork and trust. *Journal of Nursing Management, 20,* 592–598.

Roberts, M., et al. (2012). The interdepartmental ticket (IT) factor: Enhancing communication to improve quality. *Journal of Nursing Care Quality, 27,* 247–252. (Level VI)

TRANSFUSION OF BLOOD AND BLOOD PRODUCTS

Although the transfusion of blood and blood products can be a lifesaving procedure, it has risks. Such errors as the administration of the wrong blood to the wrong patient can lead to long-term health problems or even death. Nurses should use extreme caution when preparing patients for blood transfusion. Following procedures that ensure accurate patient identification and verification of blood transfusion components can help to prevent potentially fatal errors, and may be the most important step in ensuring patient safety.[1]

Transfusing blood and selected blood products

BLOOD COMPONENT	INDICATIONS	COMPATIBILITY	NURSING CONSIDERATIONS
Red blood cells (RBCs) Same RBC mass as whole blood but with 80% of the plasma removed	▪ To restore or maintain oxygen-carrying capacity in symptomatic anemia ▪ To increase RBC mass in acute anemia causes by trauma, surgical blood loss, or chemotherapy ▪ To increase RBC mass in chronic anemia with associated cardiovascular decompensation	▪ Group A receives A or O ▪ Group B receives B or O ▪ Group AB receives AB, A, B, or O ▪ Group O receives O ▪ Rh-negative recipients can only receive Rh-negative RBCs	▪ Transfuse RBCs through a sterile, pyrogen-free transfusion set with an appropriate filter. ▪ Prime the administration set with normal saline solution if using a Y-type administration set. ▪ Begin the transfusion within 30 minutes of obtaining the blood from the blood bank. ▪ Administer as the patient can tolerate, usually over 1½ to 2 hours, but complete the transfusion within 4 hours.[1] ▪ Avoid administration for anemia that's correctable with nutrition or drug therapy.
Leukocyte-reduced RBCs Same as RBCs except with nearly 70% of the leukocytes removed	▪ To restore or maintain oxygen-carrying capacity in symptomatic anemia in patients at risk for reactions caused by leukocyte antibodies ▪ To treat symptomatic anemia in immunocompromised patients ▪ To increase RBC mass in acute anemia caused by trauma, surgical blood loss, or chemotherapy in patients at risk for reactions caused by leukocyte antibodies ▪ To increase RBC mass in chronic anemia with associated cardiovascular decompensation in patients at risk for reactions caused by leukocyte antibodies	▪ Group A receives A or O ▪ Group B receives B or O ▪ Group AB receives AB, A, B, or O ▪ Group O receives O ▪ Rh-positive recipients receive Rh-positive or Rh-negative RBCs ▪ Rh-negative recipients receive only Rh-negative RBCs	▪ Transfuse the RBCs through a sterile, pyrogen-free transfusion set with an appropriate filter. ▪ Prime the administration set with normal saline solution if using a Y-type administration set. ▪ Begin the transfusion within 30 minutes of obtaining the blood from the blood bank. ▪ Administer as the patient can tolerate, usually over 1½ to 2 hours, but complete the transfusion within 4 hours.[1] ▪ Know that RBCs can be collected in special multiple-bag units so that the patient can receive a small volume of blood multiple times from the same donor. ▪ Avoid administration for anemia that's correctable with nutrition or drug therapy.
Platelets Concentrate of platelets separated from whole blood, acquired either through apheresis or pooled from multiple donors	▪ To treat bleeding caused by decreased circulating platelets or malfunctioning platelets ▪ To increase platelet count in a patient who requires an invasive procedure ▪ To prevent bleeding in a patient with a low platelet count	▪ Donor plasma ABO-compatible with recipient's RBCs when large volumes are given to adults ▪ Rh-negative recipients receive Rh-negative platelets when possible, especially in women going through childbirth	▪ Transfuse through a sterile, pyrogen-free transfusion set with an appropriate filter. (Don't use a microaggregate filter.) A leukocyte-reduction filter may be necessary if leukocyte-reduced platelets aren't available. ▪ Administration is commonly over 15 to 30 minutes and must be completed by the time indicated on the product label. ▪ Patients who don't benefit from transfusion with non-human leukocyte antigen (HLA) platelets may benefit from HLA platelets.

HOSPITAL-ACQUIRED CONDITION ALERT *The Centers for Medicare & Medicaid Services has identified blood incompatibility errors as a hospital-acquired condition* because the application of evidence-based practices can reasonably prevent such errors. *Follow evidence-based practices, such as carefully identifying the patient and blood sample for compatibility testing and participating in a two-person verification process, before blood or blood product administration* to reduce the risk of incompatibility errors.[2,3]

Health care facilities use dentification and verification processes to help prevent the transfusion of a blood product that doesn't match the patient's assigned identification number. Plasma, platelets, and blood derivatives can also cause serious transfusion reactions and should be administered with care.[1] Before administering blood or a blood product, nurses should be familiar with the different types of blood and blood products. (See *Transfusing blood and selected blood products.*)

Transfusing blood and selected blood products *(continued)*

BLOOD COMPONENT	INDICATIONS	COMPATIBILITY	NURSING CONSIDERATIONS
Plasma Noncellular portion of blood that's separated and frozen after donation; contains coagulation factors and other proteins	■ To temporarily reverse the effects of warfarin ■ For plasma exchange (especially for thrombotic thrombocytopenia) ■ To treat factor deficiency if concentrate is unavailable ■ To correct abnormal coagulation test results before invasive procedures ■ To treat liver disease with protein synthetic defect ■ To treat dilutional coagulopathy ■ To treat consumptive coagulopathy	■ Group A receives A or AB ■ Group B receives B or AB ■ Group AB receives AB ■ Group O receives O, A, B, or AB ■ Rh matching not required	■ Transfuse through a sterile, pyrogen-free transfusion set with an appropriate filter. ■ Infuse immediately after thawing.[4] ■ Administration is usually over 30 to 60 minutes.
Cryoprecipitate Also known as cryoprecipitated antihemophilic factor (AHF), noncellular blood component that's prepared by thawing fresh frozen plasma, recovering the insoluble precipitate, and then refreezing the precipitate within 1 hour of collection; contains concentrated levels of fibrinogen, Factor VIII, von Willebrand factor, Factor XIII, and fibronectin[5]	■ To treat factor deficiency when factor-specific concentrate is unavailable ■ To treat hypofibrinogenemia ■ To treat dysfibrinogenemia ■ To treat von Willebrand disease ■ To correct fibronectin deficiency	■ ABO compatibility not required but is preferred[4] ■ Rh matching not required	■ Transfuse through a sterile, pyrogen-free transfusion set with an appropriate filter. ■ Infuse immediately after thawing. May be administered through a small-gauge IV catheter. ■ Administration is usually over 15 to 30 minutes.

Equipment

Patient's medical record ■ blood or blood component administration set ■ IV pole ■ gloves ■ blood or blood product ■ preservative-free normal saline solution ■ 10-mL syringe ■ disinfectant pads ■ stethoscope ■ thermometer ■ sphygmomanometer or automated blood pressure device ■ blood request form ■ Optional: prescribed premedications, 250 mL of normal saline solution, IV catheter equipment (should include 14G to 24G catheter), blood warmer and administration set, mask, protective eyewear, gown, bar code scanning system.

Straight line and Y-type (most common) blood administration sets contain a standard 170-micron blood filter. which traps particles that are 170 microns or larger. It's designed to eliminate blood clots and cellular debris that occur during blood storage. Sometimes, however, a specialized blood filter may be required.[1] (See *Specialized blood filters,* page 786.)

Preparation of equipment

Don't obtain the blood or blood product until you're ready to begin the transfusion. The transfusion should begin within 30 minutes of obtaining the blood or blood product *to decrease the risk of bacterial growth.*[1] Prepare the equipment when you're ready to start the infusion. If the patient has a history of adverse reactions, administer premedication, as prescribed. *To ensure effectiveness,* administer oral medication 30 minutes before starting the transfusion. If IV medication is prescribed, administer it immediately before starting the transfusion.[1]

NURSING ALERT *Never store blood in a non–blood bank refrigerator. Return the blood to the blood bank refrigerator if a delay of 30 minutes or more is anticipated.*[4,5,6]

Implementation

■ Make sure that a written order is in the patient's medical record; the order should address preparation of the product and administration (including the start time and rate of infusion).[1] Confirm that the order and the medical record are labeled with the patient's first and last names and unique identification number.[6]

■ Ensure that the indication for the transfusion is documented in the patient's medical record.

■ Unless the transfusion is an emergency, confirm that the practitioner has obtained written informed consent before initiating transfusion therapy and that the consent is in the patient's medical record.[7,8,9,10]

■ Review the patient's medication regimen; *certain medications, such as antifungal agents and chemotherapy, might not be recommended for infusion during blood transfusion.*[1] Consult with the patient's practitioner if necessary.

■ Ensure that a blood sample was obtained for compatibility testing; collect a blood sample if one hasn't been collected. (See the "Venipuncture" procedure, page 821.) Note that pretransfusion testing can take 15 minutes to 1 hour, depending on the method used by your facility's blood bank. Blood samples must be collected within 3 days of red blood cell (RBC) transfusion if the patient has been pregnant within the preceding 3 months or has been transfused within the preceding 3 months, or if the patient's history is uncertain or unavailable.[1]

■ Make sure the blood bank receives a blood request form that contains the patient's first and last names, an identification number unique to the patient, the prescribed blood component and amount ordered, and the name of the responsible practitioner. (A computer-transmitted request is acceptable if it contains the required information.) Additional

EQUIPMENT

Specialized blood filters

When determined to be medically necessary, specialized filters are used to transfuse blood and blood products.[6]

FILTER TYPE	CONSIDERATIONS
Microaggregate filter	▪ Eliminates debris as small as 20 microns ▪ Use isn't warranted in routine transfusion therapy[1] ▪ Not appropriate for granulocyte infusions[1] ▪ May be indicated for use with extracorporeal membrane oxygenation circuits, preparation of intraoperative blood recovery collections, or infusion of wound drainage collections[1]
Leucocyte reduction filter	▪ Reduces the number of leukocytes by 99.9% in red blood cell and platelet units ▪ May be used to reduce the risk of transfusion complications if a prestorage leukocyte-reduced blood unit isn't available[1] ▪ Requires close following of the manufacturer's instructions for use[1]

information, such as the patient's age, gender, diagnosis, transfusion history, pregnancy history, and special blood component or service needs as well as the date and time of blood sample collection for compatibility testing, may be helpful in resolving any problems that may occur.[1]

- Gather the necessary equipment.
- Perform hand hygiene.[11,12,13,14,15,16,17]
- Confirm the patient's identity using at least two patient identifiers.[4,18]
- Explain the procedure to the patient.
- Verify that the patient's religious beliefs don't prohibit blood transfusion therapy.[1]
- Assess the patient's previous knowledge and understanding of the procedure. If the patient is disoriented or unconscious, assess the family's knowledge and understanding of the procedure.[1]
- Develop a teaching plan based on your assessment findings and then use it to explain the procedure to the patient and his family *because an informed patient and family can aid in the early detection of transfusion-related problems.* (See *Teaching about blood and blood product transfusions.*)[1]
- Put on gloves.[15,19,20,21]
- Ensure that the patient has adequate venous access with an appropriate-sized catheter (14G to 24G).[6] Verify patency by aspirating for blood return.[6,22] Insert an IV catheter if necessary. (See the "IV catheter insertion and removal" procedure, page 446.) A central venous catheter is also an acceptable option for blood transfusion;[16] be aware that catheter length affects the rate of infusion (the longer the catheter, the slower the rate of infusion).[6]
- Remove and discard your gloves.[19,21,23]
- Perform hand hygiene.[11,12,13,14,15,16,17]
- Obtain and record the patient's vital signs (temperature, pulse, respirations, and blood pressure) within 30 minutes before initiating the transfusion *to serve as a baseline for comparison.*[1]
- Question the patient about the presence of signs and symptoms that may later be mistaken for a transfusion reaction, such as chills, itching, rash, hematuria, muscle aches, and difficulty breathing.[1]
- Assist the patient to the bathroom if necessary before beginning the transfusion.[1]
- Help the patient assume a comfortable position either in a chair or bed; *providing patient comfort before the transfusion helps to reduce the number of manipulations of the blood and tubing during the course of the procedure.*[1]
- Offer the patient diversional activities, such as reading materials, television, radio, and games, *to allay anxiety during the transfusion.*[1]
- Perform hand hygiene.[11,12,13,14,15,16,17]
- Obtain the blood or blood product from the blood bank. When receiving the blood or blood product from the blood bank representative, verify the patient's two independent identifiers; ABO group and Rh type; the donor identification number, ABO group and, if required, Rh type; interpretation of crossmatch tests if required; special transfusion requirements if applicable; the expiration date and time if applicable; and the date and time of blood issue. Wear gloves or transport the blood component units in a container that prevents direct contact with the blood unit bag.[1]
- If not already wearing gloves, perform hand hygiene[11,12,13,14,15,16,17] and put on gloves and other personal protective equipment as needed *to comply with standard precautions.*[19,20,21,24]
- Use a two-person verification process in the presence of the patient *to match the blood or blood component with the practitioner's order and the patient with the blood component.*[6,25] One of the people conducting the verification must be the qualified person, usually a registered nurse, who'll administer the blood or blood component to the patient. The second person conducting the verification must be qualified to participate in the process as determined by your facility.[25] Each person must independently compare the information:[1]
- Compare the name and identification number on the patient's identification bracelet with those on the blood bag label.
- Check the blood bag identification number, ABO blood group, Rh compatibility, and interpretation of compatibility testing.
- Compare the patient's blood bank identification number with the number on the blood bag.[4]
- Check the expiration date on the blood bag, and observe for leaks, abnormal color, clots, excessive air or bubbling, and unusual odor.[1,4,6] Return expired or abnormal blood to the blood bank.[1]
- After checking all of the identifying information, sign the transfusion form to indicate that the identification was correct and that you're the person starting the transfusion; other items that may be included on the transfusion form include the name and volume of the component, the blood component's identification number, and the date and time of the transfusion.[1]
- If your facility uses a bar code scanning system, scan your identification badge, the patient's identification bracelet, and the blood component label as indicated by your facility's procedure.
- Prime the blood administration set. When using a Y-type set, use normal saline solution to prime the tubing; when using a straight set, use the blood product.[1]

NURSING ALERT *Medications should never be mixed with blood components.*[6] *If the patient requires IV medications during transfusion, start a separate IV line for the administration of medications* so that the patient can receive the therapeutic benefits of the blood component and the medication simultaneously. *Also,* because IV solutions (with the exception of Plasma-Lyte 148) aren't compatible with blood products *don't mix them with blood components.*[1,2,6]

- If you're using a blood warmer or an electronic infusion device, insert the tubing into the device and operate the device following the manufacturer's instructions for use.[1] (See *Blood warmers.*)
- Thoroughly disinfect the port of the vascular access device with a disinfectant pad using friction, and then allow it to dry.[29]

- Trace the blood administration set tubing from the patient to its point of origin before beginning the transfusion *to make sure that you're connecting the tubing to the correct port,* and then attach it to the venous access device.[22,30]
- Start the blood transfusion at a slow rate.[14]
- Stay with the patient and closely monitor him during the first 15 minutes for signs of transfusion reaction *because if a major incompatibility exists or a severe allergic reaction such as anaphylaxis occurs, signs and symptoms usually appear before the first 50 mL of the unit have been transfused.*[1]
- If a reaction occurs, immediately stop the transfusion and notify the practitioner.[1] (See the "Transfusion reaction management" procedure, page 790.)
- Obtain vital signs 15 minutes after the start of the transfusion and any time that the patient's condition warrants during the transfusion.[1]
- If no evidence of a transfusion reaction occurs within the first 15 minutes of the transfusion, increase the infusion rate to the prescribed rate.[1]
- Before leaving the patient's room, instruct him to immediately report anything unusual.[1]
- Observe the patient periodically (at least every 30 minutes) during the transfusion *to identify early signs and symptoms of a possible transfusion reaction.*[1] Closely monitor the flow rate and inspect the IV insertion site for signs of infiltration. (See *What to do if the infusion rate slows,* page 788.)
- Remove and discard your gloves and any other personal protective equipment worn.[19,21,23]
- Perform hand hygiene.[11,12,13,14,15,16,17]
- At the completion of blood product administration, obtain the patient's vital signs *to compare with baseline measurements to detect signs of a possible transfusion reaction.*[1]
- If you must administer additional units, repeat the procedure. If more than one unit can be infused within 4 hours, note that the transfusion administration set and filter can be used for up to 4 hours. (Most filters have a four-unit capacity; check the manufacturer's instructions.)[1,32]
- If additional units aren't prescribed, perform hand hygiene[11,12,13,14,15,16,17] and put on gloves,[19,20,21] and then reconnect the original IV fluid, saline lock the catheter, or discontinue the IV infusion, as prescribed.[33]
- Discard used infusion supplies in an appropriate container, and discard the blood bag, tubing, and filter in an appropriate hazardous waste container.[19,21,23,34]
- Clean and disinfect your stethoscope using a disinfectant pad.[35,36]
- Remove and discard your gloves.[19,21,23]
- Perform hand hygiene.[11,12,13,14,16,17]
- Continue to assess and monitor the patient for signs and symptoms of a delayed transfusion reaction for 1 hour after the transfusion. Teach the patient and his family about the signs and symptoms of a delayed reaction.[1,6]
- Document the procedure.[37,38,39]

Special considerations

- Note that a one-person verification process accompanied by automated identification technology, such as bar coding, is acceptable.[25]
- If necessary, using sterile technique, change the blood or blood component administration set after each unit is infused or after 4 hours. Change it immediately if you suspect contamination or if the integrity of the product or system has been compromised.[40]
- Be aware that a donor unit of blood can be split if a patient might not be able to tolerate the fluid volume of an entire unit at one time. Individual portions of the unit can be released for administration while the remainder is safely stored.[1] Consult with the blood bank if unit splitting is necessary.
- Note that the U.S. Food and Drug Administration has approved the compatibility of Plasma-Lyte 148 with blood components; it may be

Teaching about blood and blood product transfusions[1]

When developing a teaching plan, base your objectives on the information you gather during your assessment, and set criteria to evaluate whether your objectives were met. Make sure the content of your teaching plan directly relates to your objectives, and cover the following information.

Describe the sequence of events, including:

- reasons for the transfusion
- compatibility testing
- the need for IV catheter insertion (if an appropriate-sized catheter isn't already in place)
- administration of premedications (if needed and prescribed)
- vital sign and other monitoring that will take place before and during the transfusion
- activity limitations during the transfusion
- what to expect after the transfusion.

Explain the benefits of transfusion, such as:

- improving the oxygen-carrying capacity of red blood cells (RBCs) (for example, if RBCs prescribed for treating symptomatic anemia)
- providing coagulation factors to prevent or control bleeding.

Cover transfusion risks, including:

- immunologic complications, such as hemolytic and nonhemolytic reactions
- transmission of infectious disease
- fluid overload and subsequent pulmonary edema
- sepsis.

Discuss the signs and symptoms of complications the patient should be alert for, including:

- a vague, uneasy feeling
- the onset of pain (especially at the IV site, back, or chest)
- chills
- flushing
- fever
- nausea
- dizziness
- a rash
- itching
- dark or red urine.

EQUIPMENT

Blood warmers

Blood warmers may be used to prevent hypothermia, which can result from rapid infusion of large volumes of refrigerated blood.[1] Various blood and fluid warmers are available that warm blood using various mechanisms.

The blood and fluid warmer should be capable of safely delivering fluids and blood products at normothermia at both high and low flow rates;[27] the warmer must be tested and approved for use with blood components.[1] No matter what type of device is available at your facility, closely follow the manufacturer's instructions for use.

A blood warmer may be indicated for use in:

- plasma exchange transfusion
- surgery
- trauma
- cold agglutinin disease.[1,28]

TROUBLESHOOTING

What to do if the infusion rate slows

If the infusion rate slows, determine a probable cause:

- Check the IV insertion site for signs of infiltration.[1] If you observe signs of infiltration, stop the infusion immediately, disconnect the administration set, and aspirate fluid from the catheter using a small (3-mL) syringe. Remove the catheter and estimate the volume of fluid infiltrated.
- Notify the practitioner and insert a new IV catheter in a different location *to prevent an interruption in transfusion therapy.*[31]
- Assess catheter patency. If the IV catheter is no longer patent, restart a new IV catheter in a different location.[1]
- If the component is infusing by gravity, raise the height of the blood container on the IV pole.[1]
- Gently rock the unit bag back and forth two to three times *to prevent the suspended blood cells from settling.*[1]
- Change the administration set and filter *because they may have become clogged with debris.*[1]

administered before or after the infusion of blood through the same administration set (for example, as priming solution), may be added to or infused concurrently with blood components, and may be used as a diluent in the transfusion of RBCs.[1]

- If necessary, when administering blood products with a Y-type administration set, you can add normal saline solution to the bag *to dilute the cells.* To do so, close the clamp between the patient and the drip chamber and open the clamp from the blood product bag. Then lower the bag below the normal saline solution container and let 30 to 50 mL of normal saline solution flow into the bag. Finally, close the clamp to the bag, rehang the bag, rotate it gently *to mix the cells and normal saline solution,* and close the clamp to the normal saline solution.
- For rapid blood replacement, you may need to use a pressure bag or a positive-pressure electronic infusion device. Always follow the manufacturer's instructions for use. Pressure bags should be equipped with a pressure gauge, totally encase the blood bag, and exert uniform pressure against all parts of the blood container; a blood pressure cuff shouldn't be used *because it can't deliver uniform pressure.*[6]
- If the blood bag empties before the next one arrives, administer normal saline solution slowly *to keep the vein patent.* If you're using a Y-type set, close the blood-line clamp, open the clamp to the normal saline solution, and let it infuse slowly until the new unit of blood arrives. Decrease the flow rate or clamp the line before attaching the new unit of blood.
- Keep in mind that blood products must be infused within 4 hours of removal from the blood bank refrigerator.[4,6] If any blood product remains after 4 hours, discontinue the infusion and discard the remaining product, as directed.
- Keep in mind that, although some organized religions—such as Jehovah's Witnesses and Christian Scientists—prohibit transfusion therapy, most religions don't prohibit the use of blood components by their members when a medical need arises. Provide the opportunity for all patients to discuss their beliefs regarding blood transfusion.[1]
- Be aware that whole blood is rarely used. It may be used on rare occasions to restore blood volume from hemorrhage or in an exchange transfusion.

Complications

Despite improvements in crossmatching precautions, transfusion reactions can still occur during a transfusion or within 96 hours after a transfusion. Transfusion reactions typically stem from a major antigen-antibody reaction. Monitor the patient closely monitor for signs and symptoms, especially if the patient can't report the symptoms. A transfusion reaction requires prompt action *to prevent further complications and, possibly, death.*

Unlike a transfusion reaction, an infectious disease transmitted during a transfusion may go undetected until days, weeks, or even months later, when it produces signs and symptoms. Measures to prevent disease transmission include laboratory testing of blood products and careful screening of potential donors, neither of which is guaranteed. Hepatitis C accounts for most posttransfusion hepatitis cases. The tests that detect hepatitis B and hepatitis C can produce false-negative results and may allow some hepatitis cases to go undetected. The risk of transmitting human immunodeficiency virus during transfusion is rare. Blood products are tested rigorously using highly sensitive testing.[41,42] Many blood banks screen blood for cytomegalovirus (CMV). Blood with CMV is especially dangerous for an immunosuppressed, seronegative patient. Blood banks also test blood for syphilis, but refrigerating blood virtually eliminates the risk of transfusion-related syphilis.

Circulatory overload and hemolytic, allergic, febrile, and pyogenic reactions can result from any transfusion. Coagulation disturbances, citrate intoxication, hyperkalemia, acid-base imbalance, loss of 2,3-diphosphoglycerate, ammonia intoxication, and hypothermia can result from massive transfusion.

Documentation

Record the date and time of the transfusion; confirmation that informed consent was obtained; indications for the transfusion; any premedications administered; the type and amount of blood product transfused; the amount of normal saline solution infused; the patient's vital signs before, during, and after transfusion; your verification of all identification data; and the patient's response. Document any transfusion reaction and treatment. Note any patient teaching and the patient's understanding of the teaching.[1,26] (See *Documenting blood transfusions.*)

REFERENCES

1 AABB. (2012). *Primer of blood administration.* Bethesda, MD: AABB. (Level VII)

2 Jarrett, N., et al. (2013). "Evidence-based guidelines for selected and previously considered hospital-acquired conditions: Final report" [Online]. Accessed May 2015 via the Web at http://www.cms.gov/Medicare/Medicare-Fee-for-Service-Payment/HospitalAcqCond/Downloads/Evidence-Based-Guidelines.pdf

3 Centers for Medicare & Medicaid Services, Department of Health and Human Services. (2012). "Hospital-acquired conditions" [Online]. Accessed May 2015 via the Web at http://www.cms.gov/Medicare/Medicare-Fee-for-Service-Payment/HospitalAcqCond/Hospital-Acquired_Conditions.html

4 AABB, et al. (2013). *Circular of information for use of human blood and blood components.* Bethesda, MD: AABB. Accessed May 2015 via the Web at http://www.aabb.org/tm/coi/Documents/coi1113.pdf (Level VII)

5 Quraishy, N., et al. (2013). "A compendium of transfusion practice guidelines (2nd ed.)" [Online]. Accessed May 2015 via the Web at http://www.redcrossblood.org/sites/arc/files/59802_compendium_brochure_v_6_10_9_13.pdf (Level VII)

6 Standard 66. Transfusion therapy. Infusion nursing standards of practice. (2011). *Journal of Infusion Nursing, 34,* S93–S95. (Level VII)

7 The Joint Commission. (2015). Standard RI.01.03.01. *Comprehensive accreditation manual for hospitals: The official handbook.* Oakbrook Terrace, IL: The Joint Commission. (Level VII)

8 Centers for Medicare & Medicaid Services, Department of Health and Human Services. (2014). Condition of participation: Patient's rights. 42 C.F.R. § 482.13(b)(2).

9 Standard 12. Informed consent. Infusion nursing standards of practice. (2011). *Journal of Infusion Nursing, 34,* S17–S18. (Level VII)

10 American Osteopathic Association. (2014). Standard 15.01.11. *Healthcare Facilities Accreditation Program: Accreditation requirements for acute care hospitals.* Chicago, IL: American Osteopathic Association. (Level VII)
11 The Joint Commission. (2015). Standard NPSG.07.01.01. *Comprehensive accreditation manual for hospitals: The official handbook.* Oakbrook Terrace, IL: The Joint Commission. (Level VII)
12 Centers for Disease Control and Prevention. (2002). Guideline for hand hygiene in health-care settings: Recommendations of the Healthcare Infection Control Practices Advisory Committee and the HICPAC/SHEA/APIC/IDSA Hand Hygiene Task Force. *MMWR Recommendations and Reports, 51*(RR-16), 1–45. Accessed May 2015 via the Web at http://www.cdc.gov/mmwr/pdf/rr/rr5116.pdf (Level II)
13 World Health Organization. (2009). "WHO guidelines on hand hygiene in health care: First global patient safety challenge, clean care is safer care" [Online]. Accessed May 2015 via the Web at http://whqlibdoc.who.int/publications/2009/9789241597906_eng.pdf (Level IV)
14 Standard 19. Hand hygiene. Infusion nursing standards of practice. (2011). *Journal of Infusion Nursing, 34,* S26–S27. (Level VII)
15 Centers for Disease Control and Prevention. (2011). "Guidelines for the prevention of intravascular catheter–related infections" [Online]. Accessed May 2015 via the Web at http://www.cdc.gov/hicpac/pdf/guidelines/bsi-guidelines-2011.pdf (Level I)
16 Centers for Medicare & Medicaid Services, Department of Health and Human Services. (2014). Condition of participation: Infection control. 42 C.F.R. § 482.42.
17 American Osteopathic Association. (2014). Standard 07.01.21. *Healthcare Facilities Accreditation Program: Accreditation requirements for acute care hospitals.* Chicago, IL: American Osteopathic Association. (Level VII)
18 The Joint Commission. (2015). Standard NPSG.01.01.01. *Comprehensive accreditation manual for hospitals: The official handbook.* Oakbrook Terrace, IL: The Joint Commission. (Level VII)
19 Siegel, J. D., et al. (2007). "2007 guideline for isolation precautions: Preventing transmission of infectious agents in healthcare settings" [Online]. Accessed May 2015 via the Web at http://www.cdc.gov/hicpac/pdf/isolation/Isolation2007.pdf (Level II)
20 Standard 18. Infection prevention. Infusion nursing standards of practice. (2011). *Journal of Infusion Nursing, 34,* S25–S26. (Level VII)
21 Occupational Safety and Health Administration. (n.d.). "Bloodborne pathogens, standard number 1910.1030" [Online]. Accessed May 2015 via the Web at http://www.osha.gov/pls/oshaweb/owadisp.show_document?p_table=STANDARDS&p_id=10051 (Level VII)
22 Standard 61. Parenteral medication and solution administration. Infusion nursing standards of practice. (2011). *Journal of Infusion Nursing, 34,* S86–S87. (Level VII)
23 Standard 22. Safe handling and disposal of sharps, hazardous materials, and hazardous waste. Infusion nursing standards of practice. (2011). *Journal of Infusion Nursing, 34,* S28–S29. (Level VII)
24 American Osteopathic Association. (2014). Standard 07.01.10. *Healthcare Facilities Accreditation Program: Accreditation requirements for acute care hospitals.* Chicago, IL: American Osteopathic Association. (Level VII)
25 The Joint Commission. (2015). Standard NPSG.01.03.01. *Comprehensive accreditation manual for hospitals: The official handbook.* Oakbrook Terrace, IL: The Joint Commission. (Level VII)
26 AABB. (2014). *Standards for blood banks and transfusion services* (29th ed.). Bethesda, MD: AABB.
27 Smith, C. E., & Wagner, K. (2008). Principles of fluid and blood warming in trauma. *International TraumaCare, 18,* 71–79.
28 Standard 30. Blood and fluid warmers. Infusion nursing standards of practice. (2011). *Journal of Infusion Nursing, 34,* S35–S36. (Level VII)
29 Standard 27. Needleless connectors. Infusion nursing standards of practice. (2011). *Journal of Infusion Nursing, 34,* S32–S33. (Level VII)
30 U.S. Food and Drug Administration. (n.d.). "Look. Check. Connect. Safe medical device connections save lives" [Online]. Accessed May 2015 via the Web at http://www.fda.gov/downloads/MedicalDevices/Safety/AlertsandNotices/UCM134873.pdf
31 Standard 48. Infiltration and extravasation. Infusion nursing standards of practice. (2011). *Journal of Infusion Nursing, 34,* S66–S68. (Level VII)

Documenting blood transfusions

After matching the patient's name, medical record number, blood group (or type) and Rh factor (the patient's and the donor's); the crossmatch data; and the blood bank identification number with the label on the blood bag, you'll need to clearly document that you did so. The blood or blood component must be identified and documented properly by two health care professionals as well.

In the transfusion record, document:

- the date and time the transfusion was started and completed
- the name of the health care professional who verified the information
- the type and gauge of the catheter
- the total amount of the transfusion
- the patient's vital signs before and after the transfusion
- any infusion device used
- the flow rate
- any blood warming unit used.

If the patient receives his own blood, document on the intake and output record:

- the amount of autologous blood retrieved
- the amount reinfused
- laboratory data during and after the autotransfusion
- the patient's pretransfusion and posttransfusion vital signs.

Pay particular attention to the patient's:

- coagulation profile
- hemoglobin level, hematocrit, arterial blood gas values, and calcium level
- tolerance of the procedure, especially fluid status.

32 Standard 28. Filters. Infusion nursing standards of practice. (2011). *Journal of Infusion Nursing, 34,* S33–S34. (Level VII)
33 Infusion Nurses Society. (2011). *Policies and procedures for infusion nursing* (4th ed.). Boston, MA: Infusion Nurses Society.
34 Standard 35. Vascular access site preparation and device management. Infusion nursing standards of practice. (2011). *Journal of Infusion Nursing, 34,* S28–S29. (Level VII)
35 Rutala, W. A., et al. (2008). "Guideline for disinfection and sterilization in healthcare facilities, 2008" [Online]. Accessed May 2015 via the Web at http://www.cdc.gov/hicpac/pdf/guidelines/Disinfection_Nov_2008.pdf (Level I)
36 American Osteopathic Association. (2014). Standard 07.02.03. *Healthcare Facilities Accreditation Program: Accreditation requirements for acute care hospitals.* Chicago, IL: American Osteopathic Association. (Level VII)
37 The Joint Commission. (2015). Standard RC.01.03.01. *Comprehensive accreditation manual for hospitals: The official handbook.* Oakbrook Terrace, IL: The Joint Commission. (Level VII)
38 Centers for Medicare & Medicaid Services, Department of Health and Human Services. (2014). Condition of participation: Medical record services. 42 C.F.R. § 482.24(b).
39 American Osteopathic Association. (2014). Standard 10.00.03. *Healthcare Facilities Accreditation Program: Accreditation requirements for acute care hospitals.* Chicago, IL: American Osteopathic Association. (Level VII)
40 Standard 43. Administration set change. Infusion nursing standards of practice. (2011). *Journal of Infusion Nursing, 34,* S55–S57. (Level VII)
41 American Red Cross. (n.d.). "Infectious disease testing" [Online]. Accessed May 2015 via the Web at http://www.redcrossblood.org/hospitals/infectious-disease-testing
42 Centers for Disease Control and Prevention. (2012). "Blood safety: Diseases and organisms" [Online]. Accessed May 2015 via the Web at http://www.cdc.gov/bloodsafety/bbp/diseases_organisms.html (Level VII)

TRANSFUSION REACTION MANAGEMENT

A transfusion reaction is any unfavorable event that occurs in a patient during or following transfusion of blood or a blood component that can be related to the transfusion. It's estimated that about 5% to 6% of all blood transfusion recipients experience a recognizable adverse effect as a result of the transfusion.[1] Any adverse change in the patient's condition should be considered a possible indication of a transfusion reaction and calls for prompt evaluation to prevent further complications. (See *A guide to transfusion reactions.*)

Equipment

Gloves ▪ sterile cap ▪ normal saline solution ▪ IV administration set ▪ sterile urine specimen container ▪ supplies for blood collection (see the "Venipuncture" procedure, page 821) ▪ transfusion reaction report form ▪ stethoscope ▪ sphygmomanometer or automated blood pressure device ▪ pulse oximeter ▪ thermometer ▪ laboratory specimen labels ▪ laboratory request form ▪ laboratory biohazard transport bags ▪ Optional: oxygen, epinephrine, hypothermia blanket, indwelling urinary catheter and insertion kit, prescribed medications, prescribed IV fluid, resuscitation equipment.

Implementation

- Perform hand hygiene.[2,3,4,5,6,7,8]
- Put on gloves *to comply with standard precautions.*[9,10,11]
- Confirm the patient's identity using at least two patient identifiers.[12]
- If you suspect an adverse reaction, stop the transfusion immediately; don't allow the blood remaining in the filter and tubing to infuse.[1,13]
- Trace the blood administration tubing from the patient to its point of origin, disconnect it from the IV catheter, and cover the hub with a sterile cap; don't discard the administration set or the blood product.[1,14]
- Prime a new administration set with normal saline solution, attach the administration set to the IV catheter, and infuse normal saline solution at a keep-vein-open rate.[1] Trace the tubing from the patient to its point of origin *to make sure that you've connected the tubing to the correct port.*[14]
- Remain with the patient and notify the practitioner immediately.[1]
- Check the identifying information on the blood or blood product container label and other records *to make sure that the patient is receiving the correct unit of blood.*[1]
- If the patient is receiving the wrong unit of blood, notify the blood bank immediately *to prevent further mismatching.*[1,13]
- Closely monitor the patient's vital signs for indications of shock.[1] Monitor his oxygen saturation level and assess his cardiac and respiratory status frequently, as indicated by the patient's condition and the type of reaction suspected.
- Administer treatment, as prescribed, *to provide symptomatic relief.*[1,13]
- Notify the blood bank and provide a description of the clinical findings that prompted the transfusion reaction report.[1]
- Place the blood container (even if it's empty), attached IV fluids, and administration set with the related forms and labels in a laboratory biohazard transport bag[9] and return them to the blood bank *because the blood bank will test these materials to further evaluate the reaction.*[1]
- Perform a venipuncture in a different vein and obtain blood samples for laboratory testing for hemolysis and for repeat ABO group determination and direct antiglobulin testing, as ordered.[1] The practitioner may order additional laboratory testing such as blood cultures *if he suspects bacterial contamination.* The practitioner may also order blood urea nitrogen and creatinine levels *to monitor renal function* and coagulation studies, such as prothrombin time, partial thromboplastin time, fibrinogen level, and D-dimer, *to identify red blood cell destruction and to monitor for disseminated intravascular coagulation.* Report critical test results to the practitioner within the time frame determined by your facility *to prevent treatment delays.*[15]

NURSING ALERT *Limit phlebotomy and blood loss from laboratory testing.*[16]

- Collect a urine specimen *to check for the presence of hemoglobin in the urine, which is an indicator of hemolysis.*[1]
- Label all samples in the presence of the patient *to prevent mislabeling.*[12]
- Complete and send the appropriate documentation, usually a transfusion reaction form, to the laboratory along with the samples in a laboratory biohazard transport bag.[9]
- Discard used supplies in the appropriate receptacle.[9,10]
- Remove and discard your gloves.[9,10]
- Perform hand hygiene.[2,3,5,6,7,8]
- Closely monitor intake and output; insert an indwelling urinary catheter, if ordered, *to monitor urine output in a critically ill patient.*[17] Note evidence of oliguria or anuria *because hemoglobin deposition in the renal tubes can cause renal damage.*
- Make sure the patient is comfortable and provide reassurance to him and his family, as necessary.
- Perform hand hygiene.[2,3,6,7,8]
- Document the procedure.[18]

Special considerations

HOSPITAL-ACQUIRED CONDITION ALERT *The Centers for Medicare & Medicaid Services has identified blood incompatibility errors as a hospital-acquired condition* **because the application of evidence-based practices can reasonably prevent such errors.** ***Follow evidence-based practices, such as carefully identifying the patient and blood sample for compatibility testing and participating in a two-person verification process, before blood or blood product administration*** **to reduce the risk of incompatibility errors.**[19,20]

- A blood incompatibility error is considered a sentinel event by The Joint Commission. A sentinel event is an unexpected occurrence involving death or serious physical or psychological injury or the risk of death or injury. Sentinel events require immediate investigation and response. Follow your facility's process for reporting a blood incompatibility error if you suspect one.[21,22]
- Be aware that transfusion-related acute lung injury (TRALI) is the leading cause of transfusion-related mortality. Monitor the patient closely for signs and symptoms of TRALI.[1]
- Be alert for signs and symptoms of shock or cardiovascular collapse. Be prepared to intervene with emergency medications and rapid fluid administration. Follow advanced cardiac life support protocols if respiratory or cardiac arrest occurs.
- Report all fatalities from transfusion of blood or a blood product to the Food and Drug Administration (FDA). Make initial notification by e-mail (if possible) at fatalities2@fda.hhs.gov as soon as possible after the event; if e-mail isn't possible, notify by telephone (204-402-9160) or facsimile (301-595-1304, addressed to the attention of the CBER Fatality Program Manager). Send a follow-up report to the FDA by e-mail, facsimile, or express mail (Food and Drug Administration, Center for Biologics Evaluation and Research Document Control Center, 10903 New Hampshire Ave., WO71-G112, Silver Spring, MD 20993-000, Attention: CBER Fatality Program Manager).[23]

Patient teaching

Because blood transfusion reactions may occur after the transfusion is complete, teach the patient the signs and symptoms of transfusion reaction. Tell him to be alert to the possibility of a delayed reaction, and advise him to report signs and symptoms promptly.

Documentation

Record the time and date the transfusion was started, the type of blood component transfused, the unit identification number, the patient's

A guide to transfusion reactions

REACTION	CAUSES	SIGNS AND SYMPTOMS	PREVENTIVE MEASURES AND NURSING INTERVENTIONS
Acute hemolytic	▪ Administration of incompatible blood	▪ Chills ▪ Shaking ▪ Fever ▪ Pain at the IV insertion site ▪ Nausea and vomiting ▪ Chest tightness ▪ Headache ▪ Flank pain ▪ Renal failure or shock (if allowed to progress)	▪ Properly label all blood samples in the presence of the patient. ▪ Positively identify the patient and donor blood types and groups before the transfusion. ▪ Use a two-person verification process *to verify the patient and blood component.* ▪ Transfuse the blood slowly for the first 15 minutes and remain with the patient. ▪ Save the donor blood *to reattempt crossmatching with the patient's blood.* ▪ If an acute hemolytic reaction occurs, stop the transfusion immediately. ▪ Maintain patent IV access. ▪ Notify the practitioner and blood bank personnel. ▪ Monitor the patient's vital signs for indications of shock. ▪ Insert an indwelling urinary catheter, if ordered, *to monitor urine output.* ▪ Send a blood *sample to check for intravascular hemolysis* and a urine sample *to check for hemoglobin, which is also an indicator of hemolysis.* ▪ Assess for signs of disseminated intravascular coagulation. ▪ Provide supportive medical therapies, as ordered, *to reverse shock.*
Bacterial sepsis	▪ Blood product contamination	▪ Rigors ▪ Chills ▪ Fever ▪ Shock	▪ Use sterile technique when collecting and administering blood. ▪ Begin the transfusion within 30 minutes after the component is released from the blood bank. ▪ Complete the transfusion in 4 hours or less. ▪ Don't reuse the filter if the first unit of blood takes 4 hours or longer to infuse. ▪ If signs or symptoms of bacterial sepsis occur, stop the transfusion immediately. ▪ Notify the practitioner and blood bank personnel immediately. ▪ Treat the patient's fever, as prescribed. ▪ Send blood samples from the patient and blood component for culture and sensitivity testing. ▪ Administer antibiotics, as prescribed.
Febrile reactions	▪ Leukocyte or platelet antibodies ▪ Plasma protein antibodies ▪ Cytokines from donor leukocytes	▪ Fever ▪ Chills	▪ Administer acetaminophen or an antihistamine before the transfusion. ▪ Administer leukocyte-reduced red blood cells (RBCs) *because they're less likely to cause reaction.* ▪ If signs or symptoms occur, stop the transfusion immediately. ▪ Notify the practitioner and blood bank personnel.
Transfusion-related acute lung injury (TRALI)	▪ Complement and histamine release caused by granulocyte antibodies in the donor or recipient	▪ Dyspnea ▪ Pulmonary edema ▪ Normal pulmonary artery wedge pressure	▪ Administer treatment to support blood pressure, as prescribed. ▪ Administer supplemental oxygen, as prescribed. ▪ Prepare for endotracheal intubation and mechanical ventilation, if necessary.

(continued)

A guide to transfusion reactions *(continued)*

REACTION	CAUSES	SIGNS AND SYMPTOMS	PREVENTIVE MEASURES AND NURSING INTERVENTIONS
Allergic reaction	■ Allergen in donor's plasma	■ Urticaria ■ Flushing ■ Wheezing ■ Laryngeal edema	■ Administer antihistamines before the transfusion, as prescribed, if the patient tends to experience allergic reactions. ■ If the patient develops mild itching, reduce the transfusion rate. ■ If signs and symptoms are more severe than mild itching, stop the transfusion immediately. ■ Notify the practitioner and blood bank personnel. ■ Administer epinephrine, as prescribed, *to treat wheezing and anaphylactic reactions.* ■ Restart the transfusion, as ordered, if no other cause or signs and symptoms are found or if an antihistamine provides relief from itching. ■ Don't restart the transfusion if the patient has a fever, pulmonary or airway signs and symptoms, or anaphylaxis.
Transfusion-associated circulatory overload (TACO)	■ Rapid infusion of blood ■ Excessive volume of blood	■ Precordial pain ■ Dyspnea ■ Crackles ■ Cyanosis ■ Dry cough ■ Jugular vein distention	■ Administer blood components slowly. ■ Use volume-reduced platelets *to prevent fluid overload.* ■ Administer the component using an infusion pump *to maintain flow rate.* ■ Position the patient in the semi-Fowler or upright position. ■ If the patient develops signs and symptoms of TACO, stop the transfusion immediately. ■ Notify the practitioner and blood bank personnel.
Delayed hemolytic reaction (signs and symptoms occur 5 to 10 days after transfusion)	■ Production of antibodies by recipient's RBCs to antigens on transfused RBCs	■ Fever ■ RBC destruction	■ Monitor laboratory test results for anemia and reduced benefit from successive transfusions. ■ If the patient develops signs and symptoms of delayed hemolytic reaction, notify the practitioner and blood bank personnel.
Posttransfusion purpura (signs and symptoms occur 7 to 10 days after transfusion)	■ Sensitization caused by pregnancy or previous transfusion	■ Sudden, dramatic thrombocytopenia after transfusion	■ Administer high-dose immune globulin IV, as prescribed. ■ Monitor the patient's platelet count.
Graft-versus-host disease (signs and symptoms typically develop 10 to 12 days after transfusion)	■ Engrafting of T-lymphocytes from donor's component in recipient, which then react against recipient's tissue antigens	■ Fever ■ Rash ■ Diarrhea ■ Desquamation ■ Pancytopenia	■ Provide supportive care.

condition at the start of the transfusion, the patient's vital signs, and your assessment findings. Record the time the transfusion was stopped, the volume infused, the patient's condition, and the identity of the person who stopped the transfusion and observed the patient. Record any specimens sent to the laboratory for analysis, any nursing interventions performed, any treatment given, and the patient's response to treatment. Note any unexpected outcomes and interventions performed in response to those treatments. If required by your facility, complete the transfusion reaction form. Document patient and family teaching provided and their understanding of your teaching.

REFERENCES

1 AABB. (2012). *Primer of blood administration.* Bethesda, MD: AABB.

2 Centers for Disease Control and Prevention. (2002). Guideline for hand hygiene in health-care settings: Recommendations of the Healthcare Infection Control Practices Advisory Committee and the HICPAC/SHEA/APIC/IDSA Hand Hygiene Task Force. *MMWR Recommendations and Reports, 51*(RR-16), 1–45. Accessed May 2015 via the Web at http://www.cdc.gov/mmwr/pdf/rr/rr5116.pdf (Level II)

3 World Health Organization. (2009). "WHO guidelines on hand hygiene in health care: First global patient safety challenge, clean care is safer care" [Online]. Accessed May 2015 via the Web at http://whqlibdoc.who.int/publications/2009/9789241597906_eng.pdf (Level IV)

4 Centers for Disease Control and Prevention. (2011). "Guidelines for the prevention of intravascular catheter-related infections, 2011" [Online]. Accessed May 2015 via the Web at http://www.cdc.gov/hicpac/pdf/guidelines/bsi-guidelines-2011.pdf (Level I)

5 Standard 19. Hand hygiene. Infusion nursing standards of practice. (2011). *Journal of Infusion Nursing, 34,* S26–S27. (Level VII)

6 The Joint Commission. (2015). Standard NPSG.07.01.01. *Comprehensive accreditation manual for hospitals: The official handbook.* Oakbrook Terrace, IL: The Joint Commission. (Level VII)

7 Centers for Medicare & Medicaid Services, Department of Health and Human Services. (2014). Condition of participation: Infection control. 42 C.F.R. § 482.42.

8 American Osteopathic Association. (2014). Standard 07.01.21. *Healthcare Facilities Accreditation Program: Accreditation requirements for acute care hospitals.* Chicago, IL: American Osteopathic Association. (Level VII)

9 Occupational Safety and Health Administration. (n.d.). "Bloodborne pathogens, standard number 1910.1030" [Online]. Accessed May 2015 via the Web at http://www.osha.gov/pls/oshaweb/owadisp.show_document?p_table=STANDARDSp_id=10051 (Level VII)

10 Siegel, J. D., et al. (2007). "2007 guideline for isolation precautions: Preventing transmission of infectious agents in healthcare settings" [Online]. Accessed May 2015 via the Web at http://www.cdc.gov/hicpac/pdf/isolation/Isolation2007.pdf (Level II)

11 Standard 18. Infection prevention. Infusion nursing standards of practice. (2011). *Journal of Infusion Nursing, 34,* S25–S26. (Level VII)

12 The Joint Commission. (2015). Standard NPSG.01.01.01. *Comprehensive accreditation manual for hospitals: The official handbook.* Oakbrook Terrace, IL: The Joint Commission. (Level VII)

13 Standard 66. Transfusion therapy. Infusion nursing standards of practice. (2011). *Journal of Infusion Nursing, 34,* S93–S95. (Level VII)

14 U.S. Food and Drug Administration. (n.d.). "Look. Check. Connect. Safe medical device connections save lives" [Online]. Accessed May 2015 via the Web at http://www.fda.gov/downloads/MedicalDevices/Safety/AlertsandNotices/UCM134873.pdf

15 The Joint Commission. (2014). Standard NPSG.02.03.01. *Comprehensive accreditation manual for hospitals: The official handbook.* Oakbrook Terrace, IL: The Joint Commission. (Level VII)

16 Tolich, D. J., et al. (2013). Blood management: Best-practice transfusion strategies. *Nursing, 43*(1), 40–47.

17 Healthcare Infection Control Practices Advisory Committee. (2010). "Guideline for prevention of catheter-associated urinary tract infections, 2009" [Online]. Accessed May 2015 via the Web at http://www.cdc.gov/hicpac/pdf/CAUTI/CAUTIguideline2009final.pdf (Level I)

18 The Joint Commission. (2015). Standard RC.01.03.01. *Comprehensive accreditation manual for hospitals: The official handbook.* Oakbrook Terrace, IL: The Joint Commission. (Level VII)

19 Jarrett, N., et al. (2013). "Evidence-based guidelines for selected and previously considered hospital-acquired conditions: Final report" [Online]. Accessed May 2015 via the Web at http://www.cms.gov/Medicare/Medicare-Fee-for-Service-Payment/HospitalAcqCond/Downloads/Evidence-Based-Guidelines.pdf

20 Centers for Medicare & Medicaid Services, Department of Health and Human Services. (2014). "Hospital-acquired conditions" [Online]. Accessed May 2015 via the Web at http://www.cms.gov/Medicare/Medicare-Fee-for-Service-Payment/HospitalAcqCond/Hospital-Acquired_Conditions.html

21 The Joint Commission. (2012). "Sentinel event data: Event type by year 1995–2Q 2012" [Online]. Accessed May 2015 via the Web at http://www.jointcommission.org/assets/1/18/Event_Type_Year_1995_2Q2012.pdf

22 The Joint Commission. (2013). "Sentinel events (SE)" [Online]. Accessed May 2015 via the Web at http://www.jointcommission.org/assets/1/6/CAMBHC_2012_Update2_21_SE.pdf (Level VII)

23 Food and Drug Administration. (2012). "Guidance for industry: Notifying FDA of fatalities related to blood collection or transfusion" [Online]. Accessed May 2015 http://www.fda.gov/biologicsbloodvaccines/guidancecomplianceregulatoryinformation/guidances/blood/ucm074947.htm#INITIALNOTIFICATION

ADDITIONAL REFERENCES

AABB, et al. (2013). *Circular of information for use of human blood and blood components.* Bethesda, MD: AABB. (Level VII)

American Red Cross. (2013). "A compendium of transfusion practice guidelines (2nd ed.)" [Online]. Accessed May 2015 via the Web at http://www.redcrossblood.org/sites/ard/files/59802_compendium_brochure_v_6_10_9_13.pdf (Level VII).

TRANSVENOUS PACING

Usually inserted in an emergency, a temporary pacemaker consists of an external, battery-powered pulse generator and a lead or electrode system. The purpose of a transvenous pacemaker (the most common type of temporary pacemaker) is to maintain circulatory integrity by providing for standby pacing if sudden complete heart block occurs, to increase the heart rate during periods of symptomatic bradycardia and, occasionally, to control sustained supraventricular or ventricular tachycardia.

In addition to being more comfortable for the patient, a transvenous pacemaker is more reliable than a transcutaneous pacemaker. Transvenous pacing involves threading an electrode catheter through a vein into the patient's right atrium or right ventricle. Veins used for insertion include the subclavian, brachial, internal jugular, and femoral.[1] The femoral site should be used as a last resort because it's associated with an increased risk of infection. The electrode then attaches to an external pulse generator. As a result, the pulse generator can provide an electrical stimulus directly to the endocardium.

Indications for transvenous pacing include management of symptomatic bradycardia, tachyarrhythmias, and other conduction system disturbances. It may also help diagnose conduction abnormalities.

According to the 2010 American Heart Association Guidelines for Cardiopulmonary Resuscitation and Emergency Cardiovascular Care, pacing isn't recommended in cardiac arrest.[2]

Equipment

Temporary pacemaker generator with new battery ▪ guide wire or introducer ▪ electrode catheter ▪ gloves ▪ sterile gloves ▪ sterile occlusive dressing ▪ adhesive tape ▪ antiseptic solution (2% chlorhexidine-based solution) ▪ nonconducting tape or rubber surgical glove or pouch for external pulse generator ▪ emergency cardiac drugs ▪ intubation equipment ▪ defibrillator ▪ cardiac monitor with strip-chart recorder ▪ prescribed local anesthetic ▪ bridging cable ▪ percutaneous introducer tray or venous cutdown tray ▪ alligator clip (if not using fluoroscopy) ▪ sterile gowns ▪ head covers ▪ masks and goggles or masks with face shield ▪ antiseptic solution ▪ sterile fenestrated drape ▪ sutures ▪ Optional: fluoroscopy equipment, protective apron, elastic bandage or gauze strips, restraints, clippers, peripheral IV insertion equipment and IV fluids.

Preparation of equipment

Connect the patient to the cardiac monitor. Make sure intubation equipment, emergency cardiac drugs, and a defibrillator are at the patient's bedside.

Implementation

- Verify the practitioner's order.
- Gather the appropriate equipment.
- Confirm that written informed consent has been obtained is in the patient's medical record.[3,4,5,6]
- Conduct a preprocedure verification *to make sure that all relevant documentation, related information, and equipment are available and correctly identified to the patient's identifiers.*[7,8]
- Perform hand hygiene[9,10,11,12,13] and put on gloves.[14,15,16]
- Confirm the patient's identity using at least two patient identifiers.[8,17]

Sensitivity and stimulation threshold testing[1]

Sensitivity and stimulation threshold testing help determine the appropriate pacemaker rate and amount of electrical current needed to initiate depolarization of the myocardium. Testing should occur on both chambers, as appropriate. Sensitivity threshold testing isn't necessary if the patient has no intrinsic rhythm. In some facilities, critical care nurses are permitted to perform sensitivity and stimulation threshold testing; in other facilities, the practitioner must perform the testing. Frequency of testing also varies by facility. Testing typically occurs at least every 24 hours *to make sure that the pacemaker is functioning properly and that it isn't delivering high levels of energy to the myocardium.*

Performing sensitivity threshold testing

- Slowly turn the sensitivity dial counterclockwise to a higher setting until the sensing indicator light stops flashing; this occurs when the device no longer senses the patient's intrinsic rhythm.
- Gradually turn the sensitivity dial clockwise to a lower setting until the sensing light begins flashing with each complex and the pacing light stops flashing; this setting is the sensing threshold.
- Set the sensitivity dial to the setting that's one-half the value of the sensing threshold.

Performing stimulation threshold testing

- Set the pacing rate about 10 beats/minute above the patient's intrinsic rate.
- Beginning at 20 milliamperes (mA), slowly decrease the output until capture is lost.
- Gradually increase the mA until you see a 1:1 capture and the pacing light flashes; this is the stimulation threshold.
- Set the mA at least two times higher than the stimulation threshold.

- If applicable, explain the procedure to the patient and his family.
- Check the patient's history for hypersensitivity to local anesthetics or latex.
- Assess the patient's vital signs, skin color, level of consciousness (LOC), heart rate and rhythm, peripheral pulse, and emotional state *to serve as a baseline for comparison during and after the procedure.*
- If ordered, insert a peripheral IV catheter and initiate the prescribed IV infusion at the ordered rate. (See the "IV catheter insertion and removal" procedure, page 446.)
- Insert a new battery into the external pacemaker generator, and test it *to make sure it has a strong charge.* Connect the bridging cable to the generator, and align the positive and negative poles. *This cable allows slack between the electrode catheter and the generator, reducing the risk of accidental catheter displacement.*
- Place the patient in the supine position.
- If necessary, clip the hair around the insertion site.[18]
- Remove and discard your gloves[14,15] and perform hand hygiene.[9,10,11,12,13]
- Open the appropriate supply tray while maintaining a sterile field. Label all medications, medication containers, and other solutions on and off the sterile field.[19]
- Assist the practitioner in putting on a sterile gown, a mask and goggles or a mask with face shield, a head cover, and sterile gloves. If assisting, put on the same personal protective equipment.[14,15]
- Assist, as needed, with disinfecting the insertion site with an antiseptic solution and allow it to dry. If the practitioner uses fluoroscopy during the placement of leadwires, all staff should put on a protective apron and place a protective apron on the patient below the waist.
- Following maximal barrier precautions, the practitioner covers the patient from head to toe with a sterile fenestrated drape, leaving a small opening for the insertion site.
- Conduct a time-out immediately before starting the procedure *to perform a final assessment that the correct patient, site, positioning, and procedure are identified and that, as applicable, all relevant information and necessary equipment are available.*[8,20]
- After anesthetizing the insertion site, the practitioner will puncture the brachial, femoral, subclavian, or jugular vein. Then he'll insert a guide wire or an introducer and advance the electrode catheter.
- If you aren't using fluoroscopy, connect the alligator clip to the V lead of the cardiac monitor and the distal end of the electrode catheter. Set the cardiac monitor to display the V lead continuously.[1]
- As the catheter advances, watch the cardiac monitor. When the electrode catheter reaches the right atrium, you'll notice large P waves and small QRS complexes. Then, as the catheter reaches the right ventricle, the P waves will become smaller while the QRS complexes enlarge. When the catheter touches the right ventricular endocardium, expect to see elevated ST segments, premature ventricular contractions, or both.
- When the electrode catheter is in the right ventricle, it will send an impulse to the myocardium, causing depolarization. If the patient needs atrial pacing, either alone or with ventricular pacing, the practitioner may place an electrode in the right atrium.
- Meanwhile, continuously monitor the patient's cardiac status and treat any arrhythmias, as appropriate. Also assess the patient for jaw pain and earache; *these symptoms indicate that the electrode catheter has missed the superior vena cava and has moved into the neck instead.*
- When the electrode catheter is in place, attach the catheter leads to the bridging cable, lining up the positive and negative poles.
- Turn the pacemaker on and obtain settings (mode, rate, and energy level) from the practitioner. Set the pacing mode, rate, and energy level (output and milliamperes) according to the practitioner's order or as determined by sensitivity (level of intrinsic cardiac activity as sensed by electrodes) and stimulation threshold (the minimum amount of voltage necessary to initiate depolarization) testing.[1] (See *Sensitivity and stimulation threshold testing.*) Ensure that the settings are correct.
- The practitioner will then secure the catheter to the insertion site, usually by suturing.
- Assess the patient's vital signs, skin color, LOC, heart rate and rhythm, peripheral pulses, and emotional state *to determine the effectiveness of the paced rhythm.*
- Apply a sterile occlusive dressing to the site. Label the dressing with the date, the time, and your initials. Secure the pulse generator and pacemaker wires, as necessary.
- Obtain a chest X-ray, as ordered, *to detect complications associated with insertion, such as pneumothorax.*[1]
- Discard supplies in the appropriate receptacle.[14,15]
- Remove and discard your personal protective equipment.[14,15]
- Perform hand hygiene.[9,10,11,12,13]
- Document the procedure.[21,22,23]

Special considerations

- Confirm positioning of the leadwire by ultrasound, fluoroscopy, or chest X-ray.[1]
- Take steps to prevent microshock, including warning the patient not to use any electrical equipment that isn't grounded, such as landline telephones, electric shavers, televisions, and lamps.
- Other safety measures include placing a plastic cover supplied by the manufacturer over the pacemaker controls *to avoid an accidental setting change.* Also, insulate the pacemaker by covering all exposed metal parts, such as electrode connections and pacemaker terminals, with

TROUBLESHOOTING

Handling pacemaker malfunctions

Occasionally, a temporary pacemaker may fail to function properly. When this failure occurs, you need to take immediate action to correct the problem. Follow these guidelines when your patient's pacemaker fails to pace, capture, or sense intrinsic beats.

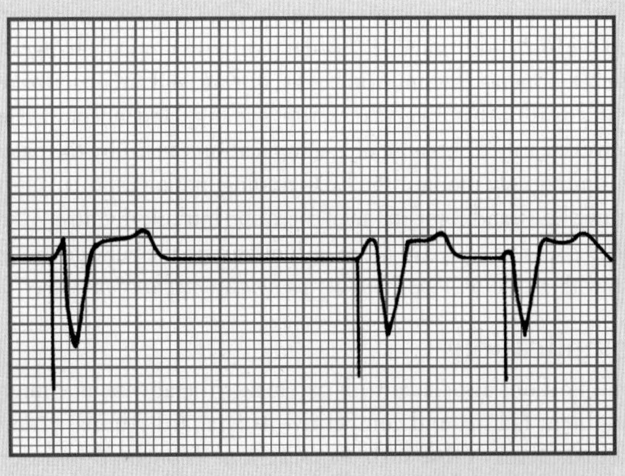

Failure to pace

Failure to pace happens when the pacemaker either doesn't fire or fires too often. The pulse generator may not be working properly, or it may not be conducting the impulse to the patient.

Nursing interventions

- If the pacing or sensing indicator flashes, check the connections to the cable and the position of the pacing electrode in the patient by X-ray. The cable may have come loose, or the electrode may have been dislodged, pulled out, or broken.
- If the pulse generator is turned on but the indicators still aren't flashing, change the battery. If that doesn't help, use a different pulse generator.
- Check the settings if the pacemaker is firing too rapidly. If they're correct or if altering them (according to your facility's guideline or the practitioner's order) doesn't help, change the pulse generator.

Failure to capture

In failure to capture, pacemaker spikes appear but the heart isn't responding. This lack of response may be caused by changes in the pacing threshold from ischemia, an electrolyte imbalance (high or low potassium or magnesium levels), acidosis, an adverse reaction to a medication, a perforated ventricle, fibrosis, or the electrode position.

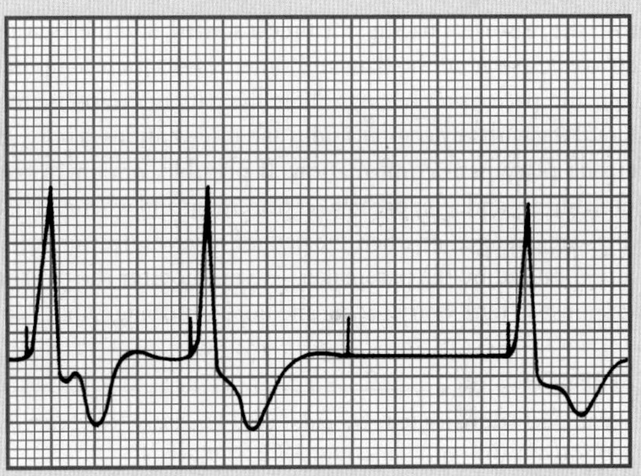

Nursing interventions

- If the patient's condition has changed, notify the practitioner and ask him for new settings.
- If pacemaker settings are altered by the patient or others, return them to their correct positions. Then make sure that the face of the pacemaker is covered with a plastic shield. Also, tell the patient or others not to touch the dials.
- If the heart isn't responding, carefully check all connections, increase the milliamperes slowly (according to your facility's protocol or the practitioner's order), or obtain a chest X-ray *to determine the electrode position.*

Failure to sense intrinsic beats

Failure to sense intrinsic beats could cause ventricular tachycardia or ventricular fibrillation if the pacemaker fires on the vulnerable T wave. This could result from the pacemaker sensing an external stimulus as a QRS complex, which could lead to asystole, or by the pacemaker not being sensitive enough, which means it could fire anywhere within the cardiac cycle.

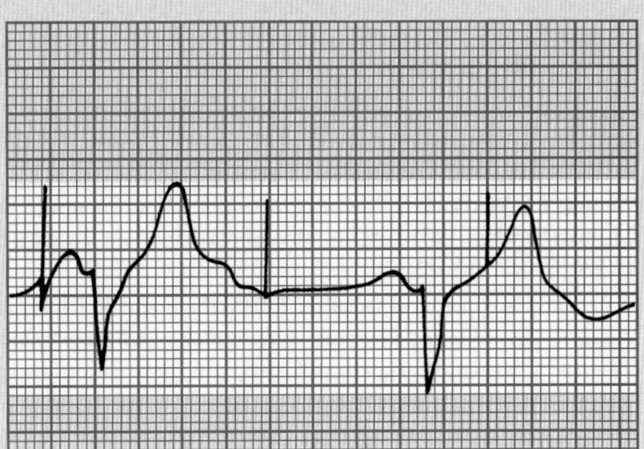

Nursing interventions

- If the pacemaker is undersensing, turn the sensitivity control completely to the right. If it's oversensing, turn it slightly to the left.
- If the pacemaker isn't functioning correctly, change the battery or the pulse generator.
- Remove items in the room causing electromechanical interference (such as razors, radios, and cautery devices). Check the ground wires on the bed and other equipment for obvious damage. Unplug each piece and see if the interference stops. When you locate the cause, notify the staff engineer and ask him to check it.
- If the pacemaker is still firing on the T wave and all else has failed, turn off the pacemaker and notify the practitioner. Make sure that atropine is available *in case the patient's heart rate drops.* Be prepared to call a code and start cardiopulmonary resuscitation.

nonconducting tape, or place the pacing unit in a dry rubber surgical glove or pouch. If the patient needs emergency defibrillation, make sure the pacemaker can withstand the procedure. If you're unsure, disconnect the pulse generator *to avoid damage.*

■ Perform a 12-lead electrocardiogram (ECG) *to serve as a baseline,* and then perform additional ECGs daily or with clinical changes. Also, if possible, obtain a rhythm strip before, during, and after pacemaker placement; any time that pacemaker settings change; and whenever the patient receives treatment because of a complication caused by the pacemaker.

■ Continuously monitor the ECG reading, noting capture, sensing, rate, intrinsic beats, and competition of paced and intrinsic rhythms.[24] If the pacemaker is sensing correctly, the sense indicator on the pulse generator should flash with each beat. (See *Handling pacemaker malfunctions,* page 795.)

Complications

Complications associated with pacemaker therapy include microshock, equipment failure, and competitive or fatal arrhythmias. Transvenous pacemakers may cause such complications as pneumothorax or hemothorax, cardiac perforation and tamponade, diaphragmatic stimulation, pulmonary embolism, thrombophlebitis, and infection. Also, if the practitioner threads the electrode through the antecubital or femoral vein, venous spasm, thrombophlebitis, or lead displacement may result.

Documentation

Record the reason for pacing, the time it started, and the locations of the electrodes. Also note the date and time, reason for a temporary pacemaker, and pacemaker settings. Note the patient's response to the procedure along with any complications and interventions taken. Document electrode placement confirmation. If possible, obtain rhythm strips before, during, and after pacemaker placement and whenever pacemaker settings are changed or when the patient receives treatment for a complication caused by the pacemaker. As you monitor the patient, record his response to temporary pacing and note any changes in his condition.

References

1 Lynn-McHale Wiegand, D. (Ed.). (2011). *AACN procedure manual for critical care* (6th ed.). St. Louis, MO: Saunders.

2 American Heart Association. (2010). 2010 American Heart Association guidelines for cardiopulmonary resuscitation and emergency cardiovascular care. *Circulation, 122,* S706–S719. (Level VII)

3 Centers for Medicare & Medicaid Services, Department of Health and Human Services. (2014). Condition of participation: Patient's rights. 42 C.F.R. § 482.13.

4 The Joint Commission. (2015). Standard RI.01.03.01. *Comprehensive accreditation manual for hospitals: The official handbook.* Oakbrook Terrace, IL: The Joint Commission. (Level VII)

5 Centers for Medicare & Medicaid Services, Department of Health and Human Services. (2014). Condition of participation: Patient's rights. 42 C.F.R. § 482.13(b)(2).

6 American Osteopathic Association. (2014). Standard 30.01.11. *Healthcare Facilities Accreditation Program: Accreditation requirements for acute care hospitals.* Chicago, IL: American Osteopathic Association. (Level VII)

7 The Joint Commission. (2015). Standard UP.01.01.01. *Comprehensive accreditation manual for hospitals: The official handbook.* Oakbrook Terrace, IL: The Joint Commission. (Level VII)

8 American Osteopathic Association. (2014). Standard 30.00.14. *Healthcare Facilities Accreditation Program: Accreditation requirements for acute care hospitals.* Chicago, IL: American Osteopathic Association. (Level VII)

9 Centers for Disease Control and Prevention (2002). Guideline for hand hygiene in health-care settings: Recommendations of the Healthcare Infection Control Practices Advisory Committee and the HICPAC/SHEA/APIC/IDSA Hand Hygiene Task Force. *MMWR Recommendations and Reports, 51*(RR-16), 1–45. Accessed May 2015 via the Web at http://www.cdc.gov/mmwr/pdf/rr/rr5116.pdf (Level II)

10 The Joint Commission. (2014). Standard NPSG.07.01.01. *Comprehensive accreditation manual for hospitals: The official handbook.* Oakbrook Terrace, IL: The Joint Commission. (Level VII)

11 World Health Organization. (2009). "WHO guidelines on hand hygiene in health care: First global patient safety challenge, clean care is safer care" [Online]. Accessed May 2015 via the Web at http://whqlibdoc.who.int/publications/2009/9789241597906_eng.pdf (Level IV)

12 American Osteopathic Association. (2014). Standard 07.01.21. *Healthcare Facilities Accreditation Program: Accreditation requirements for acute care hospitals.* Chicago, IL: American Osteopathic Association. (Level VII)

13 Centers for Medicare & Medicaid Services, Department of Health and Human Services. (2014). Condition of participation: Infection control. 42 C.F.R. § 482.42.

14 Siegel, J. D., et al. (2007). "2007 guideline for isolation precautions: Preventing transmission of infectious agents in healthcare settings" [Online]. Accessed May 2015 via the Web at http://www.cdc.gov/hicpac/pdf/isolation/Isolation2007.pdf (Level II)

15 Occupational Safety and Health Administration. (n.d.). "Bloodborne pathogens, standard number 1910.1030" [Online]. Accessed May 2015 via the Web at http://www.osha.gov/pls/oshaweb/owadisp.show_document?p_table=STANDARDS&p_id=10051 (Level VII)

16 American Osteopathic Association. (2014). Standard 07.01.10. *Healthcare Facilities Accreditation Program: Accreditation requirements for acute care hospitals.* Chicago, IL: American Osteopathic Association. (Level VII)

17 The Joint Commission. (2015). Standard NPSG.01.01.01. *Comprehensive accreditation manual for hospitals: The official handbook.* Oakbrook Terrace, IL: The Joint Commission. (Level VII)

18 The Joint Commission. (2015). Standard NPSG.07.05.01. *Comprehensive accreditation manual for hospitals: The official handbook.* Oakbrook Terrace, IL: The Joint Commission. (Level VII)

19 The Joint Commission. (2015). Standard NPSG.03.04.01. *Comprehensive accreditation manual for hospitals: The official handbook.* Oakbrook Terrace, IL: The Joint Commission. (Level VII)

20 The Joint Commission. (2015). Standard UP.01.03.01. *Comprehensive accreditation manual for hospitals: The official handbook.* Oakbrook Terrace, IL: The Joint Commission. (Level VII)

21 The Joint Commission. (2015). Standard RC.01.03.01. *Comprehensive accreditation manual for hospitals: The official handbook.* Oakbrook Terrace, IL: The Joint Commission. (Level VII)

22 Centers for Medicare & Medicaid Services, Department of Health and Human Services. (2014). Condition of participation: Medical record services. 42 C.F.R. § 482.24(b).

23 American Osteopathic Association. (2014). Standard 10.00.03. *Healthcare Facilities Accreditation Program: Accreditation requirements for acute care hospitals.* Chicago, IL: American Osteopathic Association. (Level VII)

24 Drew, B., et al. (2004). American Heart Association scientific statement: Practice standards for electrocardiographic monitoring in hospital settings. *Circulation, 110,* 2721–2746. (Level VII)

Traumatic Wound Management

Traumatic wounds include puncture wounds, abrasions, lacerations, and amputations. A puncture wound occurs when a pointed object, such as a knife, glass fragment, or nail, penetrates the skin. It can also result from a human or animal bite. A puncture wound typically doesn't cause excessive bleeding and may appear to close almost immediately; however, puncture wounds can be dangerous because of the risk of infection. Puncture wounds caused by human or animal bites are particularly prone to infection.[1]

In a traumatic abrasion, contact with a hard object, such as the road, floor, or carpet, scrapes the skin, resulting in loss of the epidermis and partial loss of the dermis of the skin. These partial-thickness wounds are typically shallow, red, painful, and highly exudative and may contain debris from the surface that caused the abrasion.[1] Occasionally, abrasions are full-thickness, involving the complete epidermis and dermis; these wounds may require debridement and skin grafting or flap coverage.[2] If they involve the head or neck, they may appear worse than they are because of the increased blood supply in these areas.[2]

A traumatic laceration is a tear in the skin that occurs from an injury. Most lacerations are located on the head or neck or an upper extremity. The most common mechanism of injury is the application of blunt force that crushes the skin against underlying bone, causing the skin to split.

A traumatic amputation is the severing of part of the body, a limb, or part of a limb.

When caring for a patient with a traumatic wound, the first priority is to assess the patient's circulation, airway, and breathing.[3] Once these are stabilized, you can address the traumatic wound. Initial management focuses on controlling bleeding, usually by applying firm, direct pressure and elevating the extremity. If bleeding continues, you may need to compress a pressure point. Assess the condition of the wound; puncture wounds may contain foreign bodies, such as fragments from the object that caused the wound or from clothing driven into the wound by the object.[1] Clean and manage the puncture wound according to the extent of the injury.

Equipment

Sterile basin ▪ normal saline solution ▪ 35-mL or 65-mL catheter-tip syringe with 19G needle or angiocatheter ▪ sterile 4″ × 4″ (10-cm × 10-cm) gauze pads ▪ gloves ▪ appropriate dressing materials ▪ fluid-impermeable pad ▪ sutures and suture kit or skin closure strips ▪ prescribed antibacterial or petroleum jelly ointment ▪ Optional: mask and goggles or mask with face shield, gown, sterile gloves, scissors, clippers, tetanus toxoid vaccine, anesthetic agent, prescribed pain medication, camera, tourniquet, supplemental oxygen, IV catheter insertion equipment, prescribed IV fluids, surgical scrub brush or sponge, sterile forceps, sterile scalpel and blade, tissue adhesive and staples, equipment for blood sample collection (needless blood collection tube holder, appropriate blood collection tubes, single-patient tourniquet), sterile roller gauze, sterile lactated Ringer solution, sterile towel, watertight bag or container and large plastic bag with ice.

Preparation of equipment

Place a fluid-impermeable pad under the area to be cleaned. Remove any clothing covering the wound. If necessary, clip hair around the wound with scissors *to promote cleaning and treatment.*

Gather needed equipment at the patient's bedside. Fill a sterile basin with normal saline solution. Make sure the treatment area has enough light *to allow close observation of the wound.* Depending on the nature and location of the wound, wear sterile or clean gloves *to avoid spreading infection.*

Implementation

- Gather the appropriate equipment.
- Perform hand hygiene.[4,5,6,7,8]
- Put on gloves and other personal protective equipment, such as a gown and a mask and goggles or mask with face shield, if spraying or splashing of body fluids is possible.[9,10,11]
- Confirm the patient's identity using at least two patient identifiers.[12]
- Check the patient's circulation, airway, and breathing. If necessary, begin cardiopulmonary resuscitation. (See the "Cardiopulmonary resuscitation" procedures.)[2]
- Explain the procedure to the patient *to allay his anxiety and enhance cooperation.*
- Remove the patient's clothing *to expose the wound* if necessary.
- Control bleeding by applying gentle pressure using a sterile gauze pad, elevating the injured area (if applicable) or, if necessary, applying compression to pressure points.[1,13,14]
- Obtain a history from the patient if able (or eye witnesses to the injury or family member) that includes the time and mechanism of injury; whether any contaminants were present; the type, size, or weight of the object, instrument, or machinery involved; whether the object was sharp or dull; the angle and speed of penetration; the environment in which the injury occurred; and tetanus immunization history. Ask about factors that may complicate wound healing, such as diabetes mellitus, peripheral vascular disease, chronic renal failure, human immunodeficiency virus infection, use of immunosuppressive medication or anticoagulants, and bleeding disorders. Inquire about allergies to medications or dressing materials.[1]
- Obtain the patient's vital signs and assess him for other injuries if appropriate.
- Perform a comprehensive pain assessment using techniques appropriate for the patient's age, condition, and ability to understand.[15]
- Administer pain medication, as needed and ordered, following safe medication administration practices.[15,16]
- Administer tetanus toxoid vaccine, as needed and ordered, following safe medication administration practices.[1,16,17]

For a traumatic puncture wound

- If the wound is minor, allow it to bleed for a few minutes before cleaning it *to help remove possible contaminates from the wound.*
- Inspect the wound and estimate its depth, the degree of contamination, and whether internal tissues were injured.[13]
- If a penetrating object remains in the wound, support the object until removal is possible. If the foreign body is in a joint or highly mobile area, splint the joint or area *to prevent further damage.*[14]
- Assist the practitioner as he inspects the wound and assesses the injured area and area distal to the injury for sensation, muscle movement, and adequate circulation *to determine whether significant nerve or vessel damage has occurred.*[1]
- If the wound is deep, assist the practitioner as he administers a local or regional anesthetic as needed *to further inspect the wound.*
- Irrigate the wound with sterile normal saline solution or tap water *to reduce the number of contaminants in the wound.*[13]
- Arrange for an X-ray, ultrasonography, or computed tomography scan, as ordered, *to locate or assess for a retained foreign body.*[1,13,14]
- Obtain consent and photograph the wound if indicated.[17]
- Clip local hair, as needed, *to prevent wound contamination*; don't clip eyebrows *because regrowth is unpredictable.*[17]
- Remove and discard your gloves,[9,10,11] perform hand hygiene,[4,5,6,7,8] and put on new gloves.[9,10,11]
- Assist the practitioner with foreign-body removal, if indicated, and wound closure using sutures or skin-closure strips.[14]
- Apply the prescribed antibacterial ointment *to help prevent infection.*
- Apply a dry, sterile dressing over the wound *to absorb drainage and help prevent bacterial contamination.*

For a traumatic abrasion

- Irrigate the wound with normal saline solution or tap water (as directed) using a 35-mL or 65-mL catheter-tip syringe with a 19G needle or angiocatheter to deliver an irrigation stream at 5 to 8 psi *to remove wound debris and bacteria.* Alternatively, if the patient is able, have him shower and clean the wound with a surgical scrub brush or sponge containing chlorhexidine (or other prescribed antiseptic solution), or if the wound is small, use a shower attachment at a faucet to clean the wound with tap water.[18]
- Obtain consent and then photograph the wound if indicated.[19]
- Assess the wound, measure the wound size, and remove any remaining debris using a surgical scrub brush or sponge containing chlorhexidine (or other prescribed antiseptic solution) if needed.[18]

Caring for a severed body part

After traumatic amputation, a surgeon may be able to reimplant the severed body part through microsurgery. The chance of successful reimplantation is much greater if the amputated part has received proper care.

If a patient arrives at the health care facility with a severed body part, first make sure that bleeding at the amputation site has been controlled. Then follow these guidelines for preserving the body part.

- Perform hand hygiene and put on sterile gloves.[9,10,11] Place several sterile gauze pads and an appropriate amount of sterile roller gauze in a sterile basin, and pour sterile normal saline or sterile lactated Ringer solution over them. *Never* use any other solution, and don't try to scrub or debride the part.
- Holding the body part in one gloved hand, carefully pat it dry with sterile gauze. Place saline-moistened gauze pads over the stump; then wrap the whole body part with saline-moistened roller gauze. Wrap the gauze with a sterile towel, if available. Then put this package in a watertight bag or container and seal it.
- Fill another plastic bag with ice and water to make an ice-water slurry and place the part, still in its watertight container, inside. Seal the outer bag. (Always protect the part from direct contact with ice—and *never* use dry ice—*to prevent irreversible tissue damage, which would make the part unsuitable for reimplantation.*) Keep this bag ice-cold until the surgeon is ready to do the reimplantation surgery.
- Label the bag with the patient's name and identification number, identification of the amputated part, the health care facility's identification number, and the date and time when cooling began.

Note: The body part must be wrapped and cooled quickly. *Irreversible tissue damage occurs after only 6 hours at ambient temperature.* However, hypothermic management seldom preserves tissues for more than 24 hours.

- If debris remains in the wound, notify the patient's practitioner *because he may need to anesthetize the site before further cleaning.* Then remove all debris from the wound *to prevent tattooing, which occurs when debris is embedded in the dermal layer.*[18]
- Arrange for an X-ray, if ordered, *to rule out the presence of a foreign body, especially if gravel or other materials are present in the wound.*
- If surgical intervention is necessary to clean the wound, prepare the patient for transfer to the operating room.
- Apply antibacterial ointment if ordered.[18]
- Cover the wound with a sterile, occlusive, low-adherent dressing *because occlusive dressings promote wound healing.*[18,20,21]

For a traumatic laceration

- Irrigate the wound with normal saline solution or tap water (as directed) using a 35-mL or 65-mL catheter-tip syringe with a 19G needle or angiocatheter to deliver an irrigation stream at 5 to 8 psi *to remove wound debris and bacteria.*[1,17,18,22,23]
- Assess the wound *to determine the severity of the wound and whether it involves muscle, tendons, nerves, blood vessels, or bones.* Determine whether your clinical findings are consistent with the patient's history.[17]
- Arrange for an X-ray, if ordered, *to assess the extent of injury or for the presence of a foreign body.*
- Obtain consent and photograph the wound if indicated.[19]
- Clip local hair, as needed, *to prevent wound contamination;* don't clip eyebrows *because regrowth is unpredictable.*[17]
- Remove and discard your gloves,[9,10,11] perform hand hygiene,[4,5,6,7,8] and put on new gloves.[9,10,11]
- Assist the practitioner as he administers a local anesthetic (for a small wound) or a regional block (for a large extremity wound) and provides wound care; he'll remove any visible foreign matter with forceps and devitalized tissue with sharp debridement *to reduce the risk of infection.*
- If indicated, prepare the patient for immediate surgical intervention *to control bleeding and treat underlying injuries.*[17]
- Assist the practitioner with wound closure (if appropriate), using sutures, tissue adhesive, staples, or skin-closure strips.[1,17] If closure must be delayed assist, assist the practitioner with packing the wound.
- Apply antibacterial ointment or petroleum jelly ointment, if ordered, *to help prevent infection.* Don't apply a topical ointment if the wound was closed with a tissue adhesive *because topical ointments loosen the adhesive and may cause wound dehiscence.*[1,17]
- Apply a dry, sterile dressing over the wound if ordered; sutured or stapled wounds should be covered with a protective, low-adherent dressing for 24 to 48 hours until adequate epithelization takes place *to protect the wound from gross contamination.*[1]

For a traumatic amputation

- Control bleeding by applying direct pressure to the wound, by elevating the injured area or, if necessary, by applying compression to pressure points. If bleeding continues, apply a tourniquet.[24]

NURSING ALERT *Keep in mind that prolonged tourniquet use can cause ischemia; assess the continued need for tourniquet use and remove it as soon as possible, preferably within 2 hours of application.*[24]

- Attach the patient to a continuous cardiac monitor, pulse oximeter, and automated blood pressure device, as indicated.
- Obtain the patient's vital signs and assess him for signs of shock, such as hypotension, tachycardia, diminished pulses, altered level of consciousness, and pallor. Assess for other injuries.[19]
- Administer supplemental oxygen, as prescribed.[19]
- Insert an IV catheter, as ordered, if the patient doesn't already have one in place. (See the "IV catheter insertion and removal" procedure, page 446.) Administer IV fluids as prescribed.[24]
- Cover the wound with sterile gauze soaked in normal saline solution and then cover the gauze with an adhesive film dressing *to prevent evaporation.* Avoid repeated wound inspection and dressing changes *because they increase the risk of infection.*[24]
- Administer antibiotics, as ordered, *to prevent infection* following safe medication administration practices.[16,19,24]
- As ordered, obtain blood samples for coagulation studies; hemoglobin, hematocrit, and electrolyte levels; and typing and crossmatching *in case blood transfusion is needed.*
- If possible, preserve the severed body part, if possible. (See *Caring for a severed body part.*)

Completing the procedure

- Reassess the patient's pain and respond appropriately.[15]
- Discard used supplies in the appropriate receptacle.[9,10,11]
- Remove and discard your gloves and any other personal protective equipment worn.[9,10,11]
- Perform hand hygiene.[4,5,6,7,8]
- Document the procedure.[25,26,27]

Special considerations

- When irrigating a traumatic wound, avoid using more than 8 psi of pressure. A 35-mL or 65-mL syringe and a 19G needle or angiocatheter deliver an irrigation stream at 8 psi *to remove wound debris and bacteria.*[19,22] *High-pressure irrigation can seriously interfere with healing, kill cells, and allow bacteria to infiltrate the tissue.*

■ Avoid cleaning a traumatic wound with alcohol *because alcohol causes pain and tissue dehydration.* Also, avoid using antiseptics for wound cleaning *because they can impede healing.* In addition, never use a cotton ball or cotton-filled gauze pad to clean a wound *because cotton fibers left in the wound can cause contamination.*

■ After cleaning a wound, the practitioner may want to debride it *to remove dead tissue and reduce the risk of infection and scarring.* If this is necessary, pack the wound with gauze pads soaked in normal saline solution until debridement.

■ Observe for signs of infection, such as warm, red skin at the site or purulent discharge. *Be aware that infection of a traumatic wound can delay healing, increase scar formation, and trigger systemic infection such as septicemia.*

■ Observe all dressings. If you note edema, adjust the dressing *to avoid impairing circulation to the area.*

Patient teaching

Teach the patient how to clean the wound and change dressings if appropriate and to report signs of infection, such as reddened skin and purulent drainage. Tell the patient when he should return for suture or staple removal if indicated; the timing of suture or staple removal varies with wound location.

Complications

Cleaning and care of traumatic wounds may temporarily increase the patient's pain. Excessive, vigorous cleaning may further disrupt tissue integrity. Localized or systemic infection can result from a traumatic puncture wound.

Documentation

Document the date and time of the procedure, wound size and condition, medication administration, specific wound care measures, and patient teaching provided and the patient's understanding of your teaching. Document the location of the wound, the type of injury, evidence collected (if appropriate), and a brief description on a body diagram, as indicated.[19]

REFERENCES

1 Capellan, O., & Hollander, J. E. (2003). Management of lacerations in the emergency department. *Emergency Medical Clinics of North America, 21,* 205–231.

2 Castana, O., et al. (2009). Traumatic injuries with deep abrasion: "A burn." *Annals of Burns and Fire Disasters, 22,* 44–47.

3 American Heart Association. (2010). 2010 American Heart Association guidelines for cardiopulmonary resuscitation and emergency cardiovascular care. *Circulation, 122,* S685–S705. (Level II)

4 The Joint Commission. (2015). Standard NPSG.07.01.01. *Comprehensive accreditation manual for hospitals: The official handbook.* Oakbrook Terrace, IL: The Joint Commission. (Level VII)

5 Centers for Disease Control and Prevention. (2002). Guideline for hand hygiene in health-care settings: Recommendations of the Healthcare Infection Control Practices Advisory Committee and the HICPAC/SHEA/APIC/IDSA Hand Hygiene Task Force. *MMWR Recommendations and Reports, 51*(RR–16), 1–45. Accessed May 2015 via the Web at http://www.cdc.gov/mmwr/pdf/rr/rr5116.pdf (Level II)

6 World Health Organization. (2009). "WHO guidelines on hand hygiene in health care: First global patient safety challenge, clean care is safer care" [Online]. Accessed May 2015 via the Web at http://whqlibdoc.who.int/publications/2009/9789241597906_eng.pdf (Level IV)

7 American Osteopathic Association. (2014). Standard 07.01.21. *Healthcare Facilities Accreditation Program: Accreditation requirements for acute care hospitals.* Chicago, IL: American Osteopathic Association. (Level VII)

8 Centers for Medicare & Medicaid Services, Department of Health and Human Services. (2014). Condition of participation: Infection control. 42 C.F.R. § 482.42.

9 Siegel, J. D., et al. (2007). "2007 guideline for isolation precautions: Preventing transmission of infectious agents in healthcare settings" [Online]. Accessed May 2015 via the Web at http://www.cdc.gov/hicpac/pdf/isolation/Isolation2007.pdf (Level II)

10 Occupational Safety and Health Administration. (n.d.). "Bloodborne pathogens, standard number 1910.1030" [Online]. Accessed May 2015 via the Web at http://www.osha.gov/pls/oshaweb/owadisp.show_document?p_table=STANDARDS&p_id=10051 (Level VII)

11 American Osteopathic Association. (2014). Standard 07.01.10. *Healthcare Facilities Accreditation Program: Accreditation requirements for acute care hospitals.* Chicago, IL: American Osteopathic Association. (Level VII)

12 The Joint Commission. (2015). Standard NPSG.01.01.01. *Comprehensive accreditation manual for hospitals: The official handbook.* Oakbrook Terrace, IL: The Joint Commission. (Level VII)

13 Katz, M. J., & Kirr, C. A. (2013). "Wound care" [Online]. Accessed May 2015 via the Web at http://www.nursingceu.com/courses/395/index_nceu.html

14 Winland-Brown, J. E., & Allen, S. (2010). Diagnosis and management of foreign bodies in the skin. *Advances in Skin and Wound Care, 23,* 471–476.

15 The Joint Commission. (2015). Standard PC.01.02.07. *Comprehensive accreditation manual for hospitals: The official handbook.* Oakbrook Terrace, IL: The Joint Commission. (Level VII)

16 American Osteopathic Association. (2014). Standard 16.01.03. *Healthcare Facilities Accreditation Program: Accreditation requirements for acute care hospitals.* Chicago, IL: American Osteopathic Association. (Level VII)

17 Forsch, R. T. (2008). Essentials of skin laceration repair. *American Family Physician, 78,* 945–951.

18 Chardon, Z. (2011). Wound & skin care: Abrasions in healthy young adults. *Nursing, 41*(5), 68–69.

19 Emergency Nurses Association. (2013). *Sheehy's emergency nursing principles and practice* (7th ed.). St. Louis, MO: Mosby.

20 Fonder, M. A., et al. (2007). Occlusive wound dressings in emergency medicine and acute care. *Emergency Medical Clinics of North America, 25,* 235–242.

21 Beam, J. W. (2008). Occlusive dressings and the healing of standardized abrasions. *Journal of Athletic Training, 43,* 600–607.

22 Baranoski, B., & Ayello, E. A. (2012). *Wound care essentials: Practice principles* (3rd ed.). Philadelphia, PA: Lippincott Williams & Wilkins.

23 Fernandez, R. , et al. (2002). Water for wound cleansing. *Cochrane Database of Systematic Reviews, 2002*(4), CD003861. (Level I)

24 Perkins, Z. B., et al. (2012). Factors affecting outcome after traumatic limb amputation. *British Journal of Surgery, 99,* 75–86. Accessed May 2015 via the Web at http://onlinelibrary.wiley.com/doi/10.1002/bjs.7766/pdf (Level V)

25 The Joint Commission. (2015). Standard RC.01.03.01. *Comprehensive accreditation manual for hospitals: The official handbook.* Oakbrook Terrace, IL: The Joint Commission. (Level VII)

26 American Osteopathic Association. (2014). Standard 10.00.03. *Healthcare Facilities Accreditation Program: Accreditation requirements for acute care hospitals.* Chicago, IL: American Osteopathic Association. (Level VII)

27 Centers for Medicare & Medicaid Services, Department of Health and Human Services. (2014). Condition of participation: Medical record services. 42 C.F.R. § 482.24(b).

TUB BATHS AND SHOWERS

Tub baths and showers provide personal hygiene, stimulate circulation, and reduce tension for the patient. They also allow you to observe skin conditions and assess joint mobility and muscle strength. If not precluded by the patient's condition or safety considerations, privacy during bathing promotes the patient's sense of well-being by allowing him to assume responsibility for his own care.

Patients who are recovering from recent surgery, who are emotionally unstable, or who have casted extremities or dressings in place usually require the practitioner's permission for a tub bath or shower.

Equipment

One or two washcloths ■ bath towels ■ bath blanket ■ skin cleaner ■ nonskid bath mat if tub lacks nonskid strips ■ nonskid shower chair for shower ■ towel mat ■ OCCUPIED sign ■ clean clothing or hospital gown ■ hospital-grade disinfectant ■ Optional: chair, shower cap, plastic bag and tape, bath oil, shampoo.

Preparation of equipment

Prepare the bathing area before the patient arrives. Close any doors or windows and adjust the room temperature *to avoid chilling the patient.* Check that the bathtub or shower is clean. Then gather bathing articles and observe appropriate safety measures.

For a bath

Position a chair next to the tub *to help the patient get in and out of the tub and to provide a seat if he becomes weak.* Place a bath blanket over the chair *to cover the patient if he becomes chilled.* If the tub doesn't have nonskid strips, place a nonskid bath mat in the tub; then fill the tub halfway with warm water and test the temperature; it should feel comfortable to the touch. Adjust water flow and temperature just before the patient gets into the tub. Place a towel mat on the floor in front of the tub *to prevent slipping.*

For a shower

Place a nonskid chair or shower chair in the locked position in the shower *to provide support.* The chair also allows the patient to sit down while washing his legs and feet *to reduce the risk of falling.* If the shower doesn't have nonskid strips, place a nonskid bath mat on the shower floor. Remove electrical appliances, such as hair dryers and heaters, from the patient's reach *to prevent electrical accidents.* Adjust water flow and temperature just before the patient gets into the shower. Place a towel mat on the floor in front of the shower *to prevent slipping.*

Implementation

- Perform hand hygiene.[1,2,3,4,5]
- Confirm the patient's identity using at least two patient identifiers.[6]
- Explain the procedure to the patient.
- Escort the patient to the bathing area, and help him undress as necessary. Offer him a shower cap if he wants to keep his hair dry. Otherwise, provide shampoo. Place all items within easy reach of the patient *to prevent reaching.*[7]
- Help the patient into the tub or shower. Encourage him to use the handrails *to prevent falling.*
- Provide washcloths and skin cleaner. If the patient has dry skin, add bath oil to the water. Wait until after he gets into the tub before adding bath oil *because oil makes the tub slick and increases the risk of falling.*
- Taking care to respect his privacy, help the patient bathe, as needed; cover the patient with a towel and wash beneath it *to alleviate embarrassment.* Watch for indications of discomfort.[8,9]
- Allow family members to assist the patient with bathing, as desired, *to minimize fear.* Allow the patient to schedule bathing according to his energy level and other preferences.[8]
- If you can safely leave the patient alone, place the call light within his reach and show him how to use it. If the patient is confused, don't leave him alone.
- Tell the patient to leave the door unlocked *for his own safety,* but assure him that you'll post an OCCUPIED sign on the door. Stay nearby in case of emergency, and check on the patient every 5 to 10 minutes.[9]
- When the patient finishes bathing, drain the tub or turn off the shower.
- *To prevent slipping,* dry the patient's feet before he steps out of the tub if bath oil was used.
- Assist the patient onto the bath mat *to prevent him from falling.* Then help him to dry off and put on a clean gown or other clothing, as appropriate.
- Escort the patient to his room or to his bed.
- Dry the floor of the bathing area well *to prevent slipping.*
- Ensure that the tub or shower and shower chair, if used, are cleaned and disinfected.[10,11]
- Dispose of soiled towels and return the patient's personal belongings to his bedside.
- Perform hand hygiene.[1,2,3,4,5]
- Document the procedure and the patient's tolerance and skin condition.[12,13,14]

Special considerations

- If you're giving a tub bath to a patient with a cast or dressing on an arm or leg, wrap the extremity in a clear plastic bag. Secure the bag with tape, being careful not to constrict circulation. Instruct the patient to dangle the arm or leg over the edge of the tub and keep it above the water.
- Encourage the patient to use safety devices, bars, and rails when bathing.
- *Because bathing in warm water causes vasodilation,* the patient may feel faint. If so, open the drain or turn off the shower. Cover the patient's shoulders and back with a bath towel. If the patient was taking a shower, assist him to a chair *to prevent injury from falling.* If the patient is able, have him cross his legs, and tighten his thigh, abdominal, and buttock muscles. *This technique increases venous return, cardiac filling pressure, and cardiac output, which increases cerebral perfusion, preventing a vasovagal reaction and fainting.*[15,16,17]

Documentation

Describe the patient's skin condition and record any discoloration or redness in your notes. Document the patient's tolerance of the procedure.

REFERENCES

1 The Joint Commission. (2015). Standard NPSG.07.01.01. *Comprehensive accreditation manual for hospitals: The official handbook.* Oakbrook Terrace, IL: The Joint Commission. (Level VII)

2 Centers for Disease Control and Prevention. (2002). Guideline for hand hygiene in health-care settings: Recommendations of the Healthcare Infection Control Practices Advisory Committee and the HICPAC/SHEA/APIC/IDSA Hand Hygiene Task Force. *MMWR Recommendations and Reports, 51*(RR-16), 1–45. Accessed May 2015 via the Web at http://www.cdc.gov/mmwr/pdf/rr/rr5116.pdf (Level II)

3 World Health Organization. (2009). "WHO guidelines on hand hygiene in health care: First global patient safety challenge, clean care is safer care" [Online]. Accessed May 2015 via the Web at http://whqlibdoc.who.int/publications/2009/9789241597906_eng.pdf (Level IV)

4 Centers for Medicare & Medicaid Services, Department of Health and Human Services. (2014). Condition of participation: Infection control. 42 C.F.R. § 482.42.

5 American Osteopathic Association. (2014). Standard 07.01.21. *Healthcare Facilities Accreditation Program: Accreditation requirements for acute care hospitals.* Chicago, IL: American Osteopathic Association. (Level VII)

6 The Joint Commission. (2015). Standard NPSG.01.01.01. *Comprehensive accreditation manual for hospitals: The official handbook.* Oakbrook Terrace, IL: The Joint Commission. (Level VII)

7 Taylor, C. R., et al. (2015). *Fundamentals of nursing: The art and science of nursing care* (8th ed.). Philadelphia, PA: Lippincott Williams & Wilkins.

8 Radar, J., et al. (2006). The bathing of older adults with dementia. *American Journal of Nursing, 106*(4), 40–48.

9 American Osteopathic Association. (2014). Standard 15.01.16. *Healthcare Facilities Accreditation Program: Accreditation requirements for acute care hospitals.* Chicago, IL: American Osteopathic Association. (Level VII)

10 Rutala, W. A., et al. (2008). "Guideline for disinfection and sterilization in healthcare facilities, 2008" [Online]. Accessed May 2015 via the Web at http://www.cdc.gov/hicpac/pdf/guidelines/Disinfection_Nov_2008.pdf (Level I)
11 American Osteopathic Association. (2012). Standard 07.02.03. *Healthcare Facilities Accreditation Program: Accreditation standards for acute care hospitals.* Chicago, IL: American Osteopathic Association. (Level VII)
12 The Joint Commission. (2015). Standard RC.01.03.01. *Comprehensive accreditation manual for hospitals: The official handbook.* Oakbrook Terrace, IL: The Joint Commission. (Level VII)
13 American Osteopathic Association. (2014). Standard 10.00.03. *Healthcare Facilities Accreditation Program: Accreditation requirements for acute care hospitals.* Chicago, IL: American Osteopathic Association (Level VII)
14 Centers for Medicare & Medicaid Services, Department of Health and Human Services. (2014). Condition of participation: Medical record services. 42 C.F.R. § 482.24(b).
15 France, C. R., et al. (2006). Blood pressure and cerebral oxygenation responses to skeletal muscle tension: A comparison of two physical maneuvers to prevent vasovagal reactions. *Clinical Physiology and Functional Imaging, 26,* 21–25.
16 Ditto, B., et al. (2003). On-site training in applied muscle tension to reduce vasovagal reactions to blood donation. *Journal of Behavioral Medicine, 26,* 53–65.
17 Marchiondo, K. J. (2010). Emergency: Recognizing and treating vasovagal syncope. *American Journal of Nursing, 110*(4), 50–53.

TUBE FEEDINGS

Gastric enteral tube feeding involves delivery of a liquid feeding formula directly to the stomach (known as *gastric gavage*). It's typically indicated for patients who can't eat normally because of dysphagia or oral or esophageal obstruction or injury. Gastric feedings also may be given to unconscious or intubated patients or to those recovering from GI tract surgery who can't ingest food orally.

Duodenal or jejunal enteral tube feeding involves delivery of a liquid feeding formula directly to the small intestine, specifically the duodenum or jejunum. Nasoduodenal or nasojejunal enteral tube feeding is indicated when the esophagus and stomach need to be bypassed or when the patient is at risk for aspiration. Jejunostomy tubes are preferred for long-term (longer than 4 weeks) administration of medications or food. Duodenal or jejunal feedings decrease the risk of aspiration because the formula bypasses the pylorus. However, jejunal feedings result in reduced pancreatic stimulation; as a result, the patient may require an elemental diet.

Enteral feedings should be started postoperatively in surgical patients without waiting for flatus or a bowel movement; current literature indicates in 24 to 48 hours.[1]

Patients usually receive gastric feedings on an intermittent schedule. However, for duodenal or jejunal feedings, most patients seem to better tolerate a continuous slow drip.

Liquid nutrient solutions come in various formulas for administration through a nasogastric tube, small-bore feeding tube, gastrostomy or jejunostomy tube, percutaneous endoscopic gastrostomy tube, or gastrostomy feeding button. Tube feeding is contraindicated in patients who have no bowel sounds or a suspected bowel obstruction, upper GI bleeding, or intractable vomiting or diarrhea.

Equipment

Feeding formula ▪ gloves ▪ alcohol pad ▪ graduated container ▪ water ▪ gavage bag with tubing and flow regulator clamp ▪ towel or fluid-impermeable pad ▪ 60-mL bulb or catheter-tipped syringe ▪ oral care supplies ▪ WARNING! FOR ENTERAL USE ONLY—NOT FOR IV USE labels ▪ Optional: IV pole, sterile water, enteral feeding pump, tubing set (for continuous administration), adapter to connect gavage tubing to feeding tubing, carbon dioxide detector designed for gastric tube placement, pH test strips, petroleum jelly, cotton-tipped applicators, prescribed promotility agent, 1″ (2.5-cm) hypoallergenic adhesive tape.

A bulb syringe or large catheter-tip syringe may be substituted for a gavage bag after the patient demonstrates tolerance for a gravity-drip infusion. The practitioner may order an infusion pump *to ensure accurate delivery of the prescribed formula.* An enteral infusion pump is generally required for small-bowel feedings[1] *to ensure accurate delivery of the prescribed formula.*

Preparation of equipment

Refrigerate formulas prepared in the dietary department or pharmacy. Refrigerate commercial formulas only after opening them. Check the formula against the practitioner's orders. Check the date on all formula container labels, discarding expired commercial formula. Use powdered formula within 24 hours of mixing.[1] Always shake the container *well to mix the solution thoroughly.*

Make sure the formula is labeled clearly with patient identification information, the type of formula, the method of administration, the date and time of preparation, and the name of the person preparing the formula if appropriate. Compare the formula label with the practitioner's order.[1]

Allow the formula to warm to room temperature before administration. *Cold formula can increase the chance of diarrhea.* Never warm it over direct heat or in a microwave *because heat may curdle the formula or change its chemical composition. Also, hot formula may injure the patient.*

Perform hand hygiene.[1,2,3,4,5,6] Open the enteral administration set and hang the gavage container on the IV pole as indicated. If available, use an administration set with a recessed spike *because an administration set with a recessed spike is less likely to become contaminated than a set with an open spike.*[1]

NURSING ALERT *Make sure the gavage container and administration set are clearly labeled with WARNING! FOR ENTERAL USE ONLY—NOT FOR IV USE.*[1]

Pour 60 mL of water into the graduated container. After closing the flow clamp on the administration set, pour the appropriate amount of formula into the gavage bag. Hang no more than a 4-hour supply at one time *to prevent bacterial growth.*[1]

If using a sterile, decanted tube-feeding formula, attach the administration set directly to the container. Sterile, decanted formula should have a hang time of 8 hours.[1]

Open the flow clamp on the administration set *to remove air from the lines. Doing so keeps air from entering the patient's stomach and causing distention and discomfort.*

Implementation

- Review the patient's medical record *to determine the appropriateness of the prescribed enteral therapy;* also check for allergies and contraindications and X-ray confirmation of tube placement.[1]
- Verify the practitioner's order, which should contain patient identifiers, the type of formula, delivery device, administration method, and rate.[1]
- Gather and prepare the necessary equipment and the enteral feeding formula.
- Perform hand hygiene.[1,2,3,4,5,6]
- Put on gloves.[7,8]
- Provide privacy.[9,10]
- Confirm the patient's identity using at least two patient identifiers.[11]
- Inform the patient that he'll receive nourishment through the tube, and explain the procedure to him. If possible, give him a schedule of subsequent feedings.
- Cover his chest with a towel or fluid-impermeable pad *to protect him and the bed linens from spills.*

■ Assess the patient's abdomen for distention, *which may indicate tube feeding intolerance.*[1]
■ Have the patient sit, or maintain the head of the bed at an elevation of at least 30 degrees (45 degrees is preferred) unless contraindicated by the patient's condition[1,12] *to prevent esophageal reflux and pulmonary aspiration of the feeding formula.* If the patient can't tolerate an elevation of this type, use a reverse Trendelenburg position unless contraindicated.[1]

For gastric feeding

■ Assess for enteral tube placement before administering the tube feeding and at 4-hour intervals.[1,12,13,14] If you suspect that the tube has migrated, don't administer the feeding; instead, notify the practitioner and prepare to obtain X-rays. To determine tube location, review routine chest and abdominal X-rays,[13,14] observe for a change in the external length of the tube by determining whether the mark placed at the tube's exit site has moved,[13,14] or observe changes in volume and appearance of feeding tube aspirates.[13,14]
■ Remove the cap or plug from the feeding tube and use a 60-mL bulb or catheter-tipped syringe to inject 5 to 10 mL of air through the tube *to clear it.* Then aspirate gastric contents (as shown below) *to be sure the tube is in the stomach.*

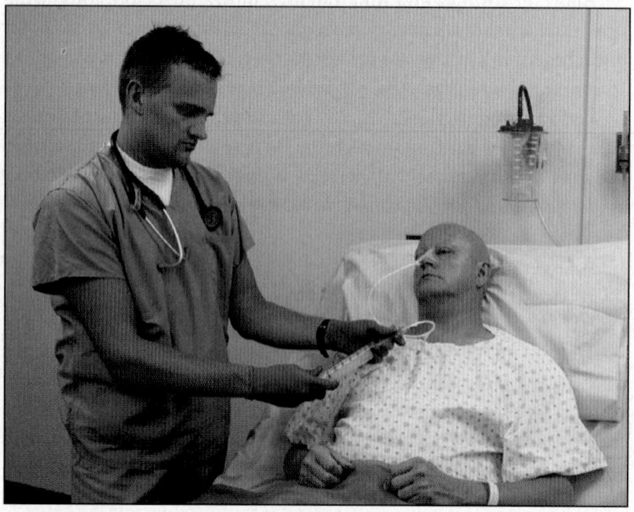

■ Measure the pH of aspirate from the tube if pH strips are available and pH measurement is performed in your facility. Fasting gastric pH is usually 5 or less, even in patients receiving gastric acid inhibitors; however, this method isn't reliable enough to exclude the need for X-ray placement verification *because gastric pH occasionally has a high pH.*[13,14]
■ Inspect the visual characteristics of the tube aspirate; fasting gastric secretions commonly appear grassy-green or clear and colorless.[13]
■ Use capnography, if available, *to detect carbon dioxide,* which indicates inadvertent tracheal insertion.[13]
■ *To assess gastric emptying,* aspirate and measure gastric residual volume (GRV). Reinstill any aspirate obtained. Hold feedings if the GRV is greater than 500 mL.[1]
■ Remove and discard your gloves.[7,8]
■ Perform hand hygiene.[1,2,3,4,5,6]
■ Put on new gloves.[7,8]
■ Thoroughly disinfect the tube hub with an alcohol pad and then allow it to dry *to prevent enteral device contamination.*[1]
■ Flush the feeding tube with 30 mL of water; use sterile water in immunocompromised or critically ill patients, especially when the safety of tap water can't be reasonably assumed.[1]
■ Connect the gavage bag tubing to the feeding tube (as shown on top right).

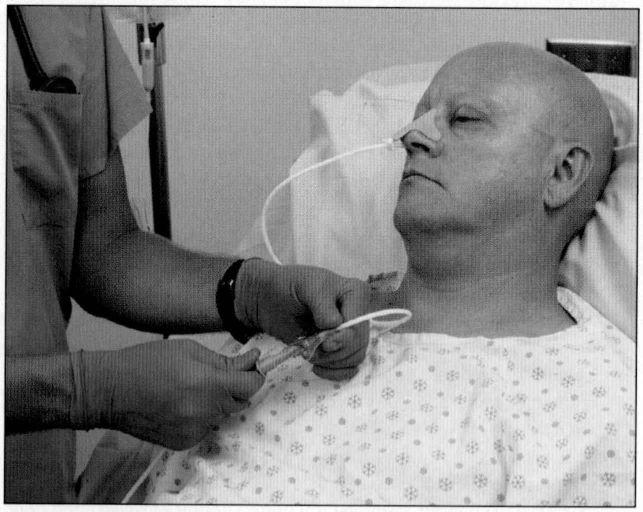

■ Trace the tubing from the patient to its point of origin *to make sure you've connected it to the proper port before beginning the tube feeding.*[15] Tape the connection *to prevent accidental disconnection of the tubing.* Route the tubing toward the patient's feet and place the enteral feeding pump toward the foot of the bed *because a standardized approach of keeping IV lines routed toward the head and enteric lines routed toward the feet prevents dangerous misconnections.* If different access sites are used, label each tubing at both the distal (near the patient connection) and proximal (near the source container) ends *to distinguish the different tubings and prevent misconnections.*[16]
■ Open the regulator clamp on the tubing, and adjust the flow rate appropriately.
■ If you're using an enteral feeding pump, thread the tube from the formula container or gavage bag through the pump according to the manufacturer's instructions. Purge the tubing of air and then attach it to the feeding tube.
■ Open the regulator clamp on the tubing, and adjust the flow rate appropriately. Make sure that the enteral feeding pump alarm limits are set according to the patient's current condition and that the alarms are turned on, functioning properly, and audible to staff.[15,18,19]
■ If you're using a bulb or catheter-tip syringe, remove the bulb or plunger (as shown below) and attach the syringe to the pinched-off feeding tube *to prevent excess air from entering the patient's stomach, causing distention.*

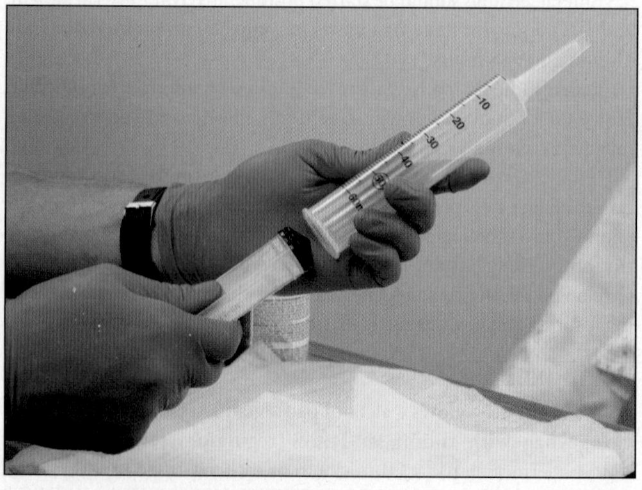

■ When you're using a bulb syringe, fill the syringe with formula and release the feeding tube *to allow formula to flow through it.* The height at which you hold the syringe will determine the flow rate. When the syringe is three-quarters empty, pour more formula into it (as shown below).

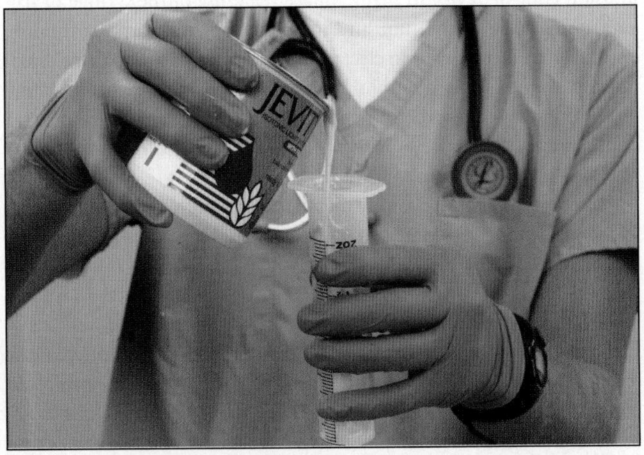

■ *To prevent air from entering the tube and the patient's stomach,* never allow the syringe to empty completely. If you're using an infusion controller, set the flow rate according to the manufacturer's instructions. Always administer a tube feeding slowly—typically 200 to 350 mL over 30 to 45 minutes, depending on the patient's tolerance and the practitioner's order—*to prevent sudden stomach distention, which can cause nausea, vomiting, cramps, and diarrhea.*
■ After administering the appropriate amount of formula, add 30 mL of water to the gavage bag or bulb syringe (as shown below) or manually flush the feeding tube using a barrel syringe.[1] *Flushing maintains the tube's patency by removing excess formula, which could occlude the tube.*

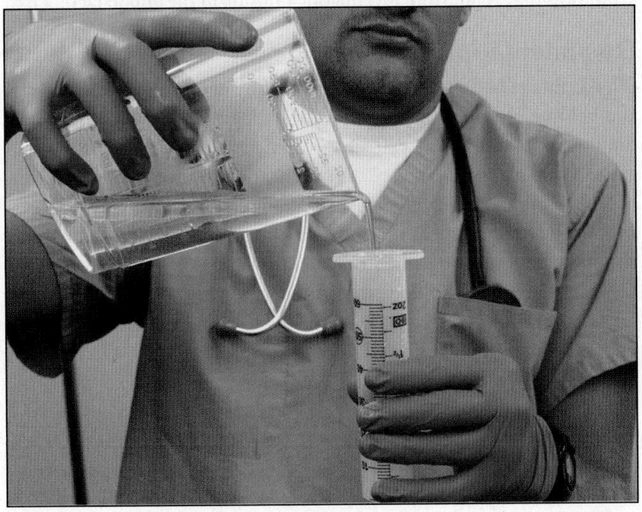

■ If you're administering a continuous feeding, flush the feeding tube with 30 mL of water every 4 hours.[1] Flush the feeding tube with 30 mL of water before and after medication administration *to help prevent tube occlusion.*
■ Measure the GRV every 4 hours for the first 48 hours. After the enteral feeding goal rate is achieved and a small-bore feeding tube is inserted, measure the GRV every 6 to 8 hours if the patient isn't critically ill; continue monitoring every 4 hours in a critically ill patient.[1]
■ Assess for GI intolerance to tube feedings at 4-hour intervals by noting abdominal distention, assessing abdominal pain, and observing for passage of flatus and stool.[1,12]
■ *To discontinue gastric feeding (depending on the equipment you're using),* close the regulator clamp on the gavage bag tubing, disconnect the syringe from the feeding tube, or turn off the enteral feeding pump.
■ Cover the end of the feeding tube with its plug or cap *to prevent leakage and contamination of the tube.*
■ Perform oral care routinely *to decrease oral bacterial colonization and the risk of aspiration pneumonia.*[7]
■ Make sure that all equipment and products are labeled with the date and time they were first used or opened.[1]

For duodenal or jejunal feeding

■ Assess for feeding tube placement before administering the feeding and at 4-hour intervals.[1,12,13,14] To do so, look for a change in the external length of the tube by determining whether the mark placed at the tube's exit site has moved, review routine chest and abdominal X-rays,[13,14] or observe changes in volume and appearance of feeding tube aspirates.[13,14]
■ Observe for changes in volume of aspirate from the feeding tube. *A large increase in volume may signal the upward dislocation of a small-bowel feeding tube into the stomach.*[12]
NURSING ALERT *Don't rely on the ausculatory method to differentiate between gastric and small-bowel placement.*[1]
■ Remove and discard your gloves.[7,8]
■ Perform hand hygiene.[2,3,4,5,6]
■ Put on new gloves.[7,8]
■ Thoroughly disinfect the tube hub with an alcohol pad and then allow it to dry *to prevent contamination.*[1]
■ Flush the enteral feeding tube with 30 mL of water; use sterile water for immunocompromised or critically ill patients.[1]
■ Connect the administration set to the feeding tube. Trace the tube from the patient to its point of origin *to make sure it's connected to the proper port before beginning the tube feeding.*[15] Tape the connection *to prevent accidental disconnection of the tubing.* Route the tubing toward the patient's feet and place the enteral feeding pump toward the foot of the bed *because a standardized approach of keeping IV lines routed toward the head and enteric lines routed toward the feet prevents dangerous misconnections.* If different access sites are used, label each tubing at both the distal (near the patient connection) and proximal (near the source container) ends *to distinguish the different tubing and prevent misconnections.*[16]
■ Open the flow clamp, and regulate the flow to the desired rate. *To regulate the rate using an enteral infusion pump,* follow the manufacturer's instructions for setting up the equipment. Most patients receive small amounts initially, with volumes increasing gradually after tolerance is established.
■ If using an enteral feeding pump, make sure that the enteral feeding pump alarm limits are set according to the patient's current condition and that the alarms are turned on, functioning properly, and audible to staff.[17,18,19]
■ Flush the tube every 4 hours with 30 mL of water (sterile water if the patient is critically ill or immunocompromised) *to maintain patency and provide hydration.*[1] Note that a needle catheter jejunostomy tube may require flushing every 2 hours *to prevent formula buildup inside the tube.* A Y-connector may also be useful for frequent flushing; attach the continuous feeding to the main port and use the side port for flushes.
■ Assess for GI intolerance to tube feedings at 4-hour intervals by noting abdominal distention, assessing abdominal pain, observing for passage of flatus and stool, and monitoring gastric residual volume as ordered.[1,12]
■ Perform oral care routinely *to decrease oral bacterial colonization and aspiration pneumonia risk.*[20]

Completing the procedure

■ Discard used equipment in appropriate receptacles.
■ Remove and discard your gloves.[7,8]
■ Perform hand hygiene.[2,3,4,5,6]
■ Document the procedure.[21,22,23]

Special considerations

- If the feeding solution doesn't initially flow through a bulb syringe, attach the bulb and squeeze it gently to start the flow. Then remove the bulb. Never use the bulb to force the formula through the tube.
- The Joint Commission issued a sentinel event alert concerning medical device alarm safety *because alarm-related events have been associated with permanent loss of function and death.* Among the major contributing factors were improper alarm settings, alarms inappropriately turned off, and alarm signals not audible to staff. Make sure that alarm limits are appropriately set and that alarms are turned on, functioning properly, and audible to staff. Follow facility guidelines for preventing alarm fatigue.[24]
- If the patient becomes nauseated or vomits, stop the feeding immediately and notify the practitioner. *The patient may vomit if his stomach becomes distended from overfeeding or delayed gastric emptying.*
- If you're using an open administration system, change the administration set at least every 24 hours. If you're using a closed system, change the system according to the manufacturer's instructions or at an interval determined by your facility.[1] Closed systems may hang for 24 to 48 hours; follow the manufacturer's guidelines.[1]
- Use petroleum jelly on dry, cracked lips. Keep in mind that dry mucous membranes may indicate dehydration, which requires increased fluid intake. Clean the patient's nostrils with cotton-tipped applicators, apply petroleum jelly along the mucosa, and assess the skin for signs of breakdown.
- During continuous feedings, assess the patient frequently for abdominal distention.[1]
- If the GRV is greater than 250 mL after a second gastric residual check, the patient may need a promotility agent. If the patient has a GRV greater than 500 mL, the feeding should be held and the patient's tolerance reassessed using an established algorithm, including performing a physical and GI assessment, evaluating glycemic control, minimizing sedation, and considering the use of a promotility agent.[1]
- Except for enteric-coated drugs and sustained-release medications, you can administer certain drugs through the feeding tube by crushing tablets or opening and diluting capsules in sterile water. Make sure to flush the tubing afterward *to ensure full instillation of the medication,* and keep in mind that some drugs can change the osmolarity of the feeding formula and cause diarrhea.
- Small-bore feeding tubes may kink, making instillation impossible. If you suspect this problem, try changing the patient's position, or withdraw the tube a few inches and restart the feeding. Never use a guide wire to reposition the tube.
- Constantly monitor the flow rate of a blended or high-residue formula *to determine if the formula is clogging the tubing as it settles. To prevent such clogging,* squeeze the bag frequently *to agitate the solution.*
- Collect laboratory specimens as ordered by the practitioner. *Glycosuria, hyperglycemia, and diuresis can indicate an excessive carbohydrate level, leading to hyperosmotic dehydration, which may be fatal.* Monitor urine and blood glucose levels *to assess glucose tolerance.* (A patient with a serum glucose level of less than 200 mg/dL and without glycosuria is considered stable.) Also monitor serum levels of electrolytes, blood urea nitrogen, and glucose as well as serum osmolality and other pertinent findings *to determine the patient's response to therapy and to assess his hydration status.*[1]
- If the tube feeding equipment isn't color-coded, label the tubing and connectors so staff members can easily identify that they are for enteral use only, not for IV use.[1,15]
- Until the patient acquires a tolerance for the formula, you may need to dilute it to half or three-quarters strength to start, and then increase it gradually, as ordered by the practitioner.
- Patients under stress or who are receiving steroids may experience a pseudodiabetic state. Assess such patients frequently *to determine the need for insulin.*

Patient teaching

Patient education for home tube feeding includes instructions on an infusion control device to maintain accuracy, use of the syringe or bag and tubing, care of the tube and insertion site, and formula mixing. Formula may be mixed in an electric blender according to package directions. Formula not used within 24 hours must be discarded. If the formula must hang for more than 4 hours, advise the patient to use a gavage or pump administration set with an ice pouch *to decrease the incidence of bacterial growth.* Tell him to use a new bag daily.

Teach the patient and family members signs and symptoms to report to the practitioner or home care nurse as well as measures to take in an emergency.

Complications

Erosion of esophageal, tracheal, nasal, and oropharyngeal mucosa can result if tubes are left in place for a long time. (See *Managing enteral tube feeding problems.*)

Using the gastric route, frequent or large-volume feedings can cause bloating and retention. Dehydration, diarrhea, and vomiting can cause metabolic disturbances. Glycosuria, cramping, and abdominal distention usually indicate intolerance.

Clogging of the feeding tube is common when using the duodenal or jejunal route. The patient may experience metabolic, fluid, and electrolyte abnormalities, including hyperglycemia, glycosuria, hyperosmolar dehydration, coma, edema, hypernatremia, and essential fatty acid deficiency.

The patient may also experience dumping syndrome, in which a large amount of hyperosmotic solution in the duodenum causes excessive diffusion of fluid through the semipermeable membrane and results in diarrhea. In a patient with low serum albumin levels, these signs and symptoms may result from low oncotic pressure in the duodenal mucosa.

Documentation

On the intake and output record, record the date, volume of formula, and volume of water. In your notes, document abdominal assessment findings (including tube exit site, if appropriate), amount of residual gastric contents, tube patency, and verification of tube placement. Also note the amount, type, and time of feeding. Discuss the patient's tolerance of the feeding, including whether the patient experienced nausea, vomiting, cramping, diarrhea, or distention.

Note the result of blood and urine tests, hydration status, and any drugs given through the tube. Include the date and time of administration set changes, oral and nasal hygiene performed, and results of specimen collections.

REFERENCES

1 Bankhead, R., et al. (2009). A.S.P.E.N. enteral nutrition practice recommendations. *Journal of Parenteral and Enteral Nutrition, 33,* 122–167. Accessed May 2015 via the Web at http://www.ismp.org/tools/articles/ASPEN.pdf (Level IV)

2 Centers for Disease Control and Prevention. (2002). Guideline for hand hygiene in health-care settings: Recommendations of the Healthcare Infection Control Practices Advisory Committee and the HICPAC/SHEA/APIC/IDSA Hand Hygiene Task Force. *MMWR Recommendations and Reports, 51*(RR-16), 1–45. Accessed January 2015 via the Web at http://www.cdc.gov/mmwr/pdf/rr/rr5116.pdf (Level II)

3 The Joint Commission. (2015). Standard NPSG.07.01.01. *Comprehensive accreditation manual for hospitals: The official handbook.* Oakbrook Terrace, IL: The Joint Commission. (Level VII)

4 World Health Organization. (2009). "WHO guidelines on hand hygiene in health care: First global patient safety challenge, clean care is safer care" [Online]. Accessed May 2015 via the Web at http://whqlibdoc.who.int/publications/2009/9789241597906_eng.pdf (Level IV)

TROUBLESHOOTING

Managing enteral tube feeding problems

COMPLICATIONS	NURSING INTERVENTIONS
Aspiration of gastric secretions	■ Elevated the head of the bed a minimum of 30 degrees, preferably 45 degrees.[1,12,13] ■ Avoid bolus tube feedings if the patient is at high risk for aspiration.[12] ■ Discontinue feeding immediately. ■ Perform tracheal suction of aspirated contents if possible. ■ Notify the practitioner if aspiration occurs. *He may order prophylactic antibiotics and chest physiotherapy.* ■ Check tube placement before feeding *to prevent complications.*[1,12,13]
Tube obstruction	■ Flush the tube with warm water. ■ Flush the tube with 30 ml of water after each feeding *to remove excess sticky formula, which could occlude the tube.*[1] ■ After ensuring proper tube placement, administer a pancreatic enzyme, as prescribed, *to unclog the tube. Ensuring proper tube placement is vital because instillation of pancreatic enzymes into the respiratory tract can lead to severe respiratory complications.* Don't use juice, coffee, soda, or meat tenderizer to unclog a tube *because the effectiveness of these substances is unproven and they may also be contraindicated by the patient's condition.*[25] ■ If necessary, replace the tube.
Oral, nasal, pharyngeal, or gastrostomy site irritation or necrosis	■ Provide frequent oral care. ■ Use petroleum jelly on cracked lips. ■ Change the tube's position. If necessary, replace the tube. ■ Provide proper skin care at the tube insertion site and use tube-anchoring devices.
Vomiting, bloating, diarrhea, or cramps	■ Reduce the flow rate. ■ Administer metoclopramide, as ordered, *to increase GI motility.* ■ Warm the formula *to prevent GI distress.* ■ Follow standard precautions when preparing and handling enteral feeding systems and accessing enteral access devices *to prevent system contamination, which increases the risk of* Clostridium difficile *infection.*[1] ■ Notify the practitioner *because he may want to reduce the amount of formula being given during each feeding, change the formula to one that's less osmotic or contains more fiber, or rule out other causes of signs and symptoms.*
Constipation	■ Provide additional fluids if the patient can tolerate them. ■ Administer a bulk-forming laxative as ordered. ■ Increase the fruit, vegetable, or sugar content of the feeding.
Electrolyte imbalance	■ Monitor electrolyte levels. ■ Notify the practitioner of elevated electrolyte levels *because he may want to adjust the formula content to correct the deficiency.*
Hyperglycemia	■ Monitor blood glucose levels. ■ Notify the practitioner of elevated levels *because he may adjust the sugar content of the formula.* ■ Administer insulin if ordered.

5 American Osteopathic Association. (2014). Standard 07.01.21. *Healthcare Facilities Accreditation Program: Accreditation requirements for acute care hospitals.* Chicago, IL: American Osteopathic Association. (Level VII)

6 Centers for Medicare & Medicaid Services, Department of Health and Human Services. (2014). Condition of participation: Infection control. 42 C.F.R. § 482.42.

7 Siegel, J. D., et al. (2007). "2007 guideline for isolation precautions: Preventing transmission of infectious agents in healthcare settings" [Online]. Accessed May 2015 via the Web at http://www.cdc.gov/hicpac/pdf/isolation/Isolation2007.pdf (Level II)

8 American Osteopathic Association. (2014). Standard 07.01.10. *Healthcare Facilities Accreditation Program: Accreditation requirements for acute care hospitals.* Chicago, IL: American Osteopathic Association. (Level VII)

9 Centers for Medicare & Medicaid Services, Department of Health and Human Services. (2014). Condition of participation: Patient's rights. 42 C.F.R. § 482.13(c)(1).

10 American Osteopathic Association. (2014). Standard 15.01.16. *Healthcare Facilities Accreditation Program: Accreditation requirements for acute care hospitals.* Chicago, IL: American Osteopathic Association. (Level VII)

11 The Joint Commission. (2015). Standard NPSG.01.01.01. *Comprehensive accreditation manual for hospitals: The official handbook.* Oakbrook Terrace, IL: The Joint Commission. (Level VII)

12 American Association of Critical-Care Nurses. (2011). "AACN practice alert: Prevention of aspiration" [Online]. Accessed May 2015 via the Web at http://www.aacn.org/WD/practice/docs/practicealerts/aacn-aspiration-practice-alert.pdf (Level VII)

Comparing skin types

Skin type	Sunburn and tanning history
I	Always burns; never tans; sensitive ("Celtic" skin)
II	Burns easily; tans minimally
III	Burns moderately; tans gradually to light brown (average Caucasian skin)
IV	Burns minimally; always tans well to moderately brown (olive skin)
V	Rarely burns; tans profusely to dark (brown skin)
VI	Never burns; deeply pigmented; not sensitive (black skin)

13 American Association of Critical-Care Nurses. (2009). "AACN practice alert: Verification of feeding tube placement (blindly inserted)" [Online]. Accessed May 2015 via the Web at http://www.aacn.org/WD/Practice/Docs/PracticeAlerts/Verification_of_Feeding_Tube_Placement_05-2005.pdf (Level VII)

14 Simons, S. R., & Abdallah, L. M. (2012). Bedside assessment of enteral tube placement: Aligning practice with evidence. *American Journal of Nursing, 112*(2), 40-46. (Level VII)

15 U.S. Food and Drug Administration. (n.d.). "Look. Check. Connect. Safe medical device connections save lives" [Online]. Accessed May 2015 via the Web at http://www.fda.gov/downloads/MedicalDevices/Safety/AlertsandNotices/UCM134873.pdf

16 The Joint Commission. (2015). "Sentinel event alert: Managing risk during transition to new ISO tubing connector standards" [Online]. Accessed May 2015 via the Web at http://www.jointcommission.org/assets/1/18/SEA_53_Connectors_8_19_14_FINAL.pdf (Level VII)

17 The Joint Commission. (2015). Standard NPSG.06.01.01. *Comprehensive accreditation manual for hospitals: The official handbook.* Oakbrook Terrace, IL: The Joint Commission. (Level VII)

18 Graham, K. C., & Cvach, M. (2010). Monitor alarm fatigue: Standardizing use of physiological monitors and decreasing nuisance alarms. *American Journal of Critical Care, 19,* 28–37.

19 American Association of Critical-Care Nurses. (2013). "AACN practice alert: Alarm management" [Online]. Accessed May 2015 via the Web at http://www.aacn.org/wd/practice/docs/practicealerts/alarm-management-practice-alert.pdf (Level VII)

20 American Association of Critical-Care Nurses. (2010). "AACN practice alert: Oral care for patients at risk for ventilator-associated pneumonia" [Online]. Accessed May 2015 via the Web at http://www.aacn.org/WD/Practice/Docs/PracticeAlerts/oral%20care%2004-2010%20final.pdf (Level VII)

21 The Joint Commission. (2015). Standard RC.01.03.01. *Comprehensive accreditation manual for hospitals: The official handbook.* Oakbrook Terrace, IL: The Joint Commission. (Level VII)

22 Centers for Medicare & Medicaid Services, Department of Health and Human Services. (2014). Condition of participation: Medical record services. 42 C.F.R. § 482.24(b).

23 American Osteopathic Association. (2014). Standard 10.00.03. *Healthcare Facilities Accreditation Program: Accreditation requirements for acute care hospitals.* Chicago, IL: American Osteopathic Association. (Level VII)

24 The Joint Commission. (2013). "Sentinel event alert: Medical device alarm safety in hospitals" [Online]. Accessed May 2015 via the Web at http://www.jointcommission.org/assets/1/18/SEA_50_alarms_4_5_13_FINAL1.PDF (Level VII)

25 Kenny, D. J., & Goodman, P. (2010). Care of the patient with enteral tube feeding: An evidence-based protocol. *Nursing Research, 59,* S22-S31.

U

ULTRAVIOLET LIGHT THERAPY

Ultraviolet (UV) light causes profound biological changes, including UV light–induced immunosuppression and temporary suppression of epidermal basal cell division followed by a later increase in cell turnover. Such skin conditions as psoriasis, mycosis fungoides, atopic dermatitis, and uremic pruritus may respond to therapy that uses timed exposure to UV light rays.

Emitted by the sun, the UV spectrum is subdivided into three bands—A, B, and C—each of which affects the skin differently. Ultraviolet A (UVA) radiation (with a relatively long wavelength of 320 to 400 nanometers [nm]) rapidly darkens preformed melanin pigment, may augment ultraviolet B (UVB) in causing sunburn and skin aging, and may induce phototoxicity in the presence of some drugs. UVB radiation (with a wavelength of 280 to 320 nm) causes sunburn and erythema. Ultraviolet C (UVC) radiation (with a wavelength of 200 to 280 nm) normally is absorbed by the earth's ozone layer and doesn't reach the ground; it's used in operating-room germicidal lamps because it kills bacteria.

The drug methoxsalen, a psoralen agent, creates artificial sensitivity to UVA by binding with the deoxyribonucleic acid in epidermal basal cells. Administered before UVA light treatment, methoxsalen photosensitizes the skin to enhance therapeutic effects. Treating skin with a photosensitizing agent such as methoxsalen and UVA is called *psoralen-plus-UVA* (PUVA) therapy, or photochemotherapy. Other drugs used in PUVA therapy include acitretin (an oral vitamin A derivative) and methotrexate.

For PUVA therapy, the initial dose is based on the patient's skin type and is increased according to the treatment protocol and as tolerated. The practitioner calculates the UVB dose based on skin type estimation or by determining a minimal erythema dose—the smallest amount of UV light needed to produce mild erythema. (See *Comparing skin types.*)

Contraindications to both PUVA and UVB therapy include lupus erythematosus and xeroderma pigmentosa; PUVA therapy is also contraindicated in those with porphyria. PUVA and UVB therapy should be used cautiously in patients with skin types I and II; a history of photosensitivity diseases, skin cancer, or arsenic ingestion; and previous skin irradiation (which can induce skin cancer); PUVA should also be used cautiously in those with a history of liver disease. All UV light therapy is also contraindicated in patients who have undergone previous ionizing chemotherapy and in those using photosensitizing or immunosuppressant drugs.

UVB therapy is considered safe according to expert opinion during pregnancy.[1] However, PUVA therapy is contraindicated in pregnant and nursing women because of the increased risk of birth defects from psoralen agents. Women of childbearing age who undergo PUVA therapy should have a pregnancy test before beginning therapy and should use a reliable form of birth control during and for 3 months after treatment.

A patient can undergo UV light therapy in a health care facility or practitioner's office, or at home. Typically set into a reflective cabinet, the light source consists of a bank of high-intensity fluorescent bulbs. (At home, the patient may use a small fluorescent sunlamp.)

Equipment

For UVA radiation

Fluorescent black-light lamp ■ high-intensity UVA fluorescent bulbs.

For UVB radiation

Fluorescent sunlamp or hot quartz lamp ■ sunlamp bulbs.

For all UV treatments

Oral or topical phototherapeutic medications if necessary ■ body-sized light chamber or smaller light box ■ dark, polarized goggles ■ sunscreen if necessary ■ hospital gown ■ towels.

Implementation

- Review the patient's health history for contraindications to UV light therapy.
- Verify the practitioner's orders *to confirm the light treatment type and dose.*
- Perform hand hygiene.[2,3,4,5,6]
- Confirm the patient's identity using at least two patient identifiers.[7]
- Ask the patient whether he's currently taking photosensitizing drugs, such as anticonvulsants, certain antihypertensives, phenothiazines, salicylates, sulfonamides, tetracyclines, tretinoin, or various cancer drugs.
- Explain the procedure to the patient. Inform the patient that UV light treatments produce a mild sunburn that will help reduce or resolve skin lesions.
- If the patient will undergo PUVA therapy, make sure that he took the prescribed psoralen agent (with food) 1½ hours before treatment.
- To begin therapy, instruct the patient to disrobe and put on a hospital gown. Have him remove the gown or expose just the treatment area once he's in the phototherapy unit.
- Make sure that the patient wears sunscreen, towels, or a hospital gown *to protect vulnerable skin areas.* All male patients receiving PUVA must wear protection over the groin area.
- Have the patient put on goggles and make sure that he wears them throughout therapy *to protect his eye from harmful UV light.*
- If the patient is having local UVB treatment, position him at the correct distance from the light source. For instance, for facial treatment with a sunlamp, position the patient's face about 12″ (30.5 cm) from the lamp. For body treatment, position the patient's body about 30″ (76 cm) from either the sunlamp or the hot quartz lamp. If he must stand for the treatment, ask him to report any dizziness *to ensure his safety.*
- If you're observing him through light-chamber windows, put on goggles.
- After delivering the prescribed UVB dose, help the patient out of the unit and instruct him to shield exposed areas of skin from sunlight for 8 hours after therapy.
- Perform hand hygiene.[2,3,4,5,6]
- Document the procedure.[8,9,10]

Special considerations

- Overexposure to UV light (sunburn) can result from prolonged treatment and an inadequate distance between the patient and light sources. It can also result from the use of photosensitizing drugs or from overly sensitive skin.
- To prevent eye damage during home therapy, the patient should use gray or green polarized lenses during UVB therapy or UV-opaque sunglasses during PUVA therapy. A patient undergoing PUVA therapy should wear these glasses for 24 hours after treatment *because methoxsalen can cause photosensitivity.*
- Before giving methoxsalen, check to ensure that baseline liver function studies have been done. Keep in mind that both drugs are hepatotoxic agents and are never given together. Liver function and blood lipid studies are required before treatment with acitretin and at regular intervals during treatment. Liver function studies and a complete blood count are required before and during methotrexate treatment.
- If the practitioner prescribes tar preparations with UVB treatment, watch for signs of sensitivity, such as erythema, pruritus, and eczematous reactions. If you apply carbonis detergens to the patient's skin before UV light therapy, remove it completely with mineral oil just before treatment begins *to let the light penetrate the skin.*

PATIENT TEACHING

Skin care guidelines

A patient who's receiving ultraviolet light treatments must know how to protect his skin from injury. Provide your patient with the following skin care tips:

- Encourage the patient to use emollients and drink plenty of fluids *to combat dry skin and maintain adequate hydration.* Warn him to avoid hot baths or showers and to use soap sparingly. *Heat and soap promote dry skin.*
- Instruct the patient to notify his practitioner before taking any medication, including aspirin, *to prevent heightened photosensitivity.*
- If the patient is receiving psoralen-plus-ultraviolet A (PUVA) therapy, review his psoralen agent dosage schedule. Explain that deviating from it could result in burns or ineffective treatment. Urge him to wear appropriate sunglasses outdoors for at least 24 hours after taking the psoralen agent. Recommend annual eye examinations *to detect cataract formation.*
- If the patient uses a sunlamp at home, advise him to let the lamp warm for 5 minutes before treatment. Stress the importance of exposing his skin to the light for the exact amount of time prescribed by the practitioner. Instruct the patient to protect his eyes with goggles and to use a dependable timer or have someone else time his therapy. Above all, urge him never to use the sunlamp when he's tired *to avoid falling asleep under the lamp and sustaining a burn.*
- Teach the patient first aid for localized burning: Tell him to apply cool water soaks for 20 minutes or until skin temperature cools. For more extensive burns, recommend tepid tap water baths after notifying the practitioner about the burn. After the patient bathes, suggest using an oil-in-water moisturizing lotion (not a petroleum jelly–based product, which can trap radiant heat).
- Tell the patient to limit natural-light exposure, to use a sunscreen when he's outdoors, and to notify his practitioner immediately if he discovers any unusual skin lesions.
- Advise the patient to avoid harsh soaps and chemicals, such as paints and solvents, and to discuss ways to manage physical and psychological stress, *which may exacerbate skin disorders.*

Patient teaching

Tell the patient to look for marked redness, blistering, peeling, or other signs of overexposure 4 to 6 hours after UVB therapy and 24 to 48 hours after UVA therapy. In either case, the erythema should disappear within another 24 hours. Tell him that mild dryness and skin peeling will occur in 1 to 2 days. Teach him appropriate skin care measures. (See *Skin care guidelines.*) Advise him to notify the practitioner if overexposure occurs. Typically, the practitioner recommends stopping treatment for a few days and then starting over at a lower exposure level.

Complications

Erythema is the major adverse effect of UVB therapy. Minimal erythema without discomfort is acceptable, but treatments are suspended if marked edema, swelling, or blistering occurs.

Erythema, nausea, and pruritus are the three major short-term adverse effects of PUVA therapy. Long-term adverse effects are similar to those caused by excessive exposure to sun—premature aging (xerosis, wrinkles, and mottled skin), lentigines, telangiectasia, increased risk of skin cancer, and cataracts if eye protection isn't used. The patient can minimize effects by using emollients, sunscreens, and cover-ups.

Documentation

Record the date and time of initial and subsequent treatments, the UV wavelength used, and the name and dose of any oral or topical medications given. Record the exact duration of therapy, the distance between the light source and the skin, and the patient's tolerance. Note safety measures used such as eye protection. Also describe the patient's skin condition before and after treatment. Note improvements and adverse reactions, such as increased pruritus, oozing, and scaling. Document how the patient tolerated the procedure.

References

1 American Academy of Dermatology. (2010). Guidelines of care for the management of psoriasis and psoriatic arthritis: Section 5. Guidelines of care for the treatment of psoriasis with phototherapy and photochemotherapy. *Journal of the American Academy of Dermatology, 62*, 114–135. (Level VII)

2 Centers for Disease Control and Prevention. (2002). Guideline for hand hygiene in health-care settings: Recommendations of the Healthcare Infection Control Practices Advisory Committee and the HICPAC/SHEA/APIC/IDSA Hand Hygiene Task Force. *MMWR Recommendations and Reports, 51*(RR-16), 1–45. Accessed May 2015 via the Web at http://www.cdc.gov/mmwr/pdf/rr/rr5116.pdf (Level II)

3 World Health Organization. (2009). "WHO guidelines on hand hygiene in health care: First global patient safety challenge, clean care is safer care" [Online]. Accessed May 2015 via the Web at http://whqlibdoc.who.int/publications/2009/9789241597906_eng.pdf (Level IV)

4 The Joint Commission. (2015). Standard NPSG.07.01.01. *Comprehensive accreditation manual for hospitals: The official handbook.* Oakbrook Terrace, IL: The Joint Commission. (Level VII)

5 American Osteopathic Association. (2014). Standard 07.01.21. *Healthcare Facilities Accreditation Program: Accreditation requirements for acute care hospitals.* Chicago, IL: American Osteopathic Association. (Level VII)

6 Centers for Medicare & Medicaid Services, Department of Health and Human Services. (2014). Condition of participation: Infection control. 42 C.F.R. § 482.42.

7 The Joint Commission. (2015). Standard NPSG.01.01.01. *Comprehensive accreditation manual for hospitals: The official handbook.* Oakbrook Terrace, IL: The Joint Commission. (Level VII)

8 The Joint Commission. (2015). Standard RC.01.03.01. *Comprehensive accreditation manual for hospitals: The official handbook.* Oakbrook Terrace, IL: The Joint Commission. (Level VII)

9 Centers for Medicare & Medicaid Services, Department of Health and Human Services. (2014). Condition of participation: Medical record services. 42 C.F.R. § 482.24(b).

10 American Osteopathic Association. (2014). Standard 10.00.03. *Healthcare Facilities Accreditation Program: Accreditation requirements for acute care hospitals.* Chicago, IL: American Osteopathic Association. (Level VII)

Additional references

Feldman, S. R. Treatment of psoriasis. (2014). In: *UpToDate*, Dellavalle, R. P., et al. (Eds.). Accessed May 2015 via the Web at http://www.uptodate.com/contents/search

Honigesmann, H. UVB Therapy (broadband and narrowband). (2013). In: *UpToDate*, Elmets, C. A. & Corona, R. (Eds.). Accessed May 2015 via the Web at http://www.uptodate.com/contents/search

Souteiro, P., et al. (2013). Catechol-O-methyltransferase activity in psoriasis patients treated with psoralen plus ultraviolet A therapy. Photodermatology, Photoimmunology & Photomedicine, 29, 227–232. (Level VI)

Stinco, G., et al. (2013). Narrow band-ultraviolet B versus clobetasol propionate foam in the treatment of vitiligo: A retrospective study. Dermatology and *Therapy, 3,* 95–105. (Level IV)

Unna boot application

Named for dermatologist Paul Gerson Unna, this nonelastic paste bandage boot can be used to treat uninfected, nonnecrotic leg and foot ulcers that result from such conditions as venous insufficiency and stasis dermatitis. A commercially prepared Unna boot is a gauze compression dressing that's impregnated with a preparation known as *Unna paste* (gelatin, zinc oxide, calamine lotion, and glycerin). The dressing wraps around the affected foot and leg. The boot's effectiveness results from compression applied by the bandage, which decreases edema, combined with moisture supplied by the paste.

The Unna boot is contraindicated in patients allergic to any ingredient used in the paste and in patients with arterial ulcers, weeping eczema, or cellulitis.

Equipment

Gauze sponge with prescribed cleaning agent ■ normal saline solution ■ commercially prepared paste bandage (impregnated with gelatin, zinc oxide, glycerin, and possibly calamine) or lightweight gauze and Unna paste ■ gloves ■ elastic bandage to cover the Unna boot ■ Optional: extra roller gauze for excessive drainage, bandage scissors, clip or tape, Doppler ultrasound equipment.

Implementation

- Gather the appropriate equipment.
- Perform hand hygiene.[1,2,3,4,5]
- Confirm the patient's identity using at least two patient identifiers.[6]
- Explain the procedure to the patient and provide privacy.[7,8]
- Put on gloves.[9,10]
- Assess the ulcer and the surrounding skin. Evaluate ulcer size, drainage, and appearance.
- Perform a neurovascular assessment of the affected foot *to ensure adequate circulation.* If you don't detect a dorsalis-pedis or posterior tibial pulse in the foot by palpation, Doppler ultrasound, or ankle-brachial index, notify the practitioner before applying the Unna boot.
- Place the patient in the supine position, elevating the leg on which you're going to place the Unna boot.
- Open all the bandage wrappers. Make sure that you have enough supplies to cover the extremity.
- Have the patient dorsiflex his foot 90 degrees.
- Clean the affected area gently with the sponge and cleaning agent *to retard bacterial growth and to remove dirt and wound debris, which may create pressure points after you apply the bandage.* Rinse with normal saline solution.
- Apply the prepared bandage in a spiral motion without tension, from just above the toes to 1″ (2.5 cm) below the knee. Be sure to cover the heel. The wrap should be snug but not tight. *To cover the area completely,* make sure each turn overlaps the previous one by one-half of the bandage width. (See *How to wrap an Unna boot.*)
- Continue wrapping the patient's leg up to the knee, using firm, even pressure. Stop the dressing 1″ (2.5 cm) below the popliteal fossa *to prevent irritation when the knee is bent.* Mold the boot with your free hand as you apply the bandage *to make it smooth and even.*
- Cover the boot with an elastic bandage *to provide external compression* and secure it in place using a clip or tape.
- Instruct the patient to remain in bed with his leg outstretched and elevated on a pillow until the paste dries (approximately 30 minutes). Observe the patient's foot for signs and symptoms of impairment, such as cyanosis, loss of feeling, and swelling. *These indicate that the bandage is too tight and must be removed.*
- Remove and discard your gloves.[9,10]
- Perform hand hygiene.[1,2,3,4,5]
- Document the procedure.[11,12,13]

Special considerations

- Leave the boot on as ordered, typically 3 to 7 days. Instruct the patient to walk on and handle the wrap carefully *to avoid damaging it.* Tell him the boot will stiffen but won't be as hard as a cast.
- Change the boot weekly or as ordered *to assess the underlying skin and ulcer healing;* also change the boot when the patient detects a loosening of the boot or anytime the wrap becomes saturated with drainage. Remove the boot by unwrapping the bandage from the knee down to the foot.
- If the boot is applied over a swollen leg, change the boot as the edema subsides—if necessary, more frequently than every 3 days.
- Don't make reverse turns while wrapping the bandage. *This could create excessive pressure areas that may cause discomfort as the bandage hardens.*
- For bathing, instruct the patient to cover the boot with a plastic bag sealed at the knee with an elastic bandage *to avoid wetting the boot. A wet boot softens and loses its effectiveness.* If the patient's safety is a concern, instruct him to take a sponge bath.
- Other two- or four-layer wraps are available that follow the same principles as an Unna boot. Some products can be removed daily, such as compression stockings, which require measurement for accurate fit after any edema has subsided.

Complications

Contact dermatitis may result from hypersensitivity to Unna paste.

Documentation

Record the date and time of application and the presence of a pulse in the affected foot. Specify which leg you bandaged. Describe the appearance of the patient's skin before and after boot application. Name the equipment used (a commercially prepared bandage or Unna paste and lightweight gauze). Describe any allergic reaction.

How to wrap an Unna boot

After cleaning and drying the patient's skin thoroughly, flex the knee. Then, starting with the foot positioned at a right angle to the leg, wrap the impregnated gauze bandage firmly—not tightly—around the patient's foot. Wrap the bandage twice around the patient's toes without tension. Make sure the dressing covers the heel. Continue wrapping upward, overlapping the dressing 50% or more with each turn. Smooth the boot with your free hand as you go (as shown below).

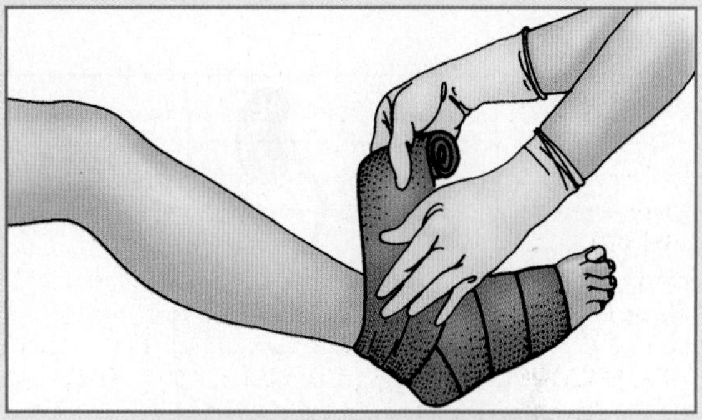

Stop wrapping about 1″ (2.5 cm) below the knee, as shown below. If necessary, make a 2″ (5-cm) slit in the boot just below the knee *to relieve constriction that may develop as the dressing hardens.*

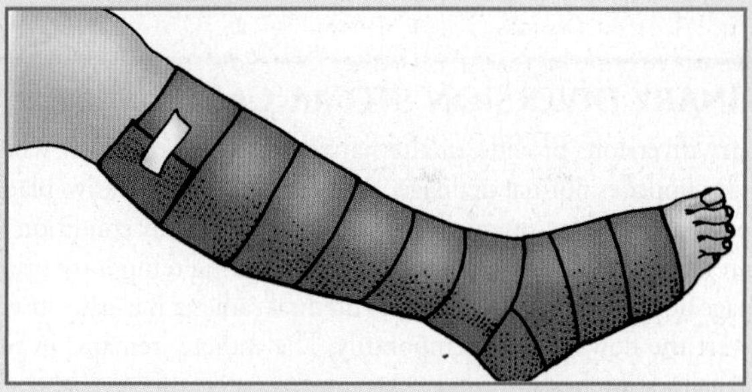

If drainage is excessive, you may wrap a roller gauze dressing over the Unna boot. As the final layer, wrap an elastic bandage in a figure-eight pattern.

REFERENCES

1 Centers for Disease Control and Prevention. (2002). Guideline for hand hygiene in health-care settings: Recommendations of the Healthcare Infection Control Practices Advisory Committee and the HICPAC/SHEA/APIC/IDSA Hand Hygiene Task Force. *MMWR Recommendations and Reports, 51*(RR-16), 1–45. Accessed May 2015 via the Web at http://www.cdc.gov/mmwr/pdf/rr/rr5116.pdf (Level II)

2 World Health Organization. (2009). "WHO guidelines on hand hygiene in health care: First global patient safety challenge, clean care is safer care" [Online]. Accessed May 2015 via the Web at http://whqlibdoc.who.int/publications/2009/9789241597906_eng.pdf (Level IV)

3 The Joint Commission. (2015). Standard NPSG.07.01.01. *Comprehensive accreditation manual for hospitals: The official handbook.* Oakbrook Terrace, IL: The Joint Commission. (Level VII)

4 American Osteopathic Association. (2014). Standard 07.01.21. *Healthcare Facilities Accreditation Program: Accreditation requirements for acute care hospitals.* Chicago, IL: American Osteopathic Association. (Level VII)

5 Centers for Medicare & Medicaid Services, Department of Health and Human Services. (2014). Condition of participation: Infection control. 42 C.F.R. § 482.42.

6 The Joint Commission. (2015). Standard NPSG.01.01.01. *Comprehensive accreditation manual for hospitals: The official handbook.* Oakbrook Terrace, IL: The Joint Commission. (Level VII)

7 American Osteopathic Association. (2014). Standard 15.01.16. *Healthcare Facilities Accreditation Program: Accreditation requirements for acute care hospitals.* Chicago, IL: American Osteopathic Association. (Level VII)

8 Centers for Medicare & Medicaid Services, Department of Health and Human Services. (2014). Condition of participation: Patient's rights. 42 C.F.R. § 482.13(c)(1).

9 Siegel, J. D., et al. (2007). "2007 guideline for isolation precautions: Preventing transmission of infectious agents in healthcare settings" [Online]. Accessed May 2015 via the Web at http://www.cdc.gov/hicpac/pdf/isolation/Isolation2007.pdf (Level II)

10 American Osteopathic Association. (2014). Standard 07.01.10. *Healthcare Facilities Accreditation Program: Accreditation requirements for acute care hospitals.* Chicago, IL: American Osteopathic Association. (Level VII)

11 The Joint Commission. (2015). Standard RC.01.03.01. *Comprehensive accreditation manual for hospitals: The official handbook.* Oakbrook Terrace, IL: The Joint Commission. (Level VII)

12 Centers for Medicare & Medicaid Services, Department of Health and Human Services. (2014). Condition of participation: Medical record services. 42 C.F.R. § 482.24(b).

13 American Osteopathic Association. (2014). Standard 10.00.03. *Healthcare Facilities Accreditation Program: Accreditation requirements for acute care hospitals.* Chicago, IL: American Osteopathic Association. (Level VII)

ADDITIONAL REFERENCES

Baranoski, S., & Ayello, E. A. (2012). *Wound care essentials: Practice principles* (3rd ed.). Philadelphia, PA: Lippincott Williams & Wilkins.

Luz, B. S., et al. (2013). Evaluating the effectiveness of the customized Unna boot when treating patients with venous ulcers. *Anais Brasileiros de Dermatologia, 88,* 41–49. (Level IV)

Types of permanent urinary diversion

The steps involved in creating an ileal conduit or a continent urinary diversion are described below.

Ileal conduit

A segment of the ileum is excised, and the two ends of the ileum that result from excision of the segment are sutured closed. Then the ureters are dissected from the bladder and anastomosed to the ileal segment. One end of the ileal segment is closed with sutures; the opposite end is brought through the abdominal wall, forming a stoma.

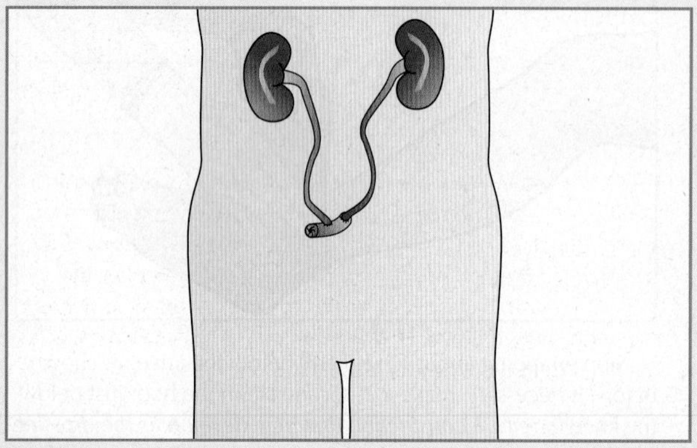

Continent urinary diversion (Indiana pouch)

The surgeon introduces the ureters into a segment of ileum and cecum. Urine is drained periodically by inserting a catheter into the stoma.

The Kock, Maine, and Florida pouches (not pictured here) are continent pouches that are also catheterizable. Another type of continent urinary diversion known as the *orthotopic neobladder* (not pictured here) is hooked back to the urethra, making a stoma unnecessary.

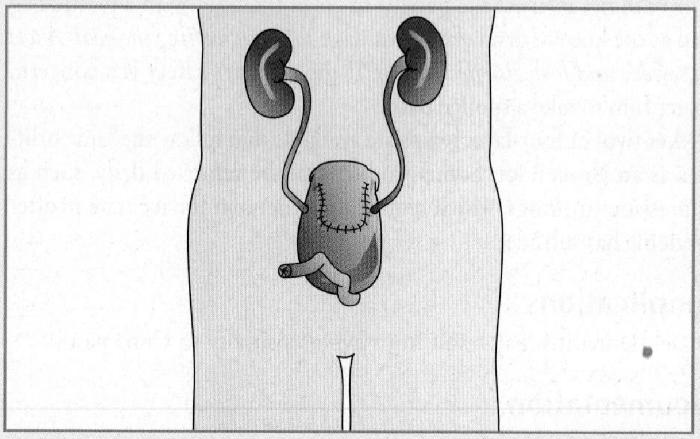

URINARY DIVERSION STOMA CARE

Urinary diversions provide an alternative route for urine flow when a disorder impedes normal drainage, as in the case of an invasive bladder tumor. A permanent urinary diversion is indicated in any condition that requires a total cystectomy. In conditions requiring temporary urinary drainage or diversion, a suprapubic or urethral catheter is usually inserted to divert the flow of urine temporarily. The catheter remains in place until the incision heals.

Urinary diversions may also be indicated for patients with neurogenic bladder, congenital anomaly, traumatic injury to the lower urinary tract, or severe chronic urinary tract infection.

Ileal conduit and continent urinary diversion are the two types of permanent urinary diversions with stomas. (See *Types of permanent urinary diversion.*) These procedures usually require the patient to wear a urine-collection appliance and to care for a newly created stoma. Evaluation by a wound, ostomy and continence nurse (WOCN) will facilitate site selection and postoperative stoma care.

Equipment

Gloves ▪ fluid-impermeable pad ▪ graduated cylinder ▪ washcloth ▪ mild soap and water ▪ absorbent, lint-free material for wicking (rolled gauze or tampon) ▪ pouching system (one-piece or two-piece, disposable or reusable, with a spout for ease of emptying; see *Urinary diversion pouching systems*) ▪ stoma measuring guide ▪ Optional: scissors, marker or pen, hair clippers, vinegar, deodorant tablets, barrier paste.

Implementation

- Gather the appropriate equipment.
- Perform hand hygiene.[1,2,3,4,5]
- Put on gloves.[6,7]
- Confirm the patient's identity using at least two patient identifiers.[8]
- Explain the procedure to the patient, and offer constant reinforcement and reassurance *to counteract negative reactions that may be elicited by stoma care; the patient or family will eventually need to perform the procedure.*
- Place the bed in the low Fowler position so the patient's abdomen is flat. *This position eliminates skin folds that could cause the appliance to slip or irritate the skin and allows the patient to observe or participate.*
- Place the fluid-impermeable pad under the patient's side, near the stoma.
- Open the drain valve of the appliance being cleaned or replaced *to empty the urine into the graduated cylinder.*
- Loosen and lift the edges of the pouch while pushing the skin back from the pouch, starting at the top of the pouch and working down to the bottom, *to remove the appliance.*[9]
- If the appliance is disposable, discard it into the waste receptacle.[10] If it's reusable, clean it with soap and lukewarm water and let it air-dry.
- *To prevent a constant flow of urine onto the skin while you're changing the appliance,* wick the urine with an absorbent, lint-free material. (See *Wicking urine from a stoma.*)
- Use water to carefully wash off any crystal deposits that may have formed around the stoma. If urine has stagnated and has a strong odor, use a very mild soap without oils, perfumes, or deodorants. Be sure to rinse the appliance thoroughly *to remove any oily residue that could cause the appliance to slip or cause skin irritation.*[9]
- Dry the peristomal area thoroughly with a gauze pad *because moisture will keep the appliance from sticking.* If necessary, remove any hair from the area with clippers *to prevent hair follicles from becoming irritated when the pouch is removed, which can cause folliculitis.*
- Inspect the stoma *for proper healing and to detect complications.* Check the color and the appearance of the suture line, and examine any moisture or drainage. Inspect the peristomal skin for redness, irritation, and intactness.
- Consult with a WOCN, if needed, when skin problems arise.
- For a pouch with an attached skin barrier (one-piece system), measure the stoma with the measuring guide. Select an opening size that matches the stoma.

■ For an adhesive-backed pouch with a separate skin barrier (two-piece), measure the stoma with the measuring guide and select the opening that matches the stoma. Trace the selected size opening onto the paper back of the skin barrier's adhesive side. Cut out the opening. (If the pouch has precut openings, which can be handy for a round stoma, select an opening no more than 1/8″ [3 mm] larger than the stoma. If the pouch comes without an opening, cut a hole 1/8″ [3 mm] wider than the measured tracing.) Many pouching systems can be fit up to the stoma edge without risk of trauma to the stoma. The cut-to-fit system works best for an irregularly shaped stoma.
■ If you're using a barrier paste, squeeze a ribbon of paste around the opening in the adhesive wafer or apply it to the peristomal skin around the stoma, making a complete circle *to provide extra skin protection and a better seal to prevent leakage.*
■ Remove the material used for wicking urine, and place it in the appropriate receptacle.[10]
■ When using a one-piece system, center it over the stoma, adhesive side down, and gently press it to the skin.
■ When using a two-piece system with a wafer, apply the wafer, then gently press the pouch opening onto the ring until it snaps into place.
■ When using a two-piece adhesive system with a coupling device, line up the adhesive portion of the pouch to the "landing zone" of the wafer. Press together *for adhesion.* You can attach the pouches used in a two-piece system to the wafer before application if the patient is still experiencing incisional discomfort.
■ Dispose of used materials in the appropriate recptacles.[10]
■ Encourage the patient to stay quietly in position for 5 minutes *to promote appliance adhesion.*
■ Remove and discard your gloves.[6,7]
■ Perform hand hygiene.[1,2,3,4,5]
■ Document the procedure.[11,12,13]

Special considerations

■ The patient's attitude toward his urinary diversion stoma plays a big part in determining how well he'll adjust to it. *To encourage a positive attitude,* help him get used to the idea of caring for his stoma and the appliance as though they're natural extensions of himself. When teaching him to perform the procedure, give him written instructions and provide positive reinforcement after he completes each step. Suggest that he perform the procedure in the morning when urine flows most slowly.
■ Help the patient choose between disposable and reusable appliances by telling him the advantages and disadvantages of each. Emphasize the importance of correct placement and of a well-fitted appliance *to prevent seepage of urine onto the skin.* When positioned correctly, most appliances remain in place for at least 3 days and for as long as 5 days if no leakage occurs. After 5 days, the appliance should be changed. With the improved adhesives and pouches available, belts aren't always necessary.
■ Because urine flows constantly, it accumulates quickly, becoming even heavier than stools. *To prevent the weight of the urine from loosening the seal around the stoma and separating the appliance from the skin,* tell the patient to empty the appliance through the drain valve when it's one-third to one-half full.
■ Instruct the patient to connect his appliance to a urine-collection container before he goes to sleep. *The continuous flow of urine into the container during the night prevents the urine from accumulating and stagnating in the* appliance.
■ Teach the patient sanitary and dietary measures that can protect the peristomal skin and control the odor that commonly results from alkaline urine, infection, or poor hygiene. Reusable appliances should be washed with soap and lukewarm water and then air-dried thoroughly *to prevent brittleness.* Soaking the appliance in vinegar and water or placing deodorant tablets in it can further dissipate stubborn odors. Generous fluid intake also helps to reduce odors by diluting the urine.

Urinary diversion pouching systems

Disposable pouching systems

Options for disposable pouching systems include a one-piece disposable system with spout closure, or a two-piece drainable, disposable pouch with a skin barrier. The one-piece system consists of a transparent or opaque, odor-proof plastic pouch with attached adhesive backing. Some pouches have microporous tape edges or belt tabs. The spout opening enables easy draining. This pouch may be permanent or temporary until the stoma size stabilizes.

The two-piece drainable, disposable pouch with a separate skin barrier permits more frequent pouch changes. Also made of transparent or opaque, odor-proof plastic, this style comes with belt tabs and usually snaps to the skin barrier with a flange mechanism. Newer two-piece pouches have an adhesive coupling. The pouch sticks to the wafer, allowing greater flexibility and comfort.

Reusable pouching system

Typically manufactured from sturdy, opaque, hypoallergenic plastic, the reusable pouch comes with a separate, custom-made faceplate and O-ring. The device has a 1- to 3-month life span, depending on how frequently the patient empties the pouch. Reusable equipment may benefit a patient who needs a firm faceplate, has sensitivity to any type of adhesive, or wishes to minimize cost.

Wicking urine from a stoma

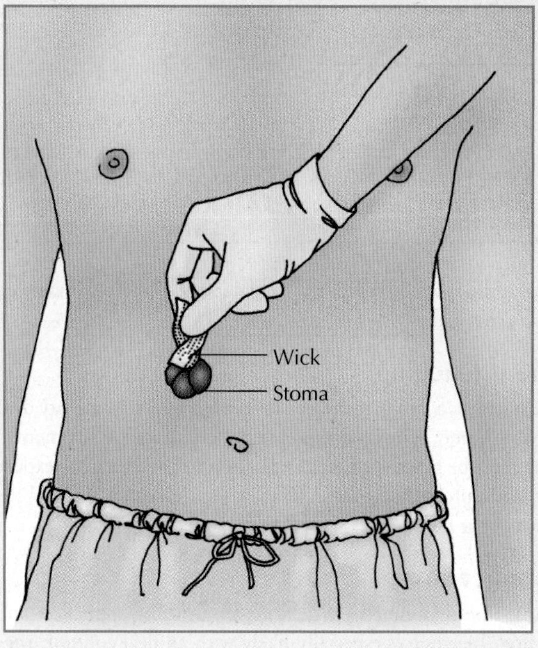

■ Tell the patient that mucus may normally be present in the urine.
■ If the patient has a continent urinary diversion, make sure you know how to meet his special needs. (See *Caring for the patient with a continent urinary diversion,* page 812.)
■ Tell the patient about ostomy support groups, the United Ostomy Association of America, and the American Cancer Society. Members of these organizations routinely visit health care facilities to explain ostomy

Caring for the patient with a continent urinary diversion

With a continent urinary diversion, an alternative to the traditional ileal conduit, a pouch created from the ascending colon and terminal ileum serves as a new bladder, which empties through a stoma. To drain urine continuously, several drains are inserted into this reconstructed bladder and left in place for 3 to 6 weeks until the new stoma heals. The patient will be discharged from the health care facility with the drains in place. He'll return to have them removed and to learn to catheterize his stoma.

First hospitalization care

■ Immediately after surgery, monitor intake and output from each drain. Be alert for decreased output, *which may indicate that urine flow is obstructed*.

■ Watch for common postoperative complications, such as infection or bleeding. Also watch for signs of urinary leakage, which include increased abdominal distention and urine appearing around the drains or midline incision.

■ Irrigate the drains as ordered.

■ Perform hand hygiene[1,2,3,4,5] and put on gloves.[6,7] Clean the area around the drains daily—first with an antiseptic swab and then with sterile water. Apply a dry, sterile dressing to the area. Use precut 4″ × 4″ (10-cm × 10-cm) drain dressings around the drains *to absorb leakage*.

■ *To increase the patient's mobility and comfort*, connect the drains to a leg bag.

Second hospitalization or outpatient care

■ After the patient's drains are removed, teach the patient how to catheterize the stoma. Begin by gathering the following equipment on a clean towel: latex-free catheter (usually #14 or #16 French), water-soluble lubricant, washcloth, stoma covering (nonadherent gauze pad or panty liner), urine-collection container, hypoallergenic adhesive tape, and an irrigating solution (optional).

■ Apply water-soluble lubricant to the catheter tip *to facilitate insertion*.

■ Remove and discard the stoma cover. Using the washcloth, clean the stoma and the area around it, starting at the stoma and working outward in a circular motion. Dry the area thoroughly.

■ Hold the urine-collection container under the catheter; then slowly insert the catheter into the stoma. Urine should begin to flow into the container. If it doesn't, gently rotate the catheter or redirect its angle. If the catheter drains slowly, it may be plugged with mucus. Irrigate it with sterile saline solution or sterile water to clear it. When the flow stops, pinch the catheter closed and remove it.

Patient teaching[14]

■ Explain that the stoma is commonly swollen in the initial postoperative period and that its size will gradually reduce over 6 to 8 weeks.

■ Teach the patient how to care for the drains and their insertion sites during the 3 to 6 weeks he'll be at home before their removal, and teach him how to attach them to a leg bag. Also teach him how to recognize the signs and symptoms of infection and obstruction.

■ After the drains are removed, teach the patient how to empty the pouch, and establish a schedule. Initially, he should catheterize the stoma and empty the pouch every 2 to 3 hours. Later, he should catheterize every 4 hours while awake and also irrigate the pouch each morning and evening, if ordered. Instruct him to empty the pouch whenever he feels a sensation of fullness.

■ Tell the patient that the catheters are reusable, but only after they've been cleaned. He should clean the catheter thoroughly with warm, soapy water; rinse it thoroughly; and hang it to dry over a clean towel. He should store cleaned and dried catheters in plastic bags. Tell him he can reuse catheters for up to 1 month before discarding them. However, he should immediately discard any catheter that becomes discolored or cracked.

■ Provide a contact telephone number for acute problems or questions.

■ Provide the patient with information on what to do when such problems as odor, urinary tract infection, and leakage occur.

■ Explain that mucus is a normal finding and what to do when there is more mucus than is normally observed. Explain that the stoma can bleed easily on contact.

■ Discuss with the patient how to manage his stoma while performing activities of daily living, such as bathing, dressing, traveling, working, engaging in hobbies, and sexual activity.

care and the types of appliances available and to help patients learn to function normally with a stoma.

Patient teaching

The patient or a family member can learn to care for a urinary diversion stoma at home. However, the patient's emotional adjustment to the stoma must be given special consideration before he can be expected to maintain it properly. Arrange for a visiting nurse or a WOCN to assist the patient at home.

Complications

Because intestinal mucosa is delicate, an ill-fitting appliance can cause bleeding. Bleeding is especially likely with an ileal conduit, the most common urinary diversion stoma, because a segment of the intestine forms the conduit.

Peristomal skin may become reddened or excoriated from too-frequent changing or improper placement of the appliance, poor skin care, or allergic reaction to the appliance or adhesive. Constant leakage around the appliance can result from improper placement of the appliance or from poor skin turgor. Other complications include mechanical injury, pressure ulcers, skin stripping injuries, mucocutaneous separation, and infections.[15]

Documentation

Record the appearance and color of the stoma and whether it's inverted, flush with the skin, or protruding. If it protrudes, note by how much it protrudes above the skin. (The normal range is ½″ to ¾″ [1.3 to 2 cm].) Record the appearance and condition of the peristomal skin, noting any redness or irritation or complaints by the patient of itching or burning as well as any nursing interventions, including consultation with the WOCN. Document any patient teaching and return demonstrations performed.

References

1 The Joint Commission. (2015). Standard NPSG.07.01.01. *Comprehensive accreditation manual for hospitals: The official handbook.* Oakbrook Terrace, IL: The Joint Commission. (Level VII)

2 Centers for Disease Control and Prevention. (2002). Guideline for hand hygiene in health-care settings: Recommendations of the Healthcare Infection Control Practices Advisory Committee and the HICPAC/SHEA/APIC/IDSA Hand Hygiene Task Force. *MMWR Recommendations and Reports, 51*(RR-16), 1–45. Accessed May 2015 via the Web at http://www.cdc.gov/mmwr/pdf/rr/rr5116.pdf (Level II)

3 World Health Organization. (2009). "WHO guidelines on hand hygiene in health care: First global patient safety challenge, clean care is safer care"

[Online]. Accessed May 2015 via the Web at http://whqlibdoc.who.int/publications/2009/9789241597906_eng.pdf (Level IV)

4 American Osteopathic Association. (2014). Standard 07.01.21. *Healthcare Facilities Accreditation Program: Accreditation requirements for acute care hospitals.* Chicago, IL: American Osteopathic Association. (Level VII)

5 Centers for Medicare & Medicaid Services, Department of Health and Human Services. (2014). Condition of participation: Infection control. 42 C.F.R. § 482.42.

6 Siegel, J. D., et al. (2007). "2007 guideline for isolation precautions: Preventing transmission of infectious agents in healthcare settings" [Online]. Accessed May 2015 via the Web at http://www.cdc.gov/hicpac/pdf/isolation/Isolation2007.pdf (Level II)

7 American Osteopathic Association. (2014). Standard 07.01.10. *Healthcare Facilities Accreditation Program: Accreditation requirements for acute care hospitals.* Chicago, IL: American Osteopathic Association. (Level VII)

8 The Joint Commission. (2014). Standard NPSG.01.01.01. *Comprehensive accreditation manual for hospitals: The official handbook.* Oakbrook Terrace, IL: The Joint Commission. (Level VII)

9 Wound, Ostomy and Continence Nurses Society. (2007). "Basic ostomy skin care: A guide for patients and health care providers" [Online]. Accessed May 2015 via the Web at http://www.ostomy.org/ostomy_info/wocn/wocn_basic_ostomy_skin_care.pdf

10 Occupational Safety and Health Administration. (n.d.). "Bloodborne pathogens, standard number 1910.1030" [Online]. Accessed May 2015 via the Web at https://www.osha.gov/pls/oshaweb/owadisp.show_document?p_id=10051&p_table=STANDARDS (Level VII)

11 The Joint Commission. (2015). Standard RC.01.03.01. *Comprehensive accreditation manual for hospitals: The official handbook.* Oakbrook Terrace, IL: The Joint Commission. (Level VII)

12 American Osteopathic Association. (2014). Standard 10.00.03. *Healthcare Facilities Accreditation Program: Accreditation requirements for acute care hospitals.* Chicago, IL: American Osteopathic Association. (Level VII)

13 Centers for Medicare & Medicaid Services, Department of Health and Human Services. (2014). Condition of participation: Medical record services. 42 C.F.R. § 482.24(b).

14 National Institute of Diabetes and Digestive and Kidney Diseases. (2013). "Urinary diversion" [Online]. Accessed May 2015 via the Web at http://kidney.niddk.nih.gov/KUdiseases/pubs/urostomy/index.aspx

15 Szymanski, K. M., et al. (2010). External stoma and peristomal complications following radical cystectomy and ileal conduit diversion: A systematic review. *Ostomy Wound Management, 56,* 28–35. (Level I)

URINE COLLECTION, 12- OR 24-HOUR TIMED

Because hormones, proteins, and electrolytes are excreted in small, variable amounts in urine, specimens for measuring these substances must typically be collected over an extended period to yield quantities of diagnostic value. A 24-hour specimen is used most commonly because it provides an average excretion rate for substances eliminated during this period. Timed specimens may also be collected for shorter periods, such as 12 hours, depending on the specific information needed.

All urine voided within the prescribed time period is collected in a suitable collection container. Depending on the intended test, a preservative may be added to the specimen collection container and the specimen may need to be kept refrigerated or on ice.[1]

Equipment

24-hour urine specimen collection container ▪ gloves ▪ specimen label ▪ laboratory request form ▪ laboratory biohazard transport bag ▪ patient-care reminders ▪ Optional: preservative, specimen collection hat, ice-filled basin, graduated container, bedpan, urinal, bedside commode.

Implementation

- Verify the practitioner's order for specimen collection.
- Check with the laboratory *to determine the proper container and preservative (if needed) for the ordered test.*[1]
- Gather the equipment. If preservative is needed, check the expiration date on the preservative container and add the preservative to the specimen container.[1]
- Perform hand hygiene.[2,3,4,5,6]
- Confirm the patient's identity using at least two patient identifiers.[7]
- Label the specimen container in the presence of the patient *to prevent mislabeling.*[7] The label should include the patient's name and identification number, the date, the start time of the collection, the time the collection should end, the test ordered, any other pertinent information, and your initials.[1]
- Explain the procedure to the patient and family, as necessary, *to enlist their cooperation and prevent accidental disposal of urine during the collection period.* Emphasize that failure to collect even one specimen during the collection period invalidates the test and requires that it be started over.
- If you are collecting a voided specimen, explain that the patient should empty his bladder just before the 24-hour collection period begins and that this specimen will be discarded. Explain that the patient should save and store all urine voided during the 12- or 24-hour collection period in one specimen collection container.[1] Instruct the patient to notify you after each void and to avoid contaminating the urine with stool or toilet tissue.
- Instruct the patient to avoid exercise and ingestion of coffee, tea, and drugs (unless directed otherwise by the practitioner) right before and during the test *to avoid altering test results.* Make sure that the patient understands the instructions and is willing to comply with the restrictions.
- Place patient-care reminders over the patient's bed, in the bathroom, and on the urinal, bedpan, bedside commode, or indwelling catheter collection bag. Include the date and the collection interval.[1]

Collecting a voided specimen

- If the patient is using the bathroom toilet, place a specimen collection hat in the toilet bowl *to collect and measure urine.*
- At the beginning of the collection period, ask the patient to void.
- Perform hand hygiene and then put on gloves.[2,3,4,5,6,8]
- Measure the amount of urine if output is being recorded.
- Discard the urine specimen *so that the patient starts the collection period with an empty bladder.*
- Note the time as the beginning time for the collection period.
- Remove and discard your gloves.
- Perform hand hygiene.[2,3,4,5,6]
- After each time the patient voids during the collection period, perform hand hygiene and put on gloves.[2,3,4,5,6,8] Measure the amount of urine if output is to be recorded. Pour the urine specimen to be saved into the specimen collection container. Then remove and discard your gloves and perform hand hygiene.[2,3,4,5,6,8]
- Keep the specimen collection container refrigerated or on ice *to preserve the specimen,* as appropriate.
- At the end of the collection period, perform hand hygiene and then put on gloves.[2,3,4,5,6,8] Ask the patient to void again, if possible, and add that specimen to the collection container.[1] Note the ending time on the specimen label.

Collecting an indwelling urinary catheter specimen

- Perform hand hygiene and then put on gloves.[2,3,4,5,6,8,9]
- Empty the drainage bag.
- Measure the amount of urine if output is being recorded.
- Discard all the urine.
- Note the time as the beginning time for the collection period.
- Put the collection bag in an ice-filled container at the bedside.
- At regular intervals during the collection period, perform hand hygiene and then put on gloves.[2,3,4,5,8,9] Empty the collection bag. Measure the amount of urine if output is being recorded. Pour the urine

specimen to be saved into the collection container. Remove and discard your gloves and perform hand hygiene.[2,3,4,5,6,8]

- Keep the collection container refrigerated or on ice *to preserve the specimen,* as appropriate.
- At the end of the collection period, perform hand hygiene and then put on gloves.[2,3,4,5,6] Collect the remaining urine from the indwelling urinary catheter collection bag and add this last specimen to the collection container. Note the ending time on the specimen label.

Completing the procedure

- Place the specimen collection container in an approved laboratory biohazard transport bag.[8]
- Remove and discard your gloves.
- Perform hand hygiene.[2,3,4,5,6]
- Immediately send the container to the laboratory with a properly completed laboratory request form.[8]
- Remove the patient-care reminders, and inform the patient and family that the specimen collection period is complete.
- Perform hand hygiene.[2,3,4,5,6]
- Document the procedure.[10,11,12]

Special considerations

- Keep the patient well hydrated before and during the test *to ensure adequate urine flow.*
- Before collection of a timed specimen, make sure the laboratory will be open when the collection period ends *to help ensure prompt, accurate results.*
- Never store a specimen in a refrigerator that contains food or medication *to avoid contamination.*
- If a specimen is accidentally discarded during the collection period, restart the procedure. Emphasize the need to save all of the patient's urine during the collection period to everyone involved in his care as well as to the patient, his family, and other visitors.
- If the patient is menstruating, postpone the test *to avoid specimen contamination.*

Patient teaching

If the patient must collect urine at home, provide written instructions for the appropriate method. Tell him that he can keep the collection container in a brown bag in his refrigerator at home, separate from other refrigerator contents.

Documentation

Record the date, time, and method of collection. Also record the name of the test, the amount of urine collected (if necessary), and the time of specimen transport to the laboratory. Note teaching provided to the patient and family and their response to it.

References

1 Fischbach, F., & Dunning, M. B. (2014). *A manual of laboratory and diagnostic tests* (9th ed.). Philadelphia, PA: Wolters Kluwer.

2 The Joint Commission. (2015). Standard NPSG.07.01.01. *Comprehensive accreditation manual for hospitals: The official handbook.* Oakbrook Terrace, IL: The Joint Commission. (Level VII)

3 World Health Organization. (2009). "WHO guidelines on hand hygiene in health care: First global patient safety challenge, clean care is safer care" [Online]. Accessed May 2015 via the Web at http://whqlibdoc.who.int/publications/2009/9789241597906_eng.pdf (Level IV)

4 Centers for Disease Control and Prevention. (2002). Guideline for hand hygiene in health-care settings: Recommendations of the Healthcare Infection Control Practices Advisory Committee and the HICPAC/SHEA/APIC/IDSA Hand Hygiene Task Force. *MMWR Recommendations and Reports, 51*(RR-16), 1–45. Accessed May 2015 via the Web at http://www.cdc.gov/mmwr/pdf/rr/rr5116.pdf (Level II)

5 Centers for Medicare & Medicaid Services, Department of Health and Human Services. (2014). Condition of participation: Infection control. 42 C.F.R. § 482.42.

6 American Osteopathic Association. (2014). Standard 07.01.21. *Healthcare Facilities Accreditation Program: Accreditation requirements for acute care hospitals.* Chicago, IL: American Osteopathic Association. (Level VII)

7 The Joint Commission. (2015). Standard NPSG.01.01.01. *Comprehensive accreditation manual for hospitals: The official handbook.* Oakbrook Terrace, IL: The Joint Commission. (Level VII)

8 Occupational Safety and Health Administration. (n.d.). "Bloodborne pathogens, standard number 1910.1030" [Online]. Accessed May 2015 via the Web at http://www.osha.gov/pls/oshaweb/owadisp.show_document?p_table=STANDARDS&p_id=10051 (Level VII)

9 Siegel, J. D., et al. (2007). "2007 guideline for isolation precautions: Preventing transmission of infectious agents in healthcare settings" [Online]. Accessed May 2015 via the Web at http://www.cdc.gov/hicpac/pdf/isolation/Isolation2007.pdf (Level II)

10 The Joint Commission. (2015). Standard RC.01.03.01. *Comprehensive accreditation manual for hospitals: The official handbook.* Oakbrook Terrace, IL: The Joint Commission. (Level VII)

11 Centers for Medicare & Medicaid Services, Department of Health and Human Services. (2014). Condition of participation: Medical record services. 42 C.F.R. § 482.24(b).

12 American Osteopathic Association. (2014). Standard 10.00.03. *Healthcare Facilities Accreditation Program: Accreditation requirements for acute care hospitals.* Chicago, IL: American Osteopathic Association. (Level VII)

URINE GLUCOSE AND KETONE TESTS

Reagent strip tests help monitor urine glucose and ketone levels and screen for diabetes. Urine ketone tests monitor fat metabolism, help diagnose carbohydrate deprivation and diabetic ketoacidosis, and help distinguish between diabetic and nondiabetic coma. Urine glucose testing isn't as accurate as blood glucose testing[1] and should be used only when blood glucose testing isn't available.

Glucose oxidase tests (such as Diastix and Clinistix strips) produce color changes when patches of reagents implanted in handheld plastic strips react with glucose in the patient's urine. Urine ketone strip tests (such as Keto-Diastix and Ketostix) are similar. Test results are read by comparing color changes with a standardized reference chart.

Equipment

Clean-catch urine collection kit ■ urine specimen container ■ gloves ■ glucose or ketone test strips ■ reference color chart.

Preparation of equipment

Check the expiration date on the reagent strips and discard them if they're expired. Allow time for refrigerated items, including reagents and patient specimens, to reach room temperature before testing, if specified in the product insert. Check and record lot numbers for test kits, test devices, and controls. (Don't mix reagents from different products or lot numbers. If you're using a new lot, set up quality control, as needed, and refer to the product insert for changes in control ranges.) Visually inspect reagent vials and the strips within them for damage, discoloration, and contamination. Prepare and store reagents according to the manufacturer's instructions. If opening a new reagent strip vial or kit, write the date opened on the outside of the vial or test kit.[2,3]

Implementation

- Verify the practitioner's order for testing.
- Gather and prepare the appropriate equipment.
- Check the patient's history for medications that may interfere with test results.
- Perform hand hygiene.[4,5,6,7,8]
- Confirm the patient's identity using at least two patient identifiers.[9]

- Explain the procedure to the patient.
- Provide the patient with a specimen container, and instruct him to collect a clean-catch, midstream urine specimen. (See the "Urine specimen collection" procedure, page 817.)
- Put on gloves.[10,11]
- Test the urine specimen immediately after the patient voids.

Glucose oxidase strip tests

- If you're using a Clinistix strip, dip the reagent end of the strip into the urine specimen for 2 seconds. *Remove excess urine* by tapping the strip against the container's rim, wait for exactly 10 seconds, and then compare its color with the standardized color chart on the test strip container. Ignore color changes that occur after 10 seconds. Record the result.
- If you're using a Diastix strip, dip the reagent end of the strip into the urine specimen for 2 seconds. *Remove excess urine* by tapping the strip against the container's rim, wait for exactly 30 seconds, and then compare the strip's color with the standardized color chart on the test strip container. Ignore color changes that occur after 30 seconds. Record the result.

Ketone strip tests

- If you're using a Ketostix strip, dip the reagent end of the strip into the urine specimen and remove it immediately. *Remove excess urine* by tapping the strip against the container's rim, and hold the strip horizontally *to prevent mixing chemicals between two reagent squares.* Wait exactly 15 seconds, and then compare the color of the strip with the standardized color chart on the test strip container. Ignore color changes that occur after 15 seconds. Record the result.
- If you're using a Keto-Diastix strip, dip the reagent end of the strip into the urine specimen and remove it immediately. *Remove excess urine* by tapping the strip against the container's rim, and hold the strip horizontally *to prevent mixing of chemicals between the two reagent squares.* Wait exactly 15 seconds, and then compare the color of the ketone part of the strip with the standardized color chart on the test strip container. After 30 seconds, compare the color of the glucose part of the strip with the color chart. Record the result.

NURSING ALERT *Always be sure to read results during the correct timeframe, especially if you're conducting more than one test at a time.* Time intervals longer than those specified in the product insert can result in false-positive, false-negative, or invalid results because of exaggerated color development, fading of reaction products, and migration beyond a visible range.[3]

Completing the procedure

- Discard the urine specimen.
- Remove and discard your gloves.
- Perform hand hygiene.[4,5,6,7,8]
- Document the procedure and the test results.[12,13,14]

Special considerations

- If you're testing a refrigerated urine specimen, allow it to warm to room temperature and mix the specimen before testing.[15]

Documentation

Record the test results according to the information on the reagent containers, or use a flowchart designed to record this information. Indicate whether the practitioner was notified of the test results. If you're teaching a patient how to perform the test, keep a record of his progress. Also, record any treatment given as a result of the testing.[12]

REFERENCES

1 Arora, S., et al. (2011). Diagnostic accuracy of point-of-care testing for diabetic ketoacidosis at emergency-department triage: β-hydroxybutyrate versus the urine dipstick. *Diabetes Care, 34,* 852–854. Accessed May 2015 via the Web at http://www.ncbi.nlm.nih.gov/pmc/articles/PMC3064039/ (Level VI)

2 Chernecky, C. C., & Berger, B. J. (2013). *Laboratory tests and diagnostic procedures* (6th ed.). St. Louis, MO: Saunders.

3 Centers for Disease Control and Prevention. (2005). Good laboratory practices for waived testing sites: Survey findings from testing sites holding a certificate of waiver under the Clinical Laboratory Improvement Amendments of 1988 and Recommendations for Promoting Quality Testing. *MMWR Recommendations and Reports, 54*(RR-13), 1–25. Accessed May 2015 via the Web at http://www.cdc.gov/mmwr/PDF/rr/rr5413.pdf (Level II)

4 The Joint Commission. (2015). Standard NPSG.07.01.01. *Comprehensive accreditation manual for hospitals: The official handbook.* Oakbrook Terrace, IL: The Joint Commission. (Level VII)

5 Centers for Disease Control and Prevention. (2002). Guideline for hand hygiene in health-care settings: Recommendations of the Healthcare Infection Control Practices Advisory Committee and the HICPAC/SHEA/APIC/IDSA Hand Hygiene Task Force. *MMWR Recommendations and Reports, 51*(RR-16), 1–45. Accessed May 2015 via the Web at http://www.cdc.gov/mmwr/pdf/rr/rr5116.pdf (Level II)

6 World Health Organization. (2009). "WHO guidelines on hand hygiene in health care: First global patient safety challenge, clean care is safer care" [Online]. Accessed May 2015 via the Web at http://whqlibdoc.who.int/publications/2009/9789241597906_eng.pdf (Level IV)

7 Centers for Medicare & Medicaid Services, Department of Health and Human Services. (2014). Condition of participation: Infection control. 42 C.F.R. § 482.42.

8 American Osteopathic Association. (2014). Standard 07.01.21. *Healthcare Facilities Accreditation Program: Accreditation requirements for acute care hospitals.* Chicago, IL: American Osteopathic Association. (Level VII)

9 The Joint Commission. (2015). Standard NPSG.01.01.01. *Comprehensive accreditation manual for hospitals: The official handbook.* Oakbrook Terrace, IL: The Joint Commission. (Level VII)

10 American Osteopathic Association. (2014). Standard 07.01.10. *Healthcare Facilities Accreditation Program: Accreditation requirements for acute care hospitals.* Chicago, IL: American Osteopathic Association. (Level VII)

11 Siegel, J. D., et al. (2007). "2007 guideline for isolation precautions: Preventing transmission of infectious agents in healthcare settings" [Online]. Accessed May 2015 via the Web at http://www.cdc.gov/hicpac/pdf/isolation/Isolation2007.pdf (Level II)

12 The Joint Commission. (2015). Standard RC.01.03.01. *Comprehensive accreditation manual for hospitals: The official handbook.* Oakbrook Terrace, IL: The Joint Commission. (Level VII)

13 Centers for Medicare & Medicaid Services, Department of Health and Human Services. (2014). Condition of participation: Medical record services. 42 C.F.R. § 482.24(b).

14 American Osteopathic Association. (2014). Standard 10.00.03. *Healthcare Facilities Accreditation Program: Accreditation requirements for acute care hospitals.* Chicago, IL: American Osteopathic Association. (Level VII)

15 Fischbach, F., & Dunning, M. B. (2014). *A manual of laboratory and diagnostic tests* (9th ed.). Philadelphia, PA: Wolters Kluwer.

ADDITIONAL REFERENCES

American Diabetes Association. (2013). Standards of medical care in diabetes—2013. *Diabetes Care, 36,* S11–S66. Accessed May 2015 via the Web at http://care.diabetesjournals.org/content/36/Supplement_1/S11.full.pdf+html (Level II)

Craven, R. F., & Hirnle, C. J. (2012). *Fundamentals of nursing: Human health and function* (7th ed.). Philadelphia, PA: Lippincott Williams & Wilkins.

URINE PH

The pH of urine—its alkalinity or acidity—reflects the kidneys' ability to maintain a normal hydrogen ion concentration in plasma and extracellular fluids. The normal hydrogen ion concentration in urine varies, ranging from 4.6 to 8.0, but it usually averages around a pH of 6.0.

The simplest procedure for testing the pH of urine consists of dipping a reagent strip (such as Combistix) into a fresh specimen of the patient's urine and comparing the resulting color change with a standardized color chart.

An alkaline pH (above 7.0), resulting from a diet low in meat but high in vegetables, dairy products, and citrus fruits, causes turbidity and the formation of phosphate, carbonate, and amorphous crystals. Alkaline urine may also result from urinary tract infection, gastric suctioning, vomiting, and metabolic or respiratory alkalosis.

An acid pH (below 7.0), resulting from a high-protein diet and a diet high in cranberries, also causes turbidity as well as the formation of oxalate, cystine, amorphous urate, and uric acid crystals. Acidic urine may also result from renal tuberculosis, phenylketonuria, alkaptonuria, pyrexia, diarrhea, starvation, diabetic ketoacidosis, renal failure, and all forms of acidosis. Low urine pH is also associated with insulin resistance and metabolic syndrome.[1]

Measuring urine pH can also help monitor some medications—including methenamine, ammonium chloride, and such diuretics as thiazides—that are active only at certain pH levels.

Equipment

Clean-catch kit urine collection kit ▪ urine specimen container ▪ gloves ▪ reagent strips that include pH indicators ▪ reference color chart.

Preparation of equipment

Check the expiration dates on the reagent strips and discard them if they're expired. Allow time for refrigerated items, including reagents and patient specimens, to reach room temperature before testing, if specified in the product insert. Check and record lot numbers for test kits, test devices, and controls. (Don't mix reagents from different products or lot numbers. If you're using a new lot, set up quality control, as needed, and refer to the product insert for changes in control ranges.) Visually inspect the reagent vials and the strips within them for damage, discoloration, and contamination. Prepare and store reagents strips according to the manufacturer's instructions. If opening a new reagent strip vial or kit, write the date opened on the outside of the vial or test kit.[2,3]

Implementation

- Gather the appropriate equipment.
- Perform hand hygiene.[4,5,6,7,8]
- Confirm the patient's identity using at least two patient identifiers.[9]
- Explain the procedure to the patient.
- Put on gloves.[10,11]
- Provide the patient with a specimen container, and instruct him to collect a clean-catch midstream specimen. (See the "Urine specimen collection" procedure, page 817.)
- Dip the reagent strip into the urine, remove it, and tap off the reagent strip against the container's rim *to remove excess urine.*
- While holding the strip horizontally *to avoid mixing reagents from adjacent test areas on the strip,* compare the color on the strip with the standardized color chart on the strip package. This comparison can be made up to 60 seconds after immersing the strip.

NURSING ALERT *Always be sure to read results during the correct timeframe, especially if conducting more than one test at a time.* Time intervals longer than those specified in the product insert can result in false-positive, false-negative, or invalid results because of exaggerated color development, fading of reaction products, and migration beyond a visible range.[2]

- If you're monitoring the patient's intake and output, measure the amount of urine.
- Discard the urine specimen.
- Remove and discard your gloves.
- Perform hand hygiene.[4,5,6,7,8]
- Document the procedure.[12,13,14]

Special considerations

- Use only a fresh urine specimen *because bacterial growth at room temperature changes urine pH.*
- Avoid letting a drop of urine run onto adjacent reagent spots on the strip *because the other reagents can change the pH result.*
- Be aware that urine collected at night is usually more acidic than urine collected during the day.

Documentation

Record the test results, time of voiding, and amount voided, if applicable. Document any patient teaching performed and the patient's comprehension of the teaching.

REFERENCES

1 Maalouf, N. M. (2011). Metabolic syndrome and the genesis of uric acid stones. *Journal of Renal Nutrition, 21,* 128–131.

2 Centers for Disease Control and Prevention. (2005). Good laboratory practices for waived testing sites: Survey findings from testing sites holding a certificate of waiver under the Clinical Laboratory Improvement Amendments of 1988 and Recommendations for Promoting Quality Testing. *MMWR Recommendations and Reports, 54*(RR-13), 1–25. Accessed May 2015 via the Web at http://www.cdc.gov/mmwr/PDF/rr/rr5413.pdf (Level II)

3 Chernecky, C. C., & Berger, B. J. (2013). *Laboratory tests and diagnostic procedures* (6th ed.). St. Louis, MO: Saunders.

4 The Joint Commission. (2015). Standard NPSG.07.01.01. *Comprehensive accreditation manual for hospitals: The official handbook.* Oakbrook Terrace, IL: The Joint Commission. (Level VII)

5 Centers for Disease Control and Prevention. (2002). Guideline for hand hygiene in health-care settings: Recommendations of the Healthcare Infection Control Practices Advisory Committee and the HICPAC/SHEA/APIC/IDSA Hand Hygiene Task Force. *MMWR Recommendations and Reports, 51*(RR-16), 1–45. Accessed May 2015 via the Web at http://www.cdc.gov/mmwr/pdf/rr/rr5116.pdf (Level II)

6 World Health Organization. (2009). "WHO guidelines on hand hygiene in health care: First global patient safety challenge, clean care is safer care" [Online]. Accessed May 2015 via the Web at http://whqlibdoc.who.int/publications/2009/9789241597906_eng.pdf (Level IV)

7 American Osteopathic Association. (2014). Standard 07.01.21. *Healthcare Facilities Accreditation Program: Accreditation requirements for acute care hospitals.* Chicago, IL: American Osteopathic Association. (Level VII)

8 Centers for Medicare & Medicaid Services, Department of Health and Human Services. (2014). Condition of participation: Infection control. 42 C.F.R. § 482.42.

9 The Joint Commission. (2015). Standard NPSG.01.01.01. *Comprehensive accreditation manual for hospitals: The official handbook.* Oakbrook Terrace, IL: The Joint Commission. (Level VII)

10 American Osteopathic Association. (2014). Standard 07.01.10. *Healthcare Facilities Accreditation Program: Accreditation requirements for acute care hospitals.* Chicago, IL: American Osteopathic Association. (Level VII)

11 Siegel, J. D., et al. (2007). "2007 guideline for isolation precautions: Preventing transmission of infectious agents in healthcare settings" [Online]. Accessed May 2015 via the Web at http://www.cdc.gov/hicpac/pdf/isolation/Isolation2007.pdf (Level II)

12 The Joint Commission. (2015). Standard RC.01.03.01. *Comprehensive accreditation manual for hospitals: The official handbook.* Oakbrook Terrace, IL: The Joint Commission. (Level VII)

13 American Osteopathic Association. (2014). Standard 10.00.03. *Healthcare Facilities Accreditation Program: Accreditation requirements for acute care hospitals.* Chicago, IL: American Osteopathic Association. (Level VII)

14 Centers for Medicare & Medicaid Services, Department of Health and Human Services. (2014). Condition of participation: Medical record services. 42 C.F.R. § 482.24(b).

ADDITIONAL REFERENCES

Craven, R. F., & Hirnle, C. J. (2012). *Fundamentals of nursing: Human health and function* (7th ed.). Philadelphia, PA: Lippincott Williams & Wilkins.

Fischbach, F., & Dunning, M. B. (2014). *A manual of laboratory and diagnostic tests* (9th ed.). Philadelphia, PA: Wolters Kluwer.

URINE SPECIMEN COLLECTION

A random urine specimen is usually collected as part of the physical examination or at various times during hospitalization. This specimen permits laboratory screening for urinary and systemic disorders; it's also used for drug screening.

Clean-catch urine specimen collection, also called the *clean-catch midstream specimen method,* is commonly used in place of random specimen collection because it provides a virtually uncontaminated specimen without the need for catheterization. Obtaining a clean-catch midstream urine specimen also provides a specimen that more accurately indicates the constituents of the urine being produced by the body. The patient first voids a small amount of urine, then collects the specimen during midstream in a sterile specimen container, and then allows the last amount of urine to be discarded.

An indwelling urinary catheter specimen—obtained by aspiration with a syringe—requires maintaining a closed urinary drainage system and using sterile collection technique to prevent catheter-associated urinary tract infections.[1,2] This method is contraindicated after genitourinary surgery.

Equipment

For a random specimen

Bedpan or urinal with cover ▪ gloves ▪ specimen container with lid ▪ specimen label ▪ laboratory request form ▪ laboratory biohazard transport bag ▪ soap ▪ water ▪ washcloth ▪ Optional: specimen collection hat, graduated container, paper towels, ice-filled basin.

For a clean-catch midstream specimen

Soap and water ▪ washcloth ▪ gloves ▪ commercial clean-catch kit containing antiseptic towelettes and a sterile specimen container with lid and label ▪ laboratory request form ▪ laboratory biohazard transport bag ▪ Optional: graduated container, specimen collection hat, bedpan, bedside commode, sterile gloves, ice-filled basin.

If a commercially prepared kit isn't used, you'll need gloves, three sterile 2″ × 2″ (5-cm × 5-cm) gauze pads or cotton balls, antiseptic solution, a sterile towel, a specimen label, and a sterile specimen container with lid.

For an indwelling catheter specimen

Gloves ▪ antiseptic pad ▪ syringe (3-mL to 20-mL, depending on the volume of urine required for the ordered test) ▪ sterile or nonsterile specimen container with lid (depending on the ordered test) ▪ specimen label ▪ laboratory request form ▪ laboratory biohazard transport bag ▪ Optional: ice-filled basin.

Implementation

- Gather the appropriate equipment.
- Verify the practitioner's order for the urine specimen.
- Perform hand hygiene.[3,4,5,6,7]
- Confirm the patient's identity using at least two patient identifiers.[8]
- Explain the procedure and its purpose to the patient and his family, if necessary, *to promote cooperation and to prevent accidental disposal of specimens.*
- Provide privacy.[9,10]

Collecting a random specimen

- Instruct the patient on bed rest to void into a clean bedpan or urinal; instruct the ambulatory patient to void into a clean bedpan or urinal or into a specimen collection hat placed in the toilet in the bathroom.
- Put on gloves.[11,12] Then pour at least 120 mL of urine into the specimen container, and cap the container securely.
- If the patient's urine output must be measured and recorded, pour the remaining urine into the graduated container. Otherwise, discard the remaining urine. If you inadvertently spill urine on the outside of the container, clean and dry it *to prevent cross-contamination.*

Collecting a clean-catch midstream specimen, female

- Tell the patient to remove all clothing from the waist down.
- Instruct the patient to clean the periurethral area (labial folds, vulva, and urinary meatus) with a washcloth using soap and water. If the patient requires assistance, put on gloves[11,12] and assist the patient with cleaning the periurethral area. Then discard the gloves and perform hand hygiene.[3,4,5,6,7]
- If appropriate, assist the patient onto a bedpan or bedside commode or walk her to the bathroom.
- Instruct the patient to sit far back on the toilet seat or bedside commode and to spread her legs.
- Perform hand hygiene.[3,4,5,6,7]
- Using sterile technique, prepare the commercial kit or create a sterile field using the sterile towel. If assisting the patient, put on sterile gloves.[11] If not using a commercial kit, pour the antiseptic over the sterile 2″ × 2″ (5-cm × 5-cm) gauze pads or cotton balls.
- Open the sterile specimen container and place the cap down with the sterile inside surface facing up. Avoid touching the inside, and also instruct the patient to avoid touching the inside of the container *to prevent contamination of the specimen.*
- Instruct the patient to spread her labial folds with the thumb and forefinger of her nondominant hand and wipe the area three times, each time with a fresh antiseptic towelette or presoaked sterile 2″ × 2″ (5-cm × 5-cm) gauze pad or cotton ball. Assist as needed.
- Tell her or assist her to wipe down one side with the first pad and discard it, to wipe the other side with the second pad and discard it, and finally to wipe down the center over the urinary meatus with the third pad and discard it.
- Stress the importance of cleaning from front to back *to avoid contaminating the genital area with fecal matter.*
- Instruct the patient to straddle the bedpan, bedside commode, or toilet *to allow labial spreading and to keep her labia separated while voiding.* Assist as needed.
- Instruct the patient to begin voiding into the bedpan, bedside commode, or toilet *because the first urine voided washes microorganisms and cellular debris out of the meatus.*[13] Then, without stopping the urine stream, the patient (or you, if assisting) should move the collection container into the urine stream, collecting 30 to 50 mL at the midstream portion of the voiding.
- After she (or you, if assisting) has collected the specimen, tell the patient to move (or you, if assisting) the container out of the continuing urine stream and to finish voiding into the bedpan, bedside commode, or toilet.
- If you weren't assisting the patient, put on gloves[11,12] and take the sterile container from the patient.
- Cap the container securely. Avoid touching the inside of the container or the lid *to prevent contamination.* If the outside of the container is soiled, clean it and wipe it dry.
- If intake and output are being recorded, measure the remaining urine (from the first and last portions of the voiding) in a graduated container. Include the amount in the specimen container when recording the total amount voided.

Collecting a clean-catch midstream specimen, male

- Tell the patient to remove all clothing from the waist down.
- Instruct the patient clean the periurethral area (tip of the penis) with a washcloth using soap and water. If the patient requires assistance, put on gloves[11,12] and assist the patient with cleaning the periurethral area.
- If appropriate, assist the patient onto a bedpan, sit him on or stand him next to a bedside commode, or walk him to the bathroom. If the patient is able to stand and is using the bathroom toilet, instruct him to stand in front of the bowl as for urination. If the patient is unable to stand, tell him to sit far back on the toilet seat or bedside commode and to spread his legs.
- Perform hand hygiene.[3,4,5,6,7]
- Using sterile technique, prepare the commercial kit or create a sterile field using the sterile towel. If assisting the patient, put on sterile gloves.[11] If not using a commercial kit, pour antiseptic solution over the sterile 2″ × 2″ (5-cm × 5-cm) gauze pads or cotton balls.
- Open the sterile specimen container and place the cap with the sterile inside surface facing up. Avoid touching the inside, and also instruct the patient to avoid touching the inside of the container *to prevent contamination of the specimen.*
- Assist or have the patient hold his penis with one hand. Have the patient use the other hand to clean the meatus and head of the penis with the antiseptic towelettes or presoaked sterile 2″ × 2″ (5-cm × 5-cm) gauze pads or cotton balls. Instruct the uncircumcised male patient to retract his foreskin *to effectively clean the meatus* and to keep it retracted during voiding. Assist as needed.
- Instruct the patient to begin voiding into the bedpan, bedside commode, or toilet *because the first urine voided washes microorganisms and cellular debris from the urethra.*[13] Then, without stopping the urine stream, the patient (or you, if assisting) should move the collection container into the stream, collecting 30 to 50 mL at the midstream portion of the voiding.
- After he (or you, if assisting) has collected the specimen, tell him to move (or you, if assisting) the container out of the continuing urine stream and to finish voiding into the bedpan, bedside commode, or toilet.
- If you weren't assisting the patient, put on gloves[11,12] and take the sterile container from the patient.
- Cap the container securely. Avoid touching the inside of the container or the lid *to prevent contamination.* If the outside of the container is soiled, clean it and wipe it dry.
- If intake and output are being recorded, measure the remaining urine (from the first and last portions of the voiding) in a graduated container. Include the amount in the specimen container when recording the total amount voided.

Collecting an indwelling catheter specimen

- Perform hand hygiene[3,4,5,6,7] and put on gloves.[11,12]
- Drain urine from the drainage tube into the collection bag.
- Disinfect the sampling port with an antiseptic pad and allow it to dry.[1]
- Attach the syringe to the port. When fresh urine appears in the tubing, aspirate the specimen into the syringe.
- Slowly transfer the specimen to the appropriate container and secure the lid.
- Dispose of the syringe in an appropriate receptacle.[11]

Completing the procedure

- Remove and discard your gloves.[11]
- Perform hand hygiene,[3,4,5,6,7] and have the patient also perform handwashing.
- Label the specimen container with the patient's name and identification number, the collection time, and the date in the presence of the patient *to avoid mislabeling.*[13]
- Place the specimen in a laboratory biohazard transport bag[14] and send it to the laboratory with the laboratory request form immediately or place it on ice if transport may be delayed. If a urine culture is to be performed, make sure you list current antibiotic therapy on the laboratory request form.[1]
- Perform hand hygiene.[3,4,5,6,7]
- Document the procedure.[15,16,17]

Special considerations

- If the specimen is to be collected at home, instruct the patient to collect the specimen in the appropriate container with a tight-fitting lid and to keep it on ice or in the refrigerator (separate from food items) for up to 24 hours. *Specimens are stable at room temperature for only 1 hour.*
- If a large volume of urine is needed for special analyses (not culture), obtain the urine specimen directly from the indwelling urinary catheter drainage bag, not the sampling port.[1]
- Be aware that some urinary drainage collection bag outlet tubes are coated with an antimicrobial agent that can interfere with the results of a urine culture if the specimen is obtained directly from the drainage bag.

Documentation

Record the time of specimen collection and when the specimen was transported to the laboratory. Specify the test as well as the appearance, odor, color, and any unusual characteristics of the specimen. If necessary, record the urine volume on the intake and output record.

REFERENCES

1 Healthcare Infection Control Practices Advisory Committee. (2010). "Guideline for prevention of catheter-associated urinary tract infections, 2009" [Online]. Accessed May 2015 via the Web at http://www.cdc.gov/hicpac/pdf/CAUTI/CAUTIguideline2009final.pdf (Level I)

2 The Joint Commission. (2015). Standard NPSG.07.06.01. *Comprehensive accreditation manual for hospitals: The official handbook.* Oakbrook Terrace, IL: The Joint Commission. (Level VII)

3 Centers for Disease Control and Prevention. (2002). Guideline for hand hygiene in health-care settings: Recommendations of the Healthcare Infection Control Practices Advisory Committee and the HICPAC/SHEA/APIC/IDSA Hand Hygiene Task Force. *MMWR Recommendations and Reports, 51*(RR-16), 1–45. Accessed May 2015 via the Web athttp://www.cdc.gov/mmwr/pdf/rr/rr5116.pdf (Level II)

4 World Health Organization. (2009). "WHO guidelines on hand hygiene in health care: First global patient safety challenge, clean care is safer care" [Online]. Accessed May 2015 via the Web at http://whqlibdoc.who.int/publications/2009/9789241597906_eng.pdf (Level IV)

5 The Joint Commission. (2015). Standard NPSG.07.01.01. *Comprehensive accreditation manual for hospitals: The official handbook.* Oakbrook Terrace, IL: The Joint Commission. (Level VII)

6 American Osteopathic Association. (2014). Standard 07.01.21. *Healthcare Facilities Accreditation Program: Accreditation requirements for acute care hospitals.* Chicago, IL: American Osteopathic Association. (Level VII)

7 Centers for Medicare & Medicaid Services, Department of Health and Human Services. (2014). Condition of participation: Infection control. 42 C.F.R. § 482.42.

8 The Joint Commission. (2015). Standard NPSG.01.01.01. *Comprehensive accreditation manual for hospitals: The official handbook.* Oakbrook Terrace, IL: The Joint Commission. (Level VII)

9 American Osteopathic Association. (2014). Standard 15.01.16. *Healthcare Facilities Accreditation Program: Accreditation requirements for acute care hospitals.* Chicago, IL: American Osteopathic Association. (Level VII)

10 Centers for Medicare & Medicaid Services, Department of Health and Human Services. (2014). Condition of participation: Patient's rights. 42 C.F.R. § 482.13(c)(1).

11 Siegel, J. D., et al. (2007). "2007 guideline for isolation precautions: Preventing transmission of infectious agents in healthcare settings" [Online]. Accessed May 2015 via the Web athttp://www.cdc.gov/hicpac/pdf/isolation/Isolation2007.pdf (Level II)

12 Craven, R. F., & Hirnle, C. J. (2012). *Fundamentals of nursing: Human health and function* (7th ed.). Philadelphia, PA: Lippincott Williams & Wilkins.
13 American Osteopathic Association. (2014). Standard 07.01.10. *Healthcare Facilities Accreditation Program: Accreditation requirements for acute care hospitals.* Chicago, IL: American Osteopathic Association. (Level VII)
14 Occupational Safety and Health Administration. (n.d.). "Bloodborne pathogens, standard number 1910.1030" [Online]. Accessed May 2015 via the Web athttp://www.osha.gov/pls/oshaweb/owadisp.show_document?p_table=STANDARDS&p_id=10051(Level VII)
15 The Joint Commission. (2015). Standard RC.01.03.01. *Comprehensive accreditation manual for hospitals: The official handbook.* Oakbrook Terrace, IL: The Joint Commission. (Level VII)
16 Centers for Medicare & Medicaid Services, Department of Health and Human Services. (2014). Condition of participation: Medical record services. 42 C.F.R. § 482.24(b).
17 American Osteopathic Association. (2014). Standard 10.00.03. *Healthcare Facilities Accreditation Program: Accreditation requirements for acute care hospitals.* Chicago, IL: American Osteopathic Association. (Level VII)

Additional references

Fischbach, F., & Dunning, M. B. (2014). *A manual of laboratory and diagnostic tests* (9th ed.). Philadelphia, PA: Wolters Kluwer.
Nettina, S. M. (2014). *Lippincott manual of nursing practice* (10th ed.). Philadelphia, PA: Wolters Kluwer.

Urine straining, for calculi

Renal calculi, or kidney stones, may develop anywhere in the urinary tract. They may be excreted with the urine or become lodged in the urinary tract, causing hematuria, urine retention, renal colic and, possibly, hydronephrosis.

Ranging in size from microscopic to several centimeters, calculi form in the kidneys when mineral salts—principally calcium oxalate or calcium phosphate—collect around a nucleus of bacterial cells, blood clots, or other particles. Other substances involved in calculus formation include uric acid, xanthine, and ammonia.

Renal calculi result from many causes, including hypercalcemia (which may occur with hyperparathyroidism, excessive dietary intake of calcium, and prolonged immobility), abnormal urine pH levels, dehydration, hyperuricemia associated with gout, and some hereditary disorders. Most commonly, calculi form as a result of urine stasis stemming from dehydration (which concentrates urine), benign prostatic hyperplasia, neurologic disorders, or urethral strictures.

Testing for the presence of calculi requires careful straining of all of the patient's urine through a gauze pad or fine-mesh sieve and, at times, quantitative laboratory analysis of questionable specimens. Such testing typically continues until the patient passes the calculi or until surgery, as ordered.

Equipment

■ Fine-mesh sieve or 4″ × 4″ (10-cm × 10-cm) gauze pad ■ graduated collection container ■ specimen label ■ gloves ■ urinal or bedpan ■ rubber band ■ laboratory request form ■ three patient-care reminders stating STRAIN ALL URINE ■ specimen container ■ biohazard laboratory transport bag.

Implementation

- Gather all necessary equipment.
- Perform hand hygiene.[1,2,3,4,5]
- Confirm the patient's identity using at least two patient identifiers.[6]
- Explain the procedure to the patient and his family, if possible, *to ensure cooperation and to stress the importance of straining all of the patient's urine.*
- Post patient-care reminders stating STRAIN ALL URINE over the patient's bed, in his bathroom, and on the collection container.
- Tell the patient to notify you after each voiding.
- If a commercial strainer isn't available, unfold a 4″ × 4″ (10-cm × 10-cm) gauze pad, place it over the top of a graduated collection container, and secure it with a rubber band.
- Leave the urinal or bedpan within the patient's reach.
- After the patient voids, put on gloves.[7,8]
- With the strainer secured over the mouth of the collection container, pour the specimen from the urinal or bedpan into the container. If the patient has an indwelling catheter in place, strain all urine from the collection bag before discarding it.
- Examine the strainer for calculi. If you detect calculi or if the filter looks questionable, notify the practitioner and place the filtrate in a specimen container.
- Label the specimen in the presence of the patient *to prevent mislabeling.*[6]
- Send the specimen to the laboratory in a biohazard laboratory transport bag with a laboratory request form.[9]
- If the strainer is intact, rinse it carefully and reuse it. If it has become damaged, discard it and replace it with a new strainer.
- Remove and discard your gloves.
- Perform hand hygiene.[1,2,3,4,5]
- Document the procedure.[10,11,12]

Special considerations

- Save and send to the laboratory any small or suspicious-looking residue in the specimen container *because even tiny calculi can cause hematuria and pain.*
- Don't leave calculi in contact with urine or other fluids *because this contact may alter the results of the analysis.*
- Be aware that calculi may appear in various colors, each of which has diagnostic value.

Patient teaching

If the patient will be straining his urine at home, teach him how to use a strainer and emphasize the importance of straining all his urine for the prescribed period.

Documentation

Document the date and time of the specimen collection as well as transport to the laboratory, if applicable. Note the characteristics of the urine and any filtrate passed. Also note pain or hematuria that occurred during voiding.

References

1 Centers for Disease Control and Prevention. (2002). Guideline for hand hygiene in health-care settings: Recommendations of the Healthcare Infection Control Practices Advisory Committee and the HICPAC/SHEA/APIC/IDSA Hand Hygiene Task Force. *MMWR Recommendations and Reports, 51*(RR-16), 1–45. Accessed May 2015 via the Web at http://www.cdc.gov/mmwr/pdf/rr/rr5116.pdf (Level II)
2 The Joint Commission. (2015). Standard NPSG.07.01.01. *Comprehensive accreditation manual for hospitals: The official handbook.* Oakbrook Terrace, IL: The Joint Commission. (Level VII)
3 World Health Organization. (2009). "WHO guidelines on hand hygiene in health care: First global patient safety challenge, clean care is safer care" [Online]. Accessed May 2015 via the Web at http://whqlibdoc.who.int/publications/2009/9789241597906_eng.pdf (Level IV)
4 American Osteopathic Association. (2014). Standard 07.01.21. *Healthcare Facilities Accreditation Program: Accreditation requirements for acute care hospitals.* Chicago, IL: American Osteopathic Association. (Level VII)
5 Centers for Medicare & Medicaid Services, Department of Health and Human Services. (2014). Condition of participation: Infection control. 42 C.F.R. § 482.42.

6 The Joint Commission. (2015). Standard NPSG.01.01.01. *Comprehensive accreditation manual for hospitals: The official handbook.* Oakbrook Terrace, IL: The Joint Commission. (Level VII)

7 American Osteopathic Association. (2014). Standard 07.01.10. *Healthcare Facilities Accreditation Program: Accreditation requirements for acute care hospitals.* Chicago, IL: American Osteopathic Association. (Level VII)

8 Siegel, J. D., et al. (2007). "2007 guideline for isolation precautions: Preventing transmission of infectious agents in healthcare settings" [Online]. Accessed May 2015 via the Web at http://www.cdc.gov/hicpac/pdf/isolation/Isolation2007.pdf (Level II)

9 Occupational Safety and Health Administration. (n.d.). "Bloodborne pathogens, standard number 1910.1030" [Online]. Accessed May 2015 via the Web at http://www.osha.gov/pls/oshaweb/owadisp.show_document?p_table=standards&p_id=10051 (Level VII)

10 The Joint Commission. (2015). Standard RC.01.03.01. *Comprehensive accreditation manual for hospitals: The official handbook.* Oakbrook Terrace, IL: The Joint Commission. (Level VII)

11 American Osteopathic Association. (2014). Standard 10.00.03. *Healthcare Facilities Accreditation Program: Accreditation requirements for acute care hospitals.* Chicago, IL: American Osteopathic Association. (Level VII)

12 Centers for Medicare & Medicaid Services, Department of Health and Human Services. (2014). Condition of participation: Medical record services. 42 C.F.R. § 482.24(b).

V

VAGINAL MEDICATION ADMINISTRATION

Vaginal medications include creams, gels, ointments, and suppositories. They can serve as a contraceptive or topical treatment for infection (caused by *Trichomonas vaginalis* or *Candida*) or inflammation.

Vaginal medications usually come with an applicator that allows placement of medication in the anterior and posterior fornices. Administration is most effective when the patient can remain lying down afterward to retain the medication.

Vaginal suppositories can also be inserted as a topical treatment for infection or inflammation. Suppositories melt when they come into contact with the vaginal mucosa, and their medication diffuses topically as effectively as creams, gels, and ointments.

Equipment

Prescribed medication ▪ applicator ▪ water-soluble lubricant ▪ gloves ▪ small sanitary pad ▪ fluid-impermeable pad ▪ washcloth ▪ soap ▪ Optional: labels.

Implementation

- Avoid distractions and interruptions when preparing and administering medications *to prevent medication administration errors.*[1,2]
- Gather the necessary equipment.
- Verify the practitioner's order.[3,4]
- Compare the medication label with the order in the patient's medical record.[3,4]
- Check the patient's medical record for an allergy or a contraindication to the prescribed medication. If an allergy or a contraindication exists, don't administer the medication; notify the practitioner.[3,4]
- Check the expiration date on the medication. If the medication is expired, return it to the pharmacy and obtain new medication.[3,4]
- Visually inspect the medication for signs of loss of integrity; if its integrity is compromised, return it to the pharmacy.[3,4]
- Discuss any unresolved concerns about the medication with the patient's practitioner.[3,4]
- Perform hand hygiene.[5,6,7,8,9]
- Confirm the patient's identity using at least two patient identifiers.[4,10]
- Provide privacy and explain the procedure to the patient.[11,12]
- If the patient is receiving the medication for the first time, teach her about potential adverse effects and discuss any other concerns related to the medication.[3,4]
- Verify that the medication is being administered to the correct patient, at the proper time, in the prescribed dose, and by the correct route and that its indication is appropriate for the patient's condition *to prevent medication administration errors.*[3,4]
- Ask the patient to void.
- If your facility uses a bar code scanning system, scan your identification badge, the patient's identification bracelet, and the medication's bar code.
- Ask the patient if she would rather insert the medication herself. If so, provide appropriate instructions.
- If you're inserting the medication, proceed with the following steps.
- Put on gloves.
- Help the patient into the lithotomy position or the supine position with the knees bent, and expose the perineum.
- Place a fluid-impermeable pad underneath the patient.
- Wash the vaginal orifice using a washcloth and warm water, wiping from front to back

Administration of vaginal creams, gels, and ointments

- Insert the plunger into the applicator. Then attach the applicator to the tube of medication.
- Gently squeeze the tube to fill the applicator with the prescribed amount of medication. Detach the applicator from the tube, and lubricate the applicator or apply a small amount of ointment to the outside of the applicator.
- Expose the vagina by spreading the labia with your fingers.
- Insert the applicator as you would a small suppository, and administer the medication by depressing the plunger on the applicator. Then remove the applicator. (See *How to insert a vaginal cream, gel, or ointment.*)
- Cover the patient *to promote dignity and comfort.*
- Remove and discard your gloves[14,15] and perform hand hygiene.[5,6,7,8,9]
- Put on gloves[14,15] and wash the applicator with soap and warm water.[16]

If the applicator can be used again, label it with the proper patient identifiers *so that it will be used only for the same patient,* and store it. Alternatively, if the applicator is disposable, discard it in the appropriate container.

Administration of a vaginal suppository

- Remove the suppository from the wrapper and lubricate it with water-soluble lubricant.
- Expose the vagina by spreading the labia.
- With an applicator or the forefinger of your free hand, insert the suppository about 2″ (5 cm) into the vagina.

Completing the procedure

- Remove and discard your gloves.[14] Perform hand hygiene.[5,6,7,8,9]
- *To prevent the medication from soiling the patient's clothing and bedding,* provide a sanitary pad.
- Help the patient return to a comfortable position, and advise her to remain in bed as much as possible for the next several hours.
- Document the procedure.[17,18,19]

Special considerations

- If possible, plan to insert vaginal medications at bedtime, *when the patient is most likely to be recumbent.*

Patient teaching

If needed, teach the patient how to insert the vaginal medication *because she may have to administer it herself after discharge.* Give her a patient-teaching sheet if one is available. Instruct the patient not to wear a tampon after inserting vaginal medication *because it would absorb the medication and decrease its effectiveness.* Also, instruct her to avoid sexual intercourse during treatment.

Complications

Vaginal medications may cause local irritation.

Documentation

Record the medication administered as well as the time and date. Note adverse reactions; the date, time, and name of the practitioner notified; prescribed interventions; and the patient's response to those interventions. Document patient teaching and the patient's understanding of your teaching.

How to insert a vaginal cream, gel, or ointment

Fill the applicator with the prescribed amount of medication. Then lubricate the applicator, hold it by the cylinder, and insert it into the vagina. *To ensure the patient's comfort,* direct the applicator down initially, toward the spine, and then up and back, toward the cervix (as shown below).

Administer the medication by depressing the plunger. Remove the applicator while the plunger is still depressed.

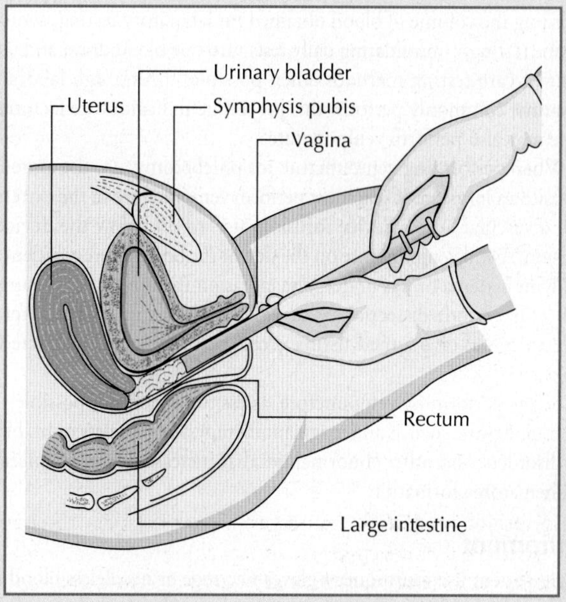

REFERENCES

1 Westbrook, J., et al. (2010). Association of interruptions with an increased risk and severity of medication administration errors. *Archives of Internal Medicine, 170,* 683–690. (Level IV)

2 Institute for Safe Medication Practices. (2012). Side tracks on the safety express: Interruptions lead to errors and unfinished...Wait, what was I doing? *Nurse Advise-ERR, 11*(2), 1–4. Accessed May 2015 via the Web at https://www.ismp.org/Newsletters/acutecare/showarticle.aspx?id=37

3 The Joint Commission. (2015). Standard MM.06.01.01. *Comprehensive accreditation manual for hospitals: The official handbook.* Oakbrook Terrace, IL: The Joint Commission. (Level VII)

4 American Osteopathic Association. (2014). Standard 16.01.03. *Healthcare Facilities Accreditation Program: Accreditation requirements for acute care hospitals.* Chicago, IL: American Osteopathic Association. (Level VII)

5 The Joint Commission. (2015). Standard NPSG.07.01.01. *Comprehensive accreditation manual for hospitals: The official handbook.* Oakbrook Terrace, IL: The Joint Commission. (Level VII)

6 Centers for Disease Control and Prevention. (2002). Guideline for hand hygiene in health-care settings: Recommendations of the Healthcare Infection Control Practices Advisory Committee and the HICPAC/SHEA/APIC/IDSA Hand Hygiene Task Force. *MMWR Recommendations and Reports, 51*(RR-16), 1–45. Accessed May 2015 via the Web at http://www.cdc.gov/mmwr/pdf/rr/rr5116.pdf (Level II)

7 World Health Organization. (2009). "WHO guidelines on hand hygiene in health care: First global patient safety challenge, clean care is safer care" [Online]. Accessed May 2015 via the Web at http://whqlibdoc.who.int/publications/2009/9789241597906_eng.pdf (Level IV)

8 American Osteopathic Association. (2014). Standard 07.01.21. *Healthcare Facilities Accreditation Program: Accreditation requirements for acute care hospitals.* Chicago, IL: American Osteopathic Association. (Level VII)

9 Centers for Medicare & Medicaid Services, Department of Health and Human Services. (2014). Condition of participation: Infection control. 42 C.F.R. § 482.42.

10 The Joint Commission. (2015). Standard NPSG.01.01.01. *Comprehensive accreditation manual for hospitals: The official handbook.* Oakbrook Terrace, IL: The Joint Commission. (Level VII)

11 American Osteopathic Association. (2014). Standard 15.01.16. *Healthcare Facilities Accreditation Program: Accreditation requirements for acute care hospitals.* Chicago, IL: American Osteopathic Association. (Level VII)

12 Centers for Medicare & Medicaid Services, Department of Health and Human Services. (2014). Condition of participation: Patient's rights. 42 C.F.R. § 482.13(c)(1).

13 The Joint Commission. (2015). Standard MM.06.01.03. *Comprehensive accreditation manual for hospitals: The official handbook.* Oakbrook Terrace, IL: The Joint Commission. (Level VII)

14 Siegel, J. D., et al. (2007). "2007 guideline for isolation precautions: Preventing transmission of infectious agents in healthcare settings" [Online]. Accessed May 2015 via the Web at http://www.cdc.gov/hicpac/pdf/isolation/Isolation2007.pdf (Level II)

15 American Osteopathic Association. (2014). Standard 07.01.10. *Healthcare Facilities Accreditation Program: Accreditation requirements for acute care hospitals.* Chicago, IL: American Osteopathic Association. (Level VII)

16 American Osteopathic Association. (2014). Standard 07.02.03. *Healthcare Facilities Accreditation Program: Accreditation requirements for acute care hospitals.* Chicago, IL: American Osteopathic Association. (Level VII)

17 The Joint Commission. (2015). Standard RC.01.03.01. *Comprehensive accreditation manual for hospitals: The official handbook.* Oakbrook Terrace, IL: The Joint Commission. (Level VII)

18 American Osteopathic Association. (2014). Standard 10.00.03. *Healthcare Facilities Accreditation Program: Accreditation requirements for acute care hospitals.* Chicago, IL: American Osteopathic Association. (Level VII)

19 Centers for Medicare & Medicaid Services, Department of Health and Human Services. (2014). Condition of participation: Medical record services. 42 C.F.R. § 482.24(b).

ADDITIONAL REFERENCES

Nettina, S. M. (2014). *Lippincott manual of nursing practice* (10th ed.). Philadelphia, PA: Wolters Kluwer.

Taylor, C., et al. (2015). *Fundamentals of nursing: The art and science of nursing care* (8th ed.). Philadelphia, PA: Wolters Kluwer.

VENIPUNCTURE

Performed to obtain a venous blood sample, venipuncture involves piercing a vein with a needle and collecting blood in an evacuated tube or syringe. If collected using a syringe, blood should be transferred cautiously to the appropriate tubes using a needleless device to prevent needlestick injury. Depressing the syringe plunger during transfer can create positive pressure, displacing the stopper and potentially resulting in exposure to the patient's blood. Using a syringe may also result in overfilling or underfilling of tubes with blood, leading to inaccurate test results.[1]

The most commonly used veins for venipuncture for phlebotomy include the median cubital, the cephalic, and the basilic veins in the antecubital area. Only the volume of blood needed for accurate testing should be obtained because phlebotomy contributes to iron deficiency and blood loss in critically ill patients. Measures to conserve the patient's blood include using low-volume blood collection tubes when possible, recording the volume of blood obtained for laboratory testing, avoiding routine testing, consolidating daily tests into one blood draw, and using point-of-care testing methods when possible.[2,3] Although laboratory personnel commonly perform this procedure in health care facilities, a nurse may also perform venipuncture.

When performing venipuncture for phlebotomy, use the extremity opposite an infusion. If you must perform venipuncture in the extremity with a vascular access device infusion, use a vein below the device or infusion. Avoid venipuncture on the side of the body where a patient has had lymphedema or has undergone radiation therapy or breast surgery with axillary node dissection. Also avoid venipuncture in an extremity with an actual or planned fistula access or that has been affected by stroke.[2,3]

Before performing venipuncture, assess the patient for possible risks of venipuncture, such as anticoagulant therapy, low platelet count, bleeding disorders, and other abnormalities that increase the risk of bleeding and hematoma formation.

Equipment

Single-patient use tourniquet ■ gloves ■ syringe or needleless blood collection tube holder ■ appropriate antiseptic swab (alcohol, tincture of iodine, chlorhexidine)[4] ■ evacuated blood collection tubes ■ venipuncture needle (21G to 23G) or winged collection device (21G, 23G, or 25G) ■ labels ■ laboratory transport bag ■ 2″ × 2″ (5-cm × 5-cm) gauze pads ■ adhesive bandage ■ Optional: needleless device, ice or cold pack, laboratory request form, sterile gloves, gown, mask with face shield or mask and goggles.

Preparation of equipment

If you're using evacuated tubes, open the needle packet or winged collection device and attach the needle or winged device to the needle holder. If you're using a syringe, attach the appropriate needle to it. Be sure to choose a syringe large enough to hold all the blood required for the test. Gather the appropriate collection tubes for the ordered laboratory tests. (See *Collection tube guide.*) Check the expiration date on the blood collection tubes; obtain a new tube if any are expired. Inspect the collection tube additives; don't use the collection tubes if additives are discolored. Gently tap collection tubes containing additives *to dislodge any material that may be adhering to the stopper.* Inspect the needle *to make sure its integrity is intact.*[1]

Implementation

- Review the patient's medical record for allergies to antiseptic, adhesive, and latex (if used in your facility). Use an alternative product if necessary *to avoid adverse reactions.*[8]
- Verify the practitioner's order.
- Check the labels *to verify the patient and testing information.* If a requisition form is also needed, verify the information.
- Gather the appropriate equipment.
- Perform hand hygiene and put on gloves or sterile gloves and other personal protective equipment needed *to comply with standard precautions.*[7,9,10,11,12,13,14,15,16]
- Confirm the patient's identity using at least two patient identifiers.[7,17]
- Tell the patient that you're about to take a blood sample; then explain the procedure *to ease his anxiety and ensure his cooperation.* Ask him if he's ever felt faint, sweaty, or nauseated when having blood drawn *to prepare to manage a vasovagal reaction in the patient at risk.*[2]
- If fasting was required for an ordered test, confirm that the patient has fasted.[2] Some tests require other dietary restrictions, so verify that such restrictions were implemented if applicable.
- If the patient is on bed rest, ask him to lie in the supine position, with his head slightly elevated and his arms at his sides. Ask the ambulatory patient to sit in a chair, and support his arm securely on an armrest or table.[7] If possible, position the patient's arm in a dependent position.[3]
- Assess the patient's veins *to determine the best puncture site and needle size.* (See *Common venipuncture sites,* page 824.) Limit 25G needles to situations in which veins are too fragile to use a larger-sized needle; however, keep in mind that improper technique may cause hemolysis.
- Assess the patient for such factors as easy bruising, increased risk of bleeding, compromised circulation, and fragile veins or skin, *which indicate that you should either not apply a tourniquet or apply it loosely.*[18]
- Apply a tourniquet, if appropriate, at an adequate location (about 2″ [5 cm] above the intended insertion site).[7] Apply the tourniquet in such a manner so that you can easily palpate an arterial pulse distal to the tourniquet *to prevent circulatory impairment.*[18]
- If the tourniquet fails to dilate the vein, have the patient open and close his fist while you lightly stroke the vein downward *to promote vascular distention.*[19] Don't have the patient pump his fist *because doing so may adversely affect test results.*[20]
- Clean the venipuncture site with an antiseptic swab according to the manufacturer's instructions and allow it to dry completely before performing venipuncture.[3,4] Don't touch the intended venipuncture site after preparation unless you're wearing sterile gloves *to prevent contamination.*[19]

NURSING ALERT *Don't use an alcohol-based antiseptic to clean the venipuncture site if you're collecting samples for blood alcohol testing.*[1]

- Immobilize the vein by pressing 1″ to 2″ (2.5 to 5 cm) below the venipuncture site with your thumb and drawing the skin taut.
- Position the needle holder or syringe with the needle bevel up and the shaft parallel to the path of the vein and at a 30-degree angle to the arm. If you're using a winged collection device attached to a needle holder, grasp the wings and position the bevel up. Insert the needle into the vein. If you're using a syringe, venous blood will appear in the hub; withdraw the blood slowly, pulling the plunger of the syringe gently *to create steady suction* until you obtain the required sample. *Pulling the plunger too forcibly may collapse the vein.* If you're using a needle holder and an evacuated tube, grasp the holder securely *to stabilize it in the vein,* and push down on the collection tube until the needle punctures the rubber stopper. Blood will flow into the tube automatically.[7]
- If you're using a winged collection set and a coagulation tube is the first specimen tube to be drawn, draw a discard tube first. The discard tube is used to fill the blood collection set tubing's dead space with blood *to ensure proper blood-to-additive ratio in the coagulation tube.* The discard tube doesn't need to be completely filled; the dead space just needs to be cleared.[1]
- Remove the tourniquet as soon as blood appears in the tube or syringe *to prevent stasis and hemoconcentration, which can impair test results.*[18] The time the tourniquet is left on the arm shouldn't exceed 1 minute.[7,20]
- When the first tube has filled to its stated volume and blood flow ceases, remove it from the holder. Continue to fill the required tubes using the correct order of draw, removing one and inserting another. Gently invert each tube and then return it to an upright position as you remove it *to help mix the additive with the sample.*[17] This counts as one complete inversion.

EQUIPMENT

Collection tube guide[1,5,6,7]

Blood collection tubes come in various sizes; they're filled by vacuum when a needle is inserted through the stopper. The tube type and the test the tube is intended for determine the amount of blood collected in each tube. The maximum draw volume for each size tube is commonly indicated by a mark (which is the same color as the stopper or closure) that you'll see at the top of the label when you hold the tube upright. Filling the tube to 50% capacity is sufficient for most testing; however, for coagulation studies, you must completely fill the tube *to ensure accurate test results.*[6]

Most tube types contain additives in varying concentrations. When performing venipuncture, make sure you obtain samples in the correct order *because contamination from the additive in the previous collection tube can cause erroneous test results.* You'll also need to mix the additive in the tube with the blood sample immediately after drawing the blood; to do so, hold the tube upright and gently invert it 180 degrees and back. The number of times you need to invert the tube varies by tube type.

The table below shows the recommended order of draw for commonly used collection tubes, the stopper or closure color, the typical laboratory studies performed, and the number of tube inversion needed to mix the sample. Consult with laboratory about less commonly ordered testing.

ORDER OF DRAW	COLLECTION TUBE TYPE	STOPPER OR CLOSURE COLOR	LABORATORY STUDIES	NUMBER OF INVERSIONS
1	Blood culture or other sterile test	▪ Blood culture bottles (no color)	▪ Blood culture	8 to 10
2	Citrate	▪ Blue stopper (tube must be filled completely)	▪ Coagulation studies	3 to 4
3	Gel, serum	▪ Red and black stopper ▪ Gold closure	▪ Serum chemistry ▪ Routine blood donor screening	5
4	No gel, serum	▪ Red stopper or closure	▪ Serum chemistry ▪ Routine blood donor screening	5 (glass), none (plastic)
5	Heparin	▪ Green stopper or closure ▪ Green and gray stopper or light green closure	▪ Plasma chemistry	8 to 10
6	EDTA	▪ Lavender stopper or closure ▪ Pink stopper or closure	▪ Whole blood hematology ▪ Routine immunohematology and blood donor screening ▪ Cross-matching (pink stopper or closure; tube contains special label for required blood bank information)	8 to 10
7	Potassium EDTA	▪ White closure	▪ Molecular diagnostic testing	8 to 10
8	Sodium fluoride	▪ Gray stopper or closure	▪ Glucose testing	8 to 10

- After you've drawn the sample, place a gauze pad over the puncture site, and slowly and gently remove the needle from the vein. When you're using an evacuated tube, remove it from the needle holder *to release the vacuum* before withdrawing the needle from the vein.
- Activate the needle protector safety device if necessary.[7]
- Apply gentle pressure to the puncture site for 2 or 3 minutes or until bleeding stops. *This prevents extravasation into the surrounding tissue, which can cause a hematoma.*[7]
- After bleeding stops, apply an adhesive bandage.[7]
- If you've used a syringe, transfer the sample to a collection tube immediately using a needleless device. Be careful to avoid foaming, *which can cause hemolysis.*[7]
- *To make sure that tube additives are properly mixed with the blood sample,* carefully invert each tube the appropriate number of times indicated by the tube's additive. Don't shake the collection tubes; *vigorous mixing may causing foaming and hemolysis.*[1,6,7]
- Label all specimens in the presence of the patient *to prevent mislabeling.*[17] Label the specimens with the patient's name and identification number, the practitioner's name, date and time of collection, and your initials if required.[7,17] If you're obtaining a blood bank specimen, sign the collection tube label if required by your facility.
- Place all tubes in a laboratory biohazard transport bag.[9]
- Discard syringes, needles, and used supplies in the appropriate containers.[9,21]
- Check the venipuncture site *to see if a hematoma has developed.* If it has, apply pressure until you are sure the bleeding has stopped; then you may apply warm soaks to the site *to help reabsorption.*[7]
- Remove and discard your gloves and any other personal protective equipment worn.[9,10,11]
- Perform hand hygiene.[10,11,12,13,14,15]
- Send the specimen tubes and the completed laboratory request form (if used in your facility) to the laboratory in a laboratory transport bag.

Common venipuncture sites

The illustrations below show the anatomic locations of veins commonly used for venipuncture. The most commonly used sites are on the forearm, followed by those on the hand.

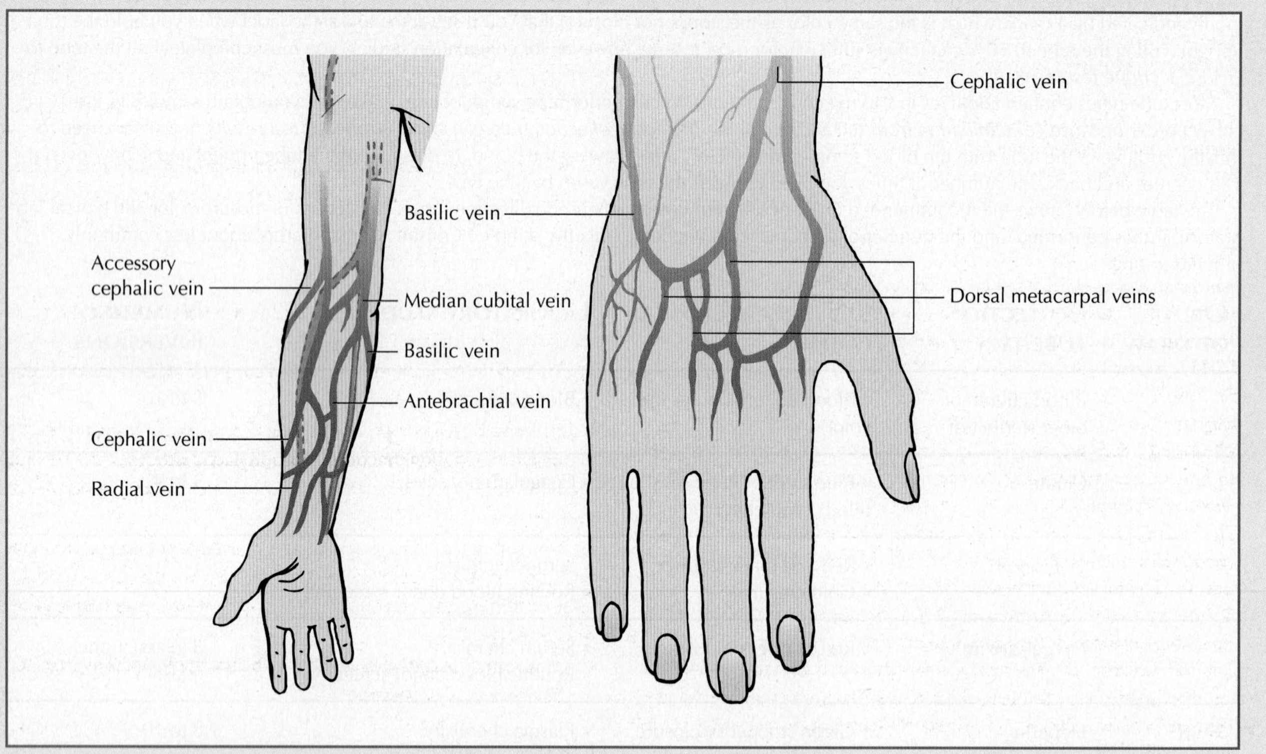

- Provide ice or a cold pack for transport if required; *coagulation studies may require ice or a cold pack for transport.*
- Document the procedure.[22,23,24]

Special considerations

- Don't collect a venous sample from an infection site *because pathogens may be introduced into the vascular system.* Likewise, avoid drawing blood from edematous areas or sites of previous hematoma or vascular injury.
- Limit your attempts at venipuncture to two; after two attempts, notify the practitioner or a specially trained phlebotomist to obtain the sample.[3,20]

Complications

A hematoma at the needle insertion site is the most common complication of venipuncture. Infection may result from poor technique.

Documentation

Record the date, time, and site of venipuncture; the name of the test; the time the sample was sent to the laboratory; the amount of blood collected; and any adverse reactions to the procedure.

References

1 Becton, Dickinson and Company. (2012). "BD Vacutainer® evacuated blood collection system: For *in vitro* diagnostic use" [Online]. Accessed May 2015 via the Web at http://www.bd.com/vacutainer/pdfs/VDP40161.pdf

2 Standard 57. Phlebotomy. Infusion nursing standards of practice. (2011). *Journal of Infusion Nursing, 34,* S77–S80. (Level I)

3 Infusion Nurses Society. (2011). *Policies and procedures for infusion nursing* (4th ed.). Boston, MA: Infusion Nurses Society.

4 Caldeira, D., et al. (2011). Skin antiseptics in venous puncture-site disinfection for prevention of blood culture contamination: Systematic review with meta-analysis. *Journal of Hospital Infection, 77,* 223–232.

5 Becton, Dickinson and Company. (2010). "BD Vacutainer® order of draw for multiple tube collections" [Online]. Accessed May 2015 via the Web at http://www.bd.com/vacutainer/pdfs/plus_plastic_tubes_wallchart_orderofdraw_VS5729.pdf

6 Johnson, L. (2013). "National Center for Competency Testing: Phlebotomy order of draw: Who, what, when, where, why, & how" [Online]. Accessed May 2015 via the Web at http://www.ncctinc.com/documents/Phlebotomy%20Order%20of%20Draw.pdf

7 Clinical Laboratory and Standards Institute (CLSI). (2007). *Procedures for the collection of diagnostic blood specimens by venipuncture* (6th ed.). Wayne, PA: CLSI.

8 Standard 25. Latex sensitivity or allergy. Infusion nursing standards of practice. (2011). *Journal of Infusion Nursing, 34,* S30. (Level I)

9 Occupational Safety and Health Administration. (n.d.). "Bloodborne pathogens, standard number 1910.1030" [Online]. Accessed May 2015 via the Web at http://www.osha.gov/pls/oshaweb/owadisp.show_document?p_table=STANDARDS&p_id=10051 (Level VII)

10 The Joint Commission. (2015). Standard NPSG.07.01.01. *Comprehensive accreditation manual for hospitals: The official handbook.* Oakbrook Terrace, IL: The Joint Commission. (Level VII)

11 Centers for Disease Control and Prevention. (2002). Guideline for hand hygiene in health-care settings: Recommendations of the Healthcare Infection Control Practices Advisory Committee and the HICPAC/SHEA/APIC/IDSA Hand Hygiene Task Force. *MMWR Recommendations and Reports, 51*(RR-16), 1–45. Accessed May 2015 via the Web at http://www.cdc.gov/mmwr/pdf/rr/rr5116.pdf (Level II)

12 World Health Organization. (2009). "WHO guidelines on hand hygiene in health care: First global patient safety challenge, clean care is safer care"

[Online]. Accessed May 2015 via the Web at http://whqlibdoc.who.int/publications/2009/9789241597906_eng.pdf (Level IV)

13 Standard 19. Hand hygiene. Infusion nursing standards of practice. (2011). *Journal of Infusion Nursing, 34,* S26. (Level I)

14 Centers for Medicare & Medicaid Services, Department of Health and Human Services. (2014). Condition of participation: Infection control. 42 C.F.R. § 482.42.

15 American Osteopathic Association. (2014). Standard 07.01.21. *Healthcare Facilities Accreditation Program: Accreditation requirements for acute care hospitals.* Chicago, IL: American Osteopathic Association. (Level VII)

16 American Osteopathic Association. (2014). Standard 07.01.10. *Healthcare Facilities Accreditation Program: Accreditation requirements for acute care hospitals.* Chicago, IL: American Osteopathic Association. (Level VII)

17 The Joint Commission. (2015). Standard NPSG.01.01.01. *Comprehensive accreditation manual for hospitals: The official handbook.* Oakbrook Terrace, IL: The Joint Commission. (Level VII)

18 Standard 31. Tourniquets. Infusion nursing standards of practice. (2011). *Journal of Infusion Nursing, 34,* S36. (Level I)

19 Standard 35. Vascular access site preparation and device placement. (2011). *Journal of Infusion Nursing, 34,* S44–46.

20 Fischbach, F., & Dunning, M. B. (2014). *A manual of laboratory and diagnostic tests* (9th ed.). Philadelphia, PA: Wolters Kluwer.

21 Standard 22. Safe handling and disposal of sharps, hazardous materials, and hazardous waste. Infusion nursing standards of practice. (2011). *Journal of Infusion Nursing, 34,* S28. (Level I)

22 The Joint Commission. (2015). Standard RC.01.03.01. *Comprehensive accreditation manual for hospitals: The official handbook.* Oakbrook Terrace, IL: The Joint Commission. (Level VII)

23 American Osteopathic Association. (2014). Standard 10.00.03. *Healthcare Facilities Accreditation Program: Accreditation requirements for acute care hospitals.* Chicago, IL: American Osteopathic Association. (Level VII)

24 Centers for Medicare & Medicaid Services, Department of Health and Human Services. (2014). Condition of participation: Medical record services. 42 C.F.R. § 482.24(b).

VENTRICULAR ASSIST DEVICE CARE

A ventricular assist device (VAD) is implanted to provide support to a failing heart. The device consists of a blood pump, cannulas, and a pneumatic or electrical drive console. It's typically implanted in the upper abdominal wall. The device provides systemic support and is designed to decrease the heart's workload and increase cardiac output in patients with ventricular failure.

Inserting a VAD involves a specific surgical procedure in which blood is diverted from a ventricle to an artificial pump. The diversion is created by inserting a cannula into either the atria or ventricles that directs blood to the pump. This pump then functions as the ventricle. An inflow cannula drains blood from the left atrium or ventricle into the pump (part of the VAD), which then pushes the blood into the aorta through the outflow cannula. (See *VAD: Help for the failing heart,* page 826.)

Candidates for a VAD include patients with massive myocardial infarction, irreversible cardiomyopathy, acute myocarditis, an inability to be weaned from cardiopulmonary bypass, valvular disease, bacterial endocarditis, heart transplant rejection, or cardiogenic shock that doesn't respond to maximal pharmacologic therapy. The device may also be used as a bridge to cardiac transplantation in patients awaiting a heart transplant.

Equipment

VAD to be inserted in the operating room ■ clippers ■ gloves ■ antiseptic solution ■ prescribed analgesics and other medications ■ thermometer ■ heparin ■ dressing supplies ■ oral and skin care supplies ■ thigh-length antiembolism stockings or sequential compression device.

Implementation

Preoperative care

- Confirm that written informed consent has been obtained and is in the patient's medical record.[1,2,3]
- Conduct a preprocedure verification *to make sure that all relevant documentation, related information, and equipment are available and correctly identified to the patient's identifiers.*[4,5]
- Perform hand hygiene.[6,7,8,9,10]
- Confirm the patient's identity using at least two patient identifiers.[3,11]
- Reinforce preoperative teaching and answer any questions the patient may have *to reduce anxiety.*
- Before surgery, explain to the patient that food and fluid intake must be restricted and that his cardiac function will be continuously monitored using an electrocardiogram, a pulmonary artery catheter, and an arterial line. Offer reassurance.
- Put on gloves.[12,13]
- If time permits, clip the hair on the patient's chest and scrub it with an antiseptic solution.[14]
- Confirm that the correct procedure has been identified for the correct patient at the correct site.[4,5]
- Administer preoperative medications, as ordered, following safe medication administration practices. A prophylactic antibiotic may be administered within 1 hour before surgical incision *to reduce the risk of surgical site infection.*
- Provide hand-off communication to the person who will be assuming care of the patient in the operating room; allow time for questions, and answer them appropriately *to prevent patient care errors associated with transitions in care.*[5,15,16]
- Remove and discard your gloves[12,13] and perform hand hygiene.[6,7,8,9,10]
- Document the procedure.[17,18,19]

Postoperative care

- When the patient returns from surgery, obtain hand-off communication from the person who was responsible for the patient's care during surgery.[15,16]
- Perform hand hygiene[6,7,8,9,10] and put on gloves.[12,13]
- Attach the patient to a continuous cardiac monitor. Make sure that the alarm limits are set appropriately for the patient's current condition and that the alarms are turned on, functioning properly, and audible to staff.[20,21,22,23]
- Frequently monitor the patient's vital signs, breath sounds, level of consciousness, peripheral circulation, and intake and output.
- Perform a comprehensive pain assessment using techniques appropriate for the patient's age, condition, and ability to understand. Administer analgesics, as ordered and needed, following safe medication administration practices.[24]
- Logroll the patient side-to-side every 2 hours *to help prevent skin breakdown.*[25]
- Provide active and passive range-of-motion exercises to the patient every 2 hours.[25]
- If the patient is intubated and on a ventilator, keep the head of the bed elevated at least 30 degrees, unless contraindicated, *to prevent ventilator-associated pneumonia.*[26,27,28]
- Monitor pulmonary artery pressures *to evaluate the effectiveness of VAD therapy.*[25]
- Monitor the patient for signs and symptoms of poor perfusion and ineffective pumping, including arrhythmias, hypotension, slow capillary refill, cool skin, oliguria or anuria, confusion, anxiety, and restlessness.
- Monitor the VAD's function and troubleshoot any problems with the VAD coordinator or practitioner. Follow the manufacturer's guidelines.
- Administer heparin, as prescribed, *to prevent thrombus formation and clotting in the pump head.*

EQUIPMENT

VAD: Help for the failing heart

A ventricular assist device (VAD) functions somewhat like an artificial heart. The major difference is that a VAD assists the heart, whereas an artificial heart replaces it. A VAD is designed to aid one or both ventricles. The pumping chambers themselves aren't usually implanted in the patient.

A permanent VAD is implanted in the patient's chest cavity, although it still provides only temporary support. The device receives power through the skin by a belt of electrical transformer coils (worn externally as a portable battery pack). It can also operate off an implanted, rechargeable battery for up to 1 hour at a time.

VADs are available as continuous flow (axial flow) or pulsatile pumps. A continuous flow pump fills continuously and returns blood to the aorta at a constant rate. A pulsatile pump may work in one of two ways: it may fill during systole and pump blood into the aorta during diastole or it may pump regardless of the patient's cardiac cycle.

Continuous flow pump

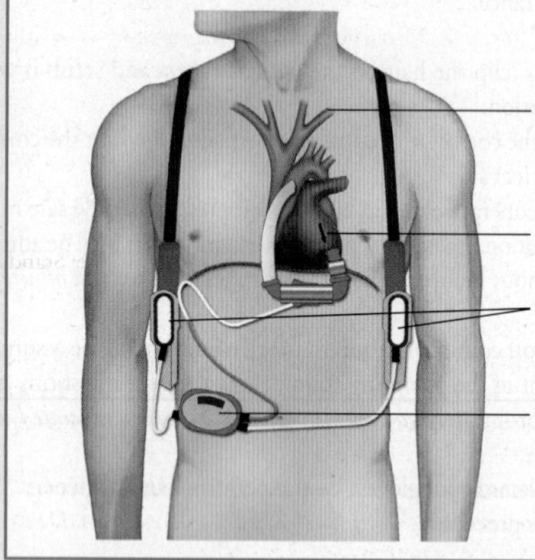

Pulsatile pump

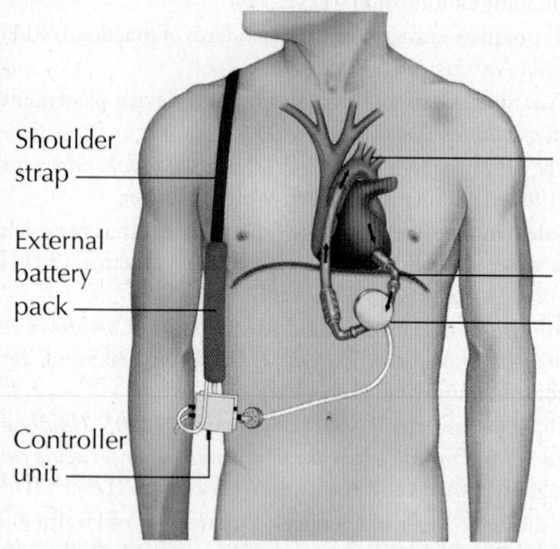

NURSING ALERT *Heparin is considered a high-alert medication* because it can cause significant harm when used in error.[29]

- Before administering heparin, have another nurse perform an independent double-check if required by your facility *to verify the patient's identity as well as to make sure that the correct medication is being administered in the prescribed concentration, that the medication's indication corresponds with the patient's diagnosis, that the dosage calculations are correct and the dosing formula used to derive the final dose is correct, that the route of administration is safe and proper for the patient, that the pump settings are correct, and that the infusion line is attached to the correct port, if applicable.*[30]
- After comparing the results of the independent double-check with the other nurse (if required), administer the medication if there are no discrepancies. If discrepancies exist, rectify them before administering the medication.[30]
- Check for bleeding, especially at the operative sites. Monitor laboratory studies, as ordered, especially complete blood count and coagulation studies.
- Assess the patient's incisions and the cannula insertion sites for signs of infection and bleeding. Monitor the patient's white blood cell count and differential daily, and take rectal or core temperatures every 4 hours.
- Change the dressings over the cannula sites at an interval determined by your facility and as needed using maximal barrier precautions *to prevent infection.*[31]
- Provide supportive care, including oral and skin care.
- Apply antiembolism stockings or a sequential compression device, as ordered, *to promote venous return and prevent venous thromboembolism.* (See the "Sequential compression therapy" and "Antiembolism stocking application" procedures, pages 687, 21.)
- Make sure prophylactic antibiotics are discontinued within 48 hours after surgery.[32]
- If the patient was receiving a beta-adrenergic blocker before surgery, collaborate with the patient's practitioner *to make sure he receives it during the perioperative period, as appropriate.*[32]
- If the patient had an indwelling urinary catheter inserted for surgery, remove the catheter on postoperative day 1 or 2 (with the day of surgery considered day 0) or as soon as the patient no longer needs it *to reduce the risk of catheter-associated urinary tract infection.*[32,33,34] (See the "Indwelling urinary catheter care and removal" procedure, page 391.)
- Remove and discard your gloves[12,13] and perform hand hygiene.[6,7,8,9,10]
- Document the procedure.[17,18,19]

Special considerations

- If ventricular function fails to improve, the patient may need a transplant. If so, provide psychological support for the patient and his family as they go through the referral process. You may also initiate the transplant process by contacting the appropriate agency.
- The psychological effects of the VAD can cause stress in the patient, his family, and his close friends. Provide emotional support and education for the patient and his family. If appropriate, refer them to other support personnel.
- After the patient is extubated and stable, encourage mobility *to help prevent atelectasis and skin breakdown.*[31]
- The Joint Commission issued a sentinel event alert concerning medical device alarm safety *because alarm-related events have been associated with permanent loss of function or death.* Among the major contributing factors were improper alarm settings, alarms inappropriately turned off, and alarm signals not audible to staff. Make sure that alarm limits are set appropriately for the patient's current condition and that alarms are turned on, functioning properly, and audible to staff. Follow facility guidelines for preventing alarm fatigue.[20]

Patient teaching

Teach the patient about the VAD device and surgery, frequency of postoperative assessments, and complications.

Complications

The VAD carries a high risk of complications, including damaged blood cells, which can increase the likelihood of thrombus formation and subsequent pulmonary embolism or stroke. Other possible complications include infection, excessive bleeding (especially immediately after implantation), acute heart failure and, rarely, device malfunction.

Documentation

Note the patient's condition following insertion of the VAD. Document the patient's vital signs, hemodynamic parameters, your assessment findings, any pump adjustments, and medications administered. Document any complications, the date and time, the name of the practitioner notified, prescribed interventions, and the patient's response to those interventions. Record your dressing changes and the condition of the insertion site. Document any patient and family teaching provided and their understanding of your teaching.

REFERENCES

1 Centers for Medicare & Medicaid Services, Department of Health and Human Services. (2014). Condition of participation: Patient's rights. 42 C.F.R. § 482.13(b)(2).

2 The Joint Commission. (2015). Standard RI.01.03.01. *Comprehensive accreditation manual for hospitals: The official handbook.* Oakbrook Terrace, IL: The Joint Commission. (Level VII)

3 American Osteopathic Association. (2014). Standard 30.01.11. *Healthcare Facilities Accreditation Program: Accreditation requirements for acute care hospitals.* Chicago, IL: American Osteopathic Association. (Level VII)

4 The Joint Commission. (2015). Standard UP.01.01.01. *Comprehensive accreditation manual for hospitals: The official handbook.* Oakbrook Terrace, IL: The Joint Commission. (Level VII)

5 American Osteopathic Association. (2014). Standard 30.00.14. *Healthcare Facilities Accreditation Program: Accreditation requirements for acute care hospitals.* Chicago, IL: American Osteopathic Association. (Level VII)

6 Centers for Disease Control and Prevention. (2002). Guideline for hand hygiene in health-care settings: Recommendations of the Healthcare Infection Control Practices Advisory Committee and the HICPAC/SHEA/APIC/IDSA Hand Hygiene Task Force. *MMWR Recommendations and Reports, 51*(RR-16), 1–45. Accessed May 2015 via the Web at http://www.cdc.gov/mmwr/pdf/rr/rr5116.pdf (Level II)

7 World Health Organization. (2009). "WHO guidelines on hand hygiene in health care: First global patient safety challenge, clean care is safer care" [Online]. Accessed May 2015 via the Web at http://whqlibdoc.who.int/publications/2009/9789241597906_eng.pdf (Level IV)

8 The Joint Commission. (2015). Standard NPSG.07.01.01. *Comprehensive accreditation manual for hospitals: The official handbook.* Oakbrook Terrace, IL: The Joint Commission. (Level VII)

9 American Osteopathic Association. (2014). Standard 07.01.21. *Healthcare Facilities Accreditation Program: Accreditation requirements for acute care hospitals.* Chicago, IL: American Osteopathic Association. (Level VII)

10 Centers for Medicare & Medicaid Services, Department of Health and Human Services. (2014). Condition of participation: Infection control. 42 C.F.R. § 482.42.

11 The Joint Commission. (2014). Standard NPSG.01.01.01. *Comprehensive accreditation manual for hospitals: The official handbook.* Oakbrook Terrace, IL: The Joint Commission. (Level VII)

12 Siegel, J. D., et al. (2007). "2007 guideline for isolation precautions: Preventing transmission of infectious agents in healthcare settings" [Online]. Accessed May 2015 via the Web at http://www.cdc.gov/hicpac/pdf/isolation/Isolation2007.pdf (Level II)

13 American Osteopathic Association. (2014). Standard 07.01.10. *Healthcare Facilities Accreditation Program: Accreditation requirements for acute care hospitals.* Chicago, IL: American Osteopathic Association. (Level VII)

14 The Joint Commission. (2015). Standard NPSG.07.05.01. *Comprehensive accreditation manual for hospitals: The official handbook.* Oakbrook Terrace, IL: The Joint Commission. (Level VII)

15 The Joint Commission. (2015). Standard PC.02.02.01. *Comprehensive accreditation manual for hospitals: The official handbook.* Oakbrook Terrace, IL: The Joint Commission. (Level VII)

16 Joint Commission Center for Transforming Healthcare. (2012). "Targeted solutions tool: Improving hand-off communications" [Online]. Accessed May 2015 via the Web at http://www.jointcommission.org/assets/1/6/TST_HOC_Persp_08_12.pdf (Level IV)

17 The Joint Commission. (2014). Standard RC.01.03.01. *Comprehensive accreditation manual for hospitals: The official handbook.* Oakbrook Terrace, IL: The Joint Commission. (Level VII)

18 American Osteopathic Association. (2014). Standard 10.00.03. *Healthcare Facilities Accreditation Program: Accreditation requirements for acute care hospitals.* Chicago, IL: American Osteopathic Association. (Level VII)

19 Centers for Medicare & Medicaid Services, Department of Health and Human Services. (2014). Condition of participation: Medical record services. 42 C.F.R. § 482.24(b).

20 The Joint Commission. (2013). "Sentinel event alert: Medical device alarm safety in hospitals" [Online]. Accessed May 2015 via the Web at http://www.jointcommission.org/assets/1/18/SEA_50_alarms_4_5_13_FINAL1.PDF (Level VII)

21 Graham, K. C., & Cvach, M. (2010). Monitor alarm fatigue: Standardizing use of physiological monitors and decreasing nuisance alarms. *American Journal of Critical Care, 19,* 28–37.

22 American Association of Critical-Care Nurses. (2013). "AACN practice alert: Alarm management" [Online]. Accessed May 2015 via the Web at http://www.aacn.org/wd/practice/docs/practicealerts/alarm-management-practice-alert.pdf (Level VII)

23 The Joint Commission. (2015). Standard NPSG.06.01.01. *Comprehensive accreditation manual for hospitals: The official handbook.* Oakbrook Terrace, IL: The Joint Commission. (Level VII)

24 The Joint Commission. (2015). Standard PC.01.02.07. *Comprehensive accreditation manual for hospitals: The official handbook.* Oakbrook Terrace, IL: The Joint Commission. (Level VII)

25 Lynn-McHale Wiegand, D. (Ed.). (2011). *AACN procedure manual for critical care* (6th ed.). St. Louis, MO: Saunders.

26 American Association of Critical-Care Nurses. (2008). "AACN practice alert: Ventilator associated pneumonia" [Online]. Accessed May 2015 via the Web at http://www.aacn.org/WD/Practice/Docs/PracticeAlerts/Ventilator%20Associated%20Pneumonia%201-2008.pdf (Level VII)

27 Association of Professionals in Infection Control and Epidemiology (APIC). (2009). "An APIC guide 2009: Guide to the elimination of ventilator-associated pneumonia" [Online]. Accessed May 2015 via the Web at http://www.apic.org/Resource_/EliminationGuideForm/18e326ad-b484-471c-9c35-6822a53ee4a2/File/VAP_09.pdf (Level IV)

28 American Osteopathic Association. (2014). Standard 07.01.02. *Healthcare Facilities Accreditation Program: Accreditation requirements for acute care hospitals.* Chicago, IL: American Osteopathic Association. (Level VII)

29 Institute for Safe Medication Practices. (2012). "ISMP's list of high-alert medications" [Online]. Accessed May 2015 via the Web at http://www.ismp.org/tools/highalertmedications.pdf

30 Institute for Safe Medication Practices. (2008). Conducting an independent double-check. *ISMP Medication Safety Alert! Nurse Advise-ERR, 6*(12), 1. Accessed May 2015 via the Web at http://www.ismp.org/newsletters/nursing/Issues/NurseAdviseERR200812.pd

31 O'Shea, G. (2012). Ventricular assist devices: What intensive care unit nurses need to know about postoperative management. *AACN Advanced Critical Care, 23,* 69–83. (Level V)

32 Centers for Medicare & Medicaid Services, & The Joint Commission. (2014). "The specifications manual for national hospital inpatient quality measures (version 4.3a)" [Online]. Accessed May 2015 via the Web at http://www.qualitynet.org/dcs/ContentServer?c=Page&pagename=QnetPublic%2FPage%2FQnetTier4&cid=1228773564870

33 Healthcare Infection Control Practices Advisory Committee. (2010). "Guideline for prevention of catheter-associated urinary tract infections,

2009" [Online]. Accessed May 2015 via the Web at http://www.cdc.gov/hicpac/pdf/CAUTI/CAUTIguideline2009final.pdf (Level I)
34 The Joint Commission. (2015). Standard NPSG.07.06.01. *Comprehensive accreditation manual for hospitals: The official handbook.* Oakbrook Terrace, IL: The Joint Commission. (Level VII)

ADDITIONAL REFERENCE

Gordon, R. J., et al. (2013). A prospective, multicenter study of ventricular assist device infections. *Circulation, 127,* 691–702. (Level IV)

VENTRICULAR DRAIN INSERTION, ASSISTING

Cerebrospinal fluid (CSF) drainage aims to reduce CSF pressure to the desired level and then to maintain it at that level. Fluid can be withdrawn from the lateral ventricle or the lumbar subarachnoid space, depending on the indication and the desired outcome, via a catheter or an external ventricular drain attached to a sterile, closed-drainage collection system. Intracranial pressure (ICP) can also be monitored by an external transducer connected to the external ventricular drainage system.[1]

To insert the ventricular drain, the practitioner inserts a ventricular catheter through a burr hole in the patient's skull using sterile technique. This procedure is usually performed in the operating room, with the patient receiving general anesthesia, but it can also be done in the emergency department or on the intensive care unit.

Strict sterile technique must be maintained throughout equipment setup, catheter insertion, and care of the ventricular drain because the catheter's location in the brain poses an increased risk of infection.[1,2] Because of the risk of resistant microorganisms, the use of prophylactic antibiotics is controversial and isn't recommended.[3]

Equipment

Overbed table ■ gloves ■ sterile gloves ■ sterile gowns ■ masks and protective eyewear ■ cardiopulmonary monitor ■ pulse oximeter ■ antiseptic solution ■ alcohol pads ■ sterile fenestrated drape ■ 3-mL syringe for local anesthetic ■ 25G ¾" (1.9-cm) needle for injecting anesthetic ■ local anesthetic (usually 1% lidocaine) ■ 18G or 20G sterile spinal needle or Tuohy needle ■ #5 French whistle-tip catheter or ventriculostomy tube ■ external ventricular drainage set (drainage tubing, drip chamber, and drainage bag) ■ suture material ■ 4" × 4" (10-cm × 10-cm) dressings ■ paper tape ■ lamp or another light source ■ IV pole ■ sterile occlusive dressing ■ twist drill and bit ■ level ■ ICP monitoring equipment with flushless transducer setup ■ pressure cable and module ■ sterile, preservative-free normal saline solution in a 30-mL or 40-mL syringe ■ sterile, nonvented caps ■ Optional: prescribed sedation or analgesia, anti-infective agent (such as an antibiotic), IV catheter insertion supplies, clippers.

Some of the equipment may be available in a prepackaged ventriculostomy tray.

Preparation of equipment

If the procedure is performed in the operating room, equipment is prepared there using sterile technique. If the procedure is performed at the bedside, open all equipment using sterile technique. Check all packaging for breaks in seals and for expiration dates.

Maintaining sterile technique, prepare the ICP monitoring equipment by priming the pressure tubing and external ventricular drainage system with preservative-free saline solution; turn the stopcocks as needed to prime the system. Remove the syringe and replace with a sterile, nonvented cap.[1] (See the "Intracranial pressure monitoring" procedure, page 424.)

Implementation

- Verify the practitioner's order.
- Confirm that written informed consent has been obtained and is in the patient's medical record.[4,5,6,7]
- Conduct a preprocedure verification *to make sure that all relevant documentation, related information, and equipment are available and correctly identified to the patient's identifiers.*[8,9]
- Review the patient's laboratory test results; *International Normalized Ratio should range from 1.2 and 1.6 in a patient with traumatic brain injury who requires emergency ventriculostomy to reduce the risk of hemorrhage.*[10] Report critical test results to the patient's practitioner within the time frame established by your facility *to prevent treatment delays.*
- Gather the necessary equipment.
- Perform hand hygiene.[11,12,13,14,15]
- Confirm the patient's identity using at least two patient identifiers.[16]
- Reinforce the practitioner's explanation of the procedure and answer the patient's questions.
- Check the patient's history for hypersensitivity to latex or the local anesthetic.
- Discuss activity restrictions that will need to be adhered to after the drain is placed.
- Provide privacy.[17,18,19]
- Attach the patient to a cardiopulmonary monitor and pulse oximeter *to monitor heart rate and rhythm and oxygen saturation level during the procedure.*[2] Make sure alarm limits are set appropriately for the patient's current condition and that alarms are turned on, functioning properly, and audible to staff.[20]
- Perform a baseline neurologic assessment, including vital signs, *to help detect alterations or signs of deterioration during and after the procedure.*
- Assess the patency of IV access or initiate IV access as needed. (See the "IV catheter insertion and removal" procedure, page 446.)
- Place the patient in the supine position with the head of the bed elevated 30 degrees. Obtain assistance if needed to immobilize the patient's head *to prevent movement during catheter insertion.*[2]
- Perform hand hygiene.[11,12,13,14,15]
- Put on a gown, a mask, protective eyewear, and gloves.[21,22]
- Set up the overbed table as a sterile field and unwrap the ventriculostomy tray using sterile technique. If the tray is unavailable, set up a sterile field and open all supplies using sterile technique.
- Label all medications, medication containers, and other solutions on and off the sterile field.[23,24]
- Adjust the height of the bed *so that the practitioner can perform the procedure comfortably.*
- Illuminate the area of the catheter insertion site.
- Assess the patient's sedation and pain management needs in collaboration with the practitioner.
- Administer medications, as indicated and prescribed, following safe medication administration practices *to ensure the patient's comfort during the procedure.*[2,25,26,27]
- Braid or clip the patient's hair, if needed, *to expose the insertion site.* If the hair was clipped, use tape or other similar sticky product *to remove residual hair clippings.*[2]
- If assisting with sterile supplies, remove and discard your gloves.[21,22]
- Perform hand hygiene.[11,12,13,14,15]
- Put on sterile gloves.[21,22]
- Assist the practitioner as needed as he cleans the insertion site with antiseptic solution and allows it to dry, drapes the site with a sterile drape, and administers a local anesthetic.
- Conduct a preprocedure verification *to make sure that all relevant documentation, related information, and equipment are available and correctly identified to the patient's identifiers.*[9,28]
- To insert the drain, the practitioner will request a twist drill and bit. After completing the ventricular drain insertion, he'll cover the insertion site with a sterile occlusive dressing and secure the catheter *to prevent accidental removal.*
- After the practitioner places the catheter, connect the monitoring system and external ventricular drainage system to the distal tip of the

catheter. Trace the tubing from the patient to the point of origin *to make sure that the tubing is connected to the correct port.* Secure connection points with tape or a connector.[29]

■ Place the external ventricular drainage system, including the drip chamber and collection bag, on an IV pole. Level the system at the level ordered by the practitioner.[1]

■ After the ventricular drain is inserted, monitor the patient's vital signs, neurologic status, and ICP at least every hour or according to the patient's condition and your facility's guidelines.

■ Make sure the drainage system tubing is secured with tape or a luer-lock connector *because loose connections can cause CSF to leak and be a potential site for infection or cause an erroneous decrease in pressure readings.*

■ Ensure that the monitoring system is free from air, *which could alter the pressure reading.*

■ Calibrate the pressure monitor according to the manufacturer's instructions.

■ Assess the waveform on the monitor and document ICP according to the practitioner's order.

■ Monitor the patient for signs and symptoms of infection or a CSF leak.

■ Discard used supplies in the appropriate receptacles.[21]

■ Remove and discard your gloves and personal protective equipment.[21,22]

■ Perform hand hygiene.[11,12,13,14,15]

■ Perform a comprehensive pain assessment using techniques appropriate for the patient's age, condition, and ability to understand.[25] Respond appropriately.

■ Perform hand hygiene.[11,12,13,14,15]

■ Document the procedure.[30,31,32]

Special considerations

■ Maintaining a continual hourly output of CSF is essential *to prevent overdrainage or underdrainage.*[1] Overdrainage can occur if the drip chamber is placed too far below the catheter insertion site. Underdrainage may indicate kinked tubing, catheter displacement, or a drip chamber placed higher than the catheter insertion site.

■ Raising or lowering the head of the bed can affect the CSF flow rate. When changing the patient's position, reposition the drip chamber.

■ Patients may experience a chronic headache during continuous CSF drainage. Reassure the patient that this symptom isn't unusual; administer analgesics, as appropriate.

■ Assess for signs and symptoms of hemorrhage, which may include headache or a change in level of consciousness and an increase in ICP.

■ Make sure ICP waveforms are being monitored at all times.

■ Moving the patient to another area of the health care facility to perform tests and procedures is discouraged *to prevent catheter dislodgement.* Check your facility's requirements for scheduling such tests and procedures at the patient's bedside.

■ Follow strict sterile technique when connecting or flushing the tubing, when taking samples from the drainage system, and during dressing changes.[1,2]

■ The Joint Commission issued a sentinel event alert concerning medical device alarm safety *because alarm-related events have been associated with permanent loss of function or death.* Among the major contributing factors were improper alarm settings, alarms inappropriately turned off, and alarm signals not audible to staff. Make sure alarm limits are set appropriately and that alarms are turned on, functioning properly, and audible to staff. Follow facility guidelines for preventing alarm fatigue.[20]

Patient teaching

Teach the patient and his family members about the reason for the drain. Explain to the patient that his activity level must be restricted. The patient may not sit up, stand, or walk when the drain is open and must ask for assistance with movement. The system must be turned off when the patient is repositioned or transferred. Instruct the patient to avoid straining, coughing, and sneezing.

Complications

Signs of excessive CSF drainage include headache, tachycardia, diaphoresis, and nausea. Acute overdrainage may result in collapsed ventricles, tonsillar herniation, and medullary compression.

NURSING ALERT *If drainage accumulates too rapidly, clamp the system, notify the practitioner immediately, and perform a complete neurologic assessment.* This complication constitutes a potential neurosurgical emergency.

Cessation of drainage may indicate clot formation. If you can't quickly identify the cause of the obstruction, notify the practitioner. If drainage is blocked, the patient may develop signs of increased ICP.

Infection may cause meningitis. *To prevent this complication,* administer antibiotics, as ordered. Maintain a sterile closed system and a dry, sterile dressing over the site.

Documentation

Record the time and date of the insertion procedure and the patient's tolerance of it. Record vital signs, neurologic assessment findings, pain assessment, and ICP.

Document the color, clarity, and amount of CSF at least every 8 hours or as required by your facility. Record hourly and 24-hour CSF output, and describe the condition of the dressing.

REFERENCES

1 Lynn-McHale Wiegand, D. (Ed.). (2011). *AACN procedure manual for critical care* (6th ed.). St. Louis, MO: Saunders.

2 American Association of Neuroscience Nurses. (2011). "Care of the patient undergoing intracranial pressure monitoring/external ventricular drainage or lumbar drainage" [Online]. Accessed May 2015 via the Web at http://www.aann.org/uploads/AANN11_ICPEVDnew.pdf (Level VII)

3 Bratton, S. L., et al. (2007). Infection prophylaxis. *Journal of Neurotrauma, 24,* S26–S31. (Level II)

4 The Joint Commission. (2015). Standard RI.01.03.01. *Comprehensive accreditation manual for hospitals: The official handbook.* Oakbrook Terrace, IL: The Joint Commission. (Level VII)

5 Centers for Medicare & Medicaid Services, Department of Health and Human Services. (2014). Condition of participation: Patient's rights. 42 C. F. R. § 482.13.

6 American Osteopathic Association. (2014). Standard 30.01.11. *Healthcare Facilities Accreditation Program: Accreditation requirements for acute care hospitals.* Chicago, IL: American Osteopathic Association. (Level VII)

7 Centers for Medicare & Medicaid Services, Department of Health and Human Services. (2014). Condition of participation: Patient's rights. 42 C.F.R. § 482.13(b)(2).

8 The Joint Commission. (2015). Standard UP.01.01.01. *Comprehensive accreditation manual for hospitals: The official handbook.* Oakbrook Terrace, IL: The Joint Commission. (Level VII)

9 American Osteopathic Association. (2014). Standard 30.00.14. *Healthcare Facilities Accreditation Program: Accreditation requirements for acute care hospitals.* Chicago, IL: American Osteopathic Association. (Level VII)

10 Bauer, D. F., et al. (2011). The relationship between INR and the development of hemorrhage with the placement of ventriculostomy. *Journal of Trauma and Acute Care Surgery, 70,* 1112–1117.

11 The Joint Commission. (2015). Standard NPSG.07.01.01. *Comprehensive accreditation manual for hospitals: The official handbook.* Oakbrook Terrace, IL: The Joint Commission. (Level VII)

12 Centers for Disease Control and Prevention. (2002). Guideline for hand hygiene in health-care settings: Recommendations of the Healthcare Infection Control Practices Advisory Committee and the HICPAC/SHEA/APIC/IDSA Hand Hygiene Task Force. *MMWR Recommendations*

and Reports, 51(RR-16), 1–45. Accessed May 2015 via the Web at http://www.cdc.gov/mmwr/pdf/rr/rr5116.pdf (Level II)

13 World Health Organization. (2009). "WHO guidelines on hand hygiene in health care: First global patient safety challenge, clean care is safer care" [Online]. Accessed May 2015 via the Web at http://whqlibdoc.who.int/publications/2009/9789241597906_eng.pdf (Level IV)

14 American Osteopathic Association. (2014). Standard 07.01.21. *Healthcare Facilities Accreditation Program: Accreditation requirements for acute care hospitals.* Chicago, IL: American Osteopathic Association. (Level VII)

15 Centers for Medicare & Medicaid Services, Department of Health and Human Services. (2014). Condition of participation: Infection control. 42 C.F.R. § 482.42.

16 The Joint Commission. (2015). Standard NPSG.01.01.01. *Comprehensive accreditation manual for hospitals: The official handbook.* Oakbrook Terrace, IL: The Joint Commission. (Level VII)

17 American Osteopathic Association. (2014). Standard 15.01.16. *Healthcare Facilities Accreditation Program: Accreditation requirements for acute care hospitals.* Chicago, IL: American Osteopathic Association. (Level VII)

18 Centers for Medicare & Medicaid Services, Department of Health and Human Services. (2014). Condition of participation: Patient's rights. 42 C.F.R. § 482.13(c)(1).

19 The Joint Commission. (2015). Standard RI.01.01.01. *Comprehensive accreditation manual for hospitals: The official handbook.* Oakbrook Terrace, IL: The Joint Commission. (Level VII)

20 The Joint Commission. (2013). "Sentinel event alert: Medical device alarm safety in hospitals" [Online]. Accessed May 2015 via the Web at http://www.jointcommission.org/assets/1/18/SEA_50_alarms_4_5_13_FINAL1.PDF (Level VII)

21 Siegel, J. D., et al. (2007). "2007 guideline for isolation precautions: Preventing transmission of infectious agents in healthcare settings" [Online]. Accessed May 2015 via the Web at http://www.cdc.gov/hicpac/pdf/isolation/Isolation2007.pdf (Level II)

22 American Osteopathic Association. (2014). Standard 07.01.10. *Healthcare Facilities Accreditation Program: Accreditation requirements for acute care hospitals.* Chicago, IL: American Osteopathic Association. (Level VII)

23 The Joint Commission. (2015). Standard NPSG.03.04.01. *Comprehensive accreditation manual for hospitals: The official handbook.* Oakbrook Terrace, IL: The Joint Commission. (Level VII)

24 American Osteopathic Association. (2014). Standard 25.01.27. *Healthcare Facilities Accreditation Program: Accreditation requirements for acute care hospitals.* Chicago, IL: American Osteopathic Association. (Level VII)

25 The Joint Commission. (2015). Standard PC.01.02.07. *Comprehensive accreditation manual for hospitals: The official handbook.* Oakbrook Terrace, IL: The Joint Commission. (Level VII)

26 American Osteopathic Association. (2014). Standard 16.01.03. *Healthcare Facilities Accreditation Program: Accreditation requirements for acute care hospitals.* Chicago, IL: American Osteopathic Association. (Level VII)

27 Centers for Medicare & Medicaid Services, Department of Health and Human Services. (2014). Condition of participation: Nursing services. 42 C.F.R. § 482.23(c).

28 The Joint Commission. (2015). Standard UP.01.03.01. *Comprehensive accreditation manual for hospitals: The official handbook.* Oakbrook Terrace, IL: The Joint Commission. (Level VII)

29 U.S. Food and Drug Administration. (n.d.). "Look. Check. Connect. Safe medical device connections save lives" [Online]. Accessed May 2015 via the Web at http://www.fda.gov/downloads/MedicalDevices/Safety/AlertsandNotices/UCM134873.pdf

30 The Joint Commission. (2015). Standard RC.01.03.01. *Comprehensive accreditation manual for hospitals: The official handbook.* Oakbrook Terrace, IL: The Joint Commission. (Level VII)

31 Centers for Medicare & Medicaid Services, Department of Health and Human Services. (2014). Condition of participation: Medical record services. 42 C.F.R. § 482.24(b).

32 American Osteopathic Association. (2014). Standard 10.00.03. *Healthcare Facilities Accreditation Program: Accreditation requirements for acute care hospitals.* Chicago, IL: American Osteopathic Association. (Level VII)

VOLUME-CONTROL SET PREPARATION

A volume-control set is similar to a standard IV administration set, with the addition of a graduated chamber immediately above the drip chamber of the tubing. This graduated chamber, which includes a separate medication port and air filter, allows administration of medications or a precise volume of fluid.

Accurate control of the flow rate prevents IV dosing errors. Controlling the dose and flow rate is particularly important when administering highly potent, irritating, or potentially toxic IV medications to children or older adults. The volume-control set design also prevents free flow of fluid and shuts off when the fluid is exhausted, preventing air from entering the IV catheter.

Despite the potential advantages, there's little evidence to support the use of volume-control sets, and research has identified medication and flushing errors associated with their use.[1]

Equipment

Volume-control set ▪ IV pole ▪ IV solution ▪ antiseptic pads (alcohol, tincture of iodine, or chlorhexidine-based) ▪ medication in labeled syringe ▪ tape ▪ label.

Although various models of volume-control sets are available, each one consists of a graduated fluid chamber (120 to 250 mL) with a spike and a filtered air line on the top and administration tubing underneath. Floating-valve sets have a valve at the bottom that closes when the chamber empties;[2] membrane-filter sets have a rigid filter at the bottom that, when wet, prevents the passage of air.

NURSING ALERT ***Make sure the volume-control set is labeled clearly when medications are added to the system. Check with the pharmacy for incompatibilities before adding the drug and always use sterile technique. Keep in mind that chemical inactivation or precipitation may occur when multiple medications are administered using the same volume-control set.***[1,3]

Preparation of equipment

Ensure the sterility of all equipment and inspect it carefully *to ensure the absence of flaws.* Take the equipment to the patient's bedside.

Prepare any ordered medication and verify compatibility of the medication and diluent before administration. Whenever possible, administer pharmacy-prepared or commercially available products.[4]

Implementation

- Verify the practitioner's order.
- Perform hand hygiene.[5,6,7,8,9,10]
- Confirm the patient's identity using at least two patient identifiers.[11]
- Explain the procedure to the patient.
- If an IV catheter is already in place, assess the insertion site for signs of infiltration and infection.[12]
- Remove the volume-control set from its box and close all the clamps.
- Remove the protective cap from the volume-control set spike, insert the spike into the IV solution container, and hang the container on the IV pole.
- Open the air vent clamp and close the upper slide clamp.
- Open the lower clamp on the IV tubing, slide it upward until it's slightly below the drip chamber, and close the clamp.
- Open the upper clamp until the fluid chamber fills with about 30 mL of solution. Then close the clamp.
- Gently squeeze the chamber.
- Release the drip chamber and let it fill about halfway with fluid.
- Open the lower clamp, prime the tubing, and close the clamp. *To use the set as a primary line,* insert the distal end of the tubing into the catheter or needleless access device.
- *To use the set as a secondary line,* thoroughly disinfect the Y-port of the primary tubing with an antiseptic pad using friction, allow it to dry, and

attach the distal end of the tubing to the Y-port of the primary tubing, following the manufacturer's instructions.

■ *To add medication,* thoroughly disinfect the injection port on the volume-control set with an antiseptic pad using friction, allow it to dry, and inject the medication (as shown below). Make sure that you follow safe medication administration practices.[13,14,15]

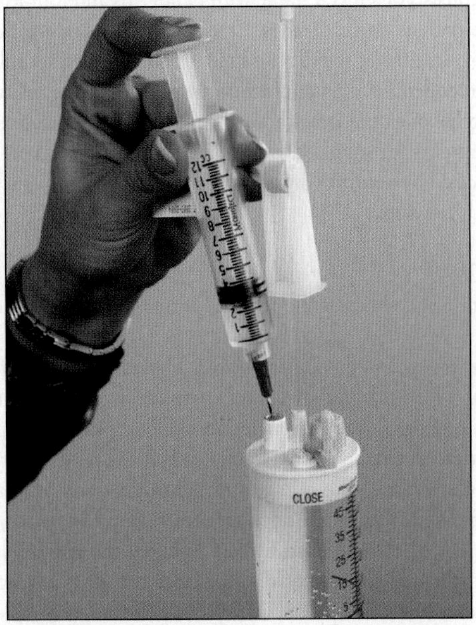

NURSING ALERT *Don't administer continuous high-alert medications as secondary infusions or connect a secondary medication to a high-alert primary continuous infusion* to avoid patient harm caused by inadvertent medication administration at incorrect or indeterminate rates.[16]

■ Place a label on the chamber, indicating the drug, dose, date, and your initials. Don't write directly on the chamber *because the plastic absorbs ink.*

■ Open the upper clamp (as shown below), fill the fluid chamber with the prescribed amount of solution, and close the clamp. Gently rotate the chamber *to mix the medication.*

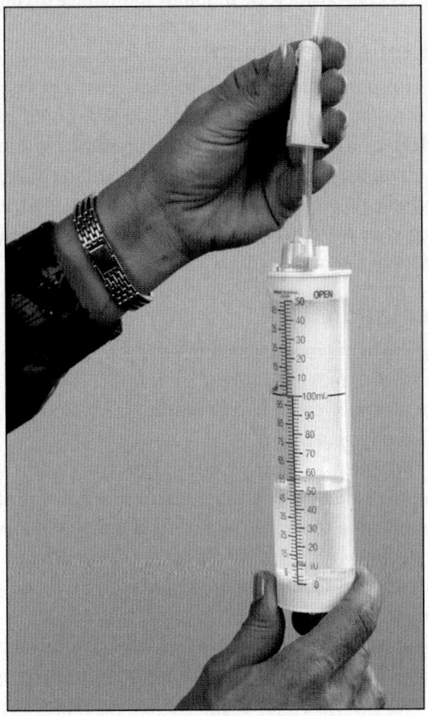

■ If using the volume-control set to deliver a secondary infusion, turn off the primary solution or lower the drip rate *to maintain an open line.* Verify that the secondary infusion is active and the primary infusion is inactive by viewing the drip chambers, as indicated.[16]

■ Trace the tubing from the patient to its point of origin *to make sure that the set is connected to the proper port.*[17,18]

■ Open the lower clamp on the volume-control set, and adjust the drip rate as ordered. After completion of the infusion, open the upper clamp and let 10 mL of IV solution flow into the chamber and through the tubing *to flush them.*

■ If you're using the volume-control set as a secondary IV line, close the lower clamp and reset the flow rate of the primary line. If you're using the set as a primary IV line, close the lower clamp, refill the chamber to the prescribed amount, and begin the infusion again.

■ Perform hand hygiene.[5,6,7,8,9,10]

■ Document the procedure.[19,20,21]

Special considerations

■ Administration sets for primary and secondary continuous infusion of fluids other than lipids or blood products should be changed no more often than every 96 hours, but at least every 7 days. Primary intermittent administration sets should be changed every 24 hours.[22,23]

■ Label any medication added to volume-control sets *to avoid the inadvertent addition of multiple, potentially incompatible medications.* Become familiar with the type or types of volume-control sets used in your facility. Although all volume-control sets work in a similar fashion, it's important to follow the manufacturer's directions for use.

■ Always check compatibility of the medication and the IV solution. If you're using a membrane-filter set, avoid administering suspensions, lipid emulsions, blood, or blood components through it.

■ If you're using a floating-valve set, the diaphragm may stick after repeated use. If it does, close the air vent and upper clamp, invert the drip chamber, and squeeze it. If the diaphragm opens, reopen the clamp and continue to use the set.

■ If the drip chamber of a floating-valve diaphragm set overfills, immediately close the upper clamp and air vent, invert the chamber, and squeeze the excess fluid from the drip chamber back into the graduated fluid chamber.

Complications

Complications of IV infusion therapy include local or systemic infection, infiltration, extravasation, air embolism, catheter occlusion or dislodgment, and circulatory overload. Improper labeling and flushing may result in drug incompatibilities or medication administration errors.

Documentation

If you add a drug to the volume-control set, record the amount and type of medication, amount of fluid used to dilute it, and date and time of infusion. Document the patient's response to the medication, patient teaching, and the patient's understanding of your teaching.

REFERENCES

1 Institute for Safe Medication Practices. (2009). "Volume control set safety" [Online]. Accessed May 2015 via the Web at http://www.ismp.org/newsletters/acutecare/issues/20090604.pdf (Level VII)

2 Recalls and field corrections-Class I: Baxter Buretrol solution sets. (2012). *Biomedical Safety and Standards, 42*(21), 161–163.

3 Foinard, A., et al. (2012). Impact of physical incompatibility on drug mass flow rates: Example of furosemide-midazolam incompatibility. *Annals of Intensive Care, 2,* 28. Accessed May 2015 via the Web at http://www.annalsofintensivecare.com/content/pdf/2110-5820-2-28.pdf

4 Standard 20. Compounding of parenteral solutions and medications. Infusion nursing standards of practice. (2011). *Journal of Infusion Nursing, 34,* S27. (Level VII)

5 The Joint Commission. (2015). Standard NPSG.07.01.01. *Comprehensive accreditation manual for hospitals: The official handbook.* Oakbrook Terrace, IL: The Joint Commission. (Level VII)

6 Standard 19. Hand hygiene. Infusion nursing standards of practice. (2011). *Journal of Infusion Nursing, 34,* S26–S27. (Level VII)

7 Centers for Disease Control and Prevention. (2002). Guideline for hand hygiene in health-care settings: Recommendations of the Healthcare Infection Control Practices Advisory Committee and the HICPAC/SHEA/APIC/IDSA Hand Hygiene Task Force. *MMWR Recommendations and Reports, 51*(RR-16), 1–45. Accessed May 2015 via the Web at http://www.cdc.gov/mmwr/pdf/rr/rr5116.pdf (Level II)

8 World Health Organization. (2009). "WHO guidelines on hand hygiene in health care: First global patient safety challenge, clean care is safer care" [Online]. Accessed May 2015 via the Web at http://whqlibdoc.who.int/publications/2009/9789241597906_eng.pdf (Level IV)

9 Centers for Medicare & Medicaid Services, Department of Health and Human Services. (2014). Condition of participation: Infection control. 42 C.F.R. § 482.42.

10 American Osteopathic Association. (2014). Standard 07.01.21. *Healthcare Facilities Accreditation Program: Accreditation requirements for acute care hospitals.* Chicago, IL: American Osteopathic Association. (Level VII)

11 The Joint Commission. (2015). Standard NPSG.01.01.01. *Comprehensive accreditation manual for hospitals: The official handbook.* Oakbrook Terrace, IL: The Joint Commission. (Level VII)

12 Standard 48. Infiltration and extravasation. Infusion nursing standards of practice. (2011). *Journal of Infusion Nursing, 34,* S66. (Level VII)

13 Standard 26. Add-on devices. Infusion nursing standards of practice. (2011). *Journal of Infusion Nursing, 34,* S31. (Level VII)

14 The Joint Commission. (2015). Standard MM.06.01.01. *Comprehensive accreditation manual for hospitals: The official handbook.* Oakbrook Terrace, IL: The Joint Commission. (Level VII)

15 Centers for Medicare & Medicaid Services, Department of Health and Human Services. (2014). Condition of participation: Nursing services. 42 C.F.R. § 482.23(c).

16 Health Technology Safety Research Team and Institute for Safe Medication Practices, Canada. (2012). "Mitigating the risks associated with multiple IV infusions: Recommendations based on a field study of twelve Ontario hospitals" [Online]. Accessed May 2015 via the Web at http://www.aami.org/htsi/infusion/wg/multiple/MultipleIVInfusions_Phase1bSummary_Recommendations%20and%20Rationale_June%202012.pdf (Level VII)

17 Standard 61. Add-on devices. Infusion nursing standards of practice. (2011). *Journal of Infusion Nursing, 34,* S86–S87. (Level VII)

18 U.S. Food and Drug Administration. (n.d.). "Look. Check. Connect. Safe medical device connections save lives" [Online]. Accessed May 2015 via the Web at http://www.fda.gov/downloads/MedicalDevices/Safety/AlertsandNotices/UCM134873.pdf

19 The Joint Commission. (2015). Standard RC.01.03.01. *Comprehensive accreditation manual for hospitals: The official handbook.* Oakbrook Terrace, IL: The Joint Commission. (Level VII)

20 Centers for Medicare & Medicaid Services, Department of Health and Human Services. (2014). Condition of participation: Medical record services. 42 C.F.R. § 482.24(b).

21 American Osteopathic Association. (2014). Standard 10.00.03. *Healthcare Facilities Accreditation Program: Accreditation requirements for acute care hospitals.* Chicago, IL: American Osteopathic Association. (Level VII)

22 Centers for Disease Control and Prevention. (2011). "Guidelines for the prevention of intravascular catheter-related infections" [Online]. Accessed May 2015 via the Web at http://www.cdc.gov/hicpac/pdf/guidelines/bsi-guidelines-2011.pdf (Level I)

23 Standard 43. Administration set change. Infusion nursing standards of practice. (2011). *Journal of Infusion Nursing, 34,* S55. (Level VII)

ADDITIONAL REFERENCES

Pierce, E. T., et al. (2013). Medication and volume delivery by gravity-driven micro-drip intravenous infusion: Potential variations during "wide-open" flow. *Anesthesia and Analgesia, 116,* 614–618.

Taylor, C., et al. (2015). *Fundamentals of nursing: The art and science of nursing care* (8th ed.). Philadelphia, PA: Wolters Kluwer.

W

WALKERS

A walker consists of a metal frame with handgrips and four legs that buttresses the patient on three sides. One side remains open. Because this device provides greater stability and security than other ambulatory aids, it's recommended for the patient with insufficient strength and balance to use crutches or a cane, or with weakness requiring frequent rest periods.

Attachments for standard walkers and modified walkers help meet special needs. For example, a walker may have a platform added to support an injured arm.

Equipment

Walker ▪ nonskid shoes or slippers ▪ Optional: platform, wheel attachments.

Various types of walkers are available. The standard walker is used by the patient with unilateral or bilateral weakness or an inability to bear weight on one leg. It requires arm strength and balance. You may add platform attachments to a standard walker for the patient with arthritic arms or a casted arm, who can't bear weight directly on his hand, wrist, or forearm. With the practitioner's approval, you may place wheels on the front legs of the standard walker to allow the extremely weak or poorly coordinated patient to roll the device forward, instead of lifting it. However, wheels are applied infrequently *because they may be a safety hazard.*

A stair walker—used by the patient who must negotiate stairs without bilateral handrails—requires good arm strength and balance. Its extra set of handles extends toward the patient on the open side. A rolling walker—used by the patient with very weak legs—has four wheels and may have a seat. A reciprocal walker—used by the patient with very weak arms—allows one side to be advanced ahead of the other.

Because research shows that 30% to 50% of patients stop using their assistive device soon after receiving it, selection of the appropriate device and thorough instruction on its benefits and use become even more important to effectively increase mobility and reduce disability.[1]

Preparation of equipment

Obtain the appropriate walker with the advice of a physical therapist, and adjust it to the patient's height. His elbows should be flexed at a 15- to 30-degree angle when standing comfortably within the walker with his hands on the grips. To adjust the length of the walker's legs, turn the walker upside down, push in the button on each shaft, and release it when the leg is in the correct position. Make sure the walker is level before the patient attempts to use it.

Implementation

- Review the patient's medical record for appropriateness of treatment, including history of falls and current fall risk.[2,3,4]
- Verify the practitioner's order, if needed.[2]
- Perform hand hygiene.[5,6,7,8,9]
- Confirm the patient's identity using at least two patient identifiers.[10]
- Make sure the patient is wearing nonskid shoes or slippers, and then help him stand within the walker and instruct him to hold the hand grips firmly and equally *to help stabilize the walker and promote safety.*[11] Make sure that the patient is standing as upright as possible. Stand behind him, closer to the involved leg.
- If the patient has one-sided leg weakness, tell him to advance the walker 6″ to 8″ (15 to 20 cm) and to step forward with the involved leg and follow with the uninvolved leg, supporting himself on his arms. Encourage him to take equal strides. If he has equal strength in both legs, instruct him to

PATIENT TEACHING

Teaching safe use of a walker

Sitting down

■ First, tell the patient to stand with the back of his stronger leg against the front of the chair, his weaker leg slightly off the floor, and the walker directly in front.
■ Tell him to grasp the armrests on the chair one arm at a time while supporting most of his weight on the stronger leg. (In the illustrations below, the patient has left leg weakness.)
■ Tell the patient to lower himself into the chair and slide backward. After he is seated, he should place the walker beside the chair.

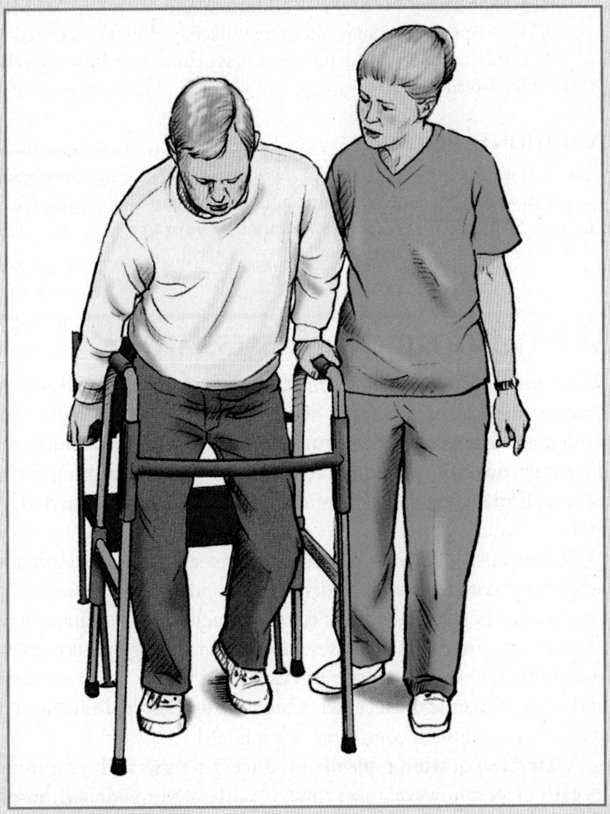

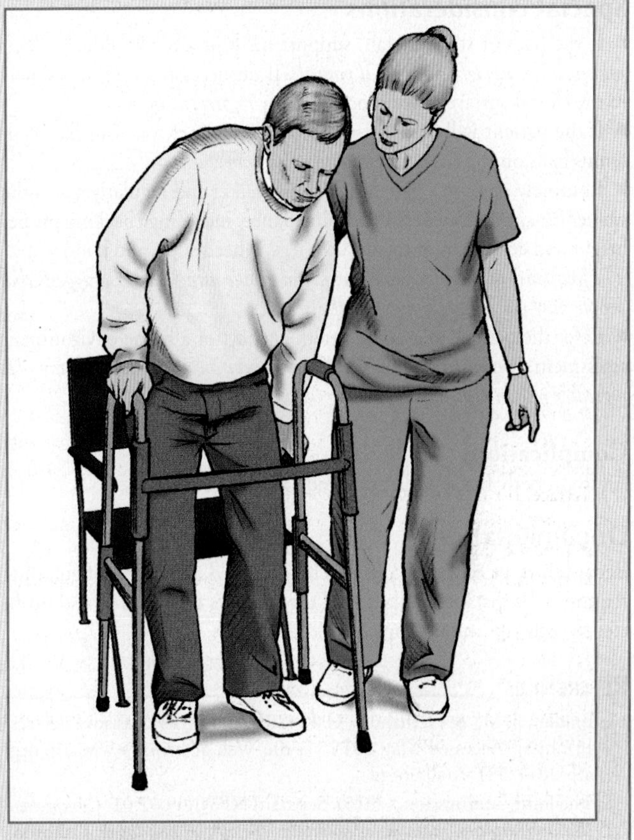

Getting up

■ After bringing the walker to the front of his chair, tell the patient to slide forward in the chair. Placing the back of his stronger leg against the seat, he should then advance the weaker leg.
■ Next, with both hands on the armrests, the patient can push himself to a standing position. Supporting himself with the stronger leg and the opposite hand, the patient should grasp the walker's handgrip with his free hand.
■ Then have the patient grasp the free handgrip with his other hand.

Walker safety tips

Go over specific measures the patient can follow to make using his walker as safe as possible. Provide him with the following list of safety tips:[15]
■ Maintain an erect posture while using the walker.
■ Maintain the rubber tips of the walker.
■ Use firm chairs with armrests if possible.
■ Don't use the walker to pull yourself up to stand.
■ Don't step too far into the walker while walking.
■ Don't lean on the walker when getting up or attempting to sit down.
■ Feel for chair arms to redistribute weight when sitting down or standing up.
■ Avoid wet surfaces; take small steps if you must walk on a wet or slippery surface.
■ Remove throw rugs or mats from your environment.
■ Don't hurry, and don't take large steps when you turn.
■ Change direction slowly and carefully.

advance the walker 6″ to 8″ (15 to 20 cm) and to step forward with either leg. If he can't use one leg, tell him to advance the walker 6″ to 8″ (15 to 20 cm) and to swing onto it, supporting his weight on his arms.
■ If the patient is using a reciprocal walker, teach him the two-point gait. Instruct the patient to stand with his weight evenly distributed between his legs and the walker. Stand behind him, slightly to one side. Tell him to simultaneously advance the walker's right side and his left foot. Then have the patient advance the walker's left side and his right foot.
■ If the patient is using a reciprocal walker, you may also teach him the four-point gait. Instruct the patient to evenly distribute his weight between his legs and the walker. Stand behind him and slightly to one side. Then have him move the right side of the walker forward. Then have the patient move his left foot forward. Next, instruct him to move the left side of the walker forward. Then have him move his right foot forward.
■ Instruct the patient to step into the walker with each step, and not to walk behind it.
■ If the patient is using a wheeled or stair walker, reinforce the physical therapist's instructions. Stress the need for caution when using a stair walker.
■ Teach the patient how to use a walker safely. (See *Teaching safe use of a walker.*)

■ Observe the patient as he returns the demonstration, and assist the patient as necessary.
■ Perform hand hygiene.[5,6,7,8,9]
■ Document the procedure.[12,13,14]

Special considerations

■ If the patient starts to fall, support his hips and shoulders *to help maintain an upright position if possible.* If unsuccessful, ease him slowly to the closest surface—bed, floor, or chair *to prevent injury.*
■ If the patient will be using the walker on carpet, you can place cut tennis balls on the rubber tips *to help ease movement.*
■ Routinely observe a patient using his walker and regularly assess the walker for appropriateness and maintenance, including checking proper height and condition of the walker's legs, wheels, tips, and hand grips.[1] *The frequency of fall injuries, especially in people using walkers, suggests that people may not use walking aids effectively.*[3]
■ Refer the patient to a home health agency for a home environment assessment, if needed, *because extrinsic or environmental factors may play a greater role in falls in people using walkers.*[3,4]

Complications

An improperly fitted walker can lead to falls and injury.

Documentation

Record the type of walker and attachments used, the degree of guarding required, the distance walked, and the patient's tolerance of and proficiency with safe ambulation.[1]

REFERENCES

1 Bradley, S. M., & Hernandez, C. R. (2011). "Geriatric assistive devices" [Online]. Accessed May 2015 via the Web at http://www.aafp.org/afp/2011/0815/p405.html

2 The Joint Commission. (2015). Standard NPSG.09.02.01. *Comprehensive accreditation manual for hospitals: The official handbook.* Oakbrook Terrace, IL: The Joint Commission. (Level VII)

3 Stevens, J. A., et al. (2009). Unintentional fall injuries associated with walkers and canes in older adults treated in U.S. emergency departments. *Journal of the American Geriatrics Society, 57,* 1464–1469.

4 American Geriatrics Society and British Geriatrics Society: Panel on Prevention of Falls in Older Persons. (2010). "Summary of the updated American Geriatrics Society/British Geriatrics Society clinical practice guideline for prevention of falls in older persons" [Online]. Accessed May 2015 via the Web at http://www.americangeriatrics.org/files/documents/health_care_pros/JAGS.Falls.Guidelines.pdf

5 The Joint Commission. (2014). Standard NPSG.07.01.01. *Comprehensive accreditation manual for hospitals: The official handbook.* Oakbrook Terrace, IL: The Joint Commission. (Level VII)

6 Centers for Disease Control and Prevention. (2002). Guideline for hand hygiene in health-care settings: Recommendations of the Healthcare Infection Control Practices Advisory Committee and the HICPAC/SHEA/APIC/IDSA Hand Hygiene Task Force. *MMWR Recommendations and Reports, 51*(RR-16), 1–45. Accessed May 2015 via the Web at http://www.cdc.gov/mmwr/pdf/rr/rr5116.pdf (Level II)

7 World Health Organization. (2009). "WHO guidelines on hand hygiene in health care: First global patient safety challenge, clean care is safer care" [Online]. Accessed May 2015 via the Web at http://whqlibdoc.who.int/publications/2009/9789241597906_eng.pdf (Level IV)

8 American Osteopathic Association. (2014). Standard 07.01.21. *Healthcare Facilities Accreditation Program: Accreditation requirements for acute care hospitals.* Chicago, IL: American Osteopathic Association. (Level VII)

9 Centers for Medicare & Medicaid Services, Department of Health and Human Services. (2014). Condition of participation: Infection control. 42 C.F.R. § 482.42.

10 The Joint Commission. (2015). Standard NPSG.01.01.01. *Comprehensive accreditation manual for hospitals: The official handbook.* Oakbrook Terrace, IL: The Joint Commission. (Level VII)

11 Taylor, C., et al. (2015). *Fundamentals of nursing: The art and science of nursing care* (8th ed.). Philadelphia, PA: Wolters Kluwer.

12 The Joint Commission. (2015). Standard RC.01.03.01. *Comprehensive accreditation manual for hospitals: The official handbook.* Oakbrook Terrace, IL: The Joint Commission. (Level VII)

13 American Osteopathic Association. (2014). Standard 10.00.03. *Healthcare Facilities Accreditation Program: Accreditation requirements for acute care hospitals.* Chicago, IL: American Osteopathic Association. (Level VII)

14 Centers for Medicare & Medicaid Services, Department of Health and Human Services. (2014). Condition of participation: Medical record services. 42 C.F.R. § 482.24(b).

15 Mayo Foundation for Medical Education and Research (MFMER). (2011). "Tips for choosing and using walkers" [Online]. Accessed May 2015 via the Web at http://www.mayoclinic.com/health/walker/HA00060&slide=3

ADDITIONAL REFERENCES

Craven, R. F., & Hirnle, C. J. (2012). *Fundamentals of nursing: Human health and function* (7th ed.). Philadelphia, PA: Lippincott Williams & Wilkins.

Nettina, S. M. (2014). *Lippincott manual of nursing practice* (10th ed.). Philadelphia, PA: Wolters Kluwer.

WATER INTOXICATION ASSESSMENT

Water intoxication occurs when the body's water and sodium levels become imbalanced as a result of excessive water intake that's accompanied by inadequate sodium intake, resulting in severe hyponatremia. This imbalance allows more water to enter the cells, causing them to swell and place excess pressure on the body's organs, especially the brain.

In patients with chronic psychiatric disorders, water intoxication may result from compulsive water drinking, or *psychogenic polydipsia.* The cause of psychogenic polydipsia is unknown, but the condition may be related to the interaction of several factors, including delusions having to do with fluid intake, adverse effects of medications, and hyperactivity of the hypothalamic thirst center. Water intoxication resulting from psychogenic polydipsia is considered self-induced.

Water intoxication typically produces no signs and symptoms in its early stages; however, over time, it causes neurologic, GI, cardiac, behavioral, and cognitive changes. The signs and symptoms of water intoxication are commonly mistaken for those of alcohol intoxication, and behavioral changes are commonly attributed to the patient's psychiatric diagnosis. (See *Signs and symptoms of water intoxication.*)

Early detection of water intoxication is crucial to prevent seizures, coma, and death, which can occur with severe hyponatremia when serum sodium concentrations are 90 to 105 mmol/L.

Equipment

Vital signs monitoring equipment (stethoscope, sphygmomanometer or electronic vital signs monitor) ■ scale ■ graduated urine collection container ■ venipuncture equipment and tubes ■ laboratory request forms ■ Optional: IV infusion equipment and fluids, prescribed medications.

Implementation

■ Review the patient's medical history, psychiatric diagnosis, and therapeutic regimen.
■ Perform hand hygiene.[1,2,3,4,5]
■ Confirm the patient's identity using at least two patient identifiers.[6]

■ Ask the patient and his family, if applicable, to describe any signs or symptoms the patient has experienced *to help identify signs and symptoms that would indicate water intoxication.*

NURSING ALERT *Be aware that patients with psychiatric disorders may not recognize signs and symptoms of water intoxication or may not admit to having them.*

■ Assess the patient for signs and symptoms of water intoxication.
■ Obtain the patient's vital signs.
■ Weigh the patient on the appropriate scale.
■ Calculate an estimated total daily fluid requirement based on the patient's body weight *to assess for excess water intake.* (See *Calculating maintenance fluid requirements.*)
■ Perform a *venipuncture to obtain baseline and serial serum sodium levels, as ordered,* and report results promptly. (See the "Venipuncture" procedure, page 821.)
■ Verify the practitioner's treatment orders.
■ Provide interventions (which may include IV administration of a hypertonic saline solution) or medications (clozapine or an oral vasopressin antagonist), as ordered.[7] Treatment may also include discontinuing contributing medications.[7,8]
■ Monitor the patient's water intake *to prevent self-induced water intoxication.*
■ Measure the patient's urine output hourly or as ordered. Immediately report an output of less than 30 mL/hour.
■ Monitor the patient, using one-to-one precautions as necessary, *to decrease excessive water intake.*
■ Provide alternative activities *to redirect the patient from drinking excessive amounts of water while awake.*
■ Continue to monitor the patient's mental status, behavior, level of consciousness, weight, vital signs, and serum sodium levels.
■ Perform hand hygiene.[1,2,3,4,5]
■ Document the procedure.[9,10,11]

Special considerations

■ If the patient has severe water intoxication, the practitioner may order IV furosemide *to promote diuresis.*

Patient teaching

Teach the patient and his family about the dangers related to excess water intake. Provide suggestions on ways for the family to redirect the patient during waking hours. If the patient demonstrates that he's willing to cooperate with restrictions, suggest alternative behaviors when he has the urge to drink excessively.

Provide the patient and his family with the patient's estimated total daily fluid requirement based on his body size *to ensure that the patient is adequately hydrated.* Review the signs and symptoms of water intoxication with the family, and instruct them to call the practitioner or seek medical attention immediately if the patient exhibits them.

Complications

Untreated or undiagnosed water intoxication can lead to seizures, coma, and death. Too-rapid replacement of saline could lead to permanent brain damage.

Documentation

Record your assessment findings and the patient's vital signs, serum sodium levels, and weight in his medical record. Also record all signs and symptoms of water intoxication, any treatment given, and the patient's response to treatment. Document the patient's estimated total daily fluid requirement and the efforts made to maintain this amount. Document intake and output. Note any teaching provided to the patient and family members and their understanding of the information.

Signs and symptoms of water intoxication

These signs and symptoms of water intoxication may occur over time.

Neurologic
■ Headache
■ Vertigo
■ Drowsiness
■ Muscle cramps
■ Blurred vision
■ Weakness
■ Tremors
■ Lethargy
■ Seizures

GI
■ Nausea
■ Repeated vomiting

Cardiac
■ Hypotension
■ Tachycardia
■ Cardiac arrhythmias
■ Heart failure

Behavioral and cognitive
■ Restlessness
■ Agitation
■ Disorientation
■ Confusion
■ Delirium

Other
■ Rapid breathing
■ Decreased urination
■ Sudden weight gain
■ Metabolic abnormalities

Calculating maintenance fluid requirements

The formula below helps you calculate the maintenance fluid requirements for your patient:

(1,500 mL for the first 20 kg) + (20 mL for each kg over 20 kg)

For example, if you have a patient who weighs 75 kg, use the formula as follows:

$$1{,}500\text{ mL} + (20\text{ mL} \times 55) = 1{,}500 + 1{,}100 = 2{,}600\text{ mL of fluid per day.}$$

REFERENCES

1 The Joint Commission. (2015). Standard NPSG.07.01.01. *Comprehensive accreditation manual for hospitals: The official handbook.* Oakbrook Terrace, IL: The Joint Commission. (Level VII)
2 Centers for Disease Control and Prevention. (2002). Guideline for hand hygiene in health-care settings: Recommendations of the Healthcare Infection Control Practices Advisory Committee and the HICPAC/SHEA/APIC/IDSA Hand Hygiene Task Force. *MMWR Recommendations and Reports, 51*(RR-16), 1–45. Accessed May 2015 via the Web at http://www.cdc.gov/mmwr/pdf/rr/rr5116.pdf (Level II)

Readiness criteria

A patient is considered ready for weaning from a ventilator when:

- his condition has resolved or improved and no longer requires ventilation
- he has an adequate natural airway or a functioning tracheostomy
- he has the ability to cough and mobilize secretions
- he has been successfully withdrawn from sedation
- he has a clear or clearing chest X-ray
- his arterial oxygen saturation is greater than 92% on fraction of inspired oxygen of less than or equal to 40% and positive end-expiratory pressure of less than or equal to 5 cm H_2O (0.49 kPa)
- his arterial blood gas values are within normal limits or have returned to baseline
- his hemoglobin is greater than 9 g/dL
- he's hemodynamically stability, has been adequately resuscitated, and has no need for vasoactive support
- he has a core body temperature greater than 96.8°F (36°C) and less than 102.2°F (39°C)
- he doesn't have any infection, acid-base or electrolyte imbalance, hyperglycemia, arrhythmias, renal failure, anemia, or excessive fatigue
- his pain is managed adequately with minimal use of pain medication.

3 World Health Organization. (2009). "WHO guidelines on hand hygiene in health care: First global patient safety challenge, clean care is safer care" [Online]. Accessed May 2015 via the Web at http://whqlibdoc.who.int/publications/2009/9789241597906_eng.pdf (Level IV)

4 Centers for Medicare & Medicaid Services, Department of Health and Human Services. (2014). Condition of participation: Infection control. 42 C.F.R. § 482.42.

5 American Osteopathic Association. (2014). Standard 07.01.21. *Healthcare Facilities Accreditation Program: Accreditation requirements for acute care hospitals.* Chicago, IL: American Osteopathic Association. (Level VII)

6 The Joint Commission. (2015). Standard NPSG.01.01.01. *Comprehensive accreditation manual for hospitals: The official handbook.* Oakbrook Terrace, IL: The Joint Commission. (Level VII)

7 Goldman, M. B. (2010). The assessment and treatment of water imbalance in patients with psychosis. *Clinical Schizophrenia and Related Psychoses, 4,* 115–123.

8 Jossiassen, R. C., et al. (2012). "Vaptans: A potential new approach for treating chronic hyponatremia in psychotic patients" [Online]. Accessed May 2015 via the Web at http://www.translationalneurosciencellc.com/uploads/1/1/8/2/11828657/2012_-_vaptans-_a_potential_new_approach.pdf

9 The Joint Commission. (2015). Standard RC.01.03.01. *Comprehensive accreditation manual for hospitals: The official handbook.* Oakbrook Terrace, IL: The Joint Commission. (Level VII)

10 Centers for Medicare & Medicaid Services, Department of Health and Human Services. (2014). Condition of participation: Medical record services. 42 C.F.R. § 482.24(b).

11 American Osteopathic Association. (2014). Standard 10.00.03. *Healthcare Facilities Accreditation Program: Accreditation requirements for acute care hospitals.* Chicago, IL: American Osteopathic Association. (Level VII)

ADDITIONAL REFERENCES

Mohr, W. K. (2013). *Psychiatric-mental health nursing: Evidence-based concepts, skills, and practices* (8th ed.). Philadelphia, PA: Lippincott Williams & Wilkins.

Nettina, S. M. (2014). *Lippincott manual of nursing practice* (10th ed.). Philadelphia, PA: Wolters Kluwer.

WEANING A PATIENT FROM A VENTILATOR

Successful weaning from a ventilator depends on the patient's ability to breathe on his own, which means that he must have a spontaneous respiratory effort for effective gas exchange, a stable cardiovascular system, and sufficient respiratory muscle strength and level of consciousness for weaning.

Weaning entails gradually reducing ventilator support until the patient can be removed from mechanical ventilation and successfully extubated. As soon as the patient's condition allows, sedation should be reduced so that the multidisciplinary team can adequately assess the patient's readiness to wean. The team should then plan to use either a facility-approved weaning protocol or an individualized weaning plan.[1]

Weaning should be initiated as soon as possible because ventilator use for longer than 24 hours increases the patient's risk of developing such complications as ventilator-associated pneumonia, GI bleeding, venous thromboembolism, and sinusitis.[1]

Equipment

Ventilator ▪ alternative oxygen delivery system ▪ practitioner-ordered or facility-approved weaning protocol ▪ pulse oximeter ▪ stethoscope ▪ blood pressure monitoring equipment ▪ thermometer ▪ disinfectant pad ▪ gloves ▪ suction equipment ▪ Optional: tracheostomy collar setup, transcutaneous partial pressure of carbon dioxide or end-tidal carbon dioxide detector, gown, mask, goggles, mask with face shield, arterial blood gas sampling equipment.

Preparation of equipment

Make sure that the alternative oxygen delivery system and suction equipment are readily available and functioning properly.

Implementation

- Verify the practitioner's order.
- Gather and prepare the appropriate equipment.
- Perform hand hygiene.[2,3,4,5,6]
- Put on gloves and other personal protective equipment as needed.[7,8]
- Confirm the patient's identity using at least two patient identifiers.[9]
- Interrupt the patient's sedative infusion according to the practitioner's order or your facility-approved weaning protocol.[10,11,12]
- Explain the procedure to the patient and his family *to help reduce anxiety and fear.*
- Assure the patient that you'll coach him through the weaning process.
- Make sure that the patient is attached to a cardiac monitor, as ordered. Make sure that the alarm limits are set appropriately for the patient's current condition and that the alarms are turned on, functioning properly, and audible to staff.[13,14,15,16]
- Perform a complete physical assessment *to evaluate patient readiness,* and discuss your results during multidisciplinary rounds.[17] (See *Readiness criteria.*)
- In collaboration with a respiratory therapist, institute a spontaneous breathing trial (SBT), as ordered or according to your facility's protocol (usually 5 to 10 minutes). *After a patient is considered ready to wean, the best method to assess whether the patient can breathe on his own is to perform an SBT.*[17]
- Instruct the patient to breath normally.[1]
- Assess the patient's vital signs, oxygenation, and mental status.

■ Monitor for signs and symptoms of intolerance, such as tachypnea, tachycardia, blood pressure elevation, and anxiety.[1,18]
■ Watch for perspiration and muscle strain in the neck and chest and paradoxical breathing patterns, including abnormal movement of the chest and abdominal muscles, inward movement of the abdomen during inspiration, and a different rate of motion between the chest and abdomen; *these signs indicate that the patient isn't tolerating the trial.*
■ If the patient doesn't tolerate the SBT, if the cardiac monitor reveals a cardiac arrhythmia, or if the patient develops chest pain, immediately return him to resting ventilator settings; then monitor his vital signs *to make sure that they return to baseline,* and notify the practitioner.[18]
■ Reassure the patient that setbacks are common. Explain that he'll have another SBT the next day if he meets the readiness criteria, and encourage him to rest.[1]
■ If the patient tolerates the SBT, follow your facility's weaning protocol (or the practitioner's order) or continue the SBT for up to 1 hour and then return to resting ventilator settings.[1] (See *After weaning.*)
■ Remove and discard your gloves and other personal protective equipment.[7,8]
■ Perform hand hygiene.[2,3,4,5,6]
■ Clean and disinfect your stethoscope using a disinfectant pad.[19,20]
■ Perform hand hygiene.[2,3,4,5,6]
■ Document the procedure.[21,22,23]

Special considerations

■ The Joint Commission has issued a sentinel event alert concerning medical device alarm safety *because alarm-related events have been associated with permanent loss of function or death.* Among the major contributing factors were improper alarm settings, alarms inappropriately turned off, and alarm signals not audible to staff. Make sure that alarm limits are set appropriately and that alarms are turned on and audible to staff. Follow facility guidelines for preventing alarm fatigue.[16]
■ Be aware that capnography may be useful during ventilator management and weaning.[24]
■ Make sure that the patient gets adequate rest and sleep *because fatigue can delay weaning from the ventilator.* Provide subdued lighting, safely muffle equipment noises, and restrict staff access to the area *to promote quiet during rest periods.*
■ Schedule weaning to fit comfortably and realistically within the patient's daily regimen. Avoid scheduling sessions after meals, baths, or lengthy therapeutic or diagnostic procedures *because the patient will be fatigued.* Have the patient help you set up the schedule *to give him some sense of control over a frightening procedure.* As the patient's tolerance for weaning increases, help him sit up in bed *to improve his breathing and sense of well-being.* Suggest diversionary activities *to take his mind off breathing.*
■ Keep in mind that setbacks are common during the weaning process, especially after long-term ventilation. Provide the patient and his family with reassurance and support.
■ Be aware that the outcome of weaning trials can range from complete, successful weaning to incomplete weaning, in which long-term partial or full mechanical ventilatory support is required, or terminal weaning, in which natural death may occur as the result of withdrawal of life support.
■ See the "Endotracheal tube care" procedure, page 283 when the patient is ready for extubation.

Complications

Hypoxia may occur if the patient isn't ready to breathe on his own or tolerate decreased ventilator settings.

After weaning[18]

Although the patient may require supplemental oxygen to achieve these goals, after being weaned, the patient should have:
■ a respiratory rate of less than 24 breaths/minute
■ heart rate and blood pressure within 15% of baseline
■ a tidal volume of 3 to 5 mL/kg
■ an arterial pH greater than 7.35
■ a partial pressure of arterial oxygen maintained at greater than 60 mm Hg (8 kPa)
■ a partial pressure of arterial carbon dioxide maintained at less than 45 mm Hg (6 kPa)
■ an oxygen saturation level maintained at greater than 90%
■ no cardiac arrhythmias
■ no accessory muscle use.

Documentation

Record your assessment findings that determined the patient's readiness to wean. Record the results after each weaning episode, including specific parameters. List all complications and nursing actions taken. If the patient was receiving pressure support ventilation or using a T-piece or tracheostomy collar, note the duration of spontaneous breathing and the patient's ability to maintain the weaning schedule. If the patient received intermittent mandatory ventilation, with or without pressure support ventilation, record the control breath rate, the time of each breath reduction, and the rate of spontaneous respirations. Also document any patient teaching provided.

References

1 Lynn-McHale Wiegand, D. (Ed.). (2011). *AACN procedure manual for critical care* (6th ed.). St. Louis, MO: Saunders.
2 Centers for Disease Control and Prevention. (2002). Guideline for hand hygiene in health-care settings: Recommendations of the Healthcare Infection Control Practices Advisory Committee and the HICPAC/SHEA/APIC/IDSA Hand Hygiene Task Force. *MMWR Recommendations and Reports, 51*(RR-16), 1–45. Accessed May 2015 via the Web at http://www.cdc.gov/mmwr/pdf/rr/rr5116.pdf (Level II)
3 The Joint Commission. (2015). Standard NPSG.07.01.01. *Comprehensive accreditation manual for hospitals: The official handbook.* Oakbrook Terrace, IL: The Joint Commission. (Level VII)
4 World Health Organization. (2009). "WHO guidelines on hand hygiene in health care: First global patient safety challenge, clean care is safer care" [Online]. Accessed May 2015 via the Web at http://whqlibdoc.who.int/publications/2009/9789241597906_eng.pdf (Level IV)
5 American Osteopathic Association. (2014). Standard 07.01.21. *Healthcare Facilities Accreditation Program: Accreditation requirements for acute care hospitals.* Chicago, IL: American Osteopathic Association. (Level VII)
6 Centers for Medicare & Medicaid Services, Department of Health and Human Services. (2014). Condition of participation: Infection control. 42 C.F.R. § 482.42.
7 Siegel, J. D., et al. (2007). "2007 guideline for isolation precautions: Preventing transmission of infectious agents in healthcare settings" [Online]. Accessed May 2015 via the Web at http://www.cdc.gov/hicpac/pdf/isolation/Isolation2007.pdf (Level II)
8 American Osteopathic Association. (2014). Standard 07.01.10. *Healthcare Facilities Accreditation Program: Accreditation requirements for acute care hospitals.* Chicago, IL: American Osteopathic Association. (Level VII)
9 The Joint Commission. (2015). Standard NPSG.01.01.01. *Comprehensive accreditation manual for hospitals: The official handbook.* Oakbrook Terrace, IL: The Joint Commission. (Level VII)

Recognizing dehiscence and evisceration

In wound dehiscence, the layers of the surgical wound separate. With evisceration, the viscera (in this case, a bowel loop) protrude through the surgical incision.

Wound dehiscence | **Evisceration of bowel loop**

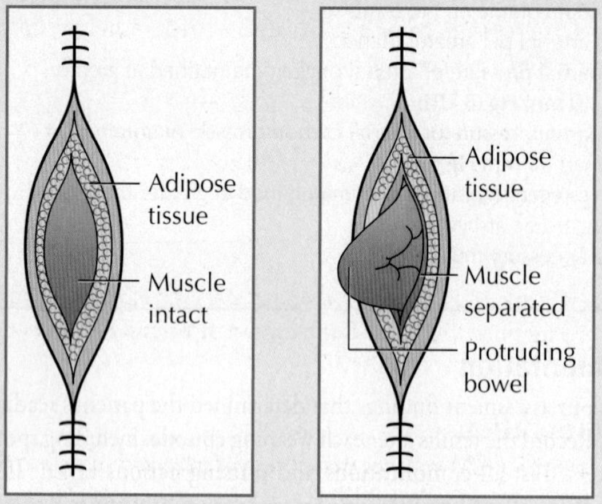

10 Association of Professionals in Infection Control and Epidemiology (APIC). (2009). "An APIC guide 2009: Guide to the elimination of ventilator-associated pneumonia" [Online]. Accessed May 2015 via the Web at http://www.apic.org/Resource_/EliminationGuideForm/18e326ad-b484-471c-9c35-6822a53ee4a2/File/VAP_09.pdf (Level IV)

11 Klompas, M., et al. (2014). Strategies to prevent ventilator-associated pneumonia in acute care hospitals: 2014 update. Infection *Control and Hospital Epidemiology, 35,* 915–936. Accessed May 2015 via the Web at http://www.jstor.org/stable/10.1086/677144 (Level II)

12 Institute for Healthcare Improvement. (2012). *How-to-guide: Prevent ventilator-associated pneumonia.* Cambridge, MA: Institute for Healthcare Improvement. (Level VII)

13 American Association of Critical-Care Nurses. (2013). "AACN practice alert: Alarm management" [Online]. Accessed May 2015 via the Web at http://www.aacn.org/wd/practice/docs/practicealerts/alarm-management-practice-alert.pdf (Level VII)

14 Graham, K. C., & Cvach, M. (2010). Monitor alarm fatigue: Standardizing use of physiological monitors and decreasing nuisance alarms. *American Journal of Critical Care, 19,* 28–37.

15 The Joint Commission. (2015). Standard NPSG.06.01.01. *Comprehensive accreditation manual for hospitals: The official handbook.* Oakbrook Terrace, IL: The Joint Commission. (Level VII)

16 The Joint Commission. (2013). "Sentinel event alert: Medical device alarm safety in hospitals" [Online]. Accessed May 2015 via the Web at http://www.jointcommission.org/assets/1/18/SEA_50_alarms_4_5_13_FINAL1.PDF (Level VII)

17 American College of Chest Physicians, American Association for Respiratory Care, American College of Critical Care Medicine. (2002). Evidence-based guidelines for weaning and discontinuing ventilatory support. *Respiratory Care, 47,* 69–90. Accessed May 2015 via the Web at http://www.aarc.org/daz/rcjournal/rcjournal/x.RCJOURNAL.COM%2002.21.07/online_resources/cpgs/ebgwdvscpg.pdf (Level VII)

18 Astle, S. M., & Smith, D. (2007). "Taking your patient off a ventilator: Following an established protocol can help you wean your patient from a respirator as soon as possible" [Online]. Accessed May 2015 via the Web at http://www.modernmedicine.com/managed-healthcare-executive/news/taking-your-patient-ventilator

19 Rutala, W. A., et al. (2008). "Guideline for disinfection and sterilization in healthcare facilities, 2008" [Online]. Accessed May 2015 via the Web at http://www.cdc.gov/hicpac/pdf/guidelines/Disinfection_Nov_2008.pdf (Level I)

20 American Osteopathic Association. (2014). Standard 07.02.03. *Healthcare Facilities Accreditation Program: Accreditation requirements for acute care hospitals.* Chicago, IL: American Osteopathic Association. (Level VII)

21 The Joint Commission. (2015). Standard RC.01.03.01. *Comprehensive accreditation manual for hospitals: The official handbook.* Oakbrook Terrace, IL: The Joint Commission. (Level VII)

22 American Osteopathic Association. (2014). Standard 10.00.03. *Healthcare Facilities Accreditation Program: Accreditation requirements for acute care hospitals.* Chicago, IL: American Osteopathic Association. (Level VII)

23 Centers for Medicare & Medicaid Services, Department of Health and Human Services. (2014). Condition of participation: Medical record services. 42 C.F.R. § 482.24(b).

24 Walsh, B. K., et al. (2011). AARC clinical practice guideline: Capnography/capnometry during mechanical ventilation: 2011. *Respiratory Care, 56,* 503–509. Accessed May 2015 via the Web at http://www.rcjournal.com/cpgs/pdf/04.11.0503.pdf (Level VII)

WOUND DEHISCENCE AND EVISCERATION MANAGEMENT

Although surgical wounds typically heal without incident, occasionally, the edges of a wound may fail to join or may separate even after they seem to be healing normally. This development, called *wound dehiscence,* may lead to an even more serious complication: evisceration, in which a portion of the viscera (usually a bowel loop) protrudes through the incision. Evisceration, in turn, can lead to peritonitis and septic shock. (See *Recognizing dehiscence and evisceration.*) Dehiscence and evisceration are most likely to occur 6 or 7 days after surgery. By then, sutures may have been removed and the patient can cough easily and breathe deeply—both of which strain the incision.

Several factors can contribute to these complications. Poor nutrition—whether from inadequate intake, obesity,[1] or a condition such as diabetes mellitus—may hinder wound healing. Chronic pulmonary or cardiac disease and metastatic cancer can also slow healing because the injured tissue doesn't get needed nutrients and oxygen. Localized wound infection may limit closure, delay healing, and weaken the incision. Stress on the incision from coughing or vomiting may cause abdominal distention or severe stretching.[2] A midline abdominal incision, for instance, poses a high risk of wound dehiscence.

Equipment

Two sterile towels ▪ 1 L of sterile normal saline solution ▪ sterile irrigation set, including a basin, a solution container, and a 50-mL catheter-tip syringe ▪ several large sterile abdominal dressings ▪ sterile, waterproof drape ▪ fluid-impermeable pads ▪ gloves ▪ sterile gloves.

If the patient will return to the operating room, be sure you also gather the following equipment: IV administration set and IV fluids, equipment for nasogastric (NG) intubation, prescribed sedative, and suction apparatus.

Implementation

- Perform hand hygiene and put on gloves.[3,4,5,6,7]
- Provide reassurance and support *to ease the patient's anxiety.* Tell him to stay in bed. If possible, stay with him while someone else notifies the practitioner and collects the necessary equipment.
- Explain the procedure to the patient *to allay his fears and enhance cooperation..*
- Place a fluid-impermeable pad under the patient *to keep the sheets dry when you moisten the exposed viscera.*
- Using sterile technique (see the "Sterile technique, basic" procedure, page 715), unfold a sterile towel *to create a sterile field.* Open the package

containing the irrigation set, and place the basin, solution container, and 50-mL syringe on the sterile field.

■ Open the bottle of sterile normal saline solution and pour about 400 mL into the solution container. Also pour about 200 mL into the sterile basin.

■ Open several large, sterile abdominal dressings and place them on the sterile field.

■ Remove and discard your gloves[8,9] and perform hand hygiene.[3,4,5,6,7]

■ Put on the sterile gloves.[8,9] and place one or two of the large sterile abdominal dressings into the basin *to saturate them with normal saline solution.*

■ Place the moistened dressings over the exposed viscera.[1,10] Then place a sterile, waterproof drape over the dressings *to prevent the sheets from getting wet.*

■ Remove and discard your gloves.[8,9]

■ Perform hand hygiene.[3,4,5,6,7]

■ Every hour, perform hand hygiene, put on sterile gloves[8,9] and moisten the dressings by withdrawing saline solution from the container through the syringe and then gently squirting the solution on the dressings.

■ When you moisten the dressings, inspect the color of the viscera. If it appears dusky or black, notify the practitioner immediately. *With its blood supply interrupted, a protruding organ may become ischemic and necrotic.*

■ Remove and discard your gloves[8,9] and perform hand hygiene.[3,4,5,6]

■ Keep the patient on absolute bed rest in the low Fowler position (no more than 20 degrees' elevation) with his knees flexed *to prevent injury and reduce stress on an abdominal incision.*[1,10]

■ Don't allow the patient to have anything by mouth *to decrease the risk of aspiration during surgery.*

■ Monitor the patient's pulse, respirations, blood pressure, and temperature frequently *to detect shock.*

Preparing the patient for return to the operating room

■ Confirm that written informed consent has been obtained and is in the patient's medical record.[11,12,13]

■ Conduct a preprocedure verification *to make sure that all relevant documentation, related information, and equipment are available and correctly identified to the patient's identifiers.*[14,15]

■ Gather the appropriate equipment.

■ Perform hand hygiene.[3,4,5,7,6]

■ Confirm the patient's identity using at least two patient identifiers.[16]

■ Begin an IV infusion, as ordered.

■ Insert an NG tube if ordered. Connect the tube to continuous or low intermittent suction, as ordered. (See the "Nasogastric tube insertion and removal" procedure, page 531.)

■ Administer preoperative medications, as ordered, following safe medication administration practices.[17,18]

■ Continue to reassure the patient while you prepare him for surgery.

■ Make sure that the operating room staff has been informed about the procedure. Provide handoff communication for the person who will assume responsibility for care of the patient during surgery. Allow time for questions and answers.[19]

Completing the procedure

■ Remove and discard your gloves[8,9] and perform hand hygiene.[3,4,5,6,7]

■ Document the procedure.[20,21,22]

Special considerations

■ When teaching a patient to cough and deep-breathe postoperatively, have him hold a pillow or bath blanket tightly against his abdomen *to equalize the internal pressure that coughing places on the incision.*

■ Depending on the circumstances, some of these procedures might not be performed at the bedside. For instance, NG intubation might make the patient gag or vomit, causing further evisceration. For this reason, the practitioner might choose to have the NG tube inserted in the operating room with the patient under anesthesia.

■ The best treatment is prevention. If you're caring for a postoperative patient who's at risk for poor healing, make sure that he gets an adequate supply of protein, vitamins, and calories. Monitor his dietary deficiencies, and discuss any problems with the practitioner and dietitian.

■ When changing wound dressings, always use sterile technique. Inspect the incision with each dressing change, and if you recognize the early signs of infection, start treatment before dehiscence or evisceration can occur. If local infection develops, clean the wound as ordered *to eliminate a buildup of purulent drainage.* Make sure bandages aren't so tight that they limit blood supply to the wound.

Complications

Infection, which can lead to peritonitis and possibly septic shock, is the most severe and most common complication of wound dehiscence and evisceration.

Documentation

Note when the problem occurred, the patient's activity preceding the problem, the patient's condition, and the time at which the practitioner was notified. Describe the appearance of the wound or eviscerated organ; the amount, color, consistency, and odor of any drainage; and any nursing actions taken. Record the patient's vital signs, the patient's response to the incident, and the practitioner's actions. Note the name and title of the person who received the handoff communication.

REFERENCES

1 Taylor, C. R., et al. (2015). *Fundamentals of nursing: The art and science of nursing care* (8th ed.). Philadelphia, PA: Wolters Kluwer.

2 Iqbal, A., et al. (2008). A study of intragastric and intravesicular pressure changes during rest, coughing, weight lifting, retching, and vomiting. *Surgical Endoscopy, 22,* 2571–2575. (Level VI)

3 Centers for Disease Control and Prevention. (2002). Guideline for hand hygiene in health-care settings: Recommendations of the Healthcare Infection Control Practices Advisory Committee and the HICPAC/SHEA/APIC/IDSA Hand Hygiene Task Force. *MMWR Recommendations and Reports, 51*(RR-16), 1–45. Accessed May 2015 via the Web at http://www.cdc.gov/mmwr/pdf/rr/rr5116.pdf (Level II)

4 World Health Organization. (2009). "WHO guidelines on hand hygiene in health care: First global patient safety challenge, clean care is safer care" [Online]. Accessed May 2015 via the Web at http://whqlibdoc.who.int/publications/2009/9789241597906_eng.pdf (Level IV)

5 The Joint Commission. (2015). Standard NPSG.07.01.01. *Comprehensive accreditation manual for hospitals: The official handbook.* Oakbrook Terrace, IL: The Joint Commission. (Level VII)

6 American Osteopathic Association. (2014). Standard 07.01.21. *Healthcare Facilities Accreditation Program: Accreditation requirements for acute care hospitals.* Chicago, IL: American Osteopathic Association. (Level VII)

7 Centers for Medicare & Medicaid Services, Department of Health and Human Services. (2014). Condition of participation: Infection control. 42 C.F.R. § 482.42.

8 Siegel, J. D., et al. (2007). "2007 guideline for isolation precautions: Preventing transmission of infectious agents in healthcare settings" [Online]. Accessed May 2015 via the Web at http://www.cdc.gov/hicpac/pdf/isolation/Isolation2007.pdf (Level II)

9 American Osteopathic Association. (2014). Standard 07.01.10. *Healthcare Facilities Accreditation Program: Accreditation requirements for acute care hospitals.* Chicago, IL: American Osteopathic Association. (Level VII)

10 Hinkle, J. L., & Cheever, K. H. (2014). *Brunner & Suddarth's textbook of medical-surgical nursing* (13th ed.). Philadelphia, PA: Wolters Kluwer.

11 The Joint Commission. (2015). Standard RI.01.03.01. *Comprehensive accreditation manual for hospitals: The official handbook.* Oakbrook Terrace, IL: The Joint Commission. (Level VII)
12 Centers for Medicare & Medicaid Services, Department of Health and Human Services. (2014). Condition of participation: Patient's rights. 42 C.F.R. § 482.13(b)(2).
13 American Osteopathic Association. (2014). Standard 30.00.11. *Healthcare Facilities Accreditation Program: Accreditation requirements for acute care hospitals.* Chicago, IL: American Osteopathic Association. (Level VII)
14 The Joint Commission. (2015). Standard UP.01.01.01. *Comprehensive accreditation manual for hospitals: The official handbook.* Oakbrook Terrace, IL: The Joint Commission. (Level VII)
15 American Osteopathic Association. (2014). Standard 30.00.14. *Healthcare Facilities Accreditation Program: Accreditation requirements for acute care hospitals.* Chicago, IL: American Osteopathic Association (Level VII)
16 The Joint Commission. (2015). Standard NPSG.01.01.01. *Comprehensive accreditation manual for hospitals: The official handbook.* Oakbrook Terrace, IL: The Joint Commission. (Level VII)
17 American Osteopathic Association. (2014). Standard 16.01.03. *Healthcare Facilities Accreditation Program: Accreditation requirements for acute care hospitals.* Chicago, IL: American Osteopathic Association. (Level VII)
18 Centers for Medicare & Medicaid Services, Department of Health and Human Services. (2014). Condition of participation: Nursing services. 42 C.F.R. § 482.23(c).
19 The Joint Commission. (2015). Standard PC.02.02.01. *Comprehensive accreditation manual for hospitals: The official handbook.* Oakbrook Terrace, IL: The Joint Commission. (Level VII)
20 The Joint Commission. (2015). Standard RC.01.03.01. *Comprehensive accreditation manual for hospitals: The official handbook.* Oakbrook Terrace, IL: The Joint Commission. (Level VII)
21 Centers for Medicare & Medicaid Services, Department of Health and Human Services. (2014). Condition of participation: Medical record services. 42 C.F.R. § 482.24(b).
22 American Osteopathic Association. (2014). Standard 10.00.03. *Healthcare Facilities Accreditation Program: Accreditation requirements for acute care hospitals.* Chicago, IL: American Osteopathic Association. (Level VII)

ADDITIONAL REFERENCES

Nettina, S. M. (2014). *Lippincott manual of nursing practice* (10th ed.). Philadelphia, PA: Wolters Kluwer.
van Ramshorst, G. H., et al. (2013). Long-term outcome study in patients with abdominal wound dehiscence: A comparative study on quality of life, body image, and incisional hernia. *Journal of Gastrointestinal Surgery, 17,* 1477–1484. (Level IV)

WOUND IRRIGATION

Irrigation cleans tissues and flushes cell debris and drainage from an open wound. Because the force of the irrigating solution stream is greater than the forces that hold the debris to the wound surface, the irrigating stream washes out the debris; research indicates that the most effected wound irrigation pressures range from 5 and 15 psi.[1]

Methods of irrigating a wound include the use of a 35-mL syringe with a 19G angiocatheter and mechanical lavage. A 35-mL syringe with a 19G angiocatheter provides irrigation pressure estimated at 8 psi; mechanical lavage delivers intermittent high-pressure irrigation that may be combined with suction to remove the irrigant and wound debris. During mechanical irrigation, the pressure shouldn't be higher than 15 psi to prevent damage to healthy tissue.[1]

Irrigation with a commercial wound cleaner helps the wound heal properly, from the inside tissue layers outward to the skin surface; it also helps prevent premature surface healing over an abscess pocket or infected tract. After irrigation, open wounds usually are packed to absorb additional drainage. The standard precautions guidelines of the Centers for Disease Control and Prevention should always be followed.[2]

Equipment

Waterproof trash container ▪ fluid-impermeable pad ▪ emesis basin ▪ gloves ▪ mask and goggles or mask with face shield ▪ gown ▪ prescribed irrigant such as sterile normal saline solution ▪ sterile container ▪ sterile gauze ▪ sterile dressing ▪ commercial wound cleaner ▪ 35-mL piston syringe with 19G angiocatheter[3] ▪ skin-protectant wipe ▪ gauze pad ▪ Optional: prescribed analgesia, wound packing, splash guard.

Preparation of equipment

Assemble all equipment in the patient's room. Perform hand hygiene.[4,5,6,7,8] Check the expiration date on each sterile package and inspect for tears. Follow the manufacturer's recommendations and your facility's guidelines regarding shelf life of solutions once they have been opened.[9]

Using sterile technique, dilute the prescribed irrigant to the correct proportions with sterile water or normal saline solution, if necessary. Let the solution stand until it reaches room temperature, or warm it to 90° to 95°F (32° to 35°C).[10]

Open the waterproof trash container and place it near the patient's bed. Position the container *to avoid reaching across the sterile field or the wound when disposing of soiled articles.*

Implementation

- Verify the practitioner's order.
- Perform hand hygiene *to prevent the spread of microorganisms.*[4,5,6,7,8]
- Confirm the patient's identity using at least two patient identifiers.[11]
- Identify any patient allergies, especially to povidone-iodine or other topical solutions or medications, latex, or tape.
- Assess the patient's condition.
- Perform a comprehensive pain assessment using techniques appropriate for the patient's age, condition, and ability to understand.[12] Provide pain medication, as ordered and needed, following safe medication administration practices *because wound care and irrigation can be painful.*[13,14]
- Provide privacy.[15,16]
- Explain the procedure to the patient *to enhance cooperation.*
- Position the patient appropriately *to gain access to the wound.*
- Place the fluid-impermeable pad under the patient *to catch any spills and avoid linen changes.*
- Place the emesis basin below the wound *so that the irrigating solution flows from the wound into the basin and drains from the clean to the dirty end of the wound.*
- If necessary, put on a gown and a mask and goggles or a mask with face shield *to protect you from splashing and contamination.*[2,17]
- Put on gloves.[2,17]
- Remove the soiled dressing and discard it in the waterproof trash container.[2]
- Remove and discard your gloves.[2,17]
- Perform hand hygiene.[4,5,6,7,8]
- Inspect the wound and surrounding tissue *to gauge the healing process and to assess for the presence of infection.*
- Establish a clean field that contains all of the equipment and supplies you'll need for irrigation and wound care.
- Pour the prescribed amount of irrigating solution into a sterile container.
- Put on gloves.[2,17]
- Fill the syringe with the irrigating solution (as shown on next page, top left) and connect the angiocatheter.

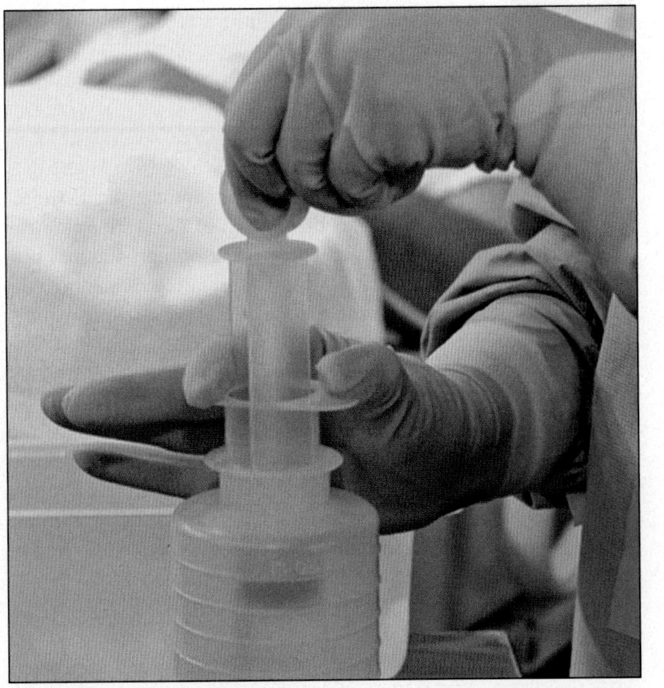

■ Gently instill a slow, steady stream of irrigating solution into the wound (as shown below) until the syringe empties. Make sure that the solution flows from the clean to the dirty area of the wound *to prevent contamination of clean tissue by exudate.* Also make sure that the solution reaches all areas of the wound.

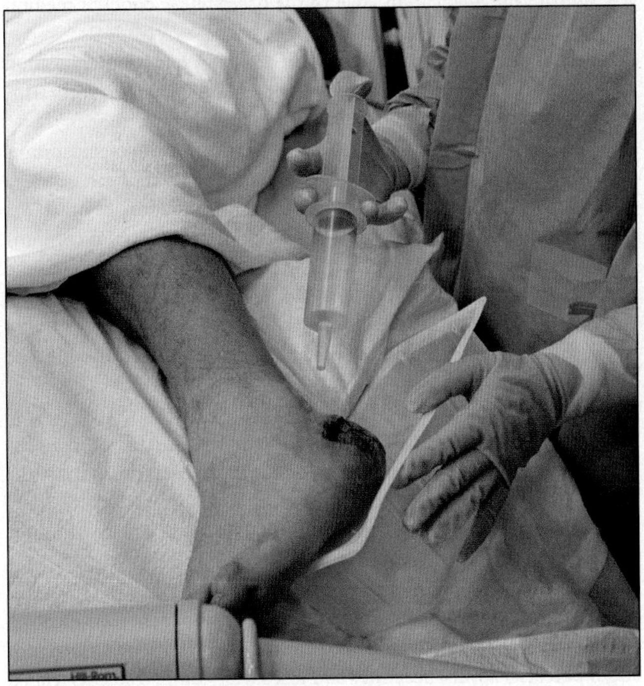

■ Refill the syringe and repeat the irrigation.
■ Continue to irrigate the wound until you've administered the prescribed amount of solution or until the solution returns clear.[18] Note the amount of solution administered.
■ Discard the syringe in a puncture-resistant sharps container.
■ Keep the patient positioned *to allow further wound drainage into the basin.*
■ Dry intact skin with a gauze pad.
■ Apply a skin-protectant wipe and allow it to dry completely *to help prevent skin breakdown and infection.*
■ Pack the wound loosely, if ordered, *to stimulate granulation.*[1]
■ Apply a sterile dressing.
■ Properly dispose of drainage and solutions, and clean or dispose of soiled equipment and supplies.[2] *To prevent contamination of other equipment,* don't return unopened sterile supplies to the sterile supply cabinet. Store them in an appropriate location in the patient's room or as directed by your facility.
■ Remove and discard your gloves and personal protective equipment in the appropriate receptacle.[2,17]
■ Perform hand hygiene.[4,5,6,7,8]
■ Reassess the patient's pain and respond appropriately.[12]
■ Perform hand hygiene.[4,5,6,7,8]
■ Document the procedure.[19,20,21]

Special considerations

■ Try to coordinate wound irrigation with the practitioner's visit *so he can inspect the wound.*
■ Use only the irrigant specified by the practitioner *because others may be erosive or otherwise harmful.*
■ Irrigate with a bulb syringe only if a piston syringe is unavailable. A bulb syringe requires caution *because it doesn't deliver enough pressure for adequate wound cleaning.* If the wound is small or not particularly deep, you may want to use just the syringe without the angiocatheter for irrigation.
■ Note that some facilities may use a splash guard for wound irrigation. *This helps decrease the risk of contaminated fluid splashing onto the linens, surrounding areas, or you.*

Patient teaching

If the wound must be irrigated at home, teach the patient or a family member how to perform the procedure using strict sterile technique. Ask for a return demonstration of the proper technique. Provide written instructions. Arrange for home health supplies and nursing visits, as appropriate. Urge the patient to call the practitioner if he detects signs of infection.

Complications

Wound irrigation increases the risk of infection and may cause excoriation and increased pain. Pressure over 15 psi causes trauma to the wound and directs bacteria back into the tissue.

Documentation

Record the date and time of irrigation, amount and type of irrigant, appearance of the wound, any sloughing tissue or exudate, amount of solution returned, skin care performed around the wound, dressings applied, and the patient's tolerance of the treatment.

REFERENCES

1 Baranoski, S., & Ayello, E. A. (2012). *Wound care essentials: Practice principles* (3rd ed.). Philadelphia, PA: Lippincott Williams & Wilkins.
2 Siegel, J. D., et al. (2007). "2007 guideline for isolation precautions: Preventing transmission of infectious agents in healthcare settings" [Online]. Accessed May 2015 via the Web at http://www.cdc.gov/hicpac/isolation/Isolation2007.pdf (Level II)
3 Wound, Ostomy and Continence Nurses Society (WOCN). (2003, revised 2010). "WOCN clinical practice guideline no. 2: Guideline for prevention and management of pressure ulcers" [Online]. Accessed March 2015 via the Web at http://guideline.gov/content.aspx?id=23868 (Level VII)

4 The Joint Commission. (2015). Standard NPSG.07.01.01. *Comprehensive accreditation manual for hospitals: The official handbook.* Oakbrook Terrace, IL: The Joint Commission. (Level VII)

5 Centers for Disease Control and Prevention. (2002). Guideline for hand hygiene in health-care settings: Recommendations of the Healthcare Infection Control Practices Advisory Committee and the HICPAC/SHEA/APIC/IDSA Hand Hygiene Task Force. *MMWR Recommendations and Reports, 51*(RR-16), 1–45. Accessed May 2015 via the Web at http://www.cdc.gov/mmwr/pdf/rr/rr5116.pdf (Level II)

6 World Health Organization. (2009). "WHO guidelines on hand hygiene in health care: First global patient safety challenge, clean care is safer care" [Online]. Accessed May 2015 via the Web at http://whqlibdoc.who.int/publications/2009/9789241597906_eng.pdf (Level IV)

7 American Osteopathic Association. (2014). Standard 07.01.21. *Healthcare Facilities Accreditation Program: Accreditation requirements for acute care hospitals.* Chicago, IL: American Osteopathic Association. (Level VII)

8 Centers for Medicare & Medicaid Services, Department of Health and Human Services. (2014). Condition of participation: Infection control. 42 C.F.R. § 482.42.

9 Wound, Ostomy and Continence Nurses Society. (2012). Clean vs. sterile dressing techniques for management of chronic wounds: A fact sheet. *Journal of Wound, Ostomy and Continence Nursing, 39*(Suppl. 2), S30–S34. (Level VII)

10 Fernandez, R., & Griffiths, R. (2008). Water for wound cleansing. *Cochrane Database of Systematic Reviews, 2008*(1), CD003861. (Level I)

11 The Joint Commission. (2015). Standard NPSG.01.01.01. *Comprehensive accreditation manual for hospitals: The official handbook.* Oakbrook Terrace, IL: The Joint Commission. (Level VII)

12 The Joint Commission. (2015). Standard PC.01.02.07. *Comprehensive accreditation manual for hospitals: The official handbook.* Oakbrook Terrace, IL: The Joint Commission. (Level VII)

13 American Osteopathic Association. (2014). Standard 16.01.03. *Healthcare Facilities Accreditation Program: Accreditation requirements for acute care hospitals.* Chicago, IL: American Osteopathic Association. (Level VII)

14 Centers for Medicare & Medicaid Services, Department of Health and Human Services. (2014). Condition of participation: Nursing services. 42 C.F.R. § 482.23(c).

15 American Osteopathic Association. (2014). Standard 15.01.16. *Healthcare Facilities Accreditation Program: Accreditation requirements for acute care hospitals.* Chicago, IL: American Osteopathic Association. (Level VII)

16 Centers for Medicare & Medicaid Services, Department of Health and Human Services. (2014). Condition of participation: Patient's rights. 42 C.F.R. § 482.13(c)(1).

17 American Osteopathic Association. (2014). Standard 07.01.10. *Healthcare Facilities Accreditation Program: Accreditation requirements for acute care hospitals.* Chicago, IL: American Osteopathic Association. (Level VII)

18 Fernandez, R., et al. (2004). The effectiveness of solutions, techniques, and pressure in wound cleansing. *JBI Reports, 2,* 231–270. (Level I)

19 The Joint Commission. (2015). Standard RC.01.03.01. *Comprehensive accreditation manual for hospitals: The official handbook.* Oakbrook Terrace, IL: The Joint Commission. (Level VII)

20 Centers for Medicare & Medicaid Services, Department of Health and Human Services. (2014). Condition of participation: Medical record services. 42 C.F.R. § 482.24(b).

21 American Osteopathic Association. (2014). Standard 10.00.03. *Healthcare Facilities Accreditation Program: Accreditation requirements for acute care hospitals.* Chicago, IL: American Osteopathic Association. (Level VII)

ADDITIONAL REFERENCES

Allen, G. (2013). "Wound irrigation" [Online]. Accessed December 2014 via the Web at http://emedicine.medscape.com/article/1895071-overview

Craven, R. F., & Hirnle, C. J. (2012). *Fundamentals of nursing: Human health and function* (7th ed.). Philadelphia, PA: Lippincott Williams & Wilkins.

Nettina, S. M. (2014). *Lippincott manual of nursing practice* (10th ed.). Philadelphia, PA: Wolters Kluwer.

Z

Z-TRACK INJECTION

The Z-track method is the preferred method for administering IM injections because it prevents leakage, or *tracking,* of medication into the subcutaneous tissue (which can cause patient discomfort and may permanently stain some tissue). Lateral displacement of the skin during the injection helps to seal the drug in the muscle. This procedure requires careful attention to technique.

Equipment

Patient's medication and medical records ■ single-use sterile syringe and needle of appropriate size (at least 1½″ [3.8 cm] recommended)[1] and gauge (self-sheathing needle recommended)[2] ■ prescribed medication ■ alcohol pads ■ Optional: gloves, ice, filter needle, 1″ (2.5-cm) tape.

The prescribed medication must be sterile. The needle may be prepackaged separately or already attached to the syringe.

Implementation

- Avoid distractions and interruptions when preparing and administering the medication *to prevent medication errors.*[3,4]
- Verify the order in the patient's medication record by checking it against the practitioner's order.[5,6,7]
- Choose the equipment appropriate to the prescribed medication and injection site, and make sure that it works properly. The needle should be straight, smooth, and free from burrs.
- Compare the medication label to the order in the patient's medical record.[5,6,7]
- Check the patient's medical record for an allergy or a contraindication to the prescribed medication. If an allergy or a contraindication exists, don't administer the medication; instead, notify the practitioner.[5,6,7]
- Check the expiration date on the medication. If the medication is expired, return it to the pharmacy and obtain new medication.[5,6,7]
- Visually inspect the solution for particles, discoloration, or other loss of integrity; don't administer the medication if its integrity is compromised.[5,6,7] Remember that for some drugs (such as suspensions), the presence of drug particles is normal. If in doubt, check with the pharmacist and the manufacturer's instructions.
- Discuss any unresolved concerns about the medication with the patient's practitioner.[5,6,7]
- Perform hand hygiene.[8,9,10,11,12]
- Carefully calculate the dose. If it's a high-alert medication that can cause significant patient harm when used in error, perform an independent double-check with another nurse if required by your facility.[13]
- Read the medication label again as you draw up the medication for injection if needed.
- Perform hand hygiene.[8,9,10,11,12]
- Confirm the patient's identity using at least two patient identifiers.[5,14]
- If the patient is receiving the medication for the first time, teach him about potential adverse reactions and discuss any other concerns related to the medication.[6]
- Verify that the medication is being administered at the proper time, in the prescribed dose, and by the correct route *to reduce the risk of medication errors.*[5,6,7]
- Provide privacy and[15,16] explain the procedure to the patient *to allay his anxiety.*
- If your facility uses a bar code scanning system, scan your identification badge, the patient's identification bracelet, and the medication's bar code.

■ Put on gloves if contact with blood or body fluids is likely or if your skin or the patient's skin isn't intact; glove use isn't necessary for routine IM injection.[17,18]
■ Select an appropriate injection site. The ventrogluteal site is used most commonly for healthy adults, although the deltoid muscle may be used for a small-volume injection (2 mL or less). Remember to always rotate injection sites for patients who require repeated injections.
■ Position and drape the patient appropriately using his bed linens, making sure the site is well exposed and that lighting is adequate.
■ After selecting the injection site, clean the skin with an alcohol pad. Move the pad outward in a circular motion to a circumference of about 2″ (5 cm) from the injection site and allow the skin to dry.[17]
■ Remove the needle sheath.
■ With the thumb and index finger of your nondominant hand, gently displace the skin and subcutaneous tissue of the injection site by pulling the skin laterally for the Z-track technique.[1]
■ Position the syringe at a 90-degree angle to the skin surface, with the needle about 2″ (5 cm) from the skin. Tell the patient that he'll feel a prick as you insert the needle. Then quickly and smoothly insert the needle through the skin and subcutaneous tissue, deep into the muscle at a 90-degree angle.
■ Support the syringe with your nondominant hand if desired. Pull back slightly on the plunger with your dominant hand *to aspirate for blood* if appropriate.

NURSING ALERT *Aspiration of blood isn't recommended when administering vaccines or toxoids by the IM route* because large blood vessels aren't present at recommended injection sites.[19]

■ Inject the drug slowly.
■ Wait 10 seconds before withdrawing the needle *to ensure dispersion of the medication.* Then withdraw the needle slowly at a 90-degree angle.[20,21]
■ Remove your finger from the skin surface, allowing the displaced skin and subcutaneous tissue to return to their normal positions *to seal the needle track,* trapping the medication in the muscle. *The needle track that forms during the procedure takes the shape of a Z, which gives the procedure its name.* Don't massage the injection site or allow the patient to wear a tight-fitting garment over the site *because it could force the medication into subcutaneous tissue.*
■ Discard the needles and syringe in an appropriate sharps container. Don't recap needles *to avoid needle-stick injuries.*[2]
■ Remove and discard your gloves if worn.[2,18]
■ Perform hand hygiene.[8,9,10,11,12]
■ Document the procedure.[22,23,24]

Special considerations

■ If the patient is receiving multiple injections or receives an injection daily, alternate injection sites.
■ Always encourage the patient to relax the muscles you'll be injecting *because injections into tense muscle are more painful and may bleed more readily.*
■ IM injections can damage local muscle cells, causing elevated serum enzyme levels (for example, of creatine kinase) that can be confused with the elevated enzyme levels resulting from damage to cardiac muscle, as in myocardial infarction. If measuring enzyme levels is important, suggest that the practitioner switch to IV administration, if appropriate, and adjust dosages accordingly.

Complications

Discomfort and tissue irritation may result from drug leakage into subcutaneous tissue. Failure to rotate sites in patients who require repeated injections can interfere with the absorption of medication. Unabsorbed medications may build up in deposits. Such deposits can reduce the desired pharmacologic effect and may lead to abscess formation or tissue fibrosis.

Documentation

Record the medication, dosage, date, time, and site of injection on the patient's medication record. Include the patient's response to the injected drug.

REFERENCES

1 Hopkins, H., & Arias, C. Y. (2013). Large-volume IM injections: A review of best practices. *Oncology Nurse Advisor, 2013,* 32–37. Accessed May 2015 via the Web at http://media.oncologynurseadvisor.com/documents/44/ona_feature0213_injections_10767.pdf

2 Occupational Safety and Health Administration. (n.d.). "Bloodborne Pathogens, standard number 1910.1030" [Online]. Accessed May 2015 via the Web at http://www.osha.gov/pls/oshaweb/owadisp.show_document?p_table=STANDARDS&p_id=10051 (Level VII)

3 Westbrook, J., et al. (2010). Association of interruptions with an increased risk and severity of medication administration errors. *Archives of Internal Medicine, 170,* 683–690. (Level IV)

4 Institute for Safe Medication Practices. (2012). Side tracks on the safety express: Interruptions lead to errors and unfinished...Wait, what was I doing? *Nurse Advise-ERR, 11*(2), 1–4. Accessed May 2015 via the Web at https://www.ismp.org/Newsletters/acutecare/showarticle.aspx?id=37

5 American Osteopathic Association. (2014). Standard 16.01.03. *Healthcare Facilities Accreditation Program: Accreditation requirements for acute care hospitals.* Chicago, IL: American Osteopathic Association. (Level VII)

6 The Joint Commission. (2015). Standard MM.06.01.01. *Comprehensive accreditation manual for hospitals: The official handbook.* Oakbrook Terrace, IL: The Joint Commission. (Level VII)

7 Centers for Medicare & Medicaid Services, Department of Health and Human Services. (2014). Condition of participation: Nursing services. 42 C.F.R. § 482.23(c).

8 The Joint Commission. (2015). Standard NPSG.07.01.01. *Comprehensive accreditation manual for hospitals: The official handbook.* Oakbrook Terrace, IL: The Joint Commission. (Level VII)

9 Centers for Disease Control and Prevention. (2002). Guideline for hand hygiene in health-care settings: Recommendations of the Healthcare Infection Control Practices Advisory Committee and the HICPAC/SHEA/APIC/IDSA Hand Hygiene Task Force. *MMWR Recommendations and Reports, 51*(RR-16), 1–45. Accessed May 2015 via the Web at http://www.cdc.gov/mmwr/pdf/rr/rr5116.pdf (Level II)

10 World Health Organization. (2009). "WHO guidelines on hand hygiene in health care: First global patient safety challenge, clean care is safer care" [Online]. Accessed May 2015 via the Web at http://whqlibdoc.who.int/publications/2009/9789241597906_eng.pdf (Level IV)

11 American Osteopathic Association. (2014). Standard 07.01.21. *Healthcare Facilities Accreditation Program: Accreditation requirements for acute care hospitals.* Chicago, IL: American Osteopathic Association. (Level VII)

12 Centers for Medicare & Medicaid Services, Department of Health and Human Services. (2014). Condition of participation: Infection control. 42 C.F.R. § 482.42.

13 Centers for Disease Control and Prevention. (2011). "Safe injection practices to prevent transmission of infections to patients" [Online]. Accessed May 2015 via the Web at http://www.cdc.gov/injectionsafety/IP07_standardPrecaution.html (Level II)

14 The Joint Commission. (2015). Standard NPSG.01.01.01. *Comprehensive accreditation manual for hospitals: The official handbook.* Oakbrook Terrace, IL: The Joint Commission. (Level VII)

15 Centers for Medicare & Medicaid Services, Department of Health and Human Services. (2014). Condition of participation: Patient's rights. 42 C.F.R. § 482.13(c)(1).

16 American Osteopathic Association. (2014). Standard 15.01.16. *Healthcare Facilities Accreditation Program: Accreditation requirements for acute care hospitals.* Chicago, IL: American Osteopathic Association. (Level VII)

17 World Health Organization. (2010). "WHO best practices for injections and related procedures toolkit" [Online]. Accessed May 2015 via the Web at http://whqlibdoc.who.int/publications/2010/9789241599252_eng.pdf

18 American Osteopathic Association. (2014). Standard 07.01.10. *Healthcare Facilities Accreditation Program: Accreditation requirements for acute care hospitals.* Chicago, IL: American Osteopathic Association. (Level VII)

19 Crawford, C. L., & Johnson J. A. (2012). To aspirate or not: An integrative review of the evidence. *Nursing, 42*(3), 20–26.

20 Nicoll, L. H., & Hesby, A. (2002). Intramuscular injection: An integrative research review and guideline for evidence-based practice. *Applied Nursing Research, 15,* 149–162.

21 Taylor, C., et al. (2015). *Fundamentals of nursing: The art and science of nursing care* (8th ed.). Philadelphia, PA: Wolters Kluwer.

22 The Joint Commission. (2015). Standard RC.01.03.01. *Comprehensive accreditation manual for hospitals: The official handbook.* Oakbrook Terrace, IL: The Joint Commission. (Level VII)

23 American Osteopathic Association. (2014). Standard 10.00.03. *Healthcare Facilities Accreditation Program: Accreditation requirements for acute care hospitals.* Chicago, IL: American Osteopathic Association. (Level VII)

24 Centers for Medicare & Medicaid Services, Department of Health and Human Services. (2014). Condition of participation: Medical record services. 42 C.F.R. § 482.24(b).

ADDITIONAL REFERENCES

Cocoman, A., & Murray, J. (2010). Recognizing the evidence and changing practices on injection sites. *British Journal of Nursing, 19,* 1170–1174. (Level V)

Craven, R. F., & Hirnle, C. J. (2012). *Fundamentals of nursing: Human health and function* (7th ed.). Philadelphia, PA: Lippincott Williams & Wilkins.

Hunter, J. (2008). Intramuscular injection techniques. *Nursing Standard, 22*(24), 35–40.

Nettina, S. M. (2014). *Lippincott manual of nursing practice* (10th ed.). Philadelphia, PA: Wolters Kluwer.

Walsh, L., & Brophy, K. (2011). Staff nurses' sites of choice for administering intramuscular injections to adult patients in the acute care setting. *Journal of Advanced Nursing, 67,* 1034–1040. (Level VI)

Zimmermann, P. G. (2010). Revisiting IM injections. *American Journal of Nursing, 110*(2), 60–61.

Index

Note: The letter i following a page number indicates an illustration; t indicates a table.

A

Abbreviations to avoid, 248t
Abdominal binder, 73–74, 73i
Abdominal paracentesis, 1–2
Abduction pillow, 15, 16i
Acute normovolemic hemodilution, 45
Adenosine, 193t
Adhesive skin closures, types of, 703i
Adjuvant chemotherapy, 164. *See also* Chemotherapeutic drugs.
Admission to unit, 2–4
  and assessment, 2
  emergency, 2, 3
  medications from home and, 3
  patient care reminders and, 3, 4
  steps in admission procedures, 2, 3
Admixture of drugs in syringe, 5–7
  cartridge-injection system, 5
  contraindications to, 5, 6
  drug incompatibility and, 6
  from multidose vial and ampule, 6
  from two ampules, 6
  from two multidose vials, 6
Adrenalin. *See* Epinephrine.
Advanced cardiac life support (ACLS), 47, 125, 192
Advance directives, 7–10
  health care proxies, 7, 9i
  living wills, 7, 8i
Adverse drug event (ADE), 678, 680
Aerosols, 577i
Airborne precautions, 10–12
  airborne infection isolation room for, 10
  CDC recommendation, 12
  conditions requiring, 11t
  high-efficiency particulate air (HEPA) filtration, 10
  powered air-purifying respirator (PAPR), 10
  respirator seal check, 12, 12i
Air-fluidized therapy beds, 13–14, 14i
  air temperature adjustment for, 13
  clinical use of, 13
  contraindications to use of, 14
Air splint, 708i
Airway clearance, tips on, 570
Alcohol-based hand rub, 345. *See also* Hand hygiene.
Alignment and pressure-reducing devices, 15–16, 16i
Allen's test, 38i
Alternating pressure pad, 59, 60i, 61
Ambulation, progressive, 639–640, 639i
American Academy of Clinical Toxicology, 336
American Association for Respiratory Care (AARC), 752
American Heart Association (AHA), 17, 48, 125, 131, 136, 196, 286, 432, 737
  algorithm for treating adult in cardiac arrest, 196i
  basic life support algorithm, 126i
  on transcutaneous pacing, 776
Amiodarone, 193t
Amniotic membrane dressing, 110, 111t
Amphetamines, 253t
Anaerobic specimen collection, 736i
Angioplasty care, 17–20. *See also* Percutaneous transluminal coronary angioplasty (PTCA).
Anticoagulant therapy, 25–26
Antiembolism stockings application, 21–23
  indications for, 21
  knee-length stocking, 21–23, 22i, 23i
  measuring for, 23i
  thigh-length stocking, 21–22, 23i
  waist-length stocking, 21–22
Apnea, 668t
Apneustic respiratory pattern, 668t
Aquadex FlexFlow ultrafiltration system, 24, 24i, 25, 27
Aquapheresis, 24–27, 26i
  anticoagulant therapy for, 25–26
  device for, 24, 24i
  double-checking high-alert medications before, 27
  hematocrit (HCT) monitor for, 26–27
  heparin infusion and, 25
Arterial blood gas (ABG) analysis, 37
  arterial puncture for, 37–39, 38i, 39i
Arterial pressure monitoring, 31–37
  abnormal waveforms, 35t
  arterial waveform, 32i
  blood sample collection and, 32, 33, 34
  changing tubing for, 32, 34
  closed system for, 32, 33–34
  direct, 31
  inserting catheter for, 32, 36
  open system for, 32, 33
  removing line for, 34
  and waveform evaluation, 32i, 35t
Arterial puncture
  for blood gas analysis, 37–39
  technique for, 39i
Arterial sheath removal, 29–30
  bleeding control following, methods for, 29
  preparing for, 29
  using manual/mechanical compression, 29
  using noninvasive hemostasis pad with manual compression, 29–30
Arterial waveform, 32
  abnormal, 35t
  components of, 32i
Arteriovenous (AV) fistulas, 353
  creation of, 354i
Arteriovenous graft, creation of, 354i
Arthroplasty, 360–362
Ascites, diagnosis of, abdominal paracentesis for, 1–2
Aspiration, 88
  bone marrow, 92–94, 93i
  precautions for, 373–375
Assessment, 40–42
  admission and, 2–3
  blood pressure, 84–87
  physical, 40–42, 41i, 42t. *See also* Physical assessment.
  temperature, 740–741
Assistive devices, at home, 15, 91
Atropine, 193t
Auscultation, 40, 42
Autologous blood recovery systems, 46i
Autologous blood transfusion
  advantages of, 43–44
  contraindications to, 44
  drawbacks of, 44
  managing problems of, 44
  perioperative, 45–46, 46i
  preoperative, 43–44
  techniques for, 44
Automated external defibrillators (AEDs), 47–49, 48i
  AHA guidelines for use of, 48
Automated vital signs monitor, 85i
Autotransfusion. *See* Autologous blood transfusion.

B

Back care, 50, 51i, 52i
Back massage, 50, 51i
  effleurage, 51i
  friction, 51i
  petrissage, 51i
Bair Hugger patient-warming system, 368i
Balloon valvuloplasty, 52
  care, 52–54
  indications for, 52
  mechanics of, 52i
  preprocedure verification, 53
Ballottement, 40, 41i
Balneotherapy. *See* Bath, therapeutic.
Bariatric beds, 56
Barthel index, 332
Barthel Self-Care Rating Scale, 332
Basic life support (BLS), 47–48
Bath, therapeutic, 742–743
  types of, 742t
  use of, 742
Bed bath, 57–58
Bed board, 59, 60
Bed equipment, supplemental, 59–61
  types of, 60i
Bed making
  with mitered corners, 65i
  for occupied bed, 61–63
  for surgical bed, 66i
  for traction bed, 62i
  for unoccupied bed, 64–67
Bedpans, 67–68
  after use of, 68
  placing, 68
Bed scale, for measuring weight, 351–352, 351i
Bedside spirometry, 69–70
Belt restraint, 669, 670

Biliary drainage catheter
  caring for, 71–72
  changing dressing of, 71–72
  clamping, 72
  emptying drainage from, 72
  managing obstruction of, 72
  placement of, 71, 71i
Binders, 73–75
  application of, 73–75
    abdominal binder, 73–74, 73i
    breast binder, 74, 74i
    Scultetus binder, 74, 74i
    T-binder, 74, 74i
  usage of, 73
Biobrane dressing, 110, 111t
Biological dressing, in burns, 110–111, 111t. *See also* Burns.
Biopsy, 92
  bone marrow aspiration and, 92–94, 93i
  skin, 697–698, 697i
Biphasic defibrillator, 195, 240, 242. *See also* Defibrillation.
Biphasic waveforms, 48i
Bispectral index monitoring, 76–77
  interpreting values in, 77i
  mechanics of, 76i
  troubleshooting sensor problems in, 77t
Bladder ultrasonography, 78–79
Blakemore-Sengstaken tube, 299i
Blebs, 700, 700i
Blood culture, sample collection for, 79–81
Blood filters, 785, 786
Blood gas sampling
  arterial, 37–39, 38i, 39i
  capillary, 114
Blood glucose, monitoring of, 81–83
Blood pressure
  classification of, 84
  cuff, positioning, 87i
  diastolic, 84
  electronic vital signs monitor, 85i
  measurement of, 84–87
    correcting problems of, 86t
  systolic, 84
Blood pressure cuff
  positioning, 87i
  selecting, 84
Blood transfusions, 783–788
  documenting, 789
  filters used in, 786
  teaching about blood and product of, 787
  types of blood components and, 784–785t
Blood warmers, 787
Body jewelry, removal of, 88–90, 89t
Body mass index (BMI), 350, 552
  calculating, 352, 552
  determining, 553i
Body mechanics, 90–91
  in lifting and carrying, 91, 91i
  principles, 90
  in pushing and pulling, 90–91, 91i
  in stooping, 91, 91i
Body surface area (BSA), estimation of, 106i
  Lund and Browder chart, 106i
  Rule of Nines, 106i
Bone marrow aspiration and biopsy, 92–94, 92i
  common sites for, 93i
Brachytherapy. *See* Radiation implant therapy.
Braden scale, 636–637t
Bradypnea, 668t
Brain tissue oxygen monitoring, 95–96
  bolt system for, 97i
  device insertion for, 97–98
  tunneled system for, 97i
Breast binder, 74, 74i
Bronchoscope, 100i
Bronchoscopy, assisting, 99–102
  indications for, 101
Buccal drug administration, 103, 104i
Burn care, 105–109. *See also* Burns.
  for arm and leg, 107
  for chest, abdomen, and back, 107
  after discharge, 108, 109
  for ear, 107
  for eye, 107–108
  for face, 107
  for hand and foot, 107
  for nose, 108
  at scene, 105
Burns
  applying dry dressing, 110
  applying wet dressing, 110
  body surface area (BSA), estimation of, 106i
    Lund and Browder chart, 106i
    Rule of Nines, 106i
  dressings for, 110–111
    biological *vs.* synthetic, 111t
  evaluating severity of, 107i
  full-thickness, 107i
  partial-thickness, 107i
  patient positioning to prevent deformity from, 108
  superficial, 107i
  wound excision, 105
Butterfly adhesive strips, 703i

C

Cadaver dressing, 111t
Canes, 112–113
  contraindications for, 112
  indications for, 112
  negotiating stairs with, 112–113
  types of, 112
  using chair with, 113
Capillary blood gas sampling, 114
Carbon monoxide oximetry, 115–116
Cardiac catheterization, 17
Cardiac monitoring, 117–120
  EASI system, 118, 118i
  identifying problems with, 120t
  lead selection for, 117, 117t
  positioning leads for
    five-lead system, 119i
    three-lead system, 119i
  types of, 118
    hardwire monitoring, 117, 118
    telemetry monitoring, 117, 118
Cardiac output measurement, 121–123
  analyzing thermodilution curves in, 124i
  setup for, 122i
  technique used for, 121, 122i
  using iced injectant for, 122
  using room-temperature injectant for, 122
Cardiopulmonary resuscitation (CPR), 47–48, 124–129, 130t, 192
  basic life support algorithm, 126i
  for child, 131–133
    establishing patent airway in, 132
    restoring heartbeat and circulation in, 131–132
    restoring ventilation in, 133
  for infant, 134–135
    restoring heartbeat and circulation in, 134–135
    restoring ventilation in, 135
  one-person, 125–128
  potential hazards of, 130t
  two-person, 128–129
  use of AED, 47–48
Cardioversion, synchronized, 136–138
  anticoagulation therapy, 136
  arrhythmias and, 136
  contraindications to, 136
Care plan, 139–140
  components of, 139
  tips for writing, 140
Care reminders, use of, 4
Cartridge-injection system, 5
Casts, 140–143
  completing, 142
  contraindications to use of, 140
  cotton-polyester, 141, 142
  cylindrical, types of, 141i
  fiberglass, 142
  petaling, 143i
  plaster, 141–142
  preparing, 140
  removing, 144–145
  use of, 140
Catheter
  central venous access, 145–152, 147t
  column-disk peritoneal, 612i
  condom, 385–386
  epidural, 295, 296i
  flanged-collar, 612i
  Foley, 394
  Groshong, 146
  indwelling urinary, 394
  pulmonary artery, 645, 646i
  suction, 712i
  Tenckhoff, 612i
Catheterization
  cardiac, 17
  femoral vein, 354i
  intermittent urinary, 409–411
  nasal balloon, 519
  self, 685–687
  subclavian vein, 354i
Cell Saver® 5+ autologous blood recovery, 45
Centers for Disease Control and Prevention (CDC)
  on hand hygiene, 343, 344
  standard precautions by, 713–715, 714t
Centers for Medicare and Medicaid Services (CMS), 669
Central venous access catheter, 145–152
  blood sampling from, 145, 146
    syringe method, 149
  changing dressing on, 146, 147–148, 151
  changing injection cap on, 146, 148
  duration of use of, 146
  flushing, 146–147, 150
  guide to, 147t

insertion of, 145, 145i, 146, 148, 151–152
pathways for, 145i
removing of, 146, 148, 151
risks of, 153–154t
usage of, 145
Central venous pressure (CVP) monitoring, 155–157
identifying hemodynamic pressure monitoring problems, 159–160t
interpreting waveforms, 158i
with transducer, 155, 156
with water manometer, 155–156, 156i
continuous, 156
intermittent, 156
Cerebrospinal fluid drainage, 160–162
lumbar drainage, 160
Ommaya reservoir and, 164, 556–559
overdrainage, 161
therapeutic uses of, 160
underdrainage, 161
ventricular drainage, 161, 161i
Cervical collar, 162–163
applying, 162–163
types of, 163i
Chair scale, for measuring weight, 350, 351i
Charting, types of
computerized, 247t
core, 247t
flow sheet, assessment, concise timely (FACT), 247t
FOCUS, 247t
Lund and Browder chart, 106i
narrative, 247t
problem-intervention-evaluation, 247t
problemoriented medical record (POMR), 247t
Charting by exception (CBE), 247t
Chattanooga Ionto™ Dual Channel Iontophoresis System, 440. *See also* Iontophoresis.
Chemical-dot thermometer, 740
Chemotherapeutic drugs
as adjuvant therapy, 164
administration of, 163–168
double-check before, 167
routes of, 164–165
adverse effects of, 168
classifying, 165
as induction therapy, 164
and managing extravasation, 167
preparation and handling, 166, 169–171
Chest physiotherapy (PT), 171–175
candidates for, 173
components of, 173
contraindications to, 173
performing percussion and vibration in, 174i
positioning patients for postural drainage, 172–173i
Chest tube
insertion, 184–186
removal, 187–188
Chest tube drainage system
monitoring and care, 175–180
checking and changing chest tube dressing, 176–177
chest tube problems, causes and interventions, 179–180t
replacing collection device, 180
setup, 181–183
dry seal–dry suction system, 182
water-seal–dry suction system, 182
water-seal–wet suction system, 181–182
Chevron method, for taping venous access site, 449i
Cheyne-Stokes respiratory pattern, 668t
Clavicle strap, 189
applying, 189–190
commercially made figure-eight strap, 189–190
elastic bandage strap, 190
types of, 189i
Clean-catch urine specimen collection, 817
Closed wound drain, 190
managing, 190–192
types of, 191i
Cocaine, 253t
Cocaine metabolite, 253t
Code management, 192–197
AHA algorithm, 196i
emergency drugs used for, 193–194t
goals of, 192
recommended priorities for, 192
Cold application, 198–199
benefits of, 198
devices for
chemical cold packs, 198, 199
cold compress/pack, 198, 199
ice bag/collar, 198, 199
K pad, 198, 199
dry, 198
moist, 198
for muscle sprain, 199
reducing pain with ice massage, 198
ColoCARE test, 319
Colostomy irrigation, 204–206
Colostomy pouch, 200–204
applying, 201–203, 202i
changing, 201–203
emptying, 200, 203
fitting, 200–201
selecting, 200
skin barrier for, 200–201, 202i
types of, 200, 201i
Column-disk peritoneal catheter, 612i
Commode, using, 68
Computerized charting system, 247t
Condom catheter, 385–386
applying, 385–386, 386i
removing, 386
Contact lens, 206–208
cleaning, 208
disinfecting, 208
inserting, 207
removing, 207–208
soft *vs.* rigid, 206–207
Contact precautions, 206–209
conditions requiring, 210–213t
Continent ileostomy, 214–216
draining pouch, 216
patient teaching for, 214, 216
postoperative care, 215
pouch construction for, 215
preoperative care, 214–215
Continuous ambulatory peritoneal dialysis (CAPD), 218–220, 218i
automated continuous-cycle system and, 219
contraindications to, 219
infusing dialysate for, 218
major steps of, 218i
temporary discontinuation of, 219–220
use of, 218
Continuous arteriovenous hemofiltration (CAVH), 219. *See also* Continuous renal replacement therapy (CRRT).
Continuous bladder irrigation, 221–223
setup for, 222i
Continuous-cycle peritoneal dialysis (CCPD), 219
Continuous passive motion (CPM) device, 224–226
Continuous positive airway pressure (CPAP), 226–228
administering, 228
by face mask, 228
by nasal mask, 226–227
by nasal pillow, 227–228
contraindications to use of, 226
mask, 575i
use of, 226
Continuous renal replacement therapy (CRRT), 229–232
in emergency, 232
preventing complications of, 232
setup for, 231i
techniques for, 230
Continuous venovenous hemodiafiltration (CVVHDF), 229
Continuous venovenous hemodialysis (CVVH-D), 229. *See also* Continuous renal replacement therapy (CRRT).
Continuous venovenous hemofiltration (CVVH), 229, 231i. *See also* Continuous renal replacement therapy (CRRT).
Core charting system, 247t
Coughing, 188
Cradle boots, 15, 16i
Credé's maneuver, 233–234, 234i
Cricothyrotomy, 235–236
needle, 235
scalpel, 235
Crutches, 237–238
fitting patient for, 237i
gaits for, 239i
types of, 237
Cuffed tube, 759, 760i
Cylindrical casts, types of, 141i
Cystostomy tube, 545
changing dressing for, 545–547

D

Debridement, sharp, 692–693
Deep-breathing exercises, 188
Defibrillation, 240–243
biphasic, 240, 242
implantable cardioverter-defibrillator (ICD), 242
implantable device for, 240, 242i
methods of current delivery in, 240
monophasic, 240, 242
paddle placement for, 240, 241i
using defibrillator, 241i
using defibrillator paddles, 242–243
using self-adhesive defibrillation pads, 241–242

Dentures, dealing with, 534, 562
Dialysis cycle, 610
Dialyzers, types of, 353, 355i
hollow-fiber, 355i
Diaphragmatic breathing, 570
Dicrotic limb, 32i
Dicrotic notch, 32i
Diltiazem, 193t
Discharge, 244–245
against medical advice, 244
planning for, 244
teaching goals for, 245
Disposable pouching systems, urinary diversion, 811
Dobutamine, 193t
Documentation, 246–247
abbreviations to avoid in, 248t
of administration of controlled substances, 372
of blood transfusions, 789
charting systems for, 247t
parenteral nutrition, 586
Dopamine, 193t
Dopppler ultrasonography
blood flow detector, 248–249
transcranial, 771–773
Dressings
amniotic membrane, 110, 111t
biobrane, 110, 111t
biological, 110–111, 111t. *See also* Burns.
cadaver, 111t
pigskin, 110, 111t
pressure-type, 632–633
synthetic, 110–111, 111t
Droplet precautions, 249–251
conditions requiring, 250–251t
Drug administration
buccal, 103–104, 104i
endotracheal, 276–277, 276i
epidural, 295–297, 296i
eye, 306
by intermittent infusion device, 400–401
intrapleural, 435–439, 436i
nasal, 516–518
oral, 564–566
safe practices, 678–680
sublingual, 103–104, 104i
Drug and alcohol specimen collection, 252–254, 253t
Drug-eluting stents, 19, 19i
Durable power of attorney for health care. *See* Health care proxy.
Dying patient, caring for, 255–257
Dying, stages of, 255

E

Eardrops, instilling, 257–258
positioning patient for, 257, 258i
Ear irrigation, 259–260
guidelines for, 260i
Ear specimen collection, 735
EASI system, 117, 118i
Edlich tube, 337i
Elastic antiembolism stockings, 21
Elastic bandage application, 261–263
techniques for
circular, 262i
figure eight, 262i
recurrent, 262i
spiral, 262i
spiral-reverse, 262i
Electrical bone growth stimulation, 263–265
direct current, 264–265
electromagnetic, 264
methods of, 264i
percutaneous, 264
Electrocardiogram (ECG)
electrode placement for, 267i, 270i, 271i
12-lead, 265–267
posterior chest lead, 269–270, 270i
right chest lead, 267–269
signal-averaged, 271–272, 271i
waveforms and components of, 266i
Electronic thermometer, 740
Electronic vital signs monitor, 85i
Emergency admissions, management of, 2, 3
Emergency department (ED) treatment, 3
Endoscopic therapy, 273–274
Endotracheal drug administration, 276–277
methods for, 276i
adapter method, 276i
syringe method, 276i
Endotracheal intubation, 278–282
advantages of, 278
blind, 279
with direct visualization, 278–279
disadvantages of, 278
nasotracheal, 278, 279
oral, 278
Endotracheal tube. *See also* Endotracheal intubation.
caring for, 283–285
managing impaired swallowing due to, 375
methods to secure, 280–281i
removing, 284
repositioning, 283–284
End-tidal carbon dioxide monitoring, 285–288
analyzing carbon dioxide levels in, 286
disposable detector for, 287
mechanics of, 285, 286i
uses for, 285
waveform in, 288i
Enemas
administration of, 289–290
cleansing, 289
retention, 289
use of, 289
Epicardial pacing, 291–293
and handling pacemaker malfunction, 294i
insertion and care, 291–292
sensitivity and stimulation threshold testing, 292
wire removal, 292
Epidural analgesic administration, 295–297, 296i
Epinephrine, 194t
Escharotomy, 105
Esophageal dysphagia, managing impaired swallowing due to, 373, 374
Esophagogastric tamponade tube, 298
care of, 298–300
insertion and removal of, 301–300
securing of, with football helmet, 302i
types of, 299i
Ethanol, 253t
Eupnea, 668t
Ewald tube, 337i
Excisional biopsy, 697. *See also* Skin biopsy.
Expiratory grunting, 667
External fixation, 303–305
advantage of, 304
devices for, 304, 304i
Eye care, 306
Eye compresses, 307–308
cold, 307, 308
warm, 307
Eye irrigation, 308–311
aftercare, 311
copious, 308, 310
devices for, 309i
moderate-volume, 308, 310
uses of, 308
Eye medications, administering, 311–313
in drop form, 312, 312i
in ointment form, 312
Eye specimen collection, 734, 735

F

Face mask, 622i
Facial nerve stimulation, 608–609
Falls, 313–316
cause of, 313
in elderly patients, 313
management of, 314–315
medications associated with, 315t
prevention of, 313–314
and promoting safety in home, 316
risk factors for, 314, 315t
Fecal immunochemical test (FIT), 318
Fecal impaction, digital removal of, 317
contraindications to, 317
side-lying position in, 317i
Fecal incontinence, 387–388
Fecal occult blood tests, 318–319
home tests, 319
Feeding, 320–325
assistive devices for, 322i
and recording fluid intake and output, 323
Feeding tube, 323–325
inserting
nasally, 324
orally, 324
managing patient with, 374–375
managing problems of, 326t
positioning, 324
removing, 324
Femoral compression, 325–327
applying device for, 326–327
after arterial access procedure, 325–326
removal of device for, 327
Femoral vein catheterization, 354i
Figure-eight strap. *See* Clavicle strap.
Flanged-collar catheter, 612i
Flashlighting technique, 772
Flow sheet, assessment, concise timely (FACT) charting system, 247t
Flutter. *See* Mucus clearance device.
FOCUS charting system, 247t
Foley catheter. *See* Urinary catheter, indwelling.
Footboard, 59
adjustable, 60i
Foot care, 328–329
for diabetes patients, 328
Foot cradle, 59, 60i

Forced expiration, 570
Forced expiratory volume (FEV), 69–70
Forced vital capacity (FVC), 69–70
Foreign-body airway obstruction management, 329–331
  for conscious adult/child, 330
  for infant, 331
  for obese/pregnant adult, 330
  for unconscious adult/child, 330–331
Full-thickness graft, 699
Functional assessment, 332

G

Gait belt, 333–335
  for ambulating patient, 334
  for transferring patient, 334
Gastric gavage, 801. *See also* Tube feedings.
Gastric lavage, 336–337
  contraindication to, 336
  tube placement in, 336
  tubes used for, 337i
  use of, 336
Gastrostomy feeding button, 338
  care of, 338–339
  reinserting, 338–339
Glasgow Coma Scale, 547, 548
Glucose oxidase strip tests, 815
Grafts, types of
  arteriovenous, 354i
  full-thickness, 699
  pedicle-flap, 699
  skin, 699
  split-thickness, 699
Groshong catheter, 146. *See also* Central venous access catheter.

H

Hair care, 339–340
Halo-vest traction, 340–343
  applying vest for, 341
  assisting with application of, 340
  caring for patient in, 341–342
  devices for, 340, 341
  use of, 340
Hand hygiene, 343–346, 344i, 345i
  failure, 346
  hand sanitizing, 345
  hand washing, 344–345
    technique for, 345i
Hand roll, 15–16, 16i
Hardwire monitoring, cardiac, 117, 118
Health care proxy, 7, 9i
Hearing aids
  care of, 346–347
  inserting of, 346
  removal of, 346
  types of, 346
Hearing loss, 346
Heat application, direct, 348–350
  by chemical hot pack, 348, 349
  dry, 348
  by electric heating pad, 348, 349
  by hot-water bottle, 348, 349
  by K pad, 348, 349
  moist, 348, 350
  by warm compress/pack, 348, 349
Height, measuring, 350–352
  overcoming problems of, 552
Heimlich maneuver, 330
Hematocrit (HCT) monitor, 26–27
Hemoccult slide test, 318
Hemodialysis, 353–358
  access sites for, 353, 354i
  dialyzers for, 355i
  discontinuing
    with double-lumen catheter, 357
    using arteriovenous access, 356–357
  indications for, 355
  initiating, 355
    using AV access, 355–356
    using double-lumen catheter, 356
  mechanics of, 353, 355i
  types of catheters for, 353, 356, 357
Hemoglobin testing, bedside, 359
Hemovac drain, 191i
High-efficiency particulate air (HEPA) respirator, 10
Hip replacement, total, 360, 361i
H method, for taping venous access site, 449i
Hour-of-sleep care, 362–363
Humidifier therapy, 363–365
  with bedside humidifier, 364, 364t, 365
  with cascade bubble diffusion humidifier, 364, 364t, 365
  with diffusion head humidifier, 364, 364t, 365
  with heated vaporizer, 364, 364t, 365
Hyperthermia-hypothermia blanket, 366–368
  automatic operation, 366
  manual operation, 366
  uses of, 366
  using cooling system, 367i
  using warming system, 368i

I

Ice massage, reducing pain with, 198
Ileostomy pouch, 200–204
  applying, 201–203, 202i
  changing, 201–203
  emptying, 200, 203
  fitting, 200–201
  selecting, 200
  skin barrier for, 200–201
  types of, 200, 201i
Ilizarov fixator, 304, 305
Impedance cardiography. *See* Thoracic electrical bioimpedance monitoring.
Implantable cardioverter-defibrillator (ICD), 242
Implanted port, 376–382, 377i
  accessing top-entry port, 377–379
  administering bolus injection by, 380
  administering continuous infusion by, 380–381
  assisting with insertion of, 377
  complications of, 382
  managing problems with, 378t
  obtaining blood sample by, 379–380
  uses of, 376
Incentive spirometry, 383–384
  complications, 384
  devices used for, 384
  and documenting flow and volume levels, 385
  guidelines for use of, 383
Incontinence device, male
  application, 385–386
  apply condom catheter, 386i
Incontinence management
  fecal, 387–388
  urinary, 388–390
Induction chemotherapy, 164. *See also* Chemotherapeutic drugs.
Indwelling urinary catheter. *See* Urinary catheter, indwelling.
Informed consent, 628
Infusion bag, changing, 492
Infusion pumps, 462i
Infusion rate
  calculation of, 462i
  control of, 461i
Injections
  intradermal, 430–432
  intramuscular (IM), 368–372
  intrathecal, 295
  IV bolus, 444–445
  subcutaneous, 721–724
  Z-track, 842–843
In-line filter, 470
Inspection, physical assessment, 40
Insulin infusion pump, 722
  closed-loop system, 722
  nonneedle delivery system, 722
  open-loop system, 722
Intermittent infusion device, 400, 401
  complications of IV therapy, 403t
  converting I.V. line to, 406
  drug administration through, 400–401
  flushing, 402–404
  inserting, 404–406
  locking, 402–404
Intermittent positive-pressure breathing (IPPB), 407–408
Intermittent urinary catheterization, 409–411
  for female patient, 409–410
  for male patient, 410–411
  use of, 409
Internal fixation, 412–414
  devices for, 412i
  uses of, 412
Intra-abdominal pressure (IAP) monitoring, 415–416
Intra-aortic balloon counterpulsation (IABC), 417–422
  contraindications for, 417
  indications for, 417
  insertion of balloon, 418–419
  interpreting waveforms in, 420, 421–422i
  mechanics of, 418, 418i
  removing balloon for, 420, 422
  surgical insertion sites for, 419i
  weaning patient from, 420
Intra-aortic balloon pump, 418i
Intracranial pressure (ICP) monitoring, 424–429
  increased ICP, management of, 429
  interpreting waveforms in, 428i
  setting up system for, 426i
  system for, 424–425, 424–425i
Intradermal injections, 430–432
  sites for, 430, 430i
  technique for, 432, 432i

Intramuscular (IM) injection, 368–372
drawing up medication for, 370
site for, 371
locating, 371i
syringe and needle selection for, 369
Intraosseous infusion, 432–434
contraindication to, 433
mechanics of, 433i
use of, 432
Intraperitoneal chemotherapy, 164. *See also* Chemotherapeutic drugs.
Intrapleural drug administration, 435–439, 436i
for administering chemotherapy, 437–438
contraindications for, 435
indications for, 435
inserting catheter for, 436, 436i
inserting chest tube for, 436–437
Intrathecal injection, 295
Iontophoresis, 440–441
Isolation garb, 441–443
face mask, 442i
removal technique, 442–443, 443i
use, 442
Isometric exercises, 593
Isoproterenol, 194t
IV bolus injection, 444–445
IV catheter. *See* Peripheral IV therapy.
IV clamps, using, 461i
IV glucose tolerance test, 83
IV line, secondary, drug infusion through, 466–467
IV pump, 462–465
IV tube, for eye irrigation, 309i

J

Jackson-Pratt drain, 191i
Jewelry, removal of, 88–90, 89t
J point, 266i
Jugular venous oxygen saturation (Sjvo2) monitoring, 471–472
criteria for, 471
inserting catheter in, 471
periods of desaturation in, 472
use of, 471

K

Katz Index of Independence in Activities of Daily Living, 332
Ketone strip tests, 815
Knee arthroplasty, postprocedure care, 473–475
Knee-length stocking, 21–23, 22i, 23i
Koch ileostomy. *See* Continent ileostomy.
Kussmaul's respiratory pattern, 668t

L

Laryngeal mask airway (LMA), 475
choosing right size of, 476t
indications for, 475
inserting, 475–478
types of, 475
use of, 475
Laser therapy, 479–480
advantages of, 479
hazard associated with, 479–480
types of, 479
Latex allergy
anesthesia induction and, 482t
diagnosis of, 481
groups at risk for developing, 481
protocol for, 481–482
screening questionnaire for, 481
signs and symptoms of, 481, 482t
Lawton Instrumental Activities of Daily Living Scale, 332, 333
12-lead electrocardiogram, 265–267
Leather restraints, 669, 670
Leg bags, 393i
Levacuator tube, 337i
Levin tube, 531, 532i
Lidocaine, 194t
Limb restraints, 669, 670
Linton tube, 299i
Lipid emulsions, 483
administration of, 483–484
contraindications to use of, 483
Liquid medications, measuring, 566
Living will, 7, 8i
Locking pliers, using, 674
Low-air-loss therapy bed, 485–486, 486i
Lumbar puncture, 487–488
contraindication to, 487
positioning for, 488i
use of, 487
Lund and Browder chart, 106i

M

Magnesium sulfate, 194t
Male incontinence device
application, 385–386
apply condom catheter, 386i
Malignant melanoma, ABCDEs of, 697i
Malnutrition, risk factors for, 554
Manual ventilation, 489–490
applying bag and mask for, 489, 491i
guidelines for using, 489–490
positive end-expiratory pressure and, 489–490
Marijuana, 253t
Marijuana metabolite, 253t
Massive infusion device, 491–493
Mechanical ventilator, 497
negative pressure, 498
positive pressure, 498
responding to alarms in, 500t
Medicated shampoos, applying, 749
Medication administration, safe practices, 678–680
accurate dosage calculations, 678
accurate medication listing, 678
administering high-alert medications, 678–679
administering scheduled medications in timely manner, 679
checking for medication contraindications, 678
"Do Not Use" list of abbreviations, 680t
handling verbal orders, 679
identifying patient, 678
verifying medication order, 678
Medication error, 678
Metered-dose inhaler (MDI), 501–502
Methoxsalen, 806
Minimal occlusive volume, 750
Minimum Data Set, 332
Minnesota esophagogastric tamponade tube, 299i
Mitt restraints, 669, 670
Mixed venous oxygen saturation monitoring, 503–504
equipment for, 504i
recalibrating monitor for, 504
Monophasic defibrillators, 240, 242, 243. *See also* Defibrillation.
Montgomery Ventrach, 756
Morgan lens, for eye irrigation, 309i
Mucus clearance device, 509–510
Muscle spasm, moist heat application for, 349, 350
Muscle sprain, cold application for, 199

N

Narrative charting system, 247t
Nasal balloon catheterization, 519
Nasal bridle, 511–513
insertion, 511–513
removing, 513
Nasal cannula, 574i
Nasal irrigation, 514–515
bulb syringe for, 514
contraindications for, 514
indications for, 514
oral irrigating device for, 514
positioning patient for, 515i
Nasal medications, administering, 516–518
in aerosol form, 516–517
in drop form, 516
in inhaler form, 516–517
positioning patient for, 517i
Nasal packing, 518–521
anterior, 520i
posterior, 519i
Nasoenteric-decompression tube, 522–523
assisting with insertion of, 522, 524–525
care of, 522–523
clearing obstruction from, 523
removing, 524–525
types of, 524
use of, 522
Nasogastric tube, 531
applications for, 531
caring for, 526–528
home use of, 535
inserting, 531–533
instilling drugs through, 528–530, 530i
removing, 533–534
suction devices for, 527i
types of, 532i
Nasopharyngeal airway, 536
care, 536–537
insertion of, 536–537, 536i
Nasopharyngeal specimen collection, 734–735, 735i
National Association of Orthopaedic Nurses, 305
National Organ Transplant Act, 567
Nebulizer therapy, 537–541
at home, 540
with in-line nebulizer, 537, 539–540
with large-volume nebulizer, 537, 538
precautions for body fluid isolation in, 537
with small-volume nebulizer, 538–539, 540
with ultrasonic nebulizer, 504, 538–540
Negative-pressure wound therapy, 541–544, 542i
contraindications for, 541

with foam packing, 541, 543
with gauze packing, 543
indications for, 541
Nephrostomy tube, 545
changing dressing for, 545–547
Neurologic assessment, 547–551
evaluating motor function in, 549–550
evaluating sensory function in, 550
examining pupils and eye movement in, 548–549, 549i
identifying warning postures and, 551i
level of consciousness and orientation in, 547–548
Nitroglycerin ointment, applying, 778i
Nonrebreather mask, 575i
Normal pulse amplitude waveform, identification of, 648i
Nosebleeds, recurrent, preventing, 521
Nutritional disorders, evaluating, 555t
Nutritional screening, 552–553

O

OASIS-C, 332
Obese patients, bariatric beds for, 56
Ommaya reservoir, 556–559
mechanics of, 556i
use of, 556
Opiates, 253t
Oral care, 560–564
in intubated patient, 562–563
performing, 561–563
supervising, 560–561
using oral irrigating device, 563
Oral drug administration, 564–566
Oral glucose tolerance test (OGTT), 83
Oral irrigating device, using, 563
Organ donor, identification, 567–568
Organ Procurement and Transplant Network, 567
Organ Procurement Organization (OPO), 567
Oronasopharyngeal suction, 569–571
nasal insertion for, 570
oral insertion for, 570
Oropharyngeal airway, 571
caring for, 571–573
inserting, 572i
Oropharyngeal dysphagia, managing impaired swallowing due to, 373–374
Outcome and Assessment Information Set (OASIS), 332
Overbed cradle, 60i
Over-the-needle cannula, 447i
Oxygen therapy, 573–577
in cardiac emergency, 573
delivery systems for, 574–577i
in home setting, 577
metabolic demand and, 573
patient monitoring during, 573
in respiratory emergency, 573

P

Pacemakers
permanent, 617–619
temporary, 294i, 796i
Pain. *See also* Pain management.
assessment of, 579
definition of, 578
Pain management, 578–581
complementary and alternative therapies for, 579
giving medications for, 578–579
providing comfort measures for, 579
providing emotional support for, 579
Palpation, 41, 41i
performing, 41i
techniques of, 41, 41i
Parenteral nutrition, 581–586
correcting common problems with, 584–585t
delivery route for, 581–582
documenting, 586
indications for, 581
laboratory monitoring of, 588
monitoring, 587–588
types of, 581, 582t
Passive range-of-motion exercises, 589–592
for ankle, 591–592
contraindications to, 589
for elbow, 591
for fingers and thumb, 591
for forearm, 591
for hip and knee, 591
indications for, 589
for neck, 589
for shoulders, 589–590
and terminology related to joint movements, 590i
for toes, 592
for wrist, 591
Passy-Muir tracheostomy and ventilator speaking valve (PMV), 756–759
Patient care reminders, use of, 3, 4i
Patient-controlled analgesia (PCA), 592–594
advantages of, 592
contraindication to, 593
Patient Self-Determination Act, 7
Pedicle-flap graft, 699
Penile sheath. *See* Condom catheter.
Percussion
blunt, 42
direct, 40, 42
indirect, 40, 43i
sounds, identification of, 42t
techniques of, 40
Percutaneous endoscopic gastrostomy (PEG) tube, 767
caring for site of, 769i
Percutaneous endoscopic jejunostomy (PEJ) tube, 767
caring for site of, 769i
Percutaneous transluminal coronary angioplasty (PTCA), 17–20
candidates, 17
ECG rhythm and vital signs, recording of, 19
preprocedure verification process and, 18
procedure, 18i
vascular stents for, 19i
Pericardial effusions, types of, 596
Pericardiocentesis, 595–597, 597i
Perineal care, 598–599
for female patients, 599
for male patients, 599
Peripheral IV therapy
access devices for, 446, 447i
applying tourniquet for, 447, 450
dressing site of, 448, 450i
inserting catheter for, 446–450
maintaining, 456–460
changing dressing, 456–457
changing solution, 457–458
changing tubing, 458
IV flow rate deviations, 459
using time tape, 458
patient teaching for, 470
preparing equipment for, 468–470
preparing site for, 447–448, 448i
removing catheter for, 449–450
risks of
air embolism, 454–455t
allergic reaction, 455t
cannula dislodgment, 452t
circulatory overload, 454t
hematoma, 453t
infiltration, 451–452t
nerve/tendon/ligament damage, 453t
occlusion, 452t
phlebitis, 451t
severed cannula, 452t
systemic infection, 454t
thrombophlebitis, 453t
thrombosis, 453t
vasovagal reaction, 454t
vein irritation/pain, 452t
venous spasm, 453t
taping site of, 449i
using in-line filter for, 470
Peripherally inserted central catheter (PICC), 600–605
administering drugs through, 600, 603–604
changing dressing for, 603
flushing, 602–603
inserting, 600, 601–602
removing, 604
troubleshooting, 606t
uses for, 600
Peripheral nerve stimulation, 608–610
Peripheral parenteral nutrition (PPN), 582. *See also* Parenteral nutrition.
Peristaltic pump, 462
Peritoneal dialysis, 610–614
catheters for, 612i
continuous ambulatory, 218–220, 218i
continuous-cycle, 219
contraindication to, 610
indications for, 610
mechanics of, 611i
setup for, 611i
Peritoneal lavage, 614–617
contraindication to, 614
interpreting results of, 616
tapping peritoneal cavity for, 615i
use of, 614
Permanent pacemaker, 617–619
candidates for, 618
codes for, 618, 618t
patient teaching for, 620
postoperative care for, 620
preoperative care for, 618–619
Personal protective equipment, 621
Phencyclidine, 253t
Physical assessment, 40–42
auscultation, 40, 42
inspection, 40

Physical assessment (*continued*)
palpation, 41, 41i
percussion, 40, 42, 42t, 43i
Piggyback port, 466
Piggyback set, 466, 467i
Pigskin dressing, 110, 111t
Piston-cylinder pump, 462
Portable syringe pump, 462
Portsmouth external fixation bar, 304
Posterior tibial nerve stimulation, 609
Postmortem care, 622–623
Postoperative care, 624–626, 626i
Pouching systems, urinary diversion, 811
Powered air-purifying respirator (PAPR), 10
Preoperative care, 628–630
Preoperative skin preparation, 631–632
hair removal for surgery, 631
Pressure dressing application, 632–633
Pressure ulcers, 633
assessing risk of developing, 633, 636–637t
common sites for, 633
preventive measures for, 633
staging, 634–635i
treatment of, 633
PR interval, 266i
Problem intervention evaluation (PIE) charting system, 247t
Problem-oriented medical record (POMR), 247t
Problemoriented medical record (POMR) charting system, 247t
Procainamide, 194t
Prone positioning, 641–643
contraindications to, 641
criteria for, 641
patient assessment before, 641
procedure before turning patient in, 641
returning patient to supine position in, 642–643
turning patient in, 642
Proning. *See* Prone positioning.
Prosthesis
applying, 665
caring for, 665
plastic, 665
Protective environment, 643–644
Psoralen plus UVA (PUVA) therapy, 806. *See also* Ultraviolet light therapy.
Psychogenic polydipsia, 834
Pulmonary artery (PA) catheter, 645, 646i
Pulmonary artery pressure (PAP) monitoring, 645–646
candidates for, 645
and square wave test, 645, 647i
taking reading of, 645
Pulmonary artery wedge pressure (PAWP) monitoring, 645–646
observing PAWP waveform, 647i
taking reading of, 645
Pulse, 649–651
apical, 650
apical-radial, 650
Doppler ultrasound detection of, 649
patterns of, 651i
radial, 650
sites for palpating, 649, 650i
Pulse amplitude monitoring, 648–649
normal pulse amplitude waveform, identification of, 648i
Pulse oximetry, 651–653
diagnosing problems with, 654
mechanics of, 651–652, 652i
using ear probe, 653
using finger probe, 652
using forehead sensor, 653
Punch biopsy, 697. *See also* Skin biopsy.
P wave, 266i

Q

QRS complex, 266i
QT interval, 266i

R

Radiation implant therapy, 654–657
complications of, 657
implant sites, 654
radioactive isotopes used in, 654, 655t
Radiation therapy, 657–658
adverse effects of, 658
doses of, 657
goals of, 657
machines used for, 657
Radioactive iodine therapy, 658–660
precautions after, 660
Radioisotopes, 655
Radiotherapy. *See* Radiation therapy.
Rancho Los Amigos Cognitive Scale, 549
Ready injectable, using, 444
Rectal ointments, applying, 660–662, 662i
Rectal suppositories, inserting, 660–662, 661i
Rectal swab specimen collection, 735
Rectal tube, inserting and removing, 662–663
Red blood cell (RBC) salvage, 46
Reduced-lead continuous 12-lead electrocardiogram (ECG) system (EASI system), 117, 118i
Residual limb
care of, 664–667
wrapping, 665i
Respiration, 667–668
measures of, 667
patterns of, 668t
Respirator, 10
seal check, 12i
use of, 10
Restraints
application of, 669–672
belt, 669, 670
CMS and Joint Commission on use of, 669
definition of, 669
leather, 669, 670
limb, 669, 670
mitt, 669, 670
orders for, 671
and tying quick-release knot, 670, 671i
use of, 669
vest, 669, 670
Retention catheter. *See* Urinary catheter, indwelling.
Reusable pouching system, urinary diversion, 811
Right chest lead ECG, 267–268
Rigid splint, 707, 708i
Ring removal, 673–675
coiled-string method for, 673
ring-cutter method for, 673–674
Rotation beds, 675–677, 676i
RotoRest™ Delta therapy system, 676i
Rule of Nines, 106i

S

Salem sump tube, 531, 532i
Saline lock. *See* Intermittent infusion device.
Scultetus binder, 74, 74i
Sedation
complications of, 507t
moderate, 505–508
Seizures
generalized, precautions for, 683
managing, 682–684
partial, 682
patients at risk for, 682
types of, 682
Self-catheterization, 685–687
for female patient, 685–686, 686i
for male patient, 685, 686i
Self-closures. *See* Binders.
Sengstaken-Blakemore tube, 299i
Sensitivity and stimulation threshold testing, 292
Sequential compression therapy, 687–689
Sexual assault examination, 690–692
anal secretion collection for, 691
blood samples collection in, 691
penile secretion collection for, 691
pubic hair collection for, 691
specimen collection for, 691
urine specimen collection for, 691
vaginal/cervical secretion collection for, 691
Sexual Assault Nurse Examiner (SANE), 690
Sharp debridement, 692–693
Shave biopsy, 697. *See also* Skin biopsy.
Shaving, 694–695
using electric razor for, 695
using safety razor for, 694–695
Shiley Phonate, 756
Short-term multilumen catheter, 147t. *See also* Central venous access catheter.
Short-term single-lumen catheter, 147t. *See also* Central venous access catheter.
Showers, 799–800
Signal-averaged electrocardiography, 271–272, 271i
Simple mask, for oxygen delivery, 574i
Sitz bath, 695–696
Skin biopsy, 697–698, 697i
Skin graft, 699
caring for, 699–701
caring for donor site, 699
evacuating fluid from, 700, 700i
types of, 699
Skin staples and clips, removing, 701–702, 702i, 703i
Slow extended daily dialysis (SLEDD), 229. *See also* Continuous renal replacement therapy (CRRT).
Smart pumps, 462, 463
Smoke evacuator, 480
Soaks, 703–704
Sotalol, 194t
Speaking valve
managing impaired swallowing due to, 375
Sphygmomanometer, 84
Spinal anesthesia, assessing level of blockade from, 625, 626i

Spiritual care, 705–707
beliefs and practices of selected religions and, 706–707
Spirometry
bedside, 69–70
incentive, 383–384
Splint, 707–709
applying, 707–709
assessing neurovascular status and, 709
rigid, 707, 708i
Split-thickness graft, 699
Sponge bath, 709–710
Sputum collection, 711–713
by expectoration, 711
by tracheal suctioning, 711–712
Square wave test, 647i
Squeeze bottle, for eye irrigation, 309i
Standard precautions, 713–715, 714t
Standing scale, for measuring weight, 350–351
Status epilepticus, 683
ST-elevation myocardial infarction (STEMI), 17
Stenting, 19
Sterile technique, 715–718
Stertor, 667
Stool specimen collection, 718–719
random, 718
timed, 718–719
Stress incontinence, 388. *See also* Urinary incontinence.
strengthening pelvic floor muscles for, 391
Stridor, 667
ST-segment, 266i
changes in, 720i
depression, 720i
elevation, 720i
monitoring, 719–721
Subclavian vein catheterization, 354i
Subcutaneous cerebrospinal fluid (CSF) reservoir. *See* Ommaya reservoir.
drugs and solutions for, 721
of heparin, 721, 724
of insulin, 721, 722i, 724
sites for, 723i
technique for, 724i
Subdermal drug implants, 725–726
Sublingual drug administration, 103
Suction catheter, attaching specimen trap to, 712i
Surgical drains, 726–727
removing, 726–727
Surgical wound management, 728–730
applying fresh gauze dressing in, 729–730
caring for wound in, 729
dressing wound with drain in, 730
removing old dressing in, 728–729
wound color and, 728
Sustained maximal inspiration, 384
Suture removal, 731, 733
methods for, 732–733i
techniques for, 731
timing of, 731
Swab specimen collection, 734–736
anaerobic, 736i
external ear, 735
eye specimen, 735
middle ear, 735
nasopharyngeal, 734–735, 735i
rectal swab, 735
throat, 734
wound, 735
Swallowing, impaired, precautions for, 373–375
Synchronized cardioversion, 136–138, 737–739
Synthetic dressing, in burns, 110–111, 111t. *See also* Burns.
Syringe feeding, 771i
Systolic peak, 32i

T

Tachypnea, 668t
T-binder, 74, 74i
Telemetry monitoring, cardiac, 117, 118, 119
Temperature, 740–741
axillary measurement of, 740
factors that influence, 740
normal range of, 740
oral measurement of, 740
rectal, 740
tympanic measurement of, 740–741
types of thermometers used to measure, 740, 741
Temporary pacemaker
correcting malfunctions in, 796i
handling malfunction in, 294i
Tenckhoff catheter, 612i
Therapeutic bath, 742–743
types of, 742t
use of, 742
Thermodilution method, for cardiac output measurement, 121–123, 124i
Thigh-length stocking, 21–22, 23i
Thoracentesis, 744–745
contraindications to, 744
positioning patient for, 744i
use of, 744
Thoracic electrical bioimpedance monitoring, 746–747
Throat specimen collection, 734
Tilt table, 747–748
Topical skin drug application, 748–750
Total parenteral nutrition (TPN), 582. *See also* Parenteral nutrition.
Tracheal cuff-pressure measurement, 750–752
Tracheal suction, 752
closed, 754i
in intubated patient, 752–755
Tracheostomy, 756, 759
caring for, 759–764
managing impaired swallowing due to, 375
tubes, 759–760, 760i
Tracheostomy and ventilator speaking valve, 756–759
Tracheotomy, 764
assisting with, 764–766, 766i
Traction, mechanical, 494–497
claw-type basic frame for, 494–495, 496i
contraindications for, 494
IV-type Balkan traction frame for, 494–495, 496i
IV-type basic frame for, 494, 495i
skeletal traction, 494
skin traction, 494
use of, 494
Traction bed, making of, 62i
Train of four (TOF) method, for monitoring neuromuscular blockade, 609–610
Transabdominal tube, 767–770
for continuous feedings, 768
for intermittent feedings, 769
site care, 768, 769i
teaching patient about syringe feedings through, 771i
Transcranial Doppler monitoring, 771–773
benefits of, 772
use of, 771
velocity waveforms in, 773i
Transcutaneous electrical nerve stimulation (TENS), 774–775
contraindications to, 774
positioning electrodes for, 775i
uses of, 774
Transcutaneous pacing, 776–777
electrode placement for, 777i
indications for, 776
Transdermal drugs, administering, 778–779
in ointment form, 779
in patch form, 779
Transdermal patch, applying, 779
Transducer system, 780–782
setting up, 780–781
zeroing, 781
Transfer of patients, within facility, 782–783
Transfusion of blood and blood products, 783–788
Transfusion reaction
guide to, 791–792
management of, 790–792
Transmission-based precautions, 714t
Transtracheal oxygen, 576i
Transvenous pacing, 793–795, 796i
sensitivity threshold testing, 794
stimulation threshold testing, 794
Trapeze and basic frame, 59, 60, 60i
Traumatic wounds, 795
abrasion, 795, 797–798
amputation, 797, 798, 798i
laceration, 797, 798
management of, 795–799
puncture wounds, 795, 797
Trochanter roll, 15, 16i
T tube. *See* Biliary drainage catheter.
Tub baths, 799–800
Tube feedings, 801–804
to duodenum, 801, 803
indications for, 801
to jejunum, 801, 803
managing problems with, 805t
to stomach, 801–802
Tubes
Blakemore-Sengstaken, 299i
chest, 184–188
cuffed, 759, 760i
cystostomy, 545
Edlich, 337i
endotracheal, 283–285
esophagogastric tamponade, 298
Ewald, 337i
feeding, 323–325
IV tube, for eye irrigation, 309i
levacuator, 337i
Levin, 531, 532i

Tubes (*continued*)
- Linton, 299i
- minnesota esophagogastric tamponade, 299i
- nasoenteric-decompression tube, 522–523
- nasogastric, 531
- nephrostomy, 545
- percutaneous endoscopic gastrostomy, 767
- percutaneous endoscopic jejunostomy, 767
- rectal, 662–663
- salem sump, 531
- tracheostomy, 759–760
- transabdominal, 767–770
- uncuffed, 759–760

T wave, 266i

Tympanic thermometer, 740

U

Ulnar nerve stimulation, 608

Ultrasonography, bladder, 78–79

Ultraviolet light therapy, 806–808
- adverse effect of, 807–808
- skin care guidelines for, 807
- skin types and, 806
- spectrum of, 806
- uses for, 806

U method, for taping venous access site, 449i

Uncuffed tube, 759–760, 760i

United Network for Organ Sharing, 256

Universal day frame, 304i

Unna paste, 801

Unna's boot, 808
- application, 808–809
- how to wrap, 809i

Urinal, 67–68
- after use of, 68
- placing, 68

Urinary catheter, indwelling, 394
- caring for, 391–393
- indications for, 394
- inserting, 394–397
  - for female patient, 395–396
  - for male patient, 396–397
- irrigating, 398–399
- removing, 391, 392
- urine drainage bags and, 393i

Urinary diversion
- caring for patient with continent, 812
- indications for, 810
- permanent, types of, 810i
- pouching systems, 811
- stoma care for, 810–812

Urinary diversion techniques, 545, 546i
- cystostomy, 546i
- nephrostomy, 546i

Urinary incontinence, 388–390
- acute, 388
- causes of, 388
- chronic, 388
- correcting, by bladder retraining, 390

Urinary sphincter implant, artificial, 389, 389i

Urine collection, timed, 813–814

Urine glucose tests, 814–815

Urine ketone tests, 814–815

Urine pH, 815–816

Urine specimen collection, 817–818
- clean-catch midstream, 817–818
- from indwelling catheter, 818
- random, 817

Urine straining, for calculi, 819

U wave, 266i

V

Vaginal medications, inserting, 820, 820i

Vaginal suppositories, administration of, 820–821

Valsalva's maneuver, 149, 151

Vascular access device. *See* Implanted port.

Vascular access port. *See* Implanted port.

Vascular stents, 19i

Vasopressin, 194t

Venipuncture, 821–824, 823t, 824i
- collection tube guide, 823t, 824i
- risks of, assessment for, 822
- sites for, 822, 824i

Venous sheath removal, 29–30

Ventilation, mechanical, 497–500, 825. *See also* Mechanical ventilator.
- negative pressure, 498
- terminology for, 498

Ventricular assist device (VAD), 825
- candidates for, 825
- caring for, 825–827
- for failing heart, 826, 826i

Ventricular drain insertion, 828–829

Venturi mask, 576i

Verapamil, 194t

Vest restraint, 669, 670

Visual pain rating scale, 580i

Vital signs
- electronic monitor, 85i
- recording of, on admission, 3

Volume-control sets, 830–831

Volumetric pumps, 462

W

Waist-length stocking, 21–22

Walkers, 832–834
- teaching safe use of, 832, 833i

Warming system, 368i

Washcloth mitt, making of, 50, 51i

Water intoxication
- assessment of, 834–835
- maintenance fluid requirements, calculation of, 835
- signs and symptoms of, 835

Water mattress, 59, 61

Weaning patient from ventilator, 836–837
- after weaning, 837
- readiness criteria, 836

Weight, measuring, 350–352
- guideline for determining healthy weights, 350, 351
- scales for, 351i

Wheezing, 667

Winged infusion set, 447i

Wong-Baker FACES pain rating scale, 580i

World Health Organization (WHO), 343
- on hand hygiene, 343, 344i

Wound dehiscence and evisceration
- managing, 838–839
- recognizing, 838i

Wound irrigation, 840–841

Wounds
- black, 728
- multicolored, 728
- puncture, 795
- red, 728
- surgical management of, 795–799
- traumatic, 795
- yellow, 728

Wound specimen collection, 735

Z

Z-track injection, 842–843

RRS1508